Approaches in Urologic Surgery

Approaches
in Urologic Surgery

G. Bartsch and S. Poisel

With 373 four-color illustrations
by Nikolaus Lechenbauer

Forewords by John P. Donohue and Donald G. Skinner

1994
Georg Thieme Verlag Stuttgart · New York
Thieme Medical Publishers, Inc. New York

Univ. Prof. Dr. Georg Bartsch
Professor and Chairman
Department of Urology
University of Innsbruck
Anichstraße 35
6020 Innsbruck
Austria

Univ. Prof. Dr. Sepp Poisel
Associate Professor
Department of Anatomy
University of Innsbruck
Müllerstraße 59
6010 Innsbruck
Austria

Translated by:
Terry C. Telger
6112 Waco Way
Fort Worth, TX 76133
USA

Library of Congress Cataloging-in-Publication Data

Bartsch, G. (Georg)
[Operative Zugangswege in der Urologie. English]
Approaches in urologic surgery/ G. Bartsch and S. Poisel ; with 373 four-color illustrations by Nikolaus Lechenbauer ; forewords by John P. Donohue and Donald G. Skinner ; [translated by Terry C. Telger].
p. cm.
Includes bibliographical references and index.
ISBN 3-13-129301-2 (GTV). – ISBN 0-86577-543-5 (TMP)
1. Genitourinary organs-Surgery-Atlases. 2. Genitourinary organs-Anatomy-Atlases. I. Poisel, S. (Sepp) II. Title.
[DNLM: 1. Urologic Diseases-surgery-atlases. 2. Urogenital System-anatomy & histology-atlases. WJ 17 B294u 1994a]
RD571.B38 13 1994
617.4 51-dc20
DNLM/DLC
for Library of Congress   94-30311
                                                                CIP

This book is an authorized translation of the German edition published and copyrighted 1994 by Georg Thieme Verlag, Stuttgart, Germany.
Title of the German edition:
Operative Zugangswege in der Urologie

© 1994 Georg Thieme Verlag,
Rüdigerstraße 14, D-70469 Stuttgart, Germany
Thieme Medical Publishers, Inc., 381 Park Avenue South, New York, N.Y. 10016

Typesetting by Druckhaus Götz GmbH,
D-71636 Ludwigsburg
(CCS-Textline [Linotronic 630])
Printed in Germany by Druckerei Grammlich,
Pliezhausen, Germany

ISBN 3-13-129301-2 (GTV, Stuttgart)
ISBN 0-86577-543-5 (TMP, New York)   1 2 3 4 5 6

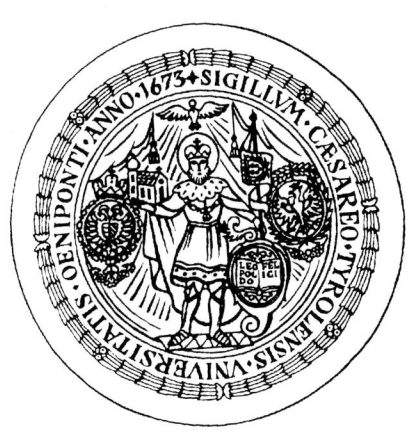

This book is dedicated to
our teachers
Hans Marberger and Werner Platzer

Preface

Extensive scientific collaboration between the Department of Urology and Department of Anatomy at the University of Innsbruck gave us the idea of pooling our experience in clinical anatomy and operative urology to achieve a synthesis of both specialties. This concept has now become a reality in this atlas of approaches in urologic surgery.

This project was further motivated by the fact that available textbooks of operative urology and topographic anatomy, taken individually, seem inadequate for the study of standardized surgical procedures on the human body. Surgical texts focus on operative techniques, pathology, and treatment, while anatomy texts are geared toward teaching requirements at the university level and give scant attention to the aspects of surgical procedures.

In the present atlas, each surgical approach is systematically illustrated by a progressive, step-by-step dissection carried out in a cadaveric specimen. Special emphasis is placed upon a clear presentation of the topographic anatomy that the surgeon will encounter. The practical value of the drawings is enhanced by the addition of instruments such as chest retractors, abdominal retractors, rake retractors, scissors, and forceps. We used a special mounting apparatus like that used in photography to position the instruments in the field so that the artist could illustrate their placement and use.

Each step of a given surgical approach was "cut" by the surgeon, "dissected" by the anatomist, and rendered by the illustrator, who worked from a Polaroid photograph to produce a rough sketch and then the finished drawing. Almost all views are presented from the perspective of the operating surgeon. Each approach is described as a complete and separate unit so that the reader will not have to leaf backward or foreword in the book.

The drawings of the surgical approaches are supplemented by anatomic drawings of the abdominal and pelvic walls and by descriptive text passages that review the anatomy of the retroperitoneal and subperitoneal spaces.

This picture atlas ist not intended as a textbook of surgery; it does not follow the "cut here, suture there" format characteristic of a surgical text. Neither do the authors claim to have covered all approaches in operative urology. We have focused our attention on approaches with which we have had personal experience. The text, deliberately concise, is intended to clarify the illustrations and is not an end in itself. We intentionally avoided an in-depth discussion of controversial issues, and we have provided statistical data only where deemed essential.

All artwork was prepared at the Department of Anatomy, employing a total of 60 cadavers. We are deeply indebted to those individuals who made this work possible through their decision to leave their physical remains to science.

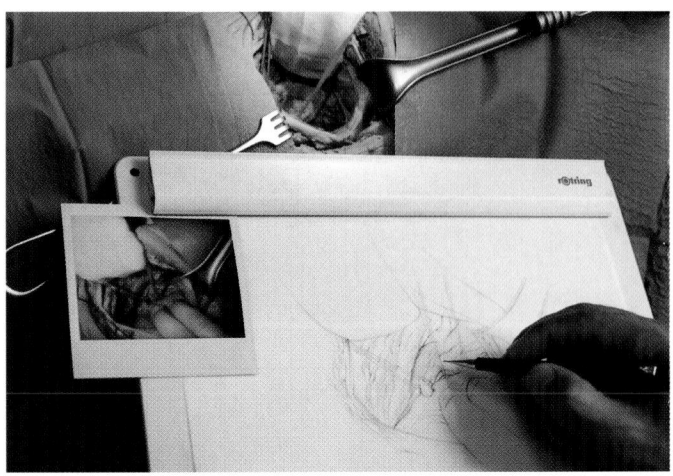

We express thanks to the chairman of the Department of Anatomy, Univ. Prof. Werner Platzer, M.D., who actively supported us with his team of scientists and laypersons at each stage during the preparation of this book.

We extend special thanks to our illustrator, Mr. Nikolaus Lechenbauer, who offered many valuable suggestions and coped with difficult deadlines, while producing his fine drawings. This book would not have been possible without his efforts.

We gratefully acknowledge support from many other sources, especially Dr. G. Hauff, Mr. A. Menge, and the staff at Thieme Medical Publishers, whose patience and professional competence contributed greatly to the production of this high-quality atlas.

We also thank our resident colleagues, Drs. Bernhard Moriggl and Heinz Wykypiel (Department of Anatomy) and Drs. Karl Colleselli and Hannes Strasser (Department of Urology), for their organizational assistance and for their help in preparing the dissections.

Innsbruck, July, 1993   Georg Bartsch
                                                               Sepp Poisel

Forewords

There has long been a need for a marriage between a classic anatomic text and a modern surgical text.

Detailed anatomic drawings and plates are notably absent in standard surgical texts (which necessarily are devoted to procedural matters in the "how-to" mode). Yet, paradoxically, exact anatomical features and their recognition form the basis or substrate of our surgical teaching.

This text is the first that I have seen that marries the present day academic anatomist and his or her department to the modern surgeon. Today's surgeons must dissect the same areas that they saw years ago as medical students, often with procedures that have been developed in the past decade. Yet they must have *detailed* knowledge of the anatomy that is impossible to convey (portray) in a typical wide-ranging "how-to" surgical text that relies on sketches or line drawings.

Furthermore, the Anatomy Department at Innsbruck University has completely updated the concepts of surgical anatomy in the pelvis, retroperitoneum, and retropubic space to include relevant anatomic details for the modern surgeon interested in the latest technical modifications of surgery, such as nerve – sparing techniques, and others. They are elegantly displayed in detailed plates worthy of the best anatomic atlas. Even more pleasing is that almost all views are presented from the perspective of the operating surgeon. Good surgeons are good anatomists; anatomy is still a growing field and a frontier for study in which more practical discoveries remain to be made. Surgeons are among the most likeley to make them. With this text Dr. Georg Bartsch and Dr. Sepp Poisel give us the opportunity to become better anatomists, which in turn makes us better surgeons.

John P. Donohue, M. D.
Professor and Chairman
Department of Urology
Indiana Univ. Hospital
Indianapolis, Indiana

Approaches in Urologic Surgery is a major surgical atlas designed to give the urologist an in-depth and detailed understanding of major surgical procedures and techniques based on anatomic relationships. This atlas reflects the unique collaboration between the Departments of Anatomy and Urology at the University of Innsbruck and has provided Professor Bartsch the basis for his personal approach to major surgical procedures. It is not comprehensive in terms of illustrating all procedures performed in urology or even all of the various surgical options available for performing a specific procedure. Rather, it represents what Professor Bartsch believes to be the optimal approaches for performing the specific surgical procedures illustrated in this atlas. The surgical techniques and approaches are based on detailed anatomic dissection and a thorough understanding of surgical anatomy. In addition, these approaches have been used extensively at the University of Innsbruck with outstanding clinical results. Thus, the reader will benefit from a philosophy a management and description of surgical techniques based on expertise developed from treatment schemes used in the authors own practice.

The illustrations are clear and presented from the surgeon's perspective supplemented by anatomic drawings showing abdominal, retroperitoneal, and pelvic wall relationships. The text is concise and allows the surgeon to easily follow and conceptualize the drawings.

This surgical atlas will become an important addition to the library of any aspiring resident or fellow contemplating a career in urologic oncology and reconstructive urologic surgery and is also for any practicing urologist seeking more effective or optimal surgical approaches for major urologic procedures.

Donald G. Skinner, M. D.
Professor and Chairman
Department of Urology
University of Southern California Medical Center
Los Angeles, California

Table of Contents

1 Abdominal Wall 1

Superficial Abdominal Muscles 2
Lateral Group 2
   External Oblique Muscle 2
   Internal Oblique Muscle 2
   Transversus Abdominis 2
Medial Group 2
   Rectus Abdominis 2
   Pyramidalis 2
Lumbar Trigone and Variations 4
Latissimus Dorsi 6
Serratus Anterior 7
Serratus Posterior Inferior 8
Intercostal Muscles 9

Diaphragm 11
   Lumbar Part of the Diaphragm 12
   Costal Part of the Diaphragm 12
   Sternal Part of the Diaphragm 12

Deep Abdominal Muscles 13
   Psoas Major 13
   Iliacus 13
   Quadratus Lumborum 13

Pelvic Floor 14
   Pelvic Diaphragm 14
   Urogenital Diaphragm 14

2 Retroperitoneal Space 17

Surgical Anatomy of the Retroperitoneal Space .. 18
   Definition, Boundaries, and Contents 18
Kidneys 20
   Position 20
   Capsules 24
   Renal Vessels 25
   Renal Nerve Supply 30
Renal Pelvis 30
Ureter 30
   Vessels and Nerves of the Ureter 30
Adrenal Gland 31
   Vessels and Nerves of the Adrenal Gland 31
Major Vessels and Nerves of the Retroperitoneal
Space 31
   Abdominal Aorta 31
   Inferior Vena Cava 32
   Lymph Vessels 33
   Nerves 33

Supracostal Approach 34
Main Indications 35
Position and Skin Incision 35

Exposure of the Lumbodorsal Fascia 36
Incision of the Lumbodorsal Fascia 40
Dissection of the Lumbodorsal Fascia and
Diaphragm from the 12th Rib 42
Incision of Gerota's Fascia 44

Transcostal Approach 45
Main Indications 46
Position and Skin Incision 46
Exposure of the 12th Rib 47
Resection of the 12th Rib 48
Exposure and Incision of the Lumbodorsal Fascia .. 48
Exposure of Gerota's Fascia 50

Foley Muscle-Splitting Approach 51
Main Indications 52
Position and Skin Incision 52
Exposure of the Superficial Muscles 53
Exposure of the Transversus Abdominis and its
Tendon of Origin 53
Exposure of Gerota's Fascia 54

Posterior Lumbotomy 55
Main Indications 56
Position and Skin Incision 56
Incision of the Superficial Layer of the
Lumbodorsal Fascia 56
Incision of the Deep Layer of the Lumbodorsal
Fascia 58
Exposure and Incision of Gerota's Fascia 58

Dorsolumbar (Nagamatsu) Approach 60
Main Indications 60
Position and Skin Incision 60
Exposure of the Deep Layer of the Lumbodorsal
Fascia 62
Division of the Lumbocostal Ligament and
Resection of Parts of the 11th and 12th Ribs 63
Separation of the Deep Lumbodorsal Fascia and
Diaphragm from the Rib Periosteum 64
Incision of Gerota's Fascia 65

Posterior Approach to the Adrenal Gland 67
Main Indications 68
Position and Skin Incision 68
Exposure and Resection of the 11th Rib 68
Incision of the Rib Bed 70
Exposure of the Adrenal Gland 71

Thoracoabdominal Approach 72
Main Indications 72
Position and Skin Incision 73
Laparotomy and Thoracotomy 74
   Modification: Thoracotomy with
   Rib Resection 76
Entry into the Retroperitoneal Space 79

Modification of the Thoracoabdominal Approach
for a Stage II or III Tumor Thrombus in the Vena
Cava 81
Cavatomy 82

Approach to the Retrocrural Lymph Nodes 84
Main Indications 85
Position and Skin Incision 85
Division of the Diaphragm 85
Exposure of the Retroperitoneal Space 86
Dissection of the Lateral Crus 88
Incision of the Aortic Aperture 90

Anterior Subcostal Approach 93
Main Indications 94
Position and Skin Incision 94
Division of the Abdominal Muscles 95
Entry into the Peritoneal Cavity 96
Dissection of the Renal Vessels 98
Dissection of the Retroperitoneal Space 100
Approach to the Adrenal Gland 102

Midline Transperitoneal Approach 105
Main Indications 106
Exposure of the Posterior Rectus Sheath 106
Position and Skin Incision 106
Entry into the Peritoneal Cavity 108
Exposure of the Retroperitoneal Space 110
Approach for a Suprahilar Lymph Node Dissection
on the Right Side 116
Incision of the Retroperitoneal Fascia 117

Paramedian Transperitoneal Approach 119
Main Indications 120
Position and Skin Incision 120
Exposure of the Rectus Sheath and Rectus Muscle .. 121
Exposure of the Posterior Rectus Sheath 122
Division of the Posterior Rectus Sheath and Parietal
Peritoneum 123

Lateral Extraperitoneal Gridiron Incision 125
Position and Skin Incision 126
Division of the Muscle 127
Entry into the Retroperitoneal Space 127

Low Lumbar Oblique Incision 129
Main Indication 130
Position and Skin Incision 130
Division of the Abdominal Muscles 132

Low Inguinal Incision 134
Main Indication 135
Position and Skin Incision 135
Division of the Abdominal Muscles 136

Extraperitoneal Paramedian Approach 138
Main Indications 139
Position and Skin Incision 139
Exposure of the Rectus Muscle 140
Dissection of the Epigastric Vessels 140

3 Pelvis 141

Anatomy of the Pelvis 142
Pelvic Part of the Ureter 142
Vessels and Nerves of the Pelvic Ureter 144
Relations of the Male Bladder to Adjacent Organs .. 146
Peritoneal Covering of the Bladder 146
Bladder and Pelvic Connective Tissue 147
Vessels and Nerves of the Bladder 149
Prostate 150
Relations of the Female Bladder to Adjacent
Organs 150

Anterior Pelvic Exenteration in the Male 151
Main Indications 152
Position and Skin Incision 152
Entry into the Peritoneal Cavity 153
Dissection of the Vesicoumbilical Plate 155
Mobilization of the Small Bowel and Ascending
Colon 157
Lymph Node Dissection by the Split-and-Roll
Technique 161
Dissection of the Lateral Bladder Pedicle (Lateral
Bladder Retinaculum) 164
Variants of the Internal Iliac Artery 166
Cul de Sac Incision 168
Exposure of the Rectovesical Septum (Posterior
Bladder Pedicle) 169
Exposure and Incision of the Endopelvic Fascia 172
Exposure of the Pubourethral Space, Entry into the
Rectourethral Space 173
Entry into the Denonvillier's Space 174
Preparation for Orthotopic Continent Ileal Reser-
voir 174

Anterior Pelvic Exenteration in the Female 176
Dissection of the Lateral Bladder Pedicle (Lateral
Bladder Retinaculum) 177
Exposure of the Posterior Bladder Pedicle 179
Opening the Posterior Vaginal Wall 180
Exposure and Incision of the Endopelvic Fascia 182

**Approach for Infrapubic Periurethral En Bloc
Resection of Female Urethral Carcinoma** 184
Main Indication 184
Position and Incision 184
Incision Around the Superior Portion of the
External Genitalia 185
Dissection of the Anterior Surface of the Symphysis . 186
En Bloc Removal of the Specimen 188

**Retropubic Approach for Radical Prosta-
tectomy** 190
Main Indication 191
Position and Skin Incision 191
Exposure of the Prevesical and Paravesical Spaces .. 192
Pelvic Lymph Node Dissection 196
Incision of the Endopelvic Fascia (Division of the
Puboprostatic Ligament) 198
Exposure of the Pubourethral Space 201

Table of Contents

Exposure and Division of the External Urethral
Sphincter (Rhabdosphincter) and Membranous
Urethra 202
Exposure of the Rectogenital Space 203
Exposure of the Vesicogenital Space 203

**Extraperitoneal Lower Abdominal Midline
Approach** 205
Main Indications 206
Position and Skin Incision 206
Exposure of the Linea Alba 207
Exposure of the Retropubic Space 208
Incision of the Bladder (Approach for a Transvesical
Prostatectomy) 210
Millin Approach 212

Pfannenstiel Incision 215
Main Indications 216
Position and Skin Incision 216
Exposure of the Rectus Muscles 216
Exposure of the Prevesical Space 219
Incision of the Bladder 220

4 Inguinal Region 221
Anatomy of the Inguinal Canal 222

Inguinal Approach 225
Main Indications 225
Position and Skin Incision 225
Exposure of the External Inguinal Ring 226
Exposure of the Internal Inguinal Ring 226

Ilioinguinal Lymph Node Dissection 229
Main Indication 229
Position and Skin Incision 229
Exposure of the Superficial Femoral (Scarpa's)
Fascia 230
Lymph Node Dissection 231
Great Saphenous Vein 232
Fascia Lata 234

5 External Genitalia 237
Pubic Approach 238
Main Indications 238
Position and Skin Incision 238
Exposure of the Superficial Dorsal Penile Vein ... 239
Exposure of the Penile Pedicle 240

Dorsal Approach to the Penis 241
Main Indications 241
Position and Skin Incision 241
Exposure of the Superficial Penile Fascia 241
Exposure of the Dorsal Neurovascular Bundle 242

Ventral Approach to the Penis 244
Main Indications 244
Position and Skin Incision 244
Mobilization of the Corpus Spongiosum 245

Approach to the Testis 246
Main Indications 246
Position and Skin Incision 246
Division of the External and Internal Spermatic
Fascia 247

**Approaches Involving the Female External Geni-
talia** 248
Main Indications 248
Position and Skin Incision 248
Exposure of the Urethrovaginal Septum 250
Bulbospongiosus Muscle Transfer 251
Gracilis Muscle Transfer 252
Transvaginal Retropubic Approach for the Pereyra-
Raz Vaginal Suspension 254

6 Perineum 255
Anatomy of the Male Urethra and Pelvic Floor .. 256

Perineal Approach to the Posterior Urethra 260
Main Indications 261
Position and Skin Incision 261
Dissection of the Central Tendon 262
Dorsal Approach Through the Perineal Body 264
Division of the Urethra 265
Dissection of the Rectourethral Septum 266
Dissection of the Prostatic Urethra (Entry into the
Pubourethral Space) 267

Transpubic Approach 268
Main Indications 269
Position and Skin Incision 269
Exposure of the Pubic Symphysis (Extraperitoneal
Midline Approach) 270
Resection of the Pubic Symphysis 272
Exposure of the Pubourethral Space 274

Perineal Approach for Radical Prostatectomy ... 275
Position and Skin Incision 276
Exposure and Division of the Central Tendon 277
Dissection of the Perineal Body, Entry into the
Rectourethral Space 278
Exposure of the Rectogenital Space 278
Exposure of the Anterior Surface of the Prostate ... 279
Exposure of the Vesicogenital and Rectogenital
Spaces 280

Posterior Sagittal Transcoccygeal Approach 282
Main Indications 282
Position and Skin Incision 282
Resection of the Coccyx 283
Incision of the Posterior Rectal Wall 284

Index 286

1 Abdominal Wall

Superficial Abdominal Muscles

(Fig. 1.**1**)

Lateral Group

External oblique muscle
Internal oblique muscle
Transversus abdominis

External Oblique Muscle

The external oblique muscle arises by eight slips from the external surfaces of the fifth through 12th ribs. Its five upper slips interdigitate with the origins of serratus anterior, its three lower slips with the origins of latissimus dorsi. Its posterior fibers descend almost vertically to the iliac crest, while the adjacent anterior fibers pass obliquely forward and medially in their downward course.

About a fingerwidth from the lateral border of the rectus abdominis muscle, the external oblique fibers terminate in an aponeurosis. The aponeuroses of both external oblique muscles unite at the *linea alba*, where they attach to the pubic symphysis and the adjacent anterior surfaces of the superior pubic ramus.

The portion of the aponeurosis between the anterior superior iliac spine and the pubic tubercle is thickened to form a tendinous band, the *inguinal ligament*. Just above and medial to the inguinal ligament is the *superficial inguinal ring*, bounded by the medial crus, lateral crus, and intercrural fibers. The latter are defined as reinforcing fibers of the external oblique aponeurosis.

Internal Oblique Muscle

The internal oblique muscle originates from the deep layer of the lumbodorsal fascia, from the intermediate line of the iliac crest, from the anterior superior iliac spine, and from the lateral portion of the inguinal ligament. Its muscular fibers fan out broadly to their sites of insertion. The uppermost posterior fibers are inserted into the inferior borders of the last three ribs. The intermediate fibers form an aponeurosis at the lateral border of the rectus abdominis muscle. This aponeurosis splits into an anterior and a posterior layer that pass around the rectus abdominis to form the rectus sheath before uniting with the contralateral aponeurotic fibers at the linea alba. The posterior rectus sheath terminates about three fingerwidths below the umbilicus at the *arcuate line* . The lower fibers of the internal oblique are continued onto the spermatic cord in males to form the *cremaster muscle*. In females, a few muscle fibers accompany the round ligament of the uterus within the inguinal canal.

Transversus Abdominis

The deepest of the three lateral abdominal muscles, the transversus abdominis arises by six slips from the internal aspects of the seventh through 12th costal cartilages, interdigitating with the slips of the costal part of the diaphragm.

Fibers also arise from the deep layer of the lumbodorsal fascia, the inner lip of the iliac crest, and the lateral part of the inguinal ligament. The transversus abdominis fibers pass in a horizontal direction and terminate in an aponeurosis along the laterally convex *semilunar line*. Above the arcuate line this aponeurosis forms the posterior layer of the rectus sheath. Below the arcuate line it unites with the anterior lamina of the internal oblique aponeurosis and helps to form the anterior layer of the rectus sheath. Each transversus aponeurosis fuses with its counterpart at the linea alba.

Medial Group

Rectus abdominis
Pyramidalis

Rectus Abdominis

The rectus abdominis muscle arises by three slips from the external surfaces of the fifth through seventh costal cartilage, from the xiphoid process, and from ligaments in this region. The muscle tapers in its straight, descending course, especially in its lower one-fourth, and inserts by a short, strong tendon into the pubic crest. The fiber mass of the rectus abdominis is interrupted by three or more transverse tendinous bands, the *tendinous intersections*, which are intimately attached to the anterior rectus sheath.

Rectus Sheath

The rectus sheath that envelops the rectus abdominis muscle is formed by the aponeuroses of the three lateral abdominal muscles. It is divided into an *anterior layer* (anterior rectus sheath) and a *posterior layer* (posterior rectus sheath). As noted above, the aponeurosis of the internal oblique muscle splits into two parts that pass behind and in front of the rectus abdominis to reach the linea alba. Above the umbilicus, or more precisely above the arcuate line, the anterior wall of the sheath consists of the external oblique aponeurosis and, deep to it, the anterior layer of the internal oblique aponeurosis. Below the level of the arcuate line, the aponeuroses of all three lateral abdominal muscles pass in front of the rectus abdominis muscle.

The posterior layer of the internal oblique aponeurosis is reinforced above the arcuate line by the aponeurosis of the transversus abdominis. Below the arcuate line, the posterior wall of the rectus sheath is formed entirely by the transversalis fascia.

Pyramidalis

The pyramidalis muscle arises broadly from the superior pubic ramus, anterior to the insertion of the rectus abdominis. It passes upward, gradually narrowing as it ascends, to insert on the linea alba. The pyramidalis is absent in approximately 20% of the population.

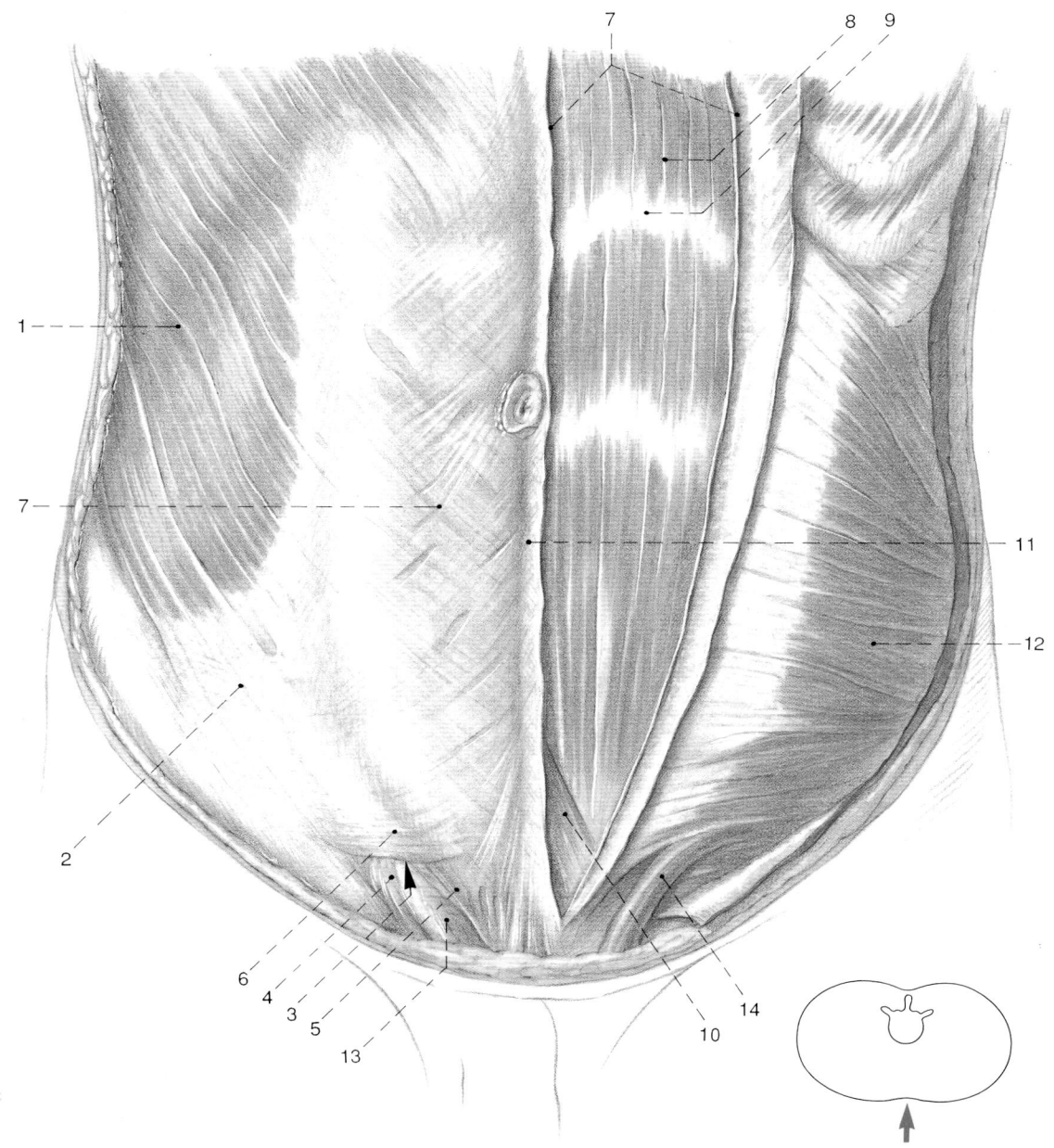

Fig. 1.**1** External view of the anterior abdominal wall. The anterior rectus sheath and external oblique muscle on the left side have been removed.

 1 External oblique muscle
 2 External oblique aponeurosis
 3 Superficial inguinal ring
 4 Lateral crus
 5 Medial crus
 6 Intercrural fibers
 7 Anterior rectus sheath
 8 Rectus muscle
 9 Tendinous intersection
10 Pyramidalis muscle
11 Linea alba
12 Internal oblique muscle
13 Spermatic cord (external spermatic fascia)
14 Spermatic cord (cremaster muscle)

Lumbar Trigone and Variations

(Fig. 1.2)

The lumbar trigone is a triangular interval bounded by the iliac crest, the posterior border of the external oblique muscle, and the anterior (lateral) border of the latissimus dorsi. The shape and size of the triangle are highly variable depending on the degree of overlap of its bordering muscles and their tendons of origin. If the musculotendinous plates overlap sufficiently, a lumbar trigone is not formed (Fig. 1.2a).

If the muscles are less prominently developed, a lumbar triangle is present. The floor of the lumbar trigone may be formed by the internal oblique, if this muscle is well developed (Fig. 1.2 b), or by the deep layer of the lumbodorsal fascia (Fig. 1.2 c). In the latter case the lumbodorsal fascia is the only solid structural component of the posterior abdominal wall in the lumbar trigone.

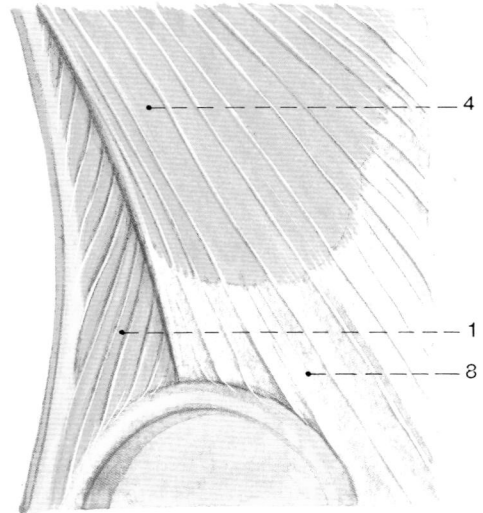

a

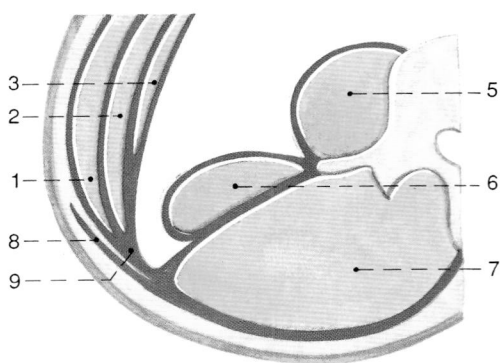

Fig. 1.2 a–c   Variations of the lumbar trigone (after von Lanz and Wachsmuth).
a Lumbodorsal fascia (superficial layer) overlies the external oblique muscle.
b Lumbodorsal fascia overlaps the internal oblique muscle.
c Lumbodorsal fascia forms a triangle (lumbar trigone) with the external oblique muscle.

1 External oblique muscle
2 Internal oblique muscle
3 Transversus abdominis
4 Latissimus dorsi
5 Psoas major
6 Quadratus lumborum
7 Erector spinae
8 Lumbodorsal fascia, superficial layer
9 Thoracolumbar fascia, deep layer

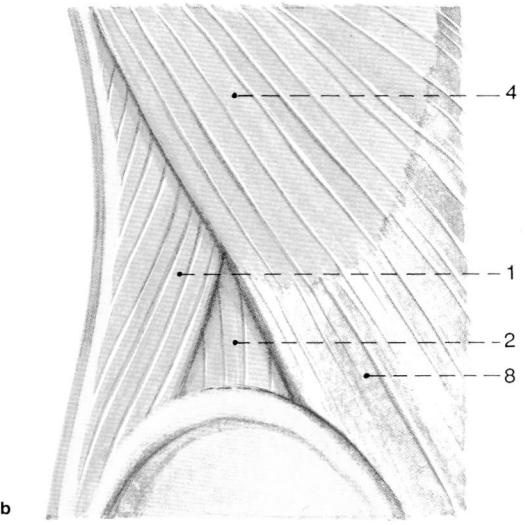

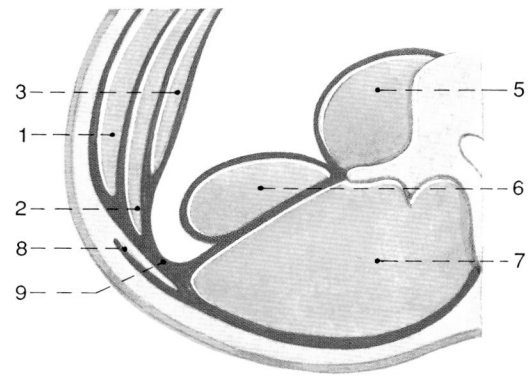

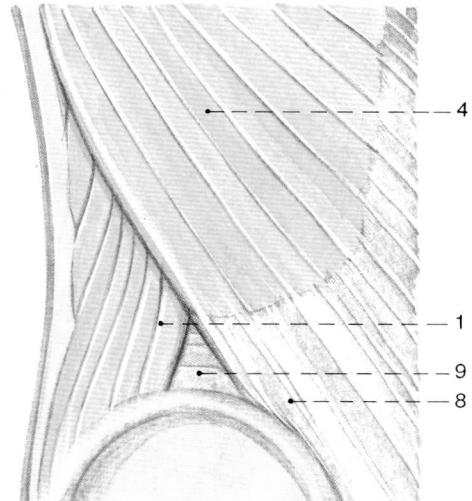

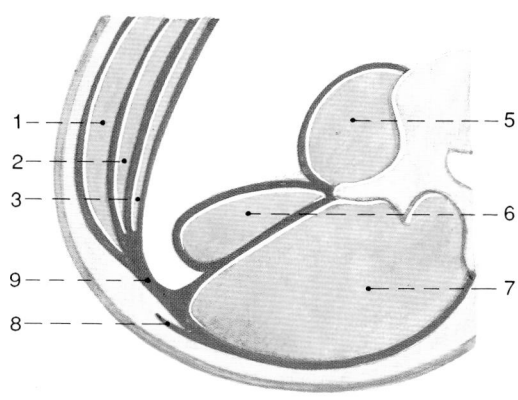

Latissimus Dorsi

(Figs. 1.**3** and 1.**4**)

The *vertebral part* of this muscle arises from the spinous processes of the fifth through 12th thoracic vertebrae and its *iliac part* from the lumbodorsal fascia and the posterior iliac crest. The *costal part* of latissimus dorsi arises from the external surfaces of the 10th through 12th ribs, and a variable *scapular part* originates from the inferior angle of the scapula. The fibers of latissimus dorsi pass laterally upward with varying degrees of obliquity to the humerus, where they insert into the crest of the lesser tubercle.

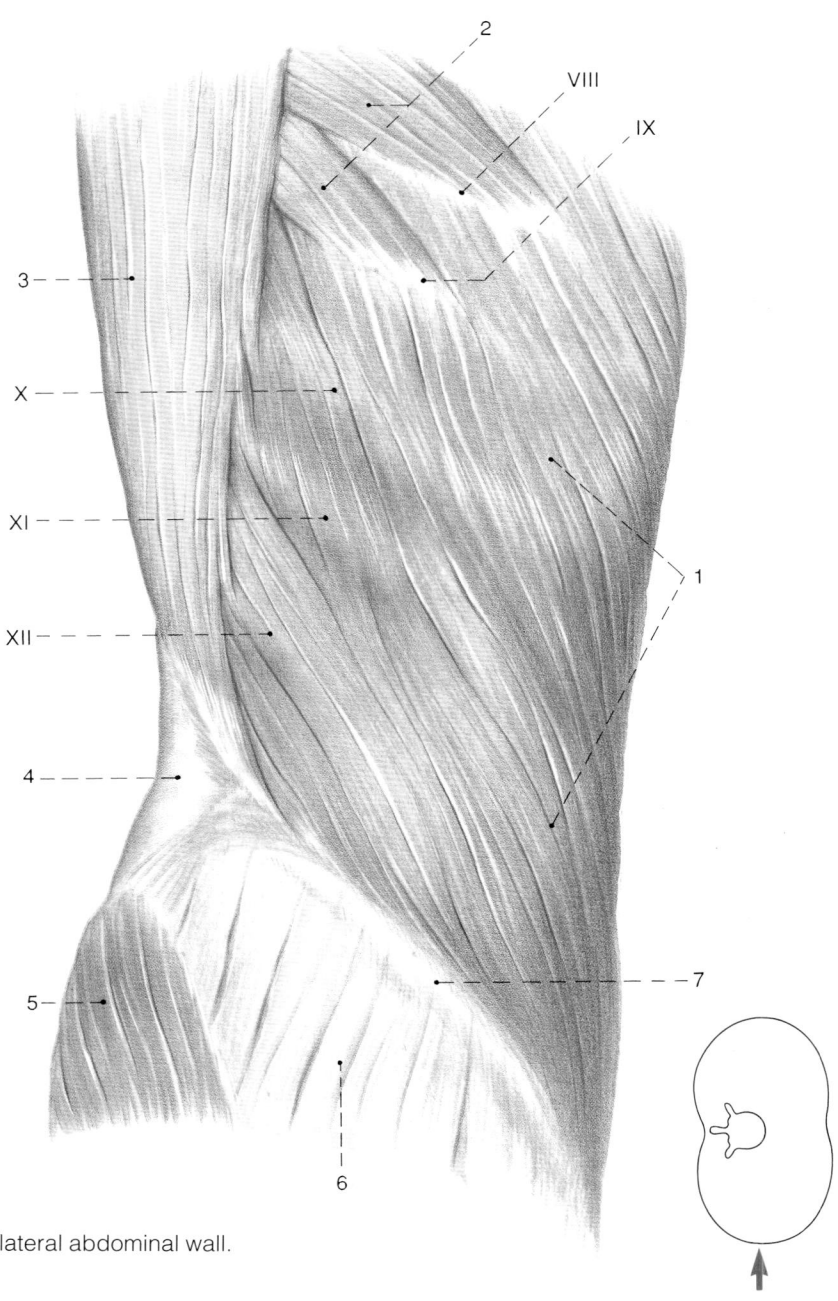

Fig. 1.**3**   External view of the lateral abdominal wall.

1 External oblique muscle
2 Serratus anterior
3 Latissimus dorsi
4 Lumbodorsal fascia
5 Gluteus maximus
6 Gluteus medius
7 Iliac crest
VIII–XII 8th through 12th ribs

Serratus Anterior

The serratus anterior muscle overlies the lateral chest wall and arises by nine and sometimes 10 slips from the outer surfaces of the upper nine (or eight) ribs. It is inserted along the entire medial border of the scapula. Its tripartite insertion consists of a *superior part* to the superior angle of the scapula, an *intermediate part* to the medial scapular margin, and an *inferior part* to the inferior angle of the scapula.

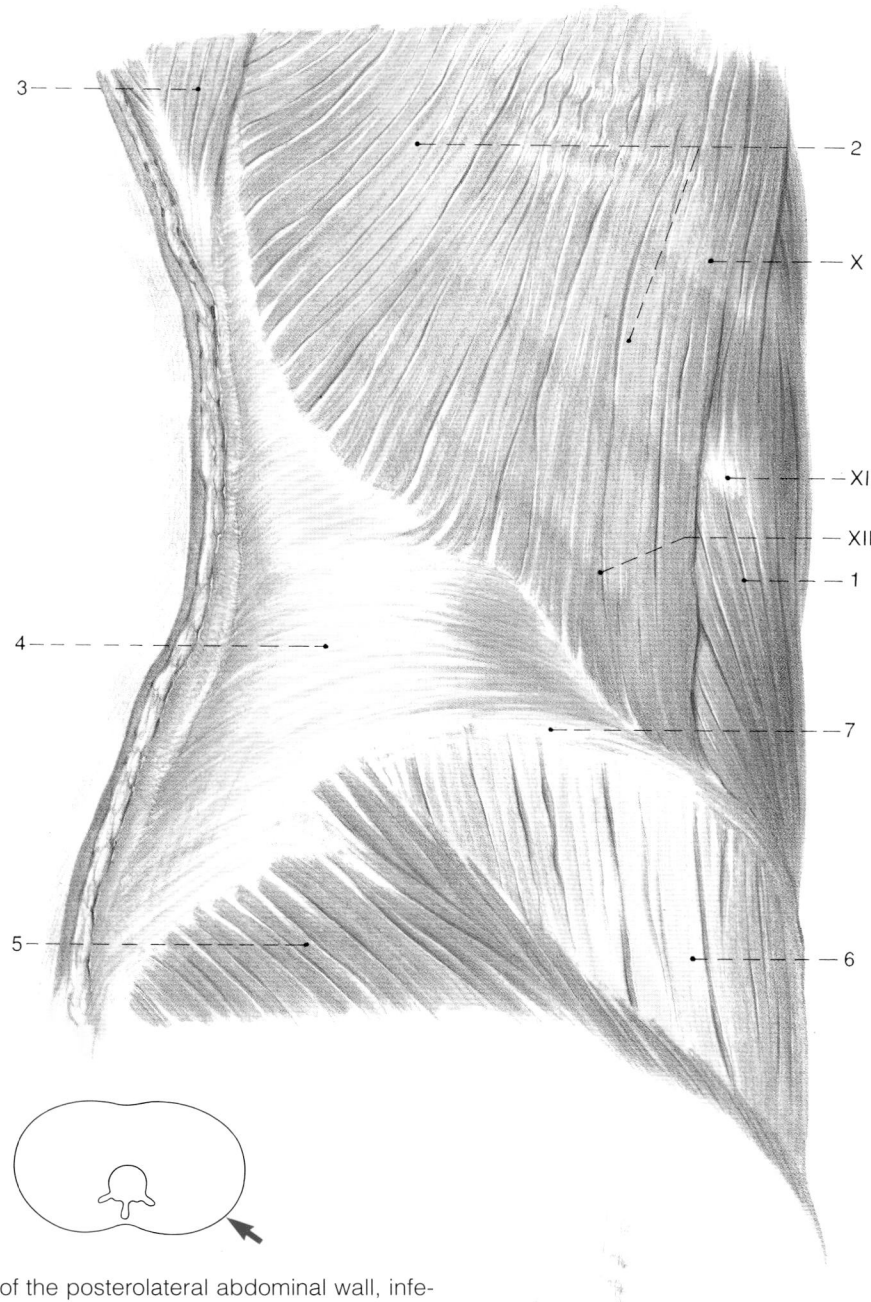

Fig. 1.**4** External view of the posterolateral abdominal wall, inferior portion.

1 External oblique muscle
2 Latissimus dorsi
3 Trapezius
4 Lumbodorsal fascia
5 Gluteus maximus
6 Gluteus medius
7 Iliac crest
X–XII 10th through 12th ribs

Serratus Posterior Inferior

(Fig. 1.5)

This muscle arises from the superficial layer of the lumbodorsal fascia at the level of the lower two thoracic vertebrae and the upper two lumbar vertebrae. It runs obliquely upward and laterally to attach by four slips to the inferior margins of the lower four ribs, somewhat lateral to their costal angles.

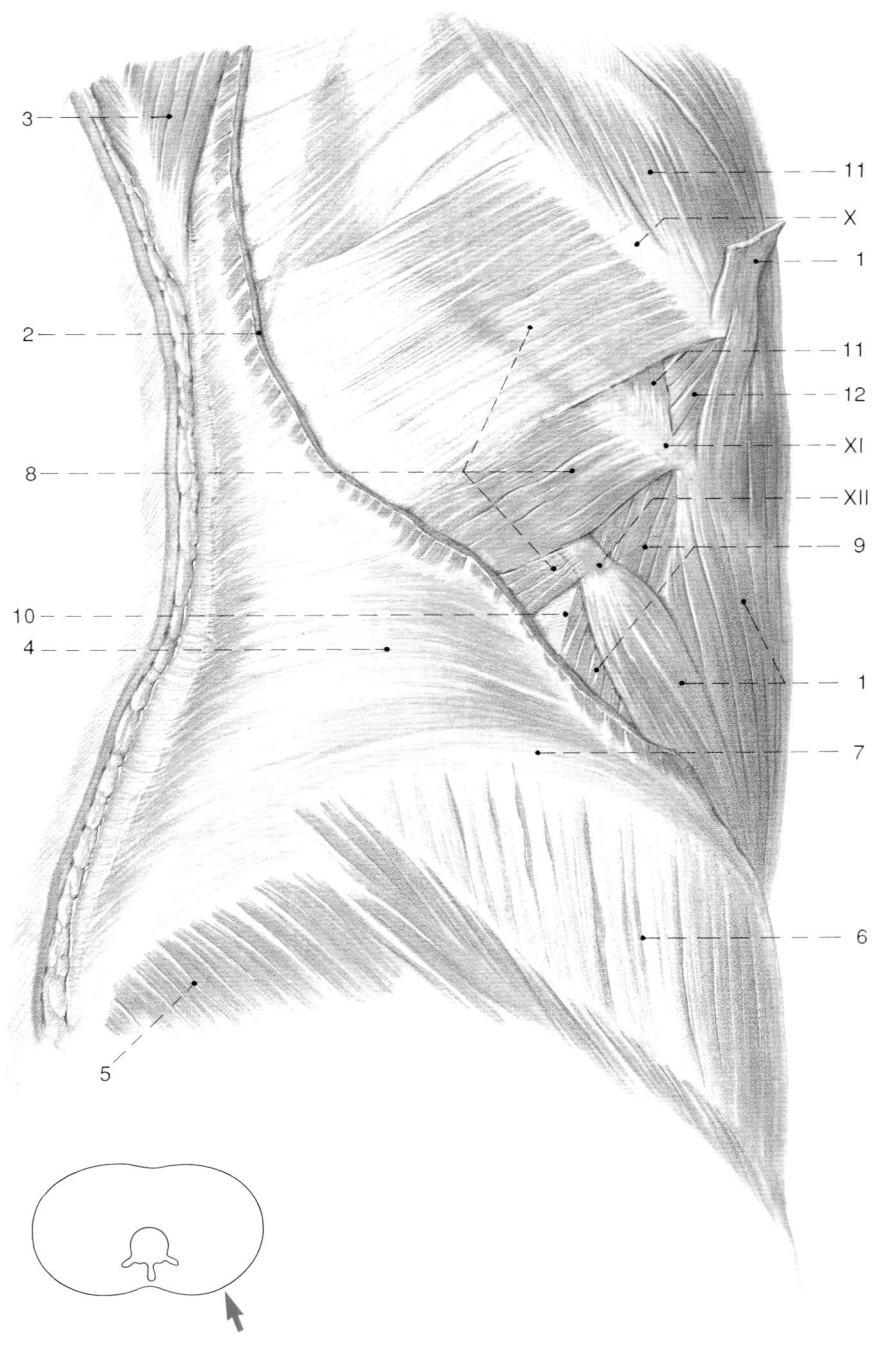

Fig. 1.5 External view of the posterolateral abdominal wall, inferior portion. The latissimus dorsi has been removed to show the origins of the external oblique muscle.

1 External oblique muscle
2 Latissimus dorsi
3 Trapezius
4 Lumbodorsal fascia

5 Gluteus maximus
6 Gluteus medius
7 Iliac crest
8 Serratus posterior inferior

9 Internal oblique muscle
10 Lumbar trigone
11 External intercostal muscle

12 Internal intercostal muscle
X–XII 10th through 12th ribs

Intercostal Muscles

These muscles partially occupy the intercostal spaces and are composed of an internal and an external layer.

The *external intercostal muscles* run forward from the costal tubercle to the margin of the rib cartilage. The external intercostals become membranous between the costal cartilages, each continuing forward to the septum as the *external intercostal membrane*. The external intercostal fibers run obliquely downward, passing laterally downward in their posterior portion and medially downward in their anterior portion.

The *internal intercostal muscles* extend obliquely forward and upward from the costal angle to the sternum. The last two internal intercostal muscles are often fused with the internal oblique muscle, showing no apparent boundary. In the intercostal space between the costal angle and vertebral column, each internal intercostal muscle is replaced by an *internal intercostal membrane*.

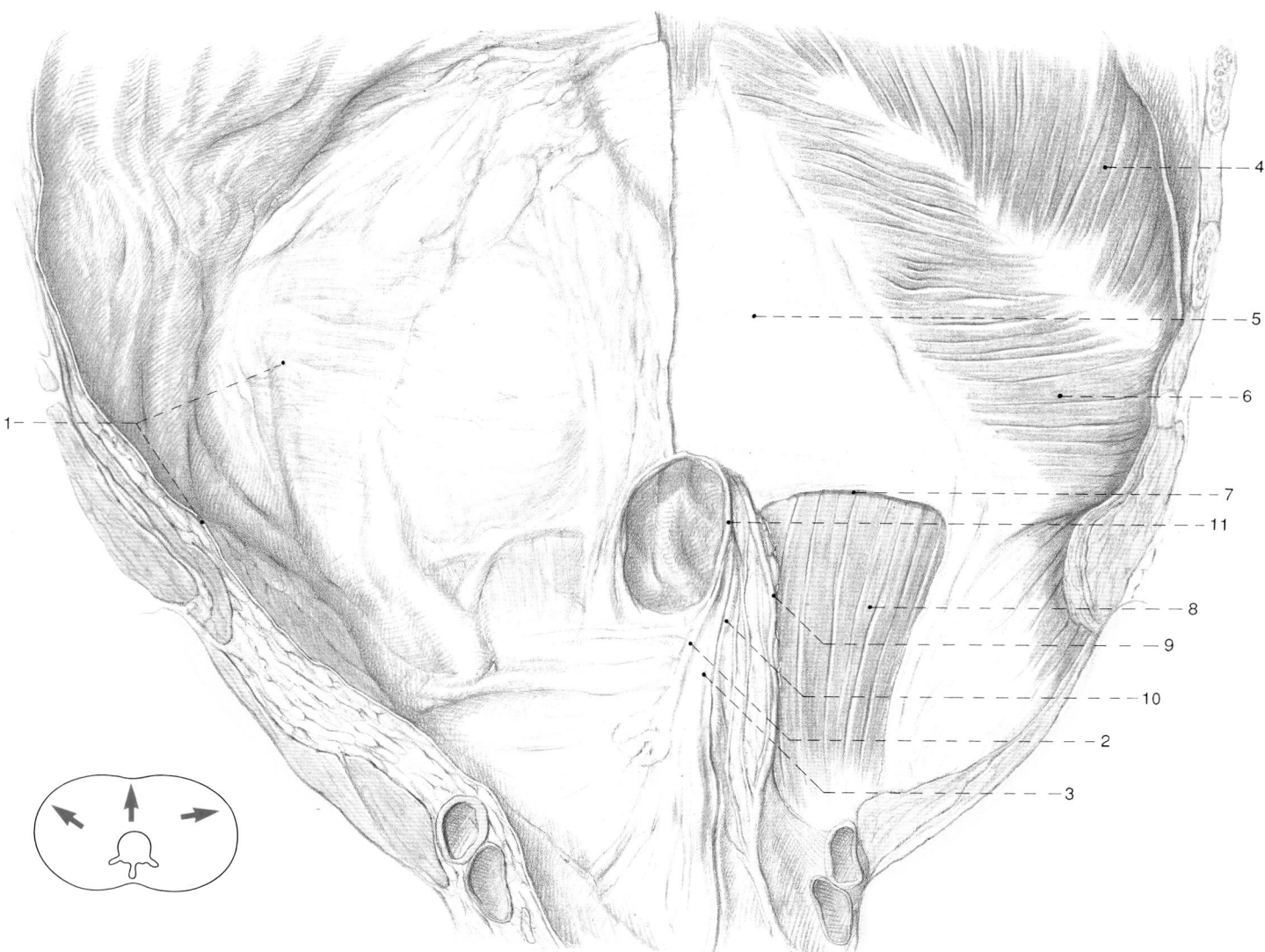

Fig. 1.**6** Internal view of the anterior abdominal wall in a specimen with an umbilical hernia. Left body half: parietal peritoneum intact. Right body half: parietal peritoneum and transversalis fascia have been removed.

1 Parietal peritoneum
2 Medial umbilical fold
3 Median umbilical fold
4 Diaphragm
5 Posterior rectus sheath
6 Transversus abdominis
7 Arcuate line
8 Rectus muscle
9 Lateral umbilical ligament
10 Median umbilical ligament
11 Hernial ring

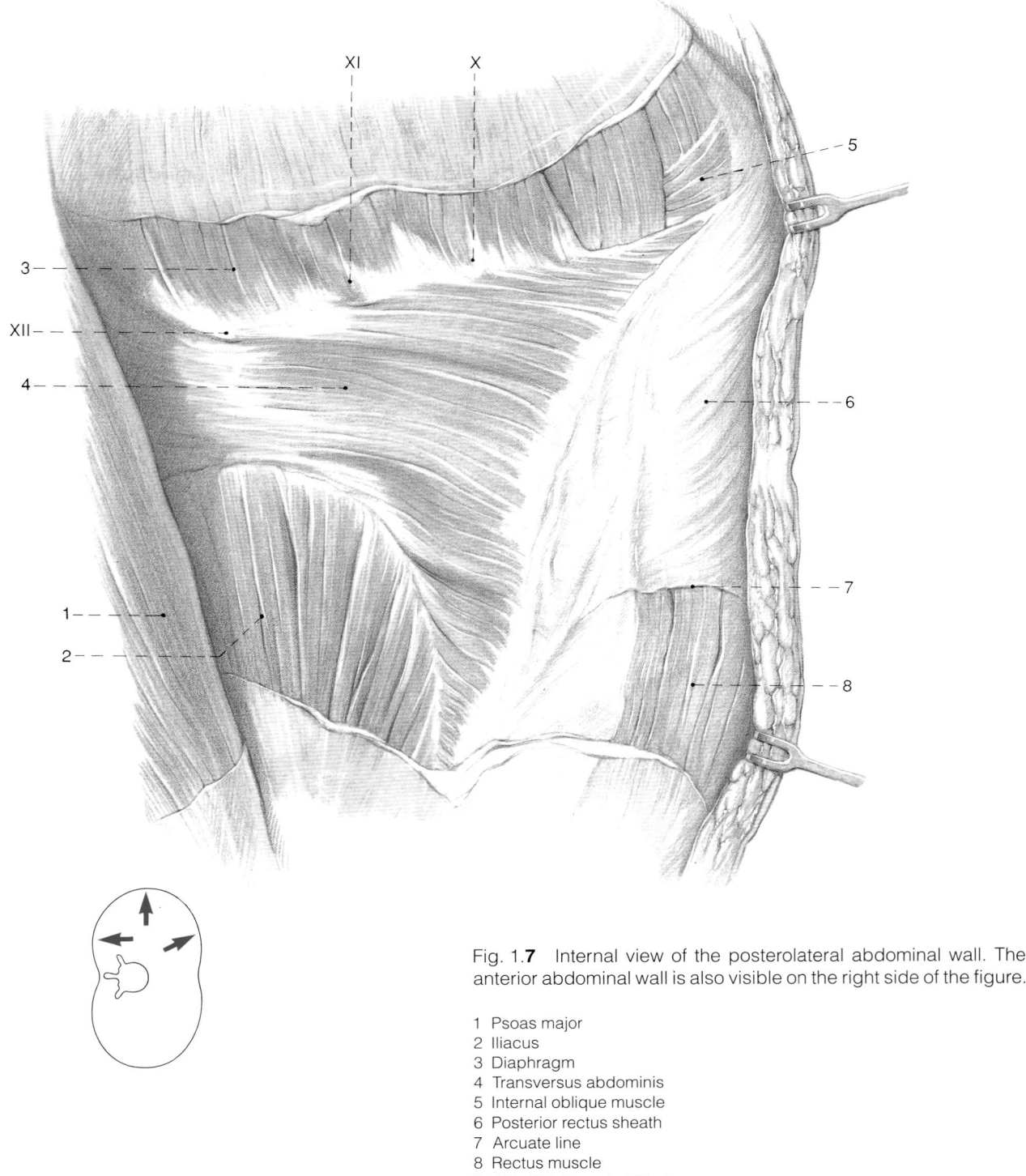

Fig. 1.**7** Internal view of the posterolateral abdominal wall. The anterior abdominal wall is also visible on the right side of the figure.

1 Psoas major
2 Iliacus
3 Diaphragm
4 Transversus abdominis
5 Internal oblique muscle
6 Posterior rectus sheath
7 Arcuate line
8 Rectus muscle
X–XII 10th through 12th ribs

Diaphragm

(Fig. 1.**8**)

The diaphragm forms a musculotendinous partition between the abdominal and thoracic cavities. Its central tendinous portion is termed the *central tendon*, and its muscular portion is divisible into a *sternal part*, a *costal part*, and a *lumbar part*.

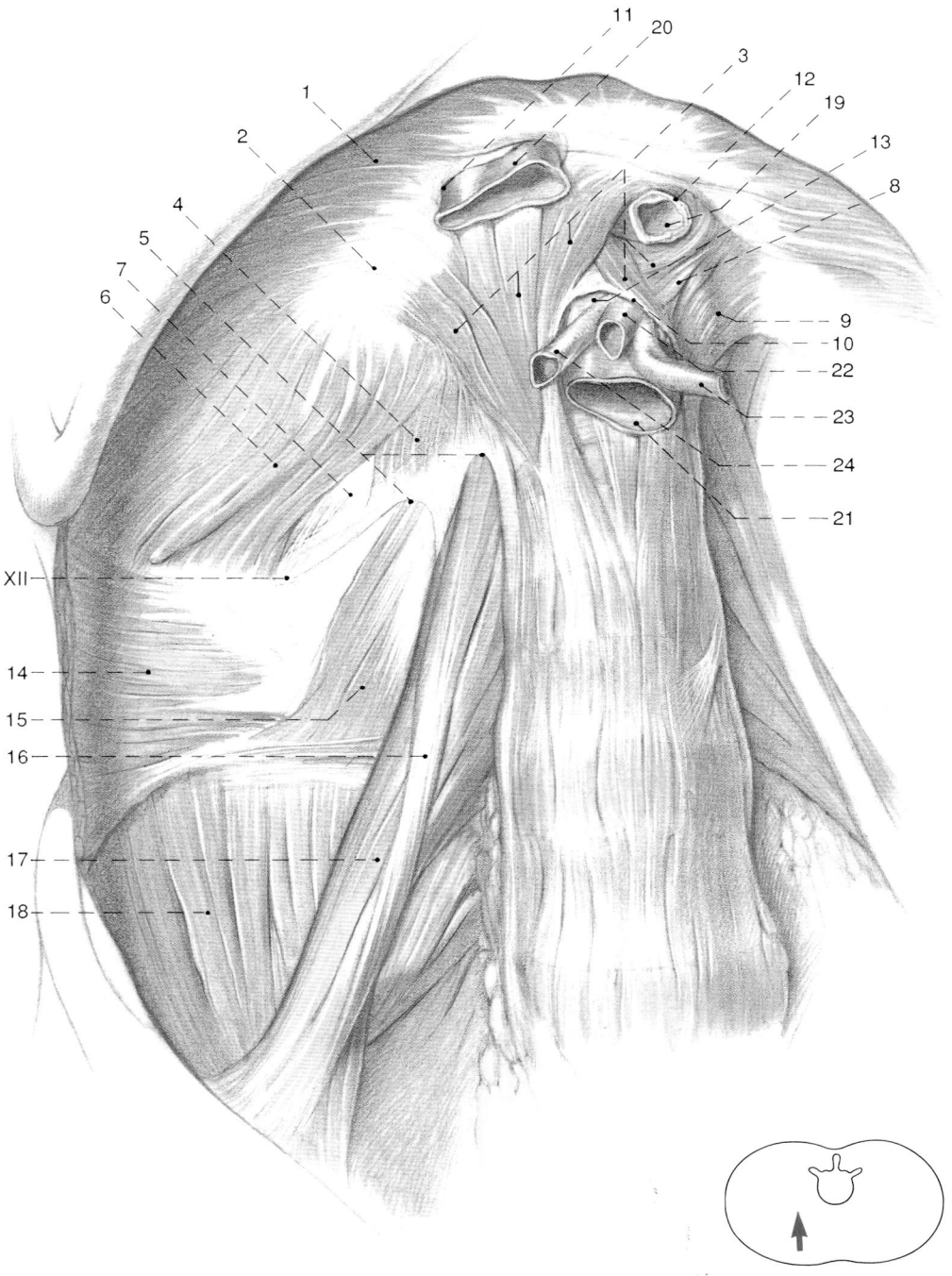

Fig. 1.**8**   Internal view of the posterosuperior abdominal wall.

1 Diaphragm	7 Lumbocostal trigone	13 Aortic hiatus	19 Esophagus
2 Central tendon	8 Lumbar part of diaphragm, left medial crus	14 Transversus abdominis	20 Inferior vena cava
3 Lumbar part of diaphragm, right medial crus	9 Lumbar part of diaphragm, left lateral crus	15 Quadratus lumborum	21 Abdominal aorta
4 Lumbar part of diaphragm, right lateral crus	10 Median arcuate ligament	16 Psoas minor	22 Celiac trunk
5 Medial and lateral arcuate ligaments	11 Vena caval foramen	17 Psoas major	23 Common hepatic artery
6 Costal part of diaphragm	12 Esophageal hiatus	18 Iliacus	24 Splenic artery

Lumbar Part of the Diaphragm

The lumbar part of the diaphragm arises by a *medial crus* and a *lateral crus*. A portion of the medial crus is sometimes split off to form an intermediate crus. The *right medial crus* arises from the anterior surfaces of the bodies of the first through fourth lumbar vertebrae, the *left medial crus* from the bodies of the first through third lumbar vertebrae. Both medial crura form the *aortic aperture* (aortic hiatus), which is bordered by the median arcuate ligament.

The *right medial crus* is composed of three muscular bundles, the first arising, as noted, from the lumbar vertebrae and merging directly with the central tendon. The second arises from the median arcuate ligament and forms the right border of the *esophageal aperture* (esophageal hiatus) of the diaphragm. The third muscular bundle, located posterior to the second, also originates from the median arcuate ligament and forms the left border of the esophageal aperture.

The *lateral crus* arises from the two tendinous arches of the medial and lateral arcuate ligaments. The medial arcuate ligament (medial lumbocostal arch or psoas arcade) extends from the lateral surface of the first (second) lumbar vertebral body to the first (second) costal process, passing over the origins of the psoas major muscle. The lateral arcuate ligament (lateral lumbocostal arch or quadratus arcade) extends from the costal process to the tip of the 12th rib, passing over the quadratus lumborum muscle. The muscle fibers run steeply upward from both tendinous arches to the central tendon.

Costal Part of the Diaphragm

The costal part of the diaphragm arises from the inner surfaces of the cartilages of the lower six ribs, interdigitating with the transversus abdominis. The muscle fibers arch to their insertion at the anterolateral border of the central tendon.

Sternal Part of the Diaphragm

This, the smallest part of the diaphragm, arises by one or more small slips from the internal surface of the xiphoid process and from the posterior layer of the rectus sheath. The muscle fibers pass almost transversely to the anterior border of the central tendon.

Deep Abdominal Muscles

Psoas major
Quadratus lumborum

Psoas Major

The superficial part of this muscle arises from the lateral surfaces of the 12th thoracic vertebra and the first four lumbar vertebrae, and its deep part from the first through fifth costal processes. It unites with the fibers of the iliacus muscle (see below) and, enveloped by the iliac fascia, inserts into the lesser trochanter of the femur as the *iliopsoas muscle*.

The *psoas minor* is a variant present in less than 50% of individuals. It arises from the 12th thoracic and first lumbar vertebrae and is attached to the iliac fascia and, via the fascia, to the iliopubic eminence.

Iliacus

The iliacus muscle arises from the iliac fossa and inserts conjointly with psoas major into the lesser trochanter of the femur. Their composite, the iliopsoas, passes through the *lacuna musculorum* (muscular compartment) beneath the inguinal ligament to reach the thigh.

Quadratus Lumborum

This flat muscle lies adjacent to the vertebral column and stretches between the 12th rib and iliac crest. It consists of two parts that cannot be completely separated from each other: a posterior part arising from the iliac crest and iliolumbar ligament and inserting into the costal processes of the first through third (or fourth) lumbar vertebrae and 12th rib, and an anterior part passing from the costal processes of the lower three or four lumbar vertebrae to the last rib.

Pelvic Floor

(Fig. 1.9)

The pelvic floor constitutes the posterior inferior boundary of the abdominal cavity. It consists of the *pelvic diaphragm* and the *urogenital diaphragm* .

Pelvic Diaphragm

The pelvic diaphragm is composed of the *levator ani* and *coccygeus* muscles.

The *levator ani* muscle group consists of the puborectalis, prerectal fibers, pubococcygeus, and iliococcygeus, which in some individuals are bounded superiorly by the sacrococcygeus and rectococcygeus muscles. The levator ani arises from the pubic bone lateral to the symphysis, from the tendinous arch of the levator ani (part of the obturator fascia), and from the ischial spine.

The most medial fibers of the puborectalis muscles form the *"levator crura,"* which bound the *levator hiatus* (genital hiatus). The prerectal fibers are attached to the perineum and separate the urogenital hiatus from the anal hiatus. The levator hiatus is traversed by the urethra in males and by the urethra and vagina in females. The rectum leaves the true pelvis behind the prerectal fibers. The pubococcygeus and iliococcygeus muscles are attached to the coccyx and anococcygeal ligament.

The *coccygeus* muscle passes from the ischial spine to the coccyx and completes the pelvic diaphragm posteriorly.

Urogenital Diaphragm

The urogenital diaphragm is a musculotendinous sheet in the subpubic angle (pubic arch in females); it closes the levator hiatus inferiorly. Its main component is the *deep transverse perineal muscle*. The urogenital diaphragm is traversed by the urethra (and the vagina in females), whose membranous portion is surrounded by the omega-shaped muscle fibers of the *urethral sphincter* (rhabdosphincter). The urogenital diaphragm is completed anteriorly by the *transverse perineal ligament*. The outer portion of the diaphragm is reinforced posteriorly and superficially by the *superficial transverse perineal muscle*.

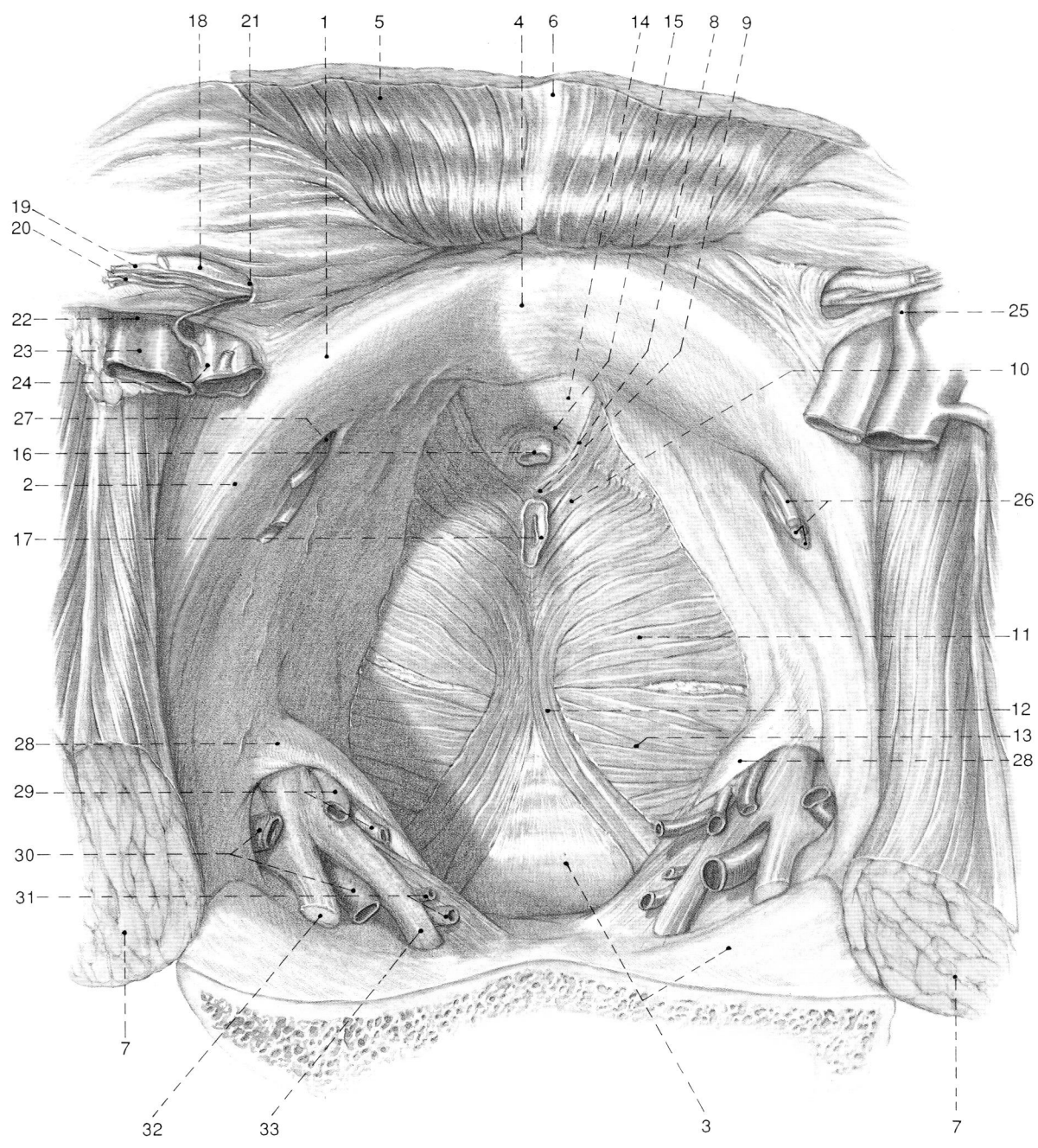

Fig. 1.**9**   Internal view of the inferior abdominal wall (pelvic floor).

1   Superior pubic ramus
2   Arcuate line
3   Sacrum
4   Pubic symphysis
5   Rectus muscle
6   Linea alba
7   Psoas major
8–13   Pelvic diaphragm
   8   Levator ani, puborectalis
   9   Prerectal fibers
  10   Pubococcygeus
  11   Iliococcygeus
  12   Sacrococcygeus and rectococcygeus
  13   Coccygeus
14, 15   Urogenital diaphragm
  14   Transverse perineal ligament
  15   Urethral sphincter

16   Male urethra
17   Rectum
18   Vas deferens
19   Genital branch of genitofemoral nerve
20   Testicular artery and pampiniform plexus
21   Deep inguinal ring
22   Lacuna vasorum
23   External iliac artery
24   External iliac vein
25   Inferior epigastric artery
26   Obturator artery, vein, and nerve
27   Obturator canal
28   Parietal pelvic fascia
29   Inferior gluteal vessels
30   Internal pudendal vessels
31   Superior gluteal vessels
32   Lumbosacral trunk
33   Ventral branch of first sacral nerve

2 Retroperitoneal Space

Surgical Anatomy of the Retroperitoneal Space

Definition, Boundaries, and Contents

The retroperitoneal space is defined as the space between the posterior parietal peritoneum and the posterior abdominal wall. It is bounded superiorly by the diaphragm, and it blends inferiorly with the connective-tissue stratum of the subperitoneal space.

The lateral boundaries of the retroperitoneal space are imprecisely defined. They are formed essentially by the close apposition of the posterior parietal peritoneum to the transversalis fascia on the inner aspect of the lateral abdominal muscles, the thin subserous connective-tissue layer forming a virtual boundary in that region.

The contents of the retroperitoneal space can be described as having either a primary or a secondary retroperitoneal location. Portions of the duodenum, pancreas, and ascending and descending colon reach the retroperitoneum secondarily. Primary retroperitoneal structures are the kidneys and renal pelves, ureters, adrenal glands, and the large nerves and vessels (Fig. 2.1).

Fig. 2.1   Topography of the organs, vessels, and nerves of the retroperitoneal space and posterior abdominal wall.

1   Right medial crus of diaphragm
2   Esophageal hiatus
3   Central tendon
4   Left lateral crus of diaphragm
5   Costal part of diaphragm
6   Right medial crus and aortic hiatus
7   Psoas major
8   Iliacus
9   Psoas minor
10 Parietal peritoneum
11 Left kidney
12 Right kidney
13 Left adrenal gland
14 Right adrenal gland
15 Left renal pelvis
16 Left ureter
17 Perirenal fat capsule
18 Esophagus
19 Abdominal aorta
20 Celiac trunk
21 Common hepatic artery
22 Left gastric artery
23 Splenic artery
24 Right inferior phrenic artery
25 Left superior suprarenal and inferior phrenic arteries
26 Middle suprarenal artery
27 Renal artery and renal plexus
28 Superior mesenteric artery
29 Testicular artery
30 Inferior mesenteric artery
31 Sigmoid artery
32 Common iliac artery
33 Inferior vena cava
34 Hepatic veins
35 Suprarenal vein
36 Renal vein
37 Testicular vein
38 Common iliac vein
39 Anterior vagal trunk
40 Posterior vagal trunk
41 Celiac plexus and ganglion and superior mesenteric plexus
42 Sympathetic trunk
43 Abdominal aortic plexus
44 Superior hypogastric plexus
45 Iliohypogastric nerve
46 Subcostal nerve
47 Ilioinguinal nerve
48 Lateral femoral cutaneous nerve
49 Genitofemoral nerve
50 Preaortic lymph nodes

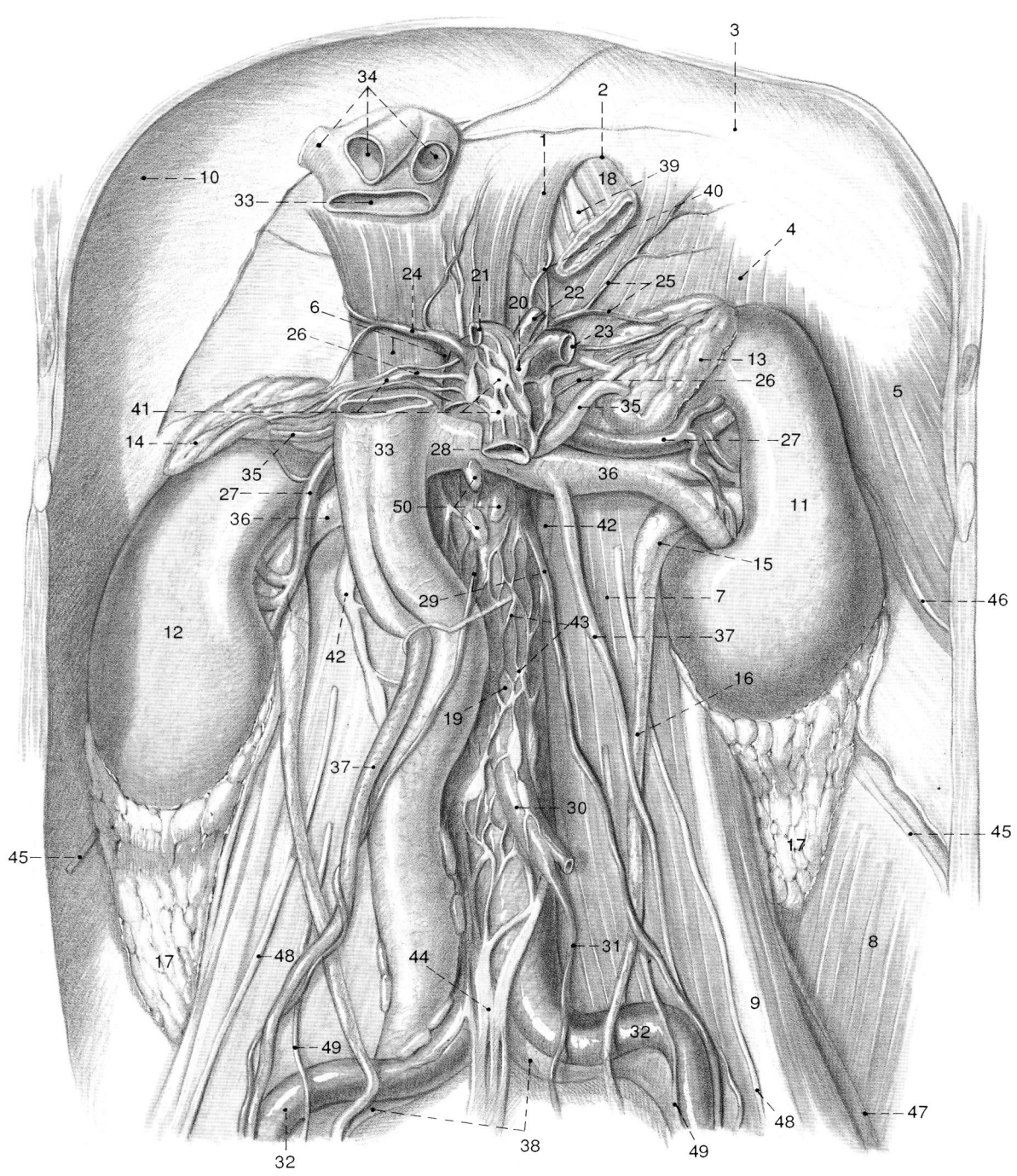

Fig. 2.**1**

Kidneys

Position

The kidneys are paired viscera that flank the vertebral column in the retroperitoneal space. Externally the kidney presents a *medial border*, a *lateral border*, an *anterior surface*, a *posterior surface*, an *upper pole*, and a *lower pole*. The medial border presents a deep fissure, the *renal hilum*, which leads into the *renal sinus*. The upper pole of the kidney is more rounded than the lower pole because of its relation to the adrenal gland.

The terms of orientation for the kidney are somewhat imprecise because the organ is oriented at an angle to the cardinal planes. The anterior suface of the kidney is angled posterolaterally from the frontal plane, so normally the renal hilum is directed anteromedially. The long axes of both kidneys are convergent superiorly, so that the upper poles of the kidneys are separated by a smaller distance (7–8 cm) than the lower poles (11–15 cm).

The level of the kidneys in relation to the vertebral column is subject to marked individual variations. Renal position is also dependent on individual body posture and the phases of respiration. Changes in renal position are more frequent and pronounced in children than in adults.

The right kidney in adults lies usually somewhat lower than the left kidney. The upper pole of the right kidney typically occupies a level between the body of the 12th thoracic vertebra and the upper third of the first lumbar vertebra. The upper pole of the left kidney is generally higher than the right upper pole by one-half the height of a vertebral body. The lower pole of the right kidney is usually level with the third lumbar vertebra, and the lower pole of the left kidney occupies a correspondingly higher position (Fig. 2.2 a).

The relation of the lower pole of the kidney to the highest point of the iliac crest is subject to the same individual variations. The right lower pole is approximately 3 cm above the iliac crest, on average, while the left lower pole is about 1 cm higher (Fig. 2.2 b).

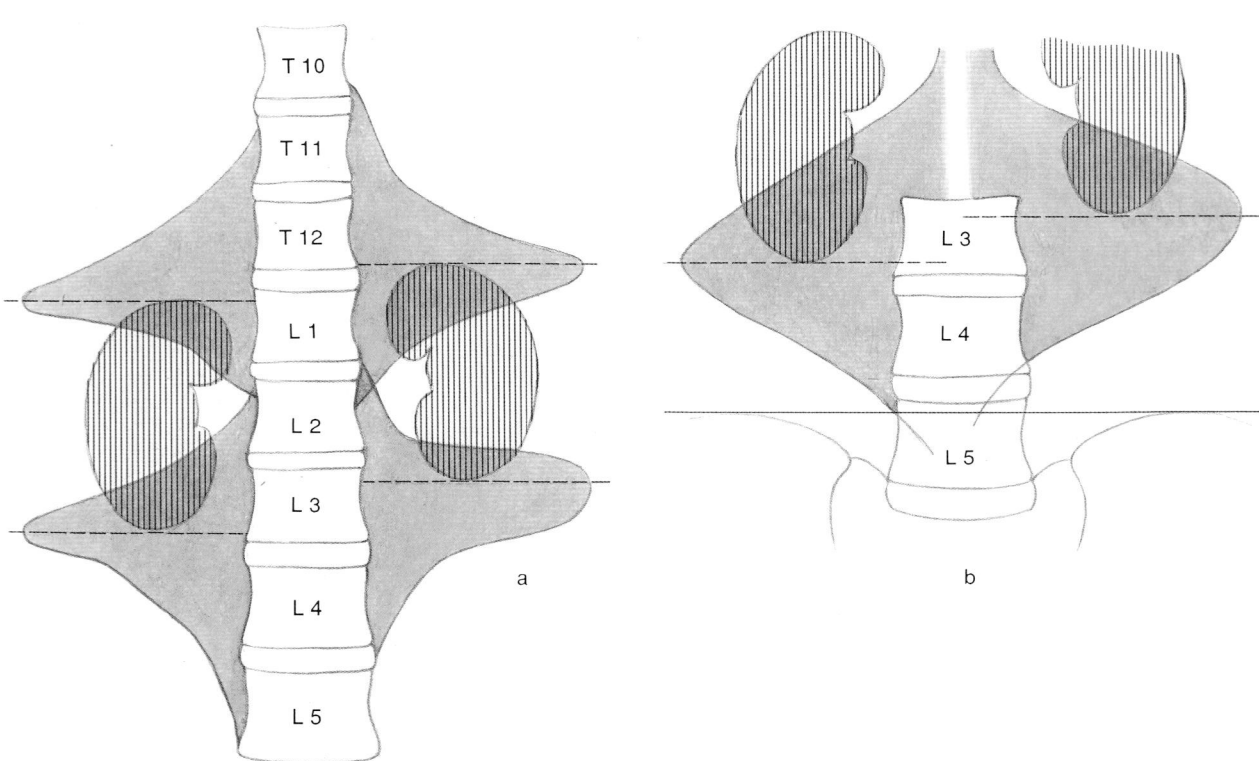

Fig. 2.**2a, b**   Range of variation in the levels of the renal poles.
a Position of the renal poles in relation to the lumbar spine.
b Position of the lower renal pole in relation to the iliac crest. The red shaded areas indicate the range of variation.

Relations

The kidneys are embedded in the perirenal fat capsule, which is separated from the outer, pararenal fat by Gerota's fascia (see below). The relations of the anterior surface of the kidney are shown in Figs. 2.**3** and 2.**4**.

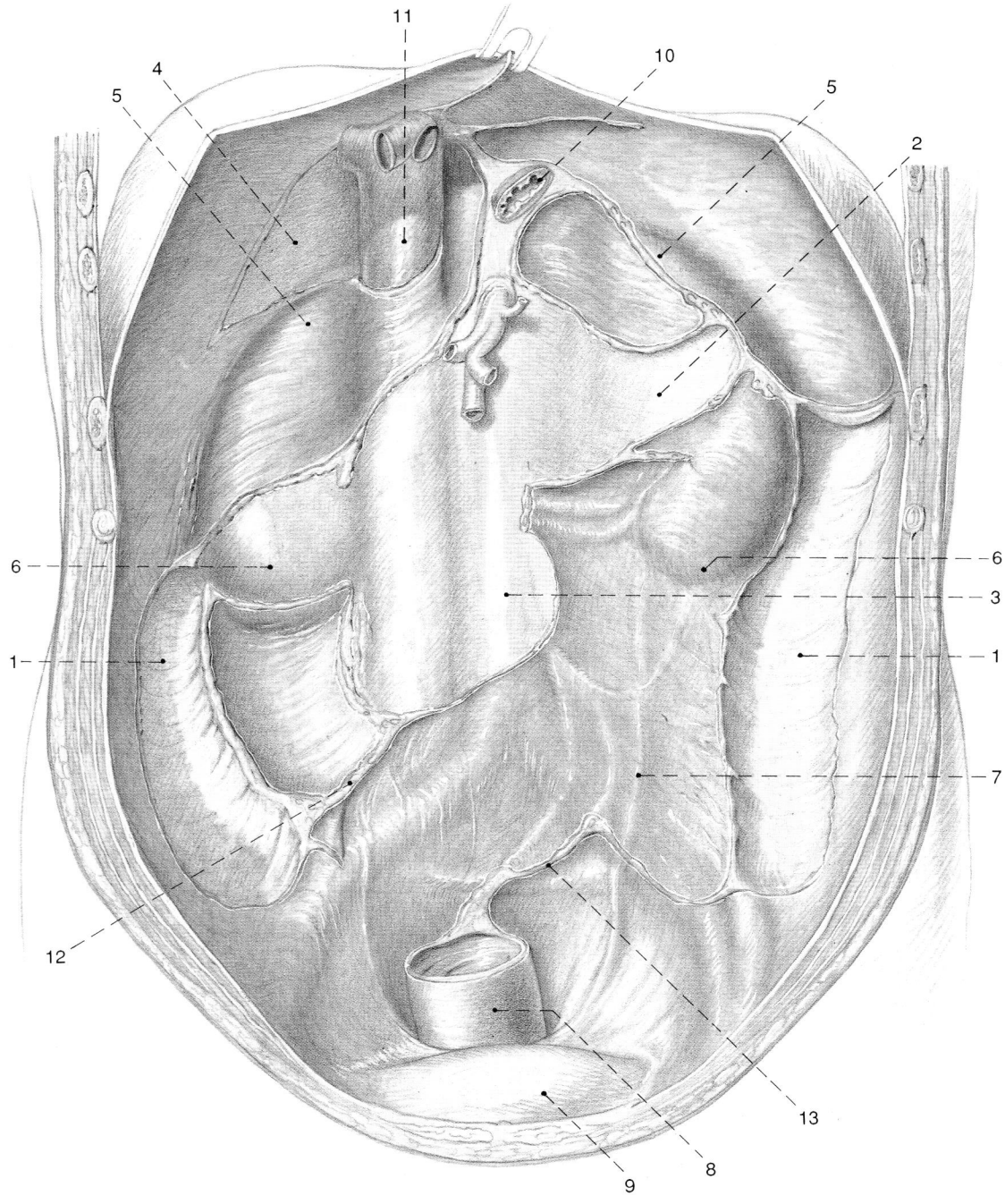

Fig. 2.**3** Relation of the kidneys to the parietal peritoneum and mesenteric roots.

1 Fibrous colic area
2 Fibrous pancreatic area
3 Fibrous duodenal area
4 Fibrous hepatic area
5 Upper pole of kidney
6 Lower pole of kidney
7 Ureteral fold

8 Rectum
9 Bladder
10 Esophagus
11 Inferior vena cava
12 Mesenteric root
13 Root of sigmoid mesocolon

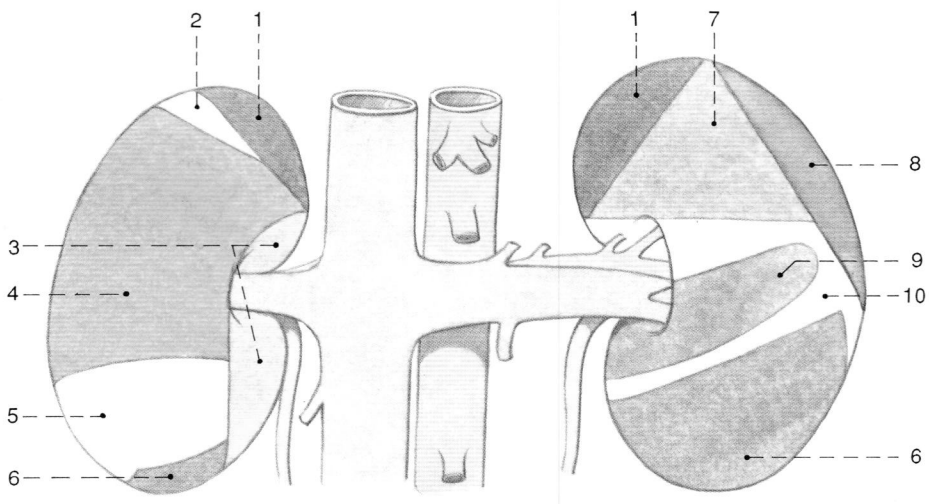

Fig. 2.**4** Contact areas of the kidneys, anterior aspect (after Pern-kopf/Platzer 1989).

1 Adrenal area
2 Fibrous hepatic area (hepatoduodenal ligament)
3 Fibrous duodenal area (descending part of duodenum)
4 Serous hepatic area
5 Fibrous colic area
6 Serous area
7 Serous gastric area
8 Serous splenic area
9 Fibrous pancreatic area
10 Fibrous colic area

The posterior relations of the kidney are virtually identical on the right and left sides (Fig. 2.**5**). The cranial half of the posterior renal surface is in contact with the diaphragm. Their area of contact depends on the renal level and so is usually greater on the left side than on the right. The kidney apposes to the lateral crus of the lumbar part of the diaphragm. Between the lumbar and costal parts of the diaphragm is a variable amuscular interval, the lumbocostal trigone, which constitutes a site of least resistance. In this area only the thin diaphragmatic fasciae separate the kidney and its fat capsule from the pleural cavity.

The caudal half of the posterior surface of the kidney is related to the quadratus lumborum muscle and the deep lumbodorsal fascia. The subcostal, iliohypogastric, and ilioinguinal nerves descend obliquely in a medial-to-lateral direction between the kidney and posterior abdominal wall.

The posterior part of the medial border of the kidney lies upon the psoas major muscle. With a normal renal position, the 12th rib passes obliquely downward and laterally to cross the upper third of the posterior renal surface. Between the 12th rib and kidney are the diaphragm and the costodiaphragmatic recess of the pleural cavity. Attention must be given to the inferior reflection of the pleura in retroperitoneal approaches to the kidney that include a rib resection.

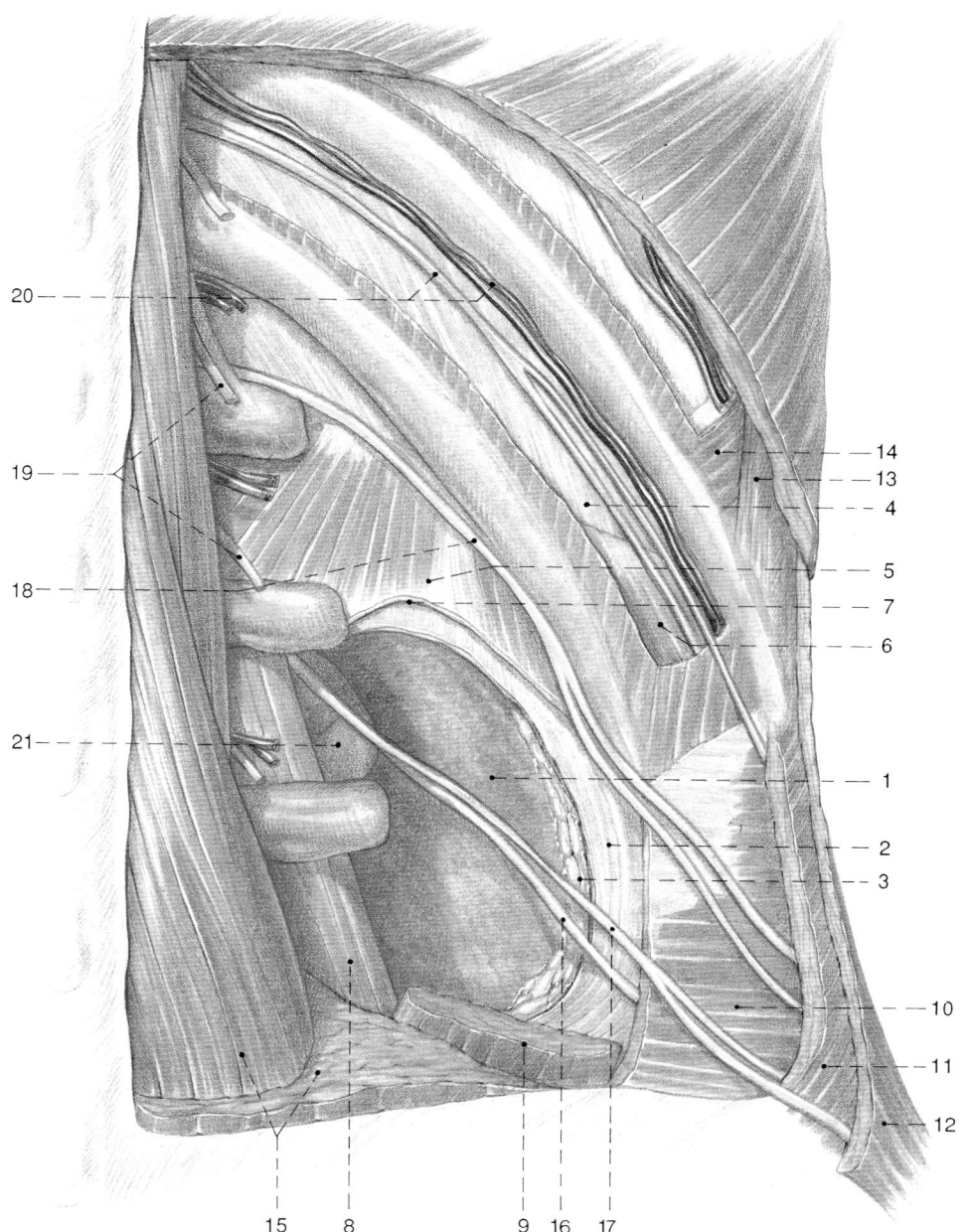

Fig. 2.**5**   Posterior relations of the right kidney.

 1 Right kidney
 2 Gerota's fascia (renal fascia)
 3 Perirenal fat capsule
 4 Parietal pleura in costodiaphragmatic recess
 5 Diaphragm, lateral crus of lumbar part
 6 Costal part of diaphragm
 7 Lateral arcuate ligament
 8 Psoas major
 9 Quadratus lumborum
10 Transversus abdominis
11 Internal oblique muscle
12 External oblique muscle
13 External intercostal muscle
14 Internal intercostal muscle
15 Erector spinae
16 Ilioinguinal nerve
17 Iliohypogastric nerve
18 Subcostal nerve
19 Dorsal branches of spinal nerve
20 Intercostal vessels and nerve
21 Renal pelvis

Capsules

Each kidney is enveloped by three capsules (Fig. 2.**6**): the fibrous capsule (capsule proper), the perirenal fat capsule, and Gerota's fascia (renal fascia, Gerota's capsule). The innermost *fibrous capsule* closely invests the renal parenchyma and is easily separated from the healthy kidney.

Surrounding the fibrous capsule is the *perirenal fat capsule*, which develops postnatally and is fully developed by puberty. The perirenal fat is connected to the inner fibrous capsule and the outer Gerota's fascia by loose connective tissue, which creates a mobile plane. The fat capsule is less

well developed on the anterior surface of the kidney than posteriorly, and it envelops the kidney and adrenal gland. Composed of structural fat, the perirenal fat capsule has the primary function of keeping the kidney in place.

The outermost renal covering is *Gerota's fascia*, which forms a "sac" enclosing the kidney, adrenal gland, and perirenal fat capsule. Gerota's fascia is functionally and structurally distinct from the fascia that envelops the muscles and is more like the connective-tissue fascia that invests the organs in the true pelvis.

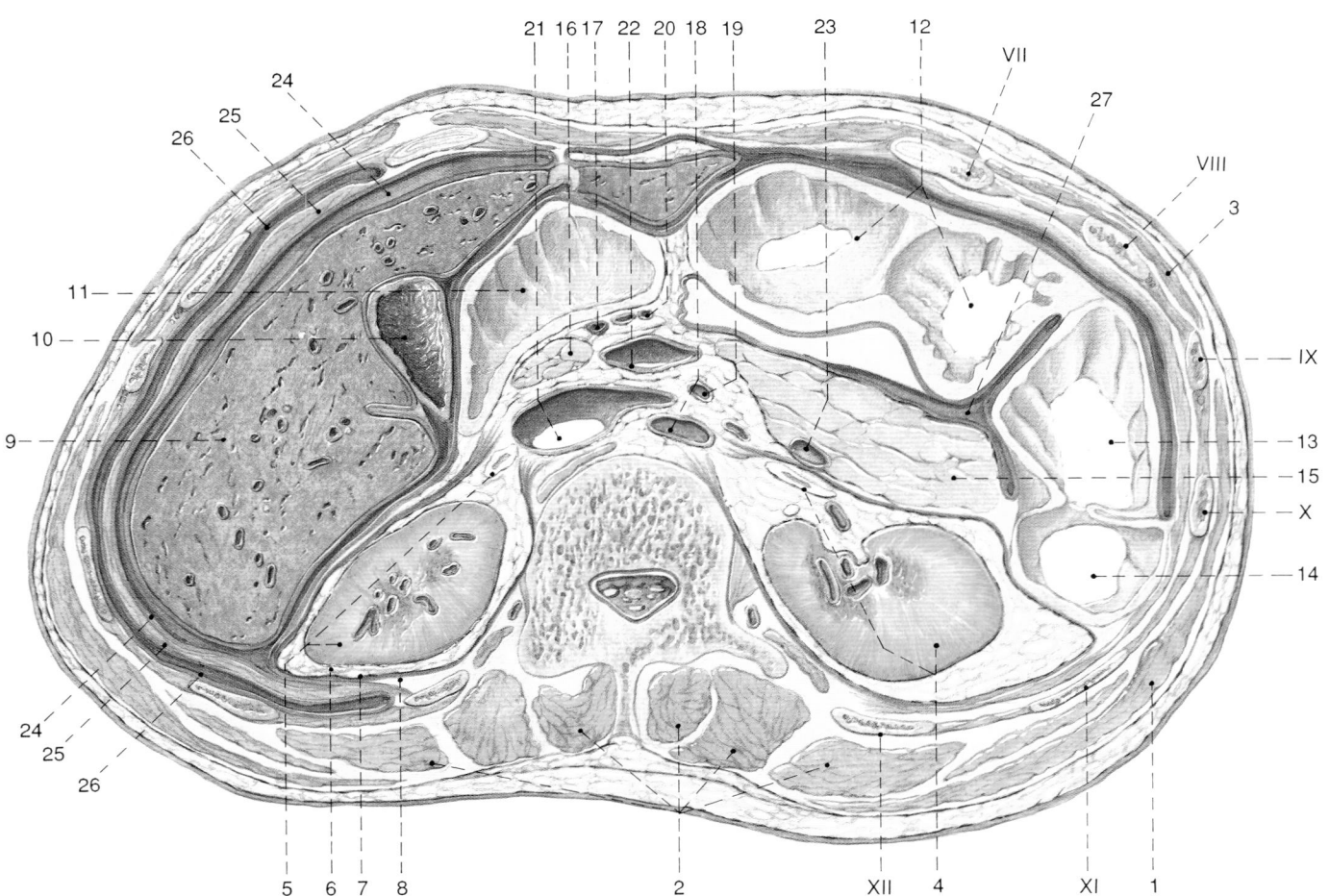

Fig. 2.**6** Transverse section through the abdomen at the level of the first lumbar vertebra (L1).

VII–XII 7th through 12th ribs	15 Tail of pancreas
1 Latissimus dorsi	16 Head of pancreas
2 Erector spinae	17 Common bile duct
3 External oblique muscle	18 Abdominal aorta
4 Left kidney and ureter	19 Superior mesenteric artery
5 Right kidney and ureter	20 Common hepatic artery
6 Fibrous capsule of kidney	21 Inferior vena cava
7 Perirenal fat capsule	22 Portal vein
8 Gerota's fascia (renal fascia)	23 Splenic vein
9 Liver	24 Peritoneal cavity
10 Gallbladder	25 Diaphragm
11 Duodenal bulb	26 Pleural cavity (costodiaphragmatic recess)
12 Pyloric part of stomach	27 Inferior recess of omental bursa
13 Transverse colon	
14 Descending colon	

Gerota's fascia consists of two layers commonly termed the prerenal (anterior) and retrorenal (posterior) fascia. The fascial layers are fused about two fingerwidths lateral to the lateral renal border and above the adrenal gland. Gerota's fascia is also attached superiorly to the fascia of the diaphragm. The two layers of Gerota's fascia are separated below the kidney to allow passage of the ureter and blood vessels. The prerenal and retrorenal layers fuse medially with the connective tissue surrounding the major blood vessels and nerves of the retroperitoneal space. The retrorenal fascia is firmly adherent to the muscular fascia of the posterior abdominal wall.

Lateral to the saclike Gerota's fascia is the *pararenal fat*, which differs from the perirenal fat capsule in that it is not composed of structural fat, so its volume is subject to marked individual and nutrition-dependent variations.

Renal Vessels

Arteries

Normally each kidney receives its blood supply from a single renal artery. Both renal arteries spring from the lateral aspect of the abdominal aorta, the right artery usually arising at a slightly lower level than the left. The origin of the renal arteries is usually situated below that of the superior mesenteric artery, between the inferior third of the first lumbar vertebra and the middle third of the second lumbar vertebra.

The right renal artery runs obliquely downward and laterally to the hilum of the kidney, passing behind the inferior vena cava. The accompanying renal vein is usually anterior to and above the artery, but in approximately 30% of cases the artery is in front of the vein (Fig. 2.**8 d,e**). Anterior to the right renal hilum and vessels is the descending portion of the duodenum.

The left renal artery is shorter than the right and usually passes to the renal hilum above and partially behind the left renal vein. The hilum and renal vessels are covered anteriorly by the body of the pancreas and the splenic vessels.

The renal arteries divide at a variable distance from the hilum into two (57%) or three (43%) main branches (anterior, posterior, and inferior) that supply corresponding portions of the renal parenchyma. The branching of the renal arteries does not follow any consistent pattern in terms of right-left or gender distribution.

Variations in the number, course, and origin of the renal artery are very common. In about 40% of cases the kidney is found to have an atypical arterial supply. The presence of accessory or aberrant renal arteries is an especially common finding. An "accessory" artery is a supernumerary artery that supplies the kidney as a separate vessel; "aberrant" arteries enter the renal parenchyma outside the hilum, generally at the upper or lower pole. Thus, an accessory artery may or may not be aberrant. An aberrant artery may arise from the renal artery itself. Possible variations of the renal arteries are illustrated in Figs. 2.**7**–2.**10**.

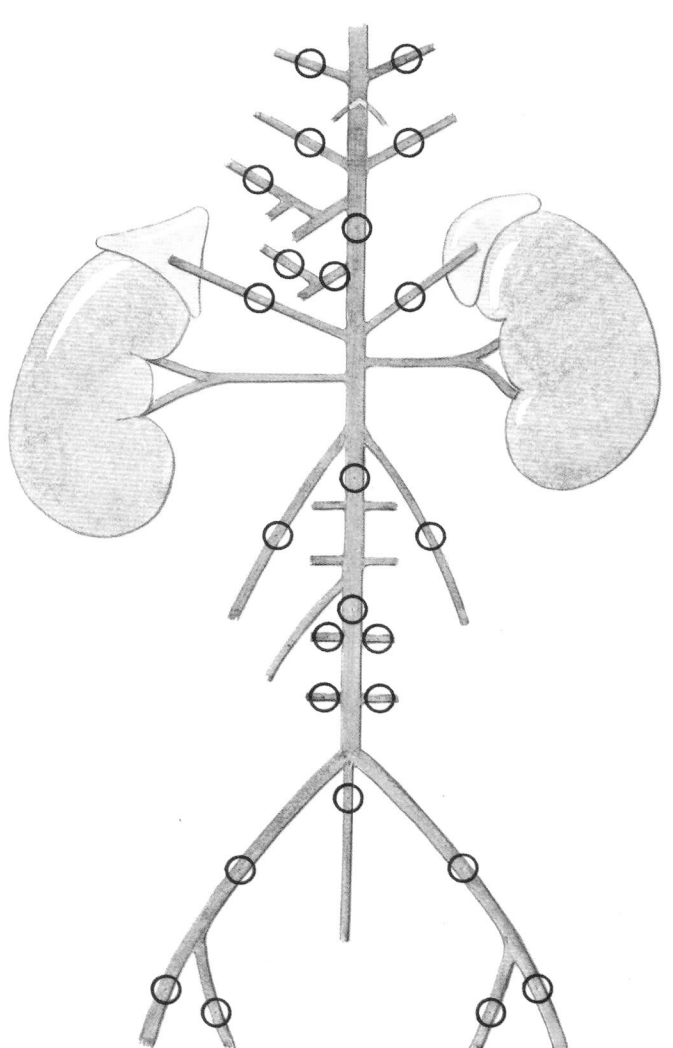

Fig. 2.**7** Schematic diagram of the abdominal aorta and kidneys. The circles indicate the potential origins of accessory (or aberrant) renal arteries.

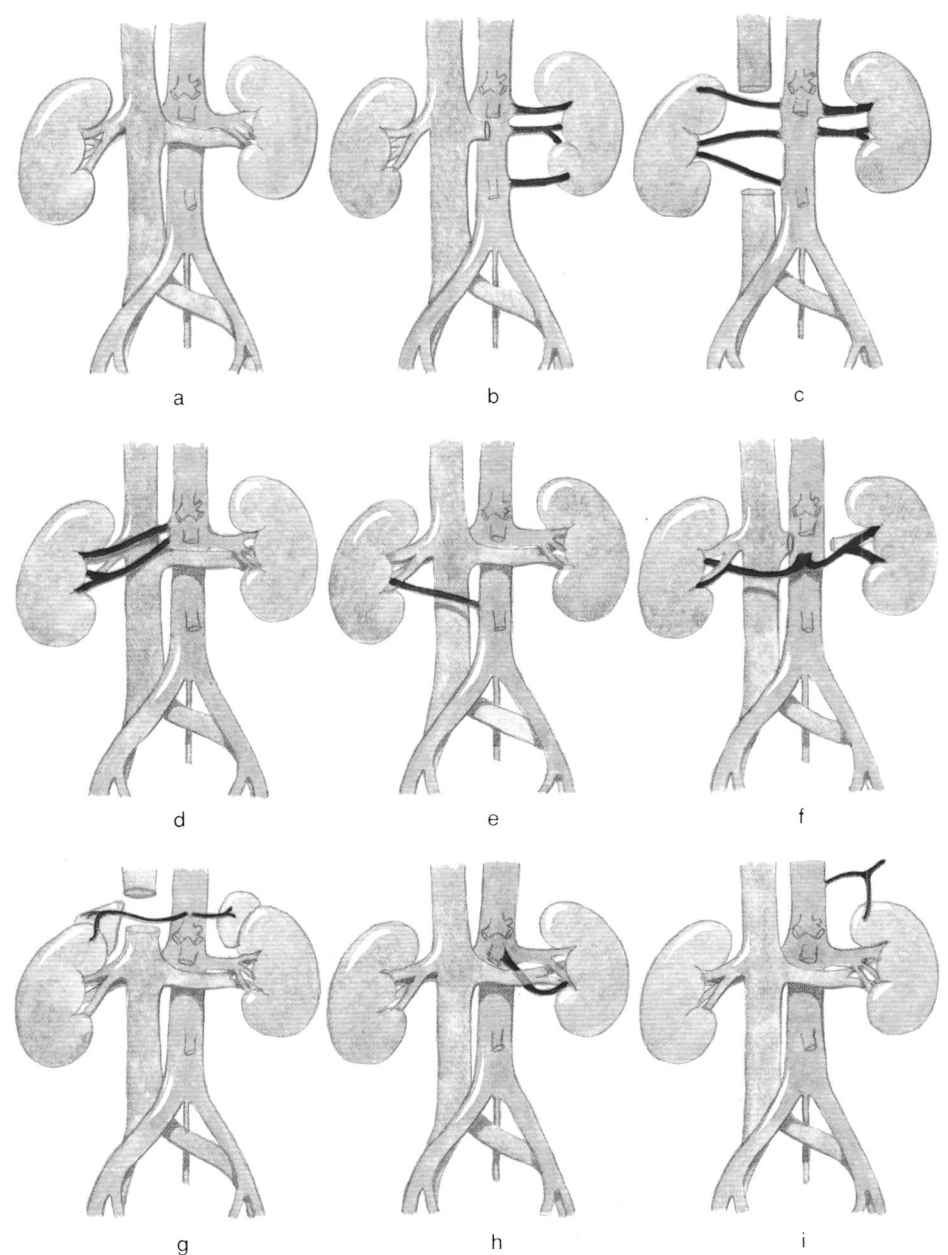

Fig. 2.**8a−i** Typical patterns of aberrant and accessory renal arteries.

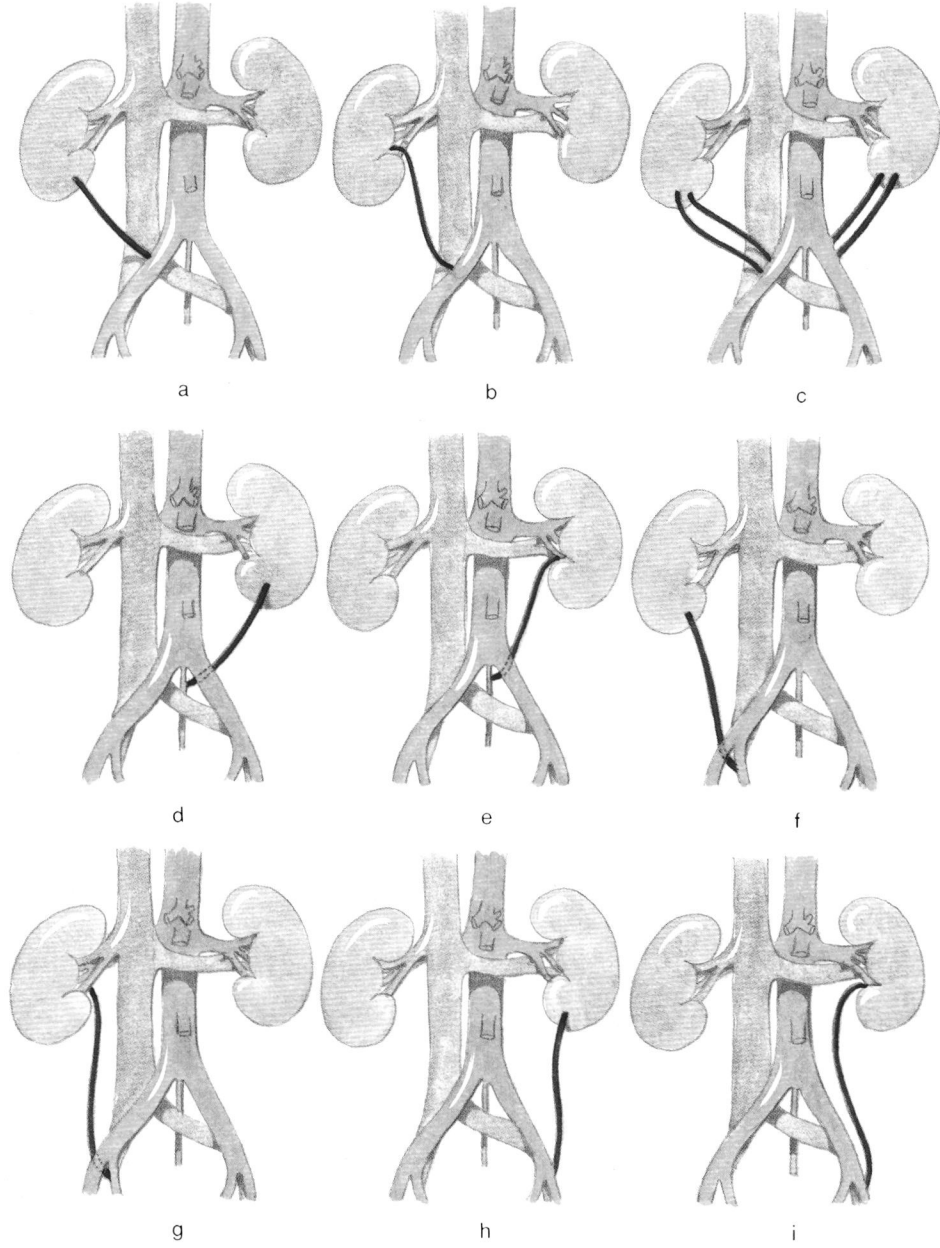

Fig. 2.**9a–i**   Typical patterns of aberrant and accessory renal arteries.

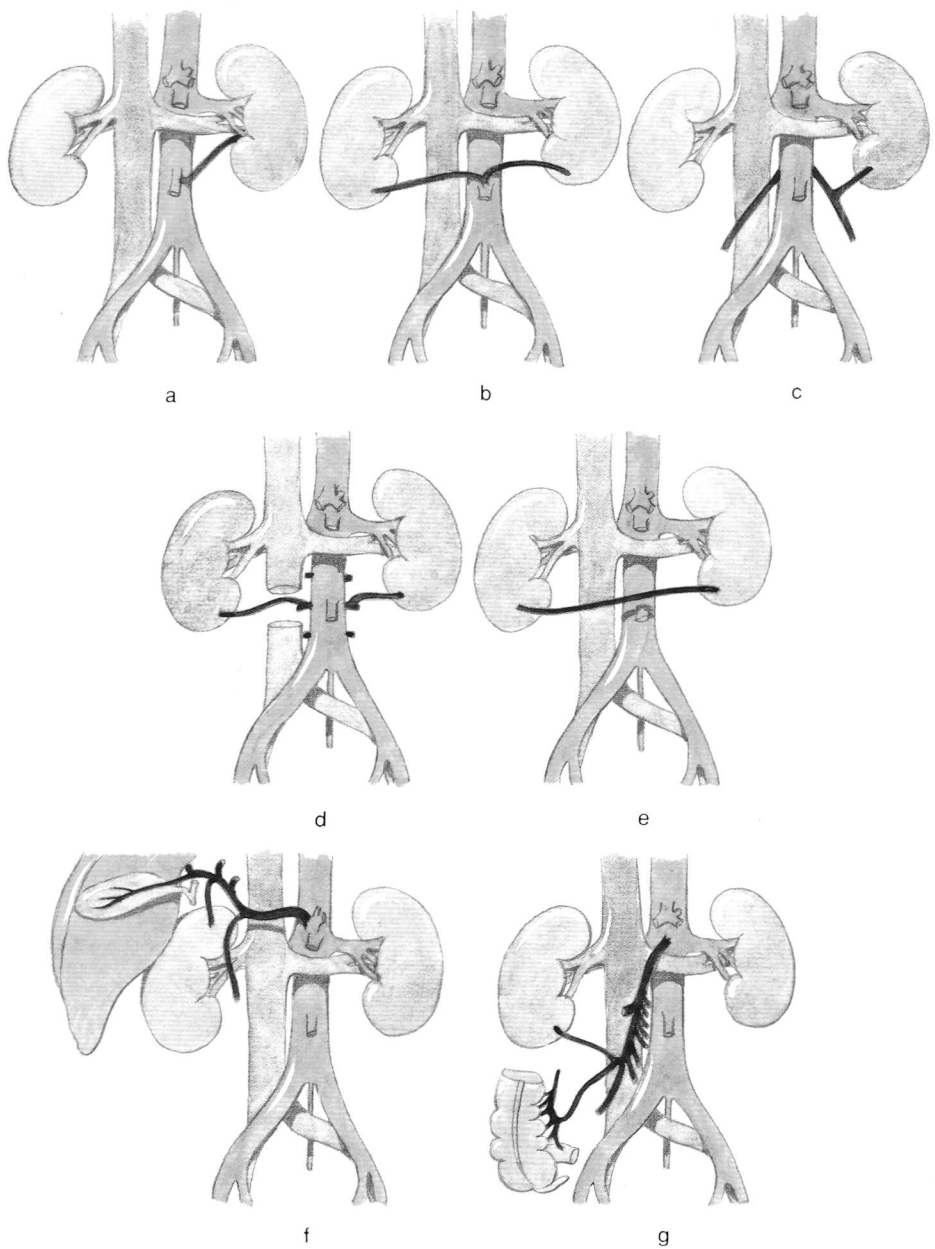

Fig. 2.**10a–i** Typical patterns of aberrant and accessory renal arteries.

Veins

The renal veins are interconnected by numerous anastomoses in the renal parenchyma and renal sinus, a pattern consistent with the general tendency for the venous system to form plexuses. The trunk of the renal vein is usually formed in the hilum by the convergence of two (53%) or three (34%) main tributaries that pass in front of the renal pelvis. A small tributary passing behind the renal pelvis occurs in approximately one-third of cases.

Outside the renal sinus, the veins are usually anterior to the renal arteries. The left renal vein frequently opens into the in-ferior vena cava at a higher level than the right renal vein. With a normally positioned inferior vena cava, the left renal vein is substantially longer (6–11 cm) than the right (2–4 cm). While the right renal vein runs a straight, direct course from the hilum to the inferior vena cava, the left vein runs medially forward and passes in front of the aorta, just below the origin of the superior mesenteric artery, before entering the inferior vena cava. Phylogenetically, the left renal vein originates as part of the cardinal venous system (see below) and consequently receives the left suprarenal and testicular (or ovarian) veins.

Lymphatics

The intrarenal lymph vessels of the kidney accompany the arteries to the renal sinus and present in the hilum as pre-vascular, retrovascular and intervascular bundles. Regional lymph nodes encountered on the right side are the right lumbar (postcaval) lymph nodes and the intermediate nodes and rarely the preaortic nodes. The renal lymphatics on the left side drain into the left lumbar lymph nodes (lateral aortic and preaortic nodes) (Fig. 2.11).

The lymph vessels draining the renal capsules pass to the lumbar lymph nodes separately from the lymph vessels of the renal parenchyma. A few lymph vessels from the renal capsule pass through the diaphragm and end in the inter-costal nodes. Anastomoses have been described between the lymph vessels of the renal capsules and those of the liver, colon, cecum, and uterine tube.

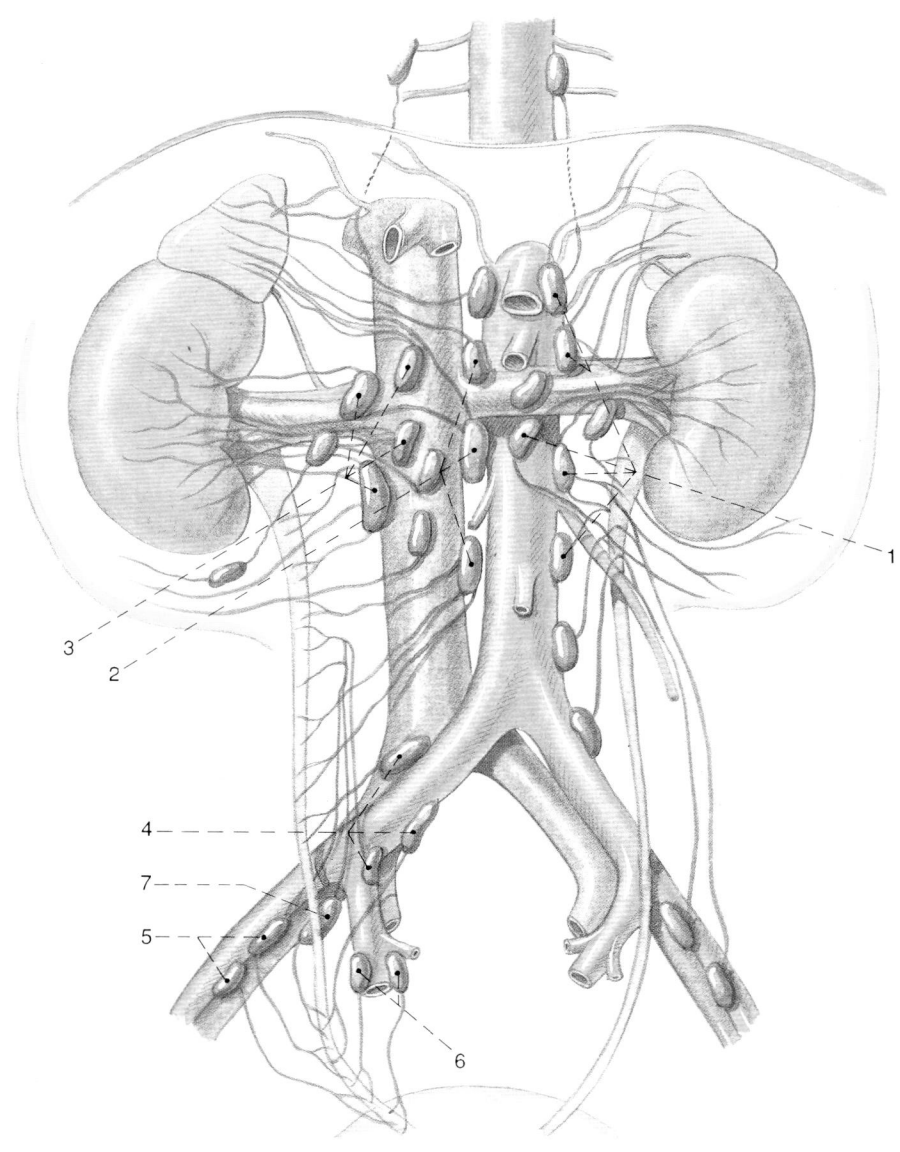

Fig. 2.**11** Lymph nodes and lymphatic vessels of the retroperi-toneal space (simplified schematic diagram after Kubik 1989).

1 Left lumbar lymph nodes (lateral aortic, preaortic, postaortic)
2 Intermediate lumbar lymph nodes
3 Right lumbar lymph nodes (lateral caval, precaval, postcaval)
4 Common iliac lymph nodes
5 External iliac lymph nodes
6 Internal iliac lymph nodes
7 Interiliac lymph nodes

Renal Nerve Supply

The kidneys derive their nerve supply from the renal plexus, which is formed by sympathetic and parasympathetic fibers from the celiac plexus and abdominal aortic plexus as well as direct fibers from the sympathetic trunk (lumbar part). The renal plexus accompanies the renal arteries to the hilum. Autonomic nerve fibers can be identified along the arteries as far as the efferent vessels of the renal glomeruli.

Renal Pelvis

The *renal pelvis* is a hollow muscular organ that forms the initial segment of the excretory portion of the urinary tract. The tension of the muscular wall of the renal pelvis varies with its momentary functional state, so the shape of the renal pelvis is variable.

The renal pelvis begins with 7–13 *minor calices* at the renal papillae. The minor calices generally unite to form two or three *major calices* that comprise the true renal pelvis (dentritic type). In some cases all of the minor calices may open directly into the renal pelvis, which then exhibits an ampule-like dilatation (ampullary type of pelvis). Forms intermediate between these extremes are common. At operation, the renal pelvis is easily accessible at the hilum through a posterior approach, except for the rare cases in which all of the pelvis is contained within the renal sinus. The only structures that cross the posterior aspect of the renal pelvis are the main posterior branch of the renal artery and the variable posterior branch of the renal vein.

The renal pelvis derives its arterial supply (see Fig. 2.1) from one or more branches of the renal artery and is drained by the renal vein. Lymphatic drainage (see Fig. 2.10) is to the lumbar lymph nodes. The nerves of the renal pelvis are derived from the renal plexus (see above).

Ureter

The renal pelvis becomes continuous with the ureter below the hilum, with no distinct ureteropelvic boundary. Their junction is at the level of the second or third lumbar vertebra.

The ureter is considered to consist of an *abdominal (proximal) part* and a *pelvic distal part* whose junction occurs at the point where the ureter is crossed by the iliac vessels.

The *abdominal (proximal) part* of the ureter passes downward and slightly medially from the renal pelvis on the fascia of the psoas major, encased within a sheath of fibro-fatty tissue. The lateral distance of the ureter from the costal processes of the lumbar vertebrae is variable. In infancy, the proximal part of the ureter is tortuous and may even exhibit proximal kinks that disappear by about one year of age.

The topographic relations of the ureters to anterior structures are different on the right and left sides owing to the asymmetric development of the abdominal viscera. At its origin the *right ureter* is overlapped by the descending part of the duodenum. In its descent it is crossed anteriorly by the right colic artery and ileocolic artery, which pass below the secondary parietal peritoneum (originally the ascending mesocolon) to the cecum and ascending colon. Finally the right ureter passes below the testicular or ovarian vessels in its retroperitoneal course. Just before entering the true pelvis, the right ureter is crossed by the root of the mesentery, giving it an indirect relation to the terminal segment of the ileum. A mobile cecum and a transversely oriented appendix also may relate anteriorly to the right ureter.

The initial part of the *left ureter* descends lateral and posterior to the superior duodenal fold, which conveys the inferior mesenteric vein to the splenic vein. As it descends further, the left ureter is crossed by the branches of the inferior mesenteric artery (left colic artery and sigmoid arteries), which lie below the secondary parietal peritoneum (originally the descending mesocolon). The left ureter, like the right, is crossed at varying levels by the testicular or ovarian vessels. Just before entering the true pelvis, the left ureter is crossed by the attachment of the sigmoid mesocolon and can be found at this level within the *intersigmoid recess*.

The right ureter is usually adherent to the peritoneum and must be separated from it at operation. The left ureter has no firm attachments to the secondary parietal peritoneum, and only the portion in the intersigmoid recess is directly apposed to the peritoneum.

Vessels and Nerves of the Ureter

The connective tissue surrounding the ureter (the adventitia) is permeated by an *arterial anastomotic network* (see Fig. 2.1) composed basically of longitudinal vessels that are interconnected by transverse anastomoses. This periureteral arterial plexus is supplied by all arteries that have a close topographic relation to the ureter. The proximal part of the ureter is consistently supplied by one or two ureteral branches from the renal artery, from the testicular or ovarian artery, and occasionally by direct branches from the abdominal aorta. At the junction of the abdominal and pelvic parts of the ureter, the plexus is supplied by branches of the iliac vessels (common iliac, external or internal iliac).

In surgical procedures on the kidney or renal pelvis, care must be taken not to injure the ureteral branches of the renal artery. They provide the essential blood supply to the proximal part of the ureter, and their caliber and connections with the periureteral plexus give them the capacity to supply the entire proximal part of the ureter.

Vascular plexuses in the muscular and submucous coats of the ureter receive blood from the adventitial plexus and contribute to the ureteral blood supply.

The *veins* draining the proximal part of the ureter essentially follow the course of the arteries. The venous drainage is directed toward the renal veins and the testicular or ovarian veins.

The *lymph vessels* draining the proximal part of the ureter (see Fig. 2.1) start at networks of lymph capillaries in the muscular wall and adventitia. They pass from the proximal ureter to the lumbar lymph nodes, on the right side draining into the lateral caval and precaval nodes and on the left into the lateral aortic and preaortic nodes. Lymphatics draining the lower portion of the proximal ureter are distributed to the common iliac nodes. Connections are generally present between these two drainage pathways.

The abdominal part of the ureter derives its *nerve supply* from the renal plexus superiorly and from the abdominal aortic plexus inferiorly. The adventitia of the ureter contains a dense network of nerve fibers that receive branches from the plexus surrounding the testicular or ovarian artery.

Adrenal Gland

The paired adrenal glands (see Fig. 2.**1**) are set upon the upper pole and anteromedial surface of the corresponding kidney. They are surrounded by the perirenal fat capsule and Gerota's fascia. Due to the close relation of the adrenal gland to the kidney and the confining "renal fascial sac," adrenal tumors can produce a distortion of the renal outline that is visible on intravenous pyelographies.

The right adrenal gland has the approximate shape of a pyramid whose base rests on the upper pole of the right kidney. The left adrenal gland is semilunar in shape and apposes to the upper part of the medial border of the left kidney. It usually extends to the renal hilum and is in contact with the renal vessels.

The posterior surface of the *right adrenal gland* is in contact with the diaphragm, and its inferior surface is related to the kidney. The anterosuperior surface of the gland is related to the bare area of the liver. Its anterior surface is behind the inferior vena cava medially, and the inferior part of its anterior surface is covered by parietal peritoneum.

The *left adrenal gland*, like the right, is only partially covered by peritoneum, which invests the upper half of its anterior surface. Thus, part of the gland projects into the omental bursa and may relate topographically to the abdominal part of the esophagus. The anteroinferior surface of the left adrenal gland is in contact with the body of the pancreas and the splenic vessels. The lateral part of the posterior surface of the gland apposes to the kidney, and the medial part is in contact with the left crus of the diaphragm.

Vessels and Nerves of the Adrenal Gland

Normally, at least three arteries contribute to the *arterial blood supply* of the adrenal gland (see Fig. 2.**1**). These are the superior, middle, and inferior suprarenal arteries, which arise respectively from the inferior phrenic artery, abdominal aorta, and renal artery.

The superior suprarenal artery normally does not supply the gland as a single vessel (see Fig. 2.**1**) but divides into 3–30 branches before entering the gland. Multiple superior suprarenal arteries also may occur. The middle suprarenal artery arises from the abdominal aorta at a variable level but always above the renal artery. The vessel may be absent or multiple (see Fig. 2.**1**). The inferior suprarenal artery enters the undersurface of the adrenal gland by several branches that may arise separately from the renal artery or from accessory or aberrant vessels.

The *venous drainage* of the adrenal gland is generally handled by a single vessel, the suprarenal vein, which leaves the glandular tissue at the anterior surface of the adrenal gland. The right suprarenal vein takes a short, direct, transverse course to the inferior vena cava. The left suprarenal vein passes over the inferior part of the anterior surface of the gland to terminate at the left renal vein.

The *lymph vessels* (see Fig. 2.**11**) from the adrenal cortex accompany the inferior phrenic and middle suprarenal arteries, and those from the adrenal medulla accompany the suprarenal vein. They terminate at the lumbar lymph nodes.

The *nerves* enter the posterior and medial aspects of the adrenal gland. The parasympathetic and sympathetic nerve fibers that form the *adrenal plexus* originate from the celiac plexus and the splanchnic nerves. Direct fibers from the sympathetic trunk can contribute to the formation of the adrenal plexus.

Major Vessels and Nerves of the Retroperitoneal Space

Abdominal Aorta
(Fig. 2.**1**)

The descending aorta enters the retroperitoneal space through the aortic aperture in the diaphragm. The thoracic duct traverses the aperture behind the aorta, and occasionally the aorta is accompanied by a splanchnic nerve.

The aorta usually enters the abdominal cavity on the median plane but deviates toward the left side as it descends further, apposed to the upper four lumbar vertebrae and intervertebral discs. It ends at the level of the fourth lumbar vertebra by dividing into its terminal branches, the common iliac arteries and the median sacral artery.

The inferior vena cava ascends to the right and slightly in front of the aorta. The left lumbar veins course between the vertebral column and aorta in a space that also contains the postaortic lymph nodes. The abdominal aorta is covered anteriorly by the autonomic aortic plexus (celiac, superior and inferior mesenteric) with corresponding ganglia and by the preaortic lymph nodes. Directly lateral to the aorta are the lateral aortic lymph nodes.

As the abdominal aorta descends, it passes behind the body of the pancreas, the left renal vein, and the horizontal (inferior) portion of the duodenum. Below the mesenteric root, the abdominal aorta is easily accessible to a transperitoneal surgical approach.

The branches of the abdominal aorta may be paired or unpaired, and the branches in both groups can be classified as visceral or parietal.

The unpaired visceral branches are as follows:
a) The celiac trunk, arising within the aortic aperture at the level of the 12th thoracic vertebra.
b) The superior mesenteric artery, arising at the level of the first lumbar vertebra.
c) The inferior mesenteric artery, arising at the level of the third lumbar vertebra.

The paired visceral branches are as follows:
a) The middle suprarenal arteries, arising at the level of the first lumbar vertebra.
b) The renal arteries, usually arising at the same level from the aorta just below the suprarenal arteries.

c) The testicular or ovarian arteries, arising at a variable level from the anterolateral aspect of the abdominal aorta and usually at different levels on the right and left sides.

The unpaired parietal branch of the abdominal aorta is one of its terminal branches, the median sacral artery.

The paired parietal branches are:
a) The inferior phrenic arteries, arising in the aortic aperture as the first branch of the abdominal aorta.
b) Four pairs of lumbar arteries, arising from the back of the aorta at the levels of the first through fourth lumbar vertebral bodies.

Inferior Vena Cava
(Fig. 2.**1**)

The inferior vena cava is formed by the union of the two common iliac veins approximately one fingerwidth below and to the right of the aortic bifurcation. The lower part of the inferior vena cava is overlapped anteriorly by the right common iliac artery and relates posteriorly to the body of the fifth lumbar vertebra.

The inferior vena cava ascends on the right side of the aorta and parallel to it until reaching the level of the lower pole of the right kidney, where it diverges slightly to the right from the abdominal aorta and travels in a groove on the posterior surface of the liver. The inferior vena cava enters the thoracic cavity through the vena cava foramen in the diaphragm (at the level of Th 10) and immediately opens into the right atrium of the heart. It is accompanied through the diaphragm by the right phrenicoabdominal branch of the phrenic nerve.

The anterior surface of the inferior vena cava is covered in its lower portion by peritoneum (primary parietal peritoneum) up to the level of the mesenteric root. As it ascends, the inferior vena cava loses its peritoneal covering (secondary retroperitoneal structure) and is apposed to the duodenum and pancreas (see Fig. 2.**3**). Ascending further in the posterior wall of the epiploic foramen, the vena cava is again covered with peritoneum and is adherent to the bare area of the liver in the groove for the inferior vena cava.

The inferior vena cava has both parietal and visceral tributaries. The parietal tributaries are as follows:

a) The common iliac veins.
b) The median sacral vein, which follows the course of the homonymous artery and may empty into the left common iliac vein.
c) The lumbar veins, whose arrangement corresponds to that of the homonymous arteries.
d) The inferior phrenic veins, which enter the inferior vena cava just before it pierces the diaphragm.

The visceral tributaries are as follows:
a) The right testicular or ovarian vein, which opens into the inferior vena cava just below the termination of the right renal vein.
b) The renal veins (discussed in connection with the kidney).
c) The right suprarenal vein (see above).
d) The hepatic veins, usually three in number, generally enter the inferior vena cava in their course through the hepatic groove for the inferior vena cava.

Variations of the inferior vena cava are fairly common and usually result from developmental anomalies (Fig. 2.**12**). The retroperitoneal venous system develops from three paired, longitudinally oriented parallel channels: the caudal cardinal vein, supracardinal vein, and subcardinal vein, which are continuous caudally with the sacrocardinal vein. Further differentiation of the venous system is characterized by a progressive asymmetry in favor of the right side, with anastomoses between the right and left cardinal veins assuming key importance.

The development of the vena caval system is shown schematically in Fig. 2.**12**. It can be seen that the caudal cardinal veins largely disappear while the supracardinal veins persist in part as the azygos and hemiazygos veins. Simply stated, the subcardinal veins develop into the inferior vena cava on the right side and into the suprarenal and testicular or ovarian veins on the left side.

Embryonic development of the inferior vena cava may be disrupted, arrested, or misdirected at any stage by extrinsic or intrinsic factors that are not yet fully understood. Each primarily formed cardinal vein (except for the lower portion of the caudal cardinal vein) may persist wholly or in part during definitive development, giving rise to such variants as a *double inferior vena cava (2.2%) or left inferior vena cava (0.2%)*. All abnormal configurations of the inferior vena caval system are based on the persistence or anomalous involution of embryonic vascular channels.

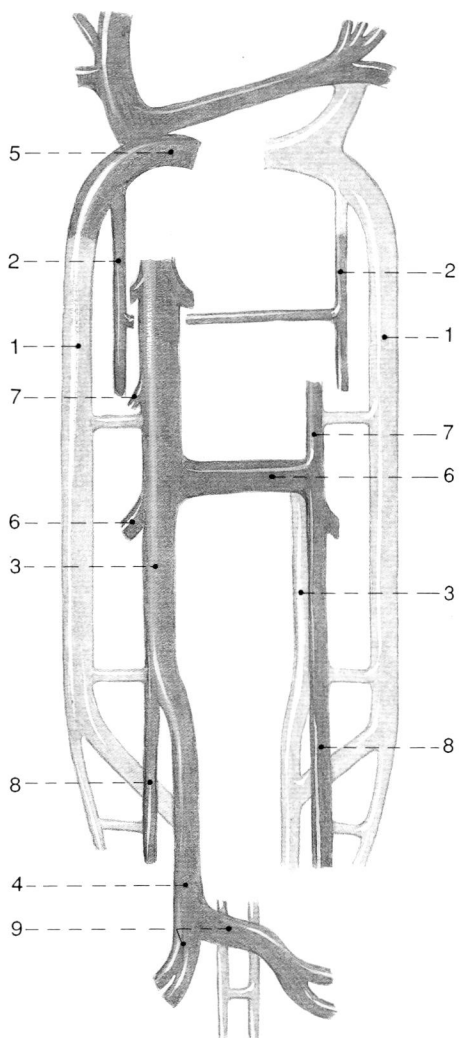

Fig. 2.**12**   Development of the vena caval system. Vessels that do not persist are colored light blue.

1 Caudal cardinal vein
2 Supracardinal vein (develops into the azygos vein on the right, the hemiazygos and accessory hemiazygos veins on the left)
3 Subcardinal vein (develops into the inferior vena cava on the right, the testicular vein on the left)
4 Sacrocardinal vein
5 Superior vena cava
6 Renal veins
7 Suprarenal veins
8 Testicular veins
9 Common iliac veins

Lymph Vessels

The *lymph vessels* and regional lymph nodes of the retroperitoneal space were discussed previously in connection with specific organs. Here we shall limit our attention to the *thoracic duct* and its tributaries.

The thoracic duct begins at the upper end of the cisterna chyli in the retroperitoneal space. The cisterna receives the lumbar and intestinal lymphatic trunks and is situated in front of the first and second lumbar vertebral bodies, behind and to the right of the abdominal aorta. The normally positioned cisterna chyli is found between the aorta and inferior vena cava, just below the left renal vein. After a short intraabdominal course the thoracic duct enters the thorax through the aortic aperture, passing behind the aorta, and ascends through the posterior mediastinum.

Nerves

The large *nerve trunks* in the retroperitoneal space are derived mainly from the abdominal portion of the autonomic nervous system.

The anterior and posterior vagal nerve trunks enter the abdominal cavity through the esophageal aperture of the diaphragm. Only the posterior vagal trunk reaches the retroperitoneal space primarily, the bulk of its fibers passing between the left adrenal gland and the left medial crus of the diaphragm to the celiac ganglion.

Two nerves belonging to the sympathetic nervous system, the greater and lesser splanchnic, enter the retroperitoneal space through an aperture in the medial crus of the diaphragm. The greater splanchnic nerve runs between the medial crus of the diaphragm and the adrenal gland to the celiac ganglion. The fibers of the lesser splanchnic nerve terminate partly in the ganglion and may have direct connections with the renal plexus.

The two sympathetic trunks enter the retroperitoneal space after passing between the medial and lateral crura of the diaphragm. Both trunks lie upon the psoas major muscles near their origin from the vertebral bodies. The left sympathetic trunk lies slightly behind and to the left of the abdominal aorta, and the right sympathetic trunk is posterior to the inferior vena cava. Connections between the right and left sympathetic trunks are generally present and course between the lumbar vertebral bodies and the aorta or inferior vena cava.

The sympathetic trunks and their ganglia send branches (the lumbar splanchnic nerves) to the preaortic plexuses and their ganglia. The lumbar portion of the sympathetic trunk blends smoothly with the sacral portion at the arcuate line.

Supracostal Approach

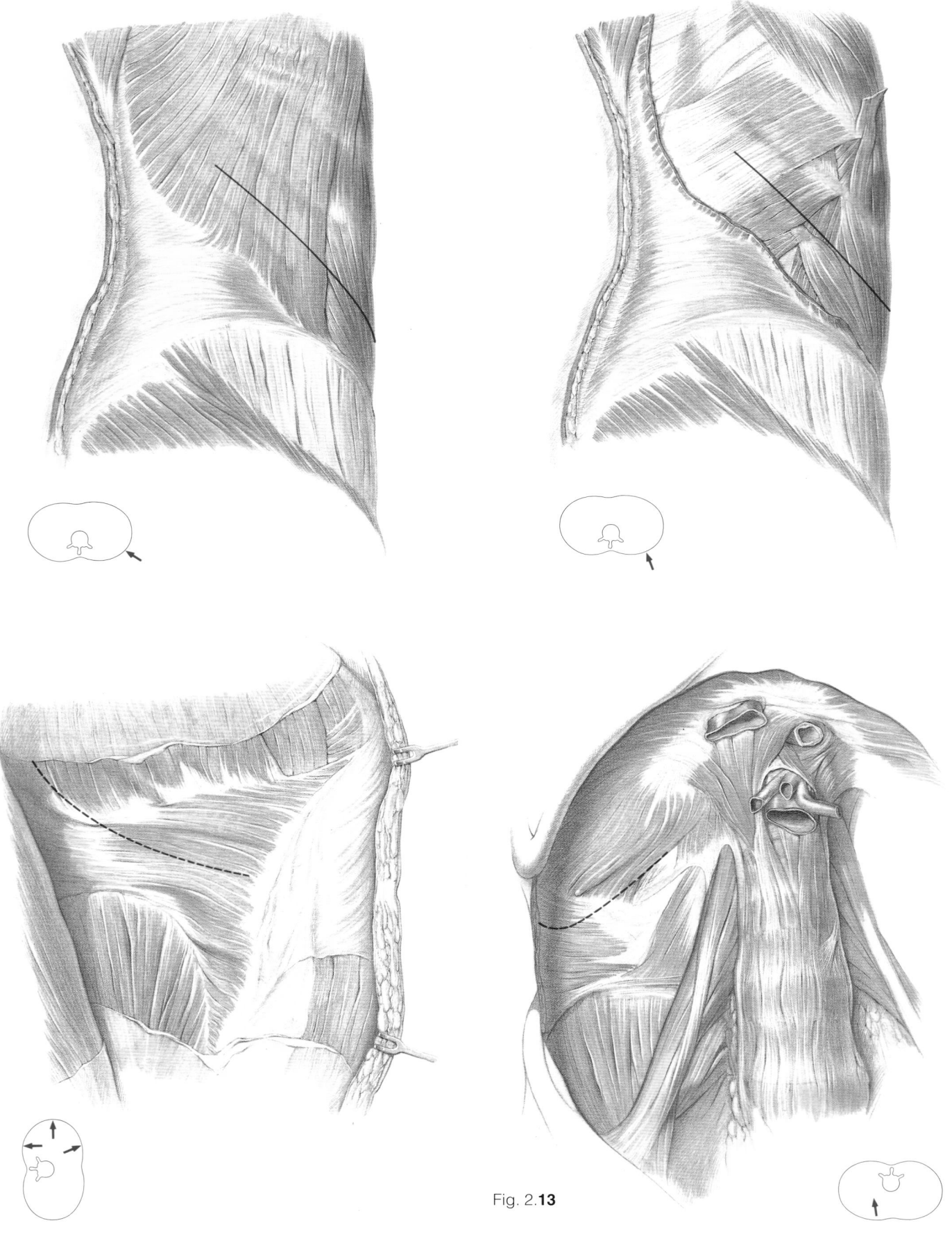

Fig. 2.**13**

Main Indications

- Procedures on the renal parenchyma
- Procedures at the ureteropelvic junction
- Nephrectomy
- Renal stone surgery

The supracostal approach affords broad exposure of the retroperitoneal space (kidney, adrenal gland, proximal ureter) while avoiding the need for rib resection. Several anatomic circumstances make this approach possible: The 11th and 12th ribs terminate freely in abdominal muscle, both ribs articulate only with the corresponding vertebral body, and the 12th rib is easily displaced downward following release of the muscles that insert on the 12th rib or arise from it.

The technique will be illustrated for a right-sided exposure.

Position and Skin Incision

The patient is positioned on the left side, and the operating table is flexed 30° at the lumbar level to hyperextend the operative area (Figs. 2.**14** , 2.**15**). The ipsilateral arm is raised toward the head, thus the distance between the costal arch and ilium is increased. The contralateral leg is flexed at the hip and knee.

The skin incision starts approximately two fingerwidths from the erector spinae muscle and passes between the 11th and 12th ribs in a gentle S-shaped curve toward the lateral border of the rectus muscle (Figs. 2.**14**, 2.**15**).

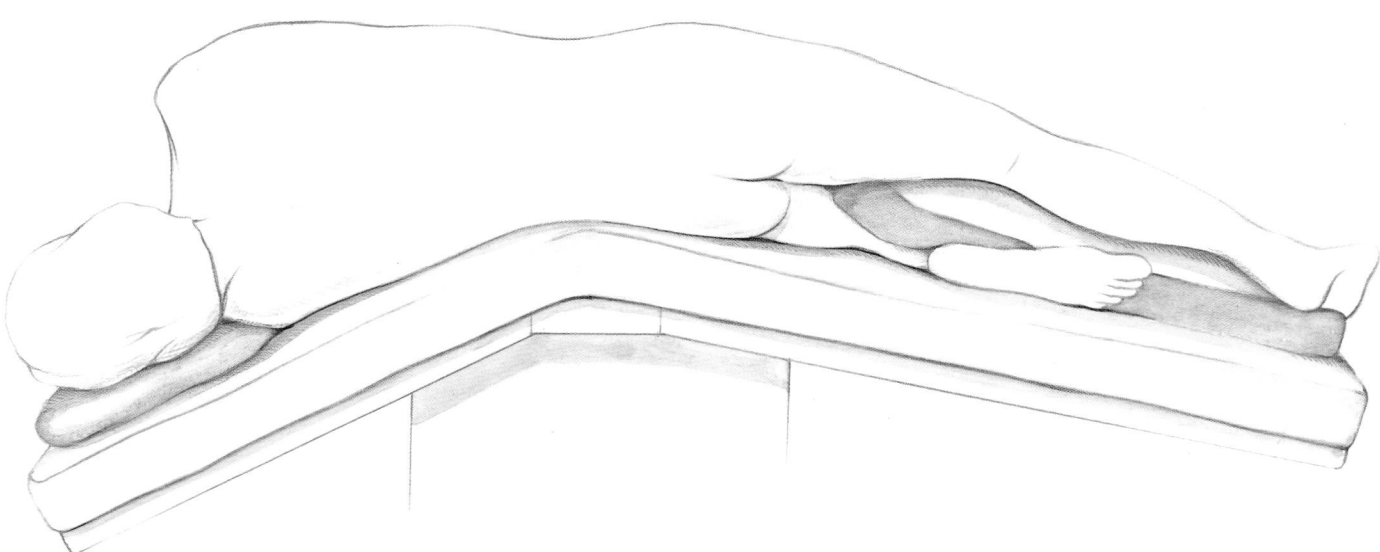

Fig. 2.**14**   Position for the supracostal approach.

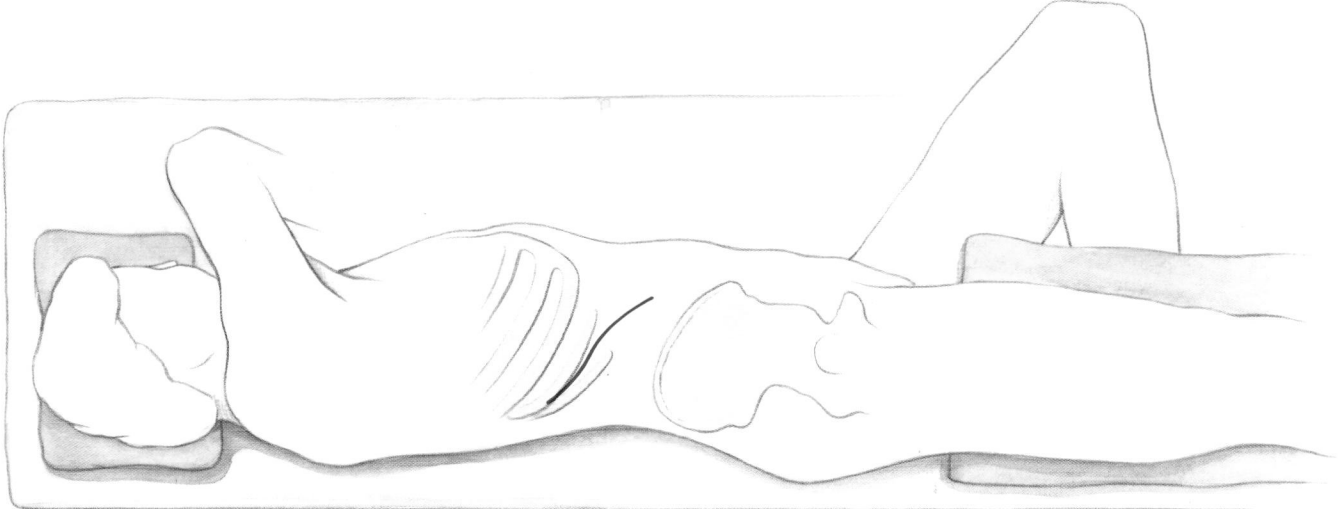

Fig. 2.**15**   Skin incision for the supracostal approach.

Exposure of the Lumbodorsal Fascia

After division of the subcutaneous fat, the thoracic fascia is divided exposing the latissimus dorsi and external oblique muscles (Fig. 2.**16**). Exposure is maintained with retractors. Individual bleeding vessels are coagulated (Fig. 2.**16**).

The muscles of the lateral chest wall are shown in Fig. 2.**17** .

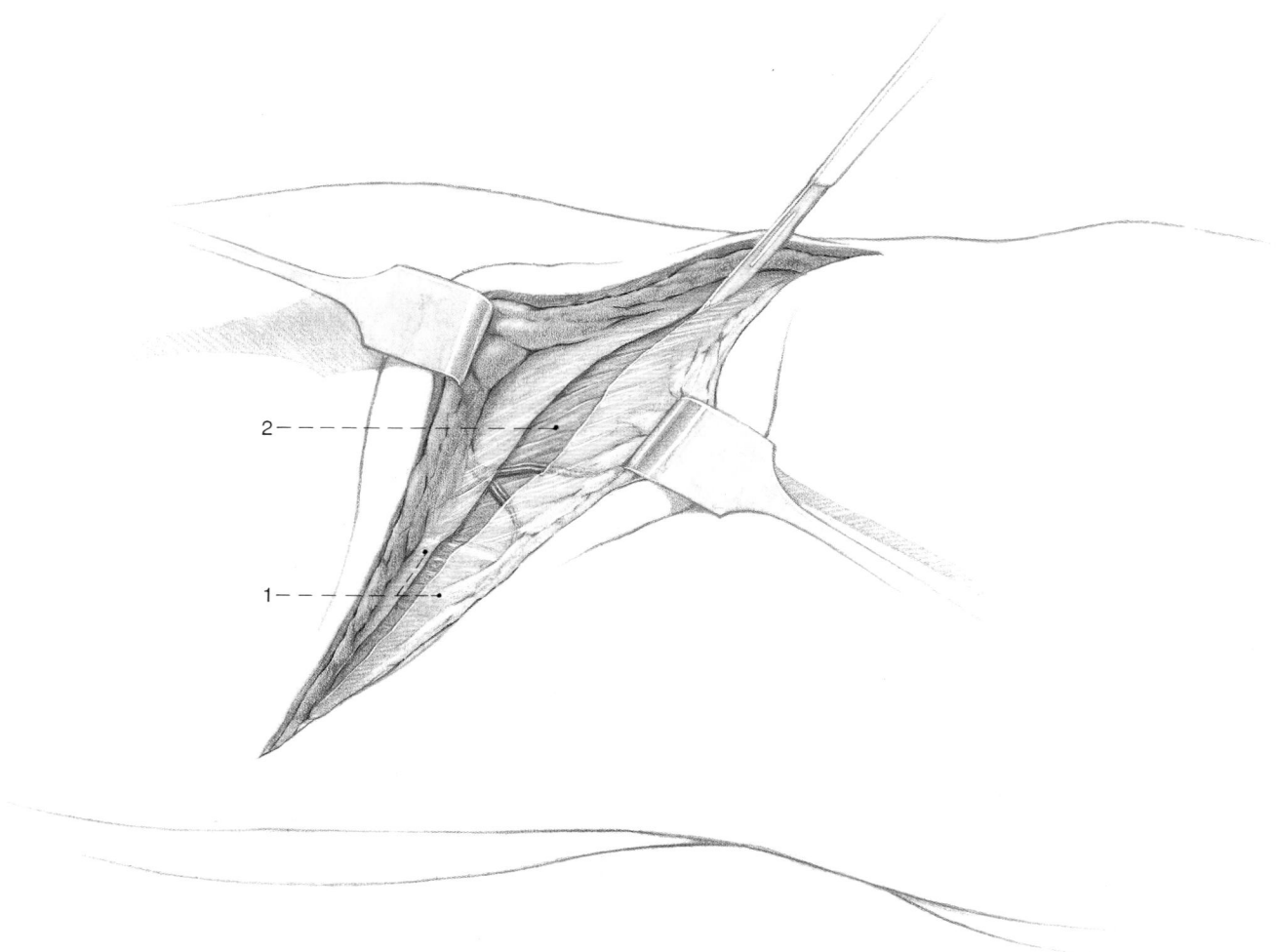

Fig. 2.**16**   Exposure of the latissimus dorsi and external oblique muscles.

1 Latissimus dorsi
2 External oblique muscle

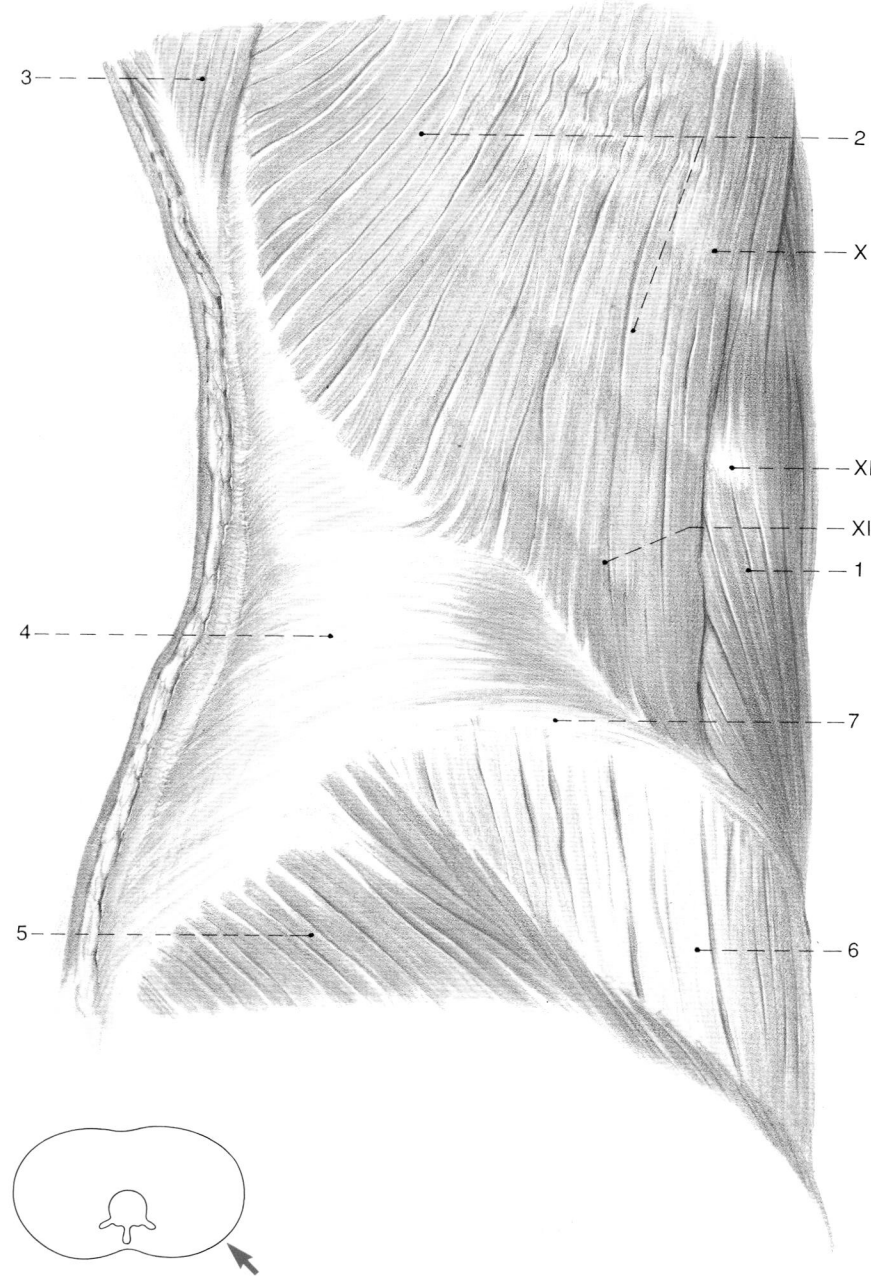

Fig. 2.**17** Muscles of the posterolateral body wall.

1 External oblique muscle
2 Latissimus dorsi
3 Trapezius
4 Lumbodorsal fascia
5 Gluteus maximus
6 Gluteus medius
7 Iliac crest
X–XII 10th through 12th ribs

The latissimus dorsi and serratus posterior inferior muscles and, anteriorly, the external oblique muscle are divided with diathermy directly on the periosteum of the 12th rib, exposing the external and internal intercostal muscles and the internal oblique muscle (Fig. 2.**18**).

Next the internal oblique is divided along the line indicated, exposing the deep layer of the lumbodorsal fascia at its junction with the fibers of transversus abdominis (Fig. 2.**19**).

The external and internal intercostal muscles are sharply dissected from the upper border of the rib with diathermy, starting at the tip of the 12th rib. This ensures that the line of incision is placed well away from the pleural cavity. After the intercostal muscles have been separated from the rib, the deep layer of the lumbodorsal fascia and the diaphragm can be identified (Fig. 2.**20**).

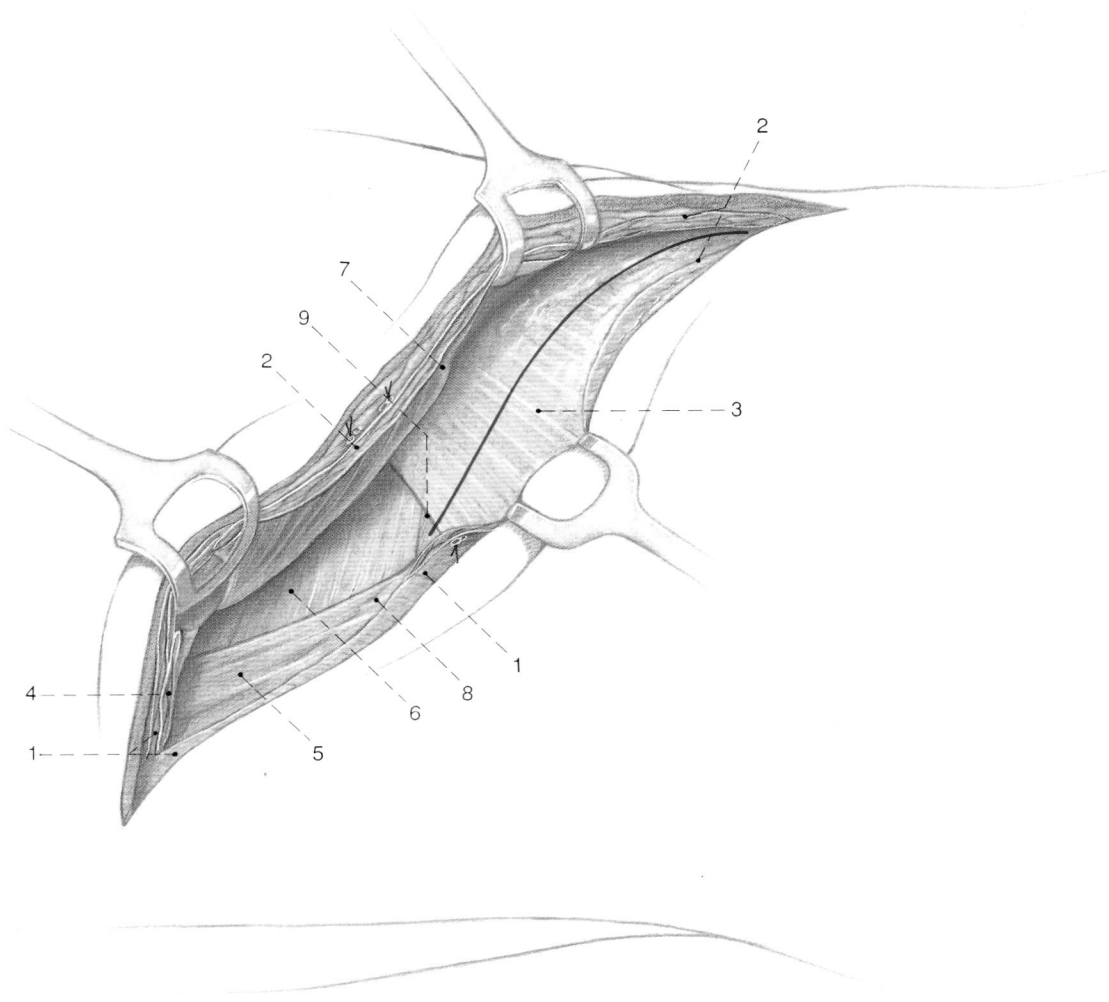

Fig. 2.**18** Exposure and division of the internal oblique and intercostal muscles.

1 Latissimus dorsi
2 External oblique muscle
3 Internal oblique muscle
4 Serratus posterior inferior
5 External intercostal muscle
6 Internal intercostal muscle
7 Tip of 11th rib
8 12th rib
9 Lumbodorsal fascia

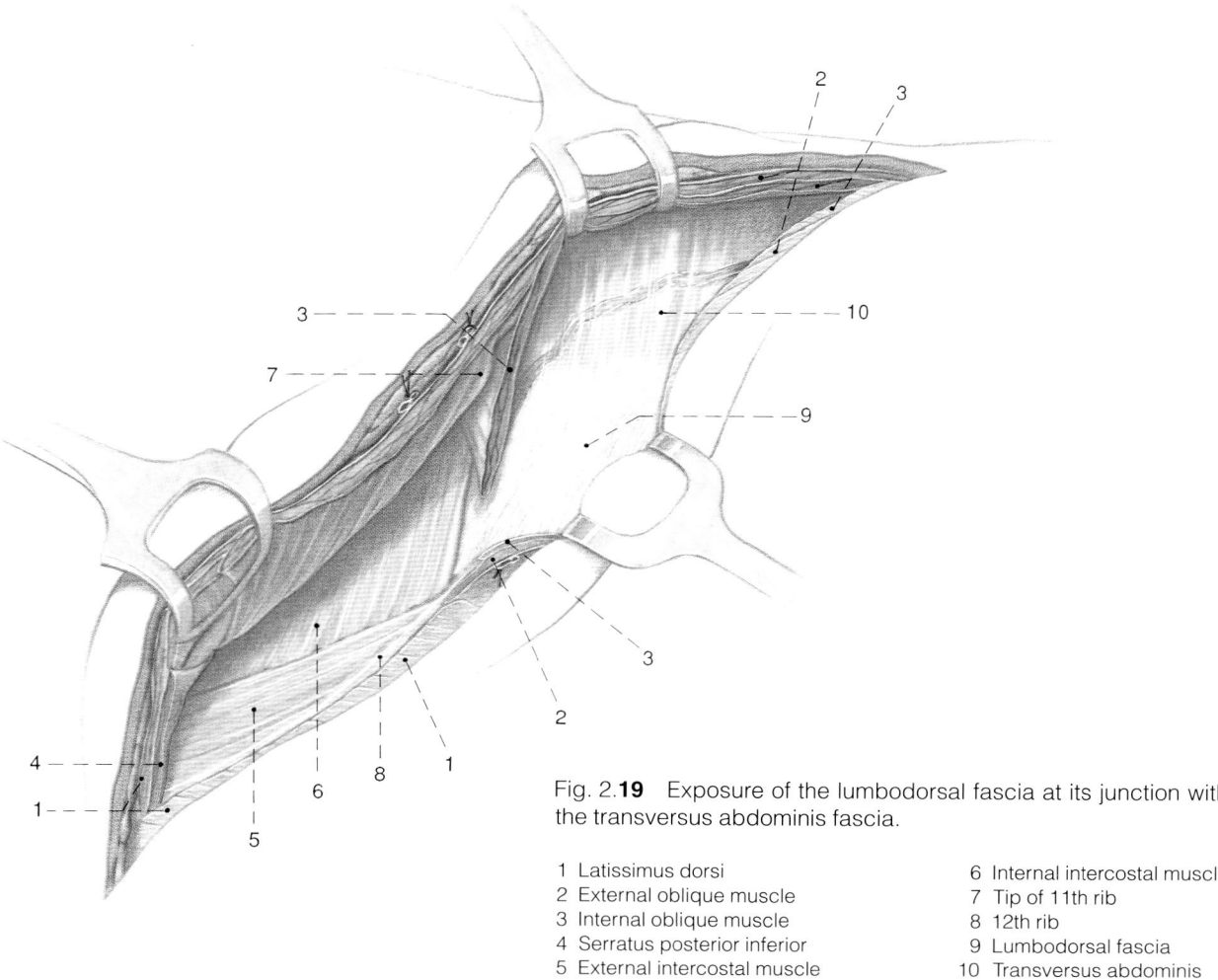

Fig. 2.**19** Exposure of the lumbodorsal fascia at its junction with the transversus abdominis fascia.

1 Latissimus dorsi
2 External oblique muscle
3 Internal oblique muscle
4 Serratus posterior inferior
5 External intercostal muscle

6 Internal intercostal muscle
7 Tip of 11th rib
8 12th rib
9 Lumbodorsal fascia
10 Transversus abdominis

Fig. 2.**20** Separation of the external and internal intercostal muscles from the 12th rib.

1 Latissimus dorsi
2 External oblique muscle
3 Internal oblique muscle
4 Serratus posterior inferior
5 External and internal intercostal muscles
6 Internal intercostal muscle

7 12th rib
8 Lumbodorsal fascia
9 Diaphragm

Incision of the Lumbodorsal Fascia

The lumbodorsal fascia is incised at the tip of the 12th rib, exposing the pararenal fat between the lumbodorsal fascia and Gerota's fascia. The lumbodorsal fascia can be opened over the fat by bluntly dissecting forward (Fig. 2.**21**).

As the 12th rib is displaced downward and forward with a retractor, the lumbodorsal fascia is dissected from the inner periosteum of the rib (Fig. 2.**22**). This affords extrapleural entry to the thoracic cavity while sparing the intercostal nerves and vessels.

The route of the approach is shown schematically in Fig. 2.**23**.

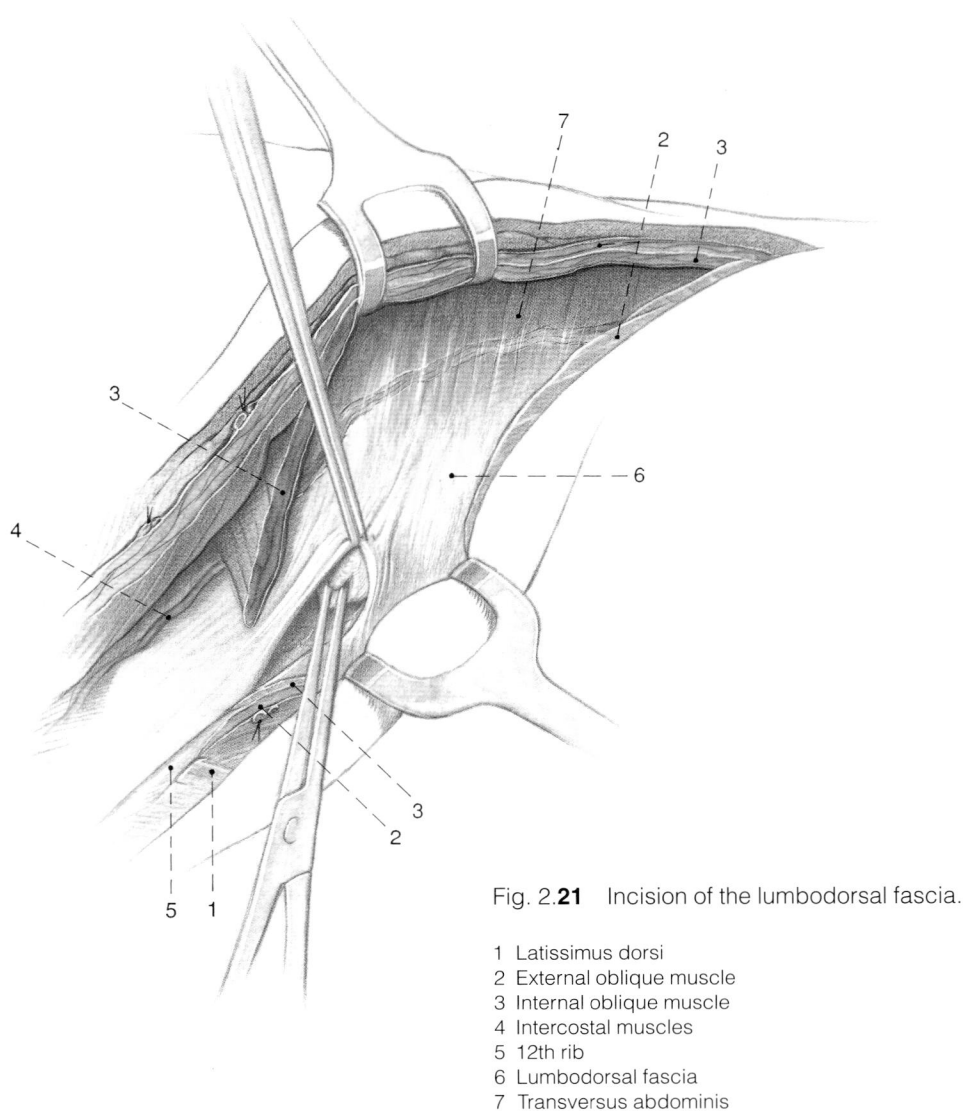

Fig. 2.**21**   Incision of the lumbodorsal fascia.

1 Latissimus dorsi
2 External oblique muscle
3 Internal oblique muscle
4 Intercostal muscles
5 12th rib
6 Lumbodorsal fascia
7 Transversus abdominis

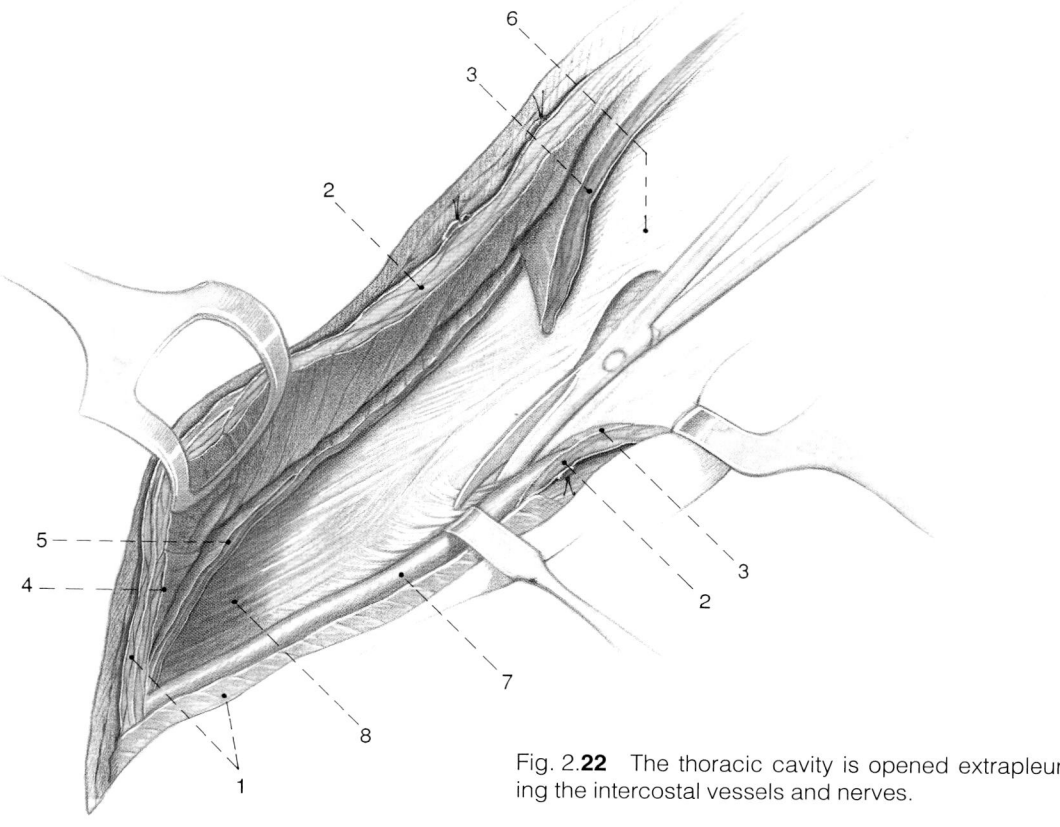

Fig. 2.**22** The thoracic cavity is opened extrapleurally, preserving the intercostal vessels and nerves.

1 Latissimus dorsi
2 External oblique muscle
3 Internal oblique muscle
4 Serratus posterior inferior
5 Intercostal muscles

6 Lumbodorsal fascia
7 12th rib
8 Diaphragm

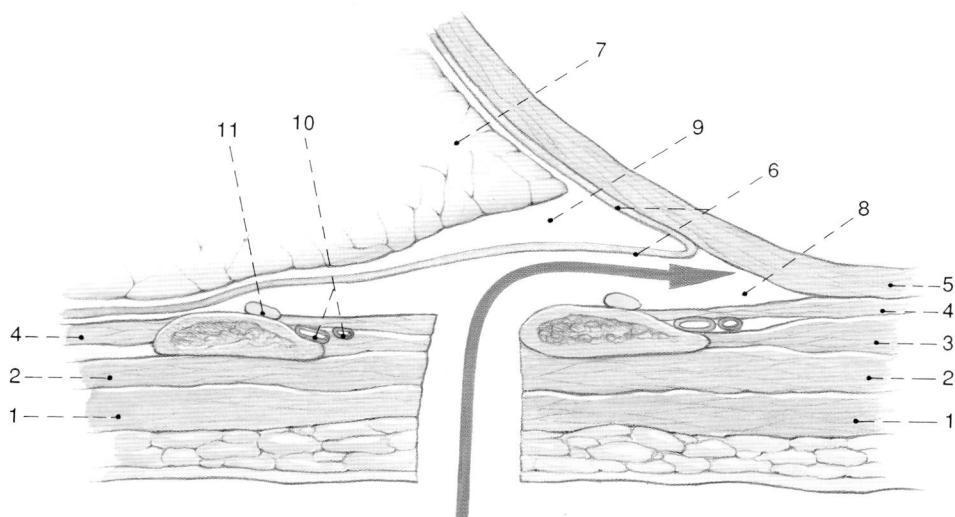

Fig. 2.**23** Schematic view of the dissection of the lumbodorsal fascia from the deep periosteum of the rib.

1 Latissimus dorsi
2 Serratus posterior inferior
3 External intercostal muscle
4 Internal intercostal muscle
5 Diaphragm
6 Parietal pleura
7 Lung

8 Thoracic cavity
9 Pleural cavity
10 Intercostal vessels
11 Intercostal nerve

Dissection of the Lumbodorsal Fascia and Diaphragm from the 12th Rib

A self-retaining chest retractor is inserted into the operative field over two packs (Fig. 2.24).

The lumbodorsal fascia and then the diaphragm are separated from the 12th rib under vision, using the finger or a small sponge stick to guide the dissection. The incision at the 12th rib can be carried over the quadratus lumborum muscle to the lateral arcuate ligament as part of the dissection, the pleural cavity and lung remaining outside the operative field (Fig. 2. 25).

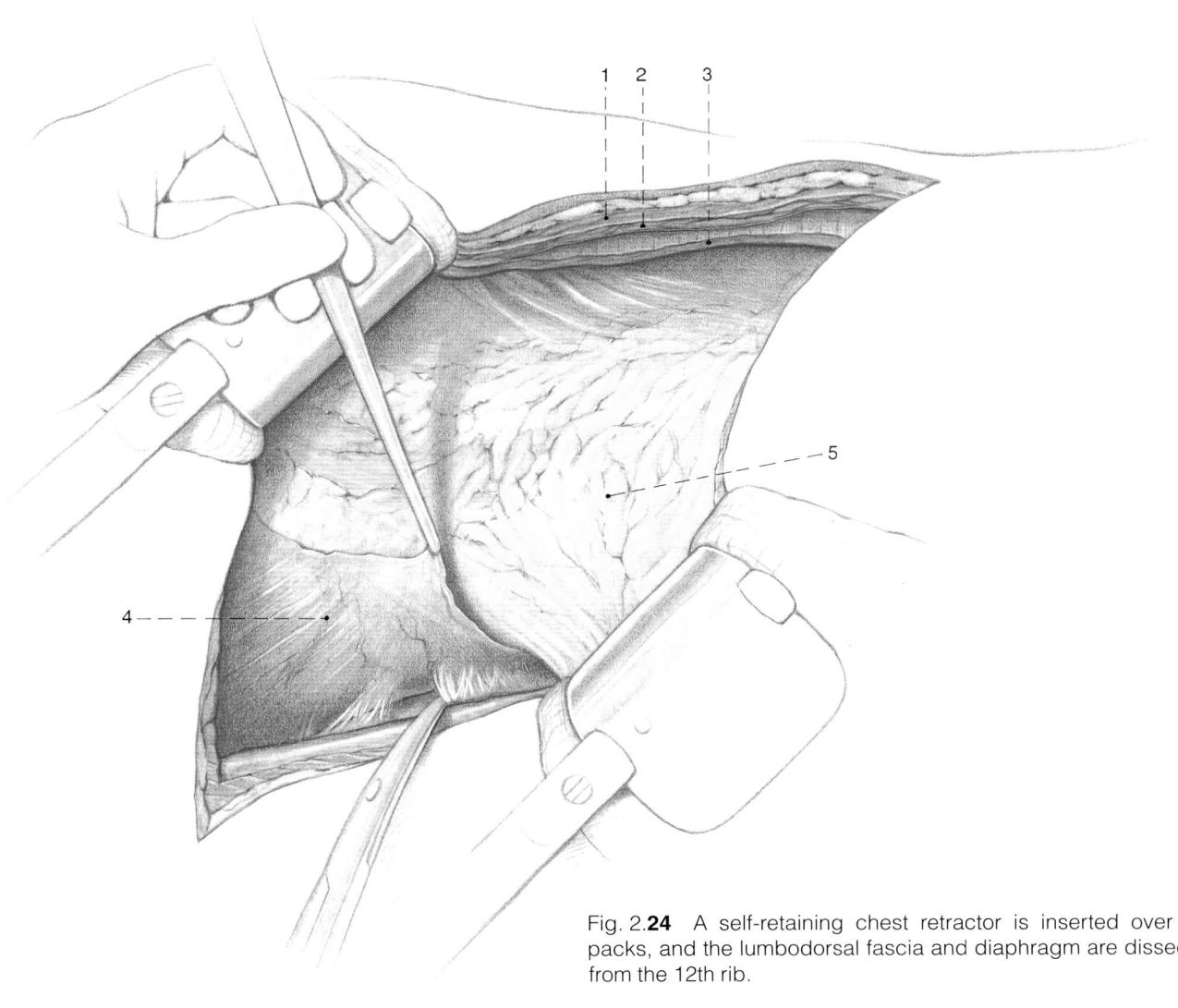

Fig. 2.24 A self-retaining chest retractor is inserted over two packs, and the lumbodorsal fascia and diaphragm are dissected from the 12th rib.

1 External oblique muscle
2 Internal oblique muscle
3 Transversus abdominis
4 Diaphragm
5 Pararenal fat

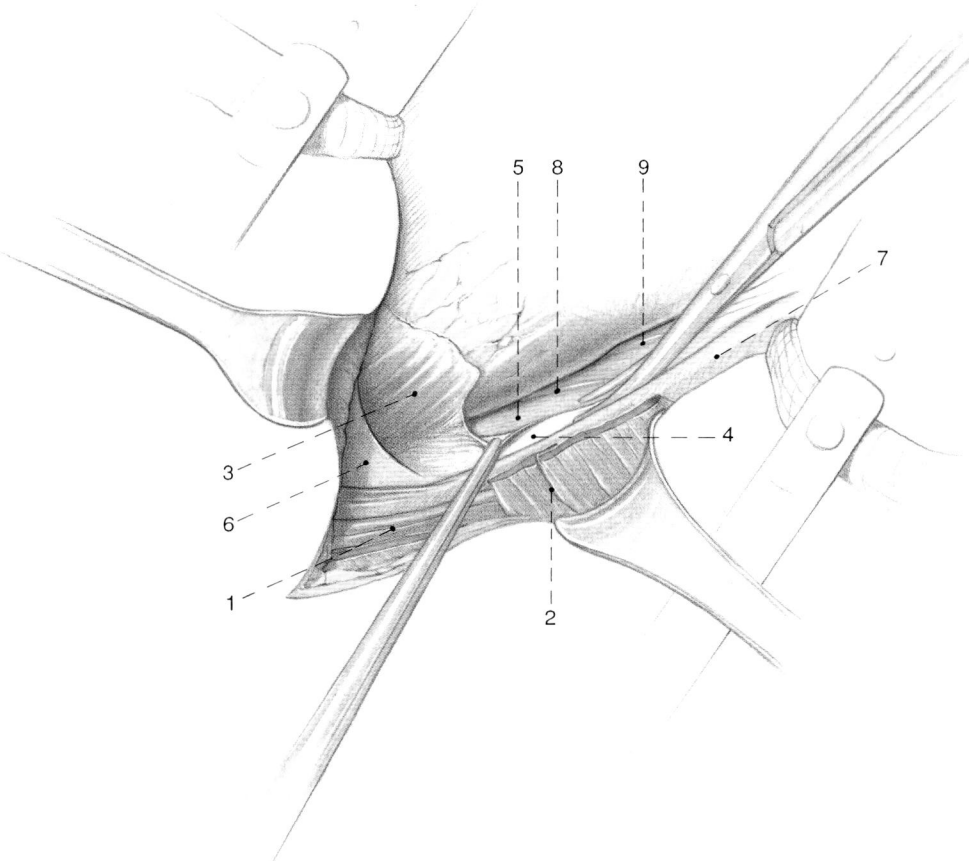

Fig. 2.**25** The pleural space and lung are outside the operative field. The quadratus lumborum muscle is visible below the lateral arcuate ligament.

1 Erector spinae
2 Serratus posterior inferior
3 Diaphragm
4 Lateral arcuate ligament
5 Quadratus lumborum
6 Parietal pleura
7 12th rib
8 Subcostal nerve
9 Ilioinguinal nerve

Incision of Gerota's Fascia

With the complete forward incision of the lumbodorsal fascia and transversus abdominis muscle, the 12th rib can be deflected downward with the chest retractor so that it is parallel to the quadratus lumborum muscle; the subcostal and iliohypogastric nerves can be identified on the muscle surface. The pararenal fat and then the peritoneum are freed up anteriorly. Gerota's fascia is opened from the posterior aspect. The pararenal fat is then exposed and dissected to provide access for dissection of the kidney and its collecting system (Fig. 2.26).

Comments

The supracostal approach is inadequate for the surgery of renal tumors. Dissection of the renal parenchyma and lower urinary tract is necessary to establish access to the renal vessels.

The supracostal approach in the 11th intercostal space is feasible only if the 12th rib is sufficiently long. Access through the 10th intercostal space differs only in that it involves freeing a greater portion of the pleura and diaphragm with the lumbodorsal fascia.

Essential elements of the supracostal approach are the primary exposure of the space between the 12th rib and the origins of the diaphragm, followed by the dissection of the lumbodorsal fascia and diaphragm from the 12th rib. The pleura lies between the chest wall and diaphragm outside the operative field; the pleural cavity is not violated.

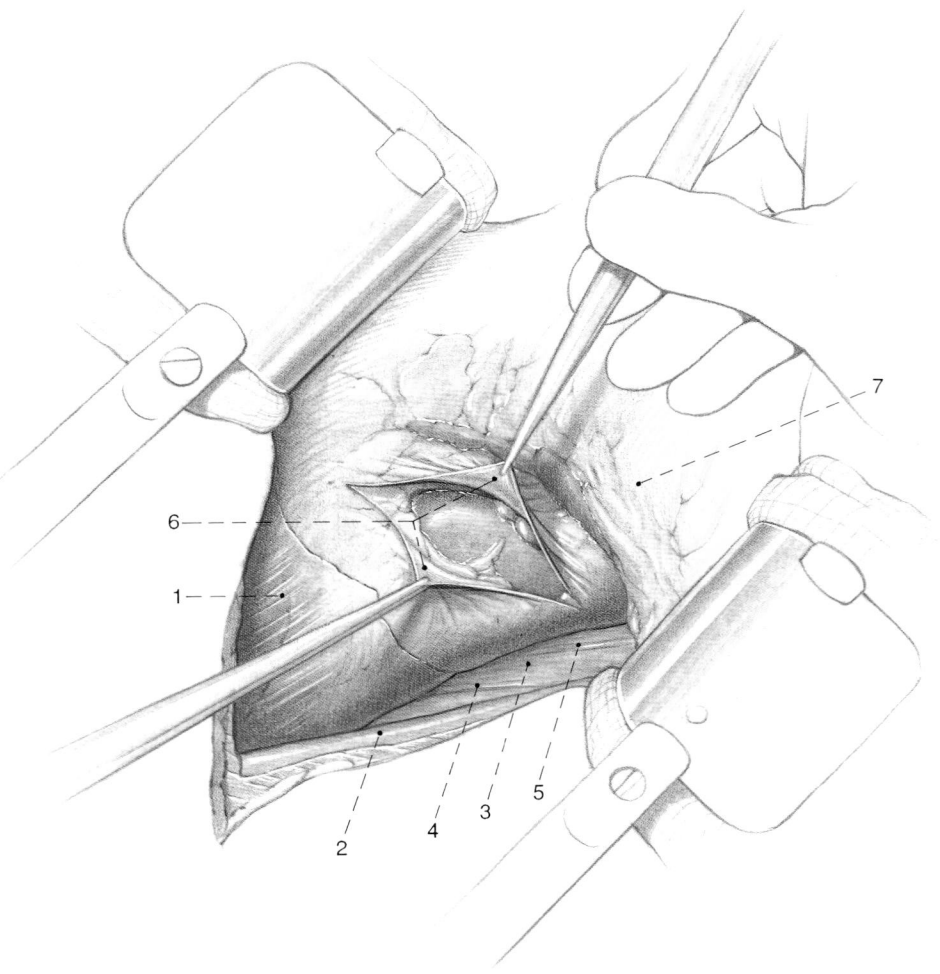

Fig. 2.**26**   Incision of Gerota's fascia.

1 Diaphragm
2 12th rib
3 Quadratus lumborum
4 Subcostal nerve
5 Iliohypogastric nerve
6 Gerota's fascia
7 Pararenal fat

Transcostal Approach

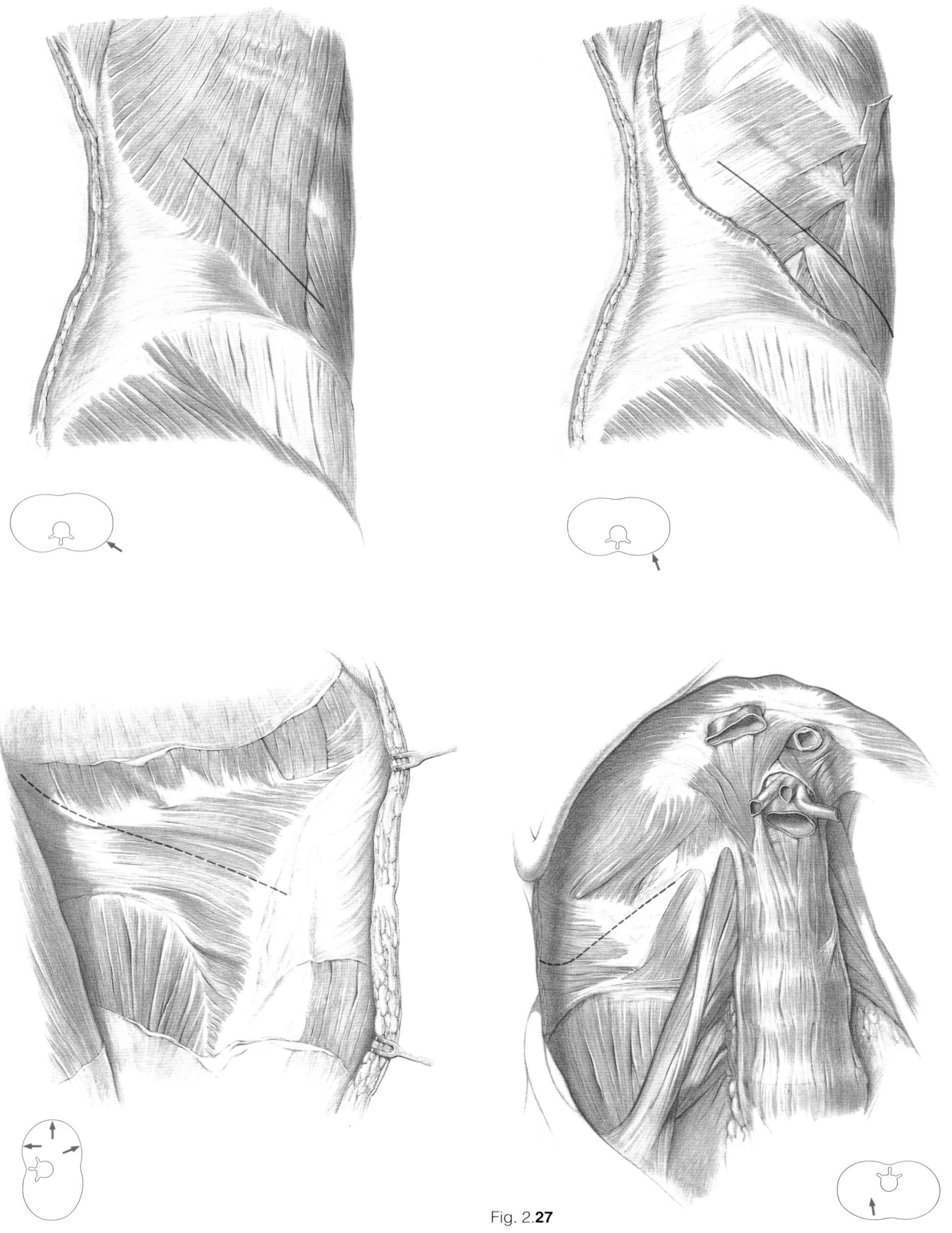

Fig. 2.**27**

Main Indications

- Procedures on the renal parenchyma
- Procedures at the ureteropelvic junction
- Nephrectomy
- Renal stone surgery

Unlike the supracostal approach, the transcostal approach can provide broad access to the retroperitoneal space (kidney, adrenal gland, proximal ureter) by resection of the 11th or 12th ribs.

The technique is illustrated for the right side.

Position and Skin Incision

The patient is positioned on the left side, and the operating table is flexed 30° at the lumbar level, as for a supracostal incision, to hyperextend the operative area (Fig. 2.**28**). The ipsilateral arm is raised; thus the distance between the costal arch and ilium is increased. The contralateral leg is flexed at the hip and knee.

The skin incision starts two fingerwidths from the erector spinae muscle and is carried over the 12th rib in a gentle S-shaped curve toward the lateral rectus muscle border, terminating at the level of the umbilicus (Fig. 2.**28**).

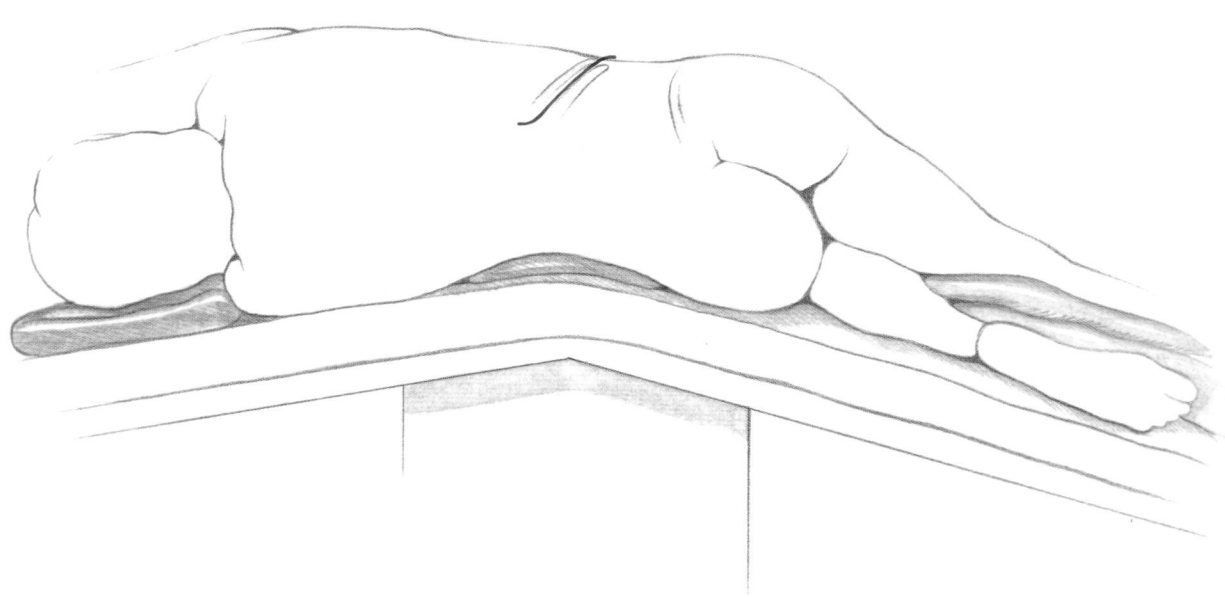

Fig. 2.**28**　Position and skin incision for the transcostal approach.

Exposure of the 12th Rib

After division of the subcutaneous fat, the thoracic fascia is transected to expose the latissimus dorsi and external oblique muscles (Fig. 2.**29**). Exposure is maintained with retractors. Individual bleeding vessels are coagulated.

The latissimus dorsi, serratus posterior inferior, and external oblique muscle anteriorly are divided directly over the periosteum of the 12th rib with diathermy, following the incision line shown in Fig. 2.**29**. The incision is opened to expose the external and internal intercostal muscles and the internal oblique muscle (Fig. 2.**30**).

The periosteum of the 12th rib is divided with diathermy along the line indicated (Fig. 2.**30**).

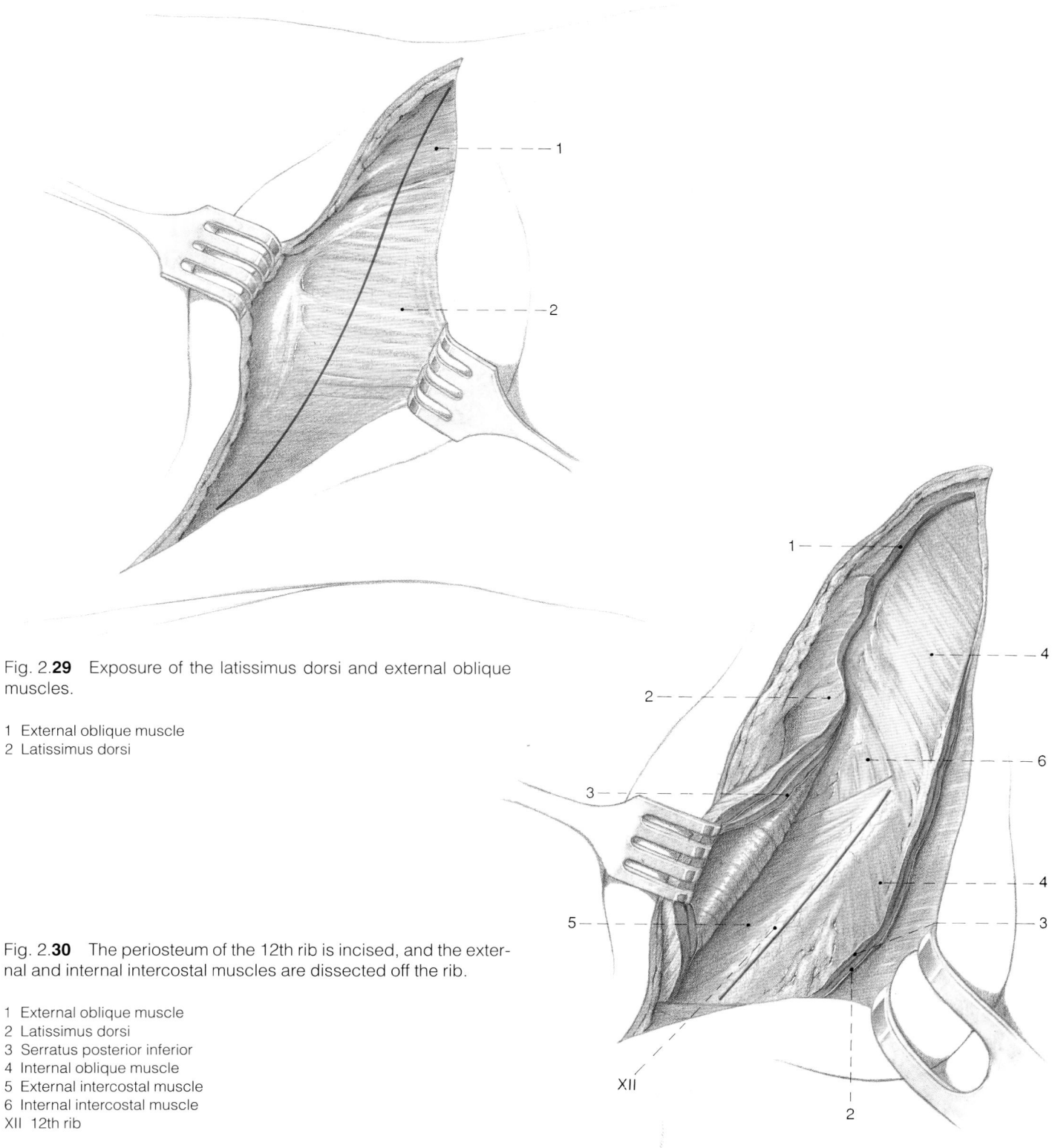

Fig. 2.**29** Exposure of the latissimus dorsi and external oblique muscles.

1 External oblique muscle
2 Latissimus dorsi

Fig. 2.**30** The periosteum of the 12th rib is incised, and the external and internal intercostal muscles are dissected off the rib.

1 External oblique muscle
2 Latissimus dorsi
3 Serratus posterior inferior
4 Internal oblique muscle
5 External intercostal muscle
6 Internal intercostal muscle
XII 12th rib

Resection of the 12th Rib

The external intercostal muscle is divided on the 12th rib and retracted upward. The periosteum is first separated from the rib with a straight periosteal elevator, and isolation of the 12th rib is completed with a curved rib stripper (Fig. 2.**31**).

The 12th rib is sectioned with rib shears as far medially as the exposure will permit, and the end of the rib is sealed with bone wax. The anterior part of the rib is freed from its fibrous attachments and removed (Fig. 2.**32**).

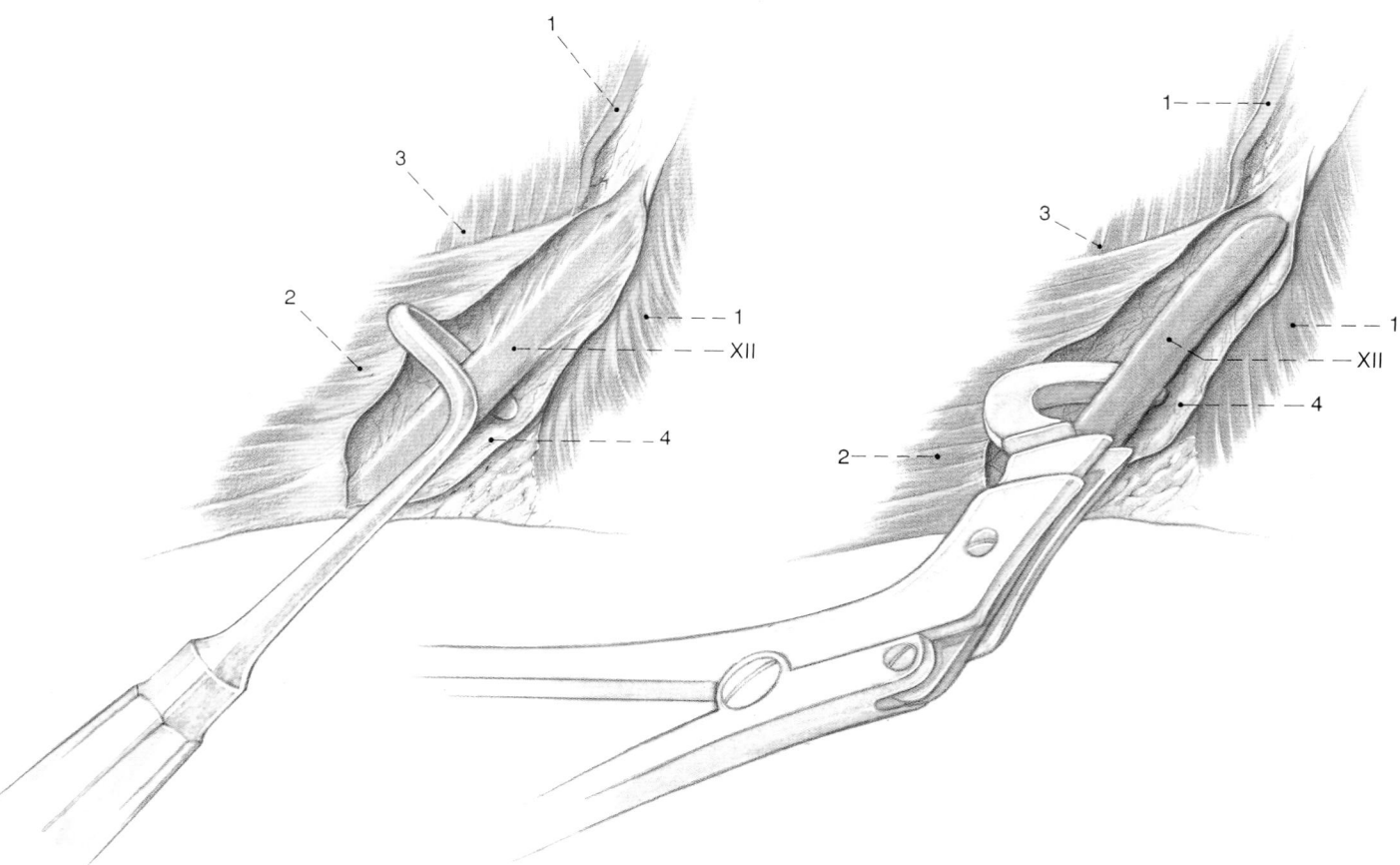

Fig. 2.**31**   Isolation of the 12th rib is completed with a curved stripper.

1 Internal oblique muscle
2 External intercostal muscle
3 Internal intercostal muscle
4 Periosteum
XII 12th rib

Fig. 2.**32**   The 12th rib is resected as far medially as possible with rib shears.

1 Internal oblique muscle
2 Intercostalis externus muscle
3 Intercostalis internus muscle
4 Periosteum
XII 12th rib

Exposure and Incision of the Lumbodorsal Fascia

The periosteal bed of the 12th rib is carefully divided with a pair of scissors, sparing the branches of the 12th intercostal neurovascular bundle that runs along the inferior border of the resected rib. During division of the external intercostal muscle at the 12th rib, care is taken to preserve the vessels that anastomose between the 11th and 12th intercostal vessels (Figs. 2.**33**, 2.**34**).

After division of the transversus abdominis, the preperitoneal fat appears in the anterior portion of the wound. The

posterior rib bed and lumbodorsal fascia are now divided to gain entry to the retroperitoneal space (Figs. 2.**33**, 2.**34**). As in the supracostal approach, the thoracic cavity is entered extrapleurally, thus preserving the intercostal vessels and nerves. This dissection is facilitated by the use of a small sponge stick.

The lumbodorsal fascia and diaphragm are freed, carrying the dissection as far as the lateral arcuate ligament over the quadratus lumborum, as in the supracostal approach. The pleural cavity and lung remain outside the operative field. In Fig. 2.**34** the lumbodorsal fascia is elevated with a forceps while the superficial muscles are held aside with retractors.

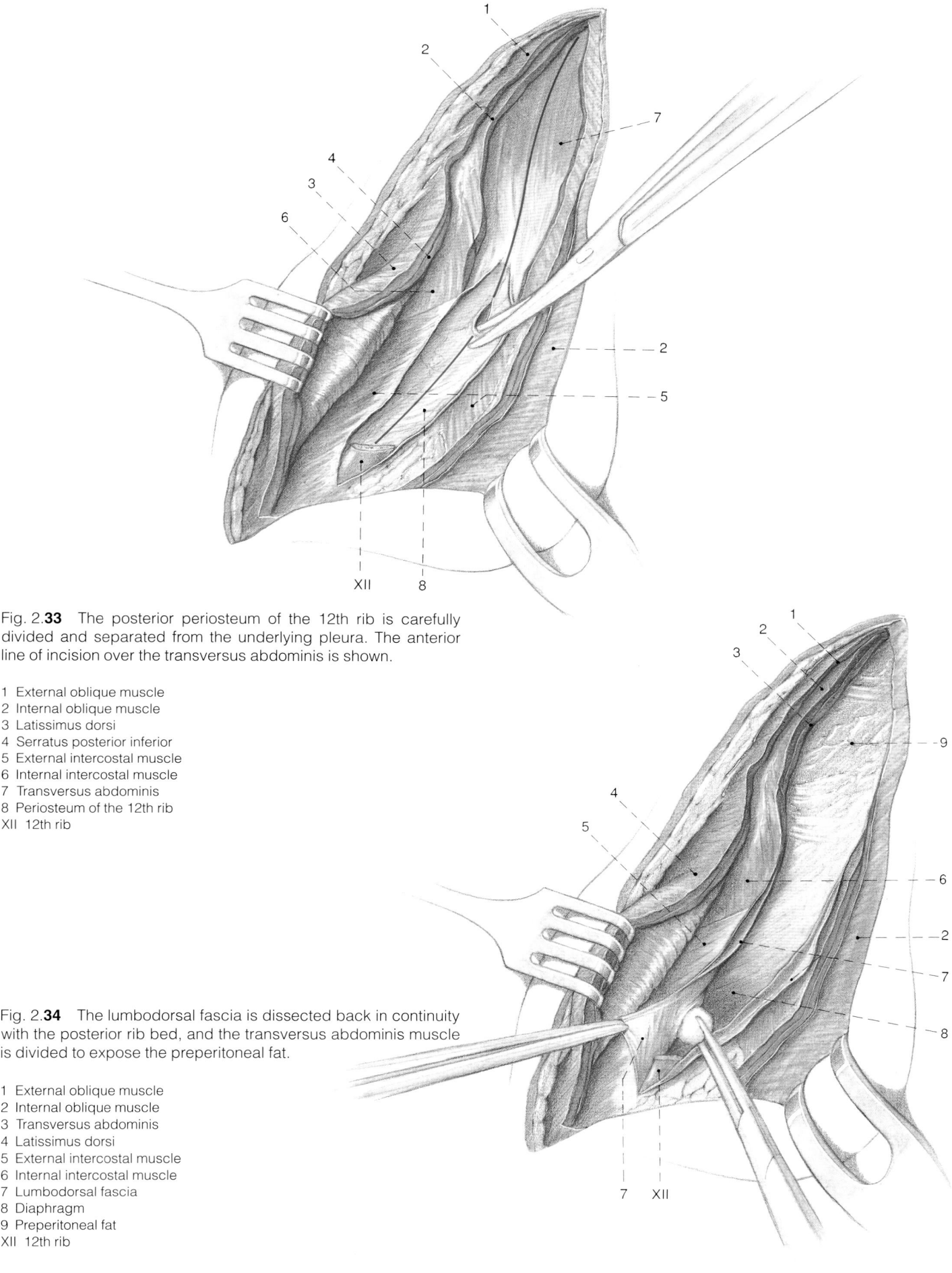

Fig. 2.**33** The posterior periosteum of the 12th rib is carefully divided and separated from the underlying pleura. The anterior line of incision over the transversus abdominis is shown.

1 External oblique muscle
2 Internal oblique muscle
3 Latissimus dorsi
4 Serratus posterior inferior
5 External intercostal muscle
6 Internal intercostal muscle
7 Transversus abdominis
8 Periosteum of the 12th rib
XII 12th rib

Fig. 2.**34** The lumbodorsal fascia is dissected back in continuity with the posterior rib bed, and the transversus abdominis muscle is divided to expose the preperitoneal fat.

1 External oblique muscle
2 Internal oblique muscle
3 Transversus abdominis
4 Latissimus dorsi
5 External intercostal muscle
6 Internal intercostal muscle
7 Lumbodorsal fascia
8 Diaphragm
9 Preperitoneal fat
XII 12th rib

Exposure of Gerota's Fascia

A chest retractor is inserted over two packs, and the retroperitoneal space is widely opened. Gerota's fascia can be seen below the pararenal fat (Fig. 2.35).

Comments

The alternative 11th rib approach, like the supracostal approach, affords broad exposure of the retroperitoneal space. Essential elements are the division of the posterior rib bed with the lumbodorsal fascia and the subsequent dissection of the lumbodorsal fascia and diaphragm. The peritoneum in the anterior part of the field and the pleura in the posterior part can be deflected downward with a finger or small sponge stick during the incision of these structures.

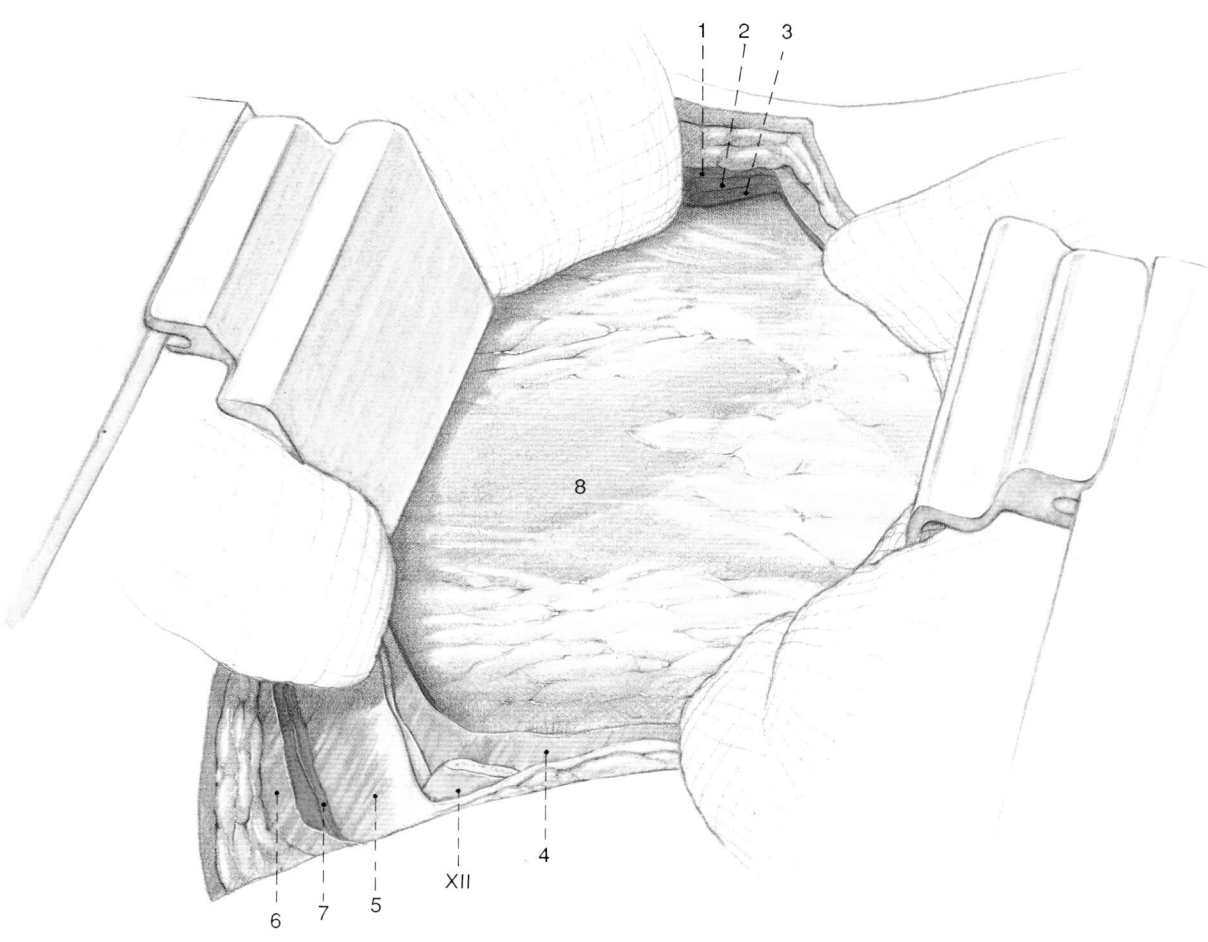

Fig. 2.**35** A self-retaining retractor is inserted, and the retroperitoneal space is exposed. The diaphragm is incised and retracted with the lumbodorsal fascia.

1 External oblique muscle
2 Internal oblique muscle
3 Transversus abdominis
4 Diaphragm
5 External intercostal muscle
6 Latissimus dorsi
7 Serratus posterior inferior
8 Gerota's fascia

Foley Muscle-Splitting Approach

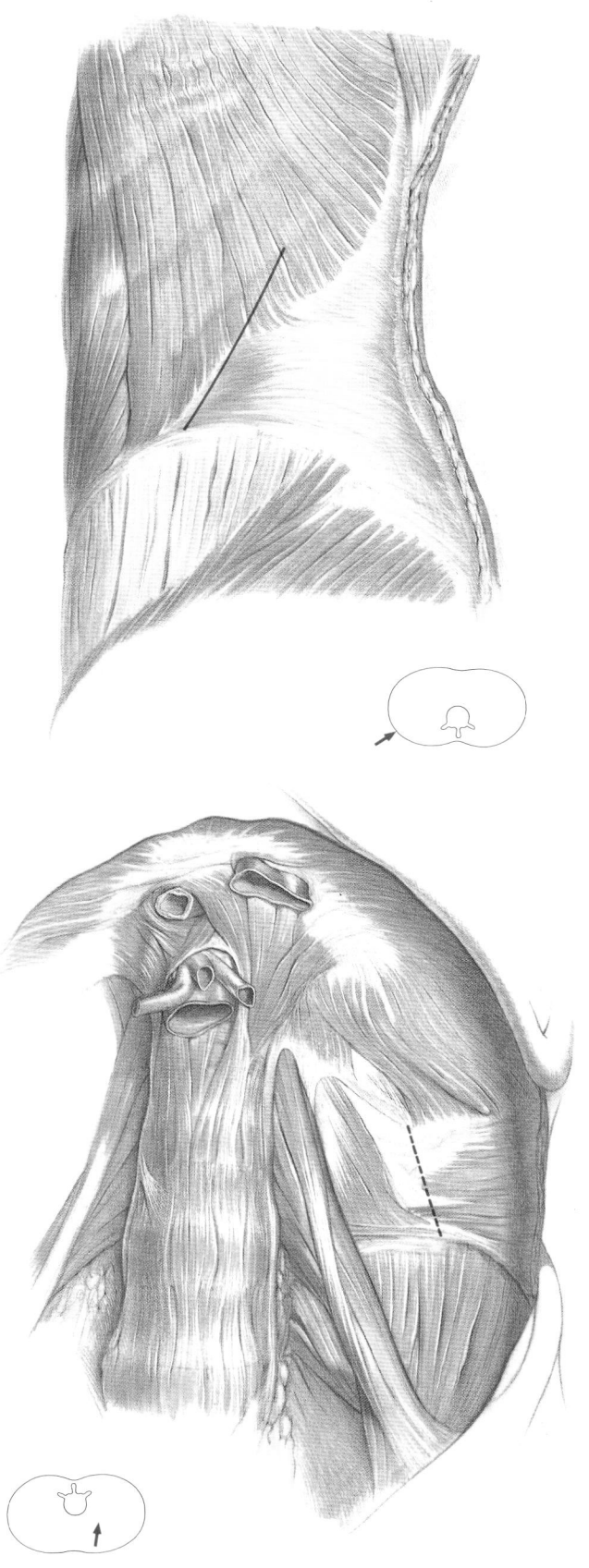

Fig. 2.**36**

Main Indications

● Procedures at the ureteropelvic junction
● Procedures on the proximal ureter

This approach gives access to the ureteropelvic junction and proximal ureter through a transfascial route. The technique is illustrated for the right side.

Position and Skin Incision

The patient is positioned on the left side, and the operating table is flexed 30° at the lumbar level to hyperextend the operative area (Figs. 2.37, 2.38). The ipsilateral arm is raised; thus the distance between the costal arch and ilium is increased. The contralateral leg is flexed at the hip and knee.

Three landmarks guide the placement of the skin incision: the inferior border of the 12th rib, the erector spinae muscle, and the iliac crest. The incision starts at the intersection of the 12th rib and erector spinae and descends toward the iliac crest (Fig. 2.38).

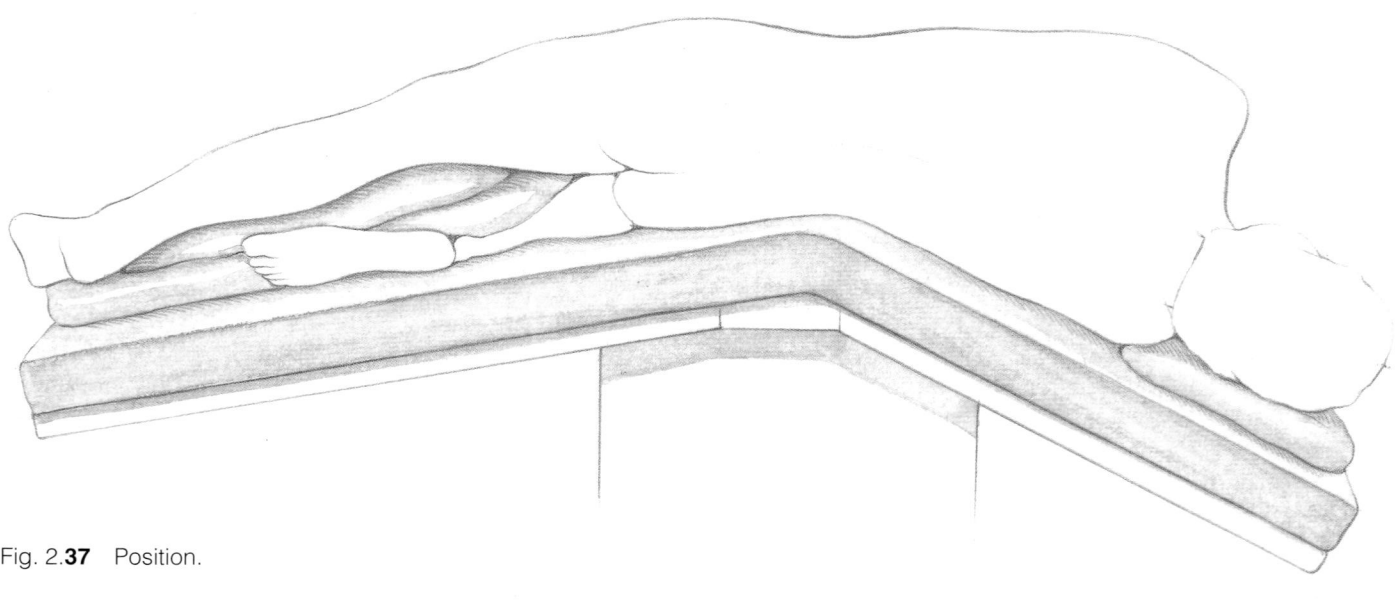

Fig. 2.**37**   Position.

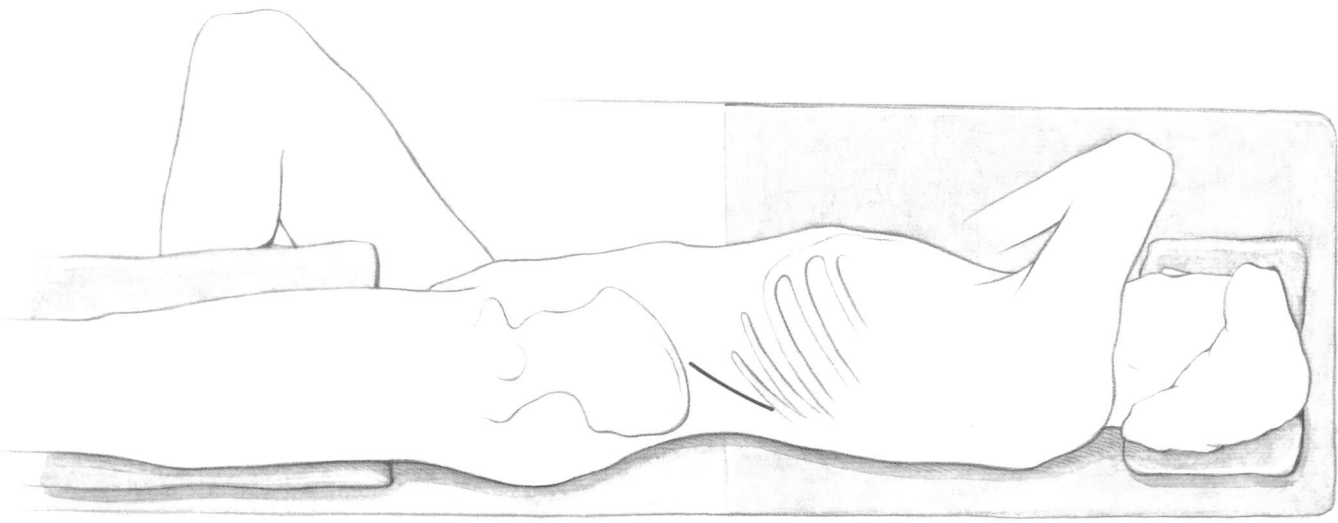

Fig. 2.**38**   Skin incision.

Exposure of the Superficial Muscles

The subcutaneous fatty tissue is divided to expose the latissimus dorsi in the posterior wound angle and the oblique abdominal muscles in the anterior wound angle. The skin and subcutaneous fat are held back with two retractors (Fig. 2.**39**). The internal oblique is exposed along the line indicated.

Exposure of the Transversus Abdominis and its Tendon of Origin

The latissimus dorsi and external oblique muscles are retracted, and a retractor is placed in the proximal part of the incision to expose the tendon of origin of the transversus abdominis and, anteriorly, the fibers of the internal oblique muscle (Fig. 2.**40**). The internal oblique is separated from the transversus abdominis along the line indicated and is retracted forward with a second retractor. The tendon of origin of transversus abdominis is incised in the direction of its fibers (Fig. 2.**41**).

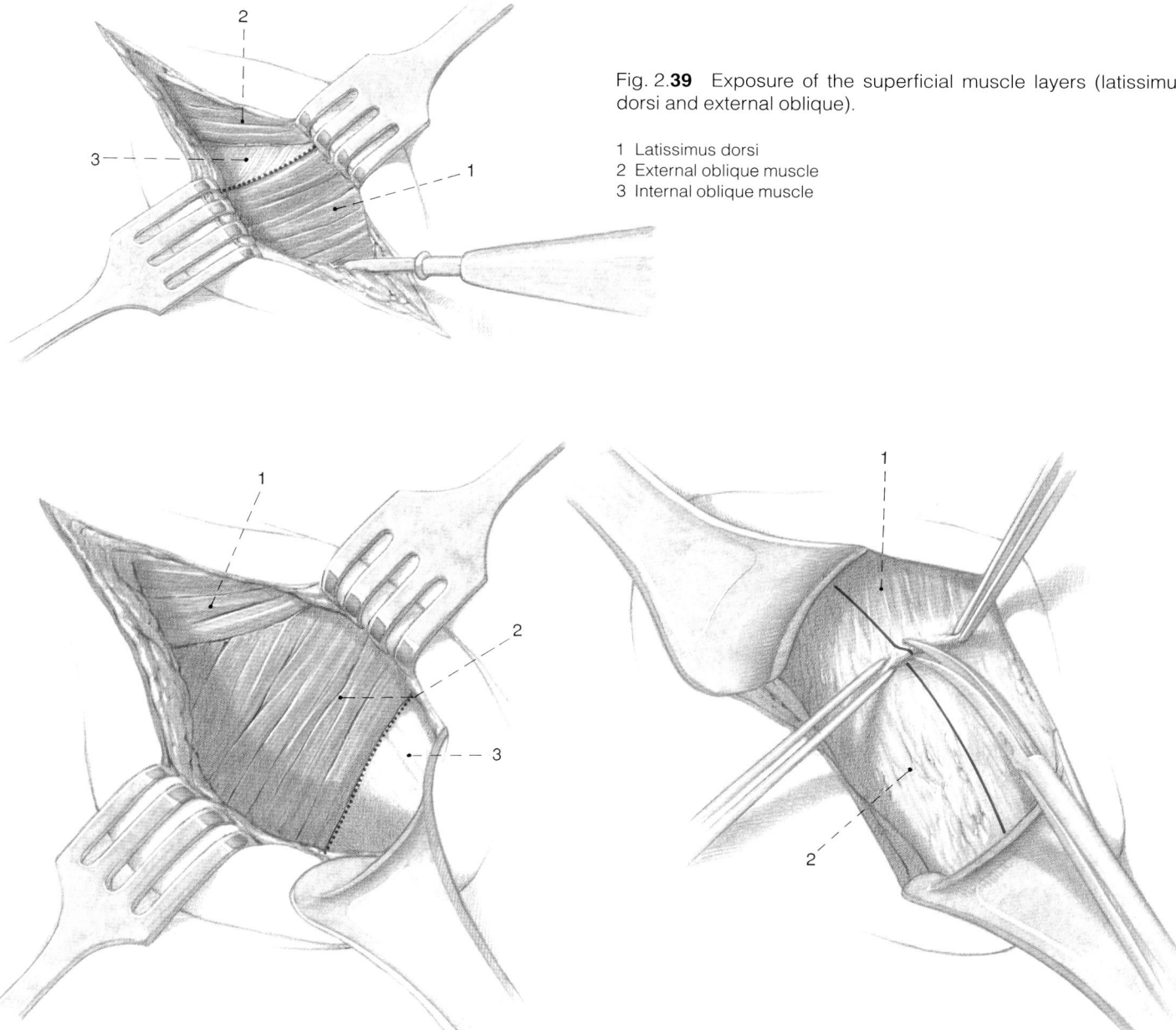

Fig. 2.**39** Exposure of the superficial muscle layers (latissimus dorsi and external oblique).

1 Latissimus dorsi
2 External oblique muscle
3 Internal oblique muscle

Fig. 2.**40** The internal oblique is separated from the transversus abdominis and its tendon of origin.

1 External oblique
2 Internal oblique
3 Transversus abdominis, tendon of origin

Fig. 2.**41** The transversus abdominis tendon of origin is incised, and the transversus muscle fibers are split.

1 Transversus abdominis muscle
2 Transversus abdominis tendon of origin

Exposure of Gerota's Fascia

After the transversus tendon of origin has been split in line with its fibers, the peritoneum is retracted medially, and Gerota's fascia is incised. The lower pole of the kidney and the proximal ureter are dissected free in the retroperitoneal space (Fig. 2.**42**). The psoas major comes into view.

Comments

This transfascial approach offers the advantage of low postoperative morbidity but gives access only to the ureteropelvic junction and proximal part of the ureter. Only the lower pole of the kidney can be visualized. Today this approach has been largely superseded by laparoscopic and endourologic procedures.

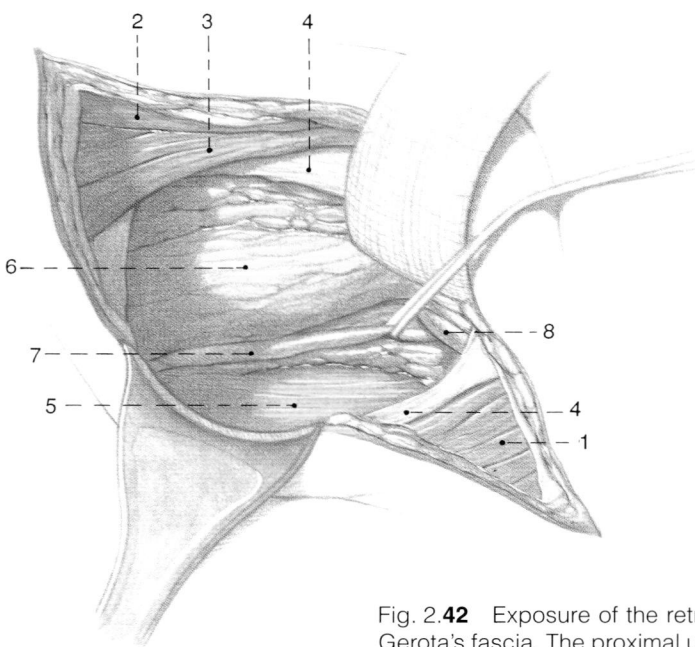

Fig. 2.**42** Exposure of the retroperitoneal space after incision of Gerota's fascia. The proximal ureter is identified.

1 Latissimus dorsi
2 External oblique muscle
3 Internal oblique muscle
4 Transversus abdominis tendon of origin
5 Psoas major
6 Parietal peritoneum
7 Ureter
8 Lower pole of kidney

Posterior Lumbotomy

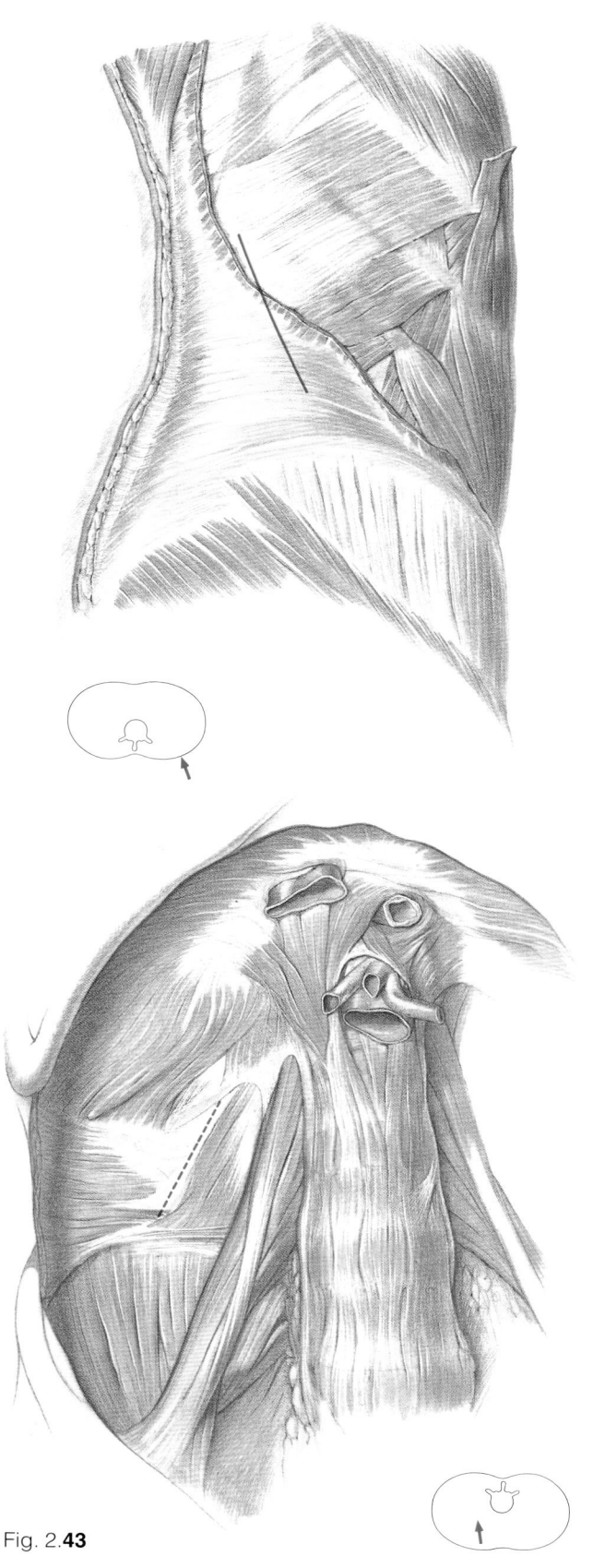

Fig. 2.**43**

Main Indications

● Procedures at the ureteropelvic junction

The posterior lumbotomy approach to the kidney has gained little acceptance compared with the supracostal approach due to its limited exposure of the kidney and retroperitoneal space. The advantage of this approach is its low postoperative morbidity (transfascial access).

The technique is illustrated for the right side.

Position and Skin Incision

The operation is performed in a modified left lateral position with the body rotated 30° forward. The operating table is mildly flexed at the lumbar level to hyperextend the operative area (Fig. 2.**44**). The ipsilateral arm is raised, as in the supracostal approach. The contralateral leg is flexed at the hip and knee.

The skin incision starts at the costal process of the first lumbar vertebra and runs directly toward the iliac crest (Fig. 2.**44**).

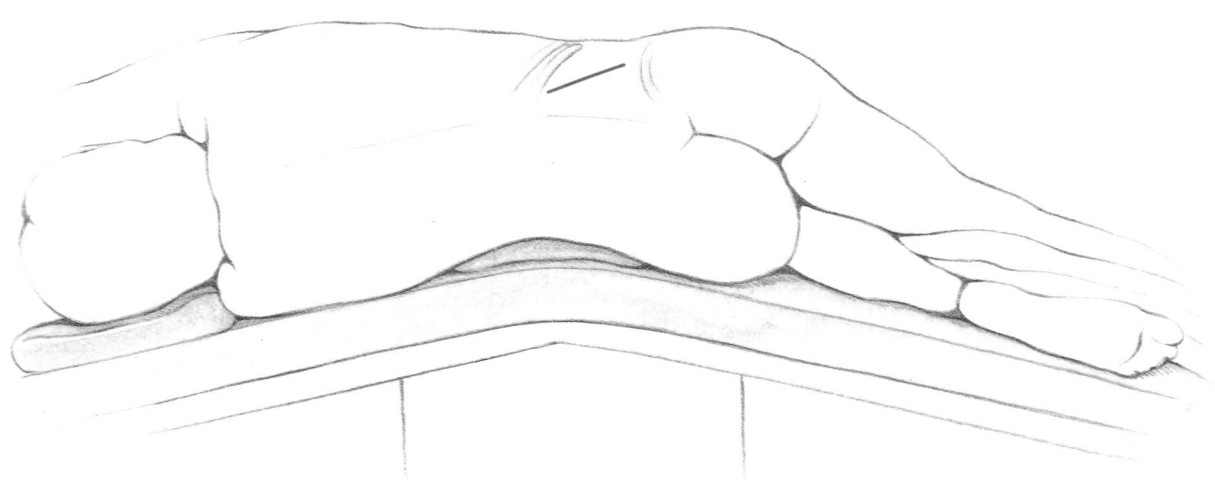

Fig. 2.**44**   Position and skin incision.

Incision of the Superficial Layer of the Lumbodorsal Fascia

The first diathermy incision (see line in figure) is made at the junction of the superficial layer of the lumbodorsal fascia with the latissimus dorsi muscle. The wound is held open with two retractors, and individual bleeding vessels are coagulated (Fig. 2.**45**).

The underlying longitudinal fibers of the erector spinae are identified. Division of the latissimus dorsi fibers is continued further downward in line with the incision. The erector spinae and latissimus dorsi are retracted to expose the deep layer of the lumbodorsal fascia (Fig. 2.**46**).

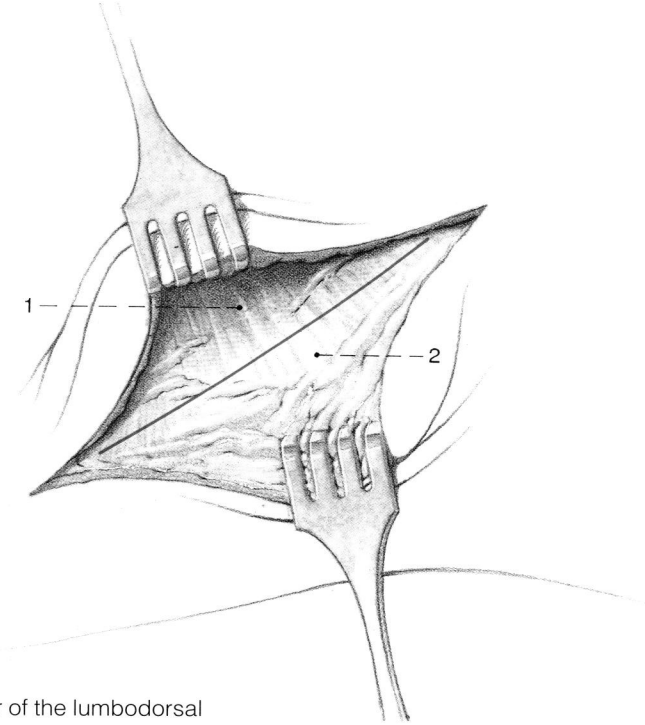

Fig. 2.**45** Incision of the superficial layer of the lumbodorsal fascia.

1 Latissimus dorsi
2 Lumbodorsal fascia, superficial layer

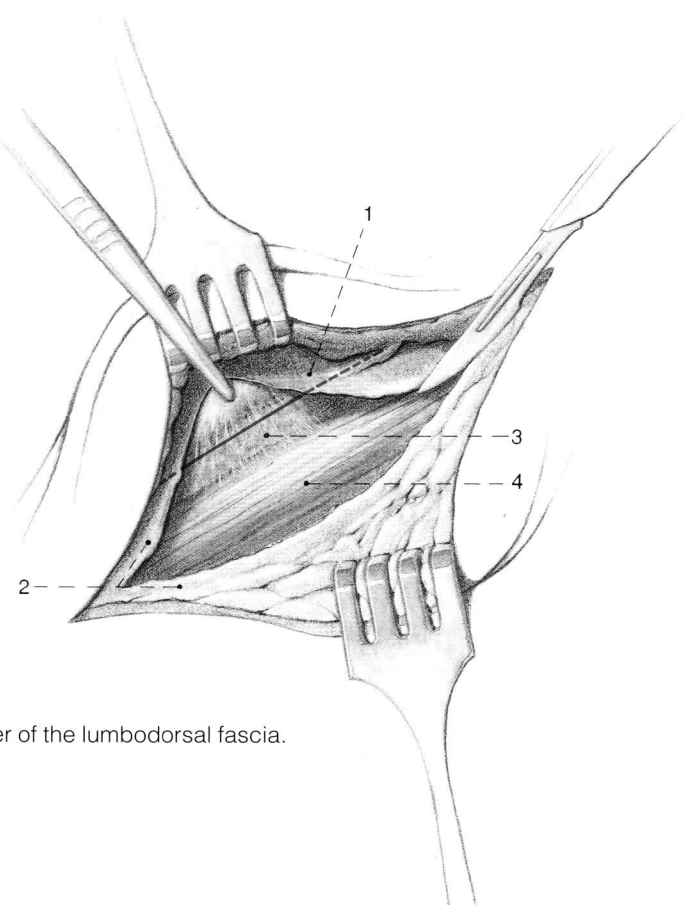

Fig. 2.**46** Exposure of the deep layer of the lumbodorsal fascia.

1 Latissimus dorsi
2 Lumbodorsal fascia, superficial layer
3 Lumbodorsal fascia, deep layer
4 Erector spinae

Incision of the Deep Layer of the Lumbodorsal Fascia

The line of incision in the deep layer of the lumbodorsal fascia is shown in Fig. 2.**46**. The incision is carried over the quadratus lumborum muscle to the iliac crest, sparing the iliohypogastric and ilioinguinal nerves coursing on the muscle (Fig. 2.**47**). The dissection is continued bluntly upward along the erector spinae to the 12th rib, dividing the lumbocostal ligament (Henle) in the upper corner of the wound (Fig. 2. **50**).

Exposure and Incision of Gerota's Fascia

The quadratus lumborum is retracted posteriorly with a blunt retractor. After meticulous transection of the deep layer of the lumbodorsal fascia, Gerota's fascia is opened giving access for dissection of the lower part of the kidney, the renal pelvis, and the ureter (Fig. 2.**48**).

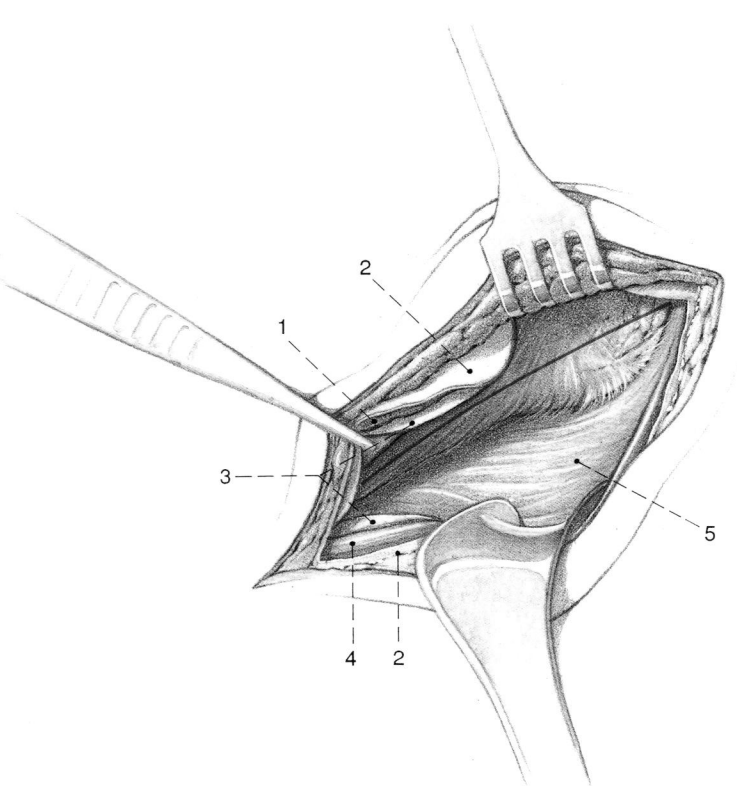
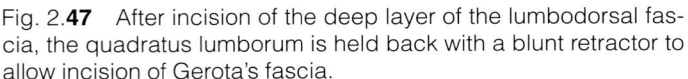

Fig. 2.**47**   After incision of the deep layer of the lumbodorsal fascia, the quadratus lumborum is held back with a blunt retractor to allow incision of Gerota's fascia.

1 Latissimus dorsi
2 Lumbodorsal fascia, superficial layer
3 Lumbodorsal fascia, deep layer
4 Erector spinae
5 Quadratus lumborum

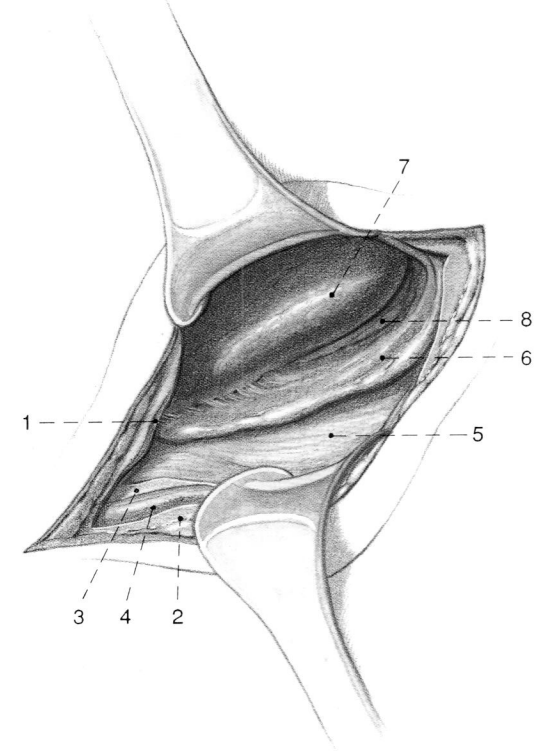

Fig. 2.**48**   Status following incision of Gerota's fascia.

1 Latissimus dorsi
2 Lumbodorsal fascia, superficial layer
3 Lumbodorsal fascia, deep layer
4 Erector spinae
5 Quadratus lumborum
6 Perirenal fat capsule
7 Lower pole of kidney
8 Ureter

Fig. 2.**50**   A dissection showing the deep layer of the lumbodorsal fascia and lumbocostal ligament. ▶

1 Latissimus dorsi
2 Lumbodorsal fascia, deep layer
3 Quadratus lumborum
4 Iliocostalis lumborum
5 External oblique muscle
6 Intercostal muscles
7 Lumbocostal ligament
8 12th rib
9 11th rib
10 Iliac crest

Comments

Figure 2.**49** shows this transfascial approach to the right kidney in a transverse section at the level of the second lumbar vertebra. The approach passes through the superficial and then the deep layer of the lumbodorsal fascia with minimal transection of muscle groups. Gerota's fascia can be opened after retraction of the quadratus lumborum.

This approach relies on an accurate dissection and incision of the deep layer of the lumbodorsal fascia, which is illustrated in a dissection of the right lumbar region (Fig. 2.**50**). The latissimus dorsi has been mobilized, and the deep layer of the lumbodorsal fascia and the external oblique and quadratus lumborum muscles are shown. The lumbocostal ligament is also visible as a continuation of the deep layer of the lumbodorsal fascia. If sufficient exposure is not obtained with this approach, a 1-cm-wide segment of the 11th and 12th ribs can be resected in continuity with the incision in the lumbocostal ligament.

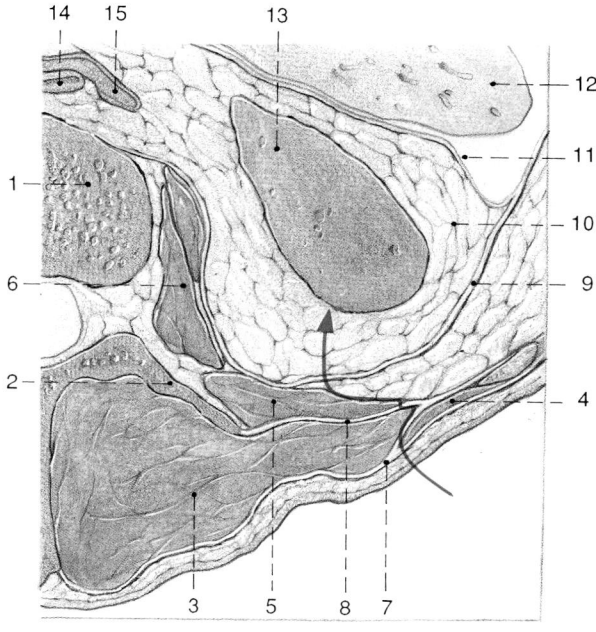

Fig. 2.**49** Schematic representation of the transfascial route of approach in a posterior lumbotomy (transverse section at the level of the second lumbar vertebra).

1 Body of second lumbar vertebra
2 Costal process of second lumbar vertebra
3 Erector spinae
4 Latissimus dorsi
5 Quadratus lumborum
6 Psoas major
7 Lumbodorsal fascia, superficial layer
8 Lumbodorsal fascia, deep layer
9 Gerota's fascia
10 Perirenal fat capsule
11 Parietal peritoneum
12 Liver
13 Right kidney
14 Renal artery
15 Renal vein

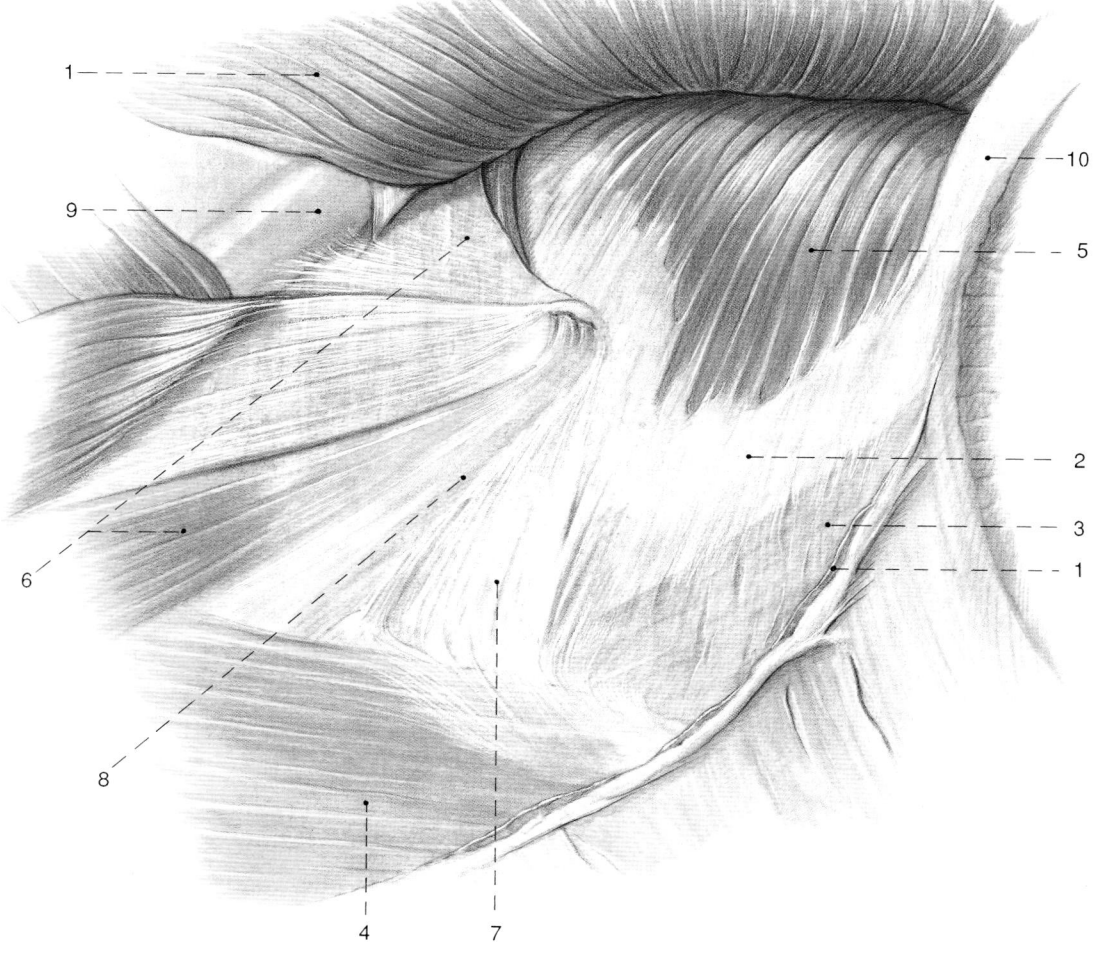

Dorsolumbar (Nagamatsu) Approach

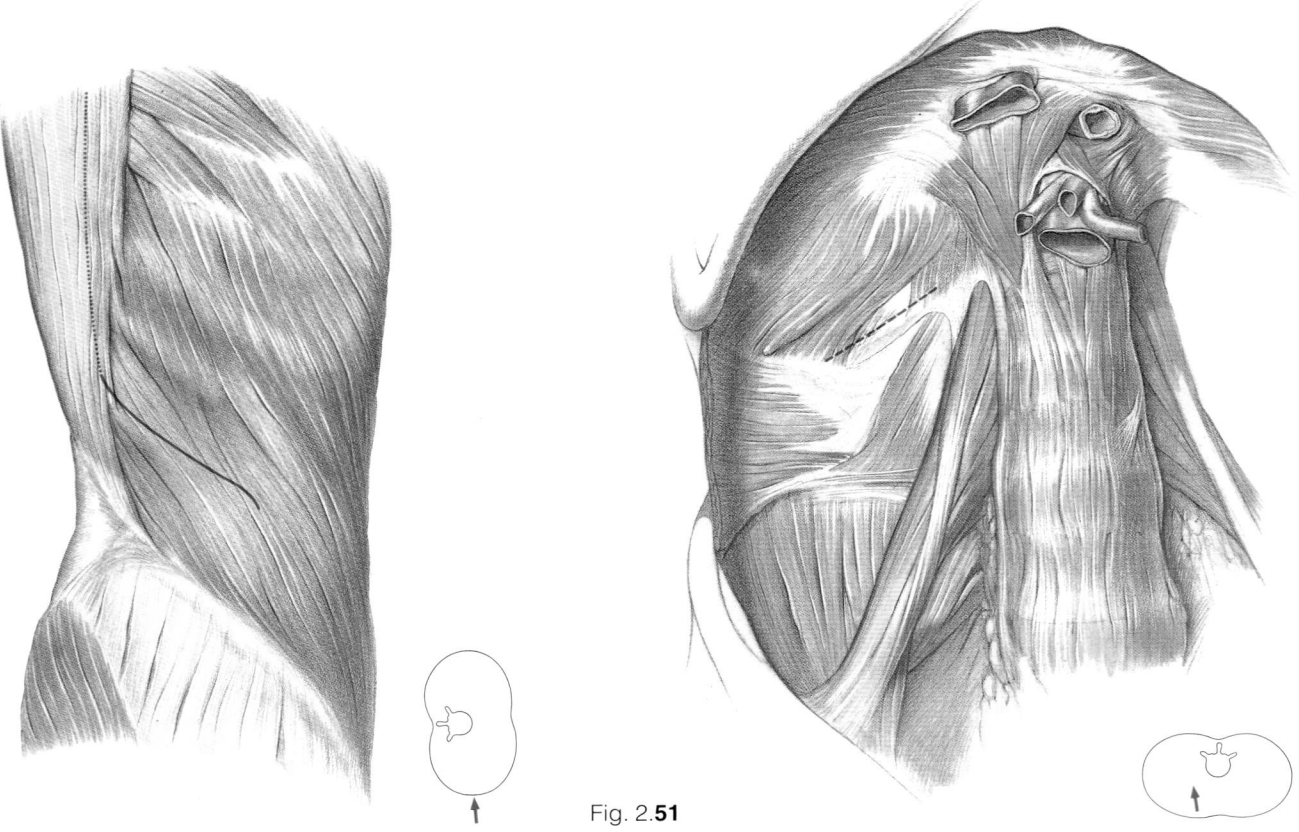

Fig. 2.**51**

Main Indications

● Procedures on the renal parenchyma
● Procedures on the adrenal gland

This posterior extraperitoneal approach, while rendering broad exposure of the retroperitoneal space, is not an acceptable alternative to the thoracoabdominal approach.

The approach can be extended anteriorly in the fashion of a subcostal incision at the 12th rib.

The technique is illustrated for the left side. Both the intercostal and subcostal variants will be described.

Position and Skin Incision

The operation is performed in right lateral position with the table tilted forward about 15° and flexed about 30° at the lumbar level to hyperextend the operative area (Fig. 2.**52**). The ipsilateral arm is raised toward the head, as in all intercostal approaches.

The skin incision starts in the ninth intercostal space and runs along the erector spinae muscle in the paravertebral line. In the intercostal approach, the incision is carried between the 11th and 12th ribs; in the subcostal approach, the incision runs forward below the border of the 12th rib. It is carried in an S-shaped curve toward the lateral border of the rectus muscle (Fig. 2.**52**).

The subcutaneous tissue is divided to expose the latissimus dorsi and external oblique muscles. Exposure is maintained by retractors (Fig. 2.**53**).

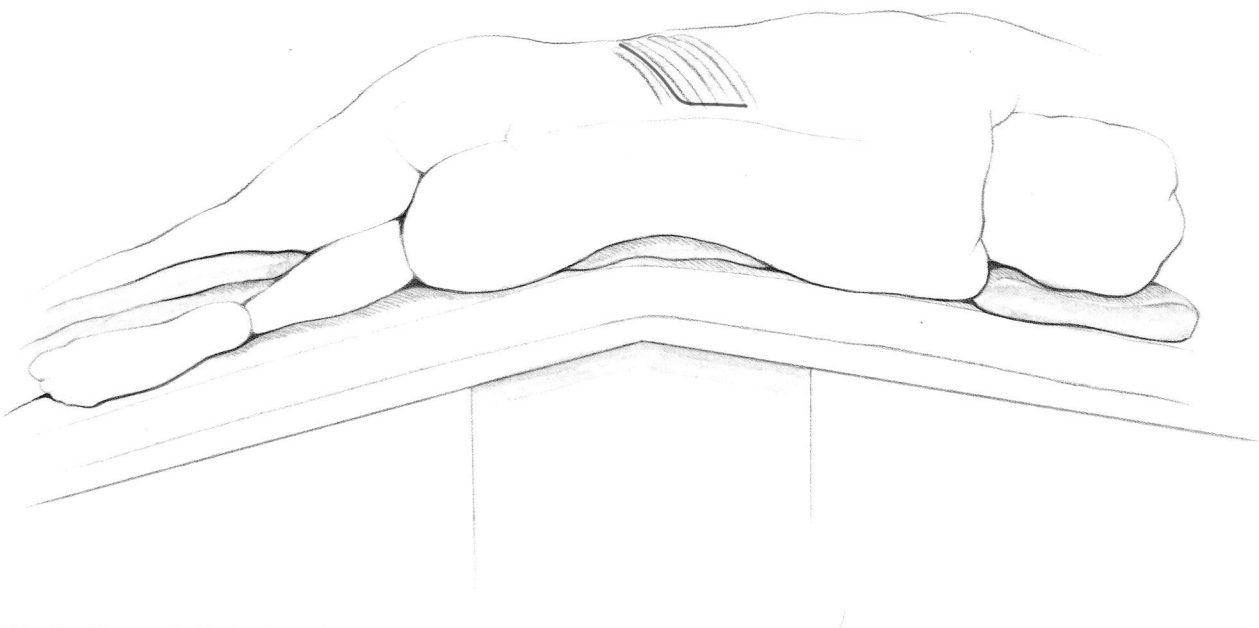

Fig. 2.**52**   Position and skin incision (intercostal route).

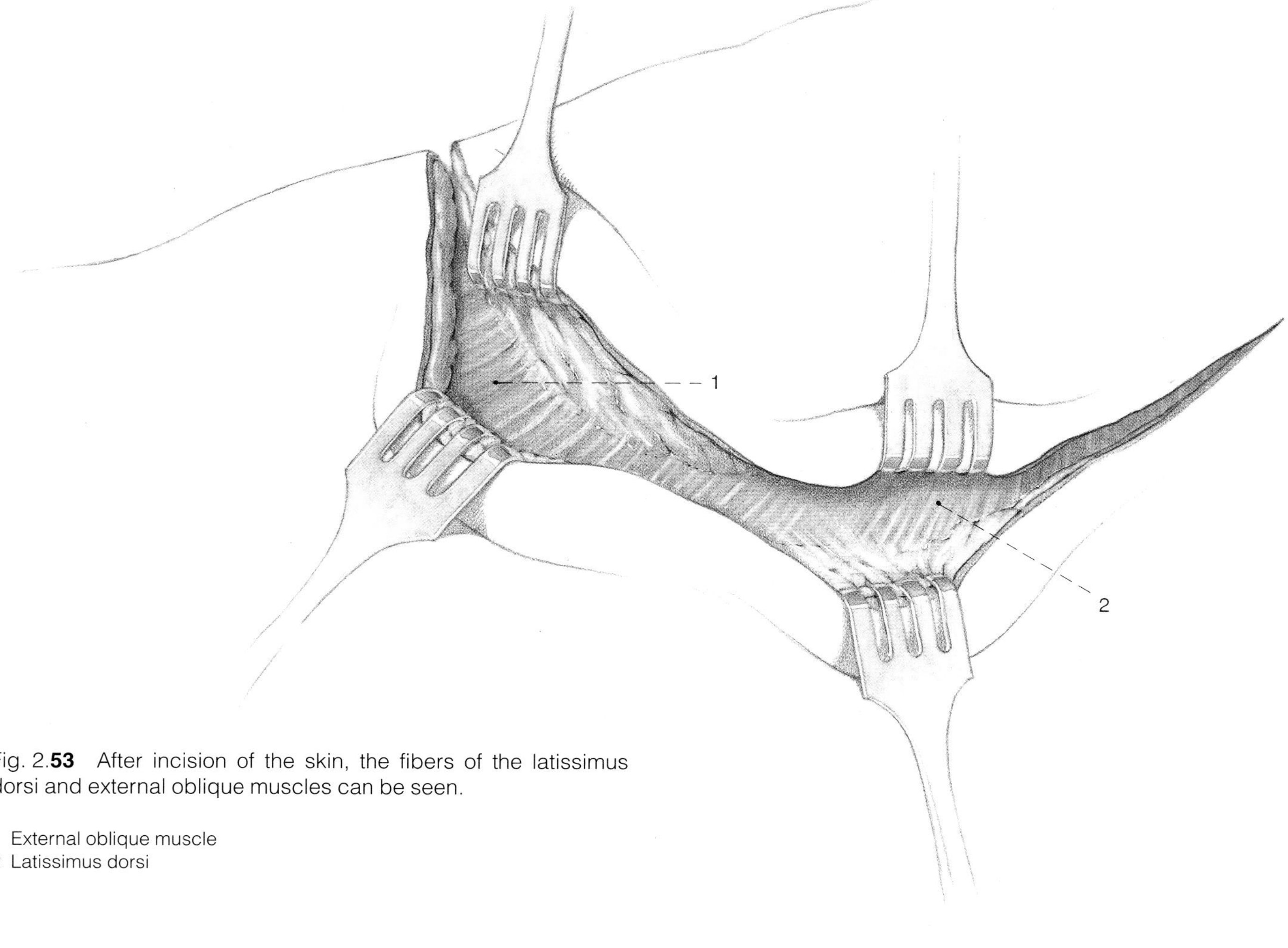

Fig. 2.**53**   After incision of the skin, the fibers of the latissimus dorsi and external oblique muscles can be seen.

1 External oblique muscle
2 Latissimus dorsi

Exposure of the Deep Layer of the Lumbodorsal Fascia

The latissimus dorsi and serratus posterior inferior are transected with diathermy over the 10th, 11th, and 12th ribs. Below the 12th rib, the external and internal oblique muscles are divided with the cautery. Individual bleeding vessels are coagulated at once. The intercostal vessels and nerves at the inferior border of the rib are preserved. The transected latissimus dorsi, serratus posterior inferior, and external and internal oblique muscles are retracted, and the deep layer of the lumbodorsal fascia is dissected (Fig. 2.**54**). The transversus abdominis muscle and lumbodorsal fascia are incised in the direction of their fibers (see incision line in Fig. 2.**54**).

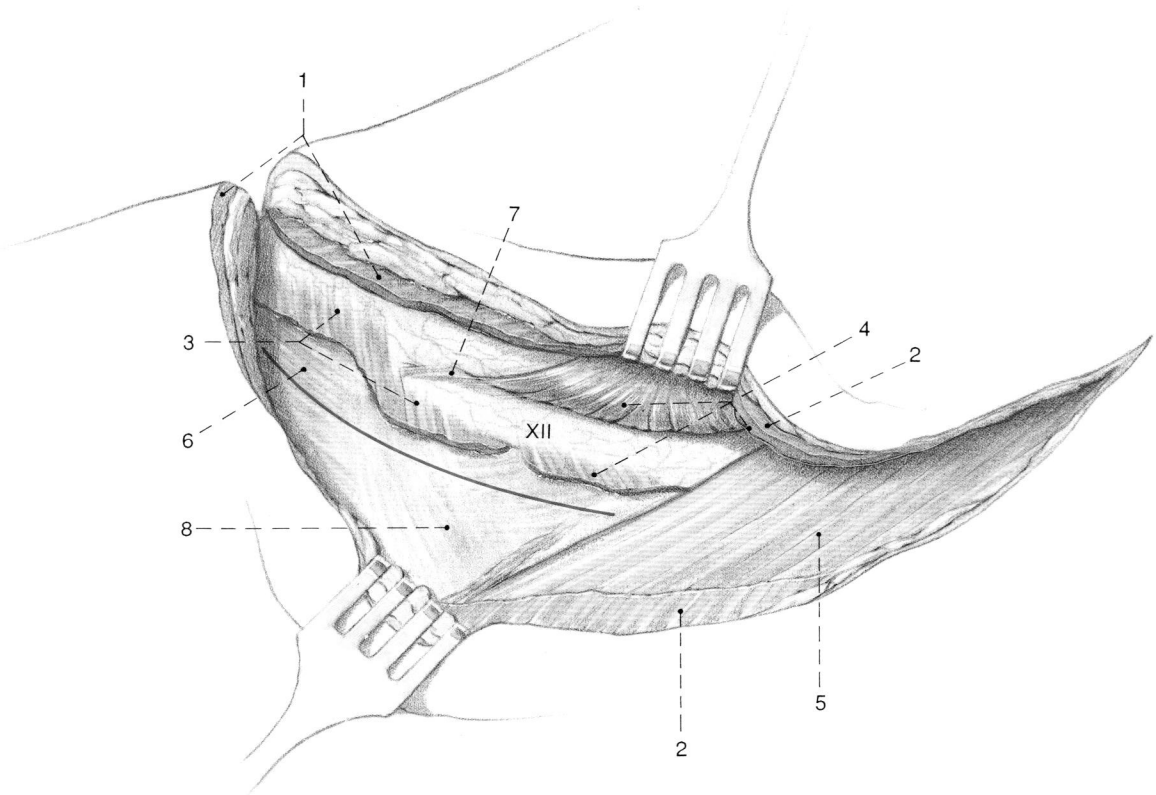

Fig. 2.**54**   Dissection of the deep layer of the lumbodorsal fascia.

1 External oblique muscle
2 Latissimus dorsi
3 Internal oblique muscle
4 Serratus posterior inferior
5 Erector spinae
6 Transversus abdominis
7 External intercostal muscle
8 Lumbodorsal fascia, deep layer
XII 12th rib

Division of the Lumbocostal Ligament and Resection of Parts of the 11th and 12th Ribs

The lumbocostal ligament is divided, carrying the incision upward and parallel to the erector spinae muscle. The upper and lower margins of the deep layer of the lumbodorsal fascia are controlled with stay sutures (Fig. 2.**55**). The periosteum of the 11th and 12th ribs is incised. It is first separated from the rib with a straight periosteal elevator, and isolation of the rib is completed with a curved rib stripper (Fig. 2.**55**). Segments 2 cm long are then resected from the 11th and 12th ribs.

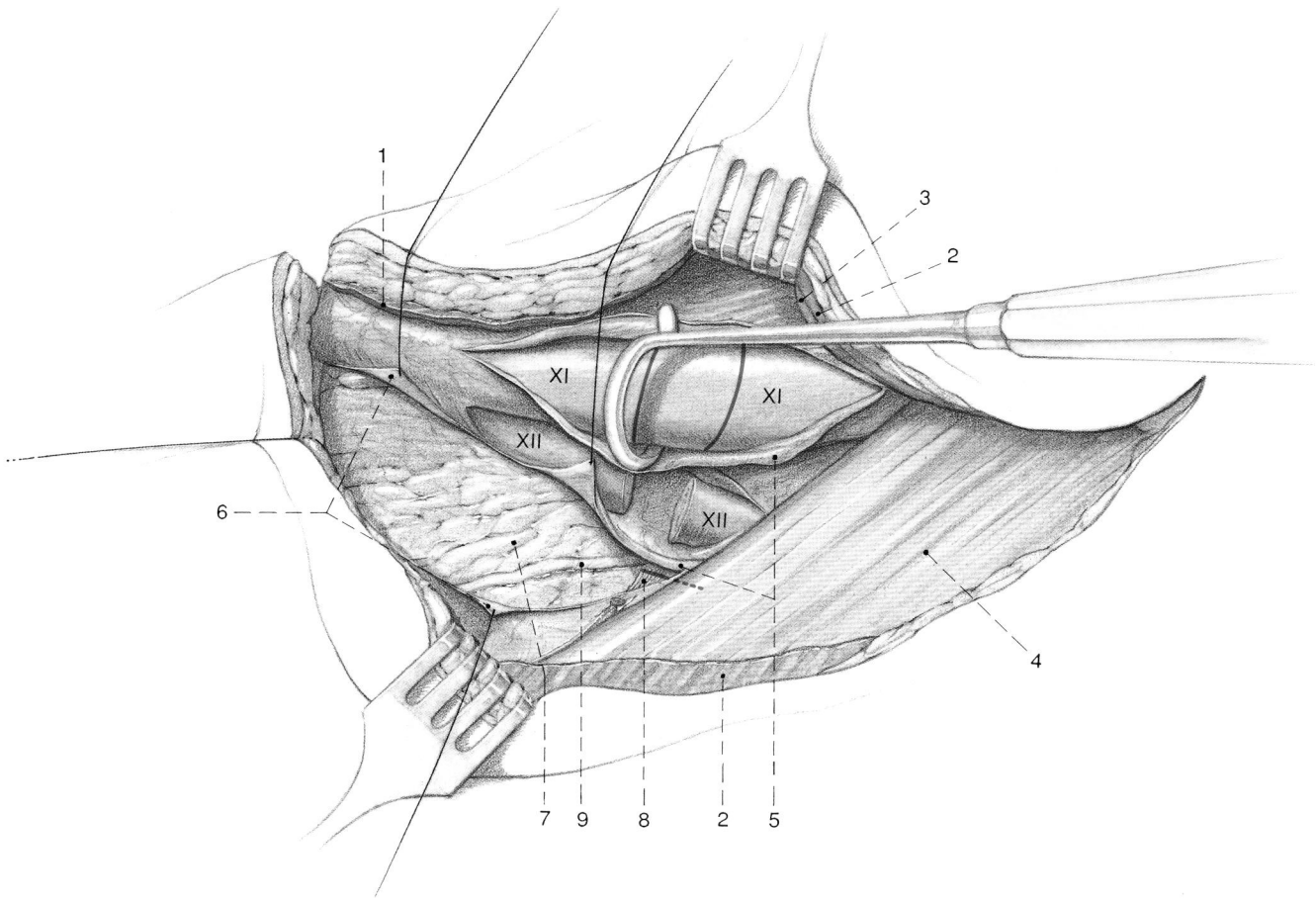

Fig. 2.**55**   The lumbocostal ligament is incised, and portions of the 11th and 12th rib are resected.

1 External oblique muscle
2 Latissimus dorsi
3 Serratus posterior inferior
4 Erector spinae
5 Periosteum
6 Lumbodorsal fascia
7 Pararenal fat
8 Lumbocostal ligament (Henle)
XI 11th rib
XII 12th rib

Separation of the Deep Lumbodorsal Fascia and Diaphragm from the Rib Periosteum

As in the supracostal approach, the deep layer of the lumbodorsal fascia is used to assist in freeing up the pleura and diaphragm (Fig. 2.**56**). The quadratus lumborum and psoas major muscles can be identified in the retroperitoneal space (Fig. 2.**56**).

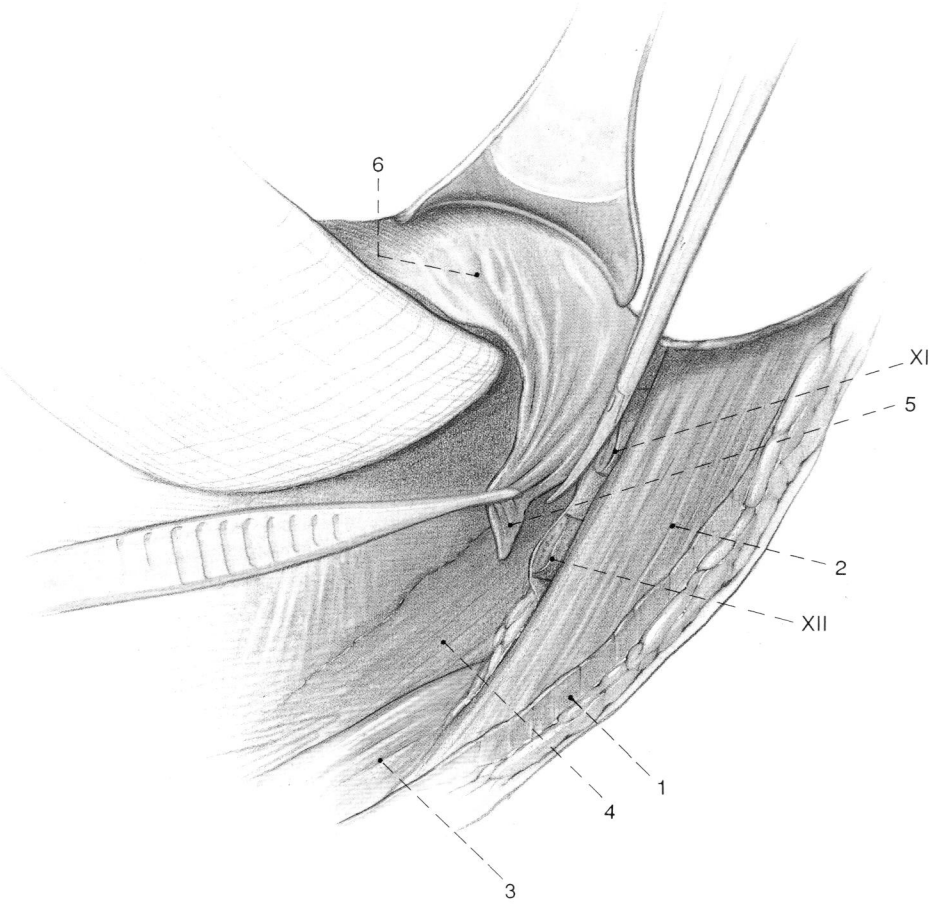

Fig. 2.**56**   Extrapleural entry into the thoracic cavity.

1 Latissimus dorsi
2 Erector spinae
3 Quadratus lumborum
4 Psoas major
5 Diaphragm
6 Parietal pleura
XI 11th rib
XII 12th rib

Incision of Gerota's Fascia

After the pararenal fat has been dissected from the lumbodorsal fascia, Gerota's fascia is grasped with two forceps and incised. The fat capsule is exposed, and a plane of cleavage is developed to expose the kidney (Fig. 2.**57**). A self-retaining retractor can be inserted at this stage in place of the manual retractors shown in the figure.

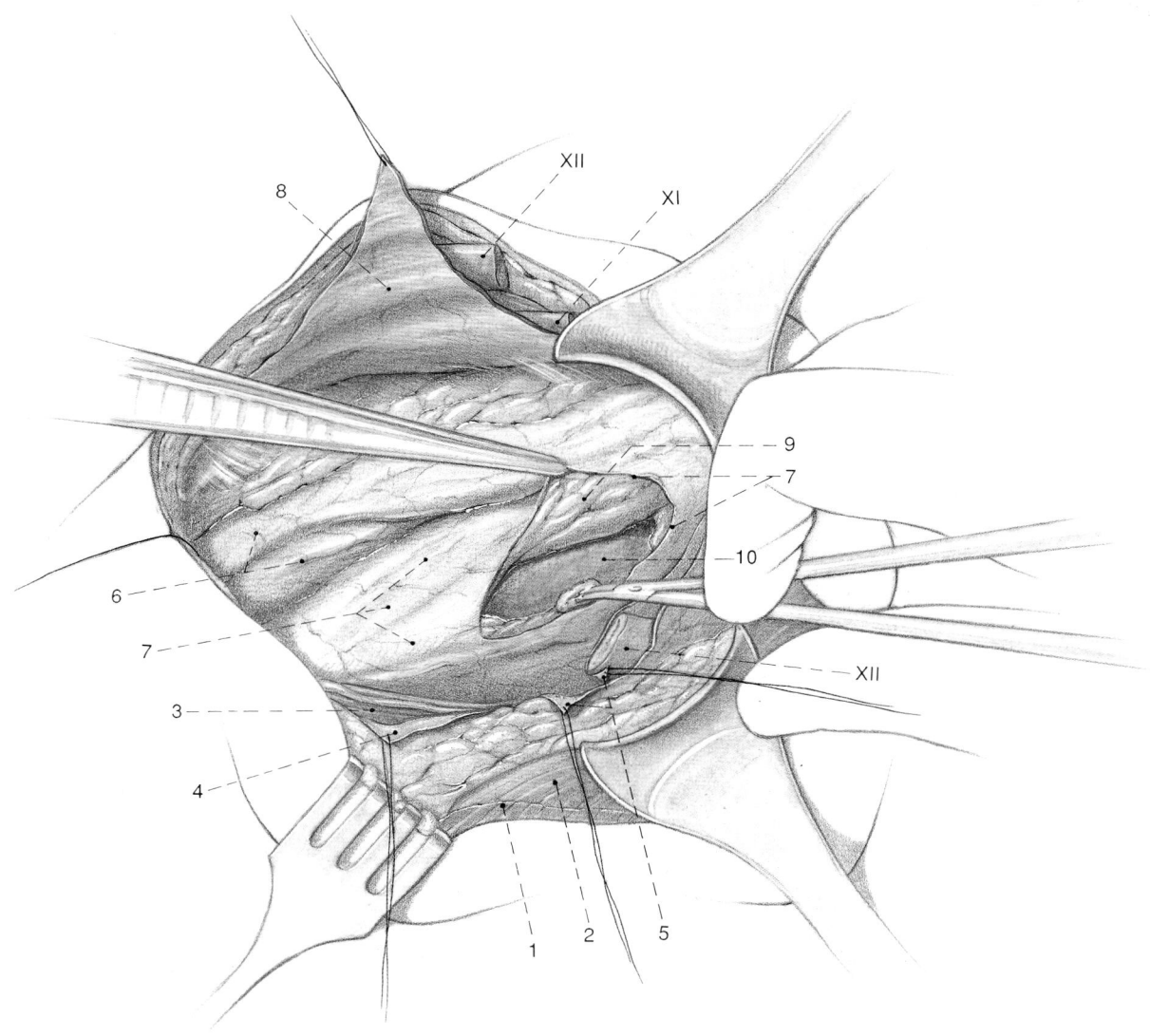

Fig. 2.**57**   Incision of Gerota's fascia.

 1 Latissimus dorsi
 2 Erector spinae
 3 Quadratus lumborum
 4 Lumbodorsal fascia, deep layer
 5 Lumbocostal ligament (of Henle)
 6 Transversalis fascia and parietal peritoneum
 7 Gerota's fascia
 8 Diaphragm
 9 Pararenal fat
10 Kidney
XI 11th rib
XII 12th rib

Further dissection exposes the kidney and the adrenal gland in the retroperitoneal space. The peritoneum and descending colon are held aside with a Deaver retractor. The renal artery and vein and the inferior suprarenal arteries are snared with tapes (Fig. 2.**58**).

Comments

The Nagamatsu approach provides broad access to the retroperitoneal space. Use of this approach requires considerable experience, however. Rib resection with preservation of the underlying periosteum and meticulous dissection of the lumbodorsal fascia and diaphragm are essential for avoiding injury to the pleural cavity.

This approach can be used for operations on the renal parenchyma and for the removal of adrenal tumors.

The approach requires clear identification of the deep layer of the lumbodorsal fascia and the lumbocostal ligament.

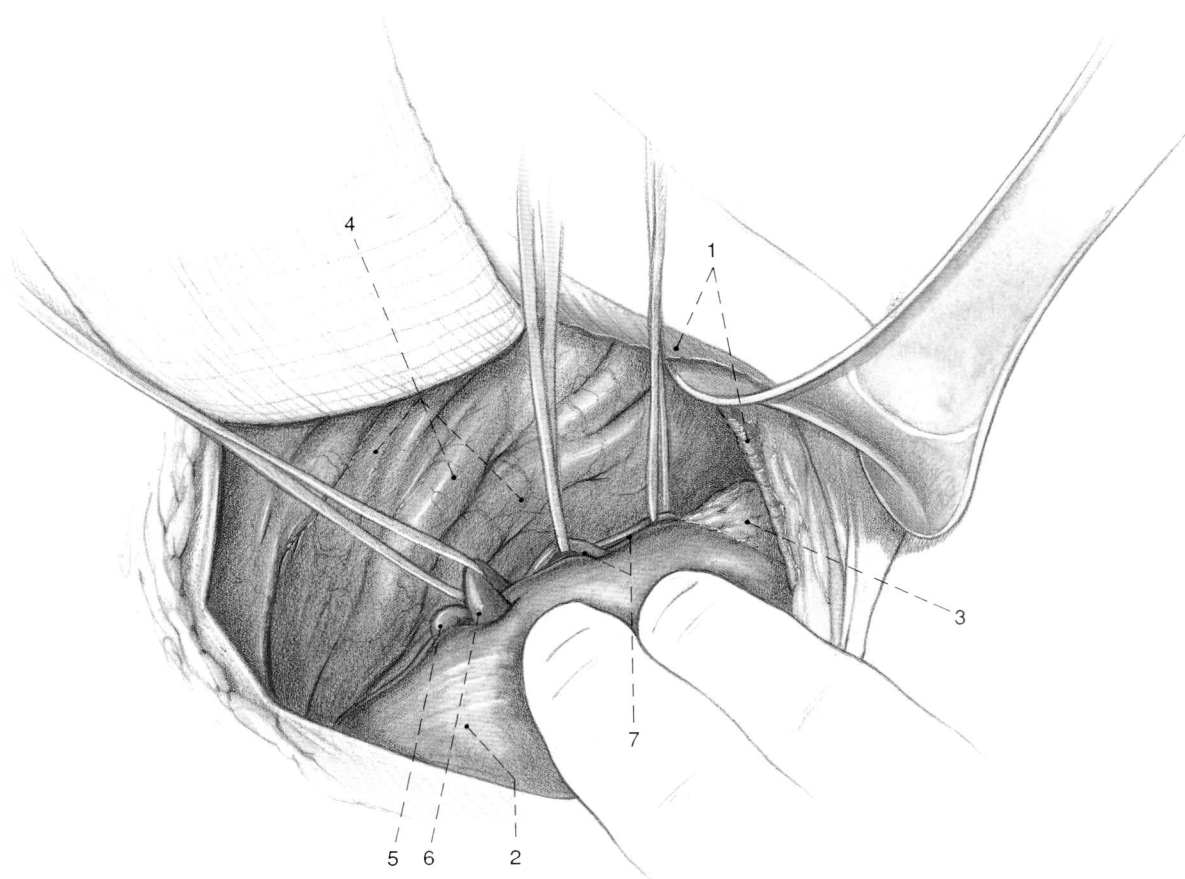

Fig. 2.**58** Exposure of the renal artery and vein. The left adrenal gland is visible in the retroperitoneal space.

1 Diaphragm
2 Kidney
3 Adrenal gland
4 Descending colon
5 Renal artery
6 Renal vein
7 Inferior suprarenal vessels

Posterior Approach to the Adrenal Gland

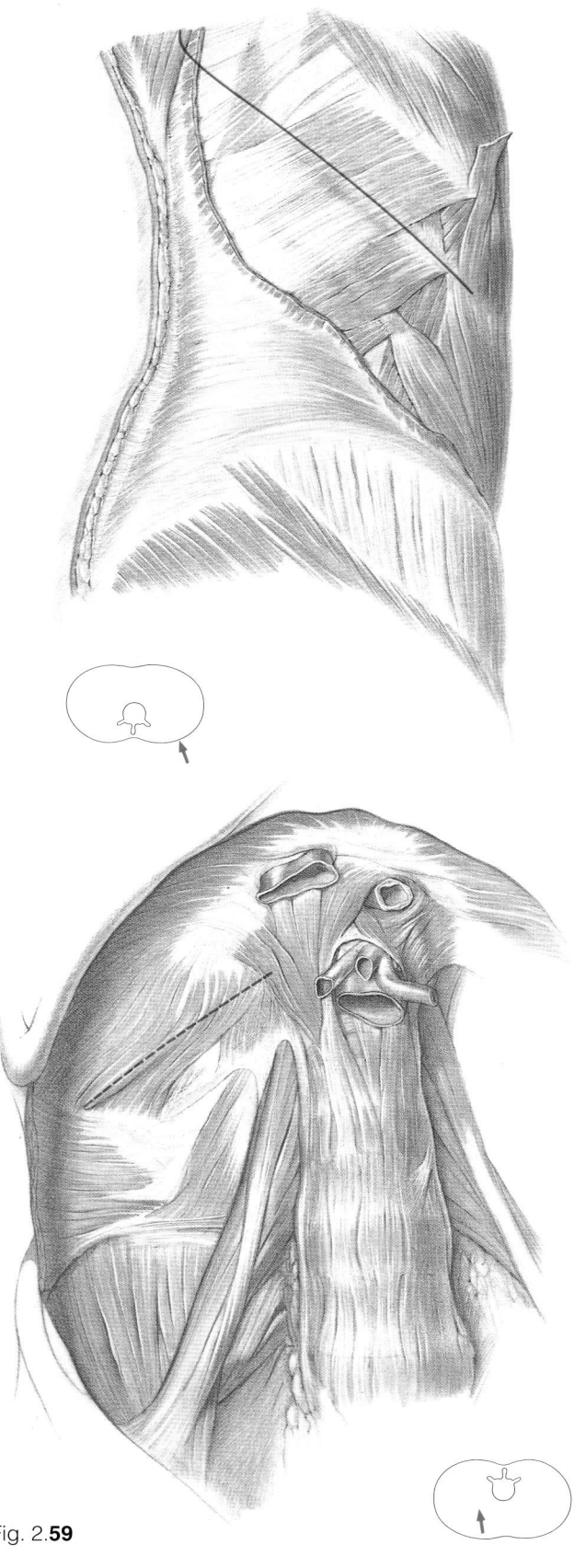

Fig. 2.**59**

Main Indications

The posterior approach is best suited for small, benign, well-localized lesions of the adrenal gland. It ensures minimal morbidity.

The techique is illustrated for the right adrenal gland.

Position and Skin Incision

The operation is performed in the prone position with the pelvis and shoulders elevated to lower the central portion of the abdominal wall. The operating table is flexed 35° at the lumbar level (Fig. 2.**60**).

The skin incision starts next to the vertebral column at the level of the 12th thoracic vertebra and extends laterally forward to a point two fingerwidths past the tip of the 11th rib (Fig. 2.**60**).

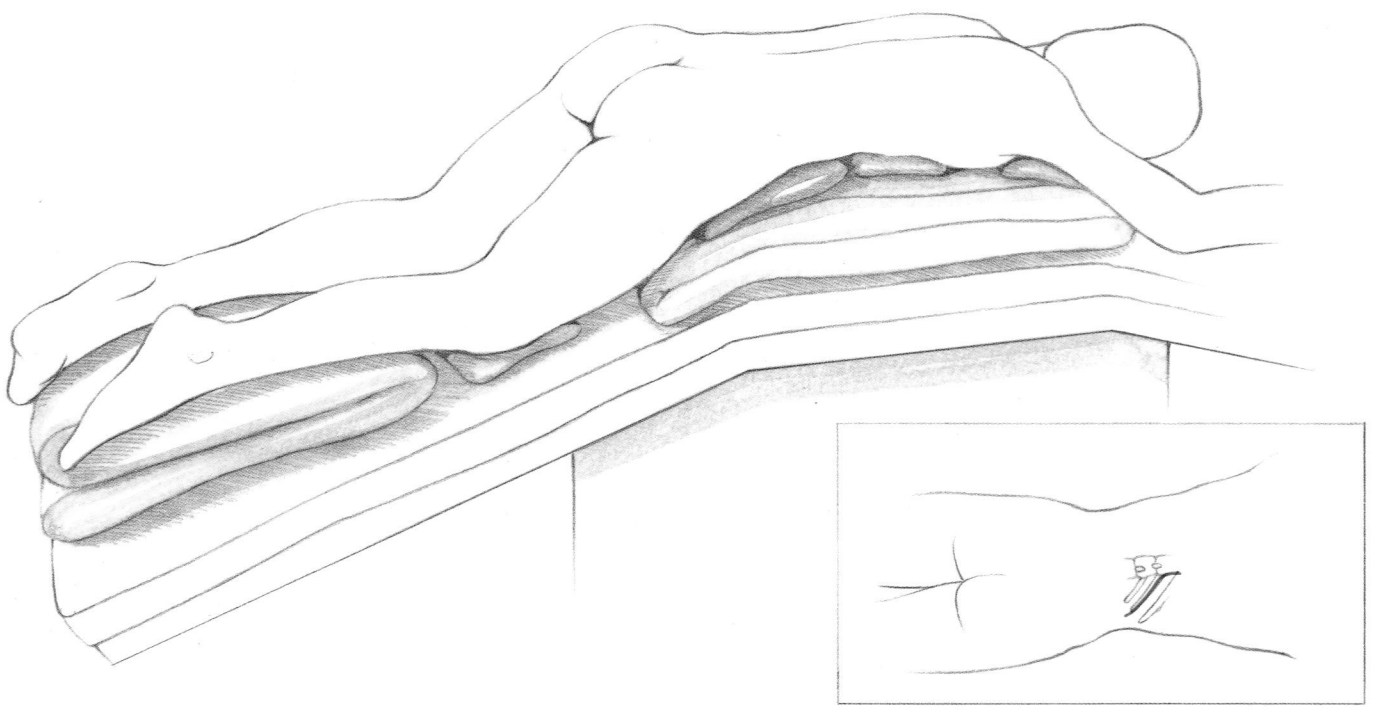

Fig. 2.**60**   Position and skin incision for the posterior approach to the adrenal gland.

Exposure and Resection of the 11th Rib

The subcutaneous fat is divided, and the thoracic fascia is exposed. The latissimus dorsi and serratus anterior muscles are identified (Fig. 2.**61**). Exposure is maintained with two retractors. The latissimus dorsi and serratus anterior are transected with a scalpel. The erector spinae muscle can be seen in the medial portion of the wound (Fig. 2.**62**).

The periosteum of the 11th rib is divided with diathermy, and the rib is progressively isolated with a straight periosteal elevator and a curved stripper. The 11th rib is resected as far medially as possible (Fig. 2.**63**).

Fig. 2.**61**   Incision of latissimus dorsi and serratus anterior.

1 Latissimus dorsi
2 Serratus anterior

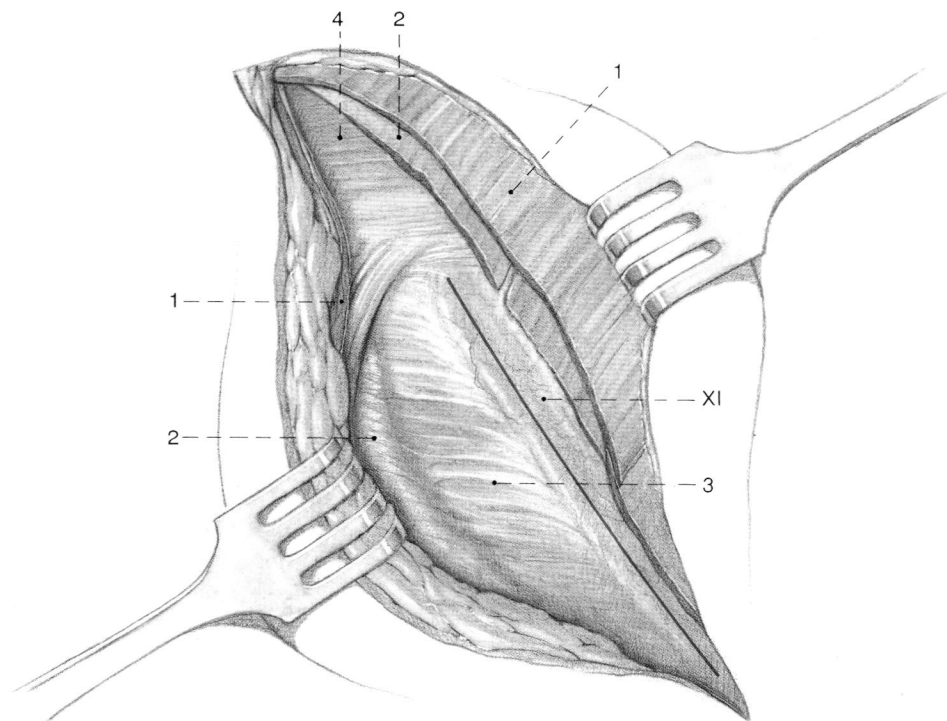

Fig. 2.**62** Exposure of the 11th rib. The transected muscles are
retracted.

1 Latissimus dorsi
2 Serratus anterior
3 External intercostal muscle
4 Erector spinae
XI 11th rib

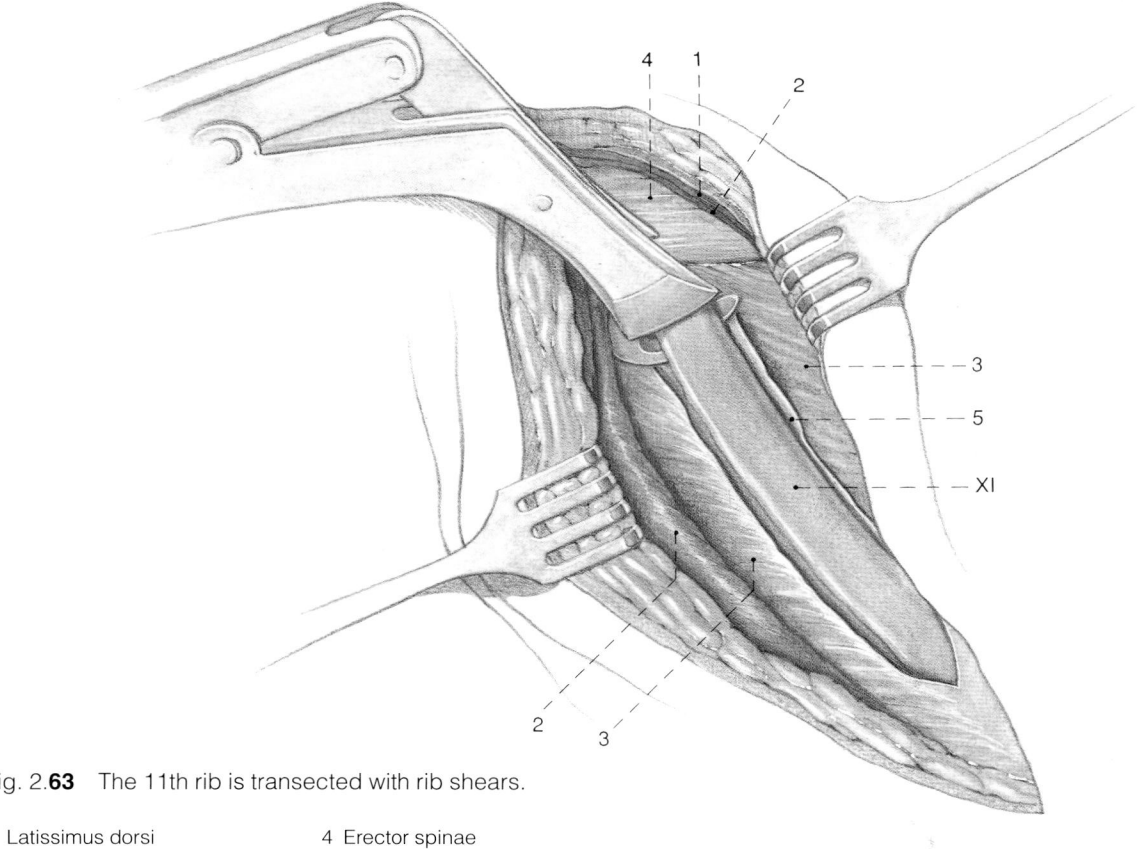

Fig. 2.**63** The 11th rib is transected with rib shears.

1 Latissimus dorsi   4 Erector spinae
2 Serratus anterior   5 Periosteum
3 External intercostal muscle   XI 11th rib

Incision of the Rib Bed

The posterior rib bed is opened with a scissors, exposing the diaphragm (Fig. 2.**64**). Care is taken to preserve the intercostal neurovascular bundle during incision of the rib bed.

Now, with the aid of a wooden tissue protector or small sponge stick, the diaphragm is carefully divided with diathermy. The plane between the diaphragm and Gerota's fascia is carefully developed, and the diaphragm is incised anteriorly and posteriorly to establish entry into the retroperitoneal space. Gerota's fascia is identified (Fig. 2.**65**).

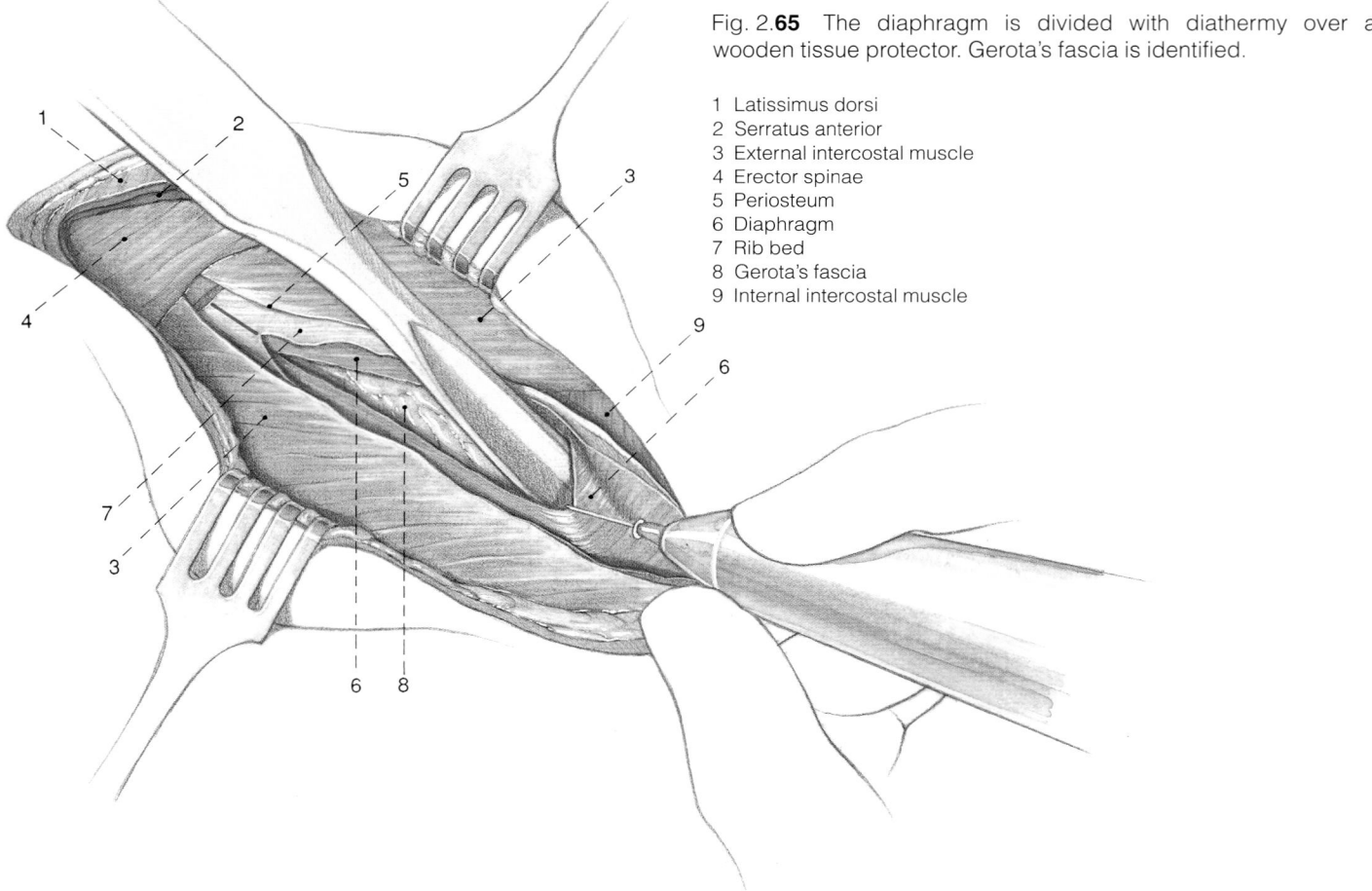

Fig. 2.**64**   The posterior rib bed is incised with scissors, exposing the diaphragm.

1   External intercostal muscle
2   Periosteum
3   Rib bed
4   Diaphragm

Fig. 2.**65**   The diaphragm is divided with diathermy over a wooden tissue protector. Gerota's fascia is identified.

1   Latissimus dorsi
2   Serratus anterior
3   External intercostal muscle
4   Erector spinae
5   Periosteum
6   Diaphragm
7   Rib bed
8   Gerota's fascia
9   Internal intercostal muscle

Exposure of the Adrenal Gland

A self-retaining retractor is inserted into the operative field over two lap packs (Fig. 2.**66**). Gerota's fascia is opened transversely, exposing the upper pole and the posterior surface of the kidney. The kidney is displaced downward, and the adrenal gland is exposed by dissection of the perirenal fat. The suprarenal vein is snared with a vascular tape (Fig. 2.**66**).

Comments

This approach is suitable for small, benign, localized tumors of the adrenal gland. It can be performed on both sides in one sitting. It is not satisfactory for the removal of large or malignant adrenal tumors with accessory vessels, which would necessitate the anterior abdominal or thoracoabdominal approach. Each of these approaches respects the vascular supply and provides better exposure of the retroperitoneal space.

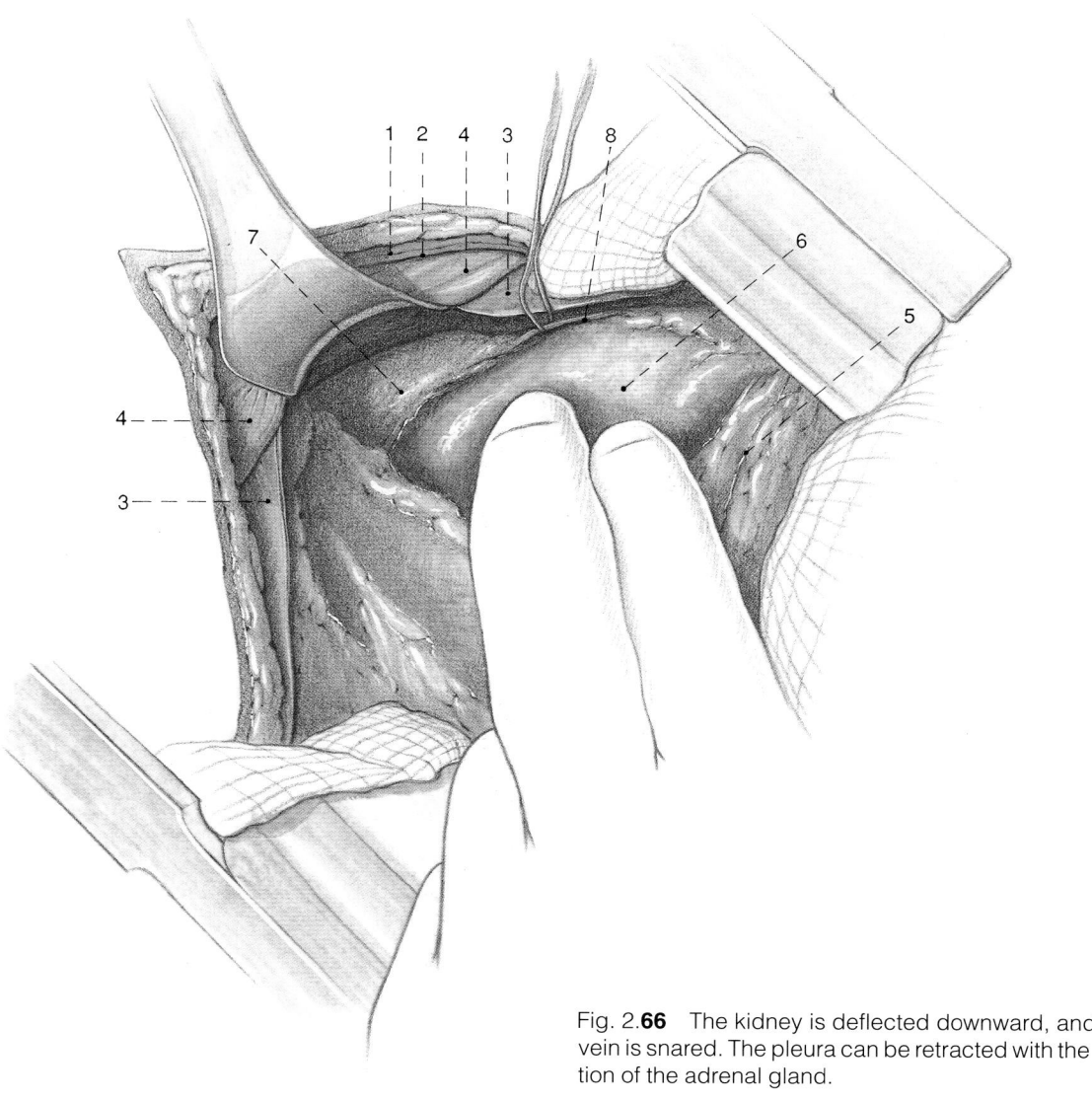

Fig. 2.**66** The kidney is deflected downward, and the suprarenal vein is snared. The pleura can be retracted with the lung for dissection of the adrenal gland.

1 Latissimus dorsi
2 Serratus anterior
3 External intercostal muscle
4 Erector spinae
5 Gerota's fascia
6 Right kidney
7 Right adrenal gland
8 Suprarenal vein

Thoracoabdominal Approach

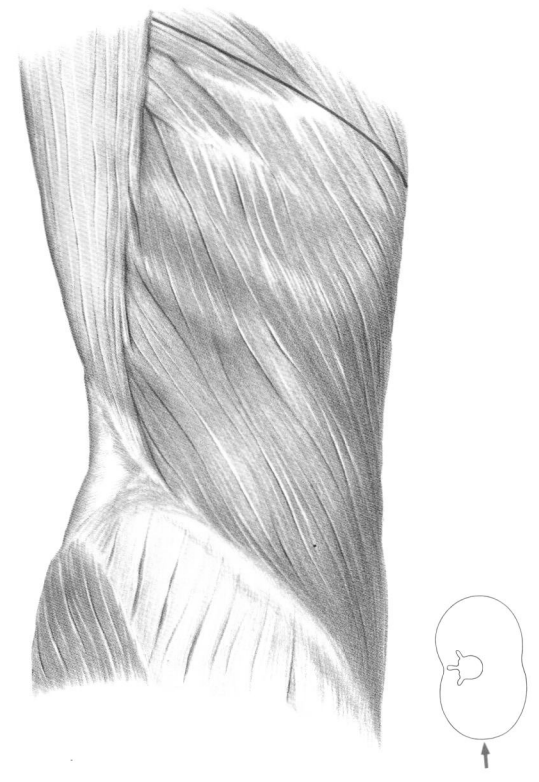

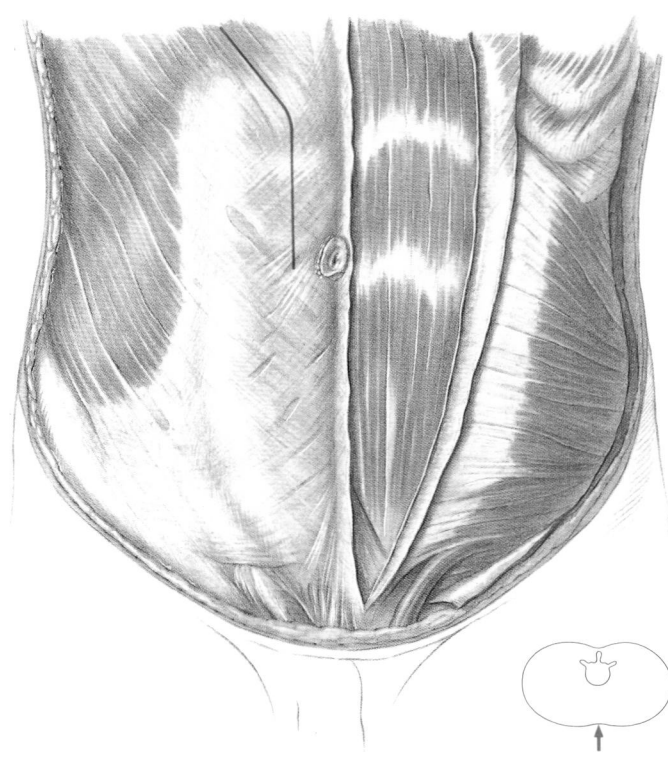

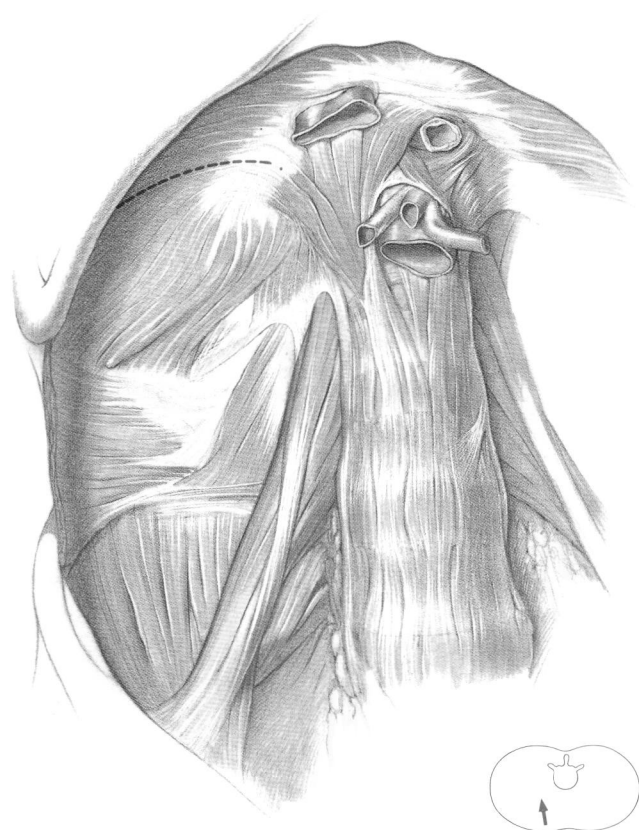

Main Indications

- Renal tumors
- Adrenal tumors
- Tumor thrombus in the vena cava
- Retroperitoneal lymph node dissection

This approach provides excellent exposure of the entire abdominal and retroperitoneal space. Since the intrathoracic portion of the inferior vena cava can also be exposed, this approach is useful for the removal of stage II and stage III tumor thrombi involving the vena cava. A modification, the primary thoracoretroperitoneal approach, is useful for lymph node dissection in patients with testicular tumors.

The technique is illustrated for the right side.

Fig. 2.**67**

Position and Skin Incision

The patient is positioned on the left side with the chest rotated about 30°40° forward at the shoulder level. The ipsilateral arm is supported above the thorax on a rest (Fig. 2.**68**). The pelvis is rotated only about 10° forward from the horizontal. The ipsilateral leg is extended, and the contralateral leg is flexed 90° at the knee. The operating table is flexed at the lumbar level to hyperextend the operative area. The costal arch forms the highest point of the operating field (Fig. 2.**68**).

In the typical seventh intercostal space approach, the skin incision is begun in the anterior axillary line and is carried down across the costal arch to the level of the umbilicus.

The subcutaneous fat is divided while individual bleeding vessels are coagulated. The fascial planes of the latissimus dorsi, serratus anterior, and external oblique are transected. The central part of the anterior rectus sheath is incised in the abdominal portion of the field (Fig. 2.**69**).

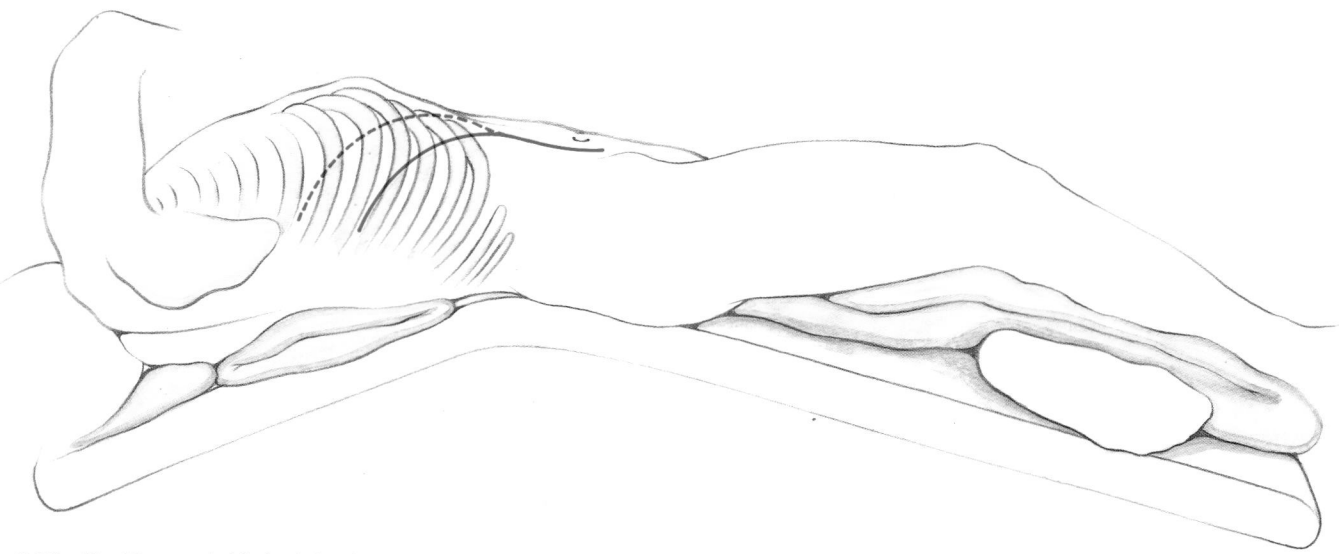

Fig. 2.**68**   Position and skin incision for the thoracoabdominal approach.

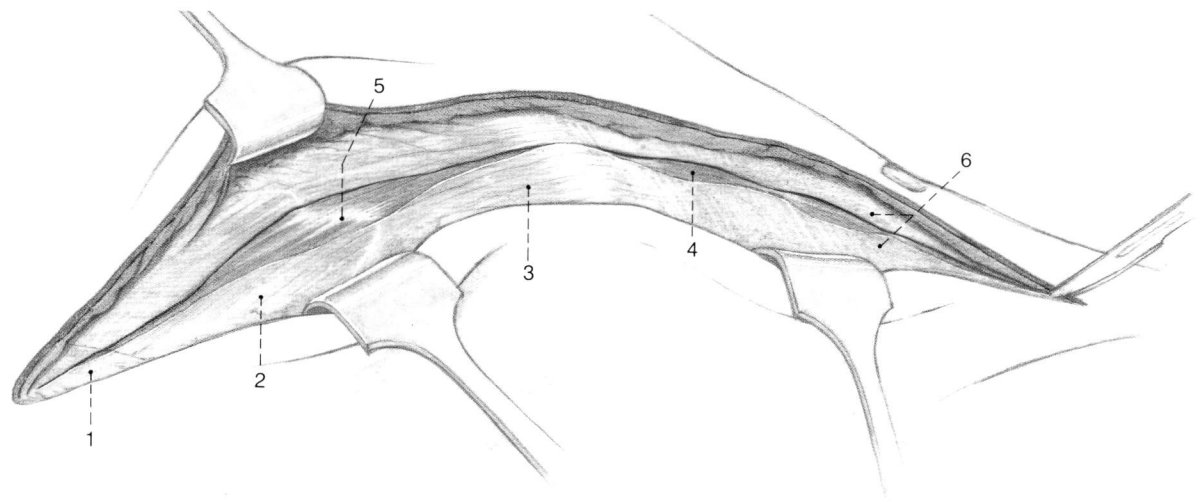

Fig. 2.**69**   The fasciae of latissimus dorsi, serratus anterior, and external oblique are divided in line with the skin incision.

1 Latissimus dorsi
2 Serratus anterior
3 External oblique muscle
4 Rectus muscle
5 Tendinous intersection
6 Anterior rectus sheath

Laparotomy and Thoracotomy

Starting at the anterior axillary line, the latissimus dorsi, serratus anterior, and external oblique muscles are transected with diathermy in line with the skin incision (Figs. 2.**70**, 2.**71**). The external and intercostal muscles are visible on the chest wall. Starting at the costal arch, the incision is first extended inferomedially, dividing the fibers of the rectus muscle in the epigastrium. The rectus abdominis is then bluntly freed laterally while sparing the nerves and vessels; this technique avoids denervation of the rectus musculature. The superior epigastric vessels are ligated. The rectus muscle is retracted laterally to expose the posterior layer of the rectus sheath. Small retractors maintain exposure in both the abdominal and thoracic portions of the field (Fig. 2.**71**).

In the abdominal part of the incision, the posterior rectus sheath is picked up with forceps on both sides along with the transversus abdominis fibers and peritoneum, and all three layers are transected to establish entry into the peritoneal cavity. The greater omentum can be identified. The abdominal cavity is opened to the level of the umbilicus (Fig. 2.**72**).

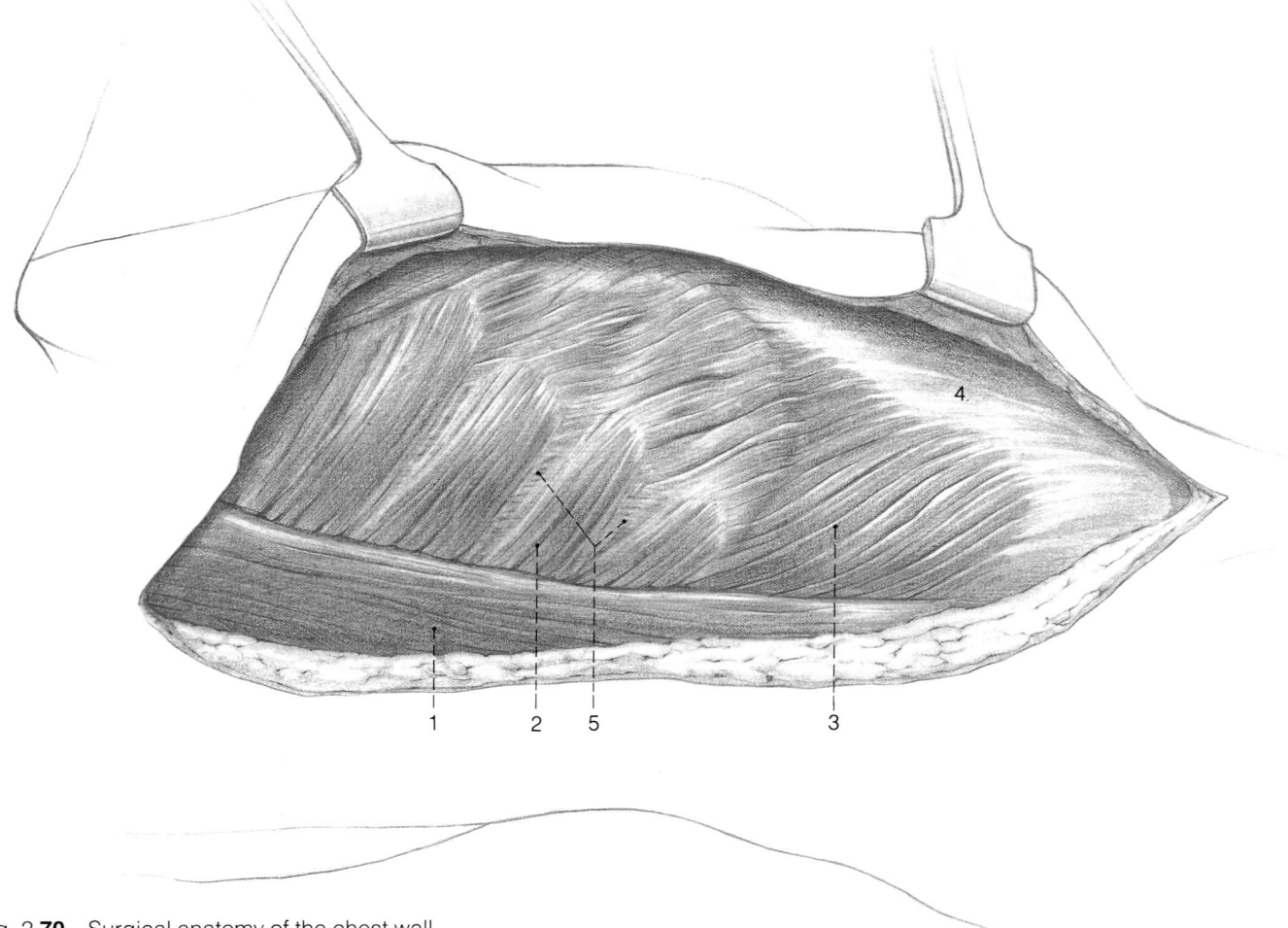

Fig. 2.**70** Surgical anatomy of the chest wall.

1 Latissimus dorsi
2 Serratus anterior
3 External oblique muscle
4 Anterior rectus sheath
5 External intercostal muscles

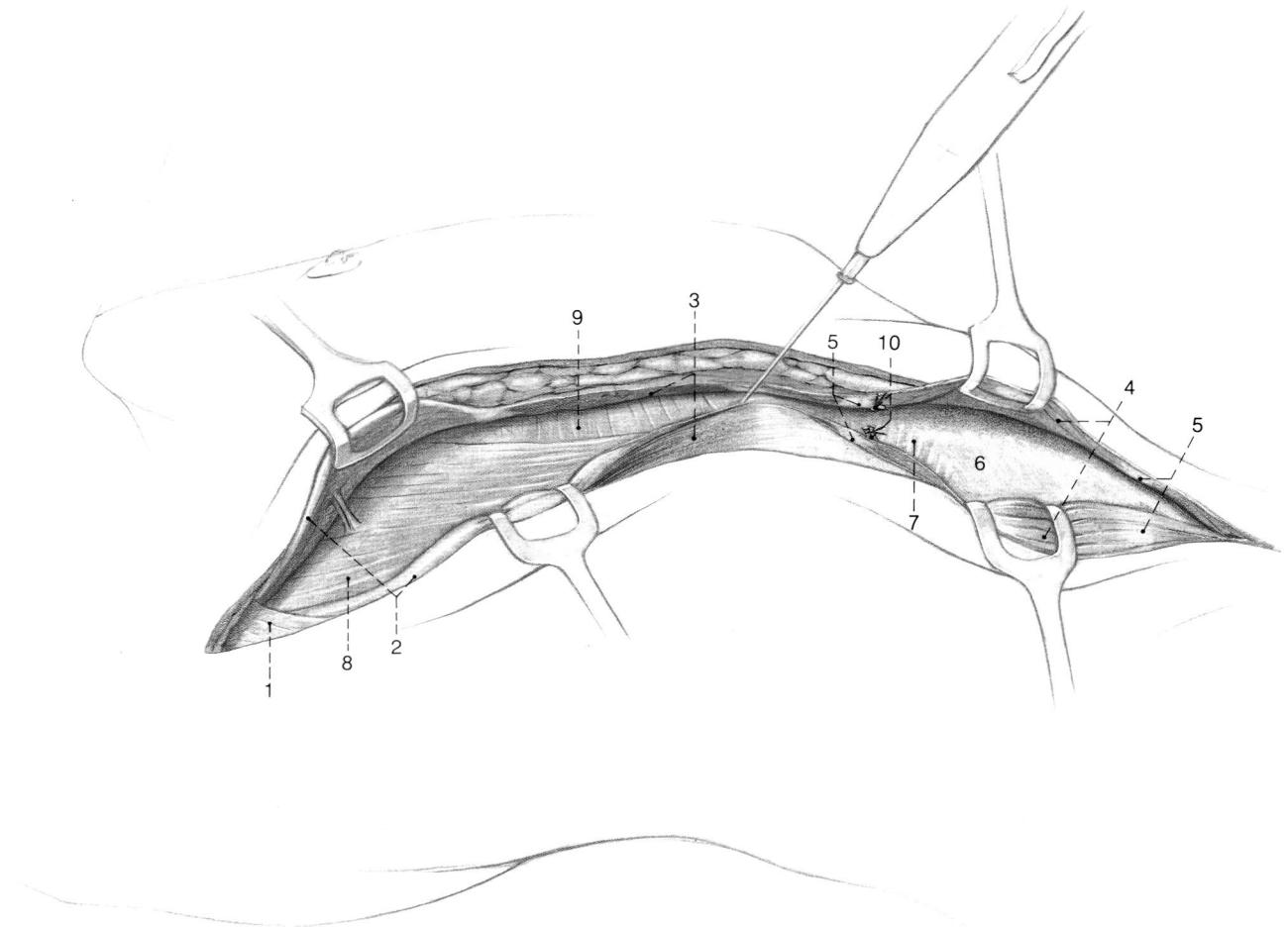

Fig. 2.**71** The serratus anterior and external oblique are transected, exposing the posterior rectus sheath.

1 Latissimus dorsi
2 Serratus anterior
3 External oblique muscle
4 Rectus muscle
5 Tendinous intersections
6 Posterior rectus sheath
7 Transversus abdominis
8 External intercostal muscle
9 Internal intercostal muscle
10 Superior epigastric vessels

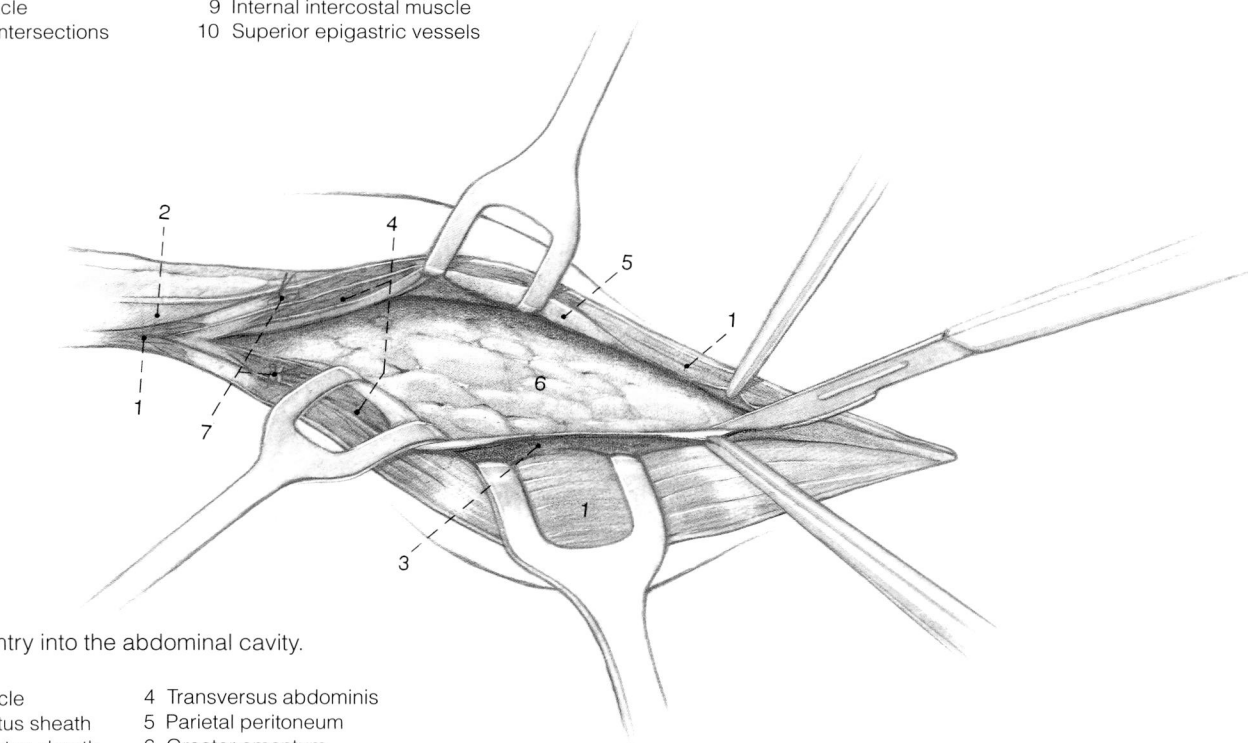

Fig. 2.**72** Entry into the abdominal cavity.

1 Rectus muscle
2 Anterior rectus sheath
3 Posterior rectus sheath
4 Transversus abdominis
5 Parietal peritoneum
6 Greater omentum

Next the thoracic cavity is entered. With a mobile thorax, the thoracotomy is performed on the intercostal plane. Entry is made through the designated interspace (7th ICS) following division of the latissimus dorsi and serratus anterior muscles. Starting at the costal arch, the internal intercostal muscles are divided with diathermy. The pleura is opened at the highest point, close to the costal arch, and the lung is deflected aside. A wooden tissue protector is inserted into the pleural cavity. The line of incision from the costal arch to the anterior axillary line should pass exactly midway between two ribs to safeguard the intercostal vessels. The external intercostal muscle is divided along with the pleura using diathermy current (Fig. 2.**73**).

Modification: Thoracotomy with Rib Resection

In this modification the periosteum of the selected rib is divided with diathermy to the osteochondral junction and separated from the rib with a straight periosteal elevator. The separation proceeds from back to front at the superior rib margin and from front to back at the inferior rib margin to respect the orientation of the intercostal muscles. A curved stripper is then used to isolate the rib from underlying attachments, and the rib is divided anteriorly at the osteochondral junction and elevated. The posterior part of the rib is transected with rib shears about two fingerwidths lateral to the costotransverse joint. The thoracic cavity is entered through the bed of the resected rib.

Division of the Costal Arch with Mayo Scissors

Before the costal arch is divided with Mayo scissors, the plane defined by the transversus abdominis and diaphragm is exposed. Once this plane has been identified, the costal arch is undermined at the osteochondral junction and divided with the Mayo scissors. With this maneuver, the underlying intercostal arteries and veins can be dealt with under direct vision (Fig. 2.**74**).

This dissection of the transversus abdominis and diaphragm is important in the primary thoracoretroperitoneal approach. In this modification, which avoids primary entry into the abdominal cavity, the approach is begun inferomedial to the costal arch, and the peritoneum is retracted medially.

After division of the costal arch, a self-retaining chest retractor is inserted. We use a type with angled, perforated blades that fit over the retracted stumps of the costal arch. The blades are slowly and carefully separated to expose the plane of dissection of the transversus abdominis and its junction with the diaphragm (Fig. 2.**75**).

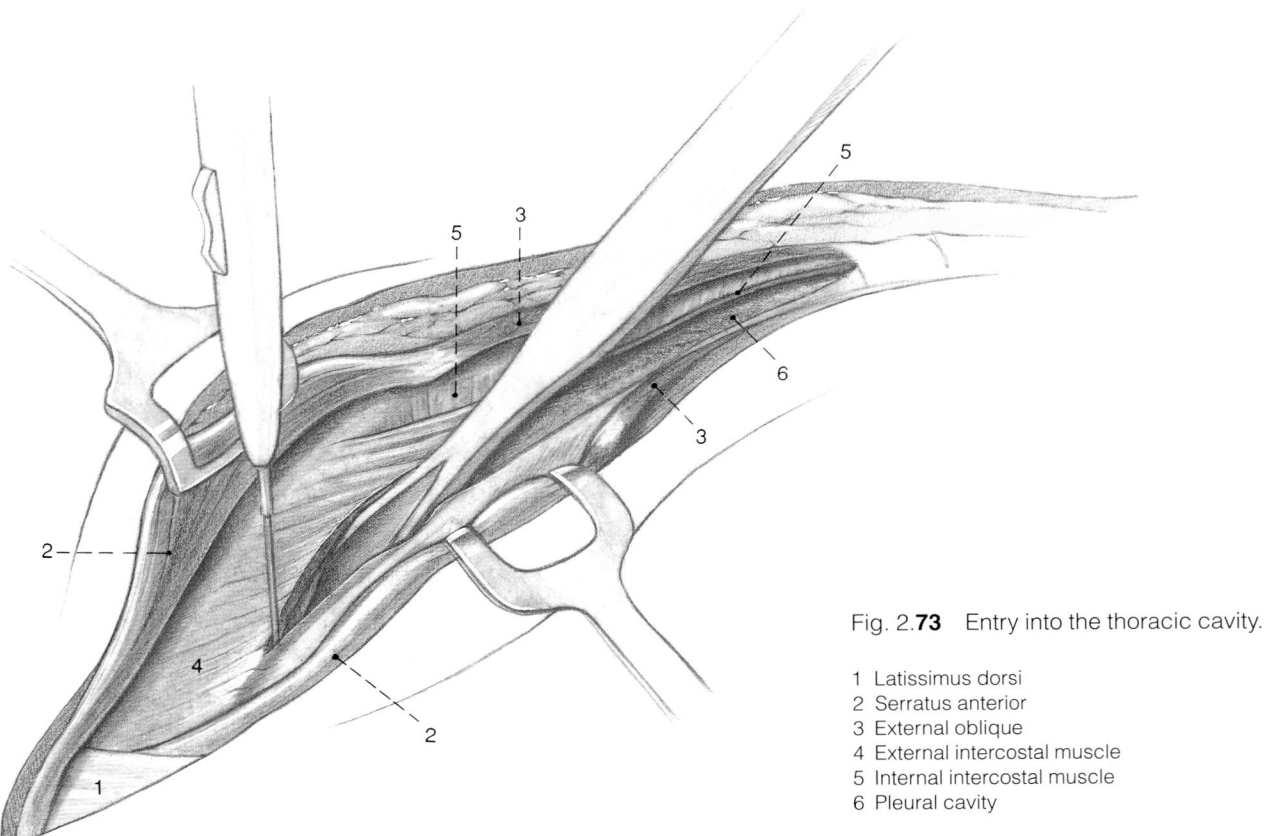

Fig. 2.**73** Entry into the thoracic cavity.

1 Latissimus dorsi
2 Serratus anterior
3 External oblique
4 External intercostal muscle
5 Internal intercostal muscle
6 Pleural cavity

Fig. 2.**74** Division of the costal arch with Mayo scissors.

1 External oblique muscle
2 Internal intercostal muscle
3 Rectus muscle
4 Transversus abdominis

5 Costal arch
6 Parietal peritoneum
7 Greater omentum
8 Pleural cavity

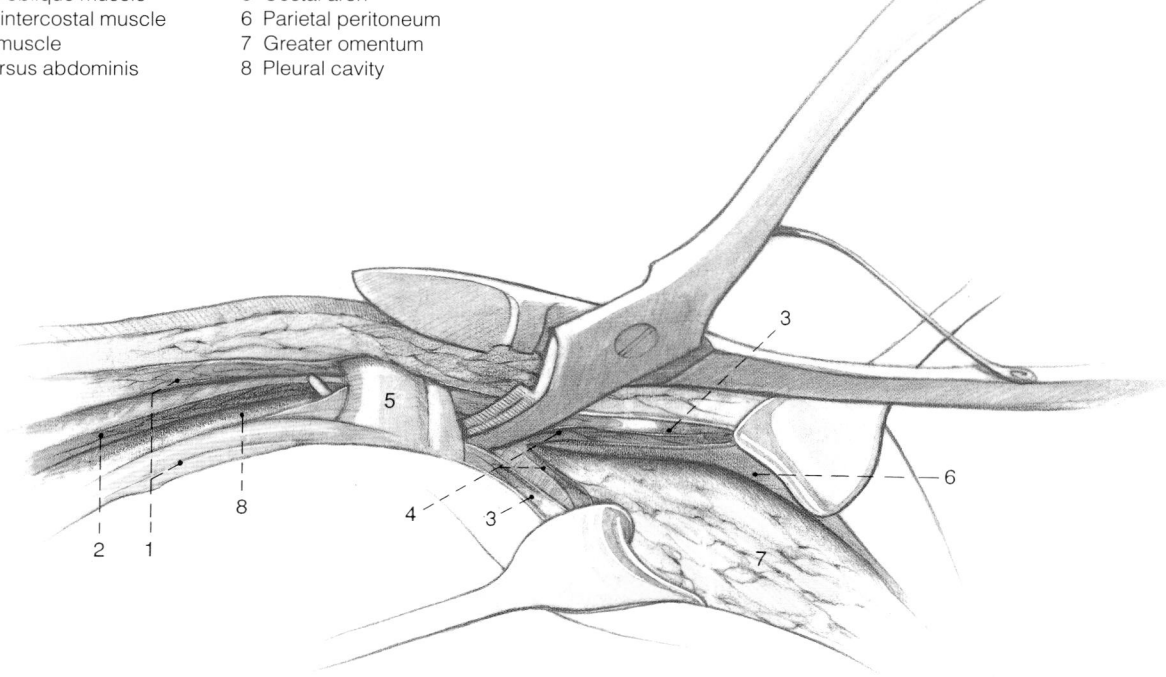

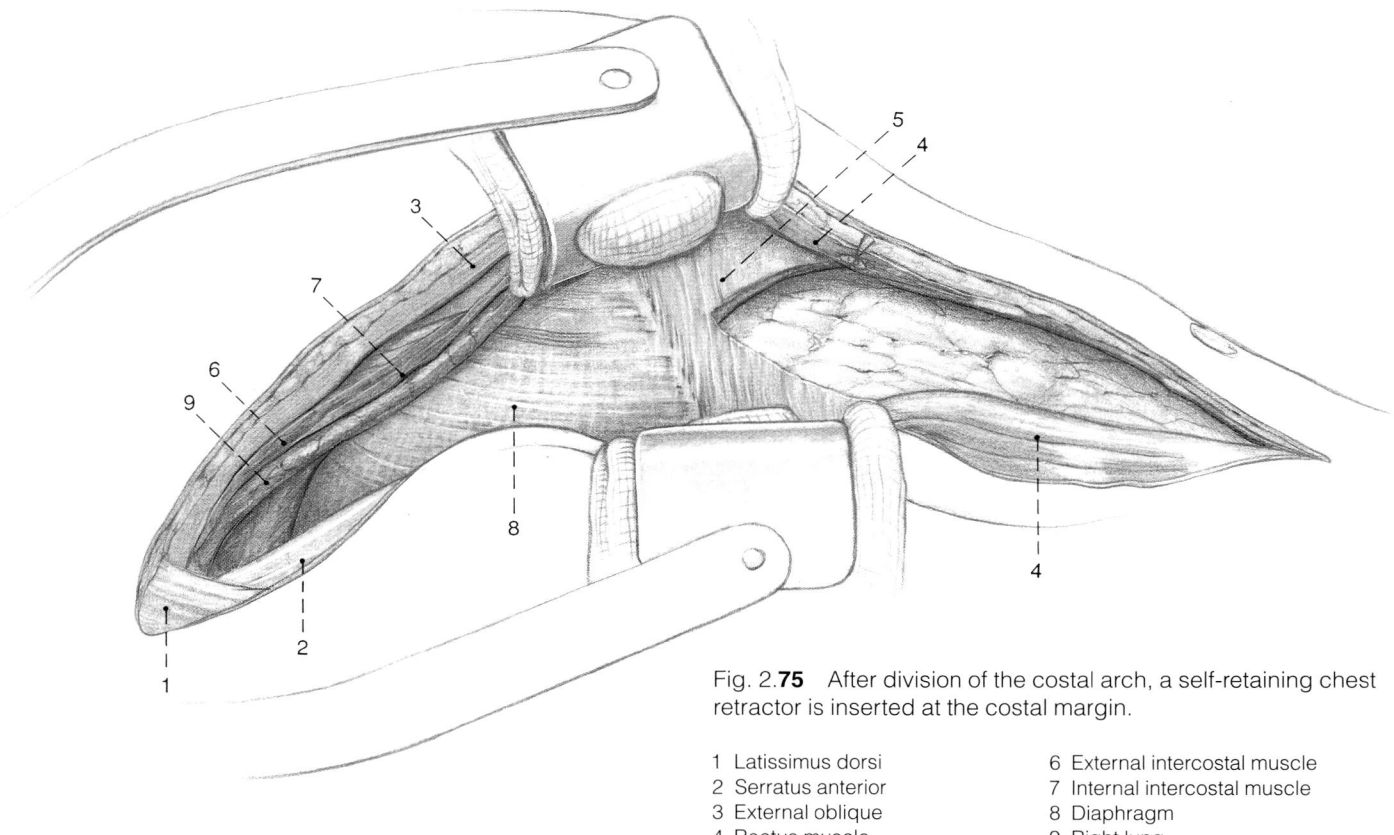

Fig. 2.**75** After division of the costal arch, a self-retaining chest retractor is inserted at the costal margin.

1 Latissimus dorsi
2 Serratus anterior
3 External oblique
4 Rectus muscle
5 Transversus abdominis

6 External intercostal muscle
7 Internal intercostal muscle
8 Diaphragm
9 Right lung

Division of the Diaphragm

After insertion of the chest retractor, the transversus abdominis fibers are divided close to the costal arch, followed by incision of the diaphragm. The diaphragm is incised as far laterally as possible to preserve the phrenic nerve branches.

Bleeding vessels are coagulated with diathermy. The right lobe of the liver can be seen. At this point the thoracoabdominal approach affords excellent exposure of the thoracic and abdominal cavities (Fig. 2.**76**).

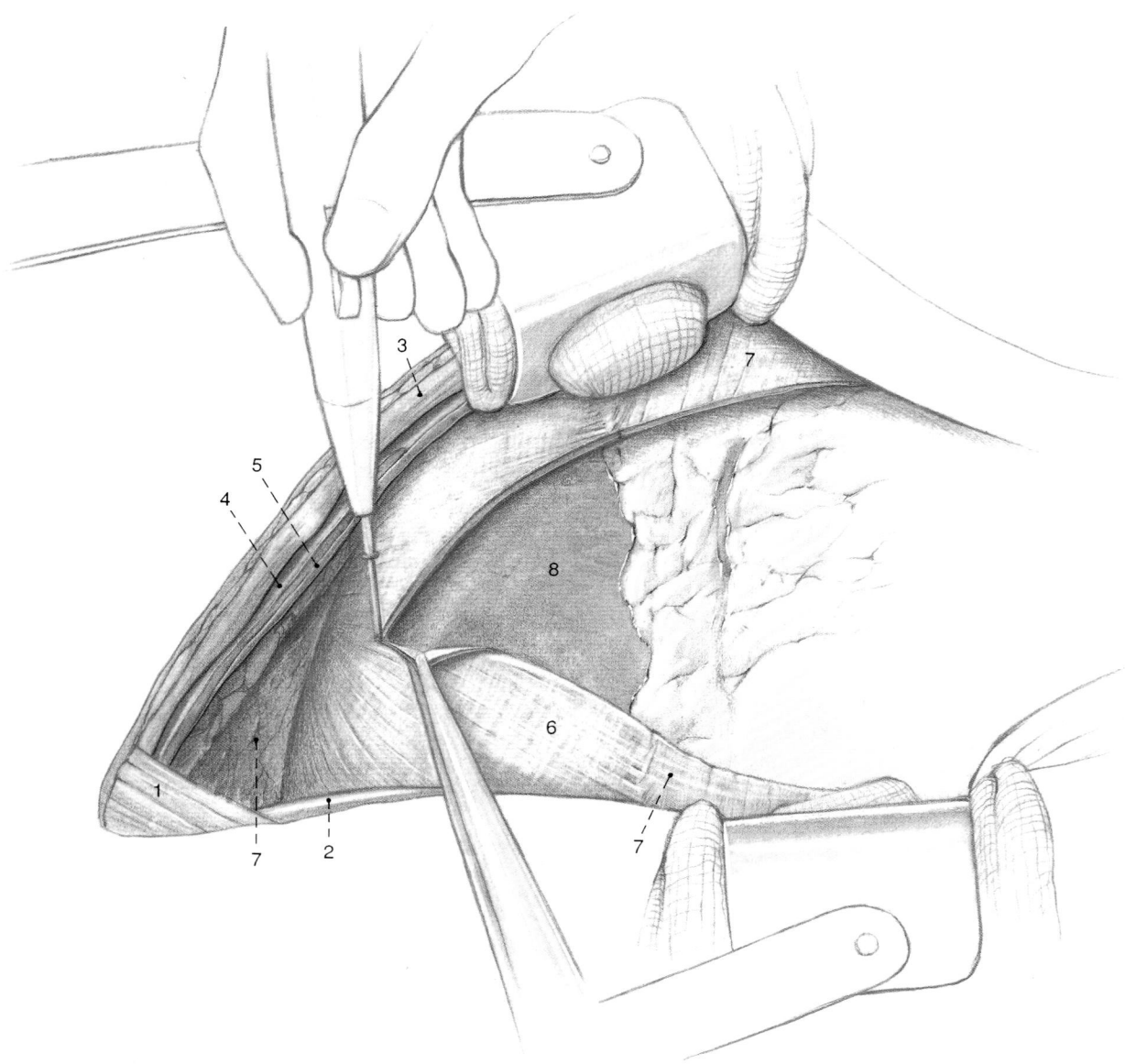

Fig. 2.**76**   Division of the diaphragm with diathermy.

1 Latissimus dorsi
2 Serratus anterior
3 External oblique muscle
4 External intercostal muscle
5 Internal intercostal muscle
6 Diaphragm
7 Transversus abdominis
8 Right lung
9 Liver

Entry into the Retroperitoneal Space

The parietal peritoneum is incised along the ascending colon. The line of incision starts at the cecum, runs along the paracolic sulcus to the right colic flexure, and continues from there to the inferior vena cava in the posterior wall of the epiploic foramen, keeping about one fingerwidth from the inferior border of the liver. The mesocolon is separated from Gerota's fascia on the fine connective-tissue plane to establish broad access to the retroperitoneal space (Fig. 2.**77**). The cecum, ascending colon, and transverse colon are held aside with padded Deaver retractors. The descending part of the duodenum is separated from Gerota's fascia with a scissors (Fig. 2.**77**).

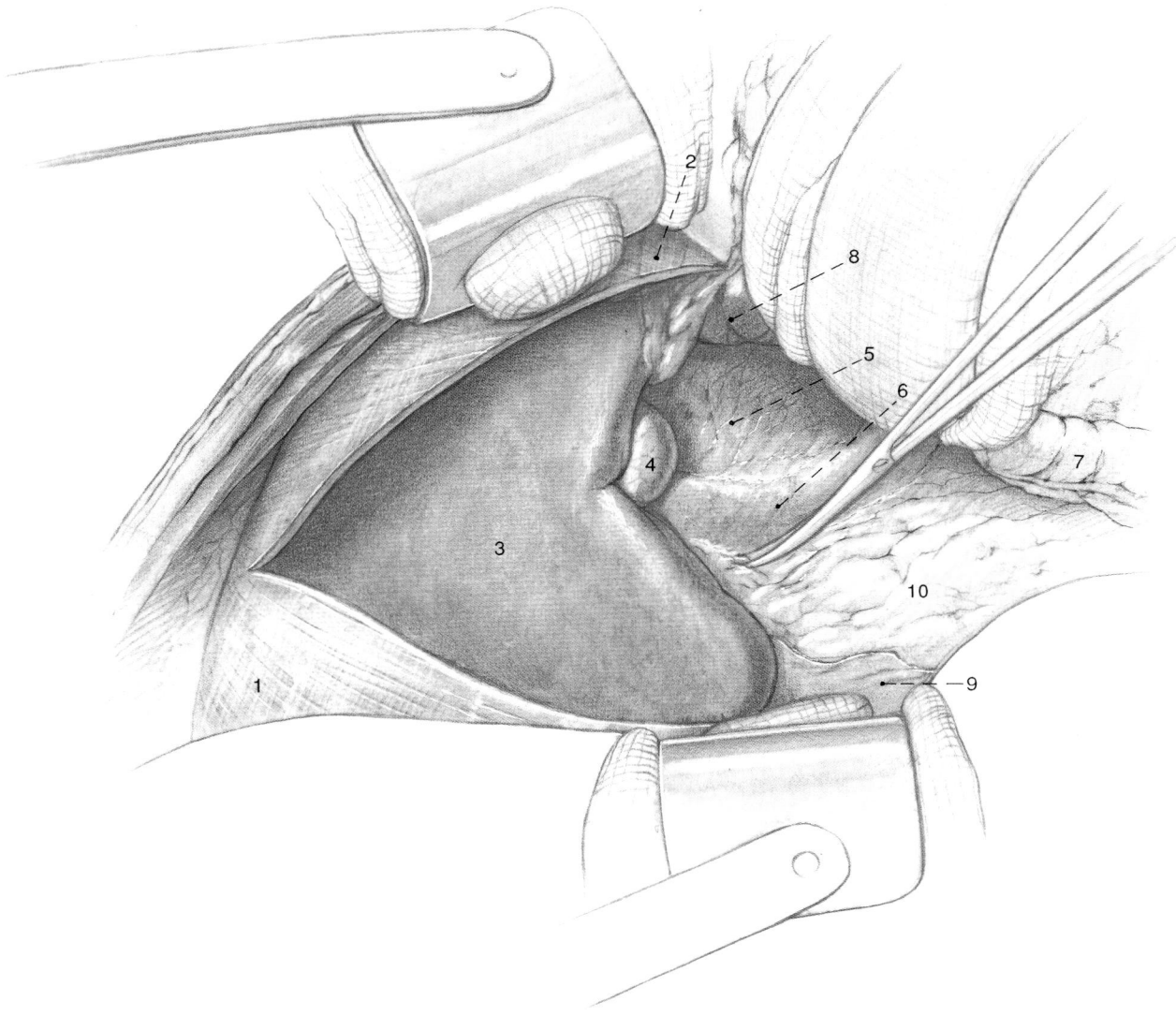

Fig. 2.**77** The descending part of the duodenum is dissected from Gerota's fascia. The line of incision in the parietal peritoneum is visible in the lateral wound angle.

1 Diaphragm
2 Transversus abdominis
3 Liver
4 Gallbladder
5 Head of pancreas
6 Duodenum, descending part
7 Ascending colon
8 Transverse colon
9 Parietal peritoneum
10 Gerota's fascia

The dissection of the descending part of the duodenum connects medially with the dissection of the head of the pancreas. As the duodenum and the head of the pancreas are mobilized, the anterior surfaces of the inferior vena cava and abdominal aorta come into view. Now the vena cava is dissected free, and the testicular (or ovarian) veins are identified. The right renal vein is isolated and snared with a vascular tape, leaving all portions of Gerota's fascia intact. After the renal artery has been identified in the aortocaval space and ligated, the renal vein may be ligated, and the entire contents of the right side of the retroperitoneal space are dissected and removed. The final ligation is that of the suprarenal vein at the inferior vena cava (Fig. 2.**78**).

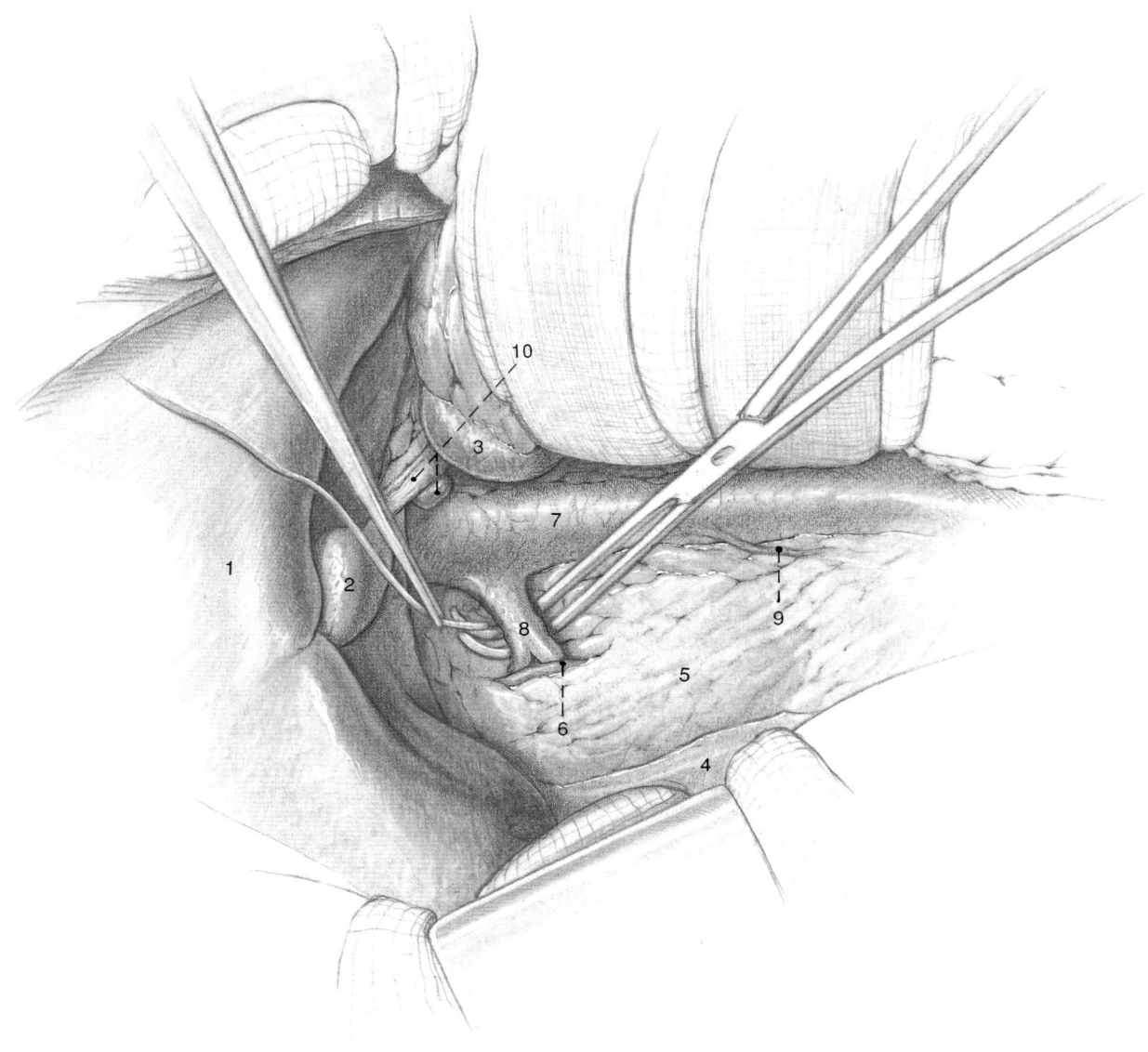

Fig. 2.**78**   The duodenum and head of the pancreas have been dissected, exposing the anterior surface of the inferior vena cava. The renal vein is snared with a vascular tape.

1 Liver
2 Gallbladder
3 Duodenum, descending part
4 Parietal peritoneum
5 Gerota's fascia
6 Right kidney, medial border
7 Inferior vena cava
8 Right renal vein
9 Right testicular vein
10 Hepatoduodenal ligament and lymph node

Modification of the Thoracoabdominal Approach for a Stage II or III Tumor Thrombus in the Vena Cava

The thoracic portion of the skin incision is placed in the fifth intercostal space (see Fig. 2.**68**).

After the abdominal cavity and chest have been opened, the incision in the mesocolon is carried along the colon and is continued along the mesentery to the duodenojejunal flexure. This line of incision permits a general mobilization of the large and small bowels, establishing access to a broad area of the retroperitoneal space. The left renal vein can be identified over the aorta and elevated to expose the superior mesenteric artery. The right renal artery is identified in the aortocaval space.

The peritoneum is dissected off the diaphragm. The right triangular ligament is incised at its attachment to the diaphragm so that the right lobe of the liver can be mobilized and deflected medially upward, exposing the hepatic veins. In this way the entire retroperitoneal course of the vena cava can be visualized (Fig. 2.**79**) together with the right adrenal gland and suprarenal vein.

Use of the fifth interspace approach also permits exposure of the intrathoracic portion of the inferior vena cava. The parietal layer of the pericardium is incised above the diaphragm. After stay sutures are preplaced on both sides, the intrathoracic part of the vena cava can be freed and encircled with a tourniquet snare (Fig. 2.**80**).

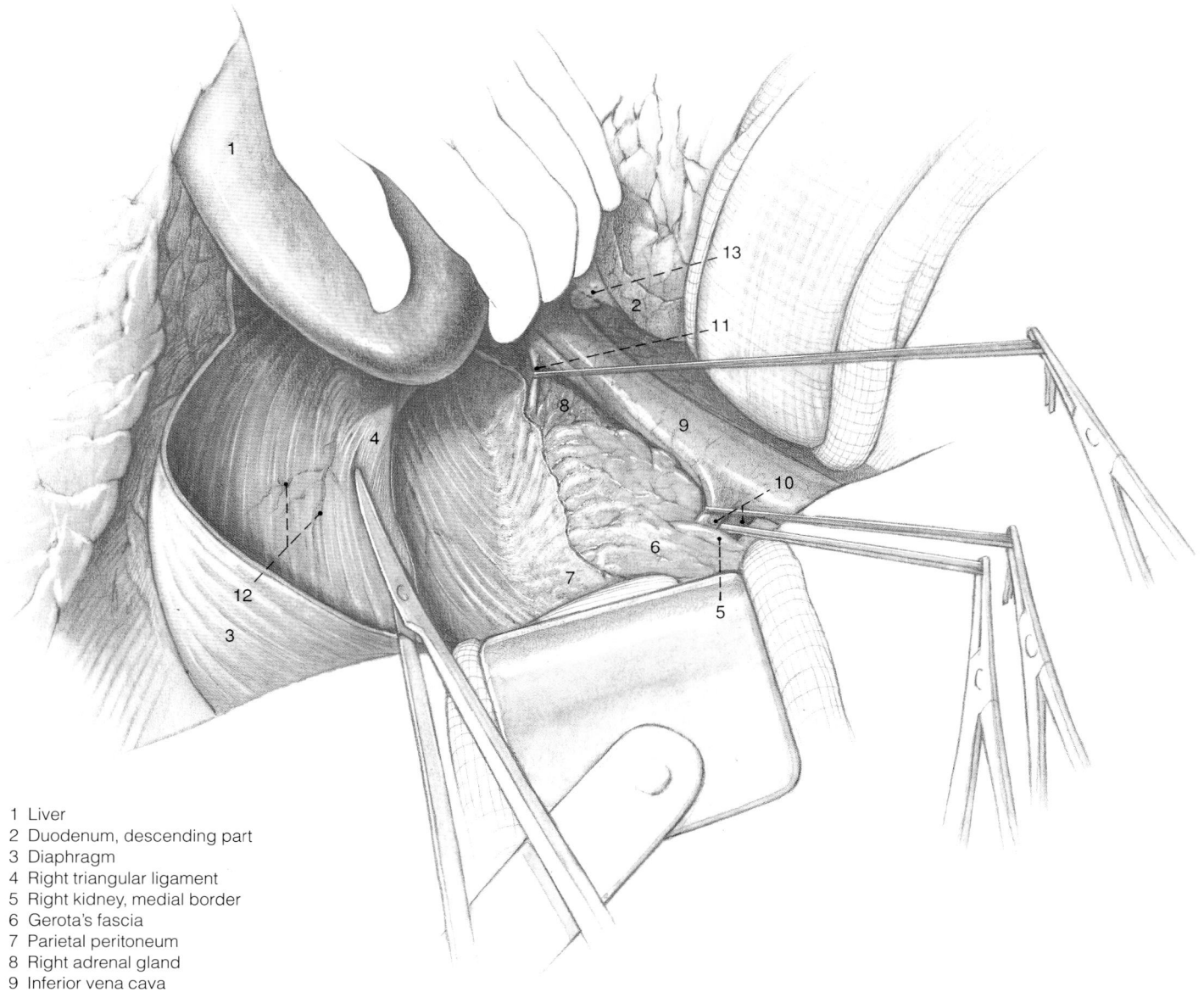

1 Liver
2 Duodenum, descending part
3 Diaphragm
4 Right triangular ligament
5 Right kidney, medial border
6 Gerota's fascia
7 Parietal peritoneum
8 Right adrenal gland
9 Inferior vena cava
10 Right renal vessels
11 Right suprarenal vein
12 Inferior phrenic vessels
13 Hepatoduodenal ligament

Fig. 2.**79** The right triangular ligament is sharply released from the diaphragm. The right adrenal gland and suprarenal vein are seen.

Cavotomy

After Gerota's fascia has been dissected from the diaphragm, the quadratus lumborum and psoas major muscles can be seen. Incision of the vena cava for the removal of tumor thrombus is preceded by the following steps: aortocaval ligation of the renal artery, tourniquet placement on the infrarenal and intrathoracic portions of the vena cava, and tourniquet placement on the left renal vein (for a right renal tumor) and hepatoduodenal ligament. The left renal vein is elevated to expose the superior mesenteric artery. Before the vena cava is opened, the blood supply is occluded by clamping the superior mesenteric artery (Fig. 2.**81**).

Comments

The thoracoabdominal approach has become standard for large renal and adrenal tumors. It affords very broad exposure of the retroperitoneal space following mobilization of the small bowel and colon. The thoracoabdominal approach is well suited for renal tumors with an associated stage II or III vena caval thrombus. It permits complete exposure of the inferior vena cava up to its intrathoracic portion, and it provides ideal access to suprahilar and retrocrural lymph nodes in patients with testicular tumors. The primary thoracoretroperitoneal approach is a useful modification for the infrahilar lymph node surgery of testicular tumors.

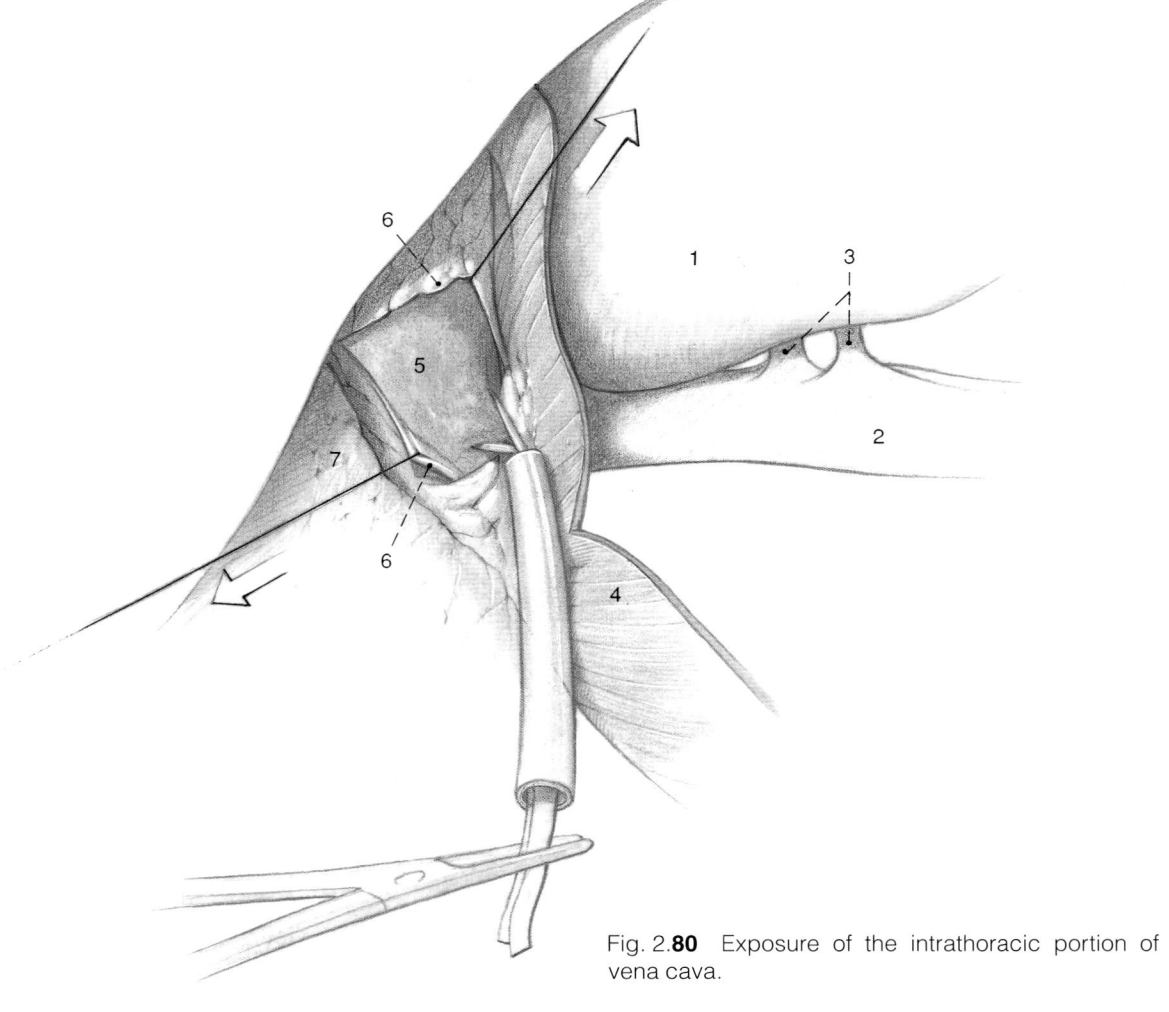

Fig. 2.**80** Exposure of the intrathoracic portion of the inferior vena cava.

1 Liver
2 Inferior vena cava
3 Hepatic veins
4 Diaphragm
5 Right atrium
6 Parietal layer of pericardium
7 Right lung

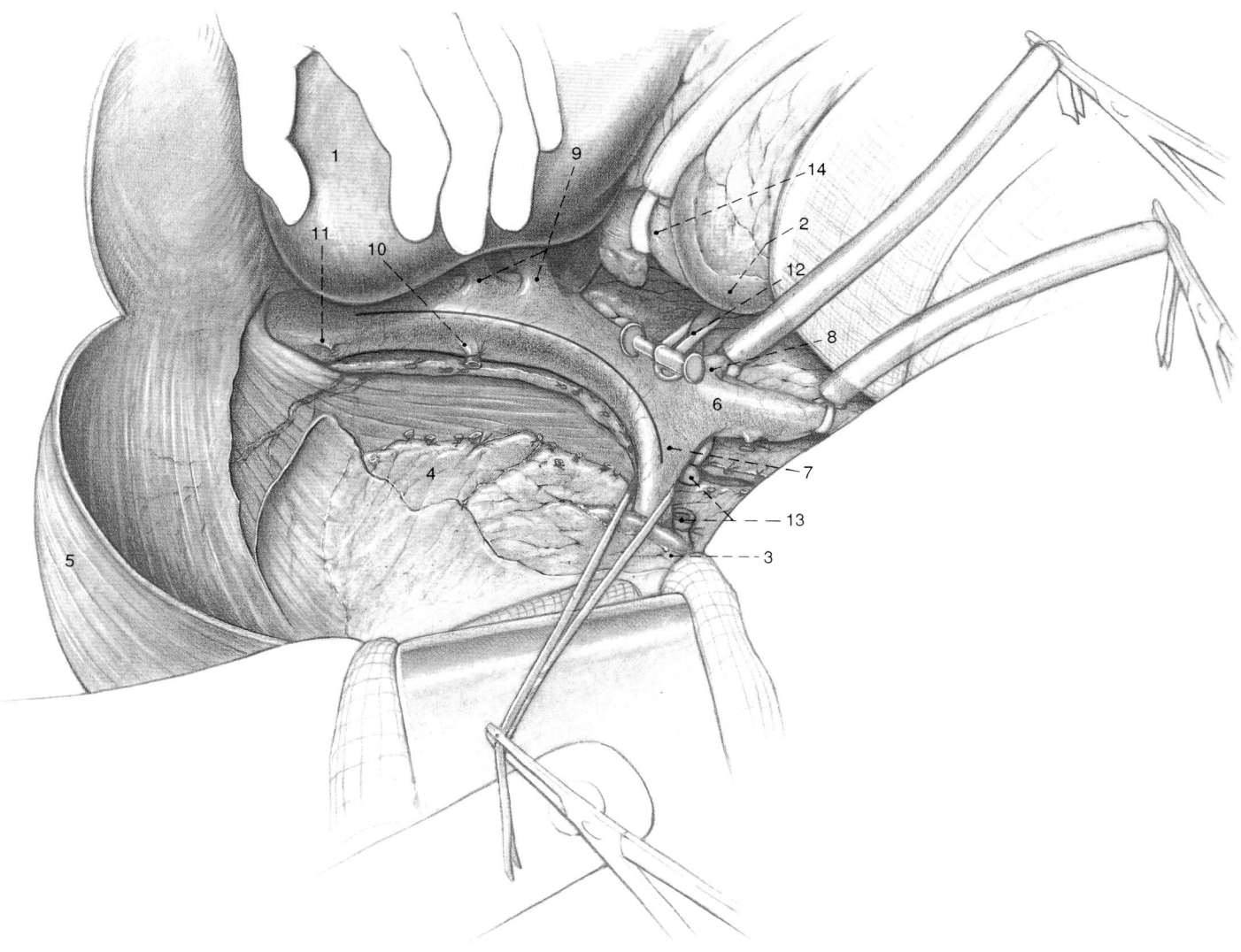

Fig. 2.**81** Preparatory steps for cavotomy.

1 Liver
2 Duodenum, descending part
3 Right kidney, medial border
4 Right adrenal gland
5 Diaphragm
6 Inferior vena cava
7 Right renal vein
8 Left renal vein
9 Hepatic veins
10 Suprarenal vein
11 Superior suprarenal vein (variant)
12 Superior mesenteric artery
13 Right renal artery
14 Hepatoduodenal ligament

Approach to the Retrocrural Lymph Nodes

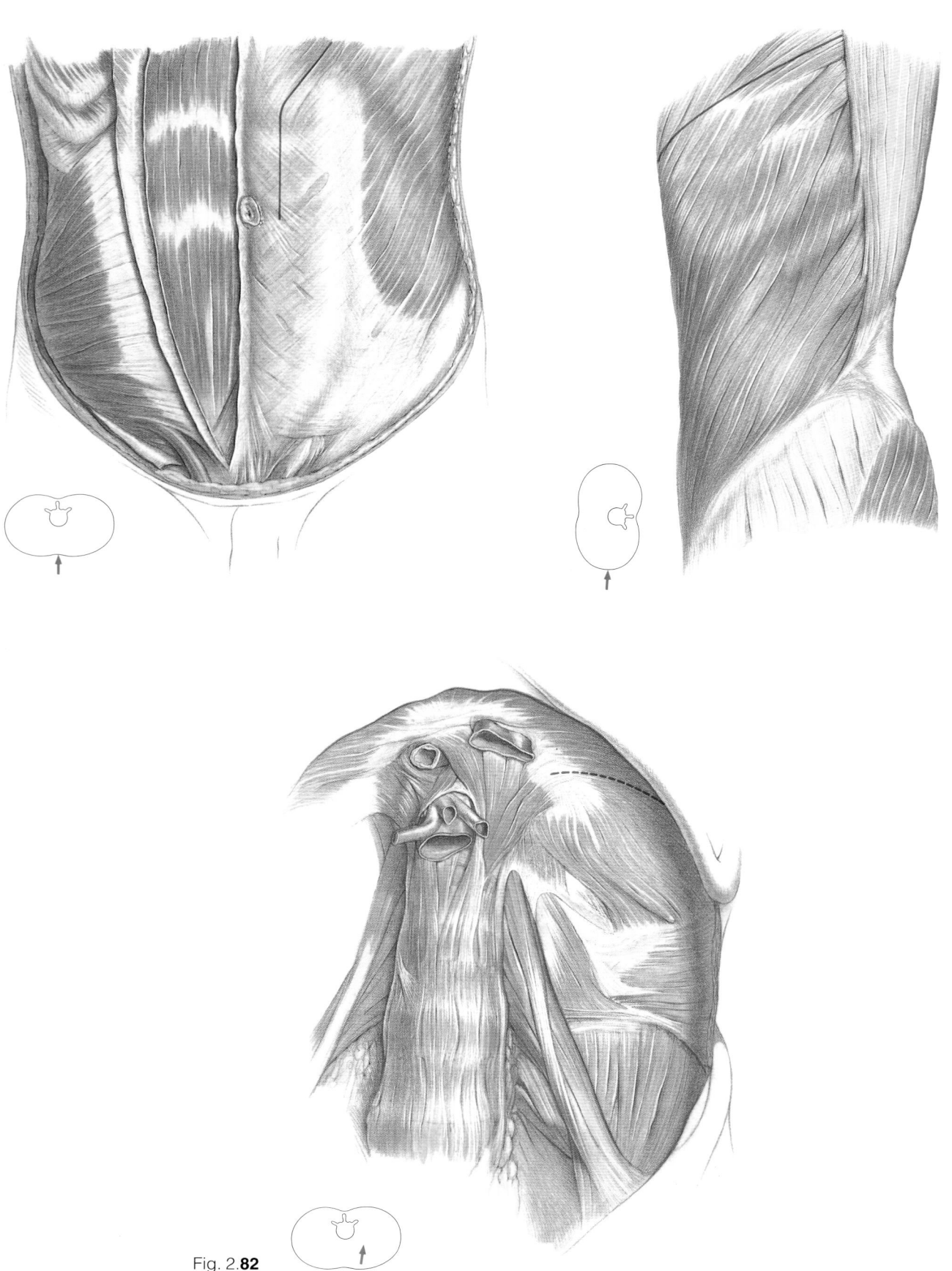

Fig. 2.**82**

Main Indications

• Metastatic involvement of retrocrural lymph nodes by testicular tumor

Position and Skin Incision

The patient is positioned on the right side with the chest rotated about 30°–40° forward at the shoulder level. The ipsilateral arm is supported above the thorax on a rest. The pelvis is rotated only about 10° forward from the horizontal. The ipsilateral leg is extended, and the contralateral leg is flexed 90° at the knee. The operating table is flexed at the lumbar level to hyperextend the operative area. The costal arch forms the highest point of the operating field.

In the standard seventh intercostal space approach, the skin incision starts in the anterior axillary line and is carried across the costal arch to the level of the umbilicus.

Division of the Diaphragm

The thoracic and abdominal cavities are opened, and exposure in both areas is maintained with self-retaining retractors. Loops of ileum, the ascending colon, the greater omentum, and the phrenicocolic ligament are visible within the abdominal cavity. The diaphragm is divided with electrocautery (Fig. 2.**83**).

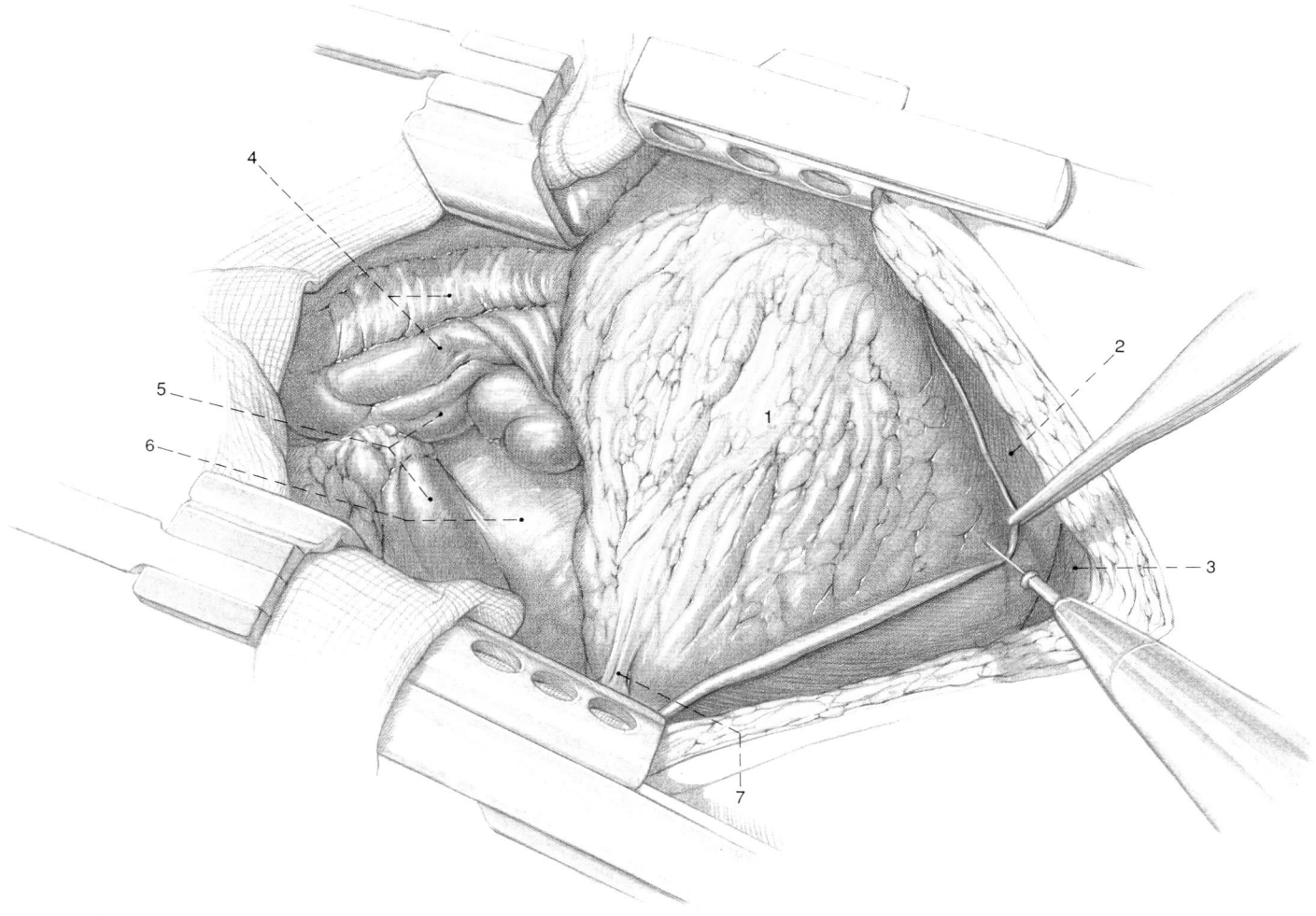

Fig. 2.**83**   The diaphragm is divided with electrocautery.

1 Greater omentum
2 Diaphragm
3 Lung
4 Ascending colon
5 Ileum
6 Parietal peritoneum
7 Phrenicocolic ligament

Exposure of the Retroperitoneal Space

The phrenicocolic ligament is divided, and the retroperitoneal space is exposed by incision of the left paracolic sulcus (Fig. 2.**84**). The descending colon and mesocolon are dissected from Gerota's fascia. The tail of the pancreas and splenic vessels are exposed in the upper portion of the field. After division of the phrenicocolic ligament, the left colic flexure can be freed and displaced medially. The bulk of the transverse colon, descending colon, and small bowel loops are retracted medially with Deaver retractors (Fig. 2.**85**).

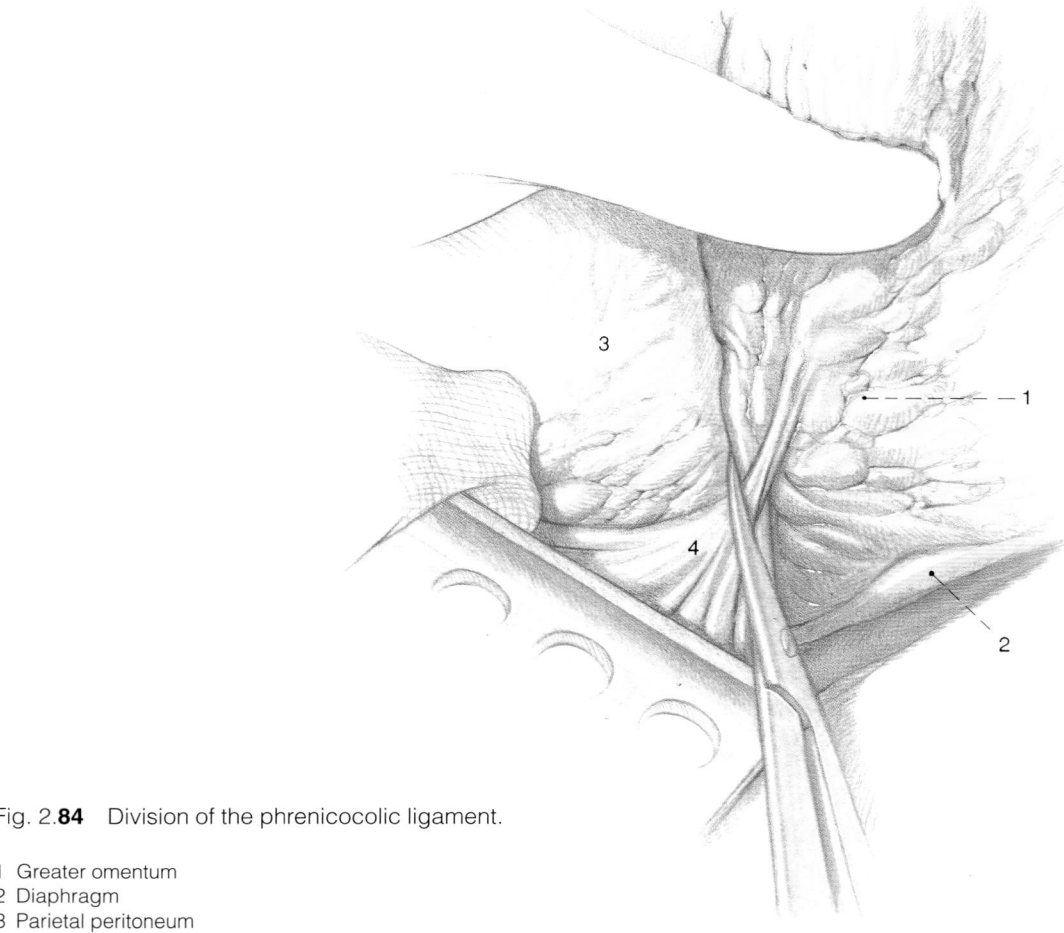

Fig. 2.**84**   Division of the phrenicocolic ligament.

1 Greater omentum
2 Diaphragm
3 Parietal peritoneum
4 Phrenicocolic ligament

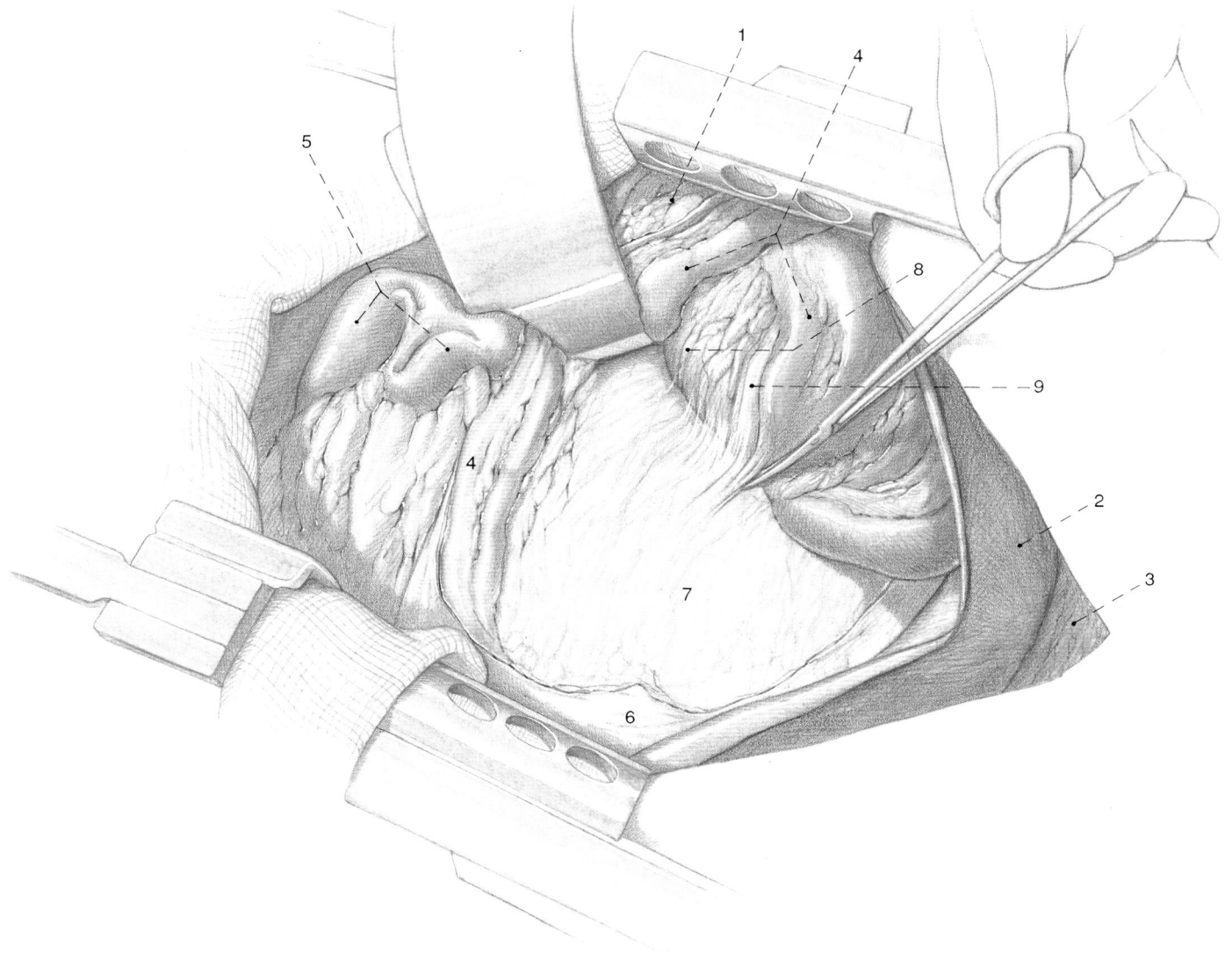

Fig. 2.**85** Exposure of the retroperitoneal space.

1 Greater omentum
2 Diaphragm
3 Lung
4 Descending colon
5 Ileum
6 Parietal peritoneum
7 Gerota's fascia
8 Tail of pancreas
9 Splenic vessels

Dissection of the Lateral Crus, Exposure of the Inferior Phrenic Artery

The left lobe of the liver and esophagus are visible in the upper aspect of the wound angle. The descending colon is retracted medially with the isolated left colic flexure. The left inferior phrenic artery and vein are identified at the lateral crus, dissected, and ligated (Fig. 2.**86**). A middle suprarenal artery from the aorta is also ligated, then the adrenal gland is freed from the lumbar part of the diaphragm and lateral crus and displaced inferolaterally (Fig. 2.**87**).

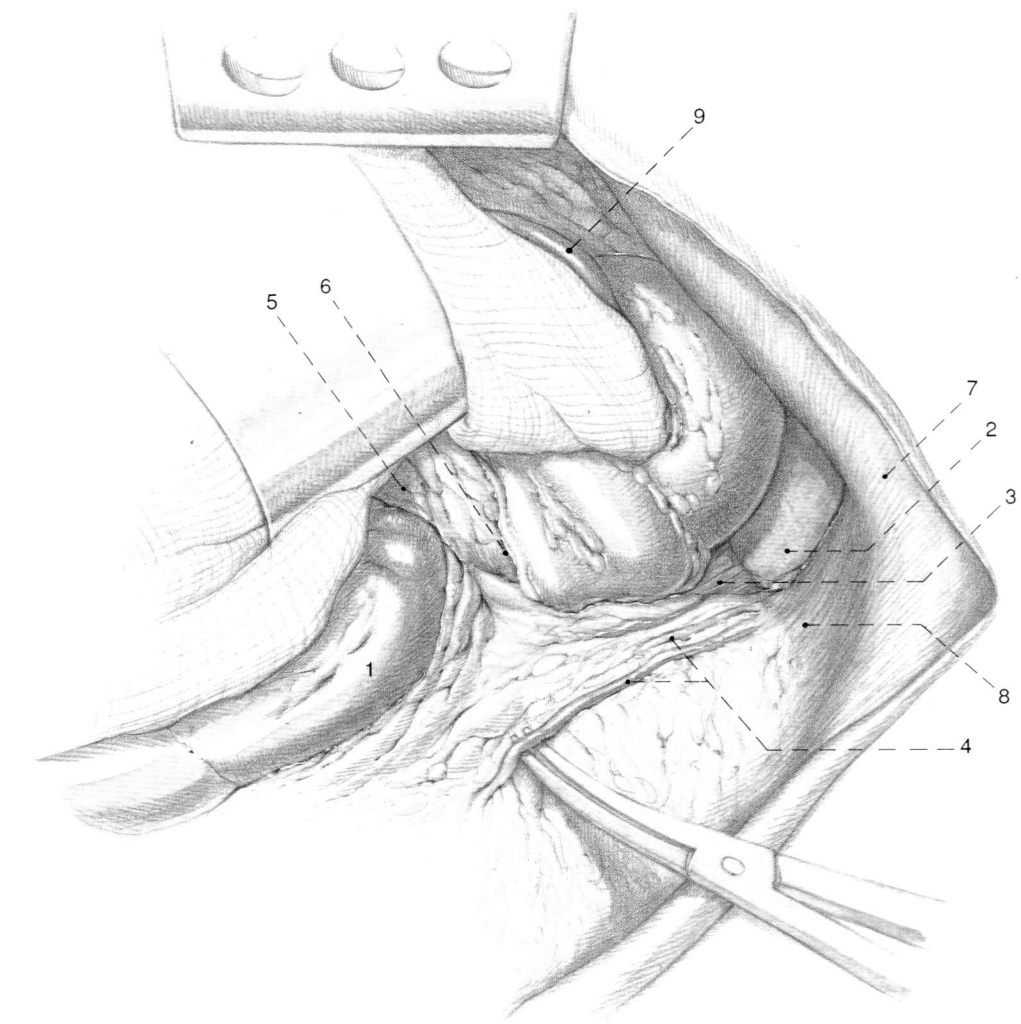

Fig. 2.**86** Exposure of the left inferior phrenic artery and vein.

1 Descending colon
2 Left lobe of liver
3 Esophagus
4 Inferior phrenic vessels
5 Tail of pancreas
6 Splenic vessels
7 Diaphragm
8 Left lateral crus
9 Spleen

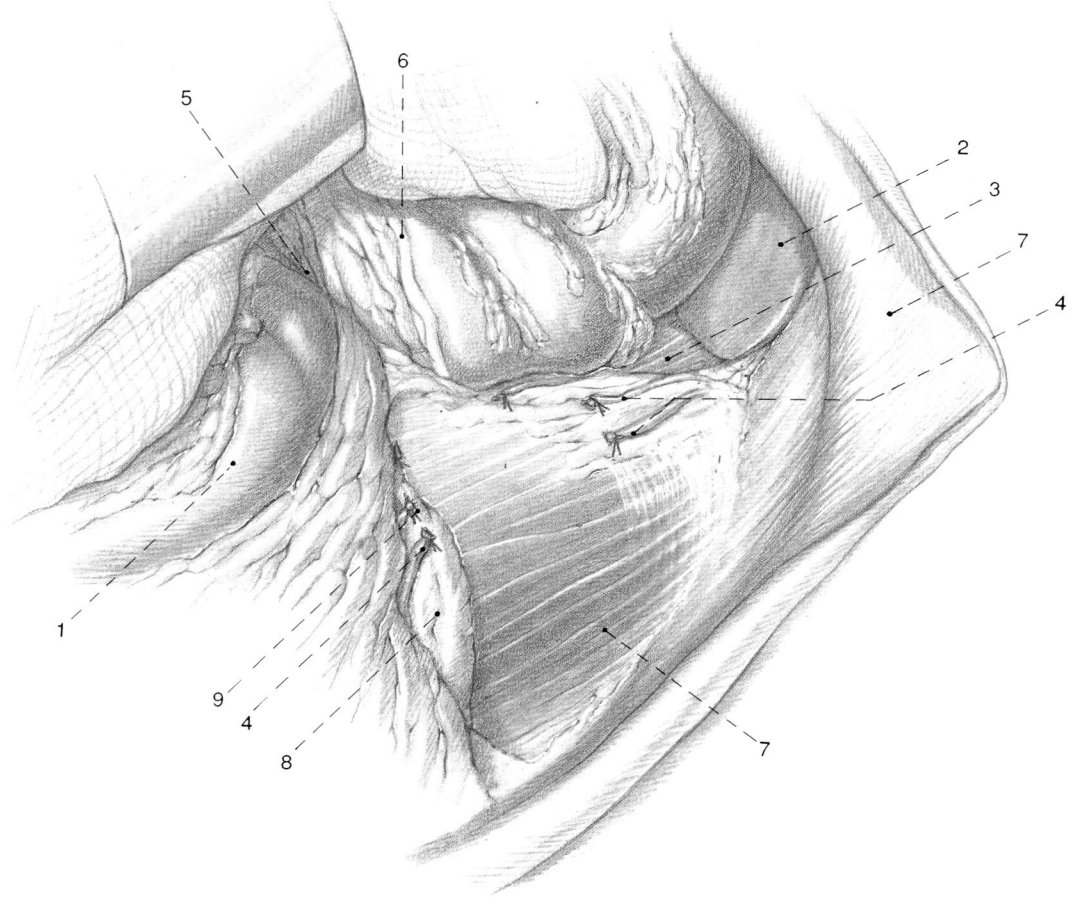

Fig. 2.**87**   The left inferior phrenic artery and vein are ligated, and the lumbar part of the diaphragm is exposed.

1 Descending colon
2 Left lobe of liver
3 Esophagus
4 Inferior phrenic vessels
5 Tail of pancreas
6 Splenic vessels
7 Diaphragm
8 Adrenal gland
9 Suprarenal vessels

Incision of the Aortic Aperture

Following exposure of the abdominal aorta, the left renal artery is identified and dissected free. After ligation of the inferior phrenic artery, the aortic aperture is incised over the abdominal aorta, starting at the median arcuate ligament. If enlarged lymph nodes are found at the celiac trunk and superior mesenteric artery, both vessels must be dissected free (Fig. 2.**88**). The incision in the aortic aperture is carried to the esophageal hiatus. The inferior phrenic artery is again ligated close to the aorta (Fig. 2.**89**).

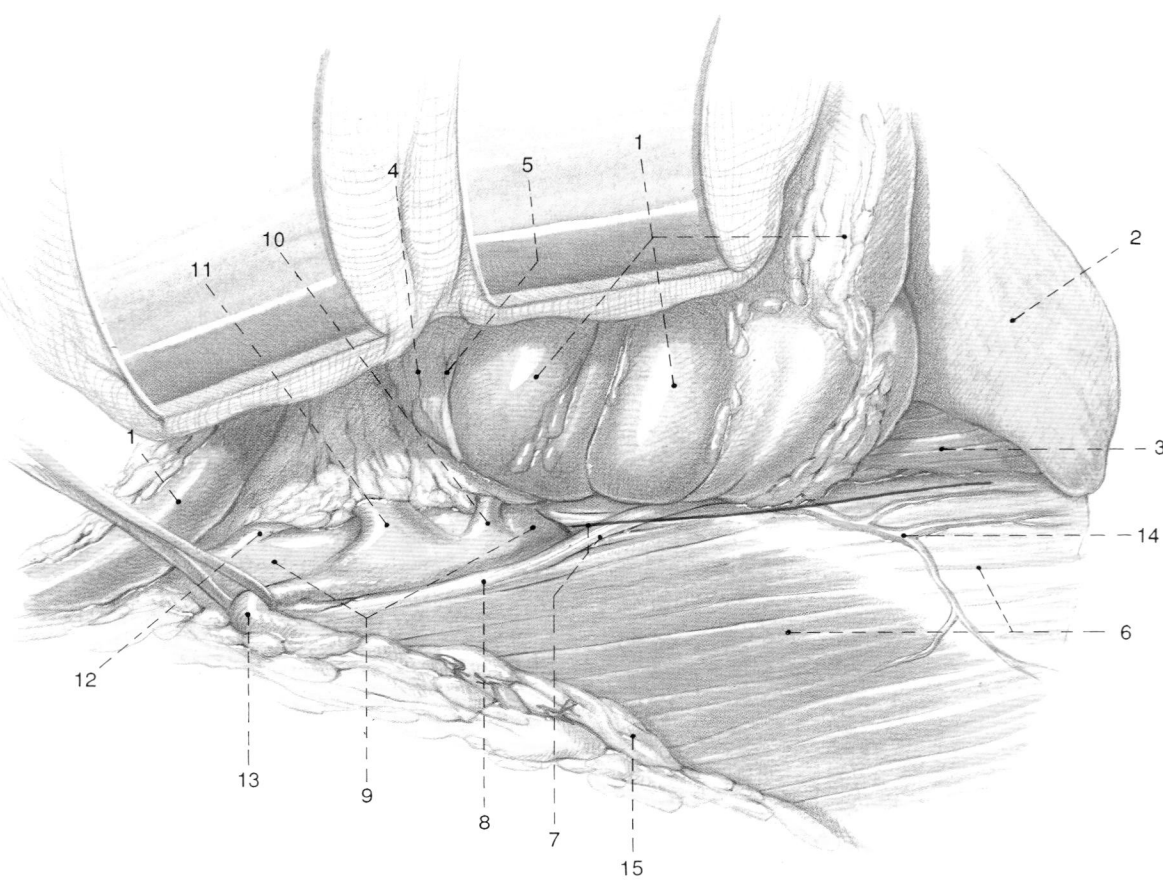

Fig. 2.**88**   Dissection of the aorta and renal artery. The line of incision from the aortic hiatus to the esophagus is shown.

1 Descending colon
2 Left lobe of liver
3 Esophagus
4 Tail of pancreas
5 Splenic vessels
6 Diaphragm
7 Aortic hiatus
8 Median arcuate ligament
9 Abdominal aorta
10 Celiac trunk
11 Superior mesenteric artery
12 Right renal artery
13 Left renal artery
14 Inferior phrenic artery
15 Adrenal gland

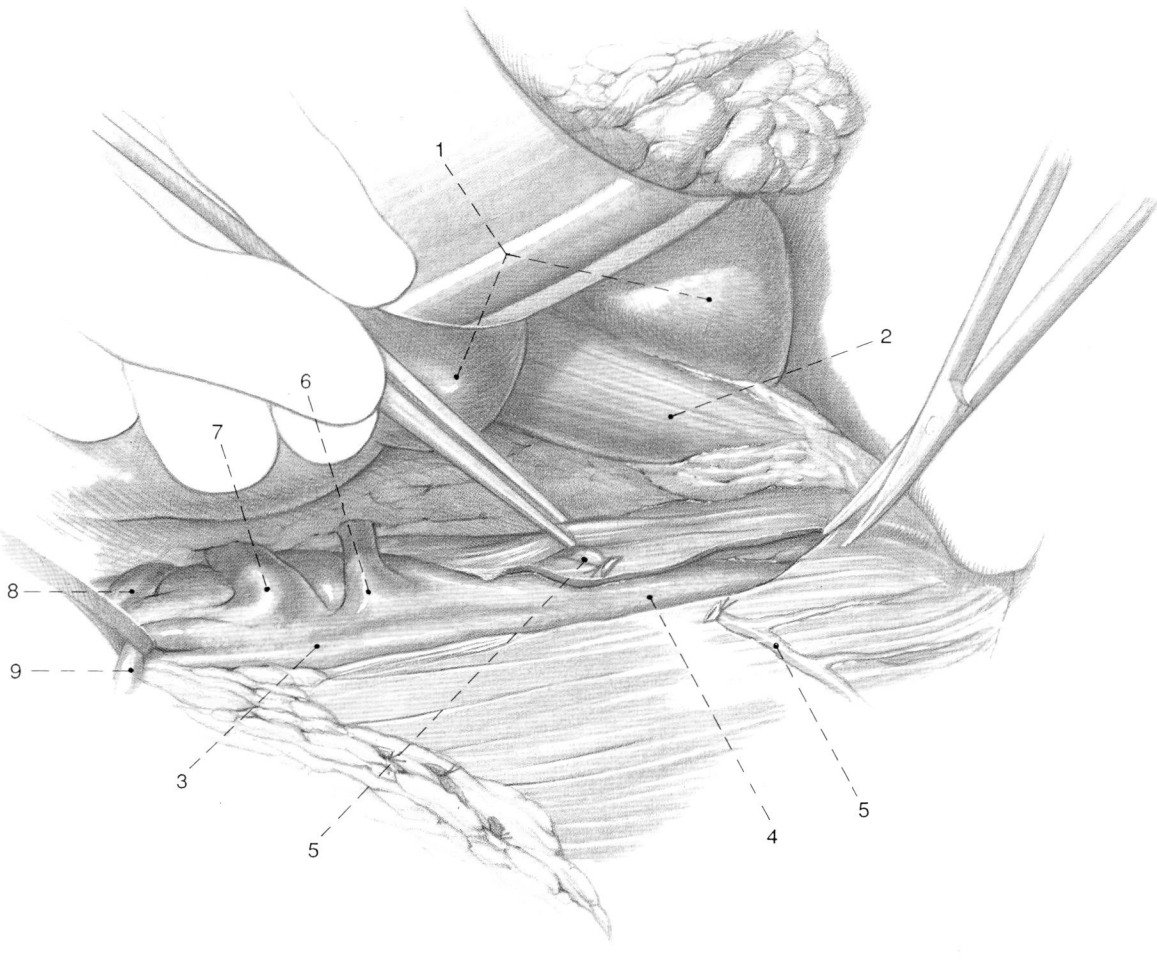

Fig. 2.**89**   Incision over the abdominal aorta.

1 Descending colon
2 Esophagus
3 Abdominal aorta
4 Thoracic aorta
5 Inferior phrenic artery
6 Celiac trunk
7 Superior mesenteric artery
8 Right renal artery
9 Left renal artery

Comments

This approach provides exposure of the retroaortic space (Fig. 2.**90**). When the aorta is mobilized, attention must be given to the last two posterior intercostal arteries and first lumbar arteries at the lateral or posterior aspect of the vessel. These arteries may give origin to the great radicular artery (of Adamkiewicz), which contributes significantly to the blood supply of the spinal cord. The segmental arteries must be preserved, therefore, especially on the left side of the body.

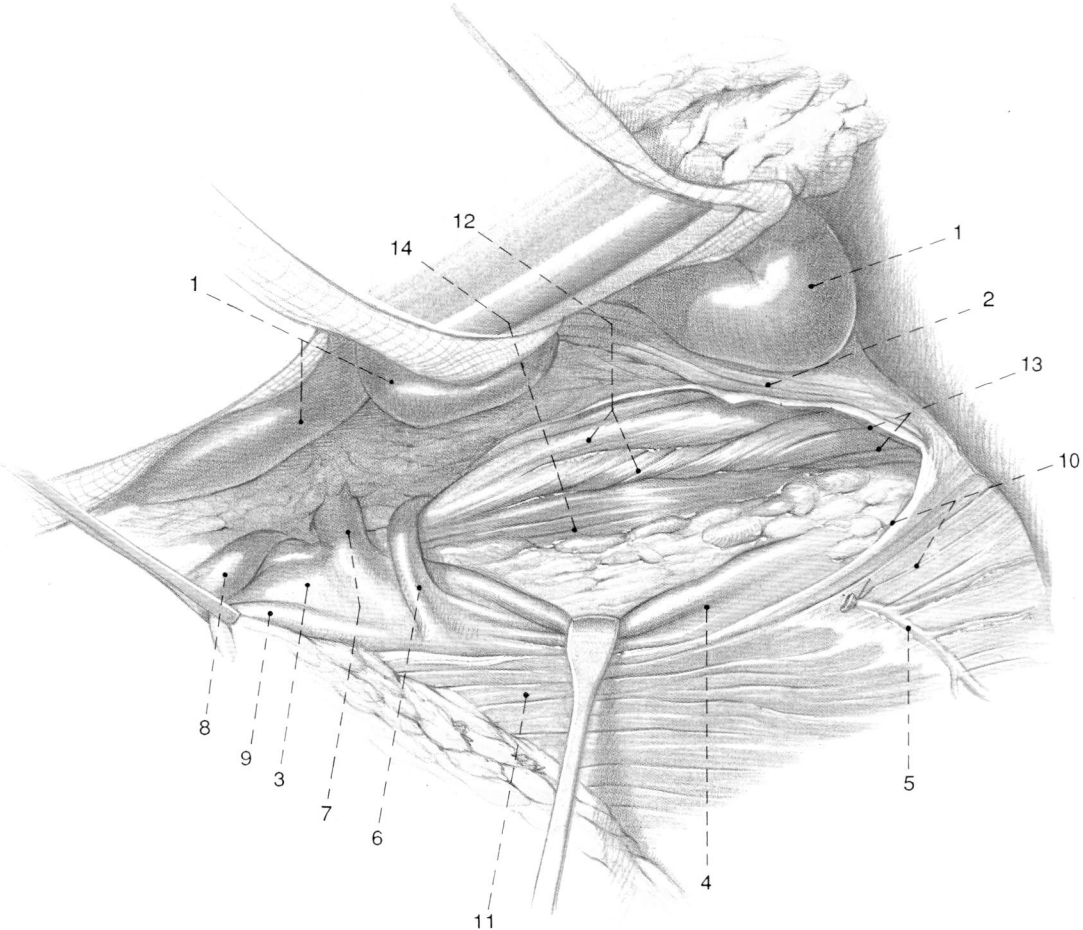

Fig. 2.**90**   Exposure of the retroaortic and retrocrural spaces.

 1 Descending colon
 2 Esophagus
 3 Abdominal aorta
 4 Thoracic aorta
 5 Inferior phrenic artery
 6 Celiac trunk
 7 Superior mesenteric artery
 8 Right renal artery
 9 Left renal artery
10 Diaphragm, left costal part
11 Diaphragm, left lumbar part
12 Diaphragm, right lumbar part
13 Diaphragm, right costal part
14 Psoas major

Anterior Subcostal Approach

93

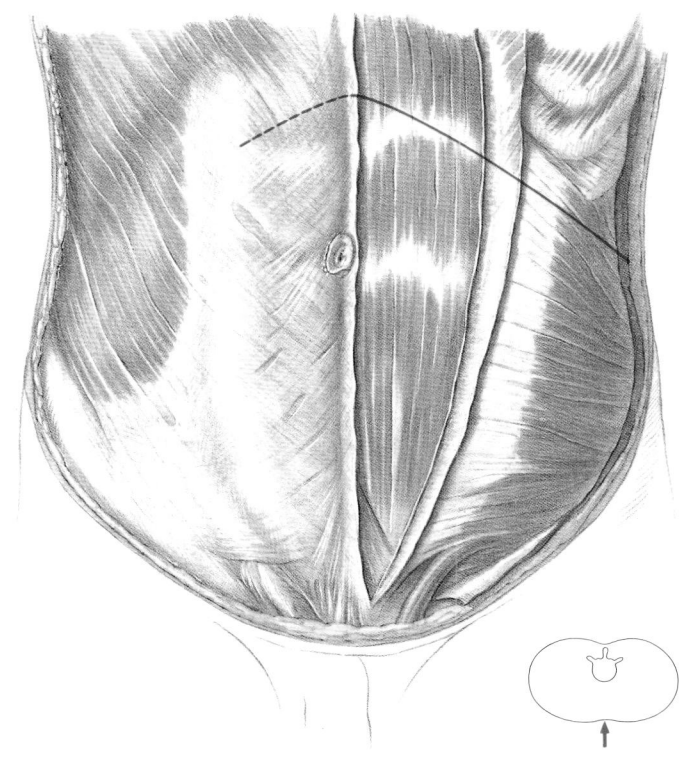

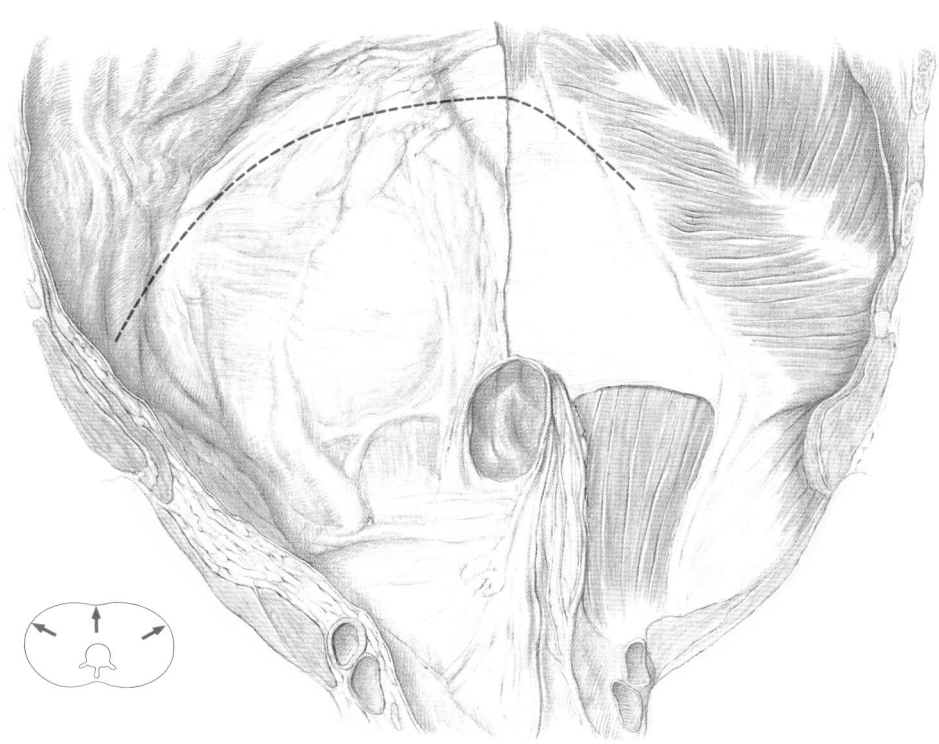

Fig. 2.**91**

Main Indications

- Tumor nephrectomy
- Adrenalectomy
- Renal trauma

Exposure of the retroperitoneal space through the abdominal route can be accomplished by the midline, the paramedian, or the anterior subcostal approach.

Position and Skin Incision

The operation is performed in a slightly hyperextended supine position.

The incision is made two fingerwidths below the costal arch. In the Kollwitz modification the incision is extended across the midline to the lateral border of the contralateral rectus muscle (Fig. 2.92).

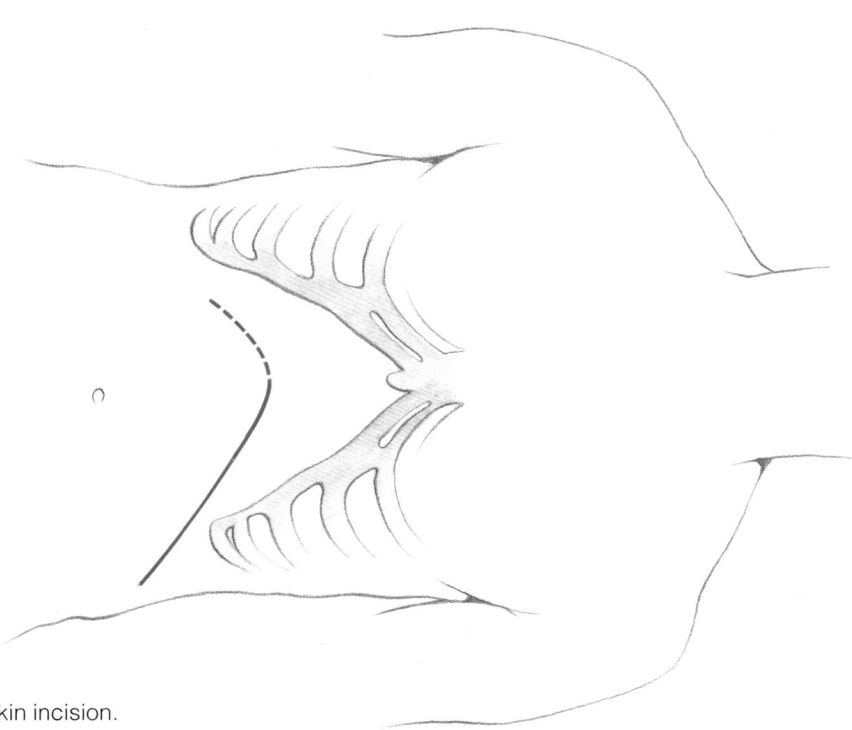

Fig. 2.**92**   Position and skin incision.

Division of the Abdominal Muscles

The subcutaneous fat is divided, and individual bleeders are coagulated. The anterior rectus sheath is transected (Fig. 2.**93**). At this point a wooden tissue protector is slipped beneath the rectus abdominis from the lateral side to the linea alba, and the muscle is divided under vision with electrocautery, simultaneously coagulating the branches of the superior epigastric artery (Fig. 2.**93**).

This incision (not shown in the figure) can be extended across the contralateral rectus muscle (Kollwitz method).

The divided rectus muscle is held aside with the anterior and posterior layers of the rectus sheath. The external oblique and then the internal oblique muscles are divided with diathermy, exposing the transversus abdominis fibers (Fig. 2.**94**).

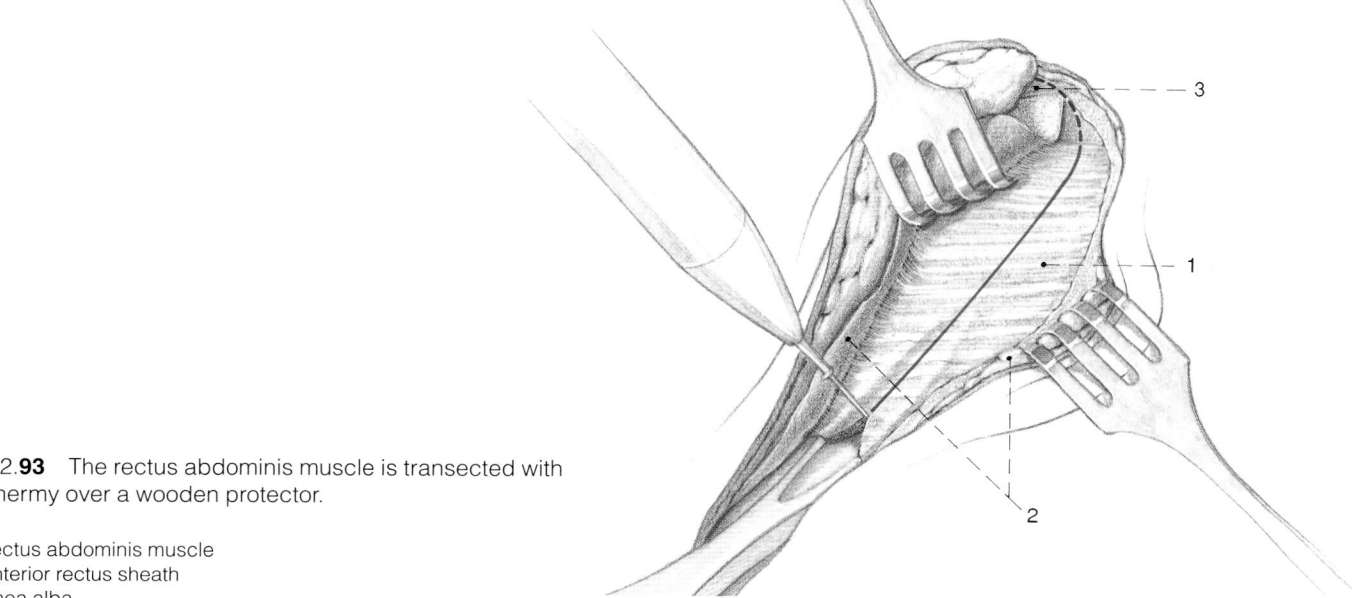

Fig. 2.**93** The rectus abdominis muscle is transected with diathermy over a wooden protector.

1 Rectus abdominis muscle
2 Anterior rectus sheath
3 Linea alba

Fig. 2.**94** The external and internal oblique muscles are divided, exposing the transversus abdominis fibers.

1 Rectus abdominis muscle
2 Anterior rectus sheath
3 Posterior rectus sheath
4 Linea alba
5 External oblique muscle
6 Internal oblique muscle
7 Transversus abdominis

Entry into the Peritoneal Cavity

After division of the transversus abdominis, the transversalis fascia and parietal peritoneum are picked up with two forceps and incised with a scalpel (Fig. 2.**95**). Following broad incision of the peritoneum, the round ligament of the liver is ligated permitting insertion of a retractor superiorly. The liver, transverse colon, and greater omentum are visible (Fig. 2.**96**).

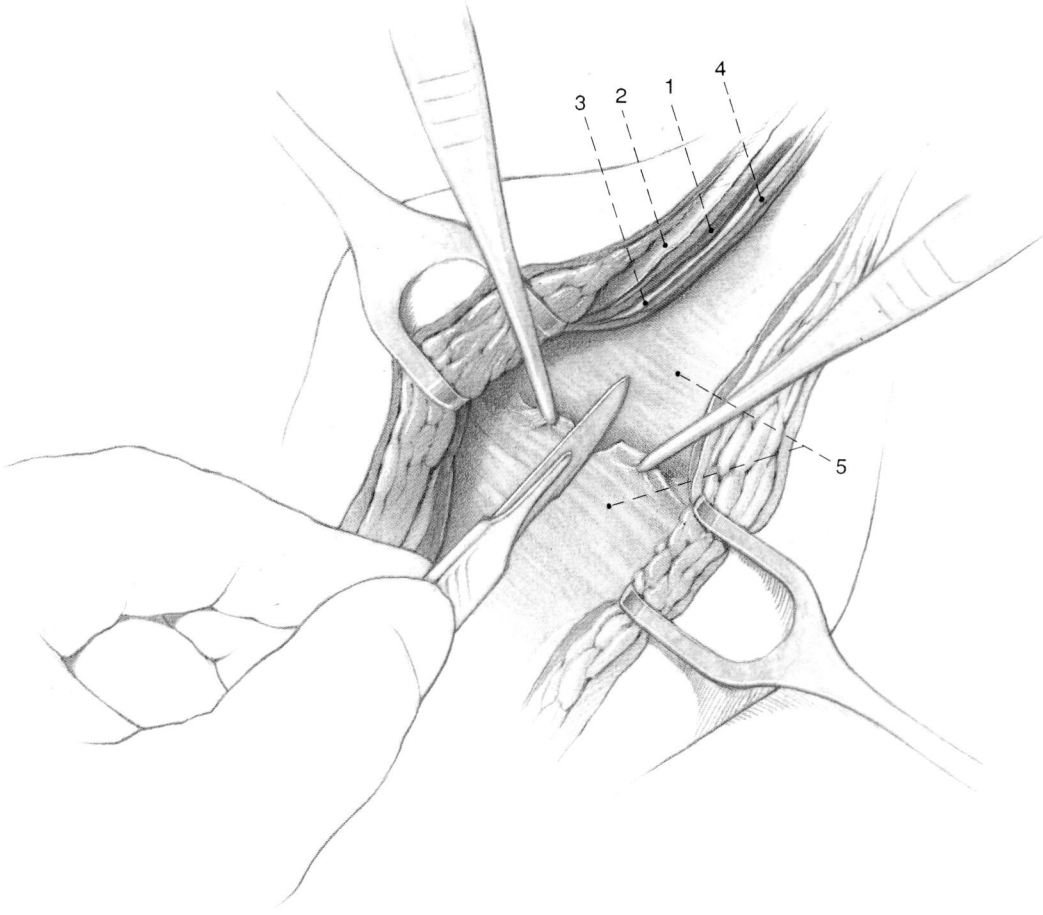

Fig. 2.**95**   Entry into the peritoneal cavity.

1 Rectus abdominis muscle
2 Anterior rectus sheath
3 Posterior rectus sheath
4 Transversus abdominis
5 Transversalis fascia and parietal peritoneum

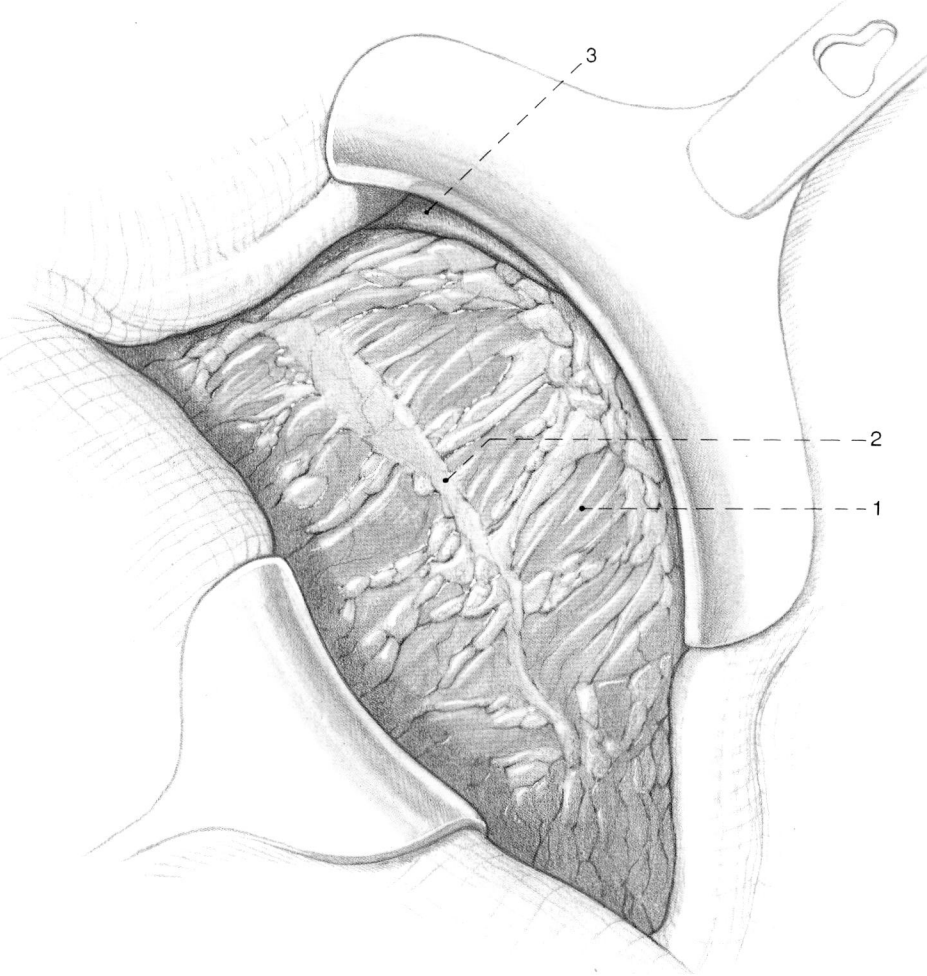

Fig. 2.**96**   A retractor is inserted superiorly.

1 Transverse colon
2 Taenia libera
3 Liver

Dissection of the Renal Vessels

For dissection of the renal vessels on the left side, the small bowel loops are packed away to the right side with Deaver retractors. The peritoneum is incised longitudinally between the aorta and inferior mesenteric vein, starting at the inferior duodenal fold (ligament of Treitz) (Fig. 2.**97**). This incision gives direct access to the vascular pedicle of the left kidney between the aorta and inferior mesenteric vein. The renal artery and vein can be dissected and snared (Figs. 2.**97**, 2. **98**).

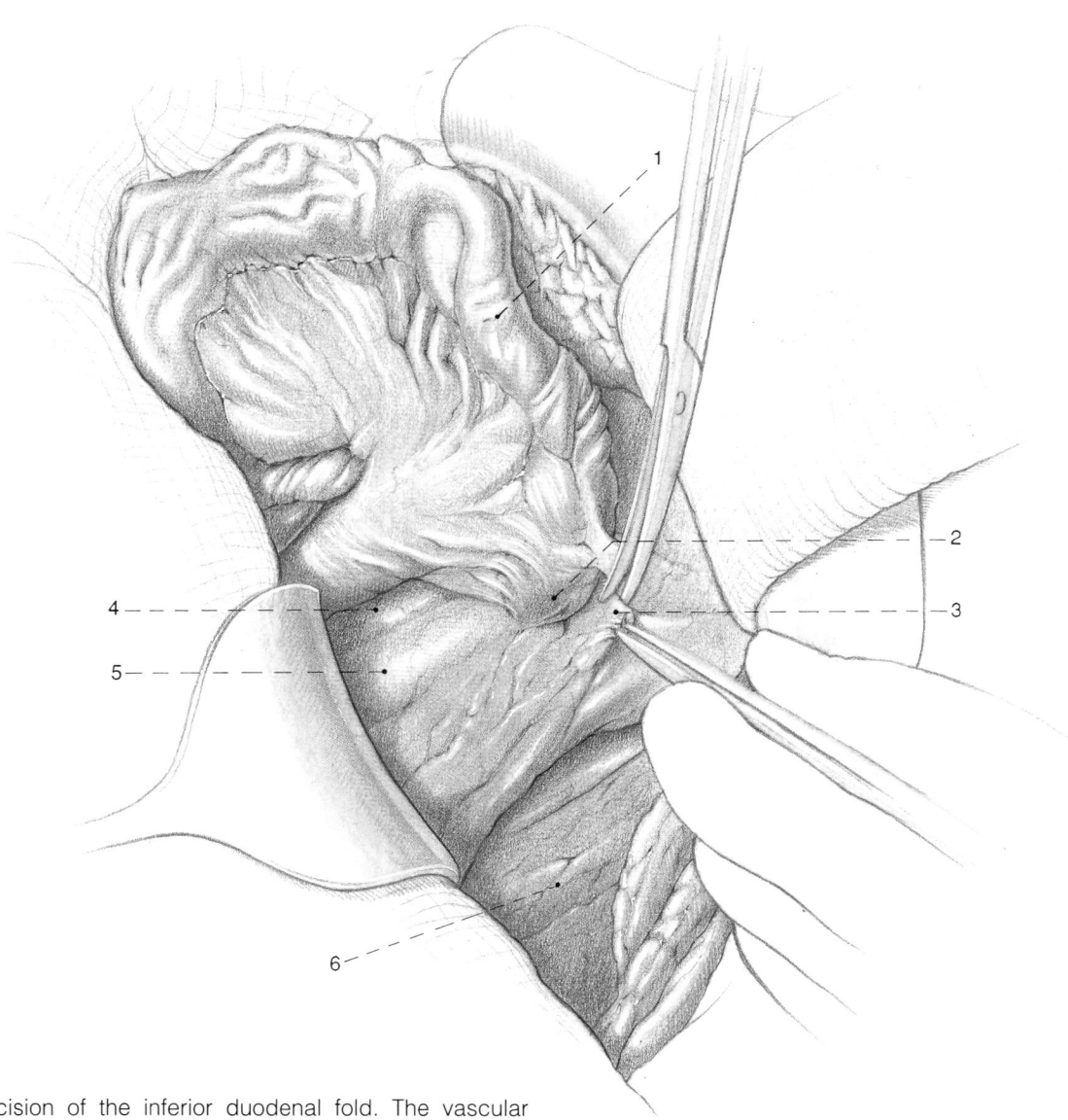

Fig. 2.**97** Incision of the inferior duodenal fold. The vascular pedicle of the kidney is approached between the aorta and inferior mesenteric vein.

1 Jejunum
2 Duodenojejunal flexure
3 Inferior duodenal fold (ligament of Treitz)
4 Inferior vena cava
5 Abdominal aorta
6 Descending colon

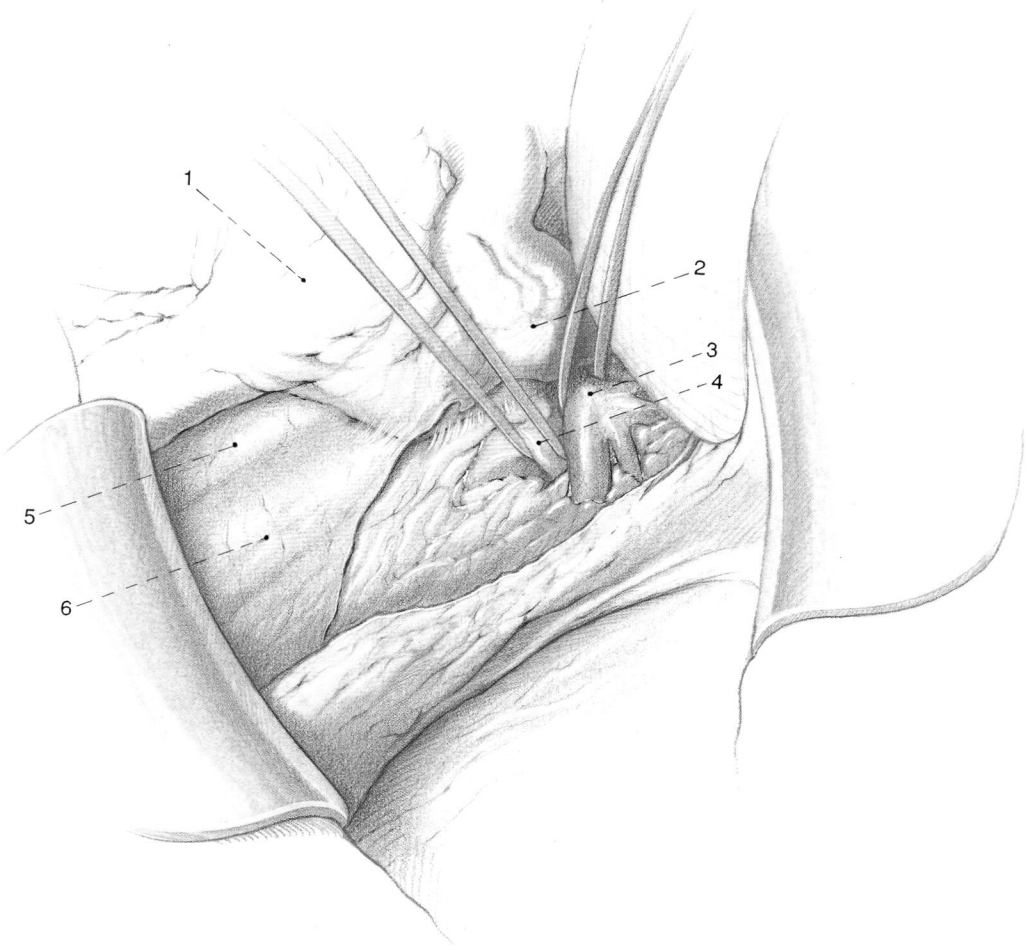

Fig. 2.**98** Exposure and isolation of the renal artery and vein.

1 Jejunum
2 Duodenojejunal flexure
3 Renal vein
4 Renal artery
5 Inferior vena cava
6 Abdominal aorta

Dissection of the Retroperitoneal Space

Incision of the left paracolic sulcus establishes access to the retroperitoneal space on the left side (Fig. 2.**99**).

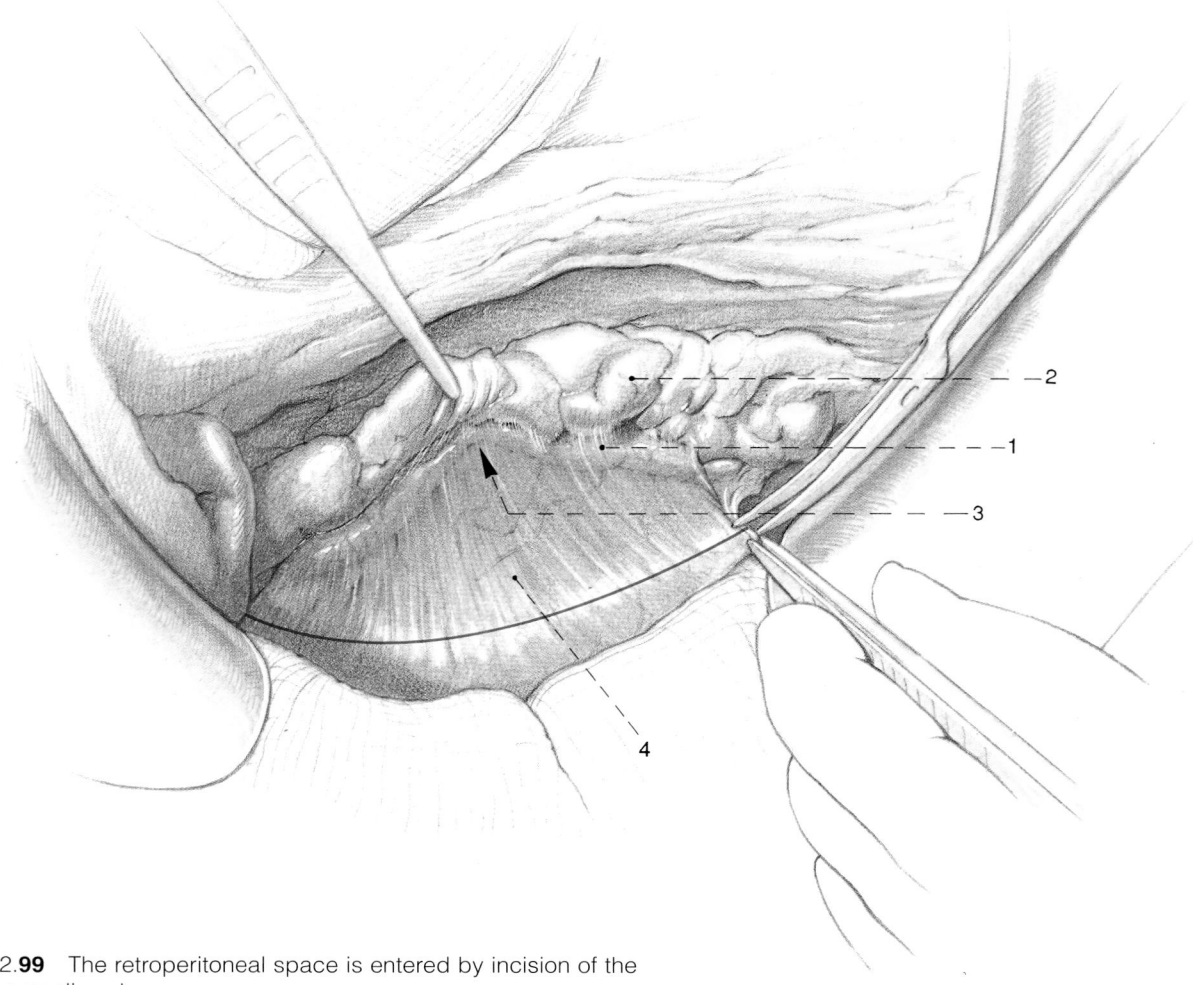

Fig. 2.**99** The retroperitoneal space is entered by incision of the left paracolic sulcus.

1 Descending colon
2 Epiploic appendices
3 Left paracolic sulcus
4 Parietal peritoneum

The descending colon and mesocolon are bluntly dissected from Gerota's fascia. The tail of the pancreas and the splenic vessels are freed up superiorly. The left colic flexure is dissected free, and the phrenicocolic ligament is isolated and divided (Fig. 2.**100**).

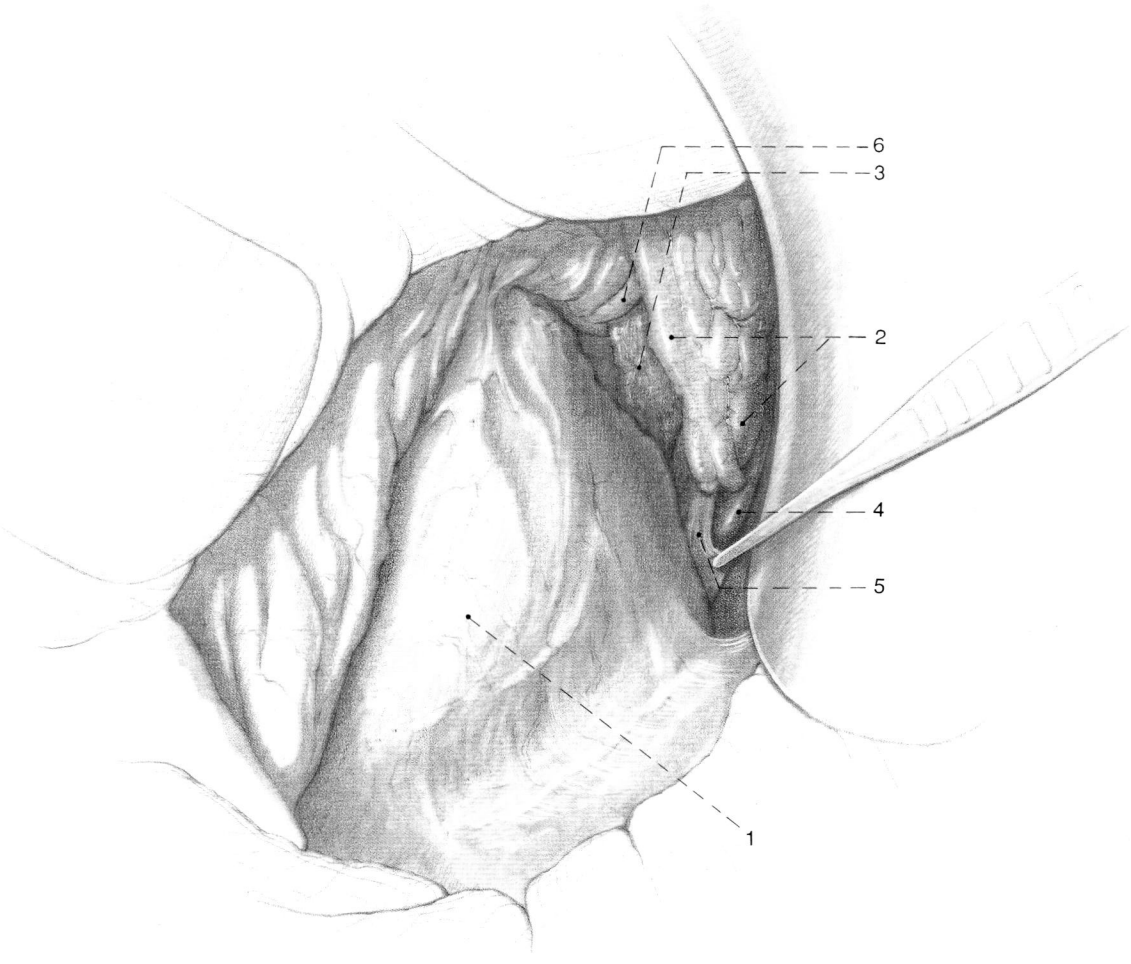

Fig. 2.**100**   Exposure of Gerota's fascia on the left side. The descending colon is dissected from the fascia with its mesentery, as are the tail of the pancreas and the splenic vessels.

1 Gerota's fascia
2 Left colic flexure
3 Tail of pancreas
4 Spleen
5 Phrenicocolic ligament
6 Splenic artery

Approach to the Adrenal Gland

The anterior subcostal approach can also provide access to the adrenal gland. Figure 2.**101** shows the isolated renal artery (swared) and vein and the snared suprarenal vein. The descending colon and part of the transverse colon are held medially with packs. The spleen and the tail of the pancreas are visible at the upper border of the field.

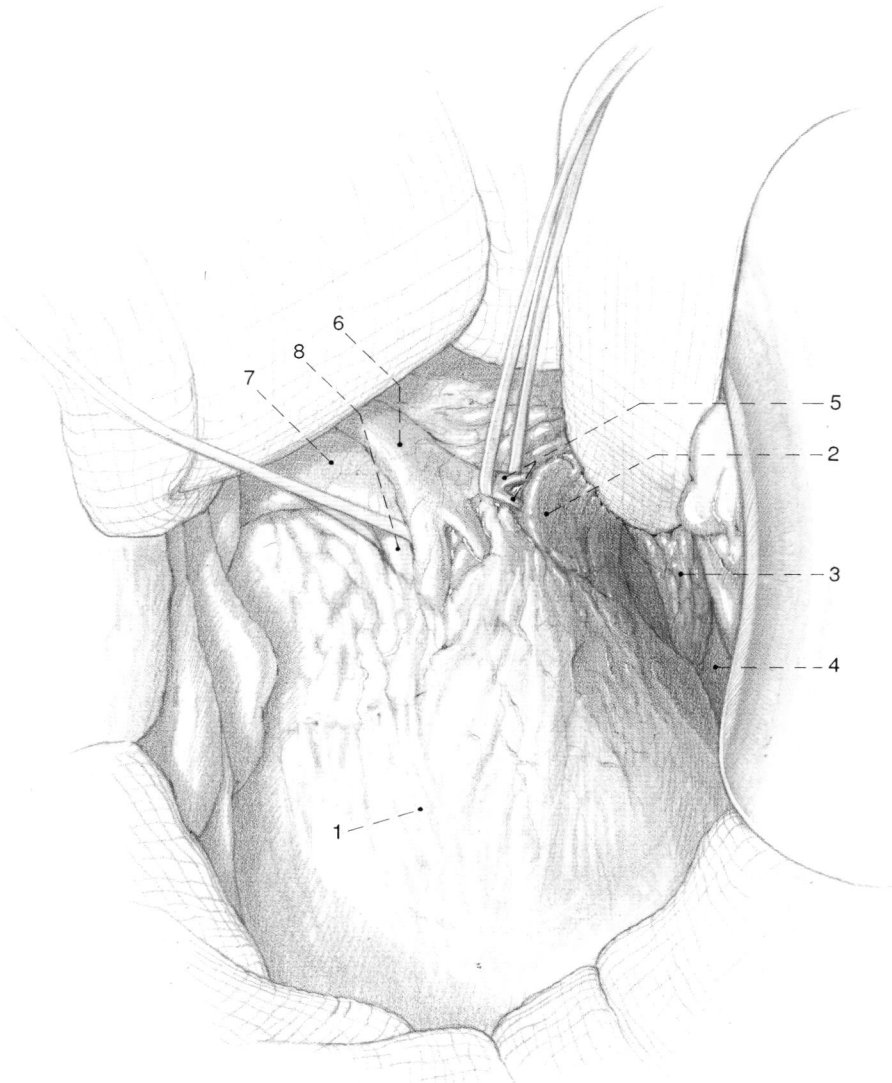

Fig. 2.**101** Access to the left adrenal gland. The suprarenal vein is snared with a tape.

1 Gerota's fascia
2 Adrenal gland
3 Tail of pancreas
4 Spleen
5 Left suprarenal vein
6 Left renal vein
7 Abdominal aorta
8 Left renal artery

Following meticulous dissection of the tail of the pancreas and splenic vessels, the entire adrenal gland can be visualized (Fig. 2.**102**). The suprarenal vein is controlled with a snare during this dissection.

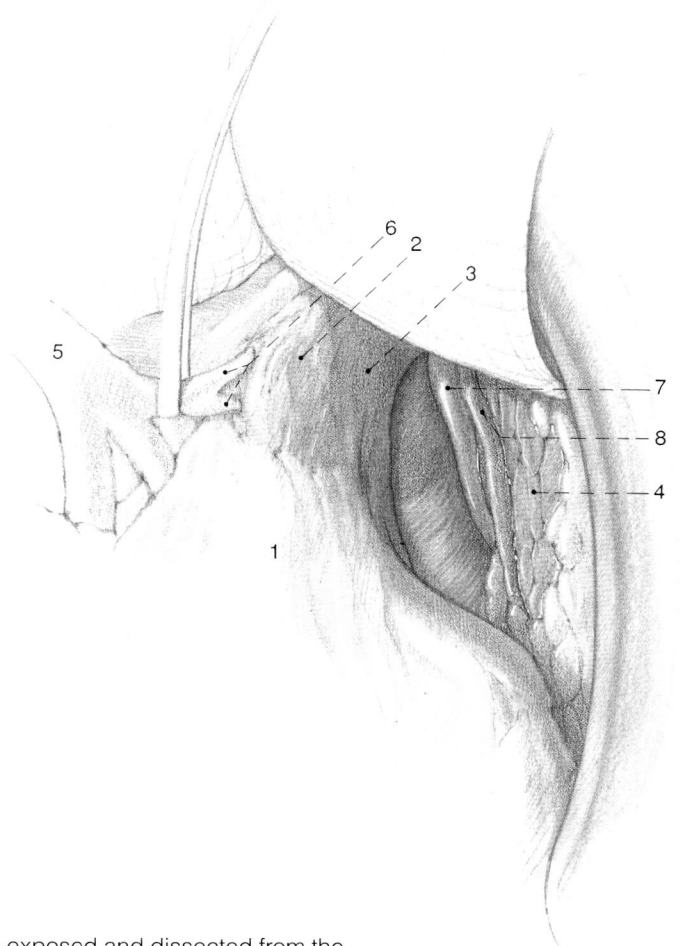

Fig. 2.**102**   The adrenal gland is exposed and dissected from the lumbar part of the diaphragm.

1 Gerota's fascia
2 Perirenal fat capsule
3 Adrenal gland
4 Tail of pancreas
5 Left renal vein
6 Left suprarenal vein
7 Splenic artery
8 Splenic vein

If a renal tumor is present, the entire contents of the left retroperitoneal space (retroperitoneal fat, kidney, adrenal gland) are removed en bloc along the abdominal aorta following ligation of the renal artery and vein.

Comments

The anterior subcostal incision can be extended to the contralateral side. The chevron incision, unlike the anterior subcostal, begins laterally at the tip of the 11th rib; it gives access to the left and right peritoneal spaces. This approach affords better exposure of the upper retroperitoneal space compared with the midline incision. The thoracoabdominal approach is preferred, however, for large renal tumors or when there is involvement of the vena cava by tumor thrombus. The chevron incision can be converted to a thoracoabdominal approach by adding a sternotomy at the midline or a lateral intercostal incision starting at the tip of the 11th rib.

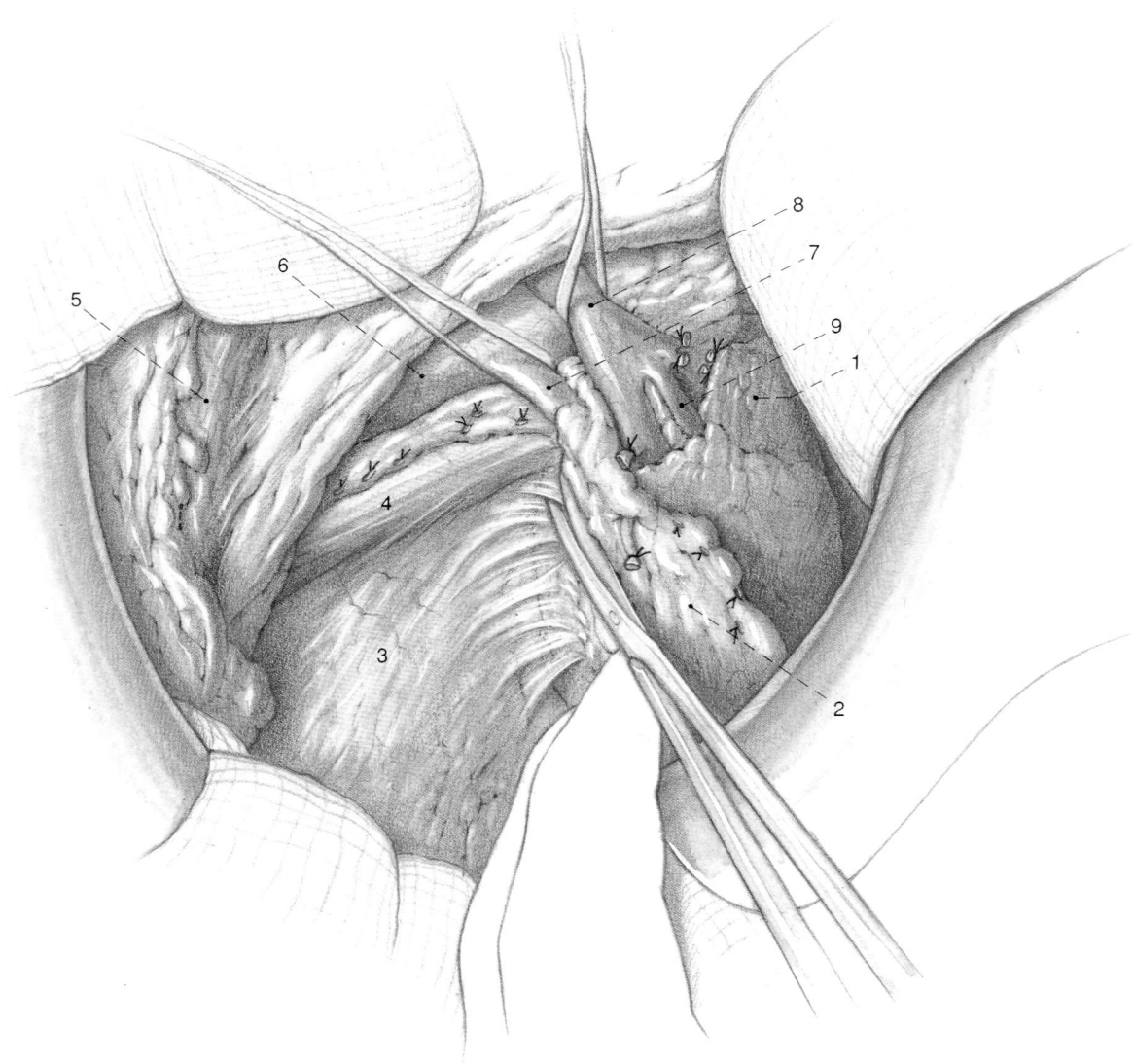

Fig. 2.**103** The entire contents of the left retroperitoneal space are removed following ligation of the left renal artery and vein.

1 Adrenal gland
2 Perirenal fat capsule
3 Renal fibrous capsule
4 Psoas major
5 Descending colon
6 Abdominal aorta
7 Renal artery
8 Renal vein
9 Suprarenal vein

Midline Transperitoneal Approach

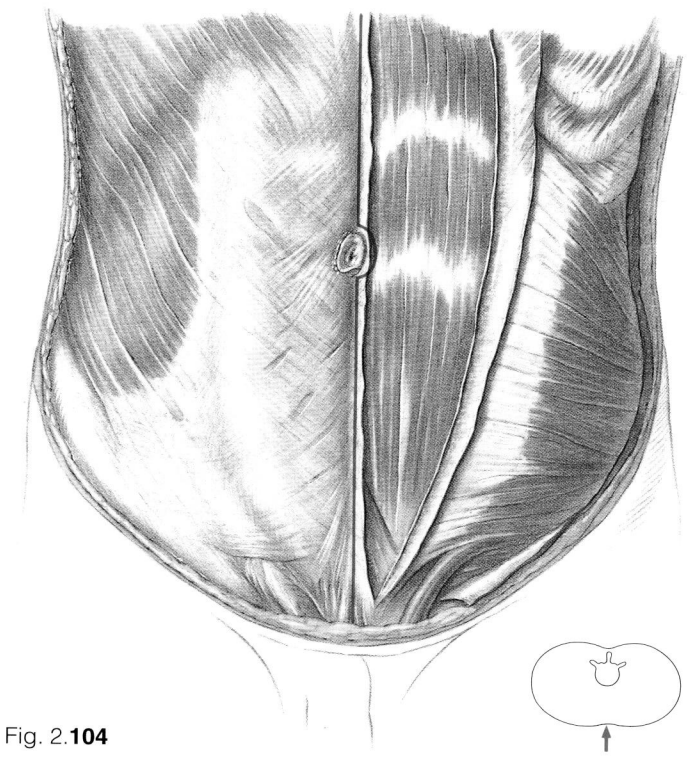

Fig. 2.**104**

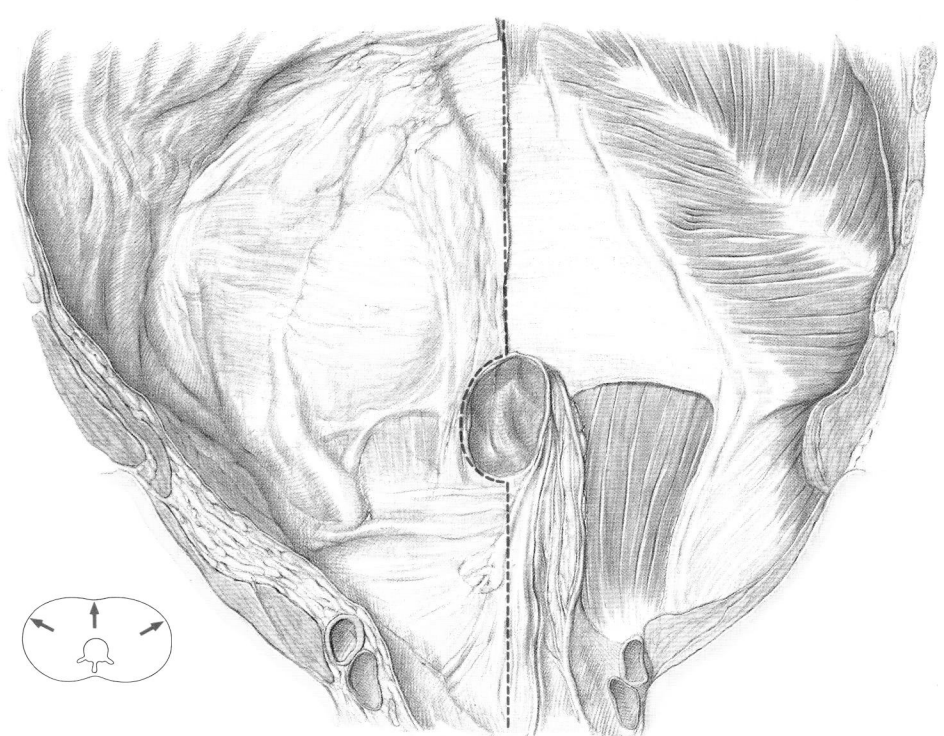

Main Indications

- Renal tumor
- Retroperitoneal fibrosis
- Horseshoe kidney
- Ectopic kidney
- Retroperitoneal lymph node dissection
- Renal trauma

This approach permits broad exposure of the retroperitoneal space. It is illustrated for a retroperitoneal lymph node dissection.

Position and Skin Incision

The patient is positioned supine with slight hyperextension of the operative area. The incision extends from the xiphoid to the pubic symphysis (Fig. 2.**105**).

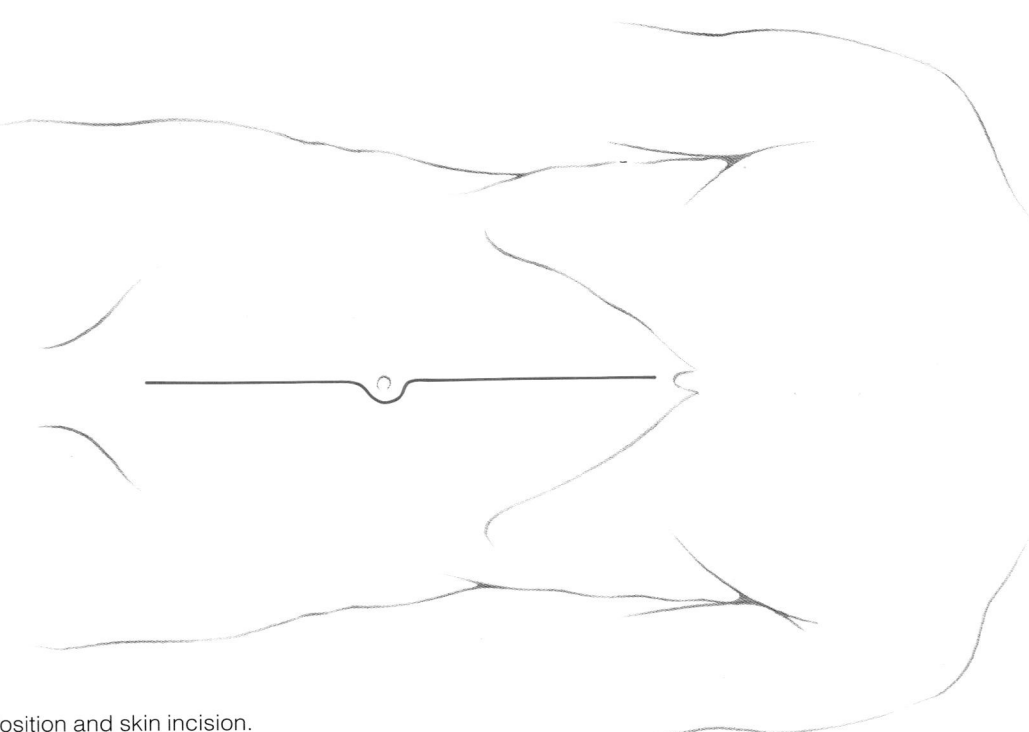

Fig. 2.**105**   Position and skin incision.

Exposure of the Posterior Rectus Sheath

After division of the subcutaneous fat, the anterior layer of the rectus sheath is incised at the linea alba (Fig. 2.**106**).

The wound is held open with retractors. The anterior rectus sheath is divided, and both rectus muscles are separated exposing the posterior rectus sheath (Fig. 2.**107**). The inferior epigastric vessels can be visualized. The posterior layer of the rectus sheath is formed by the transversalis fascia caudal to the arcuate line (Fig. 2.**107**).

Fig. 2.**107**   Exposure of the posterior rectus sheath, arcuate line, ▶
and transversalis fascia.

1 Anterior rectus sheath
2 Rectus muscle
3 Posterior rectus sheath
4 Arcuate line
5 Transversalis fascia
6 Inferior epigastric vessels

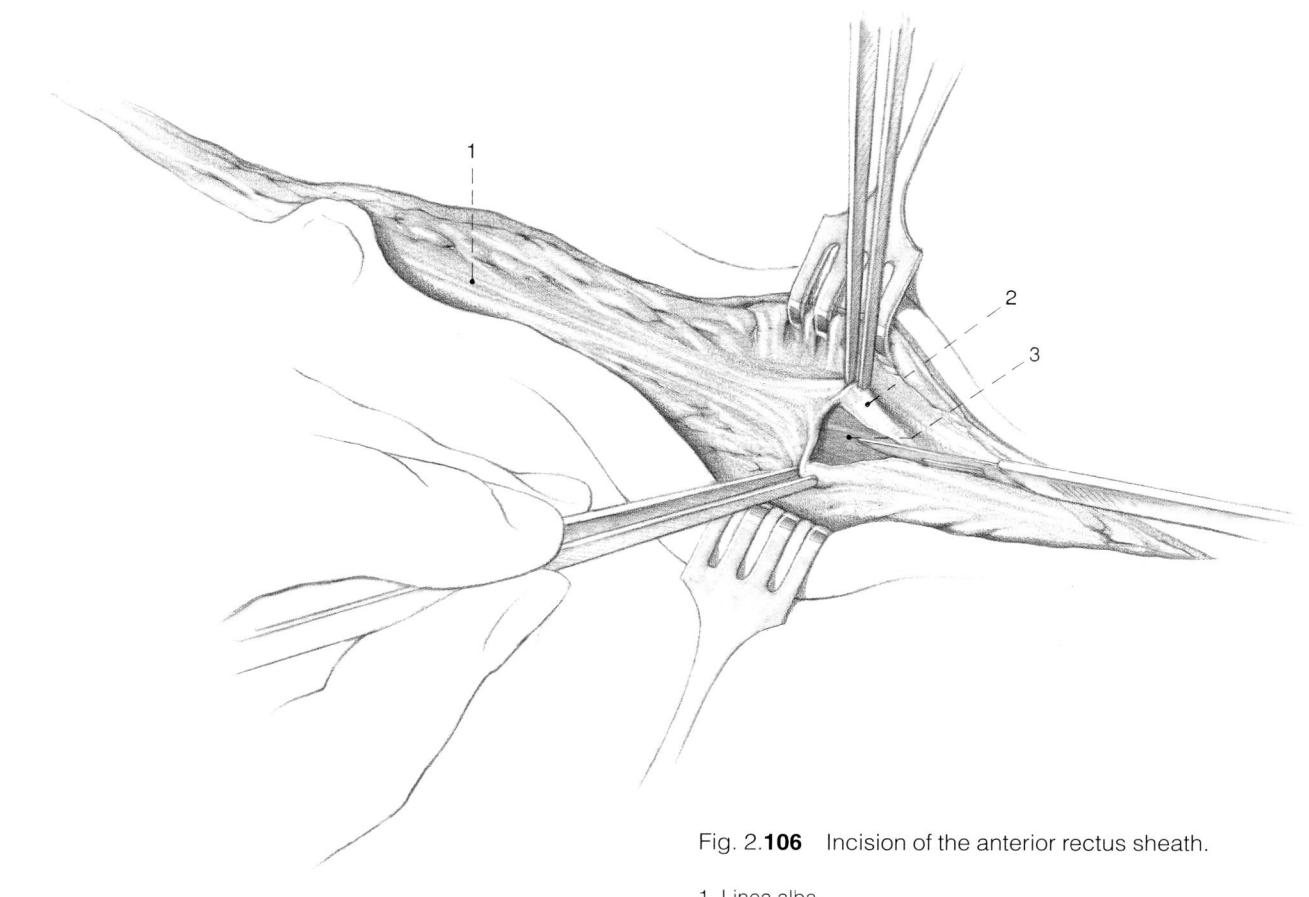

Fig. 2.**106** Incision of the anterior rectus sheath.

1 Linea alba
2 Anterior rectus sheath
3 Rectus abdominis muscle

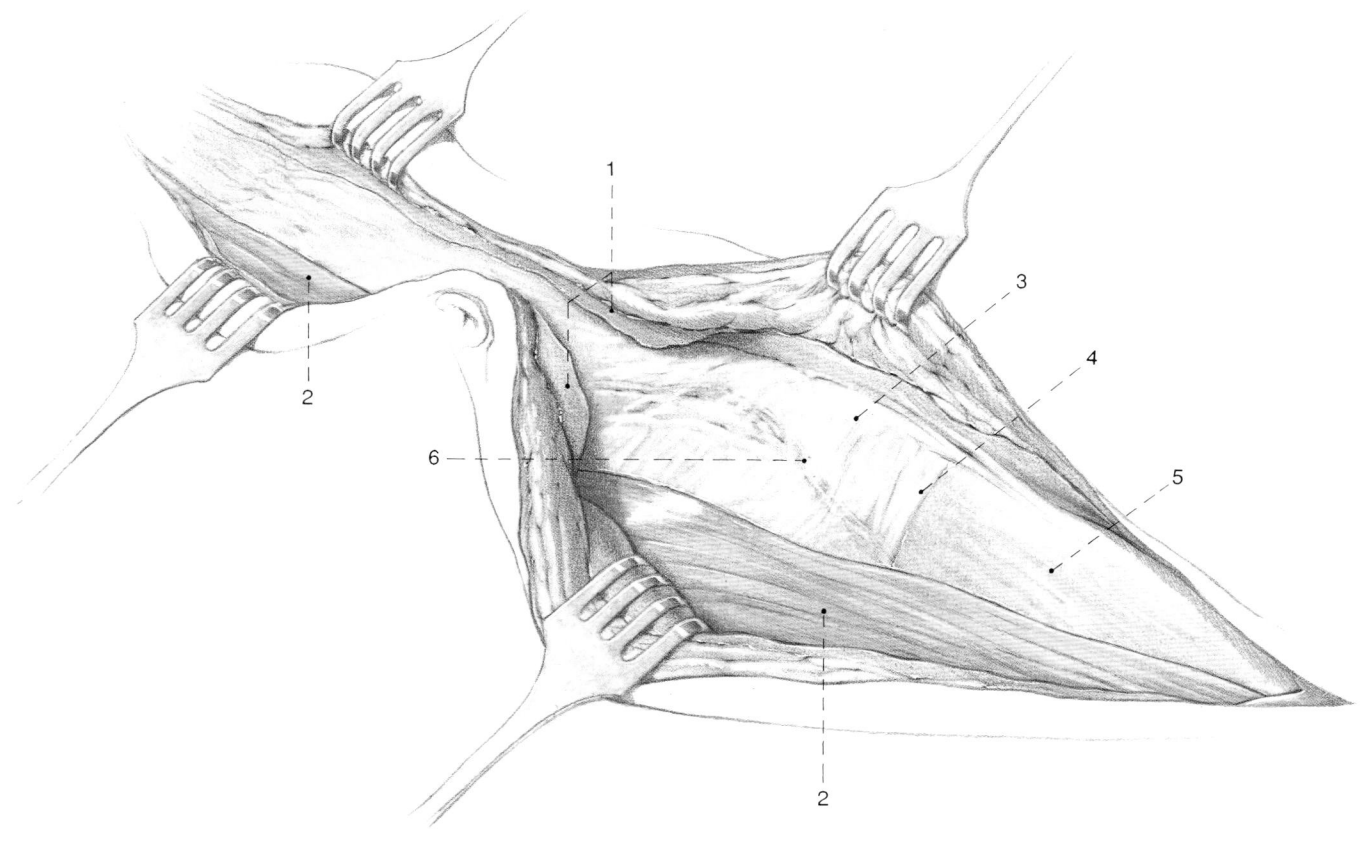

Entry into the Peritoneal Cavity

At the level of the umbilicus the posterior rectus sheath, pre-peritoneal fat, and parietal peritoneum are picked up with two forceps, and all three layers are incised with a scalpel to gain entry to the peritoneal cavity (Fig. 2.**108**).

After division of the ligamentum teres, a retractor is inserted at the upper midline, and a self-retaining chest retractor is positioned centrally to expose the liver, stomach, transverse colon, gastrocolic ligament, and greater omentum (Fig. 2.**109**).

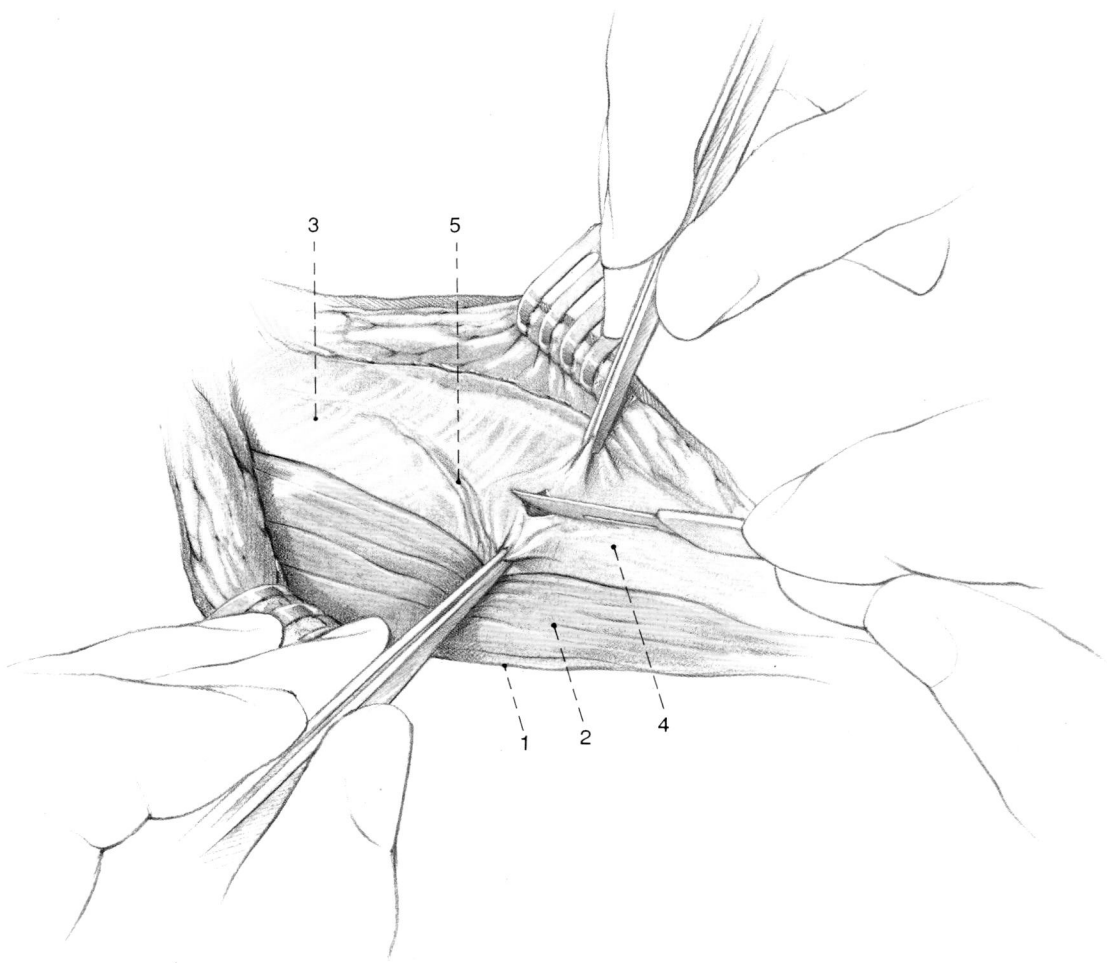

Fig. 2.**108**   Entry into the peritoneal cavity.

1 Anterior rectus sheath
2 Rectus muscle
3 Posterior rectus sheath
4 Transversalis fascia and parietal peritoneum
5 Inferior epigastric vessels

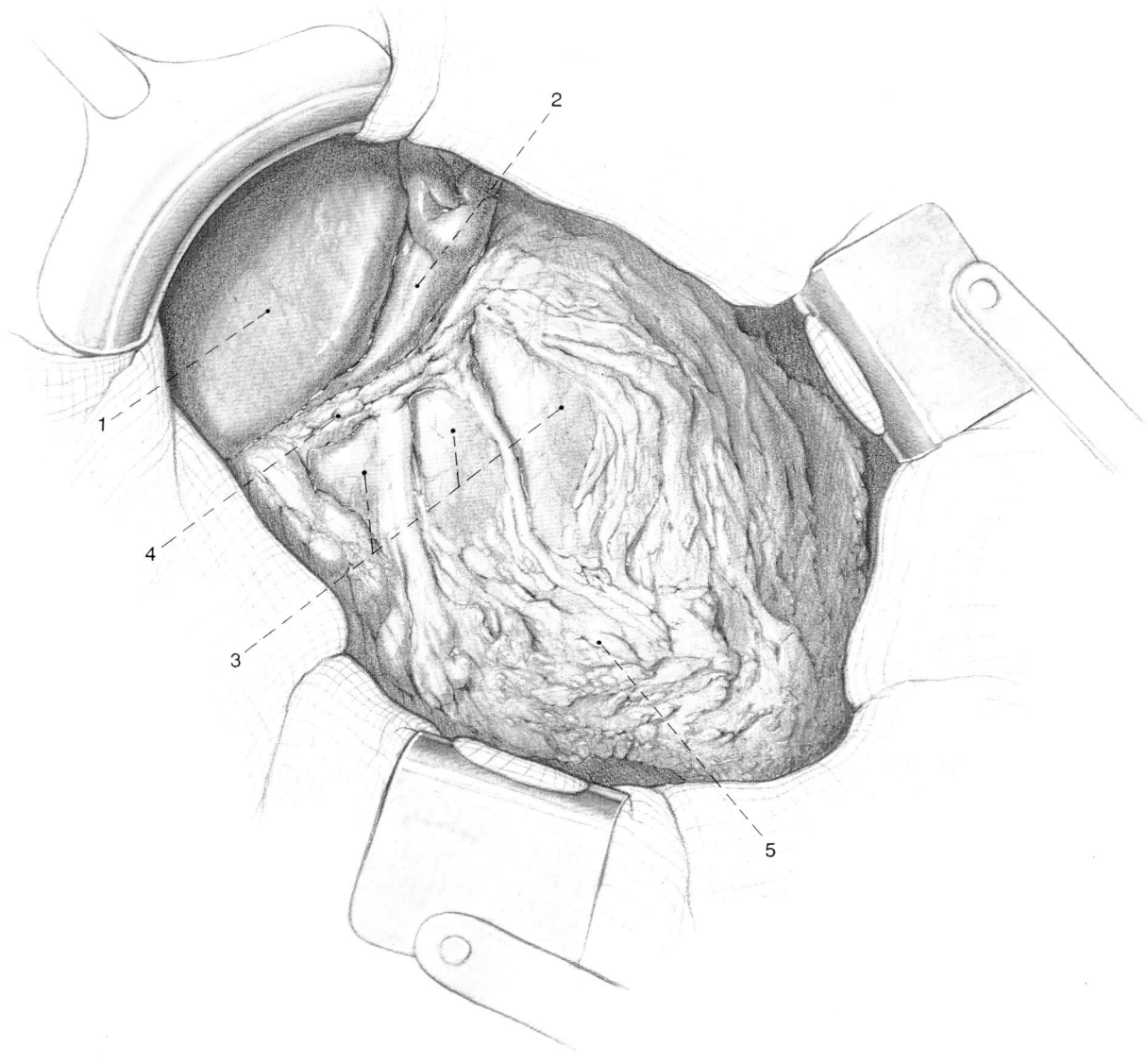

Fig. 2.**109**   Exposure is maintained with a superiorly placed
Rochard retractor and a more centrally placed chest retractor.

1 Liver
2 Stomach
3 Transverse colon
4 Gastrocolic ligament
5 Greater omentum

Exposure of the Retroperitoneal Space

Starting at the inferior duodenojejunal fold, the retroperitoneal space is opened by incising distally along the root of the mesentery while the small bowel is packed away to the right side and the descending colon and left colic flexure are retracted to the left side with Deaver retractors (Fig. 2.**110**).

Next the ascending part of the duodenum is dissected free along the line of the incision. For a suprahilar approach on the left side, the incision in the parietal peritoneum is extended further upward and to the left so that the inferior mesenteric vein can be dissected and ligated (Figs. 2.**111**, 2.**112**). This establishes broad access for the suprahilar lymph node dissection.

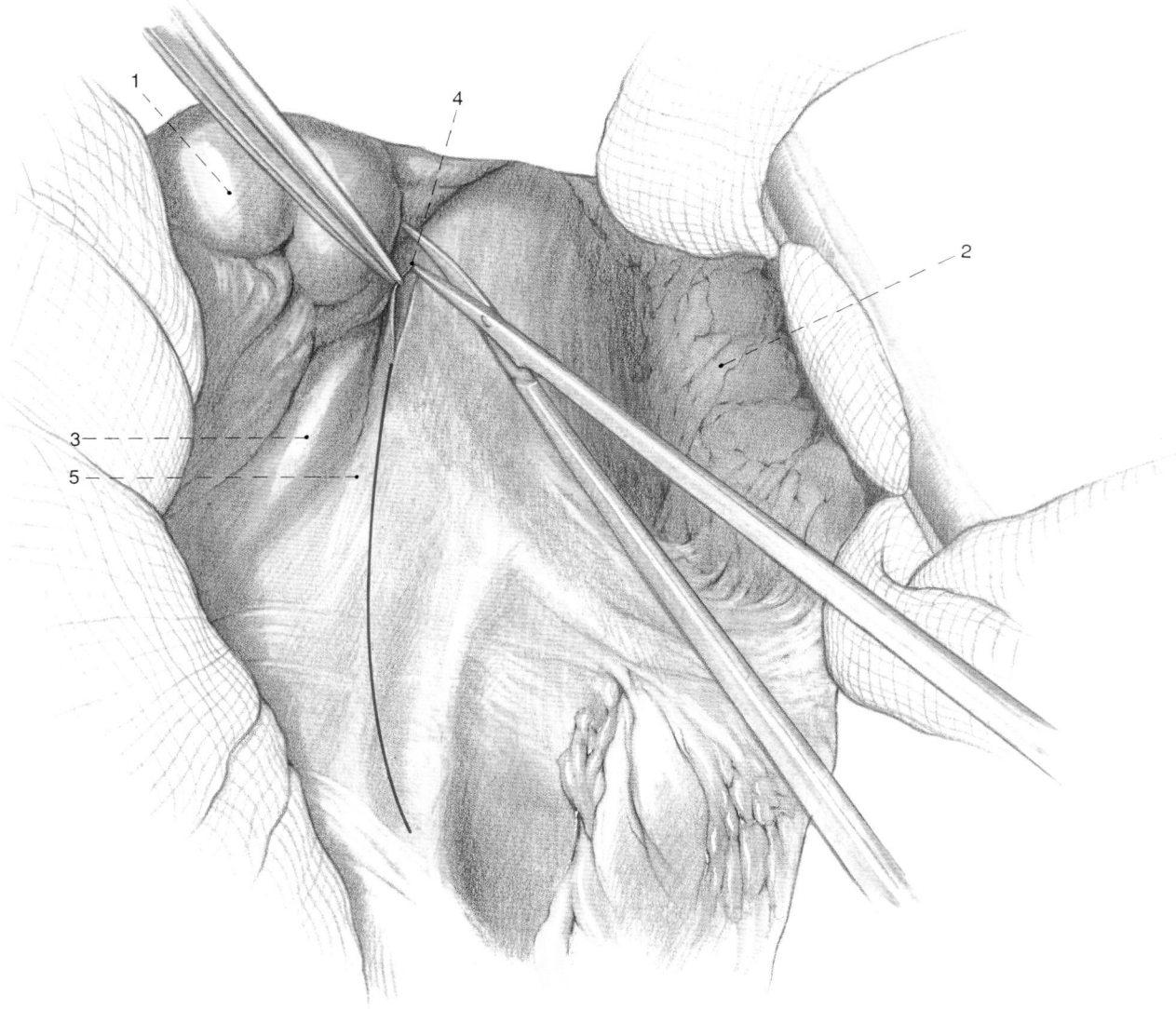

Fig. 2.**110**   The retroperitoneal space is opened along the root of the mesentery, starting at the inferior duodenojejunal fold.

1 Transverse colon
2 Sigmoid colon
3 Ascending part of duodenum
4 Inferior duodenojejunal fold
5 Root of mesentery

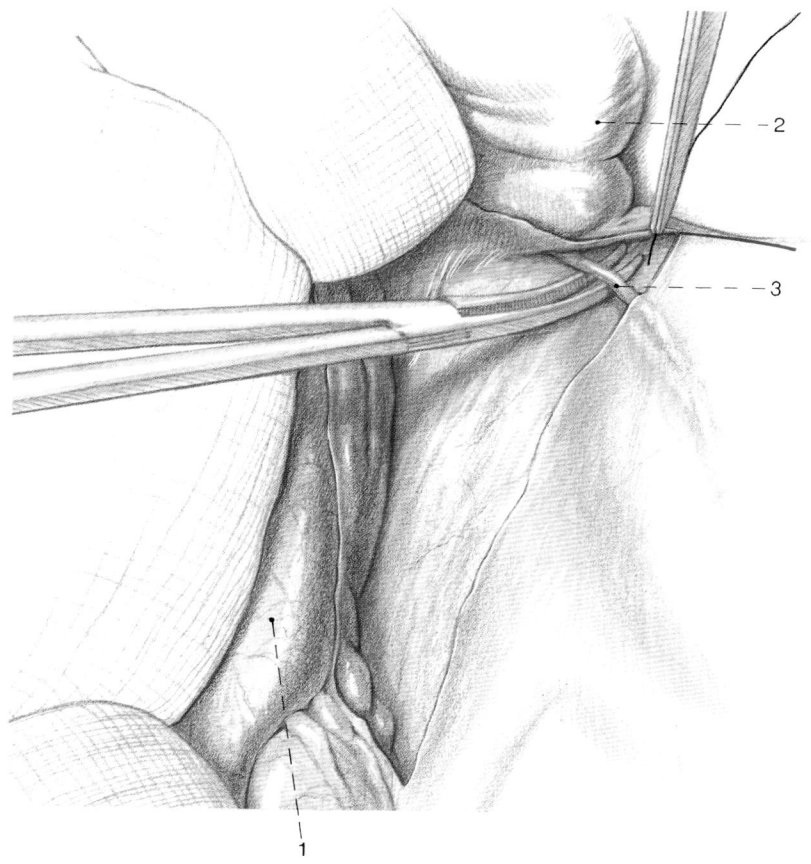

Fig. 2.**111**   Left suprahilar approach. The inferior mesenteric vein is exposed and ligated.

1 Ascending part of duodenum
2 Transverse colon
3 Inferior mesenteric vein

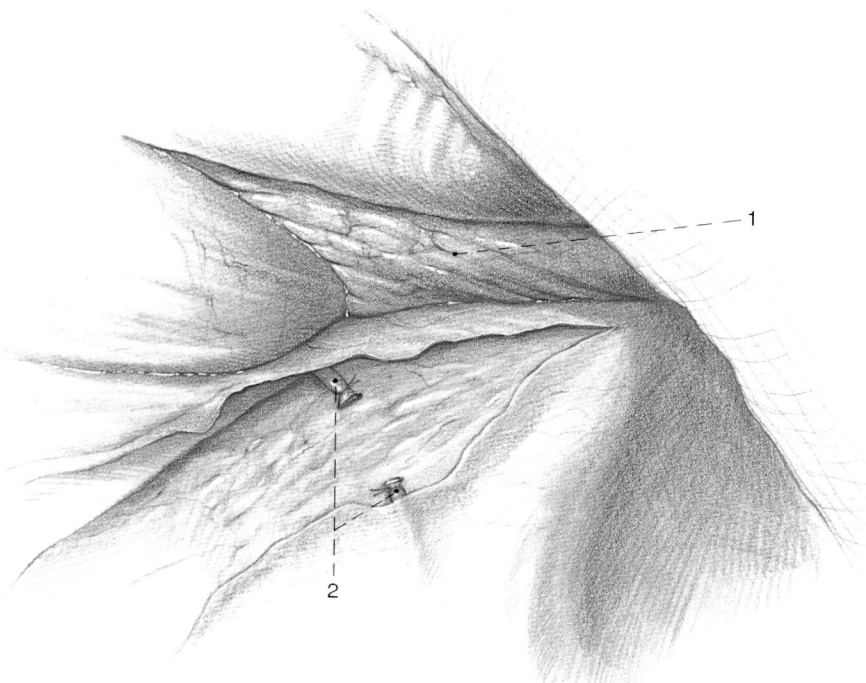

Fig. 2.**112**   Ligation of the inferior mesenteric vein.

1 Pancreas
2 Inferior mesenteric vein

The line of incision is now extended further toward the right common iliac artery from the abdominal aorta so that the cecum can be dissected from the underlying retroperitoneal connective tissue (Fig. 2.**113**).

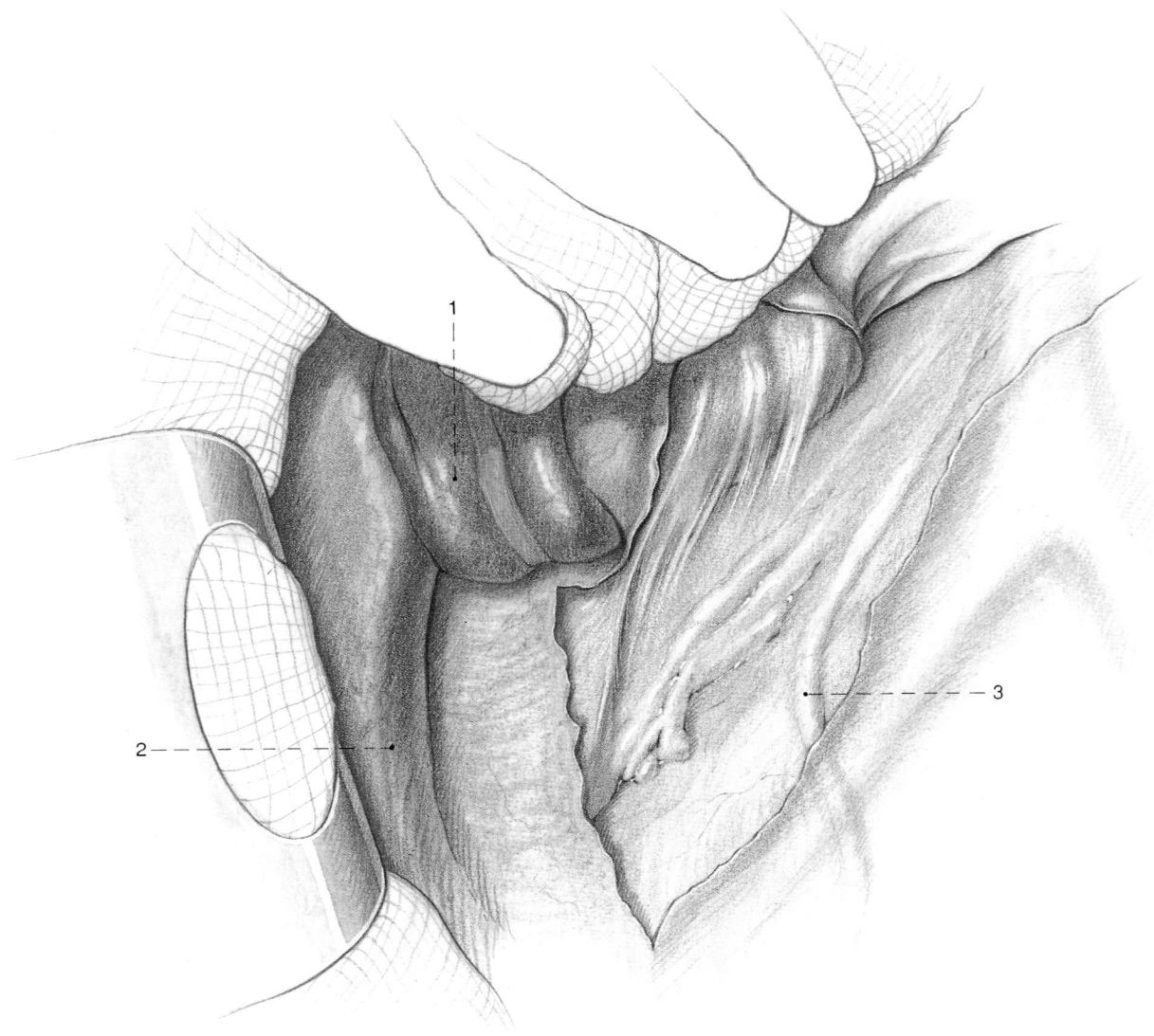

Fig. 2.**113**   The incision is extended from the abdominal aorta over the right common iliac artery.

1 Transverse colon
2 Ascending colon
3 Right ureter

The extended incision runs along the right paracolic sulcus and ends at the inferior border of the epiploic foramen (of Winslow) (Fig. 2.**114**). This provides access for dissecting the ascending colon and right colic flexure from Gerota's fascia (Fig. 2.**114**).

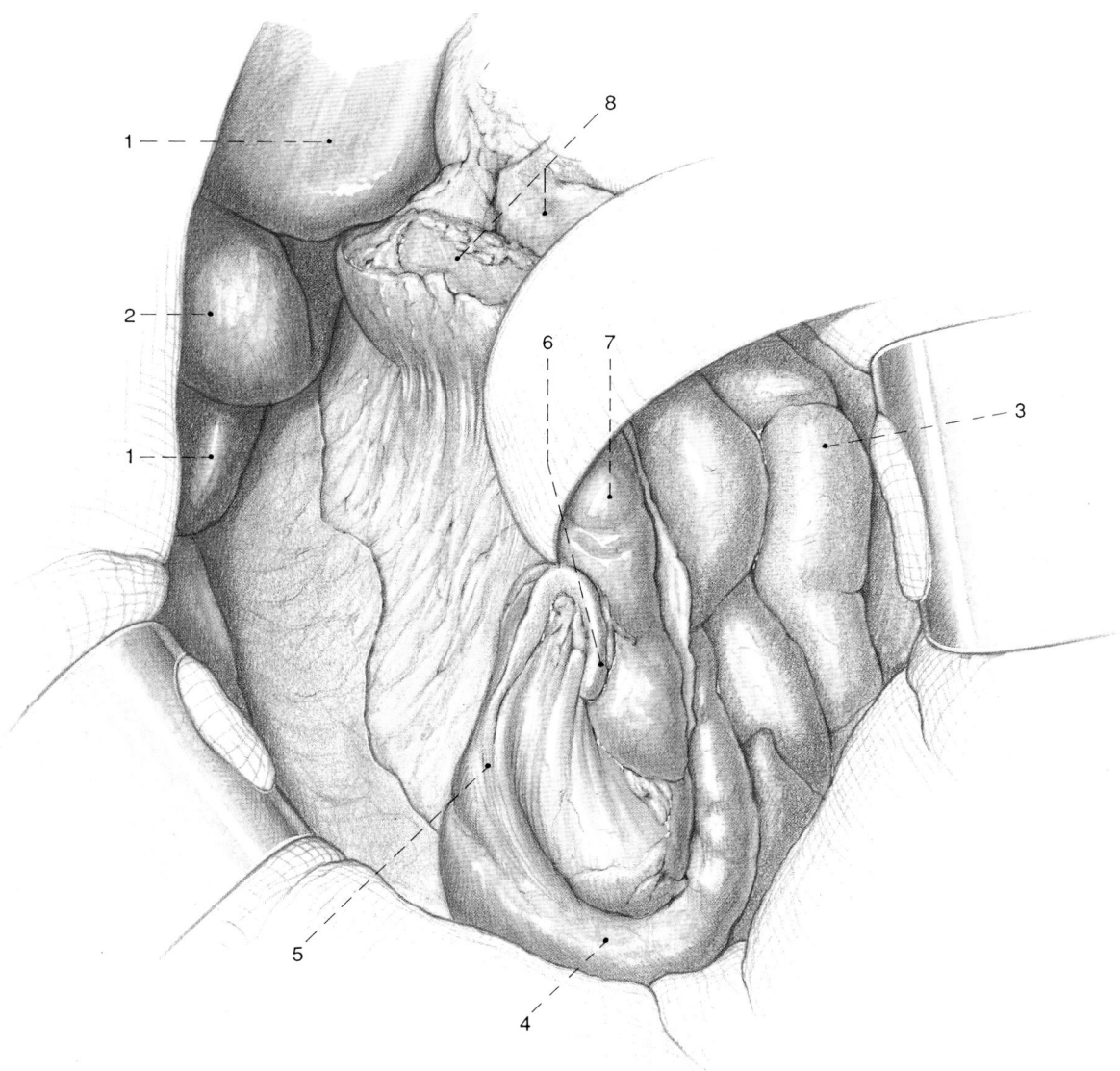

Fig. 2.**114**   The incision in the right paracolic sulcus is extended to the inferior border of the epiploic foramen.

1 Liver
2 Gallbladder
3 Jejunum
4 Terminal ileum
5 Cecum
6 Vermiform appendix
7 Ascending colon
8 Right colic flexure

This extended incision (from the inferior duodenojejunal fold to the epiploic foramen) permits the entire small bowel, cecum, ascending colon, and right colic flexure to be mobilized (and if necessary exteriorized from the abdominal cavity) (Fig. 2.**115**). The abdominal aorta and inferior vena cava are visible below fibrous and fatty tissues, respectively, at the center of the retroperitoneal space (Fig. 2.**116**).

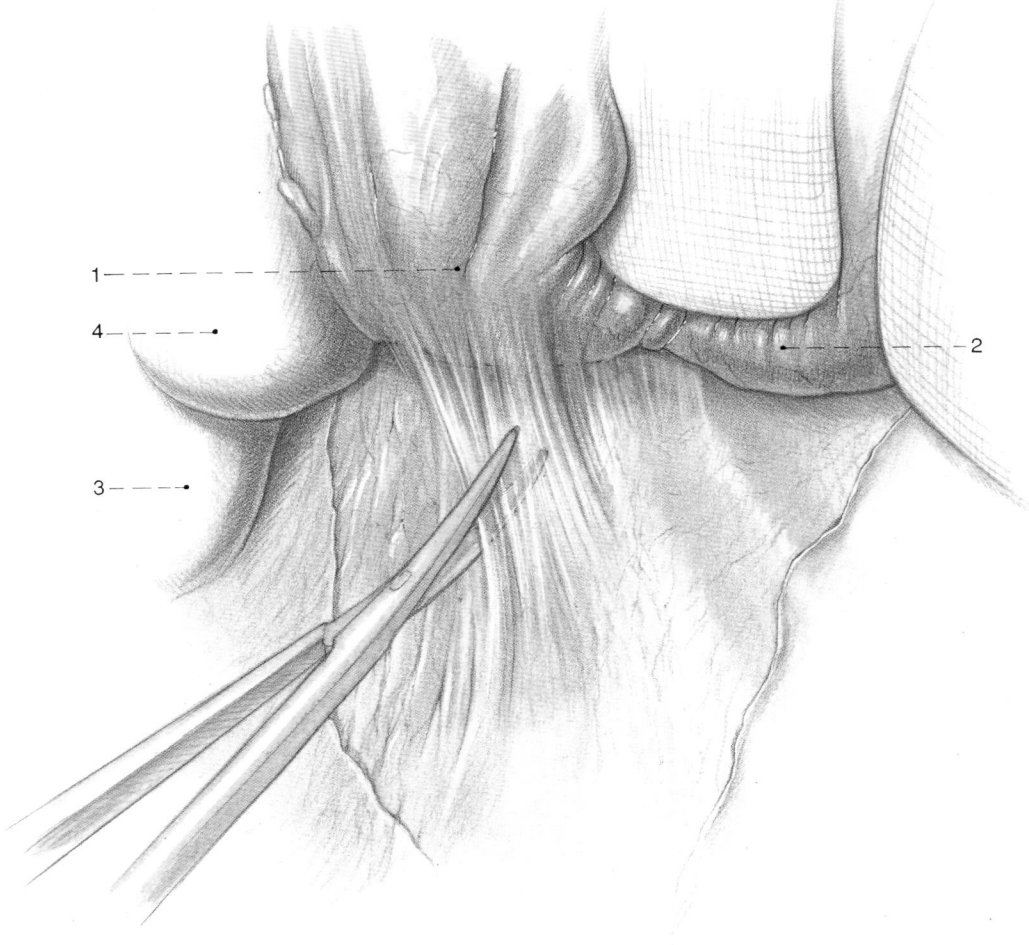

Fig. 2.**115** The ascending colon is freed from the connective tissue in the retroperitoneal space.

1 Ascending colon
2 Horizontal part of duodenum
3 Liver
4 Gallbladder

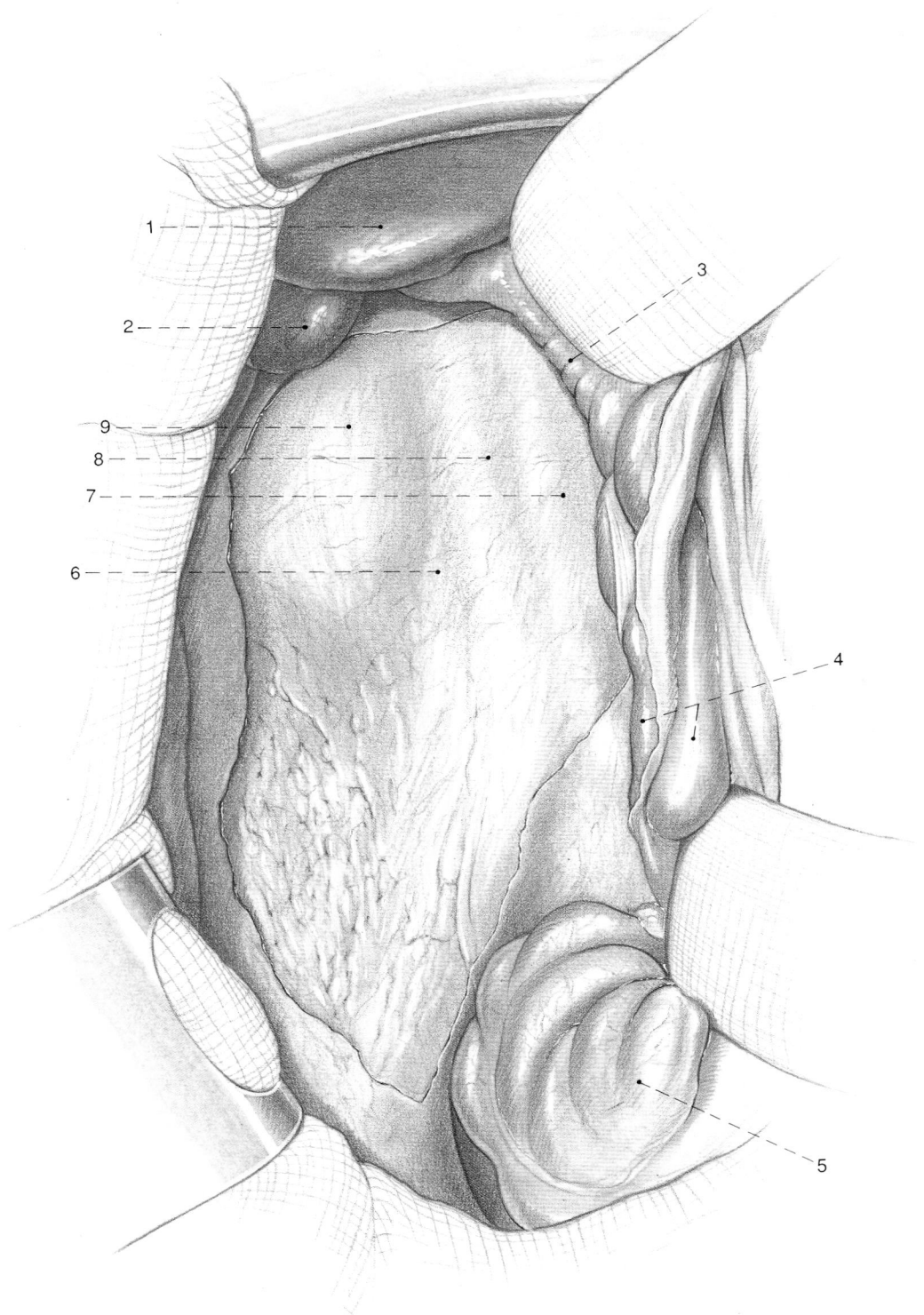

Fig. 2.**116**   View of the incision from the ligament of Treitz to the inferior border of the epiploic foramen. The entire retroperitoneal space is visible.

1 Liver
2 Gallbladder
3 Descending part of duodenum
4 Ascending colon
5 Cecum
6 Gerota's fascia
7 Abdominal aorta
8 Inferior vena cava
9 Right kidney

Approach for a Suprahilar Lymph Node Dissection on the Right Side

For a suprahilar lymph node dissection on the right side, the approach is made below the hepatoduodenal ligament. The ligament is dissected free and snared to expose the suprahilar portion of the vena cava (Fig. 2.**117**).

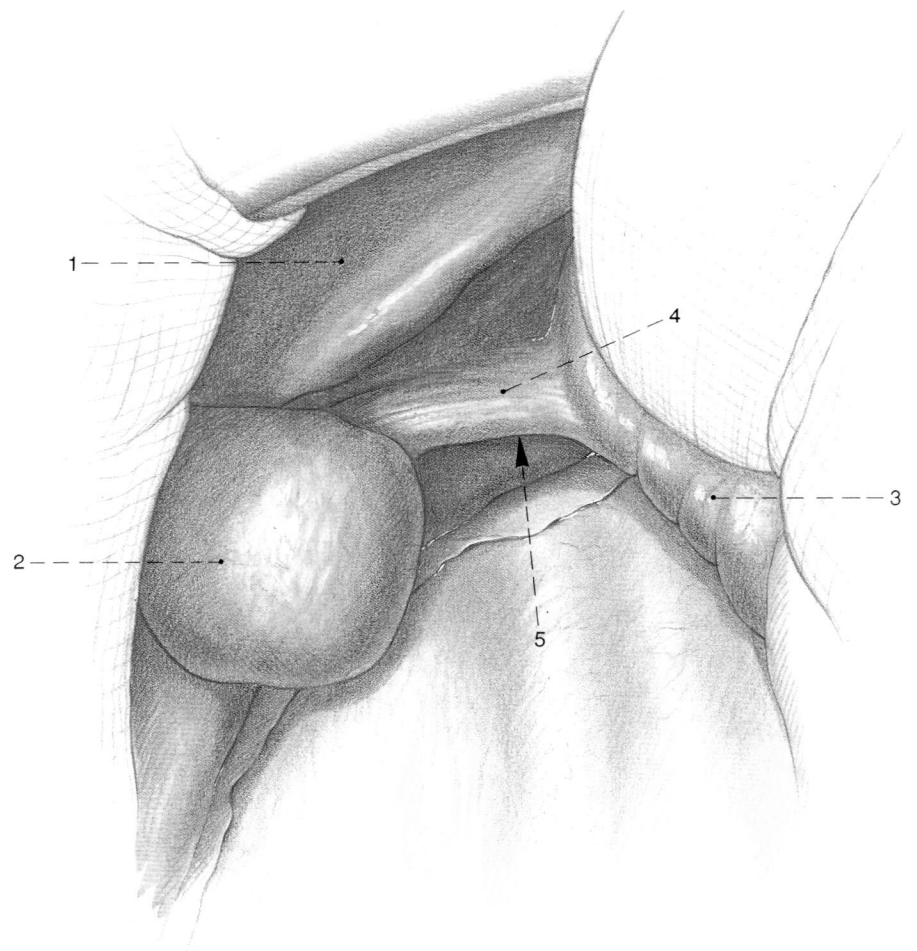

Fig. 2.**117**   Approach for a right suprahilar lymph node dissection.

1 Liver
2 Gallbladder
3 Descending part of duodenum
4 Hepatoduodenal ligament
5 Epiploic foramen

Incision of the Retroperitoneal Fascia

The fibrous and fatty tissues overlying the center of the vena cava and abdominal aorta is now opened (Fig. 2.**118**), and the lymph node dissection is carried out using a split-and-roll technique (Fig. 2.**119**).

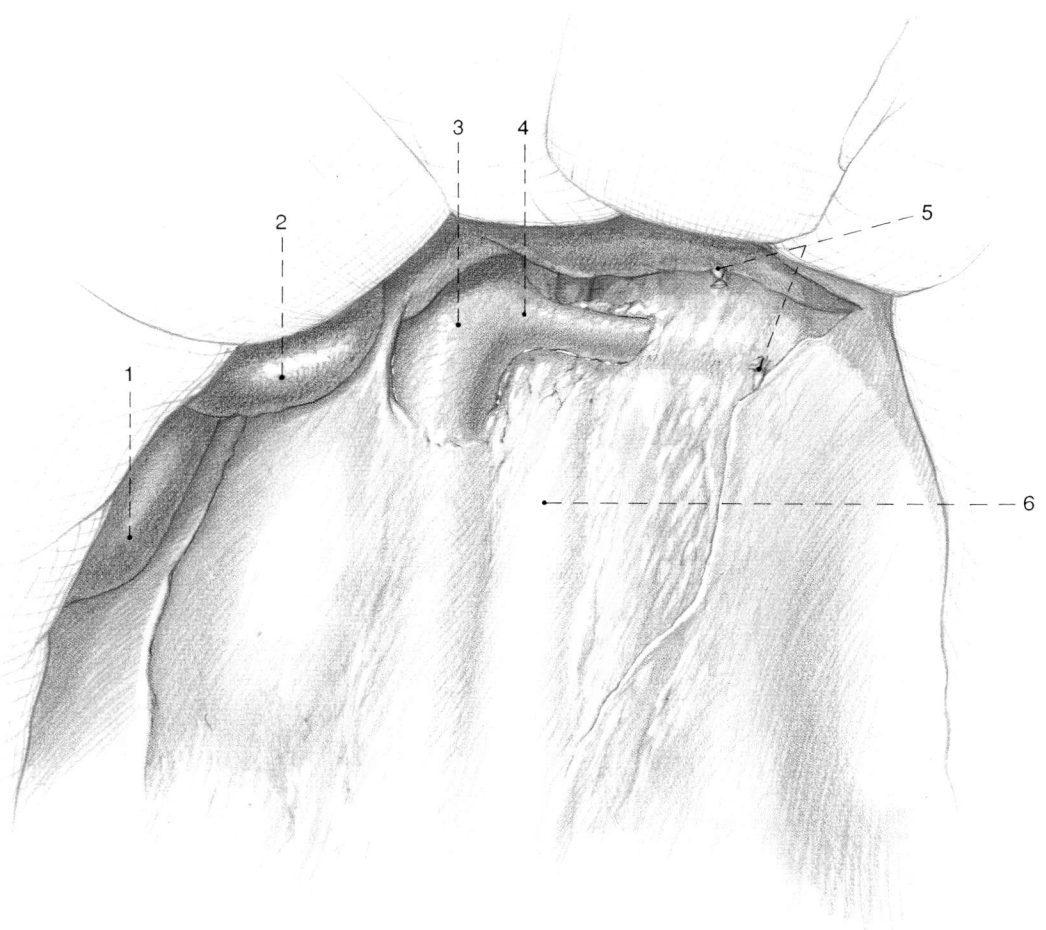

Fig. 2.**118**   The fibrous and fatty tissue covering the vena cava is opened.

1 Liver
2 Gallbladder
3 Inferior vena cava
4 Left renal vein
5 Inferior mesenteric vein
6 Abdominal aorta

Comments

This approach, especially the incision from the inferior duodenojejunal fold to the epiploic foramen, permits mobilization of the small bowel, cecum, ascending colon, and right colic flexure, allowing complete visualization of the retroperitoneal space. On the left side, the superior mesenteric artery and thus the left suprahilar retroperitoneal space can be exposed following ligation of the inferior mesenteric vein and dissection of the renal vein. The right suprahilar space is reached following exposure of the epiploic foramen.

In the modified form of the nerve-sparing lymph node dissection, it is sufficient in left-sided stage I cases to incise the inferior duodenojejunal fold as far as the right common iliac artery.

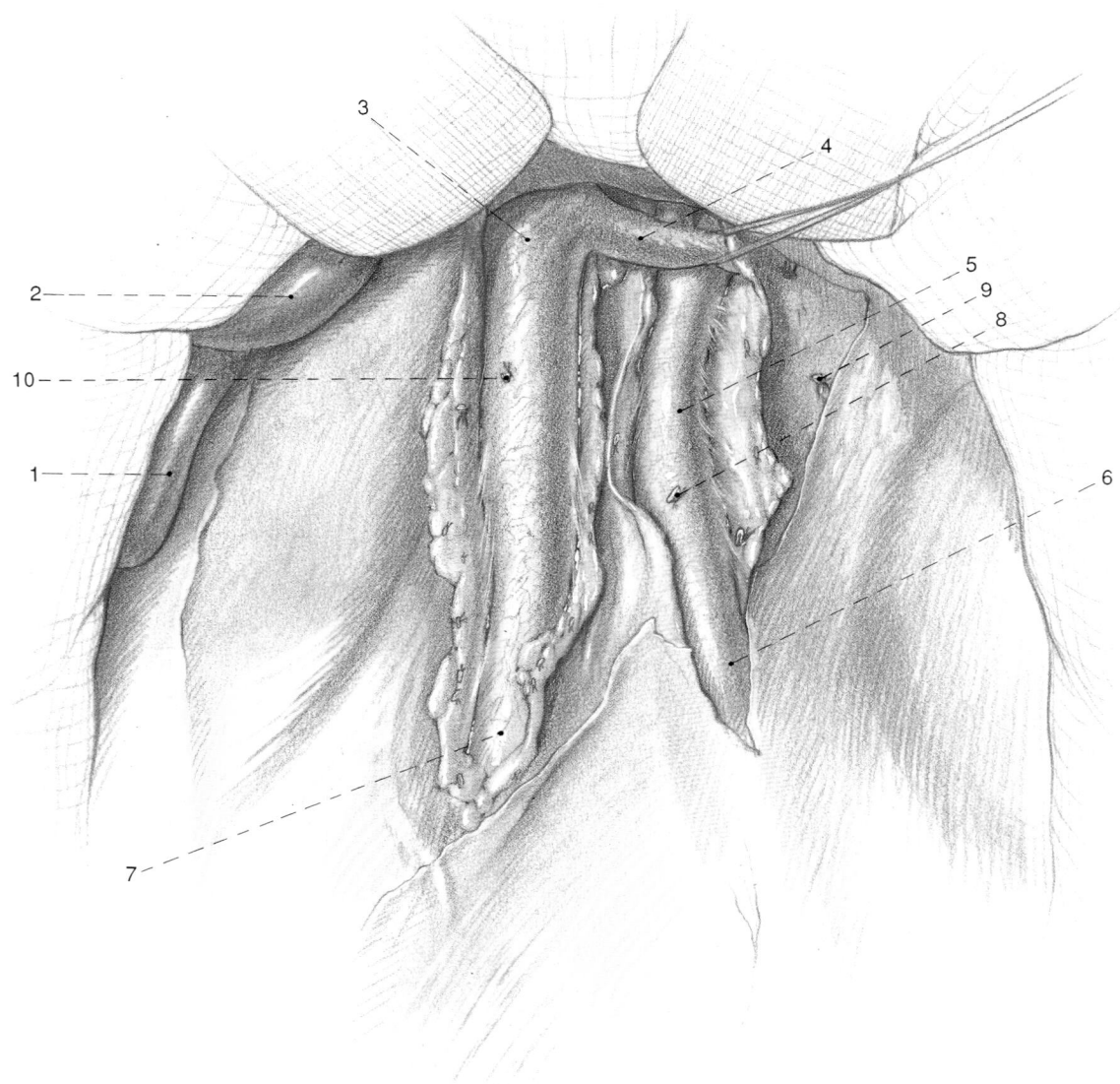

Fig. 2.**119**   Split-and-roll technique of retroperitoneal lymph node dissection.

1 Liver	8 Inferior mesenteric artery
2 Gallbladder	9 Inferior mesenteric vein
3 Inferior vena cava	10 Right testicular vein
4 Left renal vein	
5 Abdominal aorta	
6 Left common iliac artery	
7 Right common iliac vein	

Paramedian Transperitoneal Approach

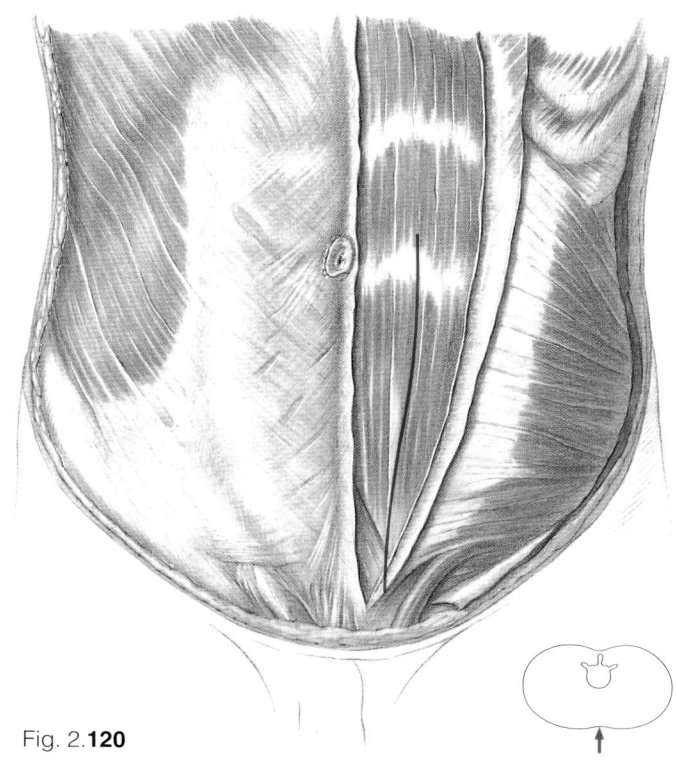

Fig. 2.**120**

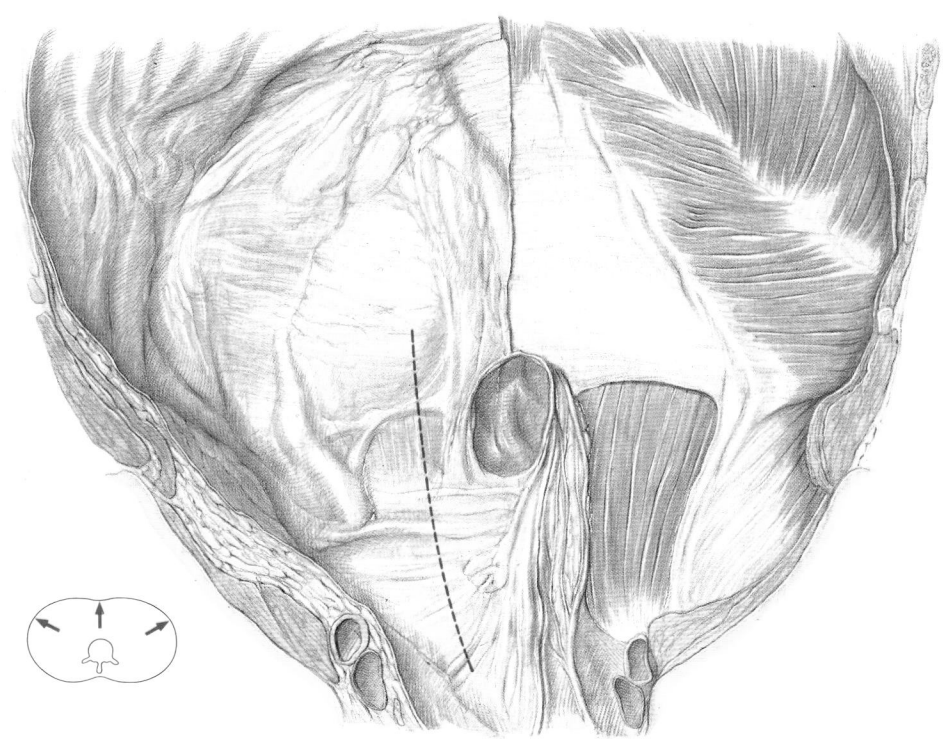

Main Indications

- Transperitoneal approach to the retroperitoneal space
- Nephrectomy
- Renovascular surgery
- Renal transplantation surgery

The paramedian approach to the retroperitoneal space is advantageous over the midline incision in that it permits wound closure in two layers. The incision may extend from the xiphoid to a point below the umbilicus or from the umbilicus to the pubic symphysis (Fig. 2.**121**). The technique is illustrated for a left paramedian incision from umbilicus to symphysis.

Position and Skin Incision

The operation is performed in a slightly hyperextended supine position. The incision extends from the umbilicus to the pubic symphysis, approximately two fingerwidths lateral to the midline (Fig. 2.**121**).

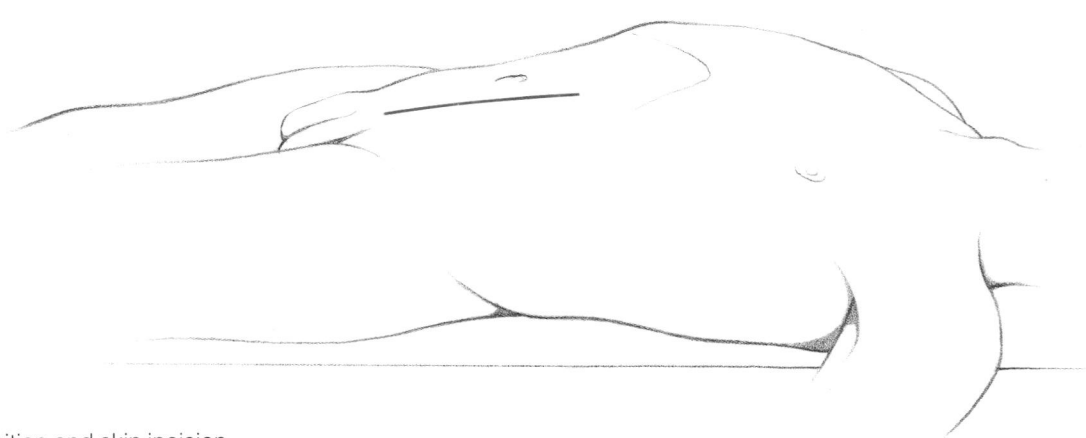

Fig. 2.**121**   Position and skin incision.

Division of the Posterior Rectus Sheath and Parietal Peritoneum

The posterior rectus sheath, preperitoneal fat, and parietal peritoneum are incised (Fig. 2.**125**). The posterior rectus sheath and parietal peritoneum are opened together in the upper part of the wound, and the parietal peritoneum is opened together with the transversalis fascia in the lower part of the wound (Fig. 2.**126**). As the peritoneal cavity is entered, the gastrocolic ligament, transverse colon, and greater omentum can be identified.

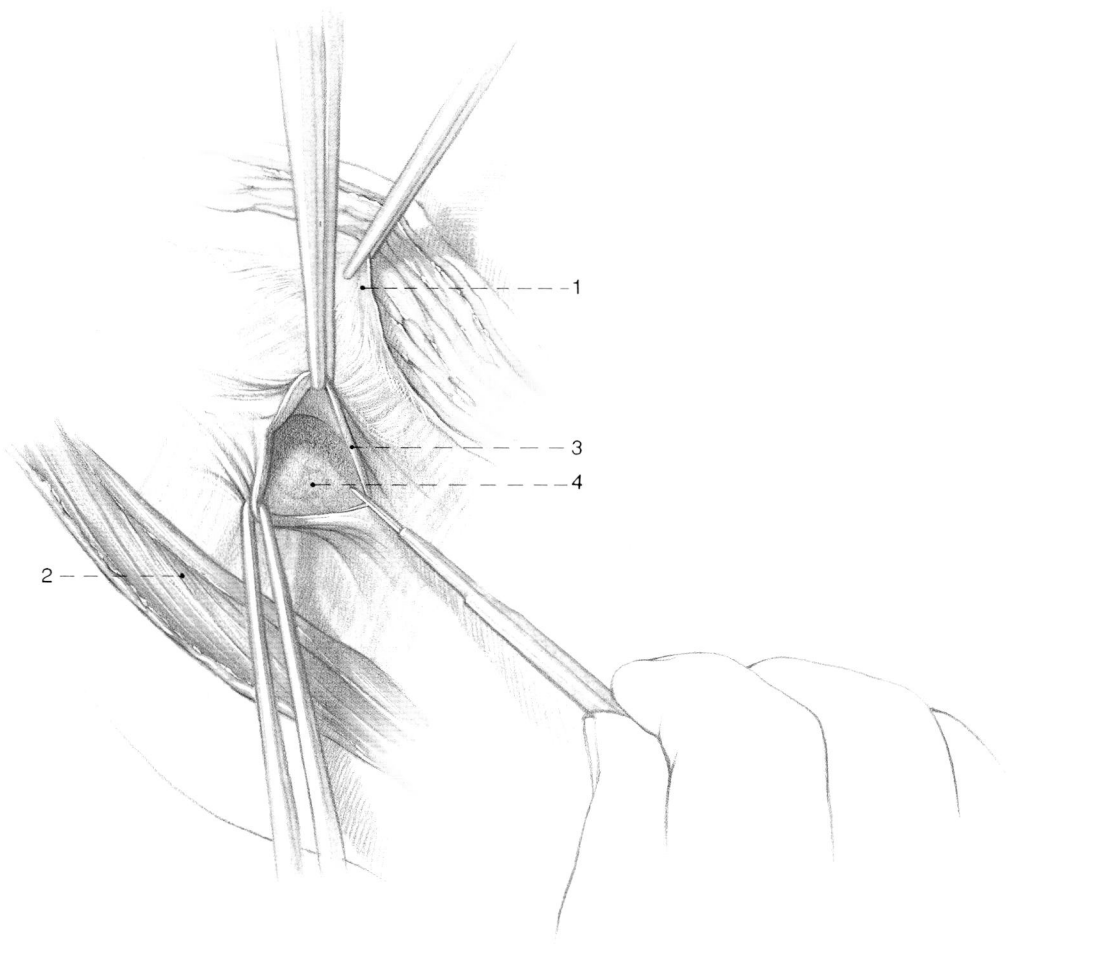

Fig. 2.**125**   Entry into the peritoneal cavity.

1 Anterior rectus sheath
2 Rectus abdominis muscle
3 Posterior rectus sheath
4 Transversalis fascia and parietal peritoneum

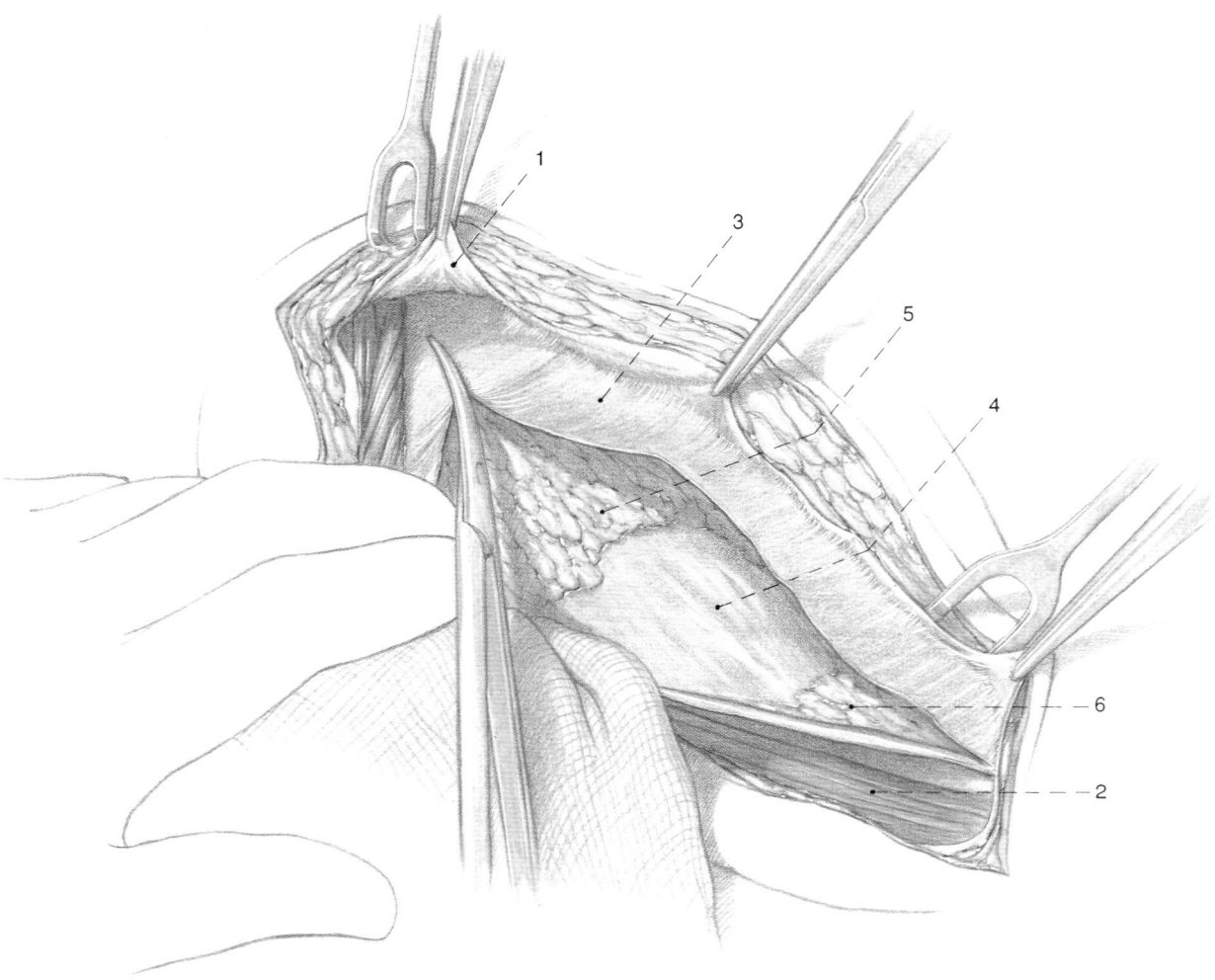

Fig. 2.**126** Division of the posterior rectus sheath and parietal peritoneum.

1 Anterior rectus sheath
2 Rectus abdominis muscle
3 Posterior rectus sheath
4 Transverse colon
5 Greater omentum
6 Gastrocolic ligament

Comments

With regard to the preparation of the rectus muscle, the approach may be made by splitting the rectus fibers or by dissecting the rectus muscle free and keeping it intact. The separation of the tendinous intersections in the latter technique involves the sacrifice of small nerves and blood vessels that approach the rectus muscle from the medial side. A rectus-splitting incision preserves these nerves and vessels but traumatizes the muscle fibers.

Lateral Extraperitoneal Gridiron Incision

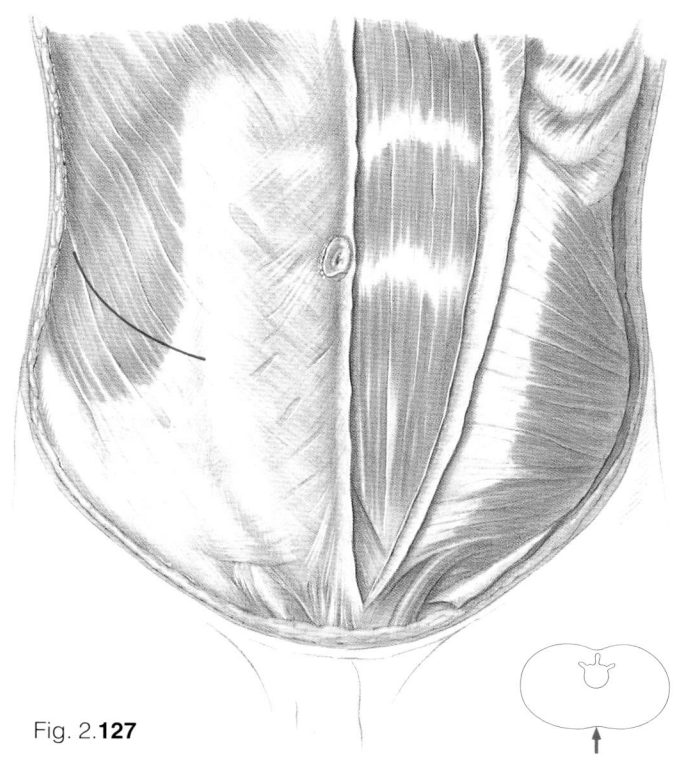

Fig. 2.**127**

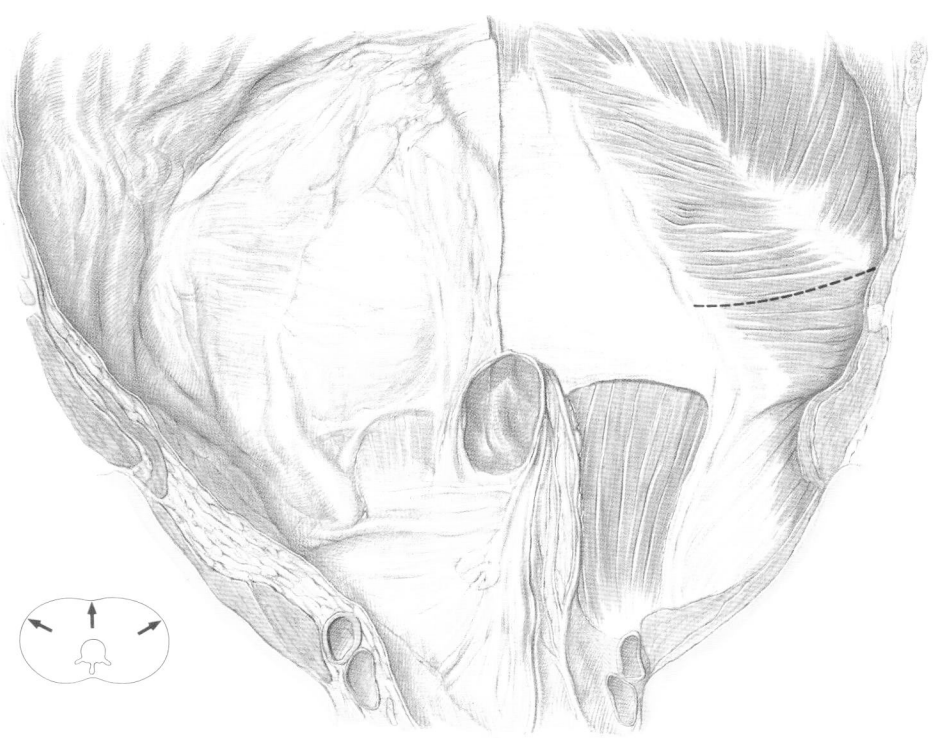

This approach is illustrated for a high ligation of the testicular vein on the right side.

Position and Skin Incision

The patient is positioned supine with the operative side slightly elevated. A reverse Trendelenburg position is used to induce venous filling.

The skin is incised along natural cleavage lines above the internal inguinal ring (Fig. 2.**128**). After division of the subcutaneous tissue, the external abdominal fascia (Camper's fascia) is exposed and transected, exposing the external oblique muscle fibers (Fig. 2.**129**).

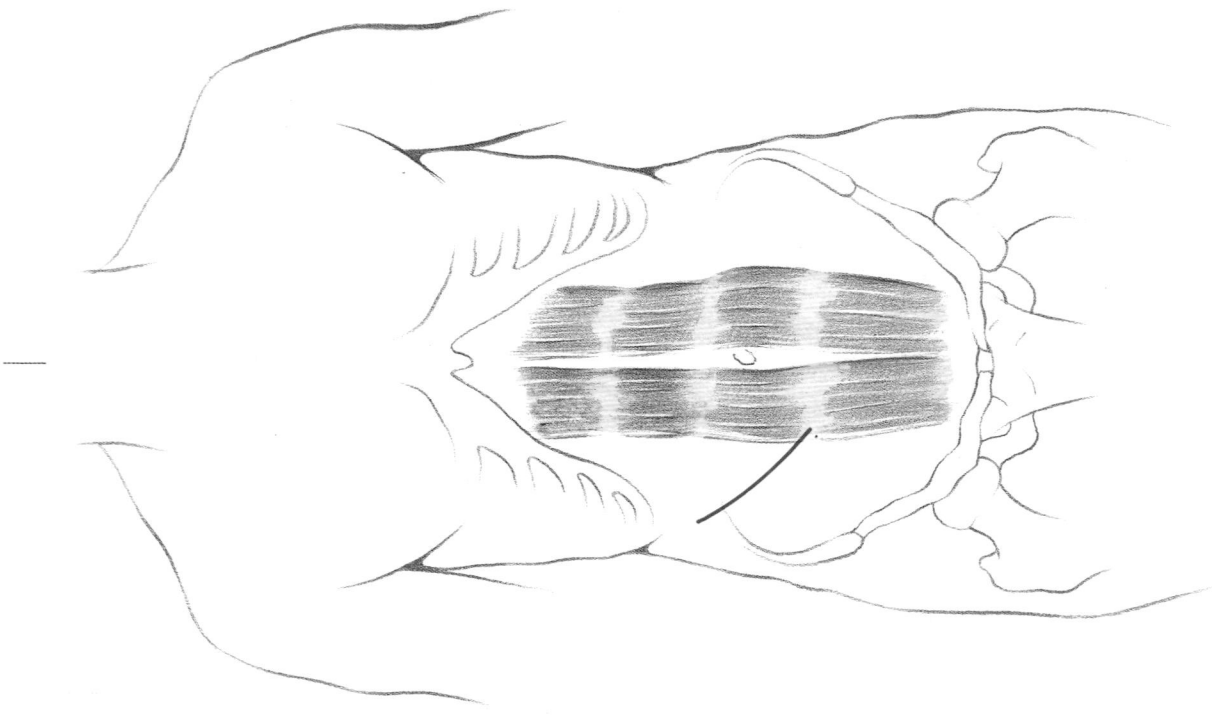

Fig. 2.**128**   Skin incision.

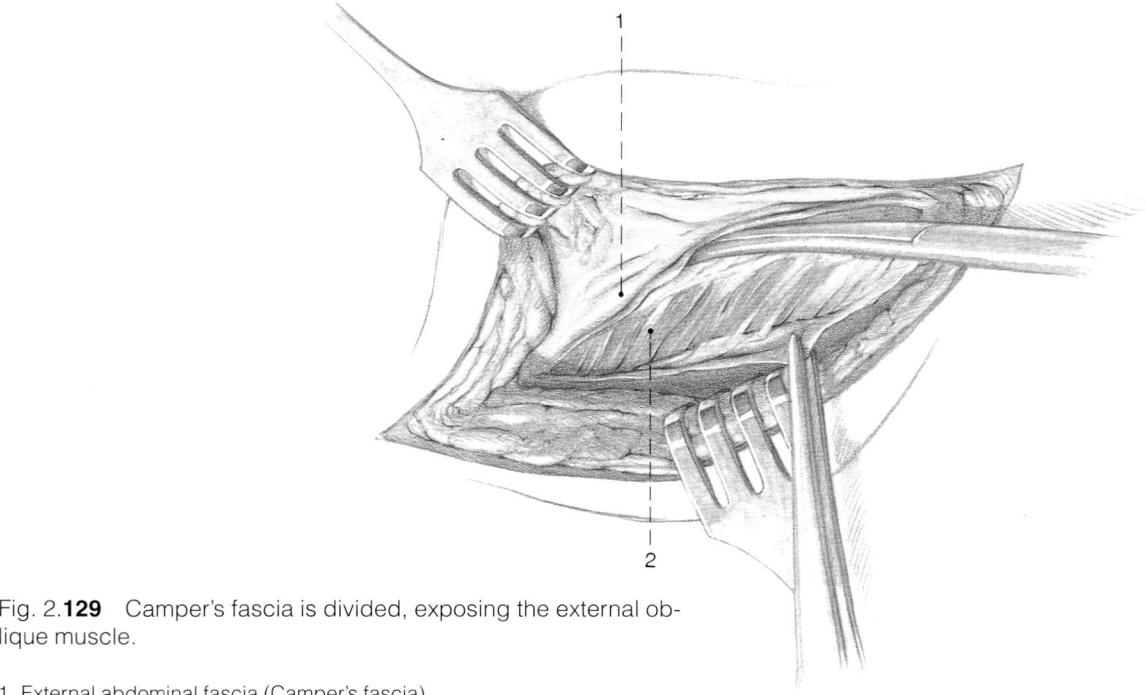

Fig. 2.**129**   Camper's fascia is divided, exposing the external oblique muscle.

1 External abdominal fascia (Camper's fascia)
2 External oblique muscle

Division of the Muscle

The external oblique muscle is divided in line with its fibers, exposing the underlying internal oblique and transversus abdominis muscles (Fig. 2.**130**). The external oblique is held aside with a retractor (Fig. 2.**130**).

Entry into the Retroperitoneal Space

Next the transversalis fascia is divided, and the transversus abdominis is incised in line with its fibers (Fig. 2.**131**). The peritoneum is freed with a small sponge stick and retracted medially with a broad, curved blade. Lateral exposure is maintained with a retractor placed over the internal oblique muscle and transversalis fascia (Fig. 2.**132**).

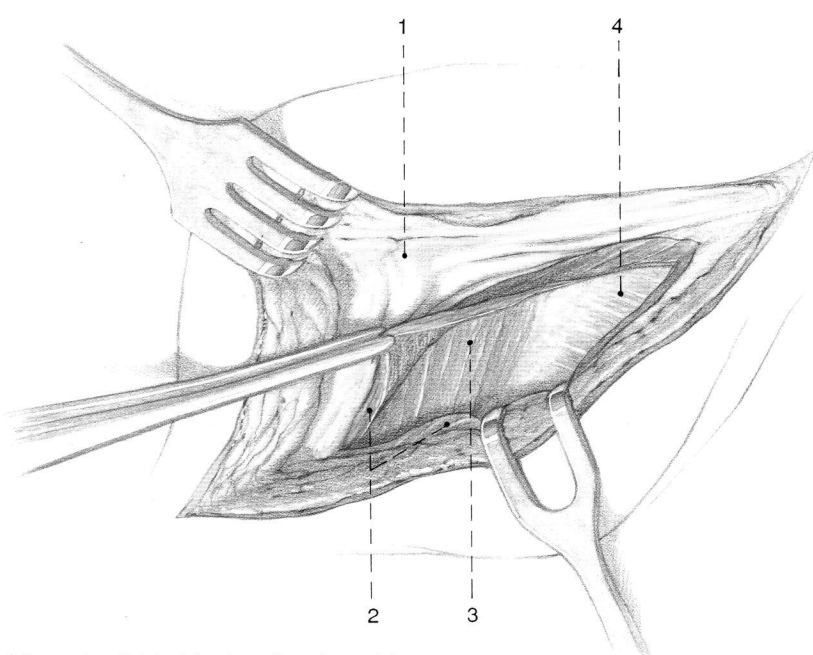

Fig. 2.**130** The external oblique is divided in the direction of its fibers.

1 External abdominal fascia (Camper's fascia)
2 External oblique muscle
3 Internal oblique muscle
4 Transversus abdominis

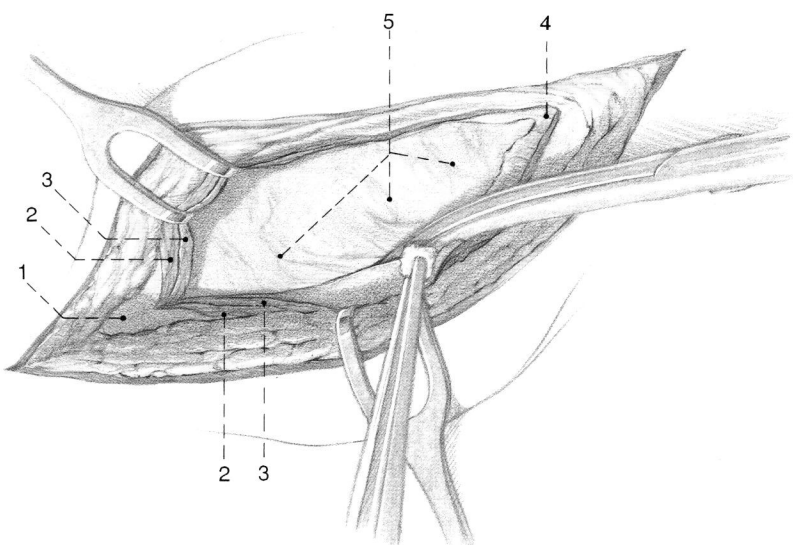

Fig. 2.**131** Exposure of the transversalis fascia following division of the transversus abdominis.

1 External abdominal fascia   3 Internal oblique muscle
   (Camper's fascia)   4 Transversus abdominis
2 External oblique muscle   5 Transversalis fascia

The retroperitoneal space is opened, and the testicular vessels are identified. Venous filling induced by the reverse Trendelenburg position aids in identifying, isolating, and ligating the veins (Fig. 2.**132**).

Comments

The artery and vein can be distinguished from each other while the patient is in the reverse Trendelenburg position.

The lumbar portion of the ureter also can be exposed through this approach. This requires greater medial dissection of the peritoneum. The ureter is found directly below the parietal peritoneum (Fig. 2.**133**).

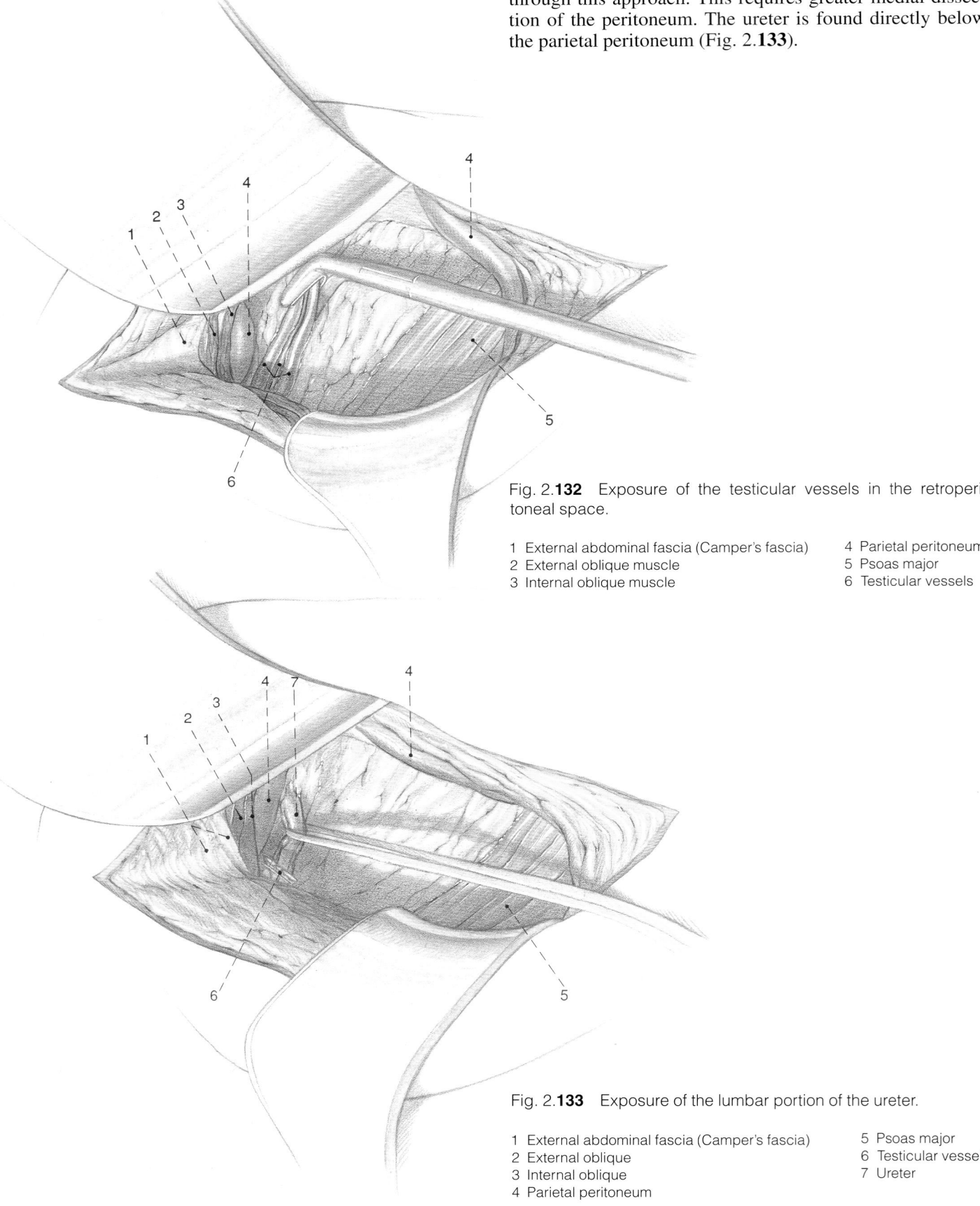

Fig. 2.**132** Exposure of the testicular vessels in the retroperitoneal space.

1 External abdominal fascia (Camper's fascia)
2 External oblique muscle
3 Internal oblique muscle
4 Parietal peritoneum
5 Psoas major
6 Testicular vessels

Fig. 2.**133** Exposure of the lumbar portion of the ureter.

1 External abdominal fascia (Camper's fascia)
2 External oblique
3 Internal oblique
4 Parietal peritoneum
5 Psoas major
6 Testicular vessels
7 Ureter

Low Lumbar Oblique Incision

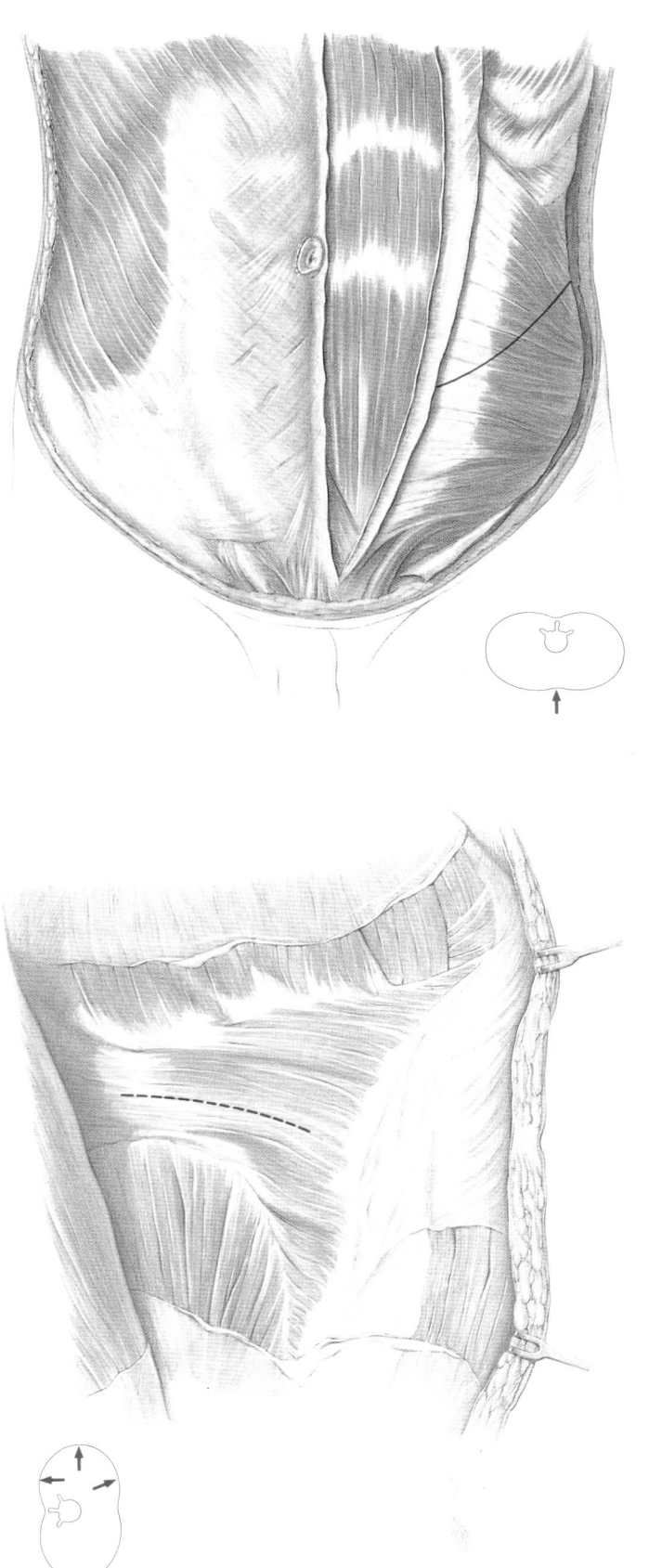

Fig. 2.**134**

Main Indication

This incision is used for exposing the lumbar portion of the ureter. The technique is illustrated for the left side.

Position and Skin Incision

The patient is positioned supine with the left side slightly elevated (Fig. 2.**135**).

The skin incision starts above the anterior superior iliac spine and runs toward McBurney's point, terminating at the border of the rectus muscle (Fig. 2.**136**).

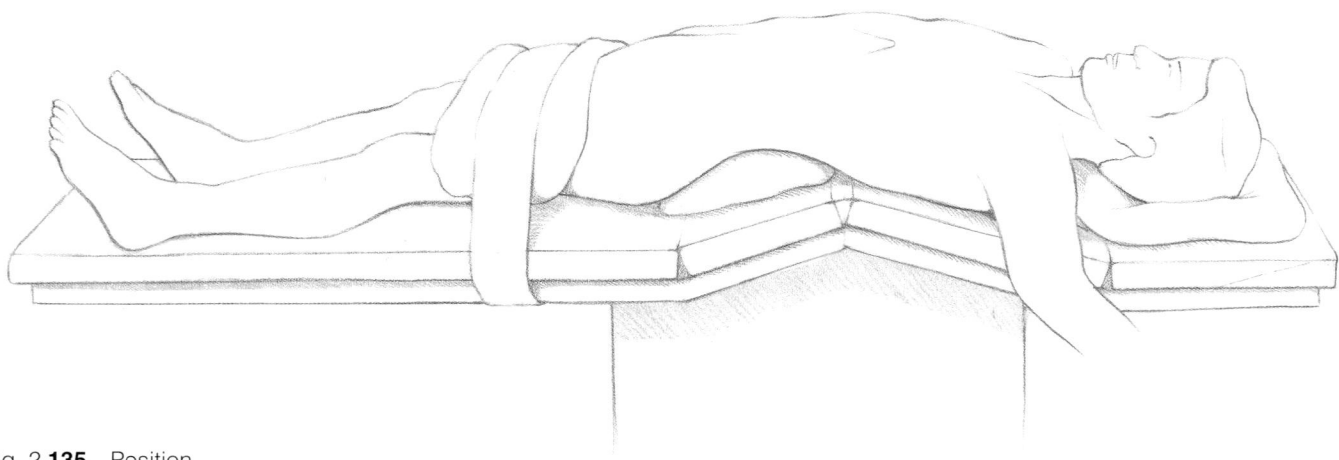

Fig. 2.**135**   Position.

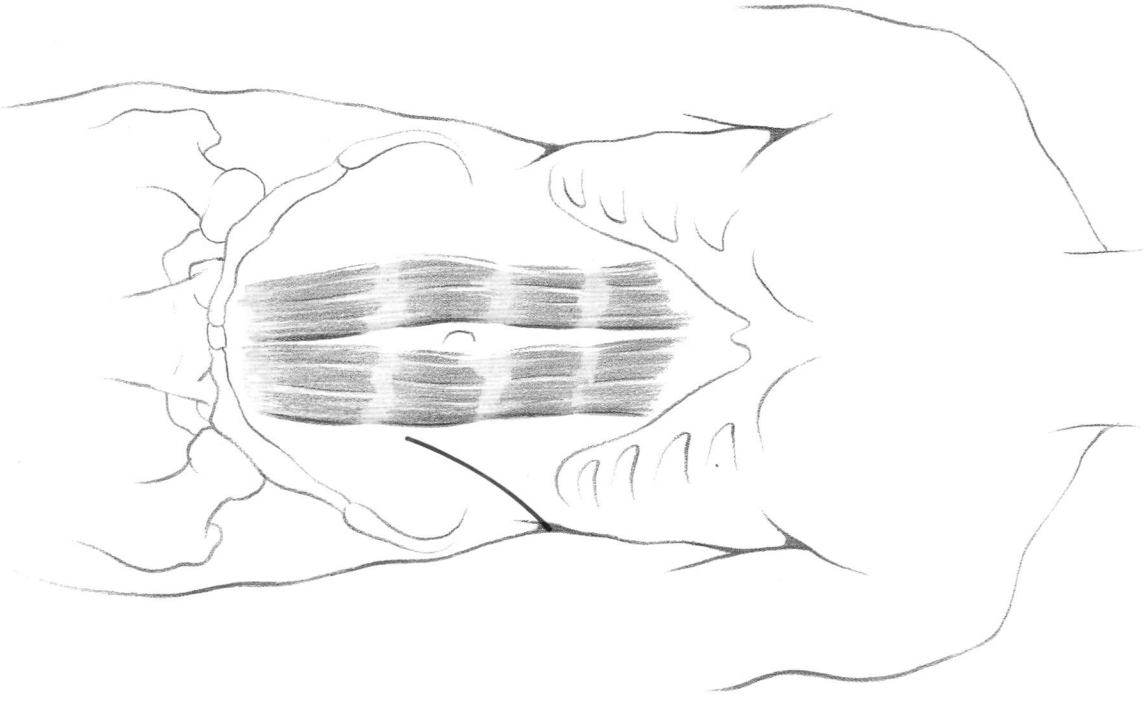

Fig. 2.**136**   Skin incision.

The subcutaneous fat is divided with diathermy to expose Camper's fascia (Fig. 2.**137**). This layer is divided, exposing the external oblique muscle fibers (Fig. 2.**138**).

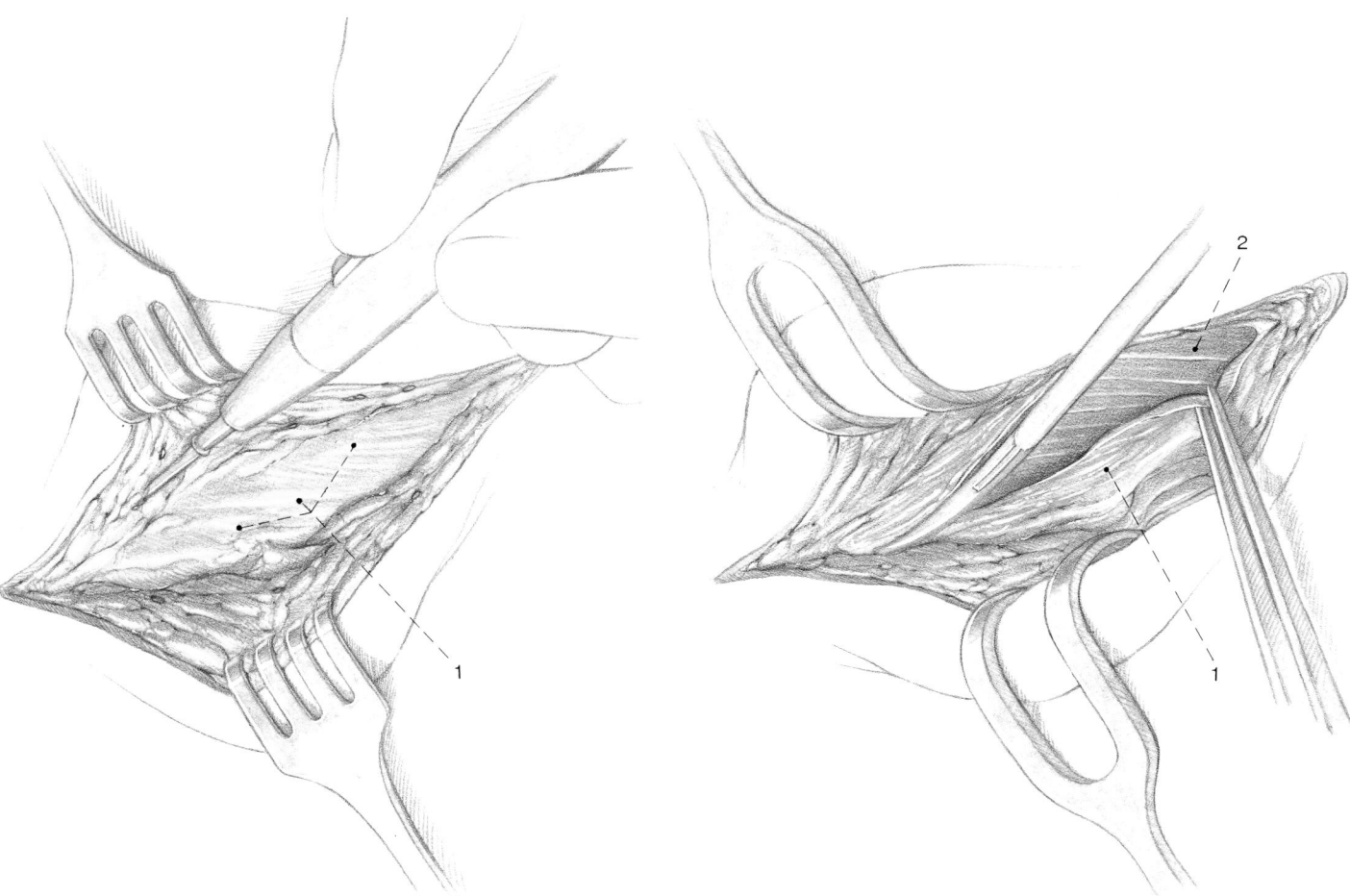

Fig. 2.**137** Exposure of Camper's fascia.

1 External abdominal fascia (Camper's fascia)

Fig. 2.**138** Incision of Camper's fascia and exposure of the external oblique muscle.

1 External abdominal fascia (Camper's fascia)
2 External oblique muscle

Division of the Abdominal Muscles

The external and internal oblique muscles are split in line with their fibers and held aside with two retractors. The transversus abdominis is incised on the line shown (Figs. 2.**139**, 2.**140**). The transversalis fascia is divided. The peritoneum is freed up medially and then retracted medially with a broad, curved blade (Fig. 2.**141**). The psoas major is identified. The lumbar portion of the ureter is dissected out of the retroperitoneal connective tissue; it is adherent to the peritoneum.

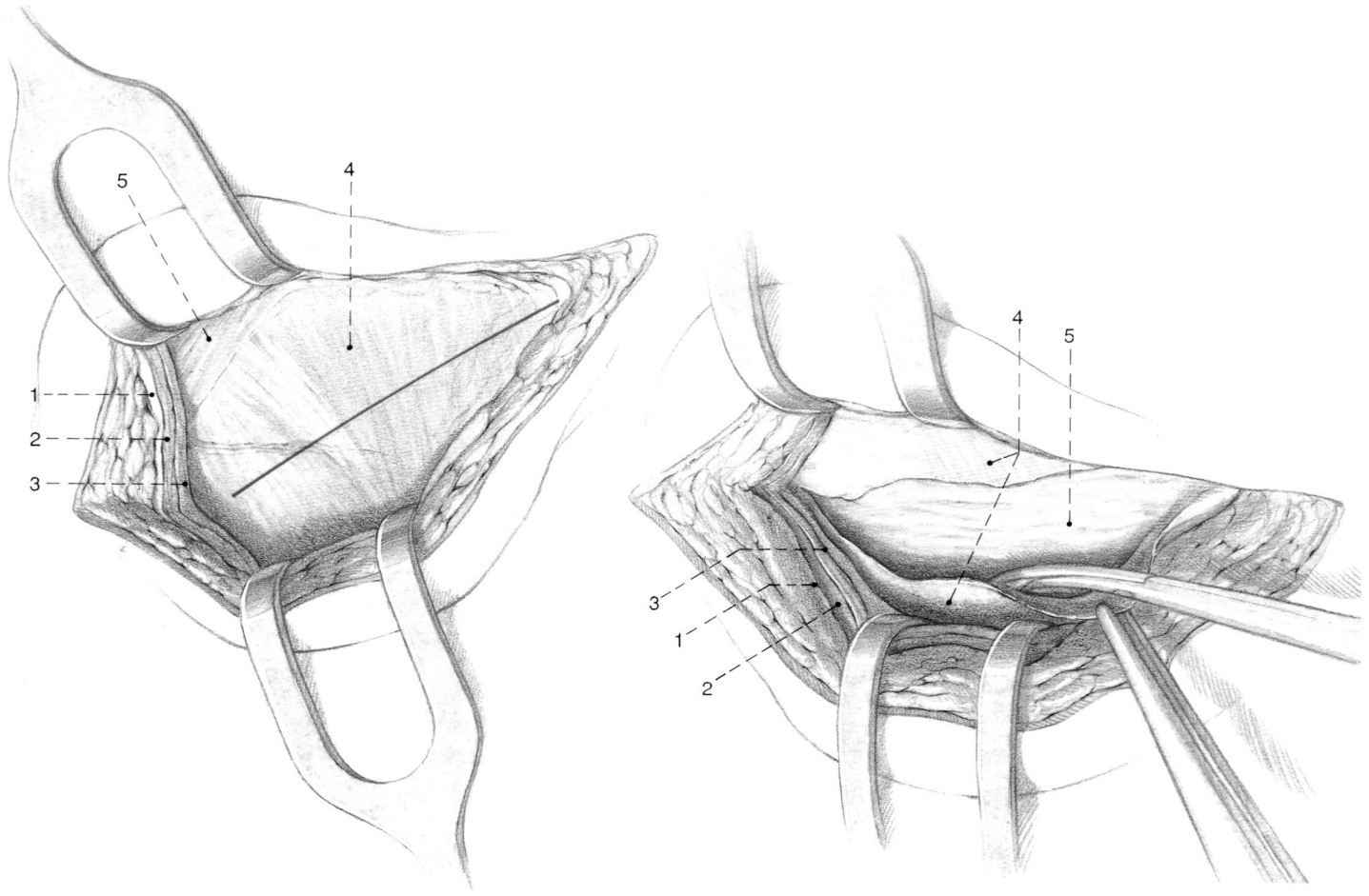

Fig. 2.**139** The external and internal oblique muscles have been divided. The line of the transversus abdominis incision is shown.

1 External abdominal fascia (Camper's fascia)
2 External oblique muscle
3 Internal oblique muscle
4 Transversus abdominis
5 Rectus abdominis muscle

Fig. 2.**140** Incision of the transversus abdominis.

1 External abdominal fascia (Camper's fascia)
2 External oblique muscle
3 Internal oblique muscle
4 Transversus abdominis
5 Transversalis fascia

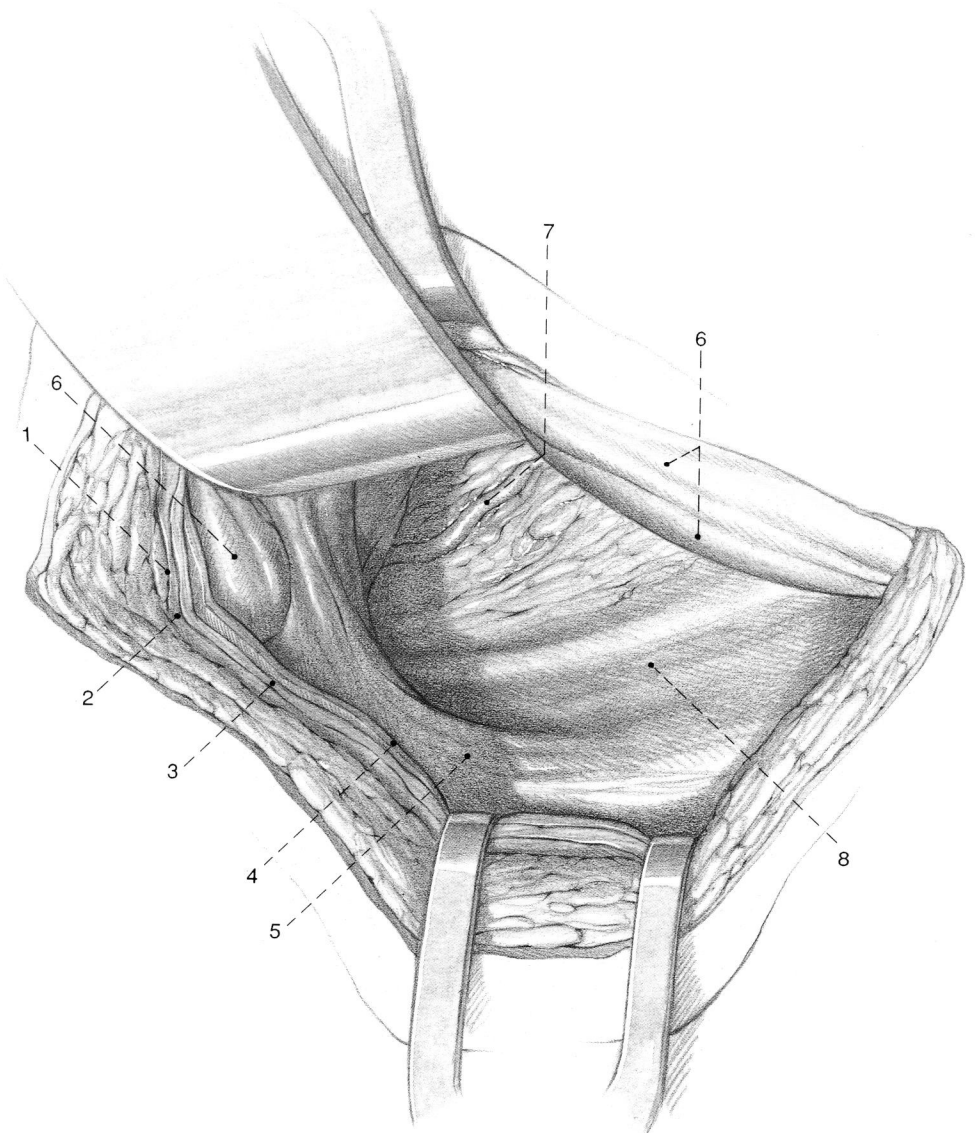

Fig. 2.**141**   Exposure of the retroperitoneal space. The lumbar portion of the ureter is dissected free.

1 External abdominal fascia (Camper's fascia)
2 External oblique muscle
3 Internal oblique muscle
4 Transversus abdominis
5 Transversalis fascia
6 Parietal peritoneum
7 Ureter
8 Psoas major

Low Inguinal Incision

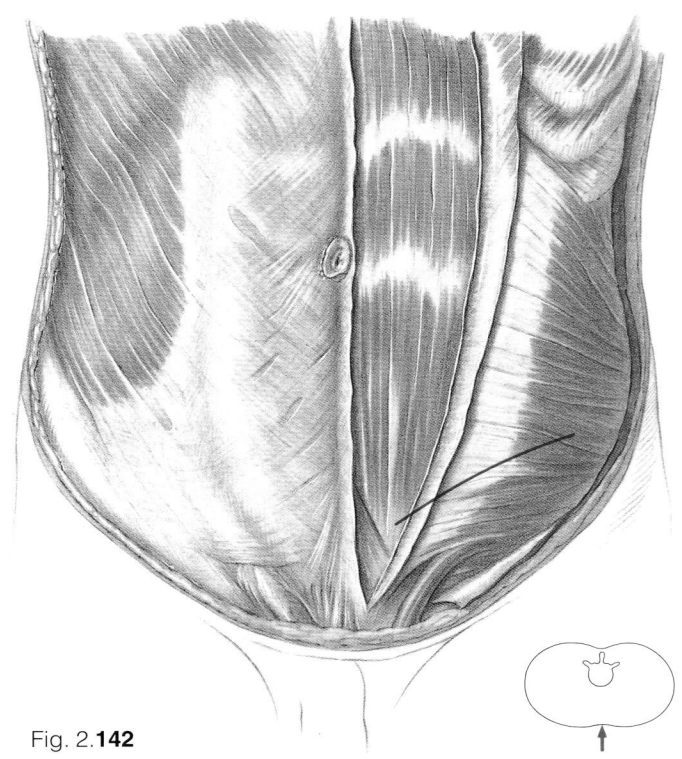

Fig. 2.**142**

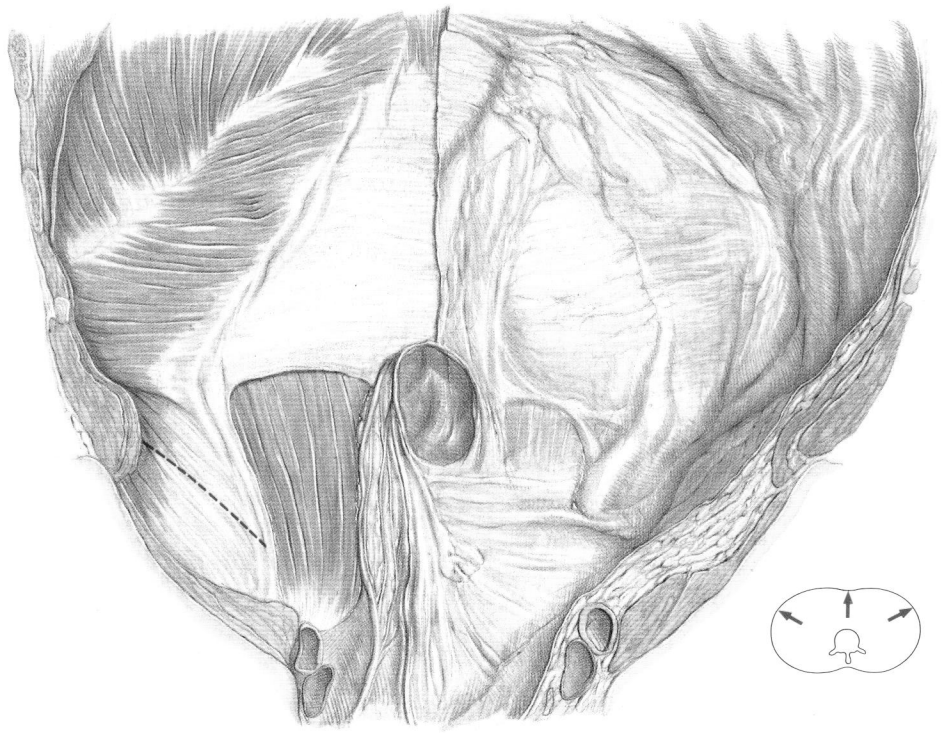

Main Indication

The low inguinal incision provides access to the pelvic portion of the ureter. The technique is illustrated for the left side.

Position and Skin Incision

The patient is positioned supine in a slight Trendelenburg position. The incision, made along cleavage lines, starts 2 cm medial to the anterior superior iliac spine and ends 2 cm above the groin at the lateral border of the rectus muscle (Fig. 2.**143**).

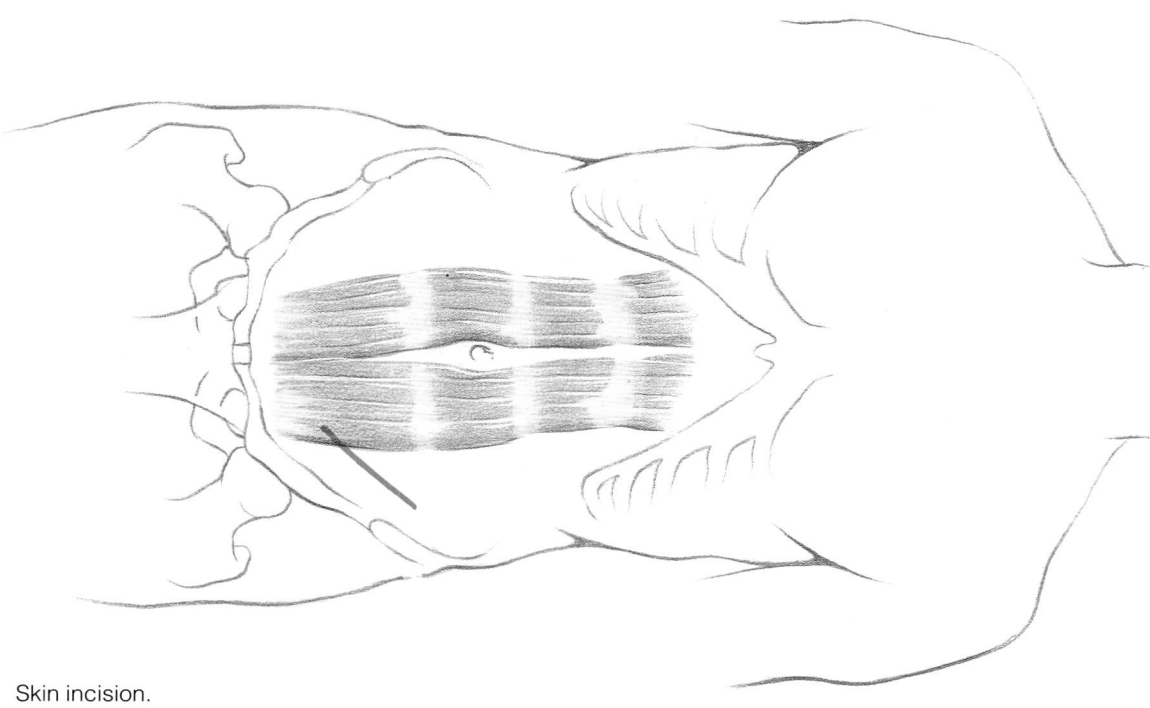

Fig. 2.**143**   Skin incision.

Division of the Abdominal Muscles

Following division of the subcutaneous fat, the aponeurosis of the external oblique muscle is exposed and transected, and the internal oblique muscle is exposed and divided in line with its fibers (Fig. 2.**144**). Exposure is maintained with two curved retractors. The transversus abdominis is divided in the direction of its fibers (Fig. 2.**145**).

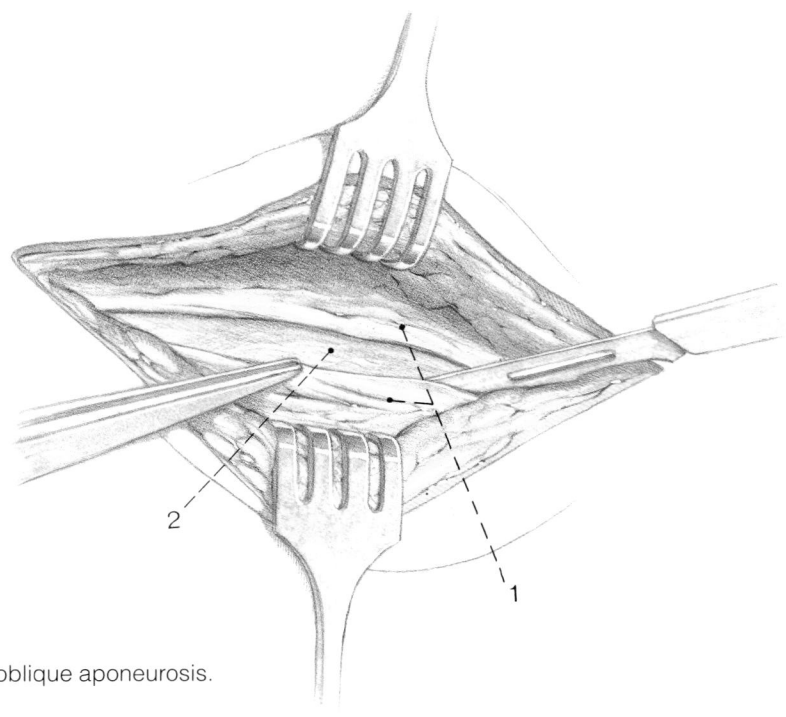

Fig. 2.**144** Exposure of the external oblique aponeurosis.

1 External oblique aponeurosis
2 Internal oblique muscle

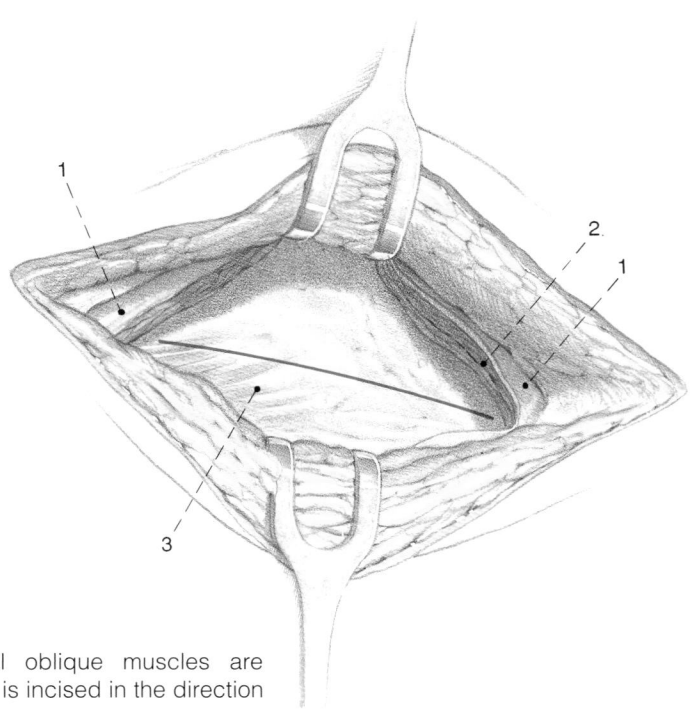

Fig. 2.**145** The external and internal oblique muscles are divided, and the transversus abdominis is incised in the direction of its fibers.

1 External oblique aponeurosis
2 Internal oblique muscle
3 Transversus abdominis

Exposure is maintained with two retractors. The peritoneum is freed up and retracted medially (Fig. 2.**146**). The ureter is identified on the undersurface of the peritoneum in its course directly below the parietal peritoneum. It is dissected from the retroperitoneal tissue at its crossing with the common iliac artery and vein (Fig. 2.**147**).

Comments

The pelvic portion of the ureter can be approached through a paraperitoneal, pararectal, transrectal, or paramedian incision. The low inguinal approach permits exposure of the ureter in its course between the common iliac artery and urinary bladder. During dissection of the ureter, care is taken to preserve all nerves, blood vessels, and lymphatics that are associated with the ureter.

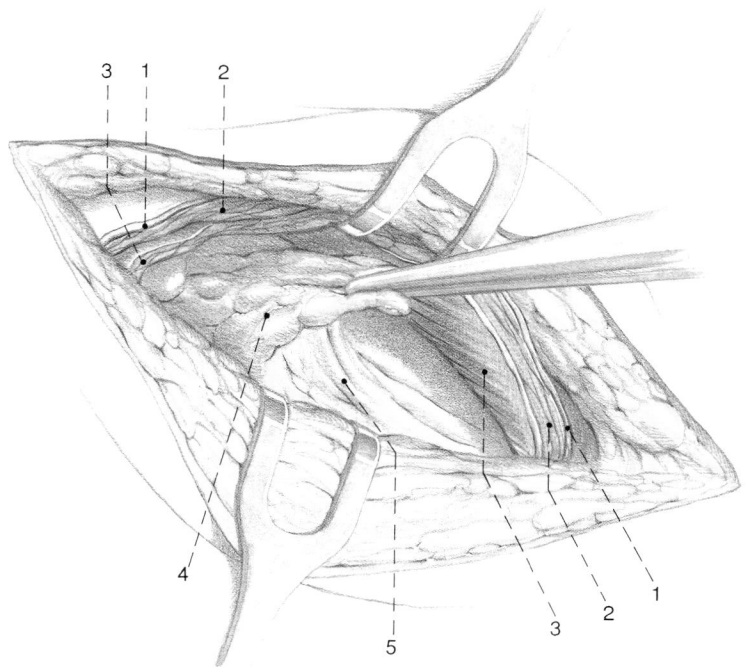

Fig. 2.**146**   The peritoneum is retracted medially, the muscles laterally.

1 External oblique aponeurosis
2 Internal oblique muscle
3 Transversus abdominis
4 Preperitoneal fat
5 Parietal peritoneum with transversalis fascia

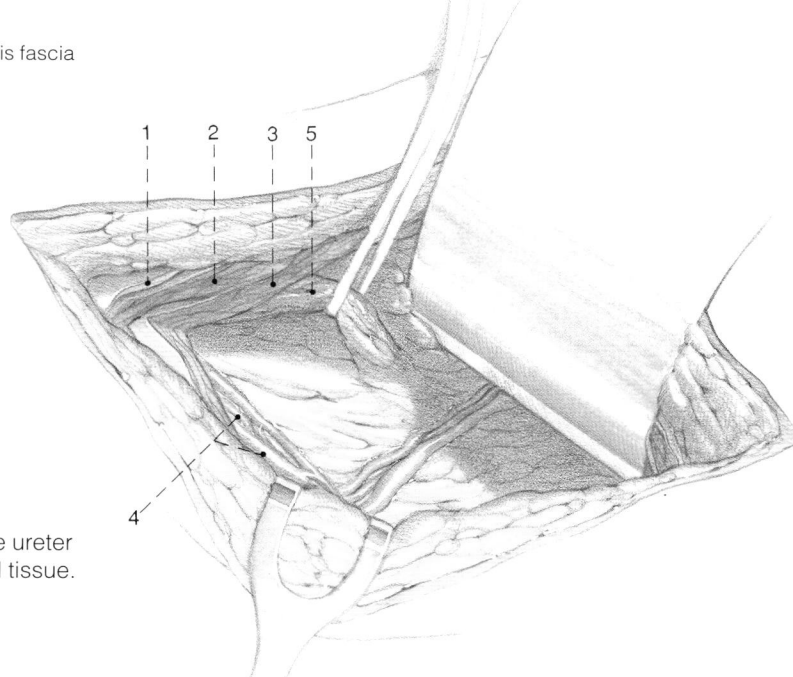

Fig. 2.**147**   The lumbar part of the ureter is isolated from the retroperitoneal tissue.

1 External oblique aponeurosis
2 Internal oblique muscle
3 Transversus abdominis
4 Testicular vessels
5 Ureter

Extraperitoneal Paramedian Approach

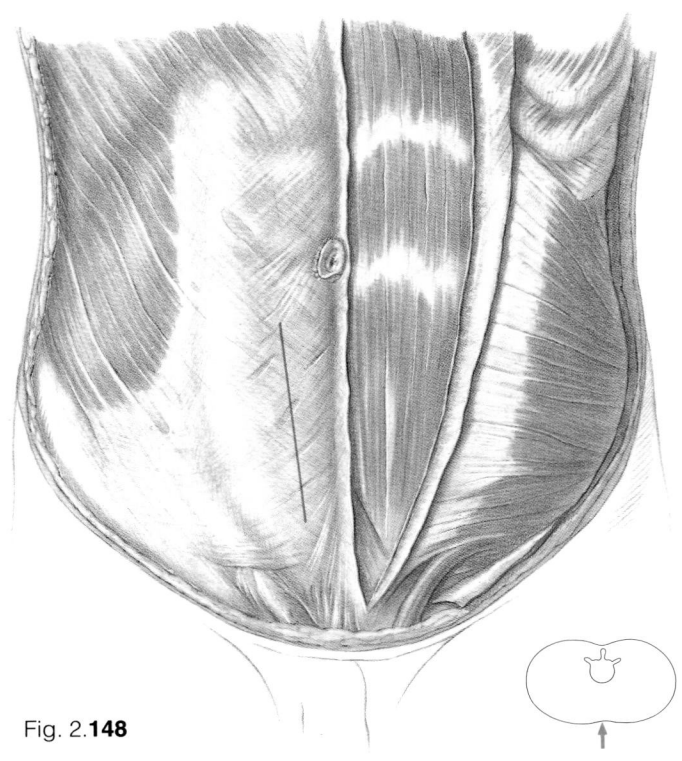

Fig. 2.**148**

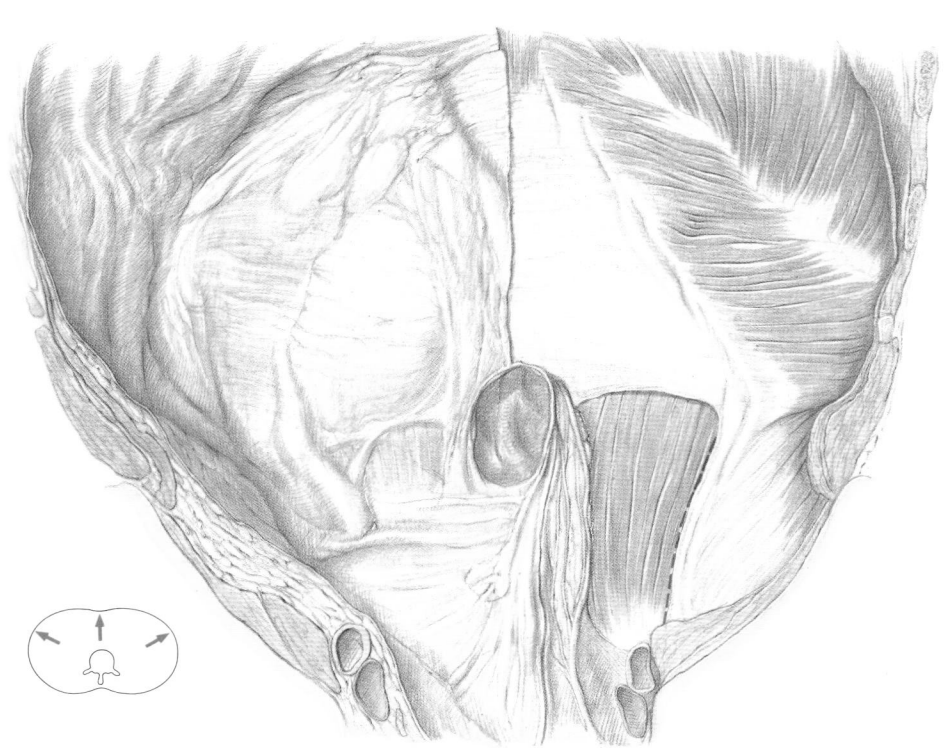

Main Indications

- Penile arterial vascularization
- Surgery of the undescended testis (autotransplantation)

The technique is illustrated for dissection of the right inferior epigastric artery and vein.

Position and Skin Incision

The patient is positioned supine. The paramedian incision is made two fingerwidths to the right of the midline, extending from the umbilicus to the superior pubic ramus (Fig. 2.**149**).

The subcutaneous fat is divided, and the anterior rectus sheath is exposed (Fig. 2.**150**).

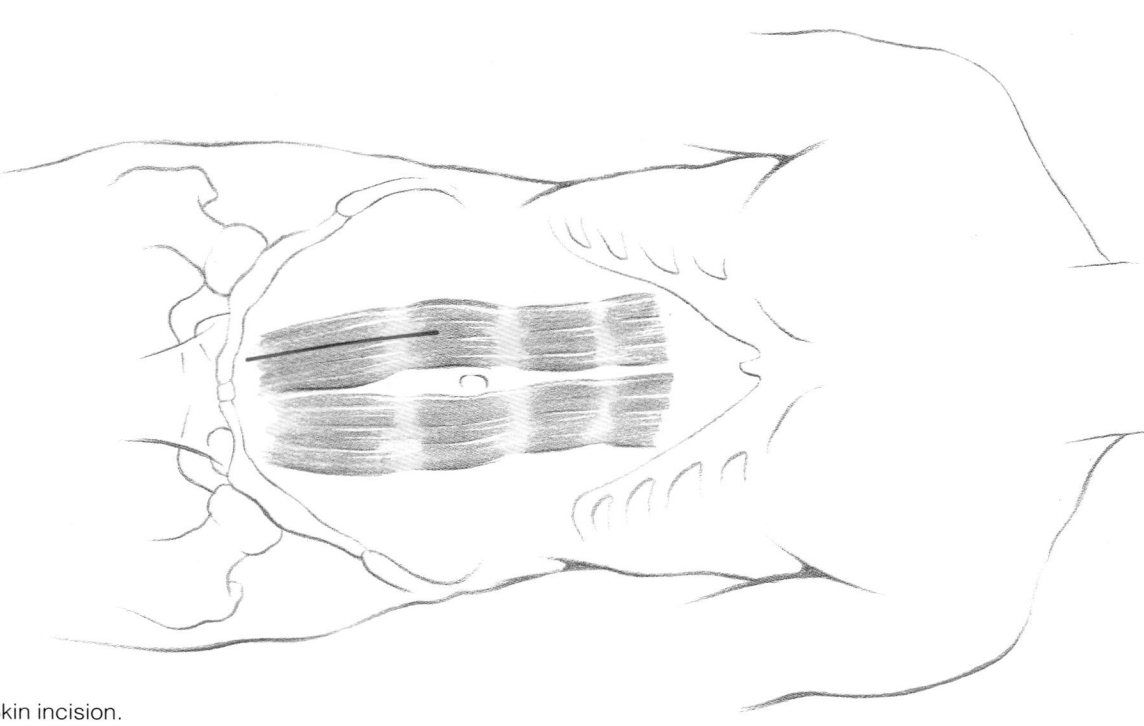

Fig. 2.**149**   Skin incision.

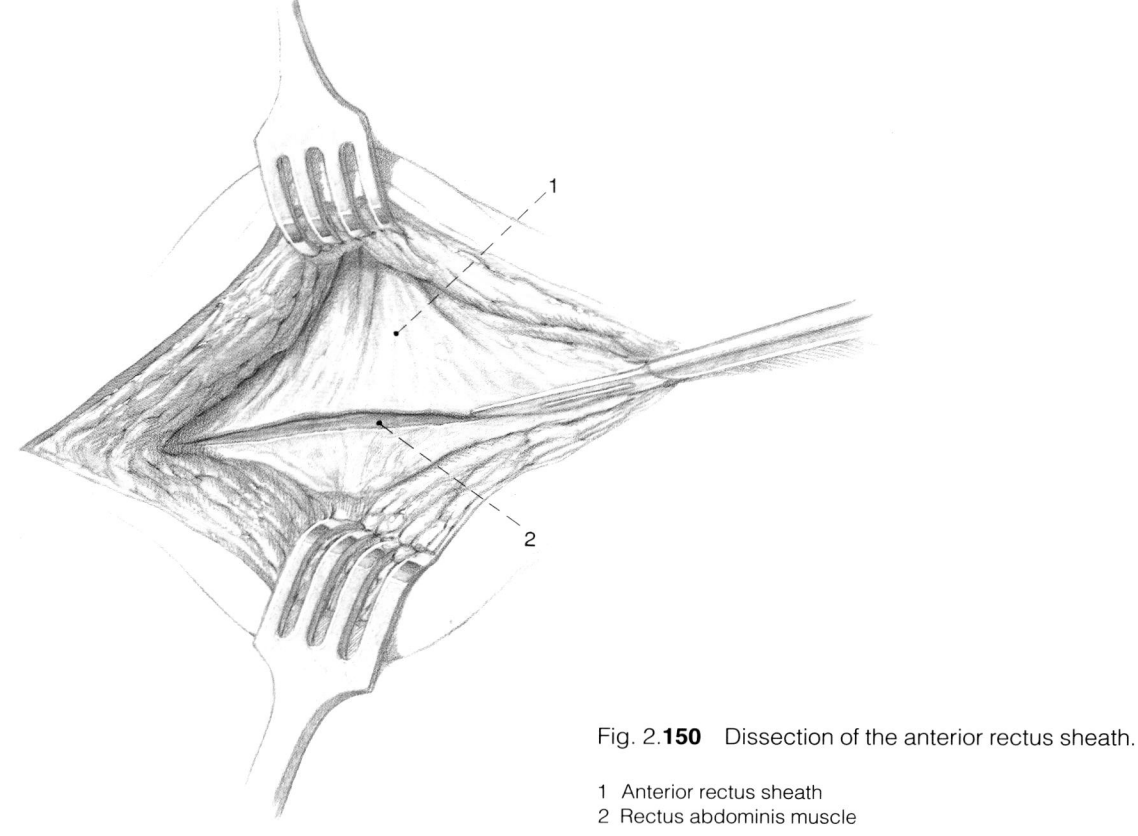

Fig. 2.**150**   Dissection of the anterior rectus sheath.

1 Anterior rectus sheath
2 Rectus abdominis muscle

Exposure of the Rectus Muscle

The rectus sheath is opened with a paramedian incision over the right rectus abdominis muscle (see Fig. 2.**150**). The rectus muscle on the right side is dissected from medially to laterally as the anterior rectus sheath is held aside with retractors (Figs. 2.**151**, 2.**152**). The dissected rectus muscle is retracted upward with adherent fat and connective tissue, leaving the posterior rectus sheath and transversalis fascia intact (Fig. 2.**152**).

Dissection of the Epigastric Vessels

The epigastric vessels (inferior epigastric artery and usually two accompanying veins) are dissected from the connective tissue at the undersurface of the rectus muscle (Fig. 2.**153**).

Comments

This approach has been illustrated for arterial reconstruction for erectile impotence. It can also be used for mobilizing an intraabdominal testis after dissection of the peritoneum from the internal inguinal ring. In this approach both the spermatic cord vessels and the vas deferens can be exposed at the internal ring.

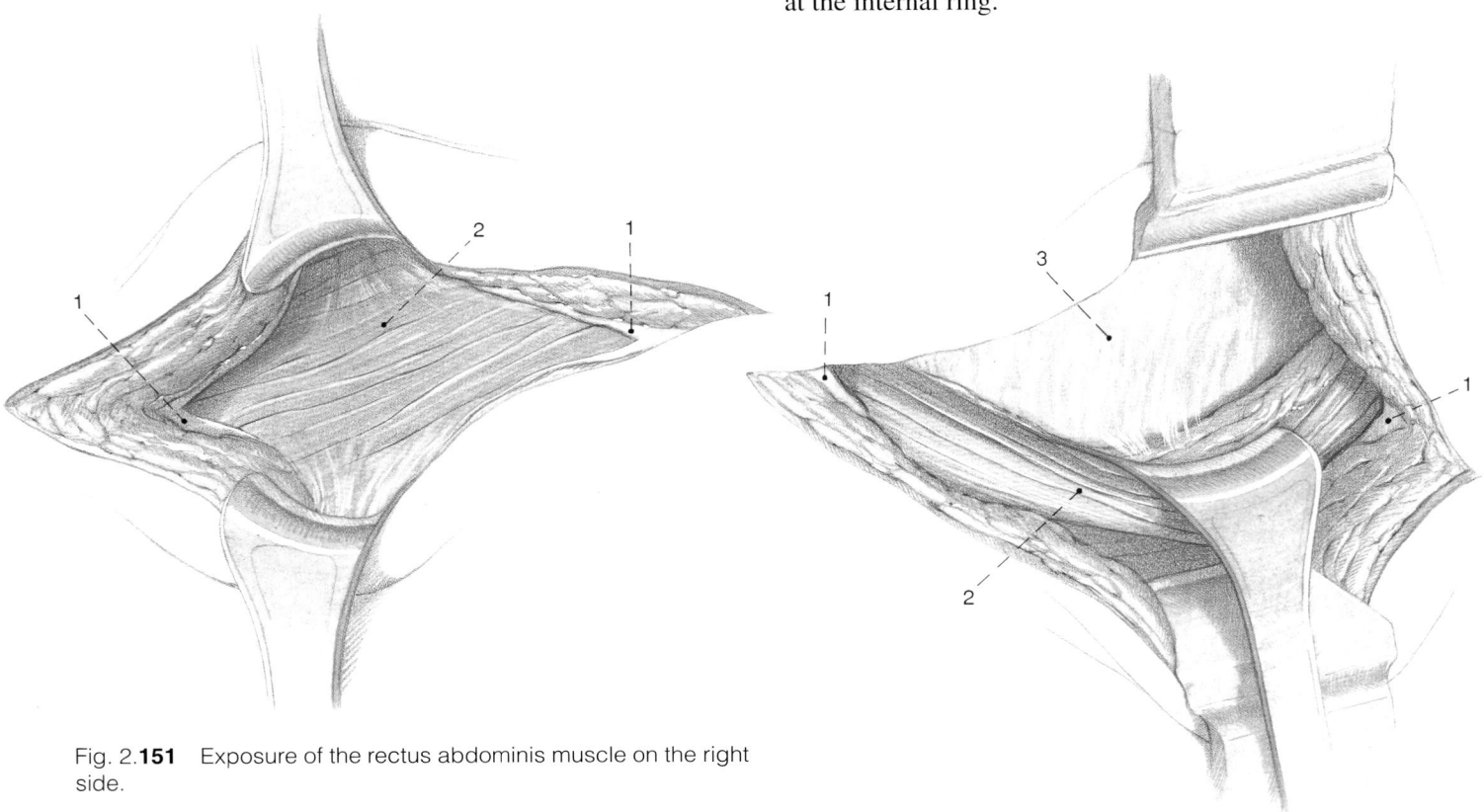

Fig. 2.**151** Exposure of the rectus abdominis muscle on the right side.

1 Anterior rectus sheath
2 Rectus abdominis muscle

Fig. 2.**152** The rectus muscle is drawn upward with a blunt retractor along with surrounding fatty and connective tissue.

1 Anterior rectus sheath
2 Rectus abdominis muscle
3 Posterior rectus sheath

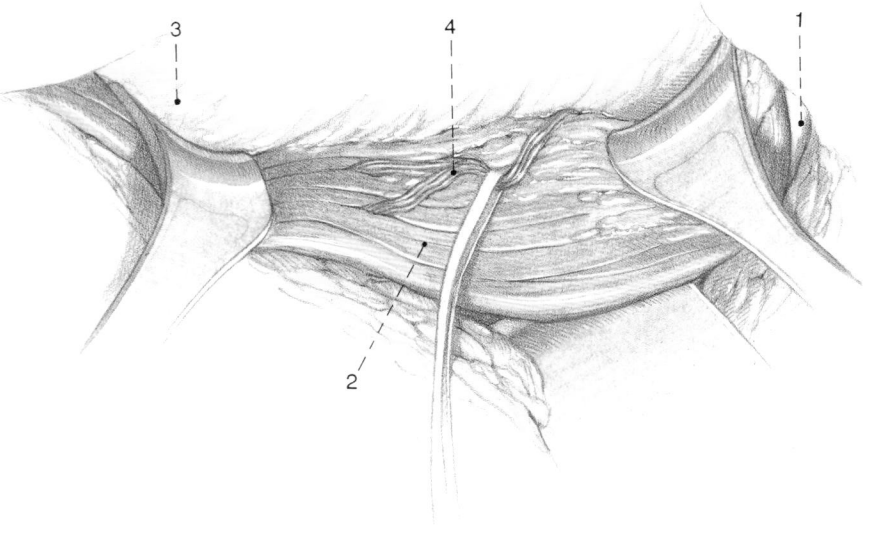

Fig. 2.**153** The inferior epigastric artery and accompanying veins are isolated and snared.

1 Anterior rectus sheath
2 Rectus abdominis muscle
3 Posterior rectus sheath
4 Epigastric vessels

3 Pelvis

Anatomy of the Pelvis

Pelvic Part of the Ureter

The pelvic (distal) part of the ureter comprises approximately half of its total length. It follows basically the same course in males and females, but its relations are gender-specific (Figs. 3.1, 3.2). The entrance of the ureter into the true pelvis is located anterior or slightly medial to the sacroiliac joint. There the ureter is related to the iliac vessels, cross-ing either the common iliac vessels or the external and internal iliac vessels depending on the position of these vessels and the level of their bifurcation. Due to the left-sided position of the abdominal aorta, the right ureter typically crosses the iliac vessels below their point of bifurcation while the left ureter generally crosses the common iliac vessels (Figs. 3.1, 3.2).

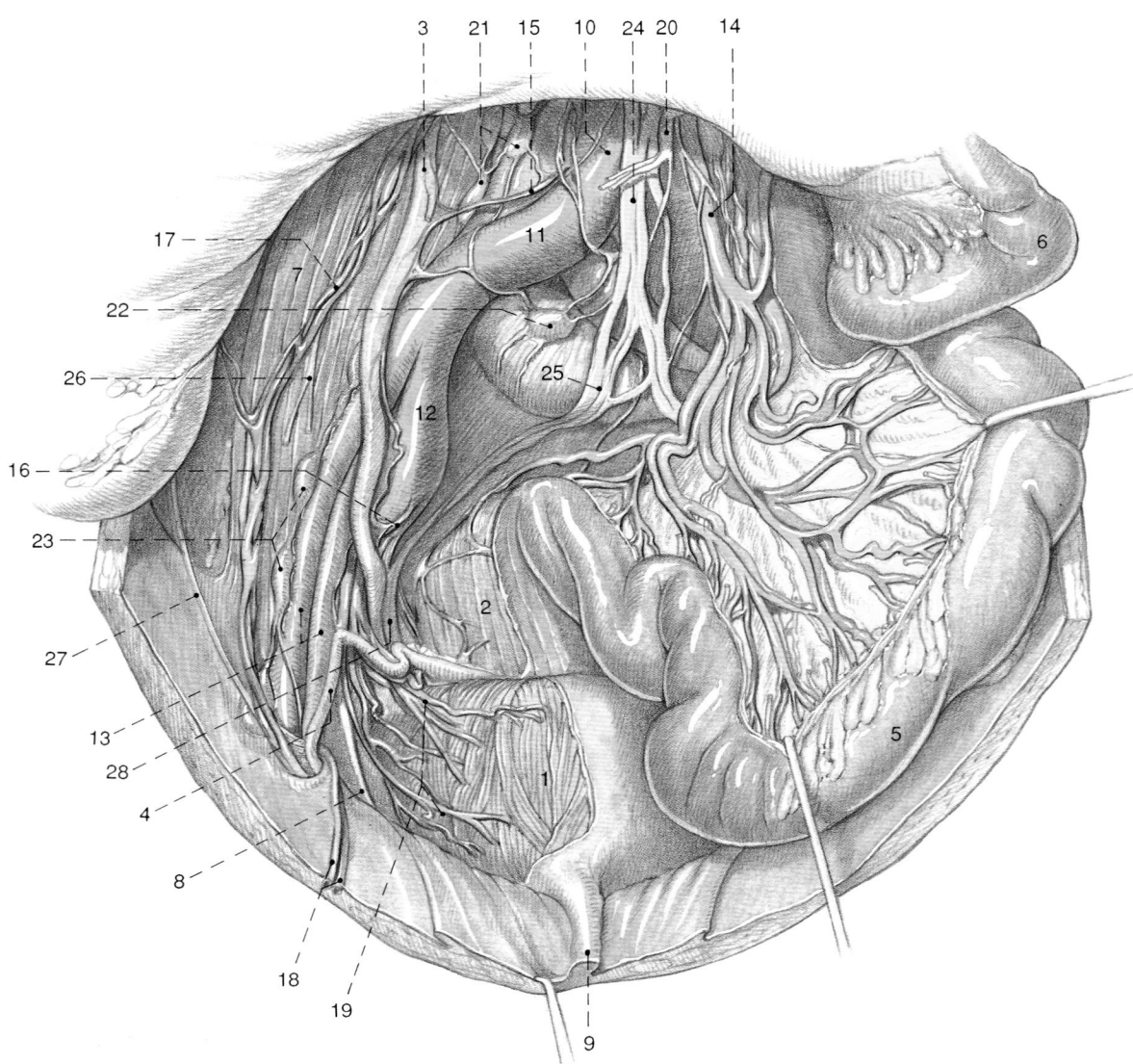

Fig. 3.1   Pelvic dissection in a male. The peritoneum has been partially removed (after Platzer).

1 Bladder	11 Common iliac artery	21 Lumbar lymph nodes
2 Rectum	12 Internal iliac artery	22 Common iliac lymph node
3 Ureter	13 External iliac vessels	23 External iliac lymph nodes
4 Vas deferens	14 Inferior mesenteric artery	24 Superior hypogastric plexus (presacral nerve)
5 Sigmoid colon	15 Ureteral branch from abdominal aorta (variant)	25 Right hypogastric nerve
6 Ileum	16 Ureteral branch from internal iliac artery	26 Genitofemoral nerve (divided)
7 Psoas major	17 Testicular artery and accompanying veins	27 Ilioinguinal nerve
8 Lateral umbilical ligament	18 Inferior epigastric vessels	28 Pelvic plexus (inferior hypogastric plexus)
9 Urachus	19 Superior vesical arteries	
10 Abdominal aorta	20 Lumbar (lymphatic) trunk	

The first part of the pelvic portion of the ureter describes an anteriorly convex arch. It lies medial to the internal iliac artery and its branches, and it crosses the obturator nerve on the lateral pelvic wall just below the parietal peritoneum (Fig. 3.1). In the female, the ureter usually passes behind the ovary on the floor of the ovarian fossa (Fig. 3.2).

After crossing the pelvic vessels, the ureter diverges from the parietal peritoneum to enter the pararectal connective tissue (paraproctium). Just before or after this point, a sheet of connective tissue leaves the ureteral adventitia to establish a direct connection between the ureter and the rectal retinaculum.

After the ureter enters the pararectal connective tissue, its topographic relations display gender-specific differences.

In the male, the ureter passes through the pararectal connective tissue from behind forward, then turns slightly medially and closely approaches the tip of the seminal vesicle (Fig. 3.5). There it crosses below the vas deferens. Surrounded by the veins of the vesical plexus, the ureter reaches and passes medially and obliquely through the bladder wall.

In the female, the ureter describes an inferiorly convex bend as it passes from the rectal retinaculum into the cardinal ligament (lateral cervical ligament). There it passes behind the uterine artery, which consistently gives off branches to the ureteral adventitia in this area. These branches travel in a thin sheet of connective tissue that is incorrectly termed the "ventral mesoureter" (Fig. 3.2).

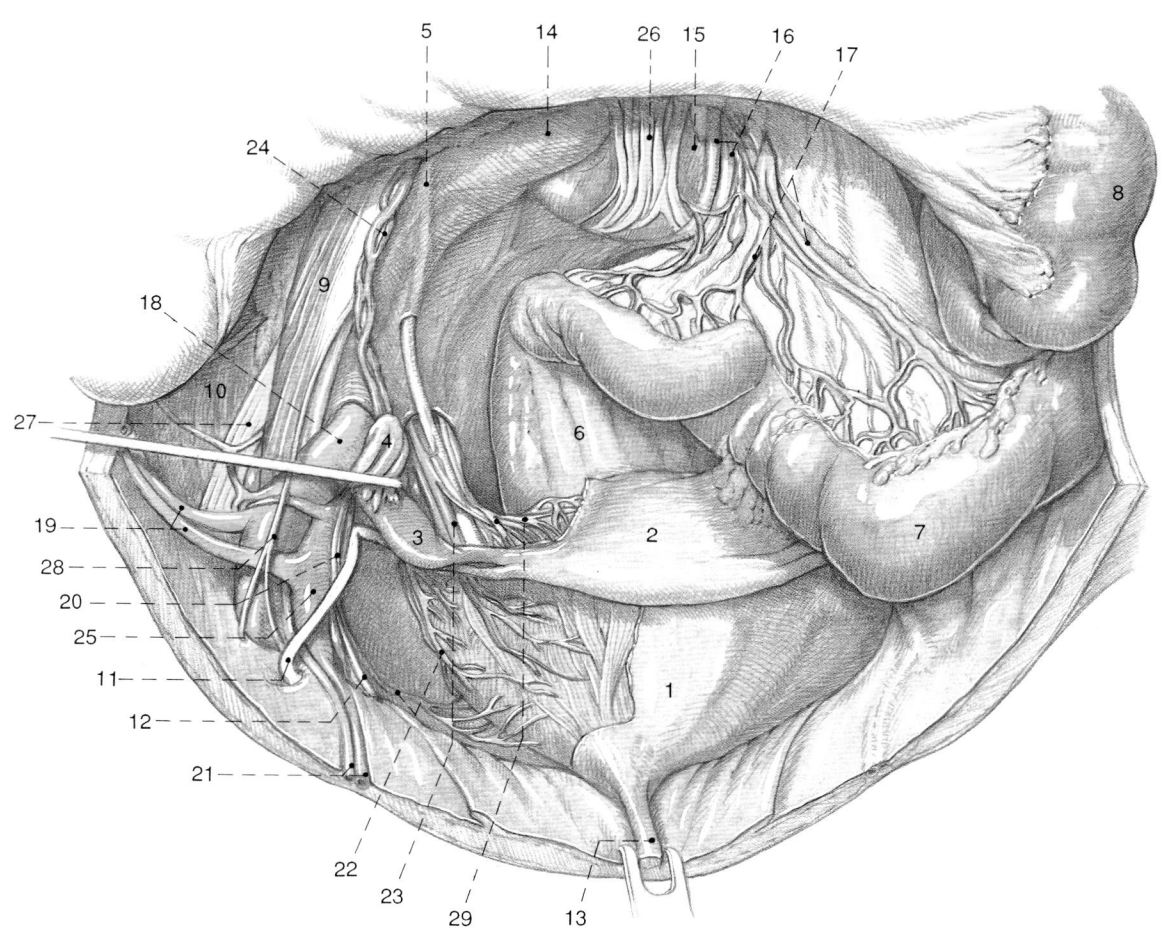

Fig. 3.2   Pelvic dissection in a female. The peritoneum has been partially removed (after Platzer).

1 Bladder	11 Round ligament of uterus	21 Inferior epigastric vessels
2 Uterus	12 Lateral umbilical ligament	22 Superior vesical arteries
3 Ovary	13 Urachus	23 Uterine artery
4 Fimbriated end of uterine tube	14 Right common iliac artery	24 Ovarian artery and accompanying veins
5 Ureter	15 Left common iliac artery	25 External iliac vein
6 Rectum	16 Superior rectal vessels	26 Superior hypogastric plexus (presacral nerve)
7 Sigmoid colon	17 Sigmoid vessels	27 Femoral nerve
8 Ileum	18 External iliac artery	28 Genitofemoral nerve
9 Psoas major	19 Deep circumflex iliac vessels	29 Uterovaginal nerve plexus
10 Iliacus muscle	20 Umbilical artery, patent section	

Generally the ureter runs about 1.5–2 cm lateral to the uterine cervix, though this distance can vary from 1 to 4 cm if the uterus occupies a paramedian position.

In its further course to the bladder, the female ureter is related to the fornix and anterior wall of the vagina. Generally the left ureter is more extensively apposed to the front of the vagina than the right ureter, so it is more vulnerable to trauma in vaginal operations. In all discussions of ureteral relations, it should be kept in mind that a distended bladder or rectum can cause displacement and even tortuosity of the ureters.

Vessels and Nerves of the Pelvic Ureter

The *arteries* of the pelvic part of the ureter form a plexus in the ureteral adventitia that, in the initial part of the pelvic ureter, is supplied by ureteral branches of the iliac vessels. These may arise from the common iliac artery or from the internal or external iliac artery. Ureteral branches from the iliolumbar and superior gluteal arteries are less commonly observed.

As the ureter descends further, its adventitial arterial plexus receives blood from the superior vesical artery, the artery of the vas deferens or uterine artery, the vaginal artery, and from the inferior vesical artery. Branches from the middle rectal artery also may reach the connective-tissue sheath of the ureter (Figs. 3.**1**, 3.**2**).

The *veins* of the pelvic part of the ureter reach the veins accompanying the arteries either directly or by way of the venous plexuses of the pelvis (vesical, prostatic, uterine, and vaginal plexuses).

The *lymph vessels* of the pelvic ureter drain into the regional lymph nodes on the pelvic wall: the external iliac, internal iliac, interiliac, and common iliac nodes.

The *nerves* of the pelvic ureter form dense networks in the adventitia, muscular wall, and mucosal layer of the ureter. They originate from the pelvic plexus, which in turn receives sympathetic fibers via the lumbar and sacral splanchnic nerves and the hypogastric plexus. Parasympathetic fibers reach the pelvic plexus via the pelvic splanchnic nerves from the sacral cord (Fig. 3.**3**).

Fig. 3.**3** Nerves in a male pelvis, viewed from the right side. ▶ Portions of the coxa have been removed (after Pernkopf/Platzer).

1 Ilium
2 Sacroiliac joint
3 Sacrum
4 Pubis
5 Ischial tuberosity
6 Sacrospinal ligament and coccygeus muscle
7 Sacrotuberal ligament
8 Piriformis muscle
9 Levator ani
10 Ischiocavernosus muscle
11 Bulbospongiosus muscle (penile bulb)
12 Common iliac artery
13 External iliac artery
14 Internal iliac artery
15 Common iliac vein
16 Vesicoprostatic venous plexus
17 Deep dorsal penile vein
18 Ureter
19 Sigmoid colon
20 Bladder
21 Prostate
22 Rectum
23 Vas deferens
24 Superior hypogastric plexus (presacral nerve)
25 Lumbosacral trunk
26 Vesical nerves
27 Dorsal penile nerve
28 Ventral branch of second sacral nerve
29 Hypogastric nerve
30 Pelvic splanchnic nerves
31 Ventral branch of fourth sacral nerve
32 Pelvic plexus (inferior hypogastric plexus)
33 Nerve of levator ani muscle
34 Cavernosal nerves of penis
35 Pudendal nerve
36 Prostatic plexus

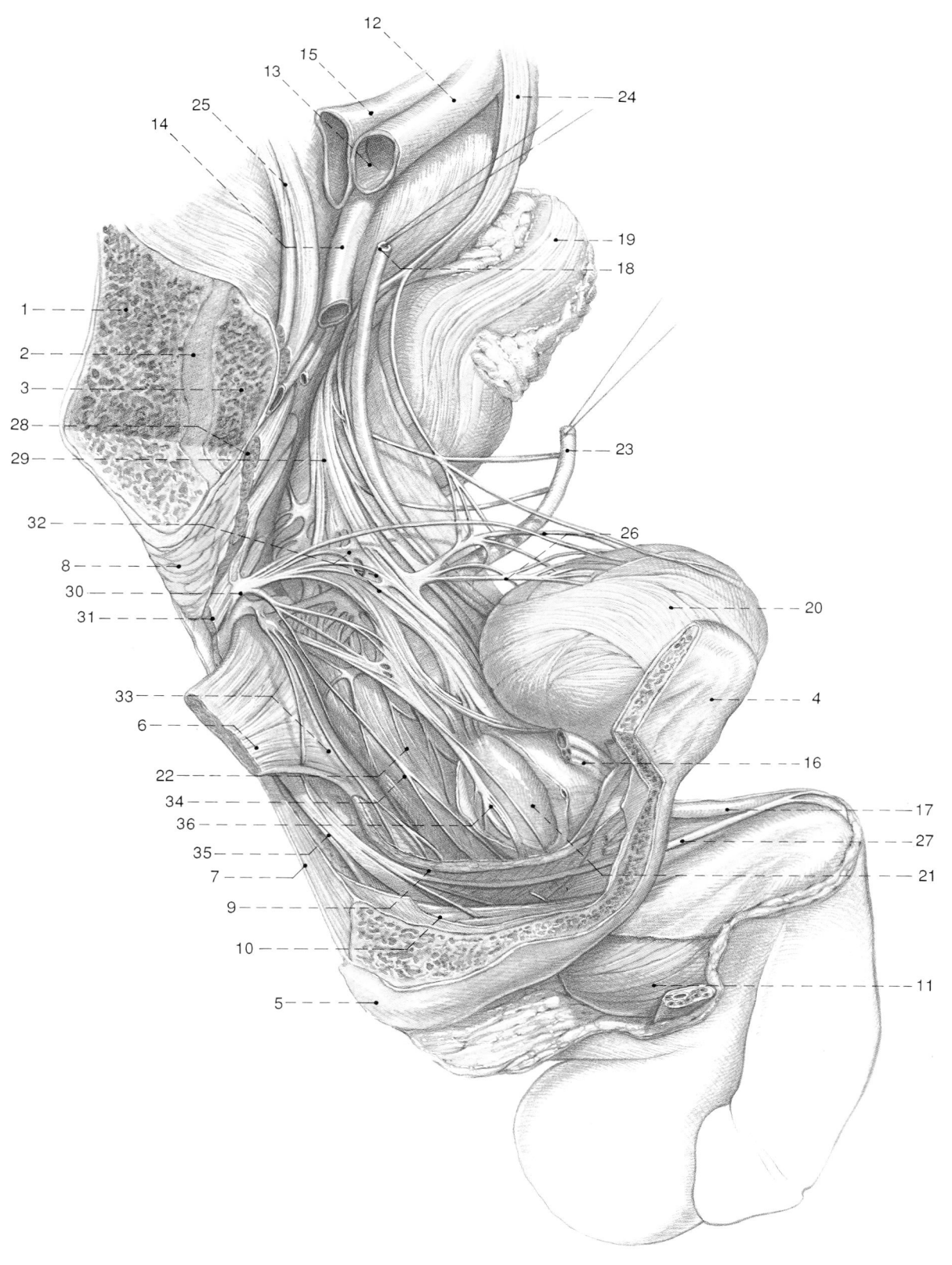

Relations of the Male Bladder to Adjacent Organs

The relations of the bladder to adjacent organs correlate closely with its relations to the pelvic connective tissue and peritoneum.

Peritoneal Covering of the Bladder

The bladder is attached to the peritoneum by loose connective tissue. This enables it to function as an expansile urinary reservoir that is mobile with respect to the peritoneum. Only a greatly distended bladder is fixed by its peritoneal covering (Fig. 3.**4**).

The parietal peritoneum is continued from the anterior abdominal wall onto the bladder apex and covers the posterior surface of the bladder to the level of the tips of the semi-nal vesicles, sometimes extending to the level of the ureteral orifices. There the peritoneum is reflected onto the anterior wall of the rectum to form the rectovesical pouch, which is the lowest point of the peritoneal cavity. The entrance to the rectovesical pouch is bounded by the two sagitally oriented rectovesical folds. These peritoneal folds are backed with connective tissue that provide posterior support for the bladder base.

The peritoneum is recessed between the bladder and anterior abdominal wall to form the supravesical fossae (Fig. 3.**4**). The right and left supravesical fossae are separated by the median umbilical fold. The supravesical fossa is bounded laterally by the medial umbilical fold. The peritoneal covering of the posterior bladder wall contains a reserve fold of peritoneum, the transverse vesical fold, that is progressively obliterated as the bladder distends.

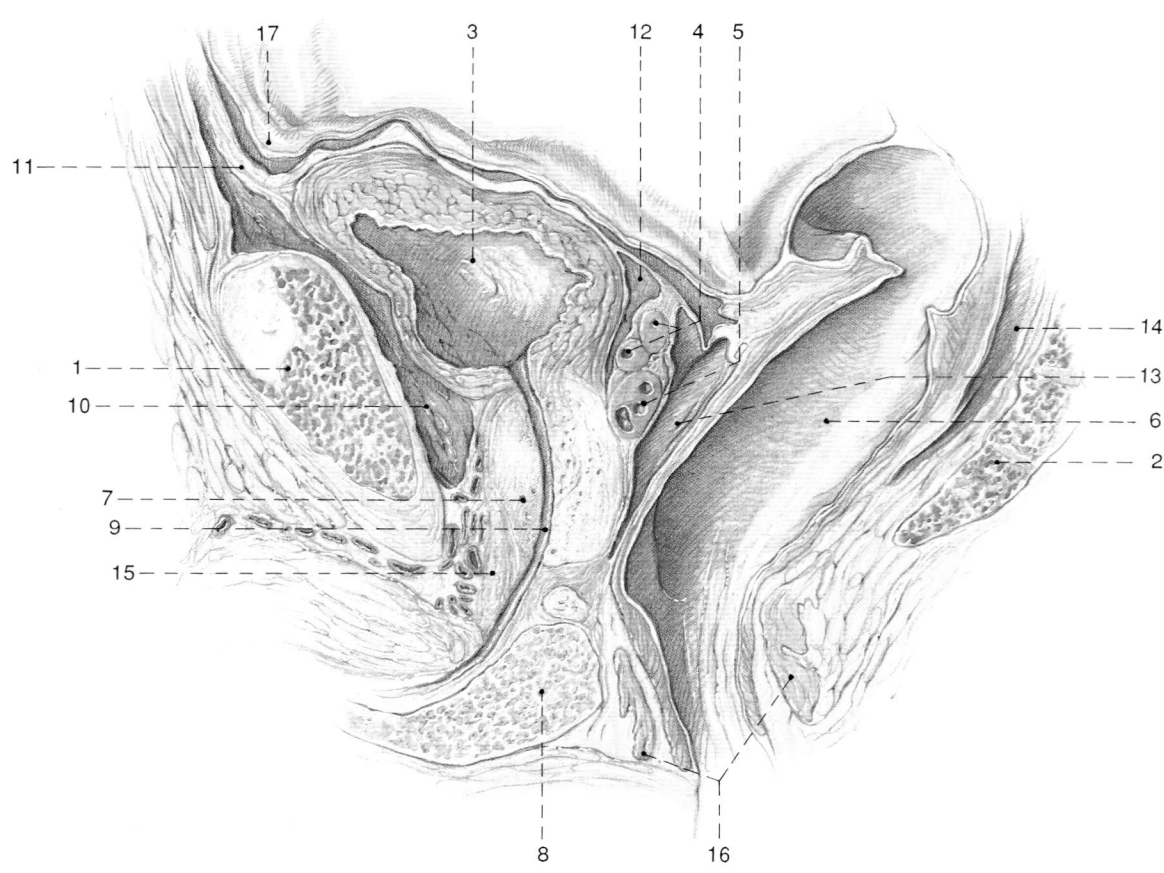

Fig. 3.**4** Midsagittal section through the pelvis. The spaces have been partially cleared of loose connective tissue.

1 Pubic symphysis	10 Prevesical (retropubic) space
2 Sacrum	11 Vesicoumbilical plate
3 Bladder	12 Vesicogenital space
4 Vas deferens	13 Rectogenital space
5 Seminal vesicle	14 Retrorectal space
6 Rectum	15 External urethral sphincter
7 Prostate	16 External anal sphincter
8 Bulb of penis	17 Supravesical fossa (parietal peritoneum)
9 Urethra, prostatic part	

Bladder and Pelvic Connective Tissue

The pelvic connective tissue consists of three main parts: the pelvic fascia (parietal and visceral), the neurovascular sheaths, and the loose connective tissue occupying the spaces of the pelvic viscera.

The *visceral pelvic fascia* is derived from the parietal pelvic fascia above the urogenital diaphragm at the site where the urethra pierces the diaphragm. The visceral fascia is reflected onto the prostate, and it invests the bladder as the *vesical fascia*.

The *neurovascular sheaths* are sheetlike condensations of intrapelvic connective tissue that invest and transmit nerves and blood vessels and additionally perform retinacular functions. Portions distributed to the bladder and prostate assist in the fixation of the bladder base. The *puboprostatic ligament* (pubovesical ligament) extends from the symphysis and adjacent portions of the pubic bone to the prostate and is continued onto the bladder neck. It binds the prostate and bladder to the anterior pelvic wall. The *paracystic connective tissue (bladder retinaculum)* passes to the bladder from the lateral pelvic wall. Between the paracystic connective tissue and *pararectal connective tissue (rectal retinaculum)*

is the *rectovesical septum*, which represents the central portion of the lateral neurovascular sheath (Fig. 3.**6**).

Loose connective tissue occupies the *spaces* between the condensations of the neurovascular sheaths and visceral fasciae. The *prevesical space* located between the anterior abdominal wall and bladder is bounded anteriorly by the transversalis fascia and posteriorly by the vesical fascia. The prevesical space is continuous inferiorly with the *retropubic space* (Figs. 3.**4**, 3.**6**, 3.**7**). This space is bounded anteriorly by the posterior surface of the pubic symphysis, posteriorly by the prostatic fascia, and inferiorly by the urogenital diaphragm.

The rectovesical and retropubic spaces communicate laterally with the *paravesical space*. This mobile tissue plane is bounded posteriorly by the paracystic connective tissue, medially by the vesical fascia, and laterally and inferiorly by the parietal pelvic fascia.

Between the rectum and bladder is the *rectovesical space*. The rectovesical septum and the seminal vesicles subdivide this space into two separate compartments termed the *vesicogenital space* and *rectogenital space* (Figs. 3.**4**–3.**6**).

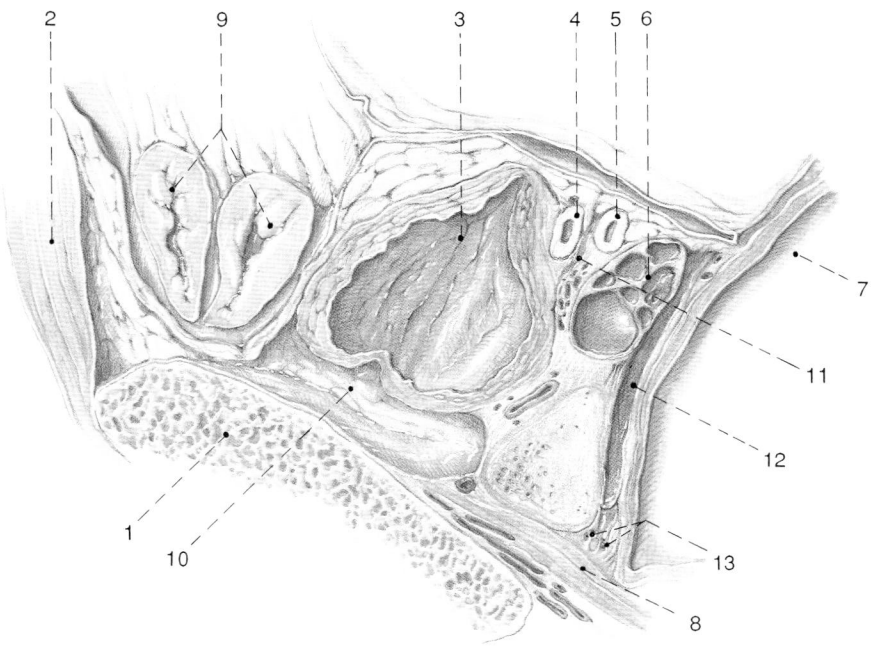

Fig. 3.**5** Paramedian section through the pelvis. The spaces have been partially cleared of loose connective tissue.

1 Pubis	10 Paravesical space
2 Rectus abdominis muscle	11 Vesicogenital space
3 Bladder	12 Rectogenital space
4 Ureter	13 Neurovascular bundle
5 Vas deferens	
6 Seminal vesicle	
7 Rectum	
8 Levator ani	
9 Ilium	

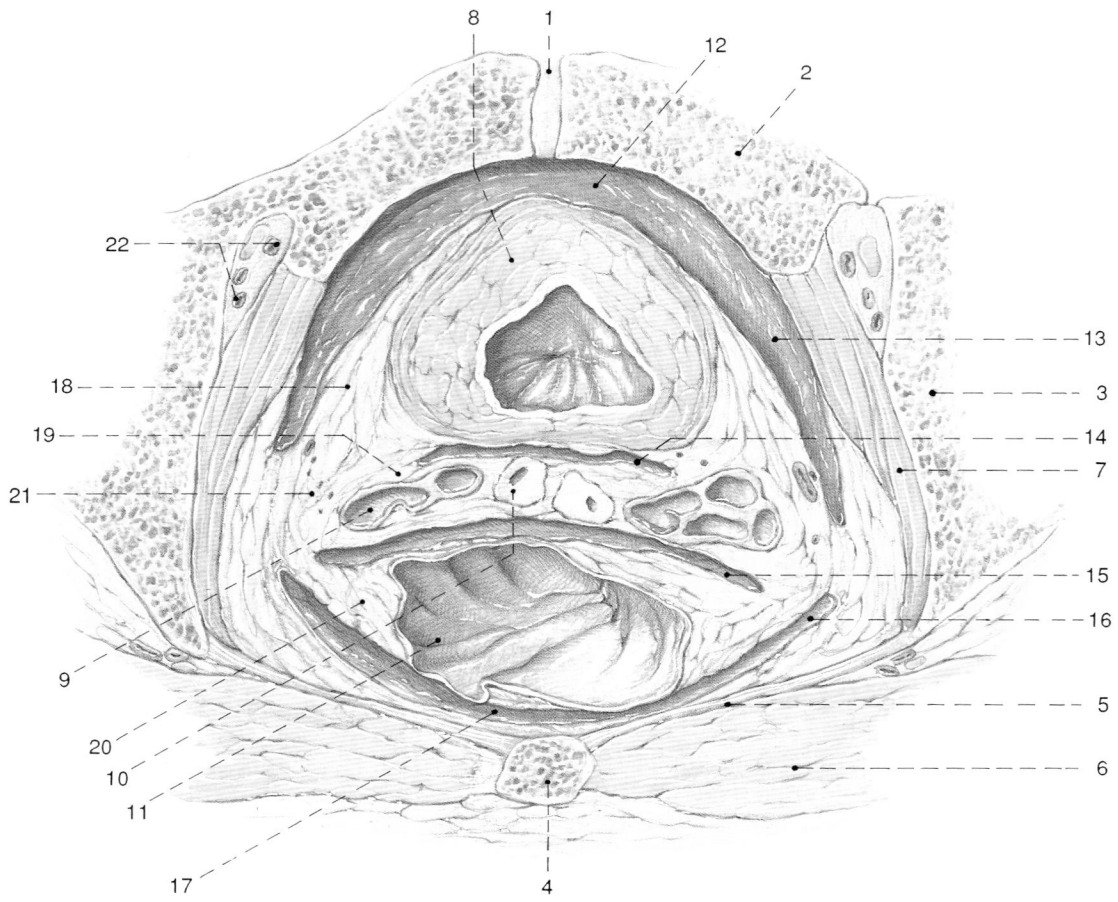

Fig. 3.**6** Transverse section through the pelvis at the level of the seminal vesicles. The spaces have been partially cleared of loose connective tissue.

1	Pubic symphysis	12	Prevesical space
2	Pubis	13	Paravesical space
3	Ischium	14	Vesicogenital space
4	Coccyx	15	Rectogenital space
5	Sacrospinal ligament	16	Pararectal space
6	Gluteus maximus	17	Retrorectal space
7	Obturator internus	18	Paracystium
8	Bladder	19	Rectovesical septum
9	Seminal vesicle	20	Paraproctium
10	Vas deferens	21	Neurovascular bundle
11	Rectum	22	Obturator canal, obturator vessels and nerve

Vessels and Nerves of the Bladder

The *arteries* of the bladder may arise directly from the internal iliac artery or from one of its visceral branches (Figs. 3.**1**, 3.**2**).

The superior vesical artery is almost always multiple. Usually there are two superior vesical arteries, their number ranging from one to four. The superior vesical arteries generally arise from the patent, unobliterated portion of the umbilical artery but occasionally are derived from the obturator artery (4.5%). They supply the base and body of the bladder and generally anastomose with the inferior vesical artery.

The inferior vesical artery is usually a direct branch of the internal iliac but may arise from a nearby vessel such as the internal pudendal artery (25%) or inferior gluteal artery (4%). It supplies the bladder base in addition to the prostate and seminal vesicles.

The *veins* of the bladder commence as intramural plexuses. The larger vessels emerging from the bladder wall form the vesical plexus, which communicates with the venous plexus of the prostate. Both plexuses drain into the internal iliac vein.

The *lymph vessels* of the bladder communicate with one another in the paravesical space and may end directly at the external iliac and interiliac lymph nodes or may reach them by way of smaller nodes (anterior, lateral, and posterior vesical nodes). Connections with the internal iliac lymph nodes are occasionally observed.

The *nerves* supplying the bladder are derived from the pelvic plexuses (Fig. 3.**3**). The parasympathetic fibers (pelvic splanchnic nerves) of these plexuses originate from the second to fourth sacral segments and supply the detrusor muscle. The sympathetic fibers reach the vesical plexus from the first two lumbar segments by way of the hypogastric plexus.

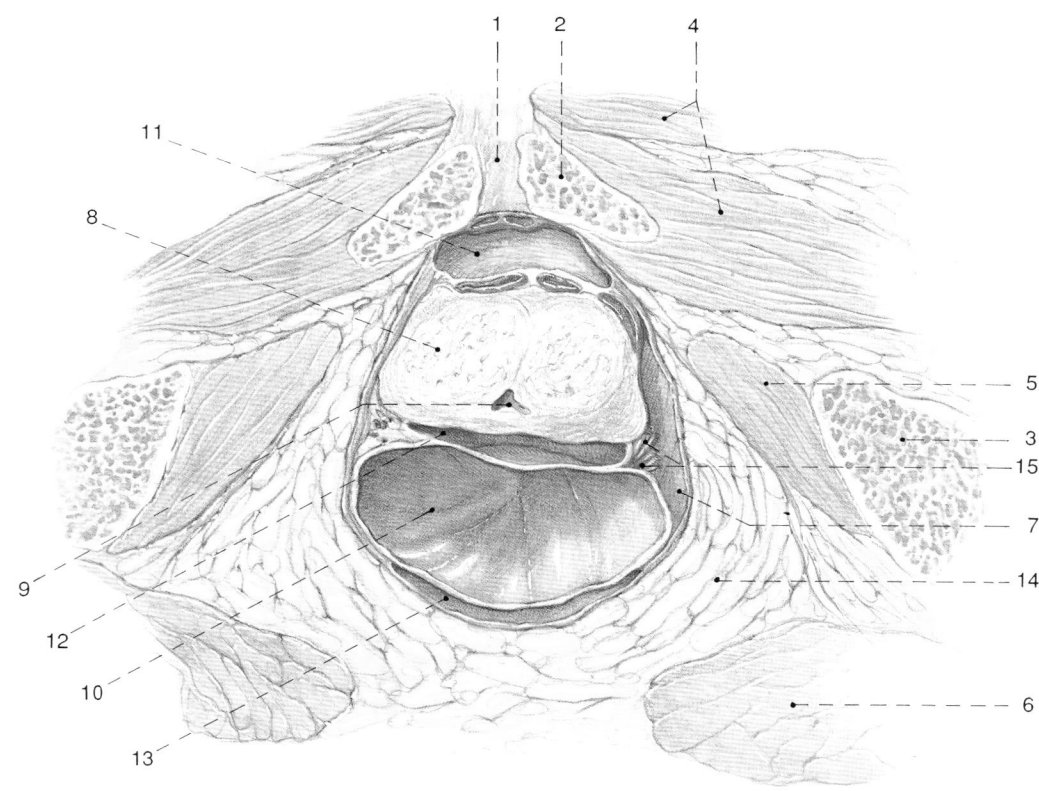

Fig. 3.**7** Transverse section through the pelvis at the level of the prostate. The spaces have been partially cleared of loose connective tissue.

1 Pubic symphysis	9 Urethra, prostatic part
2 Pubis	10 Rectum
3 Ischium	11 Pubourethral space
4 Gracilis and adductor longus	12 Rectogenital space
5 Obturator internus	13 Retrorectal space
6 Gluteus maximus	14 Ischiorectal fossa
7 Levator ani	15 Neurovascular bundle of the prostate (paraprostatic connective tissue)
8 Prostate	

Prostate

The prostate is enveloped by an external connective-tissue layer, the *prostatic capsule,* and by its visceral fascia, the *prostatic fascia.* The lateral portion of the prostatic fascia, the paraprostatic connective tissue, is well developed posteriorly to form Denonvillier's fascia. Between the prostate and rectum is the *rectoprostatic space* (Figs. 3.**4**, 3.**5**).

The rectoprostatic space communicates superiorly with the *rectovesical space,* which is subdivided by the seminal vesicles and spermatic ducts into a *rectogenital space* and a *vesicogenital space* (Figs. 3.**6**, 3.**7**). The prostate is fixed to the symphysis anteriorly by the *puboprostatic ligaments,* and it is supported posteriorly by connective tissue slips from the rectal retinaculum.

Relations of the Female Bladder to Adjacent Organs

The relations of the female bladder to the pelvic connective tissue are obviously gender-specific. The parietal fascia of the pelvic floor is reflected onto the bladder at the bladder neck to form the vesical fascia.

The pubovesical ligaments in the female pelvis, derived from the intrapelvic neurovascular-retinacular sheaths, bind the bladder to the pubic symphysis.

The paracystic connective tissue passes from the lateral pelvic wall to the bladder. Tough connective-tissue fibers are distributed to this tissue from the cardinal ligament of the uterus.

The relation of the loose connective tissue to the female bladder is the same anteriorly (prevesical space) and laterally (paravesical space) as in the male. Posteriorly, between the body of the bladder and the cervix, loose connective tissue occupies the *vesicouterine space.* The *vesicovaginal space* is located more caudally between the bladder base and the front of the vagina.

The relation of the female bladder to the pelvic connective tissue accounts in large part for its relations to adjacent organs.

The female urethra has two clinical subdivisions: a superior part and an inferior part. The superior part, comprising the cranial one-fourth of the urethra, can move relative to the vagina owing to the loose connective tissue in the *urethrovaginal space.* The inferior part lacks a true space, and in that area the vagina and urethra are fused together by their visceral fasciae. The anterosuperior portion of the female urethra is fixed by the lowermost fibers of the pubovesical ligaments, known also as the "pubourethral ligaments."

Anterior Pelvic Exenteration in the Male

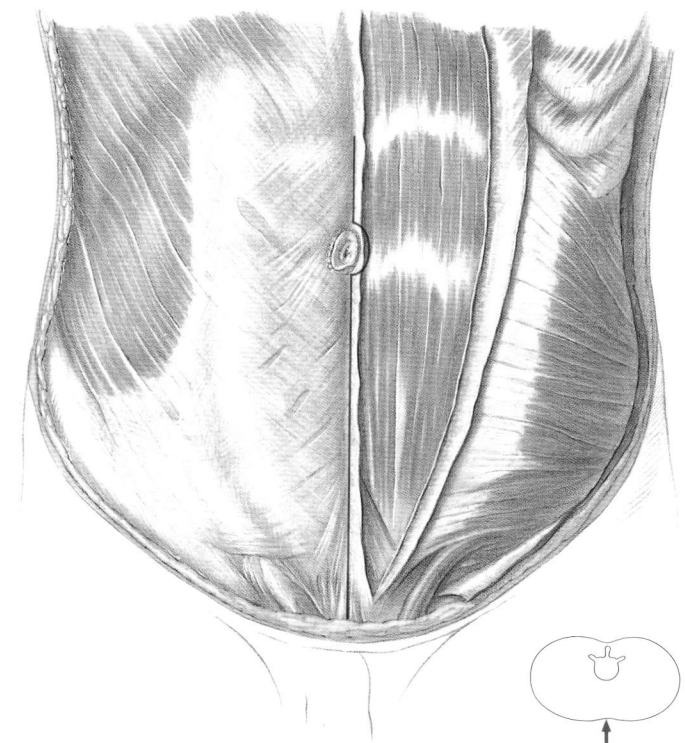

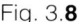

Fig. 3.**8**

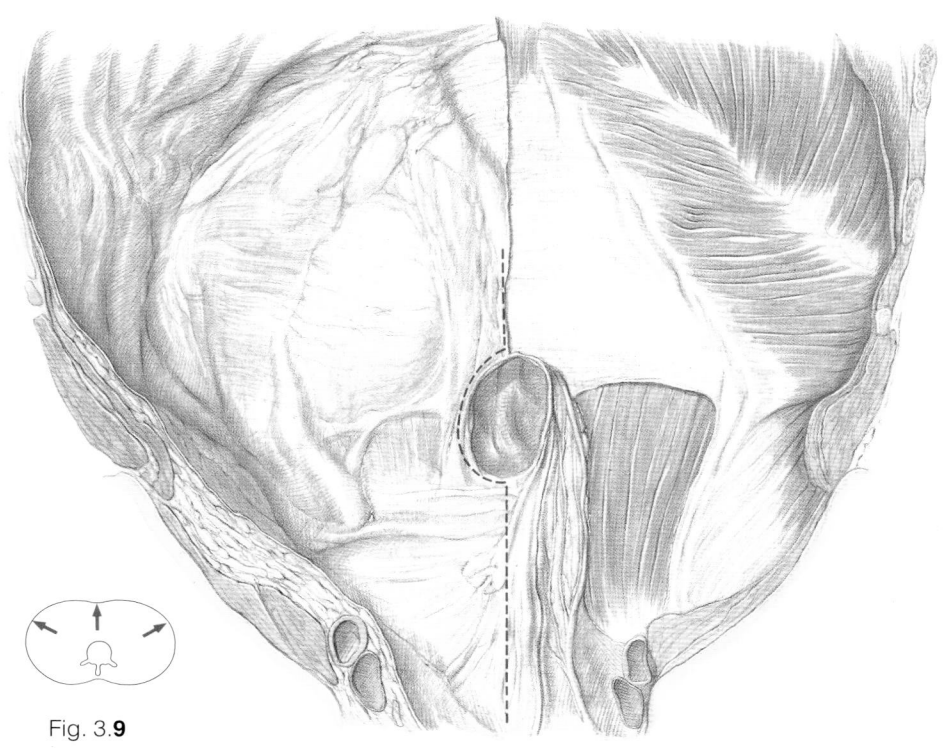

Fig. 3.**9**

Main Indications

● Invasive bladder carcinoma

Position and Skin Incision

The patient is positioned with the pelvis hyperextended (Fig. 3. **10**) to permit broad exposure of the operative field. The midline incision extends from 5 cm above the umbilicus to the pubic symphysis (Figs. 3.**10**, 3.**11**).

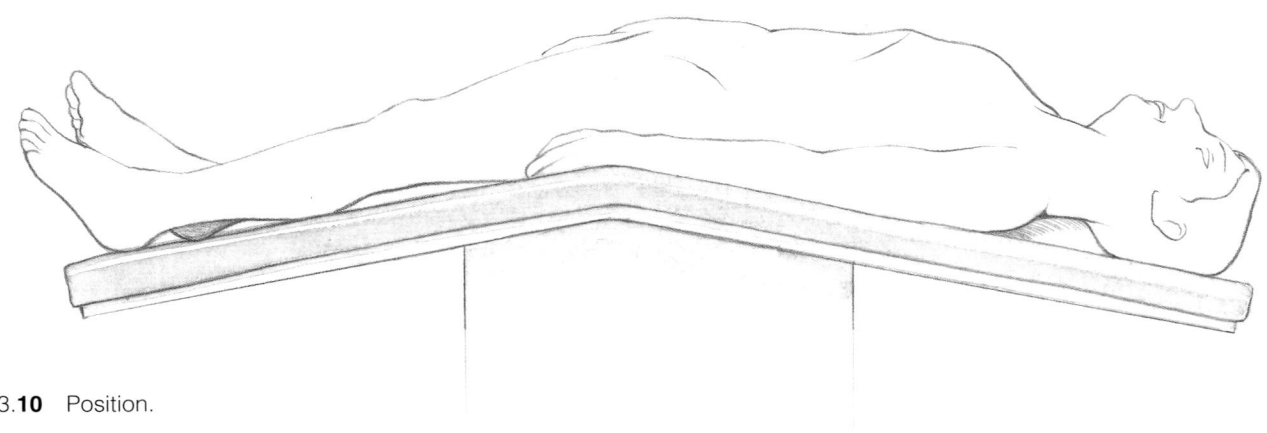

Fig. 3.**10**   Position.

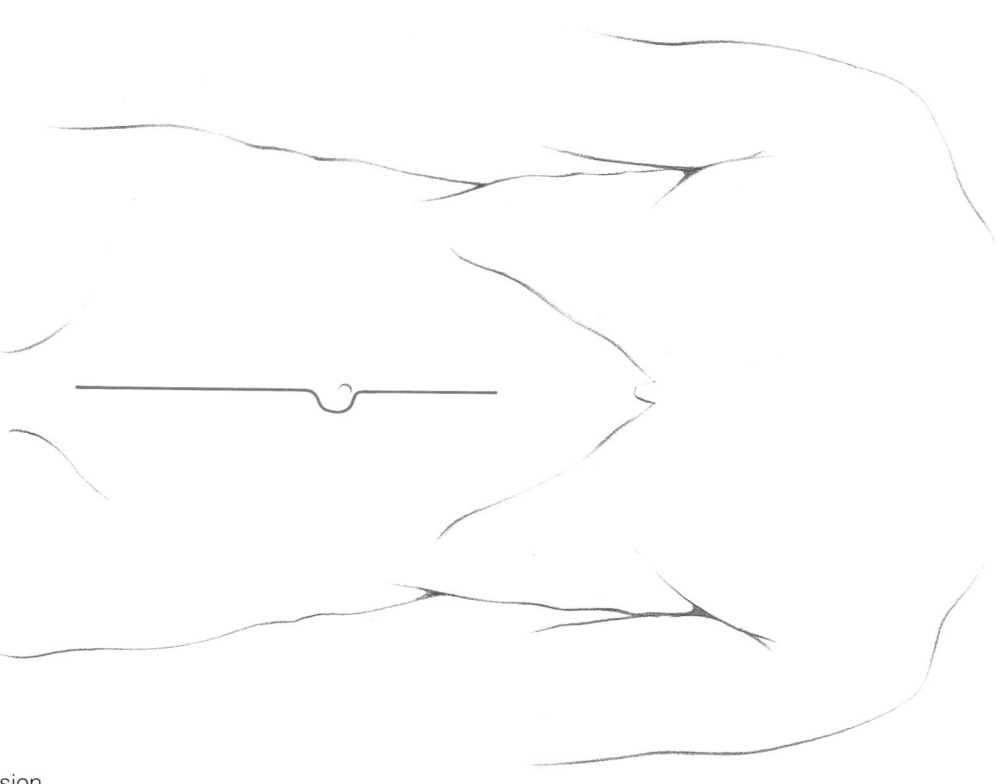

Fig. 3.**11**   Skin incision.

Entry into the Peritoneal Cavity

The subcutaneous fat is divided with diathermy, and individual bleeding vessels are coagulated at once. The anterior rectus sheath is exposed (Fig. 3.**12**).

The anterior rectus sheath is incised at the linea alba (Fig. 3. **13**). Both rectus muscles have been separated in the figure to expose the posterior rectus sheath, transversalis fascia, and arcuate line (Fig. 3.**13**). The transversalis fascia forms the posterior layer of the rectus sheath caudal to the arcuate line.

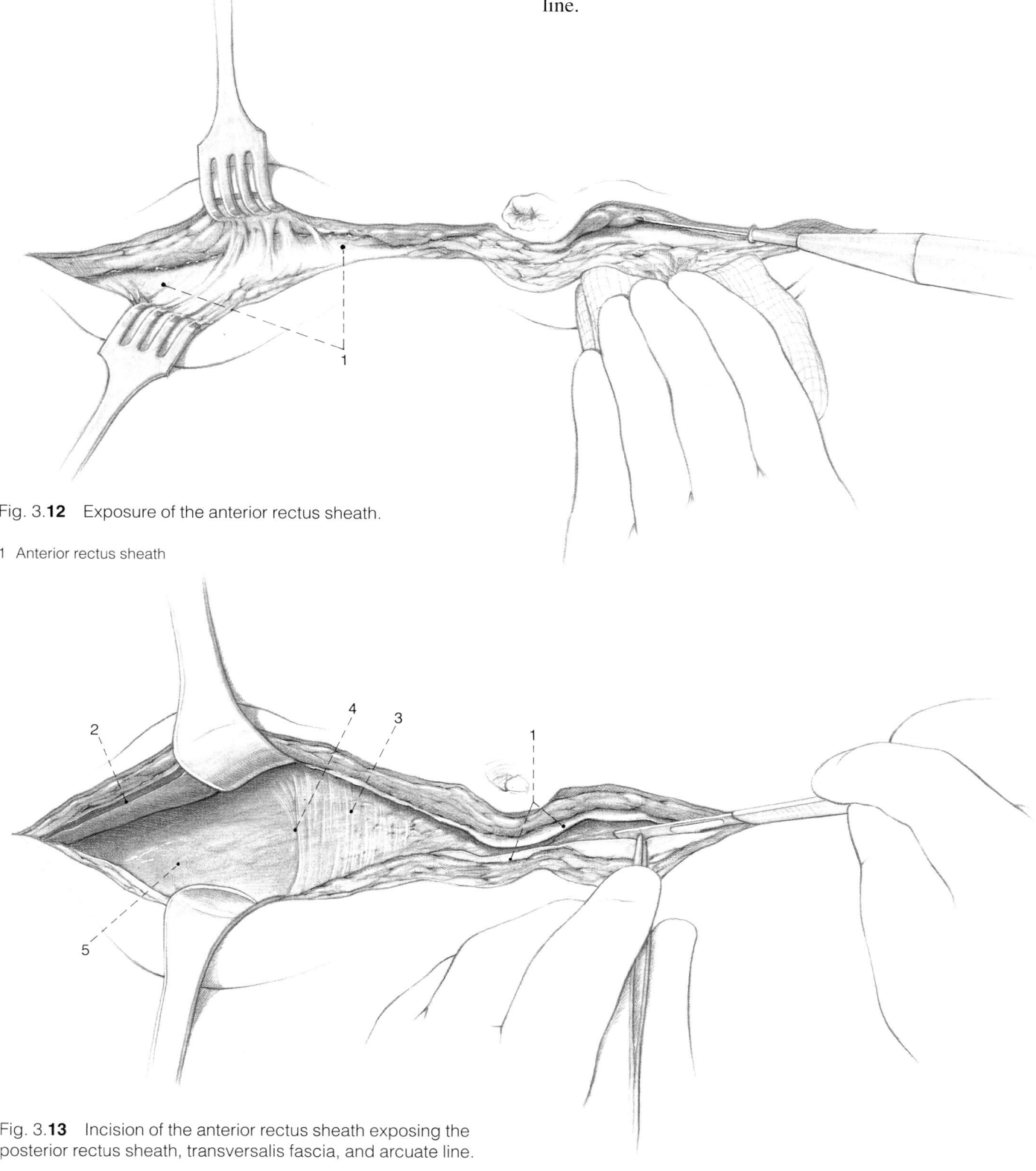

Fig. 3.**12**   Exposure of the anterior rectus sheath.

1 Anterior rectus sheath

Fig. 3.**13**   Incision of the anterior rectus sheath exposing the posterior rectus sheath, transversalis fascia, and arcuate line.

1 Anterior rectus sheath
2 Rectus abdominis muscle
3 Posterior rectus sheath
4 Arcuate line
5 Transversalis fascia (posterior rectus sheath)

The posterior rectus sheath, preperitoneal fat, and parietal peritoneum are incised to establish entry to the peritoneal cavity (Fig. 3.**14**).

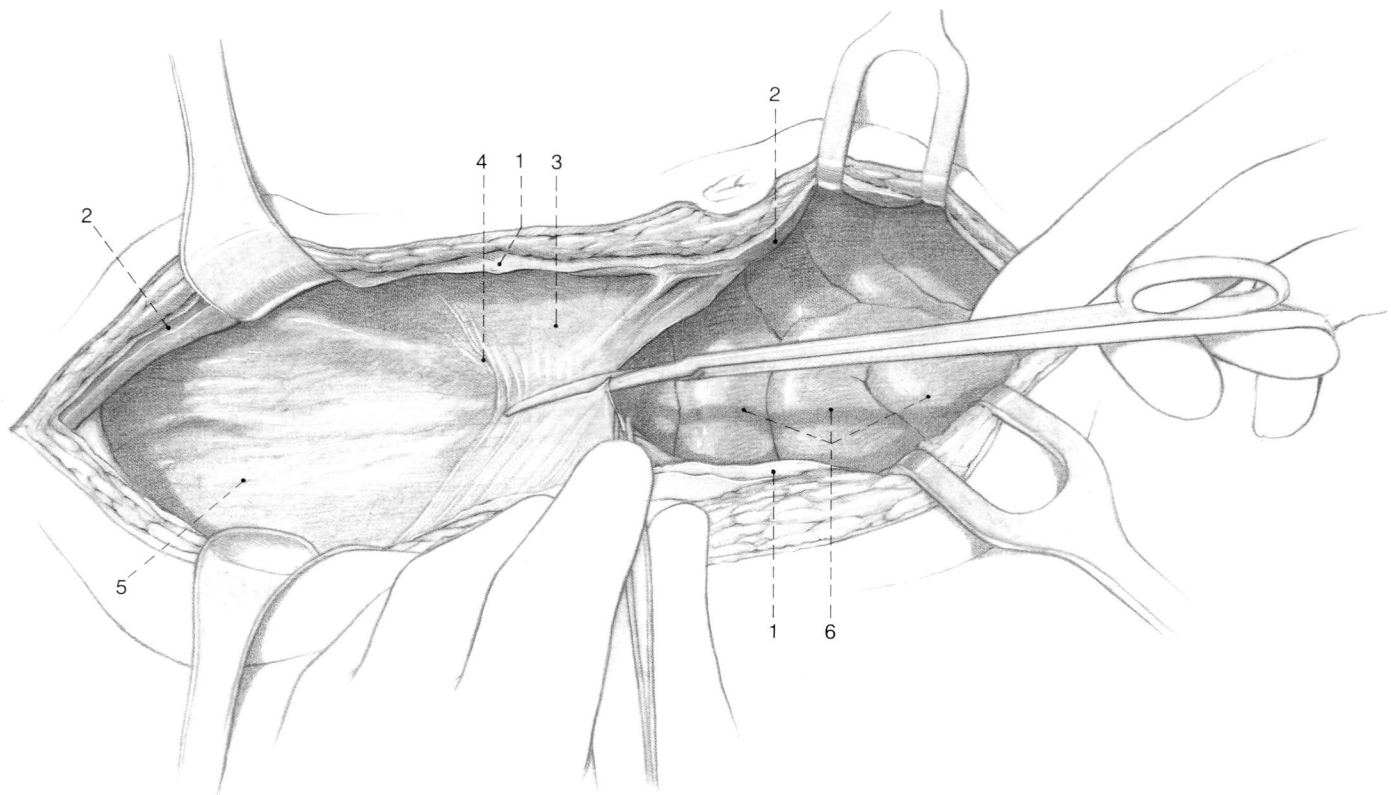

Fig. 3.**14**   Entry into the peritoneal cavity.

1 Anterior rectus sheath
2 Rectus muscle
3 Posterior rectus sheath
4 Arcuate line
5 Transversalis fascia (posterior rectus sheath)
6 Jejunum

Dissection of the Vesicoumbilical Plate

The urachus is isolated near the umbilicus and divided (Fig. 3.**15**). Entry into the peritoneal cavity at a more inferior level is established by dissecting the "vesicoumbilical plate" (medial umbilical fold, median umbilical fold, transversalis fascia, peritoneal fat, and peritoneum) downward en bloc to the lateral umbilical ligaments (Fig. 3.**16**).

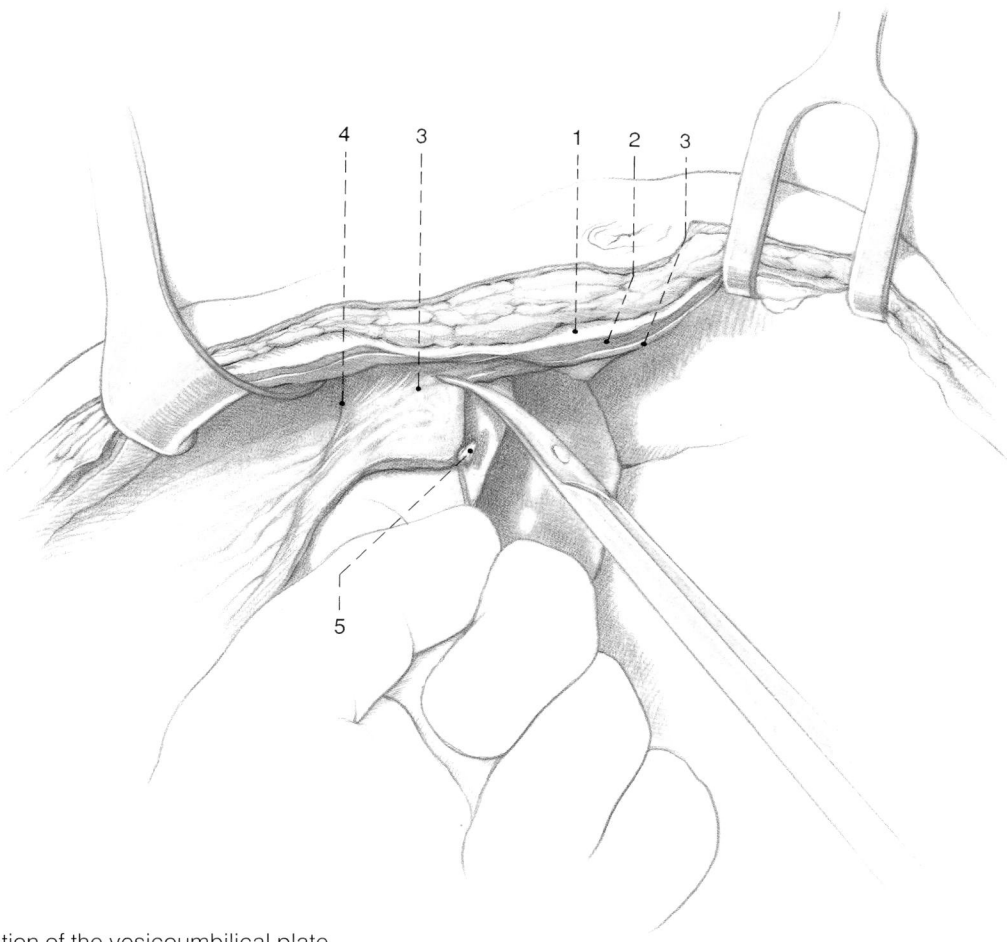

Fig. 3.**15**   Dissection of the vesicoumbilical plate.

1 Anterior rectus sheath
2 Rectus muscle
3 Posterior rectus sheath
4 Arcuate line
5 Urachus

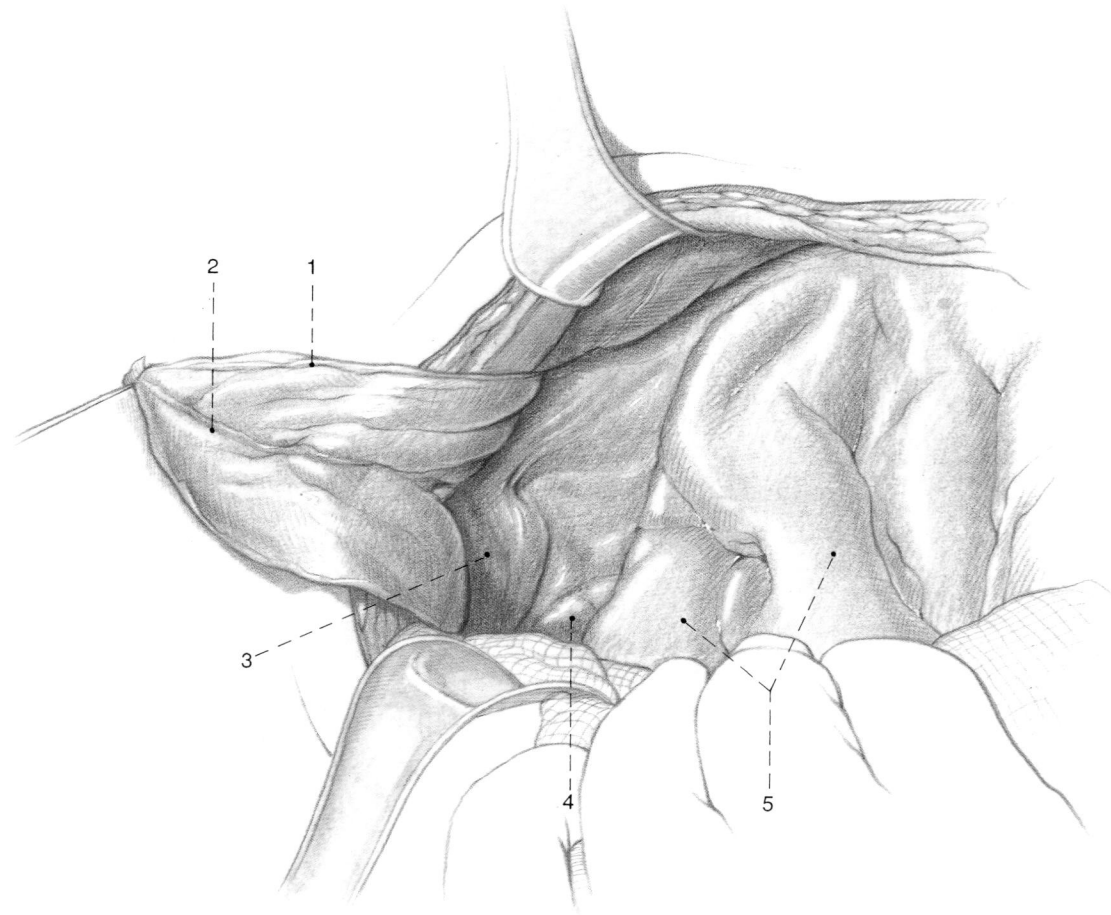

Fig. 3.**16**   The freed vesicoumbilical plate is retracted inferiorly.

1 Medial umbilical fold (umbilical ligament)
2 Median umbilical fold (urachus)
3 Bladder
4 Sigmoid colon
5 Ileum

Mobilization of the Small Bowel and Ascending Colon

The incision for entering the retroperitoneal space starts at the superior duodenojejunal fold (ligament of Treitz) and extends over the common iliac artery and vein into the right paracolic sulcus. The entire mesentery and a large portion of the colon can be circumscribed with this incision (Figs. 3.17, 3.18), the horizontal part of the duodenum forming the superior boundary of the field. All of the small bowel and ascending colon can be packed upward or to the side with a large laparotomy pad (Fig. 3.18).

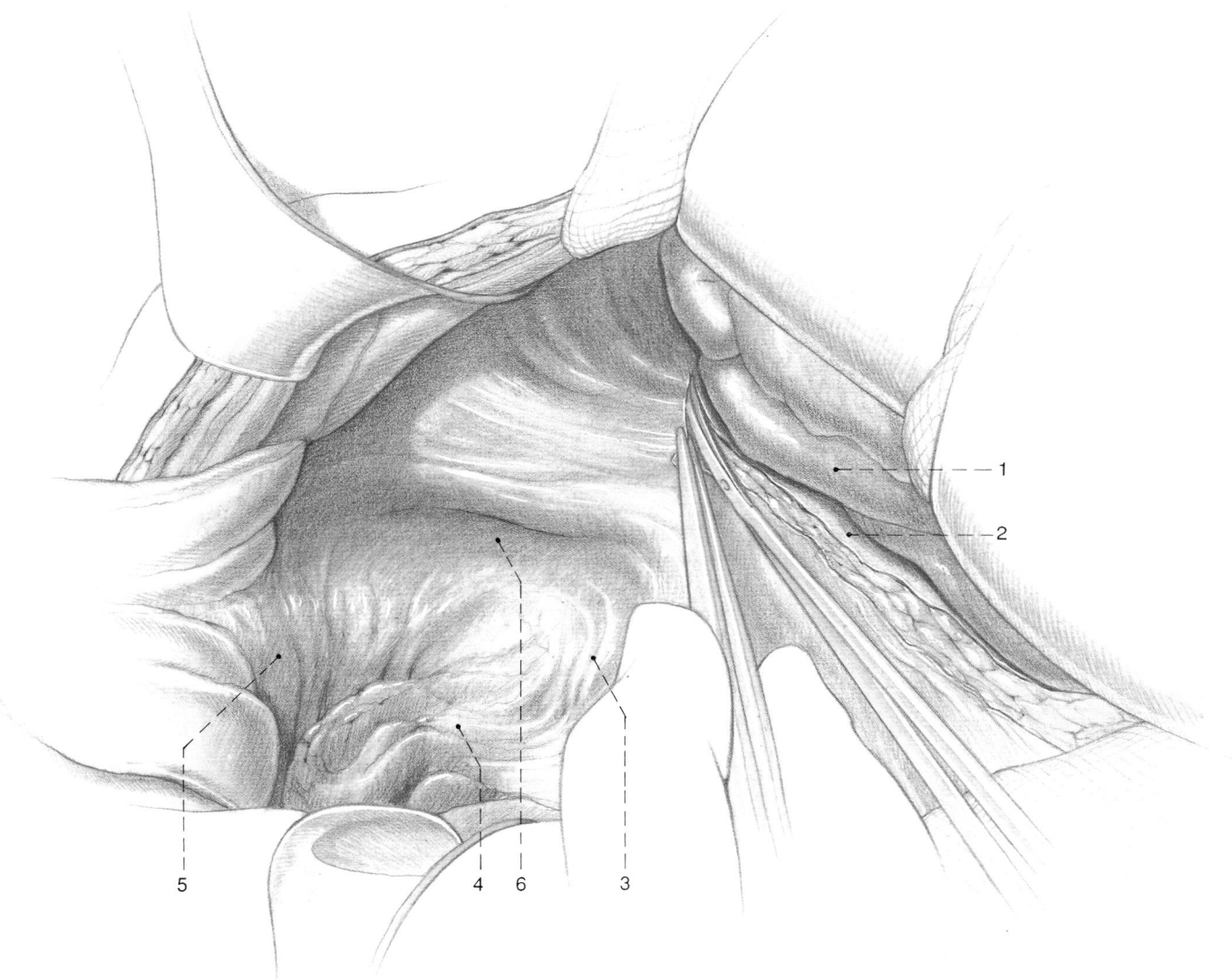

Fig. 3.17 The retroperitoneal space is opened with an incision extending from the duodenojejunal fold over the right common iliac artery and vein and around the colon.

1 Ileum
2 Parietal peritoneum
3 Rectum
4 Sigmoid colon
5 Bladder
6 Rectovesical pouch

The retroperitoneal connective tissue can be dissected over the full extent of the retroperitoneal space. The right ureter is dissected free of the retroperitoneal space and snared along with its surrounding vessels, nerves, and connective tissue. The connective tissue accompanying the ureter remains attached to collaterals of the testicular vessels (Fig. 3.**18**).

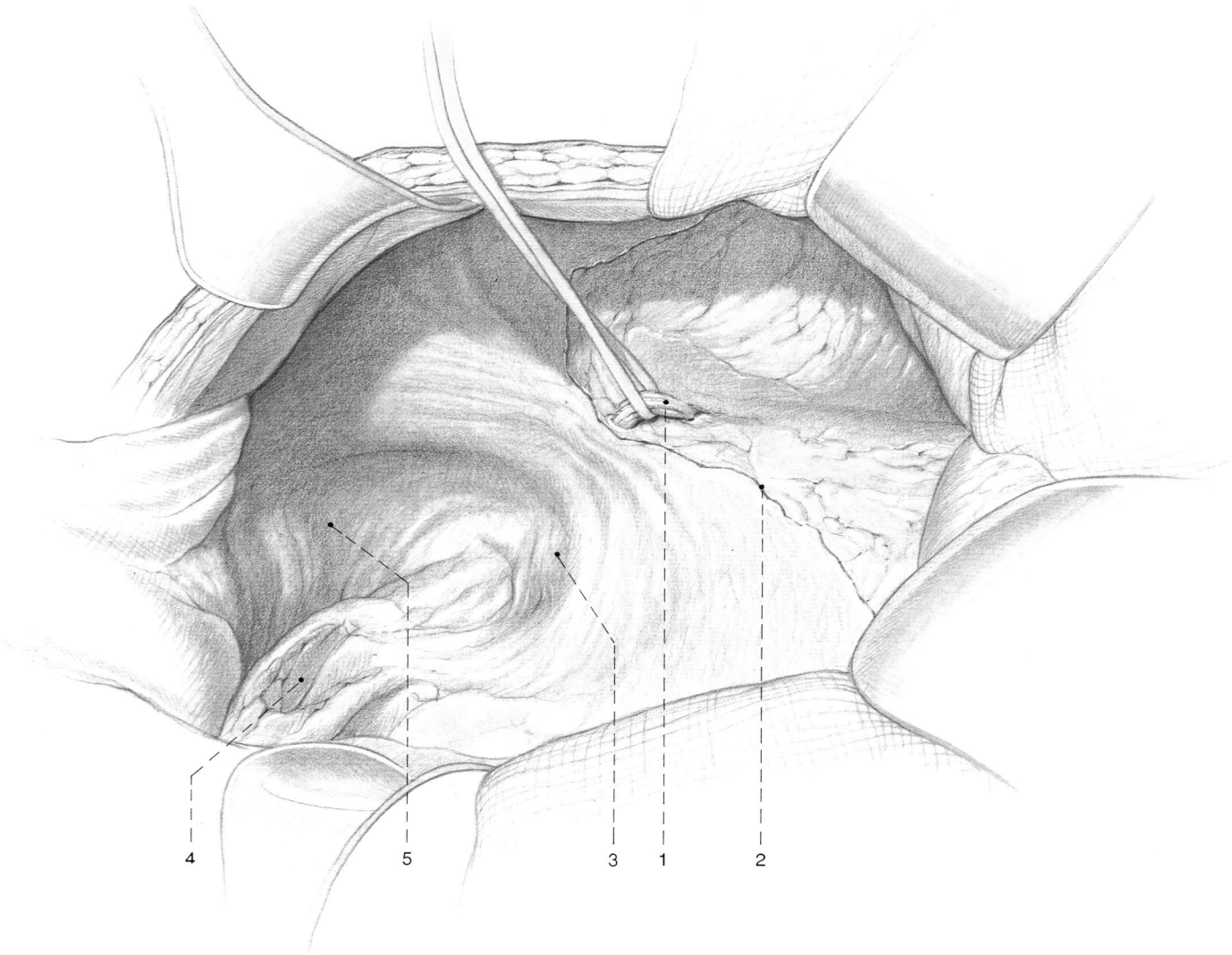

Fig. 3.**18** The incision is continued into the right paracolic sulcus, and the cecum and colon are mobilized. The right ureter is dissected free and snared.

1 Right ureter
2 Parietal peritoneum
3 Rectum
4 Sigmoid colon
5 Rectovesical pouch

For mobilization of the left ureter, the sigmoid mesocolon is incised to the level of the inferior pole of the left kidney. As on the right side, the left paracolic sulcus is opened to the level of the lower renal pole. The mesentery of the sigmoid colon is dissected free of the promontory. An incision is made in the mesentery along the abdominal aorta from the bifurcation to the origin of the inferior mesenteric artery to permit the insertion of a tape (Fig. 3.**19**).

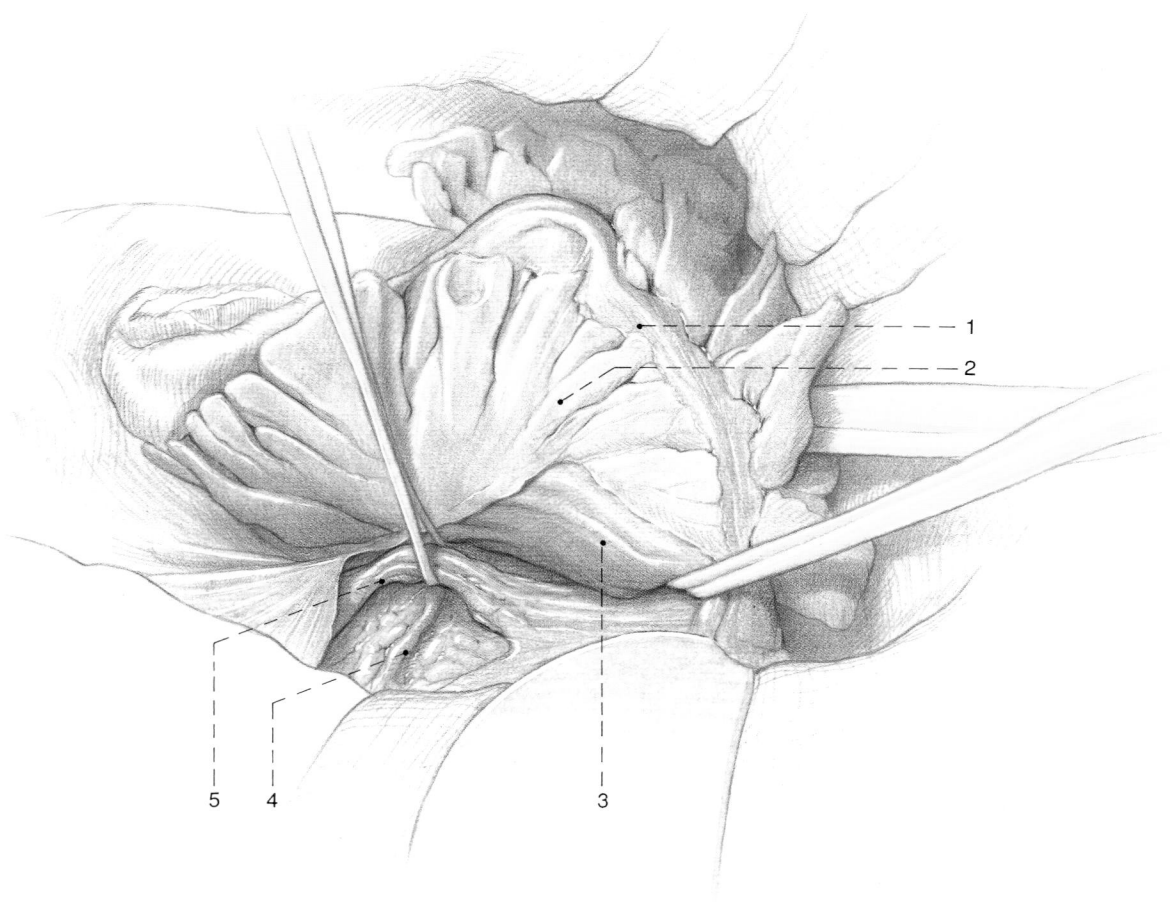

Fig. 3.**19** Approach to the left ureter. The sigmoid mesocolon is incised to the level of the lower pole of the left kidney. The mesentery of the sigmoid colon is freed from the promontory. An opening is made in the mesentery and snared with a tape. The right ureter is dissected free of the retroperitoneum.

1 Sigmoid colon
2 Sigmoid mesocolon
3 Testicular vein
4 Iliolumbar vein
5 Left ureter

At this point the descending colon and sigmoid colon lie within the operative field. The ureter is clipped 2 cm distal to its crossing with the common iliac artery and vein (Fig. 3.**20**). The upper portion of the ureter and surrounding vascular connective tissue are widely dissected out of the retroperitoneal space, leaving the ureter in continuity with the branches of the testicular vessels (Fig. 3.**20**).

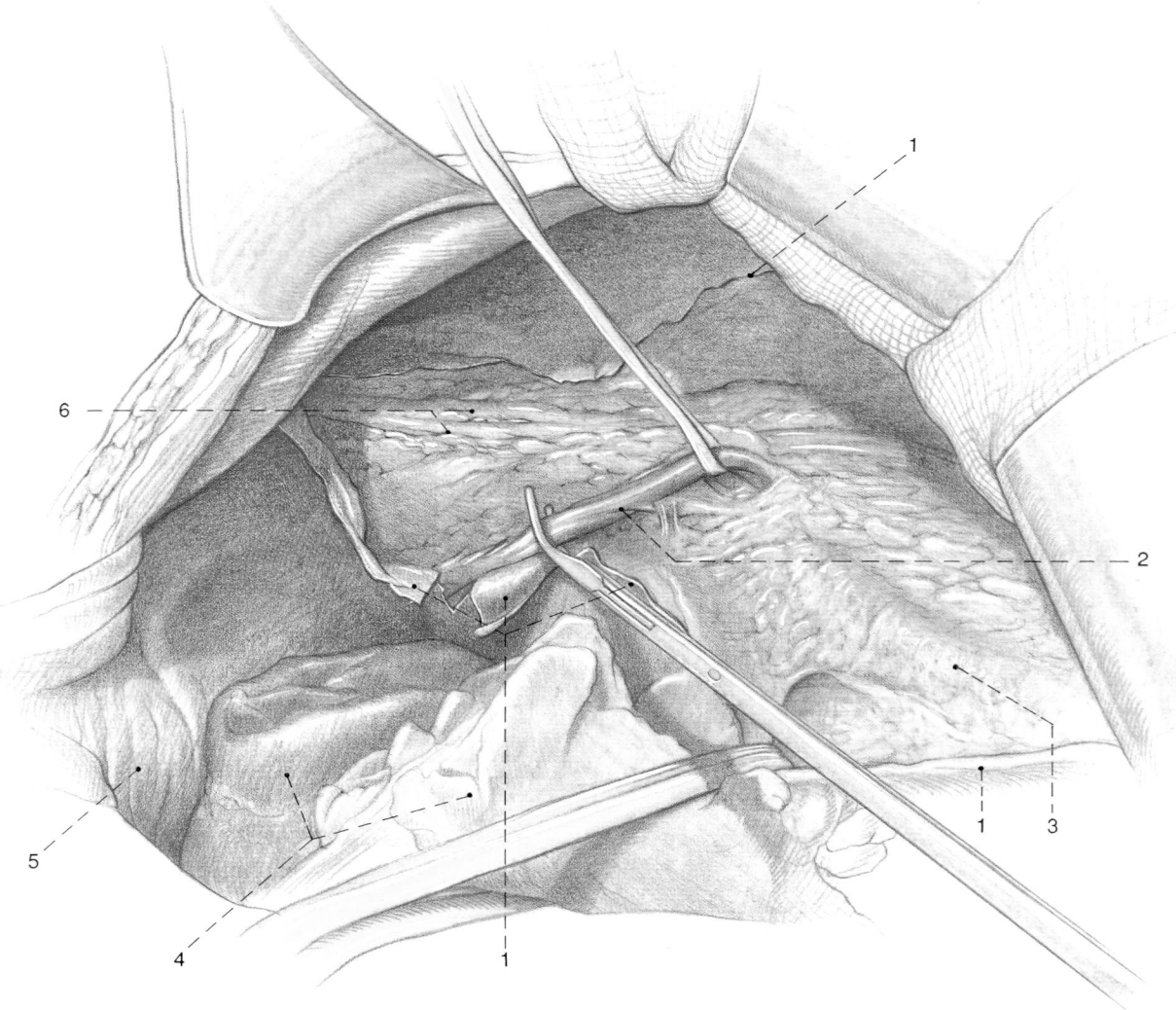

Fig. 3.**20** The right ureter is isolated and clipped past its crossing with the common iliac artery and vein.

1 Parietal peritoneum
2 Right ureter
3 Right common iliac vessels
4 Sigmoid colon
5 Bladder
6 Right testicular vein

Lymph Node Dissection by the Split-and-Roll Technique

This dissection begins 1–2 cm above the bifurcation of the abdominal aorta. The area of the dissection is bounded laterally by the genitofemoral nerve. The pelvic fat and connective tissue over the common iliac artery, external iliac artery, and external iliac vein are opened using the split-and-roll technique (Fig. 3.21). The lateral parietal peritoneum is opened forward to the femoral canal, and the right vas defer-

ens is ligated (Fig. 3.21). The external iliac artery and vein are now deflected medially with the index finger, and the lymph nodes, lymph vessels, connective tissue, and fat are mobilized downward en bloc over the internal obturator muscle (Fig. 3.22). Caution is exercised during the dissection of the obturator nerve.

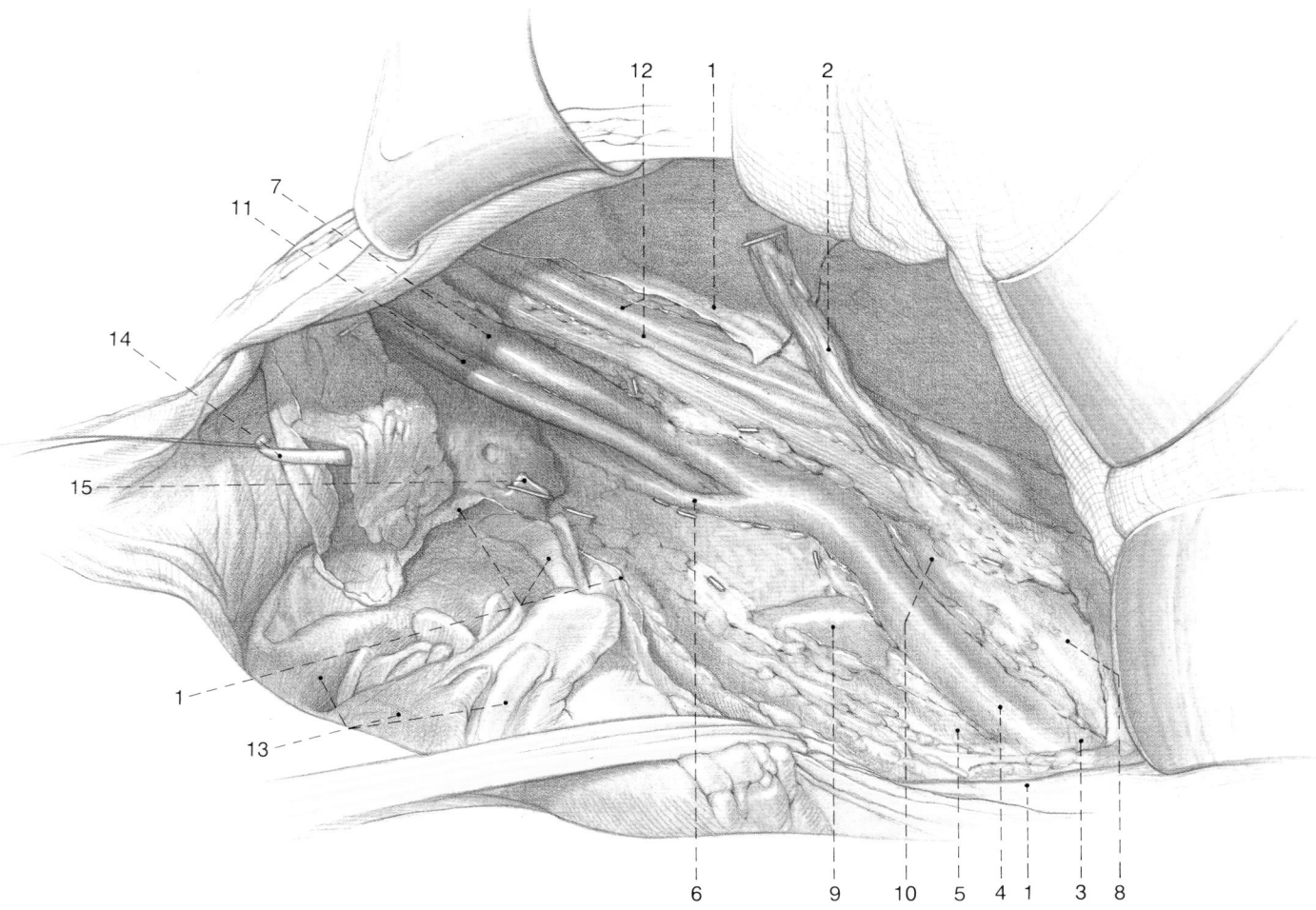

Fig. 3.21   Pelvic lymph node dissection in pelvic exenteration.

1 Parietal peritoneum	9 Left common iliac vein
2 Right ureter	10 Right common iliac vein
3 Abdominal aorta	11 Right external iliac vein
4 Right common iliac artery	12 Testicular vein
5 Left common iliac artery	13 Sigmoid colon
6 Right internal iliac artery	14 Right vas deferens
7 Right external iliac artery	15 Prevesical ureteral stump
8 Inferior vena cava	

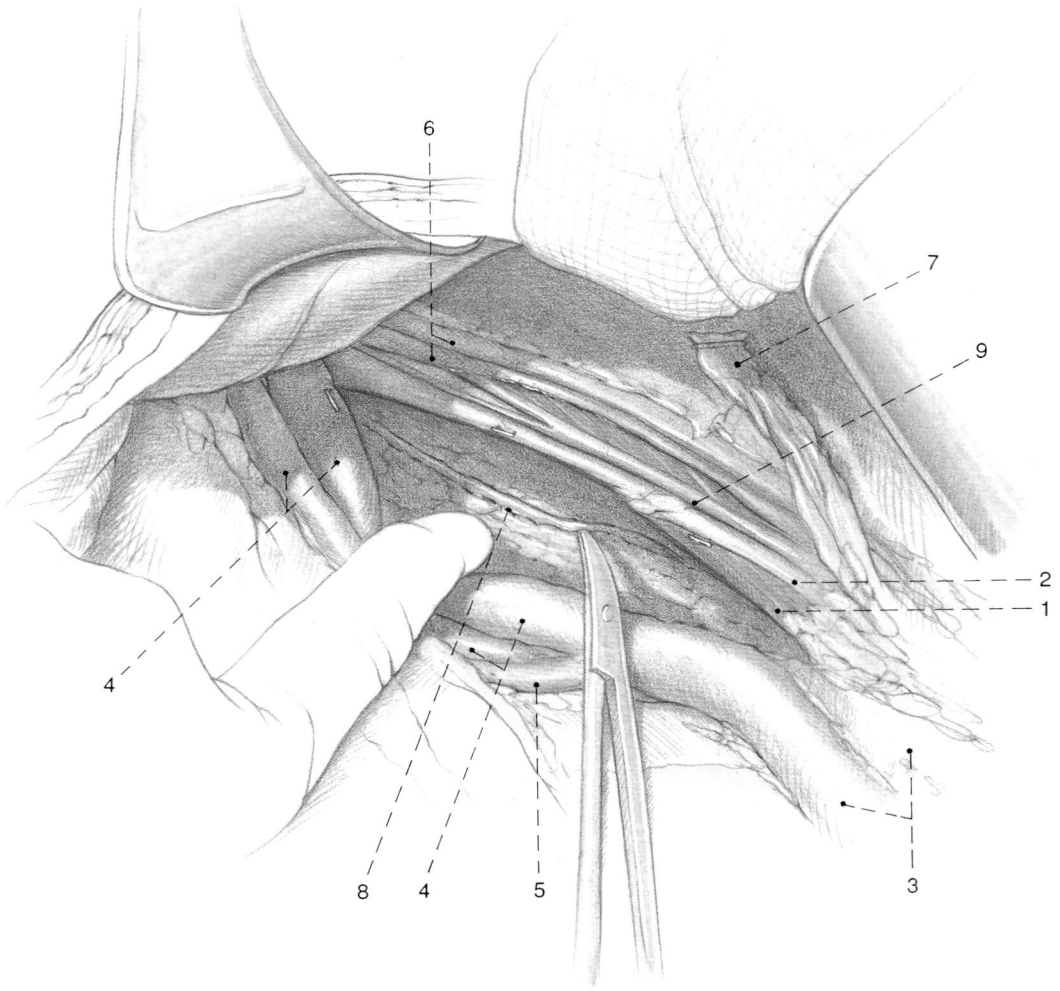

Fig. 3.**22**   Dissection of the obturator nerve on the pelvic wall.

1 Psoas major muscle
2 Psoas minor muscle
3 Right common iliac vessels
4 External iliac vessels
5 Internal iliac artery
6 Testicular vein
7 Right ureter
8 Obturator nerve
9 Genitofemoral nerve

The pectineal ligament forms the caudal boundary of the lymph node dissection (Fig. 3.**23**). The obturator vessels are isolated medial to the obturator nerve and then clipped along the endopelvic fascia (Fig. 3.**23**).

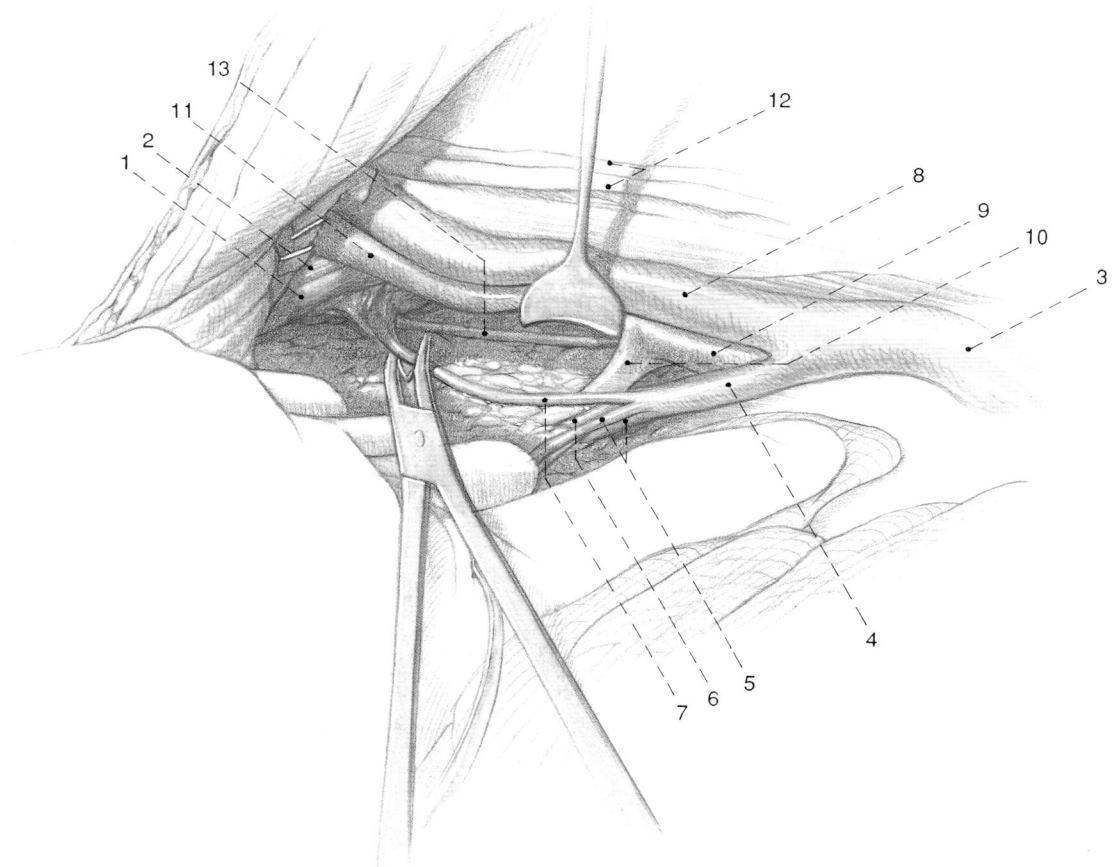

Fig. 3.**23**　The field of the lymph node dissection is bounded distally by the pectineal ligament. The obturator vessels are isolated and clipped.

 1 Superior pubic ramus
 2 Pectineal ligament
 3 Right common iliac artery
 4 Internal iliac artery
 5 Umbilical artery (patent section) and superior vesical artery
 6 Inferior vesical artery
 7 Obturator artery
 8 External iliac artery
 9 Common iliac vein
10 Internal iliac vein
11 External iliac vein
12 Testicular vein
13 Obturator nerve

Dissection of the Lateral Bladder Pedicle (Lateral Bladder Retinaculum)

The right-handed surgeon places the fourth and fifth fingers of the left hand on the bladder and medial border of the lateral paracystic connective tissue with the third finger on the internal iliac artery. The index finger is swept medially behind the internal iliac artery into the depths of the pelvis. With this maneuver the surgeon can displace the lateral retinaculum (lateral bladder pedicle) toward the bladder and the rectovesical septum (posterior bladder pedicle) toward the rectum. With the left index finger behind the lateral pedicle, the internal iliac artery is identified, followed by the anterior branches of the internal iliac artery, the lateral umbilical fold, the superior vesical artery, the inferior vesical artery, and the obturator artery. These vessels are individually isolated, identified, and ligated (Figs. 3.**24**, 3.**25**).

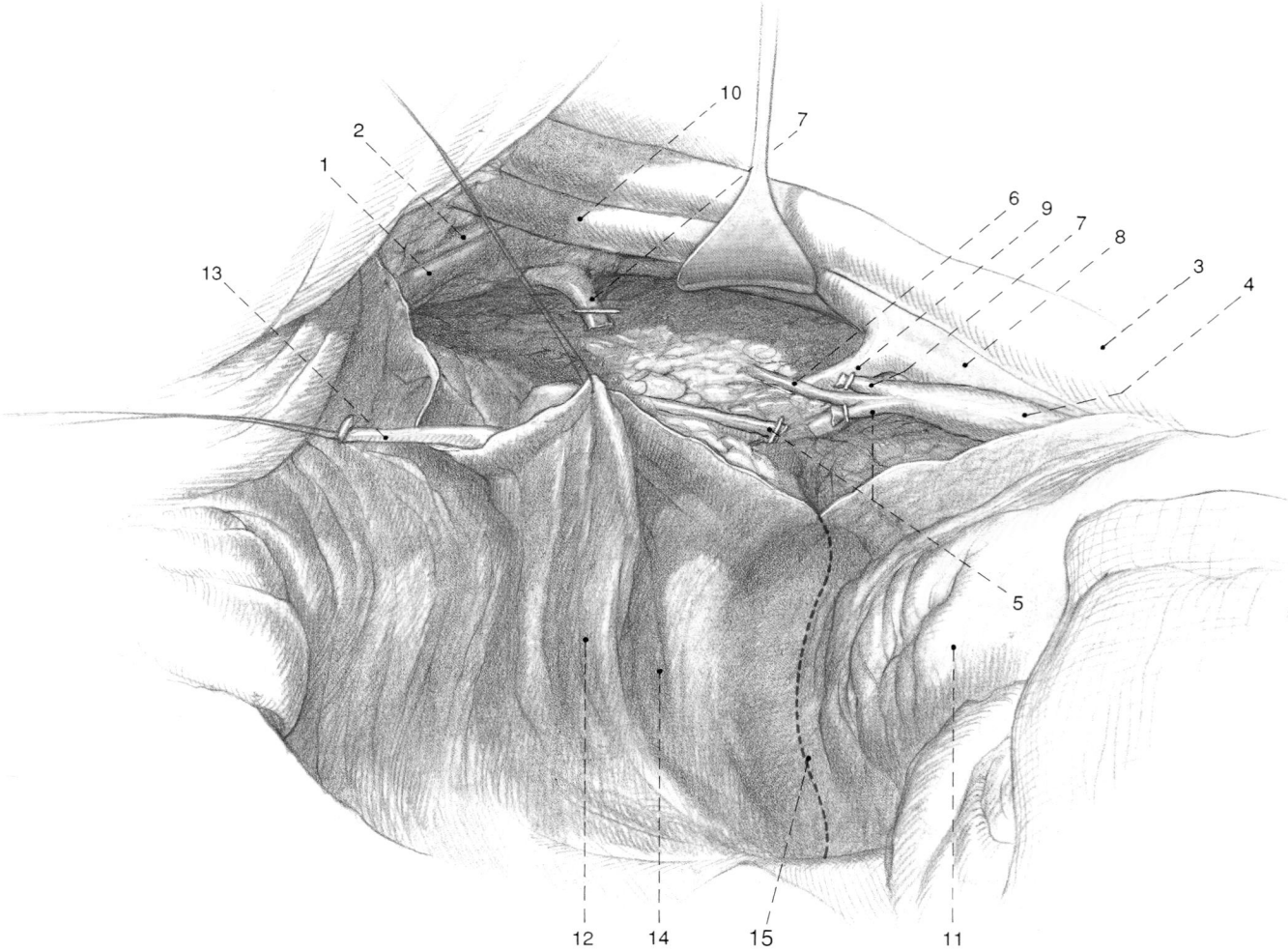

Fig. 3.**24**   Dissection of the lateral bladder pedicle.

 1 Superior pubic ramus
 2 Pectineal ligament
 3 External iliac artery
 4 Internal iliac artery
 5 Superior vesical artery
 6 Inferior vesical artery
 7 Obturator artery
 8 Common iliac vein
 9 Internal iliac vein
10 External iliac vein
11 Rectum
12 Bladder
13 Right vas deferens
14 Rectovesical pouch
15 Cul de sac

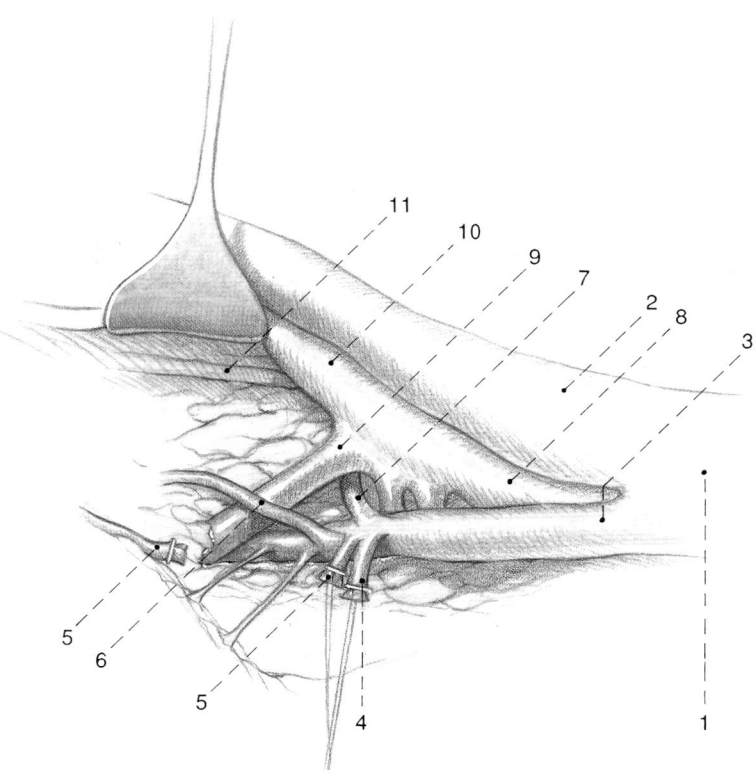

Fig. 3.**25**   Close-up view of the dissection of the lateral bladder pedicle. The obturator artery, superior vesical artery, and inferior vesical artery are identified and clipped.

 1 Common iliac artery
 2 External iliac artery
 3 Internal iliac artery
 4 Obturator artery
 5 Superior vesical artery
 6 Inferior vesical artery
 7 Superior gluteal artery
 8 Common iliac vein
 9 Internal iliac vein
10 External iliac vein
11 Obturator nerve

Variants of the Internal Iliac Artery

The branching pattern of the internal iliac artery is extremely variable. The most common variants of the parietal branches of the internal iliac artery are shown schematically in Fig. 3.**26**. The internal iliac artery usually divides at a variable level into an anterior and posterior trunk.

The origin of the obturator artery is largely independent of the primary bifurcation of the internal iliac artery.

The *obturator artery* may arise from the anterior trunk of the internal iliac artery (Fig. 3.**26 a, b, h**; 41.5%) or from the posterior trunk (Fig. 3.**26 c, f**; 13.5%). It also may arise from a common trunk for the internal pudendal and inferior gluteal arteries (Fig. 3.**26 d**; 10%). The obturator artery springs from the internal pudendal artery in about 4% of cases (Fig. 3.**26 e, i**) and from the inferior gluteal artery in 5% (Fig. 3.**26 g, k**).

In 19% of cases the obturator artery arises from the inferior epigastric artery and in 1% from the external iliac. The obturator artery is duplicated in about 5% of cases, one vessel arising from the external iliac artery and the other from the internal iliac artery or its branches.

The visceral branches of the internal iliac artery are also subject to considerable variation, as outlined below:

The *umbilical artery (patent section)* consistently gives rise to the superior vesical arteries and the artery of the vas deferens. Rarely it gives off a middle rectal artery and/or the vaginal artery.

The *inferior vesical artery* may arise directly from the internal iliac artery or one of its anterior branches. It generally anastomoses with the uterine artery (86%).

The *artery of the vas deferens* may be a direct branch of the internal iliac artery (rare) but usually arises from the umbilical artery. It is absent in 23% of cases and may give origin to a superior vesical artery.

The *middle rectal artery* is rarely absent and normally springs directly from the internal iliac. It also may arise from the vaginal artery or, very rarely, from the sacral arteries.

The *superior vesical arteries*, numbering from one to four, usually arise from the patent section of the umbilical artery but may branch from the uterine artery (9%), the artery of the vas deferens (9%), or the obturator artery (4.5%). Anastomoses between the superior and inferior vesical arteries are generally present.

The *uterine artery* is usually a direct branch of the internal iliac but may arise conjointly with the vaginal or middle rectal artery. Duplication can occur. When necessary, the uterine artery can adequately assume the supply function of the vesical arteries.

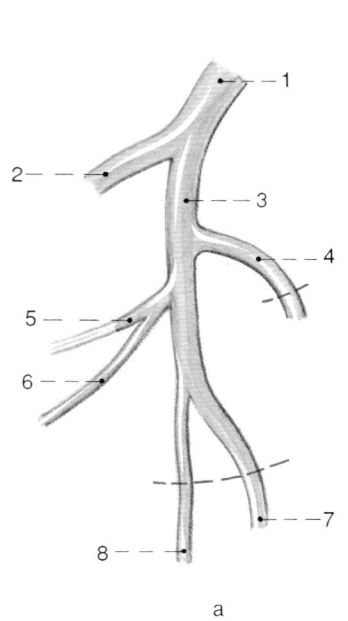

a

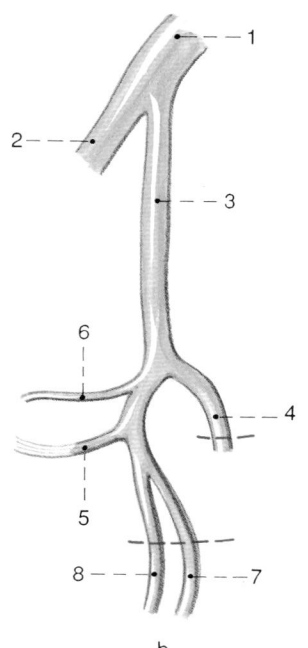

b

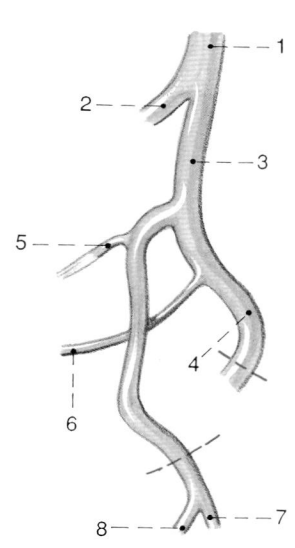

c

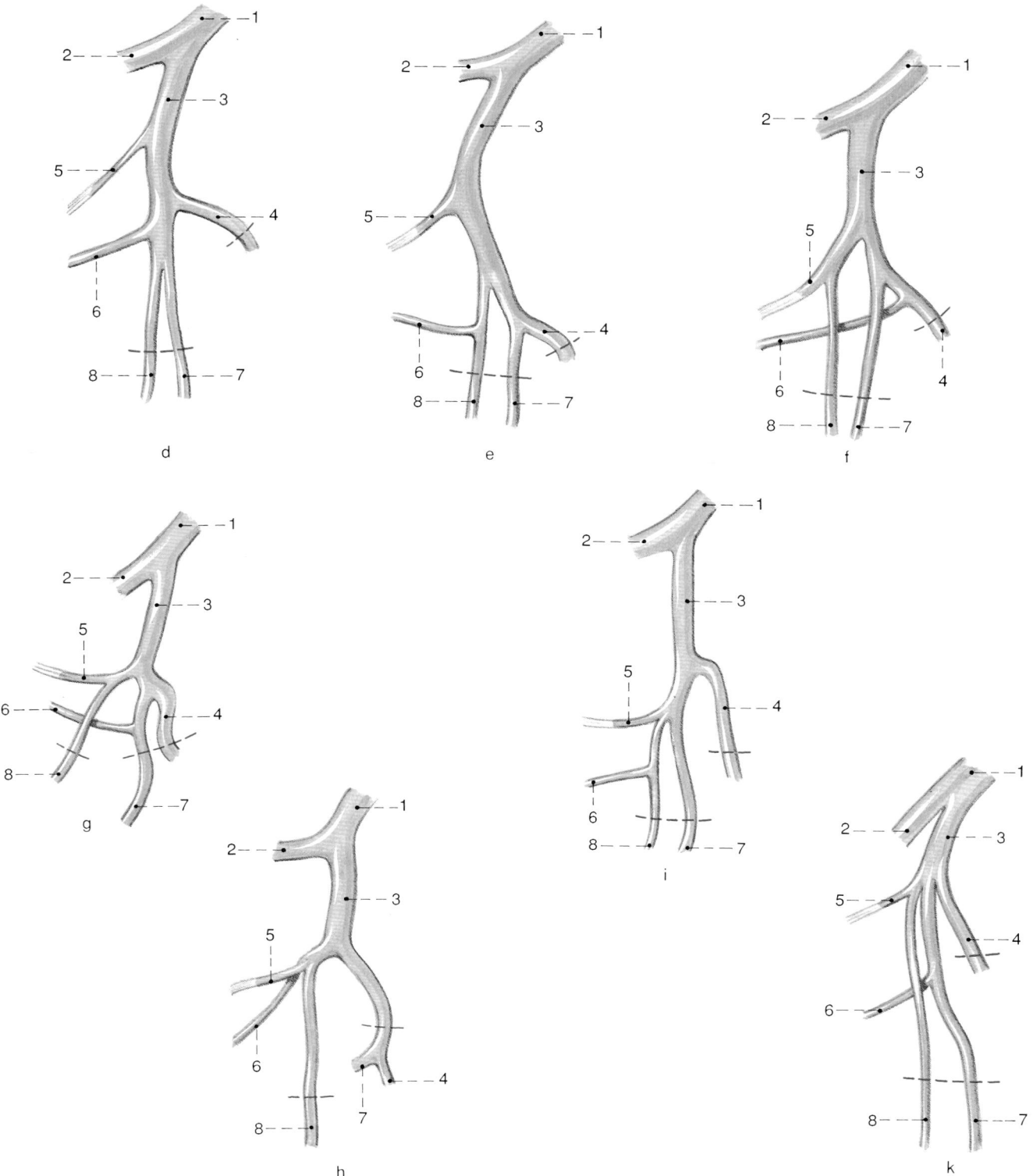

Fig. 3.**26** Variations in the branching pattern of the internal iliac artery. The broken lines indicate the supra- and infrapiriform foramina.

a, d The superior gluteal artery leaves the pelvis through the suprapiriform foramen as the terminal branch of the posterior trunk of the internal iliac artery. The internal pudendal artery and inferior gluteal artery pass through the infrapiriform foramen as the terminal branches of the anterior trunk (49%).

b, c The anterior trunk does not divide until it has passed through the infrapiriform foramen (10%).

e Both gluteal arteries and the internal pudendal artery arise by a common trunk (1.5%).

f, g The internal pudendal artery arises separately from the umbilical artery (0.5%).

g, h Both gluteal arteries form a common trunk that divides before (12%) or after (3.5%) leaving the true pelvis.

i, k The internal pudendal artery and the superior and inferior gluteal arteries arise separately in an irregular pattern (22.5%).

1 Common iliac artery
2 External iliac artery
3 Internal iliac artery
4 Superior gluteal artery

5 Umbilical artery (patent section)
6 Obturator artery
7 Inferior gluteal artery
8 Internal pudendal artery

Cul de Sac Incision

The peritoneum is incised along the pelvic wall into the rectovesical pouch (Figs. 3.**24**, 3.**27**). The line of incision runs on the anterior surface of the rectum, splitting the peritoneum directly at the line of fusion of its anterior and posterior layers. In this way the rectogenital space can be bluntly developed in continuity with the cul de sac (Fig. 3.**27**), exposing the anterior wall of the rectum and Denonvillier's fascia. The rectourethral space can also be bluntly developed in this plane from the rectogenital space to a point behind the membranous urethra.

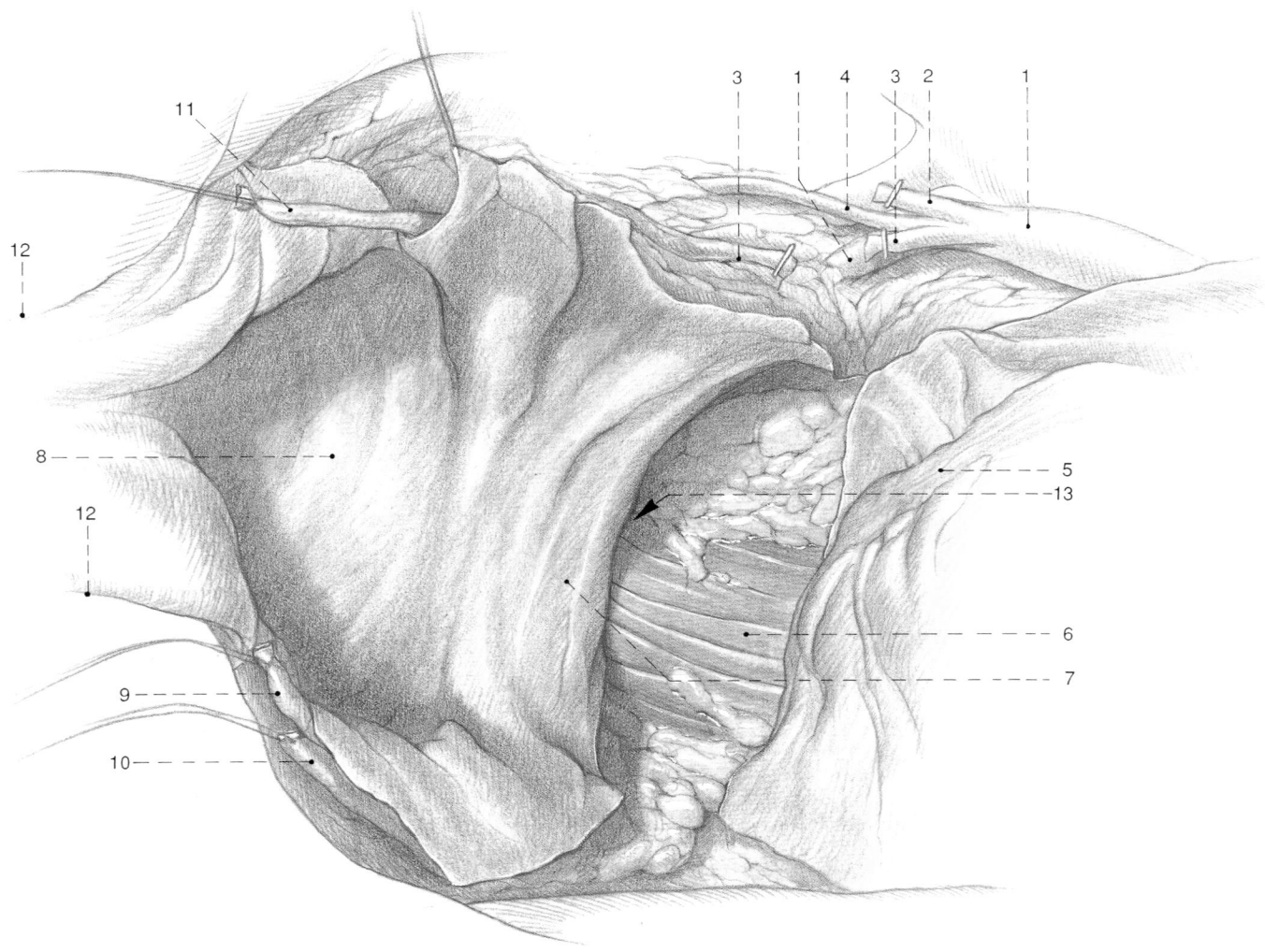

Fig. 3.**27** Incision in the cul de sac. The line of incision runs directly on the anterior surface of the rectum, cutting the peritoneum directly at the line of fusion of its anterior and posterior layers.

1 Internal iliac artery
2 Obturator artery
3 Superior vesical artery
4 Inferior vesical artery
5 Sigmoid colon
6 Rectum
7 Rectovesical pouch
8 Bladder
9 Left vas deferens
10 Left ureter
11 Right vas deferens
12 Medial umbilical fold and ligament
13 Rectogenital space

Exposure of the Rectovesical Septum (Posterior Bladder Pedicle)

The neurovascular sheath transmits the arteries and veins of the seminal vesicles and prostate in addition to the pelvic splanchnic nerves. The space between the rectal fascia and Denonvillier's fascia is developed with the right index and middle fingers (Fig. 3.28). The posterior bladder pedicle is held between the second and third fingers as the second finger presses downward on the rectum, and the posterior pedicle is progressively ligated as far as the endopelvic parietal fascia. As traction is placed on the vas deferens and ureter to enlarge the space between the rectal fascia and Denonvillier's fascia, individual portions of the posterior pedicle can be clipped or ligated under direct vision. The posterior pedicle is then progressively divided to the endopelvic parietal fascia (Figs. 3.29 3.31). The pelvic wall comes into view on the lateral side of these neurovascular bundles as they are progressively isolated and clipped or tied. The lymphadenectomy specimen on the pelvic wall is in contact medially with the bladder.

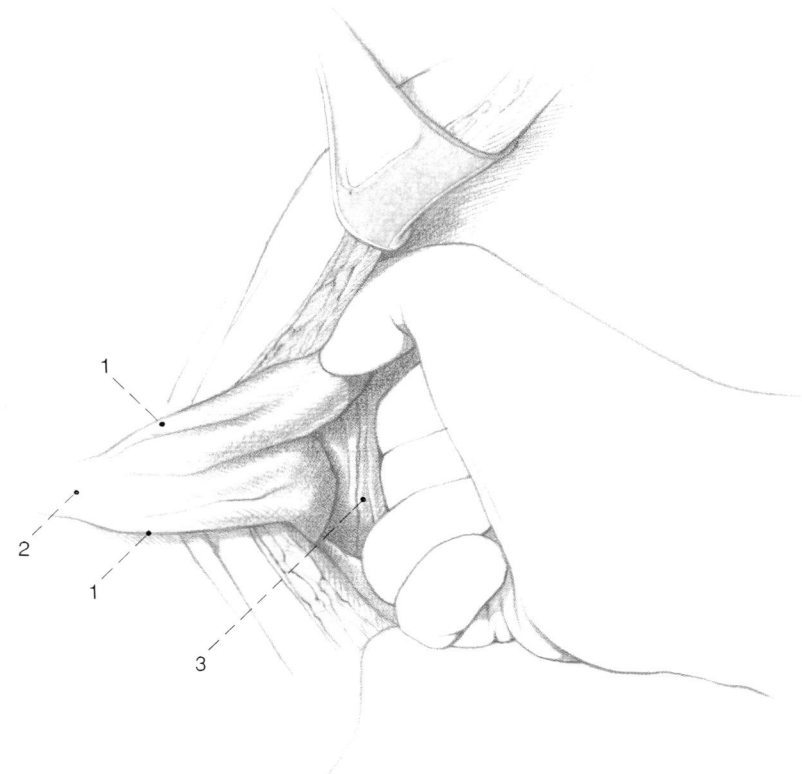

Fig. 3.**28**   The rectogenital space is bluntly developed by finger dissection.

1 Medial umbilical fold with ligament of the umbilical artery
2 Median umbilical fold with urachial ligament
3 Bladder

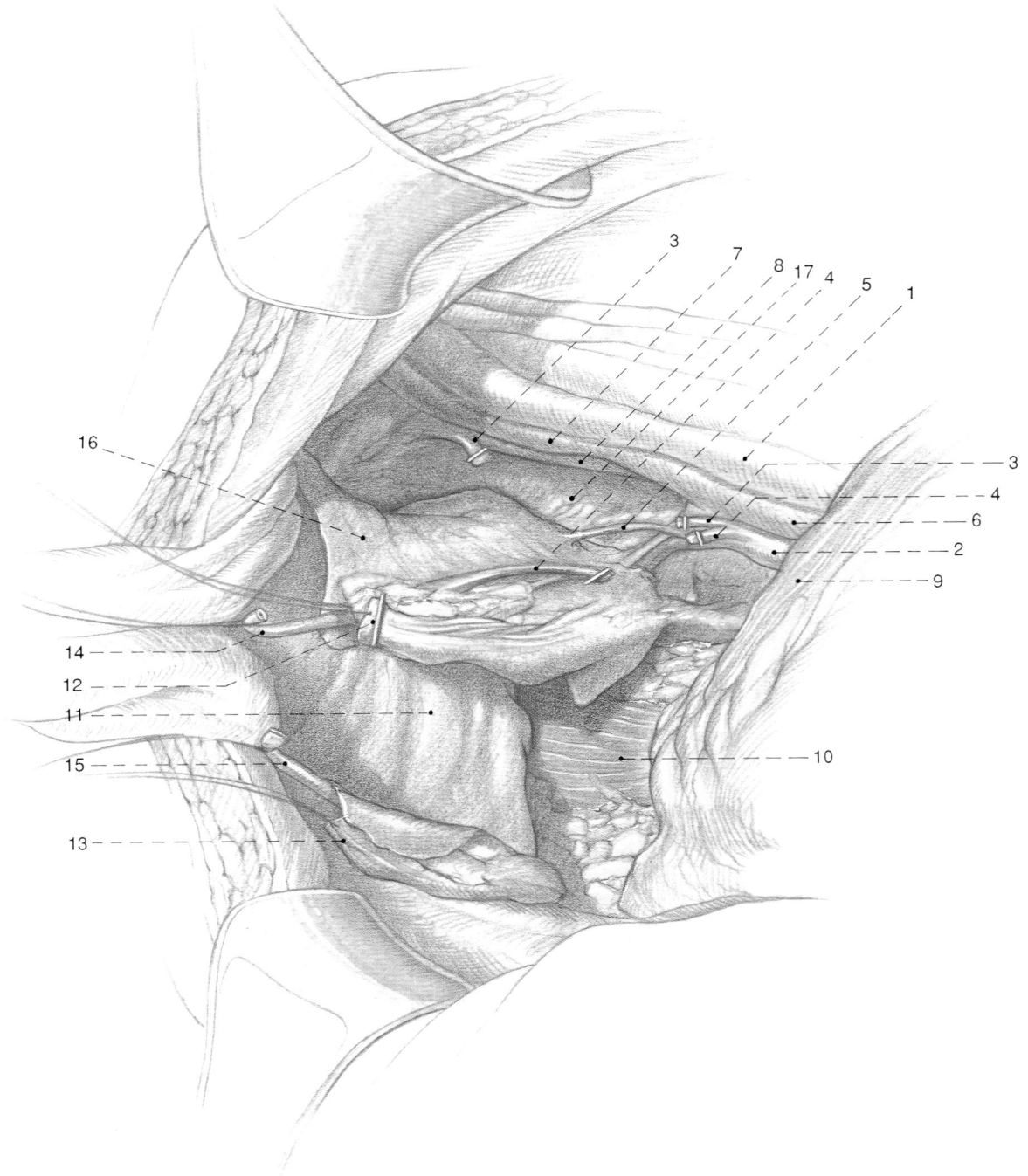

Fig. 3.**29** Exposure of the rectovesical septum (posterior bladder pedicle). The anterior branches of the internal iliac artery have been ligated, and the incision in the cul de sac has been completed. The right vas deferens and clipped ureter are retracted forward along with the freed lymph node package.

Fig. 3.**31** Exposure and incision of the endopelvic fascia (tendinous arch of the pelvic fascia). The surgical specimen is retracted forward by the vesicoumbilical plate, both vasa deferentes, and the ureters. ▶

1 External iliac artery	10 Rectum	
2 Internal iliac artery	11 Bladder	
3 Obturator artery	12 Right ureter	
4 Superior vesical artery	13 Left ureter	
5 Inferior vesical artery	14 Right vas deferens	
6 Common iliac vein	15 Left vas deferens	
7 External iliac vein	16 Parietal peritoneum	
8 Obturator nerve	17 Parietal pelvic fascia	
9 Sigmoid colon		

1 Internal iliac artery	10 Left vas deferens
2 External iliac vessels	11 Right ureter
3 Obturator artery	12 Left ureter
4 Superior and inferior vesical arteries	13 Medial umbilical fold
5 Superior vesical artery	14 Median umbilical fold
6 Superior gluteal artery	15 Rectum
7 Obturator nerve	
8 Tendious arch of pelvic fascia	
9 Right vas deferens	

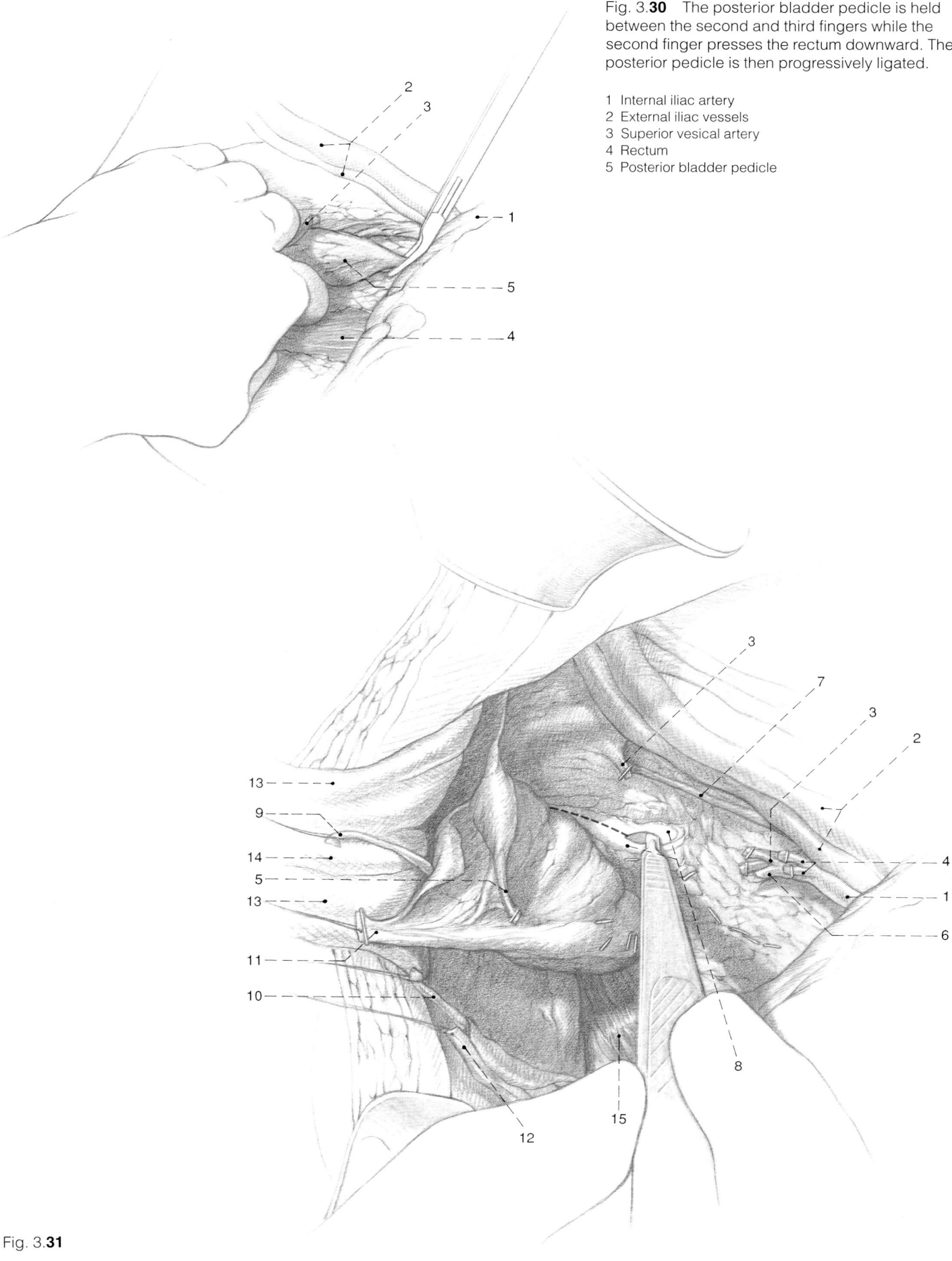

Fig. 3.**30**   The posterior bladder pedicle is held
between the second and third fingers while the
second finger presses the rectum downward. The
posterior pedicle is then progressively ligated.

1 Internal iliac artery
2 External iliac vessels
3 Superior vesical artery
4 Rectum
5 Posterior bladder pedicle

Fig. 3.**31**

Exposure and Incision of the Endopelvic Fascia

The visceral fascia of the bladder and prostate is continuous with the parietal pelvic fascia at the bladder base. This attachment, called the endopelvic fascia, is strengthened by collagenous fibers and smooth-muscle fiber tracts in the area of the symphysis to form the puboprostatic ligament, which defines the inferior boundary of the prevesical space. This reflection is progressively thinned posteriorly and finally blends with the anterior layer of the neurovascular sheath. The endopelvic fascia arises from the parietal pelvic fascia in the form of a white line, the tendinous arch of the pelvic fascia. The endopelvic fascia is incised (Fig. 3.**31**). As the fascia is incised on the right side, the right ureter, right vas deferens, and vesicoumbilical plate are retracted forward (Fig. 3.**31**). When the endopelvic fascia has been opened, the levator ani muscle is visible in the lateral portion of the true pelvis. The puboprostatic ligament is divided at its insertion on the pubic symphysis (Fig. 3.**32**).

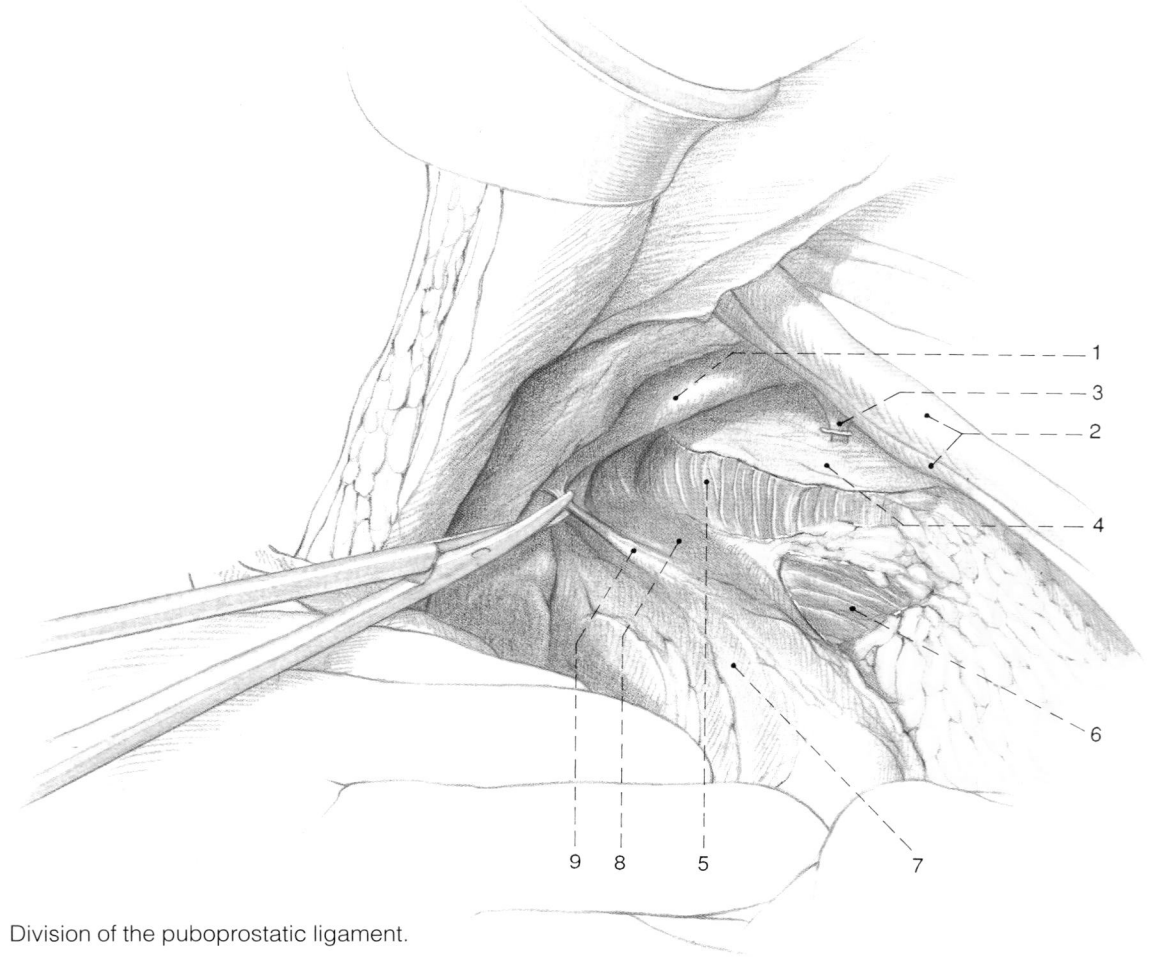

Fig. 3.**32**   Division of the puboprostatic ligament.

1 Superior pubic ramus
2 External iliac vessels
3 Obturator artery
4 Parietal pelvic fascia
5 Levator ani
6 Rectum
7 Visceral fascia of bladder
8 Prostatic fascia
9 Puboprostatic (pubovesical) ligament

Exposure of the Pubourethral Space, Entry into the Rectourethral Space

A clear view of the pubourethral space is gained by division of the puboprostatic ligament and downward deflection of the anterior surface of the prostate using a sponge stick (Fig. 3.**32**). After division of the dorsal vein complex, the rectourethral space (rectourethral septum) is opened on the anterior surface of the rectum, and the urethra is snared under vision (Fig. 3.**33**).

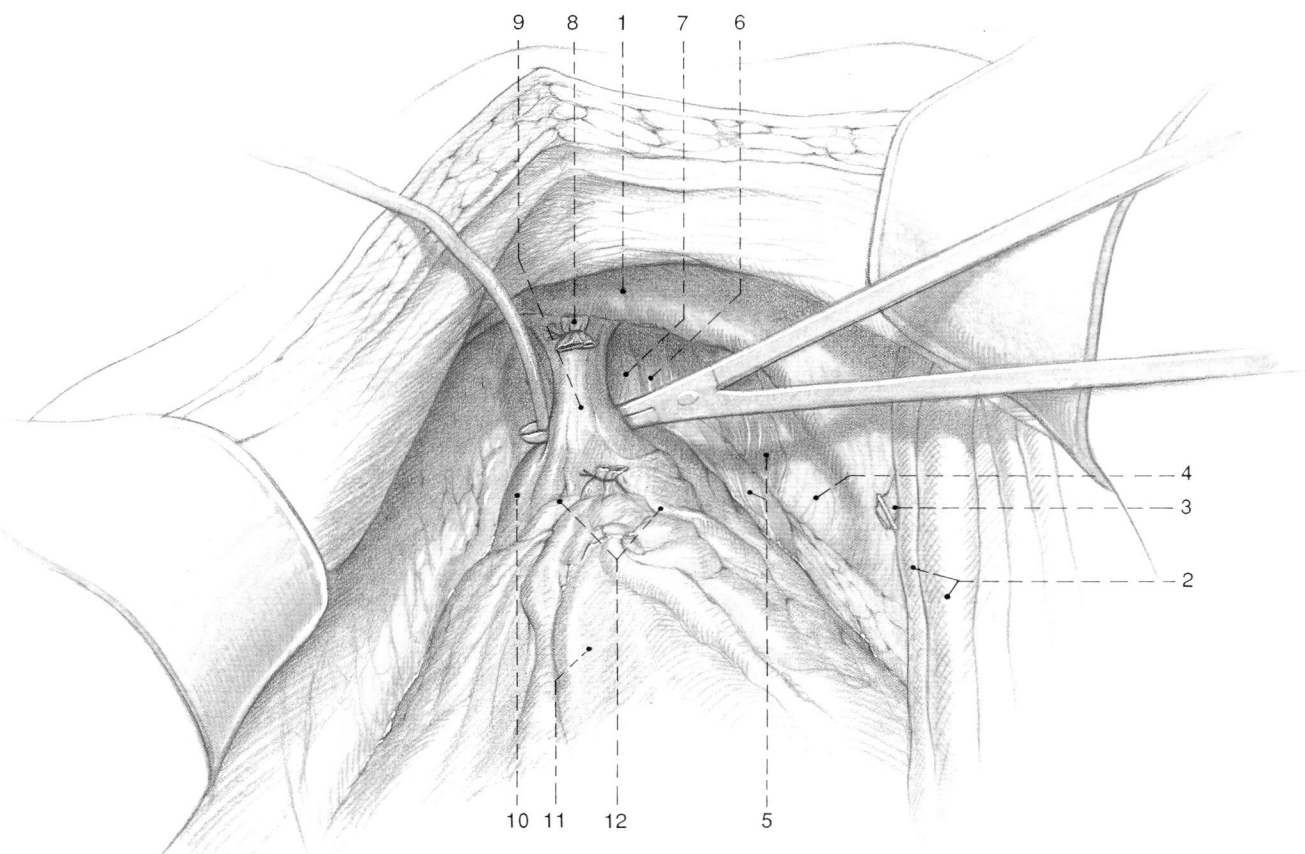

Fig. 3.**33**   The rectourethral space is opened at the anterior surface of the rectum.

1 Superior pubic ramus
2 External iliac vessels
3 Obturator artery
4 Parietal pelvic fascia
5 Levator ani
6 Puborectalis (levator crura)
7 Rectourethral septum
8 Dorsal vein complex
9 Urethra
10 Prostatic fascia
11 Bladder
12 Puboprostatic ligaments

Entry into Denonvillier's Space

The posterior surface of the prostate is bluntly dissected from the rectal fascia along with Denonvillier's fascia. Proceeding from front to back, the prostate is progressively freed from the paraprostatic connective tissue, placing individual clips or ligatures on arterial and venous vessels supplying the gland (Fig. 3.**34**). The neurovascular bundle of the prostate presents as a continuation of the rectovesical septum.

Preparation for Orthotopic Continent Ileal Reservoir

The bladder, prostate, parietal peritoneum, vesicoumbilical plate, portions of the lateral and posterior neurovascular sheaths, and the bilateral lymphadenectomy specimen are removed en bloc from the pelvis. Figure 3.**35** shows the cavity left by anterior pelvic exenteration in the male. The membranous urethra and external urethral sphincter have been engaged with traction sutures in preparation for the continent ileal reservoir. Numerous clips are visible along the lateral and posterior bladder pedicles and their anterior continuation, the paraprostatic tissue.

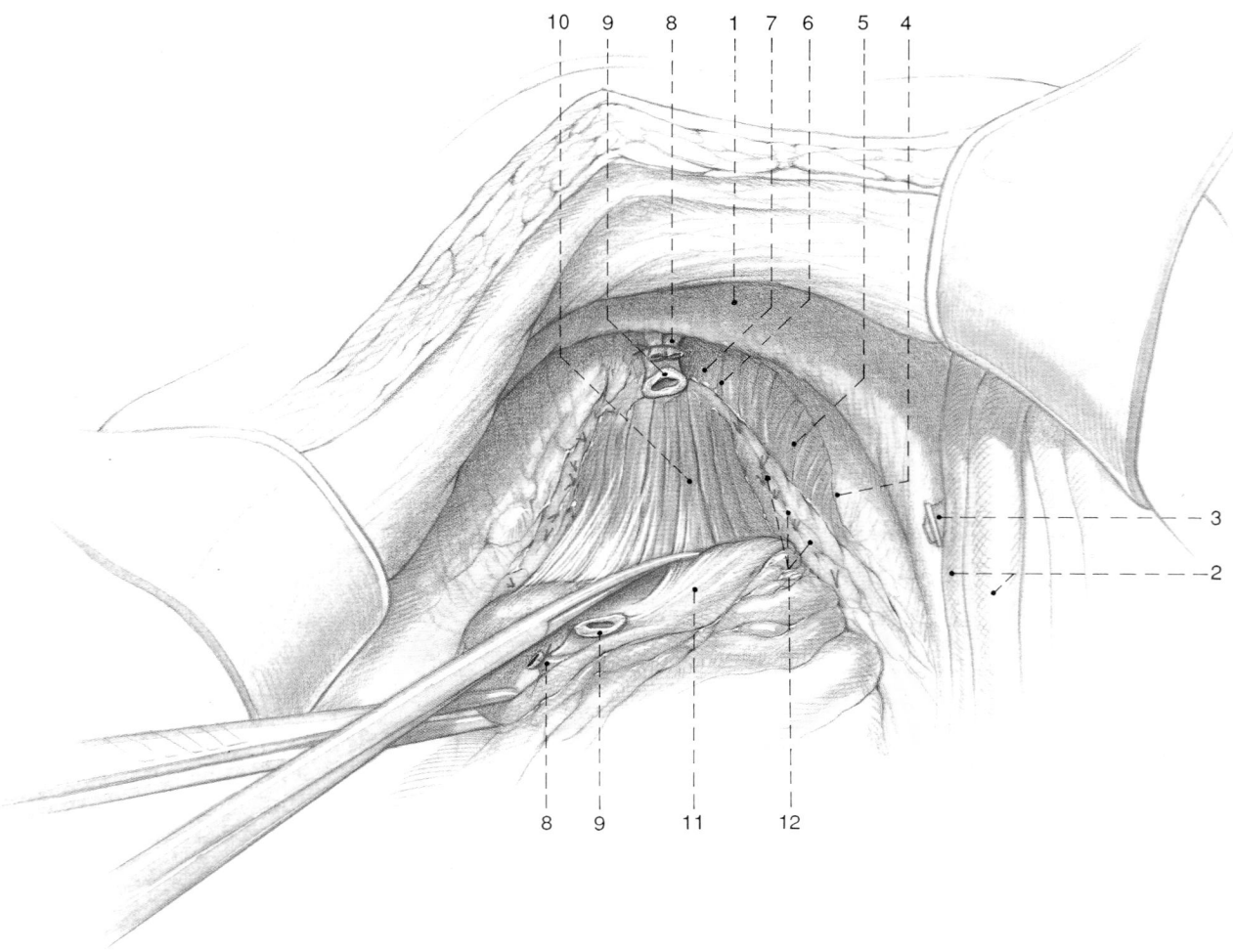

Fig. 3.**34** The posterior surface of the prostate is bluntly dissected from the rectal fascia along with Denonvillier's fascia.

1 Superior pubic ramus
2 External iliac vessels
3 Obturator artery
4 Parietal pelvic fascia (endopelvic fascia)
5 Levator ani
6 Puborectalis (levator crura)
7 Rectourethral septum
8 Dorsal vein complex
9 Urethra
10 Rectal fascia
11 Denonvillier's fascia
12 Neurovascular bundle of prostate

Comments

Entry into the true pelvis is established by mobilizing the small bowel and ascending colon and packing them into the epigastric space, creating access to the entire retroperitoneal space and pelvic cavity. An important step is the blunt separation of the lateral and posterior bladder pedicles. If the anterior branches of the internal iliac artery cannot be isolated, the trunk should be ligated past the origin of the first large posterior branch (superior gluteal artery). If Denon-villier's space cannot be entered after incision of the anterior and posterior peritoneal layers in the area of the cul de sac (e.g., following high-voltage therapy), a perineal route of approach is indicated. The rectourethral space can be approached through the central tendon and the perineal body. Denonvillier's space can be entered from the perineal aspect, much as in the perineal approach for a radical prostatectomy.

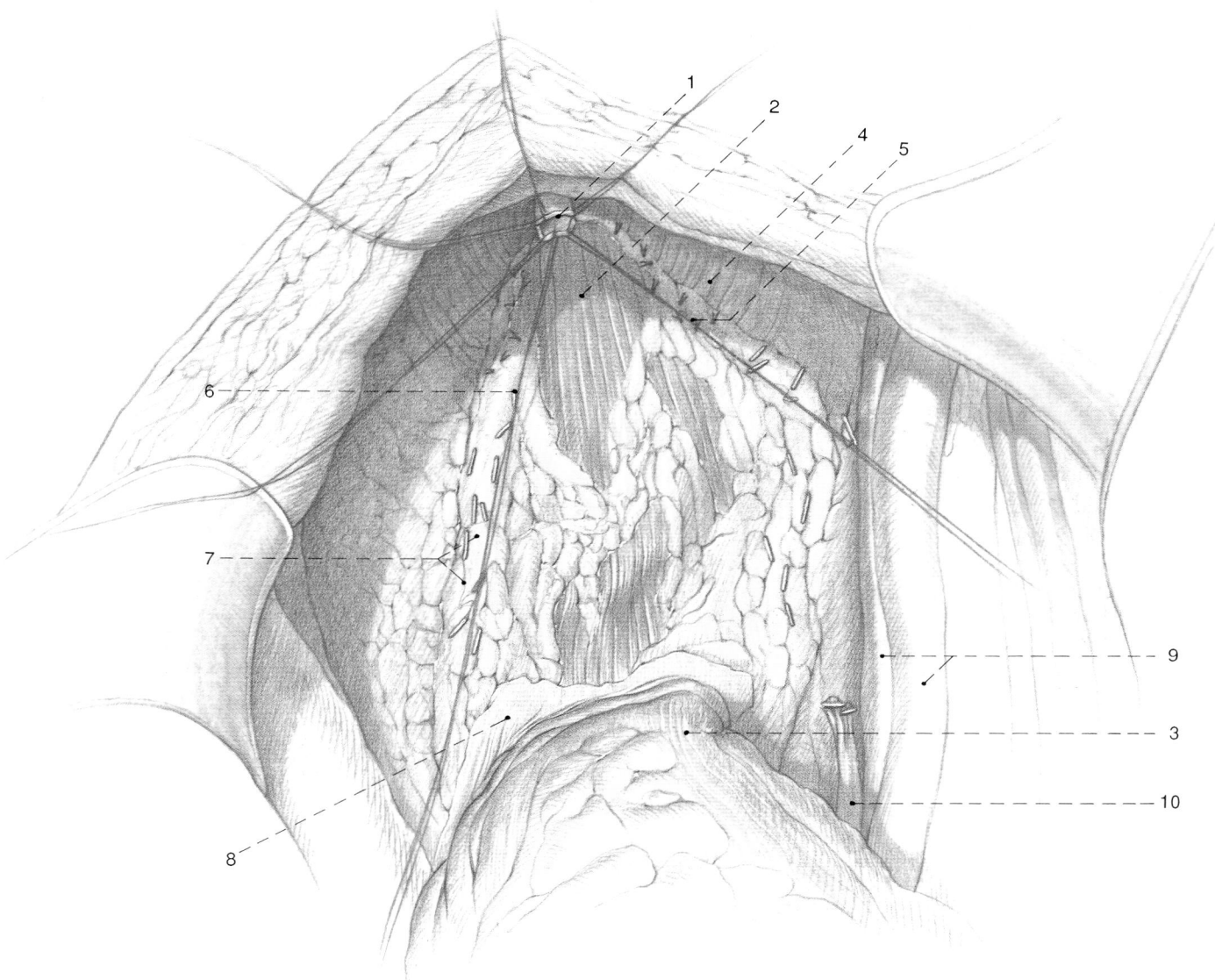

Fig. 3.**35** The bladder, prostate, parietal peritoneum, vesicoumbilical plate, and bilateral lymphadenectomy specimen are removed in continuity from the pelvis. The membranous urethra, together with the rhabdosphincter, is engaged in preparation for constructing an orthotopic continent ileal reservoir. Clips mark the lateral and posterior bladder pedicles.

1 Membranous part of urethra
2 Rectum
3 Sigmoid colon
4 Levator ani
5 Neurovascular bundle of prostate (right)
6 Neurovascular bundle of prostate (left)

7 Posterior bladder pedicle
8 Peritoneum
9 External iliac vessels
10 Internal iliac artery

Anterior Pelvic Exenteration in the Female

The **position**, **skin incision**, and **entry into the peritoneal cavity** are the same as described for anterior exenteration in the male.

The peritoneal cavity is opened and exposure maintained with a self-retaining retractor. After incision from the inferior duodenojejunal fold to the paracolic sulcus, the small bowel, cecum, and ascending colon are mobilized. The freed vesicoumbilical plate (containing the median umbilical fold, both medial umbilical folds, fat, and peritoneum) is displaced inferiorly to expose the peritoneum-covered bladder, uterus, eustachian tubes, ovaries, broad ligament and mesosalpinx, the vesicouterine pouch between the bladder and uterus, and the rectouterine pouch between the uterus and rectum (Fig. 3.**36**).

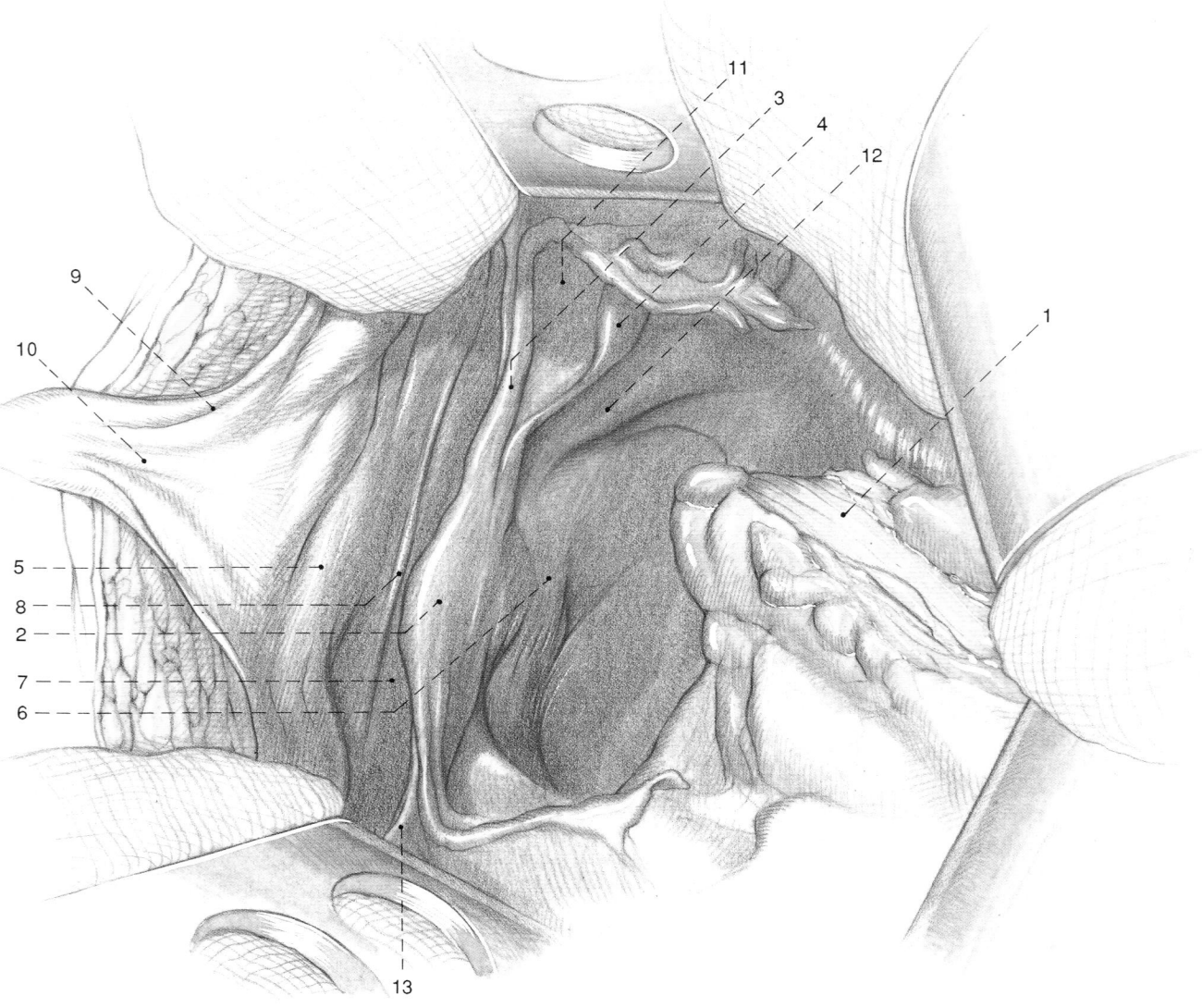

Fig. 3.**36** The peritoneum has been opened, and the vesicoumbilical plate has been freed and reflected downward.

1 Sigmoid colon
2 Uterus
3 Uterine tube
4 Ovary
5 Bladder
6 Rectouterine pouch
7 Vesicouterine pouch

8 Transverse vesical fold
9 Medial umbilical fold (ligament of umbilical artery)
10 Median umbilical fold (urachus)
11 Mesosalpinx
12 Broad ligament of uterus
13 Round ligament of uterus

Dissection of the Lateral Bladder Pedicle (Lateral Bladder Retinaculum)

Following dissection of the lymph nodes, the lateral bladder pedicle is dissected and the anterior branches of the internal iliac artery (lateral umbilical fold, obturator artery, superior and inferior vesical arteries) are clipped or ligated (Fig. 3.**37**). The ureter is clipped 1–2 cm past its crossing with the common iliac vessels, also encompassing a generous mar-

gin of vascular and connective tissue (Fig. 3.**37**). The round ligament of the uterus is ligated on the left side (Fig. 3.**38**), then a left-sided lymphadenectomy is performed as on the right side, and the dissection of the left pedicle (lateral bladder retinaculum) is carried out (Fig. 3.**37**).

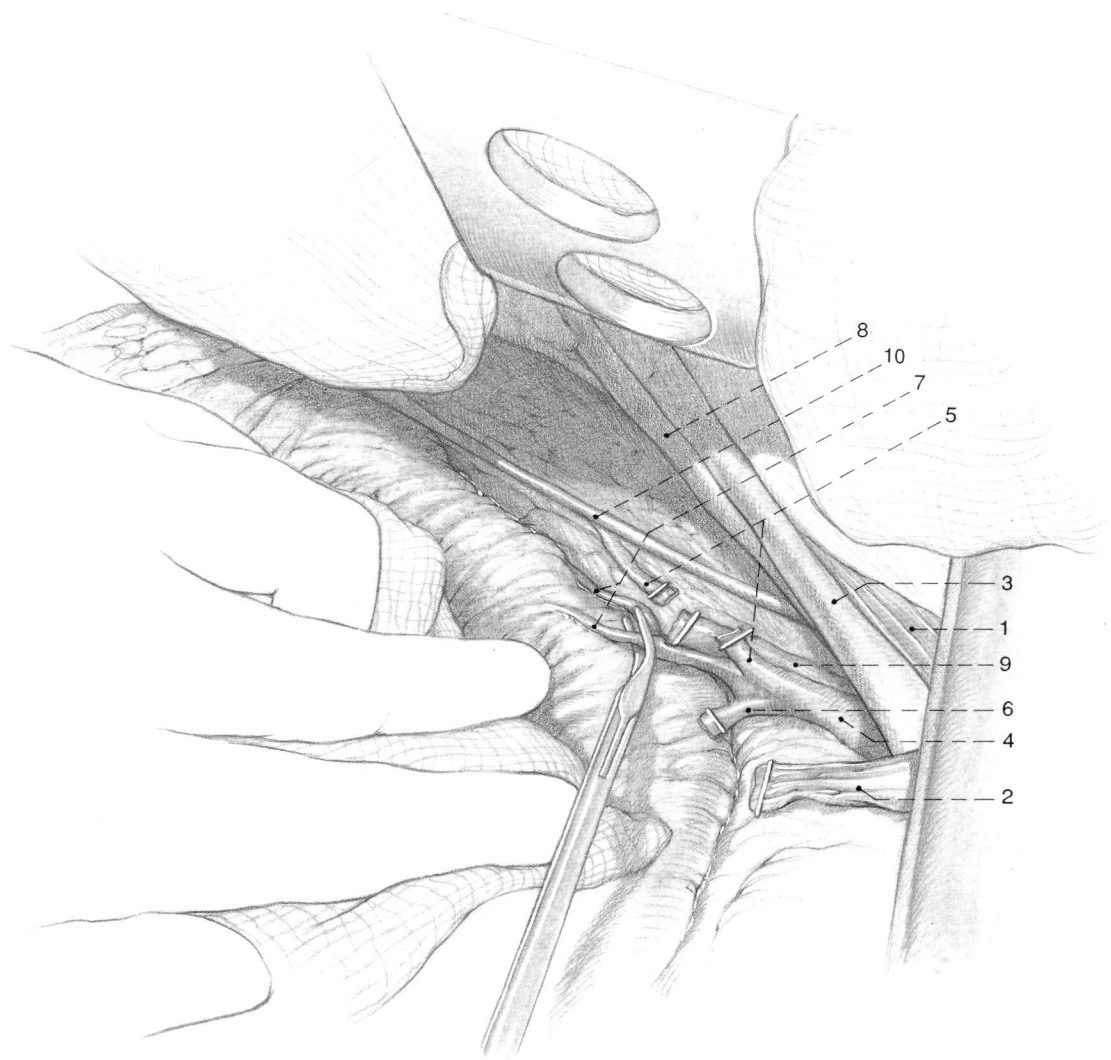

Fig. 3.**37** Dissection of the lateral bladder pedicle. The anterior branches of the internal iliac artery are isolated and clipped.

1 Psoas major
2 Ureter
3 External iliac artery
4 Internal iliac artery
5 Obturator artery
6 Superior vesical artery
7 Inferior vesical arteries
8 External iliac vein
9 Internal iliac vein
10 Obturator nerve

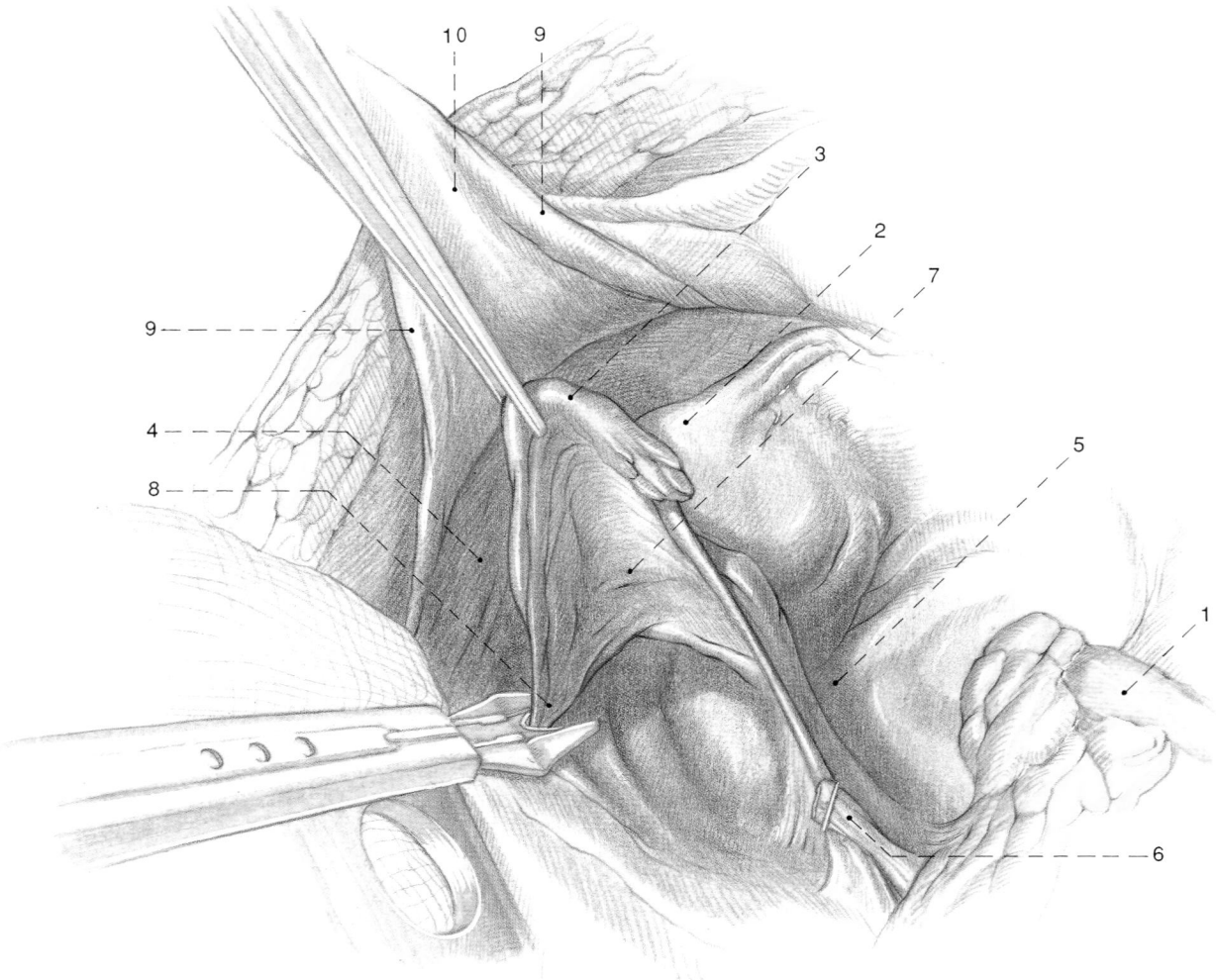

Fig. 3.**38** The uterine round ligament is ligated on the left side.

1 Sigmoid colon
2 Uterus
3 Uterine tube
4 Bladder
5 Rectouterine pouch
6 Left ureter
7 Mesosalpinx
8 Uterine round ligament
9 Medial umbilical fold (ligament of umbilical artery)
10 Median umbilical fold (urachus)

Exposure of the Posterior Bladder Pedicle

The peritoneum of the rectouterine pouch is incised from the pelvic-wall aspect (Fig. 3.**38**), and the specimen is retracted inferiorly by the vesicoumbilical plate and a uterine traction suture (Fig. 3.**39**). After division of the peritoneum over the rectum in the area of the rectouterine pouch, the posterior bladder pedicle, which includes the cardinal ligament in the female, is progressively ligated or clipped as far as the parietal pelvic fascia.

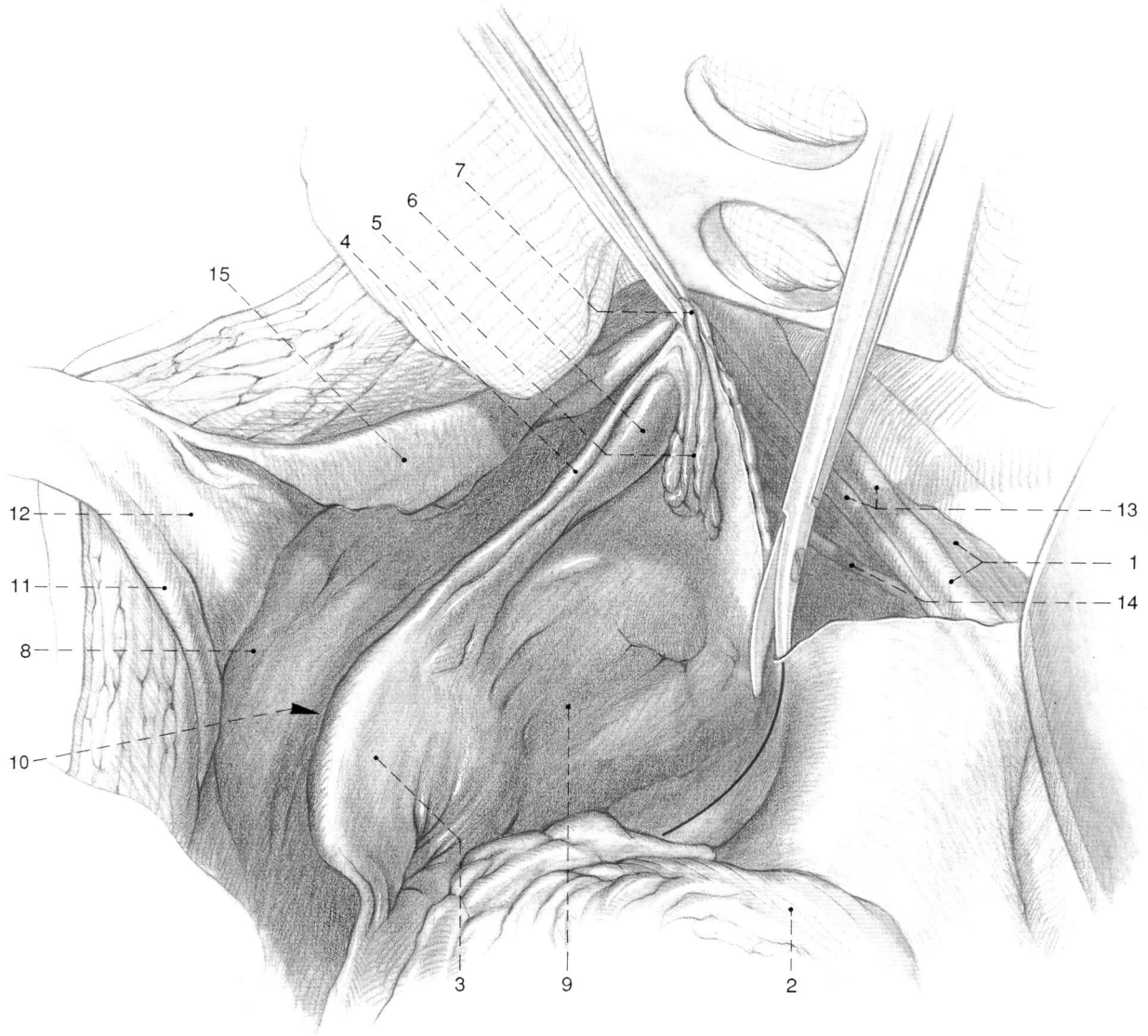

Fig. 3.**39**   Line of incision in the peritoneum. Starting at the pelvic wall, the peritoneum is divided just over the rectum in the area of the rectouterine pouch.

1 Psoas major and minor muscles	9 Rectouterine pouch
2 Sigmoid colon	10 Vesicouterine pouch
3 Uterus	11 Medial umbilical fold (ligament of umbilical artery)
4 Uterine tube	12 Median umbilical fold (urachus)
5 Fimbriated end of uterine tube	13 External iliac vessels
6 Ovary	14 Obturator nerve
7 Ovarian suspensory ligament	15 Parietal peritoneum
8 Bladder	

Opening the Posterior Vaginal Wall

The posterior bladder pedicle is clipped or ligated about 3–4 cm past the cervix, and the posterior vaginal wall is opened (Fig. 3.**40**). Much as in an anterior exenteration in the male, the remaining posterior pedicle is encircled (the second finger is in the vagina) and progressively ligated forward to the parietal pelvic fascia (Fig. 3.**41**).

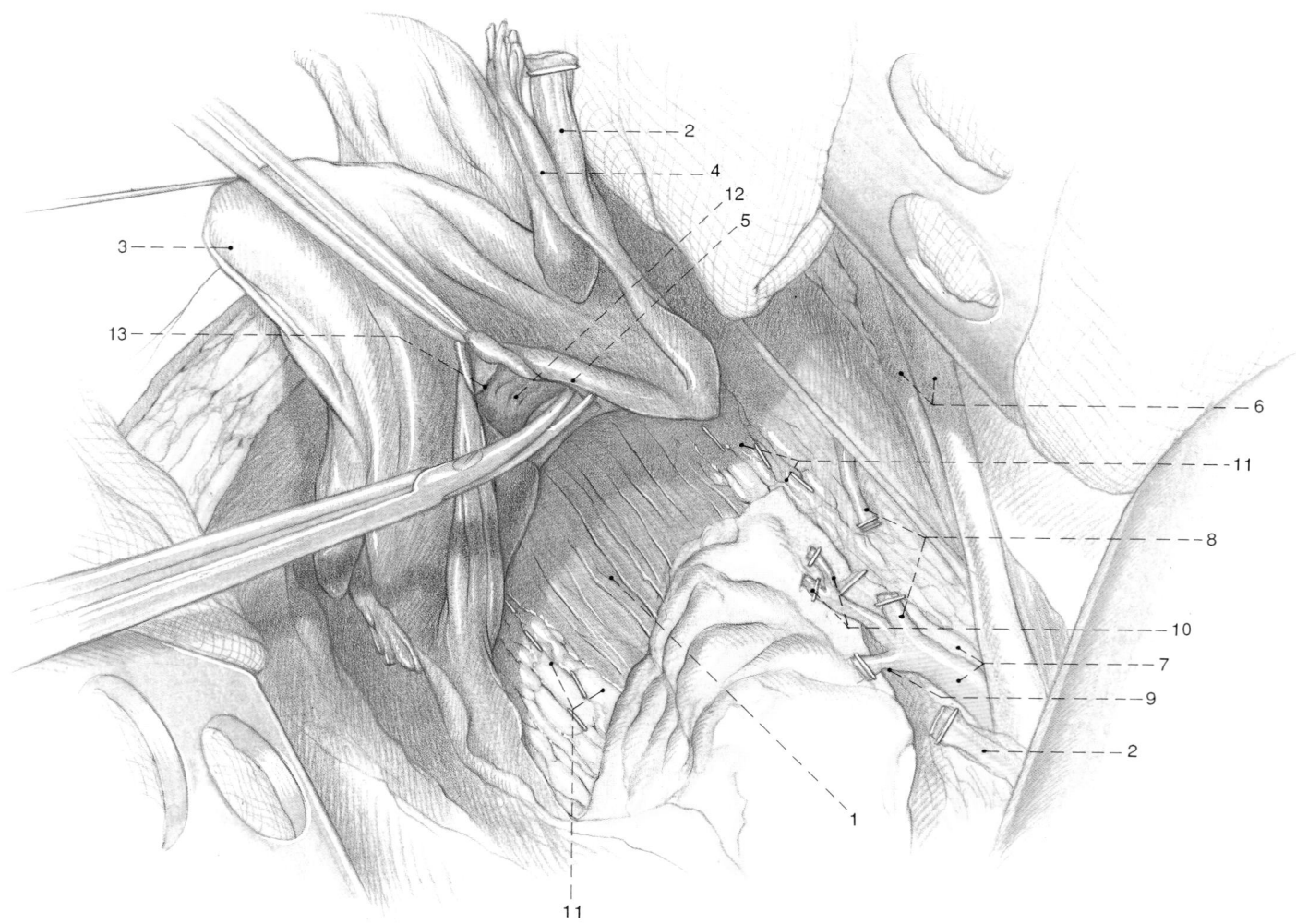

Fig. 3.**40** Exposure and division of the posterior bladder pedicle, which in the female includes the cardinal ligament. The posterior vaginal wall is opened 3–4 cm caudal to the cervix.

1 Rectum
2 Ureter
3 Uterus
4 Uterine tube
5 Parietal peritoneum of rectouterine pouch
6 External iliac vessels
7 Internal iliac vessels
8 Obturator artery
9 Superior vesical artery
10 Inferior vesical arteries
11 Parametrium (cardinal ligament), divided
12 Anterior vaginal wall
13 Posterior vaginal wall

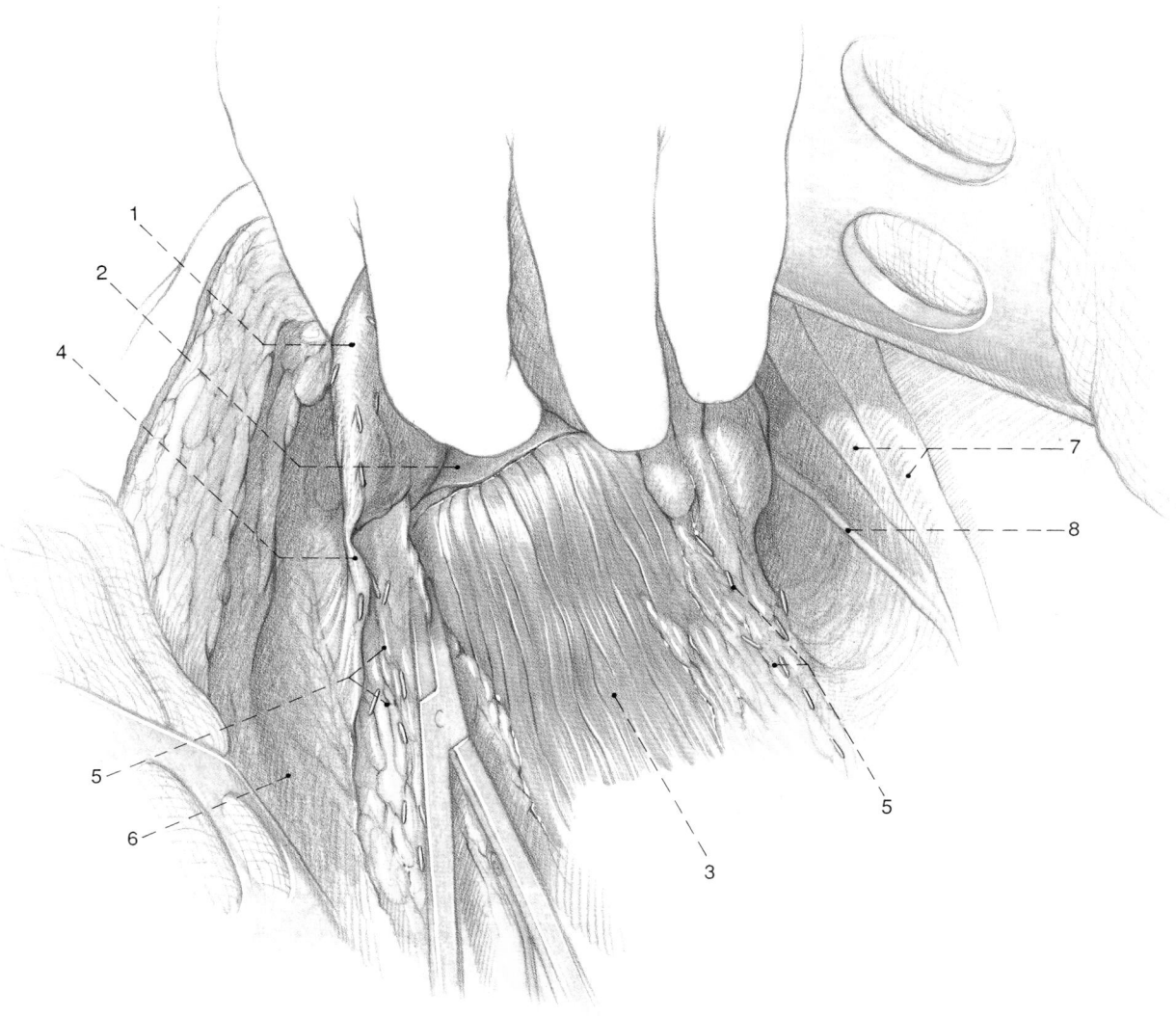

Fig. 3.**41** With the index finger in the vagina, the posterior bladder pedicle is progressively ligated as far as the endopelvic fascia.

1 Uterus
2 Posterior vaginal wall
3 Rectum
4 Endopelvic fascia, cut edge
5 Posterior bladder pedicle
6 Parietal pelvic fascia
7 External iliac vessels
8 Obturator nerve

Exposure and Incision of the Endopelvic Fascia (Tendinous Arch of the Pelvic Fascia)

The bladder is retracted downward by the vesicoumbilical plate, and the uterus is pulled cranially by its traction suture (Fig. 3.**42**). The layer of pelvic fascia reflected onto the visceral layer of the bladder is exposed and incised, and the anterior vaginal wall and urethra are removed along with the external urethral orifice (Fig. 3.**43**).

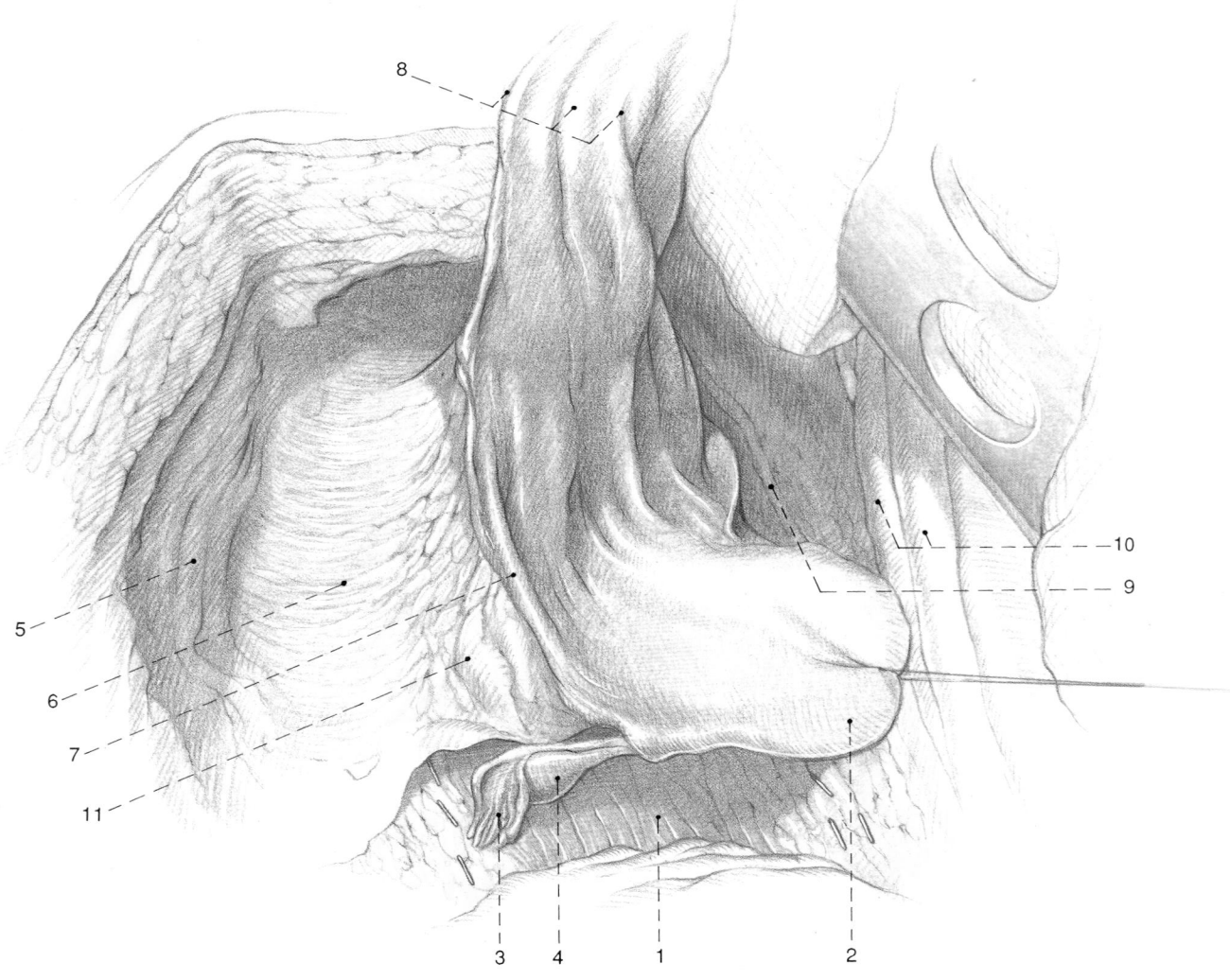

Fig. 3.**42** Exposure and incision of the endopelvic fascia. The vesicoumbilical plate is retracted downward and the uterus upward.

1 Rectum
2 Uterus
3 Fimbriated end of uterine tube
4 Ovary
5 Parietal pelvic fascia
6 Tendinous arch of pelvic fascia
7 Parietal peritoneum of vesicouterine pouch
8 Parietal peritoneum with median and medial umbilical folds
9 Obturator nerve
10 External iliac vessels
11 Visceral pelvic fascia

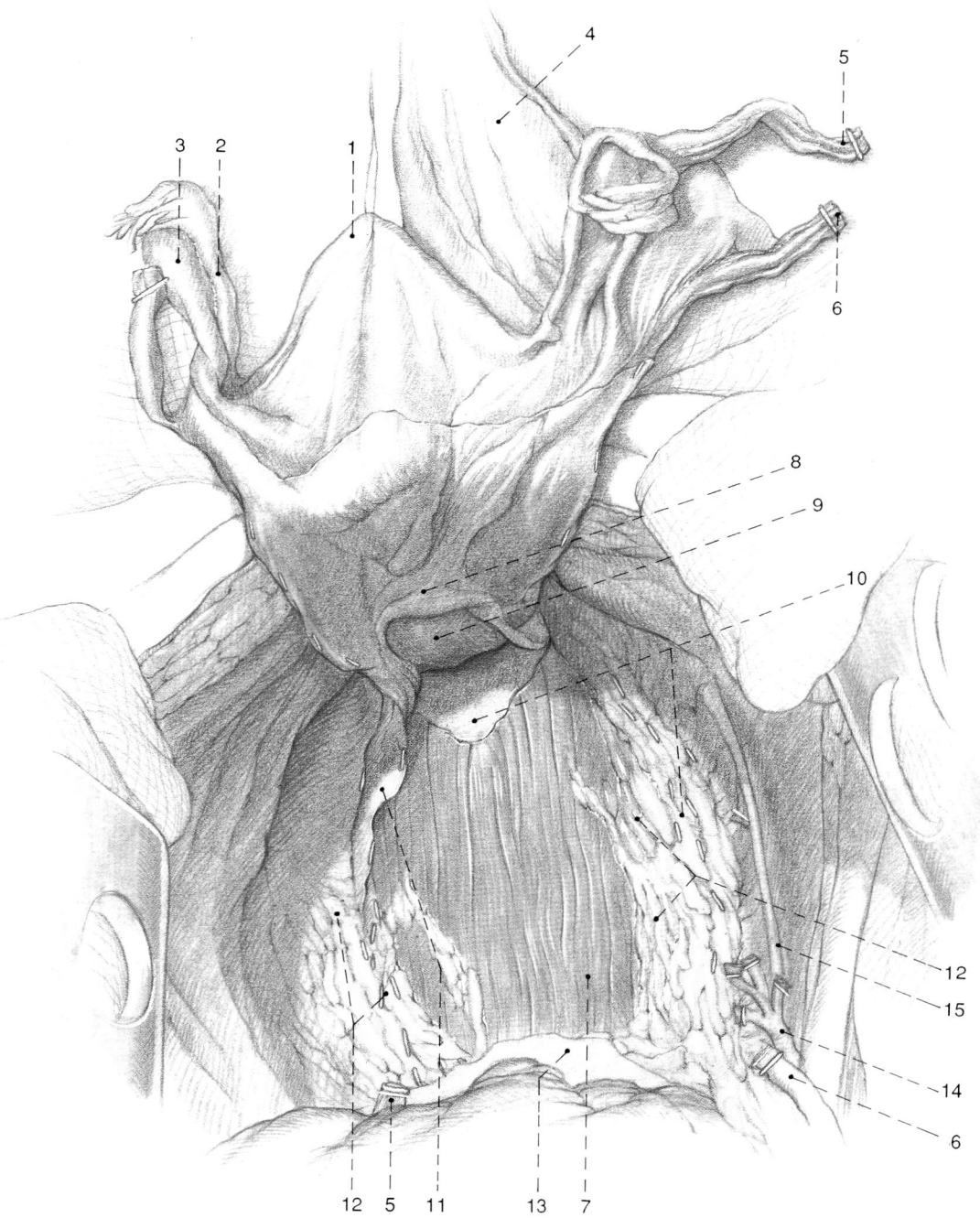

Fig. 3.**43** Further dissection of the posterior bladder pedicle, including resection of the urethra and anterior vaginal wall.

 1 Uterus
 2 Uterine tube
 3 Ovary
 4 Vesicoumbilical plate
 5 Left ureter
 6 Right ureter
 7 Rectum
 8 Posterior vaginal wall
 9 Uterine cervix, vaginal part
10 Posterior vaginal wall
11 Endopelvic fascia
12 Posterior bladder pedicle
13 Parietal peritoneum
14 Internal iliac artery
15 Obturator nerve

Approach for Infrapubic Periurethral En Bloc Resection of Female Urethral Carcinoma

Main Indication

This approach is mainly indicated for female urethral carcinoma necessitating a radical anterior pelvic exenteration that includes the inferior border of the symphysis, the anterior vaginal wall, the superior portion of the vulva, and the clitoris.

Position and Incision

The patient is placed in a hyperextended frog-legged position to expose the external genitalia and allow broad access to the pelvis.

The incision is similar to that for an anterior exenteration, but the midline incision is carried down past the symphysis to the external genitalia. The incision circumscribes half of the external genitalia along the medial aspect of the labia majora (Figs. 3.**44**, 3.**45**).

After the pelvic lymphadenectomy and anterior exenteration have been completed, the abdominal surgery is interrupted at the point where the posterior bladder pedicle is ligated 3–4 cm past the cervix and the vaginal wall is incised.

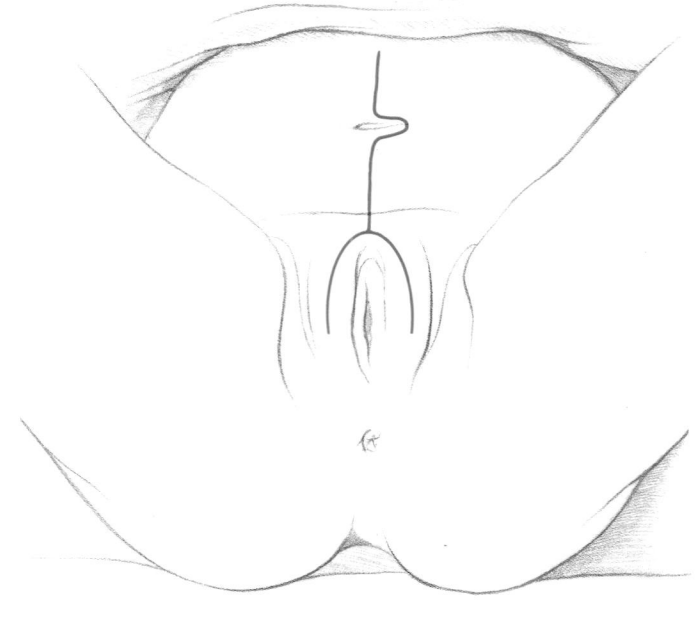

Fig. 3.**44**   Position and skin incision.

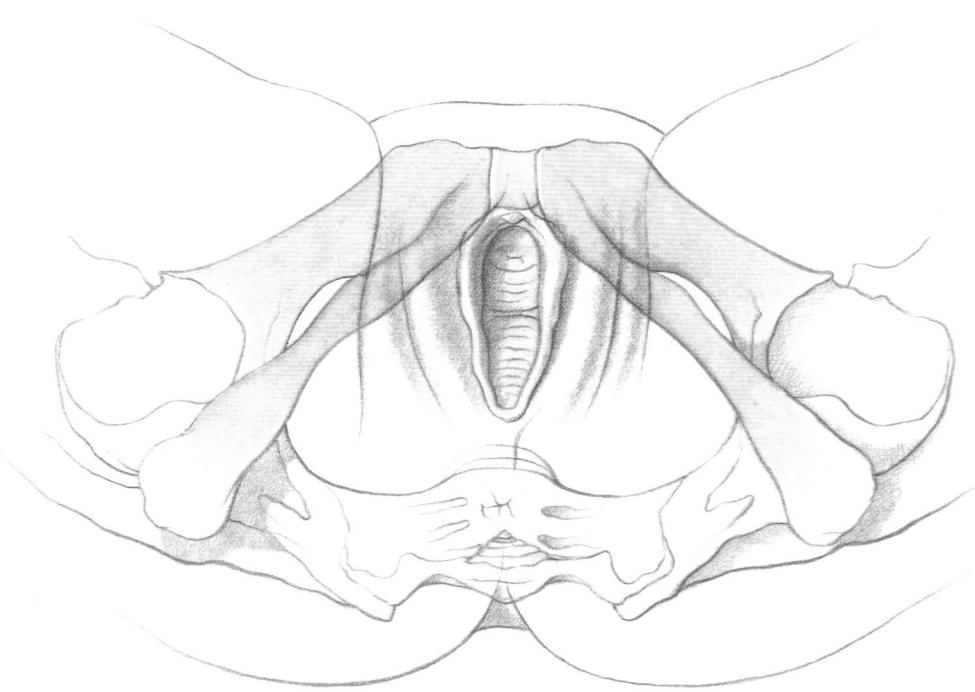

Fig. 3.**45**   Schematic relationship of the bony pelvis, urethra, and vagina.

Incision Around the Superior Portion of the External Genitalia

The line of incision is deepened with the electrocautery, removing the tissue as far as the pubic symphysis and circumscribing the upper portion of the external genitalia deep into the subcutaneous fat until the inferior pubic ramus is exposed (Fig. 3.**46**).

The crus of the clitoris is underrun and ligated (Fig. 3.**47**). Following resection of the crura, the portion of the external genitalia consisting of the labia minora, the medial portions of the labia majora, the clitoris, the bulbospongiosus muscle, and portions of the ischiocavernosus muscle are resected. Both lateral surfaces of the vaginal wall are incised, carrying the incision into the true pelvis (Fig. 3.**48**).

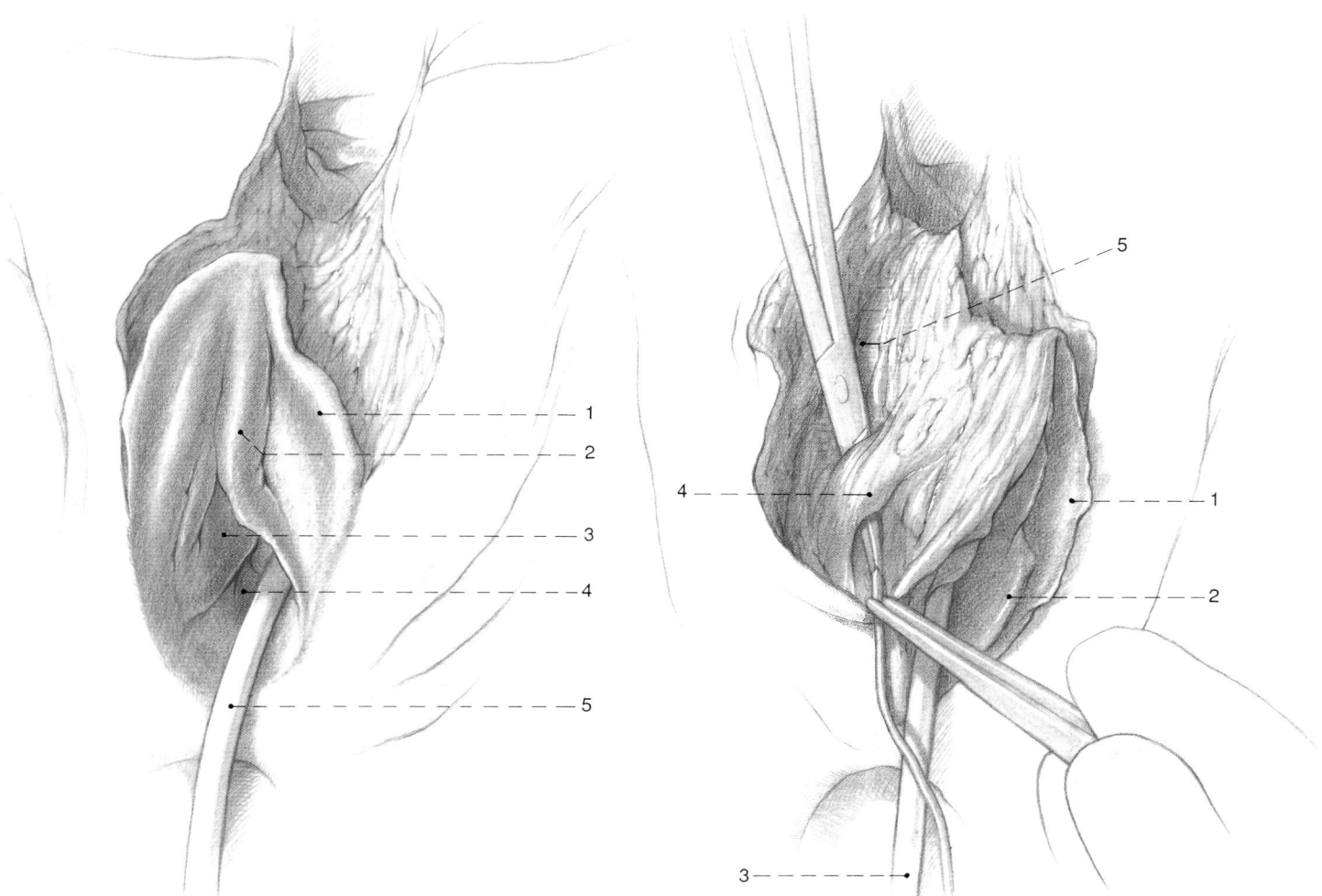

Fig. 3.**46**   Incision circumscribing the superior portion of the external genitalia.

1 Labium majus
2 Labium minus
3 Vestibule of vagina
4 Vagina
5 Catheter

Fig. 3.**47**   The crus of the clitoris is undermined and ligated.

1 Labium majus
2 Labium minus
3 Catheter
4 Crus of clitoris
5 Adductor brevis

Dissection of the Anterior Surface of the Symphysis

The origins of the adductor muscles are released from the anterior surface of the pubic symphysis and the inferior pubic ramus using a periosteal elevator. The periurethral portion of the symphysis is then removed with a Gigli saw, following the three lines of resection shown in Fig. 3.**48**. For this step a clamp is introduced into the true pelvis from the perineum through the medial part of the obturator foramen along the inferior pubic ramus. The Gigli saw is threaded behind the symphysis and brought out for sectioning each of the inferior rami. A third Gigli wire is used to saw the pubis transversely in half (Fig. 3.**49**). Then the inferior fascia of the urogenital diaphragm and the deep transverse perineal muscle are resected and removed with the bone.

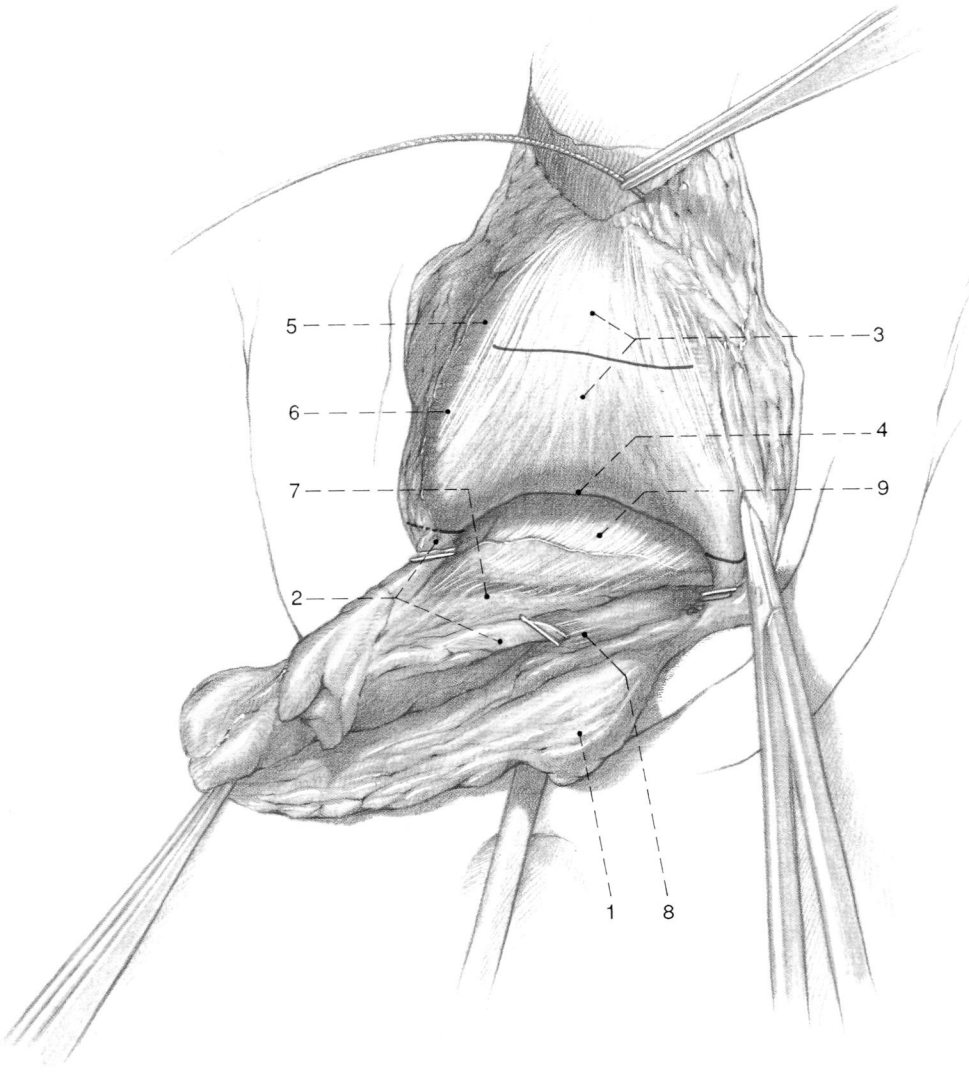

Fig. 3.**48**   The lines of resection in the pelvic bone are shown. A clamp is inserted into the true pelvis through the medial part of the obturator foramen from the perineum, and a Gigli saw is mounted within the pelvis and brought out for sectioning the periurethral bone.

1 Labium majus
2 Crus of clitoris
3 Pubic symphysis
4 Arcuate ligament of pubis
5 Adductor brevis
6 Gracilis
7 Bulbospongiosus
8 Ischiocavernosus
9 Inferior fascia of urogenital diaphragm

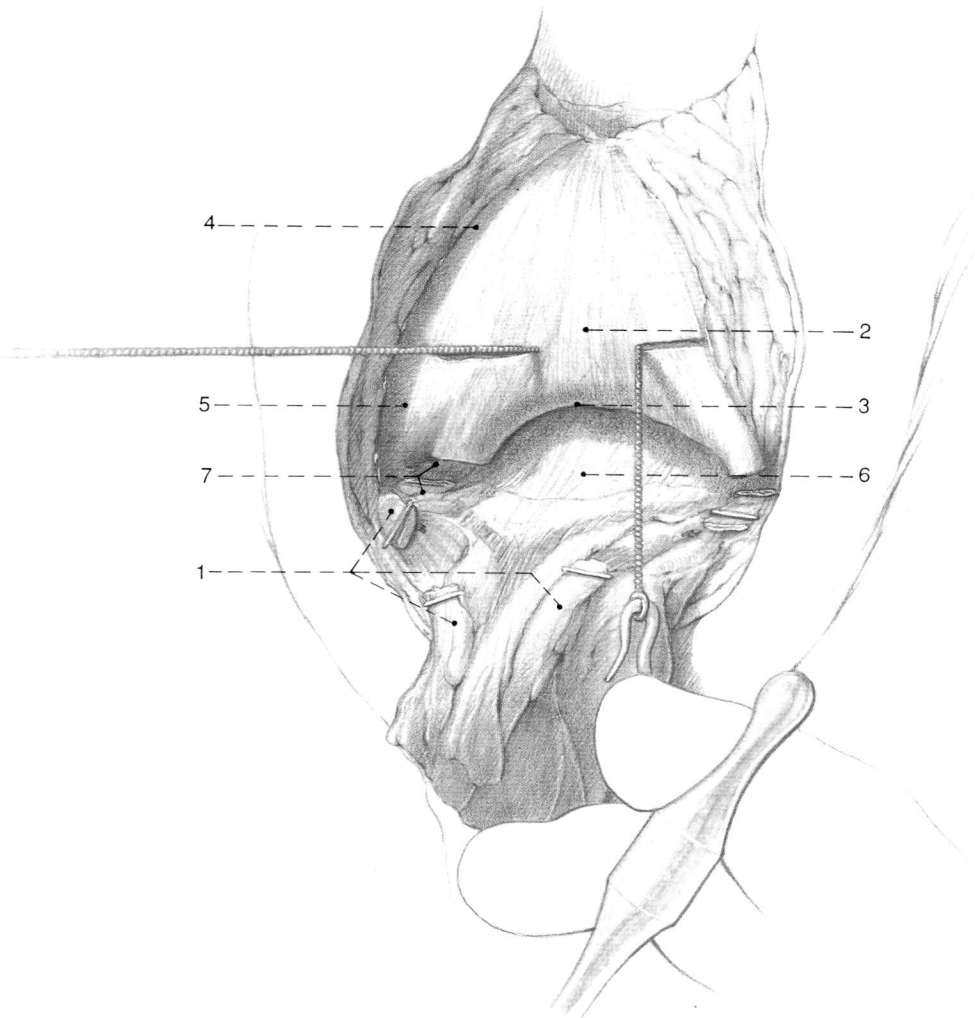

Fig. 3.**49** The pubic bone is sawed in half with a third Gigli wire. The inferior fascia of the urogenital diaphragm, deep transverse perineal muscle, and underlying urethra are resected along with the periurethral bone.

1 Crura of clitoris
2 Pubic symphysis
3 Arcuate ligament of pubis
4 Adductor brevis
5 Gracilis
6 Inferior fascia of urogenital diaphragm
7 Inferior pubic ramus

En Bloc Removal of the Specimen

Incision of the lateral vaginal wall from the outside frees up the surgical specimen, allowing an en bloc removal (Fig. 3.50). On external inspection of the wound cavity following specimen removal (Fig. 3.51), the sigmoid colon and peritoneum, the rectum, and the posterior vaginal wall are visible in the posterior portion of the pelvis. Lateral to these structures are the posterior bladder pedicles, which have been ligated to the endopelvic fascia on both sides. The obturator and levator ani muscles can be seen anterolaterally.

Comments

Applied in the setting of a radical anterior pelvic exenteration, this approach can give access for resecting the inferior border of the symphysis, the anterior vaginal wall, the upper portion of the vulva, and the clitoris (Fig. 3.52). The high incidence of recurrence of female urethral carcinoma can be significantly reduced by use of this approach. The urethra is removed with the tissue of the bulbourethral space, the surrounding bone, and a portion of the external genitalia. The pelvic floor is reconstructed externally with bilateral myocutaneous gracilis flaps and is resurfaced internally with greater omentum. The vagina is occluded as in an anterior pelvic exenteration.

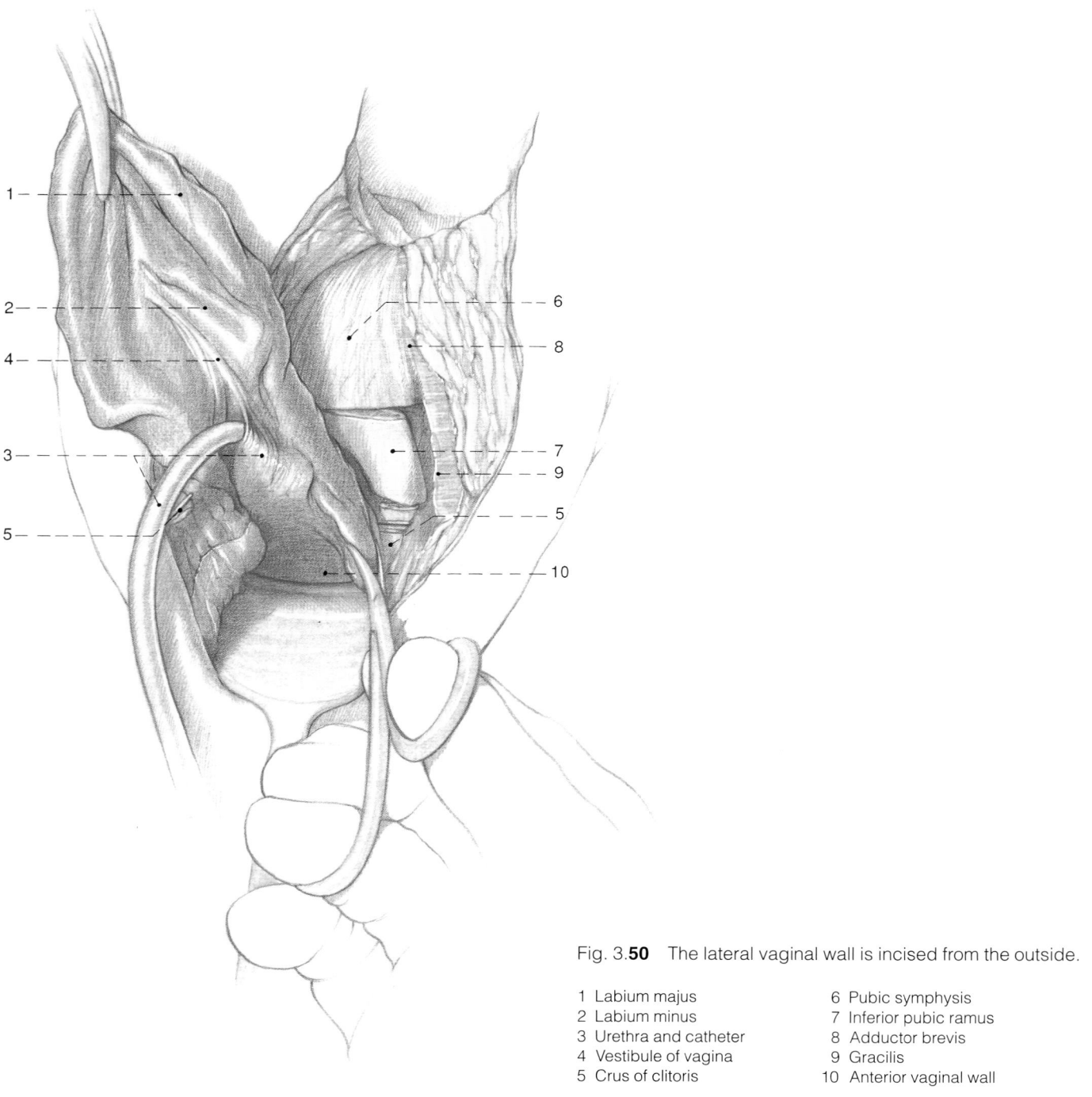

Fig. 3.50 The lateral vaginal wall is incised from the outside.

1 Labium majus	6 Pubic symphysis
2 Labium minus	7 Inferior pubic ramus
3 Urethra and catheter	8 Adductor brevis
4 Vestibule of vagina	9 Gracilis
5 Crus of clitoris	10 Anterior vaginal wall

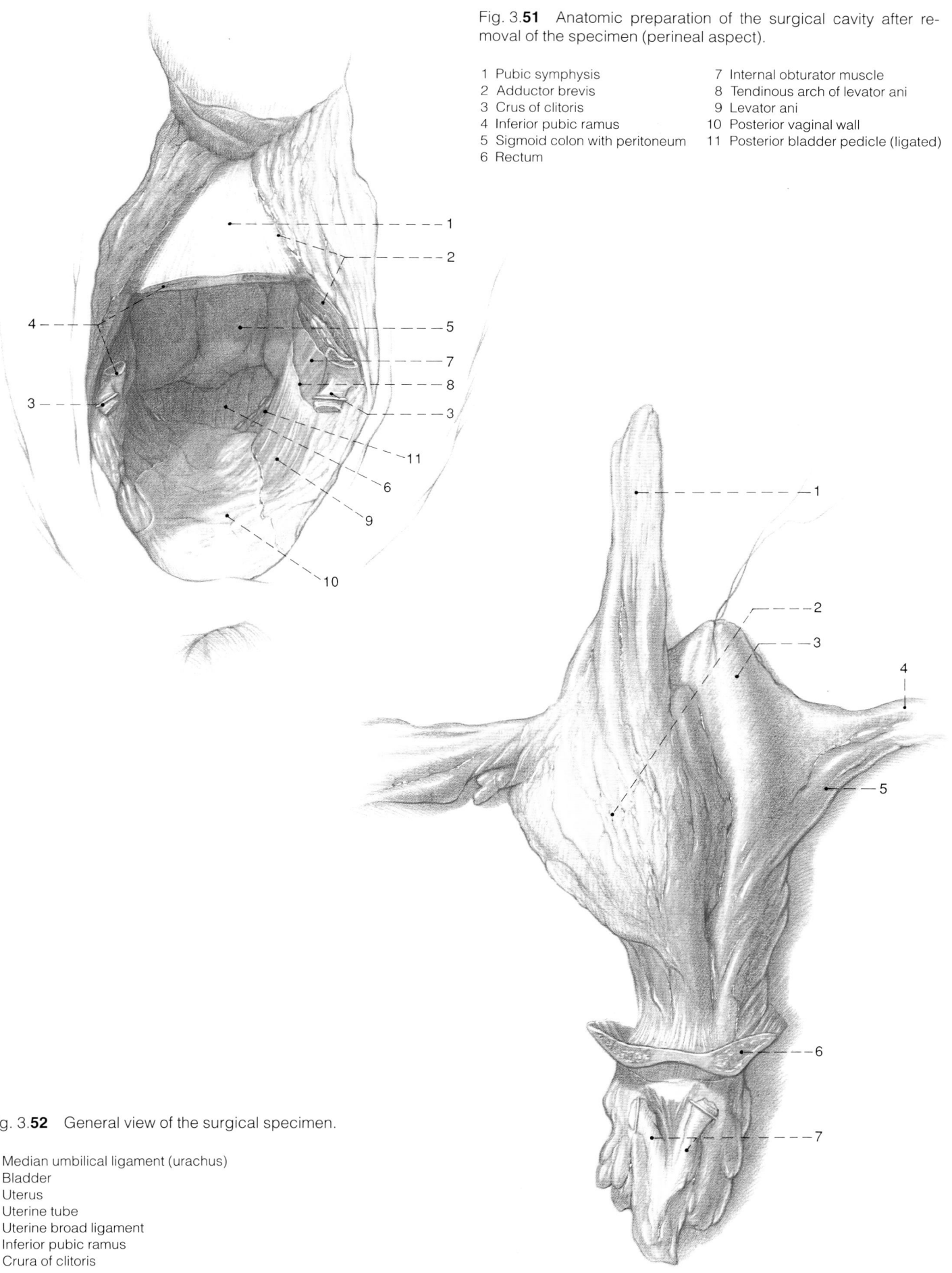

Fig. 3.**51** Anatomic preparation of the surgical cavity after removal of the specimen (perineal aspect).

1 Pubic symphysis
2 Adductor brevis
3 Crus of clitoris
4 Inferior pubic ramus
5 Sigmoid colon with peritoneum
6 Rectum
7 Internal obturator muscle
8 Tendinous arch of levator ani
9 Levator ani
10 Posterior vaginal wall
11 Posterior bladder pedicle (ligated)

Fig. 3.**52** General view of the surgical specimen.

1 Median umbilical ligament (urachus)
2 Bladder
3 Uterus
4 Uterine tube
5 Uterine broad ligament
6 Inferior pubic ramus
7 Crura of clitoris

189

Retropubic Approach for Radical Prostatectomy

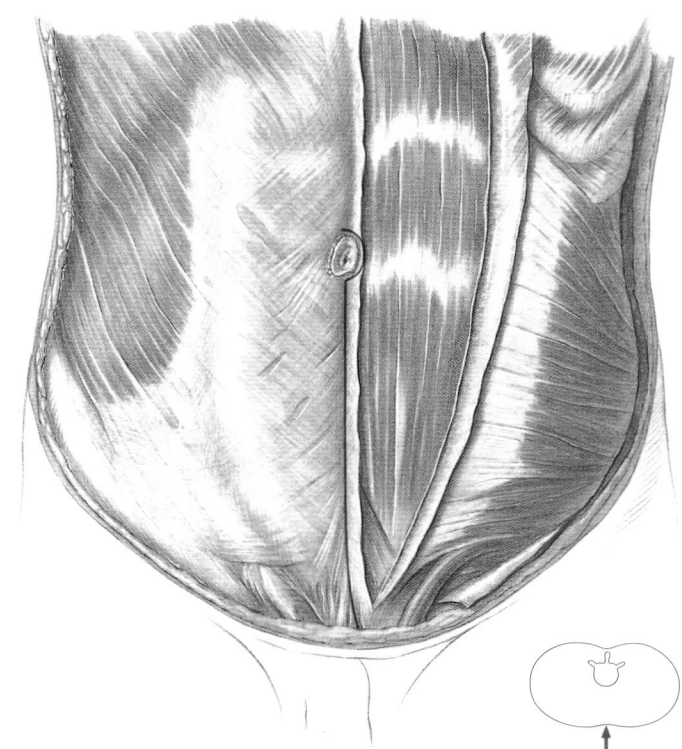

Fig. 3.**53**

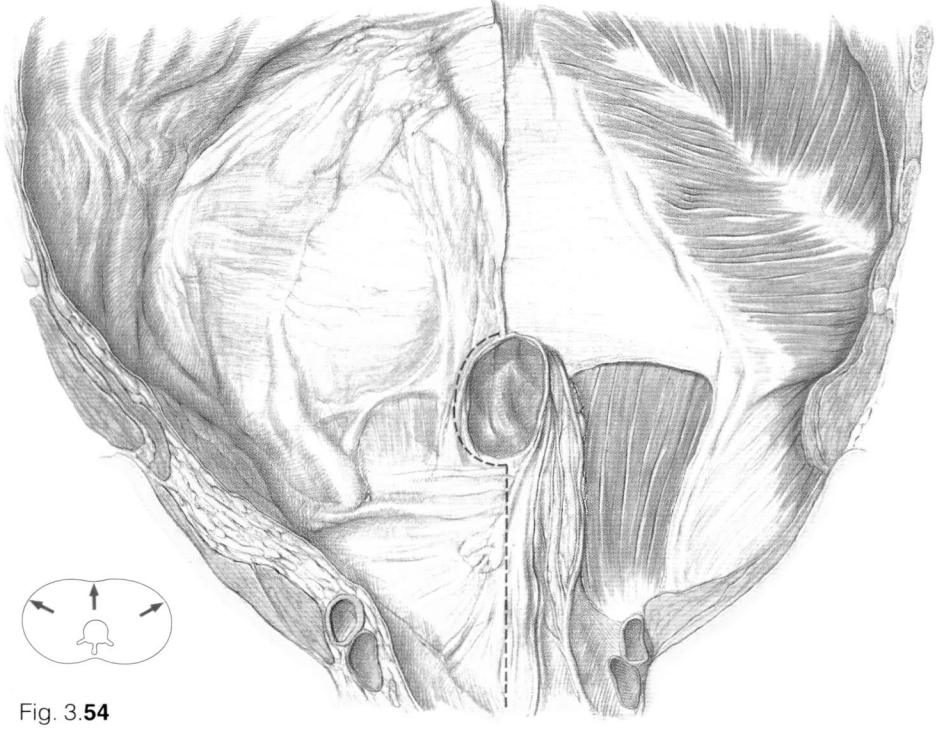

Fig. 3.**54**

Main Indication

Localized prostatic carcinoma.

Position and Skin Incision

The patient is placed in a hyperextended supine position to increase the distance from the umbilicus to the symphysis, supplemented by a mild Trendelenburg position (Fig. 3.**55**).

The lower abdominal midline incision starts above the symphysis and extends upward, skirting the left side of the umbilicus (Fig. 3.**56**).

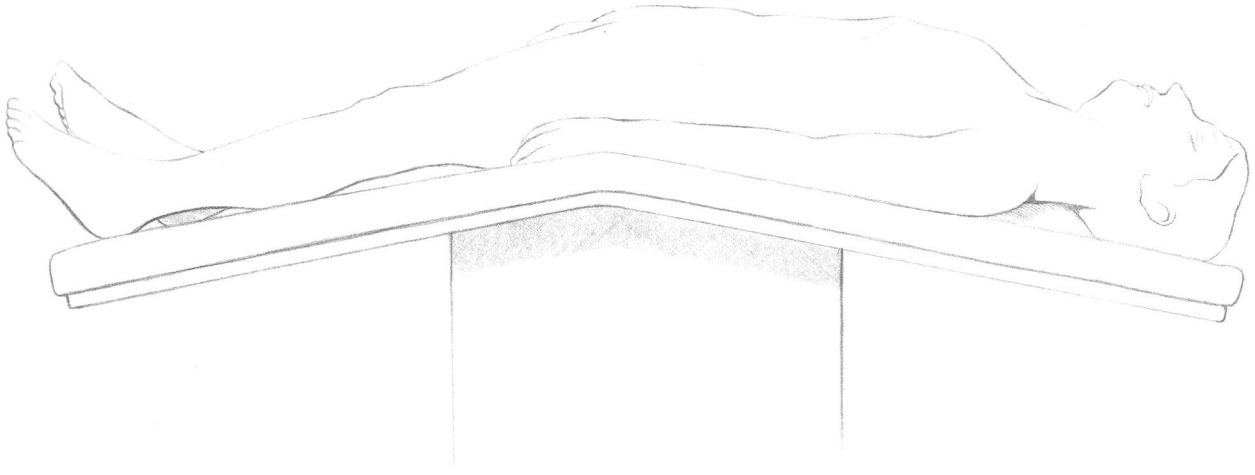

Fig. 3.**55**   Position.

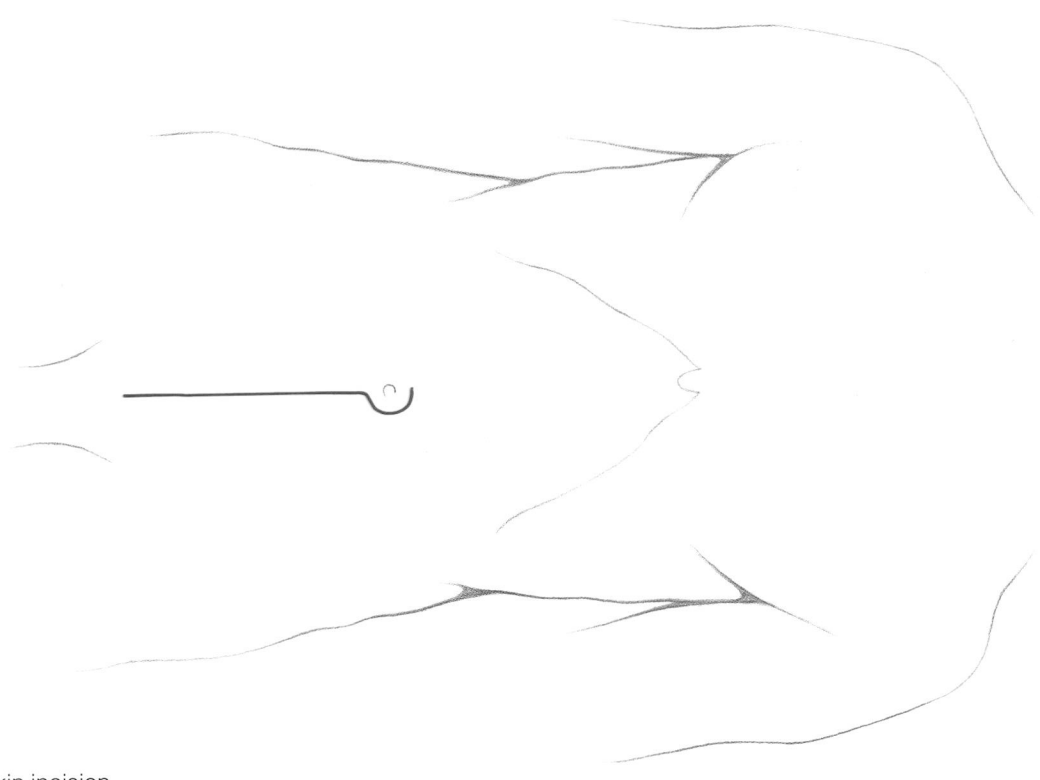

Fig. 3.**56**   Skin incision.

Exposure of the Prevesical and Paravesical Spaces

The subcutaneous tissue is divided with electrocautery, exposing the linea alba at the anterior rectus sheath (Fig. 3.**57**).

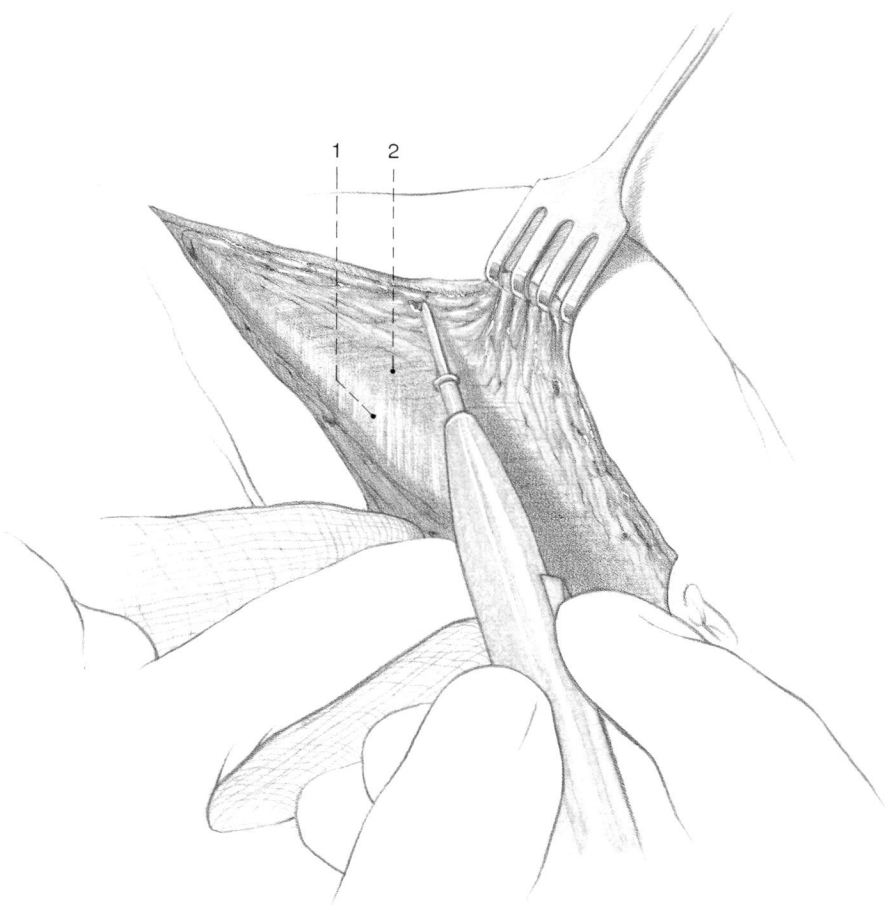

Fig. 3.**57**   Exposure of the linea alba.

1 Linea alba
2 Anterior rectus sheath

The sheath is incised, and both rectus muscles are separated at the midline exposing the posterior rectus sheath and transversalis fascia (Fig. 3.**58**).

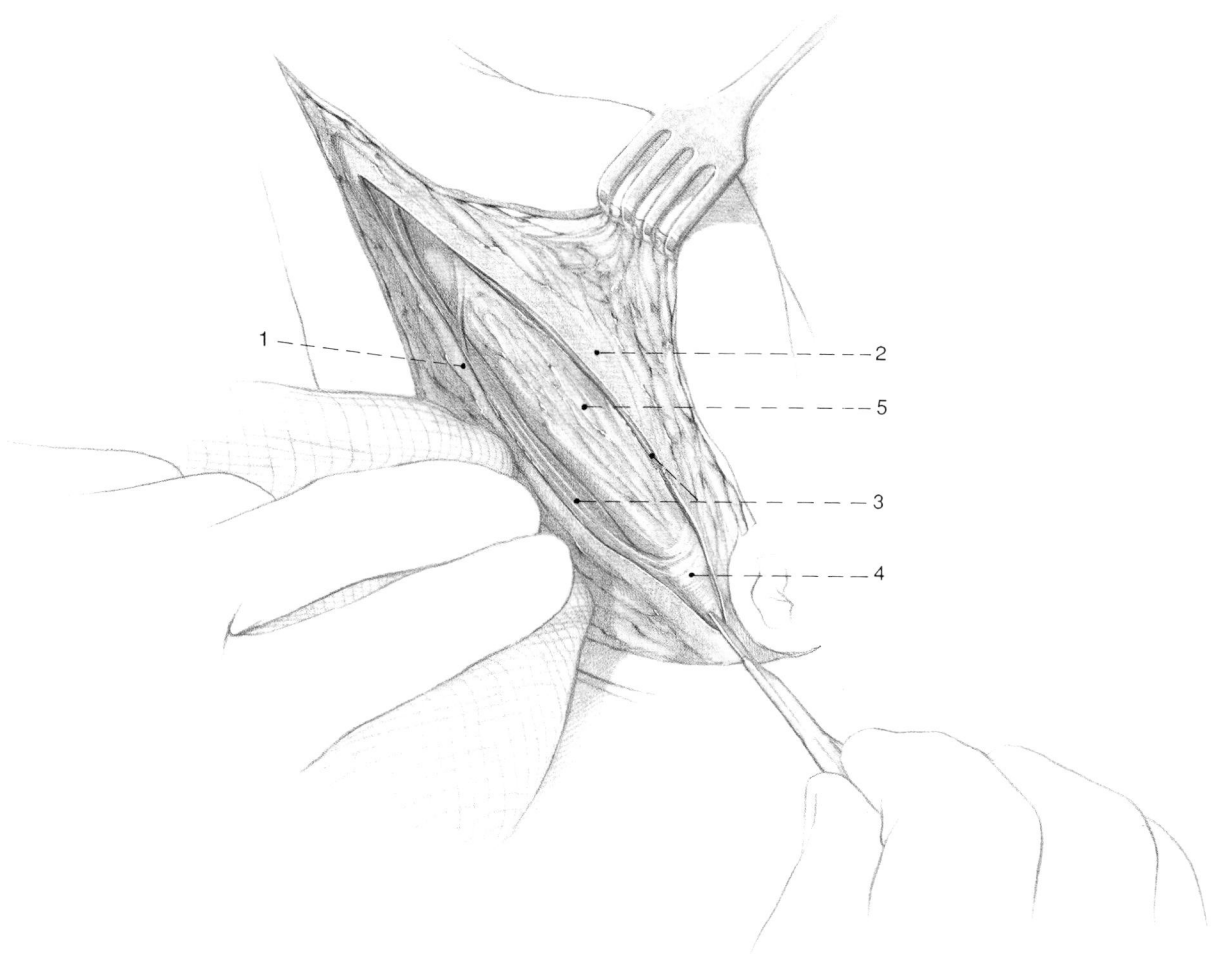

Fig. 3.**58**   Separation of the rectus muscles.

1 Linea alba
2 Anterior rectus sheath
3 Rectus muscle
4 Posterior rectus sheath
5 Transversalis fascia

The posterior rectus sheath is incised laterally to the umbilicus. After division of the transversalis fascia, the prevesical space is dissected (Fig. 3.**59**). All adherent fat and connective tissue are left on the posterior wall of the rectus muscle along with the branches of the inferior epigastric artery.

The prevesical space is opened widely, and the paravesical space is exposed. The peritoneum is dissected laterally from the external iliac vessels and the lateral abdominal wall. The parietal layer of the pelvic fascia is identified on the pelvic wall, and the visceral layer on the bladder is exposed as far as the reflection of the endopelvic fascia (tendinous arch of pelvic fascia) (Fig. 3.**60**).

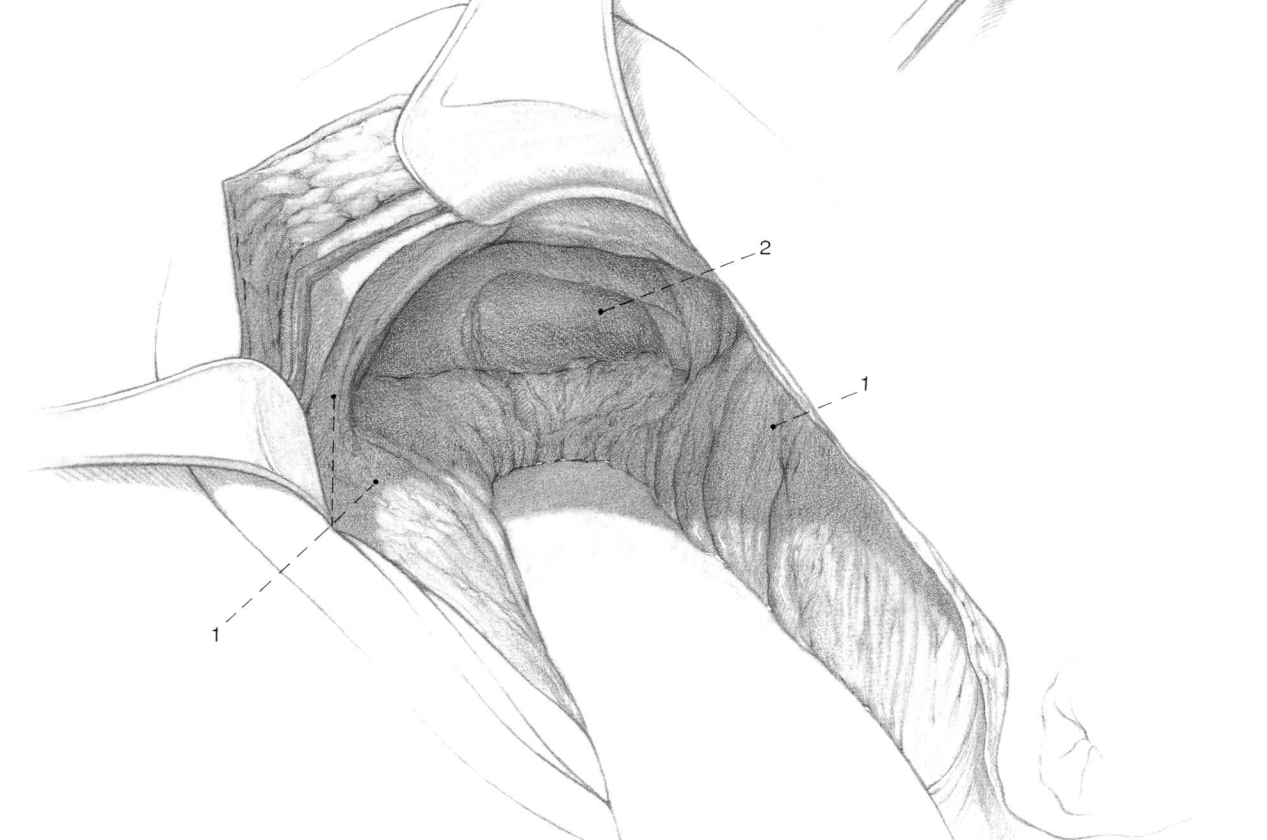

Fig. 3.**59**   Incision of the posterior rectus sheath. ▶

1 Anterior rectus sheath
2 Rectus muscle
3 Posterior rectus sheath
4 Transversalis fascia
5 Urachial ligament
6 Arcuate line

Fig. 3.**60**   Exposure of the prevesical and paravesical spaces.

1 Parietal peritoneum
2 Parietal pelvic fascia

The vas deferens is ligated at the internal inguinal ring. The parietal peritoneum is then dissected from the lateral abdominal wall on the plane defined by the retroperitoneal testicular vessels (Fig. 3.**61**).

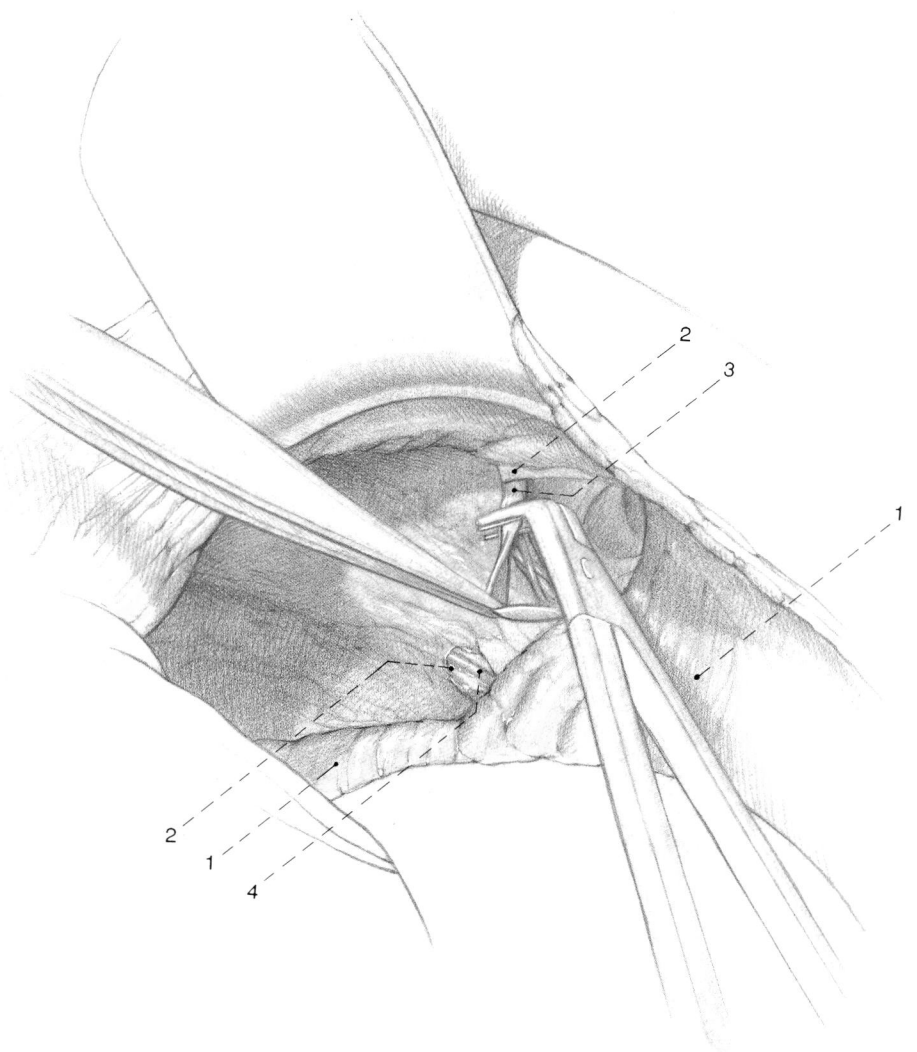

Fig. 3.**61** Division of the vas deferens and dissection of the parietal peritoneum.

1 Parietal peritoneum
2 Parietal pelvic fascia
3 Vas deferens
4 Obturator artery

Pelvic Lymph Node Dissection

The radical prostatectomy includes a modified pelvic lymph node dissection. This dissection begins at the external iliac vein, proceeds distally to the femoral canal, and ends with removal of the obturator lymph nodes (Figs. 3.**62**, 3.**63**). In contrast to the pelvic lymph node dissection in anterior exenteration, the obturator artery and vein are preserved. The obturator nerve is dissected free after removal of the lymph nodes. The internal iliac artery can be snared with a vascular tape (Fig. 3.**63**).

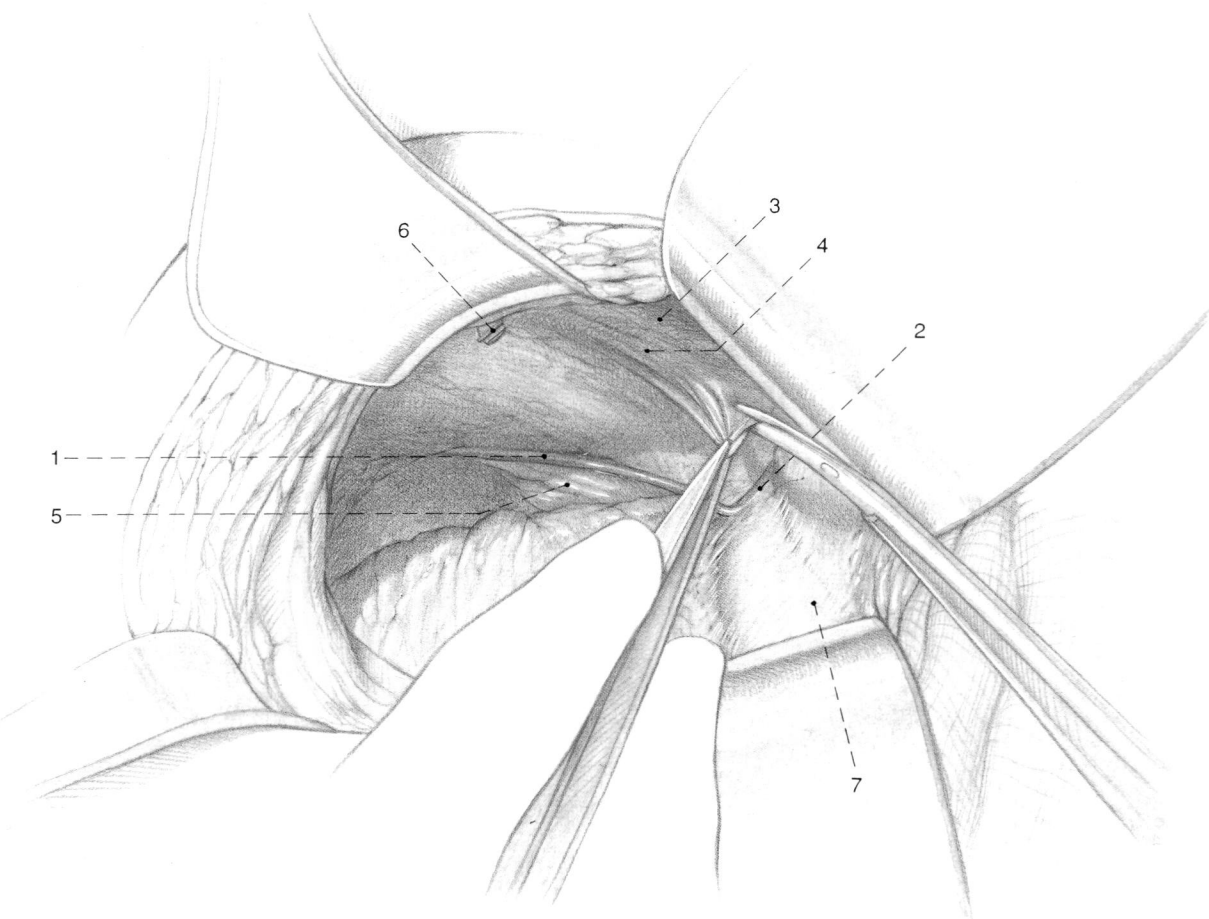

Fig. 3.**62**   Start of the pelvic lymph node dissection.

1 Obturator artery
2 Internal iliac artery
3 External iliac artery
4 External iliac vein
5 Obturator nerve
6 Right vas deferens
7 Parietal peritoneum

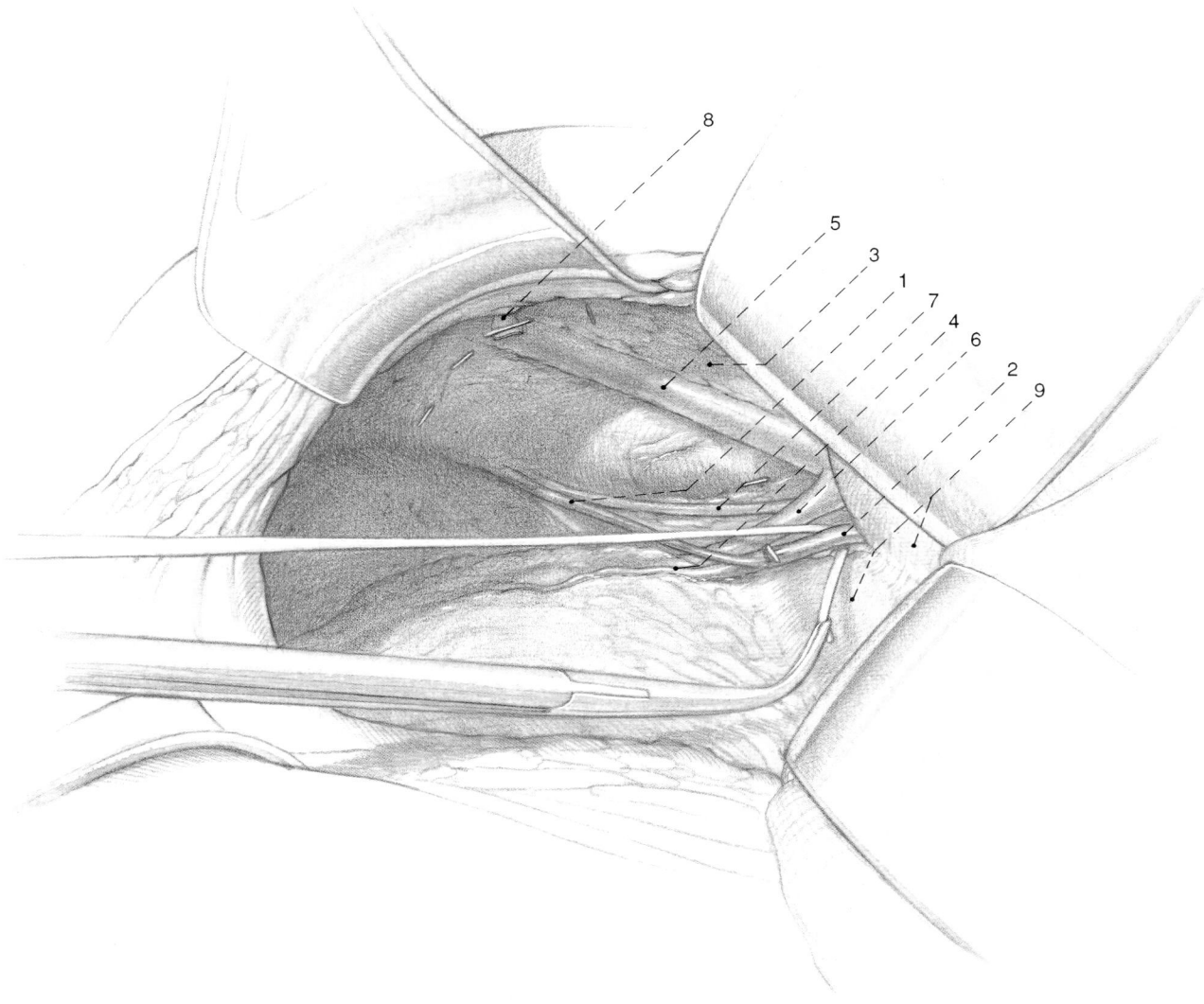

Fig. 3.**63** Status following pelvic lymph node dissection. The internal iliac artery is snared.

1 Obturator artery
2 Internal iliac artery
3 External iliac artery
4 Superior vesical artery
5 External iliac vein
6 Internal iliac vein
7 Obturator nerve
8 Vas deferens
9 Parietal peritoneum

Incision of the Endopelvic Fascia (Division of the Puboprostatic Ligament)

The bladder with its adjacent fat and visceral fascia is retracted upward with a malleable blade while traction is placed on the catheter balloon, exposing the endopelvic fascia. The endopelvic fascia is cleared of fat and connective tissue, and the reflection of the visceral layer into the parietal layer of the endopelvic fascia (tendinous arch) is exposed as far as its insertion on the pubic symphysis (Fig. 3.**64**). Incision of this fold of endopelvic fascia establishes access to the paraprostatic space (Fig. 3.**65**). Levator ani fibers are visible on the lateral side, and medially, below the endopelvic fascia, is the paraprostatic tissue containing the superficial lateral pelvic fascia and the neurovascular bundle (prostatic plexus, cavernous nerves, and prostatic ar-

teries). This space is entered by using scissors through an incision placed well laterally to avoid injury to these neurovascular structures (Fig. 3.**65**) and is carried to the lateral border of the puboprostatic ligament on each side (Fig. 3.**66**). The puboprostatic ligaments are dissected free from adjacent fat with fine forceps. Between the two ligaments lies the superficial branch of the deep dorsal penile vein, which is not covered by pelvic fascia (Fig. 3.**66**). The puboprostatic ligament is sharply released from its insertion on the pubic bone (Fig. 3.**67**) while the superficial branch of the deep dorsal penile vein is protected by deflecting it to the opposite side.

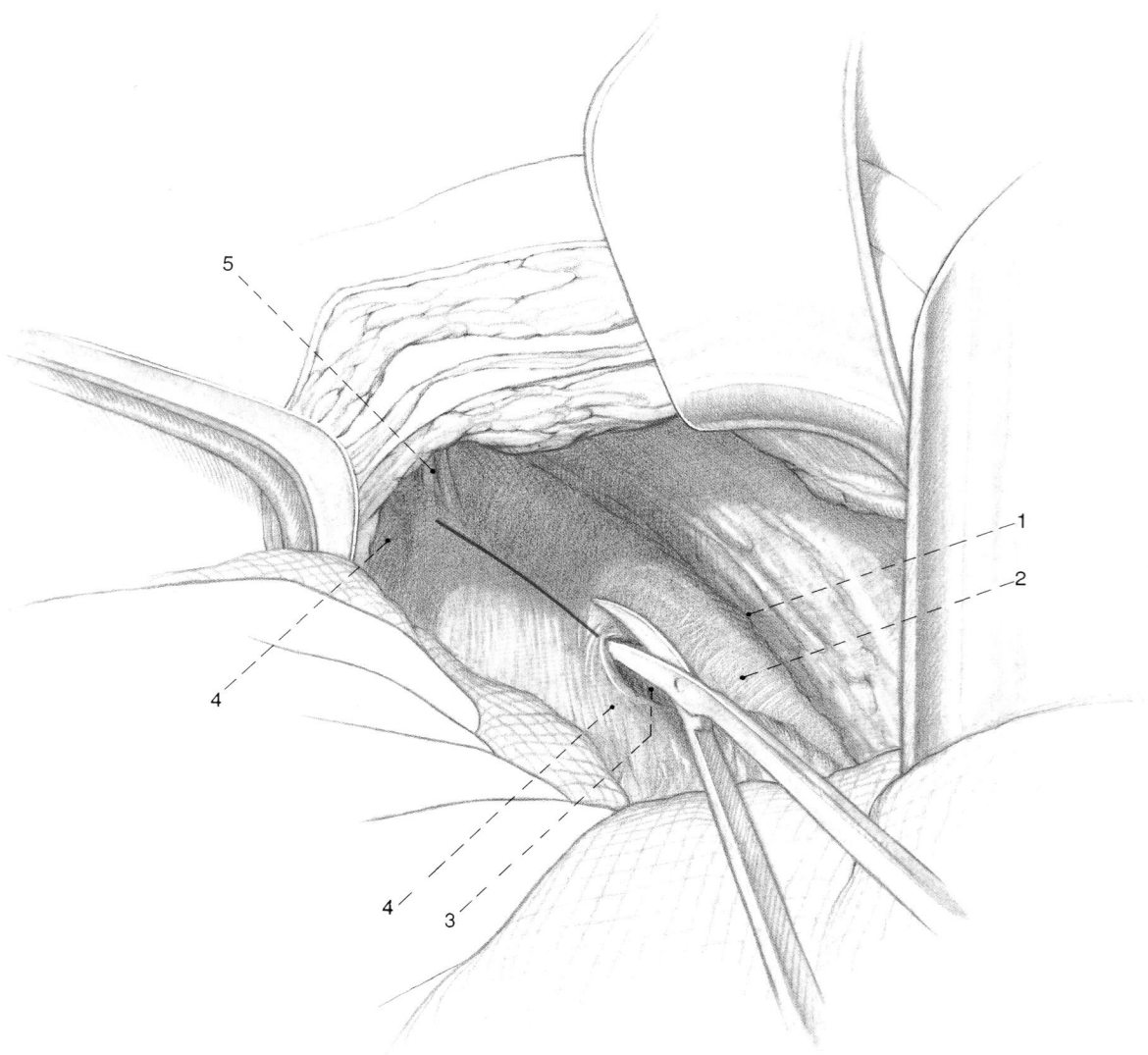

Fig. 3.**64**   Exposure of the endopelvic fascia.

1 Tendinous arch of the levator ani
2 Parietal pelvic fascia
3 Levator ani
4 Prostatic fascia (visceral pelvic fascia)
5 Puboprostatic ligament

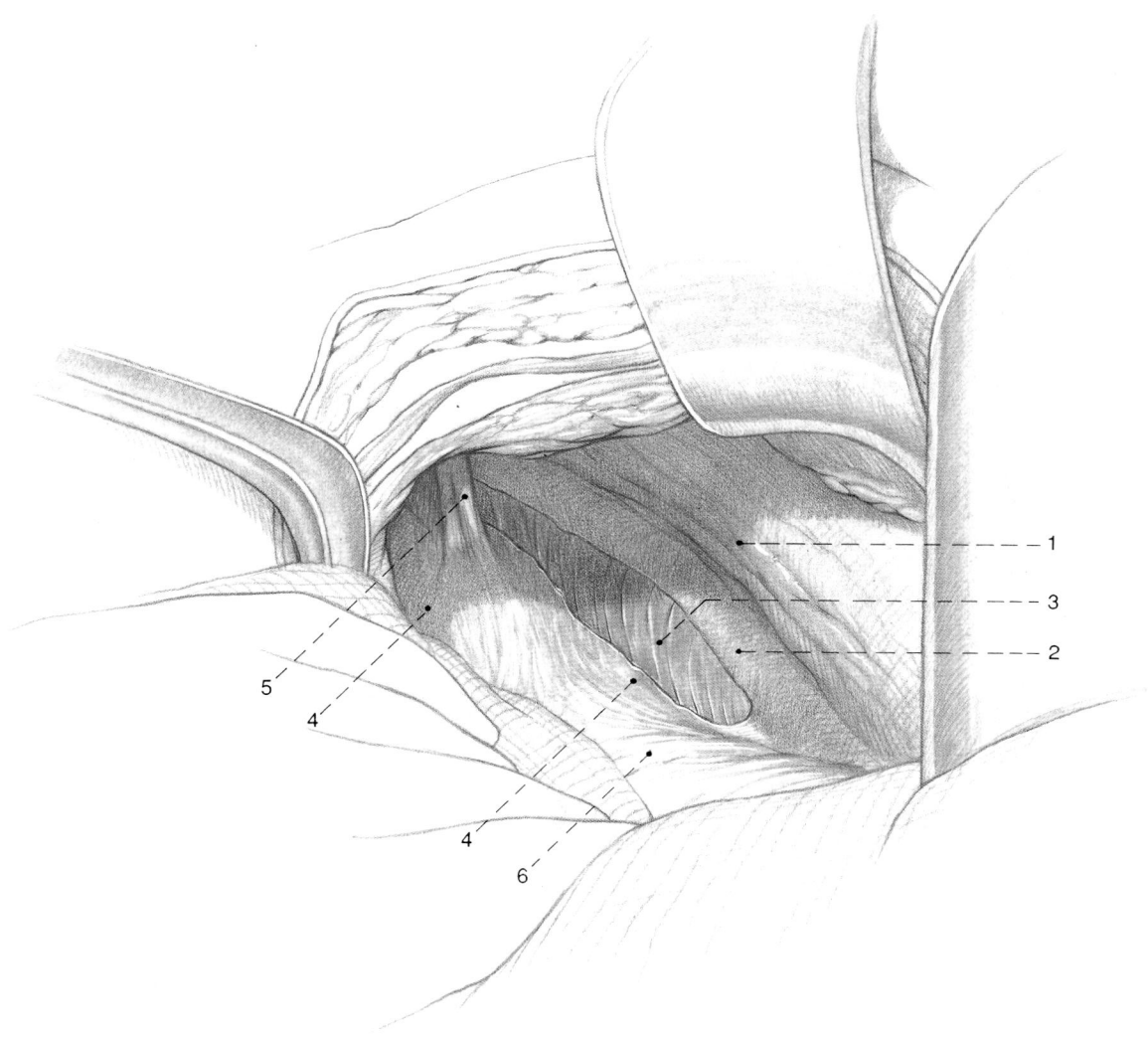

Fig. 3.**65** The endopelvic fascia is incised, exposing the levator ani laterally and the paraprostatic tissue medially.

1 Tendinous arch of levator ani
2 Parietal pelvic fascia
3 Levator ani
4 Prostatic fascia (visceral pelvic fascia)
5 Puboprostatic ligament
6 Vesical fascia

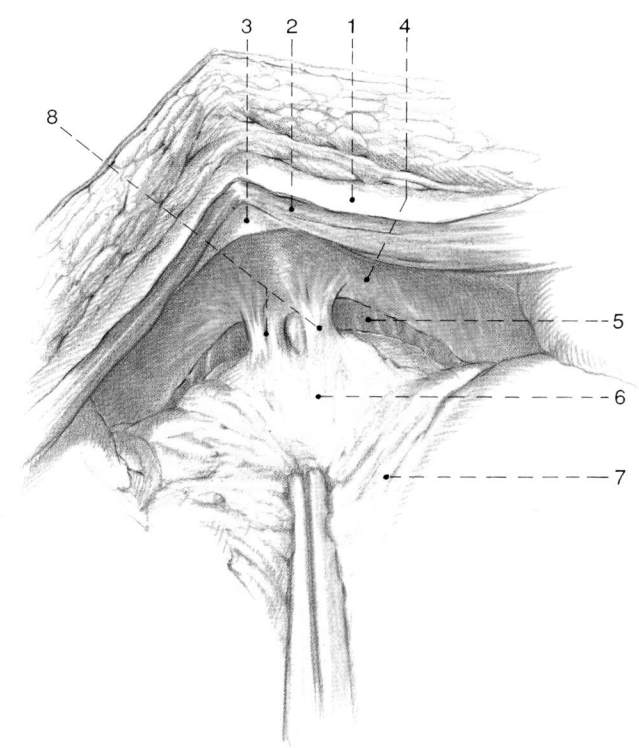

Fig. 3.**66** Anatomical dissection showing the puboprostatic ligaments. Branches of the deep dorsal penile vein are demonstrated at the center.

1 Anterior rectus sheath
2 Rectus muscle
3 Posterior rectus sheath
4 Parietal pelvic fascia
5 Levator ani (puborectalis)
6 Prostatic fascia
7 Vesical fascia
8 Puboprostatic ligaments

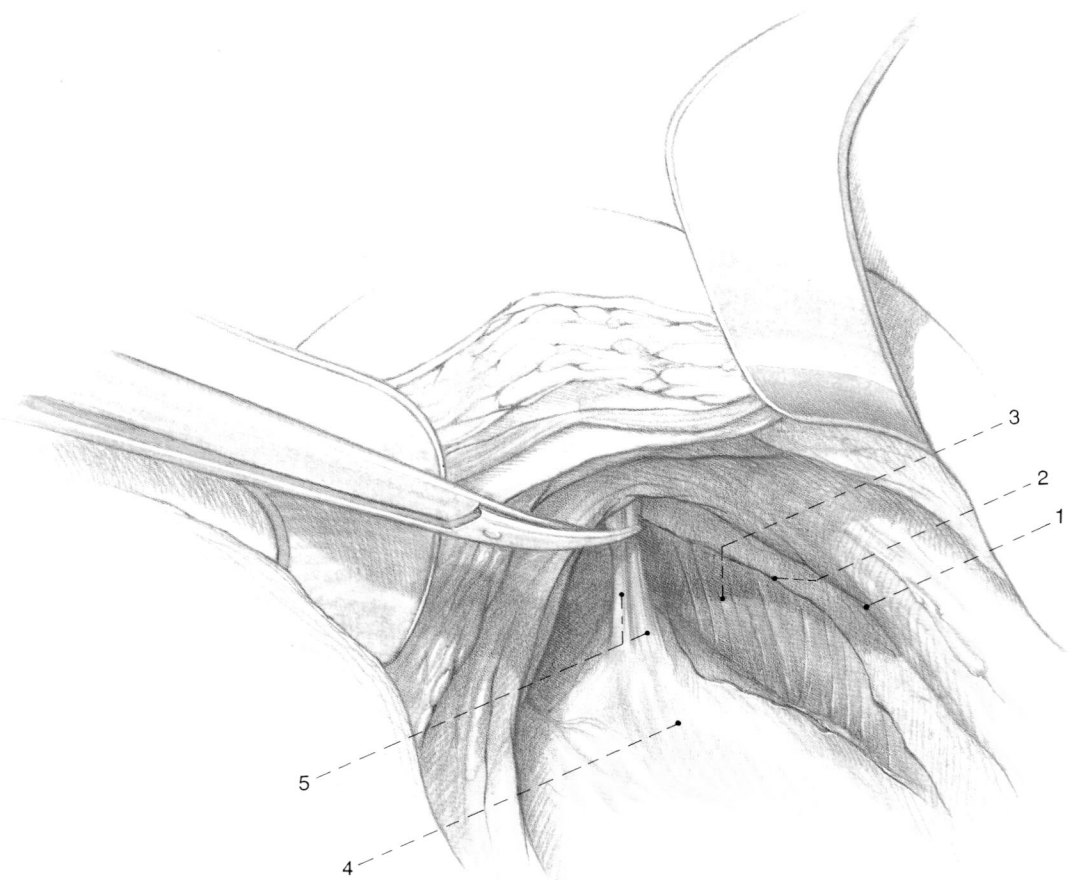

Fig. 3.**67** The puboprostatic ligament is divided at the pubic bone.

1 Tendinous arch of levator ani
2 Parietal pelvic fascia
3 Levator ani (puborectalis)
4 Prostatic fascia
5 Puboprostatic ligaments

Exposure of the Pubourethral Space

After division of the puboprostatic ligaments, the vesicoprostatic junction is deflected downward, giving access to the pubourethral space. The dorsal venous complex is identified; it contains the superficial branch, which is not covered by the pelvic fascia. By contrast, the right and left portions of the prostatic venous plexus are covered by endopelvic fascia (Figs. 3.**68**, 3.**69**). This entire complex is underrun and ligated (Fig. 3.**69**).

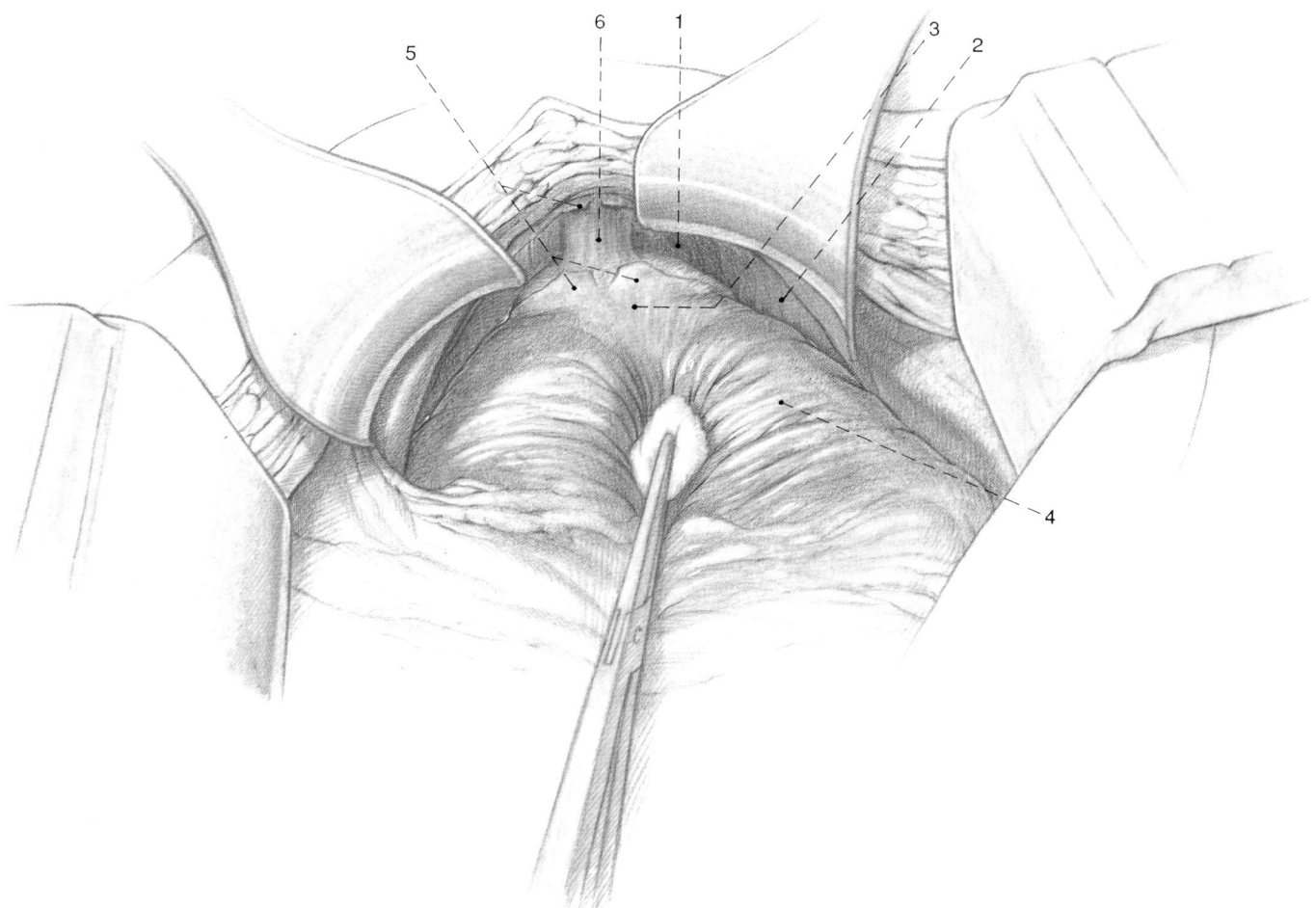

Fig. 3.**68**   Division of both puboprostatic ligaments gives access to the retropubic space and exposes the dorsal vein complex.

1 Levator ani (puborectalis)
2 Levator ani (pubococcygeus)
3 Prostatic fascia
4 Vesical fascia
5 Puboprostatic ligaments
6 Dorsal vein complex

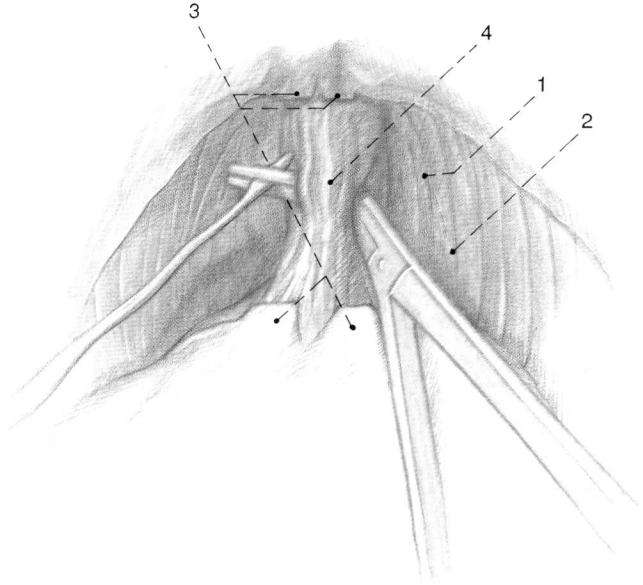

Fig. 3.**69**   The entire prostatic venous plexus ("dorsal venous complex") is underrun and ligated.

1 Levator ani (puborectalis)
2 Levator ani (pubococcygeus)
3 Puboprostatic ligaments
4 Dorsal vei complex

Exposure and Division of the External Urethral Sphincter (Rhabdosphincter) and Membranous Urethra

Following division of the dorsal venous complex, the antero-lateral aspect of the external urethral sphincter (rhabdosphincter) can be identified. It forms an omega-shaped loop anterior and lateral to the membranous urethra, its two crura inserting into the central tendon of the perineum (Fig. 3.**70**). During anatomic dissection of the pelvic floor on the internal aspect, the superior fascia of the urogenital dia-phragm can be seen along with the anterior and lateral borders of the omega-shaped urethral sphincter (rhabdosphincter). The transverse perineal ligament (preurethral ligament) presents anterior to the sphincter, and the membranous urethra is visible behind it.

The next step involves division of the external urethral sphincter and membranous urethra (Fig. 3.**71**). The first two anastomotic sutures passed forward through the membranous urethra, urethral sphincter, and endopelvic fascia are used to elevate the anterior portion of the sphincter and membranous urethra.

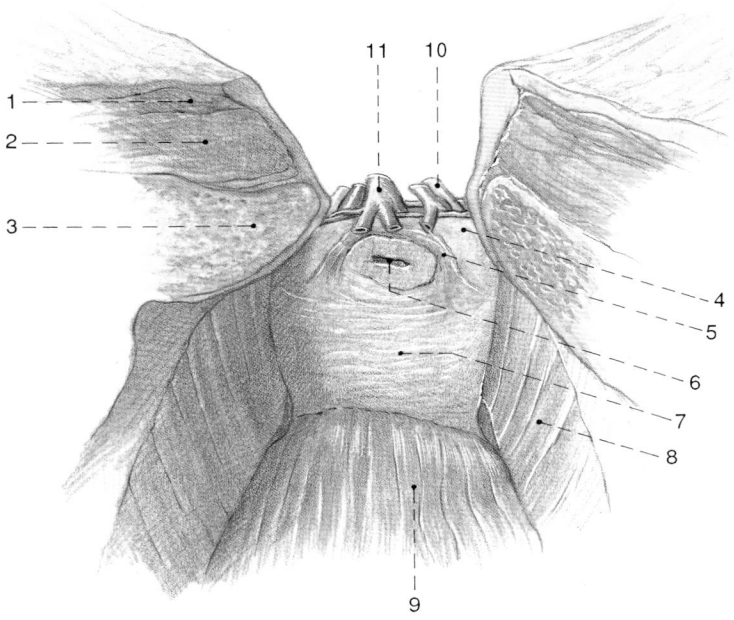

Fig. 3.**70** Anatomic preparation: The prostate is removed together with the paraprostatic tissue. The superior fascia of the urogenital diaphragm has been dissected. The urethral sphincter (rhabdosphincter), membranous urethra, and rectum can be seen. Both levator ani muscles are visible laterally.

  1 Gracilis
  2 Adductor longus
  3 Inferior pubic ramus
  4 Transverse perineal ligament
  5 External urethral sphincter
  6 Urethra
  7 Superior fascia of urogenital diaphragm
  8 Levator ani
  9 Rectum
10 Dorsal penile nerve
11 Deep dorsal penile vein

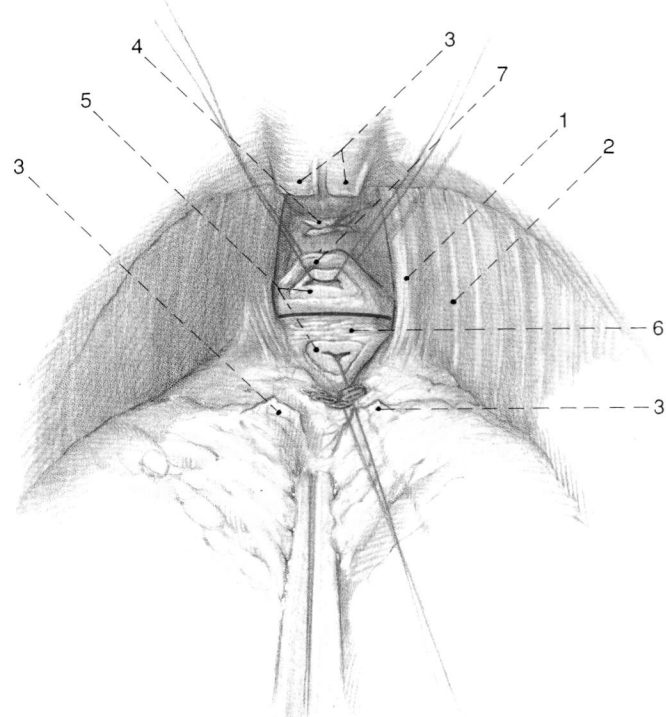

Fig. 3.**71** The urethral sphincter (rhabdosphincter) and membranous urethra are incised as far as the rectourethral septum.

1 Levator ani (puborectalis)
2 Levator ani (pubococcygeus)
3 Puboprostatic ligaments
4 Dorsal vein complex
5 Urethra
6 Rectourethral septum
7 Urethral sphincter (rhabdosphincter)

Exposure of the Rectogenital Space

The membranous urethra is divided on the line shown. The posterior prostatic fascia is divided at its attachment, the rectourethral septum (the apex of the wedge-shaped perineal body), and the rectogenital space is opened. The rectal fascia is identified at the posterior aspect of the rectogenital space (Fig. 3.72).

Exposure of the Vesicogenital Space

Now the prostate is resected with the paraprostatic tissue between the rectogenital space and levator ani muscle. The seminal vesicles and the ampullae of the spermatic ducts are dissected from the bladder detrusor, following the course of the rectogenital space. The prostate is transected at the bladder neck and dissected out of the rectogenital space.

After the prostate has been removed, the membranous urethra, the omega-shaped urethral sphincter, and the central tendon can be seen on the inner aspect of the superior fascia of the urogenital diaphragm. The deep dorsal penile vein, the dorsal penile artery, and the dorsal penile nerve course between the inner and outer fasciae of the urogenital diaphragm. The deep dorsal penile vein runs between the arcuate ligament and transverse perineal ligament, while the dorsal penile artery and nerve run directly through the tissue of the transverse perineal ligament (Fig. 3.70).

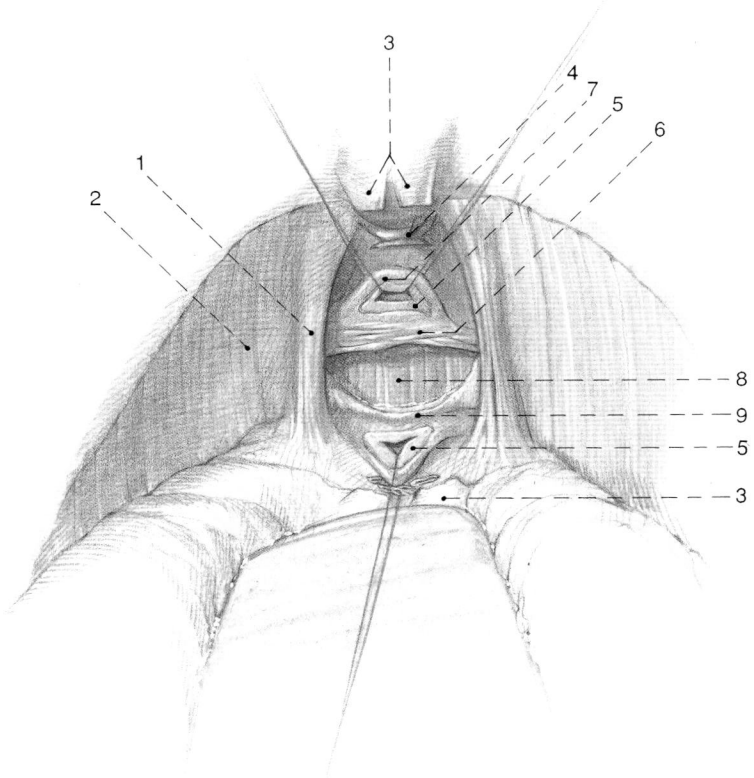

Fig. 3.**72**   The rectourethral septum is incised, Denonvillier's fascia is exposed, and the rectogenital space is entered. The rectal fascia is visible in the depths of the field.

1 Levator ani (puborectalis)
2 Levator ani (pubococcygeus)
3 Puboprostatic ligaments
4 Dorsal vein complex
5 Urethra
6 Rectourethral septum
7 Urethral sphincter (rhabdosphincter)
8 Rectum, covered by rectal fascia
9 Denonvillier's fascia

Comments

In the modification of the nerve-sparing radical prostatectomy the neurovascular bundle (base of the paraprostatic tissue) of the prostate is preserved. This bundle contains the cavernous nerves, fibers from the pelvic plexus to the membranous urethra, arterial branches to the prostate, the venous prostatic plexus and prostatic lymph vessels (Fig. 3.**73**); to approach the neurovascular bundle, the paraprostatic tissue on the lateral surface of the prostate is incised and released.

Located on the posterolateral aspect of the prostate, the neurovascular bundle is deeply embedded in the parietal layer of the fascia (= paraprostatic tissue).

The pudendal canal, covered by the levator ani, runs medial to the lower portion of the obturator internus and along the inferior pubic ramus. It is traversed by the internal pudendal artery and vein and the pudendal nerve, which pass below the levator ani and through the pelvic floor to the dorsum of the penis (Fig. 3.**74**). The pudendal nerve also gives off fibers to the external urethral sphincter (rhabdosphincter) in this area.

This relationship is important because it demonstrates the immediate proximity of the membranous urethra and rhabdosphincter to branches of the internal pudendal artery and vein and the pudendal nerve.

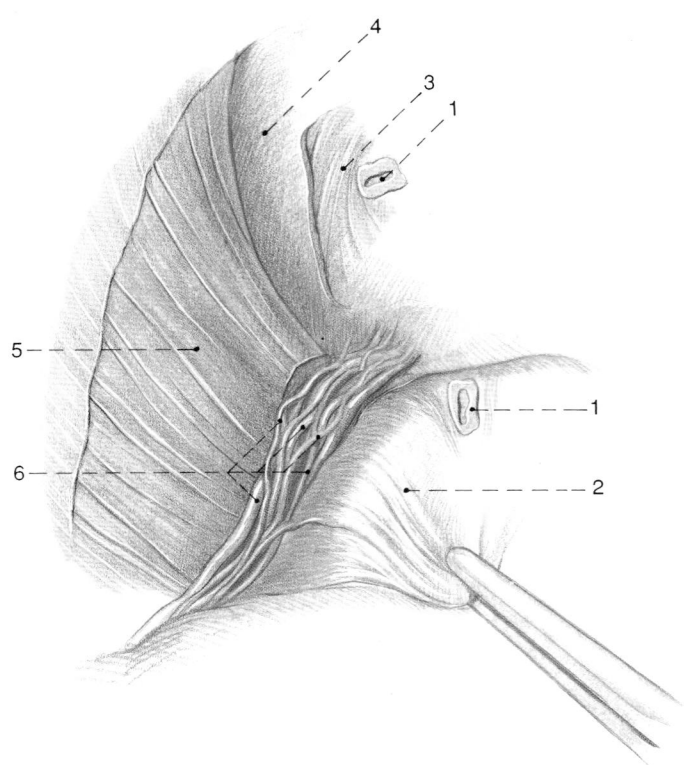

Fig. 3.**73** In this anatomic specimen the left neurovascular bundle has been dissected out of the posterolateral portion of the paraprostatic tissue.

1 Urethra
2 Prostatic fascia
3 External urethral sphincter
4 Superior fascia of urogenital diaphragm
5 Levator ani
6 Neurovascular bundle of prostate

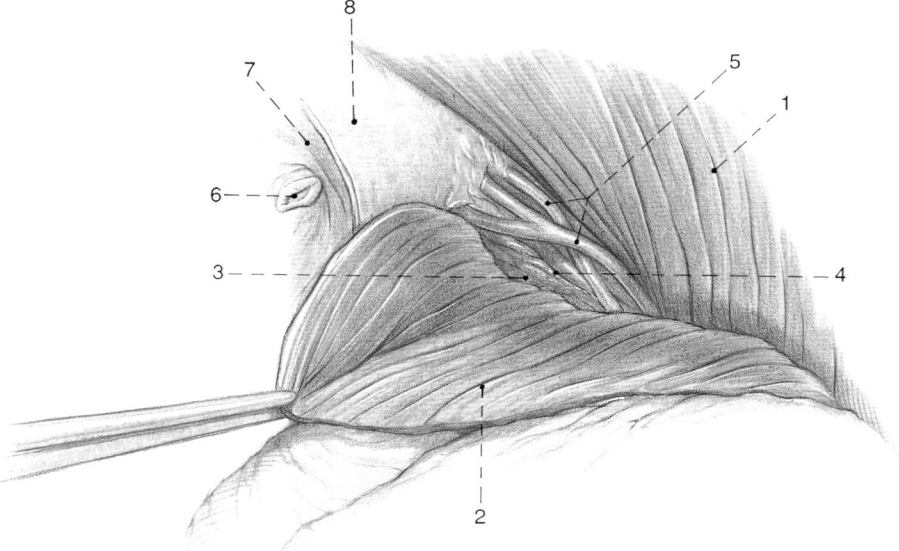

Fig. 3.**74** Anatomic exposure of the contents of the right pudendal canal (internal pudendal artery and vein, pudendal nerve).

1 Obturator internus
2 Levator ani
3 Pudendal canal (Alcock's canal)
4 Pudendal nerve
5 Internal pudendal vessels
6 Urethra
7 Urethral sphincter (rhabdosphincter)
8 Superior fascia of urogenital diaphragm

Extraperitoneal Lower Abdominal Midline Approach

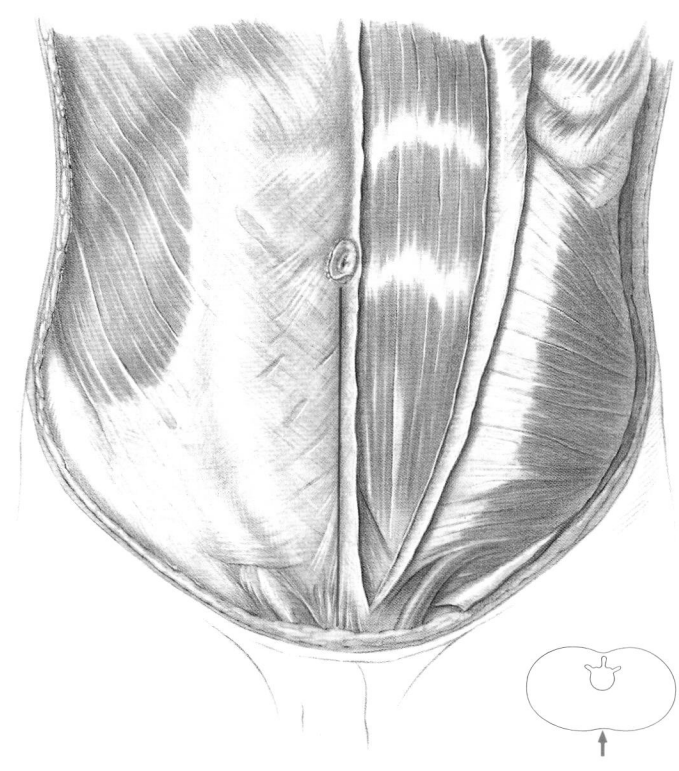

Fig. 3.**75**

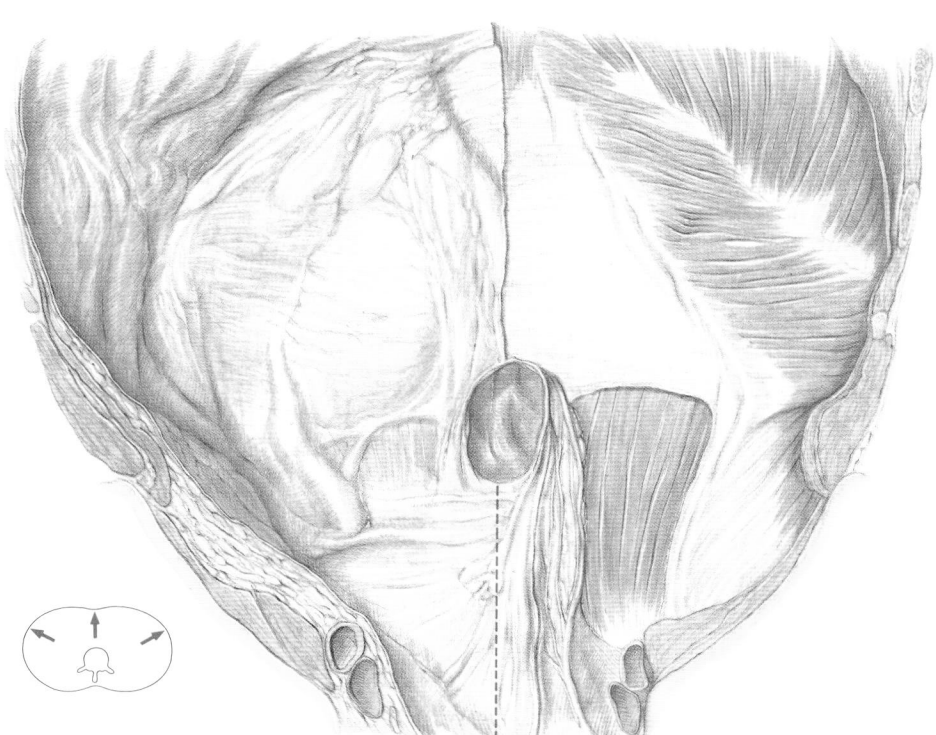

Fig. 3.**76**

Main Indications

- Surgery of the pelvic ureter
- Surgery of the urinary bladder
- Access for open prostatectomy

The approach is illustrated for an open prostatectomy.

Position and Skin Incision

The patient is positioned supine with the table slightly hyperextended at the center. The incision extends from the umbilicus to the pubic symphysis (Figs. 3.**77**, 3.**78**).

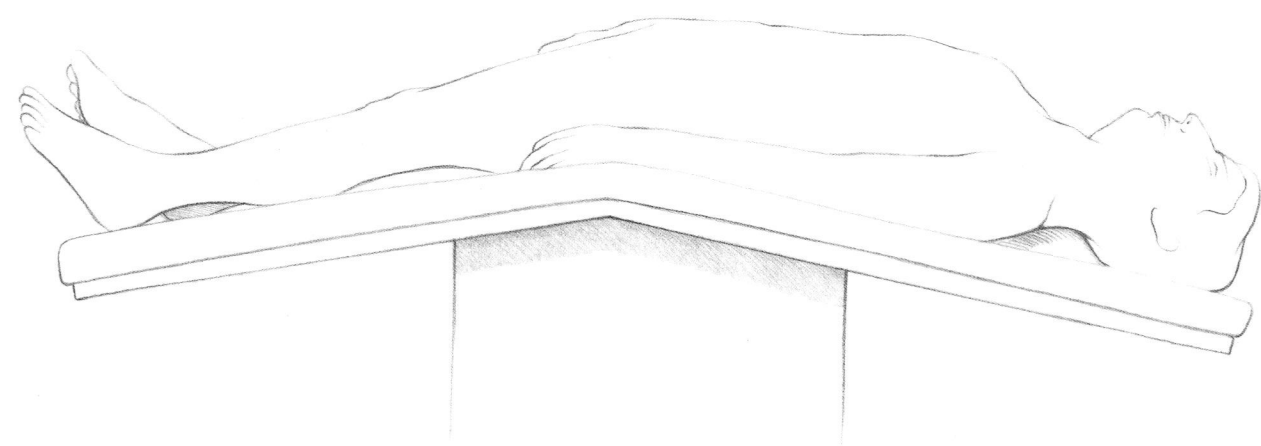

Fig. 3.**77** Position: supine with slight hyperextension.

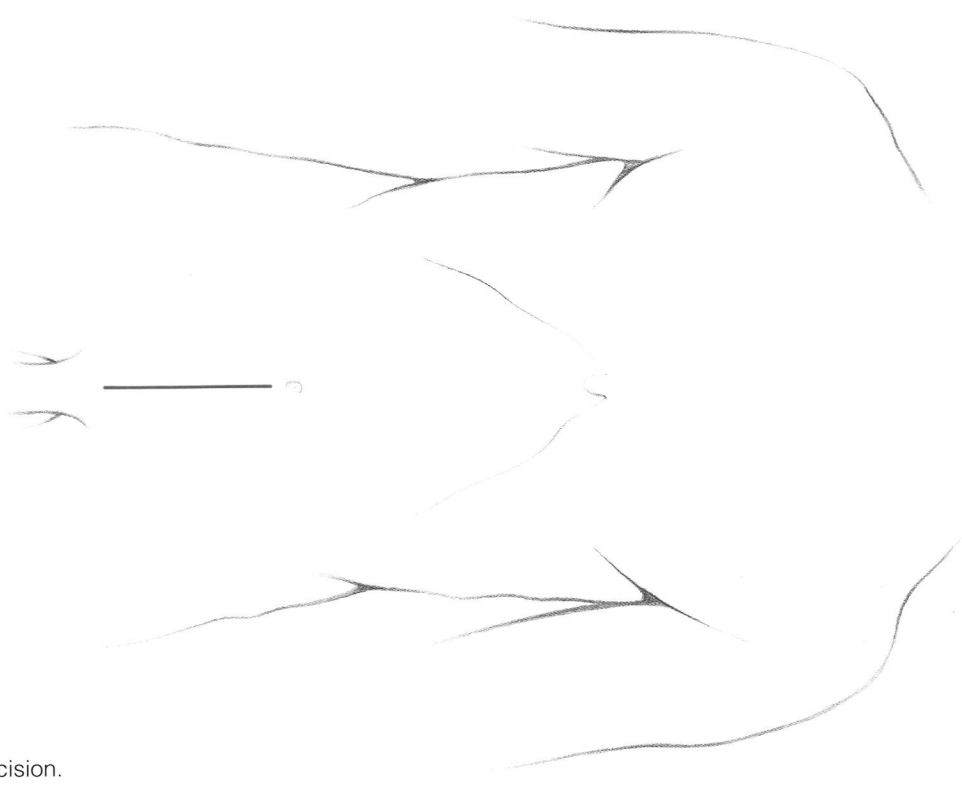

Fig. 3.**78** Line of incision.

Exposure of the Linea Alba

Following the skin incision, the subcutaneous tissue is divided and vessels are individually coagulated. The divided subcutaneous tissue is held aside with two retractors (Fig. 3.79). The anterior rectus sheath is dissected and divided. The linea alba is opened at the midline and split to its attachment on the pubic symphysis (Fig. 3.80).

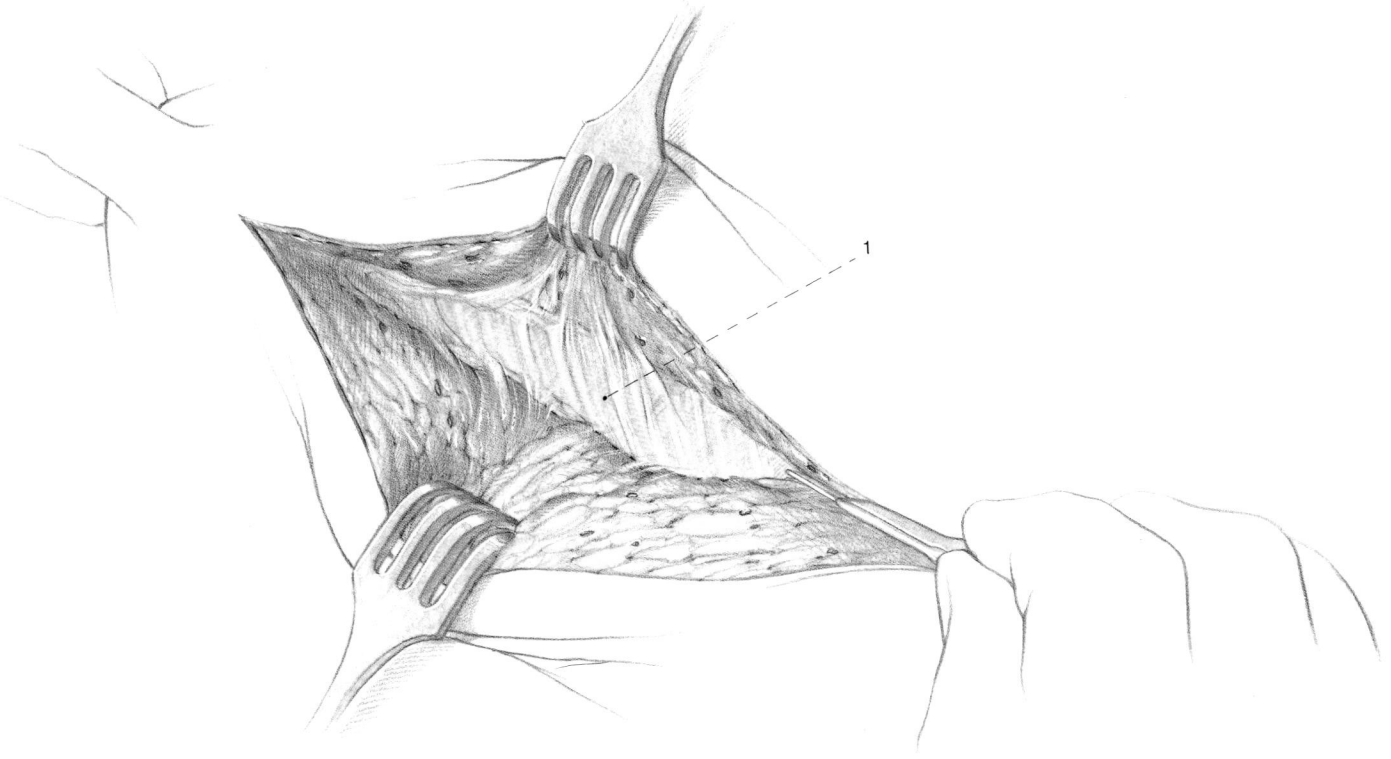

Fig. 3.**79** Exposure of the anterior rectus sheath.

1 Anterior rectus sheath

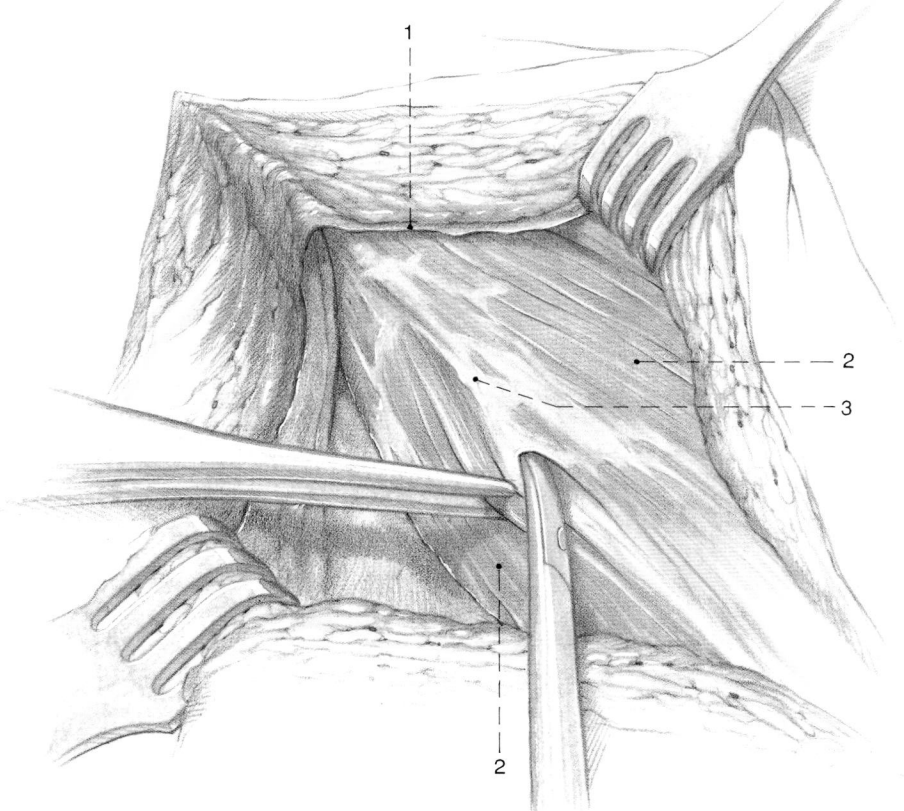

Fig. 3.**80** Division of the linea alba.

1 Anterior rectus sheath
2 Rectus muscle
3 Linea alba

Exposure of the Retropubic Space

Following division of the posterior rectus sheath and transversalis fascia on the midline, both rectus muscles are held aside with blunt retractors along with the connective tissue adherent to the undersurface of the muscles and the inferior epigastric artery and vein (Fig. 3.**81**). The parietal peritoneum and the fatty tissue in the prevesical space are dissected (Figs. 3.**81**, 3.**82**). The peritoneum is mobilized, then both rectus muscles are retracted in their sheaths. A blunt blade retracts the bladder and prevesical fat superiorly, widely opening the retropubic space (Fig. 3.**82**).

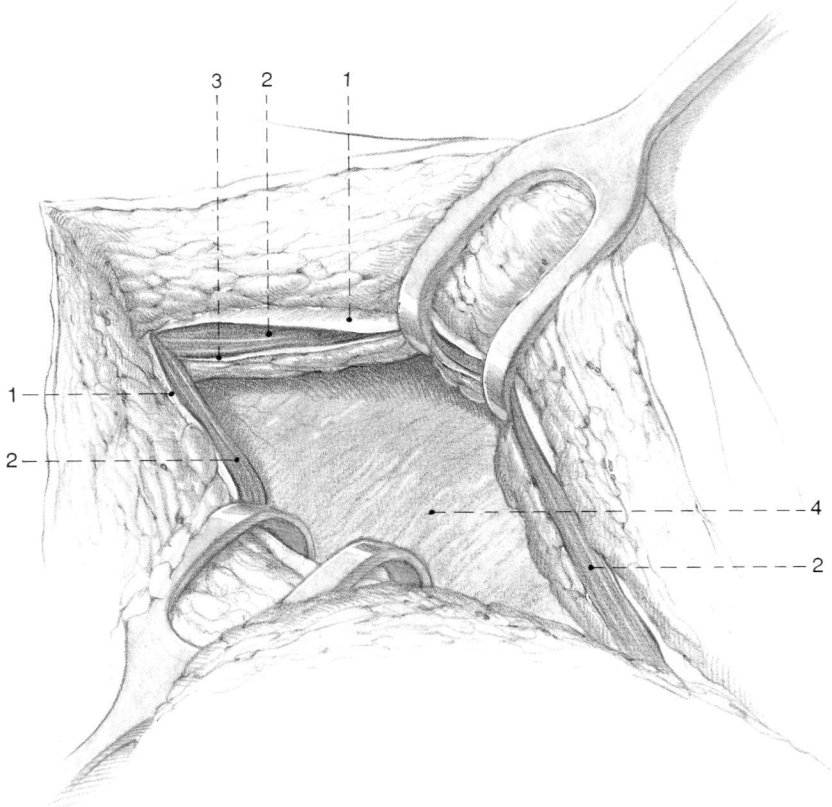

Fig. 3.**81**   Both rectus muscles and the rectus sheath are held aside with retractors.

1 Anterior rectus sheath
2 Rectus muscle
3 Posterior rectus sheath
4 Parietal peritoneum

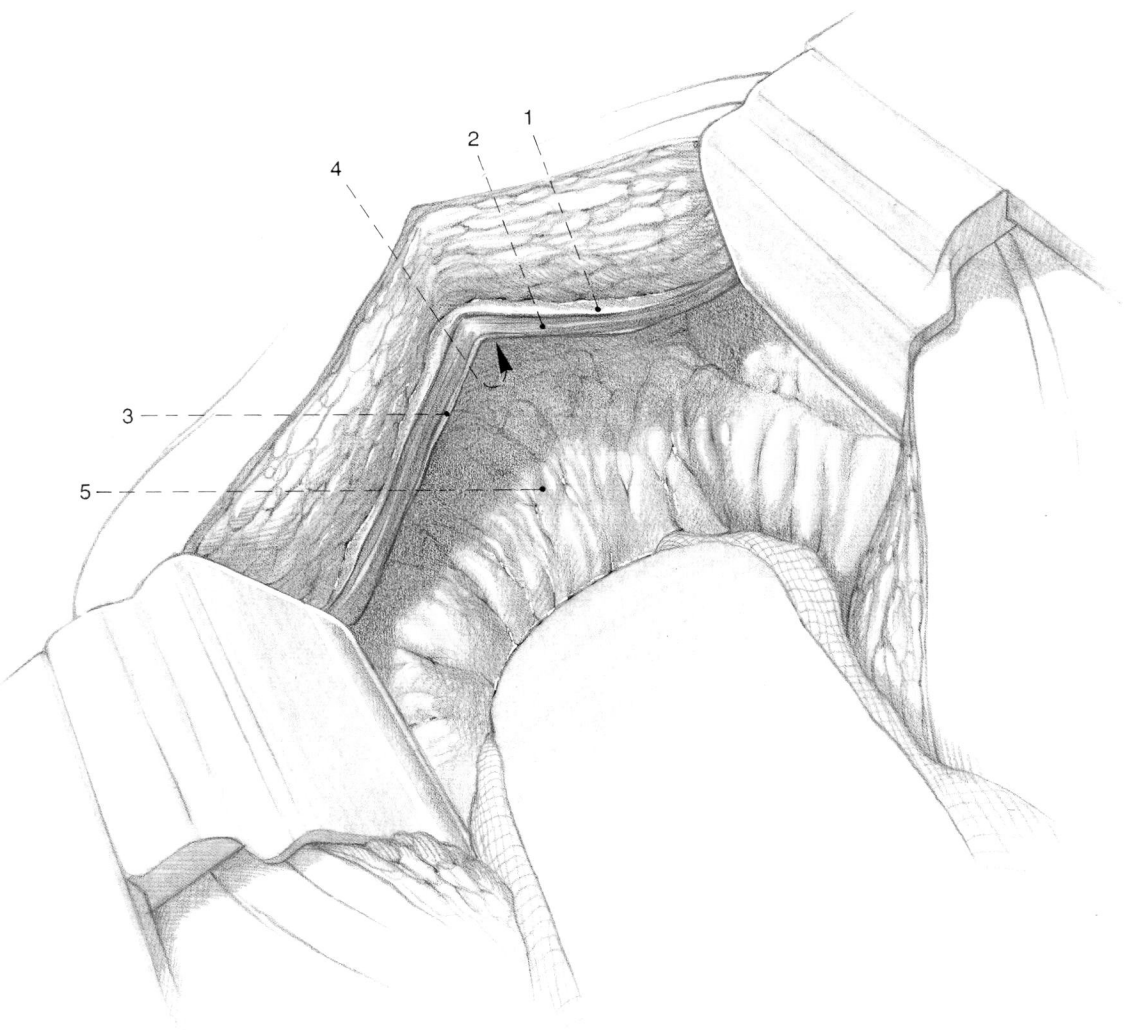

Fig. 3.**82** Exposure of the bladder and retropubic space.

1 Anterior rectus sheath
2 Rectus muscle
3 Posterior rectus sheath
4 Retropubic space
5 Vesical fascia

Incision of the Bladder (Approach for a Transvesical Prostatectomy)

The prevesical fat is removed, and two traction sutures are preplaced in the bladder wall. The bladder is then incised on the avascular midline with diathermy (Fig. 3.**83**), and the posterior bladder wall is retracted upward with a broad re-tractor blade (Fig. 3.**84**). The bladder neck is identified (Fig. 3.**84**) and circumferentially incised. The two lateral lobes of the prostate are separated at the anterior commissure and freed from the surgical capsule (Figs. 3.**84**, 3.**85**).

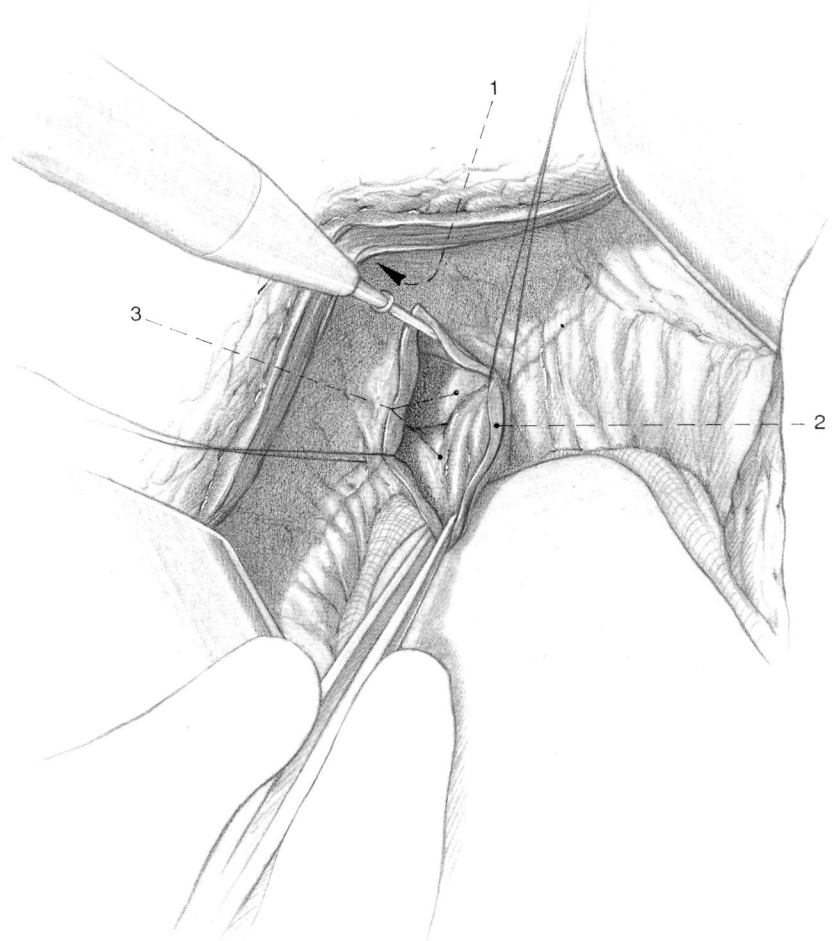

Fig. 3.**83** The bladder is opened between preplaced sutures.

1 Retropubic space
2 Bladder muscle
3 Bladder mucosa

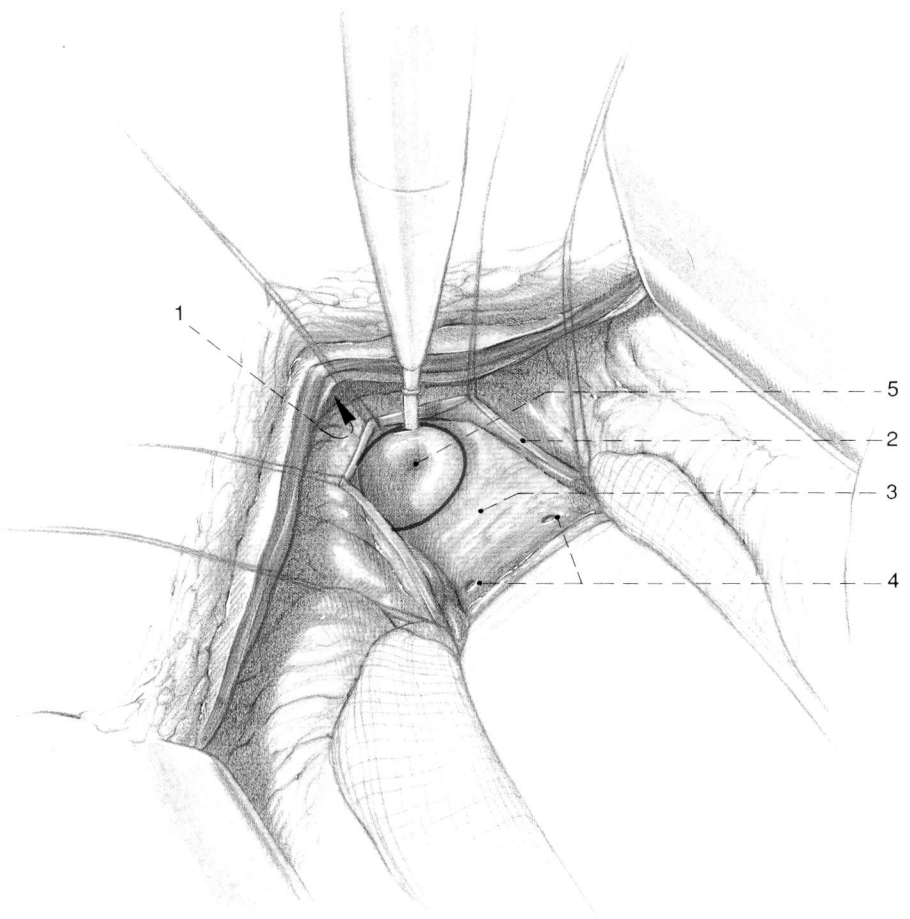

Fig. 3.**84** Circumferential incision of the bladder neck for transvesical prostatectomy.

1 Retropubic space
2 Bladder muscle
3 Bladder mucosa (trigone)
4 Ureteral orifices
5 Internal urethral orifice

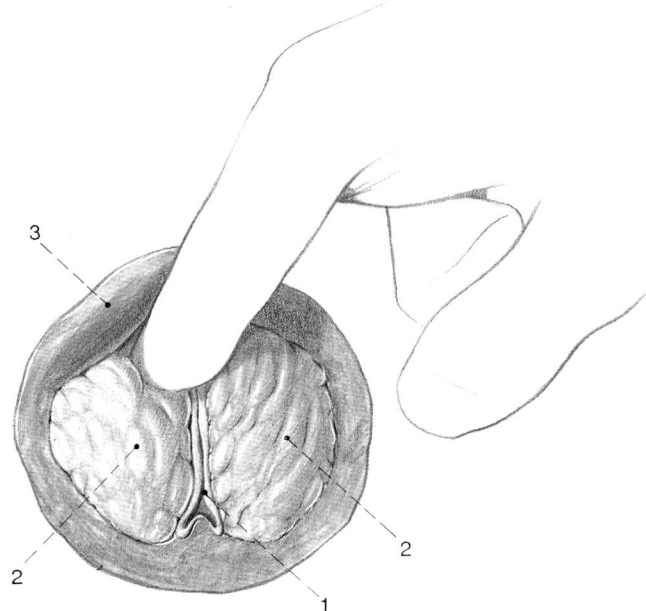

Fig. 3.**85** Separation of hyperplastic prostatic tissue from the prostatic capsule.

1 Urethra
2 Hyperplastic prostatic tissue
3 Surgical capsule

Millin Approach

The anterior wall of the bladder is retracted backward and cranially with a broad spatula retractor, widely exposing the retropubic space, the paraprostatic space, and the anterior surface of the prostate. Access to the hyperplastic prostatic tissue is gained through a transverse or vertical incision in the prostatic capsule (Fig. 3.**86**).

When a transverse incision is used, several traction sutures are placed at intervals of 1 and 2 cm below the bladder neck following ligation of the prostatic capsule. The capsule is then divided with diathermy between the rows of preplaced sutures (Fig. 3.**87**).

A cleavage plane is developed between the prostatic capsule and hyperplastic tissue (Fig. 3.**88**).

A similar technique is employed when a vertical incision is used to open the prostatic capsule (Figs. 3.**89**, 3.**90**).

Comments

The Trendelenburg position is helpful in very obese patients and facilitates access to the retropubic space. Greater attention is given to wound closure than when a Pfannenstiel incision is used due to the greater risk of hernia formation in the midline approach. The exact placement of the capsular sutures in the Millin approach will depend on the size of the prostate. A transverse incision is preferred over a vertical approach (injury to the urethral sphincter at the prostatic apex).

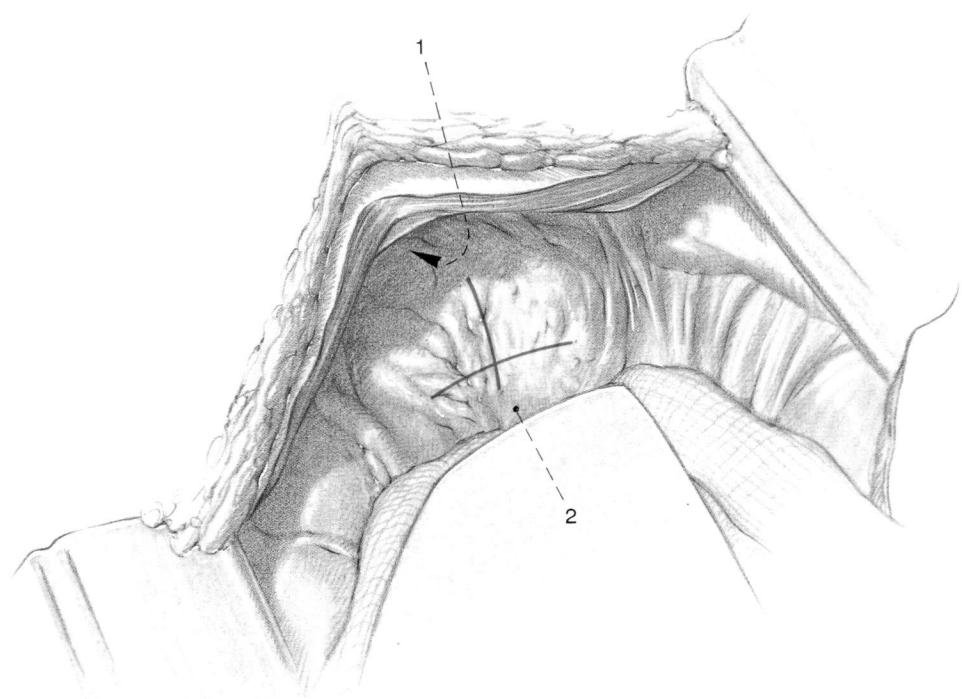

Fig. 3.**86** Millin's approach using a transverse or vertical incision.

1 Retropubic space
2 Bladder neck

Fig. 3.**87**   Ligation and incision of the prostatic capsule.

1 Retropubic space
2 Prostatic fascia
3 Prostatic capsule
4 Hyperplastic prostatic tissue

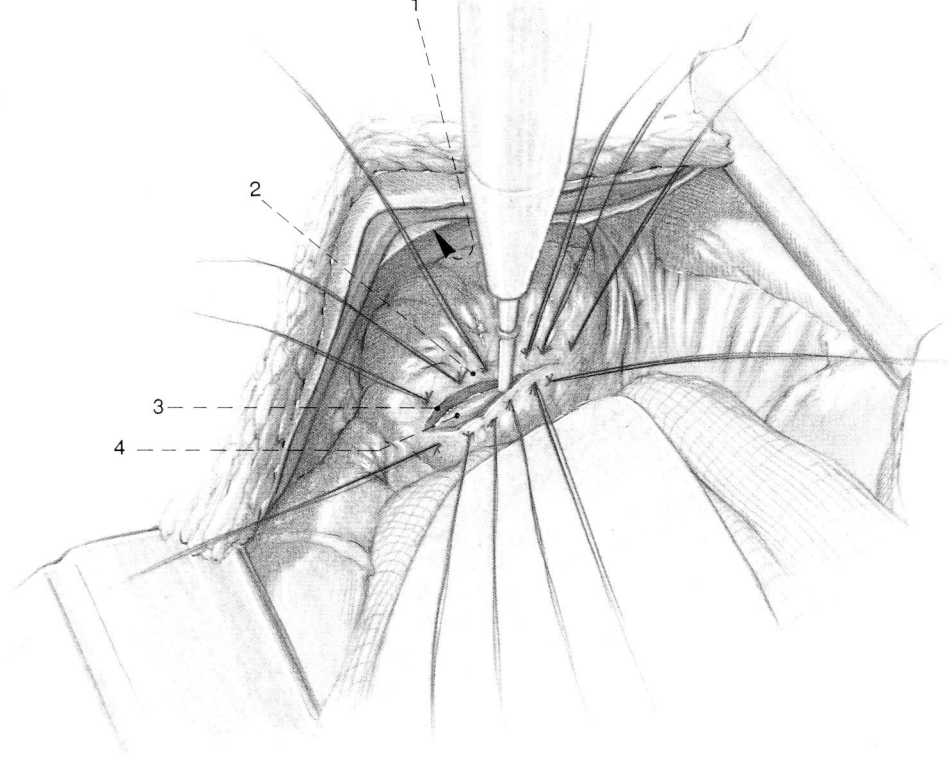

Fig. 3.**88**   The plane between the prostatic capsule and hyperplastic prostatic tissue is developed with scissors.

1 Prostatic capsule
2 Hyperplastic prostatic tissue

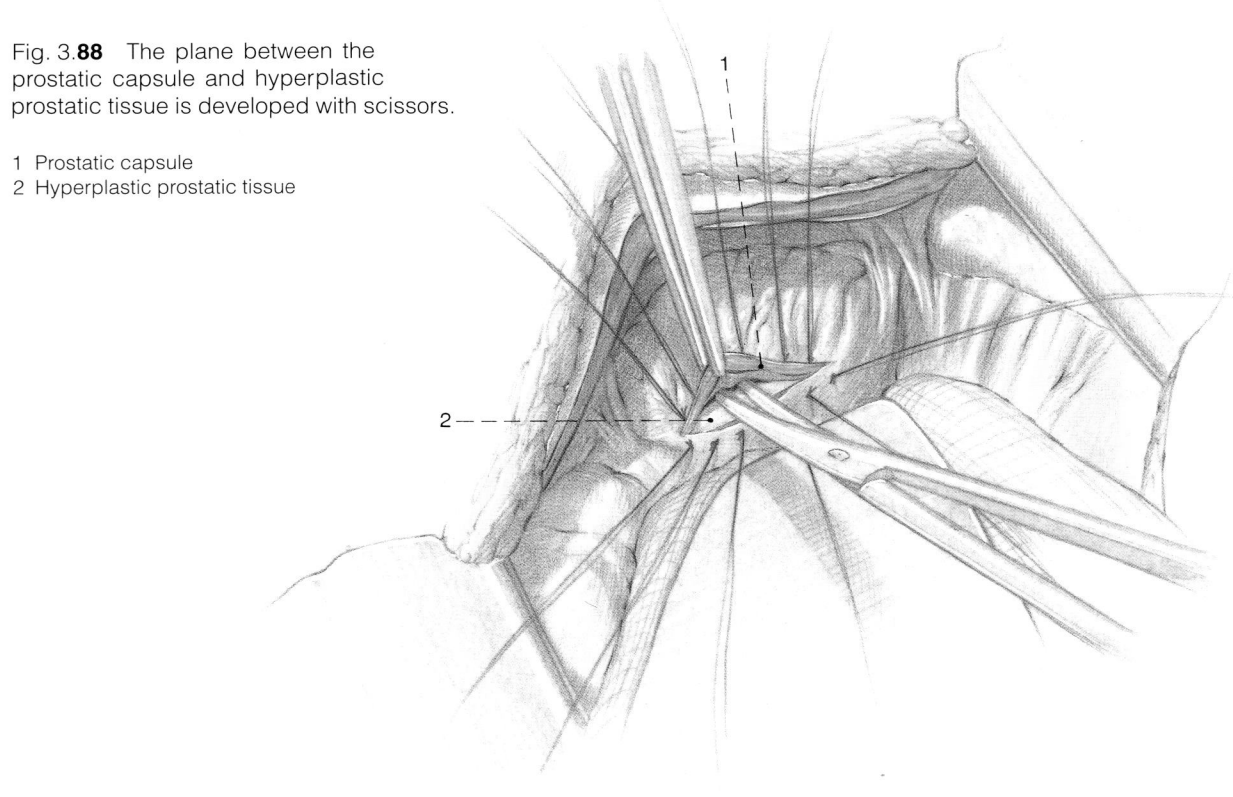

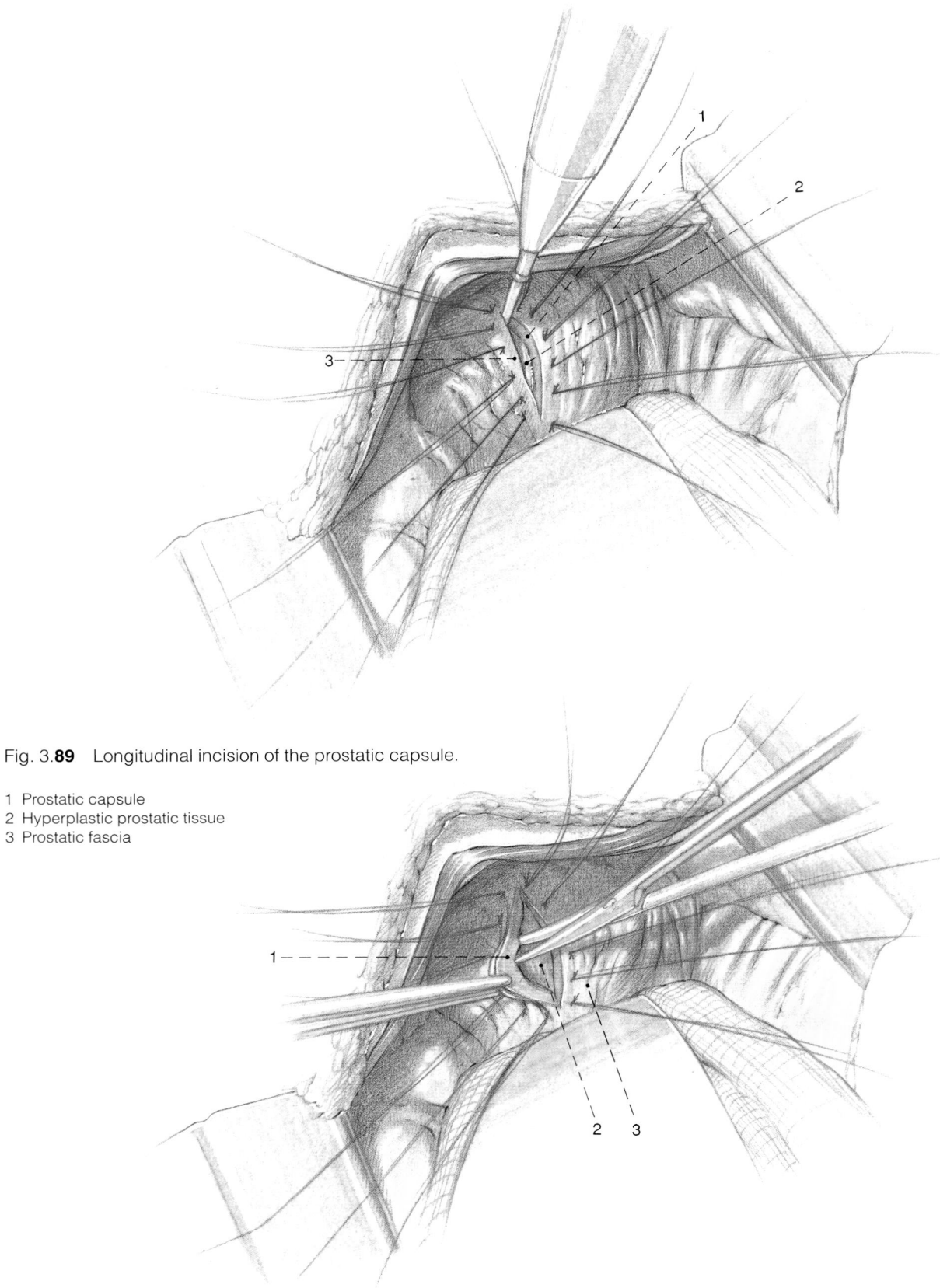

Fig. 3.**89** Longitudinal incision of the prostatic capsule.

1 Prostatic capsule
2 Hyperplastic prostatic tissue
3 Prostatic fascia

Fig. 3.**90** Development of the plane between the prostatic capsule and hyperplastic prostatic tissue.

1 Prostatic capsule
2 Hyperplastic prostatic tissue
3 Prostatic fascia

Pfannenstiel Incision

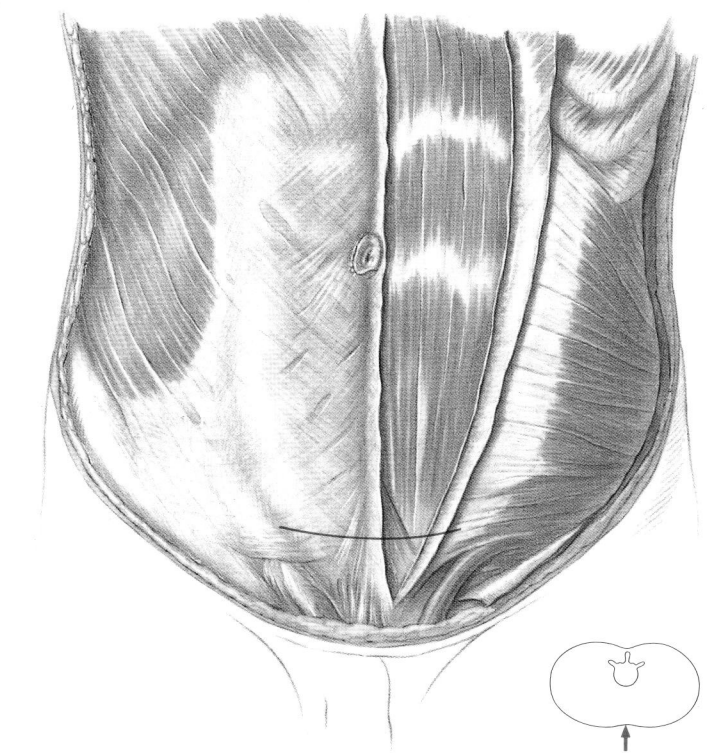

Fig. 3.**91**

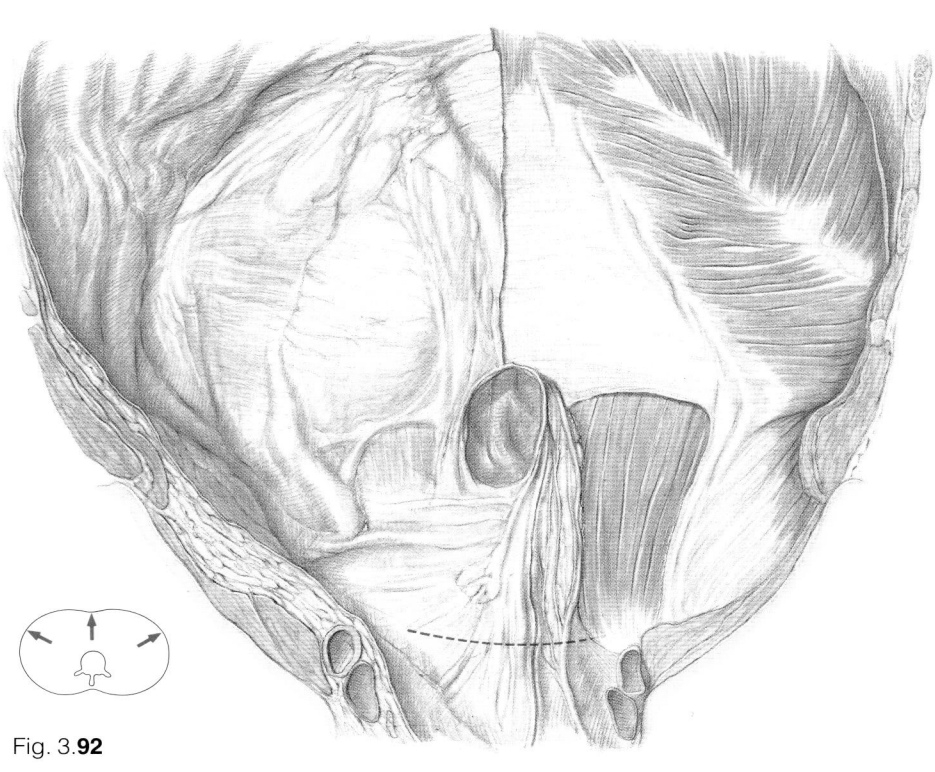

Fig. 3.**92**

Main Indications

- Surgery of the urinary bladder
- Surgery of the pelvic ureter
- Access for open prostatectomy

Position and Skin Incision

The patient is placed in a slightly hyperextended supine position. The skin is opened with a transverse incision two finger-widths above the pubic symphysis (Fig. 3.**93**).

Exposure of the Rectus Muscles

The subcutaneous fat is divided, exposing the anterior rectus sheath (Fig. 3.**94**).

The anterior rectus sheath is opened with electrocautery, extending the incision well laterally on both sides (Fig. 3.**95**). The adminiculum of the linea alba can be identified in the midline and the two rectus muscles laterally (Fig. 3.**95**).

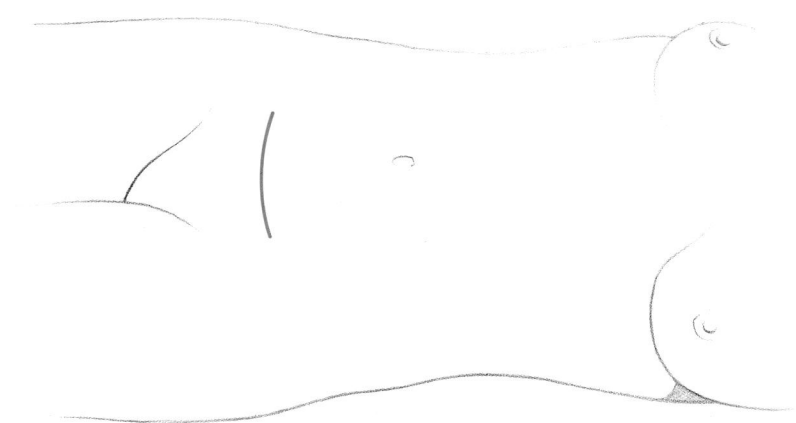

Fig. 3.**93**   Position and skin incision.

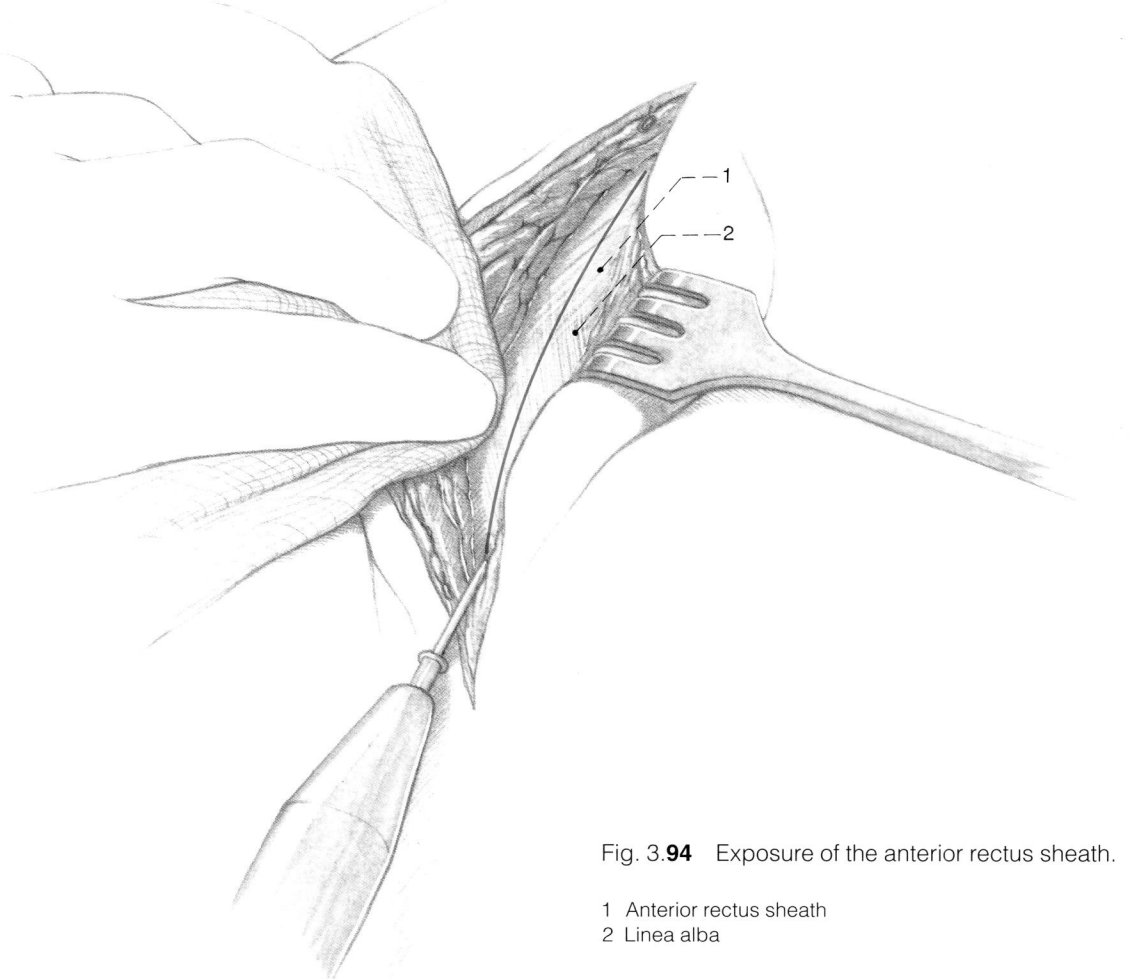

Fig. 3.**94**   Exposure of the anterior rectus sheath.

1 Anterior rectus sheath
2 Linea alba

The subcutaneous fat is retracted, and the anterior rectus sheath is picked up with two surgical forceps and dissected from the rectus muscles. The junction of the anterior and posterior layers of the rectus sheath, the linea alba, is incised on the midline, directing the incision first upward and then downward (Fig. 3.**96**).

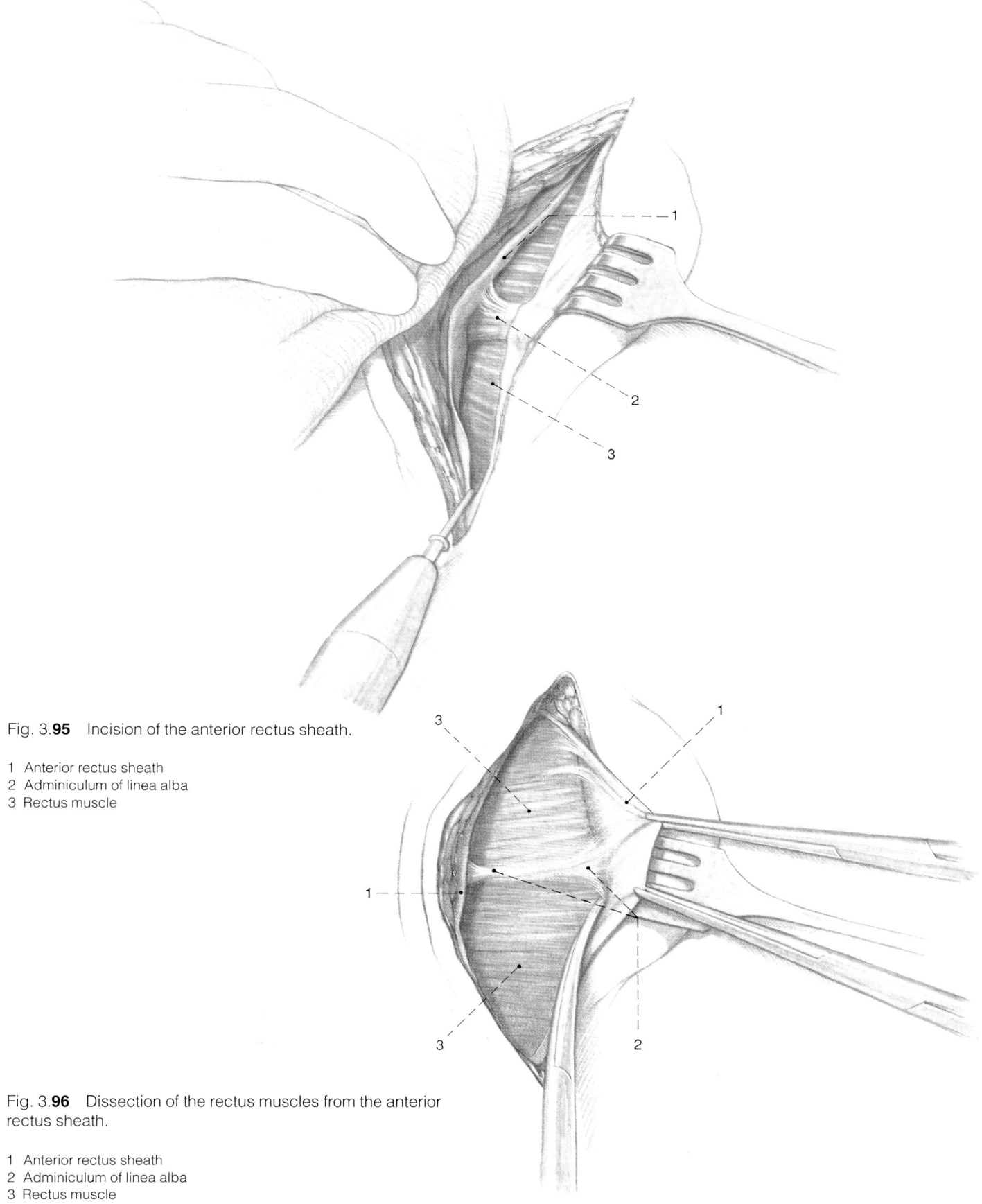

Fig. 3.**95** Incision of the anterior rectus sheath.

1 Anterior rectus sheath
2 Adminiculum of linea alba
3 Rectus muscle

Fig. 3.**96** Dissection of the rectus muscles from the anterior rectus sheath.

1 Anterior rectus sheath
2 Adminiculum of linea alba
3 Rectus muscle

The pyramidalis muscles are dissected downward from both rectus muscles as the inferior portion of the anterior rectus sheath is freed (Fig. 3.**97**).

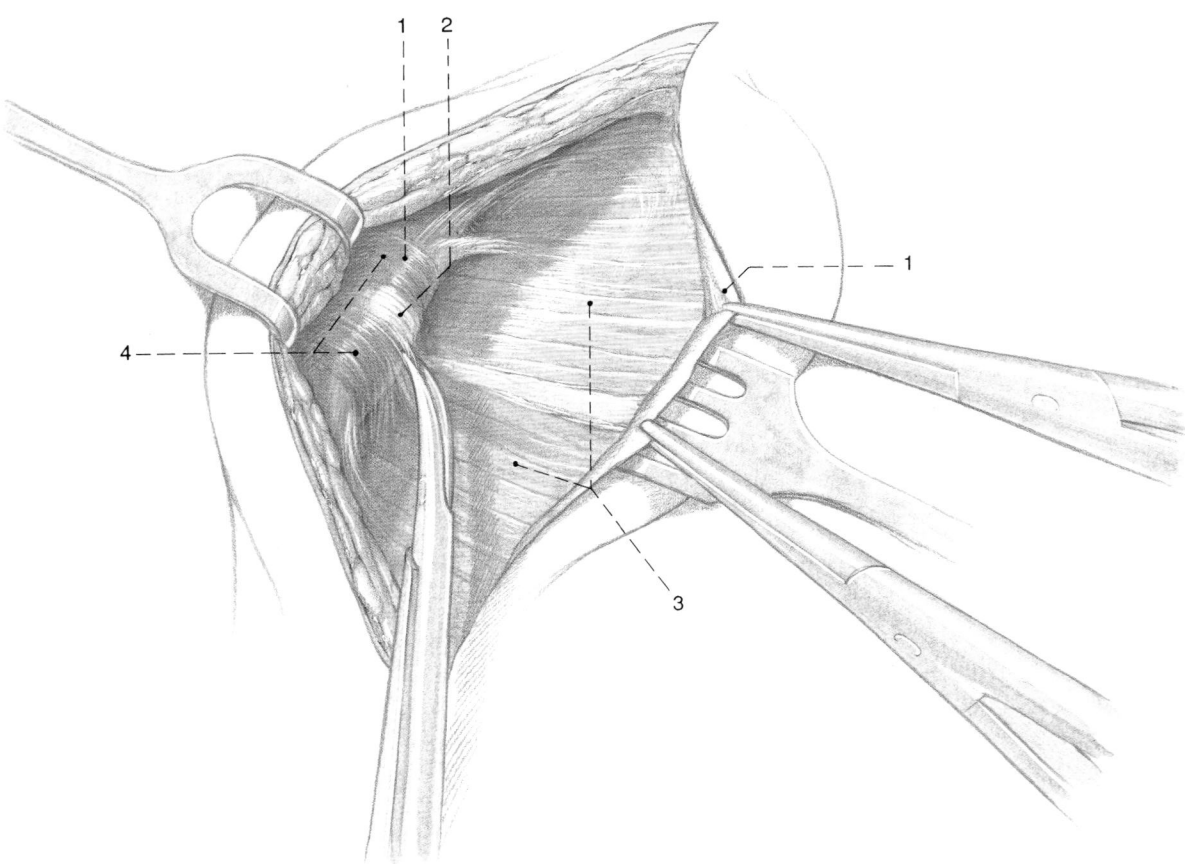

Fig. 3.**97**   Separation of the pyramidalis muscles from the rectus muscles.

1 Anterior rectus sheath
2 Linea alba
3 Rectus muscle
4 Pyramidalis muscle

Exposure of the Prevesical Space

The medial borders of the rectus muscles are now split at the midline and separated while sparing the posterior rectus sheath and the vessels and nerves supplying the rectus muscles (Fig. 3.**98**).

The transversalis fascia, subperitoneal fat, and peritoneal sac are dissected upward to develop the prevesical connective-tissue space (Fig. 3.**98**).

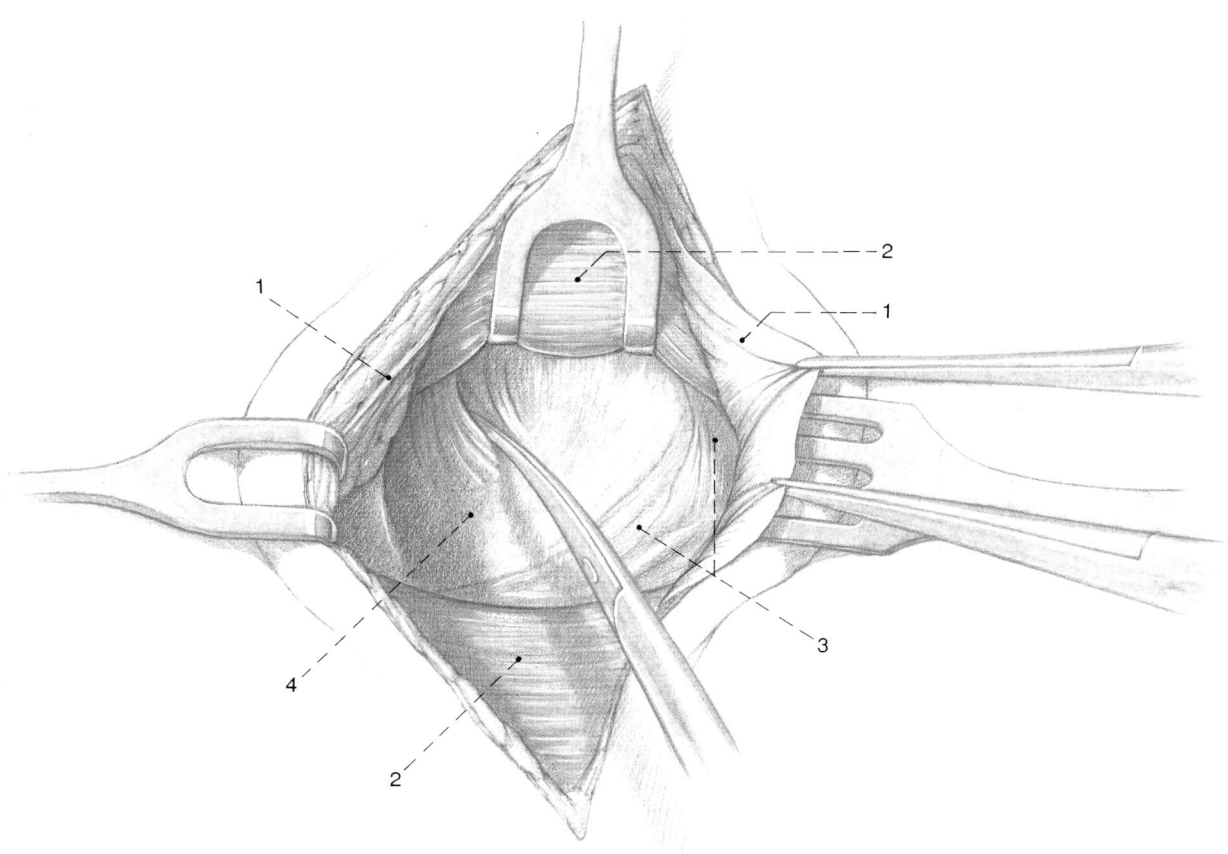

Fig. 3.**98**   Exposure of the prevesical connective-tissue space.

1 Anterior rectus sheath
2 Rectus muscle
3 Subperitoneal fat
4 Prevesical space

Incision of the Bladder

The anterior bladder wall is dissected free, and the bladder
wall is opened between two preplaced traction sutures with
scissors or diathermy (Fig. 3.**99**).

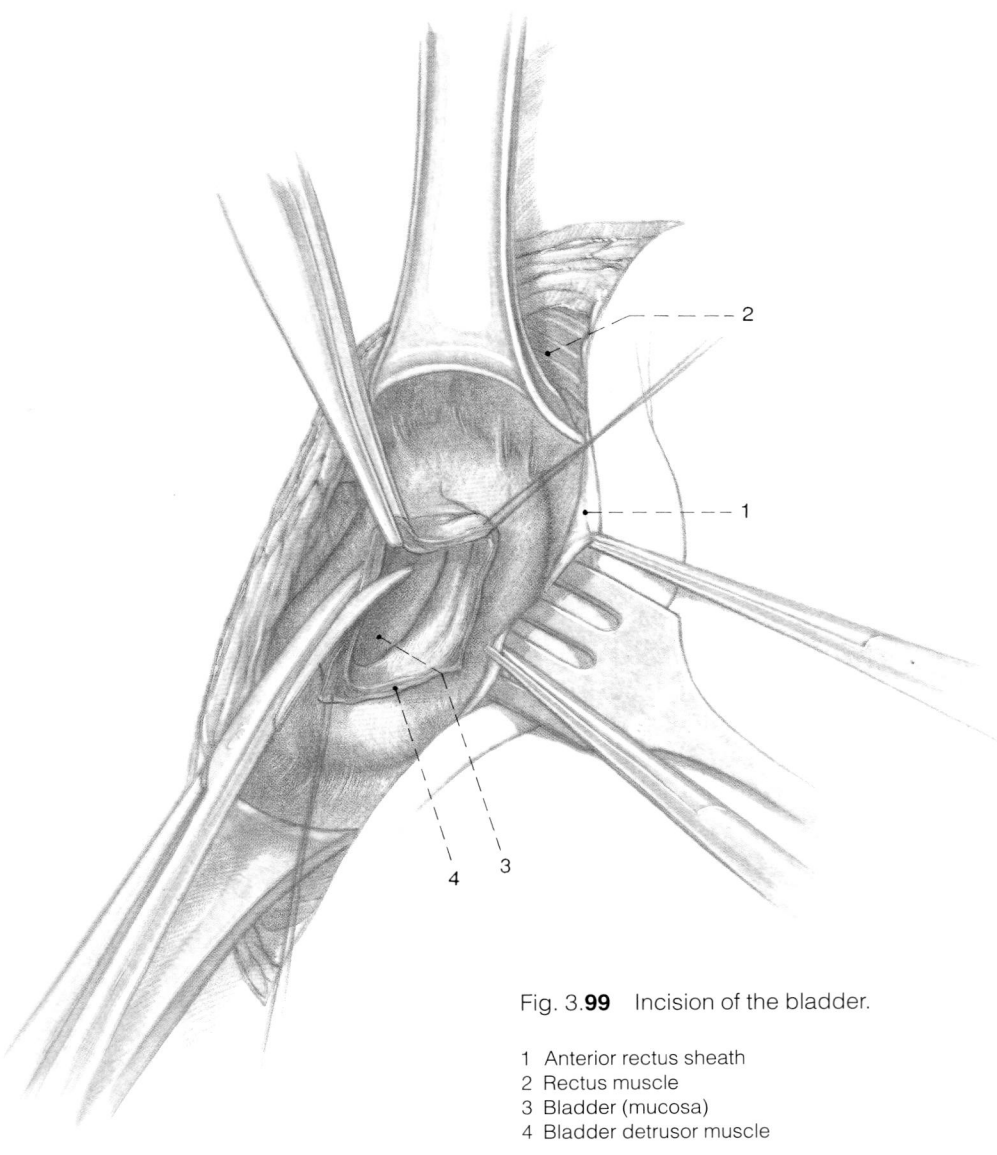

Fig. 3.**99** Incision of the bladder.

1 Anterior rectus sheath
2 Rectus muscle
3 Bladder (mucosa)
4 Bladder detrusor muscle

4 Inguinal Region

Anatomy of the Inguinal Canal

The inguinal canal obliquely traverses the abdominal wall in the medial portion of the inguinal region. The canal has a lateral to medial orientation, its lateral part being situated more deeply than its medial part. It has an average length of 4–5 cm in adult males and is about 5 mm longer in women.

The external (superficial) inguinal ring forms the external opening of the inguinal canal. Located in the external oblique aponeurosis, the ring is bounded by two thickenings in the aponeurosis termed the medial and lateral crura (Fig. 4.**1**). Both crura join at the superolateral aspect of the external ring and are sometimes reinforced in that area by transverse intercrural fibers. The development and location of these fibers are subject to marked individual variations, and the fibers can be dissected at the external inguinal ring in only 27% of the population.

The external inguinal ring is exposed by incision of the external spermatic fascia. The ring is elliptical in shape and highly variable in its size and length. In 80% of cases the superolateral border of the external ring is located above the medial half of the inguinal ligament. In the remaining 20% its boundary is more superolateral and in extreme cases may extend to the anterior superior iliac spine.

The slitlike internal opening of the inguinal canal, the internal (deep) inguinal ring, represents an evagination of the transversalis fascia. It is covered internally by parietal peritoneum, so surgical exposure of the internal ring requires incision of the peritoneum.

The layers of the lateral abdominal wall contribute in varying degrees to the substance of the inguinal canal walls. The anterior wall is formed by the external oblique aponeurosis, which is continued onto the spermatic cord as the thin external spermatic fascia. The floor of the canal is formed by the inguinal ligament.

The caudal fibers of the transversus abdominis muscle form the roof of the inguinal canal. The internal oblique muscle does not contribute to formation of the canal roof. Its caudal fibers are continued onto the spermatic cord as the cremaster muscle. The cremaster, which forms the middle coat of the spermatic cord, varies greatly in development among different individuals, and the middle covering is considered to consist of both the spermatic fascia and the cremaster muscle. Normally a definite plane of cleavage can be developed between the internal oblique and transversus abdominis muscles in the region of the inguinal canal.

The posterior wall of the inguinal canal is formed by the transversalis fascia. Medial to the internal ring this fascia is strengthened by the variable interfoveolar ligament (Hesselbach), whose fibers are derived from the transversus aponeurosis. The posterior canal wall is further strengthened by the inguinal falx (Henle's ligament). These fibers also arise from the transversus aponeurosis and blend inferiorly with the inguinal ligament and lacunar ligament. An alternate term for the inguinal falx is the conjoined tendon.

The layered dissections in Figs. 4.**1**–4.**5** serve to clarify the arrangement of the individual abdominal tissue planes in the inguinal canal. The firm subcutaneous fatty layer in the inguinal region, permeated by fibrous strands and known also as Camper's fascia, is removed to expose the external oblique aponeurosis. This aponeurosis is continued onto the spermatic cord as the external spermatic fascia (Fig. 4.**1**). Incision of the outer coat of the spermatic cord exposes the middle layer, composed of the cremasteric fascia and the cremaster muscle, which is a continuation of the internal oblique muscle. The genital branch of the genitofemoral nerve can also be identified in this plane (Fig. 4.**2**). The external oblique aponeurosis can now be split further laterally and superiorly to expose the anterior terminal branch of the iliohypogastric nerve. The middle coat of the spermatic cord is divided to expose the internal spermatic fascia, which intimately invests the cord structures (Fig. 4.**3**). Division of the caudal fibers of the internal oblique muscle uncovers the portion of the transversus abdominis that forms the roof of the inguinal canal (Fig. 4.**4**). As the last step in the dissection, the internal coat of the spermatic cord is incised to expose the cord structures themselves: the vas deferens, testicular artery, and pampiniform plexus (Fig. 4.**5**).

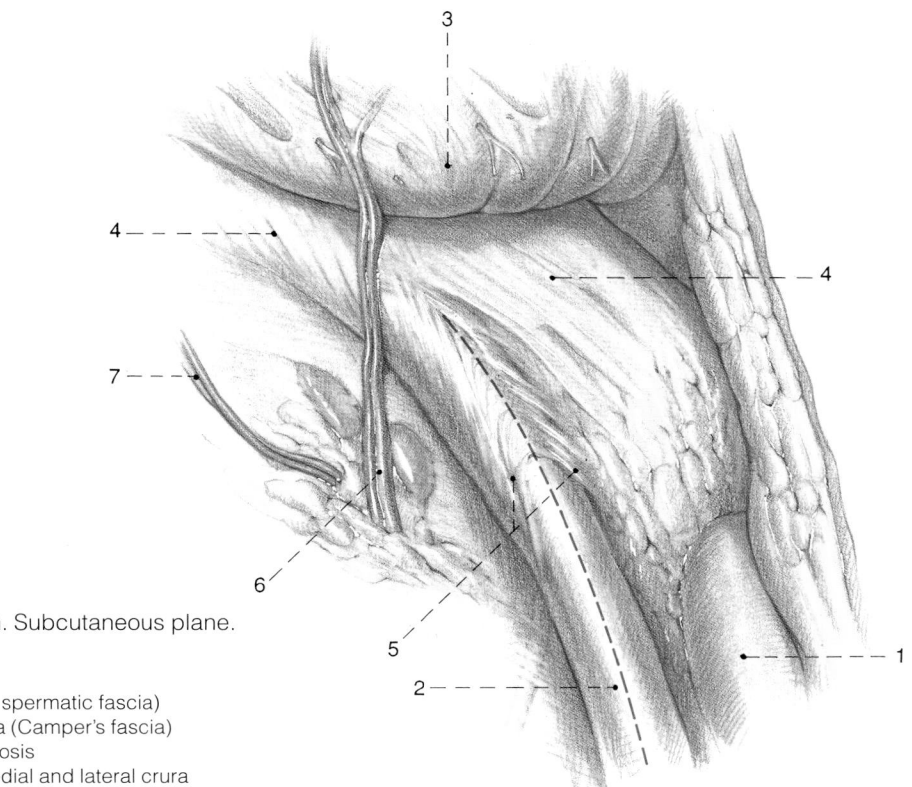

Fig. 4.**1** Inguinal region. Subcutaneous plane.

1 Penis
2 Spermatic cord (external spermatic fascia)
3 External abdominal fascia (Camper's fascia)
4 External oblique aponeurosis
5 External inguinal ring, medial and lateral crura
6 Superficial epigastric vessels
7 Superficial circumflex iliac vessels

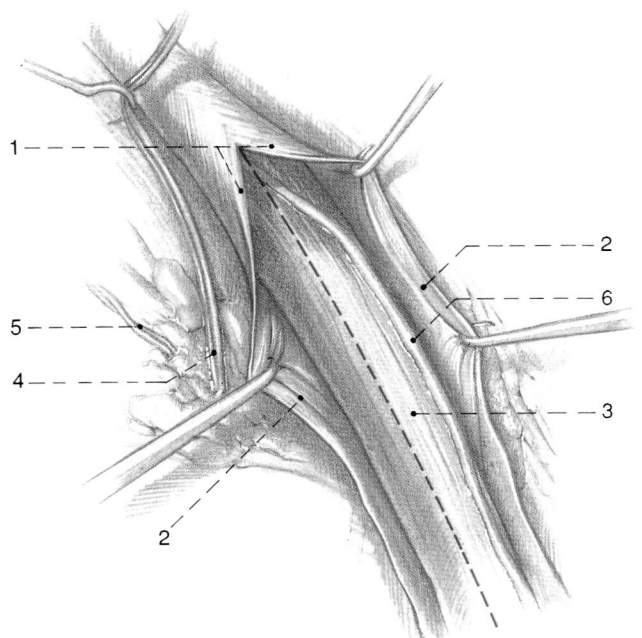

Fig. 4.**2** Spermatic cord after incision of the external spermatic fascia.

1 External oblique aponeurosis
2 External spermatic fascia
3 Cremaster muscle and cremasteric fascia
4 Superficial epigastric vessels
5 Superficial circumflex iliac vessels
6 Genital branch of genitofemoral nerve

Fig. 4.**3** Spermatic cord after incision of the cremasteric fascia.

1 External oblique aponeurosis
2 External spermatic fascia
3 Internal oblique
4 Cremaster muscle and cremasteric fascia
5 Internal spermatic fascia
6 Iliohypogastric nerve

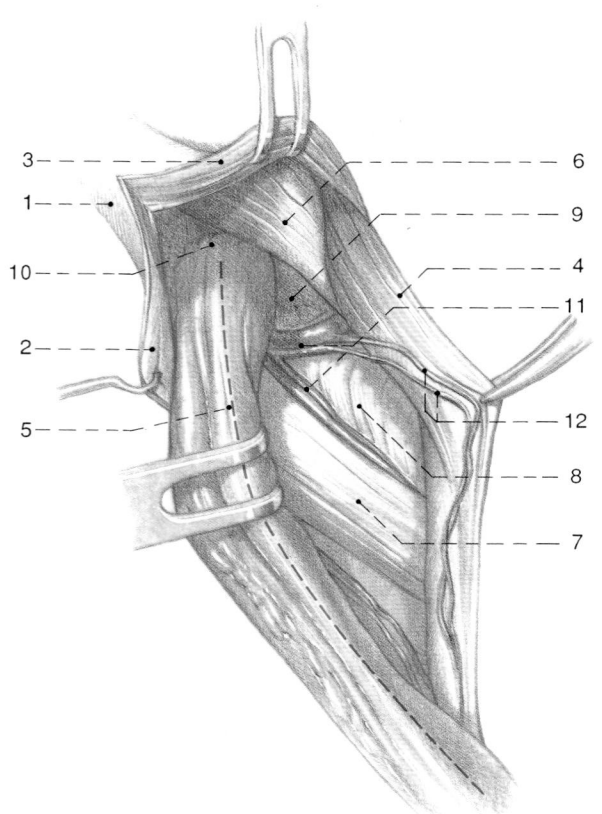

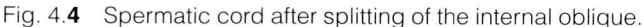

Fig. 4.**4** Spermatic cord after splitting of the internal oblique.

1 External oblique aponeurosis
2 External spermatic fascia
3 Internal oblique
4 Cremaster muscle and cremasteric fascia
5 Internal spermatic fascia
6 Transversus abdominis
7 Inguinal ligament
8 Transversalis fascia (outer surface of medial inguinal fossa)
9 Transversalis fascia (outer surface of lateral inguinal fossa)
10 Internal inguinal ring
11 Inferior epigastric vessels
12 Cremasteric vessels

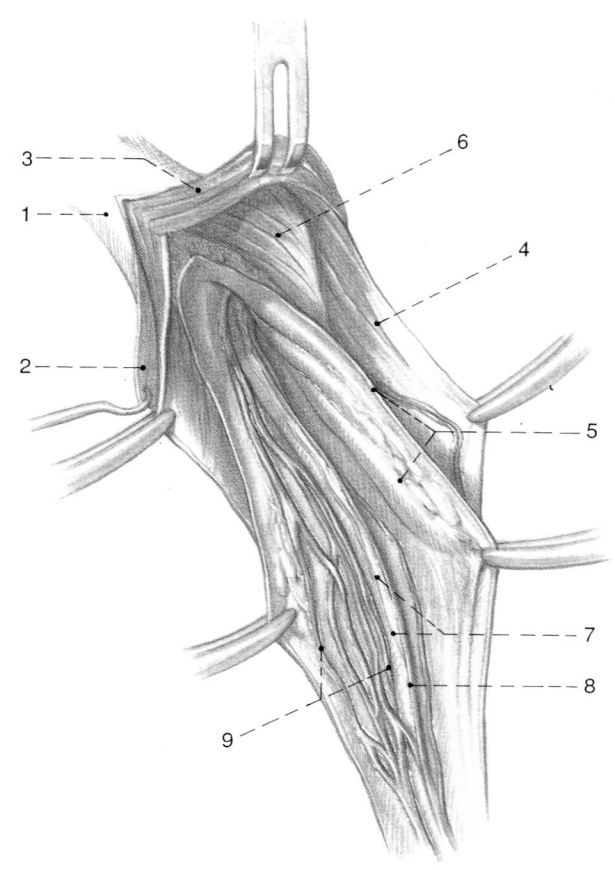

Fig. 4.**5** Spermatic cord after incision of the internal spermatic fascia.

1 External oblique aponeurosis
2 External spermatic fascia
3 Internal oblique
4 Cremaster muscle and cremasteric fascia
5 Internal spermatic fascia
6 Transversus abdominis
7 Vas deferens and artery of vas deferens
8 Testicular artery
9 Pampiniform plexus

Inguinal Approach

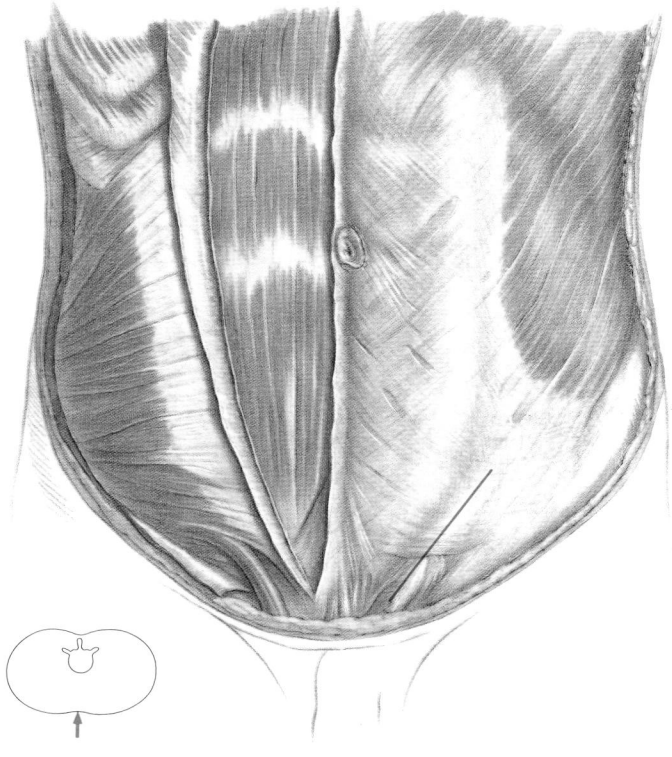

Fig. 4.**6**

Main Indications

- Undescended testis
- Semicastration for a testicular tumor
- Inguinal dissection of the pampiniform plexus

The approach is illustrated for the left side.

Position and Skin Incision

The patient is positioned supine. The incision extends obliquely over the external inguinal ring, following the fibers of the external oblique aponeurosis (Fig. 4.**7**).

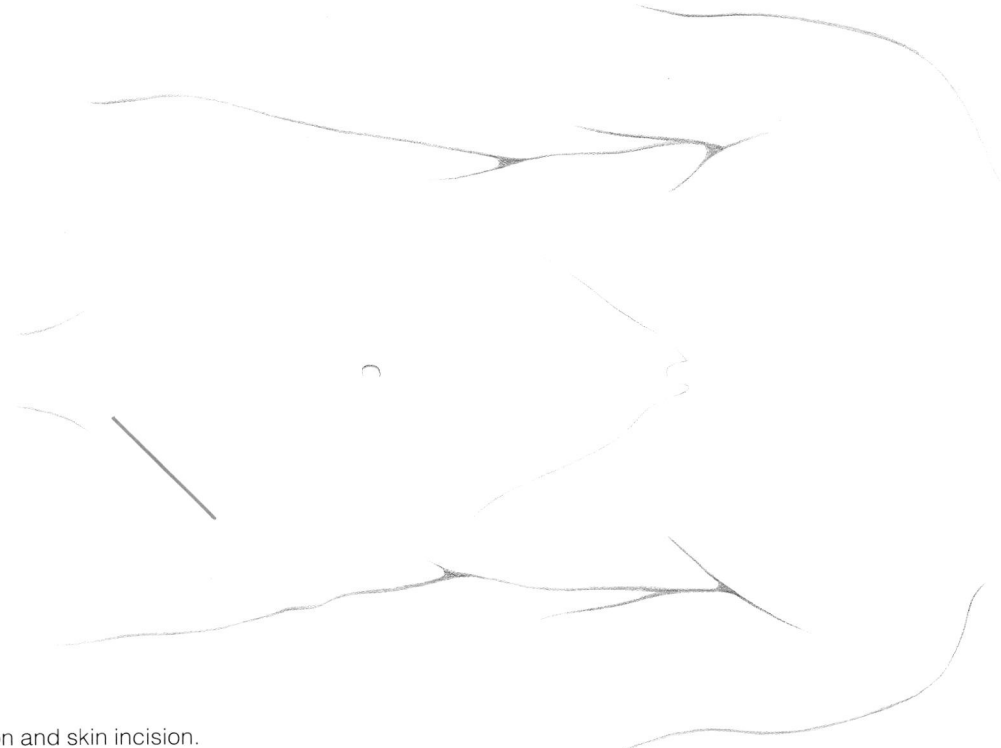

Fig. 4.**7**   Position and skin incision.

Exposure of the External Inguinal Ring

The subcutaneous fat and Camper's fascia are divided along with branches of the superficial epigastric vessels and the superficial circumflex iliac vessels. The external oblique aponeurosis is identified (Fig. 4.**8**).

Exposure of the Internal Inguinal Ring

The external oblique aponeurosis and the most anterior portion of the external spermatic fascia are divided, sparing the genital branch of the genitofemoral nerve on the cremaster muscle medially. The internal oblique muscle and cremasteric fascia are exposed (Fig. 4.**9**).

Further exposure of the inguinal canal is accomplished by incision of the cremasteric fascia and internal oblique muscle (Fig. 4.**10**). The iliohypogastric nerve and genitofemoral nerve are visible on the medial side.

The internal oblique muscle is divided exposing the transversus abdominis (Fig. 4.**11**). Following release of the cremaster muscle (whose fibers arise from the internal oblique), the spermatic cord with the surrounding internal spermatic fascia (derived from the transversalis fascia) is undermined and snared (Fig. 4.**11**). The internal fascia of the spermatic cord is dissected from the transversalis fascia to increase the length of the cord (Fig. 4.**12**). The external oblique aponeurosis and the incised internal oblique and transversus abdominis muscles are retracted upward in the proximal wound angle, allowing for further dissection of the spermatic cord, which is freed up into the internal inguinal ring (Figs. 4.**13**, 4.**14**). The inferior epigastric vessels can be seen medial to the inguinal ring.

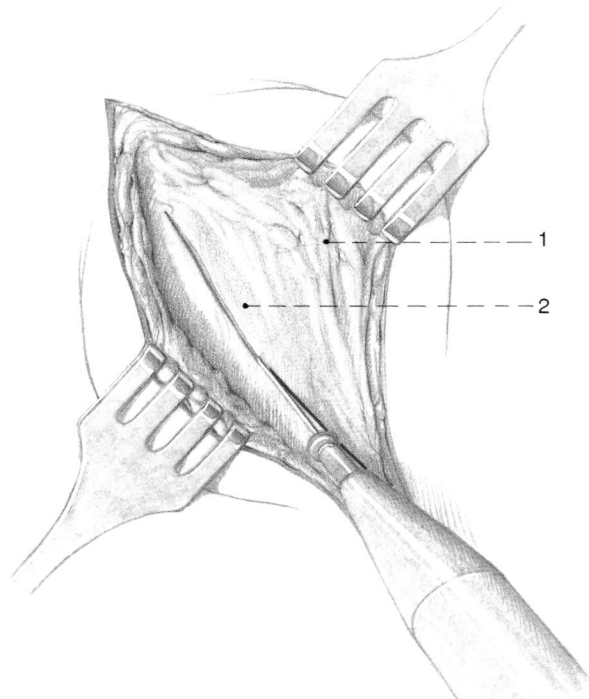

Fig. 4.**8**   Exposure of the external inguinal ring.

1 External abdominal fascia (Camper's fascia)
2 External oblique aponeurosis

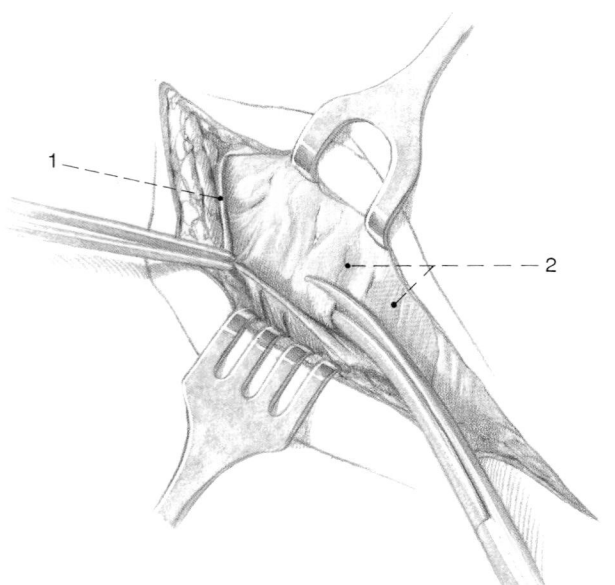

Fig. 4.**9**   Division of the external oblique aponeurosis.

1 External oblique aponeurosis
2 Internal oblique

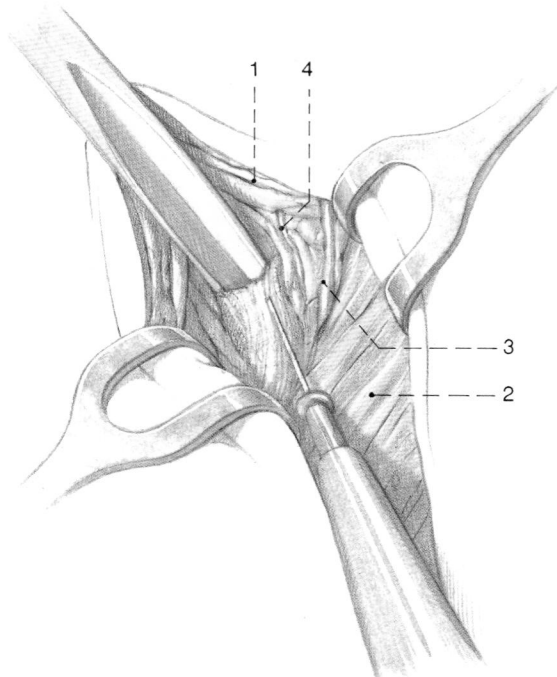

Fig. 4.**10**   The cremasteric fascia and internal oblique are divided.

1 External oblique aponeurosis
2 Internal oblique
3 Ilioinguinal nerve
4 Genitofemoral nerve

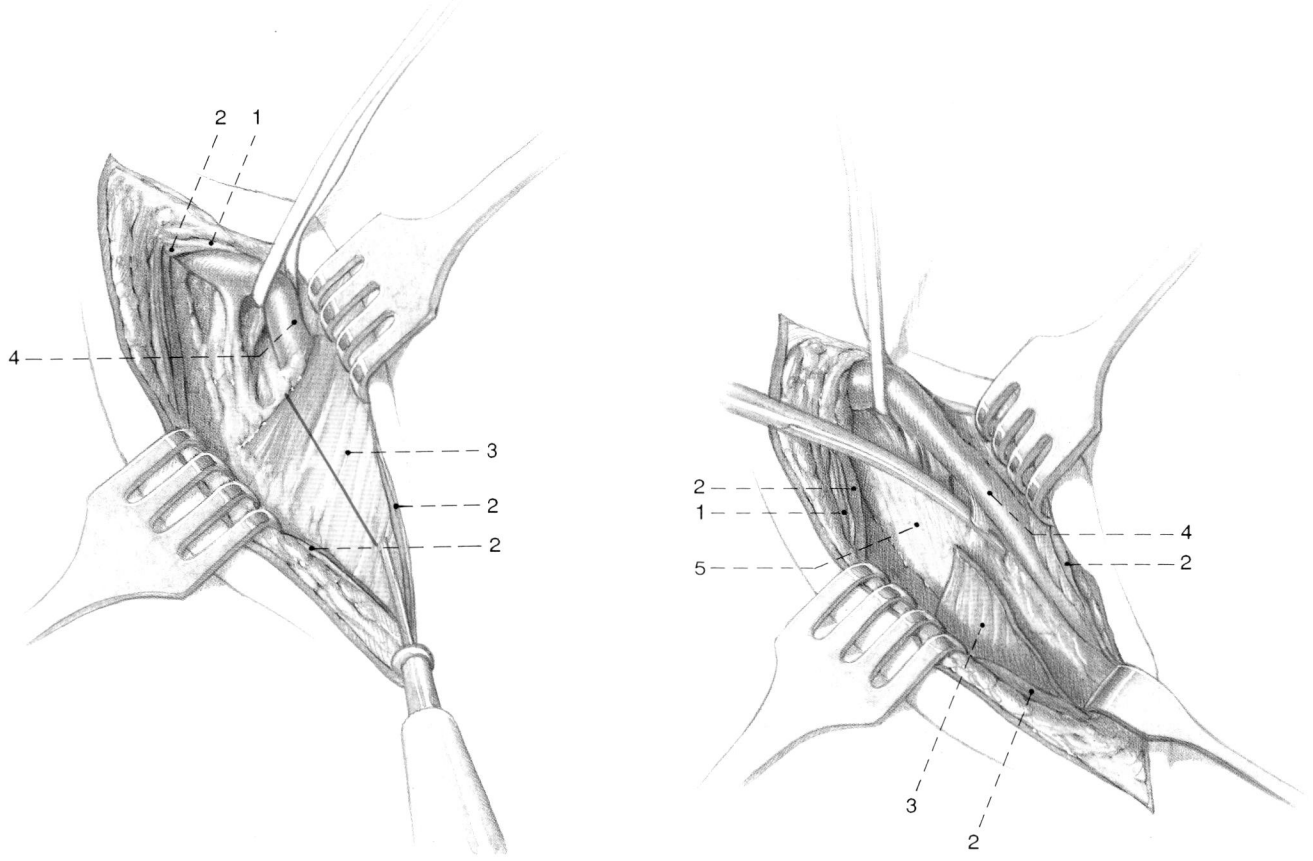

Fig. 4.**11** Mobilization of the spermatic cord and division of the transversus abdominis.

1 External oblique aponeurosis
2 Internal oblique
3 Transversus abdominis
4 Spermatic cord

Fig. 4.**12** The spermatic cord is dissected from the transversalis fascia, and the internal ring is exposed.

1 External oblique aponeurosis
2 Internal oblique
3 Transversus abdominis
4 Spermatic cord
5 Transversalis fascia

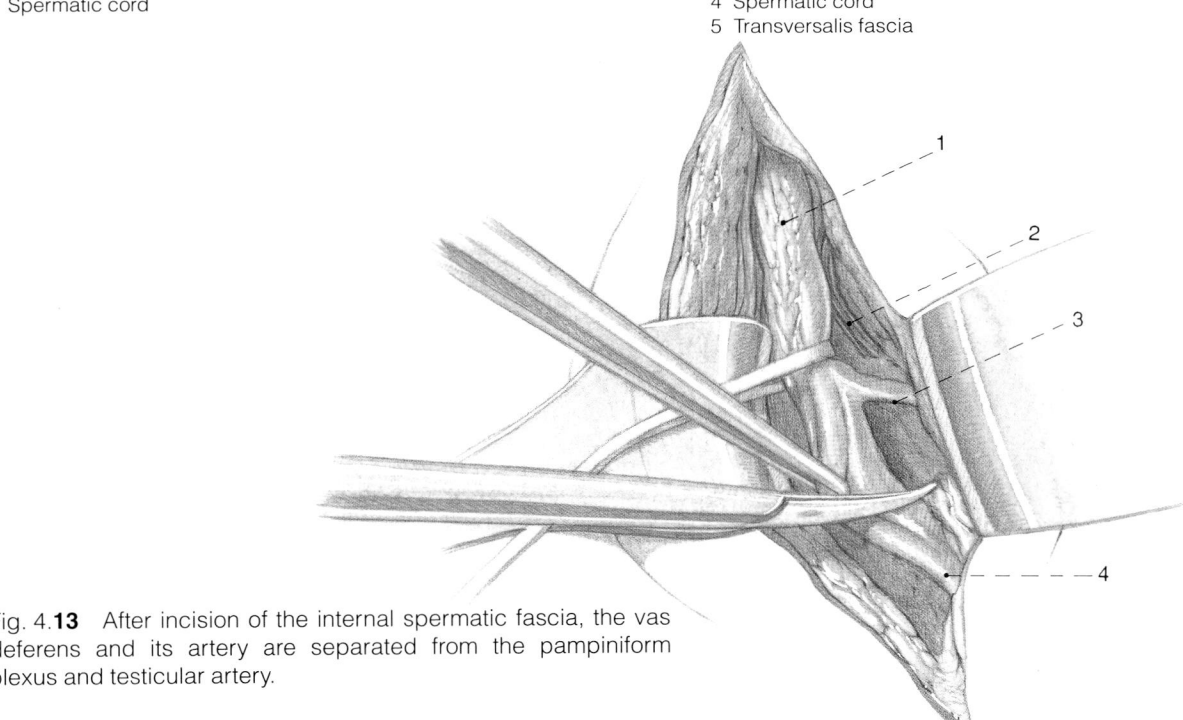

Fig. 4.**13** After incision of the internal spermatic fascia, the vas deferens and its artery are separated from the pampiniform plexus and testicular artery.

1 Spermatic cord   3 Vas deferens
2 Inferior epigastric vessels   4 Testicular vessels

Lateral to the epigastric vessels, the internal spermatic fascia is dissected free to create access for separating the vas deferens and its artery from the testicular artery and the pampiniform plexus at the internal ring (Figs. 4.**13**, 4.**14**). As the peritoneum is mobilized, dissection of the pampiniform plexus and testicular artery can be carried into the retroperitoneal space (Fig. 4.**15**).

Comments

If additional mobilization of the testis is desired, the inferior epigastric vessels may be isolated and divided. Also, the transversalis fascia can be incised in the area of the medial inguinal fossa as far as the pubic tubercle to facilitate mobilization of the testis.

The inguinal incision can be extended upward to gain access to an intraabdominal testis or an ectopic testis located in the area of the internal ring. This involves additional proximal division of the transversalis fascia. By separating the internal spermatic fascia, the surgeon can dissect the pampiniform plexus and testicular artery far into the retroperitoneal space. A funnel-shaped remnant of the vaginal process of the peritoneum can be carefully separated from the internal spermatic fascia.

For a high semicastration, incision of the internal spermatic fascia provides access for individual ligation of the vas deferens and its artery and of the pampiniform plexus and testicular artery.

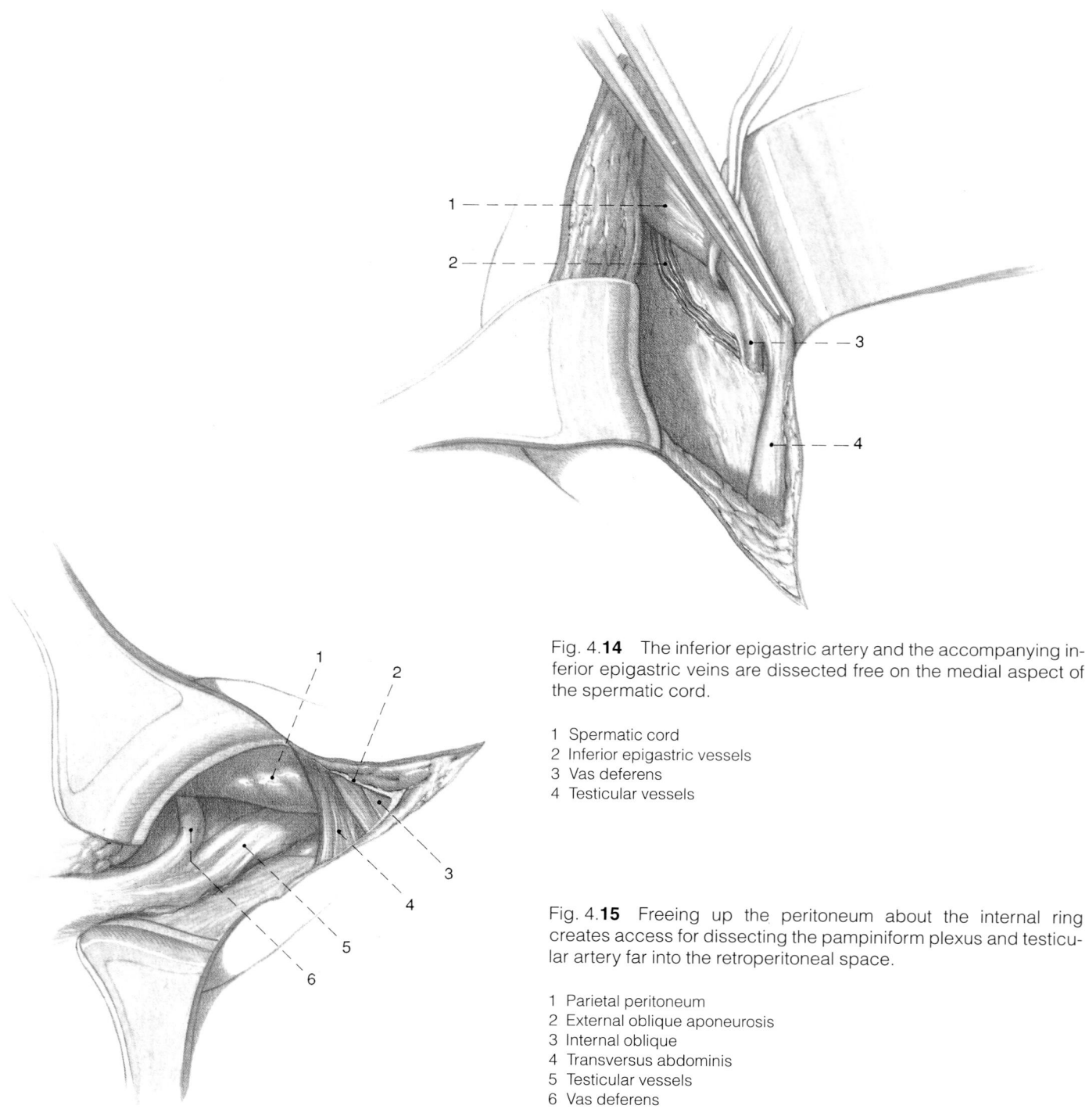

Fig. 4.**14** The inferior epigastric artery and the accompanying inferior epigastric veins are dissected free on the medial aspect of the spermatic cord.

1 Spermatic cord
2 Inferior epigastric vessels
3 Vas deferens
4 Testicular vessels

Fig. 4.**15** Freeing up the peritoneum about the internal ring creates access for dissecting the pampiniform plexus and testicular artery far into the retroperitoneal space.

1 Parietal peritoneum
2 External oblique aponeurosis
3 Internal oblique
4 Transversus abdominis
5 Testicular vessels
6 Vas deferens

Ilioinguinal Lymph Node Dissection

Main Indication

This procedure is used for dissection of the superficial and deep inguinal lymph nodes in patients with penile carcinoma.

The technique is illustrated for the right side.

Position and Skin Incision

The right hip is abducted and externally rotated. A pad is placed beneath the ipsilateral knee, and the sole of the foot on the operative side is secured against the medial side of the left lower leg (Fig. 4.16). The incision runs about 3–5 cm below the inguinal ligament, starting medially at the scrotum and curving below the inguinal ligament toward the anterior iliac spine (Fig. 4.16).

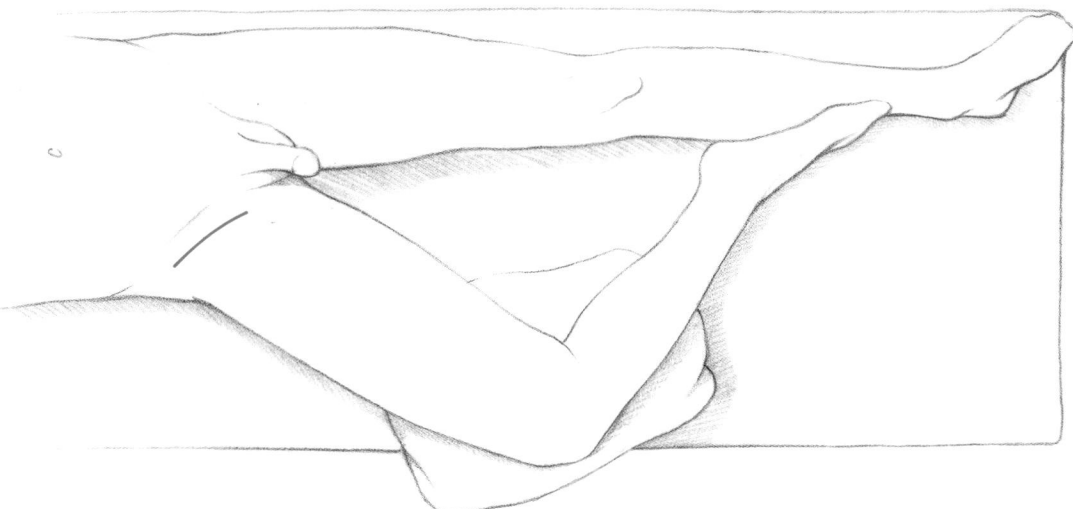

Fig. 4.16   Position and skin incision.

Exposure of the Superficial Femoral (Scarpa's) Fascia

The subcutaneous fat and Scarpa's fascia are divided, leaving subcutaneous connective tissue in both the upper and lower corners of the wound. The fatty tissue superficial to Scarpa's fascia is preserved (Fig. 4.**17**).

Superficial branches of the superficial epigastric vessels, superficial circumflex iliac vessels, and exernal pudendal vessels are spared if possible in order to preserve the blood supply to the dissected skin flap (Fig. 4.**18**).

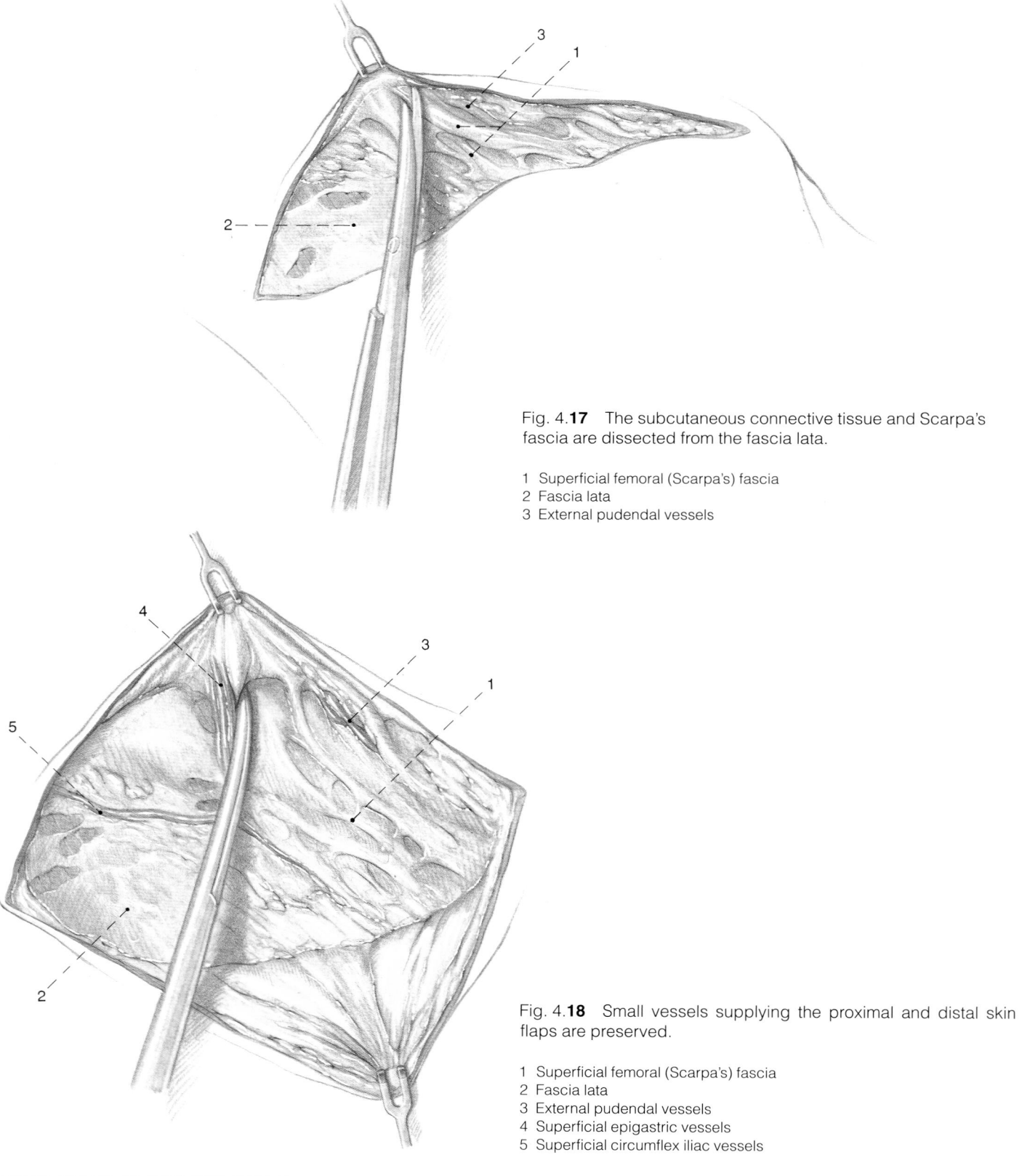

Fig. 4.**17** The subcutaneous connective tissue and Scarpa's fascia are dissected from the fascia lata.

1 Superficial femoral (Scarpa's) fascia
2 Fascia lata
3 External pudendal vessels

Fig. 4.**18** Small vessels supplying the proximal and distal skin flaps are preserved.

1 Superficial femoral (Scarpa's) fascia
2 Fascia lata
3 External pudendal vessels
4 Superficial epigastric vessels
5 Superficial circumflex iliac vessels

Lymph Node Dissection

The lymph node dissection covers an approximately square field whose superior boundary is approximately 2 cm above the inguinal ligament. It is bounded medially by the adductor longus muscle, laterally by the sartorius, and inferiorly by the apex of the femoral triangle.

The superficial inguinal lymph nodes are located below Scarpa's fascia. The lymph vessels of these nodes are connected to the deep subinguinal nodes, which are associated with the femoral artery and vein and communicate with the iliac and retroperitoneal nodes.

The removal of the superficial and deep inguinal lymph nodes comprises the superficial fascia, fascia lata, and cribriform fascia. The lymph node dissection begins in the superior wound angle. All tissue is removed from the external oblique aponeurosis distally past the inguinal ligament to the fascia lata of the thigh. If positive nodes are confirmed, the superficial epigastric vessels and superficial circumflex iliac vessels must be severed and removed with the specimen.

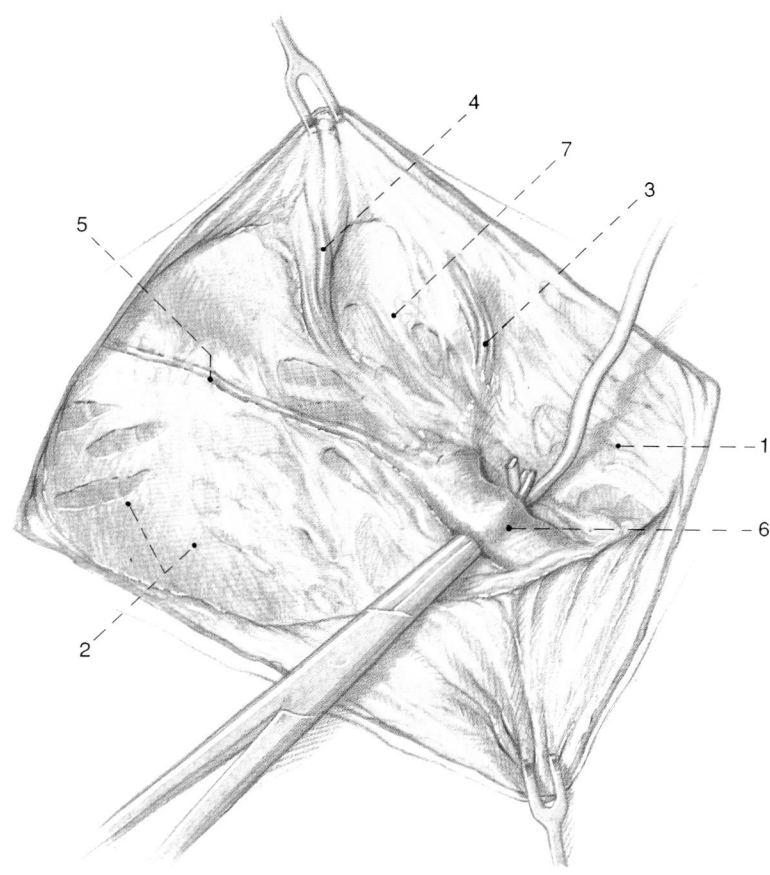

Fig. 4.**19**   The great saphenous vein is dissected free and snared.

1 Superficial femoral (Scarpa's) fascia
2 Fascia lata
3 External pudendal vessels
4 Superficial epigastric vessels
5 Superficial circumflex iliac vessels
6 Great saphenous vein
7 Cribriform fascia

Great Saphenous Vein

The great saphenous vein is dissected free from surrounding structures and snared with a vascular tape (Fig. 4.**19**).

The pattern of tributaries supplying the femoral vein in the subinguinal region (saphenous hiatus) is extremely variable.

The "typical" tributary pattern shown in Fig. 4.**20** is present in only 37% of cases. The most common variants are illustrated in Fig. 4.**21**. The largest accessory vessels observed in this region are the medial accessory saphenous vein (9%) and lateral accessory saphenous vein (48%).

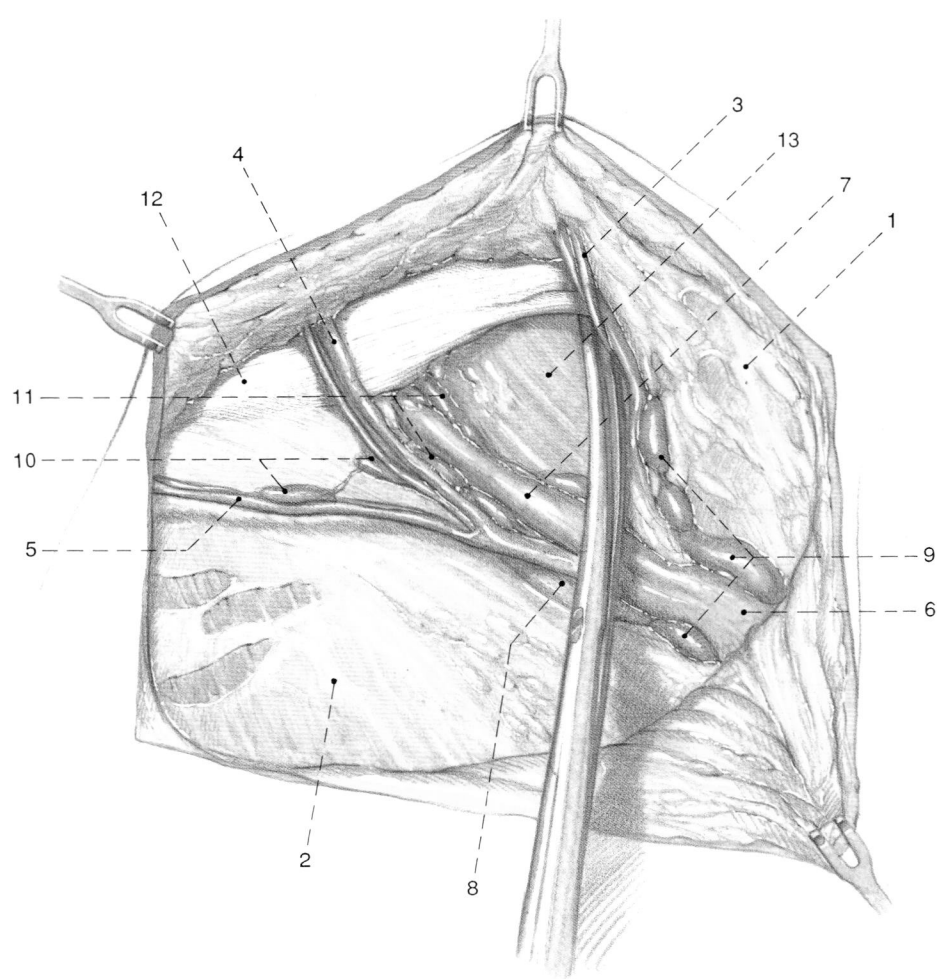

Fig. 4.**20**   The lymph node dissection is started at the external oblique aponeurosis 2 cm above the inguinal ligament.

1 Superficial femoral (Scarpa's) fascia
2 Fascia lata
3 External pudendal vessels
4 Superficial epigastric vessels
5 Superficial circumflex iliac vessels
6 Great saphenous vein
7 Femoral vein
8 Femoral artery
9 Inferior and superomedial superficial inguinal lymph nodes
    (vertical tract)
10 Superolateral superficial inguinal lymph nodes (horizontal tract)
11 Deep inguinal lymph nodes
12 External oblique aponeurosis
13 Adductor longus

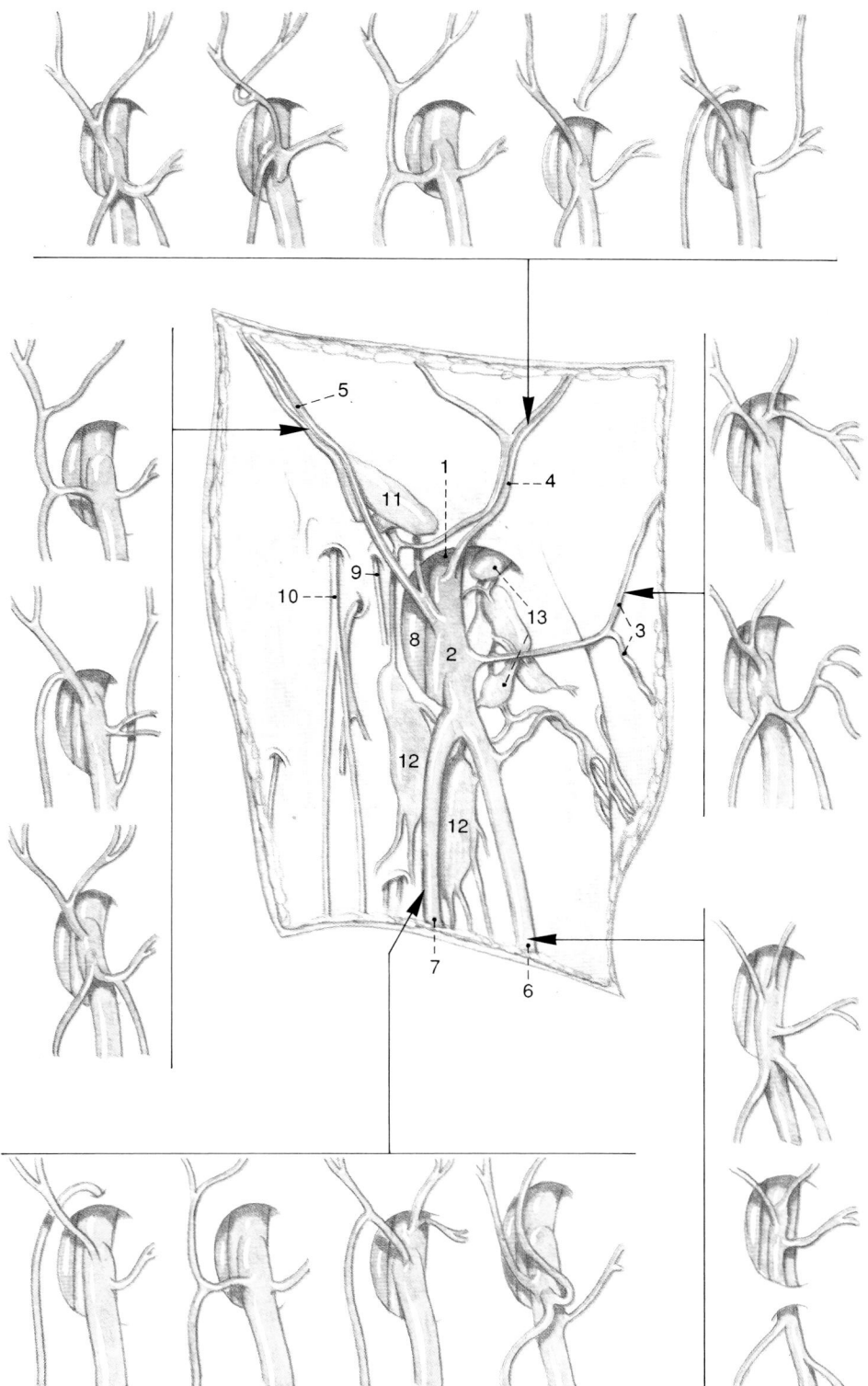

Fig. 4.**21** Variations of venous anatomy at the saphenous hiatus
in the subinguinal region (after Platzer).

1 Saphenous hiatus
2 Femoral vein
3 External pudendal veins
4 Superficial epigastric vein
5 Superficial circumflex iliac vein
6 Great saphenous vein
7 Lateral accessory saphenous vein

8 Femoral artery
9 Femoral branch of genitofemoral nerve
10 Anterior cutaneous branches of femoral nerve
11 Superolateral superficial inguinal lymph nodes (horizontal tract)
12 Inferior superficial inguinal lymph nodes (vertical tract)
13 Deep inguinal lymph nodes

Fascia Lata

The fascia lata is incised below the inguinal ligament at the lateral border of the sartorius muscle as illustrated. The fascia lata is dissected off the adductor longus starting from the medial side (Fig. 4.**22**).

The femoral artery and vein are dissected free, removing the cribriform fascia and exposing the saphenous hiatus (Fig. 4.**23**). The lymph node dissection is carried to the lateral aspect of the femoral artery. If positive nodes are found, all the fat and associated fasciae must be removed with the lymph node package together with corresponding venous and arterial branches (Fig. 4.**23**).

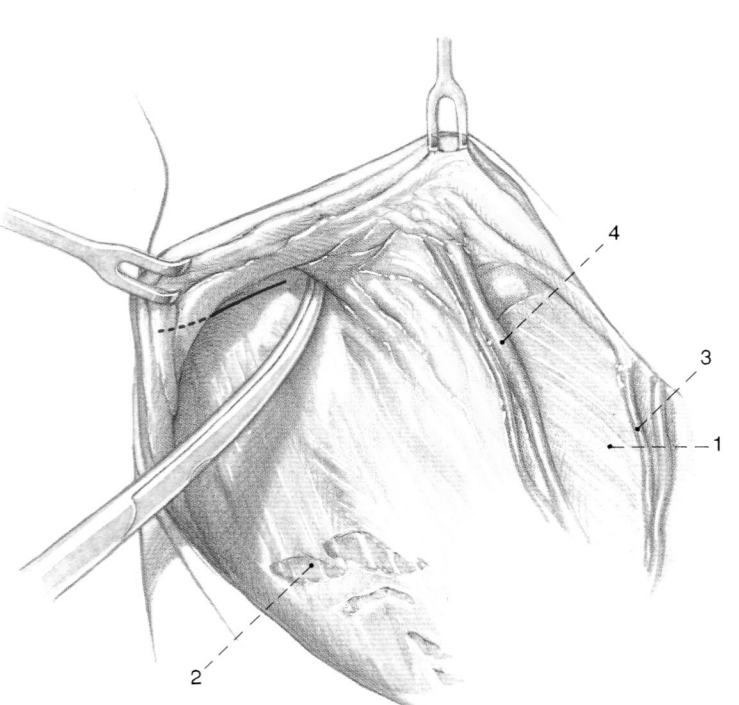

Fig. 4.**22** Lateral and medial limits of the dissection (sartorius and adductor longus muscles).

1 Adductor longus
2 Sartorius
3 External pudendal vessels
4 Superficial epigastric vessels

Fig. 4.**23** Anatomic dissection showing the vessels about the saphenous hiatus.

1 Saphenous hiatus
2 Falciform margin
3 Superior horn
4 Inferior horn
5 Adductor longus
6 Spermatic cord
7 Femoral vein
8 Great saphenous vein
9 Lateral accessory saphenous vein
10 External pudendal vessels
11 Inferior epigastric vessels
12 Superficial circumflex iliac vessels
13 Femoral artery

Comments

The great saphenous vein is isolated but is not ligated. Preservation of the great saphenous vein and, if possible, its small tributaries is helpful for reducing postoperative leg edema and decreasing the incidence of wound healing problems. The branches of the superficial epigastric vessels and external pudendal vessels should be preserved only if negative lymph nodes are confirmed. Dissection of the deep inguinal nodes must be preceded by dissection of the saphenous hiatus including its falciform margin and superior and inferior horns (Fig. 4.**23**).

A pelvic lymph node dissection also can be performed through this approach, which involves incision of the exter-

nal oblique aponeurosis followed by division of the internal oblique and transversus abdominis muscles (Fig. 4.**24**). Division of the transversalis fascia and mobilization of the peritoneum provide access to the lateral pelvic wall for dissecting the lymph nodes at the subperitoneal and retroperitoneal vessels. Dissection of the genitofemoral nerve is recommended as it provides an important landmark for identifying these structures. If a bilateral pelvic lymph node dissection is necessary, a midline extraperitoneal surgical approach will have to be carried out.

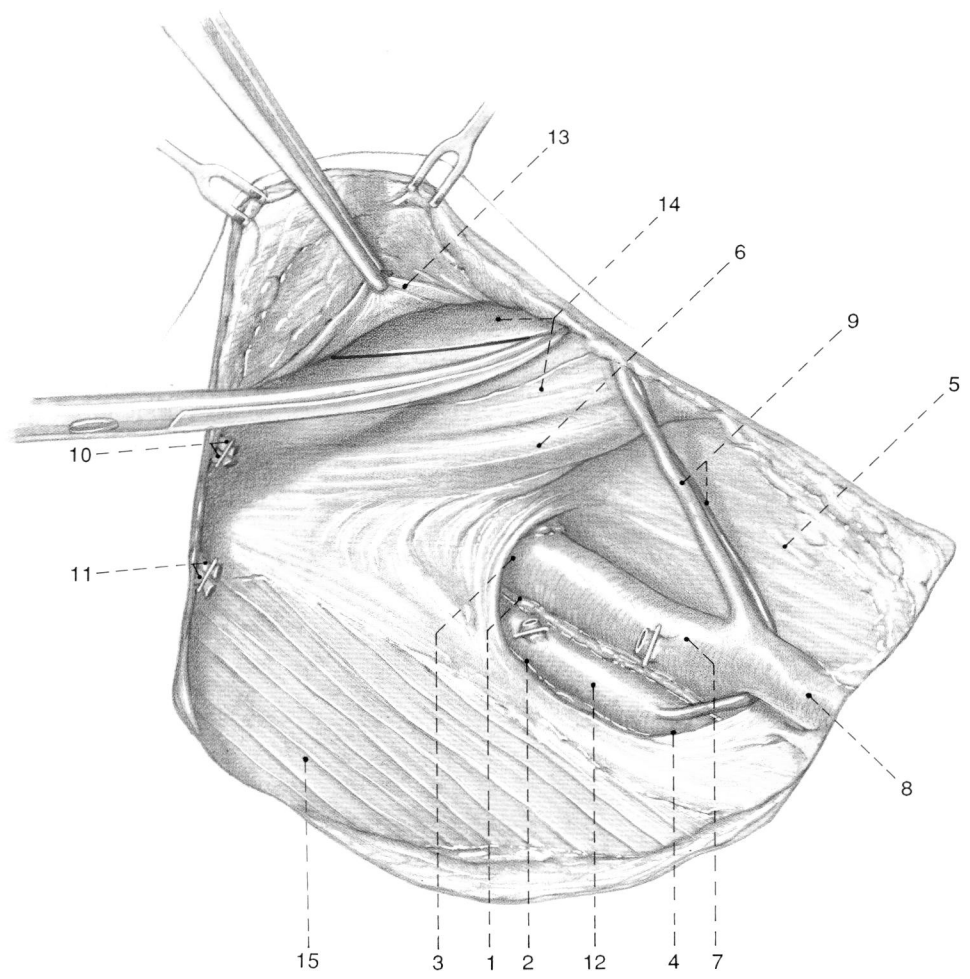

Fig. 4.**24** The approach for a unilateral pelvic lymph node dissection involves incision of the external oblique aponeurosis and then of the internal oblique and transversus abdominis muscles.

1 Saphenous hiatus
2 Falciform margin
3 Superior horn
4 Inferior horn
5 Adductor longus
6 Spermatic cord
7 Femoral vein
8 Great saphenous vein
9 External pudendal vessels
10 Inferior epigastric vessels
11 Superficial circumflex iliac vessels
12 Femoral artery
13 Camper's fascia
14 External oblique aponeurosis
15 Sartorius

5 External Genitalia

Pubic Approach

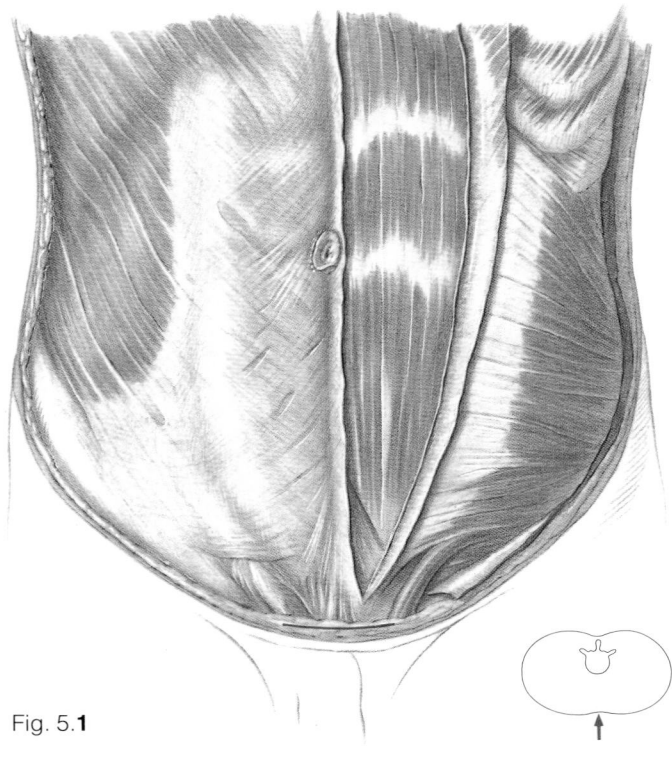

Fig. 5.**1**

Main Indications

- Penile revascularization
- Correction of venous leakage
- Prosthetic surgery

Position and Skin Incision

The patient is positioned supine. A vertical or transverse incision is made 1–2 cm above the pubic symphysis (Fig. 5.**2**).

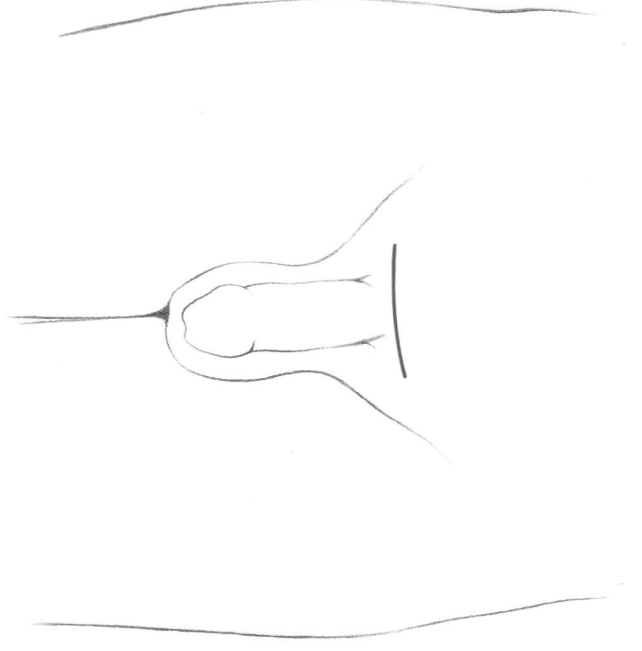

Fig. 5.**2** Position and skin incision.

Exposure of the Superficial Dorsal Penile Vein

Following division of the subcutaneous tissue and the coagulation of superficial venous branches, the superficial abdominal fascia (Camper's fascia) is identified (Fig. 5.**3**). Deep to Camper's fascia is the superficial dorsal penile vein (Fig. 5.**3**), which is dissected free and ligated (Fig. 5.**4**). Exposure is maintained with retractors.

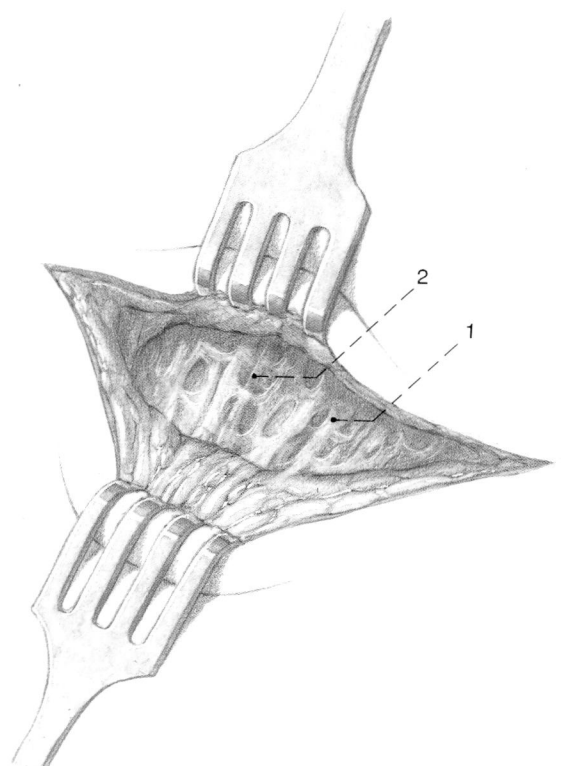

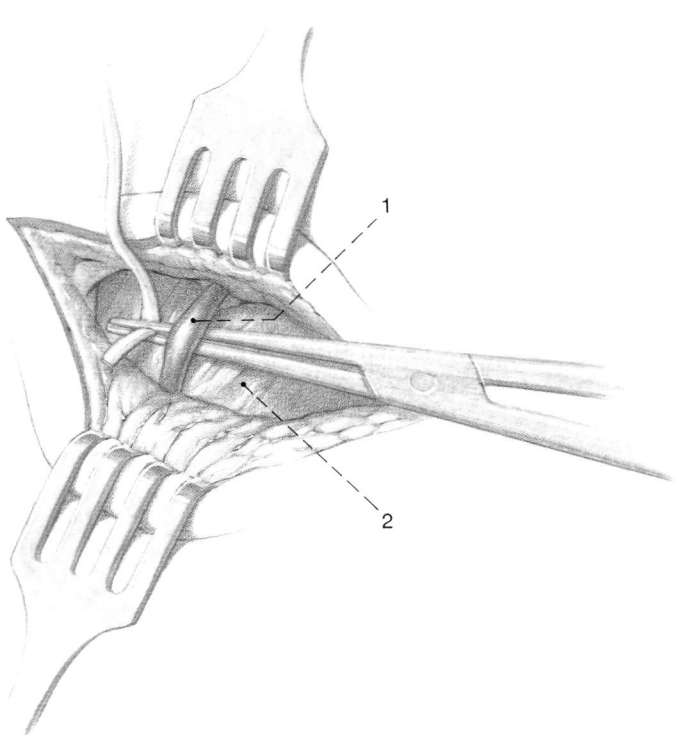

Fig. 5.**3** Exposure of the superficial abdominal fascia.

1 Superficial abdominal fascia (Camper's fascia)
2 Superficial dorsal penile vein

Fig. 5.**4** The superficial dorsal penile vein is exposed, underrun, and ligated.

1 Superficial dorsal penile vein
2 Deep penile fascia

Exposure of the Penile Pedicle

Following ligation of the superficial dorsal vein, the deep penile fascia is divided transversely, and the penile pedicle with the deep dorsal vein, dorsal artery, and dorsal nerve is exposed at the midline. The tunica albuginea of the corpus cavernosum is identified lateral to this pedicle (Fig. 5.5). The drawing illustrates the approach for penile revascularization. The inferior epigastric artery is exposed separately through an extraperitoneal paramedian approach.

Comments

Prosthetic surgery should be performed through a longitudinal incision that may be extended cranially as needed to develop the retropubic prevesical space for implantation of the reservoir.

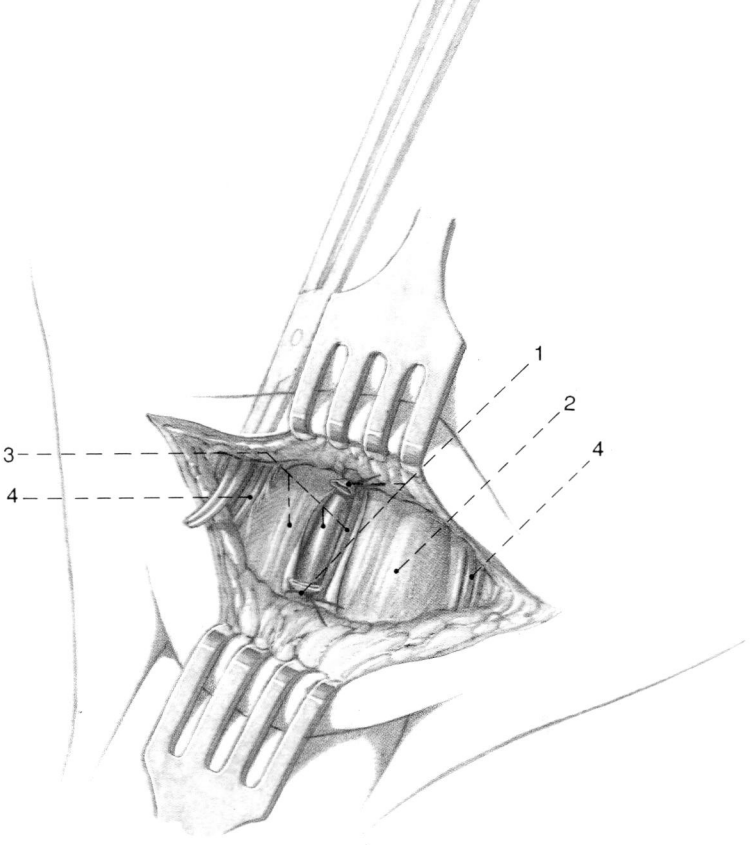

Fig. 5.**5**   The penile pedicle and deep penile fascia are exposed. A tunnel is developed for penile revascularization.

1 Superficial dorsal penile vein
2 Deep penile fascia
3 Deep dorsal penile vein, dorsal penile artery and nerve
4 External pudendal vessels

Dorsal Approach to the Penis

Main Indications

- Correction of Peyronie's Disease
- Transsexualism

Position and Skin Incision

The patient is positioned supine, and the inner layer of the prepuce is incised along the coronal sulcus (Fig. 5.**6**). The plane between the preputial and penile skin and the superficial penile fascia is developed (see Fig. 5.**7**).

Exposure of the Superficial Penile Fascia

The preputial and penile skin are dissected off the superficial penile fascia by elevation of the inner layer of the prepuce (Figs. 5.**7**, 5.**8**).

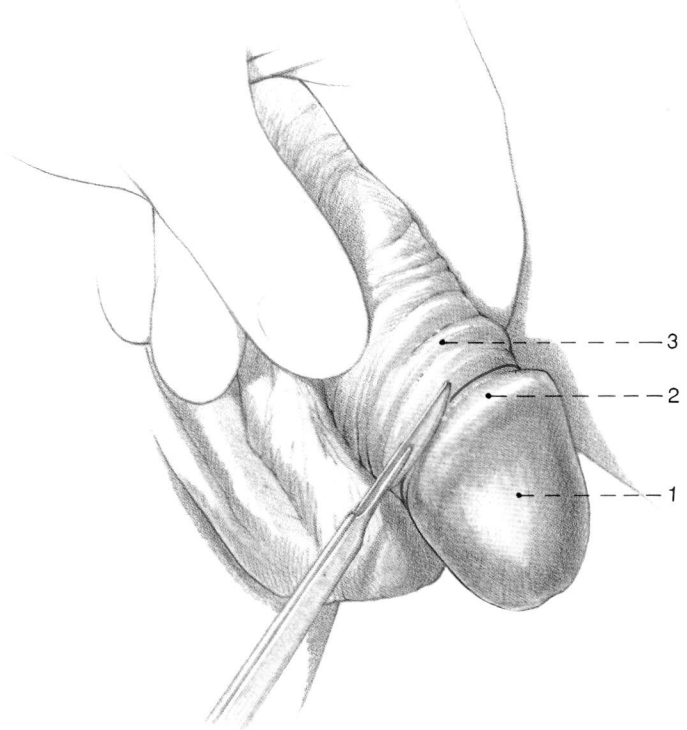

Fig. 5.**6** Line of incision along the inner layer of the prepuce.

1 Glans penis
2 Corona of glans
3 Prepuce

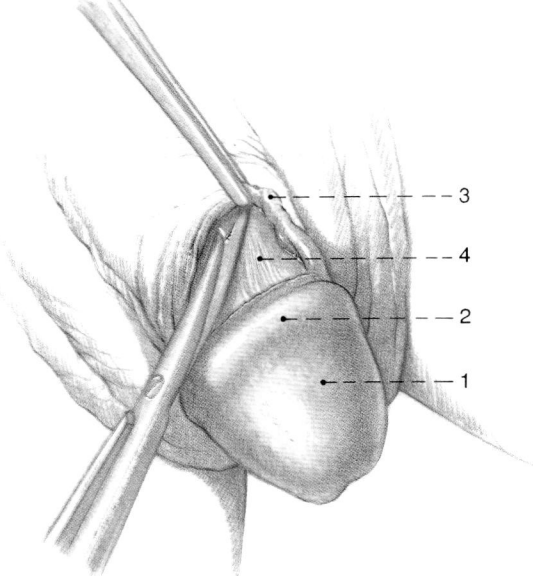

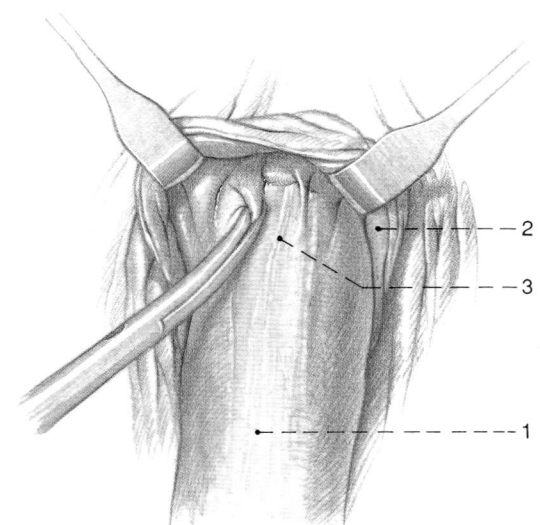

Fig. 5.**7**, 5.**8** Dissection of the preputial and penile skin from the superficial penile fascia.

1 Glans penis
2 Corona of glans
3 Prepuce
4 Superficial penile fascia

1 Superficial penile fascia
2 Prepuce
3 Superficial dorsal penile vein

Exposure of the Dorsal Neurovascular Bundle

The superficial and deep penile fasciae are dissected and incised to the tunica albuginea along the lateral side of the penis (Fig. 5.9). A counterincision is made on the opposite side, and the neurovascular bundle (deep dorsal vein, artery, and nerve) is underrun and snared with a tape (Fig. 5.10).

The anatomic dissection in Fig. 5.11 shows the structures of the dorsal neurovascular bundle: the deep dorsal penile vein, the dorsal penile artery, and the dorsal nerve of the penis, located between the deep penile fascia and the tunica albuginea (Fig. 5.11).

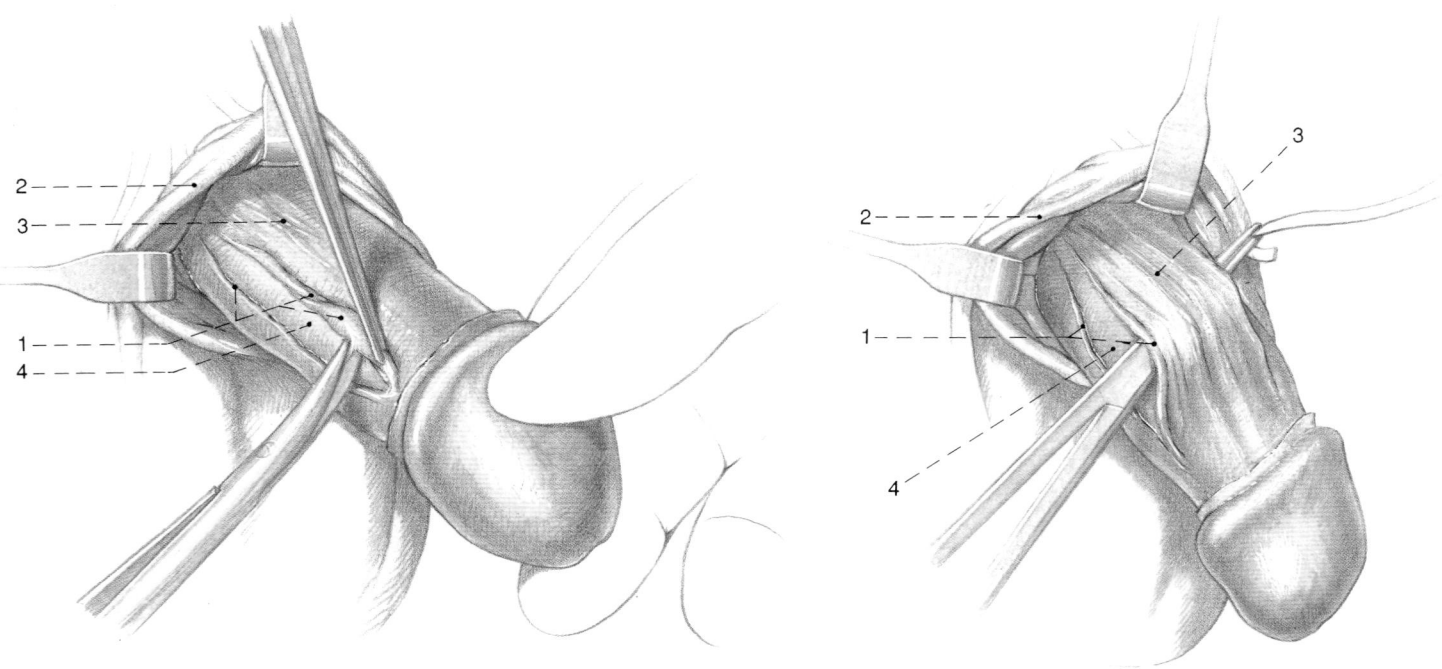

Fig. 5.9 The superficial and deep fasciae of the penis are divided down to the tunica albuginea.

1 Superficial and deep penile fasciae
2 Prepuce
3 Superficial dorsal vein of penis
4 Tunica albuginea

Fig. 5.10 The neurovascular bundle is undermined and snared with a vascular tape.

1 Superficial and deep penile fasciae
2 Prepuce
3 Superficial dorsal penile vein
4 Tunica albuginea

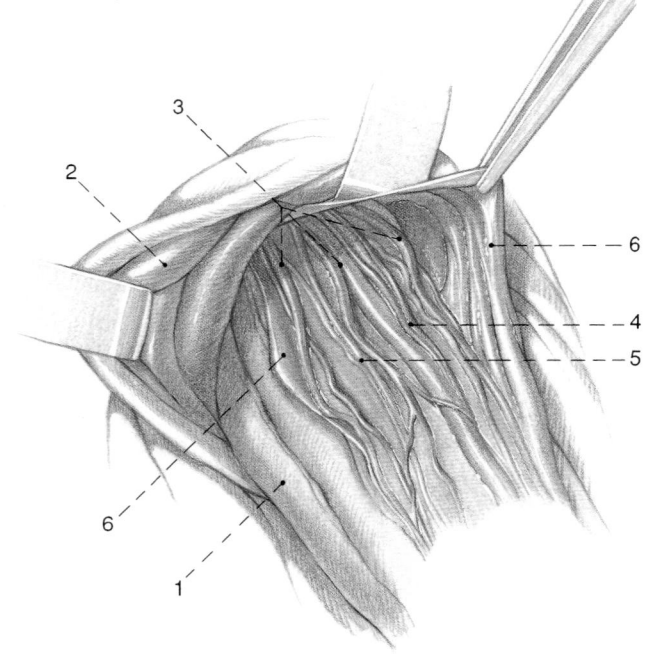

Fig. 5.11 Anatomic dissection showing the structures of the neurovascular bundle: the deep dorsal penile vein, dorsal penile artery, and dorsal penile nerve.

1 Superficial penile fascia
2 Prepuce
3 Deep dorsal penile vein
4 Dorsal penile artery
5 Dorsal penile nerve
6 Deep penile fascia

The fascial planes of the penis are shown in schematic cross section in Fig. 5.**12**.

Comments

This dorsal approach is used not only for the various corrective procedures for penile induration but also for dissecting the neurovascular bundle in nerve- and vessel-sparing clitoral reduction surgery in patients with adrenogenital syndrome. Dorsal penile exposure can be accomplished by circumferential incision or by a longitudinal or Z-shaped incision.

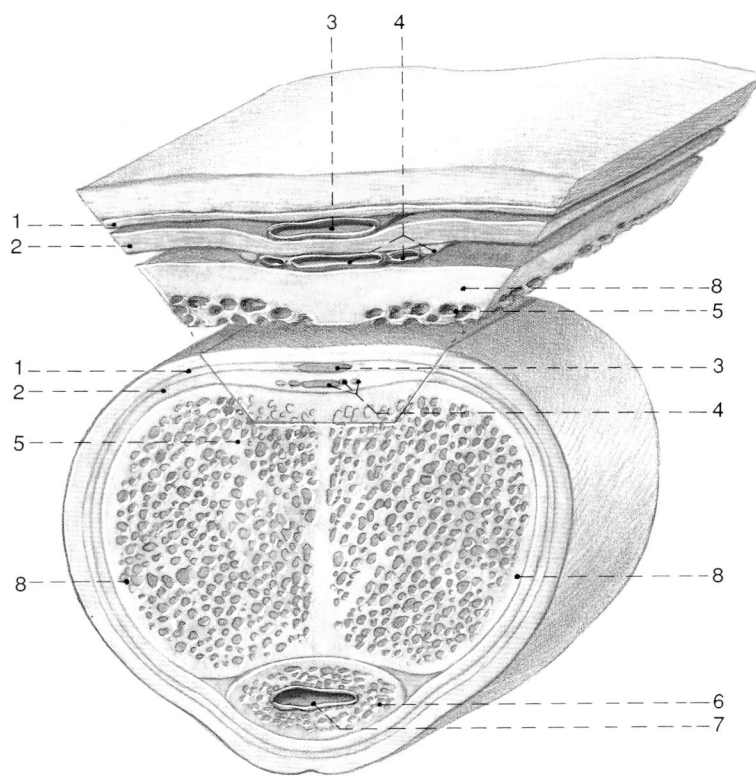

Fig. 5.**12** Schematic cross section of the penis (after Feneis).

1 Superficial penile fascia
2 Deep penile fascia
3 Superficial dorsal penile vein
4 Deep dorsal penile vein, dorsal penile artery and nerve
5 Corpus cavernosum
6 Corpus spongiosum
7 Urethra
8 Tunica albuginea

Ventral Approach to the Penis

Main Indications

- Anterior urethral surgery
- Ventral Nesbit procedure
- Correction of hypospadias
- Shunt construction between corpus cavernosum and corpus spongiosum
- Shunt construction between corpus cavernosum and great saphenous vein

Position and Skin Incision

The patient is positioned supine. The superficial penile fascia is exposed by circumcision of the prepuce (Fig. 5.13). After incision of the superficial and deep penile fasciae, the corpus spongiosum is dissected from the corpus cavernosum (Fig. 5.14).

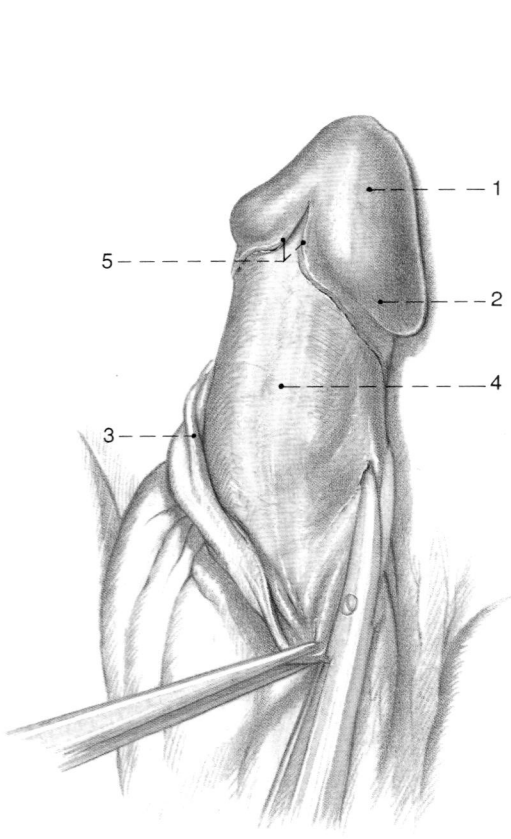

Fig. 5.**13**   The superficial penile fascia is exposed after circumcision of the prepuce.

1 Glans penis
2 Corona of glans
3 Prepuce
4 Superficial penile fascia
5 Frenulum

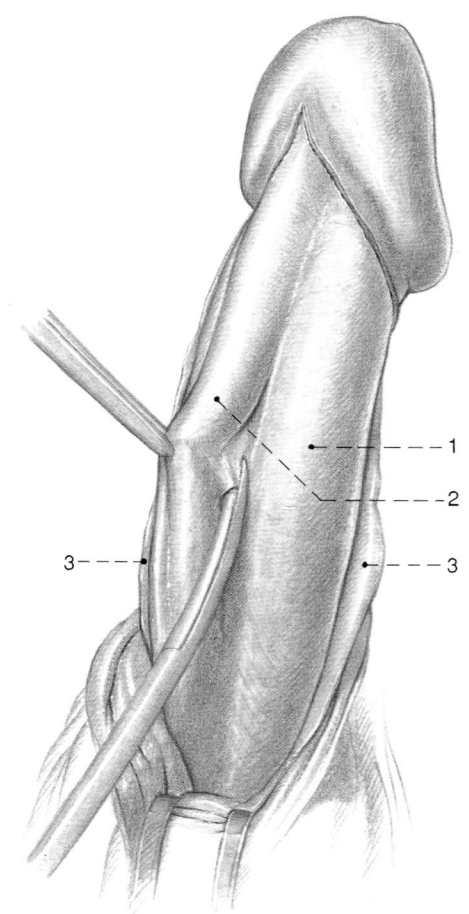

Fig. 5.**14**   The superficial and deep penile fasciae are divided, and the corpus spongiosum is separated from the corpus cavernosum.

1 Corpus cavernosum
2 Corpus spongiosum
3 Superficial and deep penile fascia

Mobilization of the Corpus Spongiosum

The corpus spongiosum is dissected free and snared with a tape (Fig. 5.**15**). The corpus spongiosum is elevated away from the corpus cavernosum, and individual anastomotic vessels are coagulated as the dissection proceeds (Fig. 5.**16**).

For treatment of a stricture, the urethra is incised into healthy tissue and is manipulated with two traction sutures for single-stage reconstruction procedures employing grafts and flaps (Fig. 5.**17**).

Comments

As the corpus spongiosum is dissected out of the urethral sulcus of the corpus cavernosum, numerous anastomoses between the circumflex penile veins and the veins of the corpus spongiosum must be divided. This dissection is performed directly on the tunica albuginea of the corpus cavernosum to avoid injury to the corpus spongiosum. This approach is also used for the correction of chordee in hypospadias. In this case the superficial and deep penile fasciae are incised far laterally to permit broad dissection of the chordee tissue from the corpus cavernosum.

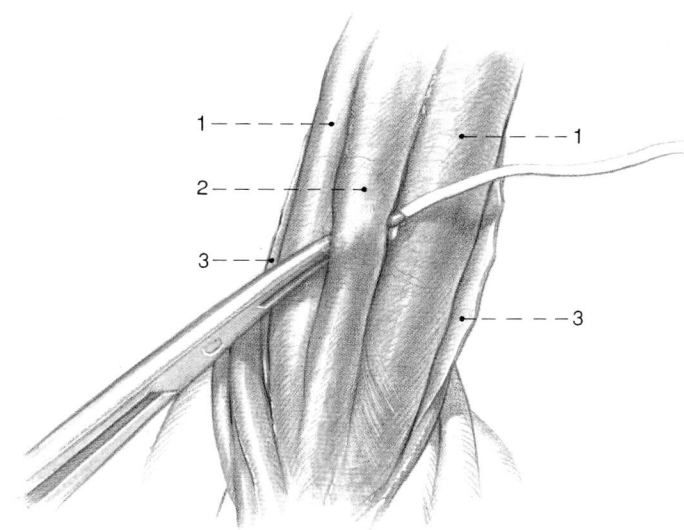

Fig. 5.**15** The corpus spongiosum is underrun and snared.

1 Corpus cavernosum
2 Corpus spongiosum
3 Superficial and deep penile fascia

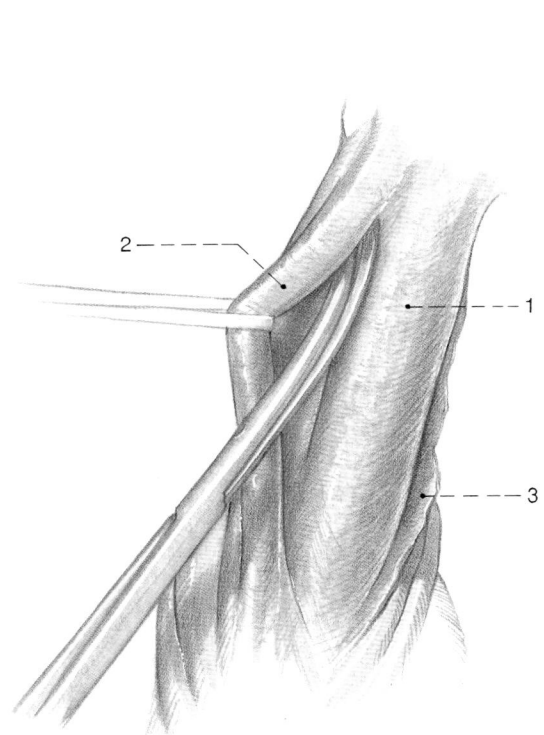

Fig. 5.**16** The corpus spongiosum is dissected out of the urethral sulcus of the corpus cavernosum.

1 Corpus cavernosum
2 Corpus spongiosum
3 Superficial and deep penile fasciae

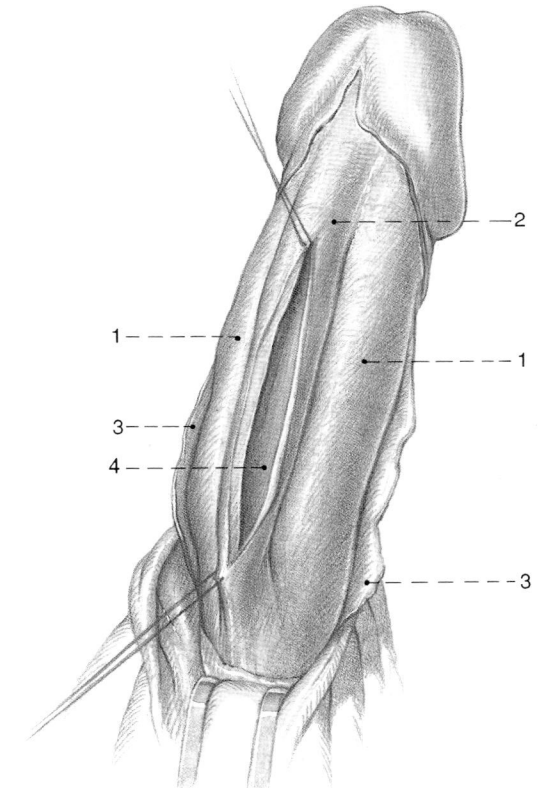

Fig. 5.**17** For a urethral stricture, the urethra is opened and engaged with traction sutures.

1 Corpus cavernosum
2 Corpus spongiosum
3 Superficial and deep penile fasciae
4 Incised anterior urethra

245

Approach to the Testis

Main Indications

- Hydrocele
- Spermatocele
- Vasovasostomy
- Epididymovasostomy
- Epididymectomy
- Testicular torsion
- Testicular biopsy
- Subcapsular orchiectomy
- Insertion of a testicular prosthesis
- Injuries of the testis and epididymis

Position and Skin Incision

The patient is positioned supine. The testis is approached through a transverse incision to preserve the vascular supply of the scrotal skin, which is incised to the tunica dartos (Fig. 5.18).

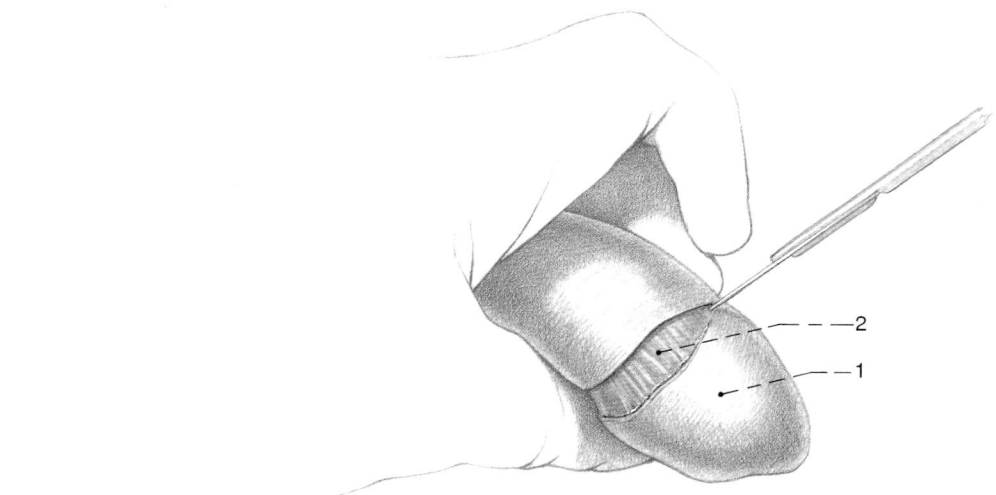

Fig. 5.**18** Transverse incision exposing the tunica dartos.

1 Scrotum
2 Tunica dartos

Division of the External and Internal Spermatic Fascia

After division of the tunica dartos, the external spermatic fascia is divided along with extensions of the cremaster muscle (Fig. 5.**19**).

The next step is the division of the internal spermatic fascia. The serous cavity of the testis is opened, exposing the tunica vaginalis (Fig. 5.**20**). The dissection in Fig. 5.**21** illustrates the arrangement of the testicular coverings: the scrotal skin, tunica dartos, external spermatic fascia, cremasteric fascia, internal spermatic fascia, and the periorchium and epiorchium of the testis and epididymis.

Comments

Aside from the very short, longitudinal incision required for a vasectomy, all approaches to the testis and epididymis are made through a transverse scrotal incision that preserves the blood supply of the scrotal skin. For a bilateral orchiectomy, the testes can be approached through the raphe and then the septum of the scrotum.

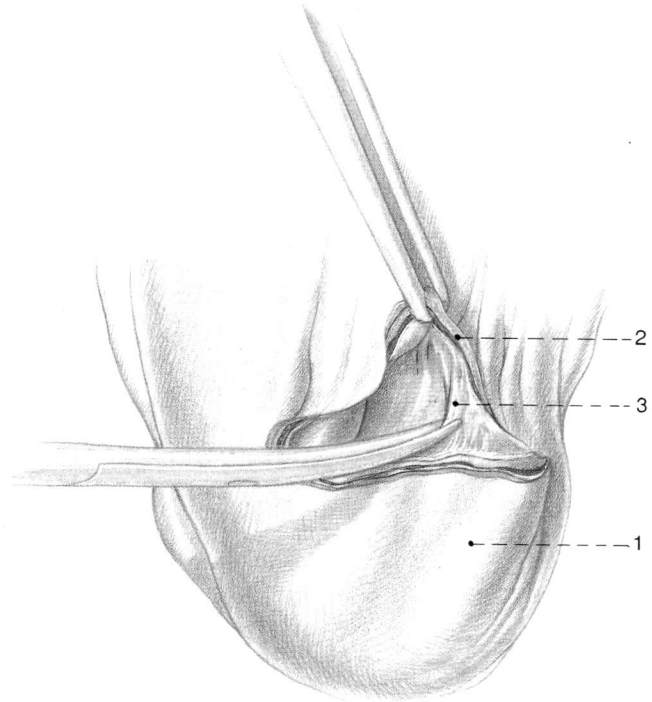

Fig. 5.**19** Division of the external spermatic fascia and cremasteric fascia.

1 Scrotum
2 Tunica dartos
3 External spermatic fascia and cremasteric fascia with cremaster muscle

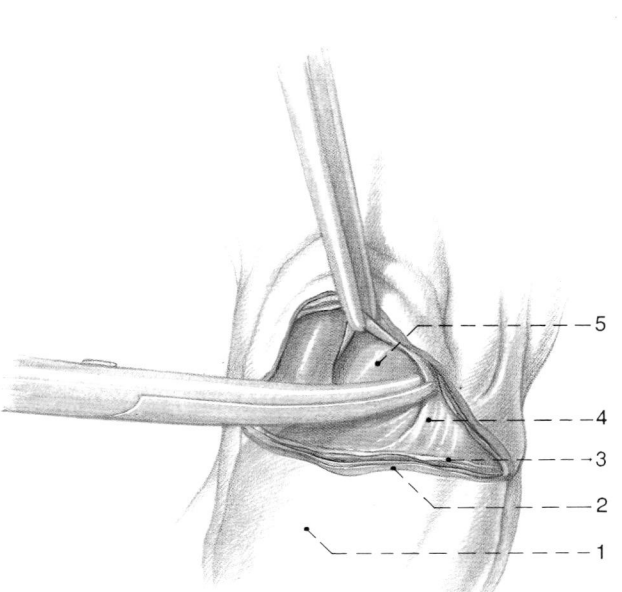

Fig. 5.**20** Division of the internal spermatic fascia.

1 Scrotum
2 Tunica dartos
3 External spermatic fascia and cremasteric fascia with cremaster muscle
4 Internal spermatic fascia
5 Tunica vaginalis, parietal layer (periorchium)

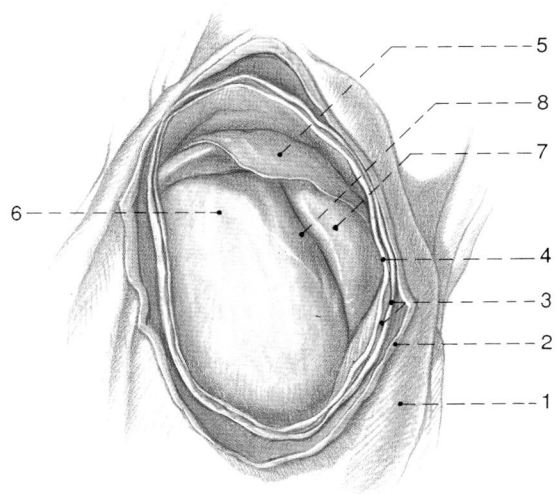

Fig. 5.**21** The coverings of the testis (anatomic dissection).

1 Scrotum
2 Tunica dartos
3 External spermatic fascia and cremasteric fascia with cremaster muscle
4 Internal spermatic fascia
5 Tunica vaginalis, parietal layer (periorchium)
6 Testis, covered by visceral layer of tunica vaginalis (epiorchium)
7 Epididymis, covered by epiorchium
8 Sinus of epididymis

Approaches Involving the Female External Genitalia

Main Indications

- Meatotomy
- Excision of a urethral caruncle
- Excision of a urethral diverticulum
- Spence-Duckett procedure
- Repair of urethral fistula

Position and Skin Incision

The patient is placed in the dorsal lithotomy position
(Fig. 5.**22**).

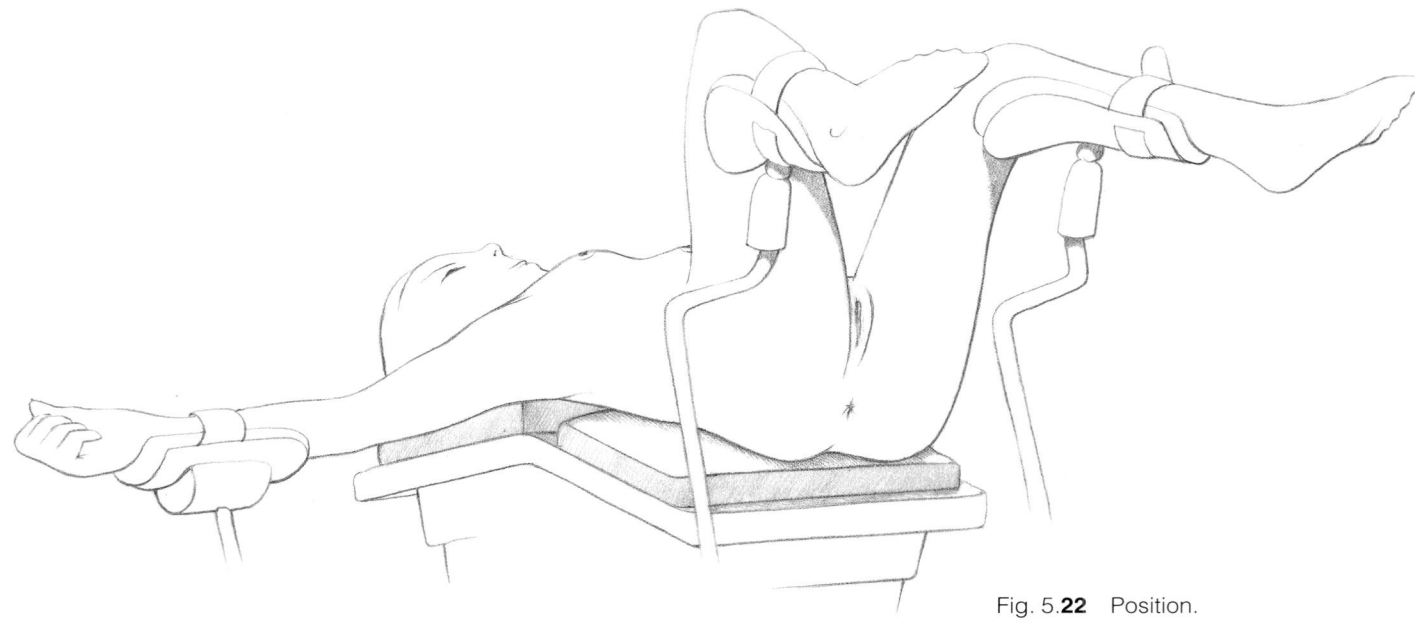

Fig. 5.**22**   Position.

The lines of incision for a meatotomy, the excision of a urethral caruncle, or the Spence-Duckett repair of a urethral diverticulum are shown in Fig. 5.**23**. In the Spence-Duckett technique, the urethrovaginal septum is incised to the proximal margin of the diverticulum. The approaches for repair of a urethral fistula or excision of a urethral diverticulum are shown in Fig. 5.**24**. A urethral catheter is introduced, and the insertion of a weighted posterior vaginal speculum facilitates the longitudinal or U-shaped incision (Fig. 5.**24**).

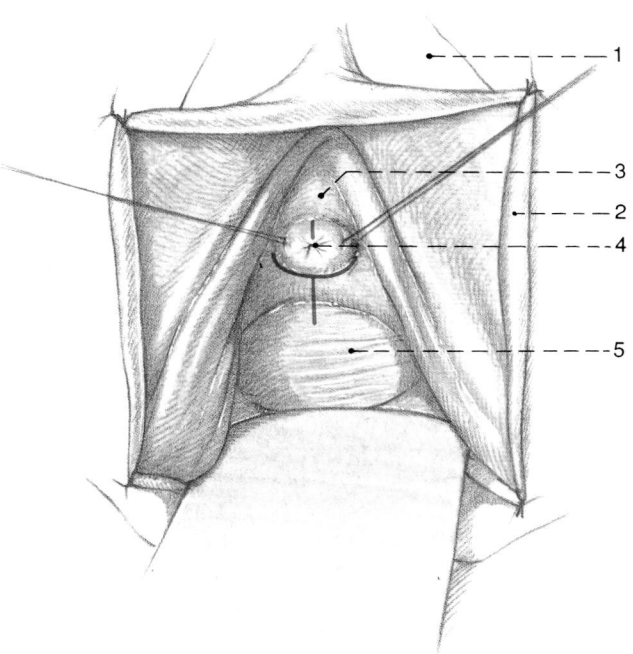

Fig. 5.**23** Incision for meatotomy, caruncle excision, or the Spence-Duckett technique.

1 Labium majus
2 Labium minus
3 Vestibule of vagina
4 External urethral orifice
5 Anterior vaginal wall

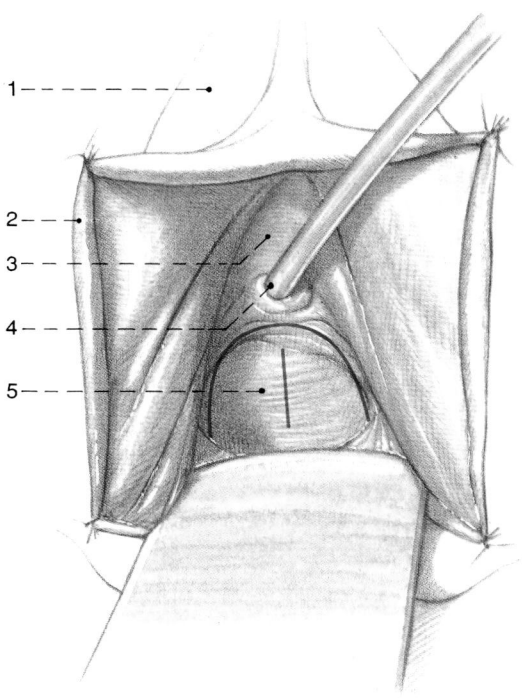

Fig. 5.**24** Incision for repair of a urethral fistula (sagittal, curved).

1 Labium majus
2 Labium minus
3 Vestibule of vagina
4 External urethral orifice
5 Anterior vaginal wall

Exposure of the Urethrovaginal Septum

During dissection of the urethral diverticulum or exposure of the urethral fistula, the urethrovaginal septum is dissected after elevation of the vaginal flap and preserved for use in closing the wound (Figs. 5. **25**, 5.**26**).

Comments

Small urethrovaginal fistulae are approached through a longitudinal incision. Larger fistulae are exposed through a U-shaped incision in the vaginal mucosa.

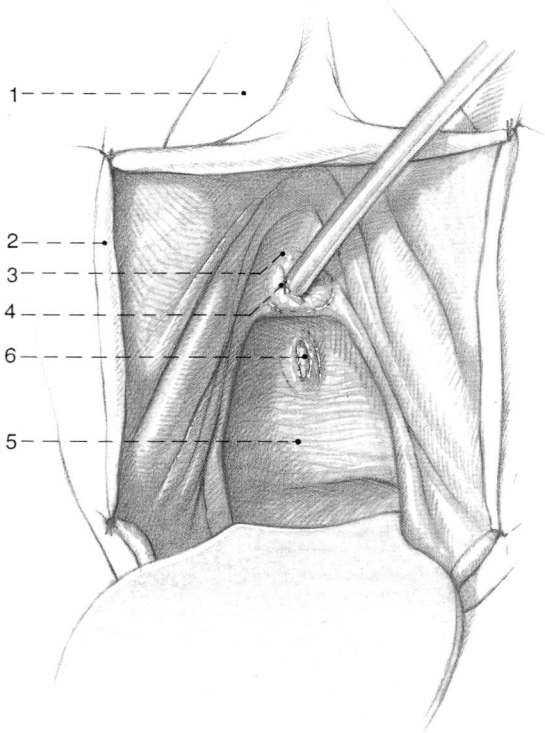

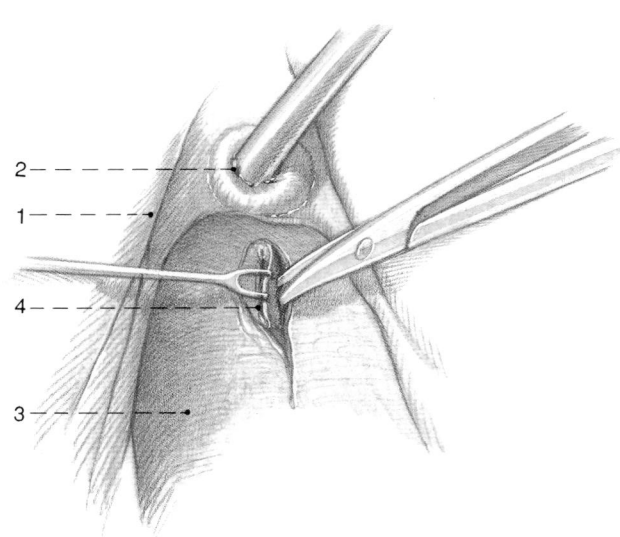

Fig. 5.**25**   A small fistula is excised through a sagittal approach.

1 Labium majus
2 Labium minus
3 Vestibule of vagina
4 External urethral orifice
5 Anterior vaginal wall
6 Urethral fistula

Fig. 5.**26**   Following incision around the fistula, a vaginal flap is developed, and the urethrovaginal septum is dissected.

1 Labium minus
2 External urethral orifice
3 Anterior vaginal wall
4 Urethral fistula

Bulbospongiosus Muscle Transfer

After closure of the fistula or excision of the urethral diverticulum, the urethrovaginal septum is sutured into place. For a large defect associated with a urethral fistula, the bulbospongiosus muscle can be transposed to cover the repair. The approach is made through an incision between the labia majora and minora (Fig. 5.27). The bulbospongiosus is dissected free from surrounding fat and ligated and transected at its insertion (Fig. 5.28). The flap is supplied by a branch of the pudendal artery at the origin of the muscle, the artery of the vestibular bulb (Fig. 5. 28). A counterincision is made on the medial side of the labium minus for tunneling the bulbospongiosus flap, together with surrounding fat and connective tissue, to the urethral defect (Fig. 5.29).

Comments

Martius, who first described the bulbospongiosus transfer, states that the muscle should not be dissected out of its surrounding fat, but that the fat should be left attached to the flap and tunneled to the urethral defect as part of the transfer.

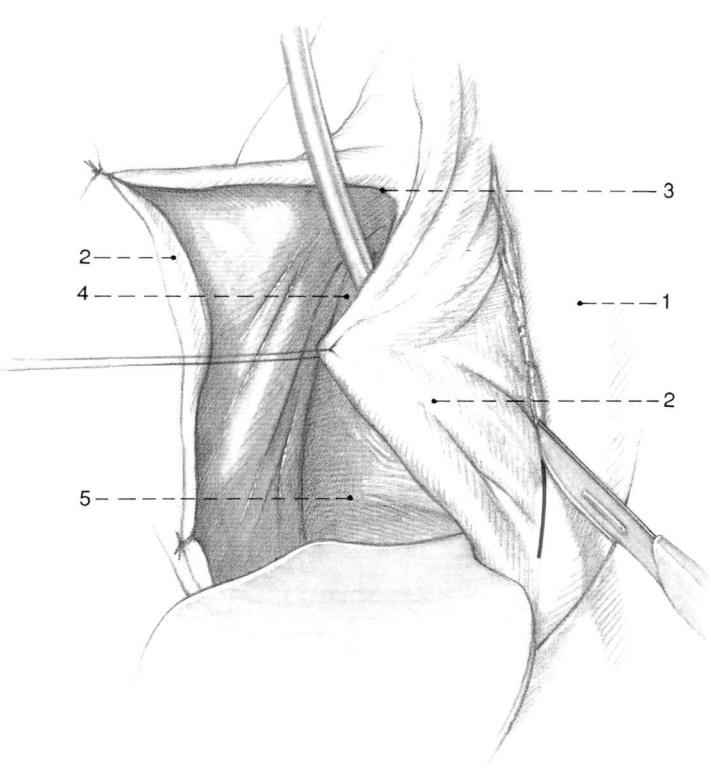

Fig. 5.**27** Approach for creating a bulbospongiosus muscle flap (Martius technique).

1 Labium majus
2 Labium minus
3 Prepuce of clitoris
4 Vestibule of vagina
5 Anterior vaginal wall

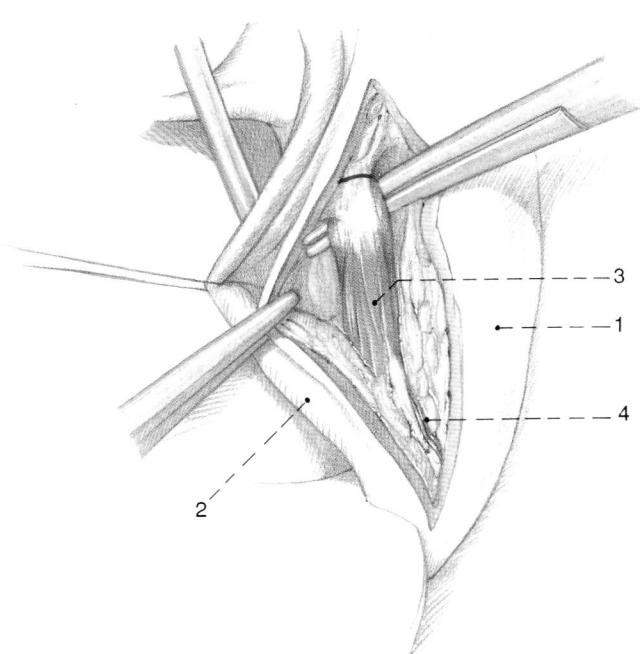

Fig. 5.**28** The bulbospongiosus muscle is divided at its insertion.

1 Labium majus   3 Bulbospongiosus
2 Labium minus   4 Artery of vestibular bulb

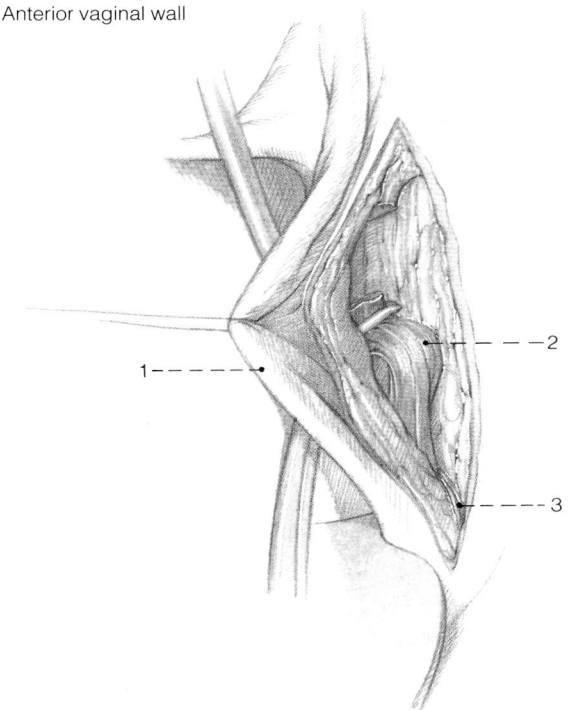

Fig. 5.**29** The vascularized bulbospongiosus flap is tunneled with surrounding fat to the urethral defect.

1 Labium minus   3 Artery of vestibular bulb
2 Bulbospongiosus

Gracilis Muscle Transfer

The gracilis muscle can be used for reconstruction of the pelvic floor or for the interpositional coverage of large actinic fistulae between the bladder, vagina, and rectum.

The gracilis inserts into the medial surface of the tibia distal to the medial condyle in the superficial pes anserinus. The incision is made over the center of the gracilis muscle (Fig. 5.30). After division of the skin and subcutaneous fat and ligation of the great saphenous vein, the gracilis is separated from the adductor longus muscle, carrying the dissection along the adductor longus to the neurovascular bundle of the gracilis (Fig. 5.31). The muscle is severed at its insertion with a tenotomy knife (Fig. 5.31).

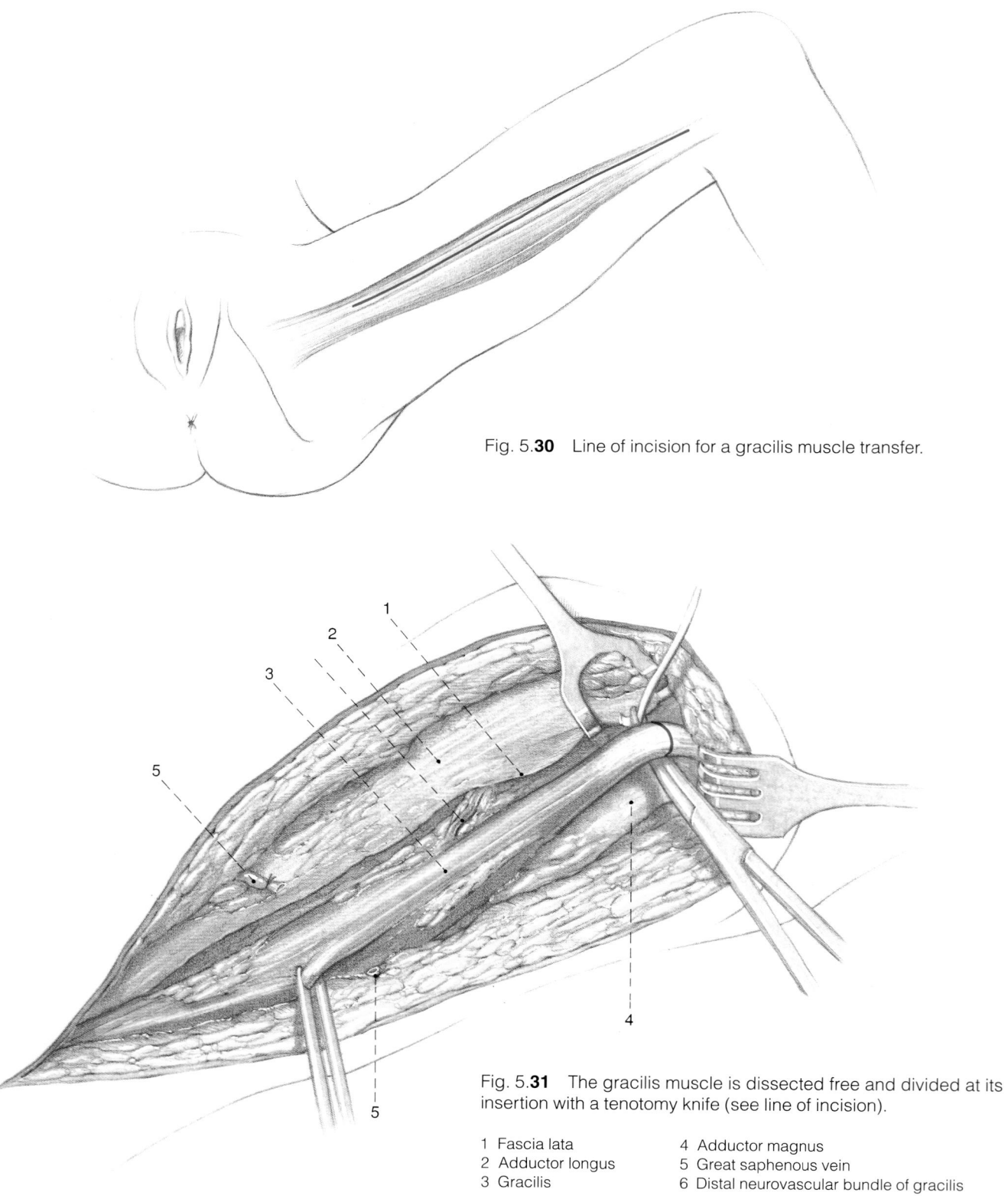

Fig. 5.**30**   Line of incision for a gracilis muscle transfer.

Fig. 5.**31**   The gracilis muscle is dissected free and divided at its insertion with a tenotomy knife (see line of incision).

1 Fascia lata	4 Adductor magnus
2 Adductor longus	5 Great saphenous vein
3 Gracilis	6 Distal neurovascular bundle of gracilis

After a counterincision is made on the medial side of the labium minus, a subcutaneous tunnel is developed in the groin, and the released gracilis is rotated into the tunnel (clockwise on the left side) without compromising its neurovascular supply. The flap receives an additional supply from the medial circumflex femoral artery in the proximal part of the muscle (Fig. 5.**32**).

Comments

This procedure can transfer well-vascularized soft tissue to the pelvic floor or between the bladder and vagina for the repair of large fistulae. Overlying skin can be used to produce a myocutaneous flap useful for concomitant bladder repair. The rectus abdominis muscle makes an acceptable alternative.

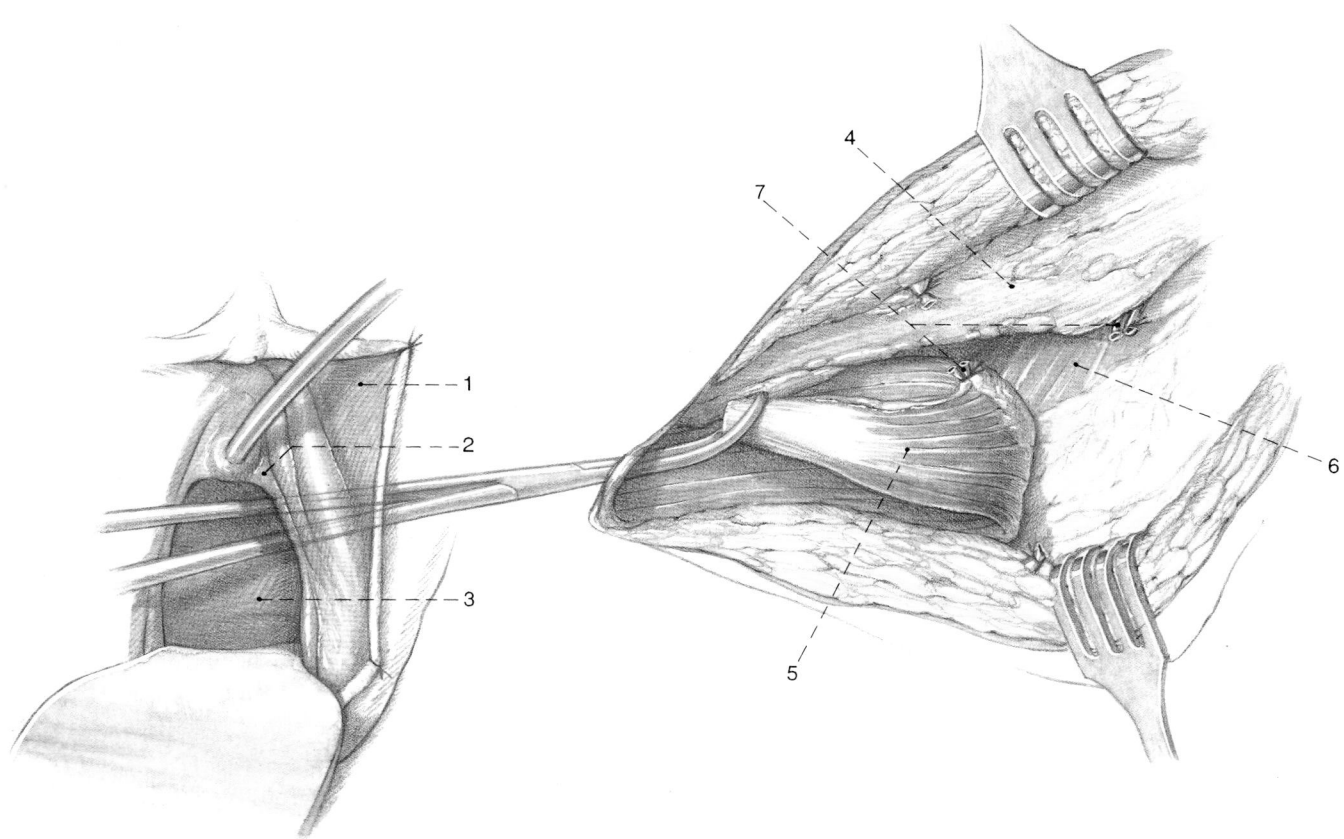

Fig. 5.**32** The gracilis muscle is tunneled to the defect through a counterincision at the labium minus.

1 Labium minus
2 Vestibule of vagina
3 Anterior vaginal wall
4 Adductor magnus
5 Gracilis
6 Adductor magnus
7 Distal neurovascular bundle of gracilis

Transvaginal Retropubic Approach for the Pereyra-Raz Vaginal Suspension

In the Pereyra-Raz technique of vaginal suspension, a vaginal flap is created with an inverted U-shaped incision whose apex is at the center of the urethra. After dissection of the urethrovaginal septum, the endopelvic fascia is divided at the pubic bone, and the index finger is passed into the retropubic space from inside the vagina. A short transverse incision is made over the symphysis, the rectus sheath is exposed, and the suspension needle is advanced along the finger into the vagina from the retropubic space (Fig. 5.33).

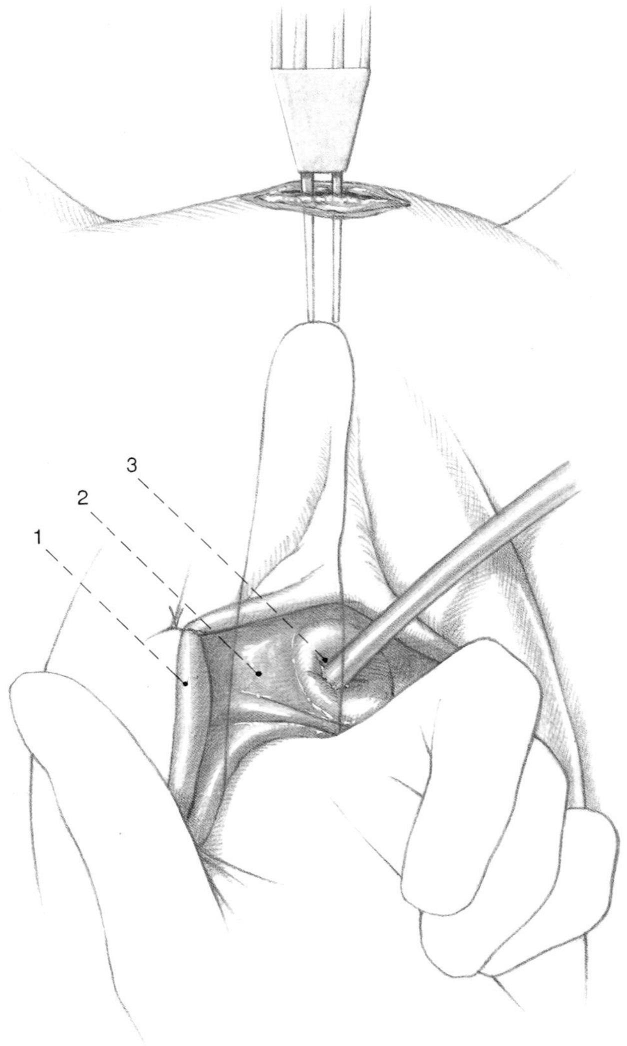

Fig. 5.**33** Approach for the Pereyra-Raz vaginal suspension procedure.

1 Labium minus
2 Vestibule of vagina
3 Urethra

6 Perineum

Anatomy of the Male Urethra and Pelvic Floor

The dissection in Fig. 6.1 demonstrates the relations of the corpus spongiosum to the pelvic floor. The corpus spongiosum is covered by the bulbospongiosus muscle and relates to the inferior aspect of the urogenital diaphragm, to which it is attached by loose connective tissue. The urogenital diaphragm consists essentially of tough, transversely oriented connective-tissue fibers, the transverse perineal ligament, which is reinforced posteriorly by deep transverse perineal muscle fibers. The superficial transverse perineal muscle completes the urogenital diaphragm superficially. All of these muscles, as well as the levator ani of the pelvic diaphragm and the external anal sphincter, converge at the central tendon of the perineum. These structures are demonstrated more clearly by removal of the corpus spongiosum at the bulb of the penis along with the bulbospongiosus muscle (Fig. 6.2).

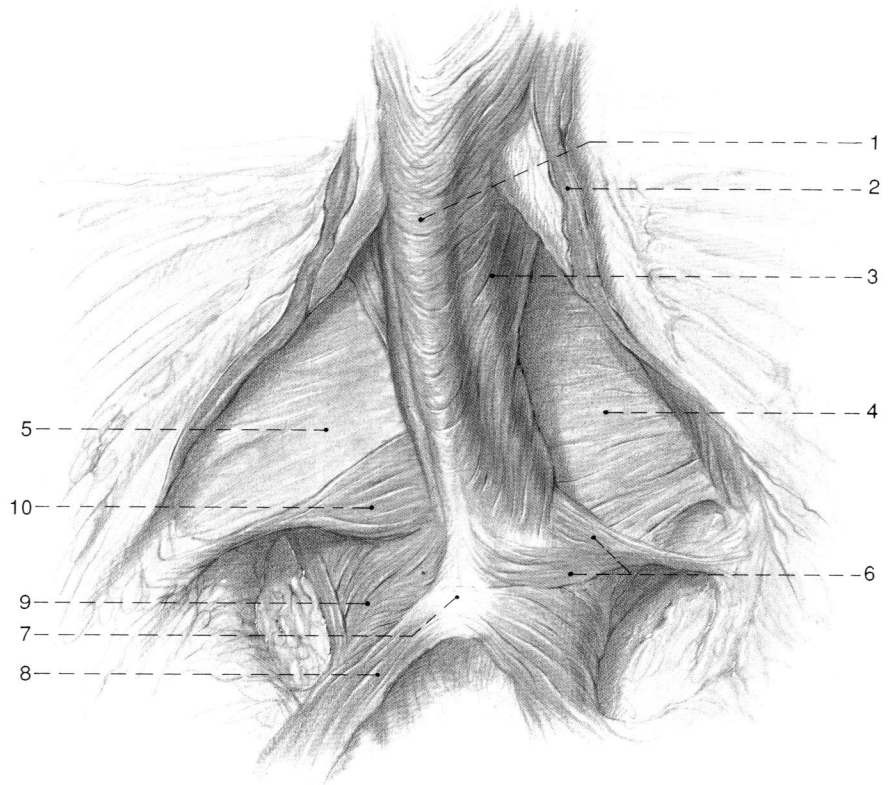

Fig. 6.1   Anatomic dissection showing the pelvic floor structures from the inferior aspect.

1 Corpus spongiosum
2 Ischiocavernosus muscle
3 Bulbospongiosus muscle
4 Urogenital diaphragm
5 Inferior fascia of urogenital diaphragm
6 Superficial transverse perineal muscle
7 Central tendon of perineum
8 External anal sphincter
9 Levator ani
10 Deep transverse perineal muscle

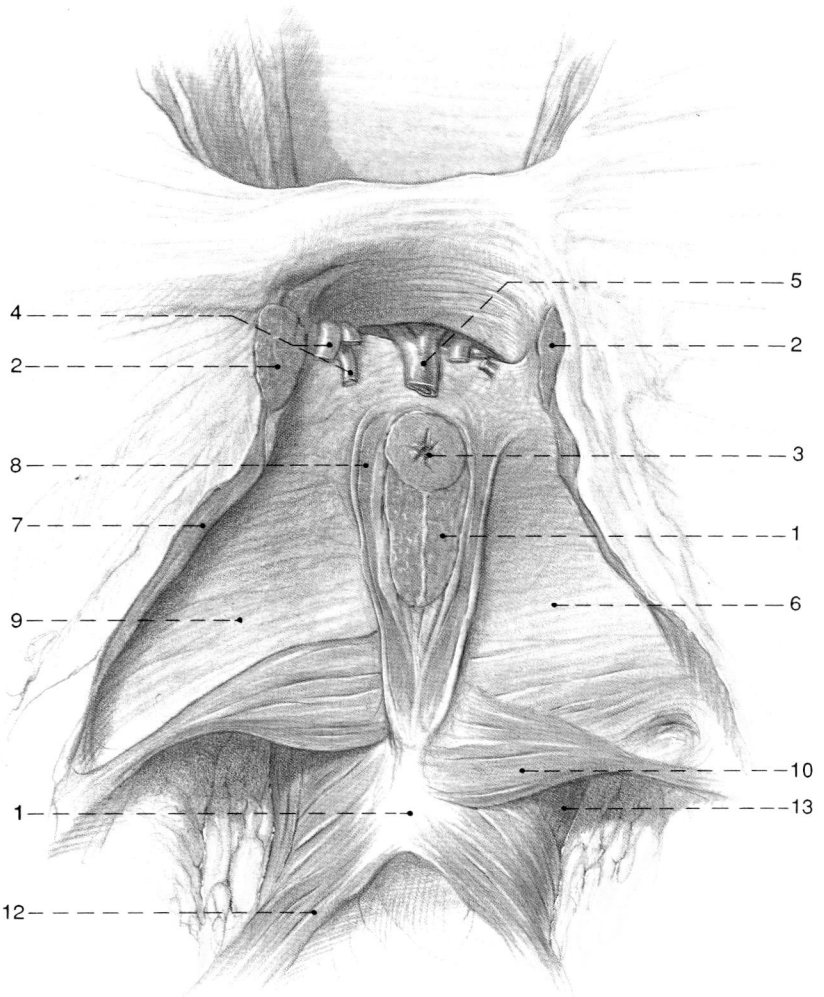

Fig. 6.**2**   Urogenital diaphragm after removal of the corpus spongiosum (anatomic dissection).

1   Corpus spongiosum (bulb)
2   Crus of penis
3   Urethra
4   Dorsal penile artery and nerve
5   Deep dorsal penile vein
6   Urogenital diaphragm
7   Ischiocavernosus muscle
8   Bulbospongiosus muscle
9   Inferior fascia of urogenital diaphragm
10   Superficial transverse perineal muscle
11   Central tendon of perineum
12   External anal sphincter
13   Levator ani

In another dissection (Fig. 6.**3**) the pubic bone has been partially removed to demonstrate the neurovascular supply of the penis (dorsal penile artery and nerve, deep dorsal penile vein). Removal of the pubic symphysis and corpora cavernosa renders a view of the urogenital diaphragm (Fig. 6.**4**).

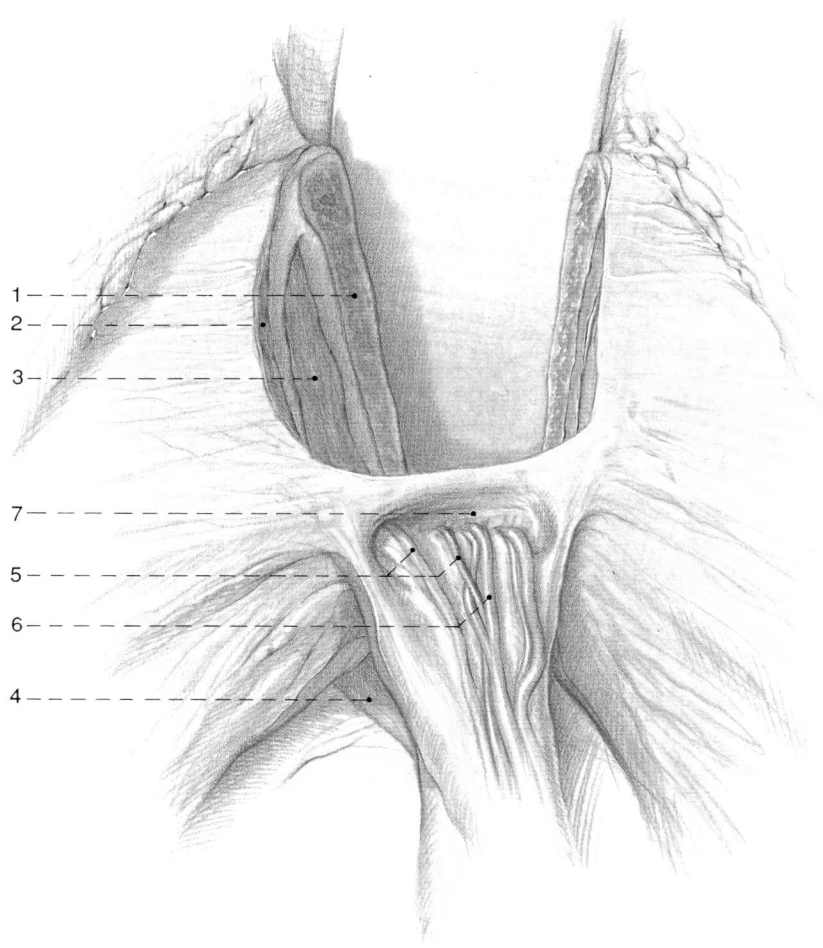

Fig. 6.**3** Dorsal neurovascular supply of the penis (anatomic dissection).

1 Superior pubic ramus
2 Gracilis
3 Adductor longus
4 Ischiocavernosus
5 Dorsal penile artery and nerve
6 Deep dorsal penile vein
7 Pubic arcuate ligament

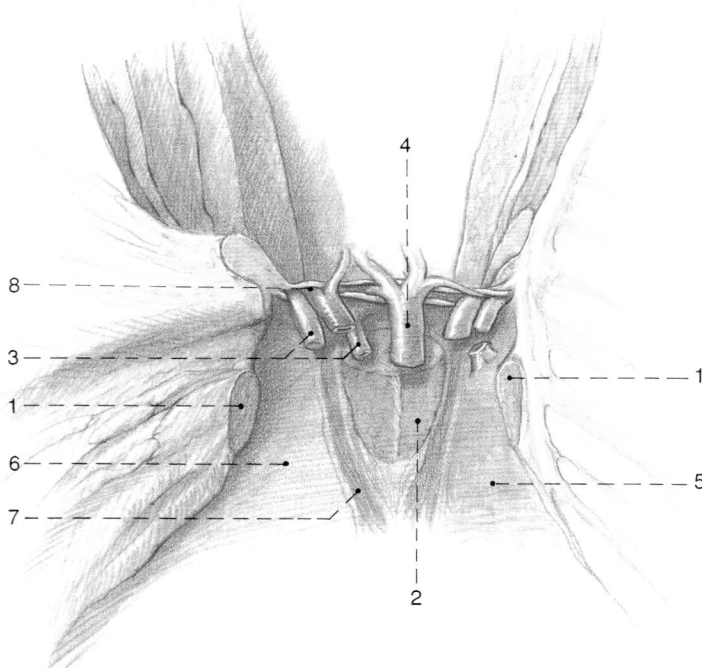

Fig. 6.**4** Appearance following resection of the corpora spongiosa and cavernosa (anatomic dissection).

1 Crus of penis
2 Bulb of penis
3 Dorsal penile artery and nerve
4 Deep dorsal penile vein
5 Urogenital diaphragm
6 Inferior fascia of urogenital diaphragm
7 Bulbospongiosus muscle
8 Superior fascia of urogenital diaphragm

Figure 6.5 shows the individual structures of the urogenital diaphragm in greater detail. Visible features include the pubic arcuate ligament, the transverse perineal ligament, and the external urethral sphincter, which forms a "horse-shoe" about the anterior and lateral aspects of the membranous urethra. The structures that pierce the urogenital diaphragm are also seen: the deep dorsal penile vein, the dorsal penile artery and nerve, and the membranous urethra. The bulb of the penis has been divided, leaving a remnant on the diaphragm.

In Fig. 6.6 the anterior circumference of the membranous urethra (from 9 to 3 o'clock) has been removed to demonstrate the lateral muscular portions of the urethral sphincter (rhabdosphincter). The artery of the bulb of the penis (bulbar artery) runs lateral to the membranous urethra. The dorsal penile artery and nerve perforate the transverse perineal ligament. The deep dorsal penile vein lies between the pubic arcuate ligament and transverse perineal ligament.

In Fig. 6.7 a grooved probe has been inserted into the urethra to open up its lumen. The probe is positioned in the lower circumference of the membranous urethra, exposing the lateral muscular portion of the external urethral sphincter.

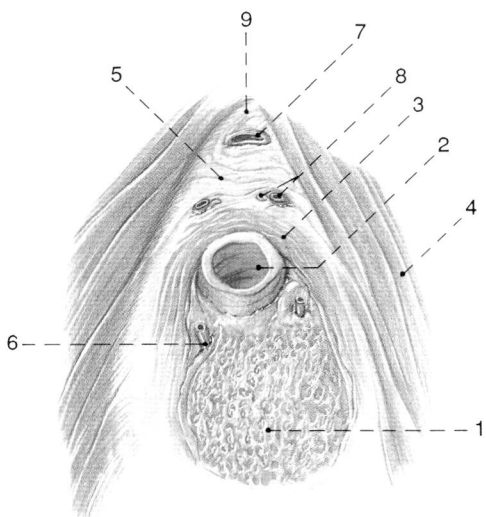

Fig. 6.5   Close-up view of the urogenital diaphragm.

1 Bulb of penis
2 Urethra
3 External urethral sphincter
4 Bulbospongiosus muscle
5 Transverse perineal ligament
6 Bulbar artery
7 Deep dorsal penile vein
8 Dorsal penile vessels and nerve
9 Pubic arcuate ligament

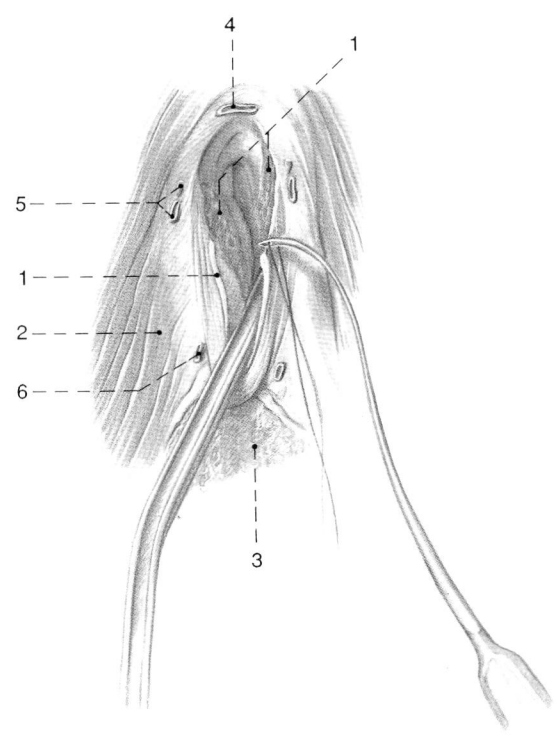

Fig. 6.7   The urethral lumen is held open with a grooved probe. The lateral muscular portion of the external urethral sphincter can be seen.

1 External urethral sphincter
2 Bulbospongiosus muscle
3 Bulb of penis
4 Deep dorsal penile vein
5 Dorsal penile vessels and nerve
6 Bulbar artery

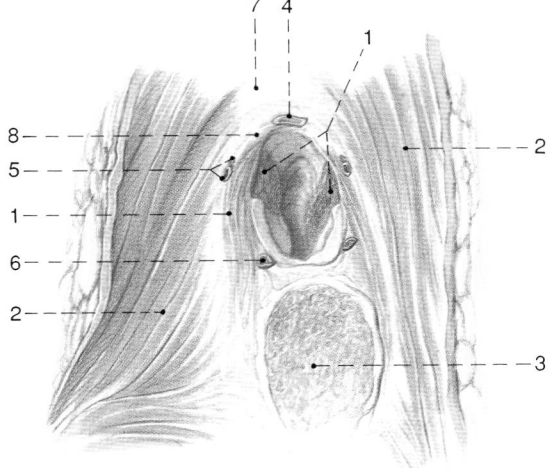

Fig. 6.6   The anterior circumference of the membranous urethra has been removed to expose the lateral muscular portion of the external urethral sphincter (rhabdosphincter).

1 External urethral sphincter
   (rhabdosphincter)
2 Bulbospongiosus muscle
3 Bulb of penis
4 Deep dorsal penile vein
5 Dorsal penile vessels and nerve
6 Bulbar artery
7 Pubic arcuate ligament
8 Transverse perineal ligament

Perineal Approach to the Posterior Urethra

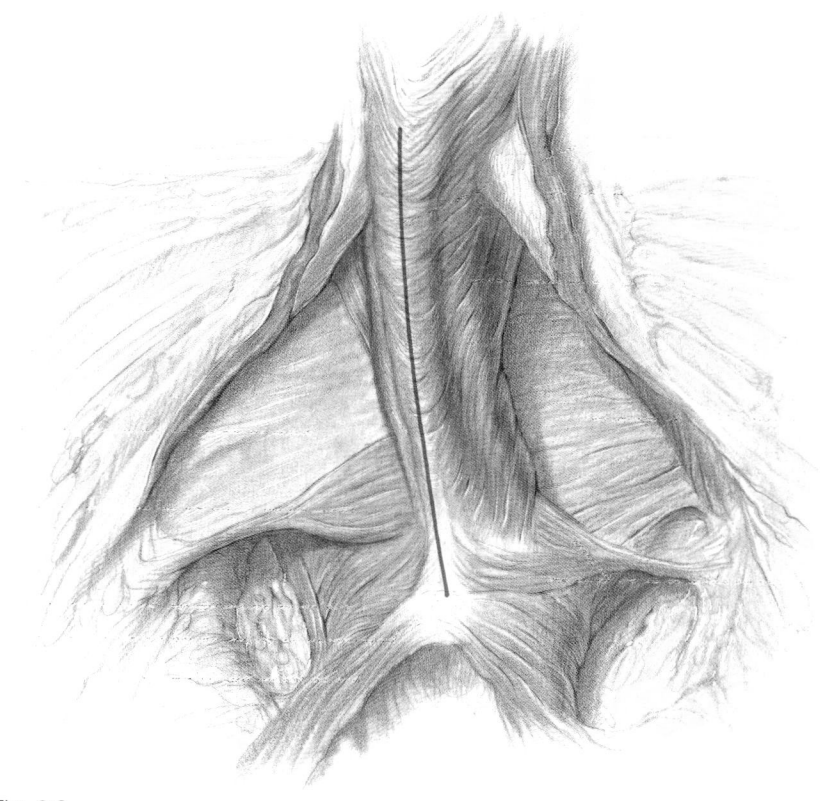

Fig. 6.**8**

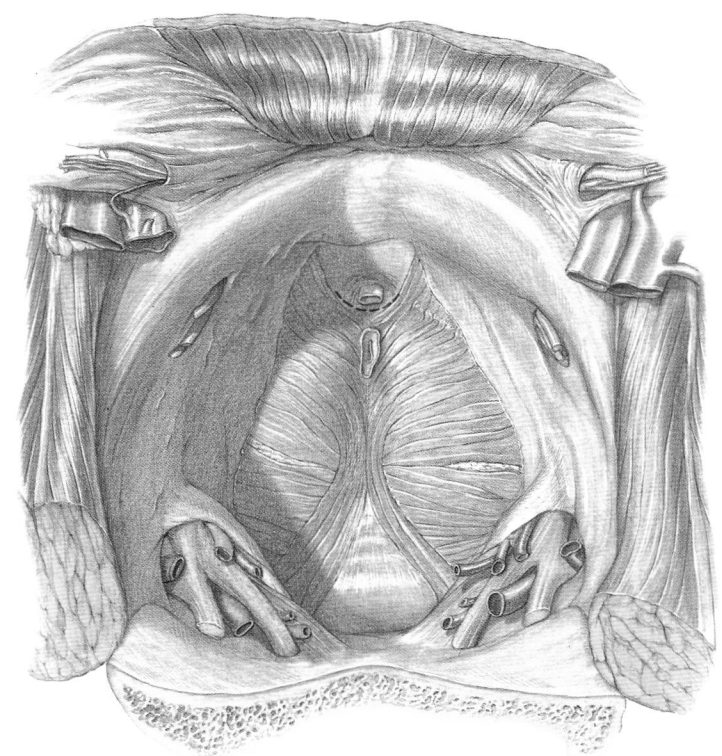

Fig. 6.**9**

Main Indications

- Stricture of the bulbar or membranous urethra
- Urethral disruption following pelvic trauma

Position and Skin Incision

The patient is placed in the standard dorsal lithotomy position for surgery of the bulbar urethra (Fig. 6.**10a**). Access to the membranous urethra for a stricture secondary to urethral disruption requires an extreme lithotomy position like that used in the perineal approach for a radical prostatectomy (Fig. 6.**10b**). Exposure of the perineal region is enhanced by adding Trendelenburg position and elevating the sacrum on a pad. The lower legs are fixed and angled toward the head.

The incision is placed strictly on the midline, extending along the scrotal raphe and over the perineum to the anal region (Fig. 6.**11**).

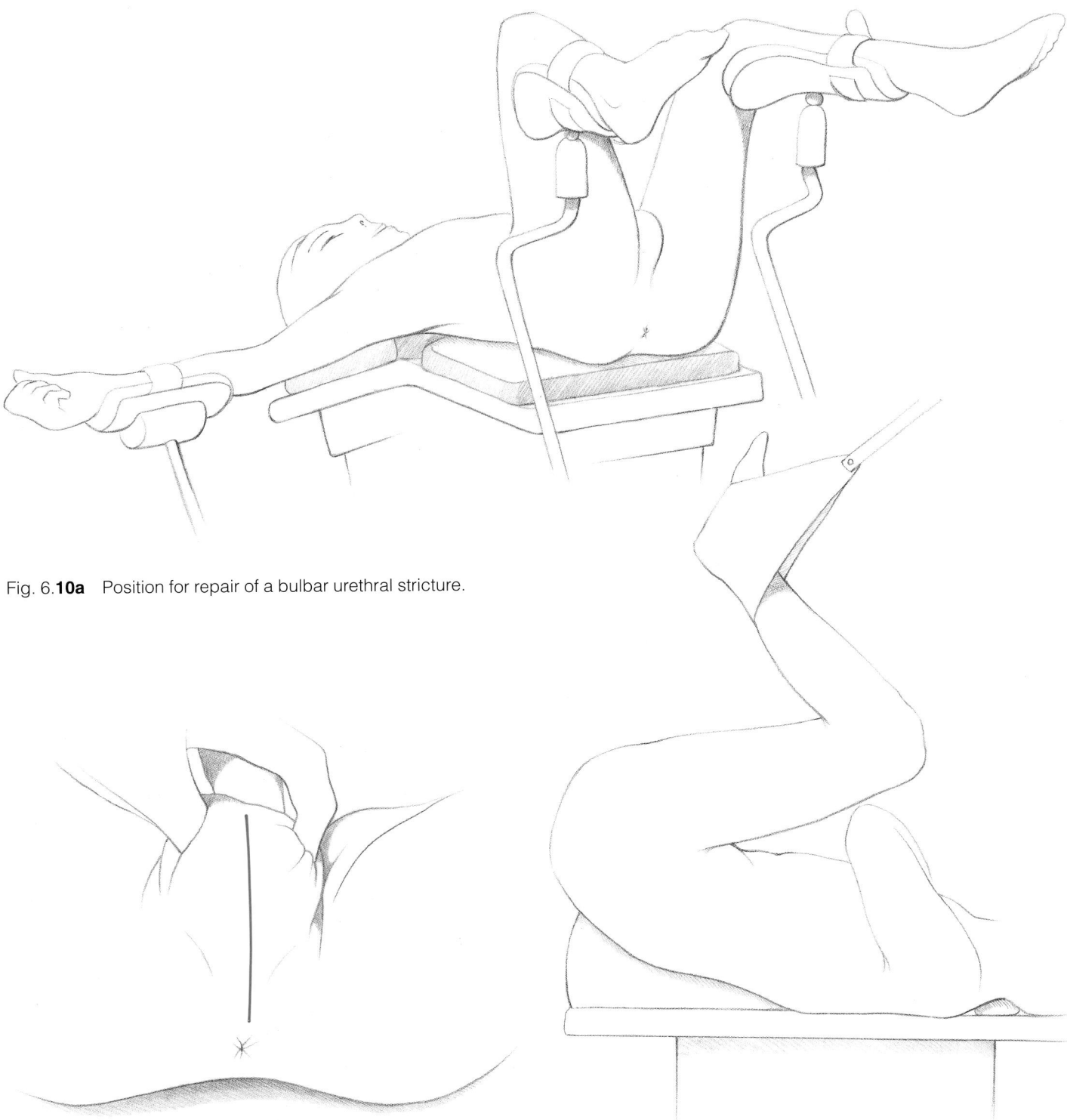

Fig. 6.**10a**   Position for repair of a bulbar urethral stricture.

Fig. 6.**11**   Line of incision.

Fig. 6.**10b**   Position for repair of a membranous urethral stricture.

Dissection of the Central Tendon

Both halves of the scrotum are held upward, and the scrotal skin, tunica dartos, and superficial perineal fascia are incised (Fig. 6.**12**). The testicular septum is incised on the midline, exposing the external spermatic fascia on both sides. In the perineal region, the superficial penile fascia is divided down to the central tendon of the perineum (Fig. 6.**13**). A Scott retractor is placed to maintain upward retraction of the skin, tunica dartos, and penile fascia (Fig. 6.**14**).

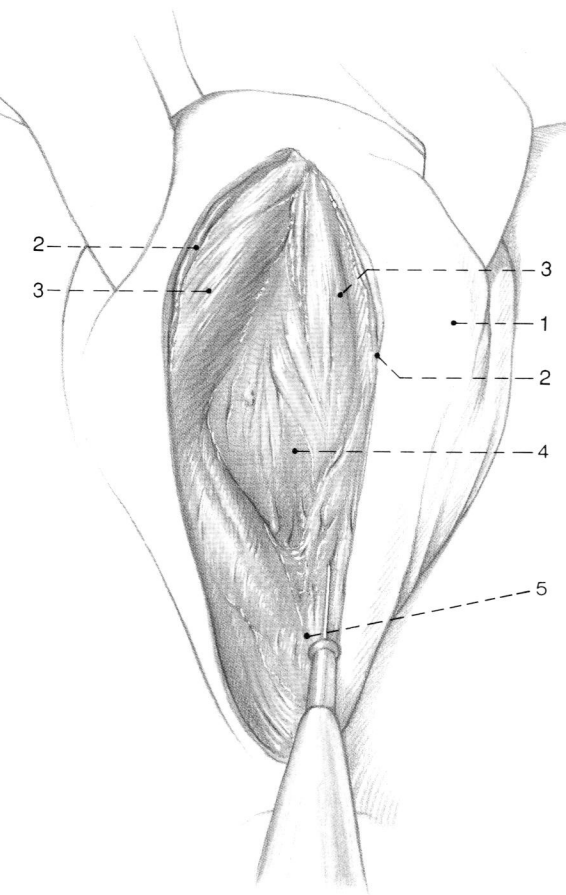

Fig. 6.**13** The testicular septum is divided.

1 Scrotum
2 Tunica dartos
3 Testis (external spermatic fascia)

4 Superficial penile fascia
5 Central tendon of perineum

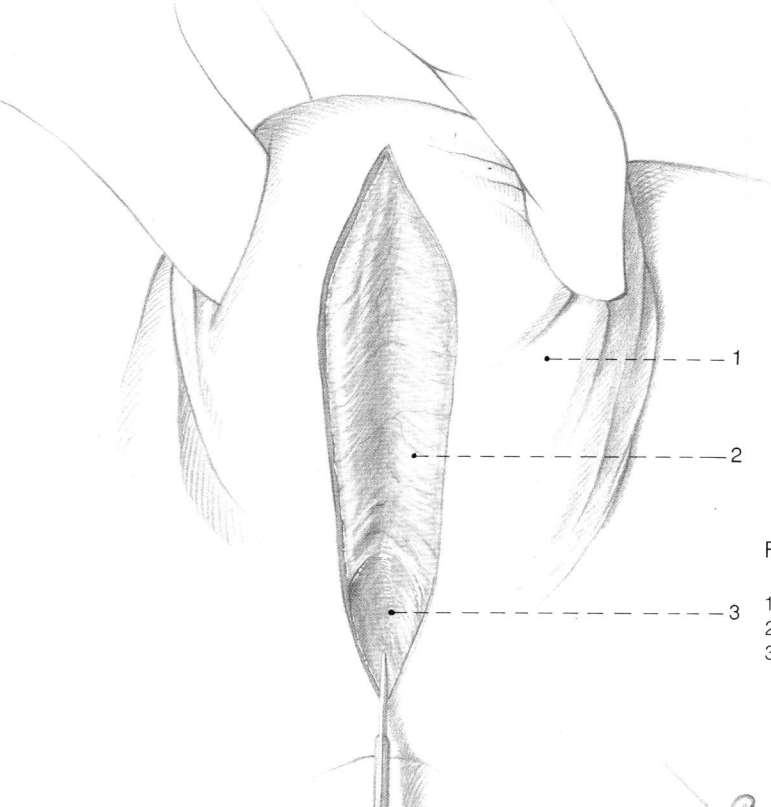

Fig. 6.**12** Division of the skin, tunica dartos, and perineal fascia.

1 Scrotum
2 Tunica dartos
3 Perineal fascia

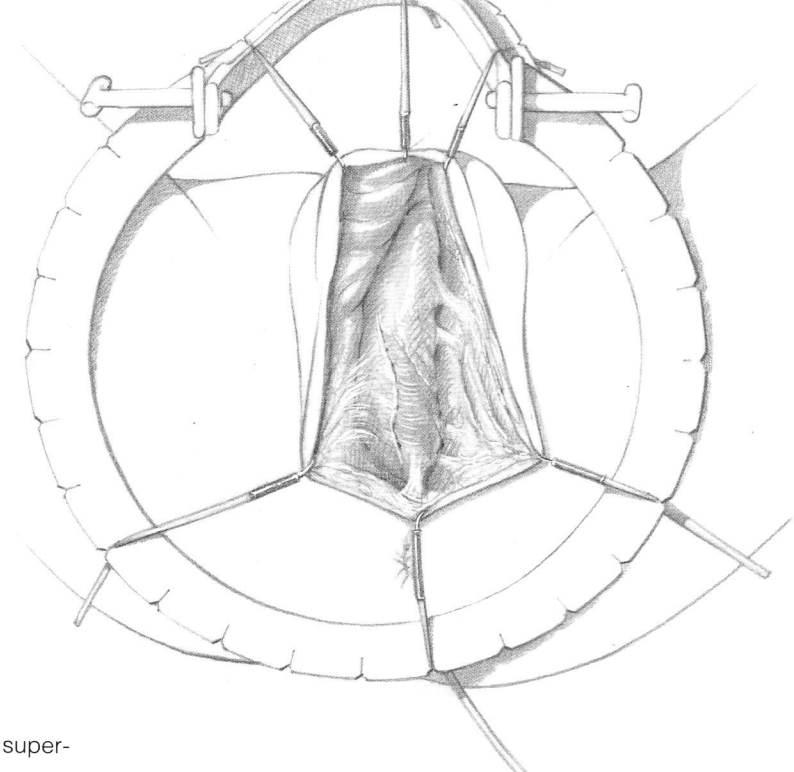

Fig. 6.**14** Upward retraction of the skin, tunica dartos, and superficial perineal fascia is maintained with a Scott retractor.

In the area of the corpus spongiosum, the midportion of the superficial penile fascia (Colles' fascia) over the bulbospongiosus muscle is incised on the line shown. The medial part of the ischiorectal fossa, the central tendon, and the external anal sphincter are exposed in the inferior wound angle (Fig. 6.15). The bulbospongiosus muscle is dissected off the corpus spongiosum from medially to laterally, and the bulb of the penis is freed from the muscular bed of the bulbospongiosus by upward traction on the corpus spongiosum. The origin of the bulbospongiosus is incised at its attachment to the central tendon. The inferior fascia of the urogenital diaphragm can be seen lateral to the dissected bulb (Fig. 6.16).

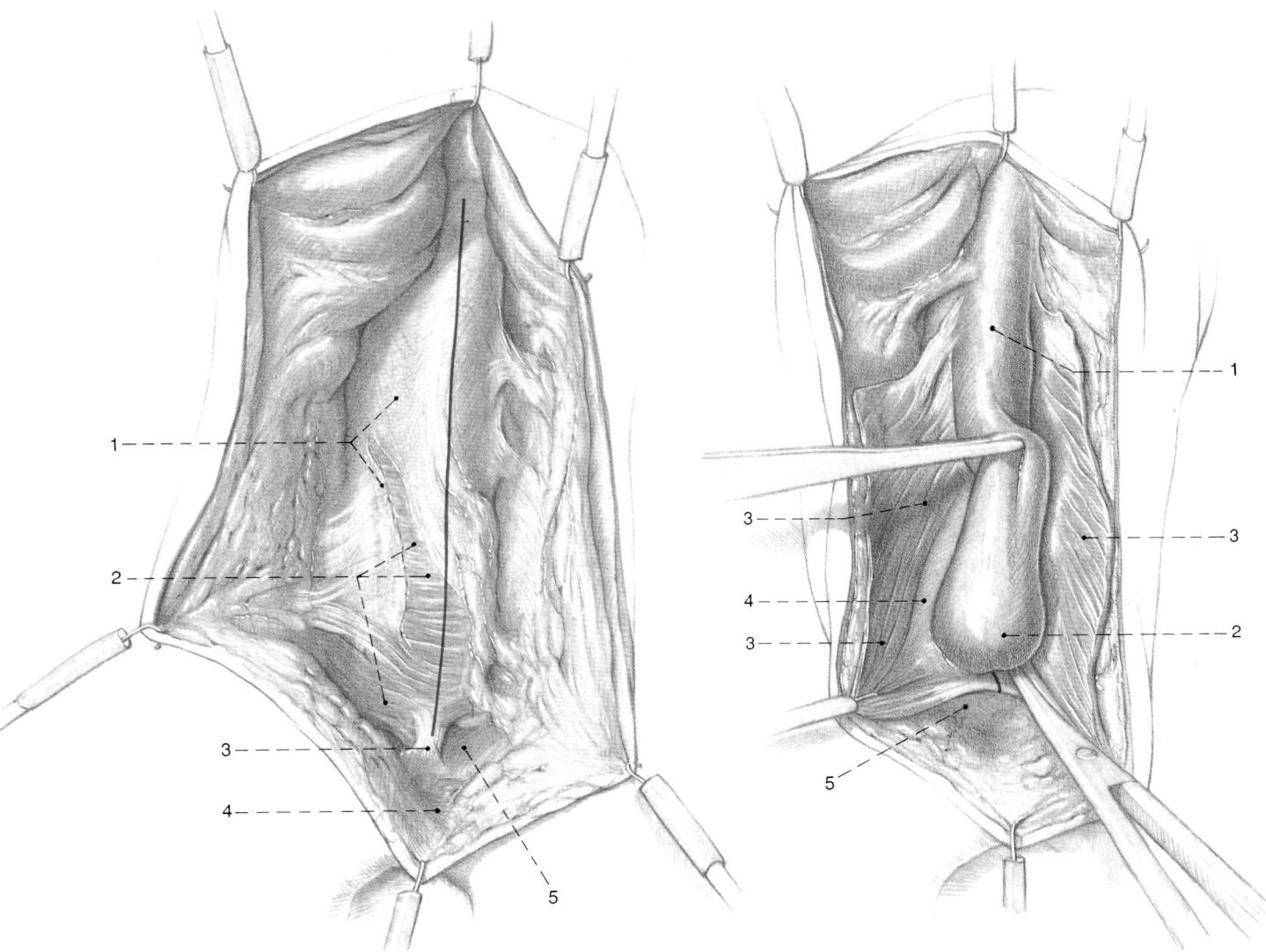

Fig. 6.15   The superficial penile fascia is opened on the midline over the bulbospongiosus muscle.

1 Superficial penile fascia
2 Bulbospongiosus muscle
3 Central tendon of perineum
4 External anal sphincter
5 Ischiorectal fossa

Fig. 6.16   The dorsal aspect of the bulb is dissected from the pelvic floor.

1 Corpus spongiosum
2 Bulb of penis
3 Bulbospongiosus muscle
4 Inferior fascia of urogenital diaphragm
5 Ischiorectal fossa

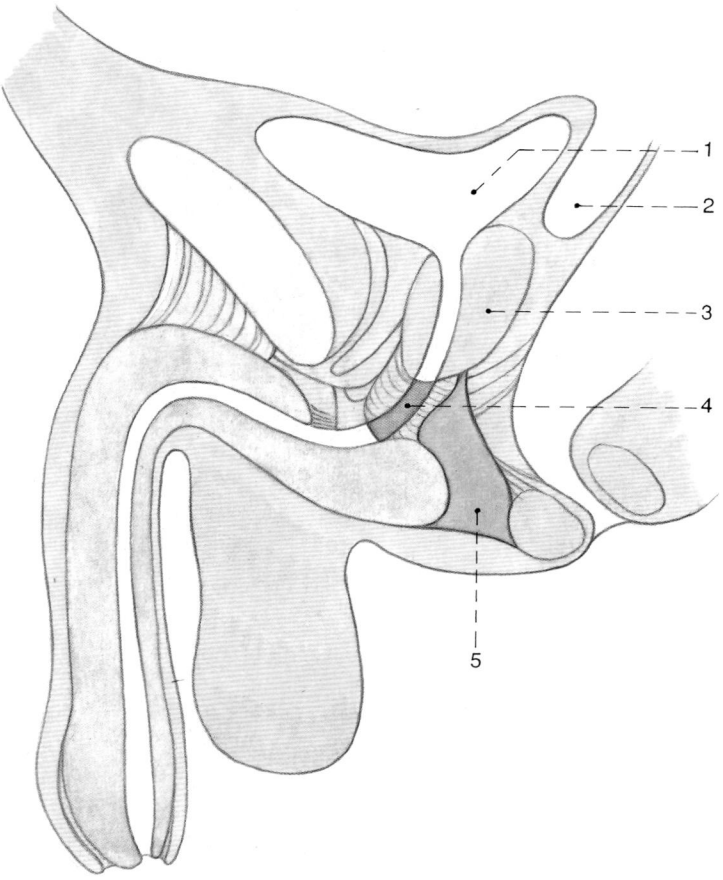

Dorsal Approach Through the Perineal Body

The dorsal approach is made through the wedge-shaped perineal body, which extends from the central tendon to the rectourethral septum (Fig. 6.**17**). The dissected bulb of the penis is held upward by its posterior surface, and individual bulbospongiosus muscle fibers are severed. The dorsal aspect of the bulb is sharply separated from the inferior urogenital fascia and the deep transverse perineal muscle (Fig. 6.**18**).

Figure 6.**19** illustrates the details of this approach. The corpus spongiosum is dissected free from the bulbospongiosus muscle, then the bulb is dissected from the pelvic floor (inferior fascia of urogenital diaphragm, deep transverse perineal muscle). The origins of the bulbospongiosus at the central tendon are divided. The bulbar artery and vein also are divided at this stage (Fig. 6.**19**).

◀ Fig. 6.**17** Scheme of the dorsal approach through the perineal body.

1 Bladder
2 Rectovesical pouch
3 Prostate
4 Membranous urethra
5 Approach to the urethra through the perineal body

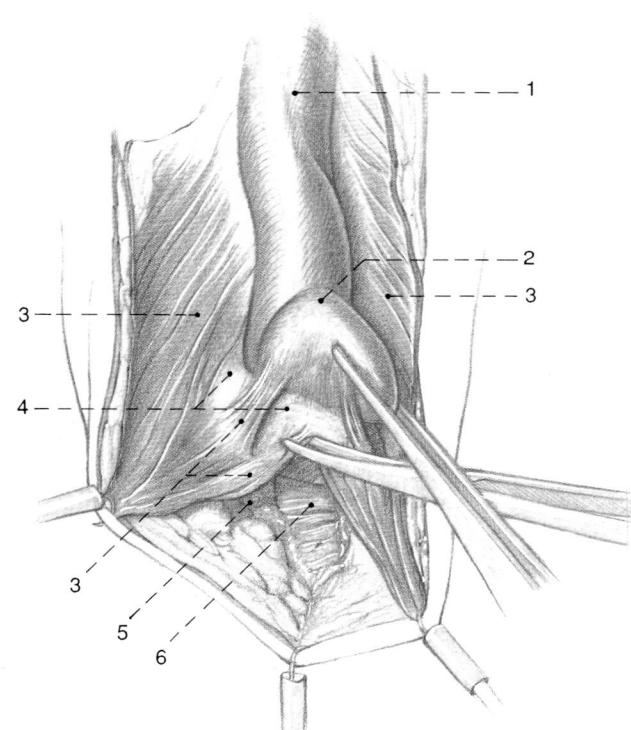

Fig. 6.**18** The bulbospongiosus muscle is removed. The tendinous origin of the bulbospongiosus is incised from front to back at the central tendon of the perineum.

1 Corpus spongiosum   4 Inferior fascia of urogenital diaphragm
2 Bulb of penis   5 Ischiorectal fossa
3 Bulbospongiosus muscle   6 External anal sphincter

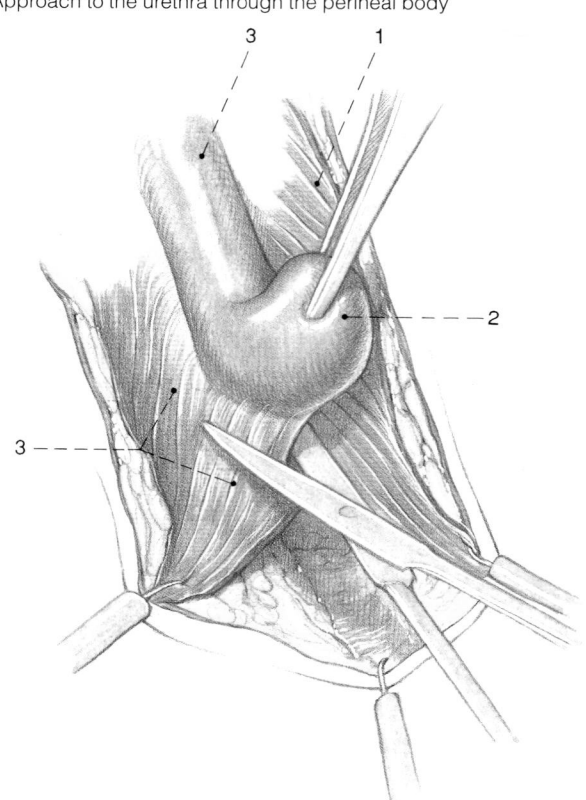

Fig. 6.**19** The bulbospongiosus fibers are detached from the dorsal aspect of the bulb.

1 Corpus spongiosum
2 Bulb of penis
3 Bulbospongiosus muscle

Division of the Urethra

The site of the stricture having been established, the mobilized penile bulb is retracted upward, and the urethra is transected at the bulbomembranous junction with scissors held parallel to the pelvic floor (Fig. 6.**20**). The corpus spongiosum is easily dissected out of the urethral sulcus of the corpus cavernosum (Fig. 6.**21**). The bulbar urethra is incised and snared.

After division of the urethra, the structures of the pelvic floor can be identified: the inferior fascia of the urogenital diaphragm, the transverse perineal ligament, and the membranous urethra (Fig. 6.**21**).

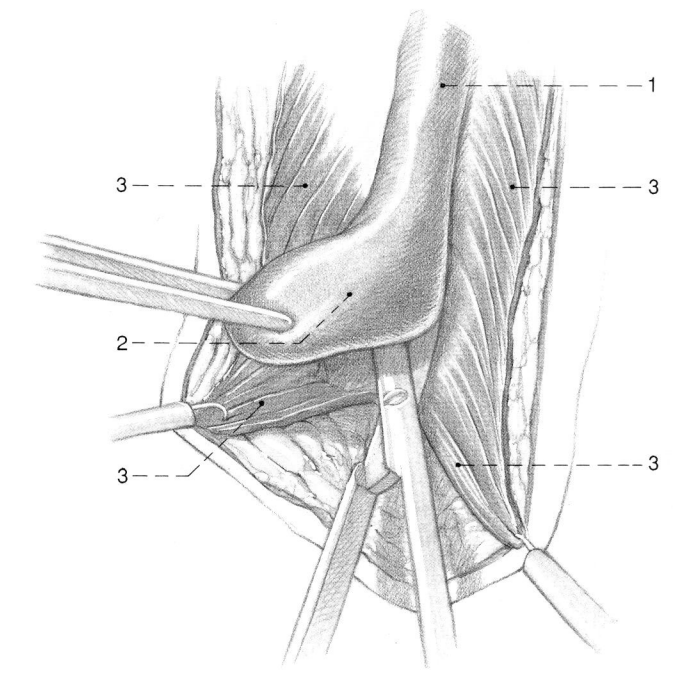

Fig. 6.**20**   Transection of the urethra through the dorsal approach. ▶
The scissors are directed parallel to the pelvic floor.

1 Corpus spongiosum
2 Bulb of penis
3 Bulbospongiosus muscle

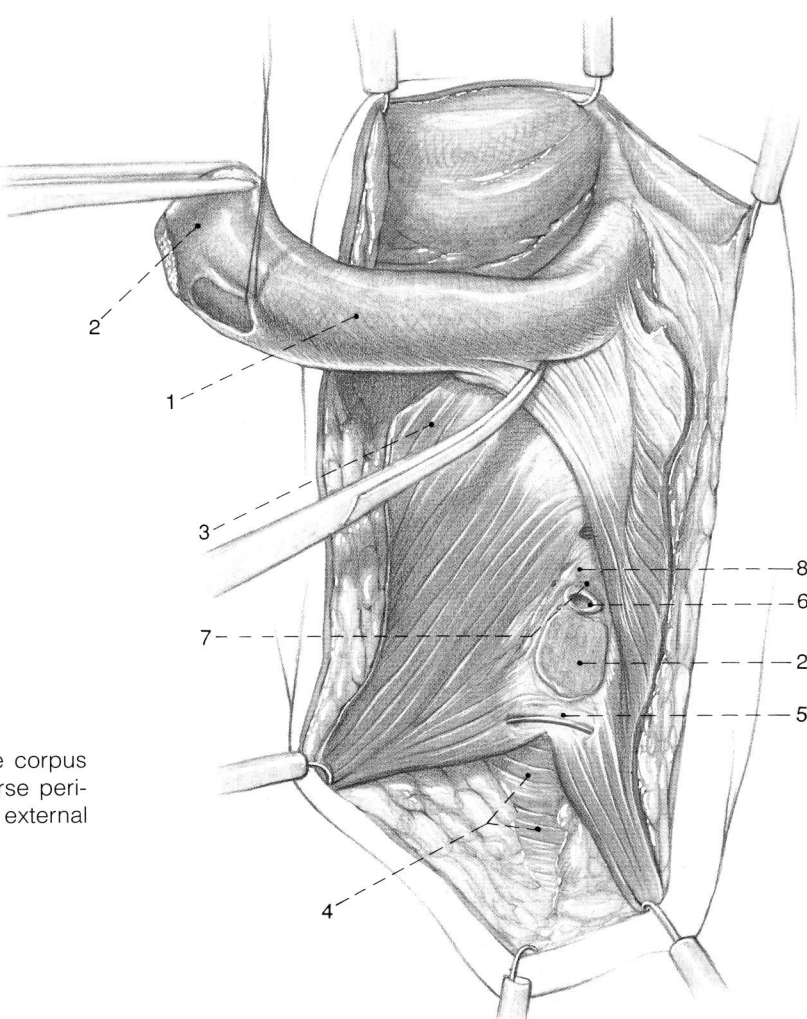

Fig. 6.**21**   The urethra is transected and freed from the corpus cavernosum, exposing the pelvic floor with the transverse perineal ligament, membranous urethra, central tendon, and external anal sphincter.

1 Corpus spongiosum
2 Bulb of penis
3 Bulbospongiosus muscle
4 External anal sphincter
5 Central tendon of perineum
6 Membranous urethra
7 External urethral sphincter
8 Transverse perineal ligament

Dissection of the Rectourethral Septum

This approach is used for the treatment of rectoprostatic fistulae or a very markedly displaced proximal prostatic urethral stump. The thick connective tissue at the apex of the perineal body is incised transversely (Fig. 6. 21).

Division of the rectourethral septum provides access for the dissection of Denonvillier's fascia (Fig. 6.22). The rectogenital septum is opened, and the posterior surface of the prostate is dissected free. A rectoprostatic fistula can be exposed by this perineal route.

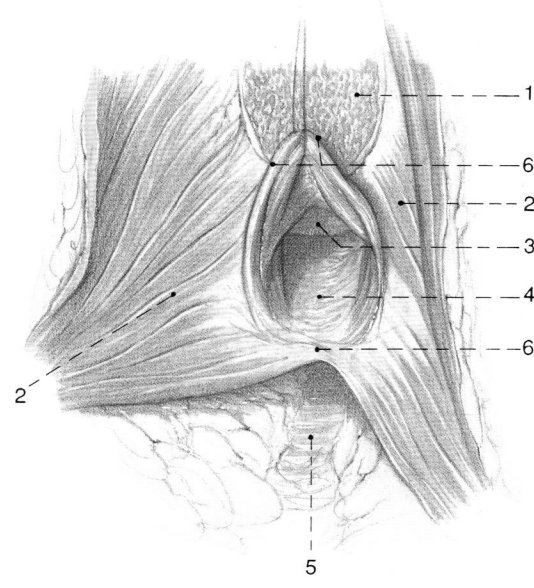

Fig. 6.**22**   Division of the rectourethral septum and exposure of Denonvillier's space. The anterior part of the central tendon is reflected upward with a traction suture.

1 Bulb of penis
2 Bulbospongiosus muscle
3 Denonvillier's fascia
4 Rectourethral septum
5 External anal sphincter
6 Central tendon

Dissection of the Prostatic Urethra (Entry into the Pubourethral Space)

The prostatic urethral stump is not mobilized. After the excision of scar tissue, a portion of the prostatic capsule and parenchyma is resected from the prostatic urethra to permit adequate opening of the urethra in preparation for its anastomosis to the stump of the bulbar urethra (Fig. 6.23).

The dissection for this approach shows the external anal sphincter, the central tendon, the bulbospongiosus muscle, and the opened prostatic urethra. Fibers of the levator ani enter the central tendon lateral to the prostate (Fig. 6.23). The sites of insertion of the levator ani and bulbospongiosus into the central tendon are particularly well demonstrated in this specimen.

Comments

Besides a simple midline incision, the approach can be made through a longitudinal midline incision that is bifurcated posteriorly in an inverted U shape toward the ischial tuberosities.

The stump of the prostatic urethra should be freed of all scar tissue on the median plane, but it should never be mobilized (to respect the anatomic course of the cavernous nerves). The length necessary for the anastomosis is gained by mobilizing the penile urethra from the corpus cavernosum. If heavy retrosymphyseal scarring has resulted from faulty primary treatment of a urethral disruption (retrosymphyseal urinoma and hematoma), the approach, in very selected patients, must be extended by adding a symphyseal resection. A short stricture of the membranous urethra following a transurethral or suprapubic prostatectomy can be managed by a bulbar sleeve anastomosis with preservation of the external urethral sphincter, as shown in the dissection (see Fig. 6.7).

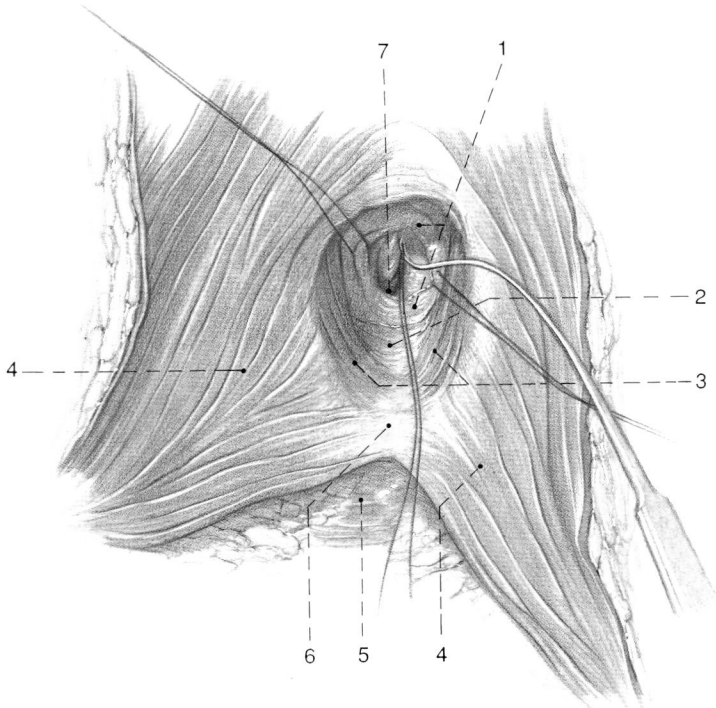

Fig. 6.23 Anastomotic sutures are preplaced in the prostatic urethra. Lateral to the prostate, the levator ani muscle bundles insert into the central tendon.

1 Prostate
2 Rectourethral septum
3 Levator ani and puborectalis muscles
4 Bulbospongiosus muscle
5 External anal sphincter
6 Central tendon
7 Prostatic urethra

Transpubic Approach

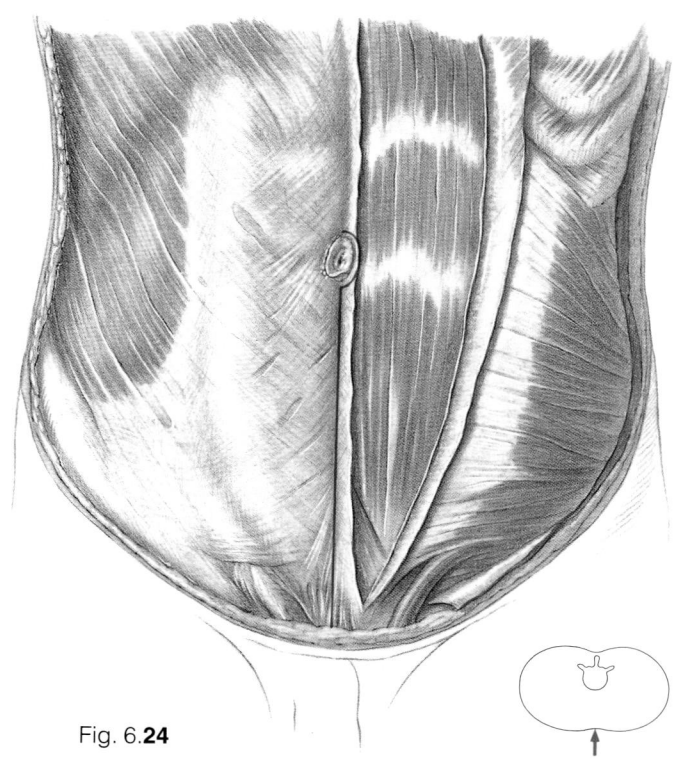

Fig. 6.**24**

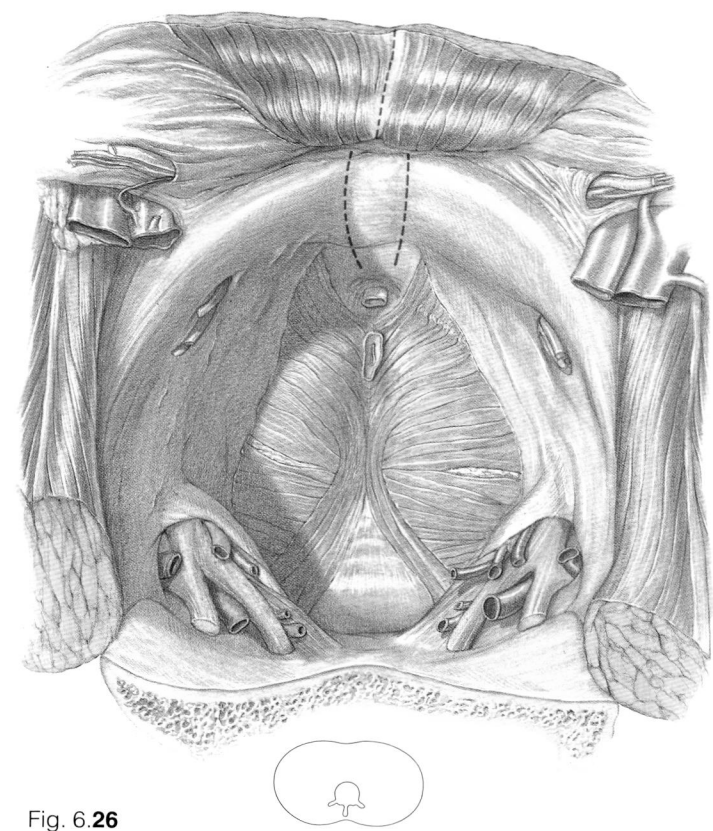

Fig. 6.**26**

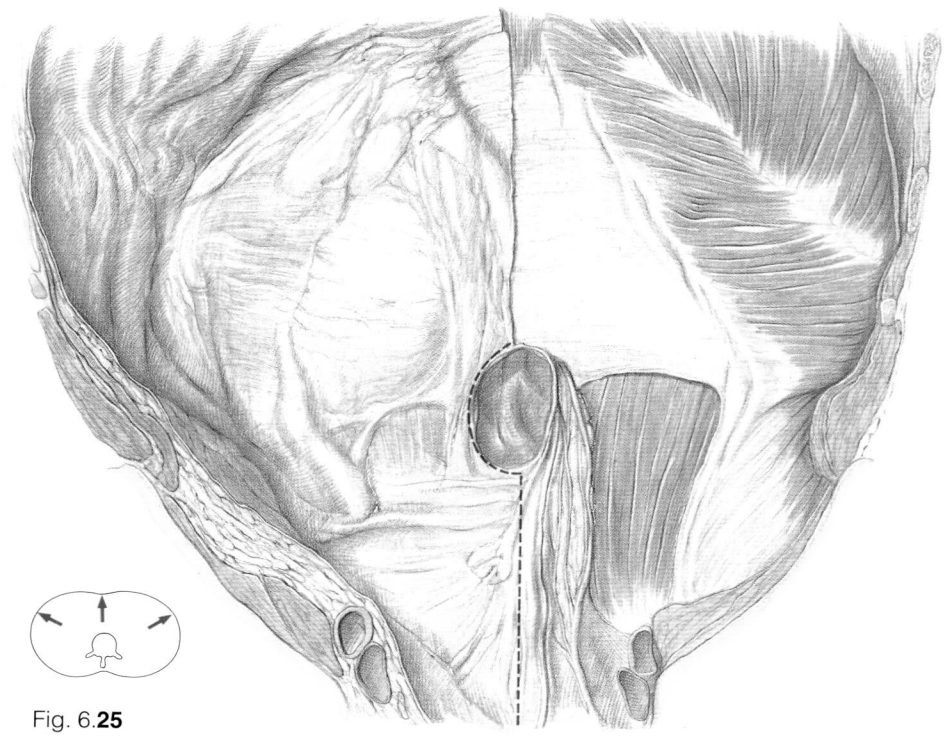

Fig. 6.**25**

Main Indications

- Posterior urethral stricture with heavy retrosymphyseal scarring
- Markedly retracted prostatic stump

Position and Skin Incision

The patient is placed in a hyperextended lithotomy position that allows for a combined perineal and transpubic approach (Fig. 6.27).

The skin incision starts above the umbilicus and extends to the base of the penis on the midline (Fig. 6.28).

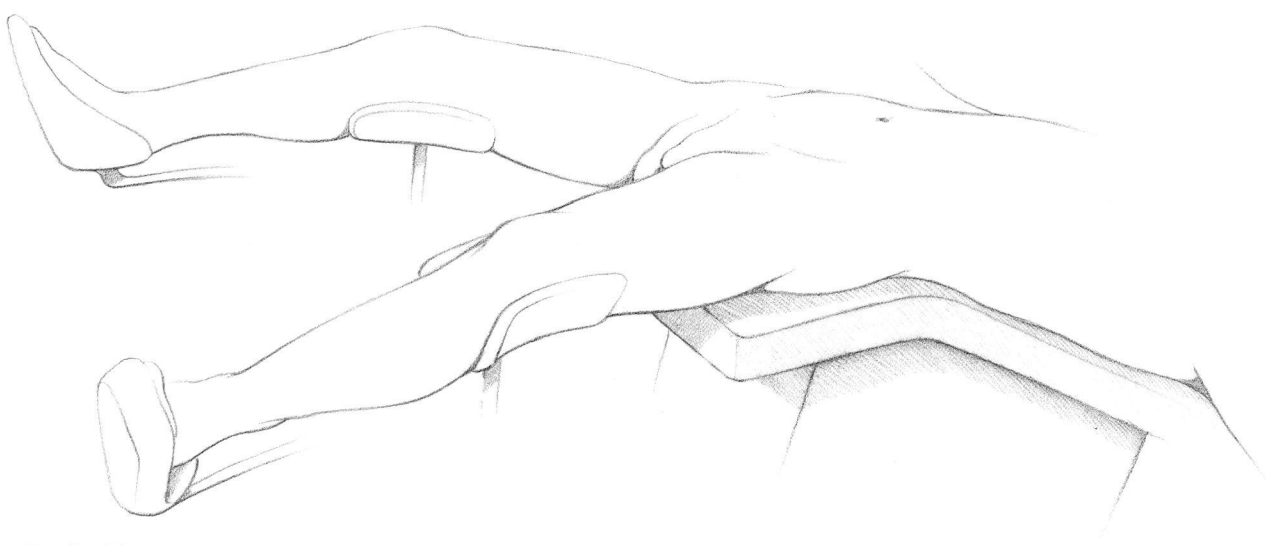

Fig. 6.27 Position.

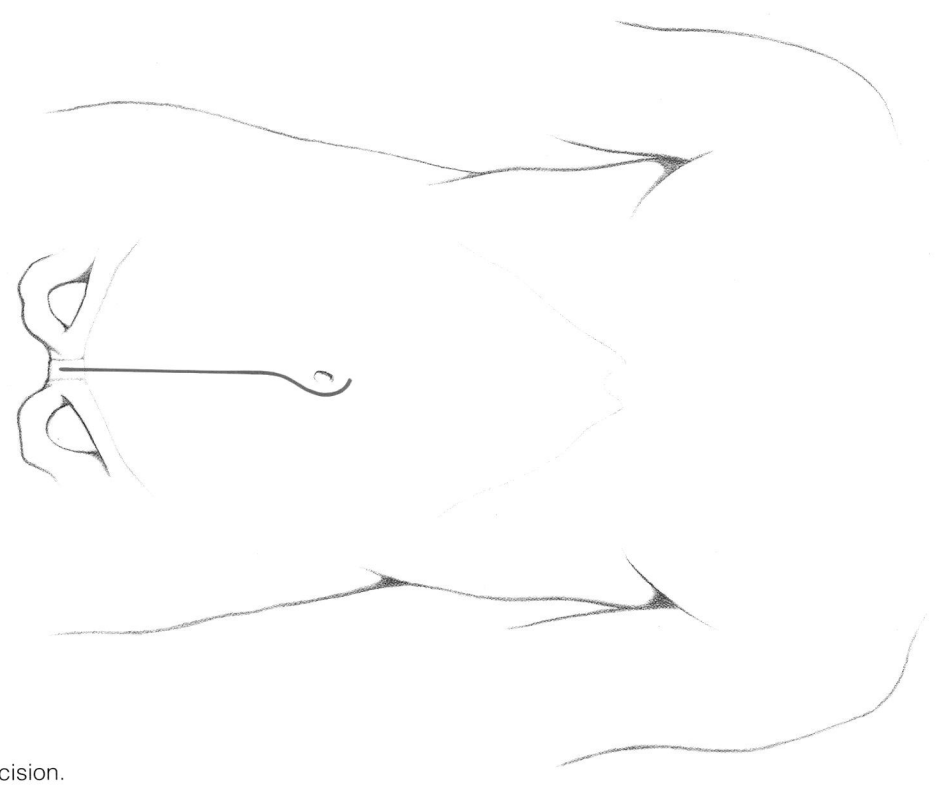

Fig. 6.28 Skin incision.

Exposure of the Pubic Symphysis (Extraperitoneal Midline Approach)

The linea alba is exposed, the anterior rectus sheath is incised, and both rectus muscles are separated at the midline. The posterior rectus sheath and transversalis fascia are opened. The prevesical space is dissected and exposed (Fig. 6.29), and the pyramidalis muscle is divided in the inferior portion of the wound (Fig. 6.29). The rectus insertion on the pubic symphysis is divided on the line indicated.

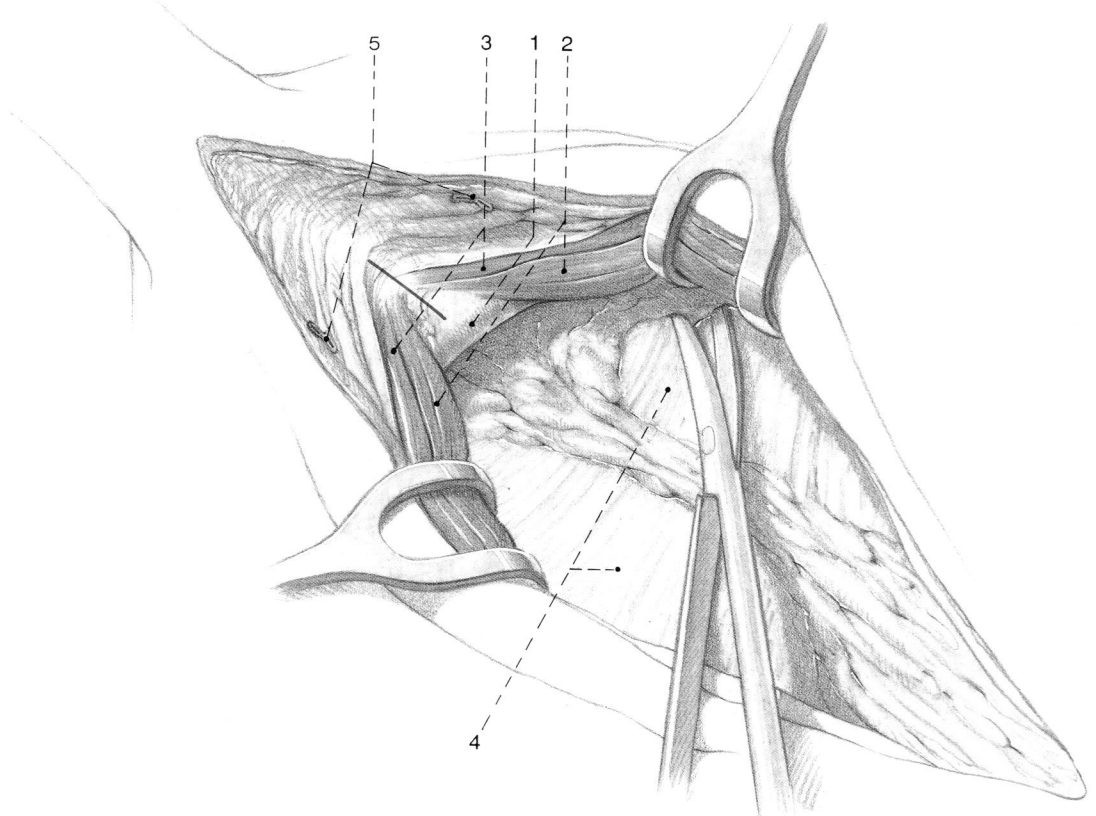

Fig. 6.29   Incision of the rectus sheath and exposure of the symphysis.

1 Pubic symphysis
2 Rectus muscle
3 Pyramidalis muscle
4 Transversalis fascia
5 External pudendal vessels

The subcutaneous fat is divided to the base of the penis, and the external pudendal vessels are ligated in the lateral part of the field (Fig. 6.**29**). Both cremaster muscles are exposed (Fig. 6.**30**). The penile suspensory ligament is divided, and the anterior surface of the pubic symphysis is exposed (Fig. 6.**30**).

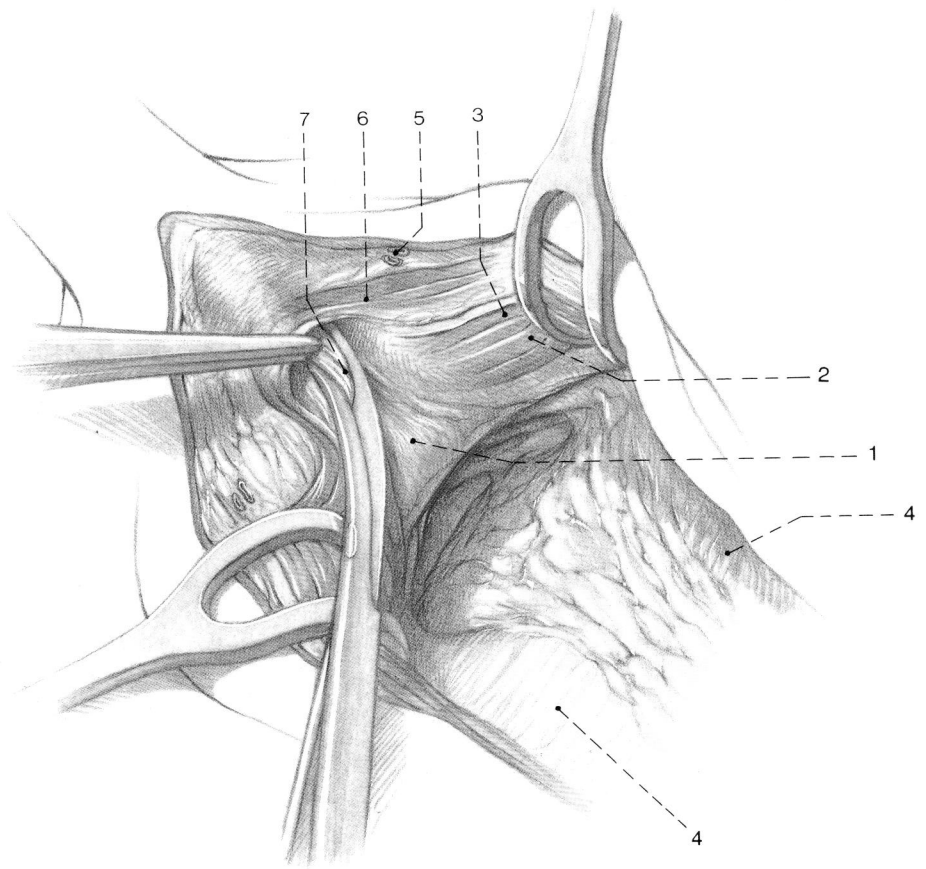

Fig. 6.**30**   The anterior surface of the symphysis is exposed, and the penile suspensory ligament is divided.

1 Pubic symphysis
2 Rectus muscle
3 Pyramidalis muscle
4 Transversalis fascia
5 External pudendal vessels
6 Cremaster muscle
7 Penile suspensory ligament

Resection of the Pubic Symphysis

The origins of the adductor muscles are released laterally to the origin of the gracilis using electrocautery or a periosteal elevator. The pelvic floor is incised far laterally between the arcuate ligament and transverse perineal ligament (Figs. **6.31**, **6.32**).

The bladder and anterior wall of the prostate are now deflected downward (sponge stick) to expose the retropubic space (Fig. **6.32**). A clamp is introduced into the lateral pelvic floor incision and advanced beneath the symphysis under vision, keeping directly on its periosteal surface (Fig. **6.32**). Then a 2-cm-wide central segment of the symphysis is removed with a Gigli saw (see resection lines).

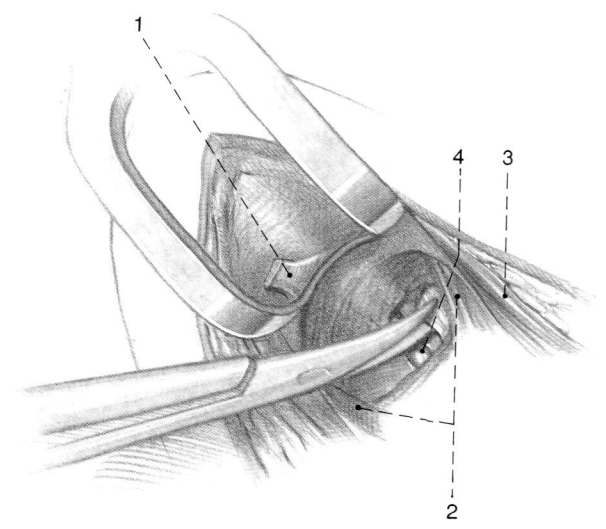

Fig. 6.**31**   Incision of the pelvic floor.

1 Penile suspensory ligament
2 Gracilis muscle
3 Cremaster muscle
4 Deep dorsal penile vein

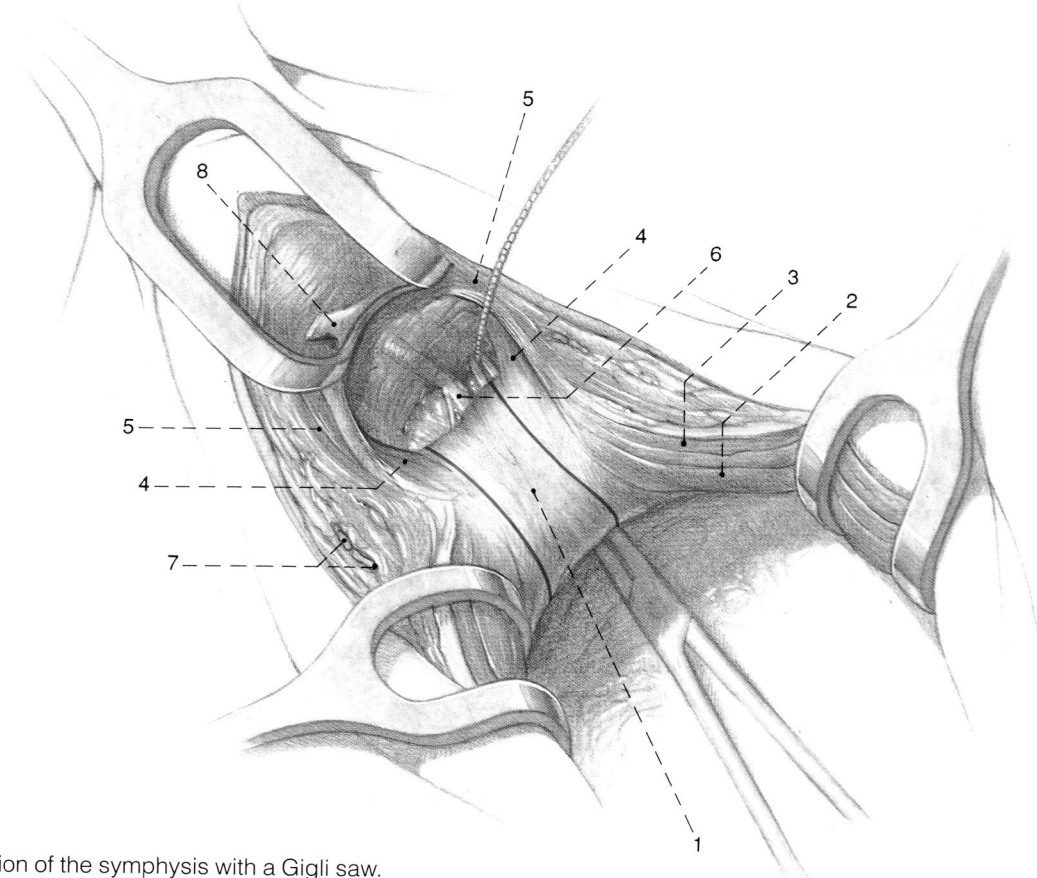

Fig. 6.**32**   Resection of the symphysis with a Gigli saw.

1 Pubic symphysis
2 Rectus muscle
3 Pyramidalis muscle
4 Gracilis muscle
5 Cremaster muscle
6 Deep dorsal penile vein
7 External pudendal vessels
8 Penile suspensory ligament

Figure 6.**33** shows the situation after partial resetion of the symphysis. The inserting fibers of the rectus and gracilis muscles and the spongiosa of the pubis are identified. Also visible are the deep dorsal penile vein, the prostatic venous plexus, and the visceral layer of the pelvic fascia of the prostate and bladder (Fig. 6.**33**).

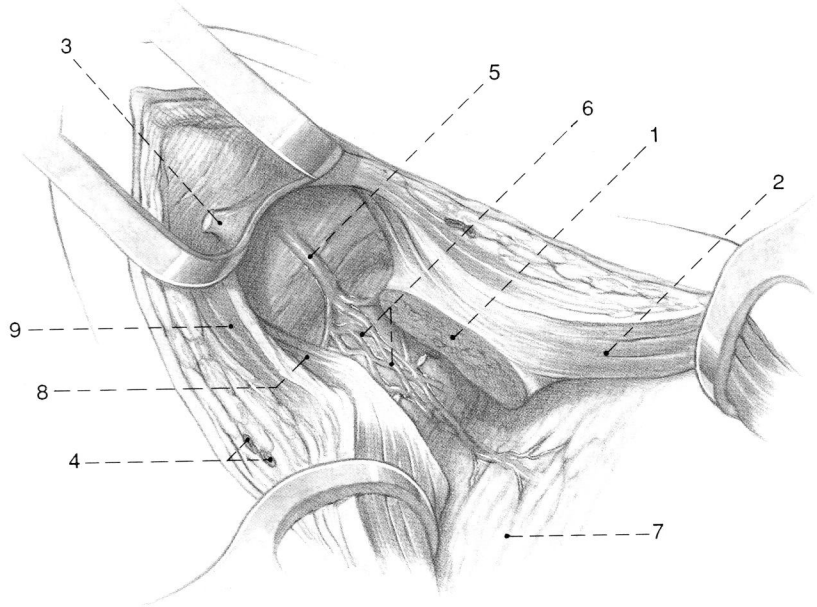

Fig. 6.**33** Appearance after resection of the symphysis. The deep dorsal penile vein and prostatic venous plexus have been dissected free.

1 Pubic bone
2 Rectus muscle
3 Penile suspensory ligament
4 External pudendal vessels
5 Deep dorsal penile vein
6 Prostatic venous plexus
7 Visceral pelvic fascia (vesical fascia)
8 Gracilis muscle
9 Cremaster muscle

Exposure of the Pubourethral Space

The dorsal vein complex is ligated, and scar tissue is excised from about the prostatic urethral stump. Following the resection of prostatic capsule and parenchyma, a satisfactory anastomotic site is prepared at the prostatic urethral stump (Fig. 6.**34**).

After the stricture site has been localized, the bulbar urethral stump is mobilized from the pubourethral space.

Comments

This combined transpubic-perineal approach is reserved for highly selected patients where there is a markedly retracted prostatic urethral stump or pronounced retrosymphyseal fibrosis.

In contrast to the dorsal approach through the perineal body, which is associated with little bleeding, the transpubic approach poses difficulties relating to the pelvic floor resection and the dissection of the dorsal vein complex. The incision in the pelvic floor must be placed well laterally to avoid injury to the deep dorsal vein, the dorsal penile artery (which pierces the transverse perineal ligament), and the dorsal penile nerve.

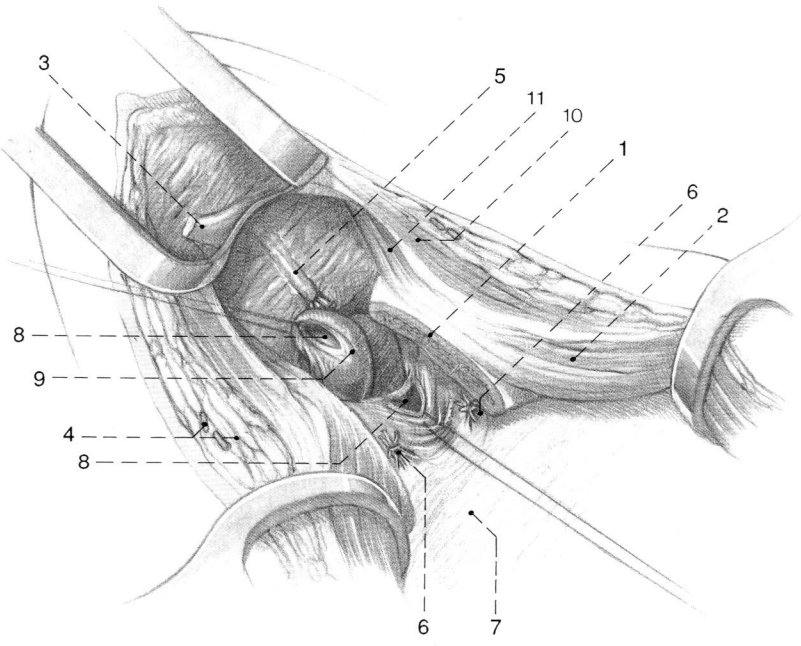

Fig. 6.**34**   Exposure of the prostatic and bulbar urethral stumps in preparation for the bulboprostatic anastomosis.

 1 Pubic bone
 2 Rectus muscle
 3 Penile suspensory ligament
 4 External pudendal vessels
 5 Deep dorsal penile vein
 6 Prostatic venous plexus
 7 Visceral pelvic fascia (vesical fascia)
 8 Anastomotic site at the prostatic urethra
 9 Bulb of penis
10 Cremaster muscle
11 Gracilis muscle

Perineal Approach for Radical Prostatectomy

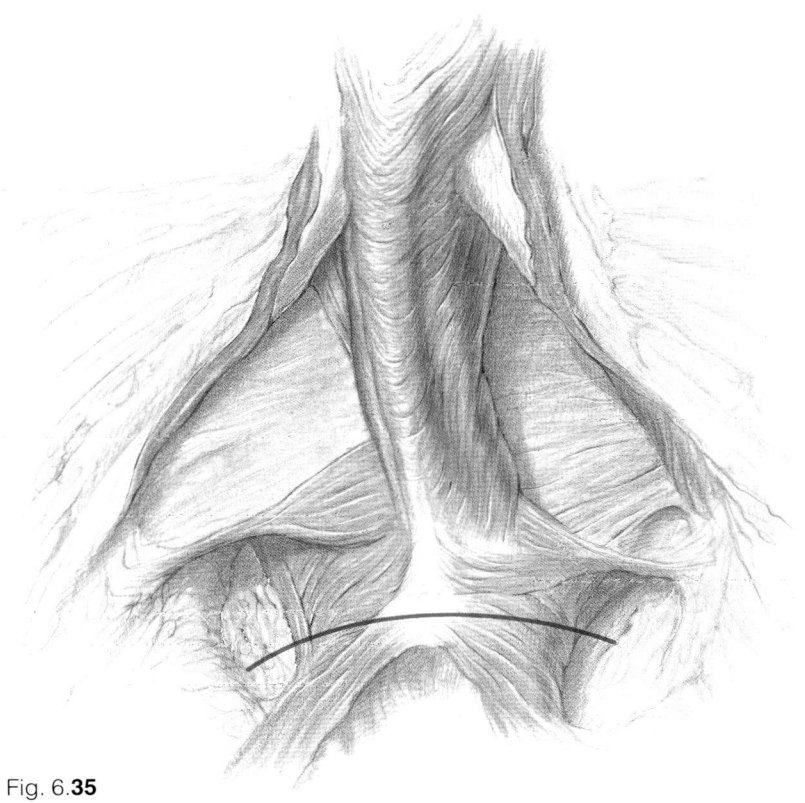

Fig. 6.**35**

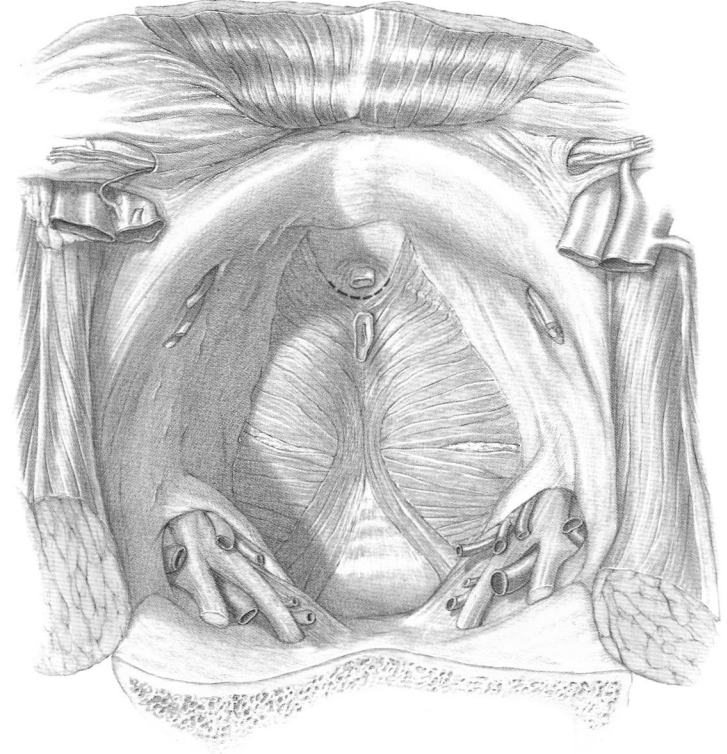

Fig. 6.**36**

Position and Skin Incision

The patient is placed in an extreme lithotomy position (Fig. 6.**37**). The sacrum is elevated on a pad, and the feet are placed in stirrups and angled toward the head.

The incision circumvents the anal region, curving from the ischial tuberosity over the center of the perineum to the opposite side (Fig. 6.**38**).

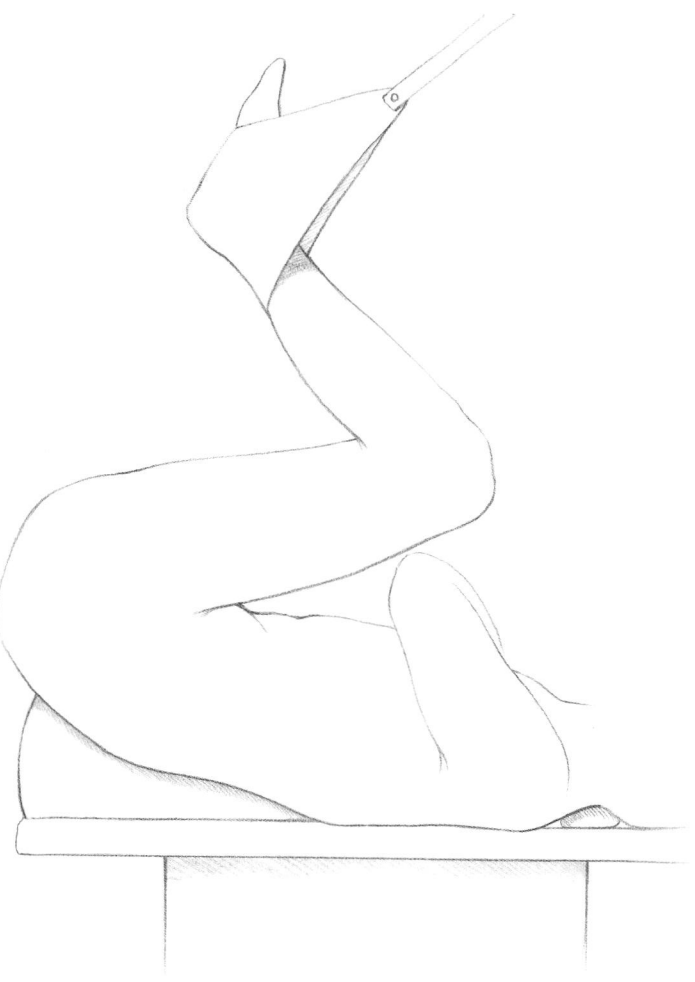

Fig. 6.**37** Position.

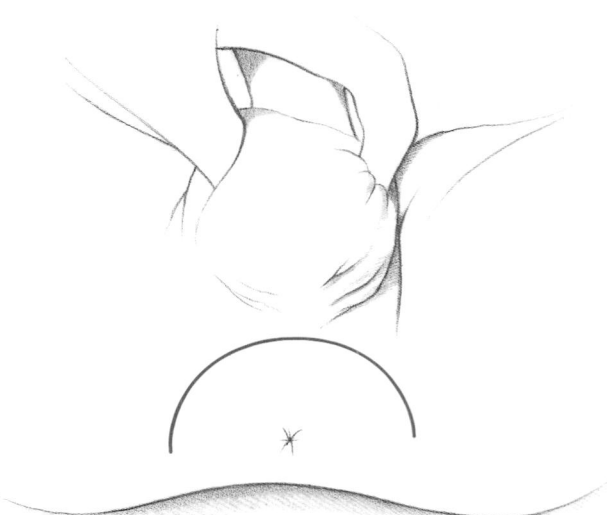

Fig. 6.**38** Skin incision.

Exposure and Division of the Central Tendon

The superficial perineal fascia is incised, and the ischiorectal fossae on both sides are progressively developed by blunt dissection (Fig. 6.**39**).

The fibromuscular structures of the central tendon are transected, preserving the superficial portion of the external anal sphincter (Fig. 6. **40**). An anatomic dissection at this stage of the approach is shown in Fig. 6.**41**. The superficial transverse perineal muscle, central tendon, and anterior rectal wall can be identified. The superficial portion of the external anal sphincter runs transversely over the rectum (Fig. 6.**41**).

Fig. 6.**39** Dissection of the ischiorectal fossa.

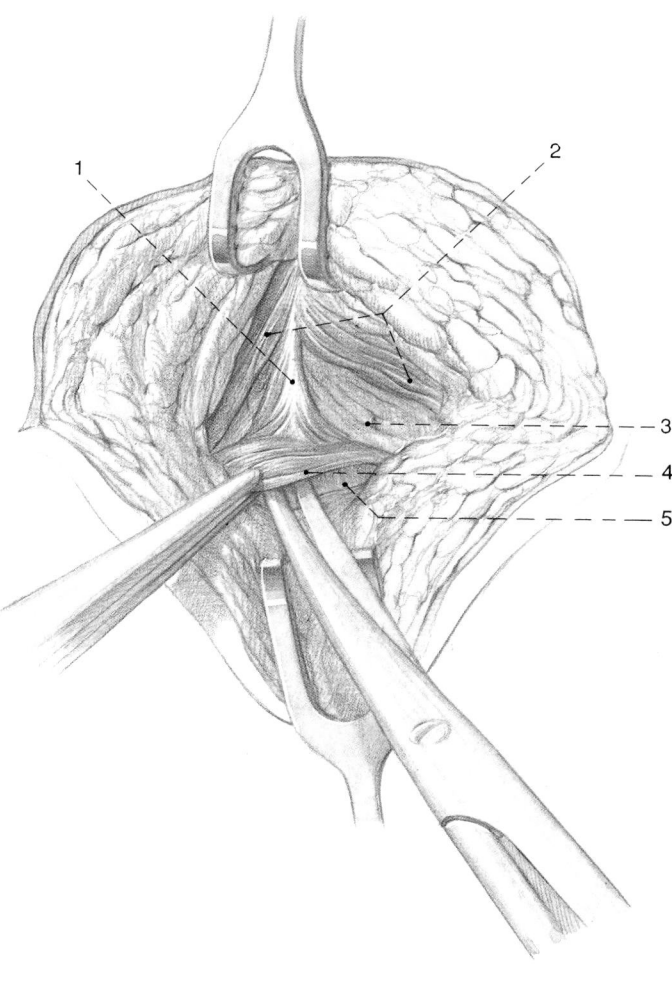

Fig. 6.**41** Dissection demonstrating the central tendon.

1 Central tendon
2 Superficial transverse perineal muscle
3 Inferior fascia of urogenital diaphragm
4 External anal sphincter
5 Rectum

Fig. 6.**40** Division of the central tendon.

1 Perineal tendinous raphe

Dissection of the Perineal Body, Entry into the Rectourethral Space

The levator ani is retracted to the side. Much as in the approach for posterior urethral surgery, the fascia on the anterior rectal wall in the area of the perineal body is exposed as far as the membranous urethra (Fig. 6.42). Numerous slips of connective tissue are divided at the apex of the central tendon (dotted line in Fig. 6.42) to gain access to the rectourethral space.

Exposure of the Rectogenital Space

The anterior rectal wall is retracted posteriorly using a special retractor. After the rectourethral space has been opened, a urethral bulb retractor is introduced (Fig. 6.43). Denonvillier's fascia is exposed at the posterior surface of the prostate and divided centrally on the line shown.

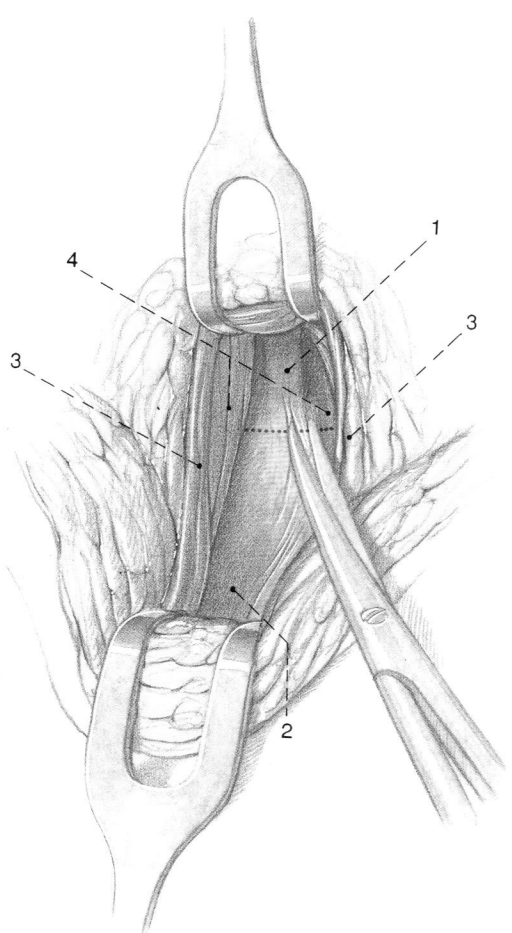

Fig. 6.**42**   The perineal body is dissected to the membranous urethra.

1 Membranous urethra
2 Rectal fascia
3 External anal sphincter
4 Levator ani

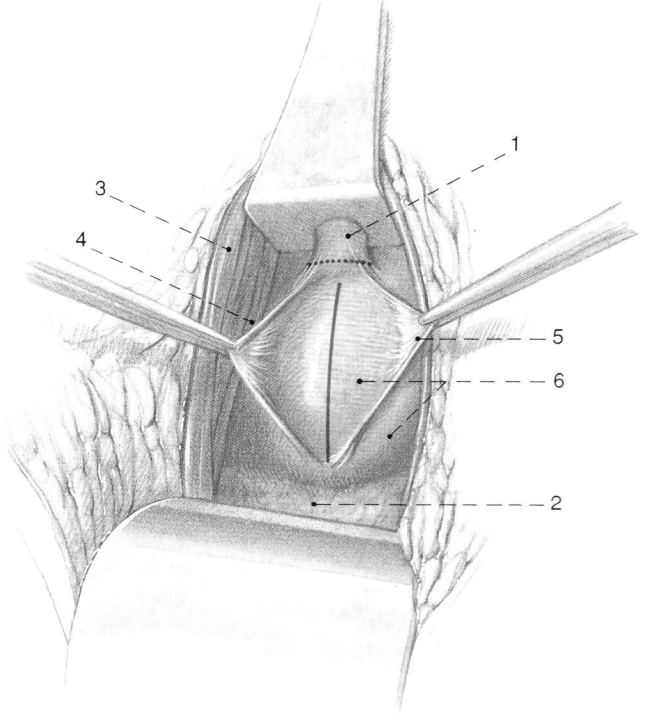

Fig. 6.**43**   Incision of the posterior layer of Denonvillier's fascia.

1 Membranous urethra
2 Rectum
3 External anal sphincter
4 Levator ani
5 Posterior layer of Denonvillier's fascia
6 Anterior layer of Denonvillier's fascia

Exposure of the Anterior Surface of the Prostate

The urethra is transected at the prostatic apex (Fig. 6.**44**). A retractor is passed into the bladder through the prostatic urethra, and the junction of the anterior surface of the prostate with the bladder is brought into view, taking care to preserve the dorsal vein complex (Fig. 6.**45**).

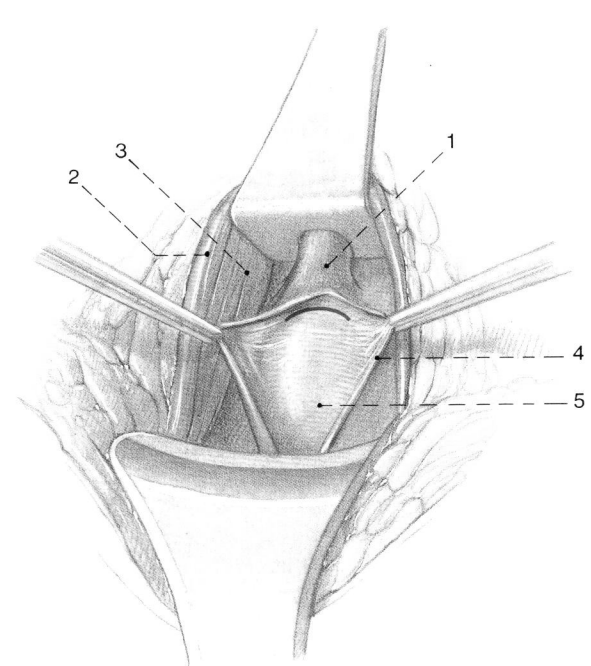

Fig. 6.**44**   Division of the urethra.

1 Membranous urethra
2 External anal sphincter
3 Levator ani
4 Posterior layer of Denonvillier's fascia
5 Anterior layer of Denonvillier's fascia

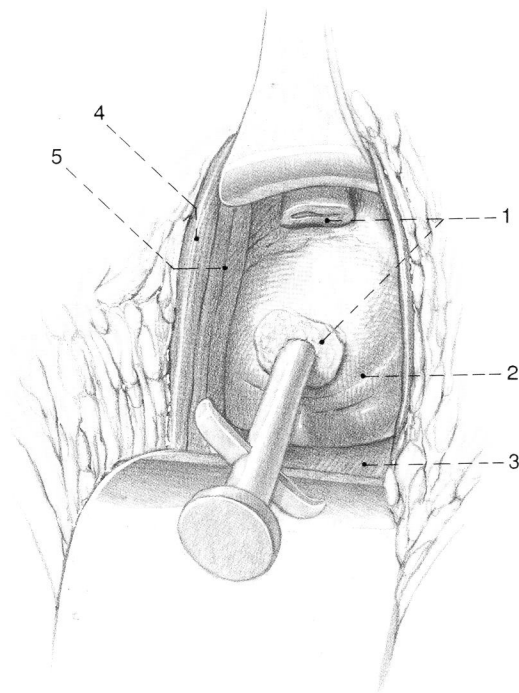

Fig. 6.**45**   Exposure of the anterior surface of the prostate.

1 Membranous urethra
2 Prostate
3 Rectum
4 External anal sphincter
5 Levator ani

Exposure of the Vesicogenital and Rectogenital Spaces

Following transection of the prostate at the bladder neck, the posterior aspect of the bladder trigone is freed and the vesicogenital space exposed. Both seminal vesicles and the ampullae of the vasa deferentia are identified. Branches of the inferior vesical artery enter the prostate lateral to the vasa deferentia (Fig. 6.**46**).

The prostate is retracted inferiorly, and both seminal vesicles are dissected out of the rectovesical space in continuity with Denonvillier's fascia between the rectum and seminal vesicle. The supplying artery at the apex of the seminal vesicle is ligated (Fig. 6.**47**).

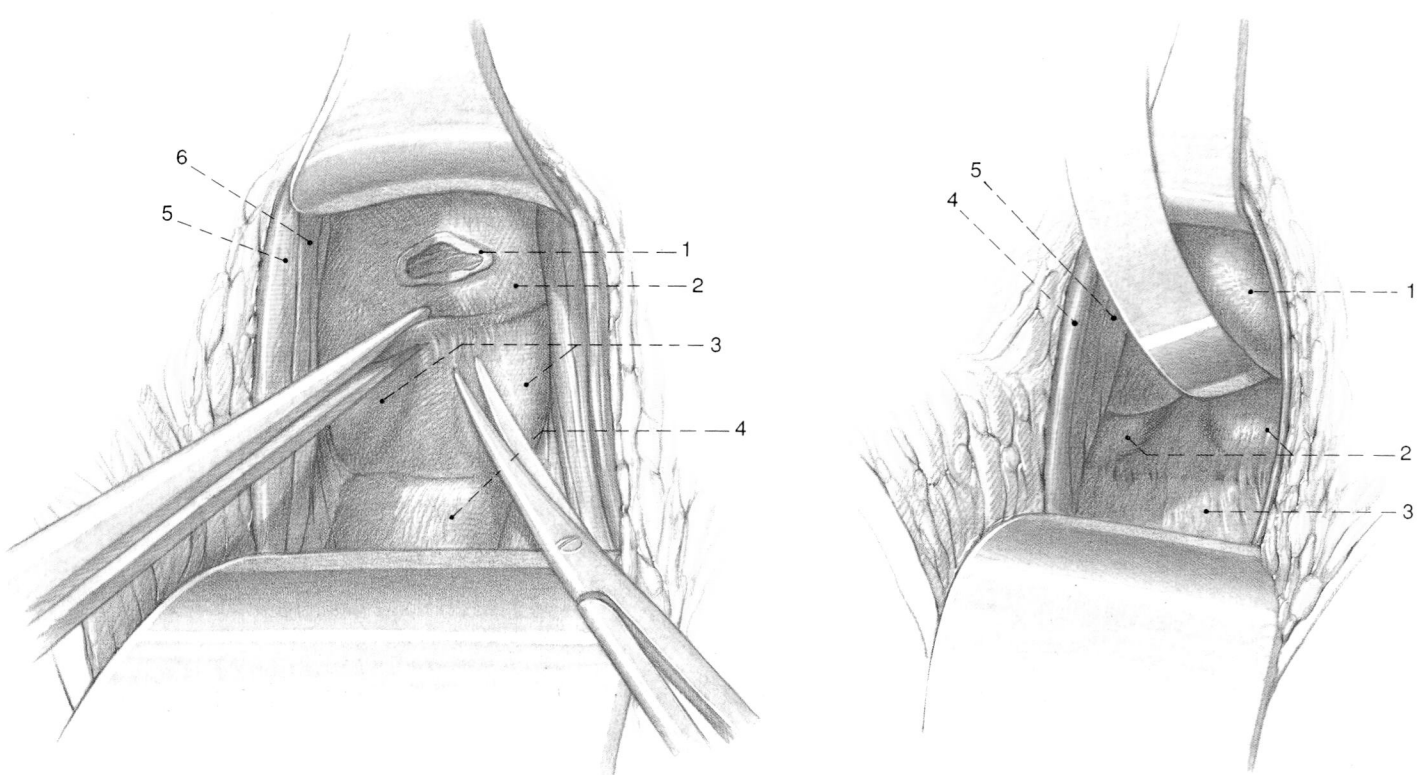

Fig. 6.**46**   Exposure of the vesicogenital space.

1 Bladder neck
2 Bladder
3 Seminal vesicle
4 Prostate
5 External anal sphincter
6 Levator ani

Fig. 6.**47**   Exposure of the rectogenital space.

1 Prostate
2 Seminal vesicle
3 Rectum
4 External anal sphincter
5 Levator ani

Comments

Either an extrasphincteric or intrasphincteric route may be used in the perineal approach.

The disadvantage of the perineal approach compared with the retropubic approach is that the perineal prostatectomy does not provide access for a pelvic lymph node dissection.

For a radical prostatectomy with curative intent, the retropubic approach is indicated. The perineal approach, by preserving the paraprostatic tissue ("lateral pelvic fascia"), avoids injury to the dorsal vein complex. In a perineal prosta-

tectomy, the prostate is removed within the paraprostatic tissue, whereas the retropubic prostatectomy removes the prostate together with all paraprostatic tissue. The retropubic approach involves incision of the paraprostatic tissue (lateral pelvic fascia) and division of the dorsal vein complex (arrow). Thus, in contrast to the perineal approach, the retropubic approach includes removal not just of Denonvillier's fascia but also of the paraprostatic tissue (lateral pelvic fascia) (Fig. 6.48).

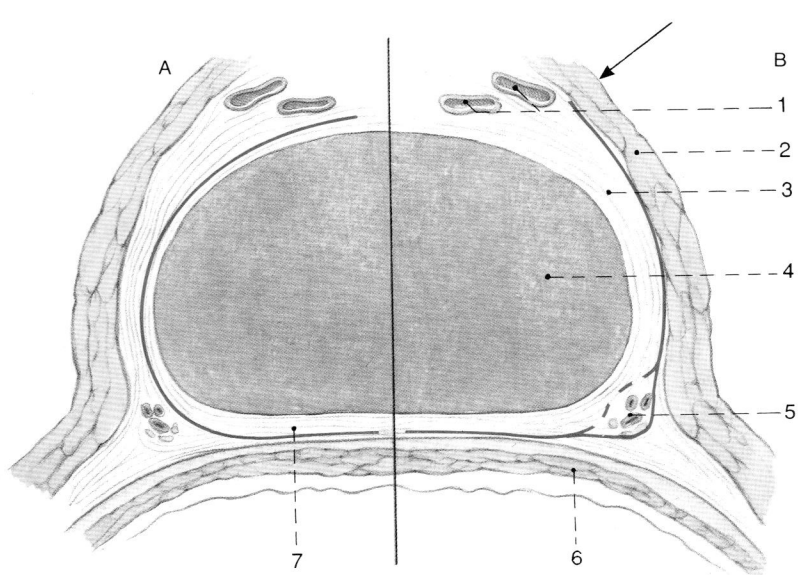

Fig. 6.**48**   Approaches for perineal (A) and retropubic (B) prostatectomy. The significance of the paraprostatic tissue (lateral pelvic fascia) in each approach is shown (... = nerve-sparing approach for a retropubic radical prostatectomy).

1 Dorsal vein complex
2 Levator ani
3 Paraprostatic tissue (lateral pelvic fascia)
4 Prostate
5 Neurovascular bundle
6 Rectum
7 Denonvillier's fascia

Posterior Sagittal Transcoccygeal Approach

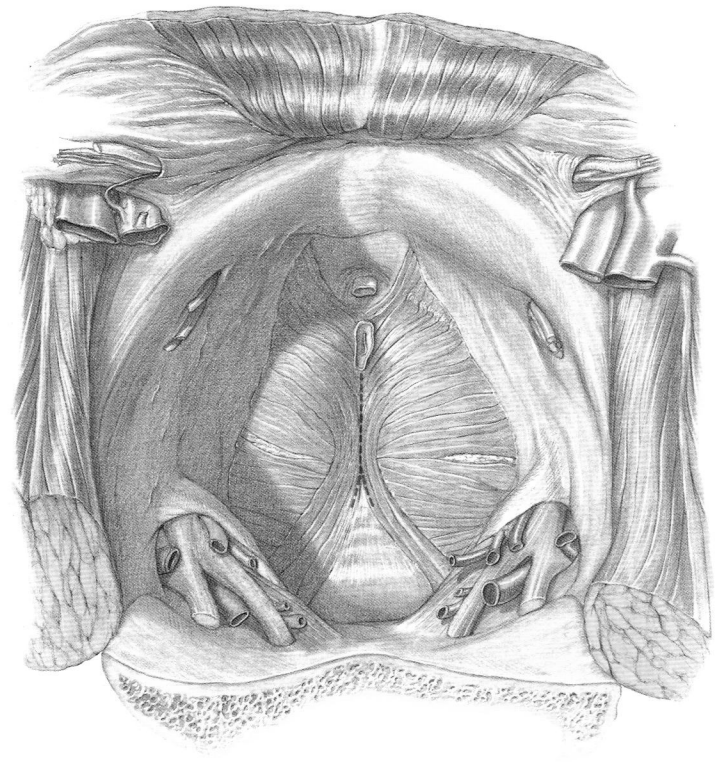

Fig. 6.**49**

Main Indications

- Imperforate anus with a rectourethral fistula
- Repair of a rectourethral fistula (Péna's approach)

Position and Skin Incision

The patient is placed in a prone position with the knees flexed. An orthopedic operating table is needed to maintain this position (Fig. 6.**50**). The incision extends from the center of the sacrum to the coccyx on the midline, circumventing the anal sphincter (Fig. 6.**51**).

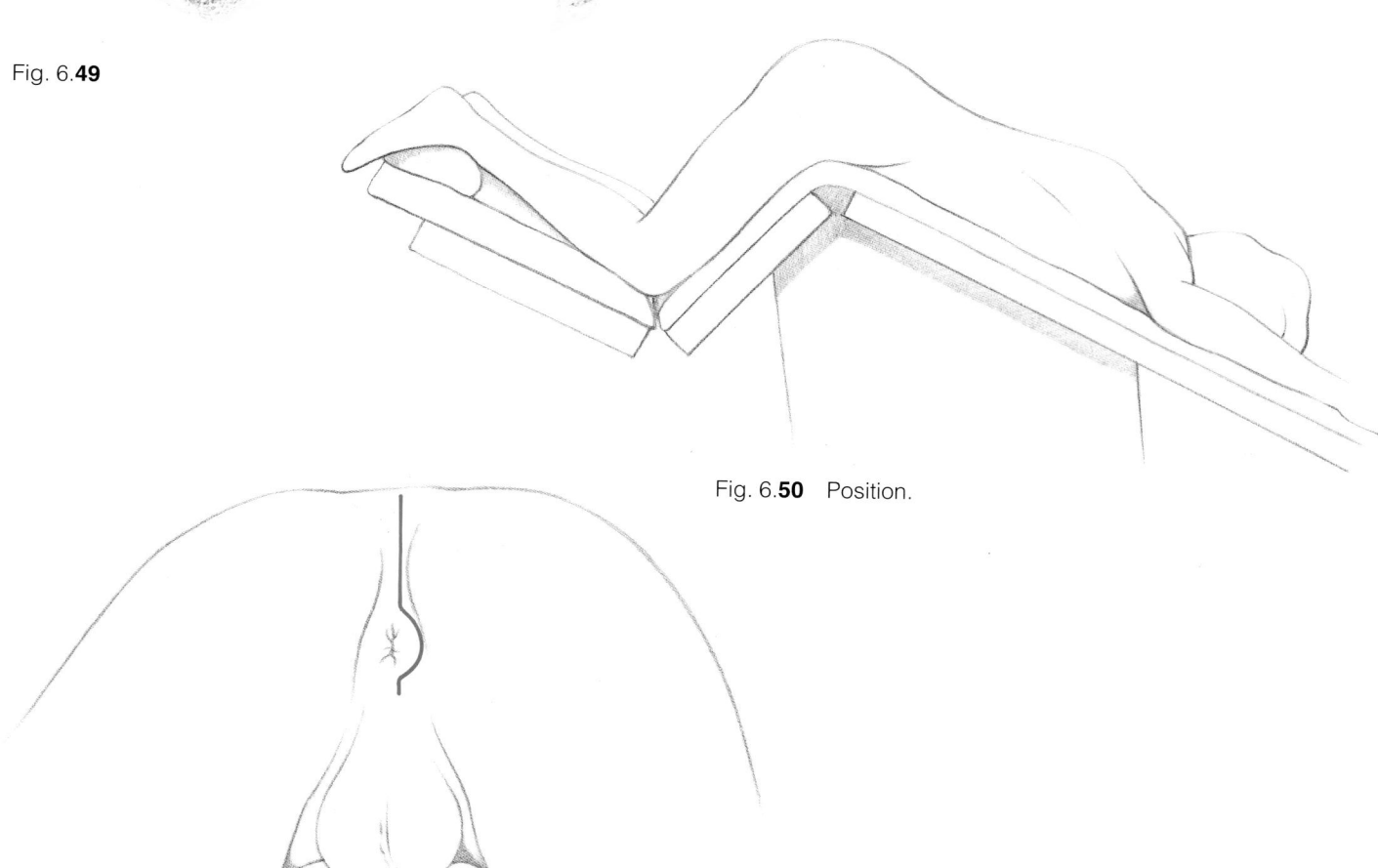

Fig. 6.**50**   Position.

Fig. 6.**51**   Skin incision.

Resection of the Coccyx

The skin and subcutaneous tissue are divided, and the fascia is divided over the median sacral crest (Fig. 6.**52**). The tendinous portion of the gluteus maximus muscle is sharply divided with scissors (Fig. 6. **53**). The rectum is freed at the tip of the coccyx by blunt finger dissection, the coccyx is elevated, and the anococcygeal ligament is divided. Finally the rectococcygeus muscle is removed, and the coccyx is resected with an osteotome (Fig. 6.**53**). In the approach for treatment of a rectourethral fistula, the external anal sphincter is preserved (Fig. 6.**53**).

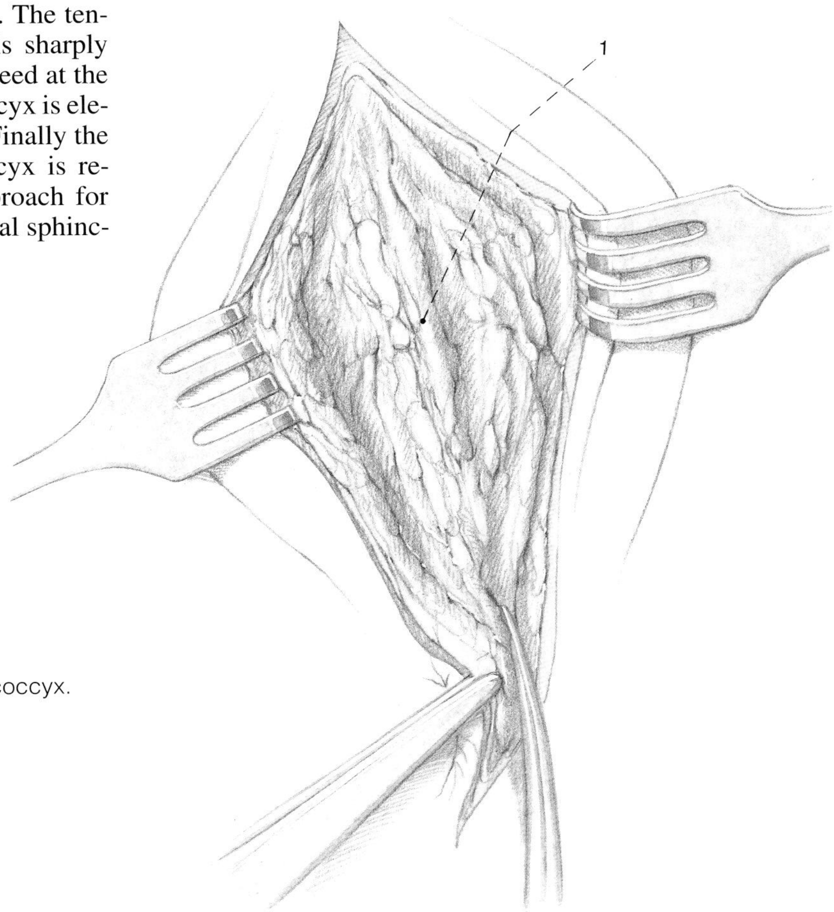

Fig. 6.**52**   Exposure of the coccyx.

1 Coccyx

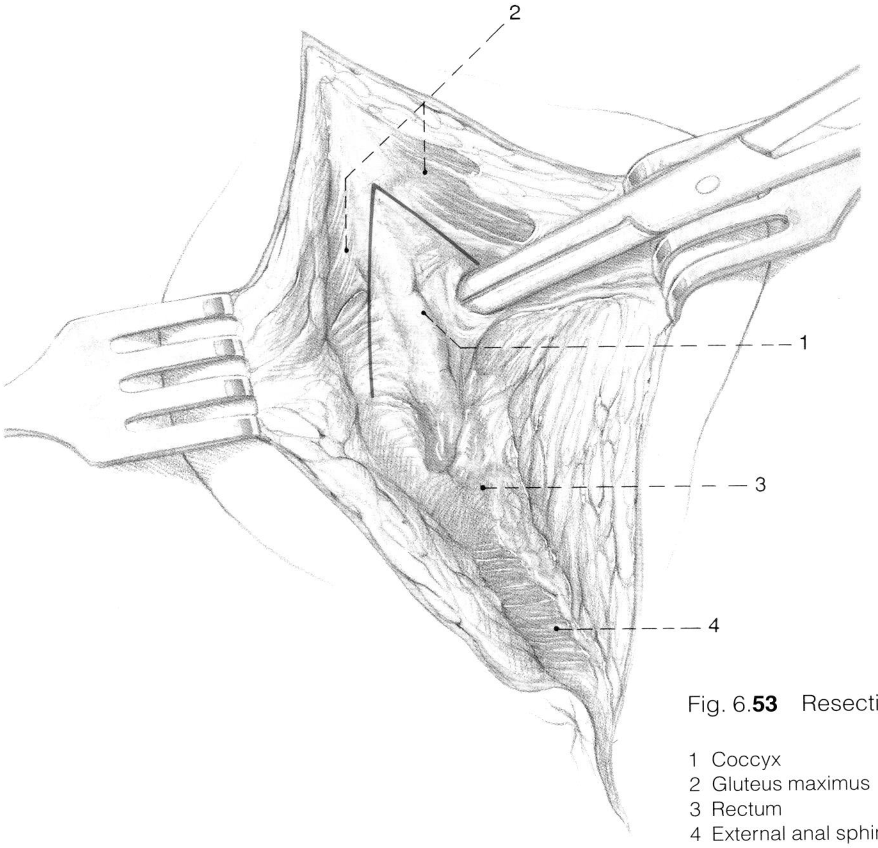

Fig. 6.**53**   Resection of the coccyx.

1 Coccyx
2 Gluteus maximus
3 Rectum
4 External anal sphincter

Incision of the Posterior Rectal Wall

The posterior rectal wall is opened between two traction sutures on the line shown (Fig. 6.54). The fistula in the anterior wall is identified and excised, and the defect is closed (Fig. 6.55).

Comments

A rectourethral fistula may be repaired through a perineal, para-anal (Young-Stone), or transanorectal (Gecelter) approach.

In the repair of a posttraumatic rectourethral fistula, the external anal sphincter can be preserved by using the approach described.

This approach can be extended transsacrally and rarely may be selected for a radical prostatectomy. In this case the coccyx and a portion of the sacrum are removed prior to dissection of the ischiorectal fossa. After separation of the levator ani, Denonvillier's fascia can be dissected on the posterior aspect of the prostate.

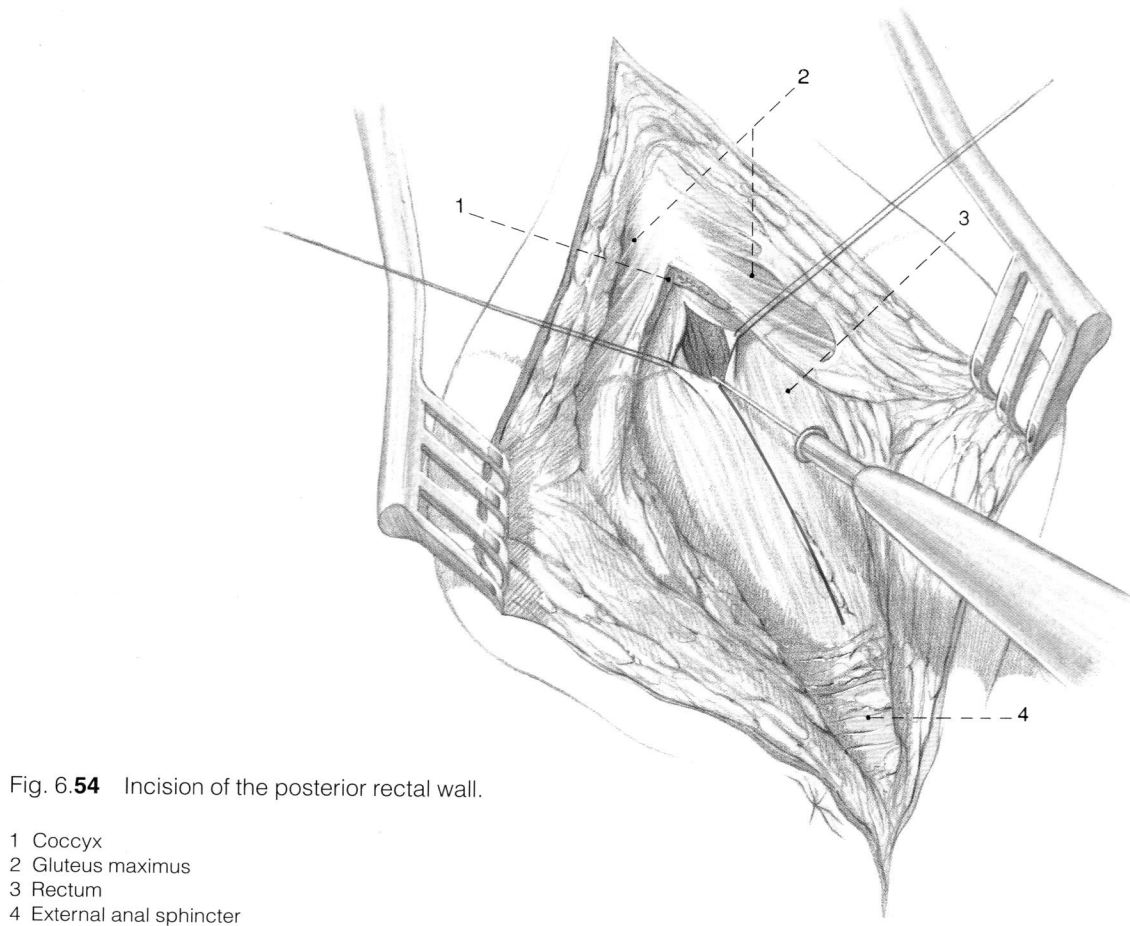

Fig. 6.**54**   Incision of the posterior rectal wall.

1 Coccyx
2 Gluteus maximus
3 Rectum
4 External anal sphincter

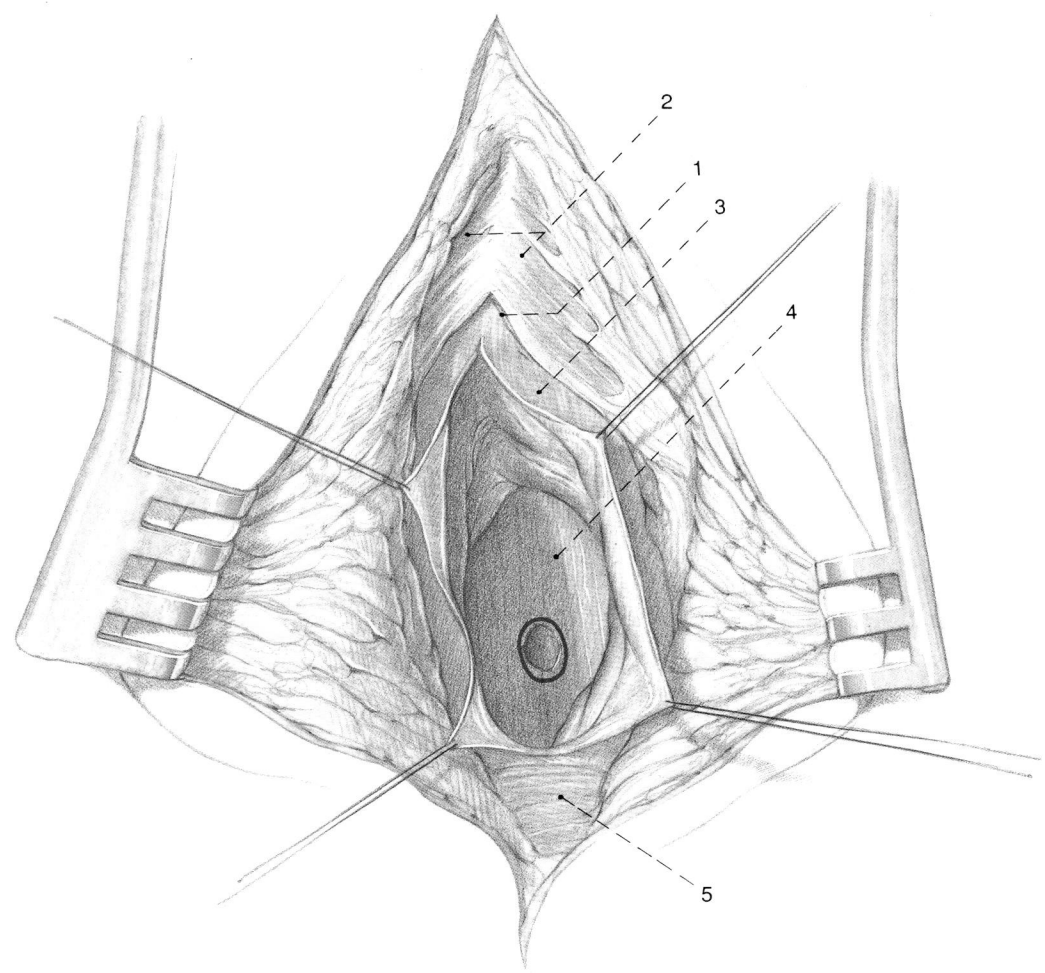

Fig. 6.**55**   Exposure of a rectourethral fistula.

1 Coccyx
2 Gluteus maximus
3 Rectum, posterior wall
4 Rectum, anterior wall
5 External anal sphincter

Index

Abbreviations used: R.S., retro-
    peritoneal space
abdominal aorta, *see* aorta
abdominal cavity in thoracolum-
    bar approach to R.S.,
    exposure/entry, 75, 78
abdominal midline approach to
    inguinal region, extraperi-
    toneal lower, 205–14
abdominal muscles, 2–10, 13, 37
    deep, 13
    superficial, 2–10
        in anterior subcostal
            approach to R.S.,
            division, 95
        in Foley muscle-splitting
            approach to R.S.,
            exposure, 53
        lateral group, 1
        in low inguinal incision,
            136–7
        in low lumbar oblique inci-
            sion, division, 132–3
        medial group, 2
        see also specific muscles
abdominal wall, 1–15
    anterior
        external view, 3
        internal view, 9
    inferior, internal view, 15
    inferior posterolateral
        external view, 7, 8
        internal view, 10
    lateral, external view, 6
    posterior, topography, 19
adductor longus, fascia lata dis-
    sected off, 234
adrenal gland, 30
    approaches, 60–71, 72–83,
        93–104
        anterior subcostal, 102–4
        posterior, 6771
    blood supply/innervation, 31
    exposure, 71
    left, 31
    right, 31
adrenal plexus, 31
adrenogenital syndrome, dorsal
    neurovascular bundle dis-
    section in, 243
anal sphincter, external, exposure,
    265
anus, imperforate, with rec-
    tourethral fistula,
    approaches, 282–5
aorta, abdominal, 31–2
    in midline transperitoneal
        approaches to R.S., inci-
        sion extending from,
        112
    in retrocrural lymph node
        approaches
        dissection, 90
        incision over, 91
aortic aperture/hiatus, 12
    in retrocrural lymph node
        approaches, incision,
        90–1
arcuate ligament (lumbocostal
    arch)
    lateral, 12
    medial, 12
arcuate line, 2
    exposure
        in midline transperitoneal
            approach to R.S., 106

in pelvic exenteration in
    males, 153
arterial supply
    adrenal, 31
    bladder, 149
    ovarian, 32
    renal, *see* renal arteries
    testicular, *see* testicular arteries
    ureteral, 30, 144
    see also specific arteries

bladder
    extraperitoneal lower abdomi-
        nal midline approach,
        205–14
    female
        anatomy/anatomical relation-
            ships, 150
        lateral pedicle/retinaculum,
            dissection, 177–8
        posterior pedicle/reti-
            naculum, exposure/
            clipping/division/liga-
            tion, 179, 180, 181
    male
        anatomy/anatomical relation-
            ships, 146–9
        cancer, pelvic exenteration,
            152–75
        incision (in approach for
            prostatectomy),
            210–11
        lateral pedicle/retinaculum,
            dissection, in males,
            164–5, 175
        posterior pedicle/reti-
            naculum, exposure/
            ligation/division,
            169–71, 175
        removal (en bloc), 174
    Pfannenstiel incision for
        approaches to, 215–20
blood vessels
    adrenal, 31
    bladder, 149
    major (of retroperitoneal
        space), 31–3
    pelvic region, 149, 201, 204
        variations in anatomy, 166–7
    renal, 25–9, 30
        in dorsolumbar/Nagamatsu
            approach to R.S.,
            exposure, 66
        in paramedian transperi-
            toneal approach to
            R.S., access to, 120
    testicular, exposure, 128
    ureteral, 30, 144
    see also neurovascular supply
        specific (types of) vessels
bowel/intestine
    large, *see* cecum; colon; rectum
    small, mobilization (in pelvic
        exenteration), 157–60,
        *see also specific parts
        of small bowel*
bulb of penis, dissection, 263, 264
bulbar artery, exposure, 259
bulbospongiosus muscle
    division, 264
    transfer, 251

cecum in pelvic exenteration,
    mobilization, 158
Camper's fascia, 222
    in lateral extraperitoneal grid-

iron incision, exposure/
    transection, 126
in low lumbar oblique incision,
    exposure/incision, 131
in pubic approach to external
    genitalia, exposure, 239
cancer
    bladder, pelvic exenteration in,
        152–75
    penile, ilioinguinal lymph node
        dissection in, 229–35
    prostatic, approach for radical
        prostatectomy, 190–204
    testicular, *see* testicles
    urethral, approach for en bloc
        resection, 184–9
capsule(s)
    prostatic, 150
        hyperplastic prostatic tissue
            separated from, 211,
            212, 213, 214
    renal, 24, *see also specific cap-
        sules*
carcinoma
    penile, ilioinguinal lymph node
        dissection in, 229–35
    prostatic, retropubic approach
        for radical prosta-
        tectomy, 190–204
    urethral, infrapubic peri-
        urethral approach for
        en bloc resection,
        184–9
caruncle, urethral, excision,
    248–54
caval vein, *see* vena cava
celiac trunk, 31
central tendons, *see* tendon
chest retraction, *see* retraction
chest wall, surgical anatomy, 74
Chevron incision, 104
circumcision of prepuce, 244
clitoral crus, undermining/liga-
    tion, 185
coccygeus, 14
coccyx, resection, 283
Colles' fascia (superficial fascia
    of penis and perineum)
    exposure, 241, 244
    incision/division, 242, 262, 263
    retraction, 262
colon
    ascending
        in midline transperitoneal
            approach to R.S., dis-
            section, 114
        in pelvic exenteration, mobi-
            lization, 157–60
    descending, in anterior sub-
        costal approach to R.S.,
        dissection, 101
    mesentery of, *see* mesenteries
conjoined tendon, 222
connective tissue, pelvic, bladder
    in relation to
    female, 150
    male, 147–8
corpus cavernosum
    corpus spongiosum and, shunt
        construction between,
        244
    great saphenous vein and,
        shunt construction
        between, 244–5
    sclerosis (= Peyronie's dis-
        ease), surgical
        approaches, 241–3

urethra transected and freed
    from, 265
corpus spongiosum
    anatomy, 256
    corpus cavernosum and, shunt
        construction between,
        244
    mobilization, 245
costal arch, division with Mayo
    scissors, 76, 77
cremaster muscle, anatomy, 2, 222
cremasteric fascia, 222, 223
    in approach to inguinal region,
        exposure/division, 226
    in approach to testes, division,
        247
crus/crura
    clitoral, undermining/ligation,
        185
    diaphragmatic
        lateral, 12, 88
        medial, 12
        in retrocrural lymph node
            approaches, dissec-
            tion, 88
    inguinal ring bounded by
        medial and lateral, 222
    levator, 14
cul de sac incision, 168

Denonvilliers' fascia (rectovesi-
    cal septum)
    anatomy, 147, 150
    in pelvic exenteration
        dissection, 174
        exposure, 169–71
    in perineal approach to poste-
        rior urethra, exposure,
        266
    in radical prostatectomy, expo-
        sure, 203, 278
Denonvilliers' space, entry, 174
    failed, 175
diaphragm, pelvic, 14
diaphragm, thoracoabdominal,
    11–12
    anatomy
        costal parts, 11, 12
        lumbar parts, 11
        sternal parts, 11, 12
    in anterior subcostal approach
        to adrenals, dissection
        of lumbar part, 103
    in dorsolumbar/Nagamatsu
        approach to R.S., sepa-
        ration from rib perios-
        teum, 64
    in retrocrural lymph node
        approaches
        division, 85
        exposure of lumbar part, 89
    in supracostal approach to
        R.S., dissection from
        12th rib, 42–3
    in thoracolumbar approach to
        R.S., dissection/divi-
        sion, 76, 78
diaphragm, urogenital
    anatomy, 14, 256, 257, 259
    inferior fascia, resection/
        removal, 186, 186
diverticulum, urethral, excision,
    248–54
dorsal approaches to penis, 241–3
dorsolumbar approaches/fascia,
    see entries under lum-
    bodorsal

duodenal fold, inferior, *see* Treitz, ligament of
duodenojejunal fold
  inferior, in midline transperitoneal approach to R.S., incisions from, 110, 114, 118
  superior, *see* Treitz, ligament of duodenum
  in midline transperitoneal approach to R.S., ascending part, dissection, 110
  in thoracolumbar approach to R.S.
    descending part, dissection, 80
    separation from Gerota's fascia, 79

endopelvic fascia
  anatomy, 172
  exposure and incision
    in pelvic exenteration, 170, 172
    in radical prostatectomy, 198–200
epididymectomy, approaches for, 246
epididymis, injury, 246–7
epididymovasostomy, approaches for, 246
epigastric vessels, dissection, 140, 228
epiploic foramen, in midline transperitoneal approach to R.S., incisions extending to, 113, 114, 118
esophageal aperture/hiatus, 12
exenteration, pelvic, *see* pelvis
extraperitoneal approach
  to inguinal region, midline, 205–14
  to pubic symphysis, midline, 270–1
  to retroperitoneal space
    lateral gridiron excision, 125–8
    paramedian, 138–40

falx, inguinal, 222
fascia
  Camper's (external/superficial abdominal), *see* Camper's fascia
  cremasteric, 222, 223
  Denonvilliers', *see* Denonvilliers' fascia
  femoral, superficial, exposure, 230
  Gerota's, *see* Gerota's fascia
  lumbodorsal/thoracolumbar, *see* lumbodorsal fascia
  pelvic (in general)
    female bladder and the, 150
    male bladder and the, 147, 150, 172
    tendinous arch of, *see* endopelvic fascia
    see also endopelvic fascia
  penile, deep
    division, 242
    exposure, 240
  penile, superficial, *see* Colles' fascia
  perineal, superficial, *see* Colles' fascia
  prostatic, 150
  rectal, prostate dissected from, 174
  retroperitoneal (in general), incision in midline transperitoneal approach to R.S., 117–18

spermatic, *see* spermatic fascia
transversalis, *see* transversalis fascia
urogenital diaphragm, inferior, resection/removal, 186, 186
vesical, 150
fascia lata, incision, 234–5
fat
  pararenal, 25
    in supracostal approach to R.S., exposure/dissection, 44
  perirenal capsule of, 24
females
  anatomy/anatomical relationships (in pelvic region), 143, 144, 150
  bladder, *see* bladder
  external genitalia, approaches, 248–58
  pelvic exenteration, anterior, 152–75
  urethra, *see* urethra
femoral fascia, superficial, exposure, 230
femoral vein, variant anatomy of tributaries supplying, 232–3
fibrous capsule of kidney, 24
fistula
  rectourethral, repair, 282–5
  urethral (in general), repair, 248–54
Foley muscle-splitting approach to R.S., 51–4
foramen
  epiploic, in midline transperitoneal approach to R.S., incision extending to, 113, 114, 118
  obturator, clamp inserted through medial part of, 186
foreskin, *see* prepuce

Gecelter approach, 284
genital hiatus, 14
genitalia, external, 237–54
  approaches to, 237–54
  superior portion, incision around, 185
Gerota's fascia/capsule, 24–5
  in anterior subcostal approach to R.S., dissection, 101
  in dorsolumbar/Nagamatsu approach to R.S., incision, 65
  in Foley muscle-splitting approach to R.S., exposure, 54
  in posterior approach to adrenals, identification, 70
  in posterior lumbotomy, exposure and incision, 58, 59
  in supracostal approach to R.S., incision, 44
  in thoracolumbar approach to R.S., separation from mesocolon and duodenum, 79
  in transcostal approach to R.S., exposure, 50
Gigli saw, pubic bone resection with, 186–7, 272
gluteal arteries, anatomical variations, 67, 166
gracilis muscle transfer, 252–3
gridiron excision, lateral extraperitoneal, 125–8

Henle's ligament, 222
hernia, umbilical, 9

hydrocele, approaches, 246–7
hypospadias, correction, 244–5

ileal reservoir, orthotopic continent, preparation for, 174, 175
iliac artery, common
  in midline transperitoneal approach to R.S., incision extending towards, 112
  in pelvic exenteration
    failure to isolate, 175
    incision extending over, 157
    ureter clipped past its crossing with, 160
iliac artery, internal
  anatomical variations, 166–7
  in pelvic exenteration, isolation/clipping of anterior branches, 177
  in radical prostatectomy, snaring, 196, 197
iliac lymph nodes, 29
iliac vein, common, in pelvic exenteration
  incision extending over, 157
  ureter clipped past its crossing with, 160
iliacus, 13
iliococcygeus, 14
iliopsoas muscle, 13
implants, *see* prosthetic surgery
inguinal ligament, 2
inguinal region, 221–35
  anatomy, 222–4
  approaches via, 134–7, 225–8
inguinal ring
  external/superficial, 2, 222
    exposure, 226
  internal/deep, 222
    exposure, 226–8
innervation, *see* nerves
intercostal approach to R.S., 60
intercostal membrane, internal, 9
intercostal muscle, 9–10
  external, 9
  internal, 9
  in supracostal approach to R.S.
    preservation, 40, 41
    separation from 12th rib, 38, 39
  in thoracolumbar approach to R.S., division, 76
  in transcostal approach to R.S., separation from 12th rib, 47
intersigmoid recess, 30
intestine, *see* bowel *and specific regions*

kidney, 20–31
  approaches to, 35–50, 59, 60–6, 72–83, 93–128
  capsules, 24, *see also specific capsules*
  contact areas, 22
  poles
    lower, 20
    upper, 20
    variations in levels, 20
  position, 20
  relations, 21–3
  see also entries under renal
Kollwitz method, 94, 95

labium minum, counterincision on medial side of, 251, 253
lacuna musculorum, 13
laparotomy, 74–9
latissimus dorsi, 6
  costal/iliac/scapular/vertebral parts, 6

in dorsolumbar/Nagamatsu approach to R.S.
  exposure, 60, 61
  transection, 62
in posterior approach to R.S. to adrenals, transection and retraction, 68, 69
in posterior lumbotomy, division/mobilization, 56, 59
in supracostal approach to R.S.
  division, 38
  exposure, 36
in thoracolumbar approach to R.S., transection, 74
  of fascial planes, 73
in transcostal approach to R.S., division, 47
levator ani (muscle group), 15
  in perineal approach to posterior urethra, exposure, 267
  in radical prostatectomy, exposure, 198, 199
levator crura, 14
levator hiatus, 14
ligament(s)
  arcuate, *see* arcuate ligament
  duodenal suspensory, *see* Treitz, ligament of
  Henle's, 222
  inguinal, 2
  lumbocostal, *see* lumbocostal ligament
  pectineal, lymph node dissection in relation to, 163
  penile suspensory, division, 271
  perineal, transverse, *see* perineal ligament
  phrenocolic, in retrocrural lymph node approaches, division, 85
  puboprostatic, *see* puboprostatic ligament
  pubourethral, 150
  pubovescical, *see* pubovesical ligament
  right triangular (of liver), incision in thoracolumbar approach to R.S., 81
  round (of uterus), ligation, 177, 178
  of Treitz, *see* Treitz, ligament of
linea alba, 2
  in midline extraperitoneal lower abdominal approach, exposure/division, 207
  in retropubic approach for radical prostatectomy, exposure, 192
liver, right triangular ligament of, incision in thoracolumbar approach to R.S., 81
lumbar arteries, 32
lumbar lymph nodes, 29
lumbar oblique incision, low, 129–33
lumbar trigone/triangle (and its variations), 4–5
lumbocostal arch, *see* arcuate ligament
lumbocostal ligament
  dissection showing, 58
  in dorsolumbar/Nagamatsu approach to R.S., division, 63
lumbodorsal (dorsolumbar approach) approach to R.S., 60–6
lumbodorsal (thoracolumbar) fascia, 56–8
  in dorsolumbar/Nagamatsu approach to R.S.

Index

lumbodorsal, exposure of deep
    layer, 62
  separation of deep layer
      from rib periosteum,
      64
  in posterior lumbotomy
    exposure of deep layer, 57
    incision of deep layer, 58, 59
    incision of superficial layer,
      56, 57, 59
  in supracostal approach to
      R.S., 36–41
    dissection from 12th rib,
      42–3
    exposure, 36–9
    incision of, 40–1
  in transcostal approach to R.S.,
      exposure and incision,
      48, 49
lumbotomy, posterior, 55–9
lymph nodes/vessels
  adrenal gland, 31
  ilioinguinal, dissection, 229–35
  pelvic, dissection/removal,
      161–3, 235
    by inguinal approach, 235
    in pelvic exenteration, 174,
      175
    in radical prostatectomy,
      196–7
  renal, 29, 30
  retrocrural
    approaches, 84–9
    metastatic involvement, 85
  retroperitoneal (in general), 29,
      30, 33
    dissection, approaches for,
      72–89, 106–18
  suprahilar, dissection, access
      for, 110, 116–18
  ureteral, 30, 144

males, 152–75, 238–47
  anatomy/anatomical relation-
      ships (in pelvic region),
      142, 143, 146–9, 256–9
  approaches in, 152–75,
      238–47, 255–85
    to external genitalia, 238–47
    for pelvic exenteration,
      152–75
  bladder, see bladder
  ureter, left, in pelvic exentera-
      tion, mobilization, 159
  ureter, right, in pelvic exentera-
      tion
    dissection, 158, 159
    isolation and clipping, 160
  urethra, see urethra
malignancy, see cancer
Martius technique, 251
Mayo scissors, costal arch divi-
      sion with, 76, 77
meatotomy, approaches for,
      248–54
men, see males
mesenteric arteries, superior/infe-
      rior, 31
mesenteric roots, kidney relations
      to, 21
mesenteric vein, inferior, in mid-
      line transperitoneal
      approach to R.S., expo-
      sure/ligation, 110, 111
mesenteries
  of colon (mesocolon)
    in anterior subcostal
        approach to R.S., dis-
        section, 101
    in pelvic exenteration, dissec-
        tion, 159

in thoracolumbar approach
    to R.S., separation
    from Gerota's fascia,
    79
  in midline transperitoneal
      approach to R.S., inci-
      sion, 110
midline approach
  extraperitoneal, see extraperi-
      toneal approach
  transperitoneal, to retroperi-
      toneal space, 105–18
Millin approach, 212–13
muscle(s)
  abdominal, see abdominal
      muscle
  pelvic diaphragm, 15
  transfers, 251–3
  urogenital diaphragm, 15
  see also specific muscles
muscle-splitting approach to R.S.,
      Foley, 51–4

Nagamatsu approach to R.S.,
      60–6
nephrectomy, approaches for,
      35–50, 93–104
nerves
  adrenal, 31
  bladder, 149
  major (of retroperitoneal
      space), 33
  pelvic region, 204
  renal, 30
  ureteral, 31, 144, 145
  see also neurovascular supply
      specific nerves
Nesbit procedure, 244–5
neurovascular supply (bundle;
      sheaths etc.) in males,
      147, 258
  in pelvic exenteration, removal
      (en bloc), 174
  to penis, exposure, 242–3, 258
  in radical prostatectomy, 204
    preservation, 204

oblique abdominal muscles (in
      general), in Foley muscle-
      splitting approach to R.S.,
      separation from transver-
      sus abdominis and retrac-
      tion, 53
oblique abdominal muscles, exter-
      nal, 2, 8
  in anterior subcostal approach
      to R.S., division, 95
  aponeurosis
    anatomy, 222
    division, 226
    ilioinguinal lymph node dis-
        section starting at,
        232
  in dorsolumbar/Nagamatsu
      approach to R.S.
    division/retraction, 62
    exposure, 60, 61
  in Foley muscle-splitting
      approach to R.S., expo-
      sure/retraction, 53
  in inguinal approach, exposure/
      division, 226
  in lateral extraperitoneal grid-
      iron incision
    division, 127
    exposure, 126
  in low inguinal incision, expo-
      sure/transection, 136
  in low lumbar oblique incision
    division, 132
    exposure, 131
  in supracostal approach to
      R.S., exposure, 36

in thoracolumbar approach to
    R.S., transection, 74, 75
  of fascial planes, 73
  in transcostal approach to R.S.,
      exposure, 47
oblique abdominal muscles, inter-
      nal
  anatomy, 2, 222
  in anterior subcostal approach
      to R.S., division, 95
  in dorsolumbar/Nagamatsu
      approach to R.S., divi-
      sion/retraction, 62
  in inguinal approach
    division, 136, 226, 235
    exposure, 136
  in lateral extraperitoneal grid-
      iron incision, exposure,
      127
  in low lumbar oblique incision,
      division, 132
  in supracostal approach to
      R.S., division, 38
obturator artery
  anatomical variations, 166
  identification and clipping,
      164, 165
obturator foramen, clamp inserted
      through medial part of,
      186
obturator nerve, dissection, 161,
      162
obturator vessels (in general),
      isolation/clipping, 163
orchiectomy, 246–7
ovarian artery, 32

pampiniform plexus, approaches
      for dissection of, 225–8
pancreas
  in anterior subcostal approach
      to R.S., dissection, 101
  in thoracolumbar approach to
      R.S., dissection, 80
paracolic sulcus
  in anterior subcostal approach
      to R.S., incision, 100
  in midline transperitoneal
      approach to R.S., inci-
      sion, 113
  in pelvic exenteration, incision
      into, 157, 158
paramedian approach to R.S.
  extraperitoneal, 138–40
  transperitoneal, 119–24
pararenal fat, see fat
parasympathetic innervation
  adrenal, 31
  bladder, 149
  ureter, 144
paravesical space, exposure for
      radical prostatectomy,
      192–5
parietal peritoneum
  bladder attachments to, 146
  in paramedian transperitoneal
      approach to R.S., divi-
      sion, 123–4
  in pelvic exenteration in males,
      incision, 154
  in radical prostatectomy, dissec-
      tion, 195
  removal (en bloc), 174, 175
pectineal ligament, lymph node
      dissection in relation to,
      163
pedicle
  of bladder, see bladder
  penile, exposure, 240
pelvic diaphragm, 14
pelvic floor
  anatomy, 14–15
  male, 256–9

bulb of penis dissected from,
      dorsal aspect of, 263
  exposure, 265
  incision, 272
pelvis (= pelvic bone), pubic por-
      tion, see symphysis
pelvis (= pelvic region), 141–220
  anatomy/anatomical relation-
      ships, 142–52, 256–9
    males, 142, 143, 146–9,
      256–9
  exenteration, anterior, 152–83
    in females, 176–83
    in males, 152–75
  lymph nodes in, see lymph
      nodes
pelvis (renal), 30
Péna's approach, 282
penile artery
  dorsal, exposure, 242, 259
  vascularization, approaches
      for, 138–40, 238–45
penile nerve, dorsal, exposure,
      242, 259
penile suspensory ligament, divi-
      sion, 271
penile vein
  deep dorsal
    dissection, 273
    exposure, 198, 199, 242,
      259, 273
  superficial dorsal, exposure/
      underrunning/ligation,
      239
penis
  approaches to, 238–45
  carcinoma, ilioinguinal lymph
      node dissection in,
      229–35
  neurovascular supply, expo-
      sure, 242–3, 258
Pereyra-Raz vaginal suspension,
      254
perineal body, see tendon
perineal ligament, transverse, 14
  exposure, 265
perineal muscles, transverse
  deep, 14
  superficial, 14
perineum, 255–85
  approaches via, 255–85
    for prostatectomy, see prosta-
        tectomy
  central tendon of, see tendon
periosteum (rib)
  of 11th rib in posterior
      approach to adrenals,
      division, 68
  of 12th rib in transcostal
      approach to R.S., inci-
      sion/division, 47, 48
  lumbodorsal fascia and dia-
      phragm separated from,
      in dorsolumbar/Naga-
      matsu approach to R.S.,
      64
perirenal fat capsule, 24
peritoneal cavity, entry
  by anterior subcostal approach,
      96–7
  by midline transperitoneal
      approach, 108–9
  by paramedian transperitoneal
      approach, 123
  in pelvic exenteration
    in females, 176
    in males, 153–4, 155
peritoneum
  bladder attachments to, 146
  parietal, see parietal peritoneum
  retraction, see retraction
  see also extraperitoneal
      approach; transperi-
      toneal approach

Peyronie's disease, surgical
approaches, 241–3
Pfannenstiel incision, 215–20
phrenic arteries, inferior, 32
in retrocrural lymph node
approaches
identification/dissection, 88
ligation, 88, 89, 90
phrenic vein, inferior, in retrocrural lymph node
approaches, identification/
dissection/ligation, 88, 89
phrenocolic ligament in retrocrural lymph node
approaches, division, 85
posterior approaches
to adrenals, 67–71
sagittal transcoccygeal, 282–5
prepuce (foreskin)
circumcision, 244
dissection, 241
incision along inner layer, 241
prerectal fibers, 14
prevesical space, 147
in Pfannenstiel incision, exposure, 219
in radical prostatectomy
division, 194
exposure, 192–5
prostate
anatomy, 149, 150
anterior surface, exposure, 279
carcinoma, 190–204
dissection from rectal fascia,
174
hyperplastic tissue, prostatic
capsule separated from,
211, 212, 213, 214
removal (= prostatectomy), see
prostatectomy
stump, approaches to markedly
retracted, 268–74
prostatectomy (prostate removal),
190–204, 210–11,
275–81
open
extraperitoneal lower abdominal midline
approach, 205–14
Pfannenstiel incision for,
215–20
in pelvic exenteration, 174, 175
radical, perineal approach,
275–81
advantages/disadvantages,
281
radical, retropubic approach,
190–204
advantages/disadvantages,
281
transvesicular approach,
210–11
prostatic urethra, dissection/divi-
sion, 267, 279
prostatic venous complex/plexus
dissection, 273
undermining and ligation, 201
prosthetic surgery
penile, approaches for, 238–45
testicular, approaches for,
246–7
psoas arcade, 12
psoas muscle
greater (psoas major), 13
smaller (psoas minor), 13
pubic approaches in males,
238–43, 268–74
external genitalia, 238–43
pubic symphysis, see symphysis
pubococcygeus, 14
puboprostatic ligament
anatomy, 147, 150, 172
division
in pelvic exenteration, 172

in radical prostatectomy,
198–200
puborectalis, 14
pubourethral ligaments, 150
pubourethral space, exposure/
entry
in pelvic exenteration, 173
in perineal approach, 267, 274
to posterior urethra, 267
in radical prostatectomy, 201
in transpubic approach, 274
pubovesical ligaments
females, 150
male equivalent, see puboprostatic ligament
pudendal artery
exposure in radical prostatectomy, 204
internal, anatomical variations,
166
pudendal nerve, exposure in radical prostatectomy, 204
pudendal vein, exposure in radical prostatectomy, 204
pyramidalis, 2
in Pfannenstiel incision, dissection, 218

quadratus arcade, 12
quadratus lumborum, 13

rectal artery, middle, anatomical
variations, 166
rectococcygeus, 14
rectogenital space, 147, 150
in pelvic exenteration, blunt
development by finger
dissection, 169
in radical prostatectomy, exposure, 203, 278, 280
rectoprostatic space, 150
rectourethral fistula, repair, 282–5
rectourethral septum
in perineal approach to posterior urethra, dissection,
266
in radical prostatectomy, incision, 203
rectourethral space (retrourethral
space), entry into, 173,
175, 278
for radical prostatectomy, 278
rectovesical septum, see Denonvilliers' fascia
rectovesical space, 150
rectum, wall/surface
anterior
Cul de Sac incision running
over, 168
retrourethral space opened
at, 173
posterior, incision, 284
rectus abdominis, 2
in midline extraperitoneal
lower abdominal
approach, retraction,
208
in paramedian extraperitoneal
approach to R.S., expo-
sure, 140
in paramedian transperitoneal
approach to R.S.
freeing, 121, 124
retraction, 122
splitting of fibers, 124
in Pfannenstiel incision, expo-
sure/dissection, 216–18
in retropubic approach for radical prostatectomy, sepa-
ration, 193
in thoracolumbar approach to
R.S., freeing/retraction,
74
rectus sheath (in general), 2
rectus sheath, anterior

in anterior subcostal approach
to R.S., transection, 95
in midline extraperitoneal
lower abdominal
approach
exposure, 207
incision, 270
in midline transperitoneal
approach to R.S., inci-
sion, 106, 107
in paramedian extraperitoneal
approach to R.S.
exposure/dissection, 139
retraction, 140
in paramedian transperitoneal
approach to R.S., expo-
sure, 122
in pelvic exenteration in males,
exposure/incision, 153
in Pfannenstiel incision, expo-
sure/incision/dissection,
216, 217, 218
in retropubic approach for radical prostatectomy, inci-
sion, 193
in thoracolumbar approach to
R.S., incision, 73
rectus sheath, posterior
in midline transperitoneal
approach to R.S., expo-
sure, 106
in paramedian transperitoneal
approach to R.S.
division, 123–4
exposure, 122
in pelvic exenteration in males
exposure, 153
incision, 154
in retropubic approach for radical prostatectomy
exposure, 193
incision, 194
in thoracolumbar approach to
R.S.
exposure, 74, 75
transection, 74
renal arteries, 25–7, 30, 31
accessory and aberrant, 25, 26,
27
in anterior subcostal approach
to R.S., exposure/isola-
tion, 98, 99
branching, 25
in dorsolumbar/Nagamatsu
approach to R.S., expo-
sure, 66
left, 25
right, 25
renal lymphatics, 29
renal nerves, 30
renal pelvis, 30
renal sinus, 20, 28
renal veins, 28, 30
in anterior subcostal approach
to R.S., exposure/isola-
tion, 98, 99
in dorsolumbar/Nagamatsu
approach to R.S., expo-
sure, 66
left, 28
right, 28
in thoracolumbar approach to
R.S., snaring, 80
renal vessels (in general), see
blood vessels
retinaculum, bladder, see bladder
retraction/retractors
abdominal/peritoneal
in low inguinal incision, 137
in subcostal approach to
R.S., 96, 97
chest
in midline transperitoneal
approach to R.S.,
108, 109

in supracostal approach to
R.S., 42
in thoracolumbar approach
to R.S., 76
in transcostal approach to
R.S., 50
rectus muscles, in midline
extraperitoneal lower
abdominal approach,
208
rectus sheath, in paramedian
extraperitoneal
approach to R.S., 140
scrotal skin/tunica dartos/
perineal fascia, 262
retroaortic space, exposure, 92
retrocrural lymph nodes, see
lymph nodes
retrocrural space, exposure, 92
retroperitoneal space, 17–140
anatomy, 18–33
approaches, 34–140
for pelvic exenteration, 157
see also specific approaches
definition/boundaries/contents,
18
retropubic approach
for Pereyra-Raz vaginal suspension, transvaginal, 254
for prostatectomy, see prostatectomy
for radical prostatectomy,
190–204
retropubic space, 147
in midline extraperitoneal
lower abdominal
approach, exposure,
208–9
retrourethral (rectourethral)
space, entry into, 173, 175
retrovesical space, 147
revascularization, penile,
approaches for, 138–40,
238–45
rhabdosphincter, see urethral
sphincter
rib(s)
avoiding resection in
approaches to R.S.,
34–44
periosteum, see periosteum
resection
in thoracolumbar approach
to R.S., thoracotomy
with, 76–8
in transcostal approach to
R.S., 45–50
see also costal arch; intercostal
approach; subcostal
approach; supracostal
approach; transcostal
approach
rib(s), 11th
Chevron incision beginning at
tip of, 104
in dorsolumbar/Nagamatsu
approach to R.S., resec-
tion of parts of, 63
in posterior approach to
adrenals
exposure and resection, 68,
69
incision in bed of, 70
in transcostal approach to R.S.,
resection, 46, 50
rib(s), 11th and 12th, in supracostal approach to R.S.,
incision between, 35
rib(s), 12th
dorsolumbar/Nagamatsu
approach to R.S., resec-
tion of parts of, 63
in supracostal approach to R.S.
diaphragm dissected from,
42–3

rib(s), 12th
    displacement, 35, 40
    intercostal muscles sepa-
        rated from, 38, 39
    lumbodorsal fascia dissected
        from, 42–3
    lumbodorsal fascia incised
        at tip of, 40
    in transcostal approach to R.S.
        exposure, 47
    resection, 46, 48
round ligament of uterus, liga-
    tion, 177, 178

sacrococcygeus, 14
saphenous hiatus
    exposure, 234
    preservation, 235
    vessels about, 234
    variant anatomy, 232, 233
saphenous vein, great, 232–3
    corpora cavernosum and, shunt
        construction between,
        244–5
    dissection/snaring, 231, 232
    variant anatomy, 232–3
sartorius muscle, fascia lata
    incised at lateral border
    of, 234
Scarpa's fascia, exposure, 230
scrotal skin, division/retraction,
    262
semilunar line, 2
seminal vesicles, transverse sec-
    tion through pelvis at
    level of, 148
serratus anterior, 7
    in posterior approach to
        adrenals, transection
        and retraction, 68, 69
    superior/intermediate/inferior
        parts, 7
    in supracostal approach to R.S.,
        division, 38
    in thoracolumbar approach to
        R.S., transection, 74, 75
    of fascial planes, 73
    in transcostal approach to R.S.,
        division, 47
serratus posterior inferior, 8
    in dorsolumbar/Nagamatsu
        approach to R.S., tran-
        section, 62
sigmoid mesocolon in pelvic
    exenteration, dissection,
    159
sinus, renal, 20, 28
skin
    preputial and penile, dissec-
        tion, 241
    scrotal, division/retraction, 262
small bowel mobilization in pel-
    vic exenteration, 157–60,
    see also specific parts of
    small bowel
SpenceDucket procedure, 248
spermatic cord, 222, 223, 224
    dissection/mobilization, 226,
    228
spermatic fascia
    exposure, 222
    incision/division, 222, 224,
    227, 247
spermatocele, approaches, 246–7
splanchnic nerves, greater and
    lesser, 33
splenic vessels in anterior sub-
    costal approach to R.S.,
    dissection, 101

split-and-roll technique of lymph
    node dissection
    in pelvic region, 161–3
    in retroperitoneal space, 117,
    118
stones, renal, approaches for,
    35–50
stricture, urethral
    dorsal approach, 264
    perineal approach, 261, 264,
    26874
    transpubic approach, 268–74
    ventral approach, 245
    subcostal approach to R.S., 60,
    95–104
    anterior, 95–104
sulcus
    paracolic, see paracolic sulcus
    urethral, of corpus caverno-
        sum, corpus spongio-
        sum dissected out of,
        245
supracostal approach to R.S.,
    34–44
suprahilar lymph nodes dissec-
    tion, access for, 110,
    116–18
suprarenal arteries, superior/
    middle/inferior, 31
suprarenal vein, 31
    in anterior approach to
        adrenals, snaring, 102,
        103
    in posterior approach to
        adrenals, snaring, 71
suspensory ligament
    duodenal, see Treitz, ligament
        of
    penile, division, 271
sympathetic innervation
    adrenal, 31
    bladder, 149
    in retroperitoneal space (in
        general), 33
    ureteral, 144
symphysis, pubic
    exposure, 270–1
    resection, 186–7, 272–3

Treitz, ligament of (inferior
    duodenal fold; suspensory
    muscle/ligament of
    duodenum)
    in anterior subcostal approach
        to R.S., incision, 98
    in midline transperitoneal
        approach to R.S., inci-
        sion, 115
    in pelvic exenteration, incision
        from, 157
triangular ligament of liver, right,
    incision in thoracolumbar
    approach to R.S., 81
tumor(s)
    adrenal, approaches, 68–71
    malignant, see cancer
    renal, approaches, 72–83,
    93–118
    testicular, see testicles
tumor thrombus in vena cava,
    approaches to, 81–3
tunica albuginea, penile fascia dis-
    sected down to, 242
tunica dartos
    exposure, 246
    retraction, 262

umbilical artery, anatomical varia-
    tions, 166

umbilical hernia, 9
ureter(s), 30–1
    anatomy, 30–1, 144, 145,
    152–5
        abdominal (proximal) part,
        301
        pelvic part, 152–5
    approaches/exposure, 129–37,
    205–20
        lumbar portion, 128, 129–33
        pelvic portion, 134–7,
        205–20
        proximal portion, 52–4
    blood supply, 30, 144
    female, 143, 144
    innervation, 31, 144, 145
    left, 30
        in pelvic exenteration, mobi-
        lization, 159
    lymph vessels, 30, 144
    male, see male
    retraction, 170, 172
    right, 30
        clipping in pelvic exentera-
        tion, 160
        dissection in pelvic exentera-
        tion, 158, 159
        traction placed on, in pelvic
        exenteration, 169
ureteropelvic junction,
    approaches to, 35–54
urethra, fistula, see fistula
urethra of females
    anatomy, 150, 184
    approaches to, 184–9, 248–54
        infrapubic periurethral, 184–9
        caruncle, excision, 248–54
        diverticulum, excision, 248–54
        resection/removal, 182, 183
        in urethral carcinoma, 184–9
urethra of males, 256–67
    anatomy, 256–9
    anterior, ventral approach to
        surgery of, 244–5
    membranous, exposure and
        division, 202
    posterior, perineal approach,
        260–7
    prostatic, dissection/division,
        267, 279
    stricture, see stricture
urethral sphincter (rhabdosphinc-
    ter), 14
    female, 14
    male, exposure, 259
        and division in radical prosta-
        tectomy, 202
urethrovaginal septum, exposure,
    250
urethrovaginal space, 150
urethrovaginal sphincter, 14
urogenital diaphragm, see dia-
    phragm, urogenital
uterine artery, anatomy, 143
    variations, 166
uterus
    retraction upward, 182
    round ligament of, ligation,
    177, 178

vagal nerve trunks, 33
vaginal suspension, PereyraRaz
    technique of, 254
vaginal wall
    lateral, incision from outside,
    188
    posterior, opening, 180–1
vas deferens

in inguinal approach, separa-
    tion from pampiniform
    plexus and testicular
    artery, 227
in pelvic exenteration
    retraction, 170, 172
    traction placed on, 169
in radical prostatectomy, liga-
    tion/division, 195
vas deferens, artery of
    anatomical variations, 166
    in inguinal approach, separa-
        tion from pampiniform
        plexus and testicular
        artery, 227
vascularization, penile,
    approaches for, 138–40,
    238–45
vasculature, see blood vessels;
    lymphatics and specific
    (type of) vessels
vasovasostomy, 246
vena cava, inferior, 32
    development, 32, 33
    fibrous/fatty tissues covering,
        opening, 117
    parietal tributaries, 32
    tumor thrombus, approaches
        to, 813
    variations, 32
    visceral tributaries, 32
vena cavotomy, 82–3
venous system/drainage
    adrenal gland, 31
    bladder, 149
    prostatic, see prostatic venous
        complex
    renal, see renal veins
    ureteral, 30, 144
    see also specific veins
ventral approaches to penis,
    244–5
vesical artery
    inferior, 149
        identification and clipping,
        164, 165
        variations in anatomy, 166
    superior, 149
        identification and clipping,
        164, 165
        variations in anatomy, 166
vesical fascia in females, 150
vesicogenital space, 147, 150
    in radical prostatectomy, expo-
        sure, 203, 280
vesicopubic ligament, see
    pubovesical ligament
vesicoumbilical plate
    in females, retraction/reflection
        downward, 176, 182
    in males
        dissection, 155–6
        removal (en bloc), 174, 175
        retraction forward, 170, 172
vesicouterine space, 150
vesicovaginal space, 150
vessels, see blood vessels; lymph
    nodes/vessels
visceral pelvic fascia, male blad-
    der and the, 147

Winslow's epiploic foramen in
    midline transperitoneal
    approach to R.S., inci-
    sions extending to, 113,
    114, 118
women, see females

Young-Stone approach, 284

D MAP PAGES

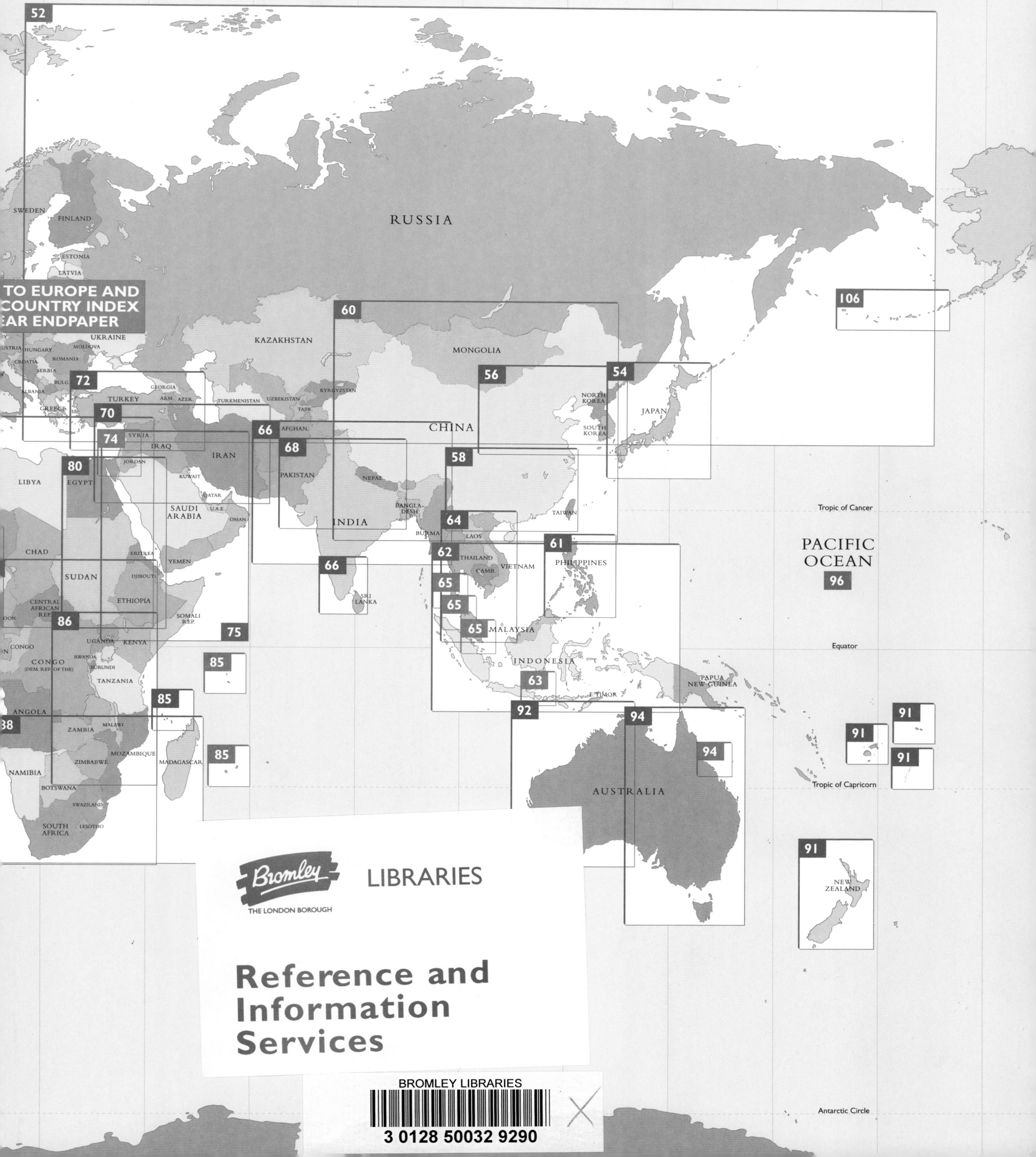

52

RUSSIA

SWEDEN
FINLAND
ESTONIA
LATVIA

**TO EUROPE AND
COUNTRY INDEX
EAR ENDPAPER**

HUNGARY
AUSTRIA
MOLDOVA
CROATIA
ROMANIA
SERBIA
ALBANIA
BULG.
GREECE

UKRAINE

KAZAKHSTAN

60

MONGOLIA

106

72

GEORGIA
TURKEY ARM. AZER.
TURKMENISTAN UZBEKISTAN
KYRGYZSTAN
TAJIK.

56

54

NORTH
KOREA

JAPAN

70

74 SYRIA
IRAQ

66 AFGHAN.

CHINA

SOUTH
KOREA

68

80
JORDAN

IRAN

KUWAIT

PAKISTAN

58

LIBYA
EGYPT

QATAR
U.A.E.
OMAN

NEPAL

BANGLA-
DESH

Tropic of Cancer

SAUDI
ARABIA

INDIA

TAIWAN

CHAD

ERITREA
YEMEN

64

BURMA
LAOS

SUDAN

DJIBOUTI

66

SRI
LANKA

62 THAILAND
CAMB. VIETNAM

61

PHILIPPINES

PACIFIC
OCEAN

96

CENTRAL
AFRICAN
REP.

ETHIOPIA

SOMALI
REP.

75

65

65

86
UGANDA KENYA

RWANDA
BURUNDI

85

65 MALAYSIA

CONGO
(DEM. REP OF THE)

TANZANIA

INDONESIA

Equator

85

63

PAPUA
NEW GUINEA

ANGOLA

ZAMBIA MALAWI

85

E TIMOR

91

91

88

ZIMBABWE

MOZAMBIQUE

85

92

94

91

NAMIBIA
BOTSWANA

MADAGASCAR

94

AUSTRALIA

Tropic of Capricorn

SWAZILAND

SOUTH
AFRICA

LESOTHO

91

NEW
ZEALAND

Bromley **LIBRARIES**

THE LONDON BOROUGH

Reference and
Information
Services

Antarctic Circle

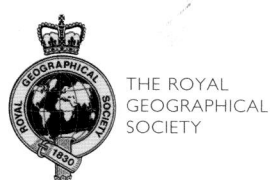

THE ROYAL
GEOGRAPHICAL
SOCIETY

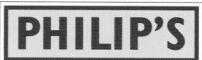

CONCISE
ATLAS
OF THE
WORLD

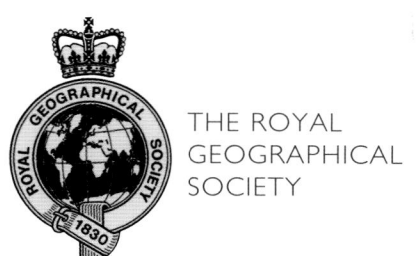

THE ROYAL GEOGRAPHICAL SOCIETY

PHILIP'S

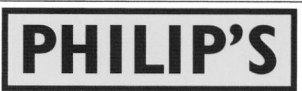

CONCISE ATLAS OF THE WORLD

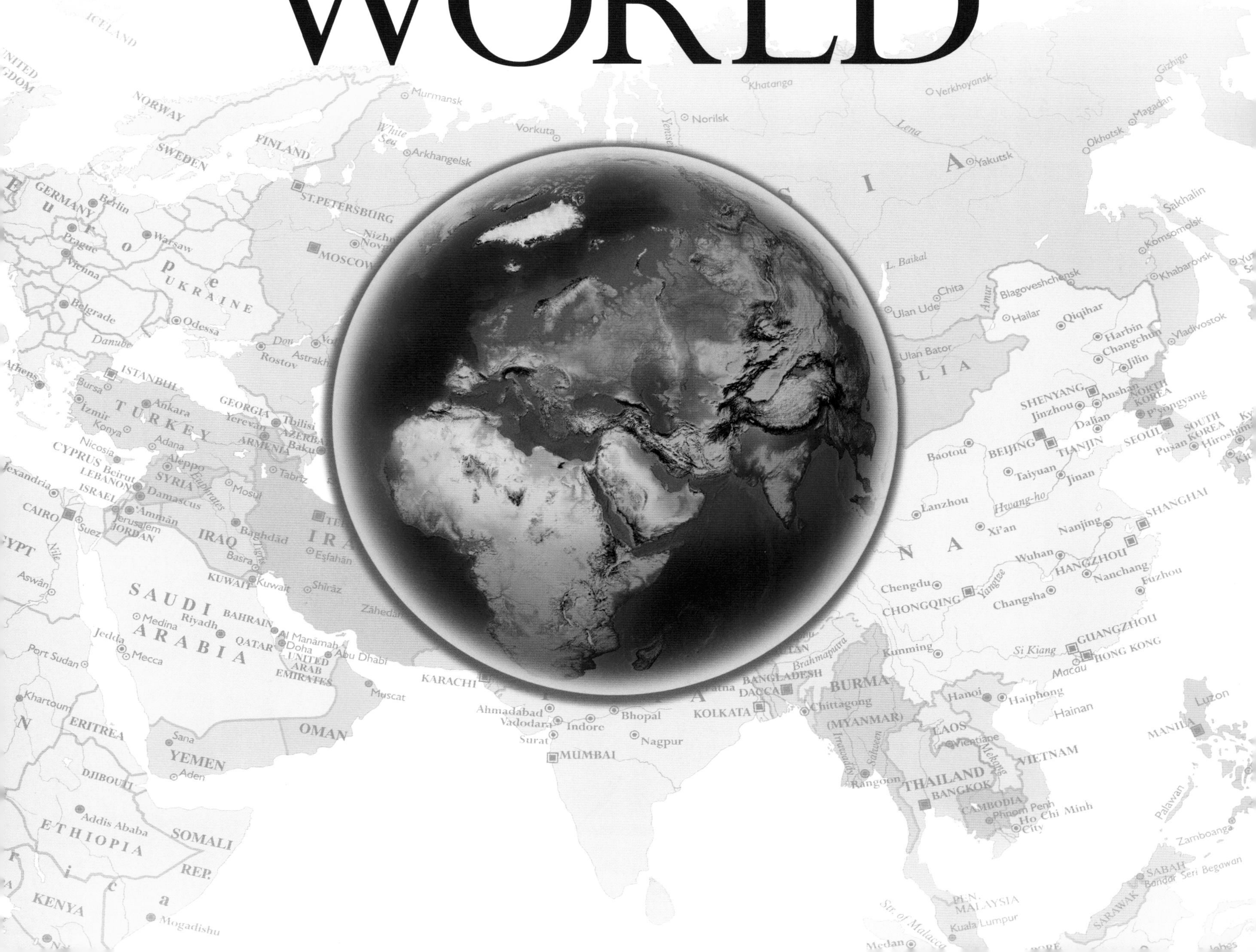

THE EARTH IN SPACE
Cartography by Philip's

Text
Keith Lye

Illustrations
Stefan Chabluk

Star Charts
Wil Tirion

PICTURE ACKNOWLEDGEMENTS
Mike Brown 46 (top left), 48 (top left), 50 (top left), 56 (top left), 60 (top left)
Corbis /William Caram 59, /Ed Eckstein 58 (bottom), /Colin Garratt; Milepost 92 1/2 60 (bottom),
/Aaron Horowitz 40 (top left), /Wolfgang Kaehler 37, /Manoocher/Webistan 48 (top right),
/Kevin R. Morris 48 (bottom), /Galen Rowell 62 (bottom), /Royalty-Free 36 (top left), 44 (top left),
47, 52 (top left), 54 (top left), 58 (top left), 62 (top left), /Peter Turnley 51, /Nik Wheeler 46
(bottom), /Tim Wright 61
Corbis Saba /Shepard Sherbell 56 (bottom)
Corbis Sygma /Thorne Anderson 63
Michael P. Doukas/USGS/CVO 32 (top left)
Akira Fujii/David Malin Images 27
Getty Images/The Image Bank /Peter Hendrie 36 (top right), /Pete Turner 55
Getty Images/Stone /James Balog 32 (bottom), /Simeone Huber 49, /Gary John Norman 52 (bottom),
/Frank Oberle 41 (top), /Dennis Oda 33, /Donovan Reese 34–5, /Michael Townsend 45
Robert Harding Picture Library /Bill Ross 57
Images Colour Library Limited 31
NASA 18 (top left), 20 (top left), 22 (top left), 24 (top left), 26 (top left), 26 (bottom), /Jacques
Descloitres, MODIS/GSFC 28 (top left), /ESA, S. Beckwith (STScI) and the HUDF Team 18 (bottom),
/GSFC 24 (top right), /Hubble Heritage Team (STScI/AURA)/R.G. French (Wellesley College)/J. Cuzzi
and J. Lissauer (NASA/Ames Research Center)/L. Dones (SwRI) 25 (bottom left), /JPL 24 (centre left),
24 (bottom left), 25 (top right), 25 (centre right), /JPL/Univ. Arizona 25 (top left), /JPL/USGS
24 (bottom right), /JSC 38 (top left), 42 (top left), /Hal Pierce/GSFC 40 (top right), /A. Stern (SwRI),
M. Buie (Lowell Observatory)/ESA 25 (bottom right), /Reto Stöckli, Robert Simmon/GSFC 17
NPA Group, Edenbridge, UK 28 (bottom), 29, (top), 29 (bottom), 64
Caroline O'Hara 34 (top left)
Christopher Rayner 30 (top left), 35 (top)
Rex Features /Sipa 50 (bottom)
Robin Scagell/Galaxy 27 (bottom)
Science Photo Library /Martin Bond 30 (bottom), /CNES, 1992 Distribution SPOT Image 43 (top),
/Luke Dodd 19, 21, /Earth Satellite Corporation 41 (bottom), /Simon Fraser 54 (bottom), /NASA 38
(bottom), 39, /David Parker 42 (bottom), /Peter Ryan 43 (bottom), /Jerry Schad 20 (bottom)
Still Pictures /François Pierrel 44 (bottom)
Tony Stone Images /Nigel Press 53

Back cover photographs:
Corbis /Royalty-Free (centre left, far right)
NPA Group, Edenbridge, UK (far left)

Published in Great Britain in 2008
by Philip's,
a division of Octopus Publishing Group Limited
www.octopusbooks.co.uk
2–4 Heron Quays, London E14 4JP
An Hachette Livre UK Company
www.hachettelivre.co.uk

Copyright © 2008 Philip's

Cartography by Philip's

ISBN 978–0–540–09253–6

A CIP catalogue record for this book is available from the British Library.

Printed in Hong Kong

Details of other Philip's titles and services can be found on our website at:
www.philips-maps.co.uk

Royal Geographical Society
with IBG

Advancing geography
and geographical learning

PHILIP'S World Atlases are published in association with THE ROYAL GEOGRAPHICAL SOCIETY (with THE INSTITUTE OF BRITISH GEOGRAPHERS).

The Society was founded in 1830 and given a Royal Charter in 1859 for 'the advancement of geographical science'. It holds historical collections of national and international importance, many of which relate to the Society's association with and support for scientific exploration and research from the 19th century onwards. It was pivotal in establishing geography as a teaching and research discipline in British universities close to the turn of the century, and has played a key role in geographical and environmental education ever since.

Today the Society is a leading world centre for geographical learning – supporting education, teaching, research and expeditions, and promoting public understanding of the subject. The Society welcomes those interested in geography as members. For further information, please visit the website at: www.rgs.org

USER GUIDE

The reference maps which form the main body of this atlas have been prepared in accordance with the highest standards of international cartography to provide an accurate and detailed representation of the Earth. The scales and projections used have been carefully chosen to give balanced coverage of the world, while emphasizing the most densely populated and economically significant regions. A hallmark of Philip's mapping is the use of hill shading and relief colouring to create a graphic impression of landforms: this makes the maps exceptionally easy to read. However, knowledge of the key features employed in the construction and presentation of the maps will enable the reader to derive the fullest benefit from the atlas.

MAP SEQUENCE

The atlas covers the Earth continent by continent: first Europe; then its land neighbour Asia (mapped north before south, in a clockwise sequence), then Africa, Australia and Oceania, North America and South America. This is the classic arrangement adopted by most cartographers since the 16th century. For each continent, there are maps at a variety of scales. First, physical relief

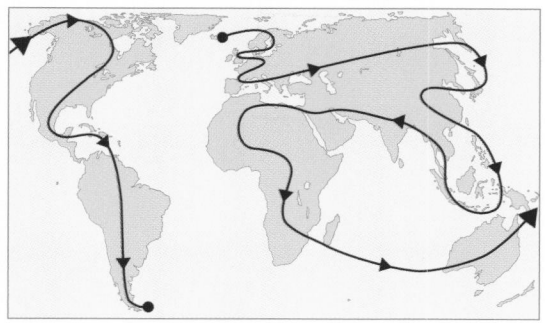

and political maps of the whole continent; then a series of larger-scale maps of the regions within the continent, each followed, where required, by still larger-scale maps of the most important or densely populated areas. The governing principle is that by turning the pages of the atlas, the reader moves steadily from north to south through each continent, with each map overlapping its neighbours.

MAP PRESENTATION

With very few exceptions (for example, for the Arctic and Antarctica), the maps are drawn with north at the top, regardless of whether they are presented upright or sideways on the page. In the borders will be found the map title; a locator diagram showing the area covered; continuation arrows showing the page numbers for maps of adjacent areas; the scale; the projection used; the degrees of latitude and longitude; and the letters and figures used in the index for locating place names and geographical features. Physical relief maps also have a height reference panel identifying the colours used for each layer of contouring.

MAP SYMBOLS

Each map contains a vast amount of detail which can only be conveyed clearly and accurately by the use of symbols. Points and circles of varying sizes locate and identify the relative importance of towns and cities; different styles of type are employed for administrative, geographical and regional place names to aid identification. A variety of pictorial symbols denote landforms such as glaciers, marshes and coral reefs, and man-made structures including roads, railways, airports and canals. International borders are shown by red lines. Where neighbouring countries are in dispute, for example in parts of the Middle East, the maps show the *de facto* boundary between nations, regardless of the legal or historical situation. The symbols are explained on the first page of the World Maps section of the atlas.

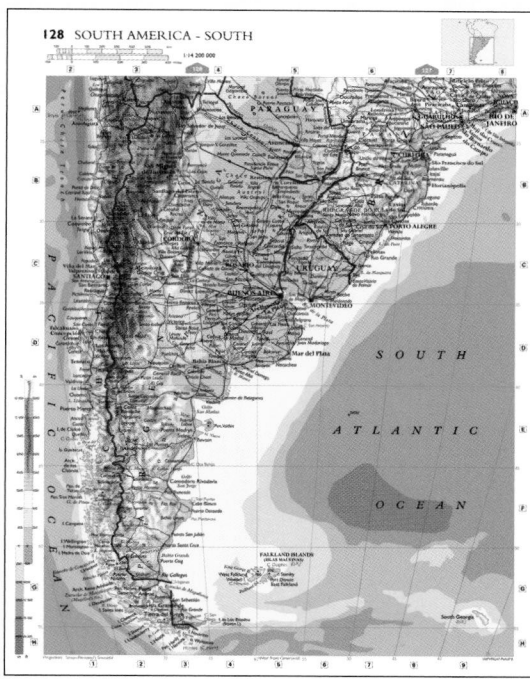

MAP SCALES

1:16 000 000
1 inch = 252 statute miles

The scale of each map is given in the numerical form known as the 'representative fraction'. The first figure is always one, signifying one unit of distance on the map; the second figure, usually in millions, is the number by which the map unit must be multiplied to give the equivalent distance on the Earth's surface. Calculations can easily be made in centimetres and kilometres, by dividing the Earth units figure by 100 000 (i.e. deleting the last five 0s). Thus 1:1 000 000 means 1 cm = 10 km. The calculation for inches and miles is more laborious, but 1 000 000 divided by 63 360 (the number of inches in a mile) shows that 1:1 000 000 means approximately 1 inch = 16 miles. The table below provides distance equivalents for scales down to 1:50 000 000.

LARGE SCALE		
1:1 000 000	1 cm = 10 km	1 inch = 16 miles
1:2 500 000	1 cm = 25 km	1 inch = 39.5 miles
1:5 000 000	1 cm = 50 km	1 inch = 79 miles
1:6 000 000	1 cm = 60 km	1 inch = 95 miles
1:8 000 000	1 cm = 80 km	1 inch = 126 miles
1:10 000 000	1 cm = 100 km	1 inch = 158 miles
1:15 000 000	1 cm = 150 km	1 inch = 237 miles
1:20 000 000	1 cm = 200 km	1 inch = 316 miles
1:50 000 000	1 cm = 500 km	1 inch = 790 miles
SMALL SCALE		

MEASURING DISTANCES

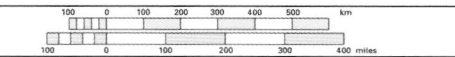

Although each map is accompanied by a scale bar, distances cannot always be measured with confidence because of the distortions involved in portraying the curved surface of the Earth on a flat page. As a general rule, the larger the map scale (that is, the lower the number of Earth units in the representative fraction), the more accurate and reliable will be the distance measured. On small-scale maps such as those of the world and of entire continents, measurement may only be accurate

along the 'standard parallels', or central axes, and should not be attempted without considering the map projection.

MAP PROJECTIONS

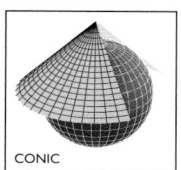
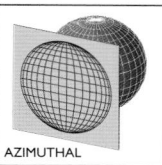
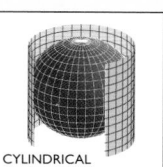

Unlike a globe, no flat map can give a true scale representation of the world in terms of area, shape and position of every region. Each of the numerous systems that have been devised for projecting the curved surface of the Earth on to a flat page involves the sacrifice of accuracy in one or more of these elements. The variations in shape and position of landmasses such as Alaska, Greenland and Australia, for example, can be quite dramatic when different projections are compared. For this atlas, the guiding principle has been to select projections that involve the least distortion of size and distance. The projection used for each map is noted in the border. Most fall into one of three categories – conic, azimuthal or cylindrical – whose basic concepts are shown above. Each involves plotting the forms of the Earth's surface on a grid of latitude and longitude lines, which may be shown as parallels, curves or radiating spokes.

LATITUDE AND LONGITUDE

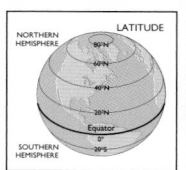
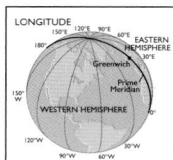
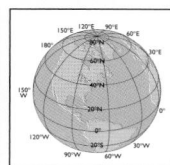

Accurate positioning of individual points on the Earth's surface is made possible by reference to the geometrical system of latitude and longitude. Latitude *parallels* are drawn west–east around the Earth and numbered by degrees north and south of the equator, which is designated 0° of latitude. Longitude *meridians* are drawn north–south and numbered by degrees east and west of the *prime meridian*, 0° of longitude, which passes through Greenwich in England. By referring to these co-ordinates and their subdivisions of minutes (1/60th of a degree) and seconds (1/60th of a minute), any place on Earth can be located to within a few hundred metres. Latitude and longitude are indicated by blue lines on the maps; they are straight or curved according to the projection employed. Reference to these lines is the easiest way of determining the relative positions of places on different maps, and for plotting compass directions.

NAME FORMS

For ease of reference, both English and local name forms appear in the atlas. Oceans, seas and countries are shown in English throughout the atlas; country names may be abbreviated to their commonly accepted form (for example, Germany, not The Federal Republic of Germany). Conventional English forms are also used for place names on the smaller-scale maps of the continents. However, local name forms are used on all large-scale and regional maps, with the English form given in brackets only for important cities – the large-scale map of Russia and Central Asia thus shows Moskva (Moscow). For countries which do not use a Roman script, place names have been transcribed according to the systems adopted by the British and US Geographic Names Authorities. For China, the Pin Yin system has been used, with some more widely known forms appearing in brackets, as with Beijing (Peking). Both English and local names appear in the index, the English form being cross-referenced to the local form.

CONTENTS

WORLD STATISTICS

COUNTRIES   10

CITIES   11

CLIMATE   12–13

PHYSICAL DIMENSIONS   14–15

THE EARTH IN SPACE

THE UNIVERSE   18–19

THE CONSTELLATIONS   20–21

STAR CHARTS   22–23

THE SOLAR SYSTEM   24–25

THE EARTH: TIME AND MOTION   26–27

THE EARTH FROM SPACE   28–29

THE DYNAMIC EARTH   30–31

EARTHQUAKES AND VOLCANOES   32–33

FORCES OF NATURE   34–35

OCEANS AND ICE   36–37

THE EARTH'S ATMOSPHERE   38–39

CLIMATE AND WEATHER   40–41

WATER AND LAND USE   42–43

THE NATURAL WORLD   44–45

THE HUMAN WORLD   46–47

LANGUAGES AND RELIGIONS   48–49

INTERNATIONAL ORGANIZATIONS   50–51

AGRICULTURE   52–53

ENERGY AND MINERALS   54–55

WORLD ECONOMIES   56–57

TRADE AND COMMERCE   58–59

TRAVEL AND COMMUNICATIONS   60–61

THE WORLD TODAY   62–63

WORLD MAPS

MAP SYMBOLS   1

THE WORLD: POLITICAL
1:84 000 000   2–3

ARCTIC OCEAN
1:31 100 000   4

ANTARCTICA
1:31 100 000   5

EUROPE

EUROPE: PHYSICAL
1:17 800 000   6

EUROPE: POLITICAL
1:17 800 000   7

SCANDINAVIA
1:5 300 000
Iceland 1:5 300 000
Færoe Islands 1:5 300 000
                                   8–9

DENMARK AND SOUTHERN SWEDEN
1:2 200 000
                                   10–11

IRELAND
1:1 800 000
                                   12

SCOTLAND
1:1 800 000
Orkney Islands 1:1 800 000
Shetland Islands 1:1 800 000
                                   13

ENGLAND AND WALES
1:1 800 000
Isles of Scilly 1:1 800 000

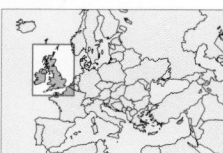

14–15

BRITISH ISLES
1:4 400 000

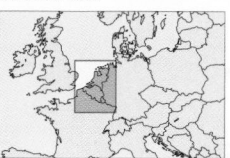

16

NETHERLANDS, BELGIUM AND LUXEMBOURG
1:2 200 000

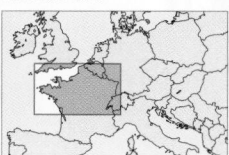

17

NORTHERN FRANCE
1:2 200 000

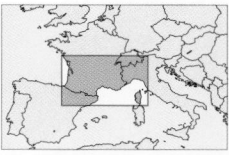

18–19

SOUTHERN FRANCE
1:2 200 000

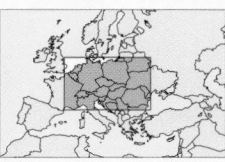

20–21

CENTRAL EUROPE
1:4 400 000

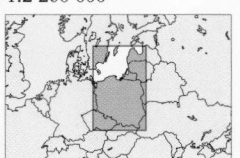

22–23

GERMANY AND SWITZERLAND
1:2 200 000

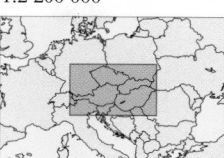

24–25

AUSTRIA, CZECH REPUBLIC
AND SLOVAK REPUBLIC
1:2 200 000

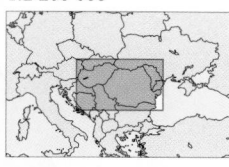

26–27

HUNGARY, ROMANIA AND THE LOWER DANUBE
1:2 200 000

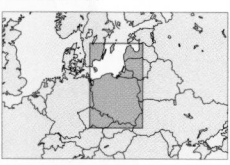

28–29

POLAND AND THE SOUTHERN BALTIC
1:2 200 000

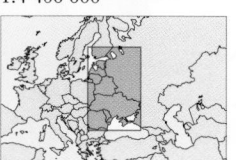

30–31

BALTIC STATES, BELARUS AND UKRAINE
1:4 400 000

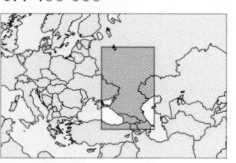

32–33

THE VOLGA BASIN AND THE CAUCASUS
1:4 400 000

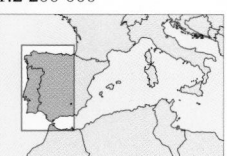

34–35

WESTERN SPAIN AND PORTUGAL
1:2 200 000

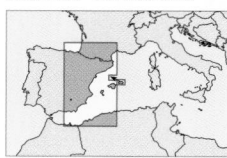

36–37

EASTERN SPAIN
1:2 200 000
Menorca 1:2 200 000

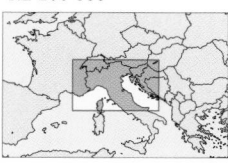

38–39

NORTHERN ITALY, SLOVENIA AND CROATIA
1:2 200 000

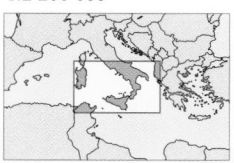

40–41

SOUTHERN ITALY
1:2 200 000

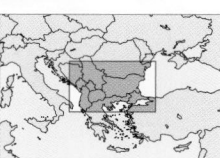

42–43

THE BALKANS
1:2 200 000

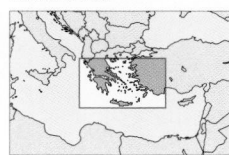

44–45

SOUTHERN GREECE AND WESTERN TURKEY
1:2 200 000

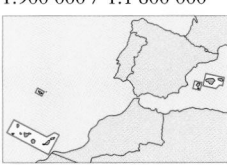

46–47

THE BALEARICS, THE CANARIES AND MADEIRA
1:900 000 / 1:1 800 000

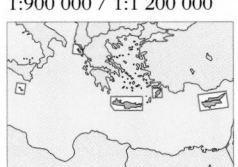

48

MALTA, CRETE, CORFU, RHODES AND CYPRUS
1:900 000 / 1:1 200 000

49

ASIA

ASIA: PHYSICAL
1:44 400 000   **50**

ASIA: POLITICAL
1:44 400 000   **51**

RUSSIA AND CENTRAL ASIA
1:17 800 000

                                                  52–53

JAPAN
1:4 400 000
Ryukyu Islands 1:4 400 000

                                                  54–55

NORTHERN CHINA AND KOREA
1:5 300 000

                                                  56–57

SOUTHERN CHINA
1:5 300 000

                                                  58–59

CHINA
1:17 800 000

                                                  60

THE PHILIPPINES
1:6 700 000

                                                  61

INDONESIA AND THE PHILIPPINES
1:11 100 000
Java and Madura 1:6 700 000
Bali 1:1 800 000

                                                  62–63

MAINLAND SOUTH-EAST ASIA
1:5 300 000
Ko Phuket 1:900 000
Ko Samui 1:900 000
Pinang 1:900 000
Singapore 1:900 000

                                                  64–65

SOUTH ASIA
1:8 900 000

                                                  66–67

NORTHERN INDIA, PAKISTAN AND NEPAL
1:5 300 000
Jammu and Kashmir 1:5 300 000

                                                  68–69

THE MIDDLE EAST
1:6 200 000

                                                  70–71

TURKEY AND TRANSCAUCASIA
1:4 400 000

                                                  72–73

THE NEAR EAST
1:2 200 000

                                                  74

ARABIA AND THE HORN OF AFRICA
1:13 300 000

                                                  75

AFRICA

AFRICA: PHYSICAL
1:37 300 000   **76**

AFRICA: POLITICAL
1: 37 300 000   **77**

NORTHERN AFRICA
1:13 300 000
The Azores 1:13 300 000
Cape Verde Islands 1:8 900 000

                                                  78–79

THE NILE VALLEY
1:7 100 000
The Nile Delta 1:3 600 000

                                                  80–81

WEST AFRICA
1:7 100 000

                                                  82–83

CENTRAL AND SOUTHERN AFRICA
1:13 300 000
Seychelles 1:2 200 000
Réunion 1:2 200 000
Mauritius 1:2 200 000
Comoros 1:7 100 000

                                                  84–85

EAST AFRICA
1:7 100 000

                                                  86–87

SOUTHERN AFRICA
1:7 100 000
Madagascar 1:7 100 000

                                                  88–89

AUSTRALIA AND OCEANIA

AUSTRALIA AND OCEANIA:
PHYSICAL AND POLITICAL
1:44 400 000   **90**

NEW ZEALAND
1:5 300 000
Fiji 1:5 300 000
Samoan Islands 1:5 300 000
Tonga 1:5 300 000
Tahiti and Moorea 1:1 100 000

91

WESTERN AUSTRALIA
1:7 100 000

92–93

EASTERN AUSTRALIA
1:7 100 000
Whitsunday Islands 1:2 200 000
Tasmania 1:7 100 000
Torres Strait 1:7 100 000

94–95

PACIFIC OCEAN
1:48 000 000   **96–97**

NORTH AMERICA

NORTH AMERICA: PHYSICAL
1:31 100 000   **98**

NORTH AMERICA: POLITICAL
1:31 100 000   **99**

CANADA
1:13 300 000

100–101

WESTERN CANADA
1:6 200 000

102–103

EASTERN CANADA
1:6 200 000

104–105

UNITED STATES
1:13 300 000
Hawai'i 1:13 300 000
Alaska 1:13 300 000

106–107

UNITED STATES – WEST
1:6 250 000

108–109

CENTRAL AND SOUTHERN CALIFORNIA
AND WESTERN WASHINGTON
1:2 200 000

110–111

UNITED STATES MIDWEST AND
NORTH-EAST
1:6 250 000

112–113

NORTH-EASTERN UNITED STATES
1:2 200 000

114–115

UNITED STATES – SOUTH
1:6 250 000

116–117

MEXICO
1:7 100 000

118–119

CENTRAL AMERICA AND THE WEST INDIES
1:7 100 000
Jamaica 1:2 700 000
Guadeloupe 1:1 800 000
Martinique 1:1 800 000
Puerto Rico 1:2 700 000
Virgin Islands 1:1 800 000
St Lucia 1:890 000
Barbados 1:890 000

120–121

SOUTH AMERICA

SOUTH AMERICA: PHYSICAL
1:31 100 000   **122**

SOUTH AMERICA: POLITICAL
1:31 100 000   **123**

SOUTH AMERICA – NORTH
1:14 200 000
Trinidad and Tobago 1:2 200 000

124–125

CENTRAL SOUTH AMERICA
1:7 100 000

126–127

SOUTH AMERICA – SOUTH
1:14 200 000

128

INDEX TO WORLD MAPS

129–224

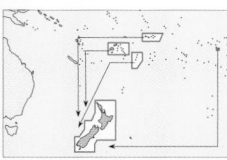

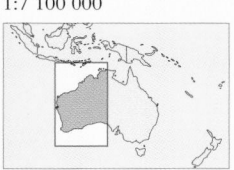

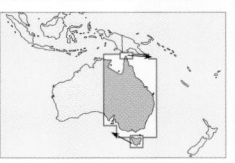

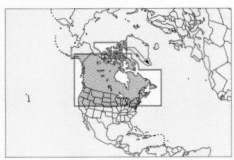

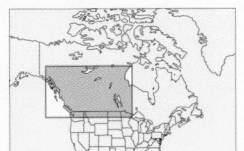

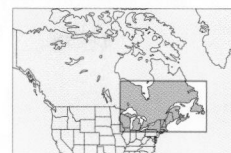

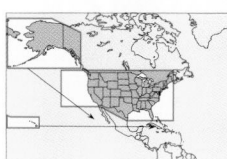

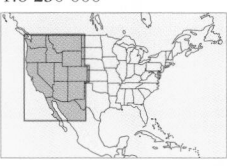

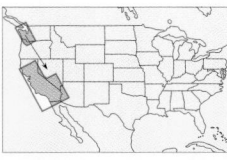

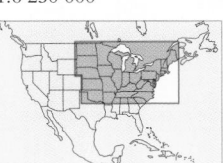

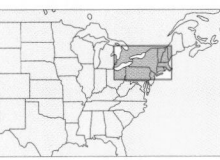

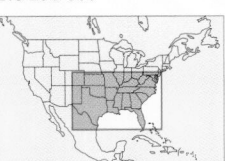

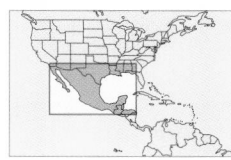

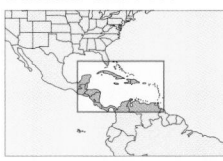

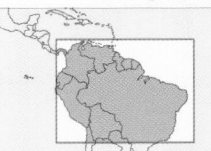

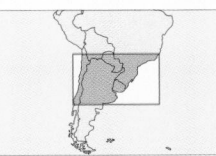

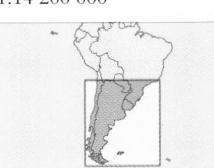

WORLD STATISTICS: COUNTRIES

This alphabetical list includes the principal countries and territories of the world. If a territory is not completely independent, the country it is associated with is named. The area figures give the total area of land, inland water and ice. The population figures are 2007 estimates where available. The annual income is the Gross Domestic Product per capita in US dollars. The figures are the latest available, usually 2007 estimates.

Country/Territory	Area km² Thousands	Area miles² Thousands	Population Thousands	Capital	Annual Income US $
Afghanistan	652	252	31,890	Kabul	800
Albania	28.7	11.1	3,601	Tirana	5,500
Algeria	2,382	920	33,333	Algiers	8,100
American Samoa (US)	0.20	0.08	58	Pago Pago	5,800
Andorra	0.47	0.18	72	Andorra La Vella	38,800
Angola	1,247	481	12,264	Luanda	6,500
Anguilla (UK)	0.10	0.04	14	The Valley	8,800
Antigua & Barbuda	0.44	0.17	69	St John's	10,900
Argentina	2,780	1,074	40,302	Buenos Aires	13,000
Armenia	29.8	11.5	2,972	Yerevan	5,700
Aruba (Netherlands)	0.19	0.07	100	Oranjestad	21,800
Australia	7,741	2,989	20,434	Canberra	37,500
Austria	83.9	32.4	8,200	Vienna	39,000
Azerbaijan	86.6	33.4	8,120	Baku	9,000
Azores (Portugal)	2.2	0.86	236	Ponta Delgada	15,000
Bahamas	13.9	5.4	306	Nassau	22,700
Bahrain	0.69	0.27	709	Manama	34,700
Bangladesh	144	55.6	150,448	Dhaka	1,400
Barbados	0.43	0.17	281	Bridgetown	19,700
Belarus	208	80.2	9,725	Minsk	10,200
Belgium	30.5	11.8	10,392	Brussels	36,500
Belize	23.0	8.9	294	Belmopan	7,800
Benin	113	43.5	9,078	Porto-Novo	1,500
Bermuda (UK)	0.05	0.02	66	Hamilton	69,900
Bhutan	47.0	18.1	2,328	Thimphu	1,400
Bolivia	1,099	424	9,119	La Paz/Sucre	4,400
Bosnia-Herzegovina	51.2	19.8	4,552	Sarajevo	6,600
Botswana	582	225	1,816	Gaborone	14,700
Brazil	8,514	3,287	190,011	Brasília	9,700
Brunei	5.8	2.2	375	Bandar Seri Begawan	25,600
Bulgaria	111	42.8	7,323	Sofia	11,800
Burkina Faso	274	106	14,326	Ouagadougou	1,200
Burma (=Myanmar)	677	261	47,374	Rangoon/Naypyidaw	1,900
Burundi	27.8	10.7	8,391	Bujumbura	800
Cambodia	181	69.9	13,996	Phnom Penh	1,800
Cameroon	475	184	18,060	Yaoundé	2,300
Canada	9,971	3,850	33,390	Ottawa	38,200
Canary Is. (Spain)	7.2	2.8	1,682	Las Palmas/Santa Cruz	19,900
Cape Verde Is.	4.0	1.6	424	Praia	7,000
Cayman Is. (UK)	0.26	0.10	47	George Town	43,800
Central African Republic	623	241	4,369	Bangui	700
Chad	1,284	496	9,886	Ndjaména	1,600
Chile	757	292	16,285	Santiago	14,400
China	9,597	3,705	1,321,852	Beijing	5,300
Colombia	1,139	440	44,380	Bogotá	7,200
Comoros	2.2	0.86	711	Moroni	600
Congo	342	132	3,801	Brazzaville	3,700
Congo (Dem. Rep. of the)	2,345	905	65,752	Kinshasa	300
Cook Is. (NZ)	0.24	0.09	22	Avarua	9,100
Costa Rica	51.1	19.7	4,134	San José	13,500
Croatia	56.5	21.8	4,493	Zagreb	15,500
Cuba	111	42.8	11,394	Havana	4,500
Cyprus	9.3	3.6	788	Nicosia	24,600
Czech Republic	78.9	30.5	10,229	Prague	24,400
Denmark	43.1	16.6	5,468	Copenhagen	37,400
Djibouti	23.2	9.0	496	Djibouti	1,000
Dominica	0.75	0.29	72	Roseau	3,800
Dominican Republic	48.5	18.7	9,366	Santo Domingo	9,200
East Timor	14.9	5.7	1,085	Dili	800
Ecuador	284	109	13,756	Quito	7,100
Egypt	1,001	387	80,335	Cairo	5,400
El Salvador	21.0	8.1	6,948	San Salvador	5,200
Equatorial Guinea	28.1	10.8	551	Malabo	4,100
Eritrea	118	45.4	4,907	Asmara	1,000
Estonia	45.1	17.4	1,316	Tallinn	21,800
Ethiopia	1,104	426	76,512	Addis Ababa	700
Faroe Is. (Denmark)	1.4	0.54	48	Tórshavn	31,000
Fiji	18.3	7.1	919	Suva	4,100
Finland	338	131	5,238	Helsinki	35,500
France	552	213	60,876	Paris	33,800
French Guiana (France)	90.0	34.7	200	Cayenne	8,300
French Polynesia (France)	4.0	1.5	279	Papeete	17,500
Gabon	268	103	1,455	Libreville	13,800
Gambia, The	11.3	4.4	1,688	Banjul	800
Gaza Strip (OPT)*	0.36	0.14	1,482	–	1,100
Georgia	69.7	26.9	4,646	Tbilisi	4,200
Germany	357	138	82,401	Berlin	34,400
Ghana	239	92.1	22,931	Accra	1,400
Gibraltar (UK)	0.006	0.002	28	Gibraltar Town	38,200
Greece	132	50.9	10,706	Athens	30,500
Greenland (Denmark)	2,176	840	56	Nuuk	20,000
Grenada	0.34	0.13	90	St George's	3,900
Guadeloupe (France)	1.7	0.66	453	Basse-Terre	7,900
Guam (US)	0.55	0.21	173	Agana	15,000
Guatemala	109	42.0	12,728	Guatemala City	5,400
Guinea	246	94.9	9,948	Conakry	1,000
Guinea-Bissau	36.1	13.9	1,473	Bissau	600
Guyana	215	83.0	769	Georgetown	5,300
Haiti	27.8	10.7	8,706	Port-au-Prince	1,900
Honduras	112	43.3	7,484	Tegucigalpa	3,300
Hungary	93.0	35.9	9,956	Budapest	19,500
Iceland	103	39.8	302	Reykjavik	39,400
India	3,287	1,269	1,129,866	New Delhi	2,700
Indonesia	1,905	735	234,694	Jakarta	3,400
Iran	1,648	636	65,398	Tehran	12,300
Iraq	438	169	27,500	Baghdad	3,600
Ireland	70.3	27.1	4,109	Dublin	45,600
Israel	20.6	8.0	6,427	Jerusalem	28,800
Italy	301	116	58,148	Rome	31,000
Ivory Coast (=Côte d'Ivoire)	322	125	18,013	Yamoussoukro	1,800
Jamaica	11.0	4.2	2,780	Kingston	4,800
Japan	378	146	127,433	Tokyo	33,800
Jordan	89.3	34.5	6,053	Amman	4,700
Kazakhstan	2,725	1,052	15,285	Astana	11,100
Kenya	580	224	36,914	Nairobi	1,600
Kiribati	0.73	0.28	108	Tarawa	1,800
Korea, North	121	46.5	23,302	Pyŏngyang	1,900
Korea, South	99.3	38.3	49,045	Seoul	24,600
Kosovo	10.9	4.2	2,127	Pristina	1,800
Kuwait	17.8	6.9	2,506	Kuwait City	55,300
Kyrgyzstan	200	77.2	5,284	Bishkek	2,000
Laos	237	91.4	6,522	Vientiane	1,900
Latvia	64.6	24.9	2,260	Riga	17,700
Lebanon	10.4	4.0	3,926	Beirut	10,400
Lesotho	30.4	11.7	2,125	Maseru	1,500
Liberia	111	43.0	3,196	Monrovia	500
Libya	1,760	679	6,037	Tripoli	13,100
Liechtenstein	0.16	0.06	34	Vaduz	25,000
Lithuania	65.2	25.2	3,575	Vilnius	16,700
Luxembourg	2.6	1.0	480	Luxembourg	80,800
Macedonia (FYROM)	25.7	9.9	2,056	Skopje	8,400
Madagascar	587	227	19,449	Antananarivo	1,000
Madeira (Portugal)	0.78	0.30	241	Funchal	22,700
Malawi	118	45.7	13,603	Lilongwe	800
Malaysia	330	127	24,821	Kuala Lumpur/Putrajaya	14,400
Maldives	0.30	0.12	369	Malé	3,900
Mali	1,240	479	11,995	Bamako	1,200
Malta	0.32	0.12	402	Valletta	23,700
Marshall Is.	0.18	0.07	62	Majuro	2,900
Martinique (France)	1.1	0.43	436	Fort-de-France	14,400
Mauritania	1,026	396	3,270	Nouakchott	1,800
Mauritius	2.0	0.79	1,251	Port Louis	11,900
Mayotte (France)	0.37	0.14	209	Mamoundzou	4,900
Mexico	1,958	756	108,701	Mexico City	12,500
Micronesia, Fed. States of	0.70	0.27	108	Palikir	2,300
Moldova	33.9	13.1	4,320	Chişinău	2,200
Monaco	0.001	0.0004	33	Monaco	30,000
Mongolia	1,567	605	2,952	Ulan Bator	2,900
Montenegro	14.0	5.4	685	Podgorica	3,800
Morocco	447	172	33,757	Rabat	3,800
Mozambique	802	309	20,906	Maputo	900
Namibia	824	318	2,055	Windhoek	5,200
Nauru	0.02	0.008	14	Yaren District	5,000
Nepal	147	56.8	28,902	Katmandu	1,100
Netherlands	41.5	16.0	16,571	Amsterdam/The Hague	38,600
Netherlands Antilles (Neths)	0.80	0.31	224	Willemstad	16,000
New Caledonia (France)	18.6	7.2	222	Nouméa	15,000
New Zealand	271	104	4,116	Wellington	27,300
Nicaragua	130	50.2	5,675	Managua	3,200
Niger	1,267	489	12,895	Niamey	700
Nigeria	924	357	135,031	Abuja	2,200
Northern Mariana Is. (US)	0.46	0.18	85	Saipan	12,500
Norway	324	125	4,628	Oslo	55,600
Oman	310	119	3,205	Muscat	19,100
Pakistan	796	307	164,742	Islamabad	2,600
Palau	0.46	0.18	21	Melekeok	7,600
Panama	75.5	29.2	3,242	Panamá	9,000
Papua New Guinea	463	179	5,796	Port Moresby	2,900
Paraguay	407	157	6,669	Asunción	4,000
Peru	1,285	496	28,675	Lima	7,600
Philippines	300	116	91,077	Manila	3,300
Poland	323	125	38,518	Warsaw	16,200
Portugal	88.8	34.3	10,643	Lisbon	21,800
Puerto Rico (US)	8.9	3.4	3,944	San Juan	19,600
Qatar	11.0	4.2	907	Doha	29,400
Réunion (France)	2.5	0.97	788	St-Denis	6,200
Romania	238	92.0	22,276	Bucharest	11,100
Russia	17,075	6,593	141,378	Moscow	14,600
Rwanda	26.3	10.2	9,908	Kigali	1,000
St Kitts & Nevis	0.26	0.10	39	Basseterre	8,200
St Lucia	0.54	0.21	171	Castries	4,800
St Vincent & Grenadines	0.39	0.15	118	Kingstown	3,600
Samoa	2.8	1.1	214	Apia	2,100
San Marino	0.06	0.02	30	San Marino	34,100
São Tomé & Príncipe	0.96	0.37	200	São Tomé	1,200
Saudi Arabia	2,150	830	27,601	Riyadh	20,700
Senegal	197	76.0	12,522	Dakar	1,700
Serbia	77.5	29.9	8,024	Belgrade	7,700
Seychelles	0.46	0.18	82	Victoria	18,400
Sierra Leone	71.7	27.7	6,145	Freetown	800
Singapore	0.68	0.26	4,553	Singapore City	48,900
Slovak Republic	49.0	18.9	5,448	Bratislava	19,800
Slovenia	20.3	7.8	2,009	Ljubljana	27,300
Solomon Is.	28.9	11.2	567	Honiara	600
Somalia	638	246	9,119	Mogadishu	600
South Africa	1,221	471	43,998	Cape Town/Pretoria	10,600
Spain	498	192	40,448	Madrid	33,700
Sri Lanka	65.6	25.3	20,926	Colombo	4,100
Sudan	2,506	967	39,379	Khartoum	2,500
Suriname	163	63.0	471	Paramaribo	7,800
Swaziland	17.4	6.7	1,133	Mbabane	4,800
Sweden	450	174	9,031	Stockholm	36,900
Switzerland	41.3	15.9	7,555	Bern	39,800
Syria	185	71.5	19,315	Damascus	4,500
Taiwan	36.0	13.9	22,859	Taipei	29,800
Tajikistan	143	55.3	7,077	Dushanbe	1,600
Tanzania	945	365	39,384	Dodoma	1,100
Thailand	513	198	65,068	Bangkok	8,000
Togo	56.8	21.9	5,702	Lomé	900
Tonga	0.65	0.25	117	Nuku'alofa	2,200
Trinidad & Tobago	5.1	2.0	1,057	Port of Spain	21,700
Tunisia	164	63.2	10,276	Tunis	7,500
Turkey	775	299	71,159	Ankara	9,400
Turkmenistan	488	188	5,097	Ashkhabad	9,200
Turks & Caicos Is. (UK)	0.43	0.17	22	Cockburn Town	11,500
Tuvalu	0.03	0.01	12	Fongafale	1,600
Uganda	241	93.1	30,263	Kampala	1,100
Ukraine	604	233	46,300	Kiev	6,900
United Arab Emirates	83.6	32.3	4,444	Abu Dhabi	55,200
United Kingdom	242	93.4	60,776	London	35,300
United States of America	9,629	3,718	301,140	Washington, DC	46,000
Uruguay	175	67.6	3,461	Montevideo	10,700
Uzbekistan	447	173	27,780	Tashkent	2,200
Vanuatu	12.2	4.7	212	Port-Vila	2,900
Venezuela	912	352	26,024	Caracas	12,800
Vietnam	332	128	85,262	Hanoi	2,600
Virgin Is. (UK)	0.15	0.06	24	Road Town	38,500
Virgin Is. (US)	0.35	0.13	108	Charlotte Amalie	14,500
Wallis & Futuna Is. (France)	0.20	0.08	16	Mata-Utu	3,800
West Bank (OPT)*	5.9	2.3	2,536	–	1,100
Western Sahara	266	103	383	El Aaiún	N/A
Yemen	528	204	22,231	Sana'	2,400
Zambia	753	291	11,477	Lusaka	1,400
Zimbabwe	391	151	12,311	Harare	500

*OPT = Occupied Palestinian Territory   N/A = Not available

WORLD STATISTICS: CITIES

This list shows the principal cities with more than 750,000 inhabitants. The figures are taken from the most recent census or estimate available, usually 2006, and as far as possible are the population of the metropolitan area or urban agglomeration (for example, greater New York, Mexico or Paris). All the figures are in thousands. Local name forms have been used for the smaller cities (for example, Thessaloniki).

AFGHANISTAN	
Kabul	3,288
ALGERIA	
Algiers	3,260
ANGOLA	
Luanda	2,839
ARGENTINA	
Buenos Aires	13,349
Córdoba	1,592
Rosario	1,312
Mendoza	1,072
San Miguel de Tucumán	837
ARMENIA	
Yerevan	1,103
AUSTRALIA	
Sydney	4,388
Melbourne	3,663
Brisbane	1,769
Perth	1,484
Adelaide	1,137
AUSTRIA	
Vienna	2,260
AZERBAIJAN	
Baku	1,856
BANGLADESH	
Dhaka	12,560
Chittagong	4,171
Khulna	1,497
Rajshahi	1,035
BELARUS	
Minsk	1,778
BELGIUM	
Brussels	1,012
BOLIVIA	
La Paz	1,533
Santa Cruz	1,352
Cochabamba	797
BRAZIL	
São Paulo	18,333
Rio de Janeiro	11,469
Belo Horizonte	5,304
Pôrto Alegre	3,795
Recife	3,527
Brasília	3,341
Salvador	3,331
Fortaleza	3,261
Curitiba	2,871
Campinas	2,640
Belém	2,097
Goiânia	1,878
Manaus	1,673
Santos	1,634
Vitória	1,602
Maceió	1,137
Natal	1,049
São Luís	982
São José dos Campos	972
João Pessoa	931
Teresina	895
Campo Grande	821
BULGARIA	
Sofia	1,093
BURKINA FASO	
Ouagadougou	870
BURMA (MYANMAR)	
Rangoon	4,107
Mandalay	927
CAMBODIA	
Phnom Penh	1,364
CAMEROON	
Douala	1,980
Yaoundé	1,727
CANADA	
Toronto	5,312
Montréal	3,640
Vancouver	2,188
Ottawa	1,156
Calgary	1,058
Edmonton	1,015
CHILE	
Santiago	5,683
CHINA	
Shanghai	14,503
Beijing	10,717
Guangzhou	8,425
Shenzhen	7,233
Wuhan	7,093
Hong Kong	7,041
Tianjin	7,040
Chongqing	6,363
Shenyang	4,720
Dongguan	4,320
Chengdu	4,065
Xi'an	3,926
Harbin	3,695
Nanjing	3,621
Guiyang	3,447
Dalian	3,073
Changchun	3,046
Zibo	2,982
Kunming	2,837
Hangzhou	2,831
Qingdao	2,817
Taiyuan	2,794
Jinan	2,743
Zhengzhou	2,590
Fuzhou	2,453
Changsha	2,451
Lanzhou	2,411
Xiamen	2,371
Shijiazhuang	2,275
Jinxi	2,268
Jilin	2,255
Wenzhou	2,212
Nanchang	2,188
Zaozhuang	2,096
Nanchong	2,046
Nanning	2,040
Linyi	2,035
Ürümqi	2,025
Yantai	1,991
Wanxian	1,963
Xuzhou	1,960
Baotou	1,920
Hefei	1,916
Suzhou	1,849
Nanyang	1,830
Tangshan	1,825
Ningbo	1,810
Datong	1,763
Yancheng	1,678
Tianmen	1,676
Shangqui	1,650
Lu'an	1,647
Wuxi	1,646
Luoyang	1,644
Hohhot	1,644
Anshan	1,611
Qiqihar	1,607
Tai'an	1,598
Daqing	1,594
Xinghua	1,587
Pingxiang	1,562
Handan	1,535
Xiantao	1,528
Zhanjiang	1,514
Weifang	1,498
Shantou	1,495
Fushun	1,456
Xianyang	1,450
Luzhou	1,447
Neijiang	1,441
Changde	1,429
Huainan	1,420
Liuzhou	1,409
Suining, Sichuan	1,401
Quanzhou	1,377
Xintai	1,334
Mianyang	1,322
Heze	1,318
Yiyang	1,318
Yueyang	1,286
Suqian	1,258
Changzhou	1,249
Huaian	1,243
Chifeng	1,238
Jingmen	1,228
Yuzhou	1,226
Zaoyang	1,210
Huzhou	1,203
Tianshui	1,199
Yongzhou	1,182
Mudanjiang	1,171
Liupanshui	1,149
Leshan	1,143
Jining, Shandong	1,143
Xiaoshan	1,130
Yixing	1,129
Zigong	1,087
Xianyang	1,072
Fuyu	1,068
Yulin	1,060
Baoding	1,042
Xinyi, Jiangsu	1,022
Zhuzhou	1,016
Jixi	1,012
Linqing	1,009
Jiamusi	1,006
Xiangfan	1,006
Zhangjiakou	1,001
Benxi	967
Xiangxiang	936
Zhangjiagang	936
Xinyu	932
Yichun, Heilongjiang	916
Yichun, Jiangxi	890
Jinzhou	888
Zhaotong	879
Yuyao	876
Anshun	864
Hengyang	853
Xuanzhou	851
Tongliao	847
Huaibei	830
Jiaxing	817
Kaifeng	810
Fuxin	807
Hunjiang	798
COLOMBIA	
Bogotá	7,594
Medellín	3,236
Cali	2,583
Barranquilla	1,918
Bucaramanga	1,069
Cartagena	1,002
Cúcuta	883
CONGO	
Brazzaville	1,173
CONGO (DEM. REP. OF THE)	
Kinshasa	6,049
Kolwezi	1,207
Lubumbashi	1,179
Mbuji-Mayi	1,024
COSTA RICA	
San José	1,217
CROATIA	
Zagreb	1,067
CUBA	
Havana	2,192
CZECH REPUBLIC	
Prague	1,171
DENMARK	
Copenhagen	1,091
DOMINICAN REPUBLIC	
Santo Domingo	2,563
Santiago de los Caballeros	804
ECUADOR	
Guayaquil	2,387
Quito	1,514
EGYPT	
Cairo	11,146
Alexandria	3,760
Shubrâ el Kheima	937
EL SALVADOR	
San Salvador	1,517
ETHIOPIA	
Addis Ababa	2,899
FINLAND	
Helsinki	1,091
FRANCE	
Paris	9,820
Lyons	1,403
Marseilles	1,382
Lille	1,029
Nice	889
Toulouse	761
Bordeaux	754
GEORGIA	
Tbilisi	1,406
GERMANY	
Berlin	3,389
Hamburg	1,740
Munich	1,263
Cologne	963
GHANA	
Accra	1,981
Kumasi	1,517
GREECE	
Athens	3,238
Thessaloniki	824
GUATEMALA	
Guatemala City	3,242
GUINEA	
Conakry	1,465
HAITI	
Port-au-Prince	2,129
HONDURAS	
Tegucigalpa	1,061
HUNGARY	
Budapest	1,693
INDIA	
Mumbai	18,336
Delhi	15,334
Kolkata	14,299
Chennai	6,915
Bangalore	6,532
Hyderabad	6,145
Ahmedabad	5,171
Pune	4,485
Surat	3,671
Kanpur	3,040
Jaipur	2,796
Lucknow	2,589
Nagpur	2,359
Patna	2,066
Indore	1,941
Vadodara	1,686
Bhopal	1,656
Coimbatore	1,628
Ludhiana	1,583
Agra	1,526
Visakhapatnam	1,468
Cochin	1,461
Nashik	1,408
Meerut	1,340
Faridabad	1,330
Varanasi	1,300
Ghaziabad	1,277
Asansol	1,272
Jamshedpur	1,246
Madurai	1,245
Jabalpur	1,234
Rajkot	1,205
Dhanbad	1,195
Amritsar	1,162
Allahabad	1,153
Vijayawada	1,093
Srinagar	1,093
Aurangabad	1,065
Bhilainagar-Durg	1,051
Solapur	1,012
Ranchi	999
Jodhpur	954
Guwahati	941
Gwalior	939
Trivandrum	918
Calicut	917
Tiruchchirapalli	913
Chandigarh	896
Hubli-Dharwad	854
Mysore	851
INDONESIA	
Jakarta	13,215
Bandung	4,126
Surabaya	2,992
Medan	2,287
Palembang	1,733
Ujung Pandang	1,284
Bandar Lampung	915
Malang	898
Tegal	898
Semarang	816
Bogor	761
IRAN	
Tehran	7,352
Mashhad	2,147
Esfahan	1,547
Tabriz	1,396
Karaj	1,235
Shiraz	1,230
Qom	1,045
Ahvaz	967
Bakhtaran	771
IRAQ	
Baghdad	5,910
Mosul	1,236
Basra	1,187
Irbil	840
IRELAND	
Dublin	1,037
ISRAEL	
Tel Aviv-Yafo	3,025
Haifa	948
ITALY	
Rome	3,348
Milan	2,953
Naples	2,245
Turin	1,660
Genoa	803
IVORY COAST (CÔTE D'IVOIRE)	
Abidjan	3,516
JAPAN	
Tokyo	12,064
Yokohama	6,427
Osaka	2,599
Nagoya	2,172
Sapporo	1,922
Kobe	1,493
Kyoto	1,468
Fukuoka	1,341
Kawasaki	1,250
Hiroshima	1,126
Kitakyushu	1,011
Sendai	1,008
Chiba	887
Sakai	792
JORDAN	
Amman	1,292
KAZAKHSTAN	
Almaty	1,156
KENYA	
Nairobi	2,818
KOREA, NORTH	
Pyŏngyang	3,351
N'ampo	1,102
Hamhung	821
KOREA, SOUTH	
Seoul	9,888
Busan	3,830
Incheon	2,884
Daegu	2,675
Daejeon	1,522
Gwangju	1,379
Seongnam	1,353
Ulsan	1,340
Ansan	984
Pucheon	900
Suwon	876
Pohang	790
KUWAIT	
Kuwait City	1,810
KYRGYZSTAN	
Bishkek	828
LATVIA	
Riga	719
LEBANON	
Beirut	2,070
LIBYA	
Tripoli	2,098
Benghazi	1,114
MADAGASCAR	
Antananarivo	1,808
MALAYSIA	
Kuala Lumpur	1,405
MALI	
Bamako	1,379
MEXICO	
Mexico City	19,013
Guadalajara	3,905
Monterrey	3,517
Toluca	1,987
Puebla	1,880
Tijuana	1,570
Ciudad Juárez	1,469
León	1,438
Torreón	1,057
San Luis Potosí	927
Mérida	919
Querétaro	913
Mexicali	840
Culiacán	799
MONGOLIA	
Ulan Bator	842
MOROCCO	
Casablanca	3,743
Rabat	1,859
Fès	1,032
Marrakesh	951
MOZAMBIQUE	
Maputo	1,316
NEPAL	
Katmandu	1,176
NETHERLANDS	
Amsterdam	1,157
Rotterdam	1,112
NEW ZEALAND	
Auckland	1,152
NICARAGUA	
Managua	1,165
NIGER	
Niamey	997
NIGERIA	
Lagos	11,135
Kano	2,884
Ibadan	2,375
Kaduna	1,329
Benin City	1,022
Ogbomosho	959
Port Harcourt	942
NORWAY	
Oslo	808
PAKISTAN	
Karachi	11,819
Lahore	6,373
Faisalabad	2,533
Rawalpindi	1,794
Gujranwala	1,466
Multan	1,459
Hyderabad	1,392
Peshawar	1,255
Islamabad	791
PANAMA	
Panamá	1,216
PARAGUAY	
Asunción	1,858
PERU	
Lima	8,180
PHILIPPINES	
Manila	10,677
Davao	1,326
POLAND	
Warsaw	1,680
Lódz	815
PORTUGAL	
Lisbon	2,761
Porto	1,309
PUERTO RICO	
San Juan	2,604
ROMANIA	
Bucharest	1,934
RUSSIA	
Moscow	10,672
Saint Petersburg	5,315
Novosibirsk	1,425
Nizhniy Novgorod	1,288
Yekaterinburg	1,281
Samara	1,140
Omsk	1,132
Kazan	1,108
Rostov	1,081
Chelyabinsk	1,067
Ufa	1,035
Volgograd	1,016
Perm	1,014
Voronezh	918
Saratov	881
Simbirsk	864
Krasnoyarsk	840
Togliatti	771
SAUDI ARABIA	
Riyadh	5,514
Jedda	3,807
Mecca	1,529
Medina	1,044
Dammam	920
SENEGAL	
Dakar	2,313
SERBIA	
Belgrade	1,116
SIERRA LEONE	
Freetown	1,007
SINGAPORE	
Singapore City	4,372
SOMALIA	
Mogadishu	1,320
SOUTH AFRICA	
Johannesburg	3,254
Cape Town	3,083
Durban	2,631
Pretoria	1,271
Vereeniging	1,027
Port Elizabeth	1,006
SPAIN	
Madrid	5,608
Barcelona	4,795
SUDAN	
Khartoum	4,518
SWEDEN	
Stockholm	1,729
Gothenburg	829
SWITZERLAND	
Zürich	1,144
SYRIA	
Aleppo	2,505
Damascus	2,317
Homs	915
TAIWAN	
Taipei	2,606
Kaohsiung	1,515
T'aichung	1,033
TANZANIA	
Dar es Salaam	2,683
THAILAND	
Bangkok	6,604
TOGO	
Lomé	1,337
TUNISIA	
Tunis	2,063
TURKEY	
Istanbul	9,712
Ankara	3,573
Izmir	2,487
Bursa	1,414
Adana	1,245
Gaziantep	862
Konya	761
UGANDA	
Kampala	1,345
UKRAINE	
Kiev	2,621
Kharkov	1,521
Dnepropetrovsk	1,122
Donetsk	1,065
Odessa	1,027
Zaporozhye	863
Lvov	794
UNITED ARAB EMIRATES	
Dubai	1,330
Abu Dhabi	928
UNITED KINGDOM	
London	8,505
Birmingham	2,280
Manchester	2,228
Liverpool	1,519
Glasgow	1,159
UNITED STATES OF AMERICA	
New York	18,718
Los Angeles	12,298
Chicago	8,814
Miami	5,434
Philadelphia	5,392
Dallas–Fort Worth	4,655
Boston	4,361
Houston	4,320
Atlanta	4,304
Washington	4,238
Detroit	4,034
Phoenix–Mesa	3,416
San Francisco	3,385
Seattle	2,989
San Diego	2,852
Minneapolis–St Paul	2,556
Tampa–St Petersburg	2,252
Denver	2,239
Baltimore	2,205
St Louis	2,159
Cleveland	1,855
Portland	1,810
Pittsburgh	1,806
Las Vegas	1,720
San Bernardino	1,690
San Jose	1,631
Cincinnati	1,599
Sacramento	1,555
Norfolk–Virginia Beach	1,460
Kansas City	1,437
San Antonio	1,436
Indianapolis	1,387
Milwaukee	1,316
Orlando	1,306
Providence	1,248
Columbus	1,236
Austin	1,107
Memphis	1,053
New Orleans	1,010
Buffalo	977
Stamford	889
Salt Lake City	888
Jacksonville	882
Louisville	864
Hartford	852
Richmond	819
Charlotte	759
URUGUAY	
Montevideo	1,353
UZBEKISTAN	
Tashkent	2,181
VENEZUELA	
Caracas	3,276
Valencia	2,330
Maracaibo	2,182
Maracay	1,138
Ciudad Guayana	966
Barquisimeto	923
VIETNAM	
Ho Chi Minh City	5,065
Hanoi	4,164
Haiphong	1,873
YEMEN	
Sana'	1,801
ZAMBIA	
Lusaka	1,450
ZIMBABWE	
Harare	1,527
Bulawayo	824

WORLD STATISTICS: CLIMATE

Rainfall and temperature figures are provided for more than 70 cities around the world. As climate is affected by altitude, the height of each city is shown in metres beneath its name. For each location, the top row of figures shows the total rainfall or snow in millimetres, and the bottom row the average temperature in degrees Celsius; the average annual temperature and total annual rainfall are at the end of the rows. The map opposite shows the city locations.

CITY	JAN.	FEB.	MAR.	APR.	MAY	JUNE	JULY	AUG.	SEPT.	OCT.	NOV.	DEC.	YEAR
EUROPE													
Athens, Greece	62	37	37	23	23	14	6	7	15	51	56	71	402
107 m	10	10	12	16	20	25	28	28	24	20	15	11	18
Berlin, Germany	42	33	41	37	54	69	56	58	45	37	44	55	571
55 m	-1	0	4	9	14	17	19	18	15	9	5	1	9
Istanbul, Turkey	87	71	63	43	33	25	24	24	44	71	85	107	655
14 m	5	6	7	11	16	20	23	23	20	16	12	8	14
Lisbon, Portugal	111	110	69	54	44	16	3	4	33	62	93	103	702
77 m	11	12	14	16	17	20	22	23	21	18	14	12	17
London, UK	54	40	37	37	46	45	57	59	49	57	64	48	593
5 m	4	5	7	9	12	16	18	17	15	11	8	5	11
Málaga, Spain	61	51	62	46	26	5	1	3	29	64	64	62	474
33 m	12	13	16	17	19	29	25	26	23	20	16	13	18
Moscow, Russia	39	38	36	37	53	58	88	71	58	45	47	54	624
156 m	-13	-10	-4	6	13	16	18	17	12	6	-1	-7	4
Odesa, Ukraine	57	62	30	21	34	34	42	37	37	13	35	71	473
64 m	-3	-1	2	9	15	20	22	22	18	12	9	1	10
Paris, France	56	46	35	42	57	54	59	64	55	50	51	50	619
75 m	3	4	8	11	15	18	20	19	17	12	7	4	12
Rome, Italy	71	62	57	51	46	37	15	21	63	99	129	93	744
17 m	8	9	11	14	18	22	25	25	22	17	13	10	16
Shannon, Ireland	94	67	56	53	61	57	77	79	86	86	96	117	929
2 m	5	5	7	9	12	14	16	16	14	11	8	6	10
Stockholm, Sweden	43	30	25	31	34	45	61	76	60	48	53	48	554
44 m	-3	-3	-1	5	10	15	18	17	12	7	3	0	7
ASIA													
Bahrain	8	18	13	8	3	0	0	0	0	0	18	18	81
5 m	17	18	21	25	29	32	33	34	31	28	24	19	26
Bangkok, Thailand	8	20	36	58	198	160	160	175	305	206	66	5	1,397
2 m	26	28	29	30	29	29	28	28	28	28	26	25	28
Beirut, Lebanon	191	158	94	53	18	3	3	3	5	51	132	185	892
34 m	14	14	16	18	22	24	27	28	26	24	19	16	21
Colombo, Sri Lanka	89	69	147	231	371	224	135	109	160	348	315	147	2,365
7 m	26	26	27	28	28	27	27	27	27	27	26	26	27
Harbin, China	6	5	10	23	43	94	112	104	46	33	8	5	488
160 m	-18	-15	-5	6	13	19	22	21	14	4	-6	-16	3
Ho Chi Minh, Vietnam	15	3	13	43	221	330	315	269	335	269	114	56	1,984
9 m	26	27	29	30	29	28	28	28	27	27	27	26	28
Hong Kong, China	33	46	74	137	292	394	381	361	257	114	43	31	2,162
33 m	16	15	18	22	26	28	28	28	27	25	21	18	23

CITY	JAN.	FEB.	MAR.	APR.	MAY	JUNE	JULY	AUG.	SEPT.	OCT.	NOV.	DEC.	YEAR
ASIA (continued)													
Jakarta, Indonesia	300	300	211	147	114	97	64	43	66	112	142	203	1,798
8 m	26	26	27	27	27	27	27	27	27	27	27	26	27
Kabul, Afghanistan	34	60	68	72	23	1	6	2	2	4	19	22	313
1,815 m	-3	-1	6	13	18	22	25	24	20	14	7	3	12
Karachi, Pakistan	13	10	8	3	3	18	81	41	13	<3	3	5	196
4 m	19	20	24	28	30	31	30	29	28	28	24	20	26
Kazalinsk, Kazakhstan	10	10	13	13	15	5	5	8	8	10	13	15	125
63 m	-12	-11	-3	6	18	23	25	23	16	8	-1	-7	7
Kolkata, India	10	31	36	43	140	297	325	328	252	114	20	5	1,600
6 m	20	22	27	30	30	30	29	29	29	28	23	19	26
Mumbai, India	3	3	3	3	18	485	617	340	264	64	13	3	1,809
11 m	24	24	26	28	30	29	27	27	27	28	27	26	27
New Delhi, India	23	18	13	8	13	74	180	172	117	10	3	10	640
218 m	14	17	23	28	33	34	31	30	29	26	20	15	25
Omsk, Russia	15	8	8	13	31	51	51	51	28	25	18	20	318
85 m	-22	-19	-12	-1	10	16	18	16	10	1	-11	-18	-1
Shanghai, China	48	58	84	94	94	180	147	142	130	71	51	36	1,135
7 m	4	5	9	14	20	24	28	28	23	19	12	7	16
Singapore	252	173	193	188	173	173	170	196	178	208	254	257	2,413
10 m	26	27	28	28	28	28	28	27	27	27	27	27	27
Tehran, Iran	46	38	46	36	13	3	3	3	3	8	20	31	246
1,220 m	2	5	9	16	21	26	30	29	25	18	12	6	17
Tokyo, Japan	48	74	107	135	147	165	142	152	234	208	97	56	1,565
6 m	3	4	7	13	17	21	25	26	23	17	11	6	14
Ulan Bator, Mongolia	3	3	3	5	10	28	76	51	23	5	5	3	208
1,325 m	-26	-21	-13	-1	6	14	16	14	8	-1	-13	-22	-3
Verkhoyansk, Russia	5	5	3	5	8	23	28	25	13	8	8	5	134
100 m	-50	-45	-32	-15	0	12	14	9	2	-15	-38	-48	-17
AFRICA													
Addis Ababa, Ethiopia	3	3	25	135	213	201	206	239	102	28	3	0	1,151
2,450 m	19	20	20	20	19	18	18	19	21	22	21	20	20
Antananarivo, Madag.	300	279	178	53	18	8	8	10	18	61	135	287	1,356
1,372 m	21	21	21	19	18	15	14	15	17	19	21	21	19
Cairo, Egypt	5	4	4	1	1	0	0	0	0	1	4	6	26
116 m	13	15	18	21	25	28	28	28	26	24	20	15	22
Cape Town, S. Africa	15	8	18	48	79	84	89	66	43	31	18	10	508
17 m	21	21	20	17	14	13	12	13	14	16	18	19	17
Jo'burg, S. Africa	114	109	89	38	25	8	8	8	23	56	107	125	709
1,665 m	20	20	18	16	13	10	11	13	16	18	19	20	16

CITY	JAN.	FEB.	MAR.	APR.	MAY	JUNE	JULY	AUG.	SEPT.	OCT.	NOV.	DEC.	YEAR
AFRICA (continued)													
Khartoum, Sudan	3	3	3	3	3	8	53	71	18	5	3	0	158
390 m	24	25	28	31	33	34	32	31	32	32	28	25	29
Kinshasa, Congo (D.R.)	135	145	196	196	158	8	3	3	31	119	221	142	1,354
325 m	26	26	27	27	26	24	23	24	25	26	26	26	25
Lagos, Nigeria	28	46	102	150	269	460	279	64	140	206	69	25	1,836
3 m	27	28	29	28	28	26	26	25	26	26	28	28	27
Lusaka, Zambia	231	191	142	18	3	3	3	0	3	10	91	150	836
1,277 m	21	22	21	21	19	16	16	18	22	24	23	22	21
Monrovia, Liberia	31	56	97	216	516	973	996	373	744	772	236	130	5,138
23 m	26	26	27	27	26	25	24	25	25	25	26	26	26
Nairobi, Kenya	38	64	125	211	158	46	15	23	31	53	109	86	958
820 m	19	19	19	19	18	16	16	16	18	19	18	18	18
Timbuktu, Mali	1	0	0	1	4	16	54	74	29	4	0	0	183
301 m	22	24	28	32	34	35	32	30	32	31	28	23	29
Tunis, Tunisia	64	51	41	36	18	8	3	8	33	51	48	61	419
66 m	10	11	13	16	19	23	26	27	25	20	16	11	18
Walvis Bay, Namibia	3	5	8	3	3	3	3	3	3	3	3	3	23
7 m	19	19	19	18	17	16	15	14	14	15	17	18	18
AUSTRALIA, NEW ZEALAND AND ANTARCTICA													
Alice Springs, Aust.	43	33	28	10	15	13	8	8	8	18	31	38	252
579 m	29	28	25	20	15	12	12	14	18	23	26	28	21
Christchurch, N.Z.	56	43	48	48	66	66	69	48	46	43	48	56	638
10 m	16	16	14	12	9	6	6	7	9	12	14	16	11
Darwin, Australia	386	312	254	97	15	3	3	3	13	51	119	239	1,491
30 m	29	29	29	29	28	26	25	26	28	29	30	29	28
Mawson, Antarctica	11	30	20	10	44	180	4	40	3	20	0	0	362
14 m	0	−5	−10	−14	−15	−16	−18	−18	−19	−13	−5	−1	−11
Perth, Australia	8	10	20	43	130	180	170	149	86	56	20	13	881
60 m	23	23	22	19	16	14	13	13	15	16	19	22	18
Sydney, Australia	89	102	127	135	127	117	117	76	73	71	73	73	1,181
42 m	22	22	21	18	15	13	12	13	15	18	19	21	17
NORTH AMERICA													
Anchorage, USA	20	18	15	10	13	18	41	66	66	56	25	23	371
40 m	−11	−8	−5	2	7	12	14	13	9	2	−5	−11	2
Chicago, USA	51	51	66	71	86	89	84	81	79	66	61	51	836
251 m	−4	−3	2	9	14	20	23	22	19	12	5	−1	10
Churchill, Canada	15	13	18	23	32	44	46	58	51	43	39	21	402
13 m	−28	−26	−20	−10	−2	6	12	11	5	−2	−12	−22	−7
Edmonton, Canada	25	19	19	22	43	77	89	78	39	17	16	25	466
676 m	−15	−10	−5	4	11	15	17	16	11	6	−4	−10	3
Honolulu, USA	104	66	79	48	25	18	23	28	36	48	64	104	643
12 m	23	18	19	20	22	24	25	26	26	24	22	19	22
Houston, USA	89	76	84	91	119	117	99	99	104	94	89	109	1,171
12 m	12	13	17	21	24	27	28	29	26	22	16	12	21

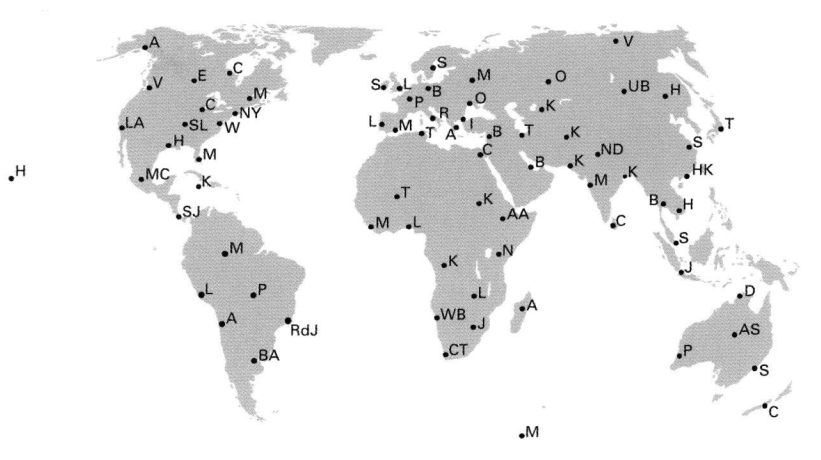

CITY	JAN.	FEB.	MAR.	APR.	MAY	JUNE	JULY	AUG.	SEPT.	OCT.	NOV.	DEC.	YEAR
NORTH AMERICA (continued)													
Kingston, Jamaica	23	15	23	31	102	89	38	91	99	180	74	36	800
34 m	25	25	25	26	26	28	28	28	27	27	26	26	26
Los Angeles, USA	79	76	71	25	10	3	3	3	5	15	31	66	381
95 m	13	14	14	16	17	19	21	22	21	18	16	14	17
Mexico City, Mexico	13	5	10	20	53	119	170	152	130	51	18	8	747
2,309 m	12	13	16	18	19	19	17	18	18	16	14	13	16
Miami, USA	71	53	64	81	173	178	155	160	203	234	71	51	1,516
8 m	20	20	22	23	25	27	28	28	27	25	22	21	24
Montréal, Canada	72	65	74	74	66	82	90	92	88	76	81	87	946
57 m	−10	−9	−3	−6	13	18	21	20	15	9	2	−7	6
New York City, USA	94	97	91	81	81	84	107	109	86	89	76	91	1,092
96 m	−1	−1	3	10	16	20	23	23	21	15	7	2	11
St Louis, USA	58	64	89	97	114	114	89	86	81	74	71	64	1,001
173 m	0	1	7	13	19	24	26	26	22	15	8	2	14
San José, Costa Rica	15	5	20	46	229	241	211	241	305	300	145	41	1,798
1,146 m	19	19	21	21	22	21	21	21	21	20	20	19	20
Vancouver, Canada	154	115	101	60	52	45	32	41	67	114	150	182	1,113
14 m	3	5	6	9	12	15	17	17	14	10	6	4	10
Washington, DC, USA	86	76	91	84	94	99	112	109	94	74	66	79	1,064
22 m	1	2	7	12	18	23	25	24	20	14	8	3	13
SOUTH AMERICA													
Antofagasta, Chile	0	0	0	3	3	3	5	3	3	3	3	0	13
94 m	21	21	20	18	16	15	14	14	15	16	18	19	17
Buenos Aires, Arg.	122	123	154	107	92	50	53	63	78	139	131	103	1,215
27 m	23	23	21	17	13	9	10	11	13	15	19	22	16
Lima, Peru	3	3	3	3	3	5	8	8	8	3	3	3	41
120 m	23	24	24	22	19	17	17	16	17	18	19	21	20
Manaus, Brazil	249	231	262	221	170	84	58	38	46	107	142	203	1,811
44 m	28	28	28	27	28	28	28	28	29	29	29	28	28
Paraná, Brazil	287	236	239	102	13	3		5	28	127	231	310	1,582
260 m	23	23	23	23	23	21	21	22	24	24	24	23	23
Rio de Janeiro, Brazil	125	122	130	107	79	53	41	43	66	79	104	137	1,082
61 m	26	26	25	24	22	21	21	21	22	23	25	25	23

WORLD STATISTICS: PHYSICAL DIMENSIONS

Each topic list is divided into continents and within a continent the items are listed in order of size. The bottom part of many of the lists is selective in order to give examples from as many different countries as possible. The order of the continents is as in the atlas, Europe through to South America. The world top ten are shown in square brackets; in the case of mountains this has not been done because the world top 30 are all in Asia. The figures are rounded as appropriate.

WORLD, CONTINENTS, OCEANS

THE WORLD	km²	miles²	%
The World	509,450,000	196,672,000	–
Land	149,450,000	57,688,000	29.3
Water	360,000,000	138,984,000	70.7
Asia	44,500,000	17,177,000	29.8
Africa	30,302,000	11,697,000	20.3
North America	24,241,000	9,357,000	16.2
South America	17,793,000	6,868,000	11.9
Antarctica	14,100,000	5,443,000	9.4
Europe	9,957,000	3,843,000	6.7
Australia & Oceania	8,557,000	3,303,000	5.7
Pacific Ocean	155,557,000	60,061,000	46.4
Atlantic Ocean	76,762,000	29,638,000	22.9
Indian Ocean	68,556,000	26,470,000	20.4
Southern Ocean	20,327,000	7,848,000	6.1
Arctic Ocean	14,056,000	5,427,000	4.2

SEAS

PACIFIC	km²	miles²
South China Sea	2,974,600	1,148,500
Bering Sea	2,268,000	875,000
Sea of Okhotsk	1,528,000	590,000
East China & Yellow	1,249,000	482,000
Sea of Japan	1,008,000	389,000
Gulf of California	162,000	62,500
Bass Strait	75,000	29,000

ATLANTIC	km²	miles²
Caribbean Sea	2,766,000	1,068,000
Mediterranean Sea	2,516,000	971,000
Gulf of Mexico	1,543,000	596,000
Hudson Bay	1,232,000	476,000
North Sea	575,000	223,000
Black Sea	462,000	178,000
Baltic Sea	422,170	163,000
Gulf of St Lawrence	238,000	92,000

INDIAN	km²	miles²
Red Sea	438,000	169,000
Persian Gulf	239,000	92,000

MOUNTAINS

EUROPE		m	ft
Elbrus	Russia	5,642	18,510
Dykh-Tau	Russia	5,205	17,076
Shkhara	Russia/Georgia	5,201	17,064
Koshtan-Tau	Russia	5,152	16,903
Kazbek	Russia/Georgia	5,047	16,558
Pushkin	Russia/Georgia	5,033	16,512
Katyn-Tau	Russia/Georgia	4,979	16,335
Shota Rustaveli	Russia/Georgia	4,860	15,945
Mont Blanc	France/Italy	4,808	15,774
Monte Rosa	Italy/Switzerland	4,634	15,203
Dom	Switzerland	4,545	14,911
Liskamm	Switzerland	4,527	14,852
Weisshorn	Switzerland	4,505	14,780
Taschorn	Switzerland	4,490	14,730
Matterhorn/Cervino	Italy/Switzerland	4,478	14,691
Mont Maudit	France/Italy	4,465	14,649
Dent Blanche	Switzerland	4,356	14,291
Nadelhorn	Switzerland	4,327	14,196
Grandes Jorasses	France/Italy	4,208	13,806
Jungfrau	Switzerland	4,158	13,642
Barre des Ecrins	France	4,103	13,461
Gran Paradiso	Italy	4,061	13,323
Piz Bernina	Italy/Switzerland	4,049	13,284
Eiger	Switzerland	3,970	13,025
Grossglockner	Austria	3,797	12,457
Mulhacén	Spain	3,478	11,411
Etna	Italy	3,340	10,958
Zugspitze	Germany	2,962	9,718
Olympus	Greece	2,917	9,570
Galdhøpiggen	Norway	2,469	8,100
Ben Nevis	UK	1,342	4,403

ASIA		m	ft
Everest	China/Nepal	8,850	29,035
K2 (Godwin Austen)	China/Kashmir	8,611	28,251
Kanchenjunga	India/Nepal	8,598	28,208
Lhotse	China/Nepal	8,516	27,939
Makalu	China/Nepal	8,481	27,824
Cho Oyu	China/Nepal	8,201	26,906
Dhaulagiri	Nepal	8,167	26,795
Manaslu	Nepal	8,156	26,758
Nanga Parbat	Kashmir	8,126	26,660
Annapurna	Nepal	8,078	26,502
Gasherbrum	China/Kashmir	8,068	26,469
Broad Peak	China/Kashmir	8,051	26,414
Xixabangma	China	8,012	26,286
Gayachung Kang	Nepal	7,897	25,909
Himalchuli	Nepal	7,893	25,896
Disteghil Sar	Kashmir	7,885	25,869
Nuptse	Nepal	7,879	25,849
Kangbachen	Nepal	7,858	25,781
Khunyang Chhish	Kashmir	7,852	25,761
Masherbrum	Kashmir	7,821	25,659
Nanda Devi	India	7,817	25,646
Rakaposhi	Kashmir	7,788	25,551
Batura	Kashmir	7,785	25,541
Namche Barwa	China	7,782	25,531
Kamet	India	7,756	25,447
Soltoro Kangri	Pakistan	7,742	25,400
Gurla Mandhata	China	7,728	25,354
Trivor	Pakistan	7,720	25,328
Kongur Shan	China	7,719	25,324
Jannu	Nepal	7,710	25,295
Tirich Mir	Pakistan	7,690	25,229
K'ula Shan	Bhutan/China	7,543	24,747
Pik Imeni Ismail Samani	Tajikistan	7,495	24,590
Demavend	Iran	5,604	18,386
Ararat	Turkey	5,165	16,945
Gunong Kinabalu	Malaysia (Borneo)	4,101	13,455
Yu Shan	Taiwan	3,997	13,113
Fuji-San	Japan	3,776	12,388

AFRICA		m	ft
Kilimanjaro	Tanzania	5,895	19,340
Mt Kenya	Kenya	5,199	17,057
Ruwenzori (Margherita)	Uganda/Congo (D.R.)	5,109	16,762
Meru	Tanzania	4,565	14,977
Ras Dashen	Ethiopia	4,533	14,872
Karisimbi	Rwanda/Congo (D.R.)	4,507	14,787
Mt Elgon	Kenya/Uganda	4,321	14,176
Batu	Ethiopia	4,307	14,130
Guna	Ethiopia	4,231	13,882
Toubkal	Morocco	4,165	13,665
Irhil Mgoun	Morocco	4,071	13,356
Mt Cameroun	Cameroon	4,070	13,353
Amba Ferit	Ethiopia	3,875	13,042
Pico del Teide	Spain (Tenerife)	3,718	12,198
Thabana Ntlenyana	Lesotho	3,482	11,424
Emi Koussi	Chad	3,415	11,204
Mt aux Sources	Lesotho/South Africa	3,282	10,768
Mt Piton	Réunion	3,069	10,069

OCEANIA		m	ft
Puncak Jaya	Indonesia	5,029	16,499
Puncak Trikora	Indonesia	4,730	15,518
Puncak Mandala	Indonesia	4,702	15,427
Mt Wilhelm	Papua New Guinea	4,508	14,790
Mauna Kea	USA (Hawai'i)	4,205	13,796
Mauna Loa	USA (Hawai'i)	4,169	13,678
Aoraki Mt Cook	New Zealand	3,753	12,313
Mt Balbi	Solomon Islands	2,439	8,002
Orohena	French Polynesia (Tahiti)	2,241	7,352
Mt Kosciuszko	Australia	2,228	7,310

NORTH AMERICA		m	ft
Mt McKinley (Denali)	USA (Alaska)	6,194	20,321
Mt Logan	Canada	5,959	19,551
Pico de Orizaba	Mexico	5,610	18,405
Mt St Elias	USA/Canada	5,489	18,008
Popocatépetl	Mexico	5,452	17,887

NORTH AMERICA (continued)		m	ft
Mt Foraker	USA (Alaska)	5,304	17,401
Iztaccihuatl	Mexico	5,286	17,343
Mt Lucania	Canada	5,226	17,146
Mt Steele	Canada	5,073	16,644
Mt Bona	USA (Alaska)	5,005	16,420
Mt Blackburn	USA (Alaska)	4,996	16,391
Mt Sanford	USA (Alaska)	4,940	16,207
Mt Wood	Canada	4,840	15,880
Nevado de Toluca	Mexico	4,670	15,321
Mt Fairweather	USA (Alaska)	4,663	15,298
Mt Hunter	USA (Alaska)	4,442	14,573
Mt Whitney	USA	4,418	14,495
Mt Elbert	USA	4,399	14,432
Mt Harvard	USA	4,395	14,419
Mt Rainier	USA	4,392	14,409
Blanca Peak	USA	4,372	14,344
Longs Peak	USA	4,345	14,255
Tajumulco	Guatemala	4,220	13,845
Grand Teton	USA	4,197	13,770
Mt Waddington	Canada	4,019	13,186
Mt Robson	Canada	3,959	12,989
Chirripó Grande	Costa Rica	3,837	12,589
Pico Duarte	Dominican Rep.	3,175	10,417

SOUTH AMERICA		m	ft
Aconcagua	Argentina	6,962	22,841
Bonete	Argentina	6,872	22,546
Ojos del Salado	Argentina/Chile	6,863	22,516
Pissis	Argentina	6,779	22,241
Mercedario	Argentina/Chile	6,770	22,211
Huascarán	Peru	6,768	22,205
Llullaillaco	Argentina/Chile	6,723	22,057
Nevado de Cachi	Argentina	6,720	22,047
Yerupaja	Peru	6,632	21,758
Nevado de Tres Cruces	Argentina/Chile	6,620	21,719
Incahuasi	Argentina/Chile	6,601	21,654
Cerro Galan	Argentina	6,600	21,654
Tupungato	Argentina/Chile	6,570	21,555
Sajama	Bolivia	6,520	21,391
Illimani	Bolivia	6,485	21,276
Coropuna	Peru	6,425	21,079
Ausangate	Peru	6,384	20,945
Cerro del Toro	Argentina	6,380	20,932
Siula Grande	Peru	6,356	20,853
Chimborazo	Ecuador	6,267	20,561
Alpamayo	Peru	5,947	19,511
Cotopaxi	Ecuador	5,896	19,344
Pico Cristóbal Colón	Colombia	5,800	19,029
Pico Bolívar	Venezuela	5,007	16,427

ANTARCTICA		m	ft
Vinson Massif		4,897	16,066
Mt Kirkpatrick		4,528	14,855
Mt Markham		4,349	14,268

OCEAN DEPTHS

ATLANTIC OCEAN	m	ft	
Puerto Rico (Milwaukee) Deep	8,604	28,232	[7]
Cayman Trench	7,680	25,197	[10]
Gulf of Mexico	5,203	17,070	
Mediterranean Sea	5,121	16,801	
Black Sea	2,211	7,254	
North Sea	660	2,165	
Baltic Sea	463	1,519	
Hudson Bay	258	846	

INDIAN OCEAN	m	ft	
Java Trench	7,450	24,442	
Red Sea	2,635	8,454	
Persian Gulf	73	239	

PACIFIC OCEAN	m	ft	
Mariana Trench	11,022	36,161	[1]
Tonga Trench	10,882	35,702	[2]
Japan Trench	10,554	34,626	[3]
Kuril Trench	10,542	34,587	[4]
Mindanao Trench	10,497	34,439	[5]
Kermadec Trench	10,047	32,962	[6]

15

PACIFIC OCEAN (continued)

	m	ft	
Peru–Chile Trench	8,050	26,410	[8]
Aleutian Trench	7,822	25,662	[9]

ARCTIC OCEAN

	m	ft
Molloy Deep	5,608	18,399

SOUTHERN OCEAN

	m	ft
South Sandwich Trench	7,235	23,737

LAND LOWS

		m	ft
Caspian Sea	Europe	−28	−92
Dead Sea	Asia	−418	−1,371
Lake Assal	Africa	−156	−512
Lake Eyre North	Oceania	−16	−52
Death Valley	North America	−86	−282
Laguna del Carbón	South America	−105	−344

RIVERS

EUROPE

		km	miles
Volga	Caspian Sea	3,700	2,300
Danube	Black Sea	2,850	1,770
Ural	Caspian Sea	2,535	1,575
Dnepr (Dnipro)	Black Sea	2,285	1,420
Kama	Volga	2,030	1,260
Don	Black Sea	1,990	1,240
Petchora	Arctic Ocean	1,790	1,110
Oka	Volga	1,480	920
Belaya	Kama	1,420	880
Dnister (Dniester)	Black Sea	1,400	870
Vyatka	Kama	1,370	850
Rhine	North Sea	1,320	820
N. Dvina	Arctic Ocean	1,290	800
Desna	Dnepr (Dnipro)	1,190	740
Elbe	North Sea	1,145	710
Wisla	Baltic Sea	1,090	675
Loire	Atlantic Ocean	1,020	635

ASIA

		km	miles	
Yangtze	Pacific Ocean	6,380	3,960	[3]
Yenisey–Angara	Arctic Ocean	5,550	3,445	[5]
Huang He	Pacific Ocean	5,464	3,395	[6]
Ob–Irtysh	Arctic Ocean	5,410	3,360	[7]
Mekong	Pacific Ocean	4,500	2,795	[9]
Amur	Pacific Ocean	4,442	2,760	
Lena	Arctic Ocean	4,402	2,735	
Irtysh	Ob	4,250	2,640	
Yenisey	Arctic Ocean	4,090	2,540	
Ob	Arctic Ocean	3,680	2,285	
Indus	Indian Ocean	3,100	1,925	
Brahmaputra	Indian Ocean	2,900	1,800	
Syrdarya	Aral Sea	2,860	1,775	
Salween	Indian Ocean	2,800	1,740	
Euphrates	Indian Ocean	2,700	1,675	
Vilyuy	Lena	2,650	1,645	
Kolyma	Arctic Ocean	2,600	1,615	
Amudarya	Aral Sea	2,540	1,578	
Ural	Caspian Sea	2,535	1,575	
Ganges	Indian Ocean	2,510	1,560	
Si Kiang	Pacific Ocean	2,100	1,305	
Irrawaddy	Indian Ocean	2,010	1,250	
Tarim–Yarkand	Lop Nor	2,000	1,240	
Tigris	Indian Ocean	1,900	1,180	

AFRICA

		km	miles	
Nile	Mediterranean	6,695	4,160	[1]
Congo	Atlantic Ocean	4,670	2,900	[8]
Niger	Atlantic Ocean	4,180	2,595	
Zambezi	Indian Ocean	3,540	2,200	
Oubangi/Uele	Congo (D.R.)	2,250	1,400	
Kasai	Congo (D.R.)	1,950	1,210	
Shaballe	Indian Ocean	1,930	1,200	
Orange	Atlantic Ocean	1,860	1,155	
Cubango	Okavango Delta	1,800	1,120	
Limpopo	Indian Ocean	1,770	1,100	
Senegal	Atlantic Ocean	1,640	1,020	
Volta	Atlantic Ocean	1,500	930	

AUSTRALIA

		km	miles
Murray–Darling	Southern Ocean	3,750	2,330
Darling	Murray	3,070	1,905
Murray	Southern Ocean	2,575	1,600
Murrumbidgee	Murray	1,690	1,050

NORTH AMERICA

		km	miles	
Mississippi–Missouri	Gulf of Mexico	5,971	3,710	[4]
Mackenzie	Arctic Ocean	4,240	2,630	
Missouri	Mississippi	4,088	2,540	

NORTH AMERICA (continued)

		km	miles
Mississippi	Gulf of Mexico	3,782	2,350
Yukon	Pacific Ocean	3,185	1,980
Rio Grande	Gulf of Mexico	3,030	1,880
Arkansas	Mississippi	2,340	1,450
Colorado	Pacific Ocean	2,330	1,445
Red	Mississippi	2,040	1,270
Columbia	Pacific Ocean	1,950	1,210
Saskatchewan	Lake Winnipeg	1,940	1,205
Snake	Columbia	1,670	1,040
Churchill	Hudson Bay	1,600	990
Ohio	Mississippi	1,580	980
Brazos	Gulf of Mexico	1,400	870
St Lawrence	Atlantic Ocean	1,170	730

SOUTH AMERICA

		km	miles	
Amazon	Atlantic Ocean	6,450	4,010	[2]
Paraná–Plate	Atlantic Ocean	4,500	2,800	[10]
Purus	Amazon	3,350	2,080	
Madeira	Amazon	3,200	1,990	
São Francisco	Atlantic Ocean	2,900	1,800	
Paraná	Plate	2,800	1,740	
Tocantins	Atlantic Ocean	2,750	1,710	
Orinoco	Atlantic Ocean	2,740	1,700	
Paraguay	Paraná	2,550	1,580	
Pilcomayo	Paraná	2,500	1,550	
Araguaia	Tocantins	2,250	1,400	
Juruá	Amazon	2,000	1,240	
Xingu	Amazon	1,980	1,230	
Ucayali	Amazon	1,900	1,180	
Uruguay	Plate	1,610	1,000	

LAKES

EUROPE

		km²	miles²
Lake Ladoga	Russia	17,700	6,800
Lake Onega	Russia	9,700	3,700
Saimaa system	Finland	8,000	3,100
Vänern	Sweden	5,500	2,100

ASIA

		km²	miles²	
Caspian Sea	Asia	371,000	143,000	[1]
Lake Baikal	Russia	30,500	11,780	[8]
Tonlé Sap	Cambodia	20,000	7,700	
Lake Balqash	Kazakhstan	18,500	7,100	
Aral Sea	Kazakhstan/Uzbekistan	17,160	6,625	
Lake Dongting	China	12,000	4,600	
Lake Ysyk	Kyrgyzstan	6,200	2,400	
Lake Orumiyeh	Iran	5,900	2,300	
Lake Koko	China	5,700	2,200	
Lake Poyang	China	5,000	1,900	
Lake Khanka	China/Russia	4,400	1,700	
Lake Van	Turkey	3,500	1,400	

AFRICA

		km²	miles²	
Lake Victoria	East Africa	68,000	26,300	[3]
Lake Tanganyika	Central Africa	33,000	13,000	[6]
Lake Malawi/Nyasa	East Africa	29,600	11,430	[9]
Lake Chad	Central Africa	25,000	9,700	
Lake Bangweulu	Zambia	9,840	3,800	
Lake Turkana	Ethiopia/Kenya	8,500	3,290	
Lake Volta	Ghana	8,480	3,270	
Lake Kariba	Zambia/Zimbabwe	5,380	2,150	
Lake Albert	Uganda/Congo (D.R.)	5,300	2,050	
Lake Nasser	Egypt/Sudan	5,250	2,030	
Lake Mweru	Zambia/Congo (D.R.)	4,920	1,900	
Lake Kyoga	Uganda	4,430	1,710	
Lake Tana	Ethiopia	3,620	1,400	
Lake Cabora Bassa	Mozambique	2,750	1,070	
Lake Rukwa	Tanzania	2,600	1,000	
Lake Mai-Ndombe	Congo (D.R.)	2,300	890	

AUSTRALIA

		km²	miles²
Lake Eyre	Australia	8,900	3,400
Lake Torrens	Australia	5,800	2,200
Lake Gairdner	Australia	4,800	1,900

NORTH AMERICA

		km²	miles²	
Lake Superior	Canada/USA	82,350	31,800	[2]
Lake Huron	Canada/USA	59,600	23,010	[4]
Lake Michigan	USA	58,000	22,400	[5]
Great Bear Lake	Canada	31,800	12,280	[7]
Great Slave Lake	Canada	28,500	11,000	[10]
Lake Erie	Canada/USA	25,700	9,900	
Lake Winnipeg	Canada	24,400	9,400	
Lake Ontario	Canada/USA	19,500	7,500	
Lake Nicaragua	Nicaragua	8,200	3,200	
Lake Athabasca	Canada	8,100	3,100	
Smallwood Reservoir	Canada	6,530	2,520	
Reindeer Lake	Canada	6,400	2,500	
Nettilling Lake	Canada	5,500	2,100	

SOUTH AMERICA

		km²	miles²
Lake Titicaca	Bolivia/Peru	8,300	3,200
Lake Poopo	Bolivia	2,800	1,100

ISLANDS

EUROPE

		km²	miles²	
Great Britain	UK	229,880	88,700	[8]
Iceland	Atlantic Ocean	103,000	39,800	
Ireland	Ireland/UK	84,400	32,600	
Novaya Zemlya (N.)	Russia	48,200	18,600	
W. Spitzbergen	Norway	39,000	15,100	
Novaya Zemlya (S.)	Russia	33,200	12,800	
Sicily	Italy	25,500	9,800	
Sardinia	Italy	24,000	9,300	
N. E. Spitzbergen	Norway	15,000	5,600	
Corsica	France	8,700	3,400	
Crete	Greece	8,350	3,200	
Zealand	Denmark	6,850	2,600	

ASIA

		km²	miles²	
Borneo	South-east Asia	744,360	287,400	[3]
Sumatra	Indonesia	473,600	182,860	[6]
Honshu	Japan	230,500	88,980	[7]
Sulawesi (Celebes)	Indonesia	189,000	73,000	
Java	Indonesia	126,700	48,900	
Luzon	Philippines	104,700	40,400	
Mindanao	Philippines	101,500	39,200	
Hokkaido	Japan	78,400	30,300	
Sakhalin	Russia	74,060	28,600	
Sri Lanka	Indian Ocean	65,600	25,300	
Taiwan	Pacific Ocean	36,000	13,900	
Kyushu	Japan	35,700	13,800	
Hainan	China	34,000	13,100	
Timor	Indonesia	33,600	13,000	
Shikoku	Japan	18,800	7,300	
Halmahera	Indonesia	18,000	6,900	
Ceram	Indonesia	17,150	6,600	
Sumbawa	Indonesia	15,450	6,000	
Flores	Indonesia	15,200	5,900	
Samar	Philippines	13,100	5,100	
Negros	Philippines	12,700	4,900	
Bangka	Indonesia	12,000	4,600	
Palawan	Philippines	12,000	4,600	
Panay	Philippines	11,500	4,400	
Sumba	Indonesia	11,100	4,300	
Mindoro	Philippines	9,750	3,800	

AFRICA

		km²	miles²	
Madagascar	Indian Ocean	587,040	226,660	[4]
Socotra	Indian Ocean	3,600	1,400	
Réunion	Indian Ocean	2,500	965	
Tenerife	Atlantic Ocean	2,350	900	
Mauritius	Indian Ocean	1,865	720	

OCEANIA

		km²	miles²	
New Guinea	Indonesia/Papua NG	821,030	317,000	[2]
New Zealand (S.)	Pacific Ocean	150,500	58,100	
New Zealand (N.)	Pacific Ocean	114,700	44,300	
Tasmania	Australia	67,800	26,200	
New Britain	Papua New Guinea	37,800	14,600	
New Caledonia	Pacific Ocean	19,100	7,400	
Viti Levu	Fiji	10,500	4,100	
Hawai'i	Pacific Ocean	10,450	4,000	
Bougainville	Papua New Guinea	9,600	3,700	
Guadalcanal	Solomon Islands	6,500	2,500	
Vanua Levu	Fiji	5,550	2,100	
New Ireland	Papua New Guinea	3,200	1,200	

NORTH AMERICA

		km²	miles²	
Greenland	Atlantic Ocean	2,175,600	839,800	[1]
Baffin Is.	Canada	508,000	196,100	[5]
Victoria Is.	Canada	212,200	81,900	[9]
Ellesmere Is.	Canada	212,000	81,800	[10]
Cuba	Caribbean Sea	110,860	42,800	
Newfoundland	Canada	110,680	42,700	
Hispaniola	Dominican Rep./Haiti	76,200	29,400	
Banks Is.	Canada	67,000	25,900	
Devon Is.	Canada	54,500	21,000	
Melville Is.	Canada	42,400	16,400	
Vancouver Is.	Canada	32,150	12,400	
Somerset Is.	Canada	24,300	9,400	
Jamaica	Caribbean Sea	11,400	4,400	
Puerto Rico	Atlantic Ocean	8,900	3,400	
Cape Breton Is.	Canada	4,000	1,500	

SOUTH AMERICA

		km²	miles²
Tierra del Fuego	Argentina/Chile	47,000	18,100
Falkland Is. (East)	Atlantic Ocean	6,800	2,600
South Georgia	Atlantic Ocean	4,200	1,600
Galapagos (Isabela)	Pacific Ocean	2,250	870

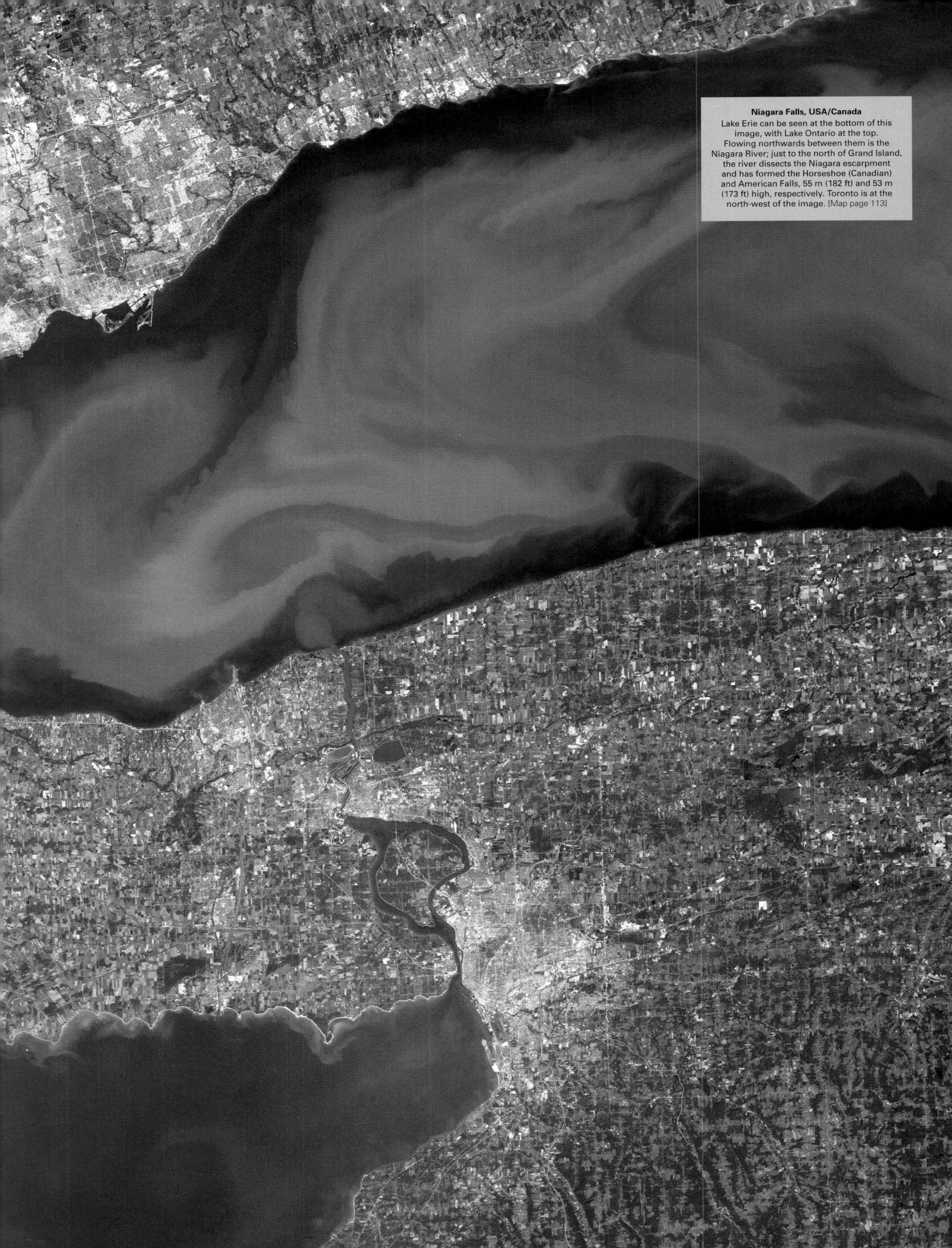

Niagara Falls, USA/Canada
Lake Erie can be seen at the bottom of this image, with Lake Ontario at the top. Flowing northwards between them is the Niagara River; just to the north of Grand Island, the river dissects the Niagara escarpment and has formed the Horseshoe (Canadian) and American Falls, 55 m (182 ft) and 53 m (173 ft) high, respectively. Toronto is at the north-west of the image. [Map page 113]

THE EARTH
IN SPACE

THE UNIVERSE

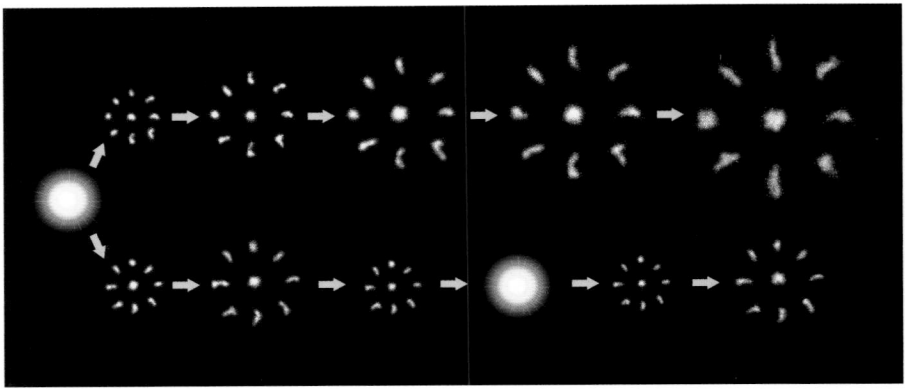

In early 2003, NASA scientists produced an image of the Universe as it was about 380,000 years after its creation. The image was produced by an American satellite called the Wilkinson Microwave Anisotropy Probe (WMAP), which was launched in June 2001.

The probe measures small variations in the cosmic microwave background (CMB) radiation, left over from the creation of the Universe. By measuring the size of hot and cold spots in the CMB, scientists have calculated how far away they are, and this data has enabled them to calculate the age of the Universe. It has also established the proportions of its three ingredients, namely 4% ordinary matter (made up of atoms), 23% of 'cold dark matter', whose nature is unknown, and 73% of the mysterious 'dark energy', which seems to be accelerating the expansion of space.

▼ *The depths of the Universe*
In this segment of sky, just one-tenth the area of the full Moon, the Hubble Space Telescope recorded an estimated 10,000 galaxies in 2003–4.

Scientists have established that our Universe was created, or 'time' began, about 13.7 billion years ago (disproving earlier estimates that ranged from 8 billion to 24 billion years), that it is flat, and that the first stars did not appear until it was 200 million years old.

THE BIG BANG

Most scientists agree that the Universe was formed by a colossal explosion, called the 'Big Bang'. In the first millionth of a second after the Big Bang, the Universe expanded from a dimensionless point of infinite mass and

▲ *The end of the Universe*
The diagram shows two theories concerning the fate of the Universe. One theory, top, suggests that the Universe will expand indefinitely, becoming an immense dark graveyard. Another theory, bottom, suggests that the galaxies will fall back until everything is again concentrated in one point in a so-called Big Crunch. This might then be followed by a new Big Bang.

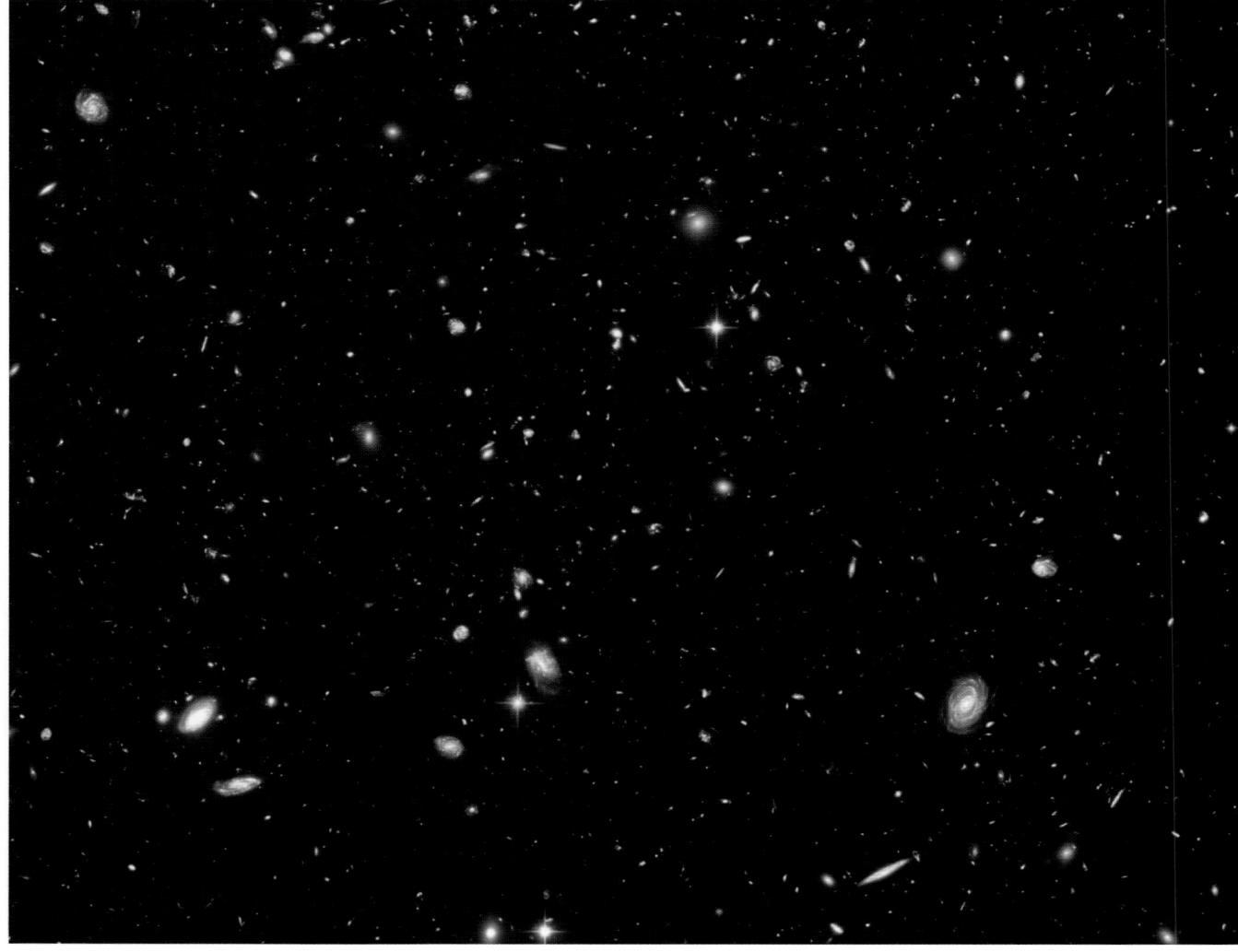

THE NEAREST STARS

The 22 nearest stars, excluding the Sun, with their distance from the Earth in light-years.*

Proxima Centauri	4.2
Alpha Centauri A	4.4
Alpha Centauri B	4.4
Barnard's Star	5.9
Wolf 359	7.8
Lalande 21185	8.3
Sirius A	8.6
Sirius B	8.6
UV Ceti A	8.7
UV Ceti B	8.7
Ross 154	9.7
Ross 248	10.3
Epsilon Eridani	10.5
HD 217987	10.7
Ross 128	10.9
L789-6	11.2
61 Cygni A	11.4
Procyon A	11.4
Procyon B	11.4
61 Cygni B	11.4
HD 173740	11.5
HD 173739	11.7

* A light-year is about 9,500 billion km [5,900 billion miles].

density into a fireball about 30 billion km [19 billion miles] across. The Universe has been expanding ever since, as demonstrated in the 1920s by Edwin Hubble, the American astronomer after whom the Hubble Space Telescope, which has also been shedding light on the origins of the Universe, was named.

The temperature at the end of the first second was perhaps 10 billion degrees – far too hot for composite atomic nuclei to exist. As a result, the fireball consisted mainly of radiation mixed with microscopic particles of matter. Almost a million years passed before the Universe was cool enough for atoms to form.

In regions where matter was relatively dense, atoms began, under the influence of gravity, to move together to form protogalaxies – masses of gas separated by empty space. The protogalaxies were dark, because the Universe had cooled. But 200 million years after its creation, stars began to form within the protogalaxies as particles were drawn together. The internal pressure produced as matter condensed created the high temperatures required to cause nuclear fusion. Stars were born and later destroyed. Each generation of stars fed on the debris of extinct ones. Each generation produced larger atoms, increasing the number of different chemical elements.

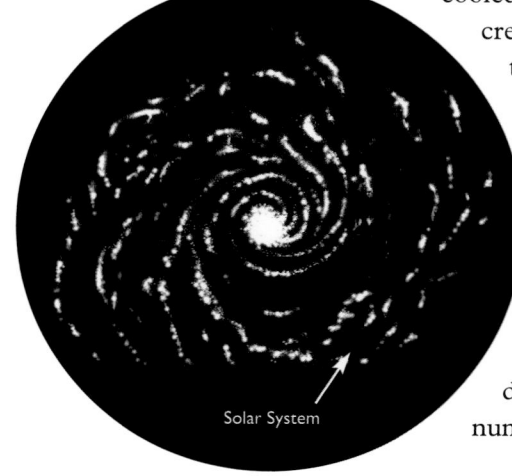

▲ *The Home Galaxy*
This schematic plan shows that our Solar System is located in one of the spiral arms of the Milky Way galaxy, a little less than 30,000 light-years from its centre. The centre of the Milky Way galaxy is not visible from Earth. Instead, it is masked by light-absorbing clouds of interstellar dust.

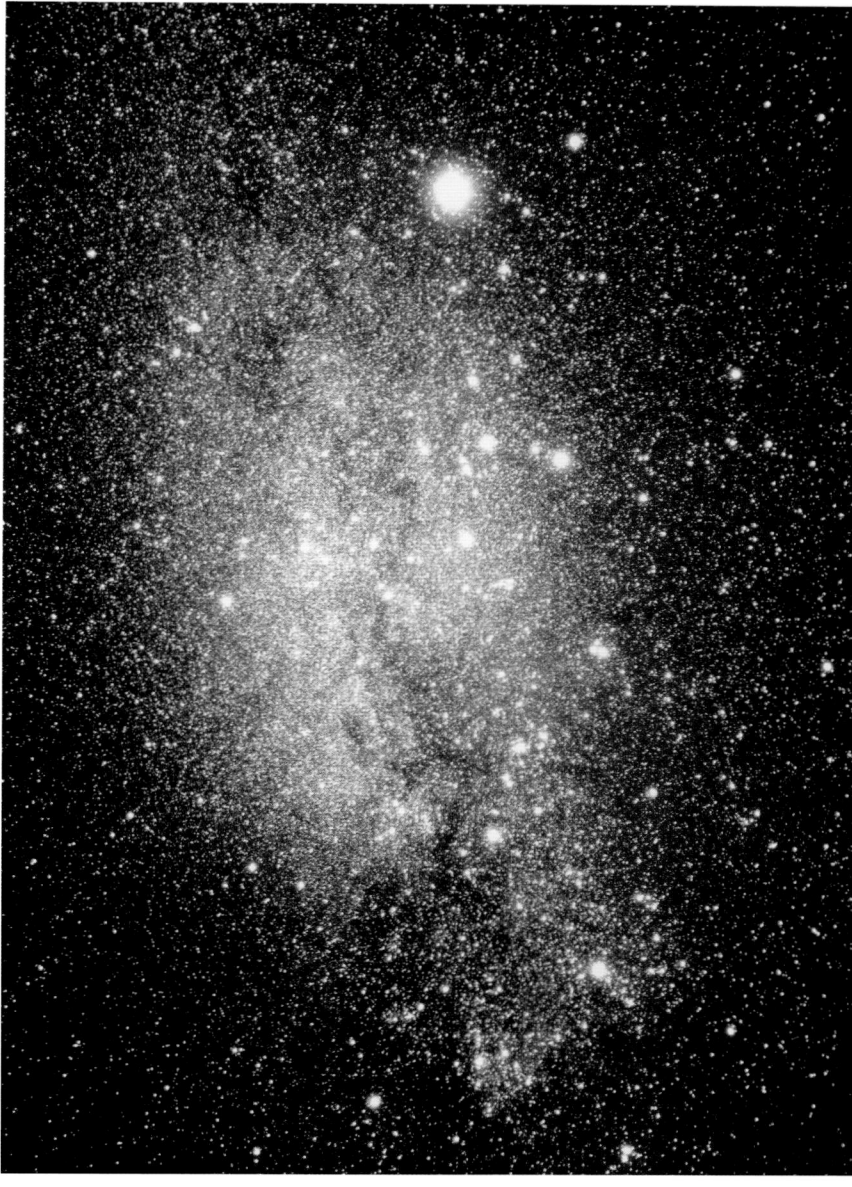

▲ *The Milky Way*
This section of the Milky Way is dominated by Sirius, the Dog Star, top centre, in the constellation of Canis Major. Sirius is the brightest star in the sky.

THE GALAXIES

At least a billion galaxies are scattered through the Universe, though the discoveries made by the Hubble Space Telescope suggest that there may be far more than once thought, and some estimates are as high as 100 billion. The largest galaxies contain trillions of stars, while small ones contain less than a billion.

Galaxies tend to occur in groups or clusters, while some clusters appear to be grouped in vast superclusters. Our Local Cluster includes the spiral Milky Way galaxy, whose diameter is about 100,000 light-years; one light-year, the distance that light travels in one year, is about 9,500 billion km [5,900 billion miles]. The Milky Way is a huge galaxy, shaped like a disk with a bulge at the centre. It is larger, brighter and more massive than many other known galaxies. It contains about 100 billion stars, which rotate around the centre of the galaxy in the same direction as the Sun does.

One medium-sized star in the Milky Way galaxy is the Sun. After its formation, about 5 billion years ago, there was enough leftover matter around it to create the planets, asteroids, moons and other bodies that together form our Solar System. The Solar System rotates around the centre of the Milky Way galaxy approximately every 225 million years.

Stars similar to our Sun are known to have planets orbiting around them. By the start of 2005, over a hundred of these extrasolar planets had been reported, and evidence from the Hubble Space Telescope suggests that the raw materials from which planets are formed is common in dusty disks around many stars. This raises one of the most intriguing questions that has ever faced humanity: if other planets exist in the Universe, are they home to living organisms?

Before the time of Galileo, people thought that the Earth lay at the centre of the Universe. But we now know that our Solar System and even the Milky Way galaxy are tiny specks in the Universe as a whole. Perhaps our planet is also not unique in its ability to support intelligent life.

THE CONSTELLATIONS

On a clear night, under the best conditions and far away from the glare of city lights, a person in northern Europe can look up and see about 2,500 stars. In a town, however, light pollution can reduce visibility to 200 stars or fewer. Over the whole celestial sphere it is possible to see about 8,500 stars with the naked eye and it is only when you look through a telescope that you begin to realize that the number of stars is countless.

SMALL AND LARGE STARS

Stars come in many sizes. Some, called neutron stars, are compact, with the same mass as the Sun but with diameters of only about 20 km [12 miles]. Larger than neutron stars are the small white dwarfs. Our Sun is a medium-sized star, but many visible stars in the night sky are giants with diameters typically 20 times that of the Sun, or supergiants with diameters from 50 to several hundred times that of the Sun.

Two bright stars in the constellation Orion are Betelgeuse (also known as Alpha Orionis) and Rigel (or Beta Orionis). Betelgeuse is an orange-red supergiant, whose diameter is about 500 times that of the Sun. Rigel is also a supergiant. Its diameter is about 50 times that of the Sun, but its luminosity is estimated to be 40,000 times that of the Sun.

The stars we see in the night sky all belong to our home galaxy, the Milky Way. This name is also used for the faint, silvery band that arches across the sky. This band, a slice through our galaxy, contains an enormous number of stars.

▼ The Plough

The Plough, or Big Dipper, seen above glowing yellow clouds lit by city lights. It is part of a larger group called Ursa Major, one of the best-known constellations of the northern hemisphere. The two bright stars to the lower right of the photograph (Merak and Dubhe) are known as the Pointers because they show the way to the Pole Star.

THE CONSTELLATIONS

The constellations and their English names. Constellations visible from both hemispheres are listed.

Andromeda	Andromeda	Delphinus	Dolphin	Perseus	Perseus
Antlia	Air Pump	Dorado	Swordfish	Phoenix	Phoenix
Apus	Bird of Paradise	Draco	Dragon	Pictor	Easel
Aquarius	Water Carrier	Equuleus	Little Horse	Pisces	Fishes
Aquila	Eagle	Eridanus	River Eridanus	Piscis Austrinus	Southern Fish
Ara	Altar	Fornax	Furnace	Puppis	Ship's Stern
Aries	Ram	Gemini	Twins	Pyxis	Mariner's Compass
Auriga	Charioteer	Grus	Crane	Reticulum	Net
Boötes	Herdsman	Hercules	Hercules	Sagitta	Arrow
Caelum	Chisel	Horologium	Clock	Sagittarius	Archer
Camelopardalis	Giraffe	Hydra	Water Snake	Scorpius	Scorpion
Cancer	Crab	Hydrus	Sea Serpent	Sculptor	Sculptor
Canes Venatici	Hunting Dogs	Indus	Indian	Scutum	Shield
Canis Major	Great Dog	Lacerta	Lizard	Serpens*	Serpent
Canis Minor	Little Dog	Leo	Lion	Sextans	Sextant
Capricornus	Sea Goat	Leo Minor	Little Lion	Taurus	Bull
Carina	Ship's Keel	Lepus	Hare	Telescopium	Telescope
Cassiopeia	Cassiopeia	Libra	Scales	Triangulum	Triangle
Centaurus	Centaur	Lupus	Wolf	Triangulum Australe	Southern Triangle
Cepheus	Cepheus	Lynx	Lynx	Tucana	Toucan
Cetus	Whale	Lyra	Lyre	Ursa Major	Great Bear
Chamaeleon	Chameleon	Mensa	Table Mountain	Ursa Minor	Little Bear
Circinus	Compasses	Microscopium	Microscope	Vela	Ship's Sails
Columba	Dove	Monoceros	Unicorn	Virgo	Virgin
Coma Berenices	Berenice's Hair	Musca	Fly	Volans	Flying Fish
Corona Australis	Southern Crown	Norma	Level	Vulpecula	Fox
Corona Borealis	Northern Crown	Octans	Octant		
Corvus	Crow	Ophiuchus	Serpent Bearer		
Crater	Cup	Orion	Hunter	*In two halves: Serpens Caput, the*	
Crux	Southern Cross	Pavo	Peacock	*head, and Serpens Cauda, the tail.*	
Cygnus	Swan	Pegasus	Winged Horse		

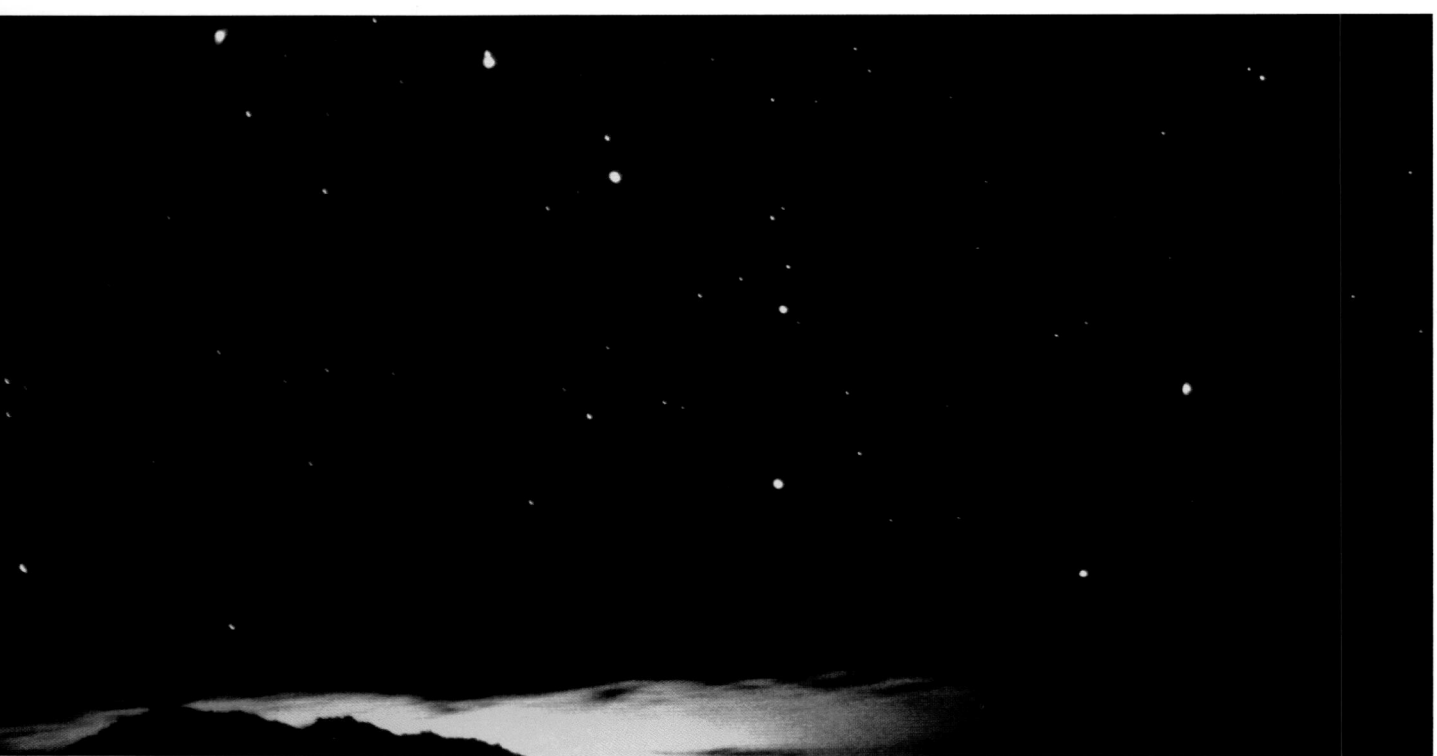

THE BRIGHTEST STARS

The 15 brightest stars visible from northern Europe. Magnitudes are given to the nearest tenth.

Sirius	−1.4
Arcturus	0.0
Vega	0.0
Capella	0.1
Rigel	0.2
Procyon	0.4
Betelgeuse	0.4
Altair	0.8
Aldebaran	0.9
Spica	1.0
Antares	1.0
Pollux	1.2
Fomalhaut	1.2
Deneb	1.2
Regulus	1.4

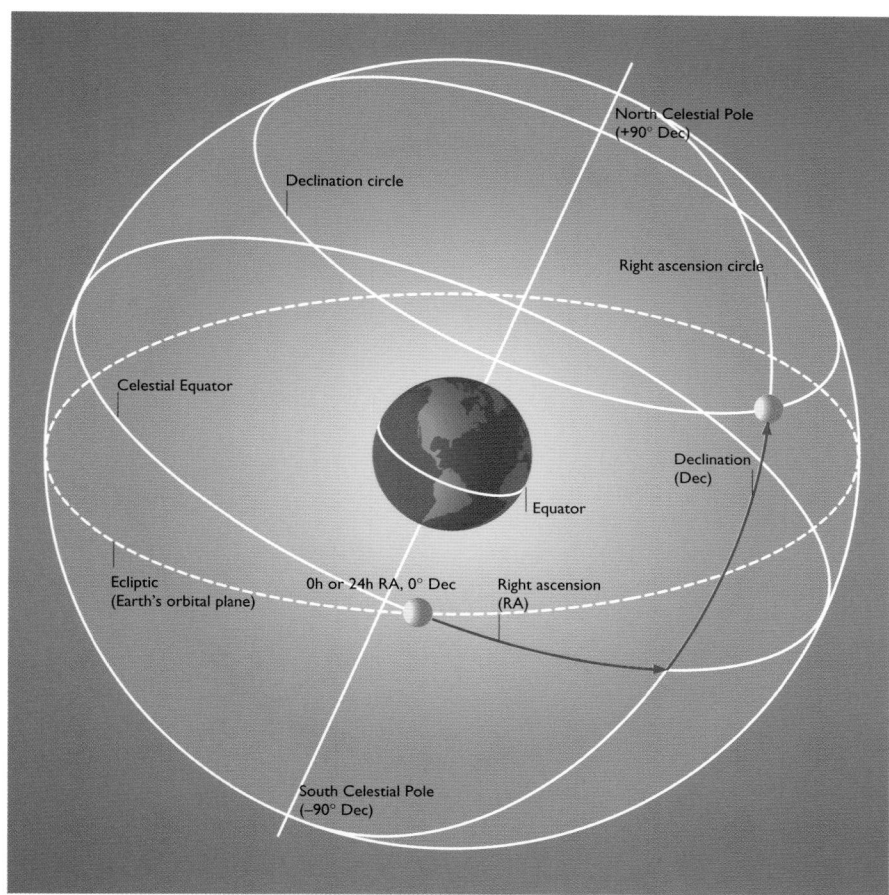

North Celestial Pole
(+90° Dec)

Declination circle

Right ascension circle

Celestial Equator

Declination
(Dec)

Equator

Ecliptic
(Earth's orbital plane)

0h or 24h RA, 0° Dec

Right ascension
(RA)

South Celestial Pole
(–90° Dec)

▲ *Celestial sphere*

*The diagram shows the imaginary
surface on which astronomical
positions are measured. The
celestial sphere appears to rotate
about the celestial poles, as though
an extension of the Earth's own
axis. The Earth's axis points
towards the celestial poles.*

The nucleus of the Milky Way galaxy cannot be seen from Earth. Lying in the direction of the constellation Sagittarius in the southern hemisphere, it is masked by clouds of dust.

THE BRIGHTNESS OF STARS

Astronomers use a scale of magnitudes to measure the brightness of stars. The brightest visible to the naked eye were originally known as first-magnitude stars, ones not so bright were second-magnitude, down to the faintest visible, which were rated as sixth-magnitude. The brighter the star, the lower the magnitude. With the advent of telescopes and the development of accurate instruments for measuring brightnesses, the magnitude scale has been refined and extended. Very bright bodies, such as Sirius, Venus and the Sun, have negative magnitudes. The nearest star is Proxima Centauri, part of a multiple star system, which is 4.2 light-years away. Proxima Centauri is very faint and has a magnitude of 11.0. Alpha Centauri A, one of the two brighter members of the system, is the nearest visible star to Earth. It has a magnitude of 1.7.

These magnitudes are known as apparent magnitudes – measures of the brightnesses of the stars as they appear to us. These are the magnitudes indicated on the star charts on pages 22–23. But the stars are at very different distances. The star Deneb, in the constellation Cygnus, for example, is 3,200 light-years away. So astronomers also use absolute magnitudes – measures of how bright the stars really are. A star's absolute magnitude is the apparent magnitude it would have if it could be placed 32.6 light-years away. So Deneb, with an apparent magnitude of 1.2, has an absolute magnitude of –8.7.

The brightest star in the night sky is Sirius, the Dog Star, with a magnitude of –1.4. This medium-sized star is 8.6 light-years distant but it gives out about 20 times as much light as the Sun. After the Sun and the Moon, the brightest objects in the sky are the planets Venus, Mars and Jupiter. For example, Venus has a magnitude of up to –4. The planets have no light of their own, however, and shine only because they reflect the Sun's rays. But while stars have fixed positions, the planets shift nightly in relation to the constellations, following a path called the ecliptic (shown on the star charts overleaf). As they follow their orbits around the Sun, their distances from the Earth vary, and therefore so also do their magnitudes.

While atlas maps record the details of the Earth's surface, star charts are a guide to the heavens. An observer at the equator can see the entire sky over the course of a year, but an observer at one of the poles can see only the stars in a single hemisphere.

▼ *The Southern Cross*

*The Southern Cross, or Crux, in the southern hemisphere,
was classified as a constellation in the 17th century.
It is as familiar to Australians and New Zealanders as
the Plough (or Big Dipper) is to people in the northern
hemisphere. The vertical axis of the Southern Cross points
towards the South Celestial Pole.*

STAR CHARTS

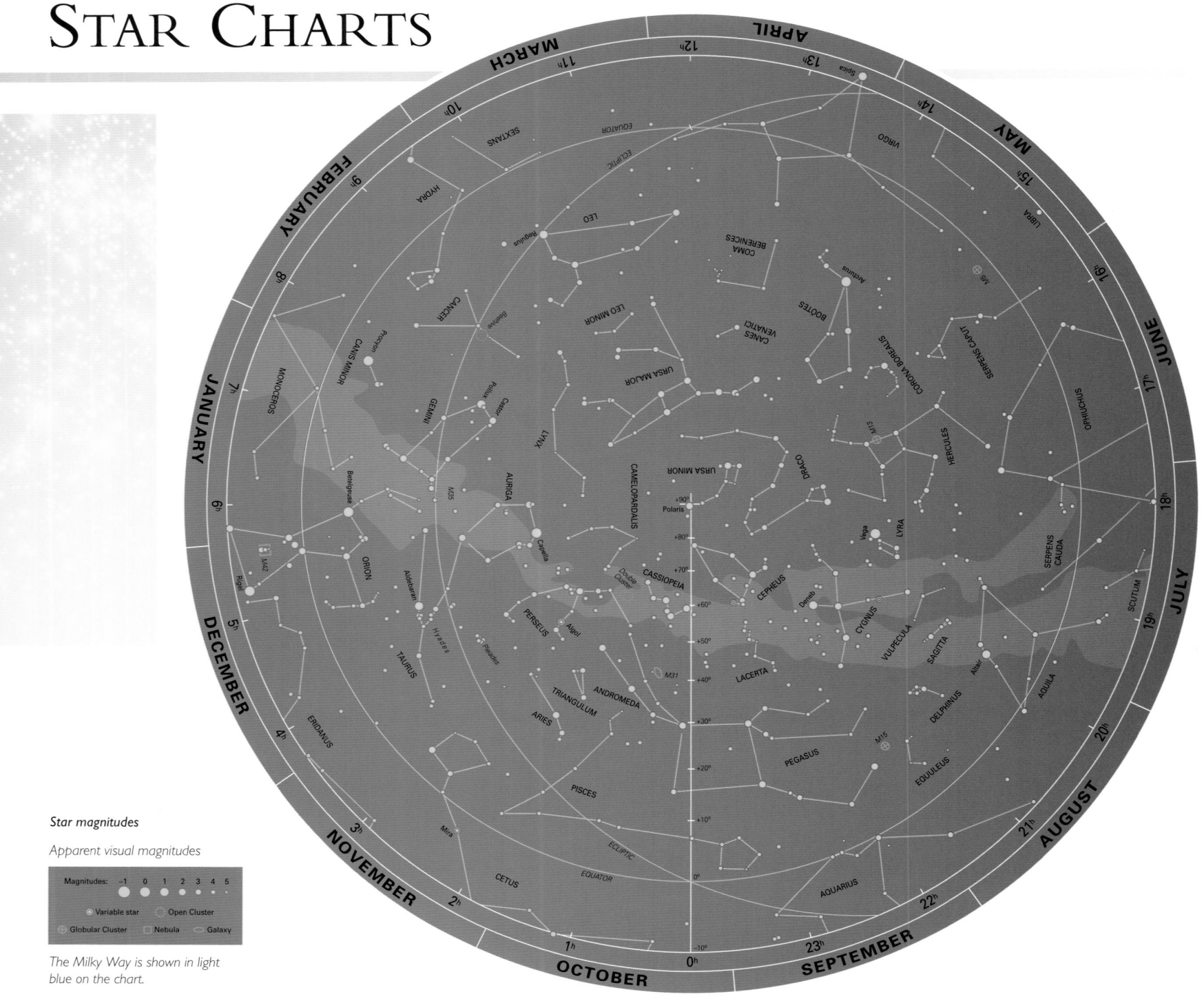

Star magnitudes

Apparent visual magnitudes

Magnitudes: −1 0 1 2 3 4 5

○ Variable star ⊕ Open Cluster
⊕ Globular Cluster ▫ Nebula ◯ Galaxy

The Milky Way is shown in light blue on the chart.

These pages show a star chart for each hemisphere. The northern hemisphere chart is centred on the North Celestial Pole, while the southern hemisphere chart is centred on the South Celestial Pole.

In the northern hemisphere, the North Pole is marked by the star Polaris, or Pole Star. Polaris lies within a degree of the point where an extension of the Earth's axis meets the sky. Polaris appears to be almost stationary, and navigators throughout history have used it as a guide. Unfortunately, the South Celestial Pole has no convenient reference point.

Star charts of the two hemispheres are bounded by the celestial equator, an imaginary line in the sky directly above the terrestrial equator. Astronomical co-ordinates, which give the location of stars, are normally stated in terms of

▲ *Star chart of the northern hemisphere*

When you look into the sky, the stars seem to be on the inside of a huge dome. This gives astronomers a way of mapping them. This chart shows the sky as it would appear from the North Pole. To use the star chart above, an observer in the northern hemisphere should face south and turn the chart so that the current month appears at the bottom. The chart will then show the constellations on view at about 11 p.m. Greenwich Mean Time. The map should be rotated clockwise 15° for each hour before 11 p.m. and anticlockwise for each hour after 11 p.m.

right ascension (the equivalent of longitude) and declination (the equivalent of latitude). Because the stars appear to rotate around the Earth every 24 hours, right ascension is measured eastwards in hours and minutes. Declination is measured in degrees north or south of the celestial equator.

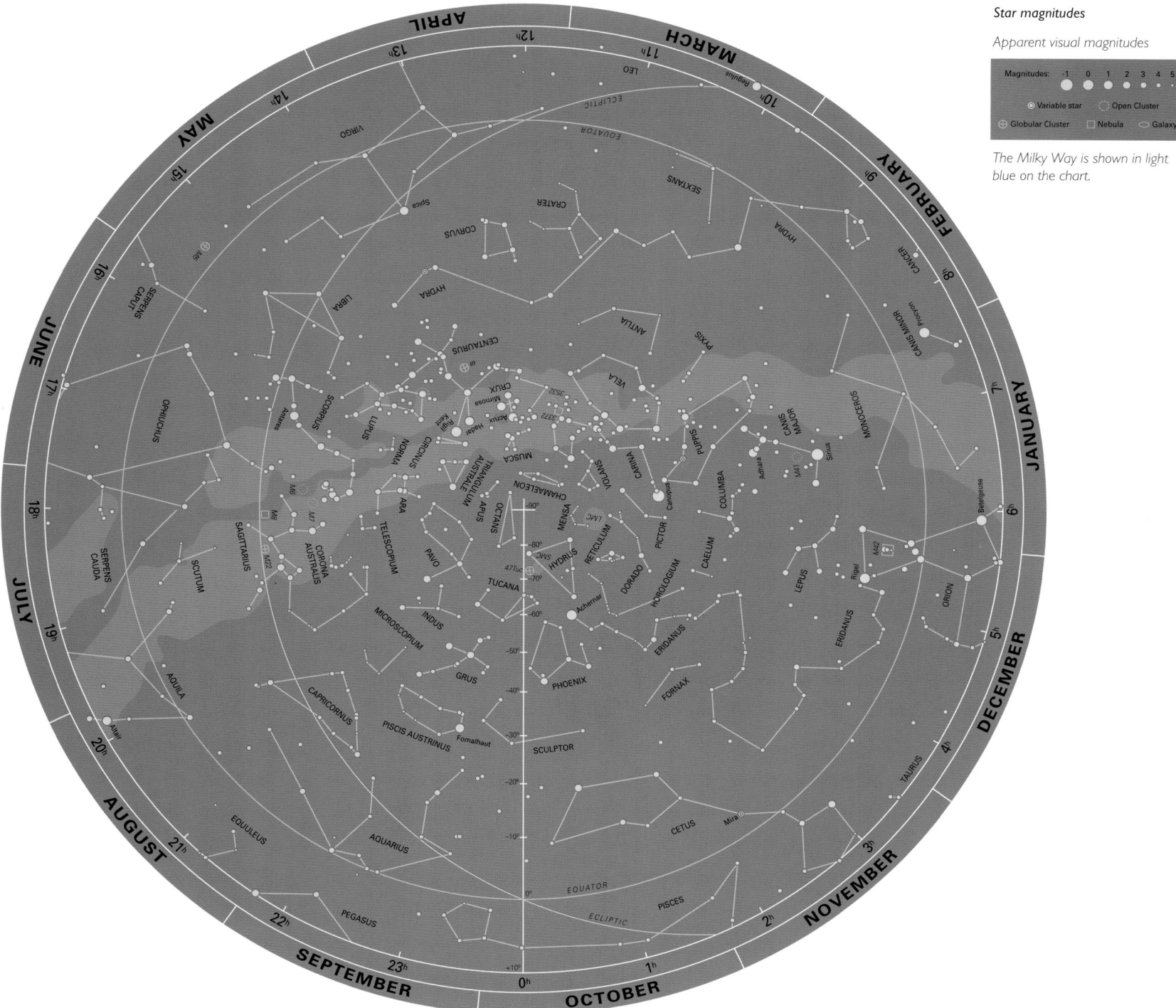

CONSTELLATIONS

Every star belongs to a particular constellation. There are 88 constellations, many of which were named by the ancient Greeks, Romans and other early peoples after animals and mythological characters, such as Orion and Perseus. More recently, astronomers invented names for constellations seen in the southern hemisphere, in areas not visible from around the Mediterranean Sea.

Some groups of easily recognizable stars form parts of a constellation. For example, seven stars form the shape of the Plough, or Big Dipper, within the constellation Ursa Major. Such groups are called asterisms.

The stars in constellations lie in the same direction in space, but normally at vastly different distances. Hence, there is no real connection

▲ *Star chart of the southern hemisphere*

Many constellations in the southern hemisphere were named not by the ancients but by later astronomers and thus have modern names. The Large and Small Magellanic Clouds (LMC, SMC) are small 'satellite' galaxies of the Milky Way. To use the chart, an observer in the southern hemisphere should face north and turn the chart so that the current month appears at the bottom. The map will then show the constellations on view at about 11 p.m. Greenwich Mean Time. The chart should be rotated clockwise 15° for each hour before 11 p.m. and anticlockwise for each hour after 11 p.m.

between them. The positions of stars seem fixed, but in fact the shapes of the constellations are changing slowly over very long periods of time. This is because the stars have their own 'proper motions', which because of the huge distances involved are imperceptible to the naked eye.

THE SOLAR SYSTEM

Our knowledge of the Solar System has increased greatly since the start of the Space Age in 1957, with the launch of the Soviet satellite Sputnik 1. Research continues and, in 2006, studies of the outer Solar System led the International Astronomical Union to reclassify Pluto as a 'dwarf planet'. It now belongs to a group of orbiting bodies, including the asteroid Ceres, and, beyond Pluto, Eris (once called UB313 or Xena), which was discovered in 2003.

Scientists believe that the Solar System was formed from a rotating disk of gas and dust, the remains of a previous generation of stars. About 5 billion years ago, a new star, the Sun, was born, containing 99.8% of the mass of our Solar System. The remaining material makes up the planets and other bodies in the Solar System.

THE PLANETS

Mercury is the closest planet to the Sun and the fastest moving. Space probes have revealed that its surface is covered by craters, and looks much like the Earth's Moon. Mercury is a hostile place, with no significant atmosphere and temperatures ranging between 400°C [750°F] by day and −170°C [−275°F] by night. It seems unlikely that anyone will ever want to visit this planet.

Venus is much the same size as Earth, but it is the hottest of the planets, with temperatures reaching 475°C [885°F], even at night. The reason for this scorching heat is the atmosphere, which consists mainly of carbon dioxide, a gas that traps heat thus creating a greenhouse effect. The density of the atmosphere is about 90 times that of Earth, and dense clouds permanently mask the planet's surface. Active volcanic regions discharging sulphur dioxide may account for the haze of sulphuric-acid droplets in the upper atmosphere. Seen from Earth, Venus is brighter than any other star or planet and is

easy to spot. It is often the first object to be seen in the evening sky and the last to be seen in the morning sky. It can even be seen in daylight.

Earth, seen from space, looks blue (because of the oceans which cover more than 70% of the planet) and white (a result of clouds in the atmosphere). The atmosphere and water make Earth the only planet known to support life. The Earth's hard outer layers, including the crust and the top of the mantle, are divided into rigid plates. Forces inside the Earth move the plates, modifying the landscape, and causing earthquakes and volcanic activity. Weathering and erosion also change the surface.

Mars has many features in common with the Earth, including an atmosphere with clouds and polar caps that partly melt in summer. Scientists once considered that it was the most likely planet on which other life might exist, but the two Viking space probes that went there in the 1970s found only a barren rocky surface, with no trace of water. But, in 2004, two NASA Mars rovers – Spirit and Opportunity – sent back evidence that Mars was once wet and potentially habitable, at least by simple microbes.

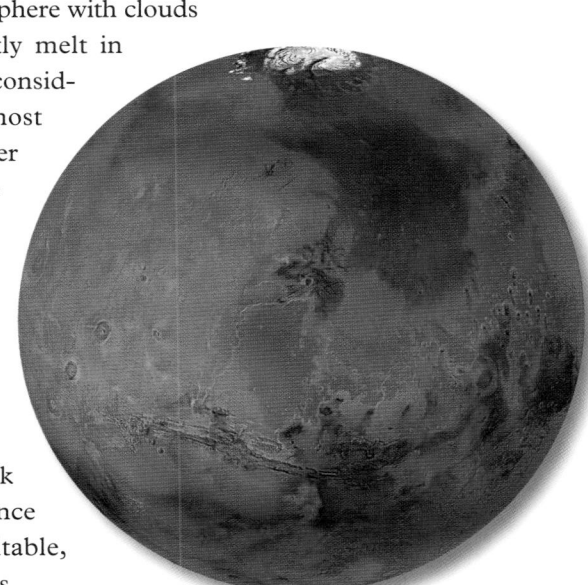

PLANETARY DATA

Planet	Mean distance from Sun (million km)	Mass (Earth=1)	Period of orbit (Earth days/yrs)	Period of rotation (Earth days)	Equatorial diameter (km)	Average density (water=1)	Surface gravity (Earth=1)	Number of known satellites*
Sun	–	332,946	–	25.38	1,392,000	1.41	27.9	–
Mercury	57.9	0.06	87.97d	58.65	4,879	5.43	0.38	0
Venus	108.2	0.82	224.7d	243.02	12,104	5.24	0.91	0
Earth	149.6	1.00	365.3d	1.00	12,756	5.52	1.00	1
Mars	227.9	0.11	687.0d	1.029	6,792	3.94	0.38	2
Jupiter	778	317.8	11.86y	0.411	142,984	1.33	2.36	63
Saturn	1,427	95.2	29.45y	0.428	120,536	0.69	0.91	60
Uranus	2,871	14.5	84.02y	0.720	51,118	1.27	0.89	27
Neptune	4,498	17.2	164.8y	0.673	49,528	1.64	1.13	13

* Number of known satellites at mid-2008

Asteroids are small, rocky bodies. Most of them orbit the Sun between Mars and Jupiter, but some small ones can approach the Earth. The largest is Ceres, 913 km [567 miles] in diameter. There may be around a million asteroids bigger than 1 km [0.6 miles].

Jupiter, the giant planet, lies beyond Mars and the asteroid belt. Its mass is almost three times as much as all the other planets combined and, because of its size, it shines more brightly than any other planet apart from Venus and, occasionally, Mars. Jupiter is made up mostly of hydrogen and helium, covered by a layer of clouds. Its Great Red Spot is a high-pressure storm. The planet also has a faint ring system. The four largest moons of Jupiter were discovered by Galileo. They are worlds in their own right: Io is the most volcanic body yet discovered; Europa and Ganymede have icy surfaces, perhaps with liquid oceans below; and Callisto has an ancient, cratered terrain. Jupiter made headline news when it was struck by fragments of Comet Shoemaker–Levy 9 in July 1994, creating huge fireballs that caused scars on the planet that remained visible for months after the event.

Saturn is structurally similar to Jupiter but it is best known for its rings. The rings measure about 270,000 km [170,000 miles] across, yet they are no more than a few hundred metres thick. Seen from Earth, the rings seem divided into three main bands of varying brightness,

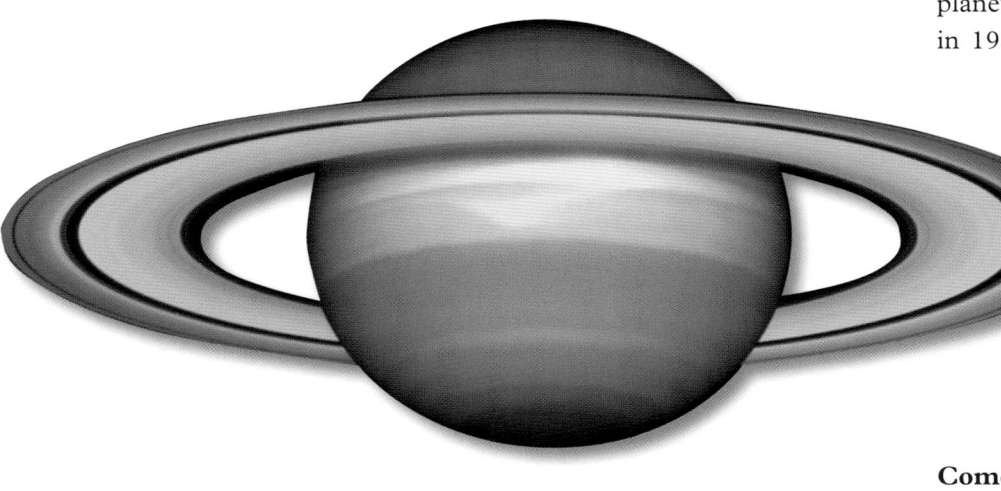

but photographs sent back by space probes showed that they are broken up into thousands of thin ringlets composed of ice particles ranging in size from a snowball to an iceberg. The origin of the rings is still a matter of debate.

Uranus was discovered in 1781 by William Herschel, who first thought it was a comet. It is broadly similar to Jupiter and Saturn in composition, though its distance from the Sun makes its surface even colder. Uranus is circled by thin rings which were discovered in 1977. Unlike the rings of Saturn, the rings of Uranus are black, which explains why they cannot be seen from Earth.

Neptune, named after the mythological sea god, was discovered in 1846 as the result of mathematical predictions made by astronomers to explain irregularities in the orbit of Uranus, its near twin. Little was known about this distant body until Voyager 2 came close to it in 1989. Neptune has thin rings, like those of Uranus. Its atmosphere features blue-green clouds and the occasional prominent dark spot.

Pluto, once regarded as the smallest planet in the Solar System, has been reclassified as a 'dwarf planet' since 2006. Discovered in 1930 by Clyde Tombaugh, the American astronomer, Pluto's orbit is odd and it sometimes comes closer to the Sun than Neptune. Pluto lies in the Kuiper Belt, a vast region beyond the orbit of Neptune. Pluto and Eris, another dwarf planet, are the largest known objects in the Kuiper Belt.

Comets are small icy bodies that orbit the Sun in highly elliptical orbits. When a comet swings in towards the Sun some of its ice evaporates, and the comet brightens and may become visible from Earth. The best known is Halley's Comet, which takes 76 years to orbit the Sun.

THE EARTH: TIME AND MOTION

The Earth is constantly moving through space like a huge, self-sufficient spaceship. First, with the rest of the Solar System, it moves around the centre of the Milky Way galaxy. Second, it rotates around the Sun at a speed of more than 100,000 km/h [60,000 mph], covering a distance of nearly 1,000 million km [600 million miles] in a little over 365 days. The Earth also spins on its axis, an imaginary line joining the North and South Poles, via the centre of the Earth, completing one turn in a day. The Earth's movements around the Sun determine our calendar, though accurate observations of the stars made by astronomers

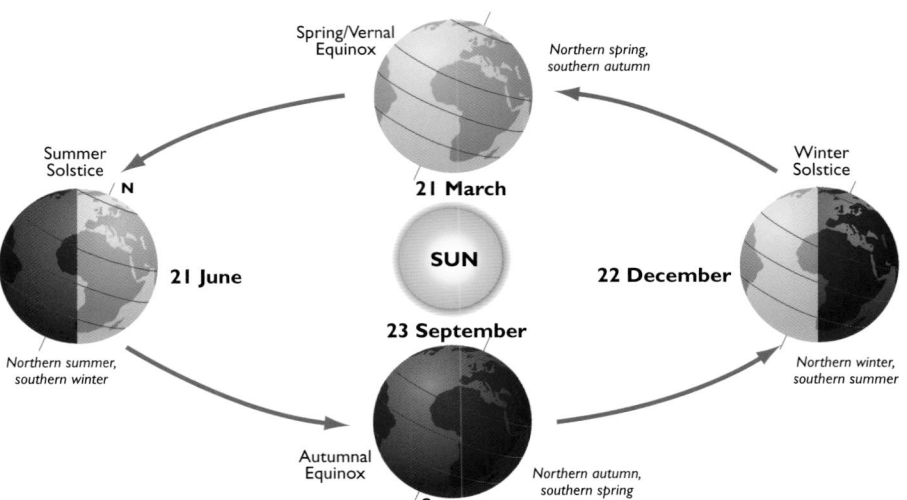

▼ **The Earth from the Moon**

In 1969, Neil Armstrong and Edwin 'Buzz' Aldrin, Jr, were the first people to set foot on the Moon. This photograph of the Earth was taken by the crew of Apollo 11 as they orbited the Moon.

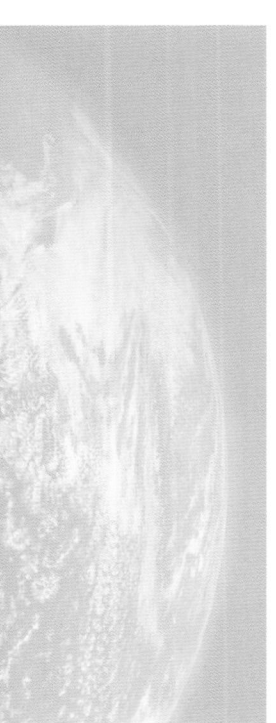

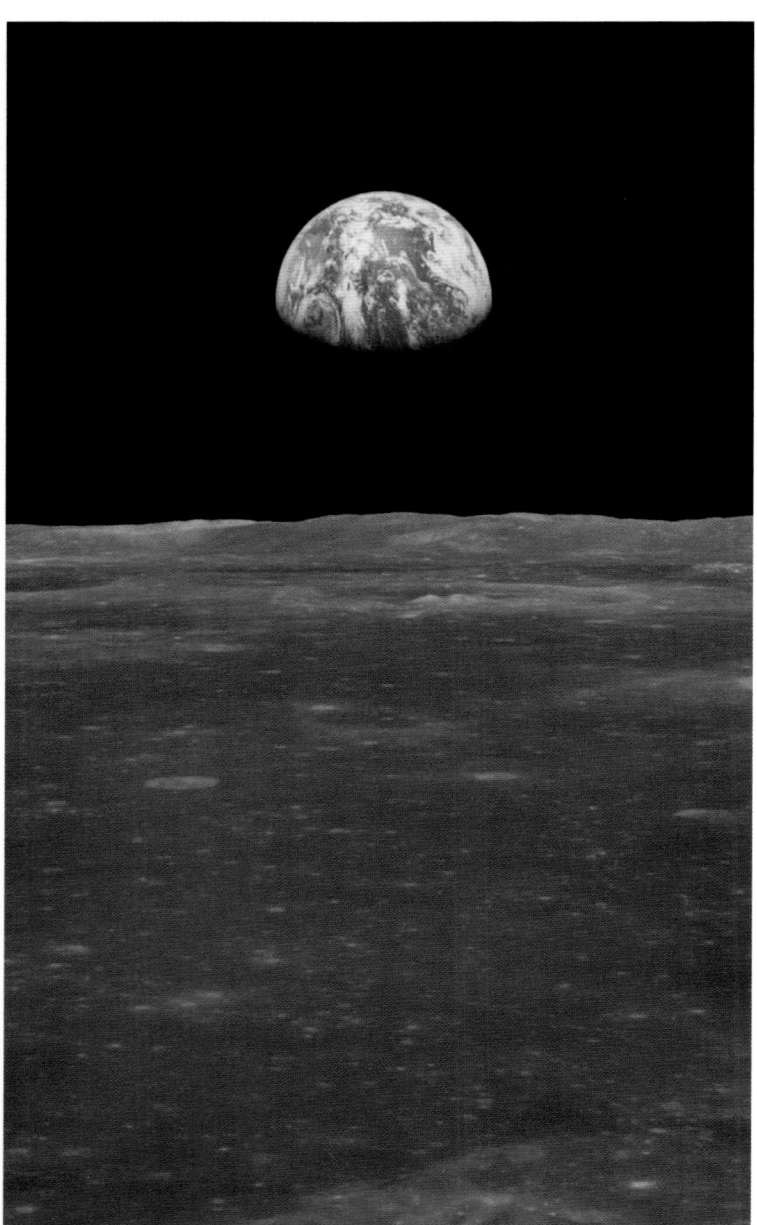

help to keep our clocks in step with the rotation of the Earth around the Sun.

THE CHANGING YEAR

The Earth takes 365 days, 6 hours, 9 minutes and 9.54 seconds to complete one orbit around the Sun. We have a calendar year of 365 days, so allowance has to be made for the extra time over and above the 365 days. This is allowed for by introducing leap years of 366 days. Leap years are generally those, such as 1992 and 1996, which are divisible by four. Century years, however, are not leap years unless they are divisible by 400. Hence, 1700, 1800 and 1900 were not leap years, but the year 2000 was one. Leap years help to make the calendar conform with the solar year.

Because the Earth's axis is tilted by approximately 23½°, the middle latitudes enjoy four distinct seasons. On 21 March, the vernal or spring equinox in the northern hemisphere, the Sun is directly overhead at the equator and everywhere on Earth has about 12 hours of daylight and 12 hours of darkness. But as the Earth continues on its journey around the Sun, the northern hemisphere tilts more and more towards the Sun. Finally, on 21 June, the Sun is overhead at the Tropic of Cancer (latitude 23½° North). This is the summer solstice in the northern hemisphere.

▲ **The Seasons**

The approximate 23½° tilt of the Earth's axis remains constant as the Earth orbits around the Sun. As a result, first the northern and then the southern hemispheres lean towards the Sun. Annual variations in the amount of sunlight received in turn by each hemisphere are responsible for the four seasons experienced in the middle latitudes.

▼ **Tides**

The daily rises and falls of the ocean's waters are caused by the gravitational pull of the Moon and the Sun. The effect is greatest on the hemisphere facing the Moon, causing a 'tidal bulge'. The diagram below shows that the Sun, Moon and Earth are in line when the spring tides occur. This causes the greatest tidal ranges. On the other hand, the neap tides occur when the pull of the Moon and the Sun are opposed. Neap tides, when tidal ranges are at their lowest, occur near the Moon's first and third quarters.

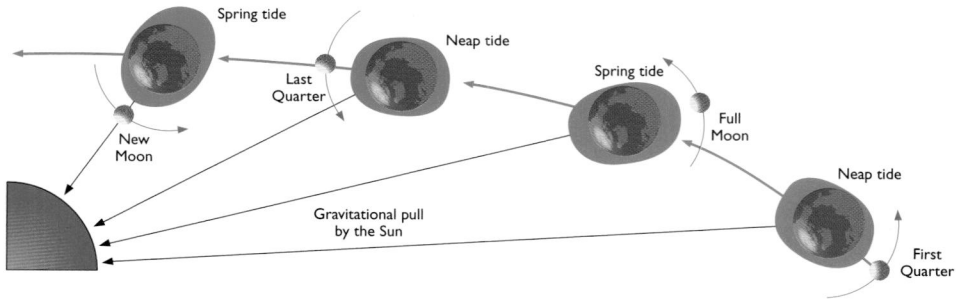

SUN DATA

DIAMETER	1.391×10^6 km
VOLUME	1.412×10^{18} km³
VOLUME (EARTH=1)	1.303×10^6
MASS	1.989×10^{30} kg
MASS (EARTH=1)	3.329×10^6
MEAN DENSITY (WATER=1)	1.409
ROTATION PERIOD:	
AT EQUATOR	25.4 days
AT POLES	about 35 days
SURFACE GRAVITY	
(EARTH=1)	28
MAGNITUDE:	
APPARENT	−26.9
ABSOLUTE	+4.71
TEMPERATURE:	
AT SURFACE	5,500°C [5,800 K]
AT CORE	15×10^6 K

MOON DATA

DIAMETER	3,475 km
MASS (EARTH=1)	0.0123
DENSITY (WATER=1)	3.34
MEAN DISTANCE FROM EARTH	384,401 km
MAXIMUM DISTANCE (APOGEE)	406,700 km
MINIMUM DISTANCE (PERIGEE)	356,400 km
SIDEREAL ROTATION AND REVOLUTION PERIOD	27.322 days
SYNODIC MONTH (NEW MOON TO NEW MOON)	29.531 days
SURFACE GRAVITY (EARTH=1)	0.165
MAXIMUM DAYTIME SURFACE TEMPERATURE	+117°C [390 K]
MINIMUM NIGHTTIME SURFACE TEMPERATURE	−163°C [110 K]

▶ *Phases of the Moon*

The Moon rotates more slowly than the Earth, making one complete turn on its axis in just over 27 days. This corresponds to its period of revolution around the Earth and, hence, the same hemisphere always faces us. The interval between one full Moon and the next (and also between new Moons) is about 29½ days, or one lunar month. The apparent changes in the appearance of the Moon are caused by its changing position in relation to the Earth. Like the planets, the Moon produces no light of its own. It shines by reflecting the Sun's rays, varying from a slim crescent to a full circle, and back again.

The overhead Sun then moves south again until, on 23 September, the autumnal equinox in the northern hemisphere, the Sun is again overhead at the Equator. The overhead Sun then moves south until, on around 22 December, it is overhead at the Tropic of Capricorn. This is the winter solstice in the northern hemisphere, and the summer solstice in the southern, where the seasons are reversed.

At the poles, there are two seasons. During half of the year, one of the poles leans towards the Sun and has continuous sunlight. For the other six months, the pole leans away from the Sun and is in continuous darkness.

Regions around the equator do not have marked seasons. Because the Sun is high in the sky throughout the year, it is always hot or warm. When people talk of seasons in the tropics, they are usually referring to other factors, such as rainy and dry periods.

DAY, NIGHT AND TIDES

As the Earth rotates on its axis every 24 hours, first one side of the planet and then the other faces the Sun and enjoys daylight, while the opposite side is in darkness.

The length of daylight varies throughout the year. The longest day in the northern hemisphere falls on the summer solstice, 21 June, while the longest day in the southern hemisphere is on 22 December. At 40° latitude, the length of daylight on the longest day is 14 hours, 30 minutes. At 60° latitude, daylight on that day lasts 18 hours, 30 minutes. On the shortest day, 22 December in the northern hemisphere and 21 June in the southern, daylight hours at 40° latitude total 9 hours and 9 minutes. At latitude 60°, daylight lasts only 5 hours, 30 minutes in the 24-hour period.

Tides are caused by the gravitational pull of the Moon and, to a lesser extent, the Sun on the waters in the world's oceans. Tides occur twice every 24 hours, 50 minutes – one complete orbit of the Moon around the Earth.

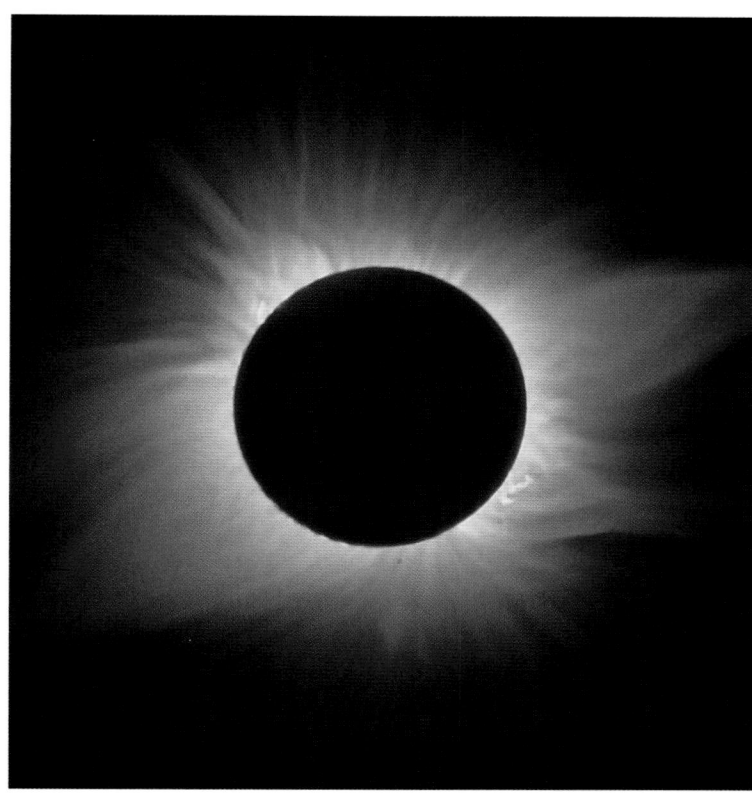

▲ *Total eclipse of the Sun*
A total eclipse is caused when the Moon passes between the Sun and the Earth. With the Sun's bright disk completely obscured, the Sun's corona, or outer atmosphere, can be viewed.

The highest tides, the spring tides, occur when the Earth, Moon and Sun are in a straight line, so that the gravitational pulls of the Moon and Sun are combined. The lowest, or neap, tides occur when the Moon, Earth and Sun form a right angle. The gravitational pull of the Moon is then opposed by the gravitational pull of the Sun. The greatest tidal ranges occur in the Bay of Fundy in Canada. The greatest mean spring range is 14.5 m [47.5 ft].

The speed at which the Earth is spinning on its axis is gradually slowing down, because of the movement of tides. As a result, experts have calculated that, in about 200 million years, the day will be 25 hours long.

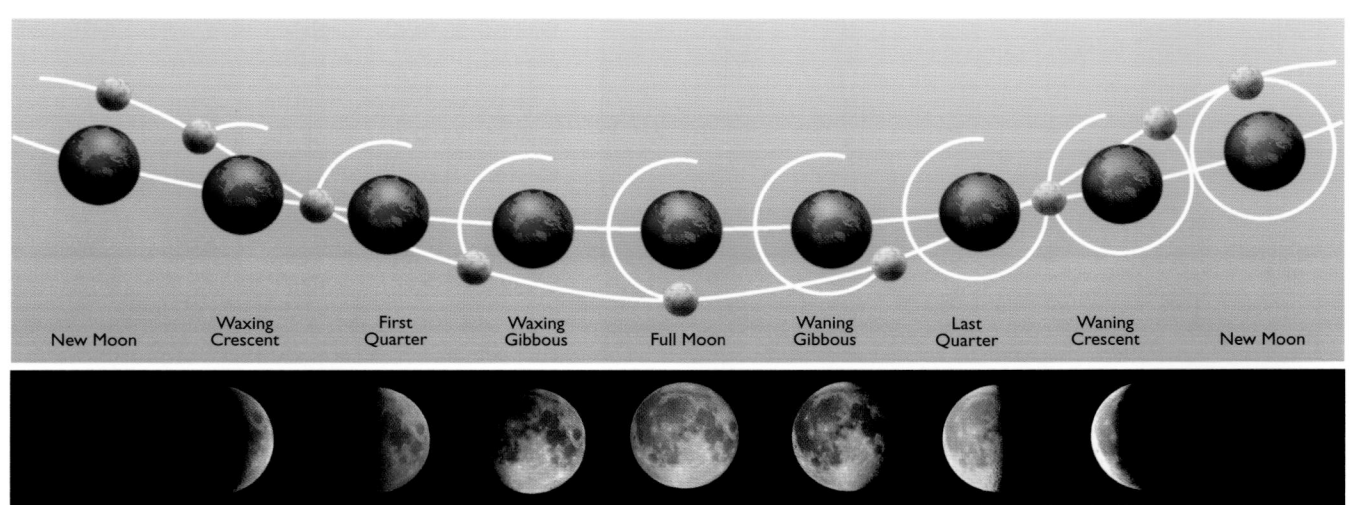

New Moon | Waxing Crescent | First Quarter | Waxing Gibbous | Full Moon | Waning Gibbous | Last Quarter | Waning Crescent | New Moon

THE EARTH FROM SPACE

Any last doubts about whether the Earth was round or flat were finally resolved by the appearance of the first photographs of our planet taken at the start of the Space Age. Satellite images also confirmed that map- and globe-makers had correctly worked out the shapes of the continents and the oceans.

More importantly, images of our beautiful, blue, white and brown planet from space impressed on many people that the Earth and its resources are finite. They made people realize that if we allow our planet to be damaged by such factors as overpopulation, pollution and irresponsible over-use of resources, then its future and the survival of all the living things upon it may be threatened.

VIEWS FROM ABOVE

The first aerial photographs were taken from balloons in the mid-19th century and their importance in military reconnaissance was recognized as early as the 1860s during the American Civil War.

Since the end of World War II, photographs

▼ Mount Etna, Sicily

The most active volcano in Europe, Mount Etna, 3,323 m [10,906 ft] high, is shown here during the 2002–3 eruption, its plume of ash and smoke spreading southwards over the Mediterranean, east of Malta.

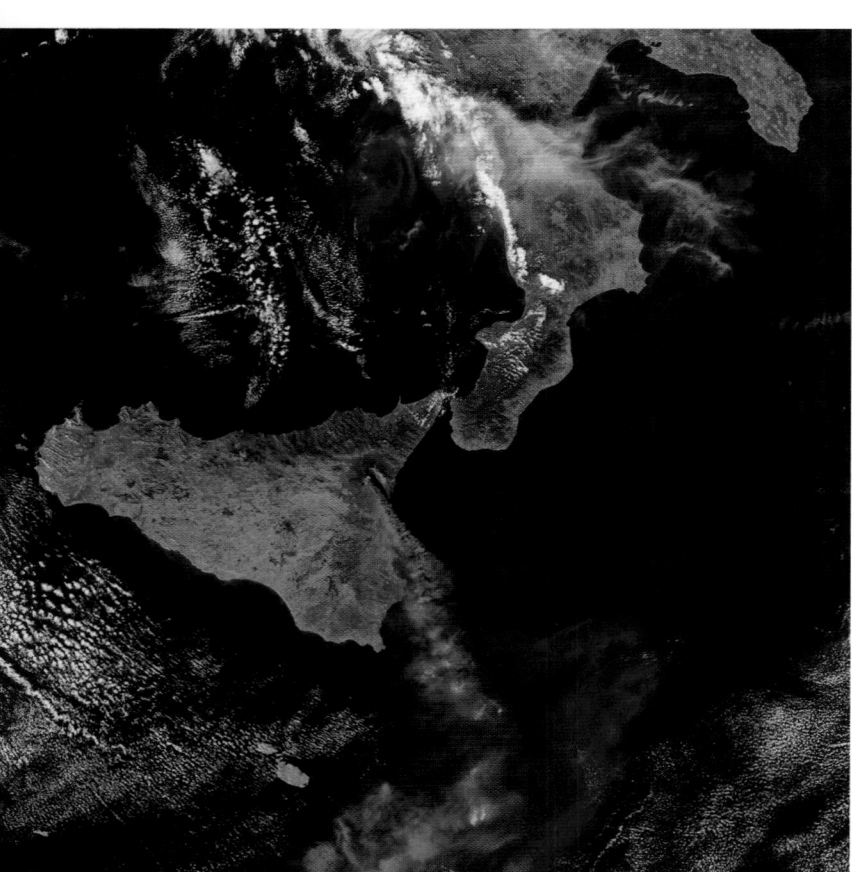

taken by aircraft have been widely used in map-making. The use of air photographs has greatly speeded up the laborious process of mapping land details and they have enabled cartographers to produce maps of the most remote parts of the world.

Aerial photographs have also proved useful because they reveal features that are not visible at ground level. For example, circles that appear on many air photographs do not correspond to visible features on the ground. Many of these mysterious shapes have turned out to be the sites of ancient settlements previously unknown to archaeologists.

IMAGES FROM SPACE

Space probes equipped with cameras and a variety of remote-sensing instruments have sent back images of distant planets and moons. From these images, detailed maps have been produced, rapidly expanding our knowledge of the Solar System.

Images from space are also proving invaluable in the study of the Earth. One of the best known uses of space imagery is the study of the atmosphere. Polar-orbiting weather satellites that circle the Earth, together with geostationary satellites, whose motion is synchronized with the Earth's rotation, now regularly transmit images showing the changing patterns of weather systems from above. Forecasters use these images to track the development and paths of hurricanes, enabling them to issue storm warnings.

Remote-sensing devices are now monitoring changes in temperatures over the land and sea, while photographs indicate the melting of ice sheets. In 2006, Indian scientists announced that satellite images showed that a once populated island in the Ganges delta had vanished, probably as a result of global warming. Such methods also reveal polluted areas and areas suffering deforestation.

In recent years, remote-sensing devices have been used to monitor the damage being done to the ozone layer in the stratosphere, which prevents most of the Sun's harmful ultraviolet radiation from reaching the surface. The discovery of 'ozone holes', where the protective layer of ozone is being thinned by chlorofluorocarbons (CFCs), chemicals used in the manufacture of such things as air conditioners and refrigerators, has enabled governments to take concerted action to save our planet from imminent danger.

EARTH DATA	
MAXIMUM DISTANCE FROM SUN (APHELION)	152,096,150 km
MINIMUM DISTANCE FROM SUN (PERIHELION)	147,099,590 km
LENGTH OF YEAR – SOLAR TROPICAL (EQUINOX TO EQUINOX)	365.24 days
LENGTH OF YEAR – SIDEREAL (FIXED STAR TO FIXED STAR)	365.26 days
LENGTH OF DAY – MEAN SOLAR DAY	24 hours, 3 minutes, 56 seconds
LENGTH OF DAY – MEAN SIDEREAL DAY	23 hours, 56 minutes, 4 seconds
SUPERFICIAL AREA	510,000,000 sq km
LAND SURFACE	149,000,000 sq km (29.2%)
WATER SURFACE	361,000,000 sq km (70.8%)
EQUATORIAL CIRCUMFERENCE	40,074 km
POLAR CIRCUMFERENCE	40,008 km
EQUATORIAL DIAMETER	12,756 km
POLAR DIAMETER	12,714 km
EQUATORIAL RADIUS	6,378 km
POLAR RADIUS	6,357 km
VOLUME OF THE EARTH	$1,083,230 \times 10^6$ cu km
MASS OF THE EARTH	5.97×10^{24} kg

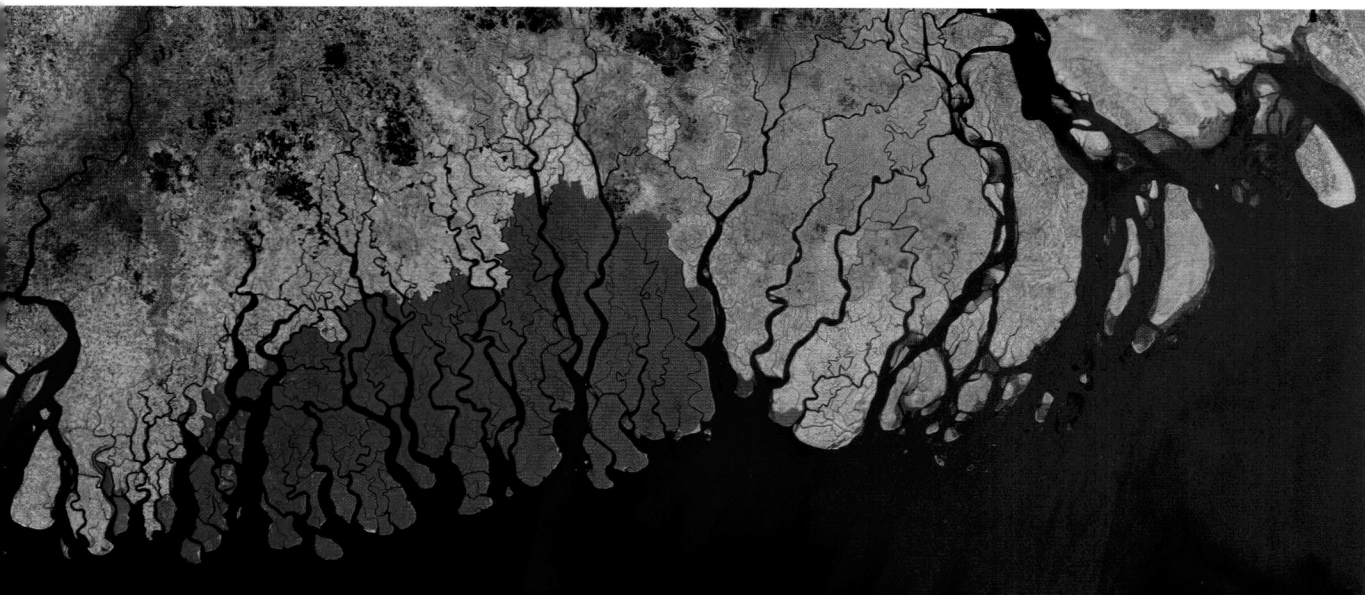

◄ *Ganges Delta, India/Bangladesh*
*Over 300 km [186 miles] wide, this
is the world's largest delta, created by
the River Ganges depositing sediment
it has carried from the Himalayas.
It is extremely vulnerable to frequent
cyclones and tidal surges, but is
densely populated because of the
fertile land. On the western side of
the image is the mouth of the Hugli,
with the elongated city of Kolkata
(Calcutta) showing as dark grey just to
the north. The large red area indicates
the presence of mangrove forests and
swamps, and is divided between the
countries of India and Bangladesh.*

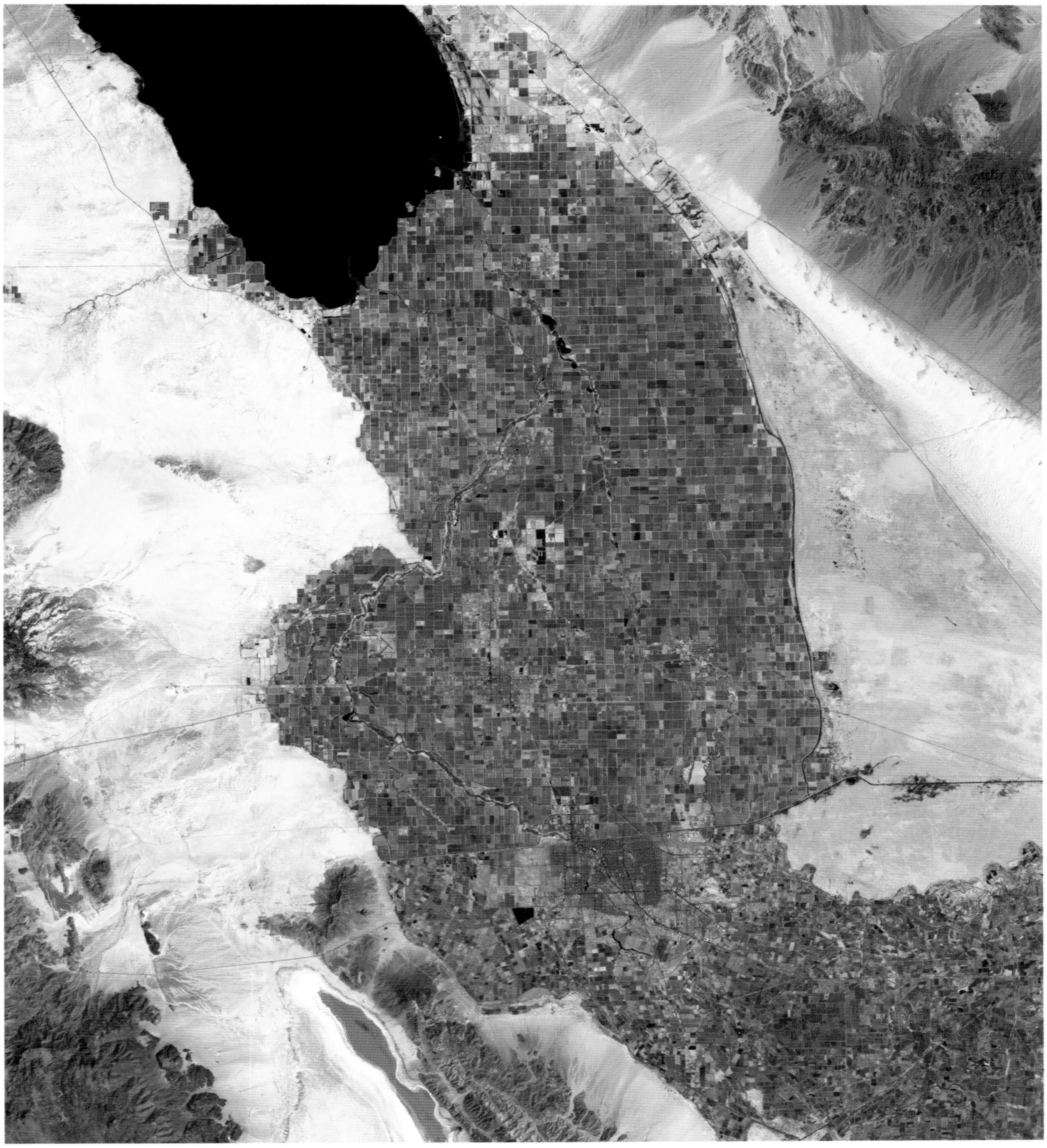

► *Imperial Valley, USA/Mexico*
*The Salton Sea is the dark area
at the top left of the image.
It was inadvertently created in
1905 during an attempt to divert
the flow of the Colorado River for
irrigation. It lies 72 m [236 ft]
below sea level and is very saline.
To the south is a large area of
productive land, showing bright
red on this image. The abrupt
colour change towards the
bottom of this area marks
the US–Mexico boundary.*

THE DYNAMIC EARTH

The Earth was formed about 4.6 billion years [4,600 million years] ago from the ring of gas and dust left over after the formation of the Sun. As the Earth took shape, lighter elements, such as silicon, rose to the surface, while heavy elements, notably iron, sank towards the centre.

Gradually, the outer layers cooled to form a hard crust. The crust enclosed the dense mantle which, in turn, surrounded the even denser liquid outer and solid inner core. Around the Earth was an atmosphere, which contained abundant water vapour. When the surface cooled, rainwater began to fill hollows, forming the first lakes and seas. Since that time, our planet has been subject to constant change – the result of powerful internal and external forces that still operate today.

THE HISTORY OF THE EARTH

From their study of rocks, geologists have pieced together the history of our planet and the life forms that evolved upon it. They have dated the oldest known crystals, composed of the mineral zircon, at 4.2 billion years. But the oldest rocks are younger, less than 4 billion years old. This is because older rocks have been recycled or weathered away by natural processes.

The oldest rocks that contain fossils, which are

▼ *Lulworth Cove, southern England*

When undisturbed by earth movements, sedimentary rock strata are generally horizontal. But lateral pressure has squeezed the Jurassic strata at Lulworth Cove into complex folds.

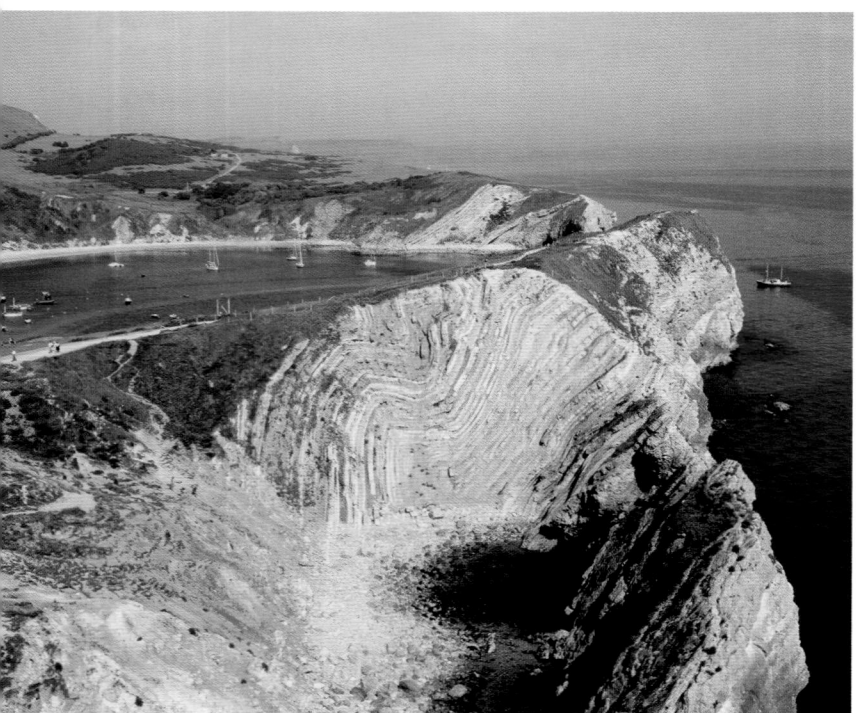

evidence of once-living organisms, are around 3.5 billion years old. But fossils are rare in rocks formed in the first 4 billion years of Earth history. This vast expanse of time is called the Precambrian. This is because it precedes the Cambrian period, at the start of which, about 590 million years ago, life was abundant in the seas.

The Cambrian is the first period in the Paleozoic (or ancient life) era. The Paleozoic era is followed by the Mesozoic (middle life) era, which witnessed the spectacular rise and fall of the dinosaurs, and the Cenozoic (recent life) era, which was dominated by the evolution of mammals. Each of the eras is divided into periods, and the periods in the Cenozoic era, covering the last 65 million years, are further divided into epochs.

THE EARTH'S CHANGING FACE

While life was gradually evolving, the face of the Earth was constantly changing. By piecing together evidence of rock structures and fossils, geologists have demonstrated that around 250 million years ago, all the world's land areas were grouped together in one huge landmass called Pangaea. Around 180 million years ago, the supercontinent Pangaea began to break up. New oceans opened up as the continents began to move towards their present positions.

Evidence of how continents drift came from studies of the ocean floor in the 1950s and 1960s. Scientists discovered that the oceans are young features. By contrast with the continents, no part of the ocean floor is more than 200 million years old. The floors of oceans older than 200 million years have completely vanished.

Studies of long undersea ranges, called ocean ridges, revealed that the youngest rocks occur along their centres, which are the edges of huge plates – rigid blocks of the Earth's lithosphere, which is made up of the crust and the solid upper layer of the mantle. The Earth's lithosphere is split into six large and several smaller plates. The ocean ridges are 'constructive' plate margins, because new crustal rock is being

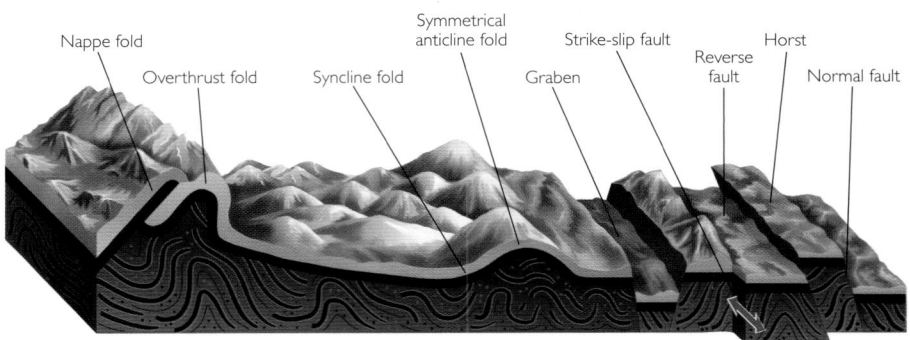

Nappe fold | Overthrust fold | Symmetrical anticline fold | Syncline fold | Strike-slip fault | Graben | Reverse fault | Horst | Normal fault

▲ *Mountain building*

Lateral pressure, which occurs when plates collide, squeezes and compresses rocks into folds. Simple symmetrical upfolds are called anticlines, while downfolds are synclines. As the pressure builds up, strata become asymmetrical and they may be tilted over to form recumbent folds. The rocks often crack under the intense pressure and the folds are sheared away and pushed forward over other rocks. These features are called overthrust folds or nappes. Plate movements also create faults along which rocks move upwards, downwards and sideways. The diagram shows a downfaulted graben, or rift valley, and an uplifted horst, or block mountain.

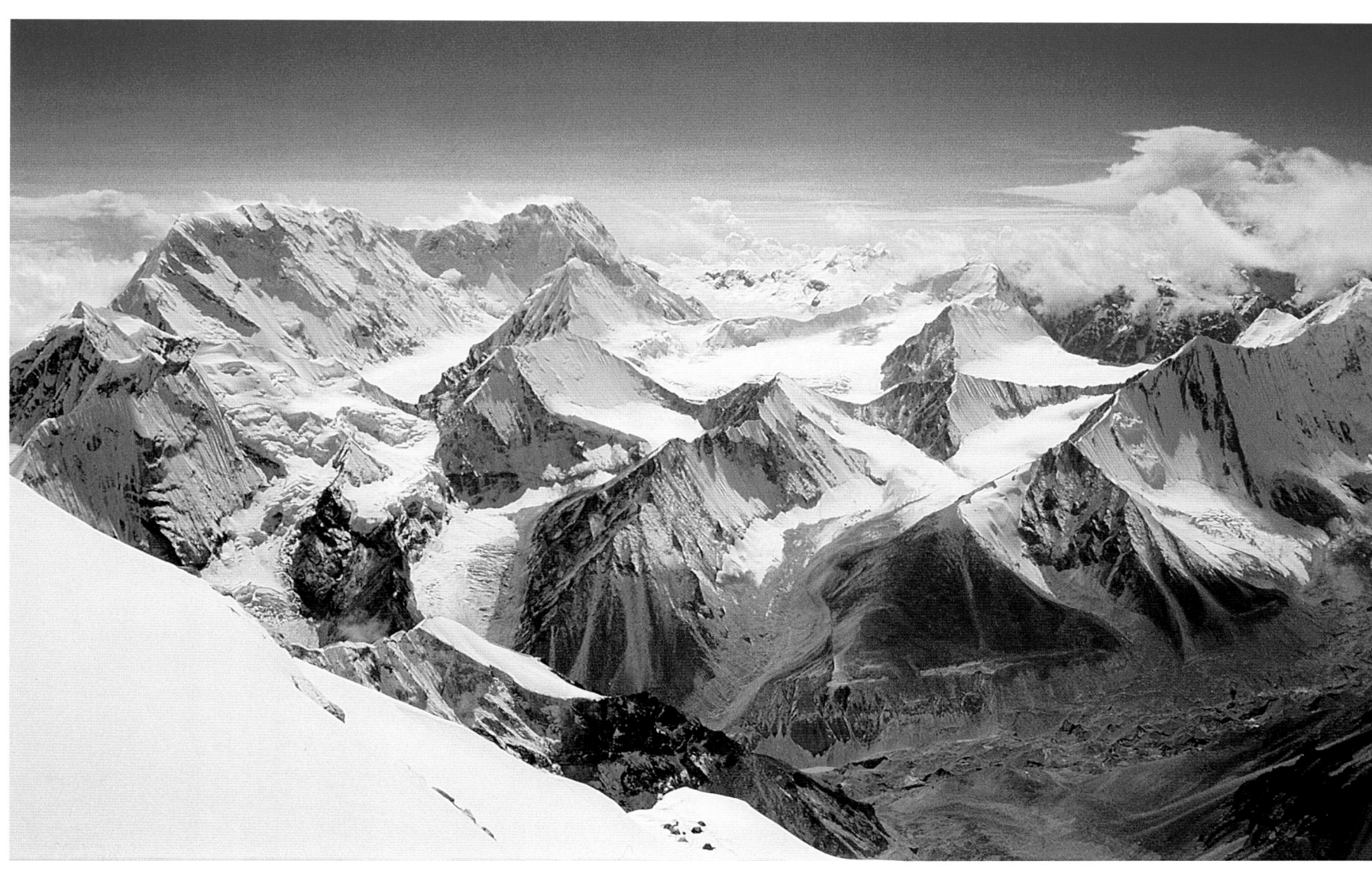

▼ *Geological time scale*

The geological time scale was first constructed by a study of the stratigraphic, or relative, ages of layers of rock. But the absolute ages of rock strata could not be fixed until the discovery of radioactivity in the early 20th century. Some names of periods, such as Cambrian (Latin for Wales), come from places where the rocks were first studied. Others, such as Carboniferous, refer to the nature of the rocks formed during the period. For example, coal seams (containing carbon) were formed from decayed plant matter during the Carboniferous period.

formed there from magma that wells up from the mantle as the plates gradually move apart. The deep-ocean trenches are 'destructive' plate edges where two plates are pushing against each other. One plate descends beneath the other into the mantle where it is melted. These areas are called 'subduction zones'.

A third type of plate edge is called a transform fault. Here two plates are moving alongside each other. The best known of these plate edges is the San Andreas fault in California, which separates the Pacific plate from the North American plate.

Slow-moving currents in the partly molten asthenosphere, which underlies the solid lithosphere, are responsible for moving the plates, a process called plate tectonics.

MOUNTAIN BUILDING

The study of plate tectonics has helped geol-ogists to understand the mechanisms that are responsible for the creation of mountains. Many of the world's greatest ranges were created by the collision of two plates and the bending of the intervening strata into huge loops, or folds. For example, the Himalayas began to rise around 50 million years ago, when a plate supporting India collided with the huge Eurasian plate. Rocks on the floor of the intervening and long-vanished Tethys Sea were squeezed up to form the Himalayan Mountain Range.

Plate movements also create tension that cracks rocks, producing long faults along which rocks move upwards, downwards or sideways. Block mountains are formed when blocks of rock are pushed upwards along faults. Steep-sided rift valleys are formed when blocks of land sink down between faults. For example, the basin and range region of the south-western United States has both block mountains and downfaulted basins, such as Death Valley.

Era	Pre-Cambrian	Lower	Paleozoic (Primary)		Upper		Mesozoic (Secondary)			Cenozoic (Tertiary, Quaternary)				
System	Pre-Cambrian	Cambrian	Ordovician	Silurian	Devonian	Carboniferous	Permian	Triassic	Jurassic	Cretaceous	Paleocene	Eocene	Oligocene	Miocene / Pliocene / Quaternary
Orogeny					CALEDONIAN FOLDING		HERCYNIAN FOLDING				LARAMIDE FOLDING	ALPINE FOLDING		

600   550   500   450   400   350   300   250   200   150   100   50

Millions of years before present

EARTHQUAKES AND VOLCANOES

On 8 October 2005, a massive earthquake occurred along the converging Indian and Eurasian plates in northern Pakistan's North-west Frontier province and Indian-ruled Kashmir. Measuring 7.6 on the Richter scale, it caused about 87,000 deaths. Thousands were injured and 3 million people were left homeless at the onset of winter. The relief work was hampered by landslides, which blocked the roads leading to remote village communities.

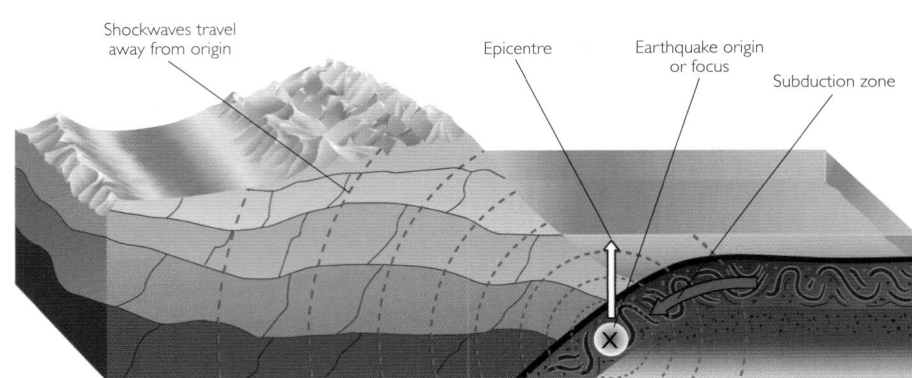

Shockwaves travel away from origin · Epicentre · Earthquake origin or focus · Subduction zone

THE RESTLESS EARTH

Earthquakes can occur anywhere, whenever rocks move along faults. But the most severe and most numerous earthquakes occur near the edges of the plates that make up the Earth's lithosphere. Japan, for example, lies in a particularly unstable region above subduction zones, where plates are descending into the Earth's mantle. It lies in a zone encircling the Pacific Ocean, called the 'Pacific ring of fire'.

▲ *Earthquakes in subduction zones*
Along subduction zones, one plate is descending beneath another. The plates are locked together until the rocks break and the descending plate lurches forwards. From the point where the plate moves – the origin – seismic waves spread through the lithosphere, making the ground shake. The earthquake in Mexico City in 1985 occurred in this way.

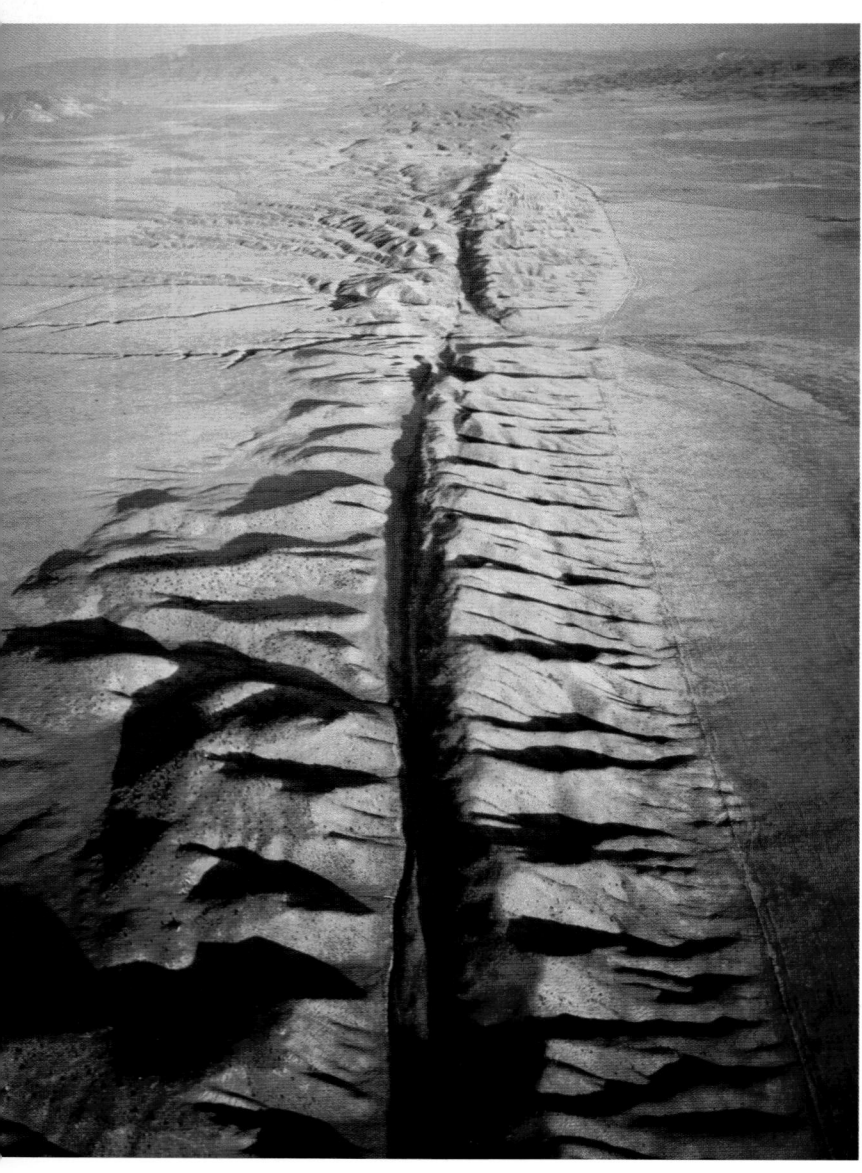

▼ *San Andreas Fault, United States*
Geologists call the San Andreas fault in south-western California a transform, or strike-slip, fault. Sudden movements along it cause earthquakes. In 1906, shifts of about 4.5 m [15 ft] occurred near San Francisco, causing a massive earthquake.

Plates do not move smoothly. Their edges are jagged and for most of the time they are locked together. However, pressure gradually builds up until the rocks break and the plates lurch forwards, setting off vibrations ranging from slight tremors to terrifying earthquakes. The greater the pressure released, the more destructive the earthquake.

Earthquakes are also common along the ocean trenches where plates are moving apart, but they mostly occur so far from land that they do little damage. Far more destructive are the earthquakes that occur where plates are moving alongside each other. For example, the earthquakes that periodically rock south-western California are caused by movements along the San Andreas Fault.

The spot where an earthquake originates is called the focus, while the point on the Earth's surface directly above the focus is called the epicentre. Two kinds of waves, P-waves or compressional waves and S-waves or shear waves, travel from the focus to the surface where they make the ground shake. P-waves travel faster than S-waves and the time difference between their arrival at recording stations enables scientists to calculate the distance from a station to the epicentre.

Earthquakes are measured on the Richter scale, which indicates the magnitude of the shock. The most destructive earthquakes are shallow-focus, that is, the focus is within 60 km [37 miles] of the surface. A magnitude of 7.0 is a major earthquake, but lower magnitude 'quakes can cause great damage if their epicentres are close to densely populated areas.

Scientists have been working for years to find effective ways of forecasting earthquakes but

NOTABLE EARTHQUAKES
(since 1900)

Year	Location	Mag.
1906	San Francisco, USA	8.3
1906	Valparaiso, Chile	8.6
1908	Messina, Italy	7.5
1915	Avezzano, Italy	7.5
1920	Gansu, China	8.6
1923	Yokohama, Japan	8.3
1927	Nan Shan, China	8.3
1932	Gansu, China	7.6
1934	Bihar, India/Nepal	8.4
1935	Quetta, India†	7.5
1939	Chillan, Chile	8.3
1939	Erzincan, Turkey	7.9
1964	Anchorage, Alaska	8.4
1968	N. E. Iran	7.4
1970	N. Peru	7.7
1976	Guatemala	7.5
1976	Tangshan, China	8.2
1978	Tabas, Iran	7.7
1980	El Asnam, Algeria	7.3
1980	S. Italy	7.2
1985	Mexico City, Mexico	8.1
1988	N. W. Armenia	6.8
1990	N. Iran	7.7
1993	Maharashtra, India	6.4
1994	Los Angeles, USA	6.6
1995	Kobe, Japan	7.2
1995	Sakhalin Is., Russia	7.5
1996	Yunnan, China	7.0
1997	N. E. Iran	7.1
1998	N. E. Afghanistan	7.0
1999	Izmit, Turkey	7.4
1999	Taipei, Taiwan	7.6
2001	El Salvador	7.7
2001	Gujarat, India	7.7
2002	Baghlan, Afghanistan	6.1
2003	Mexico	7.8
2003	Bam, Iran	6.7
2004	N. Morocco	6.5
2004	Sumatra, Indonesia	9.1
2005	N. Pakistan	7.6
2006	Java, Indonesia	6.4
2007	S. Peru	8.0
2008	Sichuan, China	7.8

† *now Pakistan*

with limited success. But in the early 2000s, some scientists claimed that they had successfully forecast eruptions by identifying tremors, called 'long-period events'. They believe these relatively minor but long-lasting tremors are caused when magma surges up underground passages but fails to reach the surface.

VOLCANIC ERUPTIONS

Most active volcanoes also occur on or near plate edges. Many undersea volcanoes along the ocean ridges are formed from magma that wells up from the asthenosphere to fill the gaps created as the plates, on the opposite sides of the ridges, move apart. Some of these volcanoes reach the surface to form islands. Iceland is a country which straddles the Mid-Atlantic Ocean Ridge. It is gradually becoming wider as magma rises to the surface through faults and vents. Other volcanoes lie alongside subduction zones. The magma that fuels them comes from the melted edges of the descending plates.

A few volcanoes lie far from plate edges. For example, Mauna Loa and Kilauea on Hawai'i are situated near the centre of the huge Pacific plate. The molten magma that reaches the surface is created by a source of heat, called a 'hot spot', in the Earth's mantle.

Magma is molten rock at temperatures of about 1,100°C to 1,200°C [2,012°F to 2,192°F]. It contains gases and superheated steam. The chemical composition of magma varies. Viscous magma is rich in silica and superheated steam, while runny magma contains less silica and steam. The chemical composition of the magma affects the nature of volcanic eruptions.

Explosive volcanoes contain thick, viscous magma. When they erupt, they usually hurl clouds of ash (shattered fragments of cooled magma) into the air. By contrast, quiet volcanoes emit long streams of runny magma, or lava. However, many volcanoes are intermediate in type, sometimes erupting explosively and sometimes emitting streams of fluid lava. Explosive and intermediate volcanoes usually have a conical shape, while quiet volcanoes are flattened, resembling upturned saucers. They are often called shield volcanoes.

One dangerous type of eruption is called a *nuée ardente*, or 'glowing cloud'. It occurs when a cloud of intensely hot volcanic gases, dust particles, and superheated steam are exploded sideways from a volcano, often following a violent explosion which hurls ash high into the air. Pyroclastic surges and flows are similar. The clouds sweep downhill, destroying all in their paths. Pyroclastic surges and flows killed many people during the Vesuvius eruption in AD 79. The bodies were later buried by ash falls.

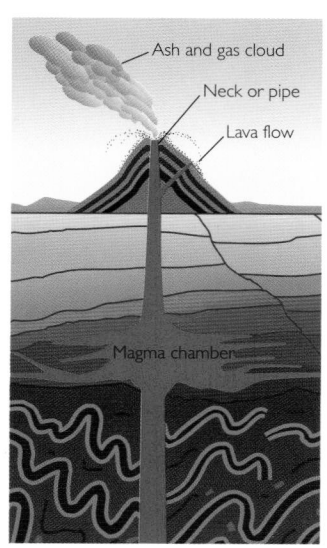

▲ *Cross-section of a volcano*
Volcanoes are vents in the ground, through which magma reaches the surface. The term volcano is also used for the mountains formed from volcanic rocks. Beneath volcanoes are pockets of magma derived from the semi-molten asthenosphere in the mantle. The magma rises under pressure through the overlying rocks until it reaches the surface. There it emerges through vents as pyroclasts, ranging in size from large lumps of magma, called volcanic bombs, to fine volcanic ash and dust. In quiet eruptions, streams of liquid lava run down the side of the mountain. Side vents sometimes appear on the flanks of existing volcanoes.

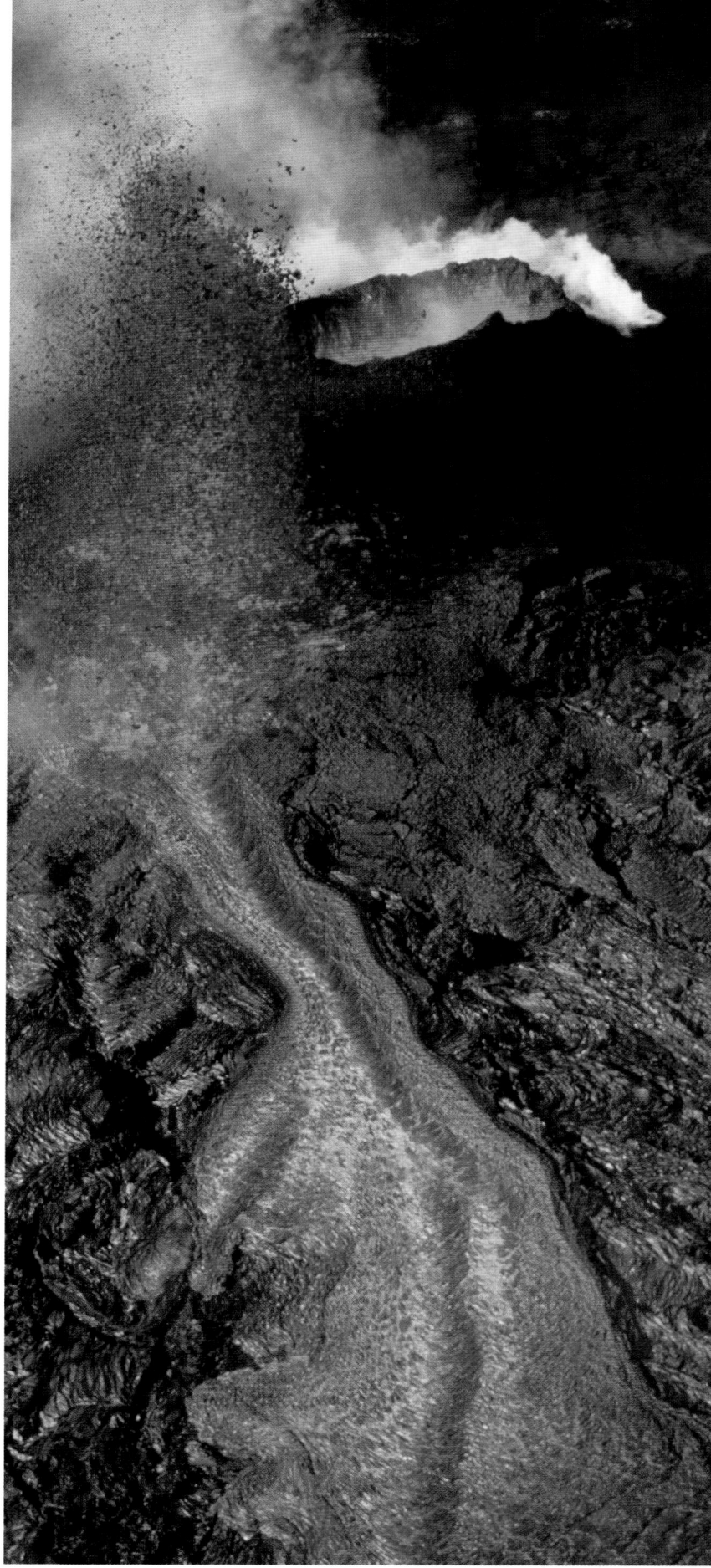

▲ *Kilauea Volcano, Hawai'i*
The volcanic Hawaiian islands in the North Pacific Ocean were formed as the Pacific plate moved over a 'hot spot' in the Earth's mantle. Kilauea on Hawai'i emits blazing streams of liquid lava.

FORCES OF NATURE

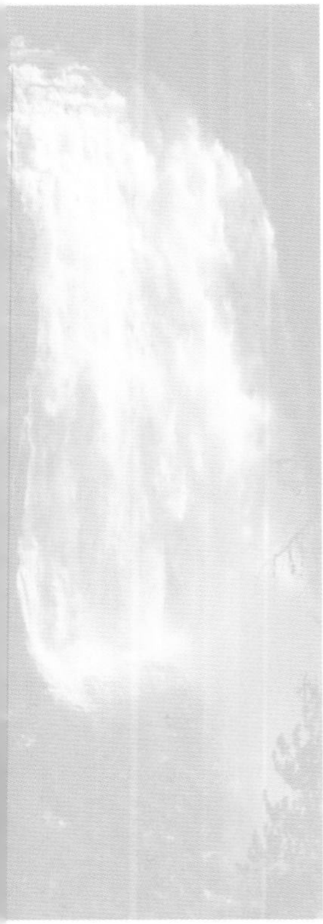

On 26 December 2004, a sudden movement of the plates beneath the Indian Ocean triggered a magnitude 9.1 earthquake. The 'quake created a tsunami, a fast-moving wave that battered the coasts of southern and south-eastern Asia, and was even felt in East Africa. Entire communities were wiped out and the death toll was about 280,000. The worst damage occurred in Indonesia, Thailand, Sri Lanka and India. Such events remind us of the great forces that operate inside our planet. But other forces are operating continuously, forever changing the landscape.

The chief forces acting on the surface of the Earth are weathering, running water, ice and winds. The forces of erosion seem to act slowly. One estimate suggests that an average of only 3.5 cm [1.4 inches] of land is removed by natural processes every 1,000 years. But over millions of years, the highest mountains are eroded away.

WEATHERING

Weathering occurs in all parts of the world, but the most effective type of weathering in any area depends on the climate and the nature of the

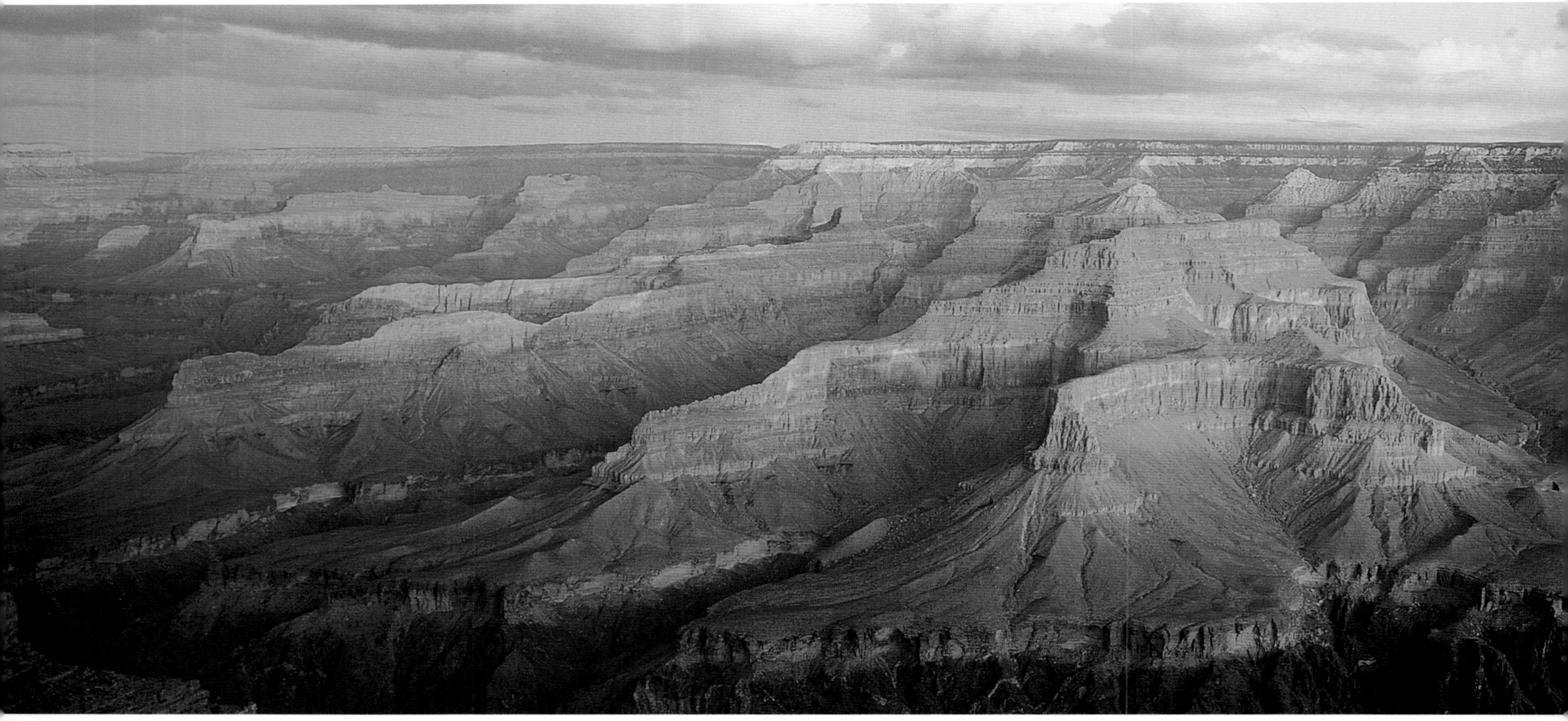

▼ *Grand Canyon, Arizona, at dusk*

The Grand Canyon in the United States is one of the world's natural wonders. Eroded by the Colorado River and its tributaries, it is up to 1.6 km [1 mile] deep and 29 km [18 miles] wide.

RATES OF EROSION

	SLOW	WEATHERING RATE	FAST
Mineral solubility	low (e.g. quartz)	moderate (e.g. feldspar)	high (e.g. calcite)
Rainfall	low	moderate	heavy
Temperature	cold	temperate	hot
Vegetation	sparse	moderate	lush
Soil cover	bare rock	thin to moderate soil	thick soil

Weathering is the breakdown and decay of rocks in situ. It may be mechanical (physical), chemical or biological.

rocks. For example, in cold mountain areas, when water freezes in cracks in rocks, the ice occupies 9% more space than the water. This exerts a force which, when repeated over and over again, can split boulders apart. By contrast, in hot deserts, intense heating by day and cooling by night causes the outer layers of rocks to expand and contract until they break up and peel away like layers of an onion. These are examples of what is called mechanical weathering.

Chemical weathering involves chemical reactions in various rocks. These reactions usually involve water. For example, rainwater containing carbon dioxide dissolved from the air or soil is a weak acid that reacts with limestone, wearing out pits, tunnels and complex networks of caves. Water also combines with some minerals, such as feldspar in granite, to create kaolin, a soft white clay.

▲ *Rates of erosion*

The chart shows that the rates at which weathering takes place depend on the chemistry and hardness of rocks, climatic factors, especially rainfall and temperature, the vegetation and the nature of the soil cover in any area. The effects of weathering are increased by human action, particularly the removal of vegetation and the exposure of soils to the rain and wind.

RUNNING WATER, ICE AND WIND

In moist regions, rivers are effective in shaping the land. They transport material worn away by weathering and erode the land. They wear out V-shaped valleys in upland regions, while vigorous meanders widen their middle courses. The work of rivers is at its most spectacular when earth movements lift up flat areas and rejuvenate the rivers, giving them a new erosive power capable of wearing out such features as the Grand Canyon. Rivers also have a constructive role. Some of the world's most fertile regions are deltas and flood plains composed of sediments periodically dumped there by such rivers as the Ganges, Mississippi and Nile.

▼ *Glaciers*

During Ice Ages, ice spreads over large areas but, during warm periods, the ice retreats. The chart shows that the volume of ice in many glaciers is decreasing. Experts estimate that, between 1850 and the early 21st century, more than half of the ice in Alpine glaciers has melted. In 2007, a scientific report stated that 80% of Europe's glaciers will vanish by the end of the 21st century because of global warming.

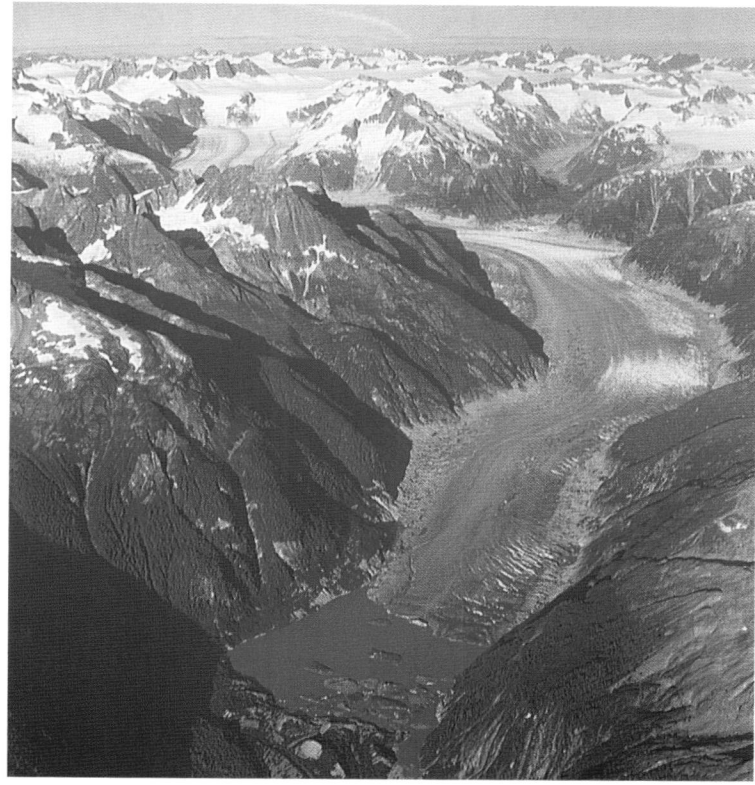

▲ *Juneau Glacier, Alaska*

Like huge conveyor belts, glaciers transport weathered debris from mountain regions. Rocks frozen in the ice give the glaciers teeth, enabling them to wear out typical glaciated land features.

ANNUAL FLUCTUATIONS FOR SELECTED GLACIERS

Glacier name and location	Changes in the annual mass balance †		
	1970–1	1990–1	2000–2001
Alfotbreen, Norway	+940	+790	−50
Careser, Italy	−650	−1,730	−1,860
Djankuat, Russia	−230	−310	−1,760
Grasubreen, Norway	+470	−520	−30
Gries, Switzerland	−970	−1,480	−902
Hintereisferner, Austria	−600	−1,325	−806
Place, Canada	−343	−990	−690
Sarennes, France	−1,100	−1,360	−1,160
Storglaciaren, Sweden	−190	+170	−115
Ürümqi, China	+102	−706	−1,170
Wolverine, USA	+770	−410	−480

† *The annual mass balance is defined as the difference between glacier accumulation and ablation (melting) averaged over the whole glacier. Balances are expressed as water equivalent in millimetres. A 'plus' indicates an increase in the depth or length of the glacier; a 'minus' indicates a reduction.*

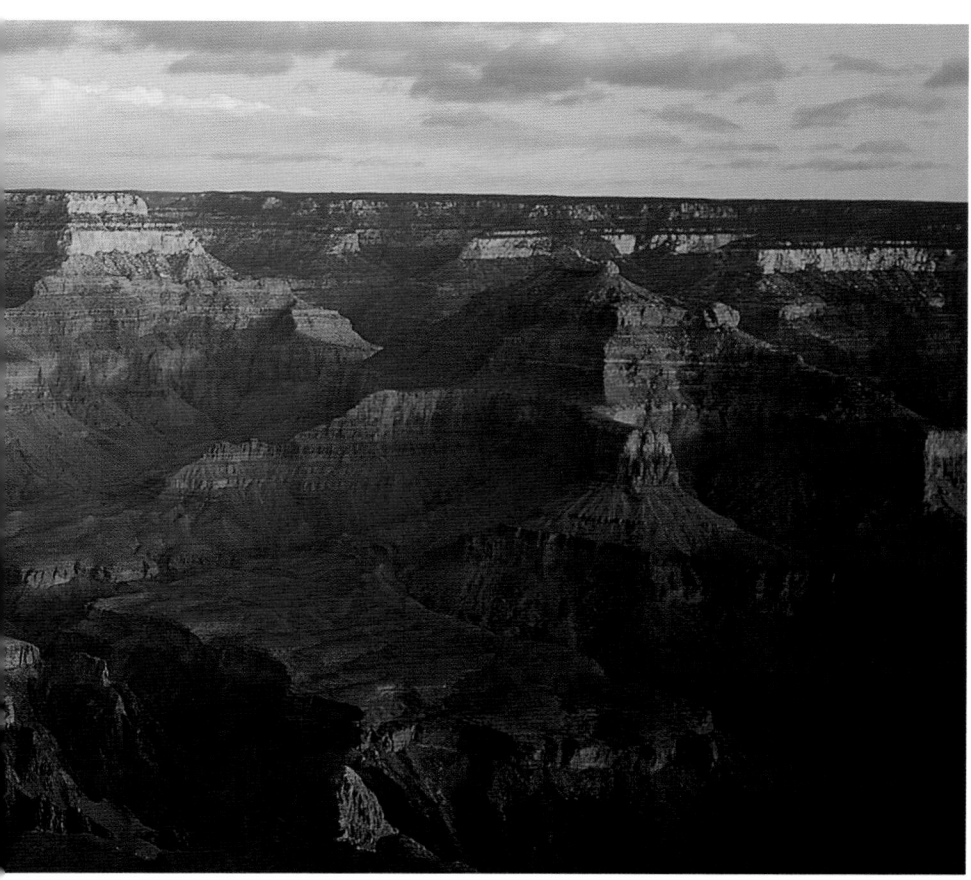

Running water in the form of sea waves and currents shapes coastlines, wearing out caves, natural arches, and stacks. The sea also transports and deposits worn material to form such features as spits and bars.

Glaciers in cold mountain regions flow downhill, gradually deepening valleys and shaping dramatic landscapes. They erode steep-sided U-shaped valleys, into which rivers often plunge in large waterfalls. Other features include cirques, armchair-shaped basins bounded by knife-edged ridges called *arêtes*. When several glacial cirques erode to form radial *arêtes*, pyramidal peaks like the Matterhorn are created. Deposits of moraine, rock material dumped by the glacier, are further evidence that ice once covered large areas.

The work of glaciers, like other agents of erosion, varies with the climate. In recent years, global warming has been making glaciers retreat in many areas, while several of the ice shelves in Antarctica have been breaking up.

Many land features in deserts were formed by running water at a time when the climate was much rainier than it is today. Water erosion also occurs when flash floods are caused by rare thunderstorms. But the chief agent of erosion in dry areas is wind-blown sand, which can strip the paint from cars, and undercut boulders to create mushroom-shaped rocks.

OCEANS AND ICE

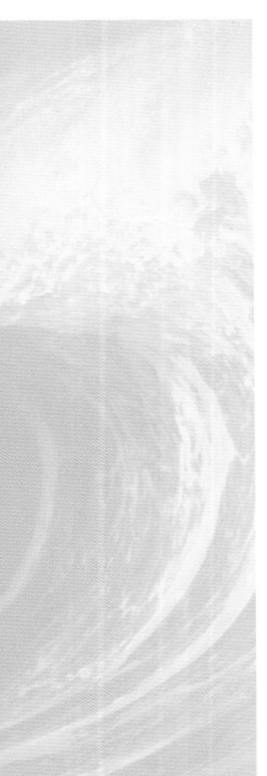

In 2005, Tim Barnett of the Scripps Institution of Oceanography presented a paper to the American Association for the Advancement of Science showing that the upper waters of the oceans had markedly warmed up in the last 65 years, dramatic evidence of global warming.

Oceanography is a major science, but, only about 50 years ago, little was known of the dark world beneath the waves. But through the use of modern technology, including echo-sounders, magnetometers, research ships equipped with huge drills, and satellites, many of the oceans' secrets have been unravelled. Scientists have visited the ocean ridges in submersibles. There, they found hot vents, or 'black smokers' – chimney-like structures made up of minerals deposited from the hot water. Around them, are swarms of bacteria – the base of a food chain that includes strange creatures, many unknown to science, such as giant worms, eyeless shrimps and white clams. These discoveries have led some to speculate that the first living organisms on Earth may have evolved in such conditions on ancient ocean floors.

The study of the ocean floor led to the discovery that the oceans are geologically young features – no more than 200 million years old. It also revealed evidence as to how oceans form and continents drift because of the action of plate tectonics.

THE BLUE PLANET

Water covers almost 71% of the Earth's surface, which makes it look blue when viewed from space. Oceanographers recognize five oceans: the Pacific, Atlantic, Indian, Southern (or Antarctic) and Arctic, but they are all interconnected. The average depth of the oceans is 3,370 m [12,238 ft], but they are divided into several zones.

Around most continents are gently sloping continental shelves, which are flooded parts of the continents. The shelves end at the continental slope, at a depth of about 200 m [656 ft]. This slope leads steeply down to the abyss. The deepest parts of the oceans are the trenches, which reach a maximum depth of 11,022 m [36,161 ft] in the Mariana Trench in the western Pacific.

Most marine life is found in the top 200 m [656 ft], where there is sufficient sunlight for plants, called phytoplankton, to grow. Below this zone, life becomes more and more scarce, though no part of the ocean, even at the bottom of the deepest trenches, is completely without living things.

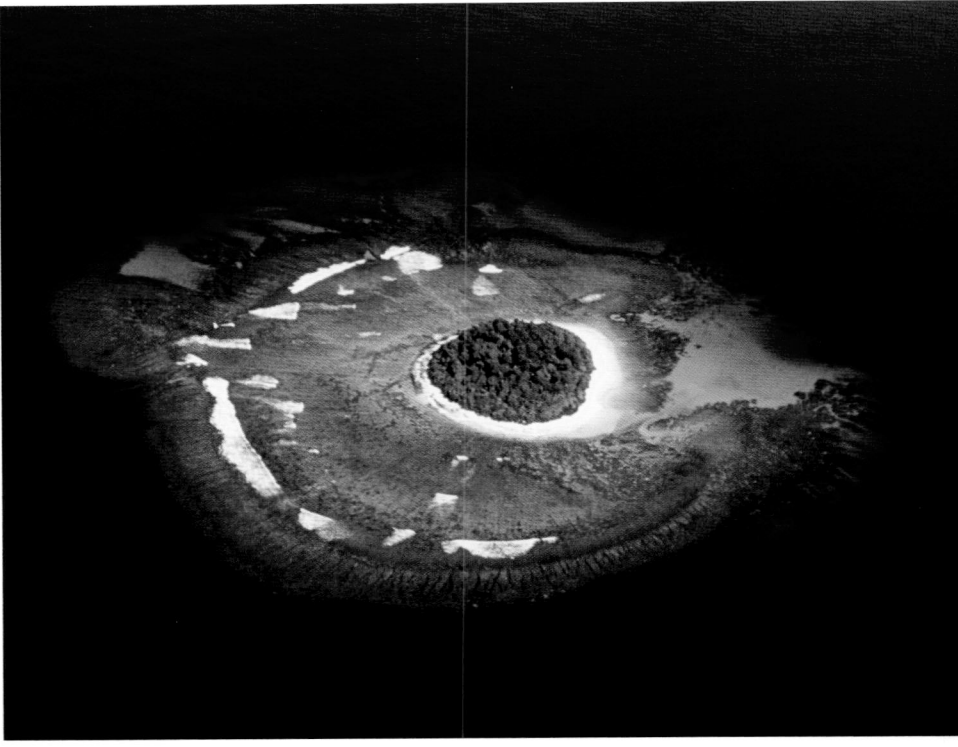

▲ *Vava'u Island, Tonga*
This small coral atoll in northern Tonga consists of a central island covered by rainforest. Low coral reefs washed by the waves surround a shallow central lagoon.

Continental islands, such as the British Isles, are high parts of the continental shelves. For example, until about 7,500 years ago, when the ice sheets formed during the Ice Ages were melting, raising the sea level and filling the North Sea and the Strait of Dover, Britain was linked to mainland Europe.

By contrast, oceanic islands, such as the Hawaiian chain in the North Pacific Ocean, rise from the ocean floor. All oceanic islands are of volcanic origin, although many of them in warm parts of the oceans have sunk and are capped by layers of coral to form ring- or horseshoe-shaped atolls and coral reefs.

OCEAN WATER

The oceans contain about 97% of the world's water. Seawater contains more than 70 dissolved elements, but chloride and sodium make up 85% of the total. Sodium chloride is common salt and it makes seawater salty. The salinity of the oceans is mostly between 3.3–3.7%. Ocean water fed by icebergs or large rivers is less saline than shallow seas in the tropics, where the evaporation rate is high. Seawater is a source of salt but the water is useless for agriculture or drinking unless it is desalinated. However, land areas get a regular

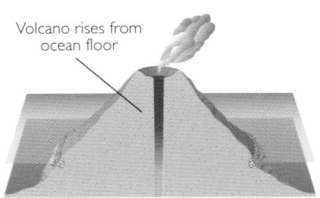

Volcano rises from ocean floor

Fringing reef

Extinct, eroding volcanic island

After subsidence, reef covers buried island

Lagoon

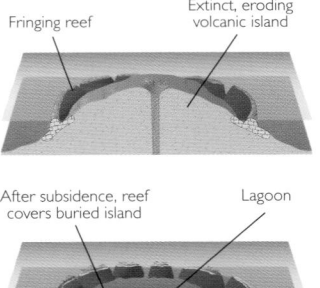

▲ *Development of an atoll*
Some of the volcanoes that rise from the ocean floor reach the surface to form islands. Some of these islands subside and become submerged. As an island sinks, coral starts to grow around the rim of the volcano, building up layer upon layer of limestone deposits to form fringing reefs. Sometimes coral grows on the tip of a central cone to form an island in the middle of the atoll.

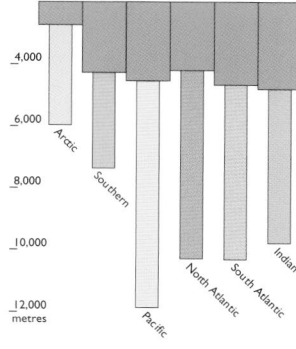

▲ The ocean depths

The diagram shows the average depths (in dark blue) and the greatest depths in the oceans. The Pacific Ocean contains the world's deepest trenches, including the Mariana Trench, where the deepest manned descent was made by the bathyscaphe Trieste in 1960. It reached a depth of 10,916 m [35,813 ft].

Relative sizes of the world's oceans:

PACIFIC 46.4%   ATLANTIC 22.9%
INDIAN 20.4%   SOUTHERN 6.1%
ARCTIC 4.2%

supply of fresh water through the hydrological cycle (see page 42).

The density of seawater depends on its salinity and temperature. Temperatures vary from –2°C [28°F], the freezing point of seawater at the poles, to around 30°C [86°F] in parts of the tropics. Density differences help to maintain the circulation of the world's oceans, especially deep-sea currents. But the main cause of currents within 350 m [1,148 ft] of the surface is the wind. Because of the Earth's rotation, currents are deflected, creating huge circular motions of surface water – clockwise in the northern hemisphere and anticlockwise in the southern hemisphere.

Ocean currents transport heat from the tropics to the polar regions and thus form part of the heat engine that drives the Earth's climates. Ocean currents have an especially marked effect on coastal climates, such as north-western Europe. Some scientists are concerned that global warming may radically alter climates by weakening currents, such as the Gulf Stream, which is responsible for the mild winters in north-western Europe.

ICE SHEETS, ICE CAPS AND GLACIERS

Of the world's two ice sheets, the largest, covering most of Antarctica, has maximum depths of 4,800 m [15,748 ft]. Its volume is about nine times greater than the Greenland ice sheet. The ice sheets, together with smaller ice caps and glaciers, account for about 2% of the world's

water. However, in many parts of the world, the ice is melting and many scientists think the cause is global warming. In March 2002, the vast Larsen ice shelf bordering the Antarctic peninsula collapsed and broke up into icebergs. Some scientists thought this was evidence of global warming, though some attributed the event to local factors.

Only about 11,000 years ago, during the final phase of the Pleistocene Ice Age, ice covered much of the northern hemisphere. The Ice Age, which began about 1.8 million years ago, was not a continuous period of cold. Instead, it consisted of glacial periods when the ice advanced and warmer interglacial periods when temperatures rose and the ice retreated.

Some scientists believe that we are now living in an interglacial period, and that glacial conditions will recur in the future. Others fear that global warming, caused mainly by pollution, may melt the world's ice, raising sea levels by up to 55 m [180 ft]. Many fertile and densely populated coastal plains, islands and cities would vanish from the map.

▼ Icebergs float past the Antarctic Peninsula

The Antarctic peninsula overlooks the Weddell Sea. The Weddell Sea and the Ross Sea are largely covered by huge ice shelves, which are extensions of the continental ice sheet. Many scientists are concerned that warmer weather is melting the ice sheets. In 2002, parts of the Larsen Ice Shelf, which adjoins the Antarctic Peninsula, collapsed and split up into icebergs.

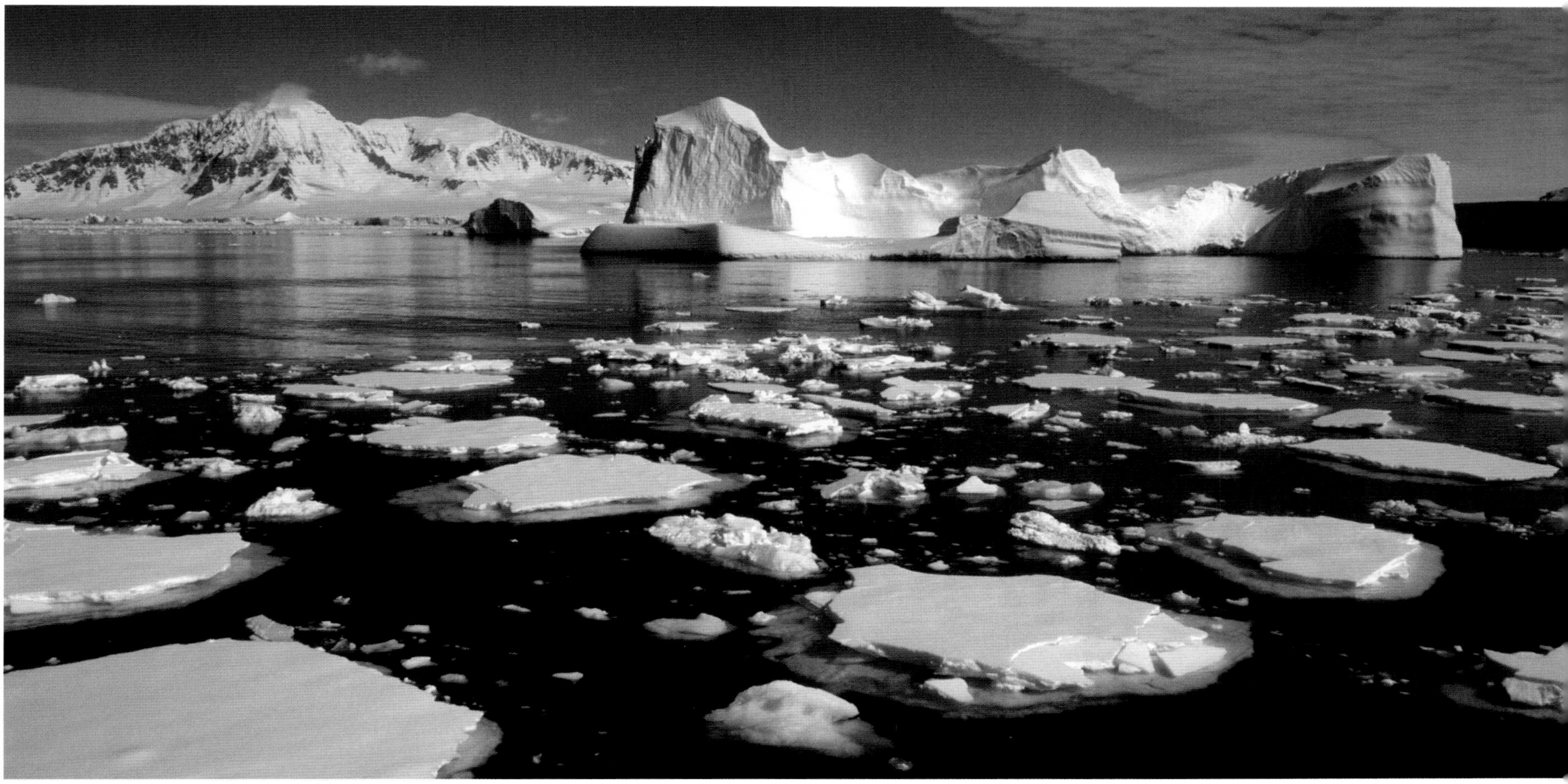

THE EARTH'S ATMOSPHERE

Since the discovery in 1985 of a thinning of the ozone layer, creating a so-called 'ozone hole', over Antarctica, many governments have worked to reduce the emissions of ozone-eating substances, notably the chlorofluorocarbons (CFCs) used in aerosols, refrigeration, air-conditioning and dry cleaning.

Following forecasts that the ozone layer would rapidly repair itself as a result of controls on these emissions, scientists were surprised in early 1996 when a marked thinning of the ozone layer over the northern hemisphere was recorded. In 2005, scientists reported that the ozone hole over Antarctica was the largest since 2000, while 2005 also saw a marked thinning of the ozone layer over the Arctic region. Scientists predicted that it might take more than 50 years before the ozone layer made a full recovery.

The ozone layer in the stratosphere blocks out most of the dangerous ultraviolet B radiation in the Sun's rays. This radiation causes skin cancer and cataracts, as well as harming plants on the land and plankton in the oceans. The ozone layer is only one way in which the atmosphere protects life on Earth. The atmosphere

also provides the air we breathe and the carbon dioxide required by plants. It is also a shield against meteors and it acts as a blanket to prevent heat radiated from the Earth escaping into space.

LAYERS OF AIR

The atmosphere is divided into four main layers. The troposphere at the bottom contains about 85% of the atmosphere's total mass, where most weather conditions occur. The troposphere is about 15 km [9 miles] thick over the equator and 8 km [5 miles] thick at the poles. Temperatures decrease with height by approximately 1°C [2°F] for every 100 m [328 ft]. At the top of the troposphere is a level called the tropopause where temperatures are stable at around –55°C [–67°F]. Above the tropopause is the stratosphere, which contains the ozone layer. Here, at about 50 km [30 miles] above the Earth's surface, temperatures rise to about 0°C [32°F].

The ionosphere extends from the stratopause to about 600 km [373 miles] above the surface. Here temperatures fall up to about 80 km [50 miles], but then rise. The aurorae, which occur in the ionosphere when charged particles

▼ *Moonrise seen from orbit*

This photograph taken by an orbiting Shuttle shows the crescent of the Moon. Silhouetted at the horizon is a dense cloud layer. The reddish-brown band is the tropopause, which separates the blue-white stratosphere from the yellow troposphere.

CIRCULATION OF AIR

▮	HIGH PRESSURE
▮	LOW PRESSURE
➡	WARM AIR
➡	COLD AIR
➡	SURFACE WINDS
☁	CLOUDS

▲ *The circulation of the atmosphere can be divided into three rotating but interconnected air systems. These systems, or cells, are responsible for redistributing heat from the warm regions to the cold, and back again.*

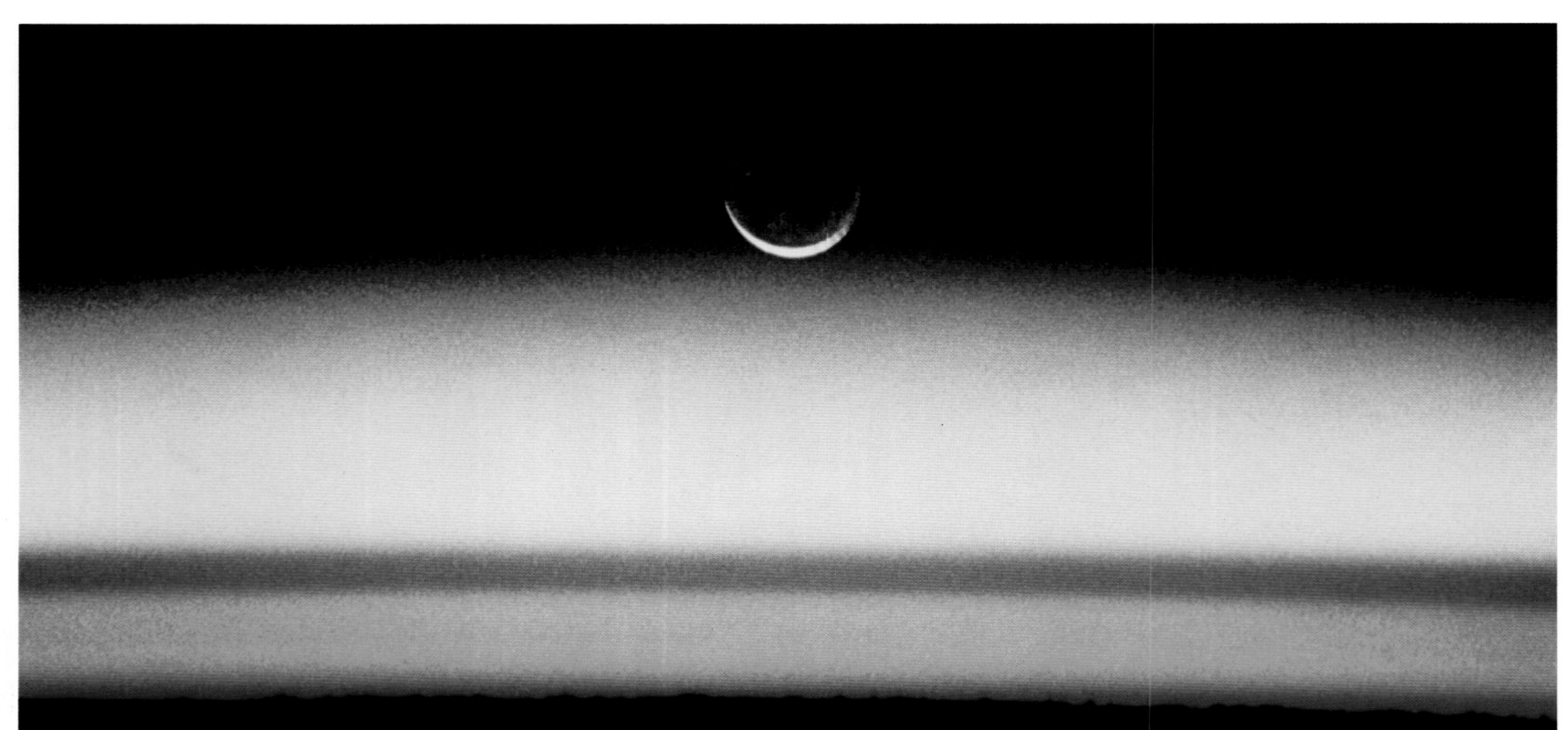

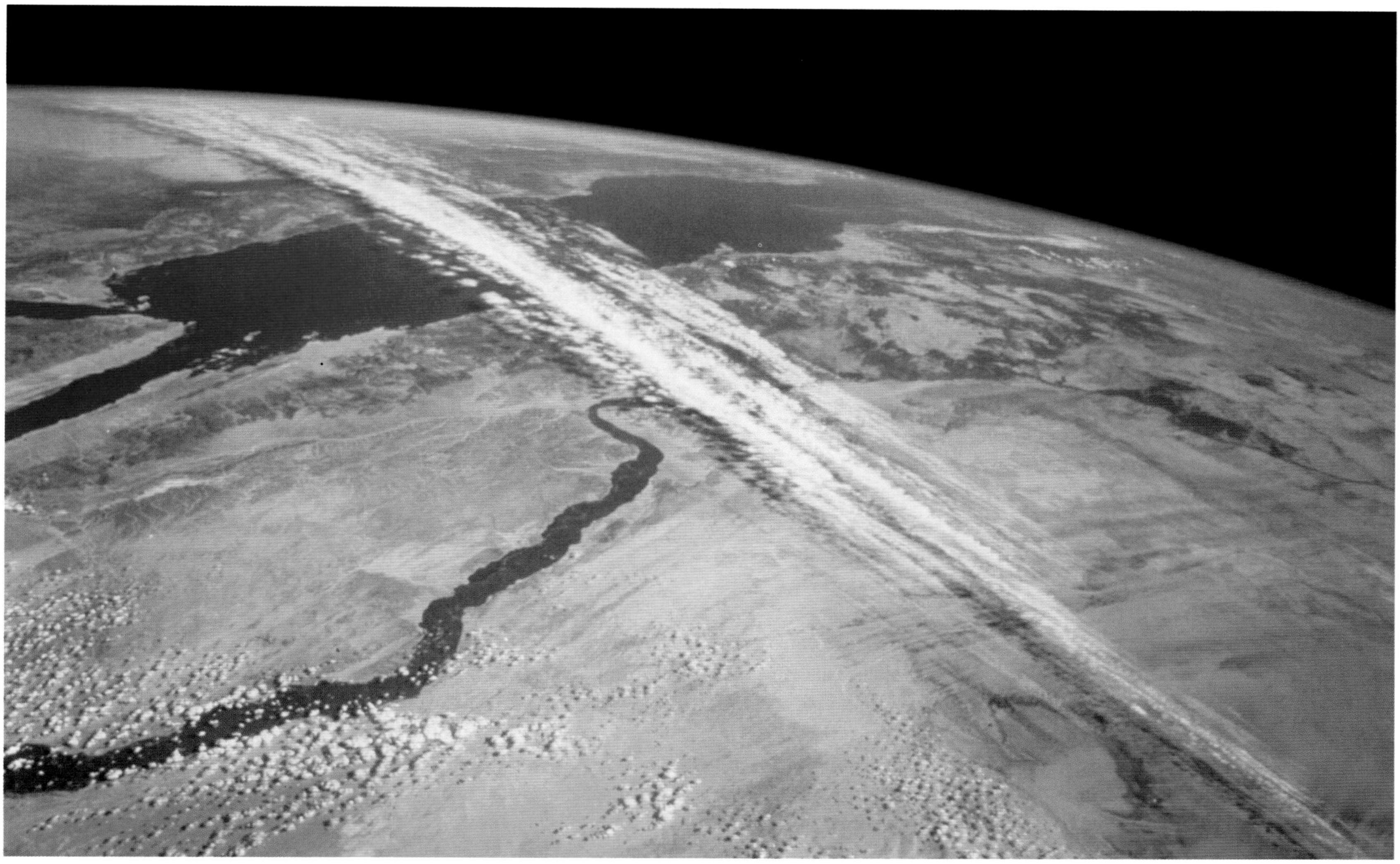

► *Classification of clouds*
Clouds are classified broadly into cumuliform, or 'heap' clouds, and stratiform, or 'layer' clouds. Both types occur at all levels. The highest clouds, composed of ice crystals, are cirrus, cirrostratus and cirrocumulus. Medium-height clouds include altostratus, a grey cloud that often indicates the approach of a depression, and altocumulus, a thicker and fluffier version of cirrocumulus. Low clouds include stratus, which forms dull, overcast skies; nimbostratus, a dark grey layer cloud which brings almost continuous rain and snow; cumulus, a brilliant white heap cloud; and stratocumulus, a layer cloud arranged in globular masses or rolls. Cumulonimbus, a cloud associated with thunderstorms, lightning and heavy rain, often extends from low to medium altitudes. It has a flat base, a fluffy outline and often an anvil-shaped top.

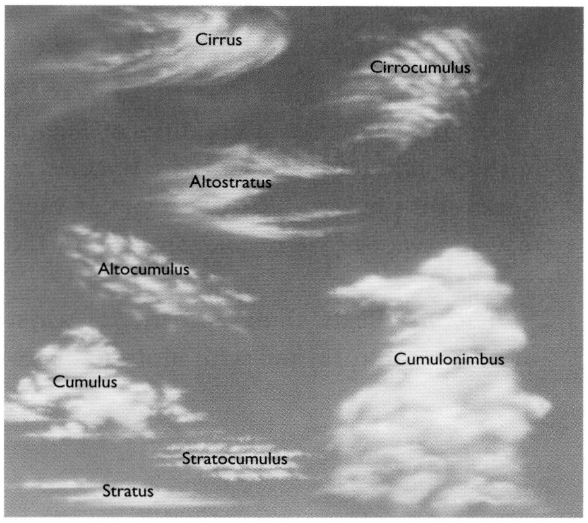

from the Sun interact with the Earth's magnetic field, are strongest near the poles. In the exosphere, the outermost layer, the atmosphere merges into space.

Circulation of the Atmosphere

The heating of the Earth is most intense around the equator where the Sun is high in the sky. Here warm, moist air rises in strong currents, creating a zone of low air pressure: the doldrums. The rising air eventually cools and spreads out north and south until it sinks downwards around latitudes 30° North and 30° South. The zones of high air pressure caused by the sinking air are called the 'horse latitudes'.

From the horse latitudes, trade winds blow back across the surface towards the equator, while westerly winds blow towards the poles. The warm westerlies finally meet the polar easterlies (cold dense air flowing from the poles). The line along which the warm and cold air streams meet is called the polar front. Depressions (or cyclones) are low-air-pressure frontal systems that form along the polar front.

▲ *Jetstream from space*
Jetstreams are strong winds that normally blow near the tropopause. Cirrus clouds mark the route of the jet stream in this photograph, which shows the Red Sea, North Africa and the Nile valley, which appears as a dark band crossing the desert.

Composition of the Atmosphere

The air in the troposphere is made up mainly of nitrogen (78%) and oxygen (21%). Argon makes up more than 0.9% and there are also minute amounts of carbon dioxide, helium, hydrogen, krypton, methane, ozone and xenon. The atmosphere also contains water vapour, the gaseous form of water, which, when it condenses around minute specks of dust and salt, forms tiny water droplets or ice crystals. Large masses of water droplets or ice crystals form clouds.

CLIMATE AND WEATHER

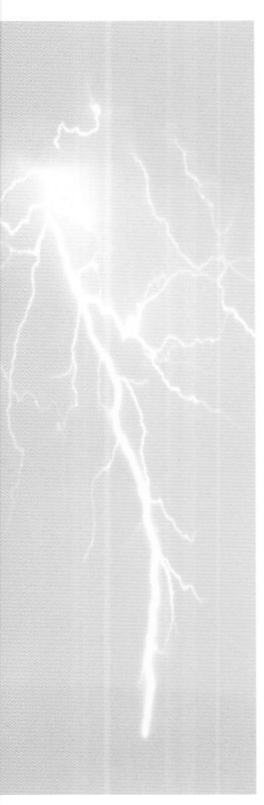

The year 2005 brought some phenomenal weather conditions. A record number of named tropical storms (26, of which 13 were classified as hurricanes) hit Central America and the United States. Hurricane Katrina devastated New Orleans in August. It was the most destructive hurricane ever to strike the United States, causing about 1,380 deaths. Heavy monsoon rain caused severe flooding in Mumbai, India, drowning around 1,000 people, while bush fires raged in Australia following severe droughts. In 2006, typhoons battered the coasts of East Asia, while flash floods drowned many people in East Africa. In 2007, the Intergovernmental Panel on Climate Change stated that many extreme weather events were the result of global warming. It also predicted a temperature rise of 4°C [7.2°F] by 2100. As a result, melting ice sheets would raise sea levels and flood coastal plains.

Climate is defined as the average weather of a place based on data obtained over a long period. By contrast, weather is the day-to-day condition of the atmosphere. In some areas, the weather is stable; in other areas, especially the middle latitudes, it is highly variable.

CLIMATIC FACTORS

Climate depends basically on the unequal heating of the Sun between the equator and the poles. But ocean currents and terrain also affect climate. For example, despite their northerly positions, Norway's ports remain ice-free in winter. This is because of the warming effect of the North Atlantic Drift, an extension of the Gulf Stream which flows across the Atlantic Ocean from the Gulf of Mexico.

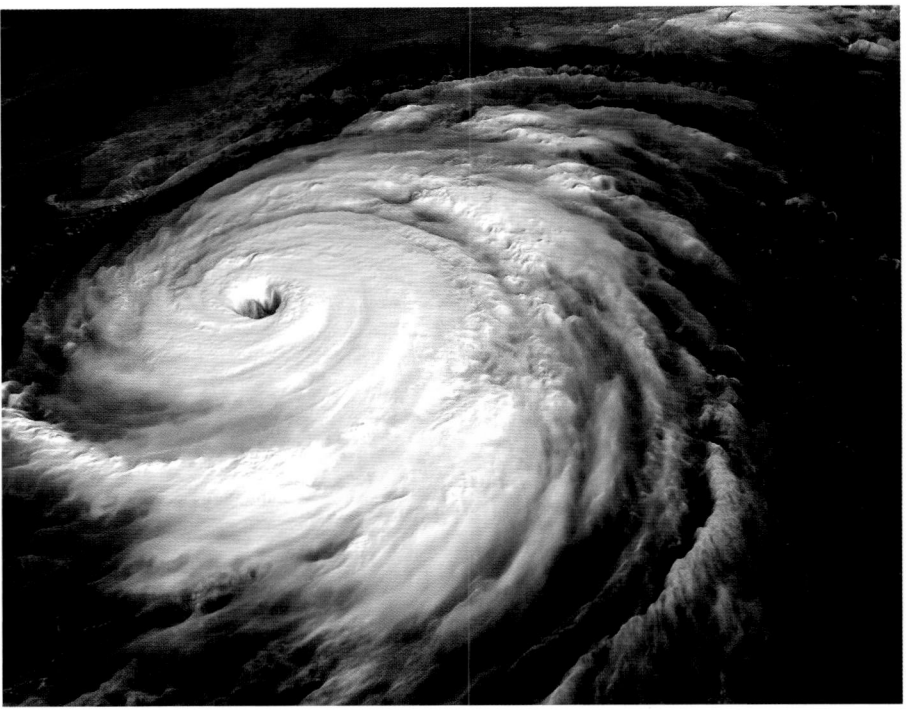

▲ *Satellite image of Hurricane Floyd in 1999*
Hurricanes form over warm oceans north and south of the equator. Their movements are tracked by satellites, enabling forecasters to issue advance warnings. North American forecasters identify them with boys' and girls' names.

By contrast, the cold Benguela current which flows up the coast of south-western Africa cools the coast and causes arid conditions. This is because the cold onshore winds are warmed as they pass over the land. The warm air can hold more water vapour than cold air, giving the winds a drying effect.

The terrain affects climate in several ways. Because temperatures fall with altitude, high-

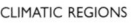

CLIMATIC REGIONS

Tropical rainy climates
All mean monthly temperatures above 18°C [64°F].

⬛ RAINFOREST CLIMATE

⬛ MONSOON CLIMATE

⬛ SAVANNA CLIMATE

Dry climates
Low rainfall combined with a wide range of temperatures.

⬛ STEPPE CLIMATE

⬛ DESERT CLIMATE

Warm temperate rainy climates
The mean temperature is below 18°C [64°F] but above −3°C [26°F], and that of the warmest month is over 10°C [50°F].

⬛ DRY WINTER CLIMATE

⬛ DRY SUMMER CLIMATE

⬛ CLIMATE WITH NO DRY SEASON

Cold temperate rainy climates
The mean temperature of the coldest month is below 3°C [37°F] but the warmest month is over 10°C [50°F].

⬛ DRY WINTER CLIMATE

⬛ CLIMATE WITH NO DRY SEASON

Polar climates
The temperature of the warmest month is below 10°C [50°F], giving permanently frozen subsoil.

⬛ TUNDRA CLIMATE

⬛ POLAR CLIMATE

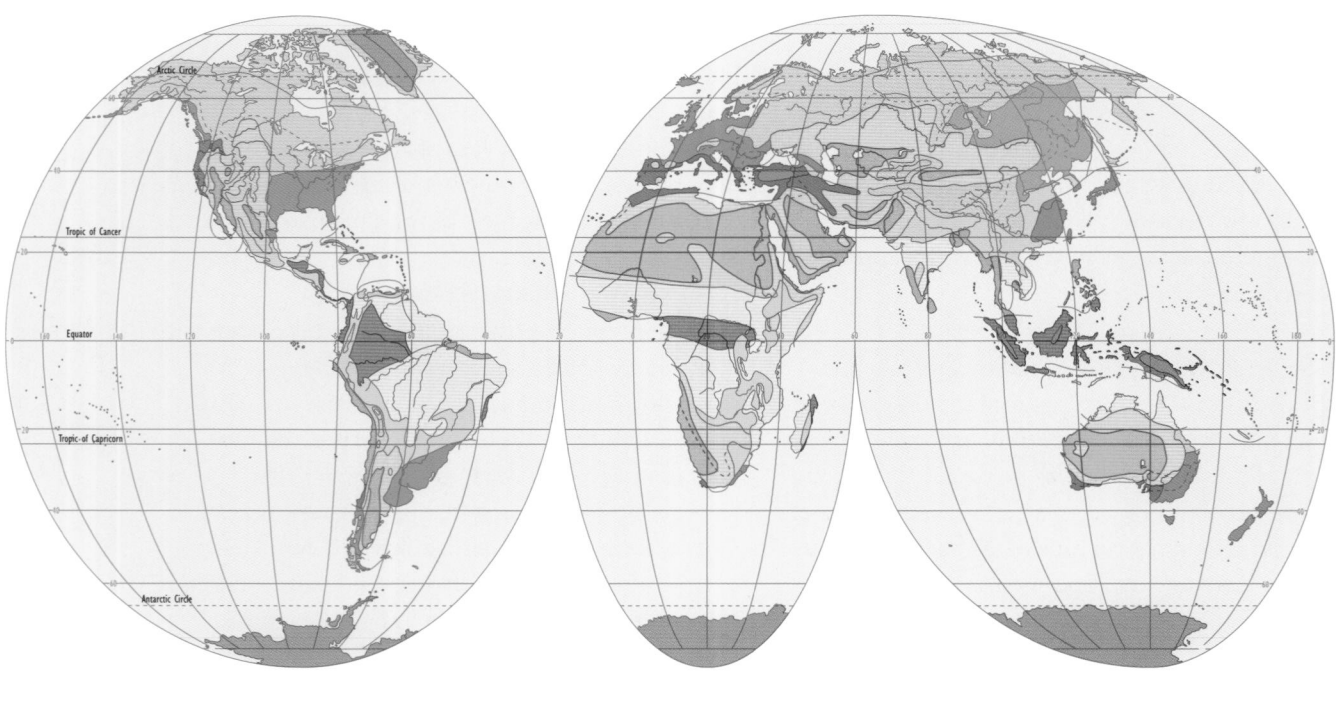

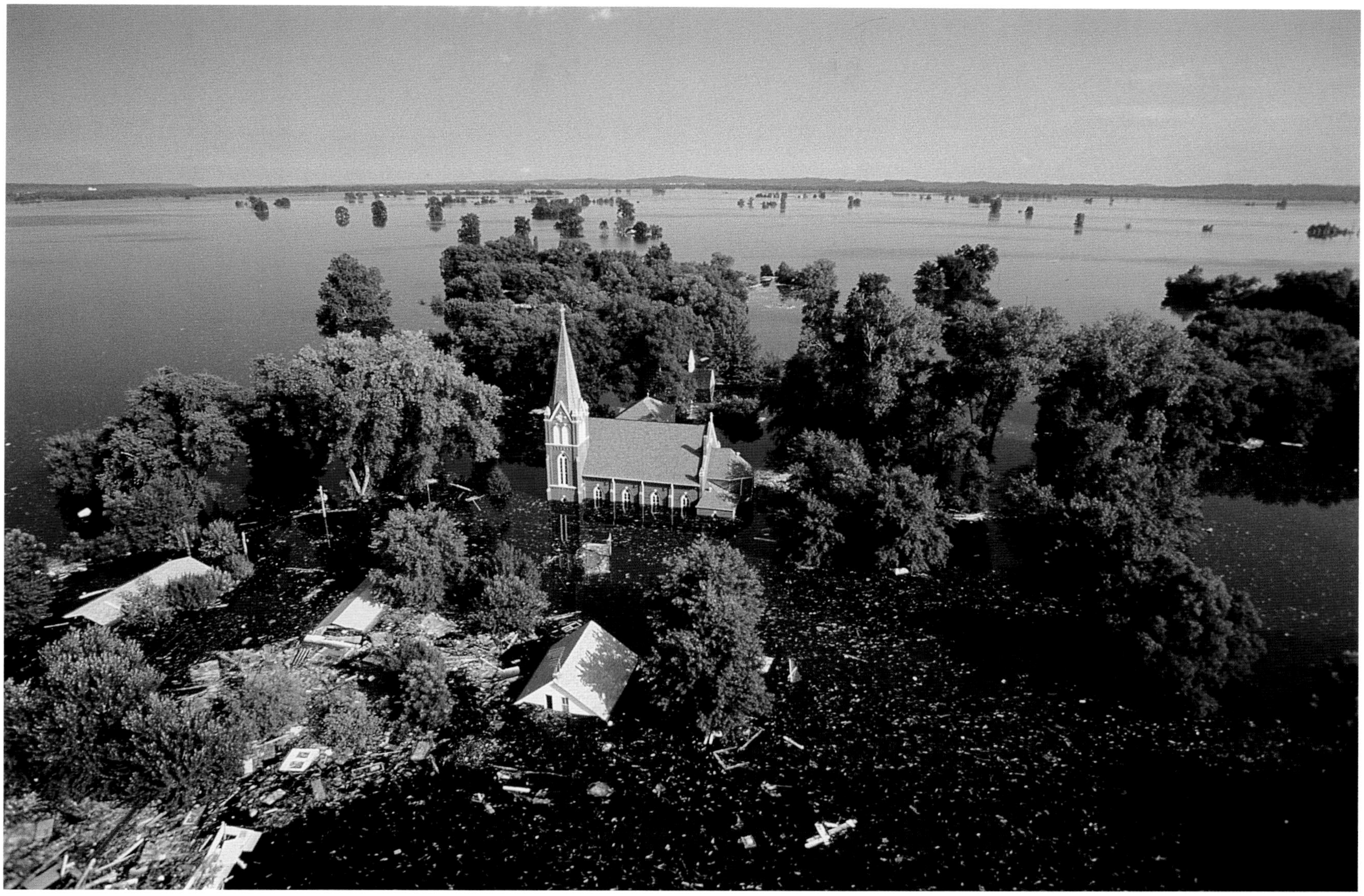

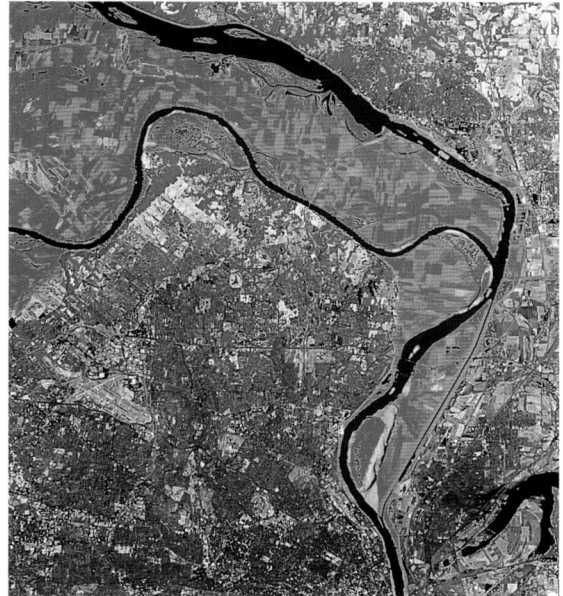

▶ *Floods in St Louis, USA*

The satellite image, right, shows the extent of the floods at St Louis at the confluence of the Mississippi and the Missouri rivers in June and July 1993. The floods occurred when very heavy rainfall raised river levels by up to 14 m [46 ft]. The floods reached their greatest extent between Minneapolis in the north and a point approximately 150 km [93 miles] south of St Louis. In places, the width of the Mississippi increased to nearly 11 km [7 miles], while the Missouri reached widths of 32 km [20 miles]. In all, more than 28,000 sq km [10,800 sq miles] were inundated and hundreds of towns and cities were flooded. Damage to crops was estimated at $8 billion. The US was hit again by flooding in early 1997, when heavy rainfall in North Dakota and Minnesota caused the Red River to flood. Many scientists believe that recent extreme weather events are probably linked to global warming.

lands are cooler than lowlands at the same latitude. Terrain also affects rainfall. When moist onshore winds pass over mountain ranges, they are chilled as they are forced to rise and the water vapour they contain condenses to form clouds, which bring rain and snow. Beyond the mountains, the air descends and is warmed. These drying winds create rain-shadow (arid) regions on the lee side of mountains.

▲ *Flood damage in the United States*

In June and July 1993, the Mississippi River basin suffered record floods. The photograph shows a sunken church in Illinois. The flooding along the Mississippi, Missouri and other rivers caused great damage, amounting to about $12 billion. At least 48 people died in the floods.

CLIMATIC REGIONS

The two major factors that affect climate are temperature and precipitation, including rain and snow. In addition, seasonal variations and other climatic features are also taken into account. Climatic classifications vary because of the weighting given to various features. Yet most classifications are based on five main climatic types: tropical rainy climates; dry climates; warm temperate rainy climates; cold temperate rainy climates; and very cold polar climates. Some classifications also allow for the effect of altitude. The main climatic regions are sub-divided according to seasonal variations and also to the kind of vegetation associated with the climate. With rain throughout the year, rainforest climates differ from monsoon and savanna climates, which have dry seasons, while desert climates differ from steppe climates, which have enough moisture for grasses to grow.

WATER AND LAND USE

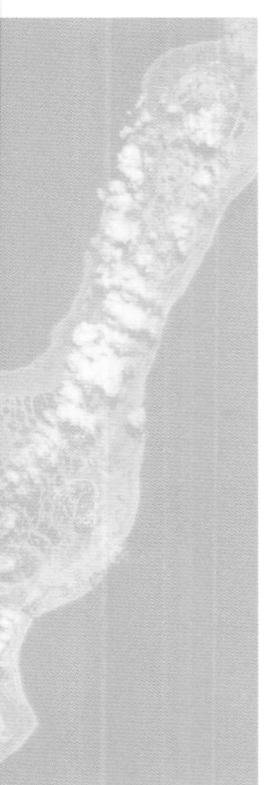

All life on land depends on fresh water. Yet about 80 countries now face acute water shortages. The world demand for fresh water is increasing by about 2.3% a year and this demand will double every 21 years. About a billion people, mainly in developing countries, do not have access to clean drinking water and around 10 million die every year from drinking dirty water. This problem is made worse in many countries by the pollution of rivers and lakes.

UN experts predict that water is becoming the most pressing environmental and development issue facing the world. By 2003, heavily populated regions in 26 countries were suffering serious water shortages. In 20 years, this number

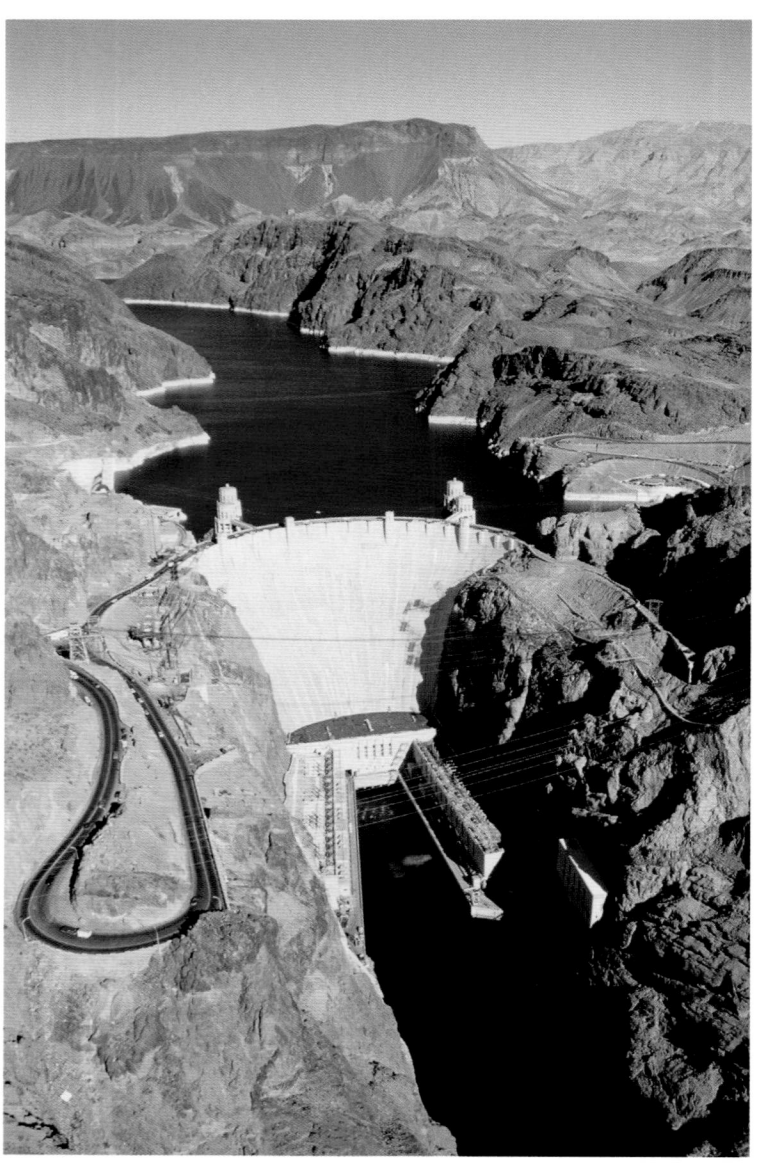

▼ *Hoover Dam, United States*
The Hoover Dam in Arizona controls the Colorado River's flood waters. Its reservoir supplies domestic and irrigation water to the south-west, while a hydroelectric plant produces electricity.

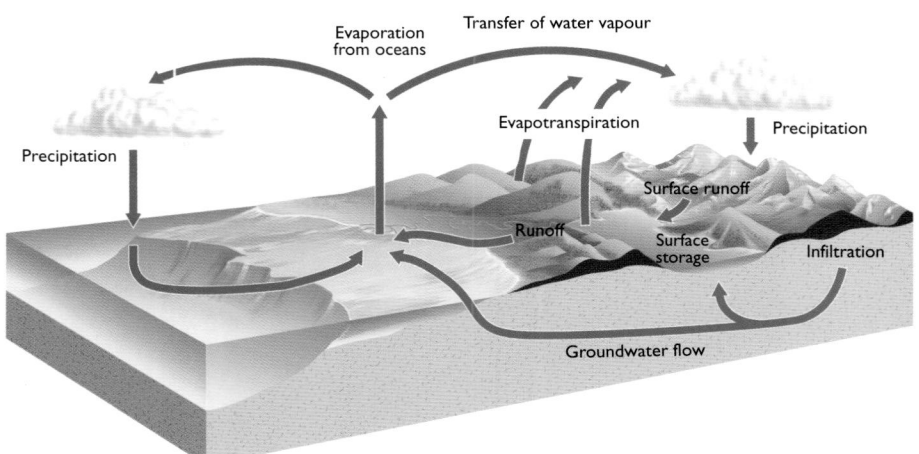

will probably rise to 65. In 2006, the United Nations estimated that nearly 2 million children die every year due to lack of clean water and proper sanitation. Some 1.1 billion people do not have proper sanitation and 2.6 billion suffer from inadequate sewerage. Other major problems include the uneven distribution of water and its inefficient and wasteful use.

THE WORLD'S WATER SUPPLY
Of the world's total water supply, 99.4% is in the oceans or frozen in bodies of ice. Most of the rest circulates through the rocks beneath our feet as groundwater. Water in rivers and lakes, in the soil and in the atmosphere together make up only 0.013% of the world's water.

The freshwater supply on land is dependent on the hydrological, or water, cycle which is driven by the Sun's heat. Water is evaporated from the oceans and carried into the air as invisible water vapour. Although this vapour averages less than 2% of the total mass of the atmosphere, it is the chief component from the standpoint of weather.

When air rises, water vapour condenses into visible water droplets or ice crystals, which eventually fall to earth as rain, snow, sleet, hail or frost. Some of the precipitation that reaches the ground returns directly to the atmosphere through evaporation or transpiration via plants. Much of the rest of the water flows into the rocks to become groundwater, or across the surface into rivers and, eventually, back to the oceans, so completing the hydrological cycle.

WATER AND AGRICULTURE
In 2005, a US study revealed that about 40% of the world's land is used to grow crops or to graze cattle. The biggest recent changes have occurred in the Amazon basin, where tropical forest is being felled to create land for growing soybeans.

▲ *The hydrological cycle*
The hydrological cycle is responsible for the continuous circulation of water around the planet. Water vapour contains and transports latent heat, or latent energy. When the water vapour condenses back into water (and falls as rain, hail or snow), the heat is released. When condensation takes place on cold nights, the cooling effect associated with nightfall is offset by the liberation of latent heat.

WATER DISTRIBUTION
The distribution of planetary water, by percentage.

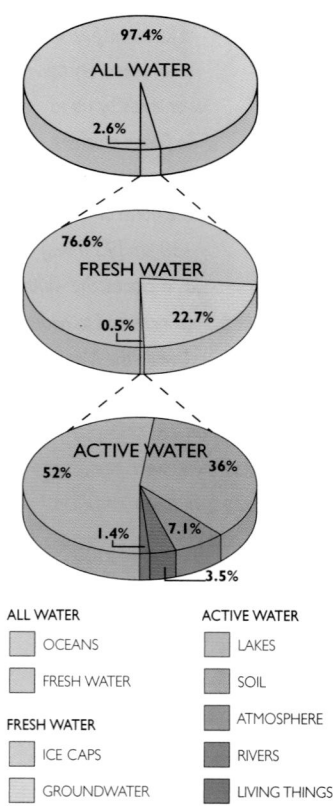

ALL WATER	ACTIVE WATER
OCEANS	LAKES
FRESH WATER	SOIL
FRESH WATER	ATMOSPHERE
ICE CAPS	RIVERS
GROUNDWATER	LIVING THINGS
ACTIVE WATER	

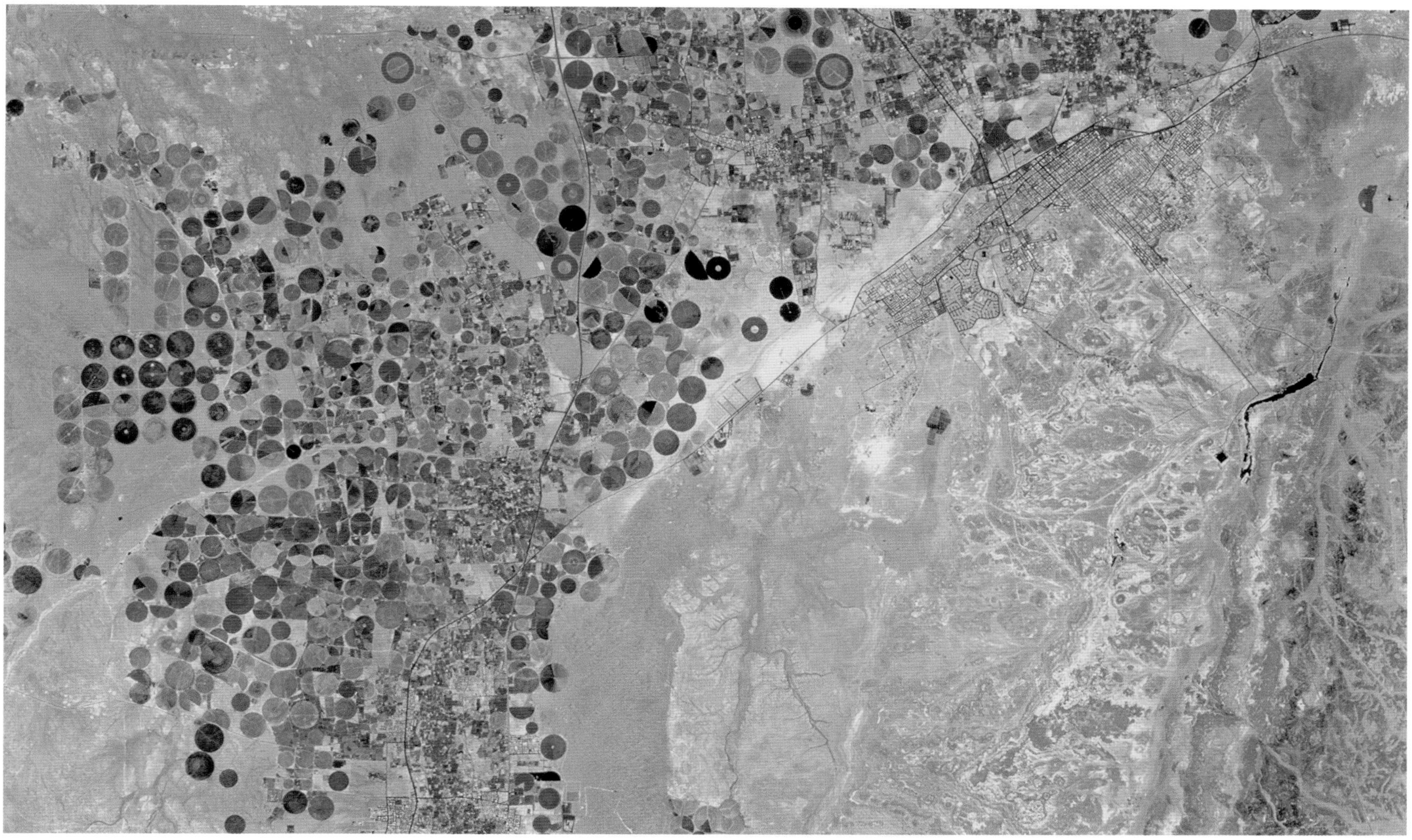

▲ Irrigation in Saudi Arabia

▶ **Irrigation boom**

The photograph shows a pivotal irrigation boom used to sprinkle water over a wheat field in Saudi Arabia. Irrigation in hot countries often takes place at night so that water loss through evaporation is reduced. Irrigation techniques vary from place to place. In monsoon areas with abundant water, the fields are often flooded, or the water is led to the crops along straight furrows. Sprinkler irrigation has become important since the 1940s. In other types of irrigation, the water is led through pipes which are on or under the ground. Underground pipes supply water directly to the plant roots and, as a result, water loss through evaporation is minimized.

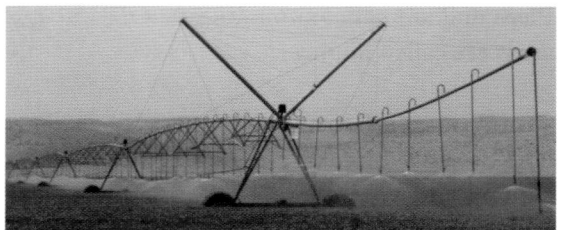

▲ **Irrigation in Saudi Arabia**

Saudi Arabia is a desert country that gets its water from oases, which tap groundwater supplies, and desalination plants. The sale of oil has enabled the arid countries of south-western Asia to develop their agriculture. In the above satellite image, vegetation appears as brown and red circles, generated by centre-pivot irrigation systems.

The study pointed out that the world is running out of fertile land, because large areas are too dry, too cold or too mountainous for farming. Although the demand for food increases every year, problems arise when attempts are made to increase the area of farmland. The soils and climate of tropical forests or semi-arid regions are not ideal for farming and often lead to the deterioration of fragile environments. To increase food supply, farmers must concentrate on making existing agriculture more productive.

To grow crops, farmers need fertile, workable land, an equable climate, and an adequate supply of fresh water. In some areas, the water supply comes directly from rain, but many other regions depend on irrigation.

Irrigation involves water conservation through the building of dams which hold back storage reservoirs. In some areas, irrigation water comes from underground aquifers, layers of permeable and porous rocks through which groundwater percolates. But in many cases, the water in the

aquifers has been there for thousands of years, having accumulated at a time when the rainfall was much greater than it is today. As a result, these aquifers are not being renewed and will, one day, dry up.

Other sources of irrigation water are desalination plants, which remove salt from seawater and pump it to farms. This is a highly expensive process and is employed in areas where water supplies are extremely low, such as the island of Malta, or in the oil-rich desert countries around the Persian Gulf, which can afford to build huge desalination plants.

LAND USE BY CONTINENT (2006)

	Forest	Permanent pasture	Permanent crops	Arable	Non-productive
N. & C. America	26.0%	16.4%	0.7%	12.0%	45.0%
S. America	50.5%	26.4%	0.8%	6.1%	16.0%
Europe	46.0%	8.3%	0.8%	12.9%	32.0%
Africa	21.8%	31.1%	0.9%	6.7%	39.5%
Asia	17.8%	35.8%	2.1%	16.4%	28.0%
Oceania	23.3%	47.8%	0.4%	5.9%	23.0%

THE NATURAL WORLD

In 2007, the International Union for the Conservation of Nature published its Red List, stating that 16,306 animal and plant species are threatened with extinction, 800 species more than in 2004, while 41,415 species are endangered, including one-fourth of the world's mammals, one-third of all reptiles, one in eight birds and 75% of the world's assessed plants. Human activities are the main cause of this devastating reduction in our planet's bio-diversity, which might lead to the loss of the unique combinations of genes that could be vital in improving food production or in the manufacture of drugs to combat disease.

Extinctions of species have occurred through-out Earth's history, but today the extinction rate is estimated to be about 10,000 times the natural average. Some scientists have even compared it with the mass extinction that wiped out the dinosaurs 65 million years ago. However, the main cause of today's high extinction rate is not some natural disaster, such as the impact of an asteroid a few kilometres across, but it is the result of human actions. In some areas, such

▼ *Rainforest in Rwanda*

Rainforests are the most threatened of the world's biomes. Effective conservation policies must demonstrate to poor local people that they can benefit from the survival of the forests.

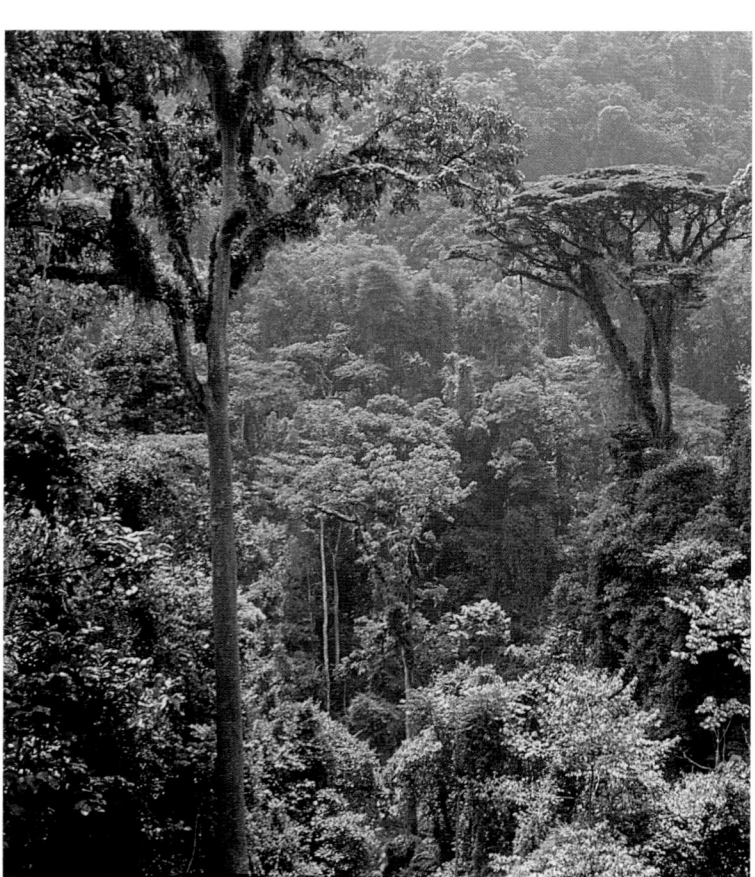

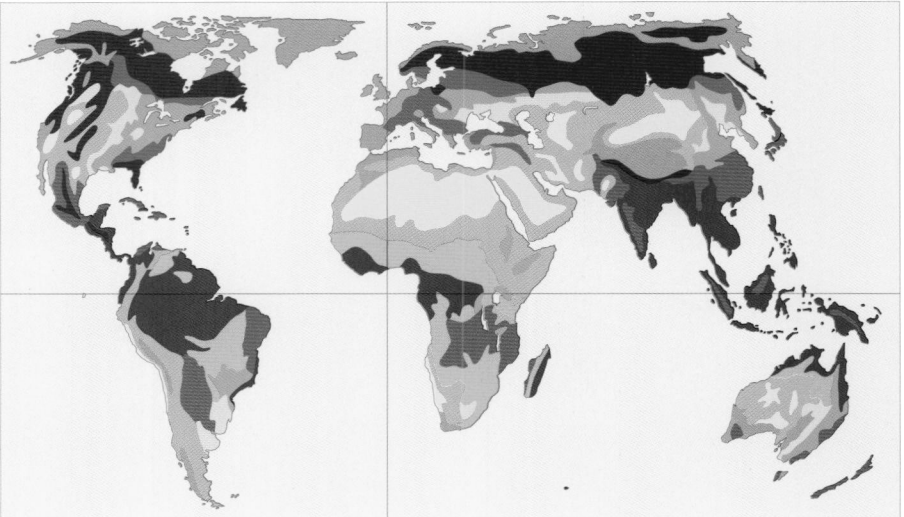

as Western Europe, the natural habitats were destroyed long ago. The greatest damage is now occurring in tropical rainforests, which contain more than half of the world's known species.

Modern technology has enabled people to live comfortably almost anywhere on Earth. But most plants and many animals are adapted to particular climatic conditions, and they live in association with and dependent on each other. Plant and animal communities that cover large areas are called biomes.

THE WORLD'S BIOMES

The world's biomes are defined mainly by climate and vegetation. They range from the tundra, in polar regions and high mountain regions, to the lush equatorial rainforests.

The Arctic tundra covers large areas in the polar regions of the northern hemisphere. Snow covers the land for more than half of the year and the subsoil, called permafrost, is per-manently frozen. Comparatively few species can survive in this harsh, treeless environment. The main plants are hardy mosses, lichens, grasses, sedges and low shrubs. However, in summer, the tundra plays an important part in world animal geography, when its growing plants and swarms of insects provide food for migrating animals and birds that arrive from the south.

The tundra of the northern hemisphere merges in the south into a vast region of needle-leaf evergreen forest, called the boreal forest or taiga. Such trees as fir, larch, pine and spruce are adapted to survive the long, bitterly cold winters of this region, but the number of plant and animal species is again small. South of the boreal forests is a zone of mixed needleleaf evergreens and broadleaf deciduous trees, which shed their leaves in winter. In warmer areas, this

NATURAL VEGETATION

- TUNDRA & MOUNTAIN VEGETATION
- NEEDLELEAF EVERGREEN FOREST
- MIXED NEEDLELEAF EVERGREEN & BROADLEAF DECIDUOUS TREES
- BROADLEAF DECIDUOUS WOODLAND
- MID-LATITUDE GRASSLAND
- EVERGREEN BROADLEAF & DECIDUOUS TREES & SHRUBS
- SEMI-DESERT SCRUB
- DESERT
- TROPICAL GRASSLAND (SAVANNA)
- TROPICAL BROADLEAF RAINFOREST & MONSOON FOREST
- SUBTROPICAL BROADLEAF & NEEDLELEAF FOREST

▲ *The map shows the world's main biomes. The classification is based on the natural 'climax' vegetation of regions, a result of the climate and the terrain. But human activities have greatly modified this basic division. For example, the original deciduous forests of Western Europe and the eastern United States have largely disappeared. In recent times, human development of some semi-arid areas has turned former dry grasslands into barren desert. Scientists predict that temperatures will rise by 4°C [7.2°F] by 2100, radically altering existing biomes. For example, many experts believe that global warming is currently threatening half of the Arctic tundra.*

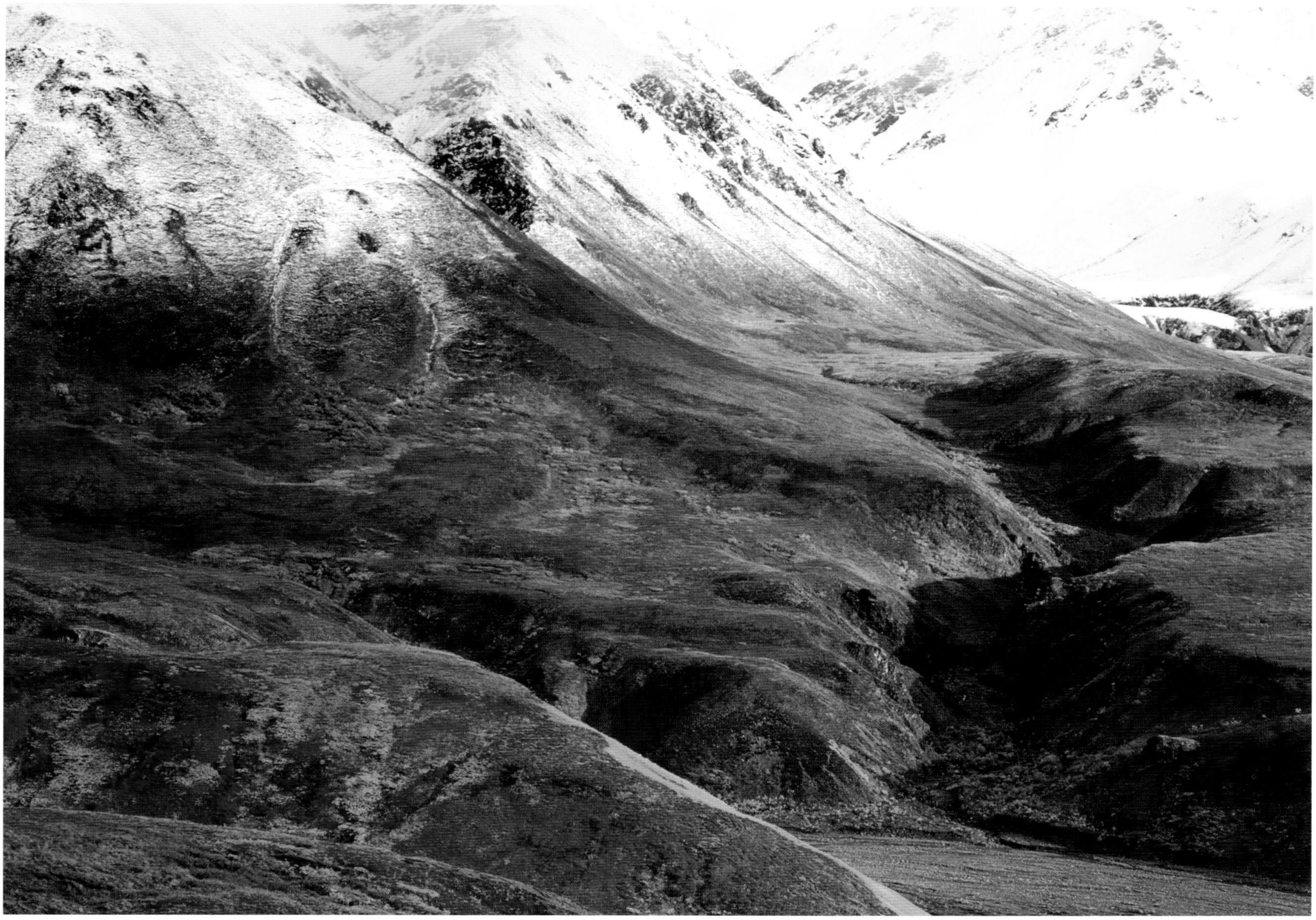

▼ *The net primary production of eight major biomes is expressed in grams of dry organic matter per square metre per year. The tropical rainforests produce the greatest amount of organic material. The tundra and deserts produce the least.*

NET PRIMARY PRODUCTION OF EIGHT MAJOR BIOMES

- ■ TROPICAL RAINFORESTS
- ■ DECIDUOUS FORESTS
- ■ TROPICAL GRASSLANDS
- ■ CONIFEROUS FORESTS
- ■ MEDITERRANEAN
- ■ TEMPERATE GRASSLANDS
- ■ TUNDRA
- ■ DESERTS

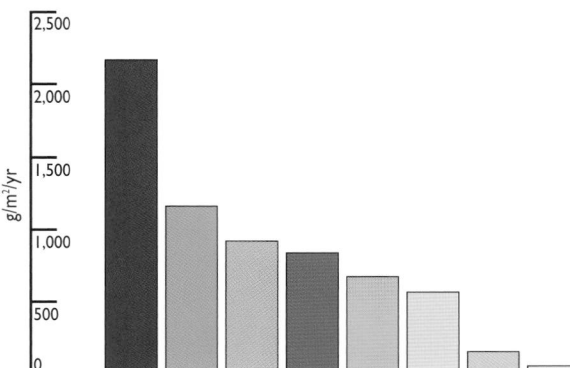

mixed forest merges into broadleaf deciduous forest, where the number and diversity of plant species is much greater.

Deciduous forests are adapted to temperate, humid regions. Evergreen broadleaf and deciduous trees grow in Mediterranean regions, with their hot, dry summers. But much of the original deciduous forest has been cut down and has given way to scrub and heathland. Grasslands occupy large areas in the middle latitudes, where the rainfall is insufficient to support forest growth. The moister grasslands are often called prairies, while drier areas are called steppe.

▲ *Tundra in subarctic Alaska, United States*
The Denali National Park, Alaska, contains magnificent mountain scenery and tundra vegetation that flourishes during the brief summer. The park is open between 1 June and 15 September.

The tropics also contain vast dry areas of semi-desert scrub that merges into desert, as well as large areas of tropical savanna, which is grassland, ranging from luxuriant to sparse, with scattered shrubs and trees, whose growth is limited by a marked dry season. Savanna regions support a wide range of animals.

Tropical and subtropical regions contain three types of forest biomes. The tropical rainforest, the world's richest biome measured by its plant and animal species, experiences rain and high temperatures throughout the year. Similar forests occur in monsoon regions, which have a season of very heavy rainfall. They, too, are rich in plant species, though less so than the tropical rainforest. A third type of forest is the subtropical broadleaf and needleleaf forest, found in such places as south-eastern China, south-central Africa and eastern Brazil.

THE HUMAN WORLD

Every minute, the world's population increases by more than 100. Predictions of future growth vary. In 1999, UN demographers stated that the population, which passed the 6 billion mark in October 1999, would reach 8.9 billion by 2050. It would level out after 2200, when it would peak at 11 billion. But, in 2004, UN demographers predicted that the world's population would peak at 9.1 billion in 2050 and then could start to decline. In 2006, the UN predicted that, by 2050, 50 countries, many of them in Europe, would have fewer people than they have today. But the populations of most developing countries – the least able to afford the high costs arising from a population explosion – will continue to increase rapidly.

▼ Quito, capital city of Ecuador
In common with world trends, the annual growth rate in the population of Ecuador is declining, while urbanization is increasing rapidly.

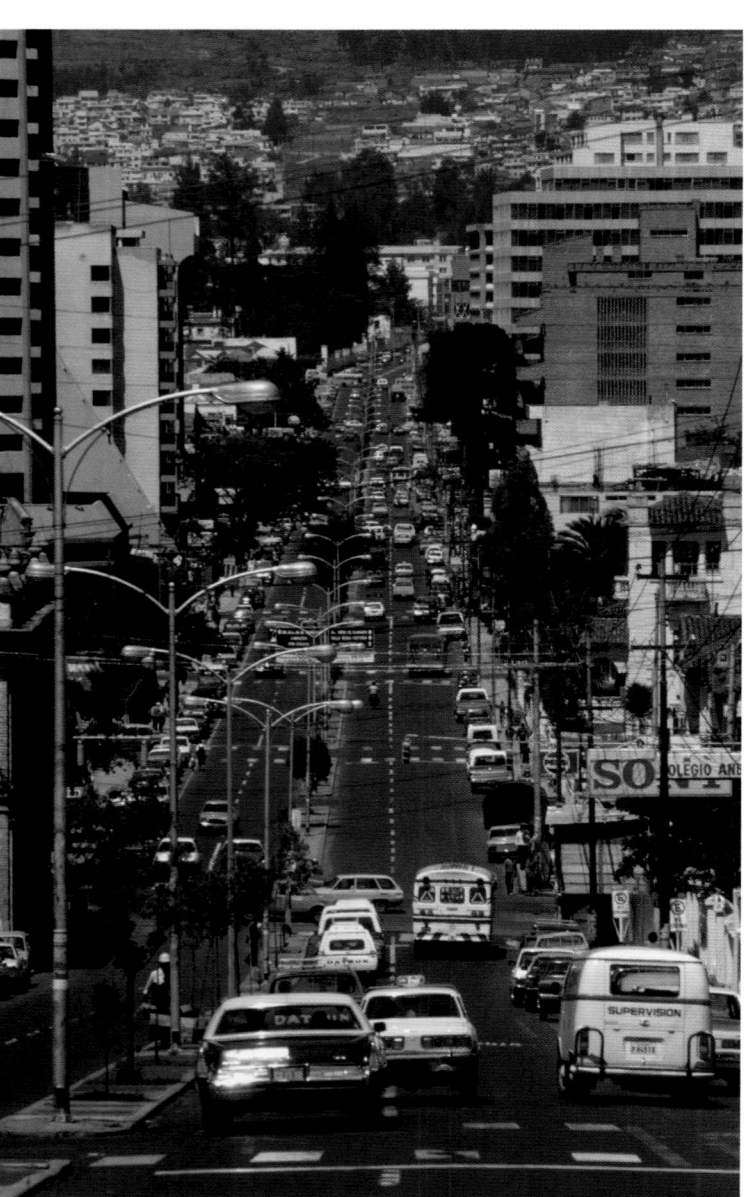

Average world population growth rates are expected to decline from 1.6% per year in 1975–2001 to 1.1% in 2001–15. This is partly due to a decline in fertility rates – that is, the number of births to the number of women of child-bearing age – especially in developed countries where, as income has risen, the average size of families has fallen.

Declining fertility rates were also evident in many developing countries. Even Africa shows signs of such change, though its population is expected to triple before it begins to fall. Population growth is also dependent on death rates, which are affected by such factors as famine, disease and the quality of medical care.

THE POPULATION EXPLOSION

The world's population has grown steadily throughout most of human history, though certain events triggered periods of population growth. The invention of agriculture, around 10,000 years ago, led to great changes in human society. Before then, most people had obtained food by hunting animals and gathering plants. Average life expectancies were probably no more than 20 years and life was hard. However, when farmers began to produce food surpluses, people began to live settled lives. This major milestone in human history led to the development of the first cities and early civilizations.

From an estimated 8 million in 8000 BC, the world population rose to about 300 million by AD 1000. Between 1000 and 1750, the rate of world population increase was around 0.1% per year, but another period of major economic and social change – the Industrial Revolution – began in the late 18th century. The Industrial Revolution led to improvements in farm technology and increases in food production. The world population began to increase quickly as industrialization spread across Europe and into North America. By 1850, it had reached 1.2 billion. The 2 billion mark was passed in the 1920s, and then the population rapidly doubled to 4 billion by the 1970s.

POPULATION FEATURES

Population growth affects the structure of societies. In developing countries with high annual rates of population increase, the large majority of the people are young and soon to become parents themselves. For example, in Kenya, which had until recently an annual rate of population growth of around 4%, about 42% of the population is under 15 years of age, as

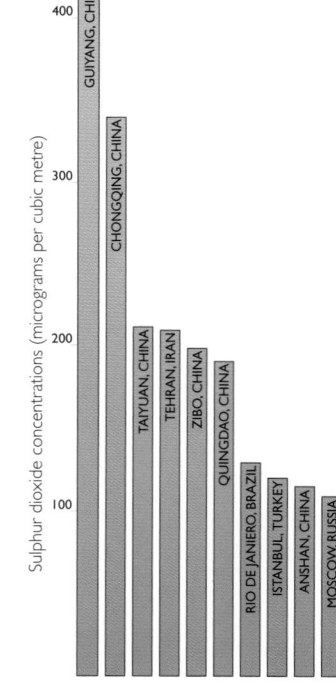

▲ Urban air pollution
This diagram shows the world's most polluted cities. Sulphur dioxide is an air pollutant which contributes to acid rain and can damage human health. The WHO threshold of sulphur dioxide concentrations is 150 micrograms per cubic metre.

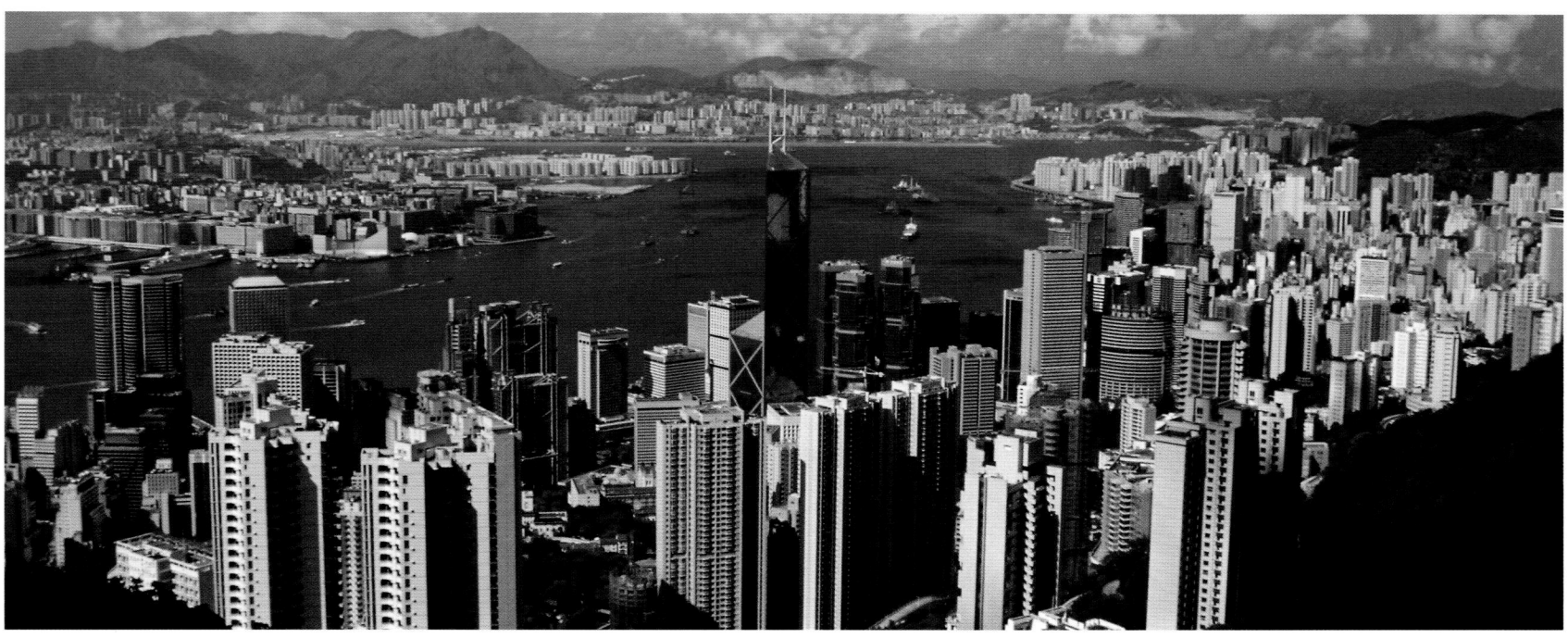

compared with 21% in the United States. Most developed countries have a fairly even spread across the age groups.

Such differences are reflected in average life expectancies. In a rich country, such as the USA, the average life expectancy in 2006 was 78 years (75 for men and 80 for women; women live longer, on average, than men). As a result, an increasing proportion of the people are elderly and retired. The reverse applies in many poor countries, where average life expectancies are below 60 years. In the early 21st century, life expectancies were falling in parts of southern Africa because of the spread of HIV and AIDS. However, overall, the world population is ageing. In 2003, demographers predicted that the average age of the world's people will rise from 28 to 40 years.

Paralleling the population explosion has been a rapid growth in the number and size of cities. Urban areas contained about half of the world's people in 2007. This proportion is expected to rise to nearly two-thirds by 2025.

Urbanization occurred first in areas under-

POPULATION CHANGE
The projected population change for the years 2004–2050.

- OVER 125% POPULATION GAIN
- 100–125% POPULATION GAIN
- 50–100% POPULATION GAIN
- 25–50% POPULATION GAIN
- 0–25% POPULATION GAIN
- LOSS OR NO CHANGE
- NO DATA AVAILABLE

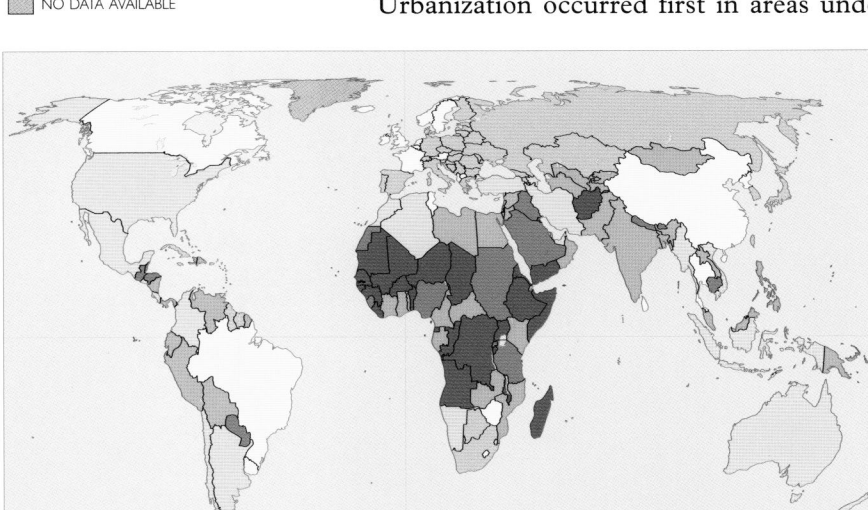

▲ *Hong Kong's business district*
By contrast with the picturesque old streets of Hong Kong, the business district of Hong Kong City, on the northern shore of Hong Kong Island, is a cluster of modern high-rise buildings. The glittering skyscrapers reflect the success of this tiny region, which has one of the strongest economies in Asia.

going the industrialization of their economies, but today it is also a feature of the developing world. In developing countries, people are leaving impoverished rural areas hoping to gain access to the education, health and other services available in cities. But many cities cannot provide the facilities necessitated by rapid population growth. By 2007, about a billion people lived in slums, where pollution, crime and disease are features of daily life.

The population explosion poses another problem for the entire world. No one knows how many people the world can support or how consumer demand will damage the fragile environments on our planet. The British economist Thomas Malthus argued in the late 18th century that overpopulation would lead to famine and war. But an increase in farm technology in the 19th and 20th centuries, combined with a green revolution, in which scientists developed high-yield crop varieties, has greatly increased food production since Malthus' time.

However, some modern scientists argue that overpopulation may become a problem in the 21st century. They argue that food and water shortages leading to disastrous famines will result unless population growth can be halted. Such people argue in favour of birth-control programmes. China, one of the two countries with more than a billion people, introduced a one-child family policy. Its action has slowed the growth of China's huge population.

LANGUAGES AND RELIGIONS

In 2008, 89-year-old Marie Smith, the last person able to speak the Eyak language, died. Eyak became an extinct language, though before her death, she had compiled an Eyak dictionary and grammar guide. Eyak is one of about 20 native Alaskan languages, many of which are under threat of extinction. Experts regularly report the disappearance of languages. Some predict that up to 90% of the world's languages will not exist by the end of the 21st century.

Improved transport and communications are partly to blame, because they bring people from various cultures into closer and closer contact. Many children no longer speak the language of their parents, preferring instead to learn the language used at their schools. The pressures on children to speak dominant rather than minority languages are often great. In the first part of the 20th century, Native American children were punished if they spoke their native language.

The disappearance of a language represents the extinction of a way of thinking, a unique expression of the experiences and knowledge of a group of people. Language and religion together give people an identity and a sense of belonging. However, there are others who argue that the disappearance of minority languages is a step towards international understanding and economic efficiency.

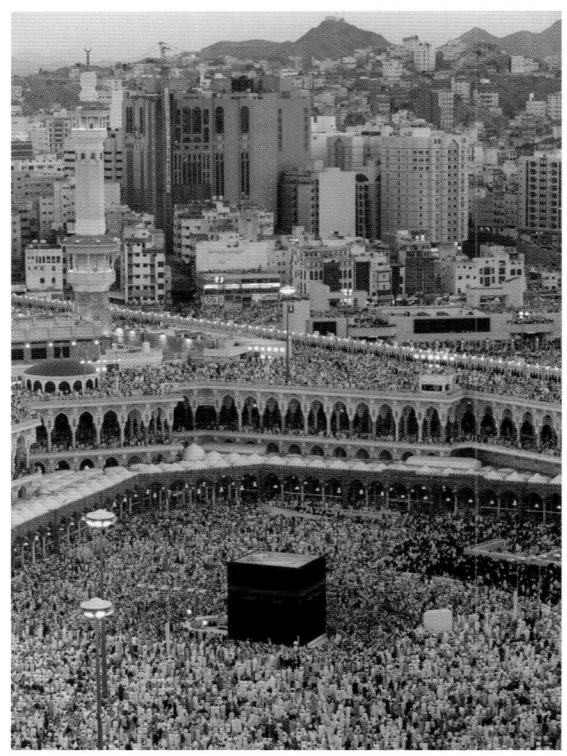
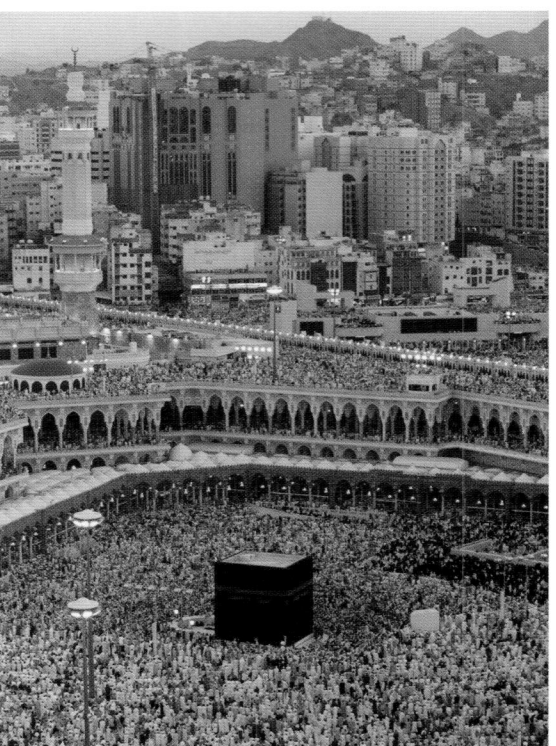

THE WORLD'S LANGUAGES

Definitions of what is a language or a dialect vary and, hence, estimates of the number of languages spoken around the world range from about 3,000 to 6,000. But whatever the figure, it is clear that the number of languages far exceeds the number of countries.

◄ *The Kaaba, Makkah (Mecca), Saudi Arabia*

Islam is a major world religion. It was first preached by the Prophet Muhammad who was born in Makkah (or Mecca) in Saudi Arabia in about AD 570. Its holiest shrine is the Kaaba, a black, square building in the Great Mosque in Makkah. Every adult Muslim must, if possible, make at least one pilgrimage (or hajj) to Makkah. More than a million Muslims make the pilgrimage every year. The pilgrims walk or run around the Kaaba seven times, praying or reciting verses from the Koran, the sacred book of the Muslims.

RELIGIOUS ADHERENTS

Number of adherents to the world's major religions, in millions (2006).

Christianity	2,100
Roman Catholic	1,050
Protestant	396
Orthodox	240
Anglican	73
Others	341
Islam	1,070
Sunni	940
Shi'ite	120
Others	10
Secular/Atheist/Agnostic/ Non-religious	1,100
Hinduism	900
Chinese folk	394
Buddhism	376
Ethnic religions	300
New religions	103
Sikhism	23
Spiritism	15
Judaism	14
Baha'i	7
Confucianism	6
Jainism	4
Shintoism	4

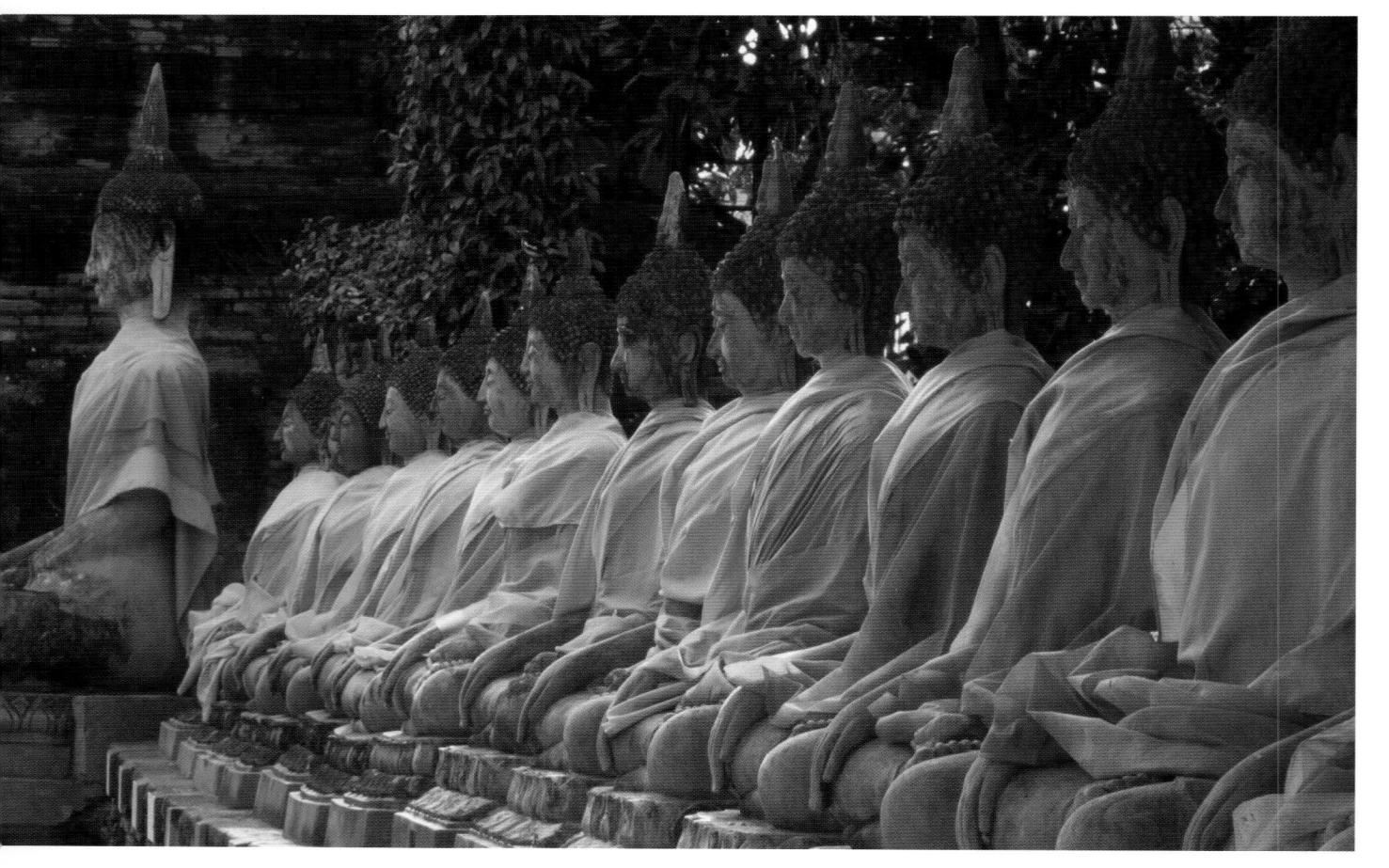

◄ *Statues of the Buddha, Wat Yai Chai Mongkol, Thailand*

Buddhism is a major religion in South-east Asia, Sri Lanka and Japan. The statues of the Buddha in the photograph are swathed in saffron robes. They surround the main chedi, or Golden Mount Pagoda, at Wat Yai Chai Mongkol, a World Heritage site near the ancient city of Ayutthaya, north of Bangkok.

Countries with only one language tend to be small. For example, in Liechtenstein, everyone speaks German. By contrast, more than 820 languages have been identified in Papua New Guinea, whose population is only about 5.8 million people. Hence, many of its languages are spoken by only small groups of people. In fact, scientists have estimated that about a third of the world's languages are now spoken by less than 1,000 people. By contrast, more than half of the world's population speak just seven languages.

The world's languages are grouped into families. The Indo-European family consists of languages spoken between Europe and the Indian subcontinent. The growth of European empires over the last 300 years led several Indo-European languages, most notably English, French, Portuguese and Spanish, to spread throughout much of North and South America, Africa, Australia and New Zealand.

English has become the official language in many countries which together contain more than a quarter of the world's population. It is now a major international language, surpassing in importance Mandarin Chinese, a member of the Sino-Tibetan family, which is the world's leading first language. Without a knowledge of English, businessmen face many problems when conducting international trade, especially with the United States or other English-speaking countries. But proposals that English, French, Russian or some other language should become a world language seem unlikely to be acceptable to a majority of the world's peoples.

MOTHER TONGUES
First-language speakers of the
major languages, in millions.

- MANDARIN CHINESE 873M
- HINDI 366M
- SPANISH 322M
- ENGLISH 309M
- PORTUGUESE 176M
- BENGALI 171M
- RUSSIAN 145M
- JAPANESE 122M
- GERMAN 95M
- WU CHINESE 77M

OFFICIAL LANGUAGES:
% OF WORLD POPULATION

English	27.0%
Chinese	19.0%
Hindi	13.5%
Spanish	5.4%
Russian	5.2%
French	4.2%
Arabic	3.3%
Portuguese	3.0%
Malay	3.0%
Bengali	2.9%
Japanese	2.3%

▶ *Polyglot nations*

The graph shows countries of the world with more than 200 languages. Although it has only about 5.8 million people, Papua New Guinea holds the record for the number of languages spoken.

Brazil (200)
Congo (DR) (216)
China (241)
Australia (275)
Cameroon (280)
Mexico (297)
India (427)
Nigeria (516)
Indonesia (742)
Papua New Guinea (820)

WORLD RELIGIONS

Religion is another fundamental aspect of human culture. It has inspired much of the world's finest architecture, literature, music and art. It has also helped to shape human cultures since prehistoric times and is responsible for the codes of ethics by which most people live.

The world's major religions were all founded in Asia. Judaism, one of the first faiths to teach that there is only one god, is one of the world's oldest. Founded in south-western Asia, it influenced the more recent Christianity and Islam, two other monotheistic religions which now have the great-

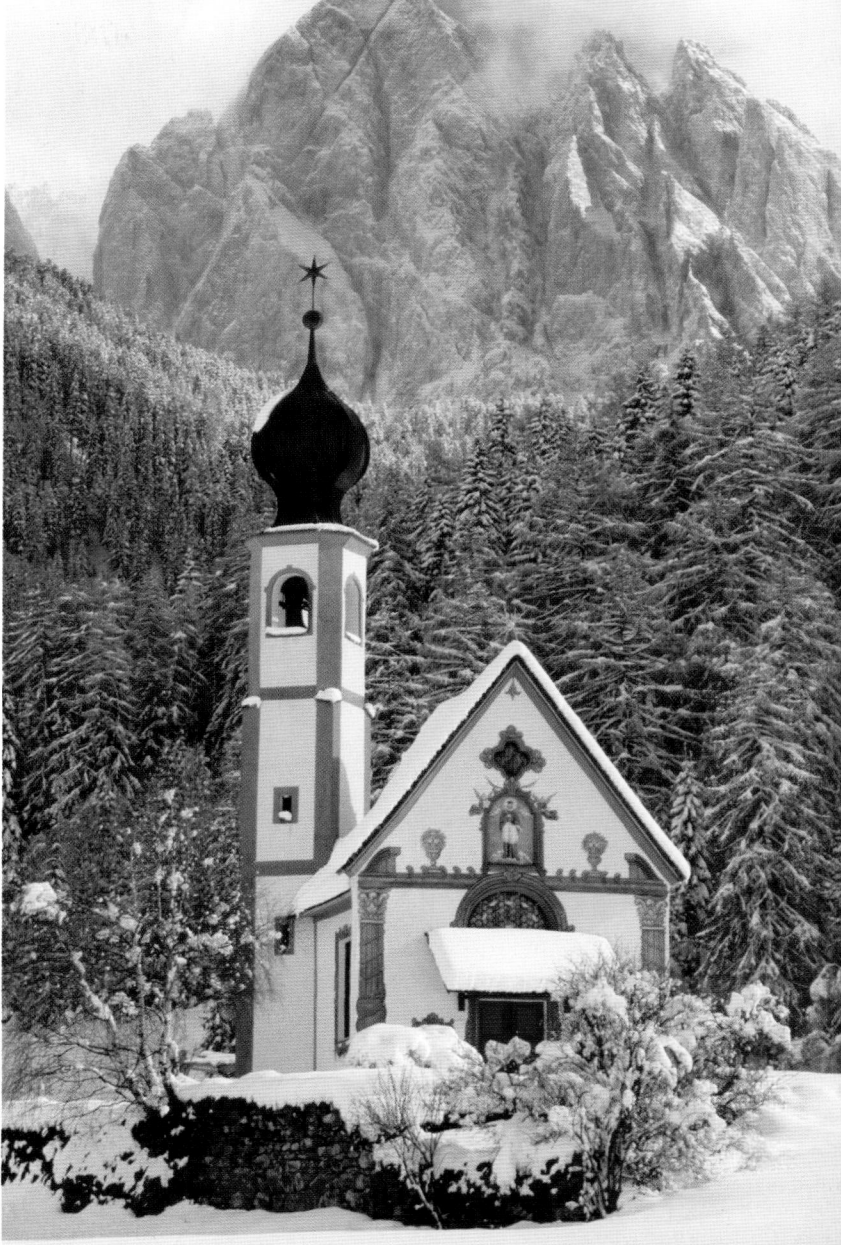

▲ *The Church of San Giovanni, Dolomites, Italy*
Christianity has done much to shape Western civilization. Christian churches were built as places of worship, but many of them are among the finest achievements of world architecture.

est number of followers. Hinduism, the third leading faith in terms of the numbers of followers, originated in the Indian subcontinent and most Hindus are now found in India. Another major religion, Buddhism, was founded in the subcontinent partly as a reaction to certain aspects of Hinduism. But unlike Hinduism, it has spread from India throughout much of eastern Asia.

Religion and language are powerful creative forces. They are also essential features of nationalism, which gives people a sense of belonging and pride. But nationalism is often also a cause of rivalry and tension. Cultural differences have led to racial hatred, the persecution of minorities, and to war between national groups.

INTERNATIONAL ORGANIZATIONS

Twelve days before the surrender of Germany and four months before the final end of World War II, representatives of 50 nations met in San Francisco to create a plan to set up a peace-keeping organization, the United Nations. Since its birth on 24 October 1945, its membership has grown from 51 to 192 by 2007.

Its first 60 years have been marked by failures as well as successes. For example, because of the UN policy of neutrality, the Blue Berets, as UN troops are called, have been sometimes forced to stand by when atrocities have occurred. As a result, the UN Secretary-General announced a reform plan in 2005.

THE WORK OF THE UN

The United Nations has six main organs. They include the General Assembly, where member states meet to discuss issues concerned with peace, security and development. The Security Council, containing 15 members, is concerned with maintaining world peace. The Secretariat, under the Secretary-General, helps the other organs to do their jobs effectively, while the Economic and Social Council works with specialized agencies to implement policies concerned with such matters as development, education and health. The International Court of Justice, or World Court, helps to settle disputes between member nations. The sixth organ of the UN, the Trusteeship Council, was designed to bring 11 UN trust territories to independence. Its task has now been completed.

The specialized agencies do much important

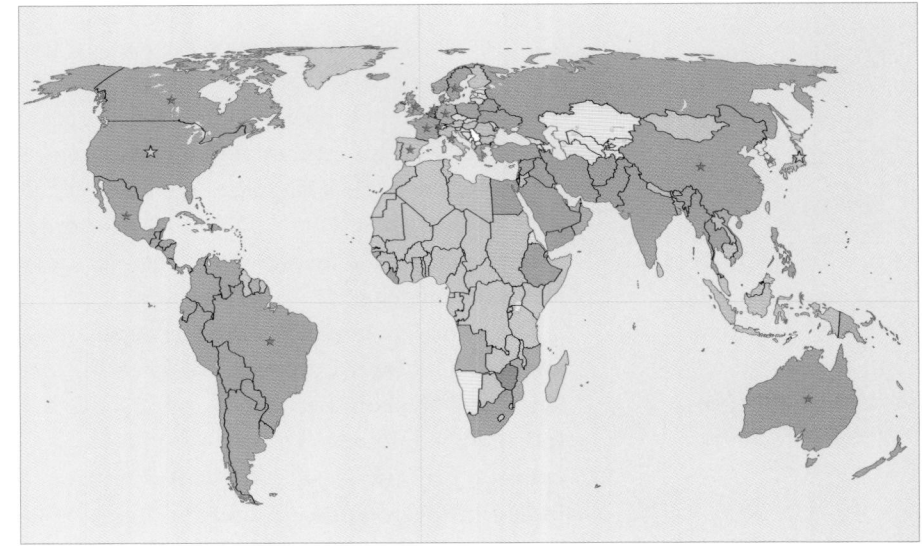

work. For example, UNICEF (United Nations International Children's Fund) has provided health care and aid for children in many parts of the world. The ILO (International Labour Organization) has improved working conditions in many areas, while the FAO (Food and Agricultural Organization) has worked to improve the production and distribution of food. Among the other agencies are organizations to help refugees, to further human rights, and to control the environment. The latest agency, set up in 1995, is the WTO (World Trade Organization), which took over the work of GATT (General Agreement on Tariffs and Trade).

OTHER ORGANIZATIONS

In a world in which nations have become increasingly interdependent, many other organizations have been set up to deal with a variety of problems. Some, such as NATO (the North Atlantic Treaty Organization), are defence alliances. In the early 1990s, the end of the Cold War suggested that NATO's role might be finished, but the civil war in the former Yugoslavia showed that it still has a role in maintaining peace and security.

Other organizations encourage social and economic co-operation in various regions. Some are NGOs (non-governmental organizations), such as the Red Cross and its Muslim equivalent, the Red Crescent. Other NGOs raise funds to provide aid to countries facing major crises, such as famine.

Some major international organizations aim at economic co-operation and the removal of trade barriers. For example, in 2003, the European Union had 15 members, of which 12 had adopted a single currency, the euro, on 1 January 2001. On 1 May 2004, another ten countries in

MEMBERS OF THE UNITED NATIONS
Year of joining:

- 1940s
- 1950s
- 1960s
- 1970s
- 1980s
- 1990s
- 2000s
- NON–MEMBERS

★ 1% – 10% CONTRIBUTION TO FUNDING

☆ OVER 10% CONTRIBUTION TO FUNDING

INTERNATIONAL AID AND GNI
Aid provided as a percentage of GNI, with total aid in brackets (2006).

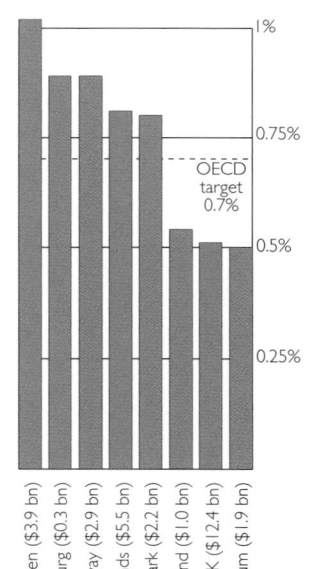

▼ *UN peace-keeping missions*

In the 1990s, a UN peace-keeping mission worked to restore peace to Bosnia-Herzegovina, following the Dayton Peace Accord of 1995. By 2005, hopes of long-term stability were high and refugees were returning home in large numbers.

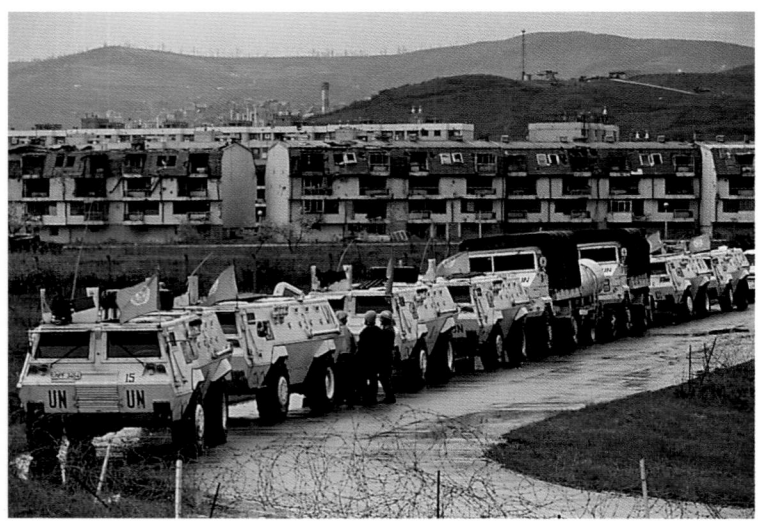

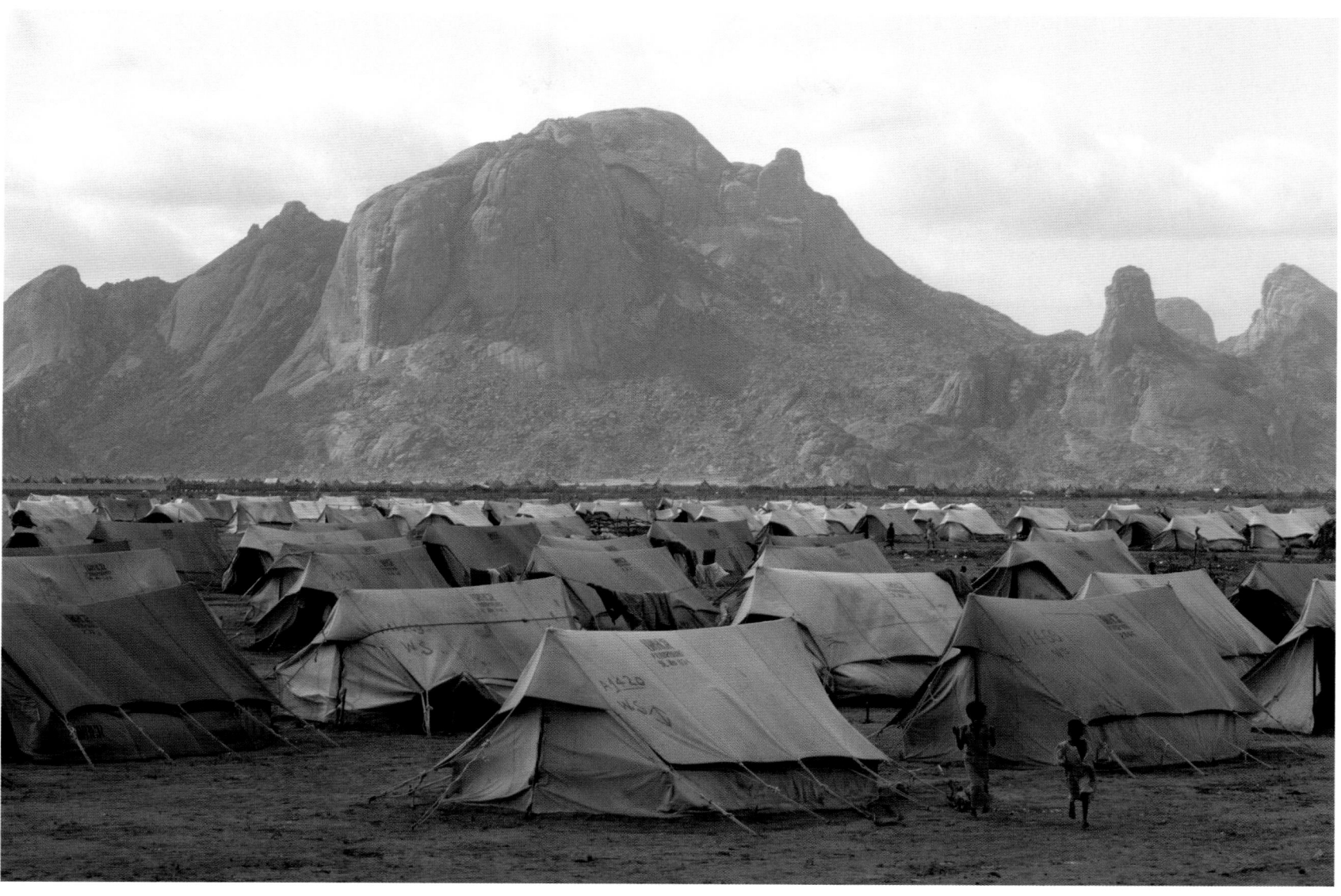

eastern and southern Europe joined the EU; Bulgaria and Romania were admitted in 2007.

Other groupings include ASEAN (the Association of South-east Asian Nations) which aims to reduce trade barriers between its members (Brunei, Burma [Myanmar], Cambodia, Indonesia, Laos, Malaysia, the Philippines, Singapore, Thailand and Vietnam). APEC (the Asia-Pacific Co-operation Group), founded in 1989, aims to create a free-trade zone between the countries

▲ *Refugee camp, Sudan*

In the late 20th and early 21st centuries, many people in the Horn of Africa and Sudan were displaced by war. Here, and in other parts of the world, refugees from war depend largely on aid from international organizations and NGOs.

of eastern Asia, North America, Australia and New Zealand by 2020. Meanwhile, Canada, Mexico and the United States have formed NAFTA (the North American Free Trade Agreement), while other economic groupings link most of the countries in Latin America. Another grouping with a more limited but important objective is OPEC (the Organization of Oil-Exporting Countries). OPEC works to unify policies concerning trade in oil on the world markets.

Some organizations exist to discuss matters of common interest between groups of nations. The Commonwealth of Nations, for example, grew out of links created by the British Empire. In North and South America, the OAS (Organization of American States) aims to increase understanding in the Western hemisphere. The African Union (formerly the Organization of African Unity) has a similar role in Africa, while the Arab League represents Arab nations.

COUNTRIES OF THE EUROPEAN UNION

Country	Total land area (sq km)	Total population (2007 est.)	Year of accession to the EU	Country	Total land area (sq km)	Total population (2007 est.)	Year of accession to the EU
Austria	83,859	8,200,000	1995	Latvia	64,600	2,260,000	2004
Belgium	30,528	10,392,000	1958	Lithuania	65,200	3,575,000	2004
Bulgaria	110,912	7,323,000	2007	Luxembourg	2,586	480,000	1958
Cyprus	9,251	788,000	2004	Malta	316	402,000	2004
Czech Republic	78,866	10,229,000	2004	Netherlands	41,526	16,571,000	1958
Denmark	43,094	5,468,000	1973	Poland	323,250	38,518,000	2004
Estonia	45,100	1,316,000	2004	Portugal	88,797	10,643,000	1986
Finland	338,145	5,238,000	1995	Romania	238,391	22,276,000	2007
France	551,500	60,876,000	1958	Slovak Republic	49,012	5,448,000	2004
Germany	357,022	82,401,000	1958	Slovenia	20,256	2,009,000	2004
Greece	131,957	10,706,000	1981	Spain	497,548	40,448,000	1986
Hungary	93,032	9,956,000	2004	Sweden	449,964	9,031,000	1995
Ireland	70,273	4,109,000	1973	United Kingdom	241,857	60,776,000	1973
Italy	301,318	58,148,000	1958				

AGRICULTURE

In 1798, the British economist Thomas Robert Malthus published his view that populations would outgrow food supply, leading to famine and war. His forecasts proved incorrect because intensive farming and new technology greatly increased production. Furthermore, while only 7% of the world's land was used for crops or grazing in 1700, a study based on satellite data in 2005 showed that currently around 40% of the land is used for some kind of agriculture. In rich countries, food is cheaper than ever, and obesity, not food shortages, has become a major health issue. However, malnutrition is still rife in Africa, where local farmers cannot compete with the flood of subsidized food from rich countries.

From the 1950s, the 'green revolution' greatly increased food production. By using new crop varieties, irrigation, and the extensive use of

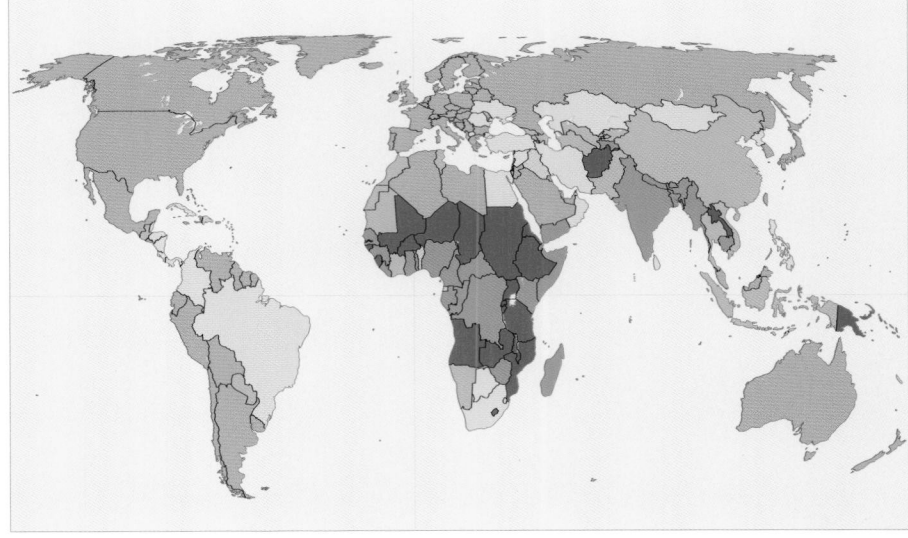

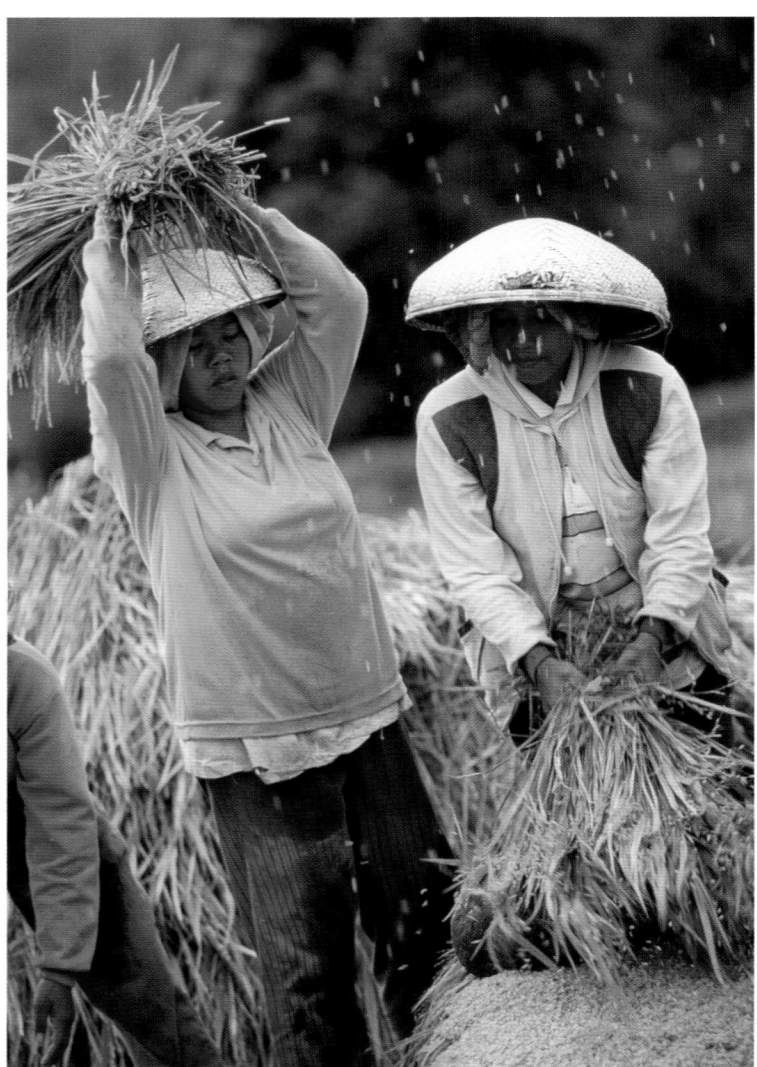

▼ *Rice harvest, Bali, Indonesia*

More than half of the world's people eat rice as their basic food. Rice grows well in tropical and subtropical regions, such as in Indonesia, India and south-eastern China.

fertilizers and pesticides, India, once a food importer, became self-sufficient in food. However, the increasing use of farmland to produce biofuels, which help to reduce global warming, may cause serious food shortages.

In the early 2000s, many people placed hopes in the use of genetically modified crops. Supporters argued that GM crops could be one of the greatest advances ever in farming. But critics of GM crops voiced serious environmental and health concerns.

FOOD PRODUCTION

Agriculture, which supplies most of our food, together with materials to make clothes and other products, is the world's most important economic activity. But its relative importance has declined in comparison with manufacturing and service industries. As a result, the end of the 20th century marked the first time for 10,000 years when the vast majority of the people no longer had to depend for their living on growing crops and herding animals.

However, agriculture remains the dominant economic activity in many developing countries in Africa and Asia. For example, in the early 21st century, 80% or more of the people of Bhutan, Burundi and Rwanda depended on farming for their living.

Many people in developing countries eke out the barest of livings by nomadic herding or shifting cultivation, combined with hunting, fishing and gathering plant foods. A large proportion of farmers live at subsistence level, producing little more than they require to provide the basic needs of their families.

The world's largest food producer and exporter is the United States, although agriculture employs around 1.6% of its total workforce.

IMPORTANCE OF AGRICULTURE

Agricultural workforce as a percentage of the total workforce (2006).

- OVER 80%
- 60–80%
- 40–60%
- 20–40%
- UNDER 20%
- NO DATA AVAILABLE

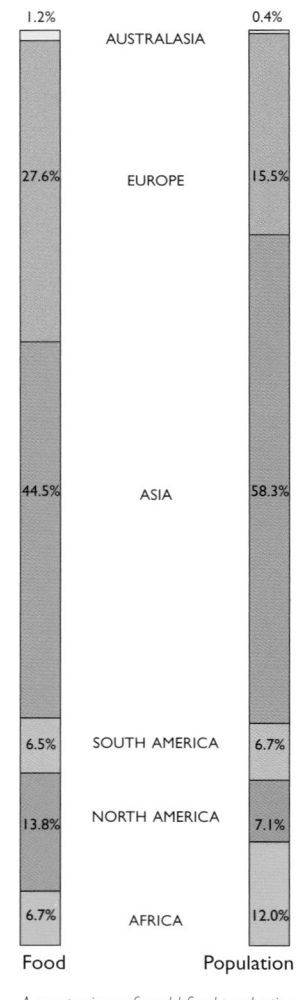

Food		Population
1.2%	AUSTRALASIA	0.4%
27.6%	EUROPE	15.5%
44.5%	ASIA	58.3%
6.5%	SOUTH AMERICA	6.7%
13.8%	NORTH AMERICA	7.1%
6.7%	AFRICA	12.0%

A comparison of world food production and population by continent.

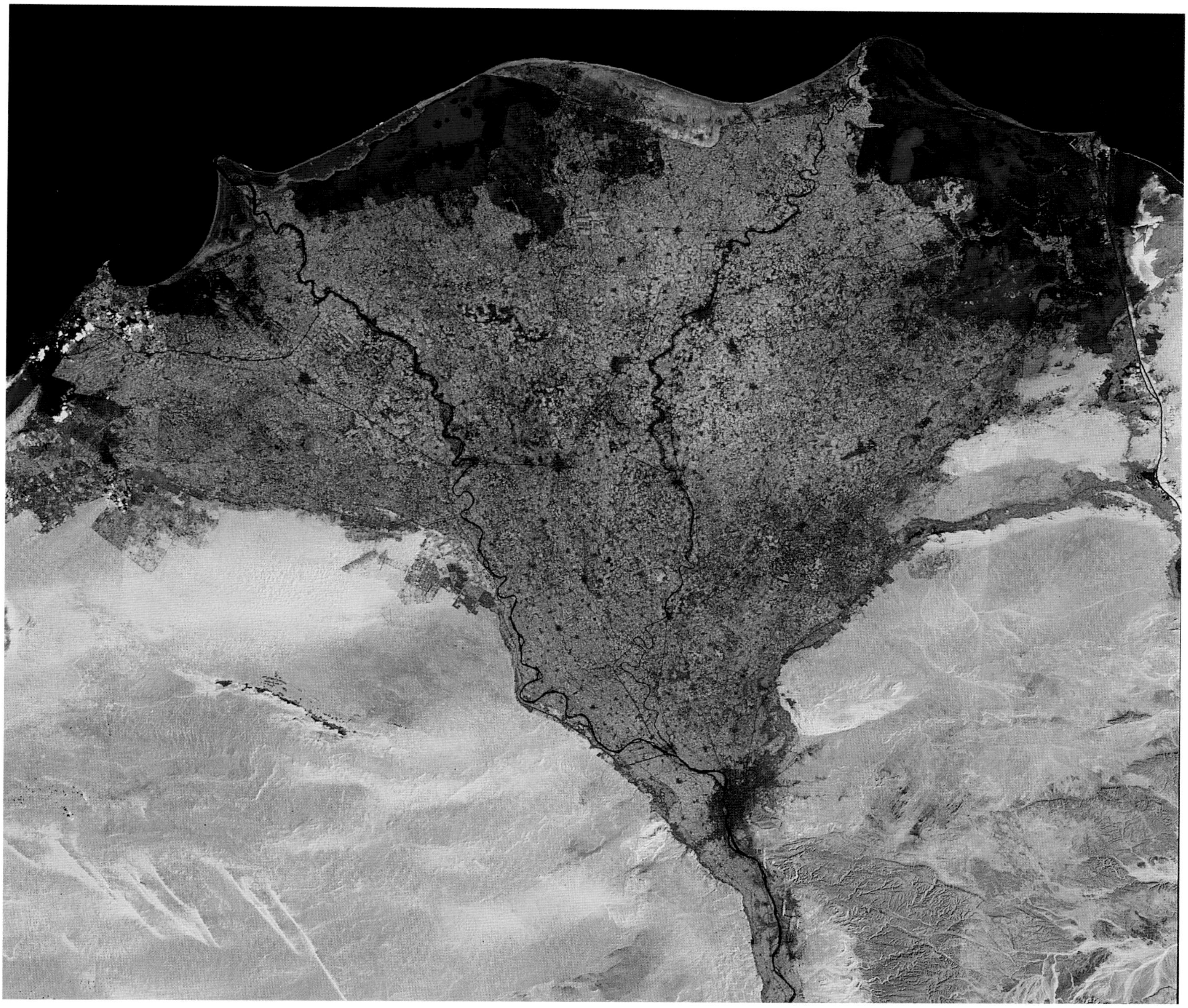

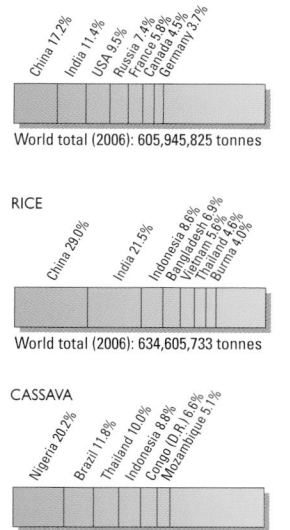

WHEAT

China 17.2%
India 11.4%
USA 9.5%
Russia 7.4%
France 5.9%
Canada 4.5%
Germany 3.7%

World total (2006): 605,945,825 tonnes

RICE

China 29.0%
India 21.5%
Indonesia 8.6%
Bangladesh 6.9%
Vietnam 5.6%
Thailand 4.6%
Burma 4.0%

World total (2006): 634,605,733 tonnes

CASSAVA

Nigeria 20.2%
Brazil 11.8%
Thailand 10.0%
Indonesia 8.8%
Congo (D.R.) 6.6%
Mozambique 5.1%

World total (2006): 226,337,396 tonnes

The high production of the United States is explained by its use of scientific methods and mechanization, which are features of agriculture throughout the developed world.

INTENSIVE OR ORGANIC FARMING

In the early 21st century, some people were beginning to question the dependence of farmers on chemical fertilizers and pesticides. Many people became concerned that the widespread use of chemicals was seriously polluting and damaging the environment.

Others objected to the intensive farming of animals to raise production and lower prices. For example, the suggestion in Britain in 1996 that BSE, or 'mad cow disease', might be passed on to people causing CJD (Creuzfeldt-Jakob Disease) caused widespread alarm. Such

▲ *Landsat image of the Nile delta, Egypt*

Most Egyptians live in the Nile valley and on its delta. Because much of the silt carried by the Nile now ends up on the floor of Lake Nasser, upstream of the Aswan Dam, the delta is now retreating and seawater is seeping inland. This eventuality was not foreseen when the Aswan High Dam was built in the 1960s.

factors, combined with the debate about the safety issues surrounding GM foods, have caused much concern.

Some farmers have returned to organic farming, which is based on animal-welfare principles and the banning of chemical fertilizers and pesticides. Organic foods are more expensive to produce than those produced by intensive farming, but an increasing number of consumers are demanding them.

ENERGY AND MINERALS

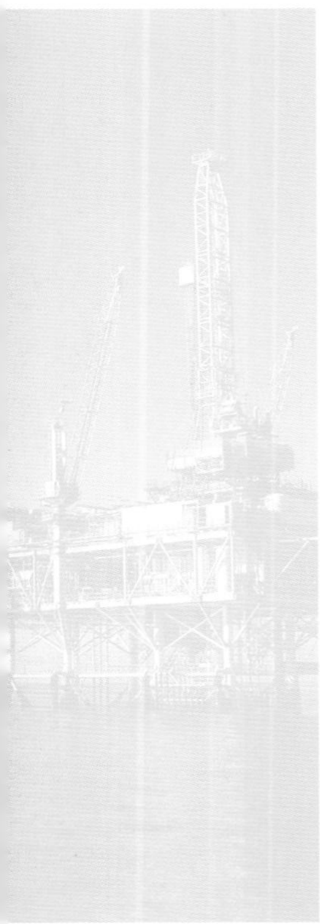

In August 2004, a serious accident occurred when a pipe carrying superheated steam exploded at Mihama nuclear power plant, 80 km [50 miles] north of Kyoto, Japan. Four people were killed and seven injured. No nuclear contamination occurred, but the accident further weakened public confidence in the industry. Nuclear power provides about 17% of the world's electricity, though concerns about safety and high costs cloud its future. But, while some nations are committed to phasing out nuclear energy, others are considering further development of nuclear power plants, as the reserves of fuels, which cause global warming, start to run low.

FOSSIL FUELS

Huge amounts of energy are needed for heating, generating electricity and for transport. In the

▼ *Wind farms in California, United States*
Wind farms using giant turbines can produce electricity at a lower cost than conventional power stations. But in many areas, winds are too light or too strong for wind farms to be effective.

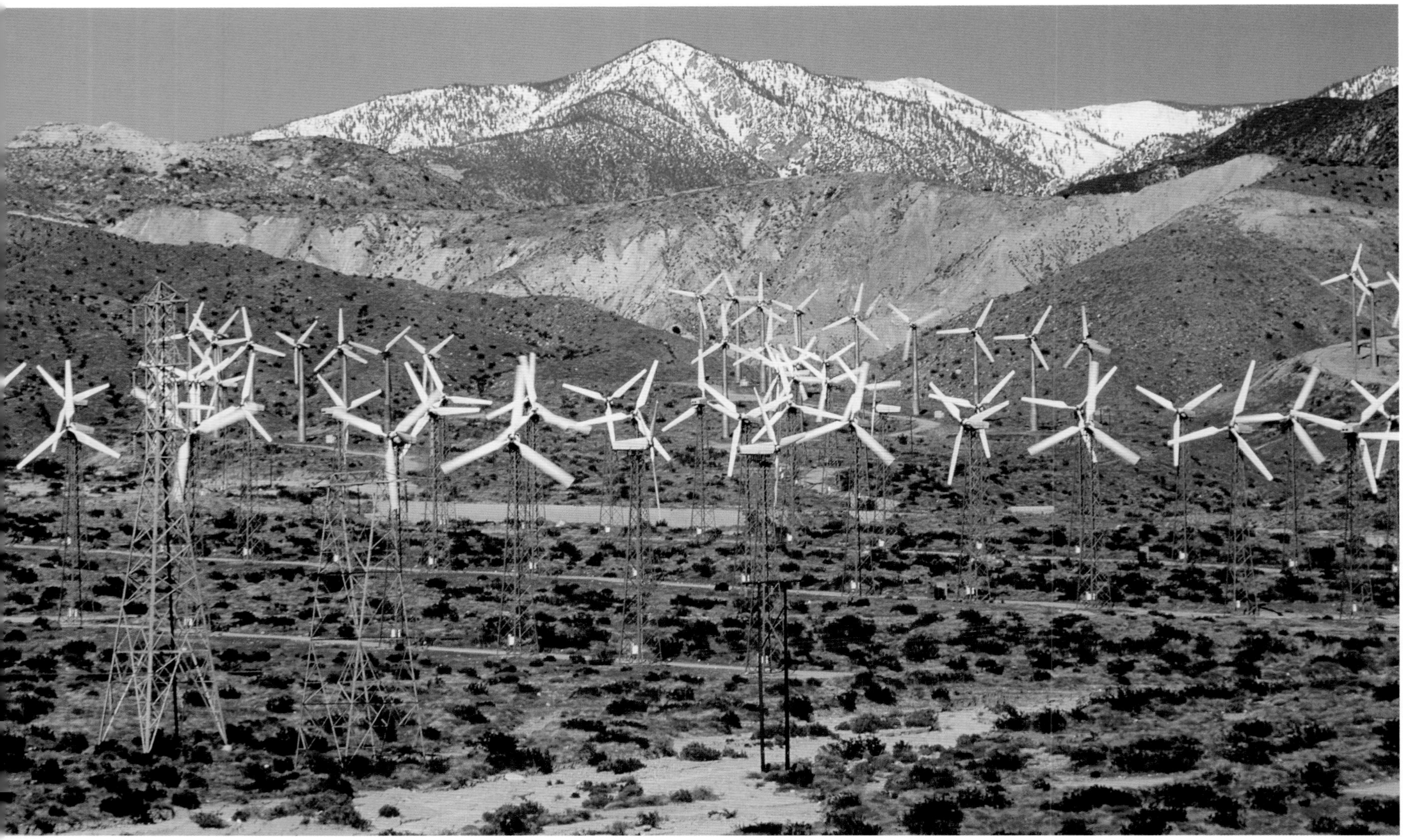

early years of the Industrial Revolution, coal, formed from organic matter buried beneath the Earth's surface, was the leading source of energy. It remains important as a raw material in the manufacture of drugs and other products, and also as a fuel, despite the fact that burning coal causes air pollution and gives off carbon dioxide, an important greenhouse gas.

However, oil and natural gas, which came into wide use in the 20th century, are cheaper to produce and easier to handle than coal, while, kilogram for kilogram, they give out more heat. Oil is especially important in moving transport, supplying about 97% of the fuel required.

In the 1990s, proven reserves of oil were sufficient to supply the world, at current rates of production, for 43 years, while supplies of natural gas stood at about 66 years. Coal reserves are more abundant and known reserves would last 200 years at present rates of use. Although these figures must be regarded with caution, because they do not allow for future discoveries, it is clear that fossil fuel reserves will one day run out.

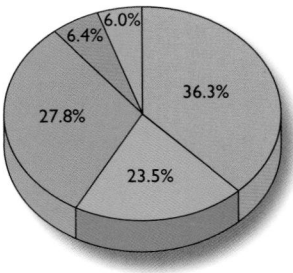

WORLD ENERGY CONSUMPTION
- OIL
- GAS
- COAL
- HYDRO
- NUCLEAR

▲ *The diagram shows the proportion of world energy consumption in 2006 by form. Total energy consumption was 10,878 million tonnes of oil equivalent. Wood, peat and animal wastes, plus renewable forms, such as wind power, are locally important but they comprise only 0.8% of the total.*

SELECTED MINERAL PRODUCTION STATISTICS
(percentage of world total output, 2006)

Bauxite		Diamonds	
Australia	34.7%	Australia	29.4%
Brazil	11.9%	Congo (D.R.)	28.2%
China	11.3%	Russia	17.6%
Guinea	8.6%	S. Africa	10.6%
Jamaica	8.4%	Botswana	9.4%

Gold		Iron ore	
S. Africa	10.8%	China	30.8%
Australia	10.4%	Brazil	17.8%
USA	10.4%	Australia	16.0%
China	9.6%	India	8.9%
Peru	8.4%	Russia	6.2%

Manganese		Zinc	
S. Africa	20.0%	China	25.0%
Brazil	14.5%	Australia	14.0%
Gabon	14.1%	Peru	12.1%
Australia	13.6%	Canada	7.3%
China	10.9%	USA	7.3%

▼ MINERAL DISTRIBUTION

The map shows the richest sources of the most important minerals. Major mineral locations are named. Undersea deposits, most of which are considered inaccessible, are not shown.

▽ GOLD
⬭ SILVER
◆ DIAMONDS
▽ TUNGSTEN
● IRON ORE
■ NICKEL
⏷ CHROME
▲ MANGANESE
□ COBALT
▲ MOLYBDENUM
■ COPPER
▲ LEAD
● BAUXITE
▽ TIN
◆ ZINC
⏷ MERCURY

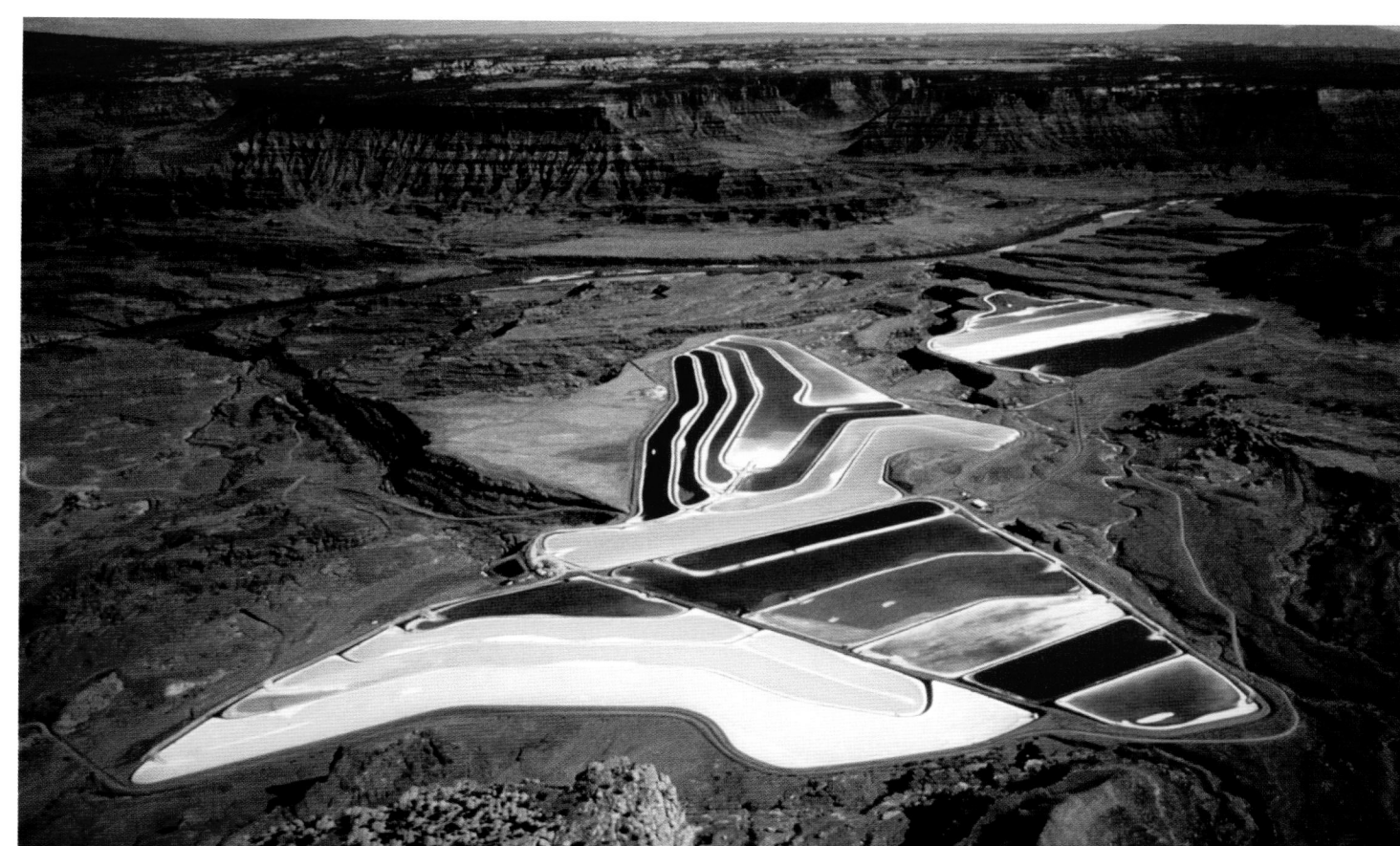

▲ *Potash mines in Utah, United States*

Potash is a mineral used mainly to make fertilizers. Much of it comes from mines where deposits formed when ancient seas dried up are exploited. Potash is also extracted from salt lakes.

ALTERNATIVE ENERGY

Other sources of energy are therefore required. Besides nuclear energy, the main alternative to fossil fuels is water power. The costs of building dams and hydroelectric power stations are high, though hydroelectric production is comparatively cheap. But the creation of reservoirs uproots people and destroys natural habitats. Water power is also suitable only in areas with plenty of rivers and steep slopes, such as Norway.

In Brazil, alcohol made from sugar has been used to fuel cars. Initially, this government-backed policy met with success. However, it proved to be expensive and the production of ethanol-fuelled cars was halted until Brazil struck a deal with Germany in the early 2000s.

In 2006, President George W. Bush announced that ethanol production in the United States should increase in the next 10 years to reduce his country's dependency on imported oil.

Other forms of energy, which are renewable and cleaner than fossil fuels, are winds, sea waves, the rise and fall of tides, and geothermal power. While renewable energy sources are attractive, some experts doubt whether they can provide sufficient energy on their own.

MINERALS FOR INDUSTRY

In addition to energy, manufacturing industries need raw materials, including minerals, and these natural resources are also being used in such huge quantities that some experts have predicted shortages of some of them before long.

Manufacturers depend on supplies of about 80 minerals. Some, such as bauxite (aluminium ore) and iron, are abundant, but others are scarce or are found only in deposits that are uneconomical to mine. Many experts advocate a policy of recycling scrap metal, including aluminium, chromium, copper, lead, nickel and zinc. This practice would reduce pollution and conserve the energy required for extracting and refining mineral ores.

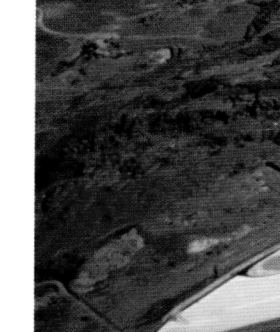

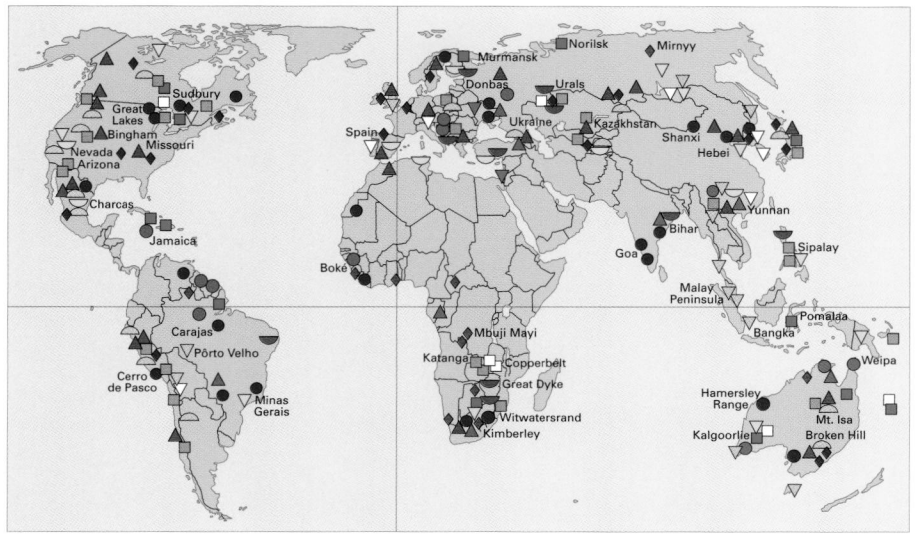

WORLD ECONOMIES

In 2006, Burundi had a per capita GNI (Gross National Income) of US$100, as compared with Norway, whose per capita GNI was $68,440, according to the World Bank. These figures indicate the vast gap between the economies and standards of living of the two countries.

The GNI includes the GDP (Gross Domestic Product), which consists of the total output of goods and services in a country in a given year, plus net exports – that is, the value of goods and services sold abroad less the value of foreign goods and services used in the country in the same year. The GNI divided by the population gives a country's GNI per capita. In low-income developing countries, agriculture makes a high contribution to the GNI. For example, in Ethiopia, 48% of the country's GDP came from agriculture. On the other hand, industry was small-scale and contributed only 10.9% of the GDP. By comparison, in high-income economies, the percentage contribution of manufacturing far exceeds that of agriculture.

▼ *Hard-disk assembly factory*

The manufacture of computer equipment and computer software is a fairly new industrial phenomenon. In Asia, high-tech industries have developed quickly, helping relatively poor developing countries to achieve rapid economic growth.

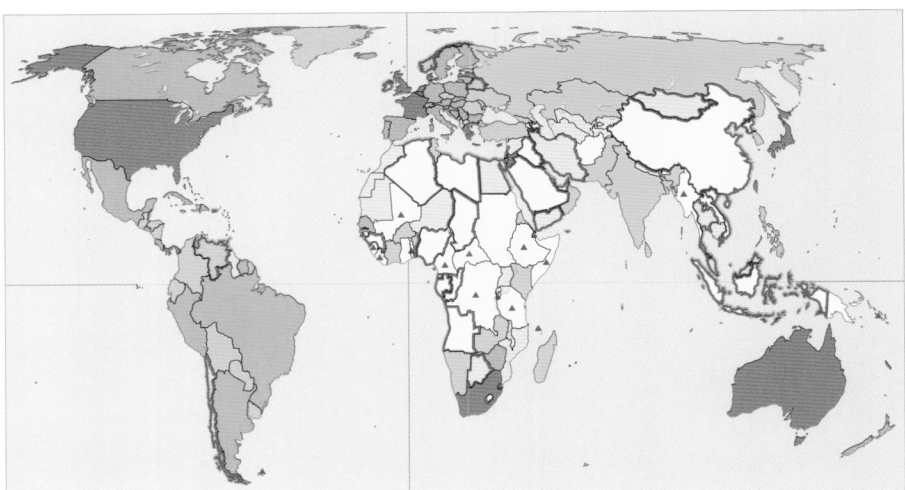

INDUSTRIALIZATION

The Industrial Revolution began in Britain in the late 18th century. Before that time, most people worked on farms. But with the Industrial Revolution came factories, using machines that could manufacture goods much faster and more cheaply than those made by cottage industries that already existed.

The Industrial Revolution soon spread to several countries in mainland Europe and the United States and, by the late 19th century, it had reached Canada, Japan and Russia. At first, industrial development was based on such areas as coalfields or ironfields. But in the 20th

IMPORTANCE OF THE SERVICE INDUSTRY
Percentage of total GDP from the service sector (2007).

- OVER 70%
- 60–70%
- 50–60%
- 40–50%
- UNDER 40%
- NO DATA AVAILABLE
- OVER 40% OF TOTAL GDP FROM THE INDUSTRIAL SECTOR
- OVER 40% OF TOTAL GDP FROM THE AGRICULTURAL SECTOR

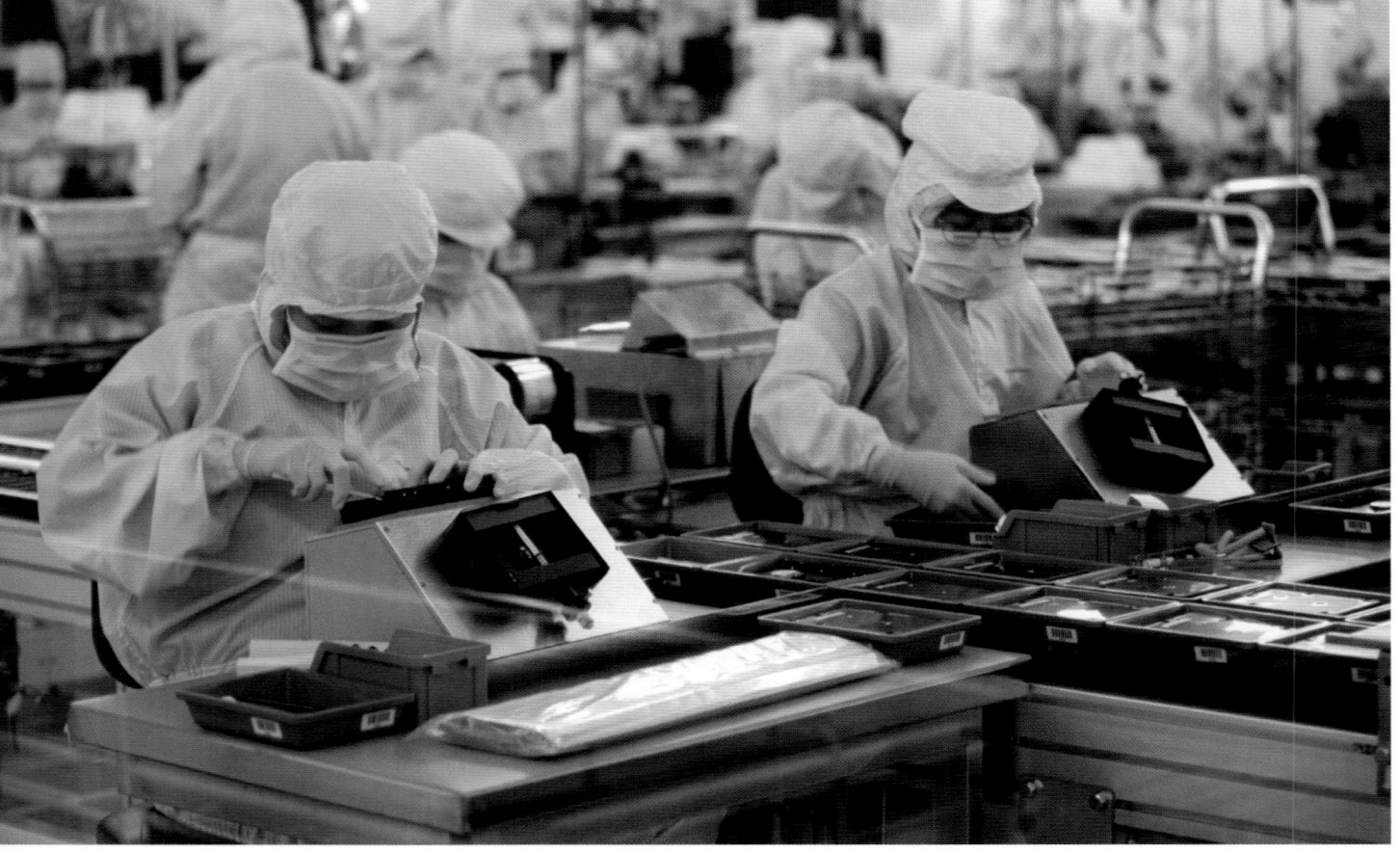

GROSS NATIONAL INCOME PER CAPITA IN US$ (2006)	
1 Luxembourg	$71,240
2 Norway	$68,440
3 Switzerland	$58,050
4 Denmark	$52,110
5 Iceland	$49,960
6 Ireland	$44,830
7 United States	$44,710
8 Sweden	$43,530
9 Netherlands	$43,050
10 Finland	$41,360
11 United Kingdom	$40,560
12 Austria	$39,750
13 Japan	$38,630
14 Belgium	$38,460
15 Germany	$36,810
16 Canada	$36,650
17 France	$36,560
18 Australia	$35,860
19 Italy	$31,990
20 Kuwait	$30,630

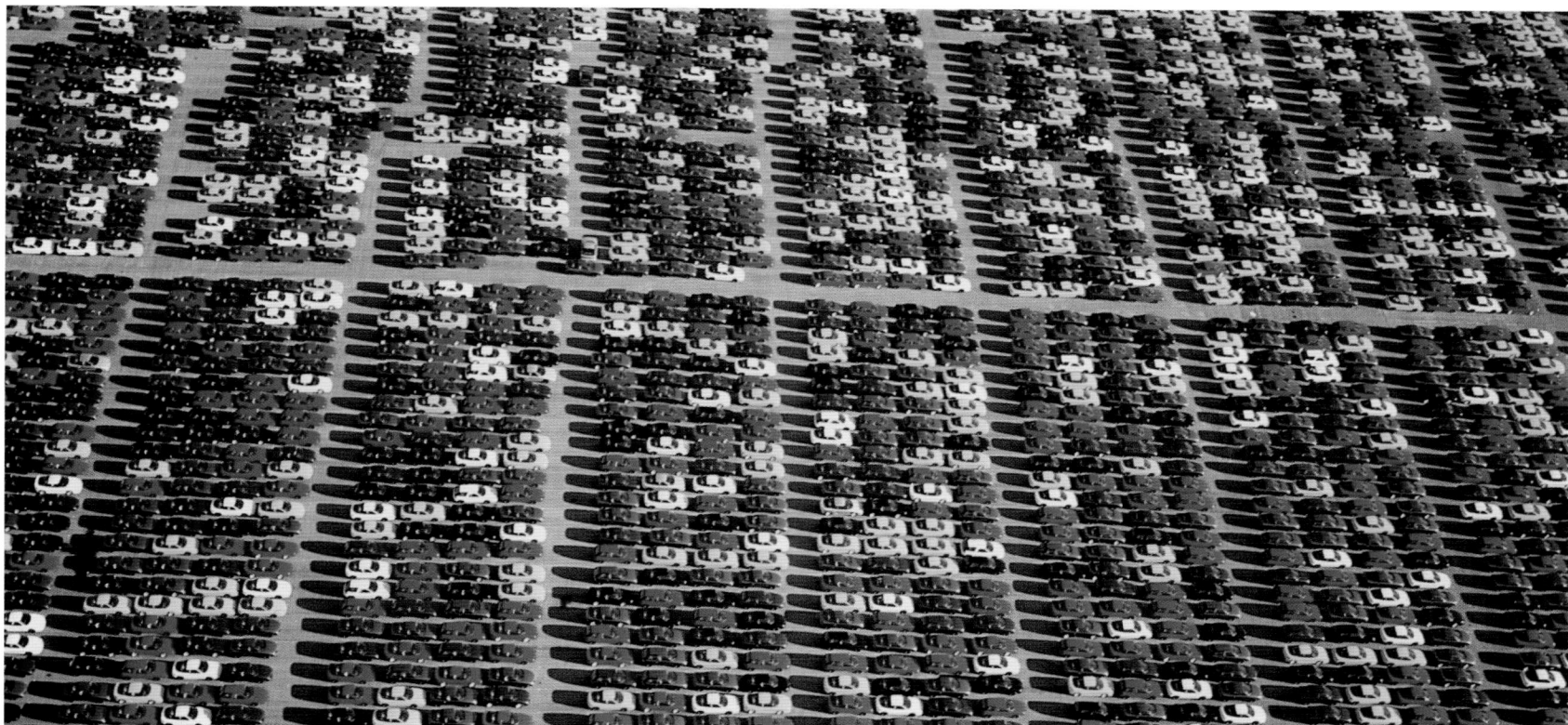

century, the use of oil, which is easy to transport along pipelines, made it possible for industries to be set up anywhere.

Some nations, such as Switzerland, became industrialized even though they lacked natural resources. They depended instead on the specialized skills of their workers. This same pattern applies today. Some countries with rich natural resources, such as Mexico (with a per capita GNI in 2006 of US$7,830), lag far behind Japan ($38,630) and Malta ($15,310), which lack resources and have to import many of the materials they need to sustain their manufacturing industries.

SERVICE INDUSTRIES

Experts often refer to high-income countries as industrial economies. But manufacturing employs only one in six workers in the United States, one in five in Britain, and one in three in Germany and Japan.

▲ *New cars awaiting transportation, Los Angeles, USA*
Cars are the most important single manufactured item in world trade, followed by vehicle parts and engines. The world's leading car producers are Japan, the United States, Germany and France.

In most developed economies, the percentage of manufacturing jobs has fallen in recent years, while jobs in service industries have risen. In Britain, between 1970 and the early 2000s, the proportion of jobs in manufacturing fell by about two-thirds, while jobs in the service sector rose by more than a half. Similar, if less rapid, changes have taken place in most industrial economies. Service industries now account for well over half of the jobs in the generally prosperous countries which make up the OECD (Organization for Economic Co-operation and Development). Instead of being called the 'industrial' economies, these countries might be better named the 'service' economies.

Service industries offer a wide range of jobs and many of them require high educational qualifications. These include finance, insurance and high-tech industries, such as computer programming, entertainment and telecommunications. Service industries also include marketing and advertising, which are essential if the cars and television sets made by manufacturers are to be sold. Another valuable service industry is tourism; in some countries, such as the Gambia, it is the major foreign-exchange earner. Trade in services plays a crucial part in world economies. Service industries now account for more than a fifth of world trade.

THE WORKFORCE
Percentage of men and women over 15 years old in employment, selected countries.

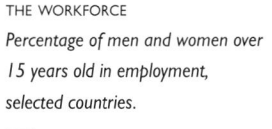

MEN
WOMEN

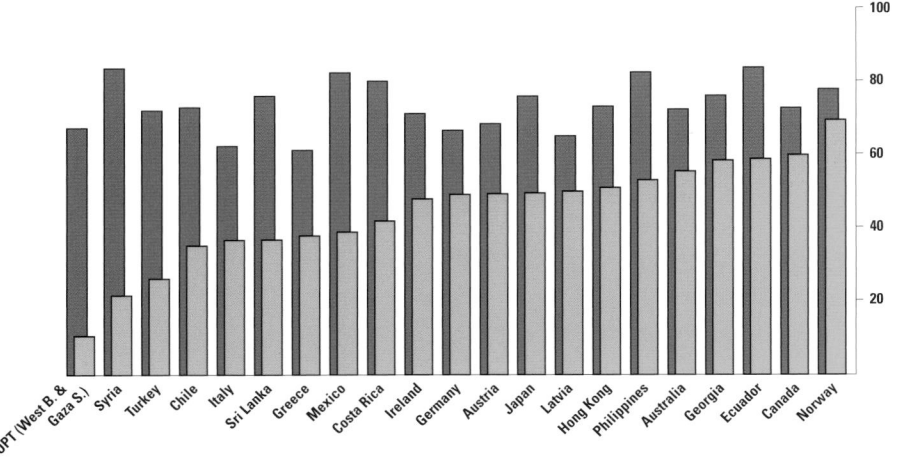

TRADE AND COMMERCE

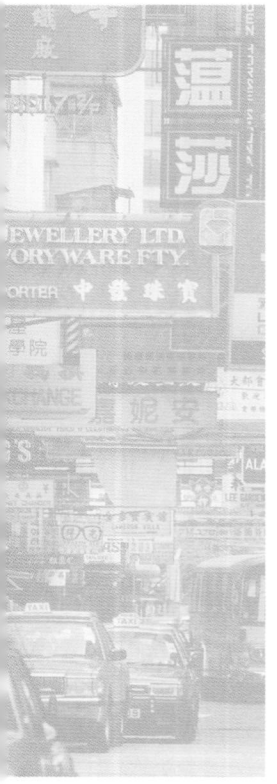

The establishment of the WTO (World Trade Organization) on 1 January 1995 was the latest step in the long history of world trade. The WTO was set up by the eighth round of negotiations, popularly called the 'Uruguay round', conducted by the General Agreement on Tariffs and Trade (GATT). This treaty was signed by representatives of 125 governments in April 1994. The membership reached 150 when Vietnam joined in January 2007.

GATT was first established in 1948. Its initial aim was to produce a charter to create a body called the International Trade Organization. This body never came into being. Instead, GATT, acting as an *ad hoc* agency, pioneered a series of agreements aimed at liberalizing world trade by reducing tariffs on imports and other obstacles to free trade.

▼ *New York City Stock Exchange, United States*

Stock exchanges, where stocks and shares are sold and bought, are important in channelling savings and investments to companies and governments. The world's largest stock exchange is in Tokyo, Japan.

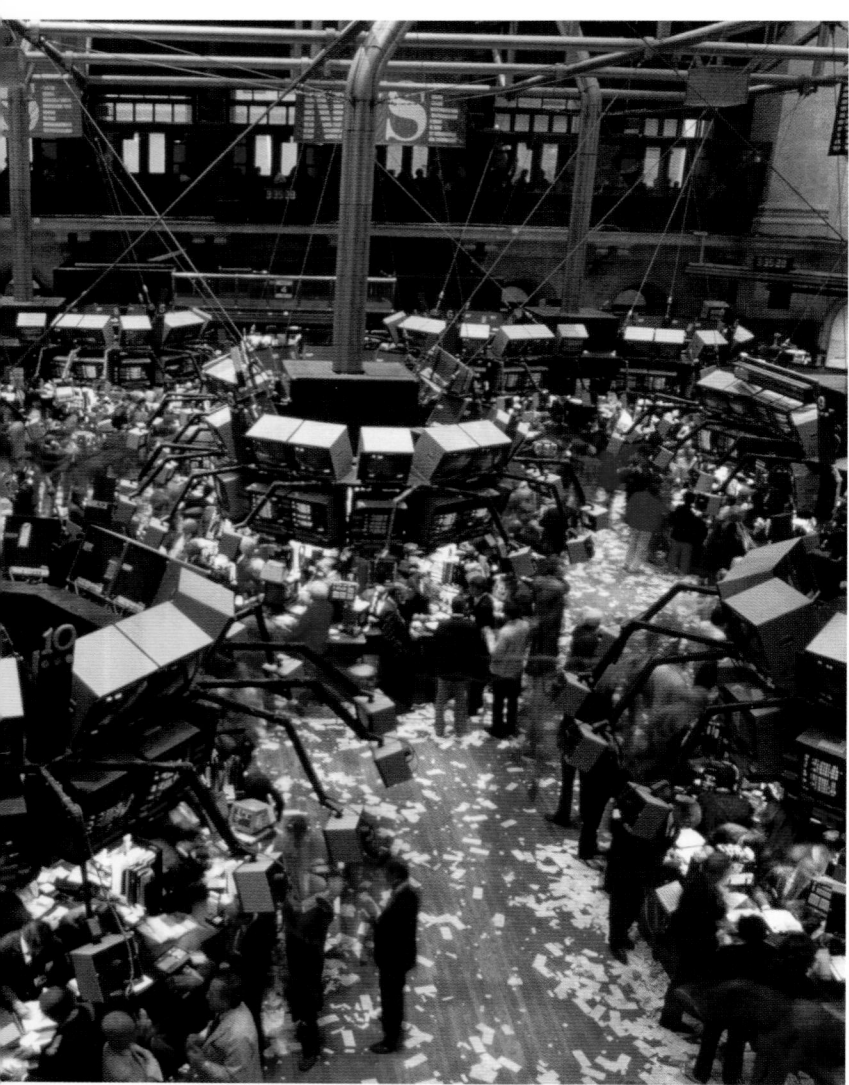

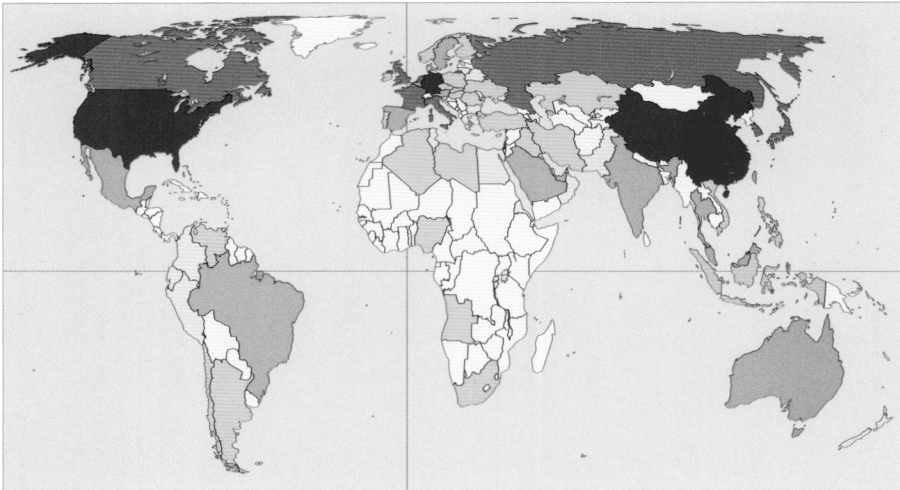

GATT's objectives were based on the belief that international trade creates wealth. Trade occurs because the world's resources are not distributed evenly between countries, and, in theory, free trade means that every country should concentrate on what it can do best and purchase from others goods and services that they can supply more cheaply. In practice, however, free trade may cause unemployment when imported goods are cheaper than those produced within the country.

Trade is sometimes an important factor in world politics, especially when trade sanctions are applied against countries whose actions incur the disapproval of the international community. For example, in the 1990s, world-wide trade sanctions were imposed on Serbia because of its involvement in the civil war in Bosnia-Herzegovina.

CHANGING TRADE PATTERNS

The early 16th century, when Europeans began to divide the world into huge empires, opened up a new era in international trade. By the 19th century, the colonial powers, who were among the first industrial powers, promoted trade with their colonies, from which they obtained unprocessed raw materials, such as food, natural fibres, minerals and timber. In return, they shipped clothes, shoes and other cheap items to the colonies.

From the late 19th century until the early 1950s, primary products dominated world trade, with oil becoming the leading item in the latter part of this period. Many developing countries still depend heavily on the export of one or two primary products, such as coffee or iron ore, but overall the proportion of primary products in world trade has fallen since the 1950s. Today the most important elements

WORLD TRADE

Percentage share of total world exports by value (2007).

- ■ OVER 5%
- ■ 2.5–5%
- ■ 1–2.5%
- ■ 0.25–1%
- □ 0.1–0.25%
- □ UNDER 0.1%

The world's leading trading nations, according to the combined value of their exports and imports, are the United States, Germany, Japan, France and the United Kingdom.

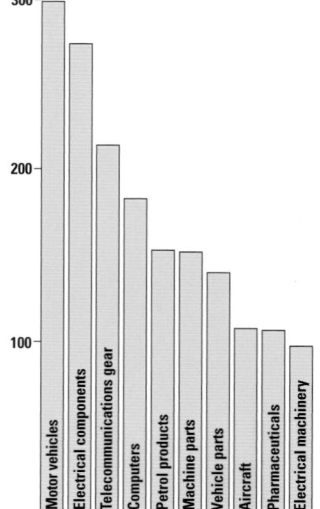

TRADED PRODUCTS

The diagram shows major manufactures traded by value in billions of US$. Manufactures in total comprise 74% of the world's total trade, the value of which was $13,870 billion in 2007.

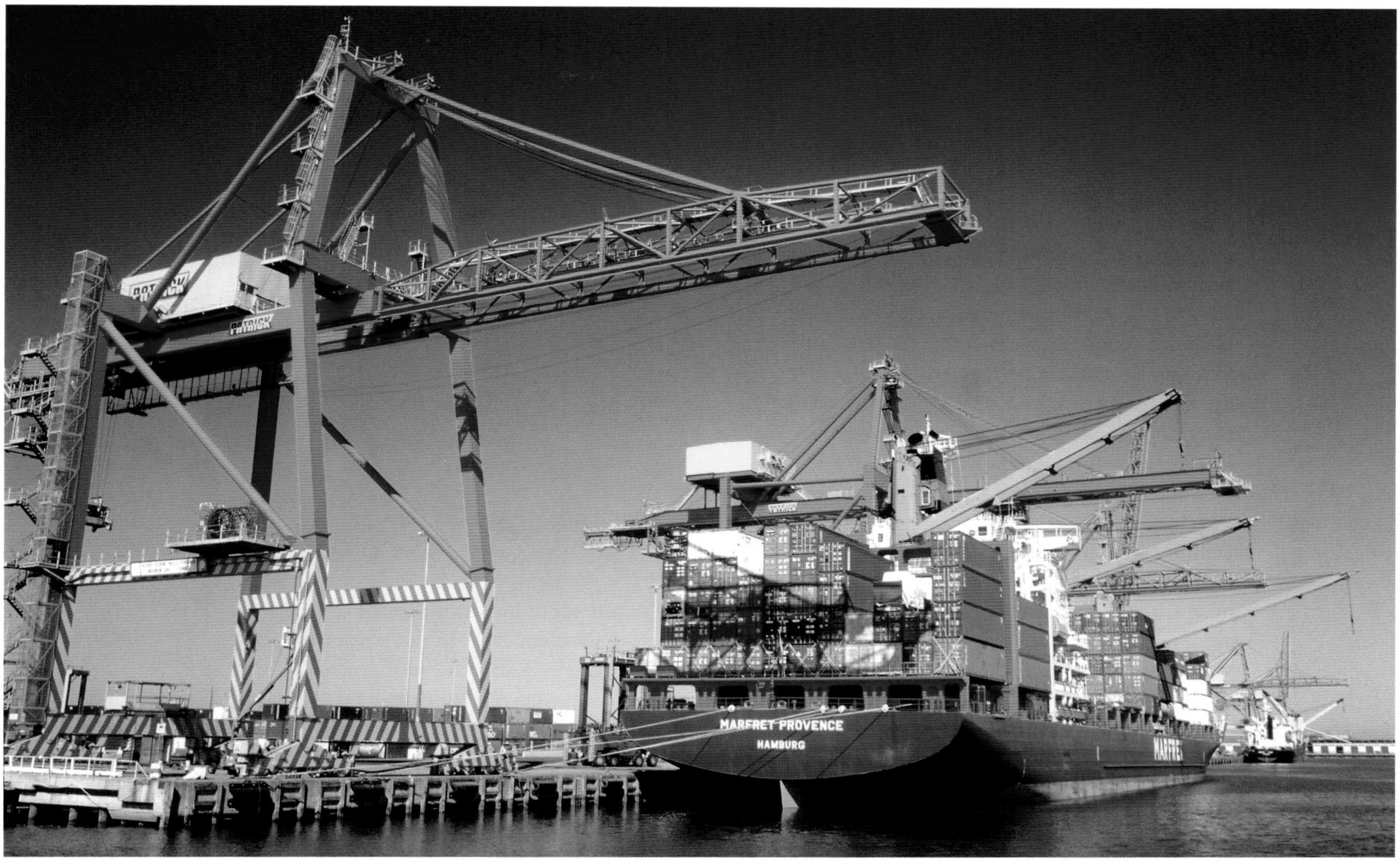

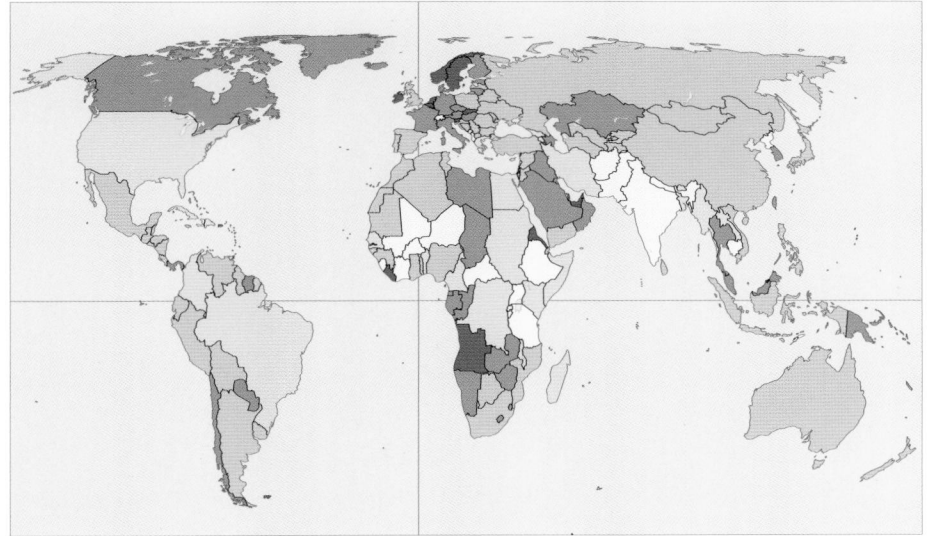

in world trade are manufactures and semi-manufactures, exchanged mainly between the industrialized nations.

DEPENDENCE ON TRADE
Value of exports as a percentage of GDP (2007).

- OVER 50% GDP FROM EXPORTS
- 25–50% GDP FROM EXPORTS
- 10–25% GDP FROM EXPORTS
- 5–10% GDP FROM EXPORTS
- UNDER 5% GDP FROM EXPORTS
- NO DATA AVAILABLE

THE WORLD'S MARKETS

Private companies conduct most of world trade, but government policies affect it. Governments which believe that certain industries are strategic, or essential for the country's future, may impose tariffs on imports, or import quotas to limit the volume of imports, if they are thought to be undercutting the domestic industries.

For example, the United States has argued that

▲ *Melbourne, Australia*

World trade depends on transport. Containerization, introduced in the 1950s, reduced the risk of damage to cargo and cut the time and cost of loading and unloading.

Japan has greater access to its markets than the United States has to Japan's. This might have led the United States to resort to protectionism, but instead the United States remains committed to free trade despite occasional disputes.

Other problems in international trade occur when governments give subsidies to its producers, who can then export products at low prices. Another difficulty, called 'dumping', occurs when products are sold at below the market price in order to gain a market share. One of the aims of the newly-created WTO is the phasing out of government subsidies for agricultural products, though the world's poorest countries will be exempt from many of the WTO's most severe regulations.

Governments are also concerned about the volume of imports and exports, and most countries keep records of international transactions. When the total value of goods and services imported exceeds the value of goods and services exported, then the country has a deficit in its balance of payments. Large deficits can weaken a country's economy.

TRAVEL AND COMMUNICATIONS

By the early 21st century, millions of people were linked to an 'information super-highway' called the Internet. Equipped with a personal computer, an electricity supply, a telephone and a modem, people are able to communicate with others all over the world. People can now send messages by e-mail (electronic mail), they can engage in electronic discussions, contacting people with similar interests, and engage in 'chat lines', which are the latest equivalent of telephone conferences.

These new developments are likely to affect the working lives of people everywhere, enabling them to work at home whilst having many of the facilities that are available in an office. The Internet is part of an ongoing and astonishingly rapid evolution in the fields of communications and transport.

TRANSPORT

Around 200 years ago, most people never travelled far from their birthplace, but today we are much more mobile. Cars and buses now provide convenient forms of transport for many millions of people, huge ships transport massive cargoes around the world, and jet airliners can transport high-value goods as well as holiday-makers to almost any part of the world.

Land transport of freight has developed greatly since the start of the Industrial Revolution.

▼ *Eurostar travel*

High-speed Eurostar services connect London to Paris and Brussels via the $15 billion Channel Tunnel, linking the UK to mainland Europe. Only 13 years after the tunnel opened in 1994, Eurostar carried about 8.2 million passengers per year.

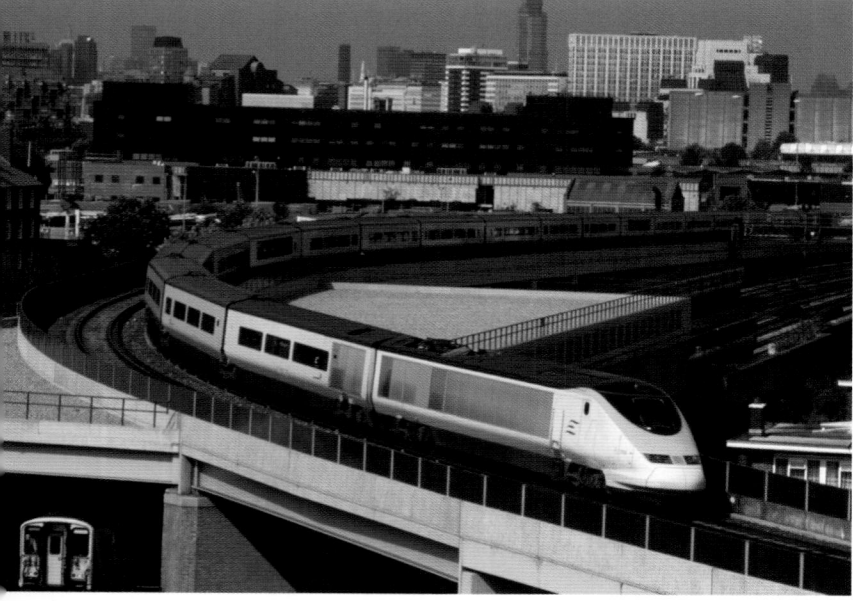

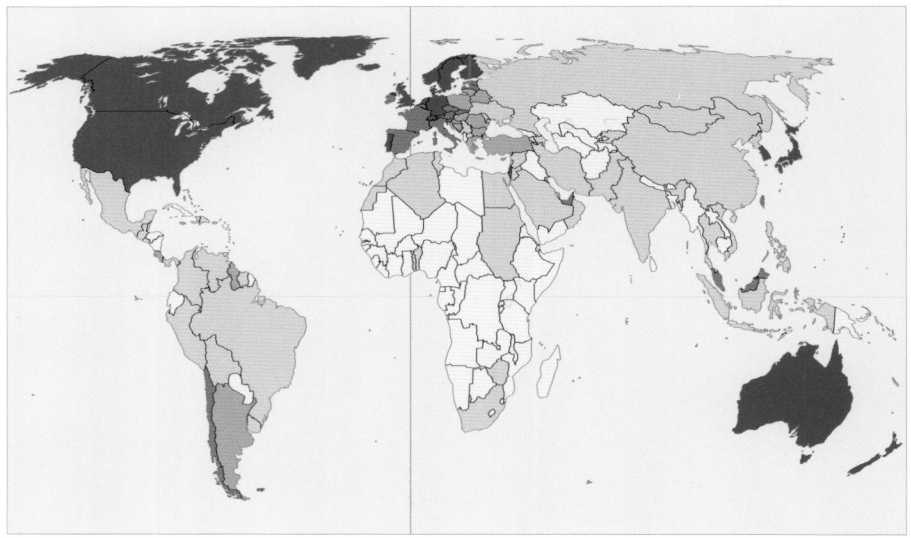

Canals, which became important in the 18th century, could not compete with rail transport in the 19th century. Rail transport remains important, but, during the 20th century, it suffered from competition with road transport, which is cheaper and has the advantage of carrying materials and goods from door to door.

Road transport causes pollution and the burning of fuels creates greenhouse gases that contribute to global warming. Yet privately owned cars are now the leading form of passenger traffic in developed nations, especially for journeys of less than around 400 km [250 miles]. Car owners do not have to suffer the inconvenience of waiting for public transport, such as buses, though they often have to endure traffic jams at peak travel times.

Ocean passenger traffic is now modest, but ships carry the bulk of international trade. Huge oil tankers and bulk grain carriers now ply the oceans with their cargoes, while container ships carry mixed cargoes. Containers are boxes built to international standards that contain cargo. Containers are easy to handle, and so they

INTERNET USERS

Percentage of the total population using the Internet (2005).

- OVER 60%
- 40–60%
- 20–40%
- 5–20%
- UNDER 5%
- NO DATA AVAILABLE

SELECTED NEWSPAPER CIRCULATION FIGURES (2006)

France		**Russia**	
Le Monde	314,000	Argumenty i Fakty	2,611,000
Le Figaro	322,000	Pravda	729,000
		Izvestia	246,000
Germany			
Bild	3,867,000	**Spain**	
Süddeutsche Zeitung	442,000	El Pais	435,000
India		**United Kingdom**	
The Times of India	1,680,000	The Sun	3,032,000
The Hindustan Times	1,108,000	Daily Mail	2,342,000
		Daily Mirror	1,542,000
Italy		The Daily Telegraph	896,000
Corriere della Sera	685,000	Daily Express	759,000
La Repubblica	622,000		
La Stampa	307,000	**United States**	
		USA Today	2,270,000
Japan		The Wall Street Journal	2,043,000
Yomiuri Shimbun	14,067,000	The New York Times	1,087,000
Asahi Shimbun	12,121,000	Los Angeles Times	776,000

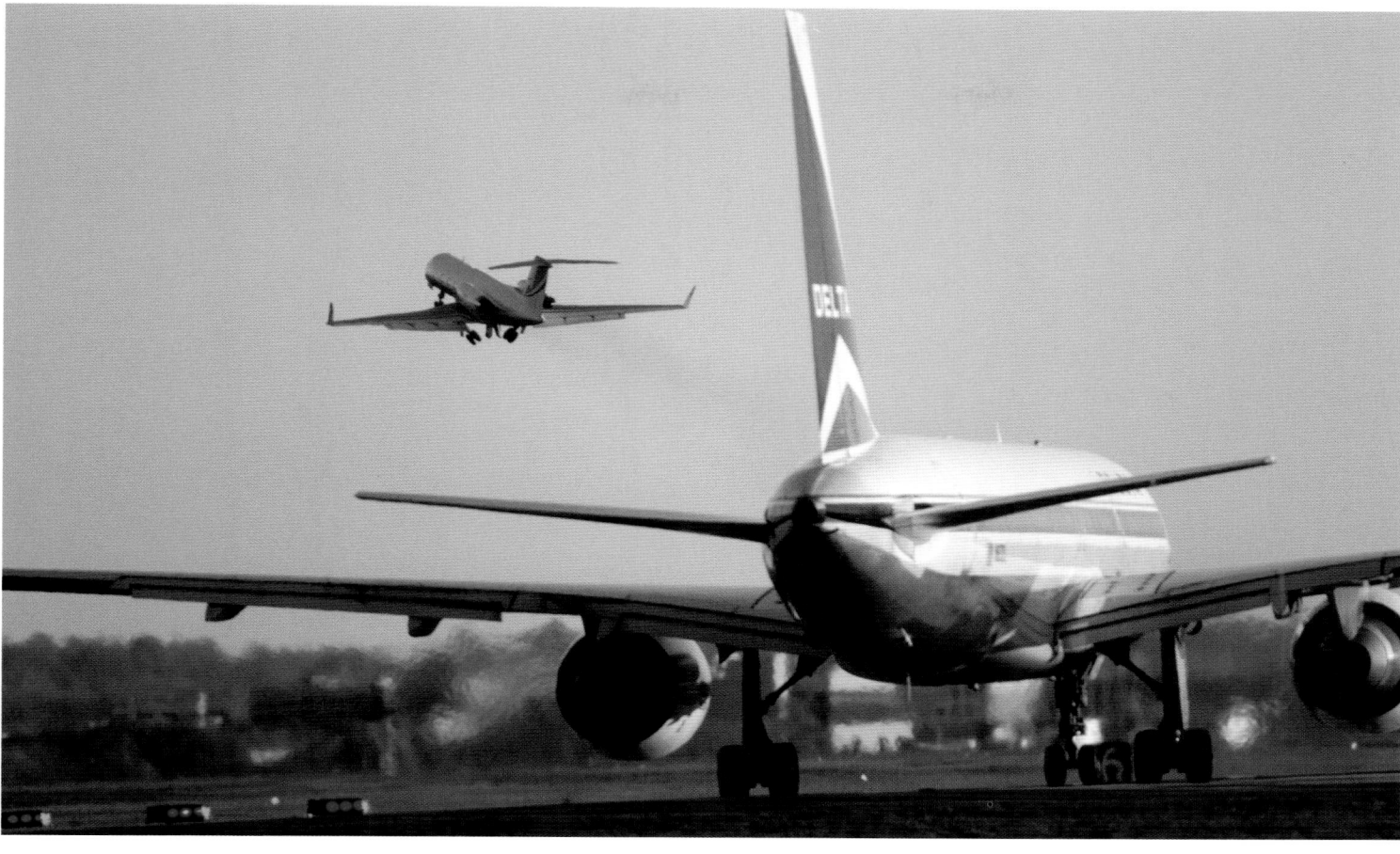

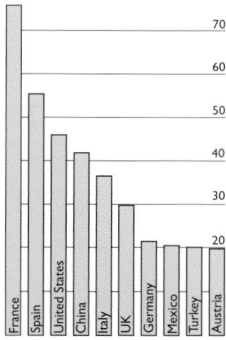

TOP TOURIST DESTINATIONS

International tourist arrivals in millions (2005)

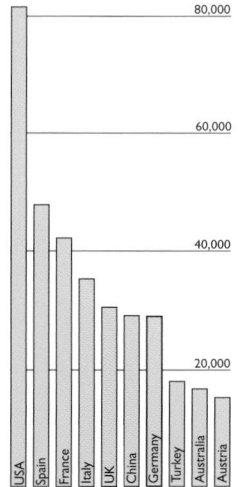

Countries receiving the most from overseas tourism, US\$ million (2005).

reduce shipping costs, speed up deliveries and cut losses caused by breakages. Most large ports now have the facilities to handle containers.

Air transport is suitable for carrying goods that are expensive, light and compact, or perishable. However, because of the high costs of air freight, it is most suitable for carrying passengers along long-distance routes around the world. Through air travel, international tourism has become a major industry, despite anxieties about aircraft pollution that contributes to global warming.

COMMUNICATIONS

After humans first began to communicate by using the spoken word, the next great stage in the development of communications was the invention of writing around 5,500 years ago.

The invention of movable type in the mid-15th century led to the mass production of books and, in the early 17th century, the first newspapers. Newspapers now play an important part in the mass communication of information, although today radio and, even more important, television have led to a decline in the circulation of newspapers in many parts of the world.

The most recent developments have occurred in the field of electronics. Artificial communications satellites now circle the planet, relaying radio, television, telegraph and telephone signals. This enables people to watch events on the far side of the globe as they are happening. Electronic equipment is also used in many other ways, such as in navigation systems used in air,

▲ *Commercial jet airliners, Washington, DC, United States*
Air travel has transformed world tourism. However, the terrorist attacks by suicide bombers on the United States on 11 September 2001 led to greater security checks at airports. Falls in passenger numbers were another consequence of the hijackings.

sea and space, and also in modern weaponry, as shown vividly in the television coverage of Middle Eastern conflicts in the 21st century.

THE AGE OF COMPUTERS

One of the most remarkable applications of electronics is in the field of computers. Computers are now making a huge contribution to communications. They are able to process data at incredibly high speeds and can store vast quantities of information. For example, the work of weather forecasters has been greatly improved now that computers can process the enormous amount of data required for a single weather forecast. They also have many other applications in such fields as business, government, science and medicine.

Through the Internet, computers provide a free interchange of news and views around the world. But the dangers of misuse, such as the exchange of pornographic images, have led to calls for censorship. Censorship, however, is a blunt weapon, which can be used by authoritarian governments to suppress the free exchange of information that the new information superhighway makes possible.

THE WORLD TODAY

The early years of the 20th century witnessed the exploration of Antarctica, the last uncharted continent. Today, less than 100 years later, tourists are able to take cruises to the icy southern continent, while almost no part of the globe is inaccessible to the determined traveller. Improved transport and images from space have made our world seem smaller.

A DIVIDED WORLD

Between the end of World War II in 1945 and the late 1980s, the world was divided, politically and economically, into three main groups: the developed countries or Western democracies, with their free enterprise or mixed economies; the centrally planned or Communist countries; and the developing countries or Third World.

This division became obsolete when the former Soviet Union and its old European allies, together with the 'special economic zones' in eastern China, began the transition from centrally planned to free-enterprise economies. This left the world divided into two broad camps: the prosperous developed countries and the poorer developing countries. The simplest way of distinguishing between the groups is with reference to their per capita GNIs (Gross National Incomes).

The World Bank divides the developing countries into three main groups. At the bottom are the low-income economies, including India and most of sub-Saharan Africa. This group has a population of more than 2.3 billion. However, according to the World Bank, the average per

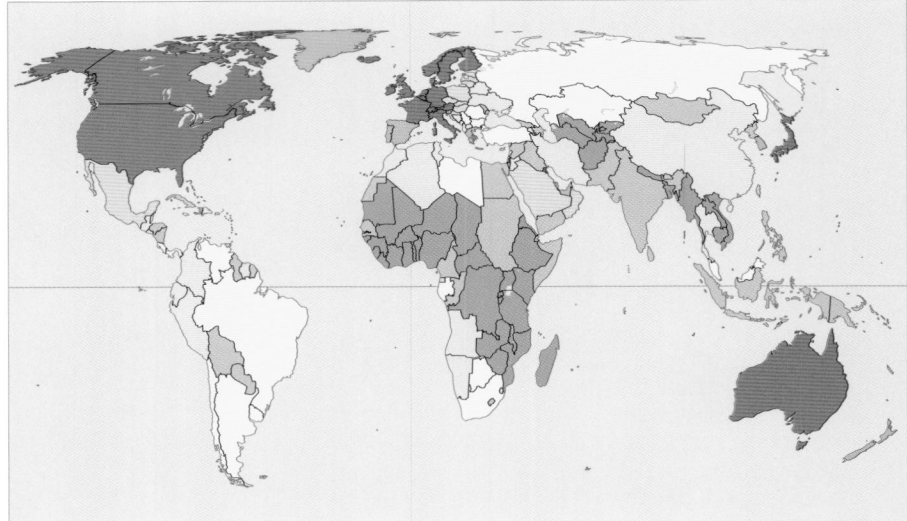

capita Gross National Income in 2006 was only US$649, with some countries as low as $100. Two other groups, with a combined population of around 3 billion people, are the lower-middle-income economies, with an average per capita GNI of $2,038, and the upper-middle-income economies with an average per capita GNI of $5,913. The high-income economies, with around 1 billion people, have an average (and rising) per capita GNI of $36,508.

ECONOMIC AND SOCIAL CONTRASTS

Other factors, such as rates of population growth, are also important. The low- and middle-income economies have a population growth of about 2%, while the average growth rate in the high-income economies is about 1%. While the populations of low- and middle-income economies are young, youths make up less than one-fifth of the populations of high-income economies, while over-65s make up one-seventh.

Stark contrasts exist worldwide in the quality of life. Generally, the people in Western Europe

▼ *East African tourism*

Improved transport, including the use of four-wheel drive vehicles, has led to a boom in tourism in many developing regions, such as East Africa. But terrorist incidents may slow down the development of tourism in some areas.

GROSS NATIONAL INCOME PER CAPITA
The value of total income divided by the population (2006).

- OVER 400% OF WORLD AVERAGE
- 200–400% OF WORLD AVERAGE
- 100–200% OF WORLD AVERAGE
- 50–100% OF WORLD AVERAGE
- 25–50% OF WORLD AVERAGE
- 10–25% OF WORLD AVERAGE
- UNDER 10% OF WORLD AVERAGE
- NO DATA AVAILABLE

RICHEST COUNTRIES (GNI PER CAPITA, 2006)

Luxembourg	US$71,240
Norway	US$68,440
Switzerland	US$58,050
Denmark	US$52,110
Iceland	US$49,960

POOREST COUNTRIES (GNI PER CAPITA, 2006)

Burundi	US$100
Congo (Dem. Rep.)	US$130
Liberia	US$130
Ethiopia	US$170
Guinea-Bissau	US$190

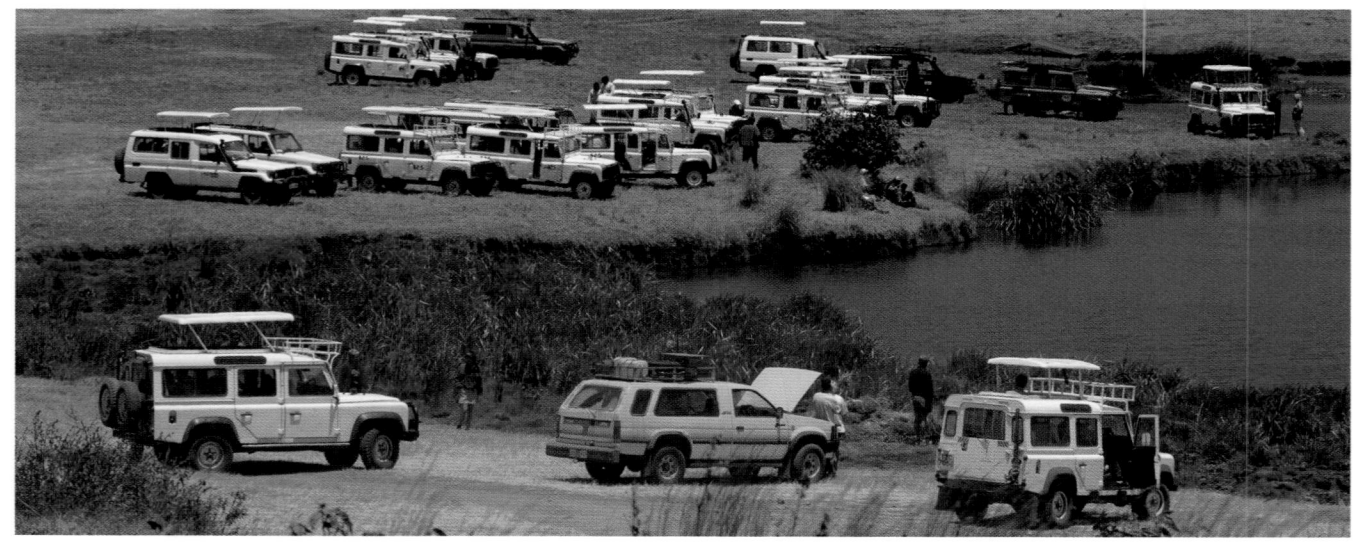

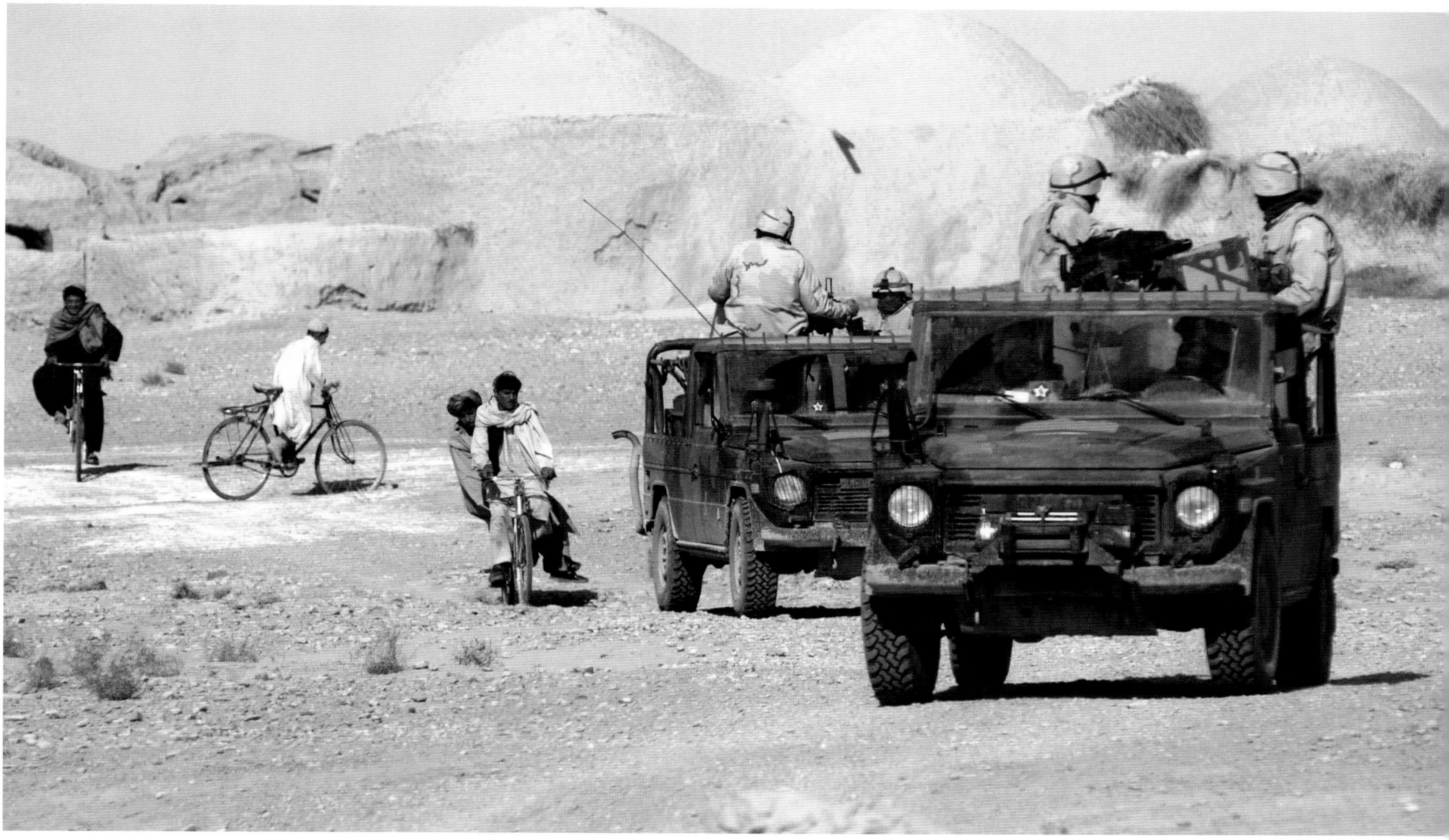

and North America are better fed, healthier, and have more cars and better homes than the people in low- and middle-income economies.

In 2006, the World Health Organization stated that, due partly to AIDS and partly to poverty, average life expectancy at birth in Zimbabwe had fallen to 37 years for men and 34 years for women. By contrast, the average life expectancy in Japan was 82 years. Illiteracy rates in low-income economies are also substantially lower for women than for men, whereas, in high-income countries, illiteracy is rare for both sexes.

FUTURE DEVELOPMENT

In the last 50 years, despite all the aid supplied to developing countries, much of the world still suffers from poverty and economic backwardness. Some countries are even poorer now than they were a generation ago.

However, several factors suggest that poor countries may find progress easier in the 21st century. For example, technology is now more readily transferable between countries, while improved transport and communications make it easier for countries to take part in the world economy. But industrial development could lead to an increase in global pollution. Hence, any strategy for global economic expansion must also take account of environmental factors.

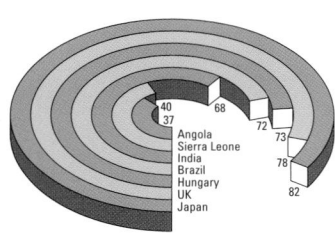

▲ *Years of life expectancy at birth, selected countries (2007).*
The chart shows the contrasting range of average life expectancies at birth for a range of countries, including both low-income and high-income economies. Generally, improved health services are raising life expectancies. On average, women live longer than men, even in the poorer developing countries.

▲ *Operation Enduring Freedom, Afghanistan*
A joint patrol of US Marines and Army soldiers is seen here patrolling through the village of Cem, Afghanistan, some 10 km [6 miles] from the airport near Kandahar, in January 2002.

A WORLD IN CONFLICT

The end of the Cold War held out hopes of a new world order. But ethnic, religious and other rivalries have subsequently led to appalling violence in places as diverse as the Balkan peninsula, Israel and the Palestinian territories, and Rwanda–Burundi. Then, on 11 September 2001, the attack on those symbols of the economic and military might of the United States – the World Trade Center and the Pentagon Building – demonstrated that nowhere on Earth is safe from attack by extremists prepared to sacrifice their lives in pursuit of their aims.

The dangers posed by terrorist groups or rogue states has forced many countries into new alliances. International co-operation is also vital in combating global warming, which some experts believe is the greatest danger now threatening the world. Unless effective action is taken, they warn that the world faces such problems as falls in food production, the spread of diseases, increasing extreme weather phenomena, and the flooding of coastal plains.

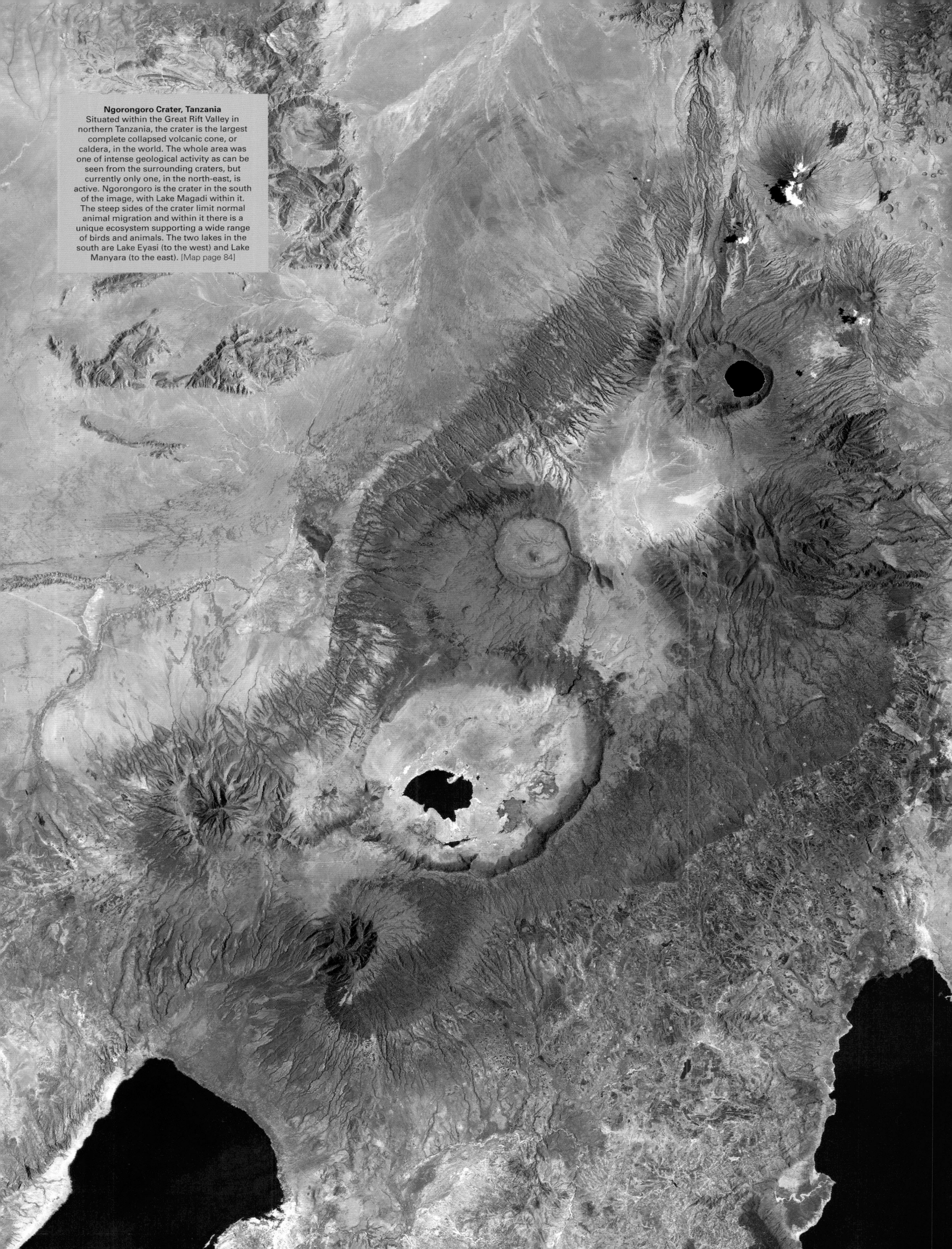

Ngorongoro Crater, Tanzania
Situated within the Great Rift Valley in northern Tanzania, the crater is the largest complete collapsed volcanic cone, or caldera, in the world. The whole area was one of intense geological activity as can be seen from the surrounding craters, but currently only one, in the north-east, is active. Ngorongoro is the crater in the south of the image, with Lake Magadi within it. The steep sides of the crater limit normal animal migration and within it there is a unique ecosystem supporting a wide range of birds and animals. The two lakes in the south are Lake Eyasi (to the west) and Lake Manyara (to the east). [Map page 84]

WORLD MAPS

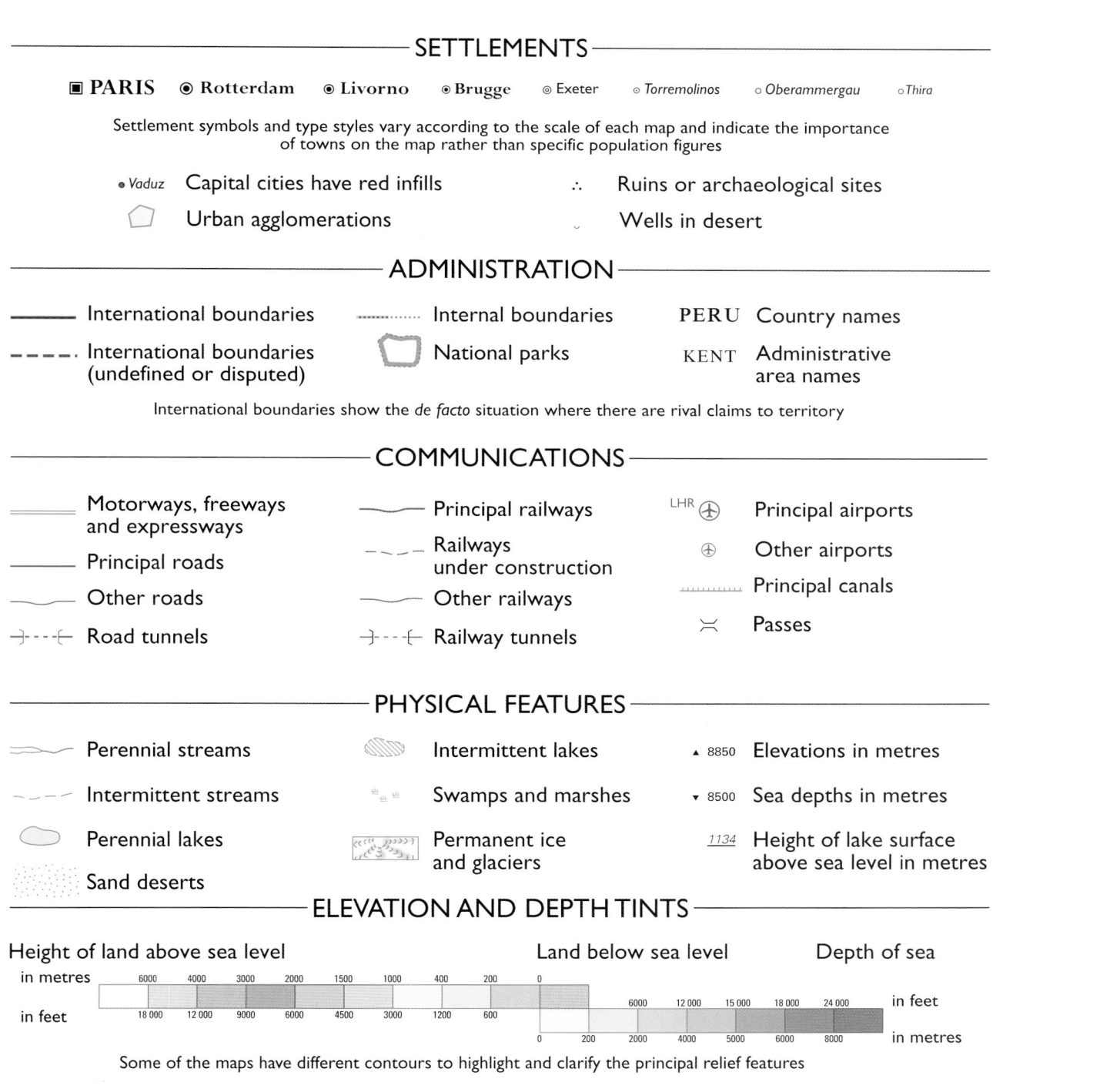

SETTLEMENTS

■ **PARIS**   ◉ **Rotterdam**   ◉ **Livorno**   ◉ Brugge   ◉ Exeter   ○ Torremolinos   ○ Oberammergau   ○ Thira

Settlement symbols and type styles vary according to the scale of each map and indicate the importance of towns on the map rather than specific population figures

• Vaduz   Capital cities have red infills   ∴   Ruins or archaeological sites

⬠   Urban agglomerations   ⌣   Wells in desert

ADMINISTRATION

——— International boundaries   ·········· Internal boundaries   PERU   Country names

- - - - · International boundaries   ⬠ National parks   KENT   Administrative
(undefined or disputed)   area names

International boundaries show the *de facto* situation where there are rival claims to territory

COMMUNICATIONS

═══ Motorways, freeways   ——— Principal railways   ^LHR ✈ Principal airports
and expressways

——— Principal roads   - _ _ - Railways   ⊕ Other airports
under construction

——— Other roads   ——— Other railways   ·········· Principal canals

+---+ Road tunnels   +---+ Railway tunnels   ⌒ Passes

PHYSICAL FEATURES

〜 Perennial streams   ⬭ Intermittent lakes   ▲ 8850 Elevations in metres

- 〜 - Intermittent streams   ⬭ Swamps and marshes   ▼ 8500 Sea depths in metres

⬭ Perennial lakes   ⬭ Permanent ice   *1134* Height of lake surface
and glaciers   above sea level in metres

⬚ Sand deserts

ELEVATION AND DEPTH TINTS

Height of land above sea level   Land below sea level   Depth of sea

in metres	6000	4000	3000	2000	1500	1000	400	200	0						
in feet	18 000	12 000	9000	6000	4500	3000	1200	600		6000	12 000	15 000	18 000	24 000	in feet
									0	200	2000	4000	5000	6000	8000	in metres

Some of the maps have different contours to highlight and clarify the principal relief features

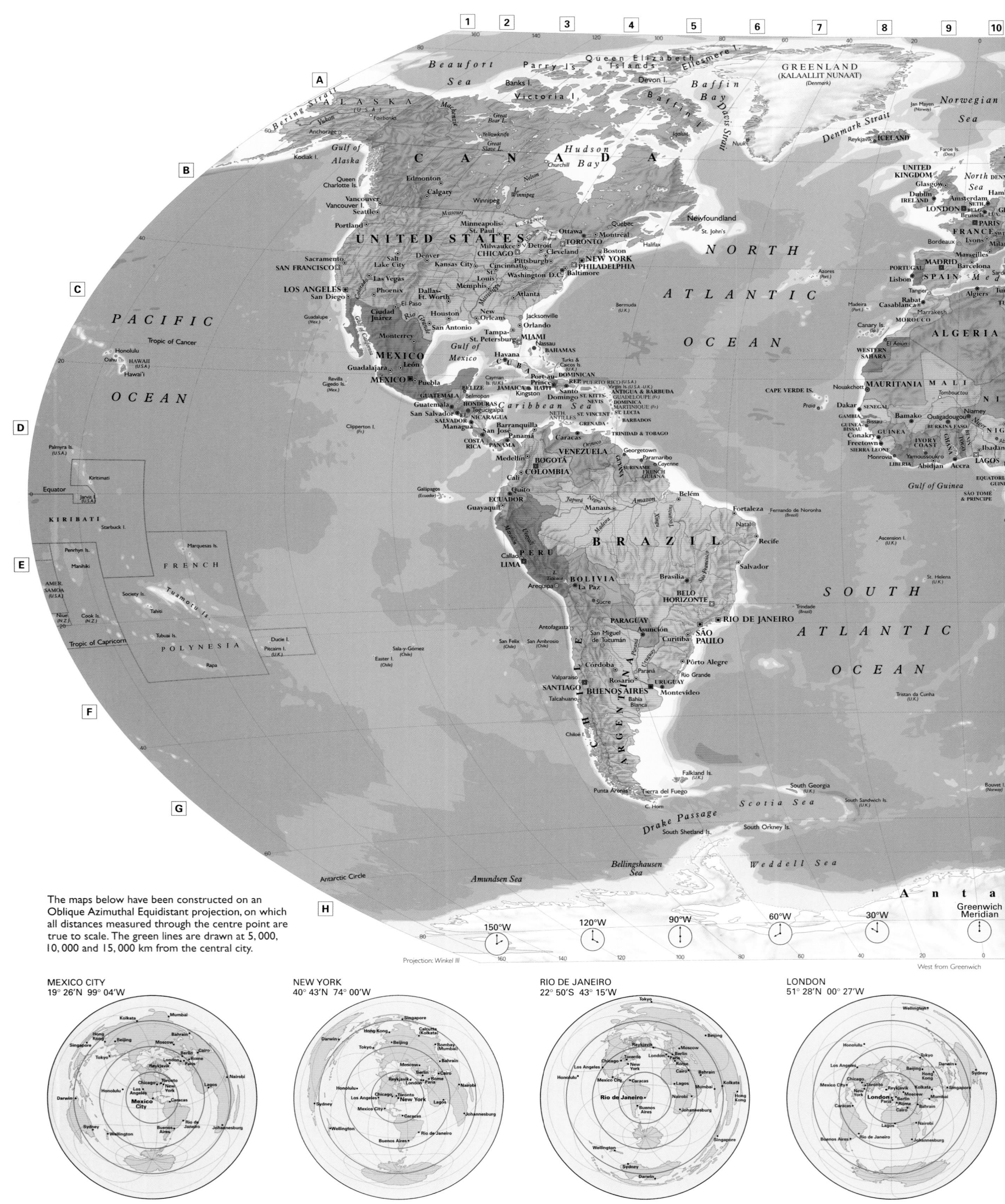

The maps below have been constructed on an Oblique Azimuthal Equidistant projection, on which all distances measured through the centre point are true to scale. The green lines are drawn at 5,000, 10,000 and 15,000 km from the central city.

Projection: Winkel III

West from Greenwich

MEXICO CITY
19° 26'N 99° 04'W

NEW YORK
40° 43'N 74° 00'W

RIO DE JANEIRO
22° 50'S 43° 15'W

LONDON
51° 28'N 00° 27'W

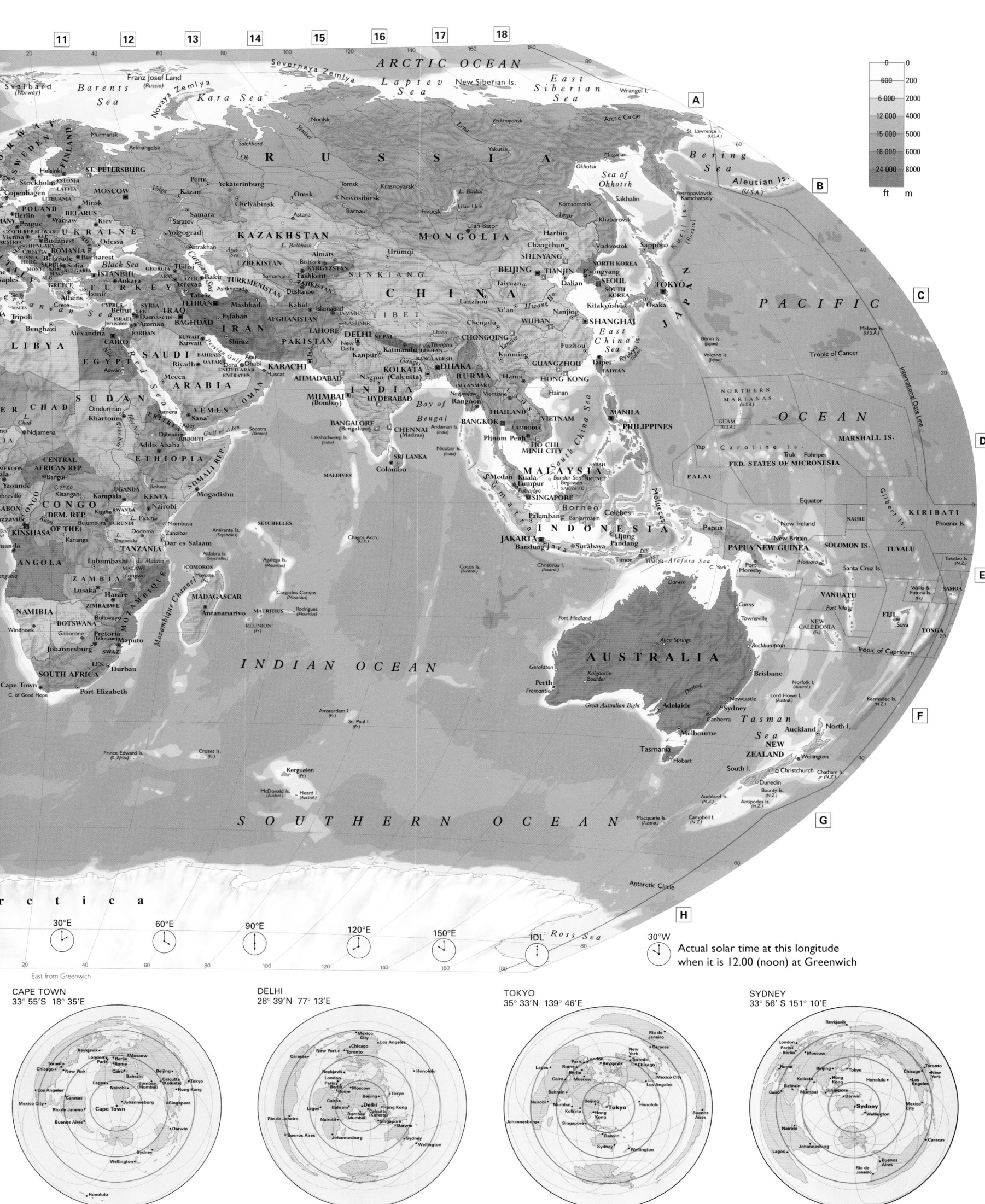

CAPE TOWN
33° 55'S 18° 35'E

DELHI
28° 39'N 77° 13'E

TOKYO
35° 33'N 139° 46'E

SYDNEY
33° 56' S 151° 10'E

COPYRIGHT PHILIP'S

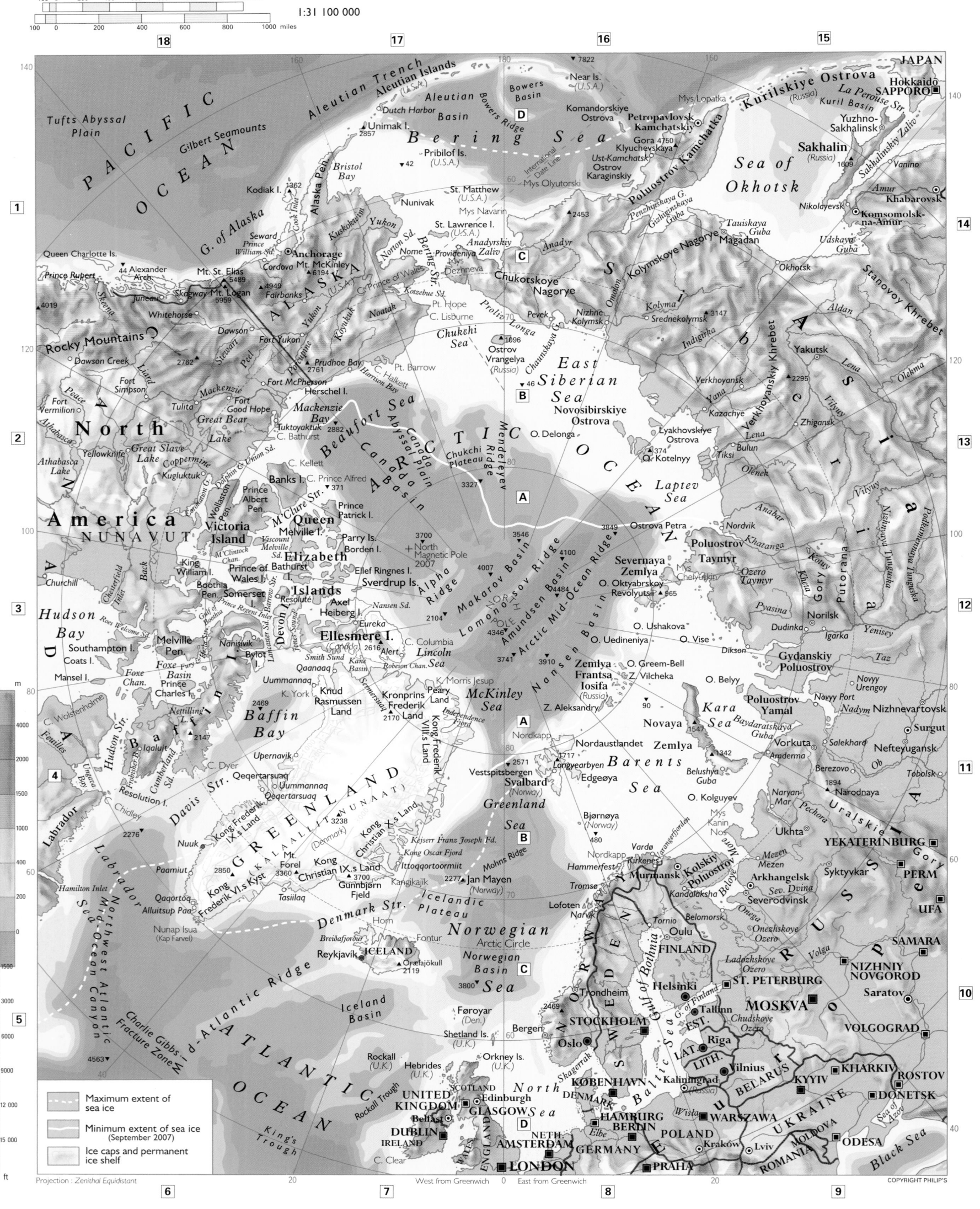

100   0   200   400   600   800   1000   1200   1400 km

100   0   200   400   600   800   1000 miles

1:31 100 000

Tufts Abyssal Plain

PACIFIC OCEAN

Gilbert Seamounts

Aleutian Trench

Aleutian Islands (U.S.A.)

Aleutian Basin

Bowers Ridge

Bowers Basin

Near Is. (U.S.A.)

▼7822

Komandorskiye Ostrova

Mys Lopatka

Kurilskiye Ostrova (Russia)

La Perouse Str.

JAPAN

Hokkaidô

SAPPORO

Kuril Basin

Yuzhno-Sakhalinsk

International Date Line

Dutch Harbor

Unimak I.

2857

Bering Sea

180

Petropavlovsk-Kamchatskiy

Gora 4750

Klyuchevskaya

Poluostrov Kamchatka

Sakhalin (Russia)

1609

Vanino

Sea of Okhotsk

Pribilof Is. (U.S.A.)

▼42

60

Mys Navarin

Ust-Kamchatsk

Ostrov Karaginskiy

Amur

Khabarovsk

Kodiak I. 1362

Bristol Bay

St. Matthew (U.S.A.)

2453

Anadyrskiy Zaliv

Penzhinskaya G.

Gizhiginskaya Guba

Tauiskaya Guba

Magadan

Nikolayevsk

Komsomolsk-na-Amur

G. of Alaska

Nunivak

Nome

St. Lawrence I. (U.S.A.)

Anadyr

Okhotsk

Udskaya Guba

Stanovoy Khrebet

Seward

Prince William Sd.

Cook Inlet

Cordova

Anchorage

Mt. McKinley 6194

Norton Sd.

Bering Str.

Providenniya

Mys Dezhneva

Chukotskoye Nagorye

S

Kolymskoye Nagorye

Queen Charlotte Is.

44 Alexander Arch.

Mt. St. Elias 5489

Skagway Mt. Logan 5959

Fairbanks

4949

Prince of Wales

Kotzebue Sd.

Pt. Hope

C. Lisburne

Proliv Longa

Pevek

Nizhne Kolymsk

Kolyma

3147

Yakutsk

Lena

Olekma

ALASKA

Prince Rupert

Juneau

4019

Yukon

Koyukuk

Noatak

Chukchi Sea

1096

Ostrov Vrangelya (Russia)

Chaunskaya G.

Srednekolymsk

Verkhoyansk

2295

Verkhoyanskiy Khrebet

Zhigansk

Rocky Mountains

Whitehorse

Dawson

Stewart

Prudhoe Bay 2761

Fort McPherson

Herschel I.

Pt. Barrow

Harrison Bay

C. Halkett

▼46

East Siberian Sea

Indigirka

Yana

Kazachye

Tiksi

Olenek

North America

Dawson Creek

Fort Nelson

Liard

Peace

Fort Simpson

Mackenzie

Great Bear Lake

Fort Good Hope

Tulita

Tuktoyaktuk

Mackenzie Bay

C. Bathurst

2882

Beaufort Sea

Canada Abyssal Plain

Canada Basin

Novosibirskiye Ostrova

Lyakhovskiye Ostrova

374

Kotelnyy

Bulun

Lena

A

Fort Vermilion

Athabasca

Yellowknife

Great Slave Lake

Coppermine

Kugluktuk

C. Kellett

Banks I.

C. Prince Alfred ▼371

Chukchi Plateau

Mendeleyev Ridge

3327

ARCTIC OCEAN

Laptev Sea

Ostrova Petra

Nordvik

Kharanga

S i b e r i a

Athabasca Lake

Dolphin & Union Sd.

Prince Albert Pen.

Prince Patrick I.

Borden I.

3700

North Magnetic Pole 2007

3546

3849

Severnaya Zemlya

Poluostrov Taymyr

Mys Chelyuskin

Ozero Taymyr

Gory Putorana

America

NUNAVUT

Victoria Island

M'Clure Str.

Queen

Melville I.

Parry Is.

4007

4100

Oktyabrskoy Revolyutsii

965

Pyasina

Norilsk

King William I.

Prince of Bathurst

Elizabeth

Ellef Ringnes I.

Sverdrup Is.

Alpha Ridge

NORTH

Makarov Basin

Lomonosov Ridge

Amundsen Basin

Arctic Mid-Ocean Ridge

Nansen Basin

Poluostrov Gydanskiy

Dudinka

Igarka

Yenisey

Churchill

Boothia Pen.

Somerset

Prince of Wales I.

Islands

Axel Heiberg I.

2104

POLE

4346

44484

O. Ushakova

O. Vise

Dikson

Hudson Bay

Gulf of Boothia

Resolute

Devon I.

Nansen Sd.

Ellesmere I. (Canada)

2616

C. Columbia

Lincoln Sea

3741

3910

Zemlya Frantsa Iosifa (Russia)

O. Greem-Bell

Z. Vilcheka

O. Belyy

O. Uedineniya

Novyy Urengoy

Novyy Port

Nadym

Southampton I.

Melville Pen.

Nanisivik

Bylot

Alert

K. Morris Jesup

Peary Land

McKinley Sea

90

Z. Aleksandry

Novaya

1547

Kara Sea

Poluostrov Yamal

Baydaratskaya Guba

Nizhnevartovsk

Coats I.

Foxe Chan.

Fury

Qaanaaq

Smith Sund

Kane Basin

Knud Rasmussen Land

Kronprins Frederik Land

Independence Fjord

Kong Frederik VIII's Land

80

Nordkapp

80

2571

Zemlya

Longyearbyen

Edgeøya

Barents Sea

Amderma

Vorkuta

Berezovo

Surgut

Neftyugansk

Mansel I.

Prince Charles I.

Nettilling L.

2469

2147

Baffin Bay

Uummannaq

K. York

1717

Vestspitsbergen

Svalbard

Nordaustlandet

Belushya Guba

1894 Narodnaya

Ob

Tobolsk

Foxe Basin

Iqaluit

Upernavik

C. Dyer

Davis Str.

Qeqertarsuaq

Uummannaq

Qeqertarsuaq

GREENLAND

(KALAALLIT NUNAAT) (Denmark)

3238

Kong Frederik IX's Land

Kong Christian X's Land

Kejser Franz Joseph Fd.

Kong Oscar Fjord

Ittoqqortoormiit

Greenland Sea

B

Jan Mayen (Norway)

2277

Mohns Ridge

480

O. Kolguyev

Mys Kanin Nos

Varangerfjorden

Vardø

NORWAY

Naryan-Mar

Pechora

Ukhta

Gory Uralskie

YEKATERINBURG

PERM

UFA

Resolution I.

Chidley

Labrador

2276

Nuuk

Kong Frederik VI's Kyst

Mt. Forel 3360

Kong Christian IX's Land

3700

Gunnbjørn Fjeld

Kangikajik

2850

B

Icelandic Plateau

Nordkapp

Hammerfest

Kirkenes

Tromsø

Murmansk

Kolskiy Poluostrov

Arkhangelsk

Sev. Dvina

Severodvinsk

Mezen

Mezen

60

SAMARA

Labrador Sea

Mid-Atlantic Ridge

Northwest Atlantic Mid-Ocean Canyon

Paamiut

Qaqortoq

Alluitsup Paa

Tasiilaq

Denmark Str.

Horn

Fontur

2277

Icelandic Plateau

Norwegian Basin

C

Lofoten

Narvik

Bodø

2469

Trondheim

SWEDEN

Oulu

Gulf of Bothnia

FINLAND

Helsinki

ST. PETERBURG

Onezhskoye Ozero

Ladozhskoye Ozero

Volga

NIZHNIY NOVGOROD

Saratov

RUSSIA

Nunap Isua (Kap Farvel)

Breiðafjörður

Reykjavík ICELAND

Öræfajökull 2119

3800

Norwegian Sea

Oslo

STOCKHOLM

Tallinn

EST.

MOSKVA

VOLGOGRAD

Iceland Basin

Føroyar (Den.)

Bergen

40

Shetland Is. (U.K.)

North Sea

Skagerrak

Baltic Sea

Riga

LAT.

LITH.

Vilnius

Chudskoye Ozero

KHARKIV

ROSTOV

Rockall (U.K.)

Hebrides (U.K.)

Orkney Is. (U.K.)

ATLANTIC OCEAN

Charlie Gibbs Fracture Zone

4563

Mid-Atlantic Ridge

King's Trough

Scotland

Edinburgh

GLASGOW

D

Kaliningrad (Russia)

KØBENHAVN

DENMARK

HAMBURG

BERLIN

POLAND

WARSZAWA

BELARUS

KYYIV

UKRAINE

ODESA

DONETSK

Rockall Trough

UNITED KINGDOM

Belfast

DUBLIN

IRELAND

England

LONDON

AMSTERDAM

GERMANY

NETH.

Elbe

PRAHA

Wisła

Kraków

Lviv

MOLDOVA

ROMANIA

Sea of Azov

Black Sea

C. Clear

Projection: Zenithal Equidistant

West from Greenwich

0

East from Greenwich

COPYRIGHT PHILIP'S

ft m

12 000 4000

6000 2000

4500 1500

3000 1000

2000 600

1000 400

600 200

0

500 150

1000 3000

2000 6000

3000 9000

4000 12 000

5000 15 000

m ft

Maximum extent of sea ice

Minimum extent of sea ice (September 2007)

Ice caps and permanent ice shelf

1:31 100 000

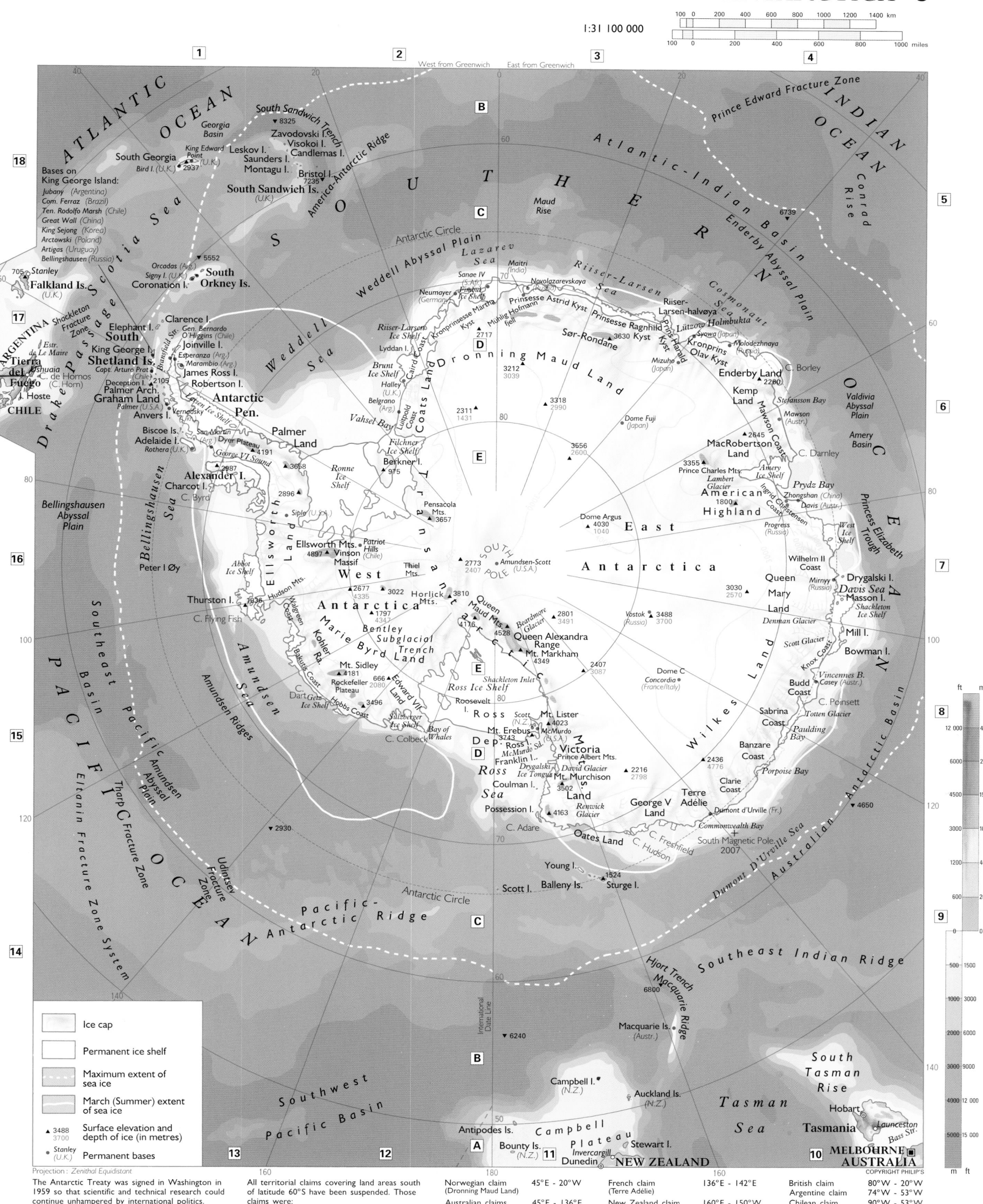

Legend

- Ice cap
- Permanent ice shelf
- Maximum extent of sea ice
- March (Summer) extent of sea ice
- ▲ 3488 / 3700 Surface elevation and depth of ice (in metres)
- • Stanley (U.K.) Permanent bases

Projection : Zenithal Equidistant

COPYRIGHT PHILIP'S

The Antarctic Treaty was signed in Washington in 1959 so that scientific and technical research could continue unhampered by international politics.

All territorial claims covering land areas south of latitude 60°S have been suspended. Those claims were:

Norwegian claim (Dronning Maud Land)	45°E – 20°W	French claim (Terre Adélie)	136°E – 142°E	British claim	80°W – 20°W
Australian claims	45°E – 136°E / 142°E – 160°E	New Zealand claim (Ross Dependency)	160°E – 150°W	Argentine claim	74°W – 53°W
				Chilean claim	90°W – 53°W

Bases on King George Island:
Jubany (Argentina)
Com. Ferraz (Brazil)
Ten. Rodolfo Marsh (Chile)
Great Wall (China)
King Sejong (Korea)
Arctowski (Poland)
Artigas (Uruguay)
Bellingshausen (Russia)

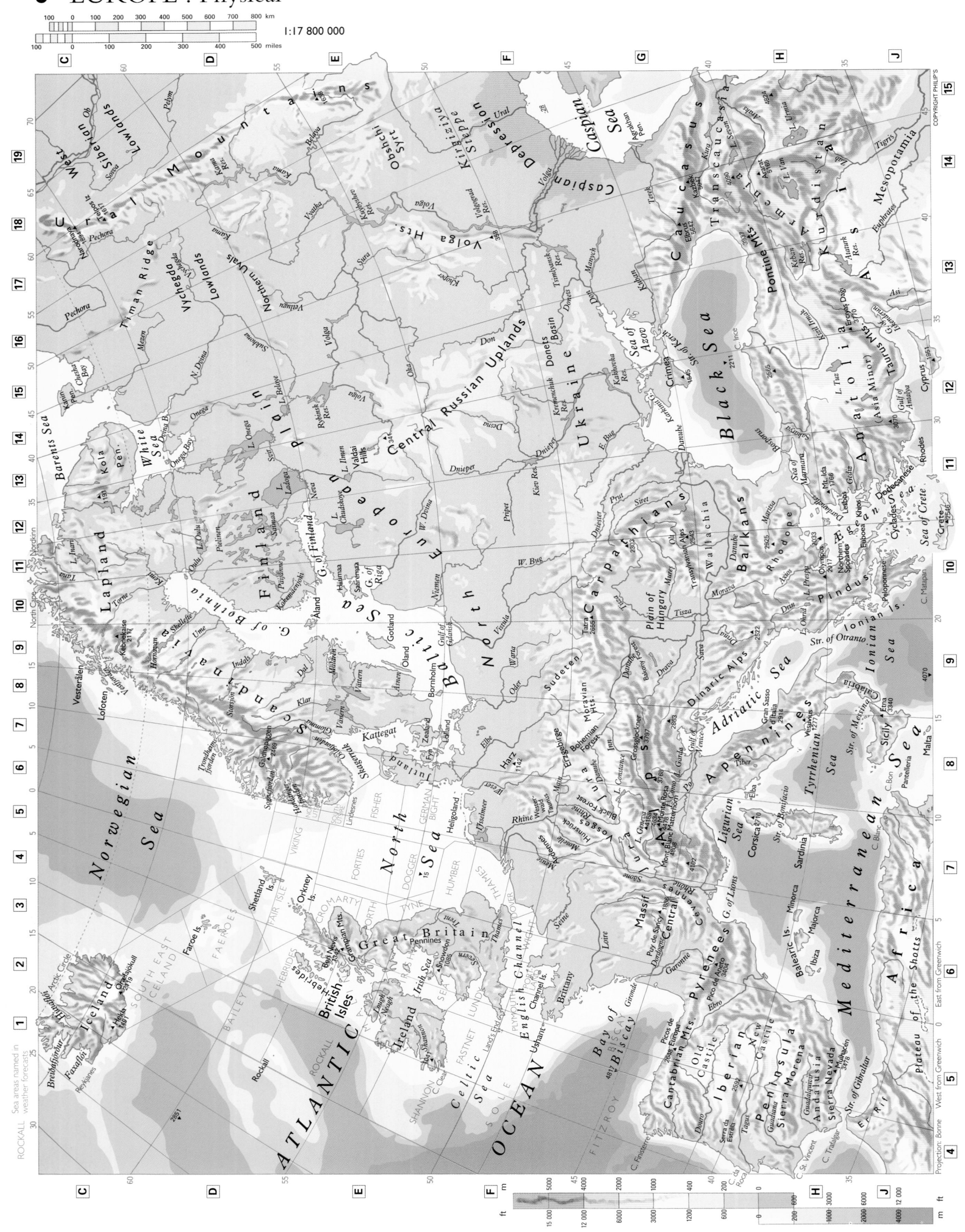

1:17 800 000

COPYRIGHT PHILIP'S

Projection: Bonne

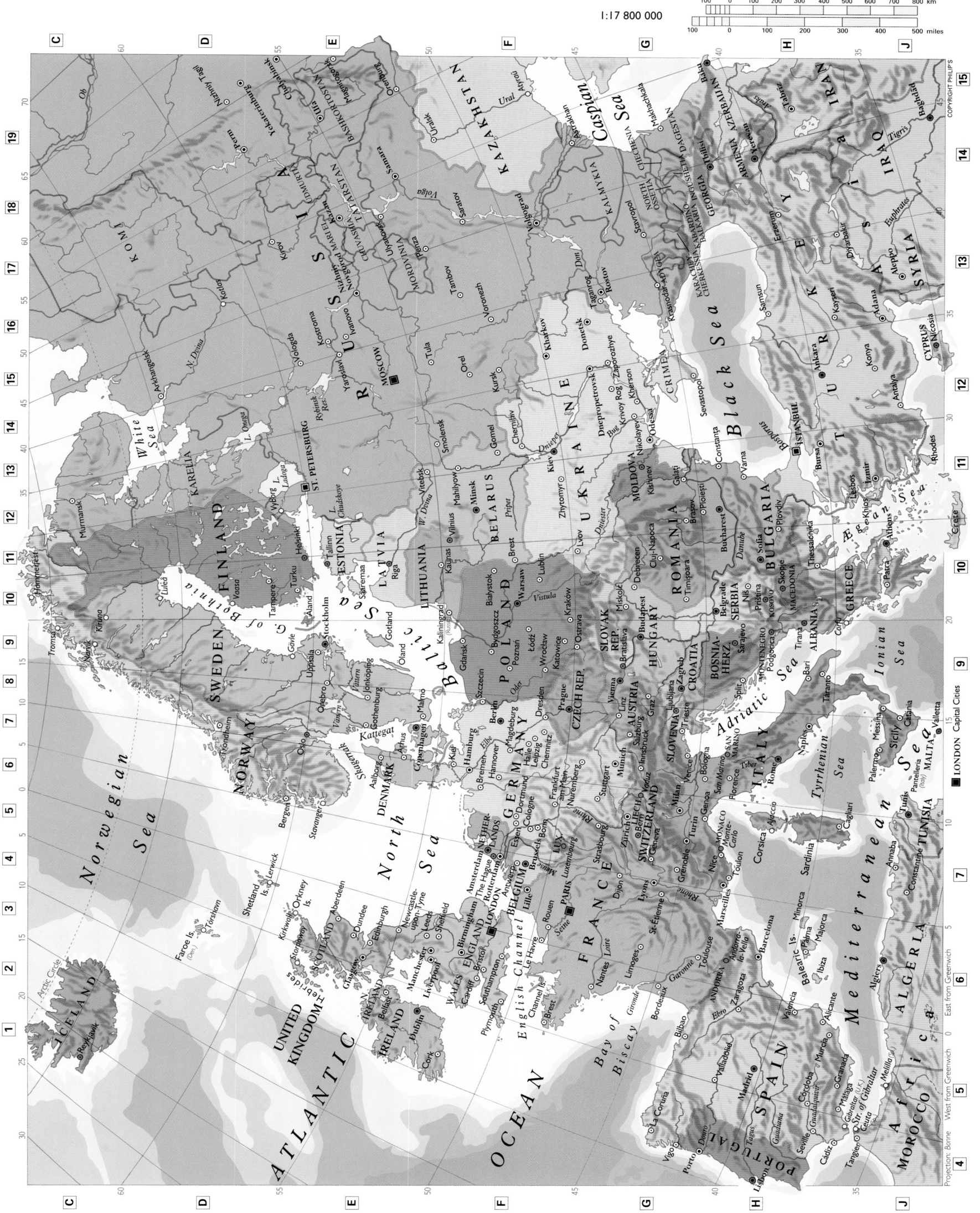

1:5 300 000

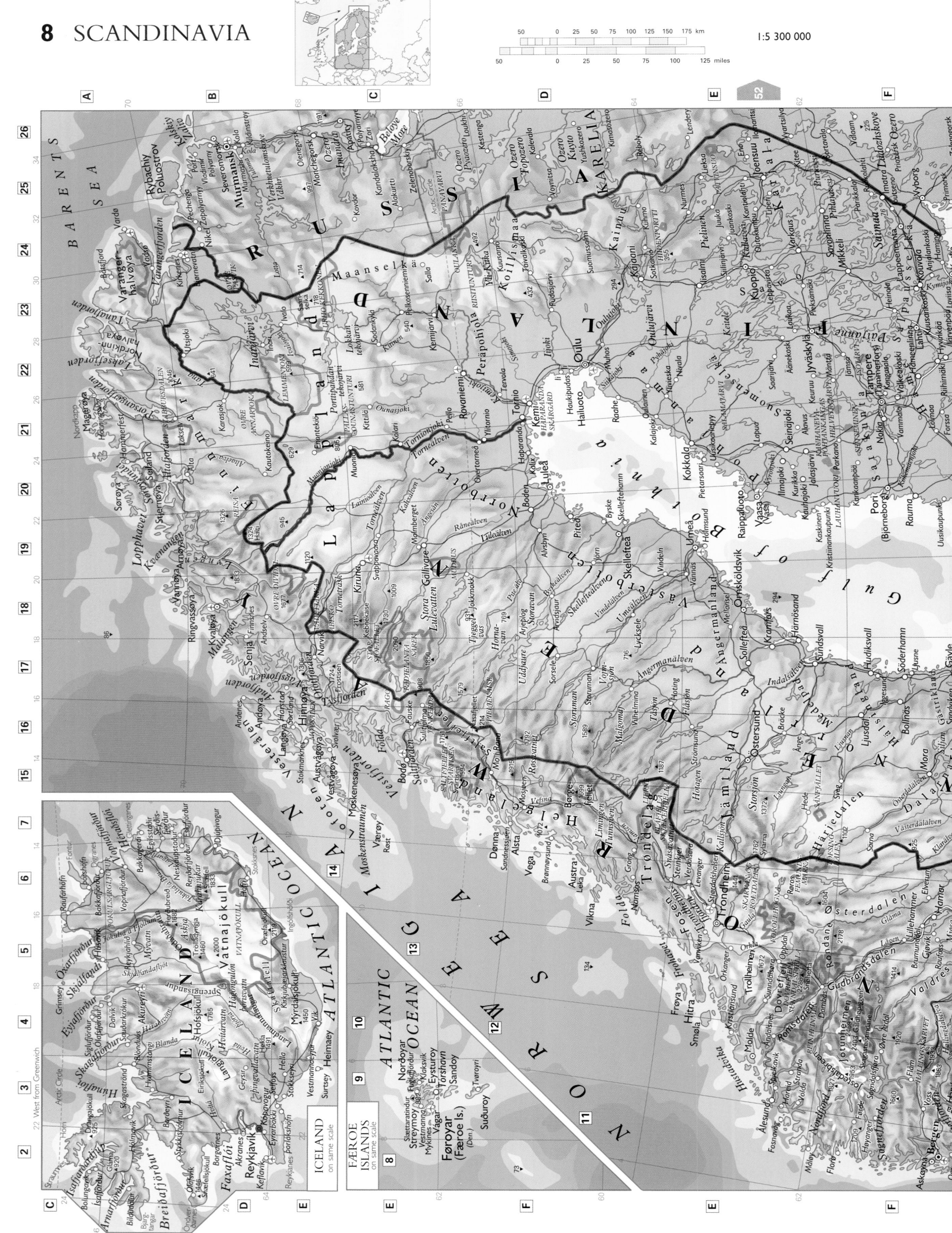

50 0 25 50 75 100 125 150 175 km

50 0 25 50 75 100 125 miles

52

ICELAND
on same scale

FÆROE
ISLANDS
on same scale

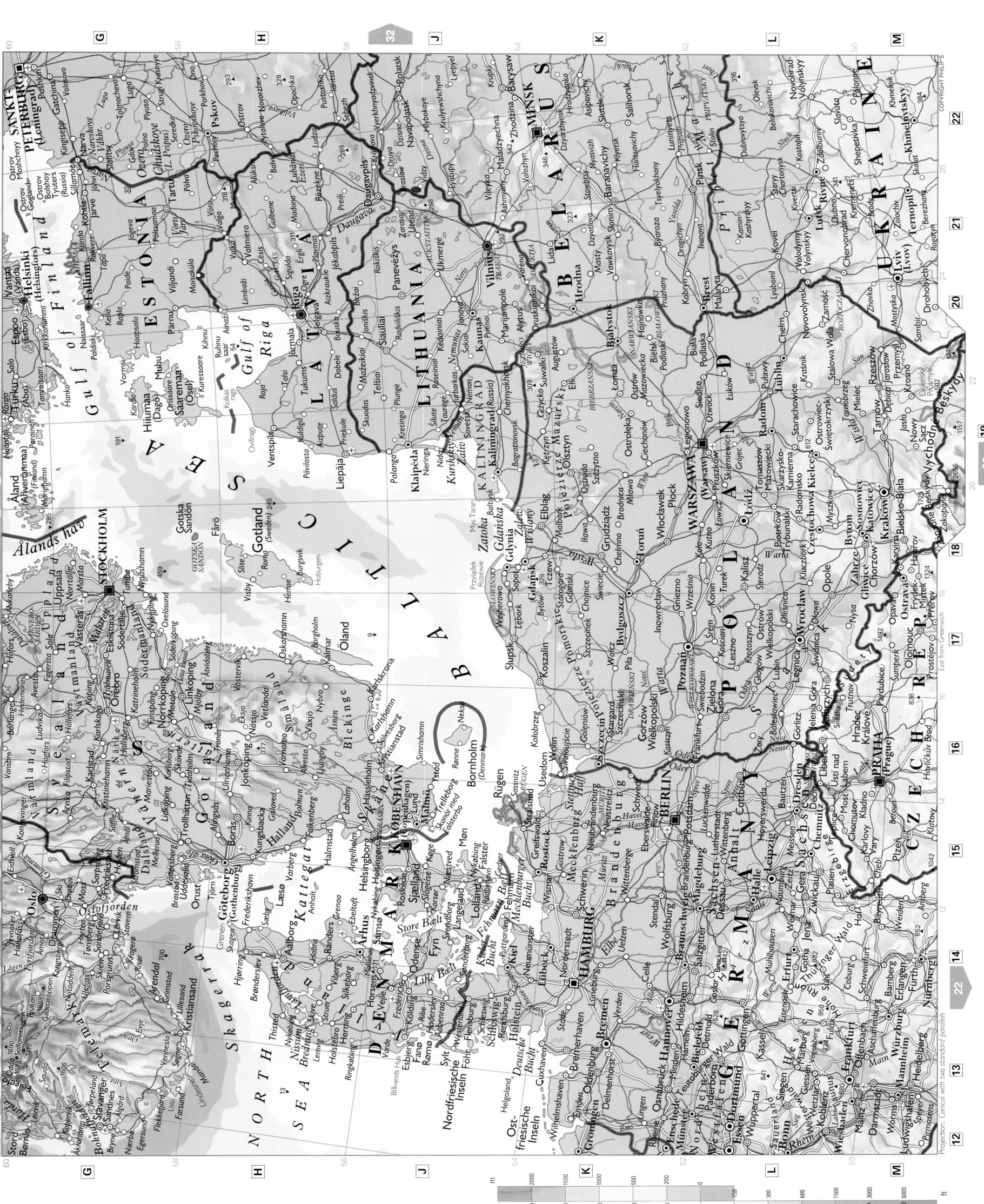

Projection: Conic with two standard parallels

East from Greenwich

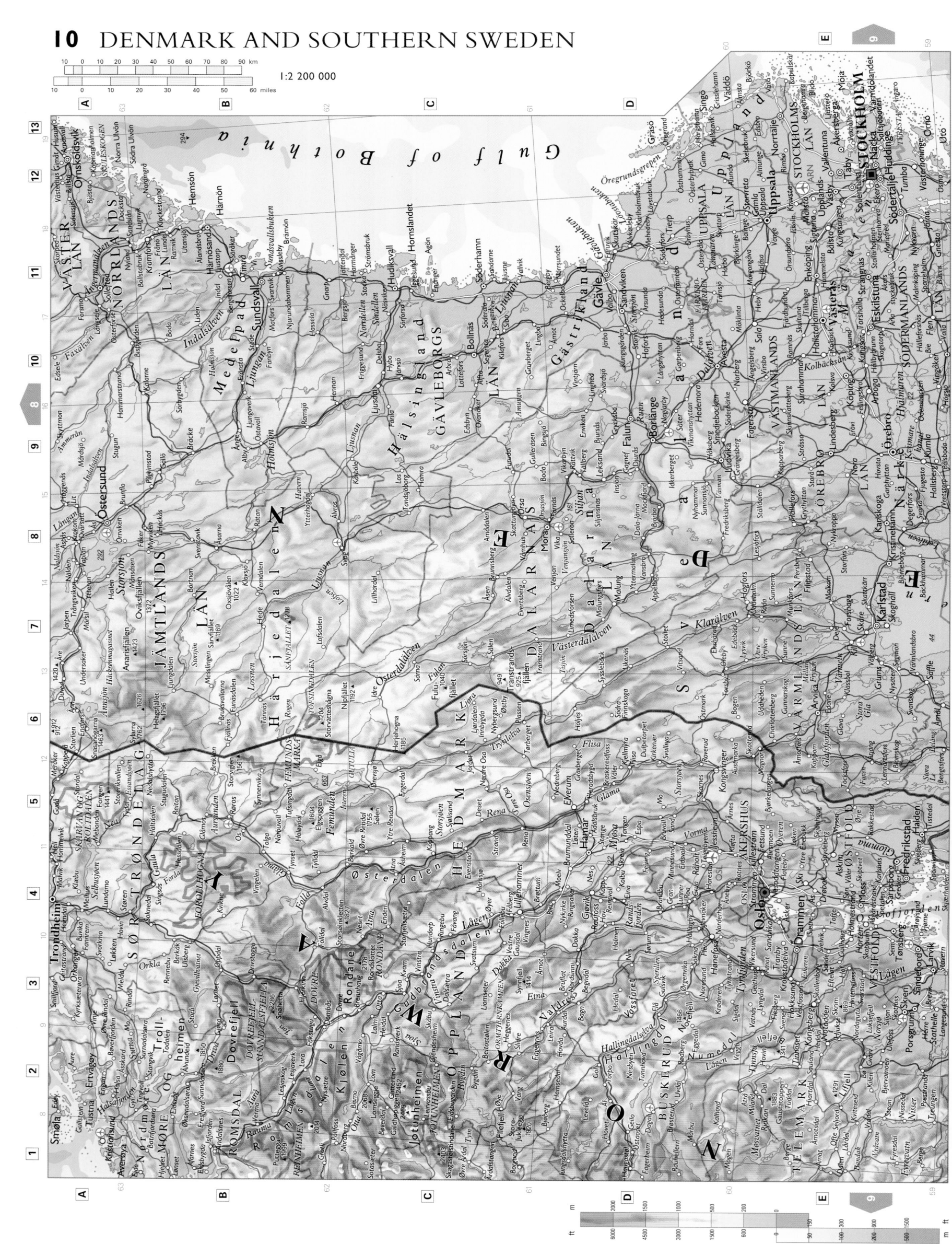

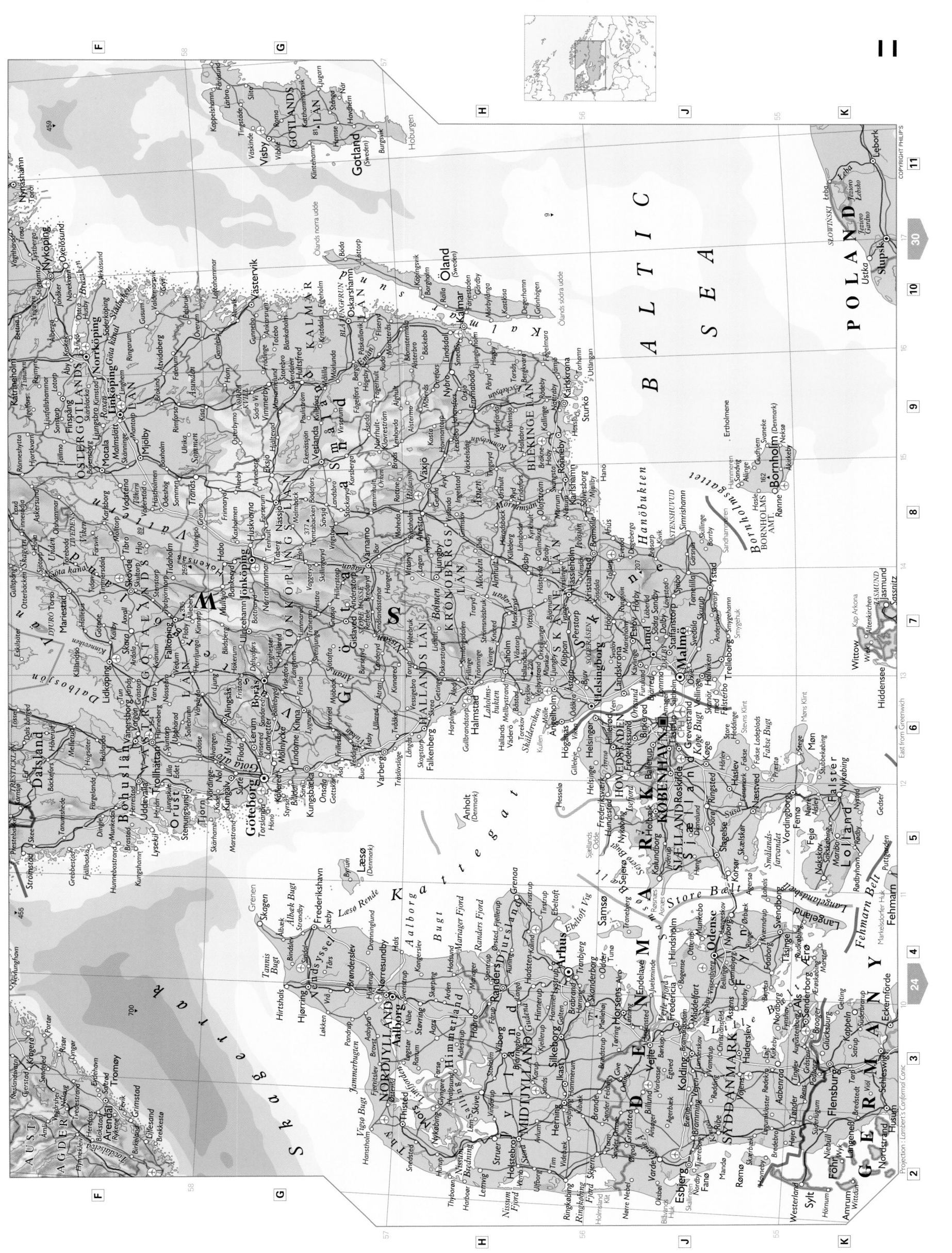

12 IRELAND

1:1 800 000

10 0 10 20 30 40 50 60 70 80 km
10 0 10 20 30 40 50 miles

Projection: Lambert's Conformal Conic

West from Greenwich

COPYRIGHT PHILIP'S

ATLANTIC OCEAN

IRISH SEA

CELTIC SEA

North Channel

St. George's Channel

Firth of Clyde

SCOTLAND Kintyre

WALES

NORTHERN IRELAND

IRELAND

Ulster

Leinster

Munster

Connacht

Provinces and Counties

DONEGAL, LONDONDERRY, ANTRIM, TYRONE, FERMANAGH, ARMAGH, MONAGHAN, DOWN, CAVAN, LEITRIM, SLIGO, MAYO, ROSCOMMON, LONGFORD, MEATH, LOUTH, WESTMEATH, OFFALY, KILDARE, DUBLIN, WICKLOW, GALWAY, CLARE, LIMERICK, TIPPERARY, LAOIS, CARLOW, KILKENNY, WEXFORD, KERRY, CORK, WATERFORD

Cities and Towns

Londonderry, Belfast, Dublin, Dun Laoghaire, Cork, Limerick, Galway, Waterford, Sligo, Dundalk, Drogheda, Wexford, Tralee, Killarney, Ennis, Clonmel, Kilkenny, Carlow, Athlone, Mullingar, Monaghan, Cavan, Longford, Roscommon, Castlebar, Westport, Donegal, Letterkenny, Coleraine, Ballymena, Larne, Newry, Armagh, Omagh, Enniskillen, Dungannon, Lisburn, Bangor, Newtownards, Downpatrick, Portadown, Craigavon, Lurgan, Banbridge, Kells, Navan, Naas, Bray, Greystones, Arklow, Gorey, Enniscorthy, New Ross, Rosslare, Youghal, Midleton, Cobh, Kinsale, Bandon, Clonakilty, Skibbereen, Bantry, Macroom, Mallow, Fermoy, Mitchelstown, Cashel, Tipperary, Thurles, Roscrea, Nenagh, Birr, Tullamore, Portlaoise, Abbeyleix, Mountmellick, Edenderry, Kildare, Newbridge, Athy, Carrick-on-Suir, Dungarvan

Physical Features

Carrauntoohil, Macgillycuddy's Reeks, Mweelrea, Croagh Patrick, Nephin, Errigal, Slieve League, Lugnaquilla, Galtymore, Keeper Hill, Mt. Leinster, Slievenamon, Mangerton

Lough Neagh, Lough Erne, Lower L. Erne, Upper L. Erne, Lough Corrib, Lough Mask, Lough Conn, Lough Carra, Lough Derg, Lough Ree, Lough Gara, Lough Key, Lough Allen, Lough Melvin, Lough Arrow, L. Sheelin, L. Oughter, L. Gowna, L. Ramor, L. Leane, L. Currane, Carlingford L., Strangford L., Belfast L., Lough Foyle

Rivers: Shannon, Liffey, Boyne, Suir, Nore, Barrow, Blackwater, Lee, Bann, Foyle, Moy, Erne, Slaney, Brosna, Inny

Donegal Bay, Galway Bay, Clew Bay, Dingle Bay, Bantry Bay, Tralee Bay, Dundalk Bay, Waterford Harbour, Wexford Harbour, Cork Harbour, Youghal B., Sligo Bay, Blacksod Bay, Broad Haven, Killary Harbour, Kenmare River, Bertraghboy Bay, Mouth of the Shannon

Malin Hd., Horn Hd., Bloody Foreland, Erris Hd., Achill Hd., Slyne Hd., Loop Hd., Mizen Hd., Brow Hd., Old Head of Kinsale, Carnsore Pt., Hook Hd., Wicklow Hd., Howth Hd., Fair Hd., Benbane Hd., Mull of Kintyre, Mull of Oa

Inishowen Pen., Mullet Pen., Dingle Pen., Ards Pen., Hook Hd.

Islands: Achill I., Aran Is., Aran I., Tory I., Clare I., Inishturk, Inishbofin, Inishmore, Inishmaan, Inisheer, Valencia I., Great Blasket I., Dursey I., Bear I., Whiddy I., Sherkin I., Clear I., Rathlin I., Lambay I., Ireland's Eye, Saltee Is., Fastnet Rock, Great Skellig, Rathlin O'Birne I., Inishtrahull, Inishmurray

Mountains and ranges: Sperrin Mts., Mts. of Antrim, Mourne Mts., Wicklow Mts., Comeragh Mts., Knockmealdown Mts., Galty Mts., Silvermine Mts., Slieve Bloom, Slieve Aughty, Nephin Beg Range, Partry Mts., Derryveagh Mts., Blue Stack Mts., Ox Mts., Slieve Mish, Caha Mts., Boggeragh Mts., Nagles Mts., Burren

Giants Causeway, Glenveagh, Glenariff

Heights (m): 752, 683, 806, 819, 765, 601, 544, 380, 672, 683, 676, 554, 577, 683, 852, 926, 754, 796, 920, 722, 694, 529, 429, 646, 707, 775, 953, 853, 1041, 519, 368, 345, 269, 123, 115

Tory I., Inishfree B., Aran I., The Rosses, Dunglow, Crohy Hd., Gweebarra B., Dawros Hd., Loughros More B., Rossan Pt., St. John's Pt., Killala B., Mutton I., Kilkee, Ballybunion, Kerry Hd., Smerwick Harbour, Brandon B.

CONNEMARA, THE BURREN, GOLDEN VALE, Bog of Allen

1:1 800 000

10 0 10 20 30 40 50 60 70 80 km
10 0 10 20 30 40 50 miles

Key to Scottish unitary authorities on map
1 CITY OF ABERDEEN
2 DUNDEE CITY
3 WEST DUNBARTONSHIRE
4 EAST DUNBARTONSHIRE
5 CITY OF GLASGOW
6 INVERCLYDE
7 RENFREWSHIRE
8 EAST RENFREWSHIRE
9 NORTH LANARKSHIRE
10 FALKIRK
11 CLACKMANNANSHIRE
12 WEST LOTHIAN
13 CITY OF EDINBURGH
14 MIDLOTHIAN

ORKNEY IS. on same scale

ORKNEY
North Ronaldsay
Papa Westray
Westray
Eday
Sanday
Rousay
Stronsay
Shapinsay
Brough Hd.
Stromness
Mainland
Kirkwall
St. Mary's
Burray
Hoy
Scapa Flow
Burwick
South Ronaldsay
Dunnet Hd.
Stroma
Pentland Firth
Duncansby Head
John o' Groats
Thurso
Sinclair's Bay

SHETLAND IS. on same scale

Muckle Flugga
Unst
Haroldswick
Yell
Fetlar
Yell Sound
Ulsta
Out Skerries
Esha Ness
Sullom Voe
Whalsay
St. Magnus Bay
Voe
Papa Stour
Walls
Lerwick
Foula
Scalloway
Bressay
West Burra
Boddam
Sumburgh Hd.

SCOTLAND

ATLANTIC OCEAN

NORTH SEA

NORTHERN IRELAND
Belfast

ENGLAND
Newcastle-upon-Tyne

WESTERN ISLES
Butt of Lewis
Flannan Is.
Stornoway
Broad Bay
Eye Peninsula
Lewis
Harris
Tarbert
Scarp
Taransay
Toe Hd.
North Uist
Lochmaddy
Baleshare
Grimsay
Benbecula
Ardivachar Pt.
South Uist
Lochboisdale
Barra
Castlebay
Vatersay
Sandray
Barra Hd.
Eriskay

Hebrides
North Minch
Little Minch
Sound of Harris

C. Wrath
Durness
Cape Wrath
Handa
Reay Forest
Sutherland
Caithness
Dunnet Hd.
Thurso
Halkirk
Wick
John o' Groats
Stroma
Pentland Firth
Scapa Flow
Hoy
Burwick
Noss Hd.
Sinclair's Bay
Lybster
Ord of Caithness
Helmsdale
Brora
Golspie
Dornoch
Tarbat Ness
Tain
Bonar Bridge

L. Laxford
L. Assynt
Ben More Assynt 998
L. Shin
Lairg
Oykel
Brora
L. Broom
Ullapool
Greenstone Pt.
Gruinard B.
L. Ewe
L. Maree 1053
Gairloch
L. Torridon
Applecross
Raasay
Rona
Scalpay
Portree
Skye
Dunvegan
Cuillin Hills 992
Cuillin Sound
L. Bracadale
Sleat
Kyle of Lochalsh
Glenelg
Mallaig
Arisaig
L. Morar
L. Shiel
L. Moidart
Rhum (Rùm)
Eigg
Muck
Canna
Coll
Tiree
Passage of Tiree
Staffa
Ulva
Iona
Mull
Ben More 966
Tobermory
Morvern
Sound of Mull
Lismore
Kerrera
Oban
Seil
Luing
Scarba
Colonsay
Oronsay
Islay
Bowmore
Port Ellen
Rhinns Pt.
Mull of Oa
Jura
Sound of Jura
Gigha
Kintyre
Campbeltown
Mull of Kintyre
Ailsa Craig

NORTH WEST HIGHLANDS
Ben Hope 927
Ben More 961
Ben Dearg 1081
Ben Wyvis 1045
Carn Eige 1182
Glen Affric
Glen Moriston
Fort Augustus
Glen Garry
L. Arkaig
L. Lochy
Loch Ness
Inverness
Dingwall
Strathpeffer
Muir of Ord
Beauly
Nairn
Forres
Elgin
Lossiemouth
Buckie
Cullen
Banff
Macduff
Fraserburgh
Peterhead
Buchan Ness
Cruden Bay
Ellon
Oldmeldrum
Inverurie
Kintore
Dyce
Aberdeen
Girdle Ness
Peterculter
Banchory
Stonehaven
Inverbervie
Montrose
Brechin
Forfar
Arbroath
Carnoustie
Monifieth
Firth of Tay
Dundee
Tayport
Leuchars
St. Andrews
Fife Ness
Anstruther
Leven
Buckhaven
Kirkcaldy
Firth of Forth
North Berwick
Dunbar
St. Abb's Head
Eyemouth
Berwick-upon-Tweed

HIGHLAND
MORAY
ABERDEENSHIRE
Huntly
Turriff
Aberchirder
Keith
Dufftown
Rothes
Aberlour
Charlestown of Aberlour
Tomintoul
Grantown-on-Spey
Aviemore
Kingussie
Newtonmore
Cairn Gorm 1309
CAIRNGORMS
Braemar
Ballater
Aboyne
Alford
Westhill
Don
Dee

Ben Nevis 1342
Fort William
Kinlochleven
Glen Coe
Ballachulish
Rannoch Moor
Ben Cruachan 1126
Crianlarich
Ben More 1174
Ben Lawers 1214
L. Rannoch
L. Tay
Pitlochry
Blair Atholl
Forest of Atholl
Aberfeldy
Dunkeld
Kirriemuir
Blairgowrie
Coupar
Alyth
Perth
Scone
Crieff
Comrie
Auchterarder
Gleneagles
Ben Vorlich 983
Callander
Aberfoyle
LOCH LOMOND TROSSACHS
L. Katrine
QUEEN ELIZABETH
Loch Lomond
Inveraray
Lochgilphead
Tarbert
L. Fyne
L. Awe
ARGYLL AND BUTE
Helensburgh
Dunoon
Rothesay
Bute
Largs
Dumbarton
Alexandria
Greenock
Gourock
Port Glasgow
Paisley
GLASGOW
Clydebank
Kirkintilloch
Cumbernauld
Airdrie
Coatbridge
Motherwell
Hamilton
East Kilbride
Wishaw
Carluke
Lanark
Biggar
Peebles
STIRLING
Stirling
Dunblane
Bridge of Allan
Bannockburn
Denny
Falkirk
Grangemouth
Bo'ness
Alloa
Dollar
Dunfermline
Cowdenbeath
Glenrothes
Falkland
Cupar
Kinross
L. Leven
FIFE
Auchtermuchty
Ochil Hills
Sidlaw Hills
Strathmore
KINROSS
PERTH AND KINROSS
ANGUS
Laurencekirk
N. Esk
S. Esk
Inverbervie

EDINBURGH
Livingston
Dalkeith
Bonnyrigg
Penicuik
Pentland Hills
Moorfoot Hills
Musselburgh
Haddington
EAST LOTHIAN
Lammermuir Hills
Duns
SCOTTISH BORDERS
Galashiels
Melrose
Selkirk
Kelso
Coldstream
Jedburgh
Hawick
Moffat
Langholm
Lockerbie
Gretna
Annan
DUMFRIES & GALLOWAY
Dumfries
Lochmaben
Lochar
Dalbeattie
Castle Douglas
Kirkcudbright
Gatehouse of Fleet
Newton Stewart
Wigtown
Whithorn
Stranraer
Portpatrick
Cairnryan
L. Ryan
Luce Bay
Burrow Hd.
Mull of Galloway
Solway Firth
GALLOWAY
New Galloway
Merrick 844
SOUTH LANARKSHIRE
Strathaven
Cumnock
Sanquhar
Dalmellington
Maybole
Girvan
Ayr
Prestwick
Troon
Irvine
Saltcoats
Ardrossan
Kilwinning
Kilmarnock
Dalry
EAST AYRSHIRE
NORTH AYRSHIRE
SOUTH AYRSHIRE
Arran
Brodick
Goat Fell 874
Kilbrannan Sound
Firth of Clyde
CLYDE
MUIRSHIEL
Broad Law 840

CUMBRIA
Carlisle
Brampton
Haltwhistle
Hexham
NORTHUMBERLAND
Alnwick
Almouth
Amble
Morpeth
Blaydon
Gateshead
Stanley
Consett
Crook
DURHAM
Bishop Auckland
Barnard Castle
Penrith
Appleby-in-Westmorland
Kielder Water
Cheviot Hills
The Cheviot 816
Cheviot
Wooler
Bamburgh
Holy I.
Farne Is.
Flodden
Tweed
Teviot

Projection: Lambert's Conformal Conic

West from Greenwich

COPYRIGHT PHILIP'S

ft / m
3000 / 1000
1500 / 500
600 / 200
300 / 100
0
150 / 50
300 / 100
600 / 200
1500 / 500
3000 / 1000
m / ft

1:1 800 000

10 0 10 20 30 40 50 60 70 80 km
10 0 10 20 30 40 50 miles

Key to English unitary authorities on map

25 HARTLEPOOL
26 DARLINGTON
27 STOCKTON-ON-TEES
28 MIDDLESBROUGH
29 REDCAR AND CLEVELAND
30 BLACKPOOL
31 BLACKBURN WITH DARWEN
32 HALTON
33 WARRINGTON
34 KINGSTON UPON HULL
35 NORTH EAST LINCOLNSHIRE
36 STOKE-ON-TRENT
37 TELFORD AND WREKIN
38 DERBY CITY
39 CITY OF NOTTINGHAM
40 LEICESTER CITY
41 RUTLAND
42 PETERBOROUGH
43 MILTON KEYNES
44 LUTON
45 NORTH SOMERSET
46 CITY OF BRISTOL
47 BATH AND NORTH EAST SOMERSET
48 SWINDON
49 READING
50 WOKINGHAM
51 WINDSOR AND MAIDENHEAD
52 SLOUGH
53 BRACKNELL FOREST
54 THURROCK
55 SOUTHEND-ON-SEA
56 MEDWAY
57 PLYMOUTH
58 TORBAY
59 POOLE
60 BOURNEMOUTH
61 SOUTHAMPTON
62 PORTSMOUTH
63 BRIGHTON AND HOVE

Key to Welsh unitary authorities on map

15 SWANSEA
16 NEATH PORT TALBOT
17 BRIDGEND
18 RHONDDA CYNON TAFF
19 MERTHYR TYDFIL
20 CAERPHILLY
21 BLAENAU GWENT
22 TORFAEN
23 CARDIFF
24 NEWPORT

NORTH SEA

IRISH SEA

North Channel

SCOTLAND

NORTHERN IRELAND

ISLE OF MAN

[Numerous place names including: Edinburgh, Glasgow, Newcastle-upon-Tyne, Sunderland, Middlesbrough, Hartlepool, York, Leeds, Bradford, Manchester, Liverpool, Sheffield, Derby, Nottingham, Lincoln, Kingston upon Hull, Scarborough, Carlisle, Blackpool, Chester, Stoke-on-Trent, Berwick-upon-Tweed, etc.]

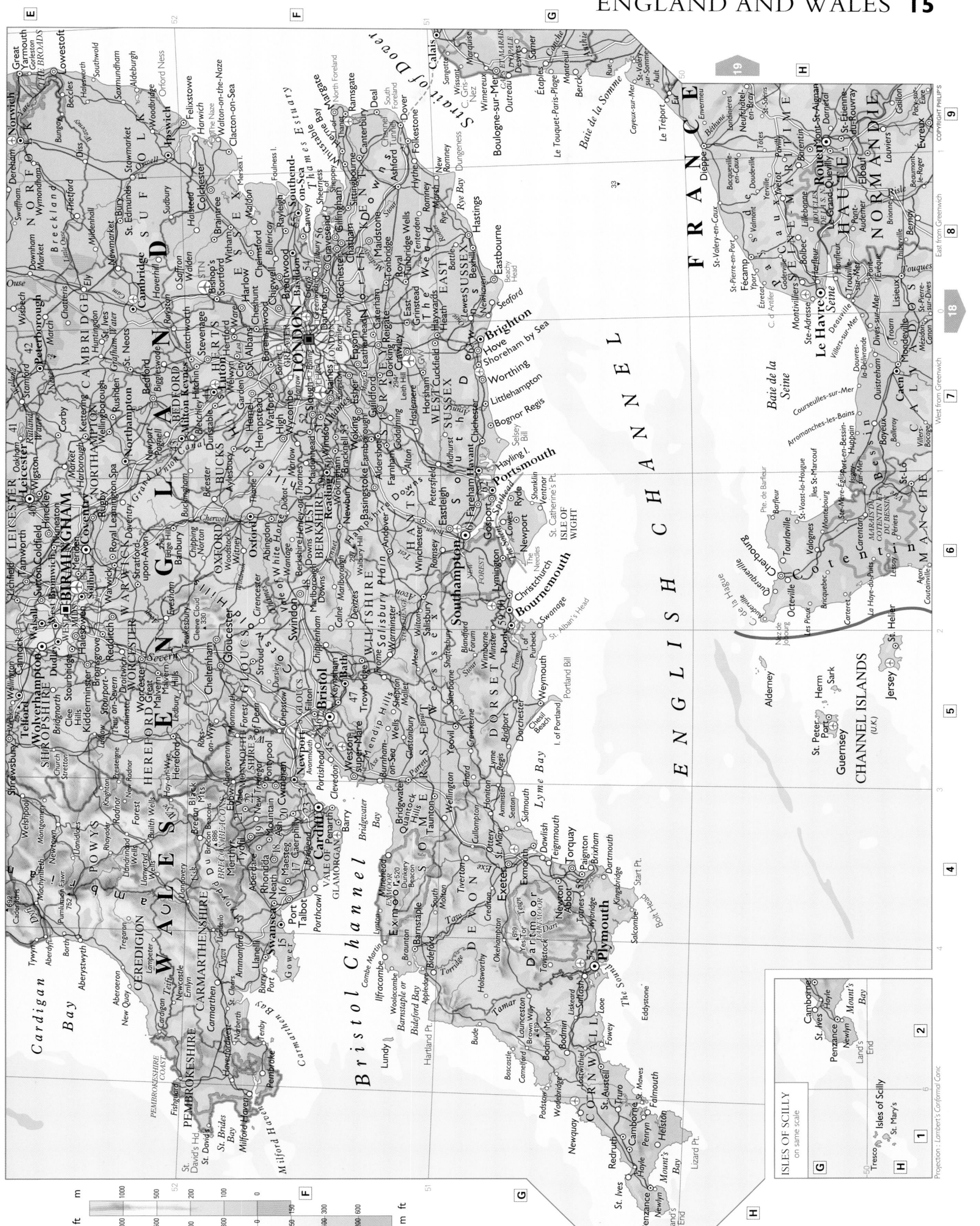

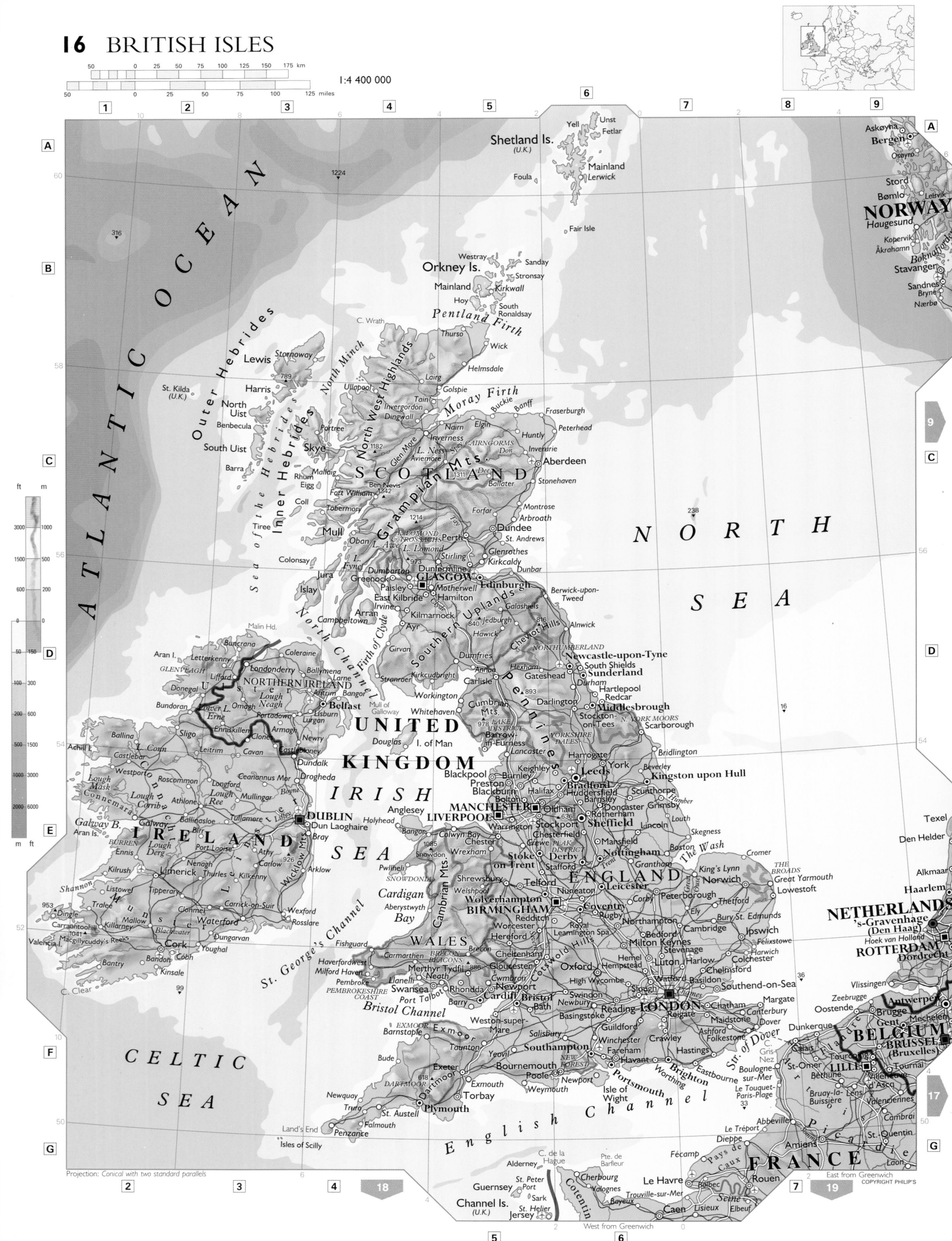

1:4 400 000

50   0 25 50 75 100 125 150 175 km
50   0   25   50   75   100 125 miles

ATLANTIC OCEAN

NORWAY

Shetland Is. (U.K.)
Yell
Unst
Fetlar
Mainland
Lerwick
Foula
Fair Isle

Askøyna
Bergen
Osøyro
Stord
Bømlo
Leirvik
Haugesund
Kopervik
Åkrahamn
Boknafjorden
Stavanger
Sandnes
Bryne
Nærbø

Orkney Is.
Westray
Sanday
Stronsay
Mainland
Kirkwall
Hoy
South Ronaldsay

NORTH SEA

C. Wrath
Pentland Firth
Thurso
Wick
Helmsdale

Lewis
Stornoway
North Minch
Harris
St. Kilda (U.K.)
789
Ullapool
Lairg
Golspie
Tain
Invergordon
Dingwall
Moray Firth
Buckie
Banff
Fraserburgh
Peterhead

North Uist
Benbecula
South Uist
Barra
Portree
Skye
Glen More
L. Ness
1182
Nairn
Elgin
Aviemore
CAIRNGORMS
Huntly
Inverurie
Inverness
Don
Aberdeen

Rhum
Eigg
Mallaig
Fort William
Ben Nevis
1342
1311
Dee
Ballater
Stonehaven

Coll
Tobermory
1214
Forfar
Arbroath
Montrose

Tiree
Mull
Oban
Perth
Dundee
St. Andrews

Colonsay
L. Awe
973
L. Lomond
Stirling
Glenrothes
Kirkcaldy

Jura
L. Fyne
Dumbarton
GLASGOW
Dunfermline
Edinburgh
Berwick-upon-Tweed

Islay
Greenock
Paisley
Motherwell
Hamilton
East Kilbride
Kilmarnock
Irvine
Galashiels
816
Jedburgh
840
Hawick
CHEVIOT HILLS

Campbeltown
Firth of Clyde
Arran
Ayr
Southern Uplands
Girvan
Dumfries
Alnwick

Malin Hd.
North Channel
Stranraer
Kirkcudbright
Annan
Carlisle
NORTHUMBERLAND
Newcastle-upon-Tyne
South Shields
Sunderland

Buncrana
Coleraine
Ballymena
Larne
Mull of Galloway
Workington
Whitehaven
Cumbrian Mts.
978
LAKE DISTRICT
Durham
Hartlepool
Redcar
Gateshead
Hexham
893
Darlington
Middlesbrough
Stockton-on-Tees

Aran I.
Letterkenny
Londonderry
Lifford
NORTHERN IRELAND
Lough Neagh
Antrim
Belfast
Lisburn
Bangor

Donegal
GLENVEAGH
Omagh
Ulster
Portadown
Armagh
Lurgan
Newry

Bundoran
Lower L. Erne
Enniskillen
Clones
Douglas
I. of Man
Barrow-in-Furness
Lancaster
N. YORK MOORS
Scarborough
YORKSHIRE DALES

Achill
Ballina
Sligo
Leitrim
Cavan
Castleblaney
Dundalk
UNITED
KINGDOM
IRISH SEA
Bridlington

Castlebar
L. Corn
Roscommon
Longford
Mullingar
Boyne
Drogheda
Ceanannus Mor
KINGDOM

Lough Mask
Lough Corrib
Connemara
Westport
Ballinasloe
Athlone
Tullamore
Navan
Liffey
DUBLIN
Dun Laoghaire
Bray
Anglesey
Holyhead
Blackpool
Preston
Blackburn
Burnley
Harrogate
York
Beverley
Kingston upon Hull

Galway B.
Galway
Aran Is.
BURREN
Ennis
Lough Derg
Birr
Athy
Carlow
926
Wicklow Mts.
Arklow
Bangor
Colwyn Bay
Chester
Crewe
Leeds
Bradford
Huddersfield
Halifax
Bolton
Barnsley
Doncaster
Grimsby
Humber

Limerick
Nenagh
Thurles
Kilkenny
Snowdon
1085
Wrexham
Snowdonia
MANCHESTER
LIVERPOOL
Oldham
Stockport
Warrington
Sheffield
Chesterfield
Lincoln
Louth
Skegness
Boston
The Wash

Tralee
Listowel
Tipperary
Clonmel
Carrick-on-Suir
Waterford
Wexford
Rosslare
Pwllheli
636
Cardigan Bay
Aberystwyth
PEAK DISTRICT
Stoke-on-Trent
Derby
Nottingham
Mansfield
Stafford
Telford
Shrewsbury
Welshpool
Cambrian Mts.
Grantham
King's Lynn
Norwich
Cromer
THE BROADS
Great Yarmouth
Lowestoft

953
Dingle
Carrauntoohill
1041
Macgillycuddy's Reeks
Killarney
Mallow
Blackwater
Clonakilty
Dungarvan
Youghal
99

WALES
BRECON BEACONS
886
Brecon
Carmarthen
Haverfordwest
Milford Haven
Pembroke
PEMBROKESHIRE COAST
Fishguard
St. George's Channel

Valencia
Bandon
Kinsale
Cork
Cóbh

C. Clear

CELTIC SEA

Newquay
Truro
St. Austell
Falmouth
Penzance
Land's End
Isles of Scilly

ENGLAND
Leicester
Coventry
Rugby
Nuneaton
BIRMINGHAM
Wolverhampton
Redditch
Royal Leamington Spa
Corby
Peterborough
Northampton
Bedford
Ely
Bury St. Edmunds
Thetford
Milton Keynes
Cambridge
Ipswich
Stevenage
Hereford
Worcester
Gloucester
Cheltenham
COTSWOLD HILLS
Oxford
Luton
Harlow
Colchester
Harwich
Felixstowe

Merthyr Tydfil
Neath
Rhondda
Llanelli
Swansea
Port Talbot
Barry
Cwmbran
Newport
Cardiff
Bristol
Bath
Newbury
Reading
LONDON
Basildon
Southend-on-Sea
Chatham
Margate
Canterbury
Maidstone

Weston-super-Mare
Salisbury
Swindon
High Wycombe
Hemel Hempstead
Watford
Slough
Guildford
Reigate
Ashford
Folkestone
Dover
Str. of Dover

Bristol Channel
Barnstaple
Bude
Exmoor
Taunton
Yeovil
Winchester
Fareham
Southampton
Bournemouth
Poole
Newport
Isle of Wight
Portsmouth
Havant
Crawley
Brighton
Worthing
Eastbourne
Hastings

DARTMOOR
618
Dartmoor
Exeter
Exmouth
Torbay
Plymouth
Weymouth
NEW FOREST
33

ENGLISH CHANNEL

Alderney
C. de la Hague
Pte. de Barfleur
Guernsey
St. Peter Port
Sark
Cherbourg
Valognes
Cotentin
Bayeux
Caen
Lisieux
Elbeuf
Fécamp
Pays de Caux
Rouen
Seine
Trouville-sur-Mer
Le Havre
Dieppe
St. Valéry
Le Tréport
Abbeville
Amiens
FRANCE

Channel Is. (U.K.)
St. Helier
Jersey

NETHERLANDS
Texel
Den Helder
Alkmaar
Haarlem
's-Gravenhage (Den Haag)
ROTTERDAM
Dordrecht
Hoek van Holland

Vlissingen
Zeebrugge
Oostende
Brugge
Gent
Mechelen
Antwerpen
BELGIUM
BRUSSEL (Bruxelles)
LILLE
Tournai

Dunkerque
Calais
Gris Nez
Boulogne-sur-Mer
St.-Omer
Béthune
Lens
Bruay-la-Buissière
Le Touquet-Paris-Plage
Tourcoing
Roubaix
Valenciennes
Picardie
Cambrai
St. Quentin
Laon

East from Greenwich
COPYRIGHT PHILIP'S
West from Greenwich

Projection: Conical with two standard parallels

1:2 200 000

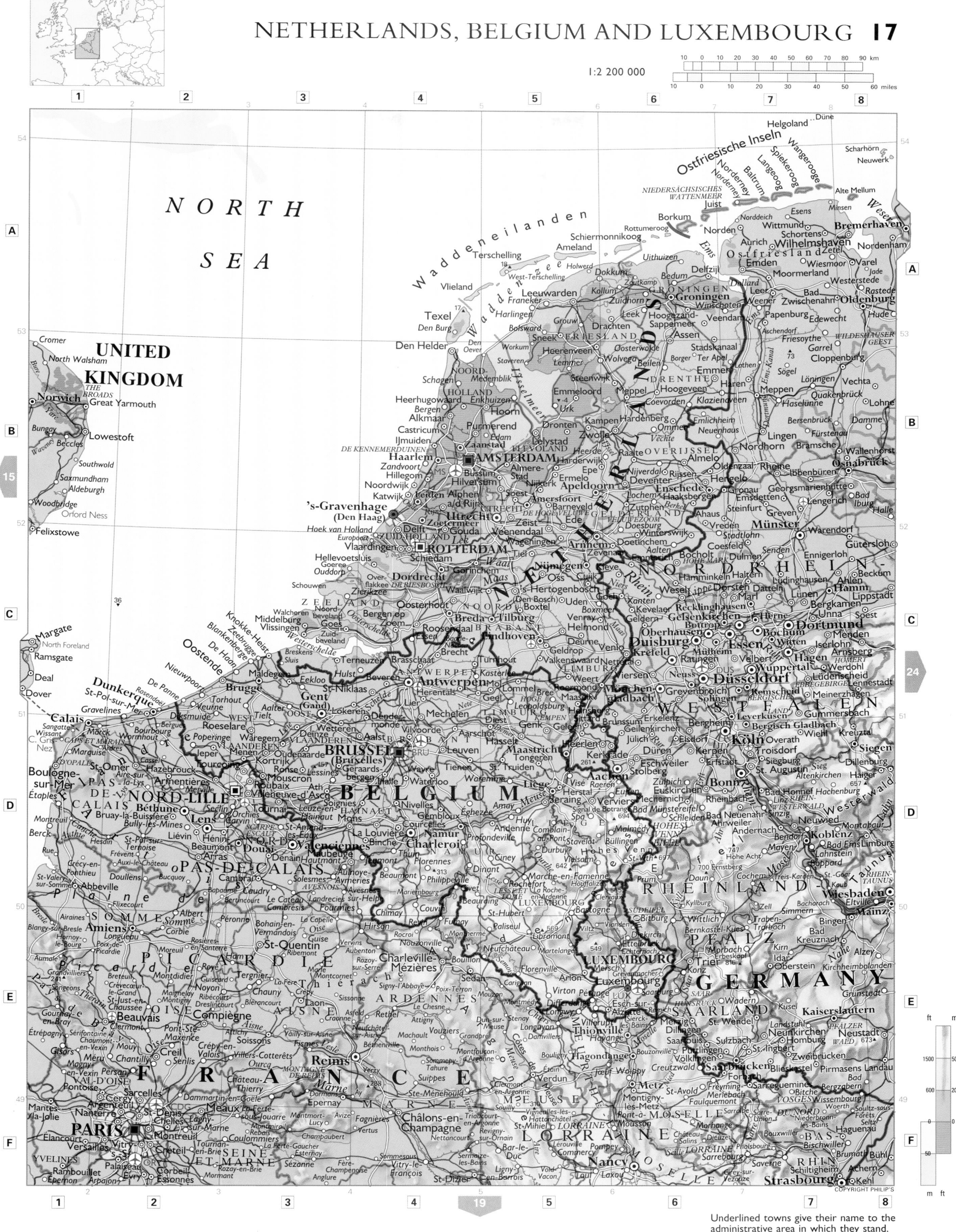

Underlined towns give their name to the
administrative area in which they stand.

1:2 200 000

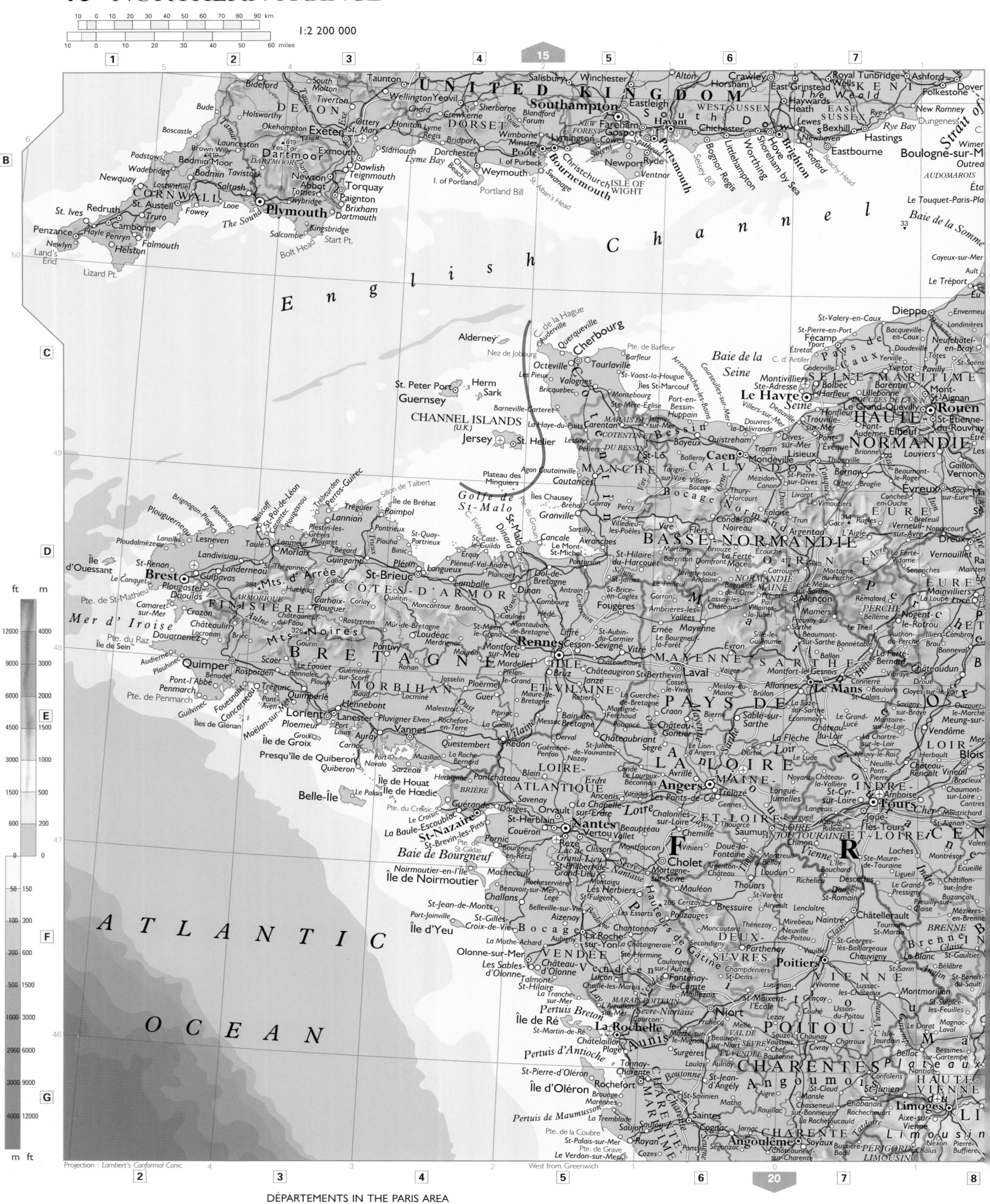

Projection : Lambert's Conformal Conic

DÉPARTEMENTS IN THE PARIS AREA
1 Ville de Paris   3 Val-de-Marne
2 Seine-St-Denis   4 Hauts-de-Seine

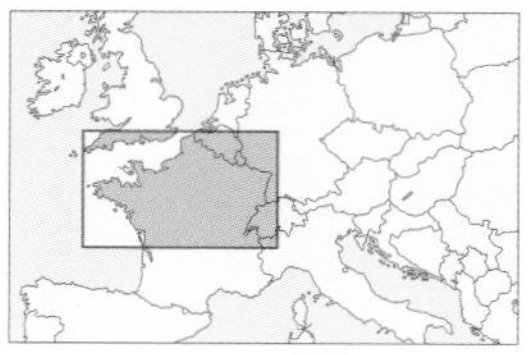

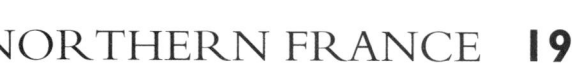

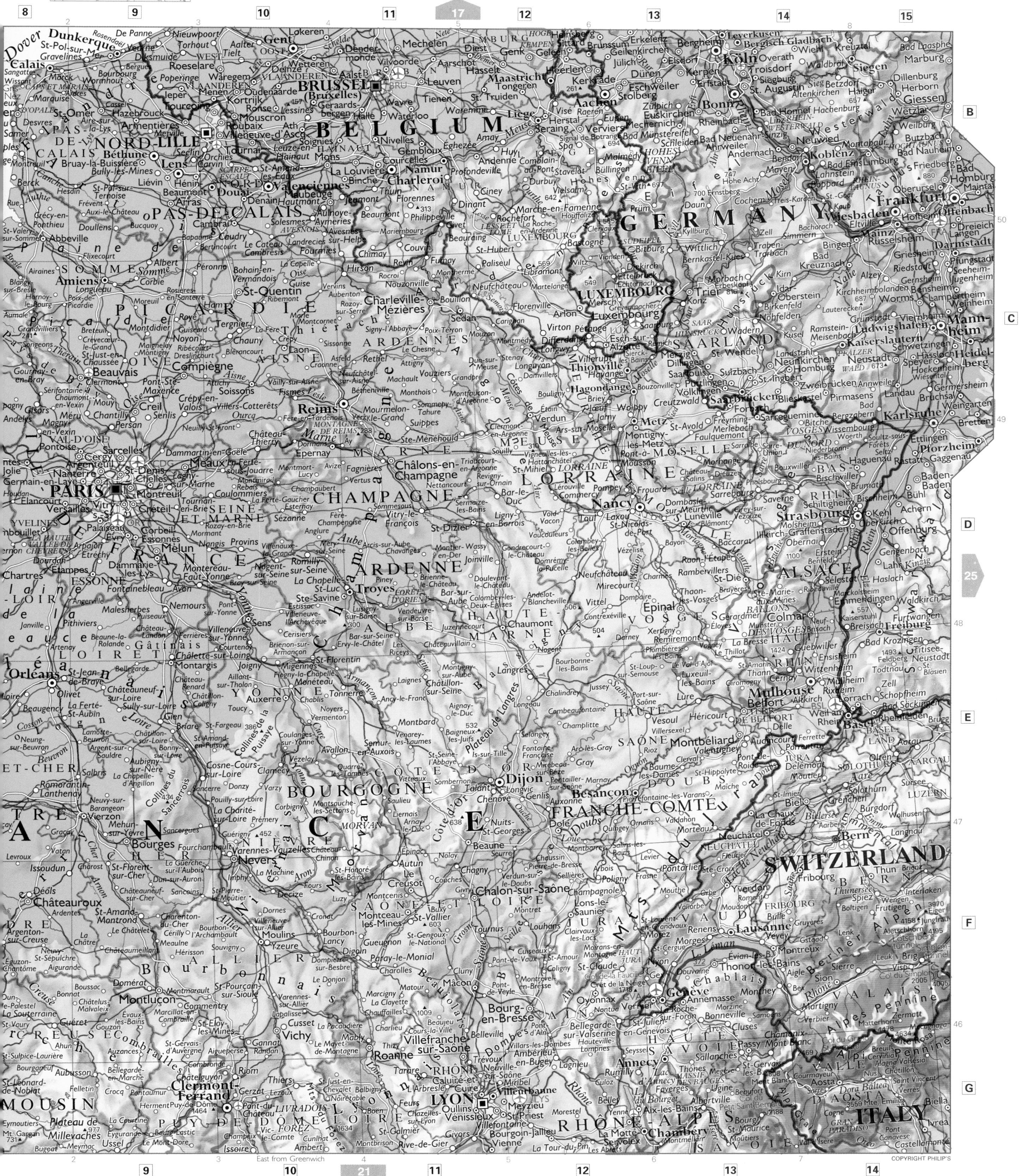

Underlined towns give their name to the administrative area in which they stand.

East from Greenwich

COPYRIGHT PHILIP'S

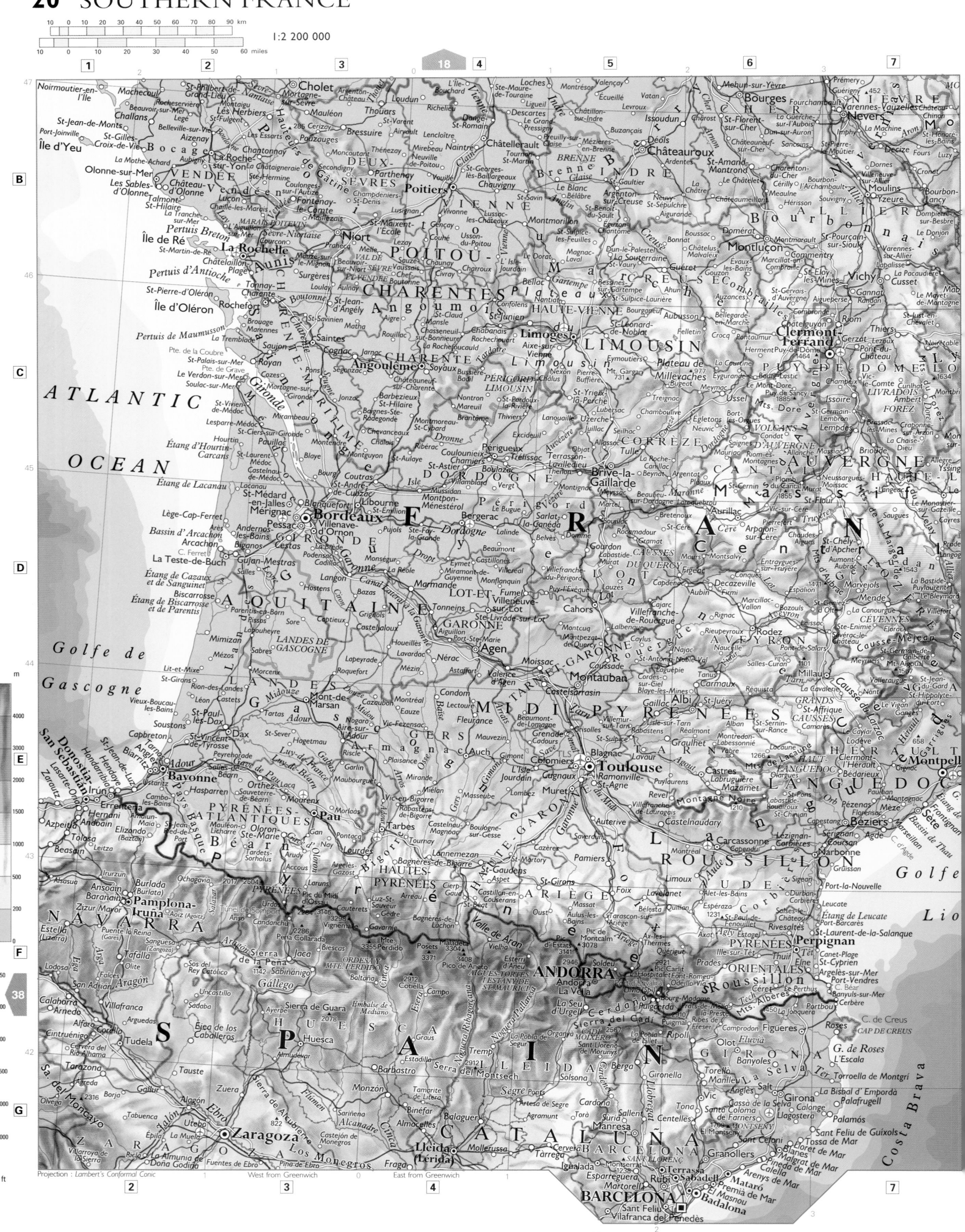

1:2 200 000

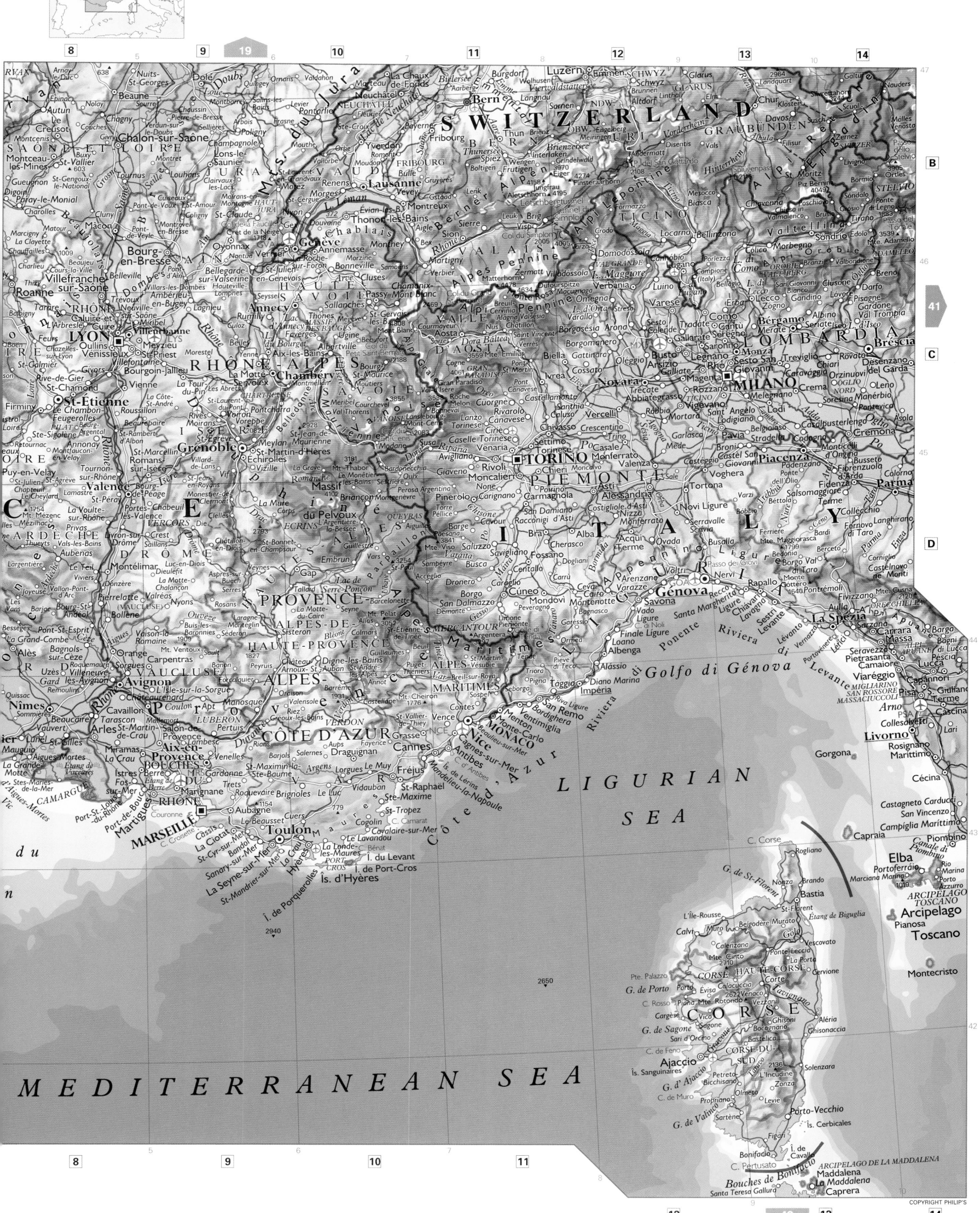

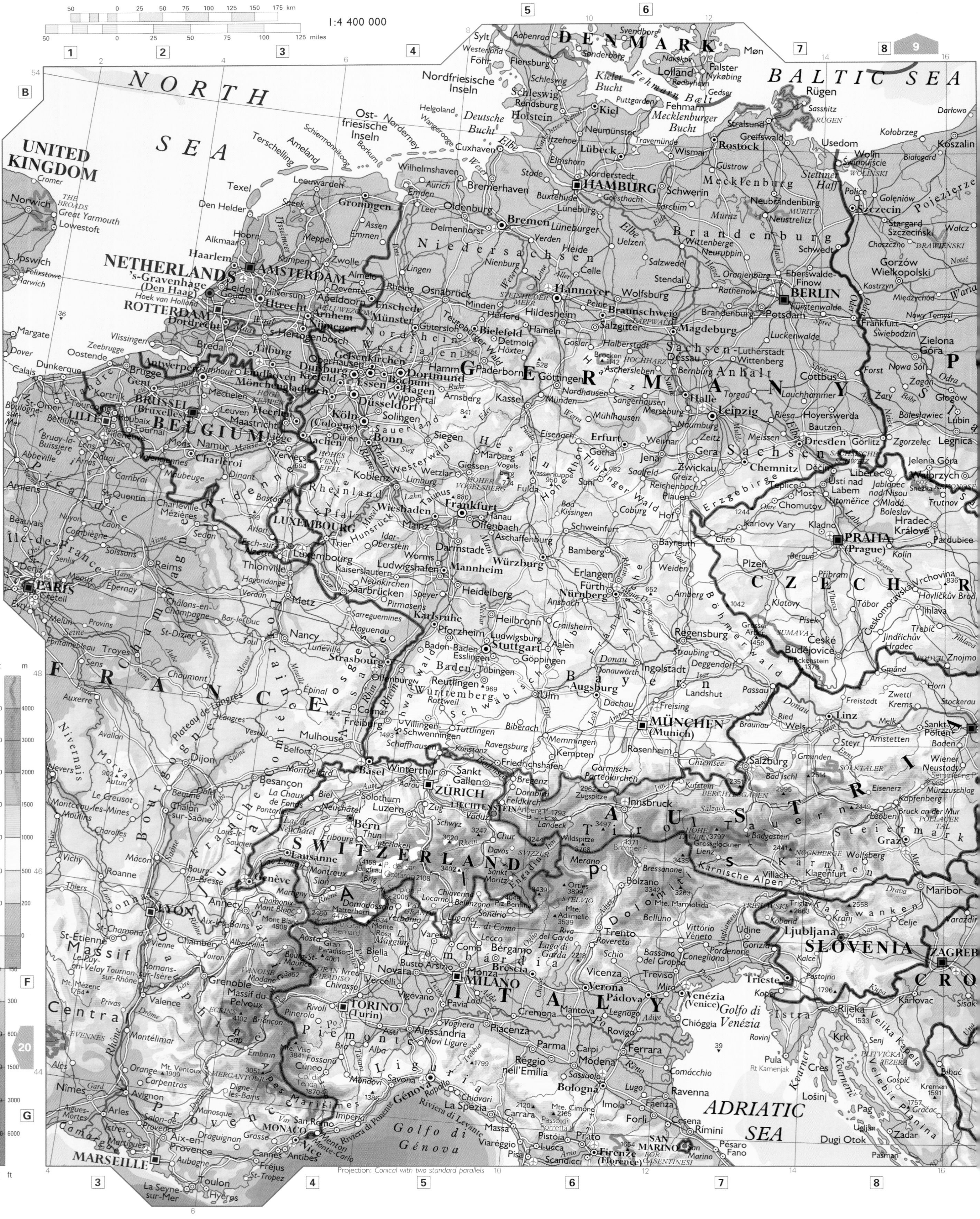

1:4 400 000

50 0 25 50 75 100 125 150 175 km
50 0 25 50 75 100 125 miles

NORTH SEA

BALTIC SEA

DENMARK

UNITED KINGDOM

NETHERLANDS

BELGIUM

LUXEMBOURG

GERMANY

FRANCE

SWITZERLAND

ITALY

AUSTRIA

CZECH

POLAND

SLOVENIA

CROATIA

ADRIATIC SEA

Projection: Conical with two standard parallels

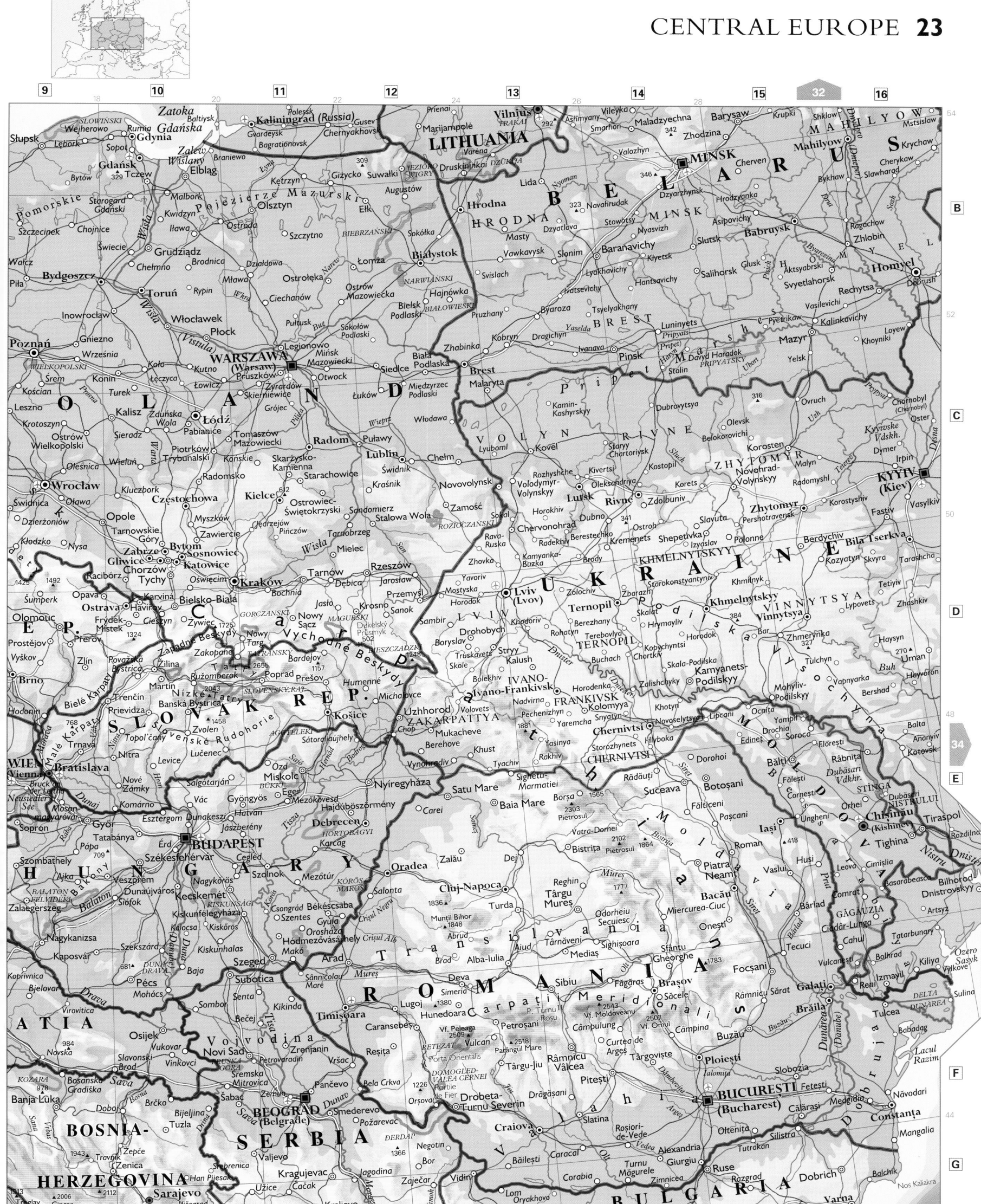

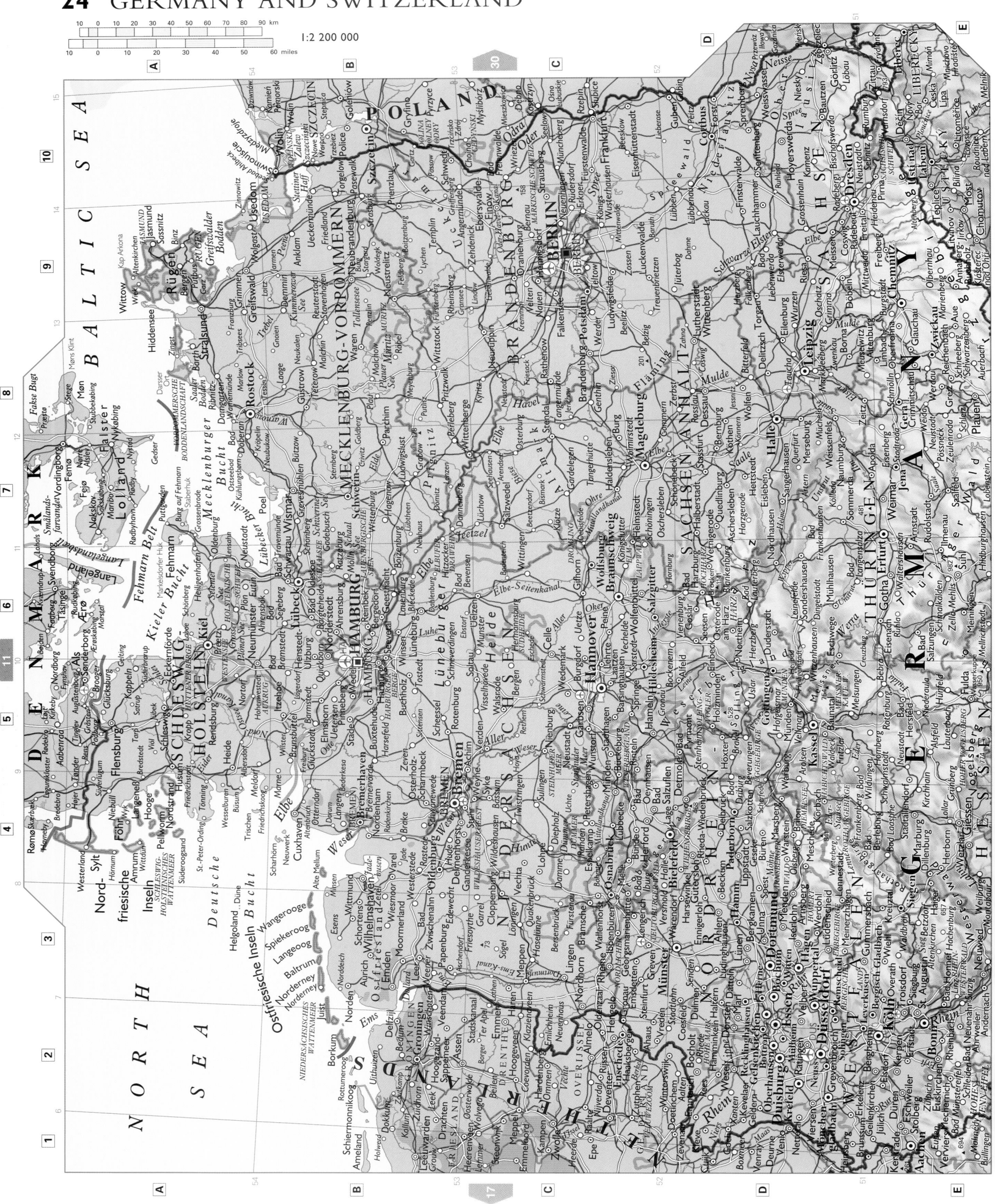

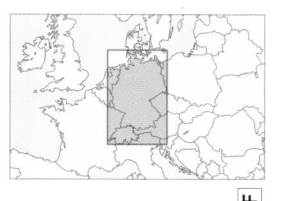

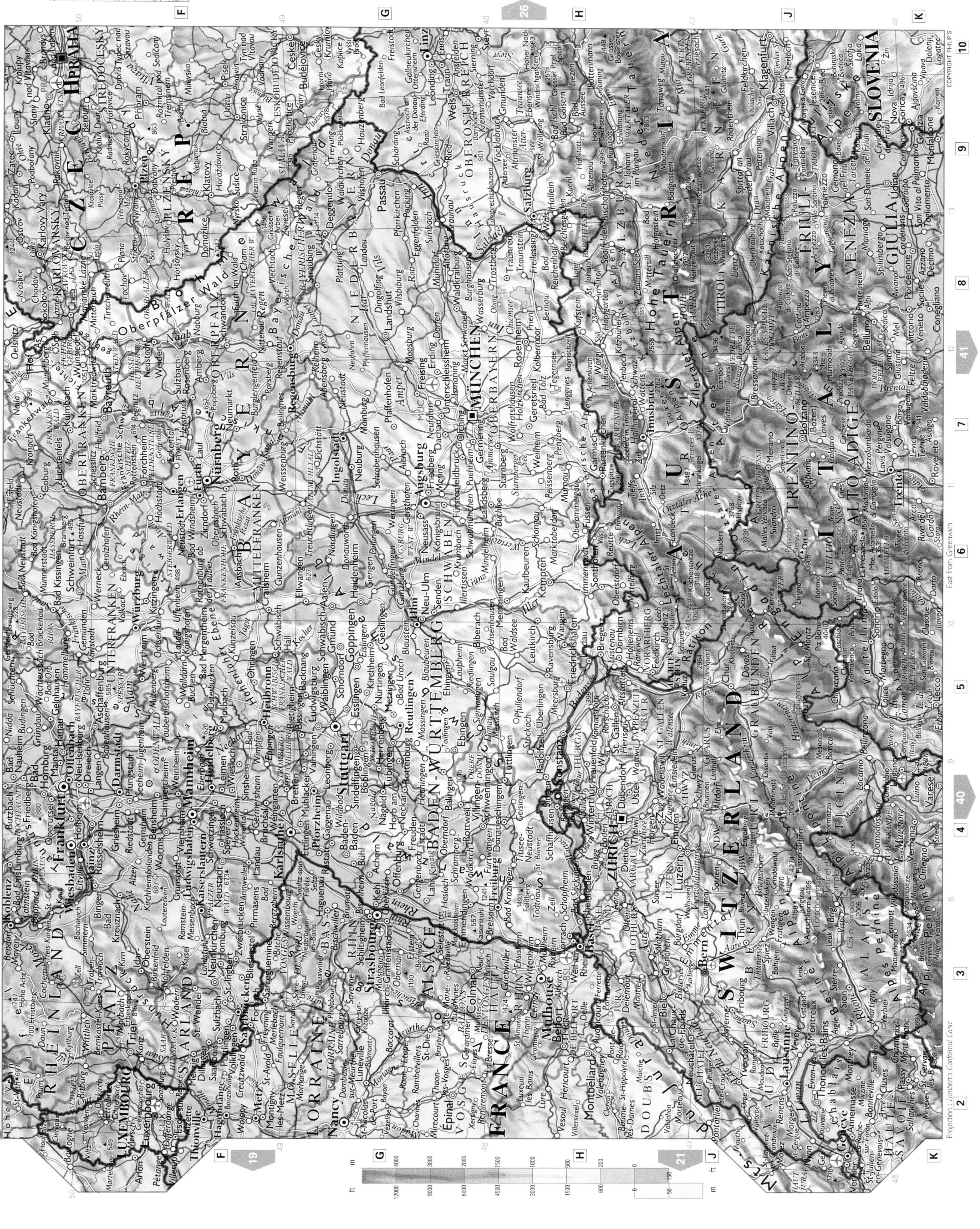

Underlined towns give their name to the administrative area in which they stand.

Projection: Lambert's Conformal Conic

East from Greenwich

COPYRIGHT PHILIP'S

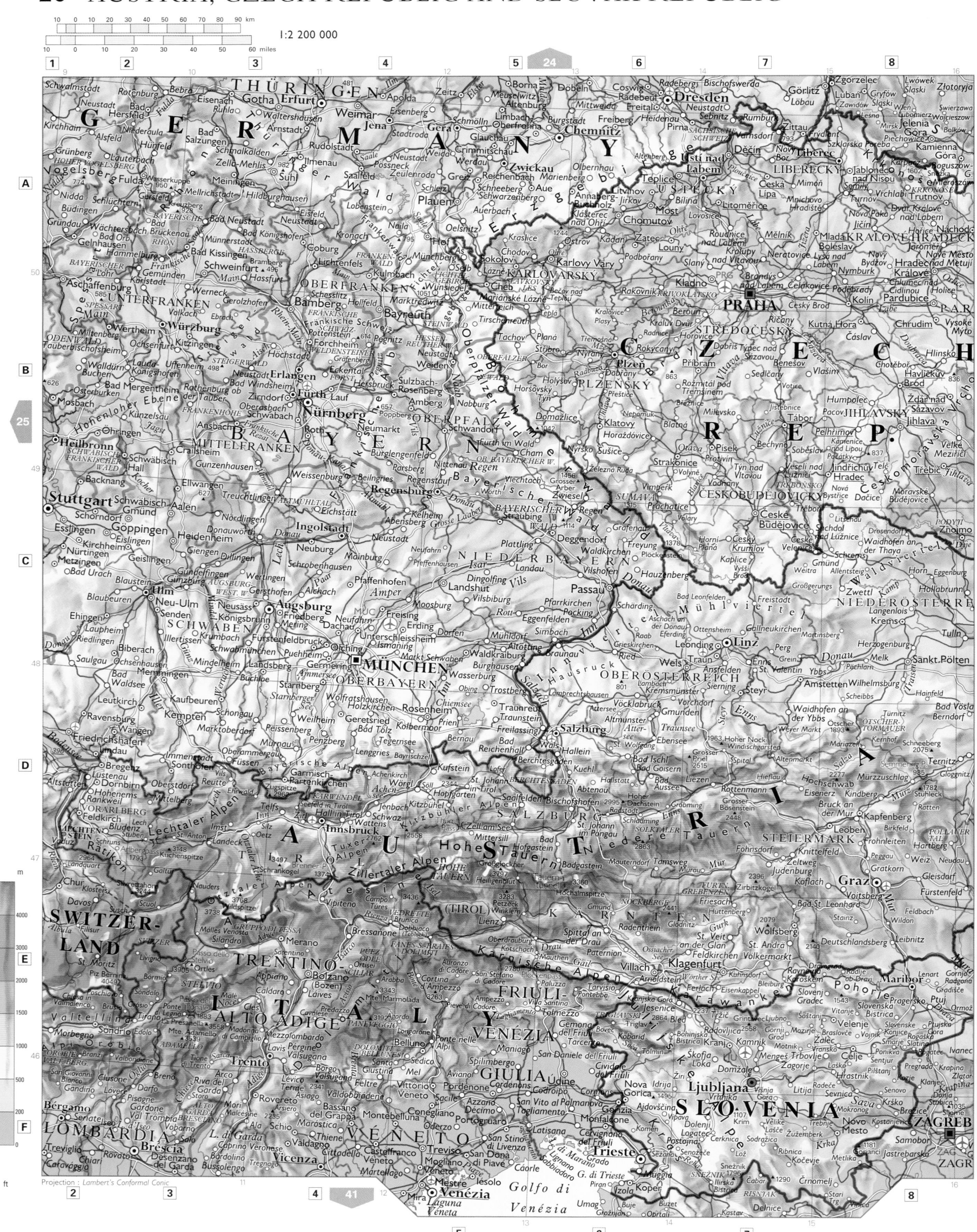

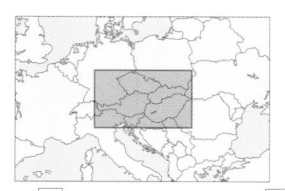

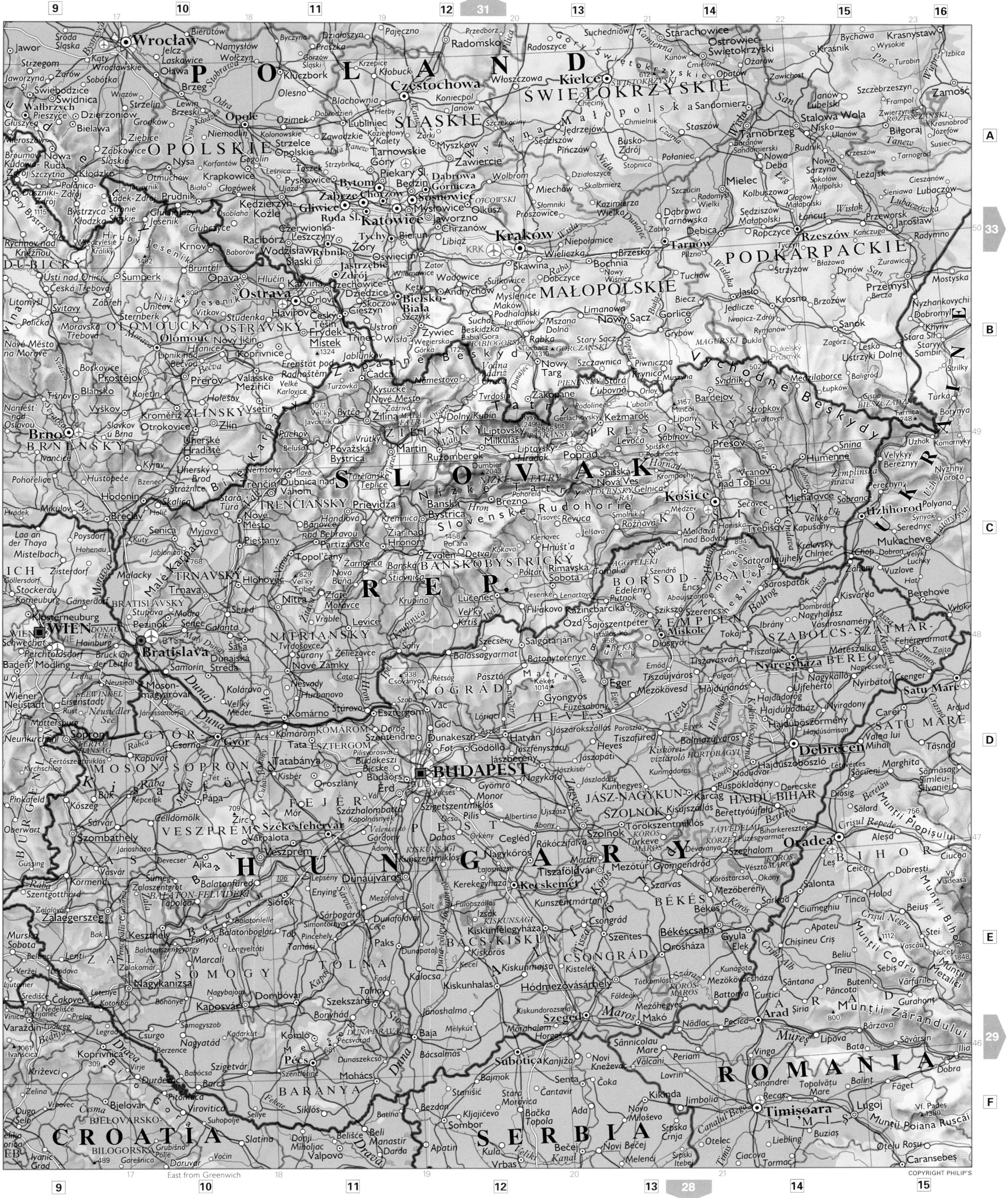

Underlined towns give their name to the administrative area in which they stand.

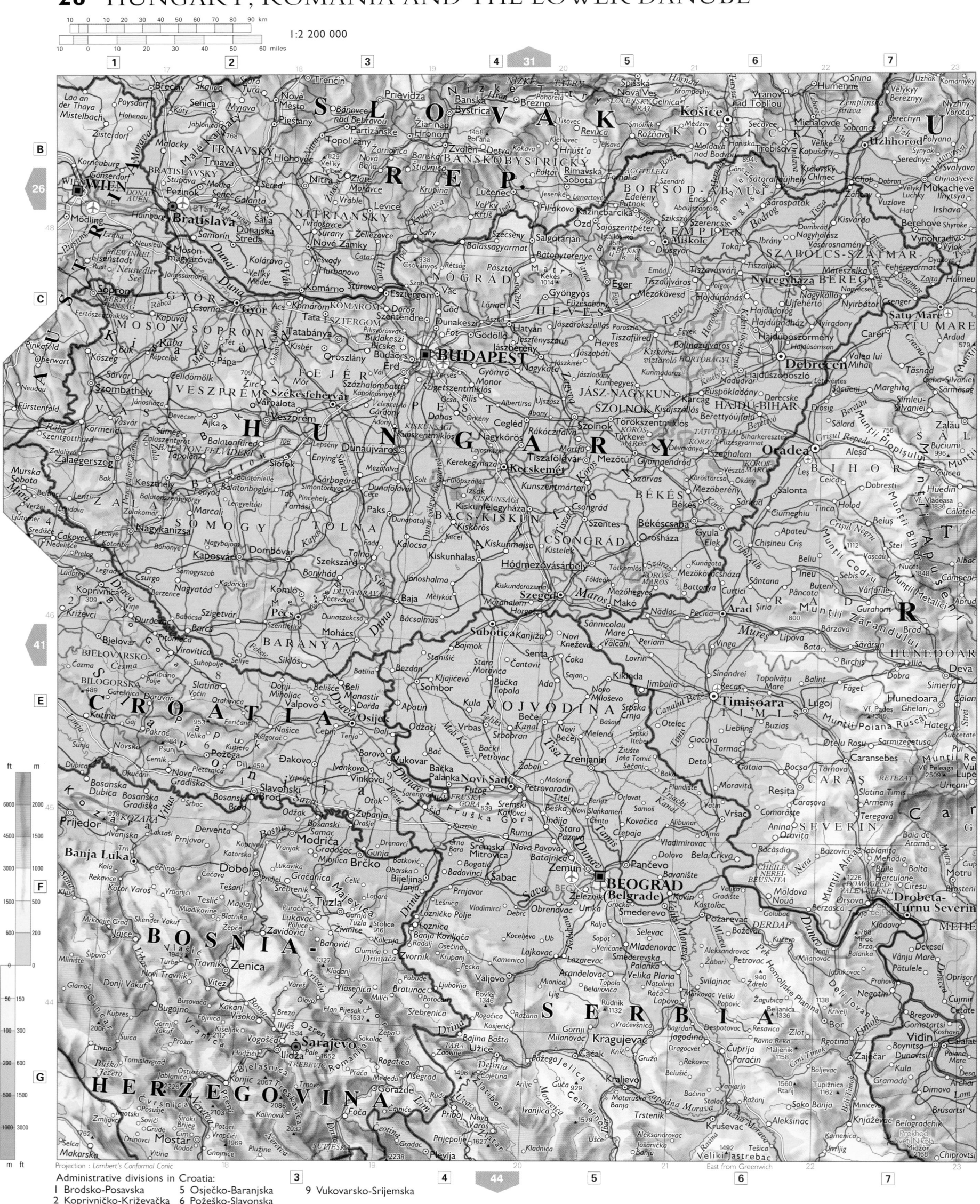

1:2 200 000

Administrative divisions in Croatia:
1 Brodsko-Posavska   5 Osječko-Baranjska   9 Vukovarsko-Srijemska
2 Koprivničko-Križevačka   6 Požeško-Slavonska
4 Medimurska   8 Virovitičko-Podravska

East from Greenwich

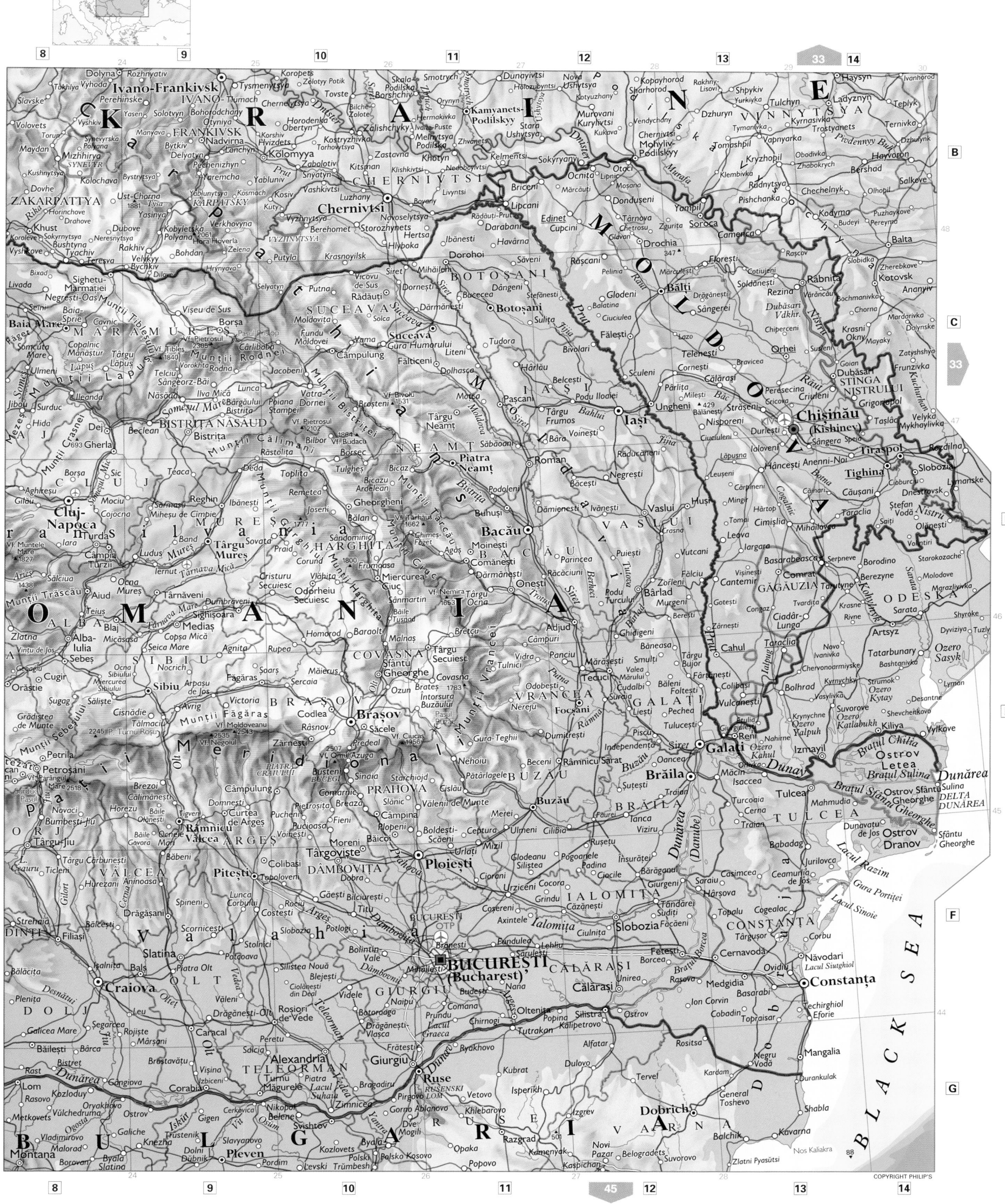

1:2 200 000

10 0 10 20 30 40 50 60 70 80 90 km
10 0 10 20 30 40 50 60 miles

SWEDEN

LATVIA

LITHUANIA

KALININGRAD (Russia)

POLAND (WARMIŃSKO-MAZURSKIE, POMORSKIE, ZACHODNIO-POMORSKIE, KUJAWSKO-)

Gulf of Riga

BALTIC SEA

Irbes saurums (Kura kurk)

Gotland (Sweden)

Öland (Sweden)

Bornholm (Denmark) BORNHOLMS AMT.

Hanöbukten

Bornholmsgattet

Zatoka Gdańska

Kurshskiy Zaliv

Zalew Wiślany

Neman / Nemunas

Selected place names:

Riga, Jūrmala, Jelgava, Tukums, Talsi, Ventspils, Liepāja, Kuldīga, Saldus, Dobele, Mažeikiai, Šiauliai, Telšiai, Plungė, Kretinga, Klaipėda, Palanga, Šilutė, Tauragė, Kaunas, Marijampolė, Kaliningrad, Gusev, Chernyakhovsk, Sovetsk, Baltiysk, Gdynia, Sopot, Gdańsk, Elbląg, Malbork, Olsztyn, Ostróda, Koszalin, Słupsk, Lębork, Wejherowo, Władysławowo, Hel, Puck, Tczew, Grudziądz, Starogard, Ełk, Suwałki, Hrodna, Augustów, Białystok, Szczecin, Stargard, Świnoujście, Wolin

Jönköping, Visby, Kalmar, Karlskrona, Västervik, Växjö

Grid references: A B C D E / 1–11

Underlined towns give their name to the
administrative area in which they stand.

COPYRIGHT PHILIP'S

Projection: Lambert's Conformal Conic

East from Greenwich

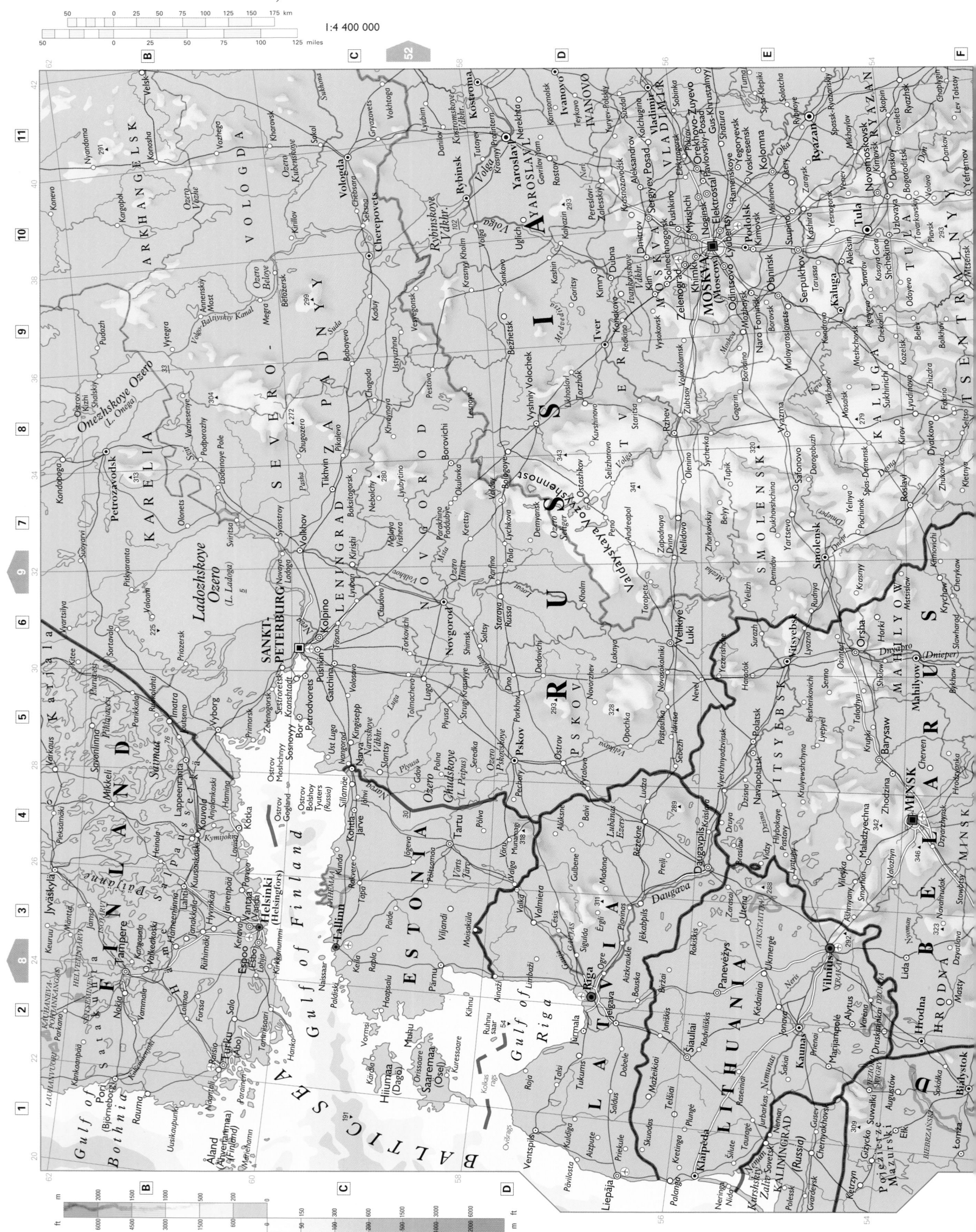

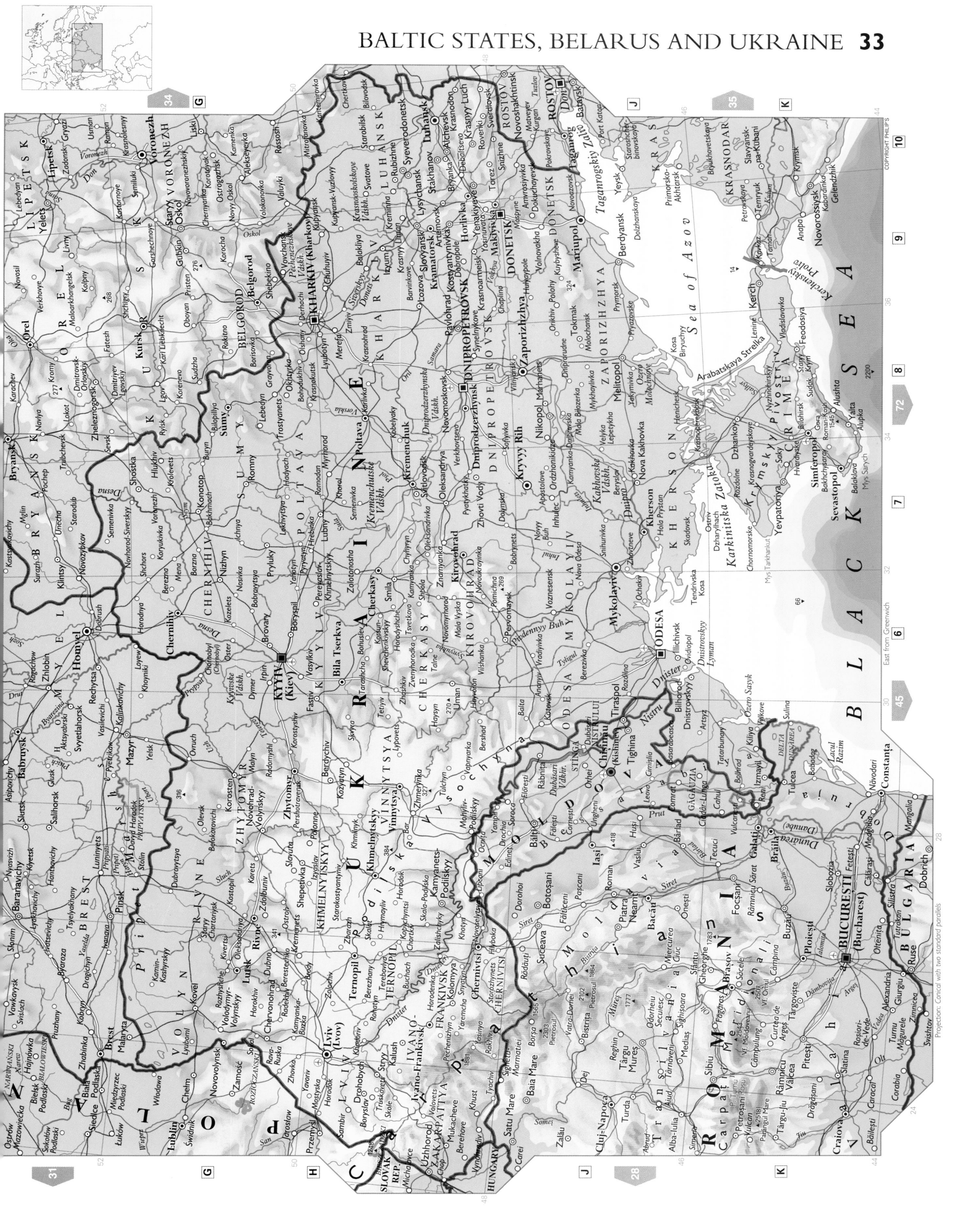

Projection: Conical with two standard parallels

East from Greenwich

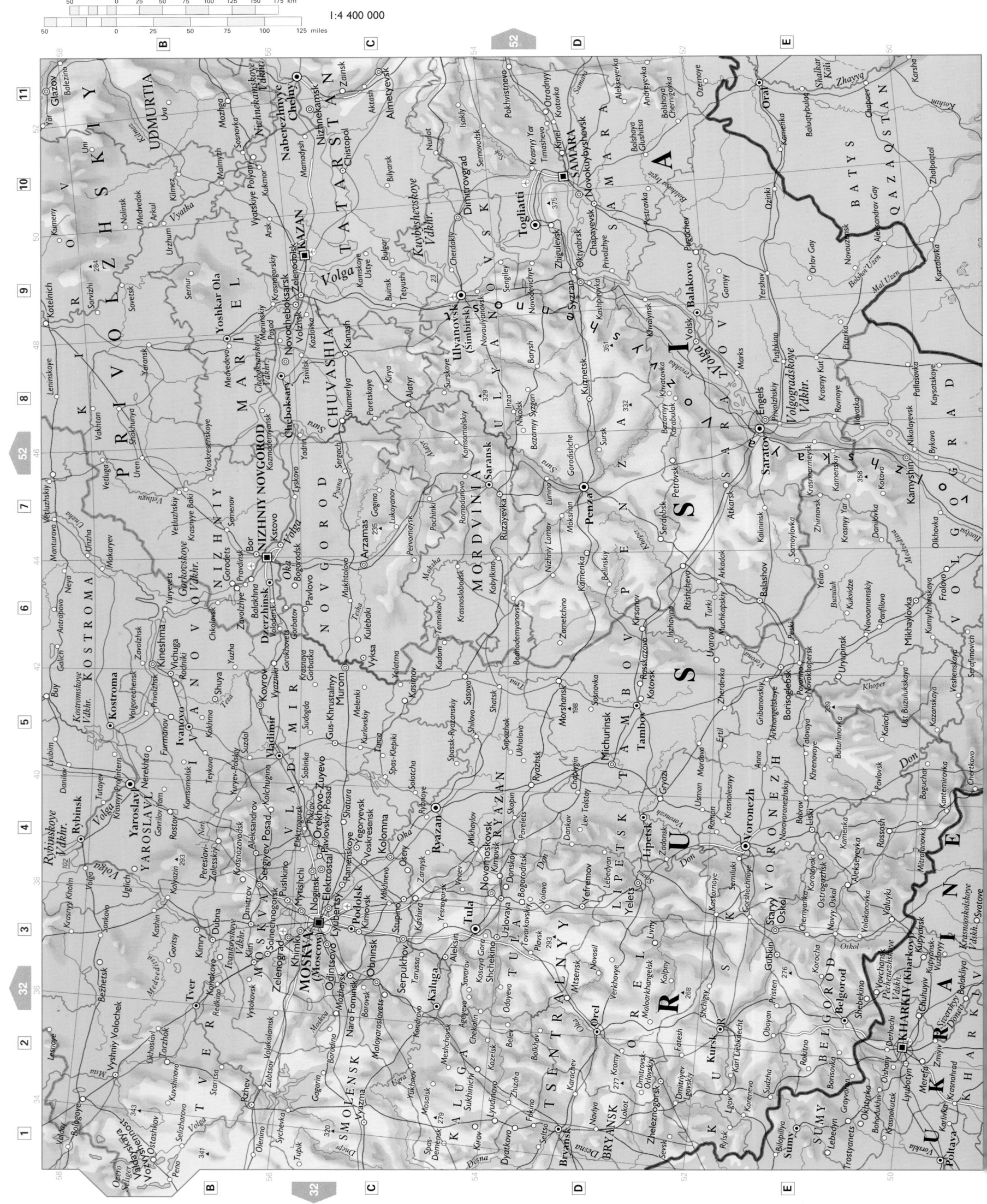

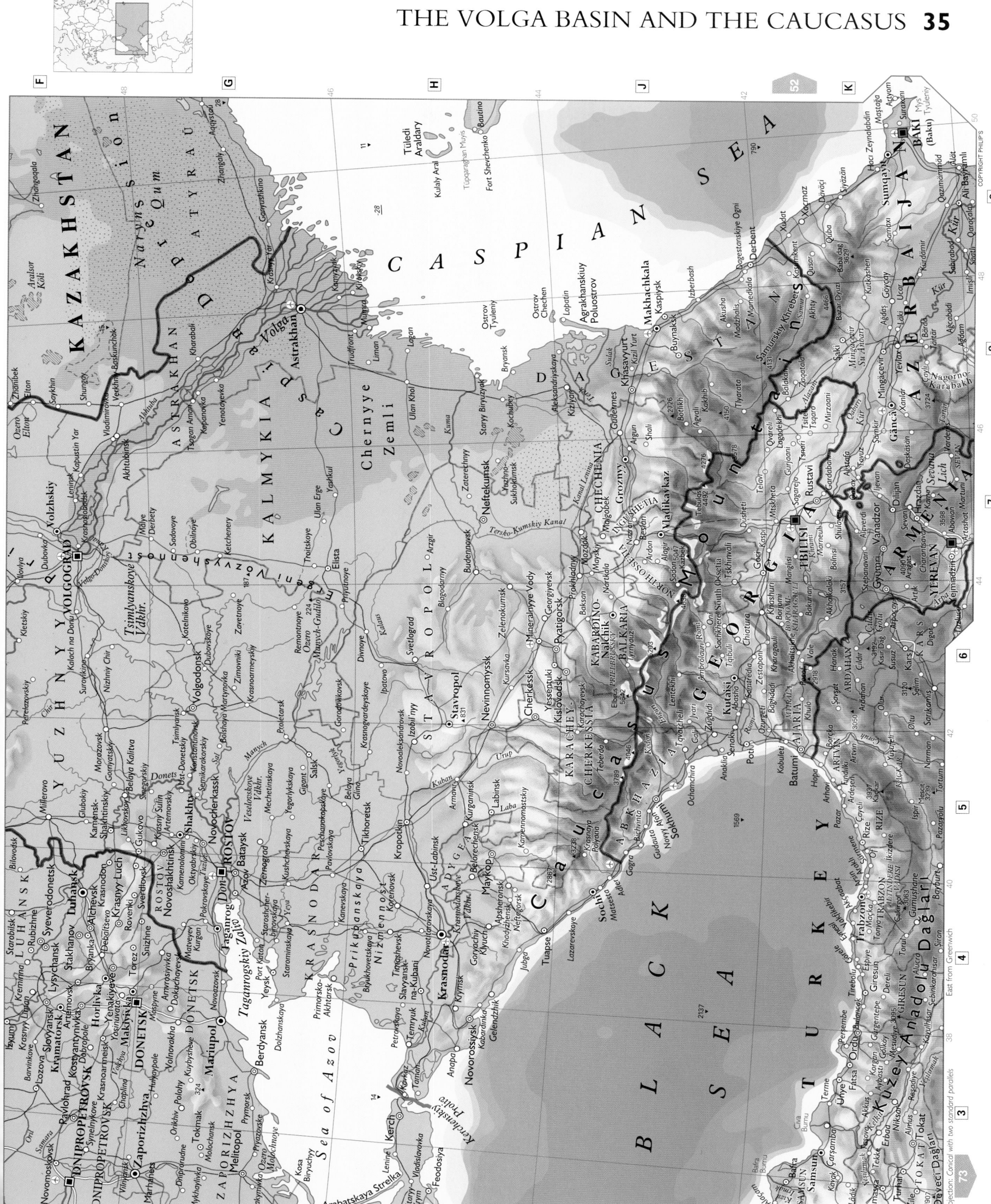

1:2 200 000

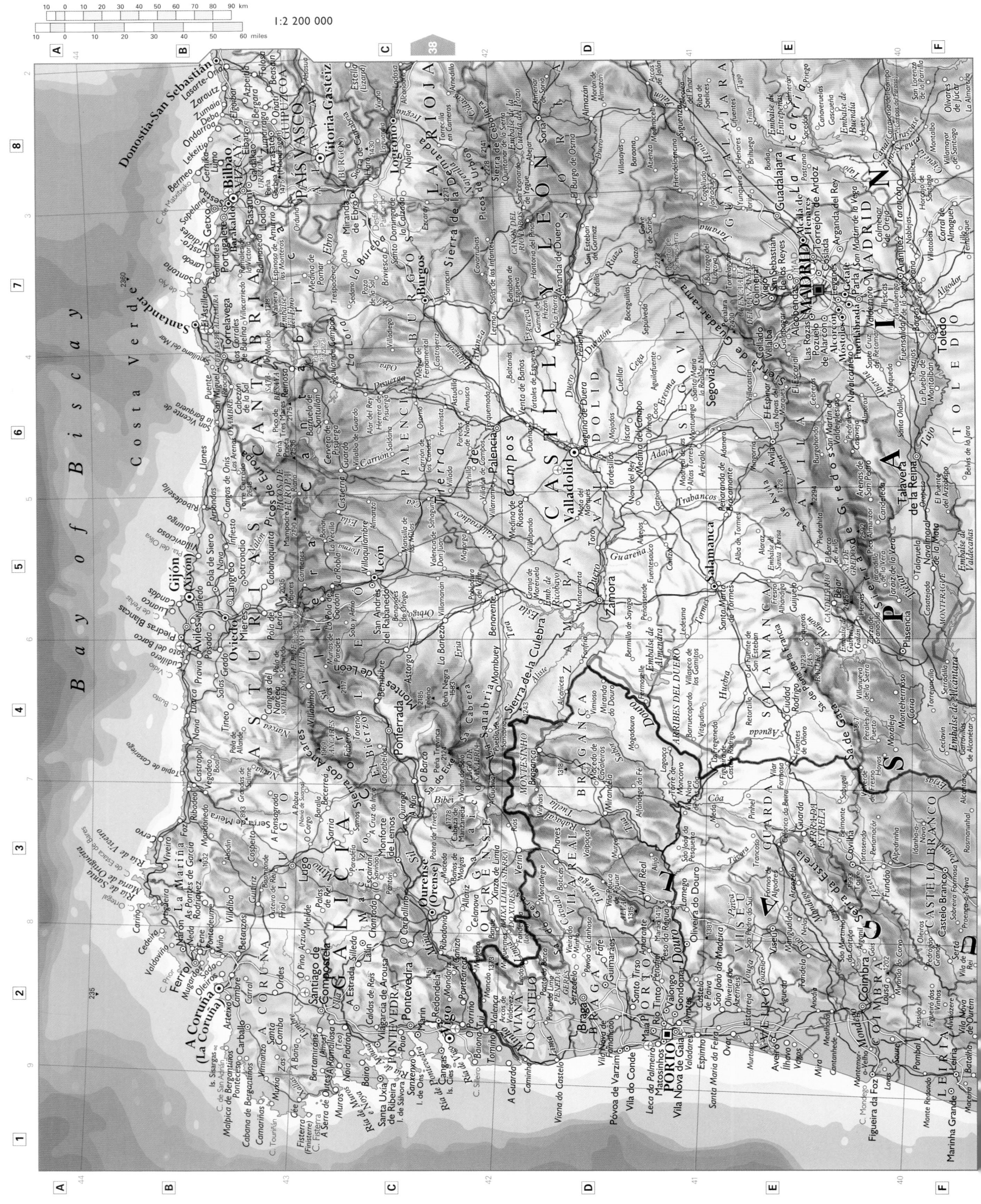

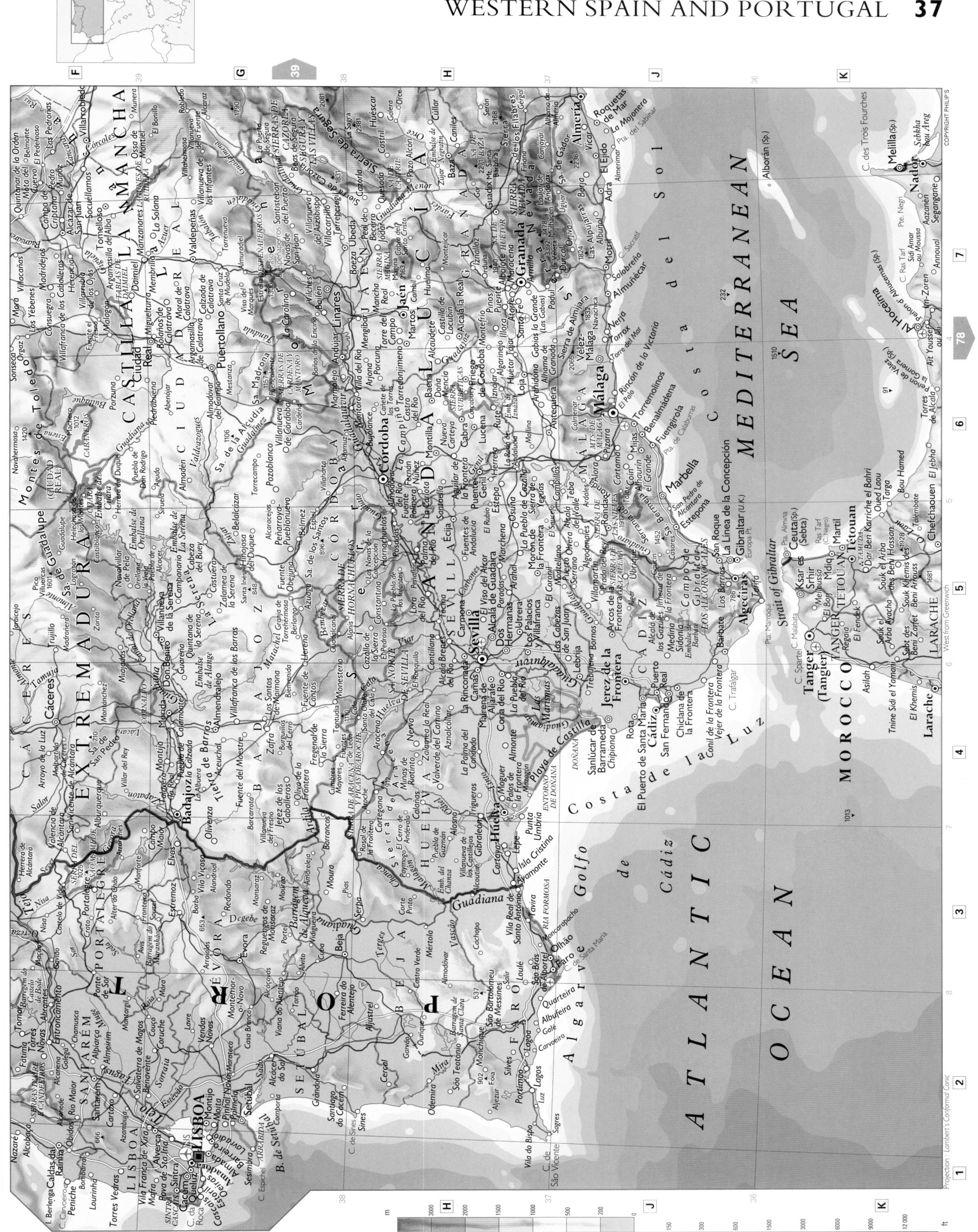

1:2 200 000

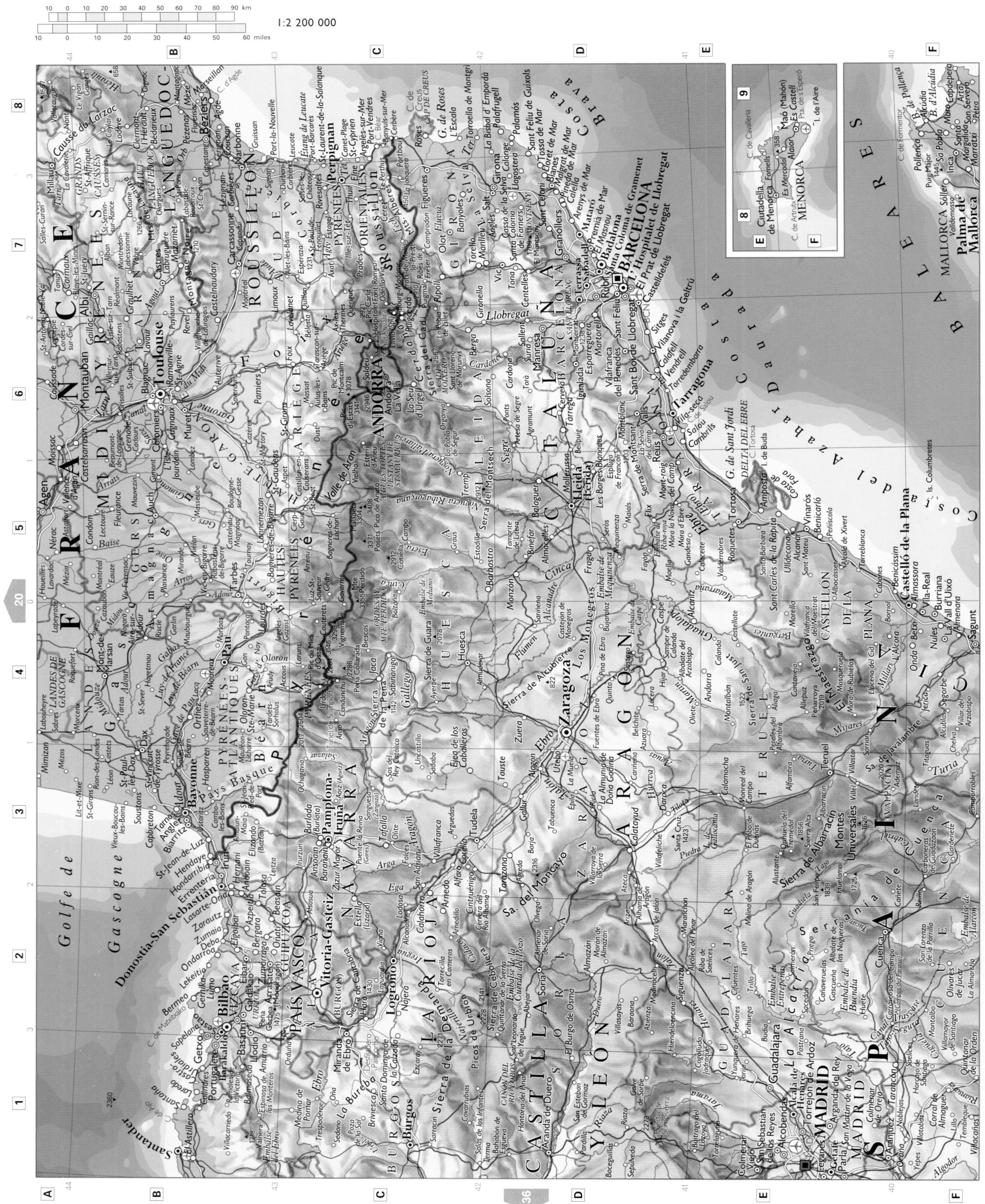

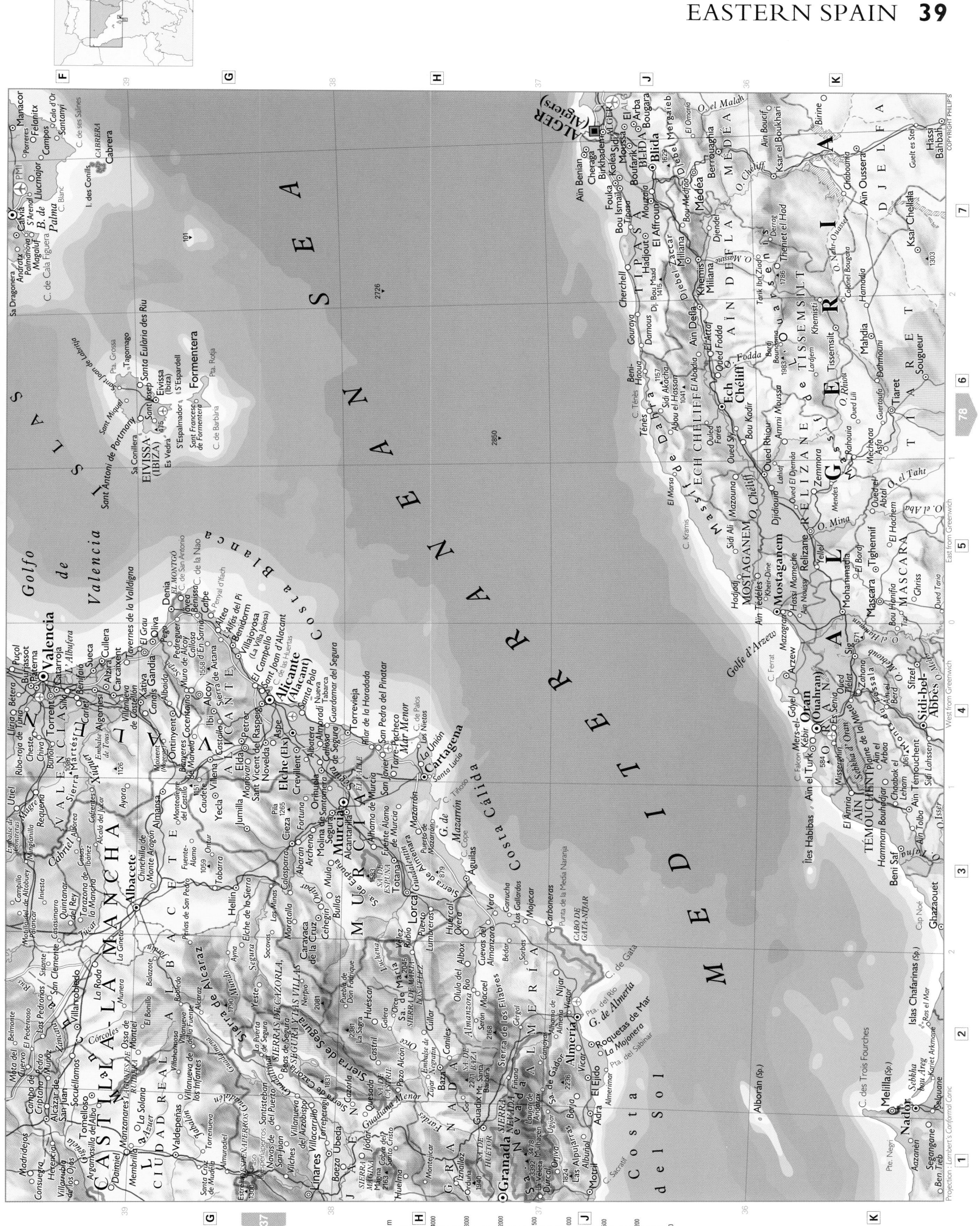

SEA

MEDITERRANEAN

BALEARIC ISLANDS

Cabrera

Manacor
Porreres
Felanitx
Campos
C. de ses Salines
Andratx
Calvià
S'Arenal
B. de
Palma
C. de Cala Figuera
Santanyi
C. Blanc
I. des Conills
Sa Dragonera
Palmanova
Magaluf
Llucmajor
PMI

Formentera
Santa Eularia des Riu
Pta. Grossa
Tagomago
Sant Joan de Labritja
Sant Miquel
Sant Antoni de Portmany
Sa Conillera
EIVISSA
(IBIZA)
Eivissa
(Ibiza)
Sant Josep
Es Vedra
S'Espalmador
Sant Francesc
de Formentera
C. de Barbària
Pta. Rotja

Golfo
de
Valencia

VALENCIA
Puçol
Burjassot
Paterna
Llíria
Bétera
Torrent
Catarroja
Benifaió
Sueca
Alzira
Cullera
Carcaixent
Villanueva de
Castellón
Alberic
Alcira
Xàtiva
Gandia
Oliva
Denia
El Grau
Pego
El Montgó
C. de San Antonio
Calpe
Penyal d'Ifach
Benissa
C. de la Nao
Altea
Benidorm
La Vila Joiosa
(Villajoyosa)
L'Alfàs del Pi
El Campello
Sant Joan d'Alacant
Alicante
(Alacant)
Santa Pola
C. de les Huertes
Elche
(Elx)
Crevillent
Albatera
Callosa
Pilar de la Horadada
Torrevieja
Guardamar del Segura
Mar Menor
San Pedro del Pinatar
Torre Pacheco
San Javier
Los Alcázares
La Unión
Cartagena
C. de Palos
Los Nietos
Santa Lucía

Murcia
Alcantarilla
Alhama de Murcia
Fuente Álamo
Mazarrón
Puerto de
Mazarrón
G. de
Mazarrón
C. Cope
Águilas
Costa Cálida

Costa Blanca

Albacete
Chinchilla de
Monte Aragón
Almansa
Alpera
Caudete
Villena
Yecla
Jumilla
Cieza
Calasparra
Caravaca
de la Cruz
Cehegín
Bullas
Mula
Alcantarilla
Abarán
Archena
Fortuna
Molina de
Segura
Lorca
Totana
Aledo
Puerto
Lumbreras
Vélez
Rubio
Huércal
Overa
Cuevas del
Almanzora
Vera
Garrucha
Mojácar
Carboneras
Punta de la Media Naranja
CABO DE
GATA-NÍJAR
C. de Gata

Almería
G. de Almería
Roquetas de Mar
La Mojonera
Pta. del Sabinar

CASTILLA-LA MANCHA

CIUDAD REAL

GRANADA
Granada
SIERRA NEVADA
Mulhacén
Guadix
Baza
Huéscar
Orce
Cúllar
Galera
Castril
La Sagra

ALMERÍA
Tabernas
Sorbas
Níjar

Costa del Sol

Motril
Adra
El Ejido
Berja
Órgiva

ALGER
(Algiers)
Cherchell
Tipasa
Koléa
Blida
Boufarik
Médéa
Miliana
Khemis

ALGERIE

ORAN
Oran
(Ouahran)
Mers-el-Kébir
Arzew
Mostaganem
Relizane
Mascara
Sidi-bel-Abbès
Tlemcen
Ghazaouet

Melilla (Sp.)
Nador

Projection: Lambert's Conformal Conic

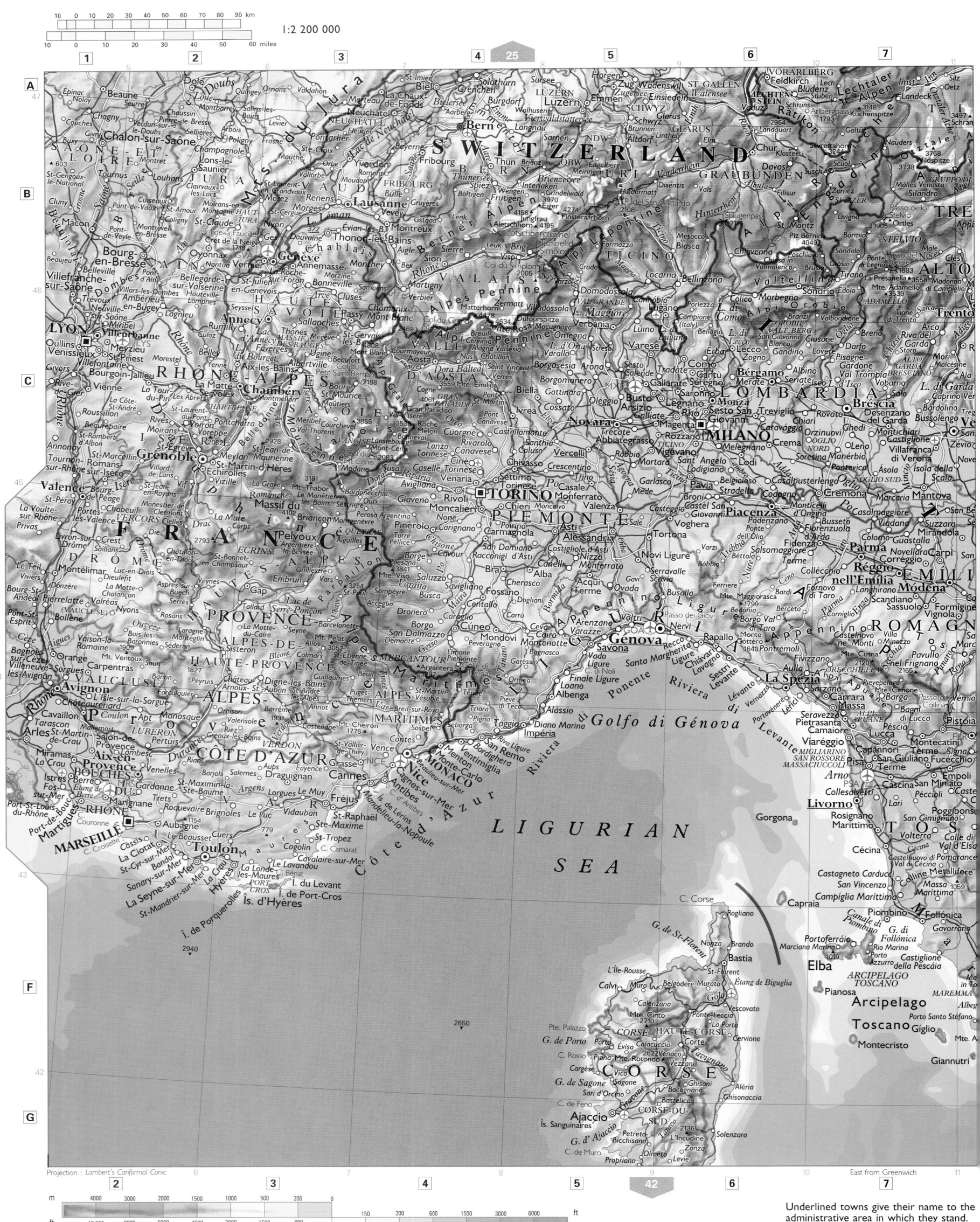

Underlined towns give their name to the administrative area in which they stand.

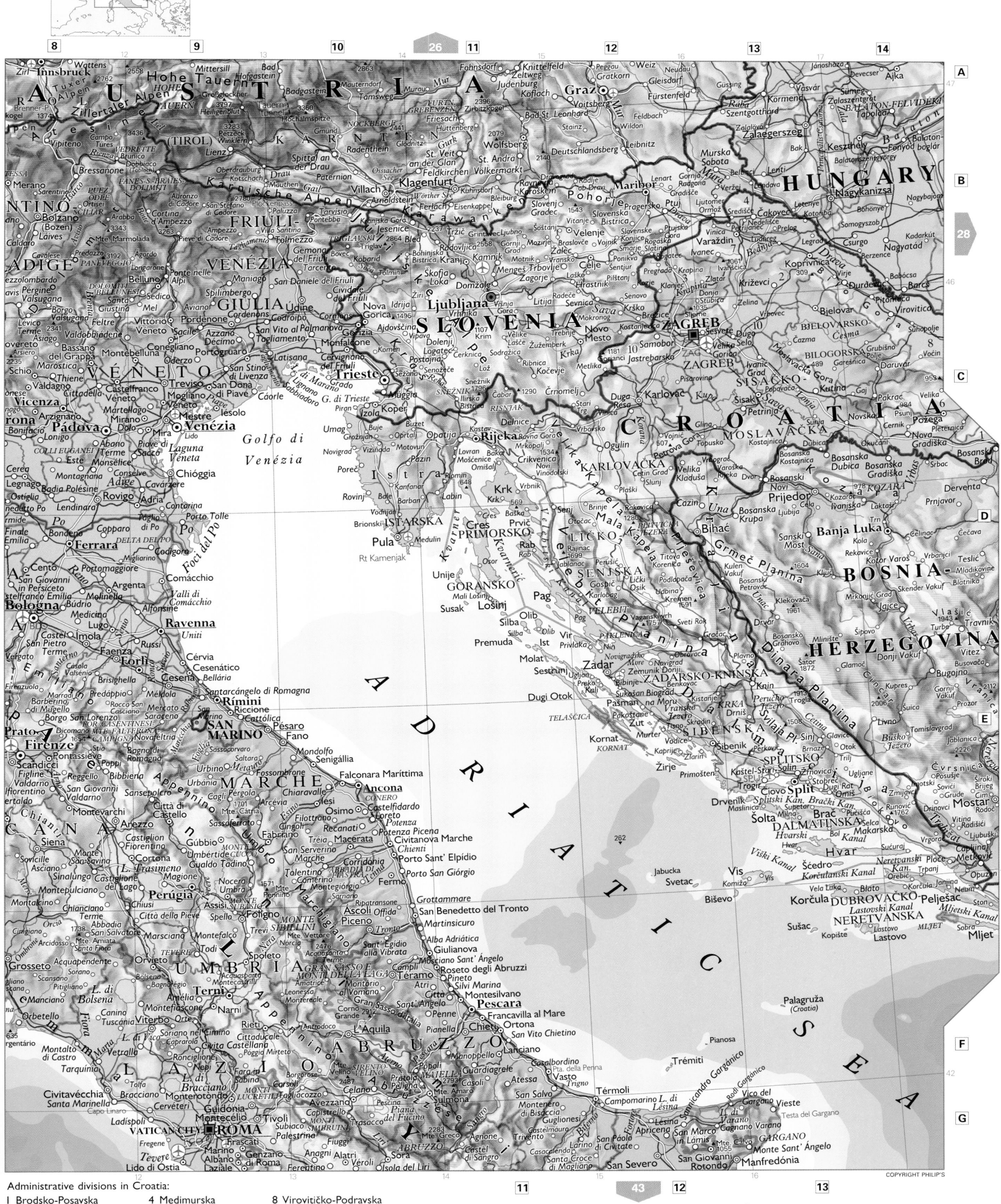

Administrative divisions in Croatia:

1 Brodsko-Posavska
2 Koprivničko-Križevačka
3 Krapinsko-Zagorska

4 Medimurska
6 Požeško-Slavonska
7 Varaždinska

8 Virovitičko-Podravska
10 Zagreba čka

1:2 200 000

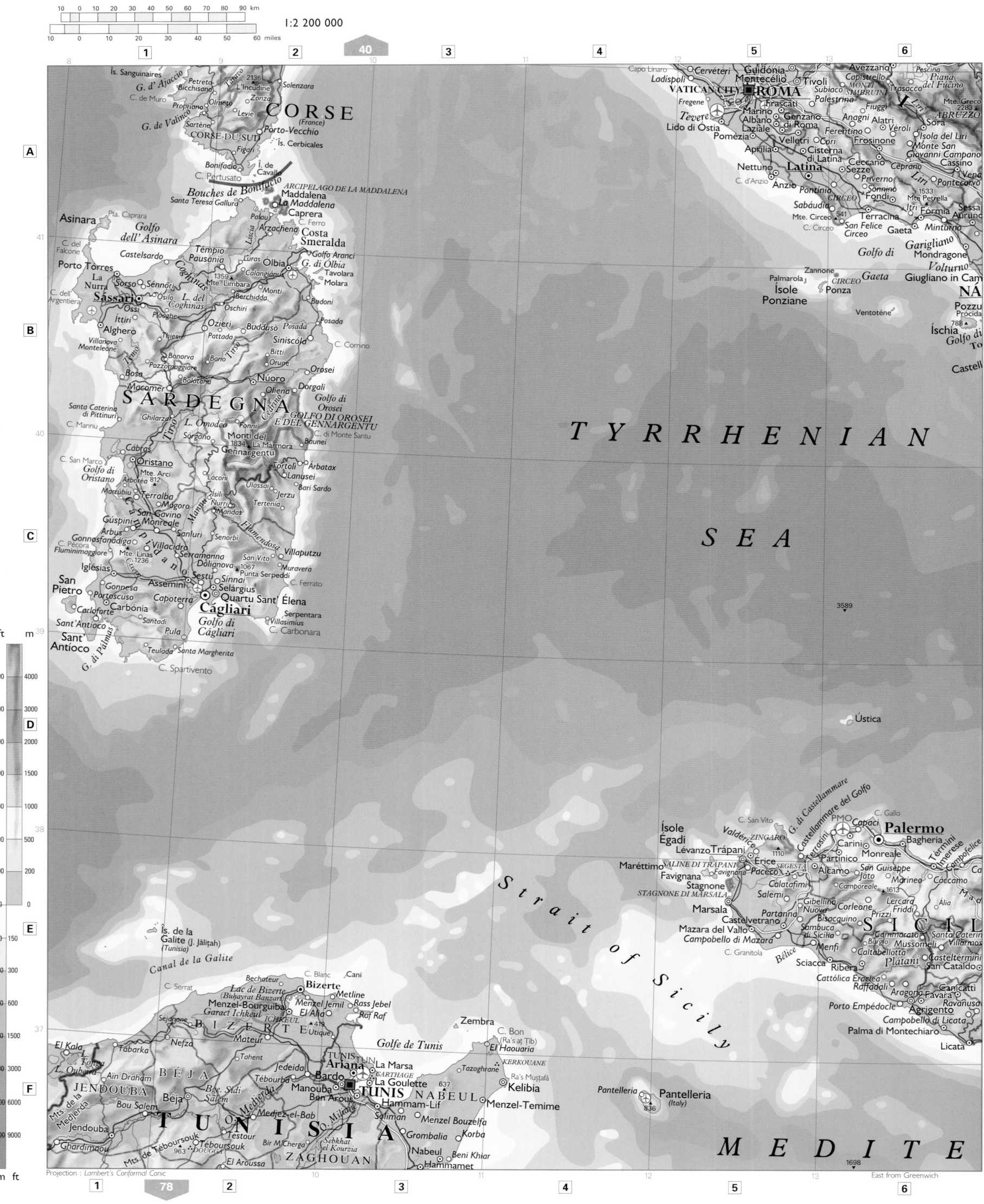

CORSE (France)

CORSE-DU-SUD

ARCIPELAGO DE LA MADDALENA

SARDEGNA

Golfo dell' Asinara

Sassari

GOLFO DI OROSEI E DEL GENNARGENTU

Monti del Gennargentu

Oristano

Golfo di Oristano

Cágliari

Golfo di Cágliari

TYRRHENIAN

SEA

3589

Ústica

G. di Castellammare del Golfo

Palermo

Bagheria

Ísole Égadi

Trápani

Erice

LE SALINE DI TRÁPANI

STAGNONE DI MARSALA

Marsala

Castelvetrano

Mazara del Vallo

Campobello di Mazara

SICILI

Strait of Sicily

Porto Empédocle

Agrigento

Campobello di Licata

Palma di Montechiaro

Licata

Pantelleria

Pantelleria (Italy)

836

Bizerte

BIZERTE

Canal de la Galite

Golfe de Tunis

TUNIS

Ariana

Bardo

Tunis

NABEUL

Kelibia

Menzel-Temime

TUNISIA

ZAGHOUAN

Nabeul

Hammamet

1698

M E D I T E

Projection : Lambert's Conformal Conic

East from Greenwich

VATICAN CITY · **ROMA**

Latina

Golfo di Gaeta

CIRCEO

Ísole Ponziane

Ponza

Ventotene

ABRUZZO

Piana del Fúcino

NÁ

Pózzu

Prócida

Íschia

Golfo di To

Castell

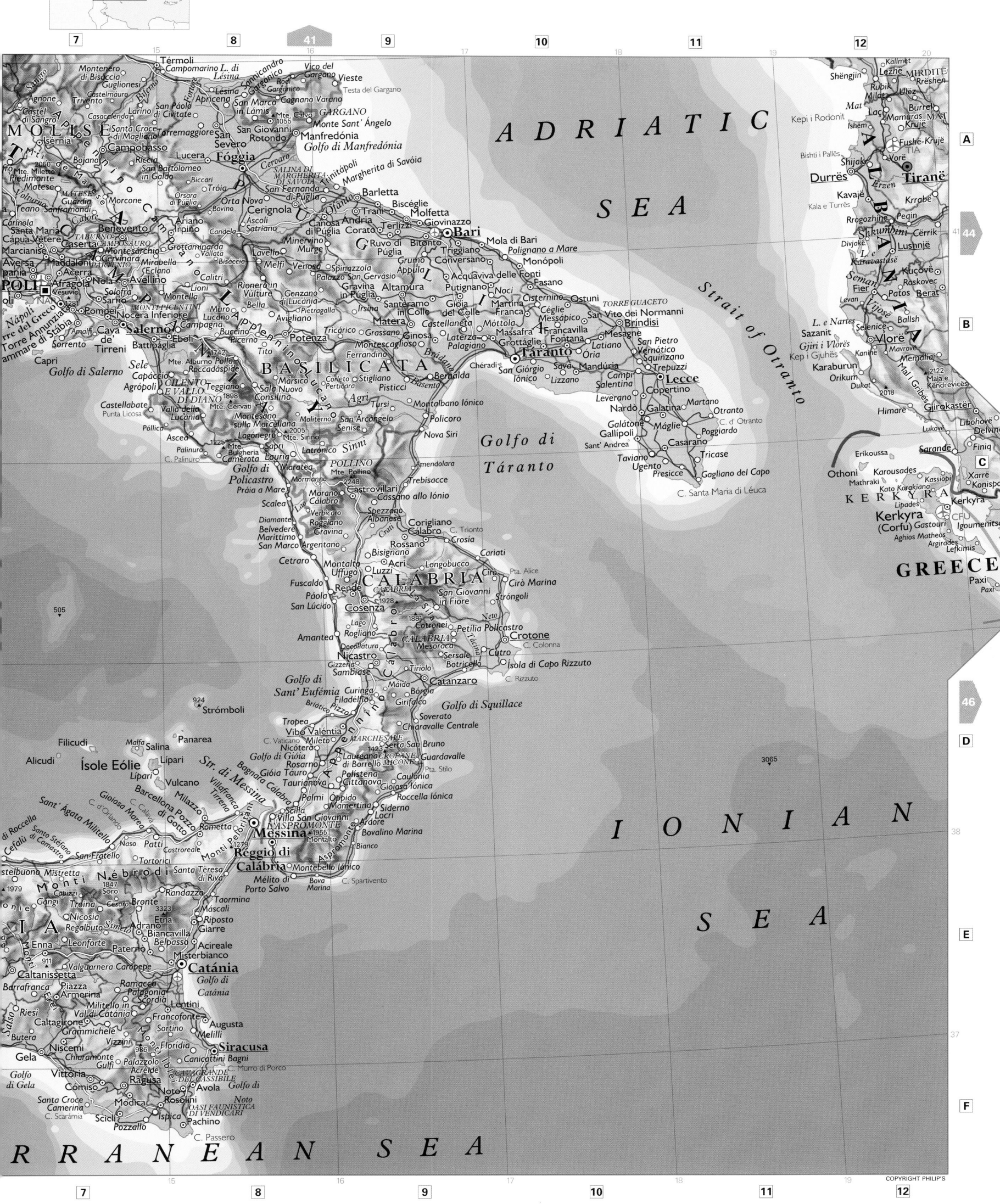

Underlined towns give their name to the
administrative area in which they stand.

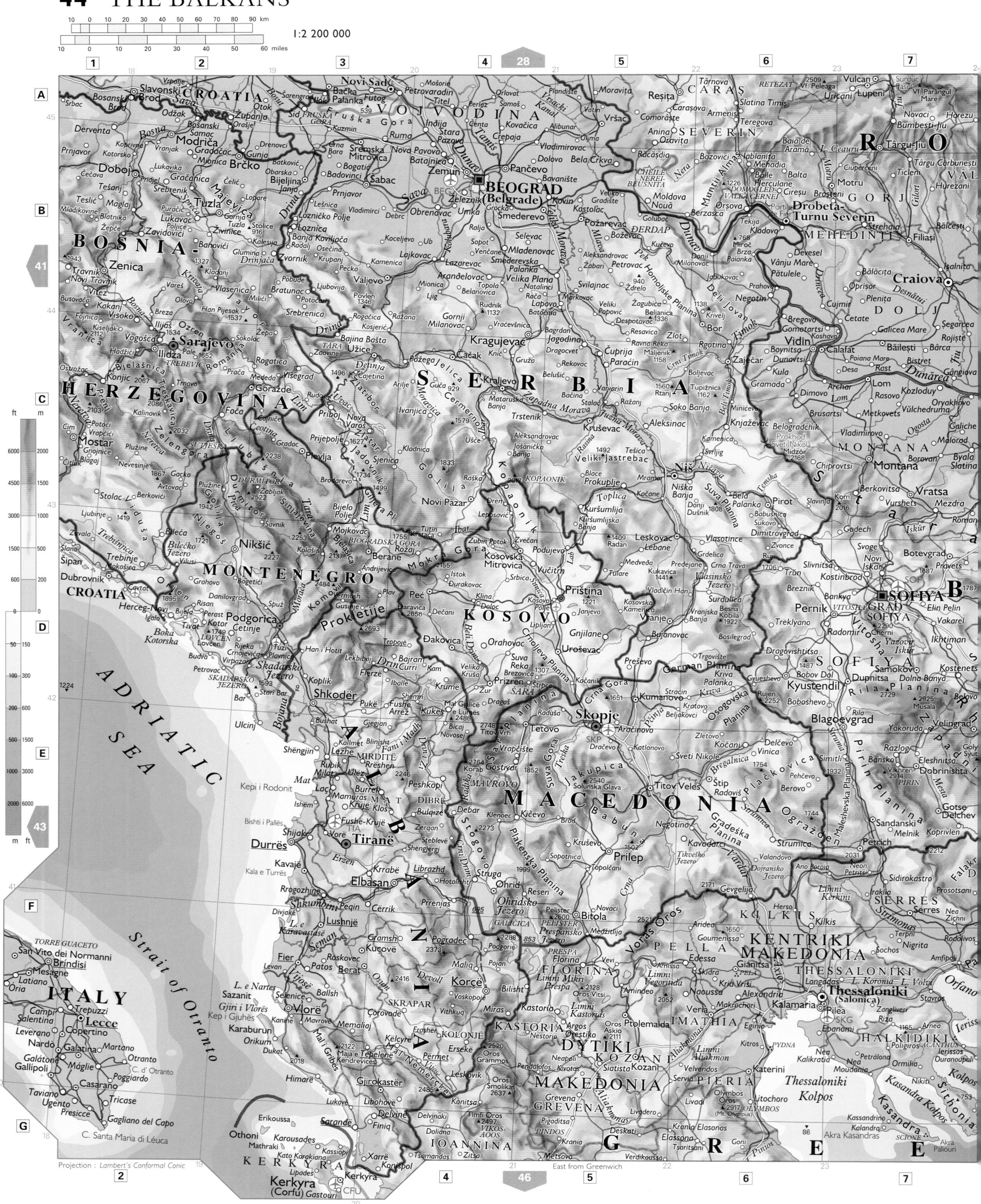

Projection : Lambert's Conformal Conic

East from Greenwich

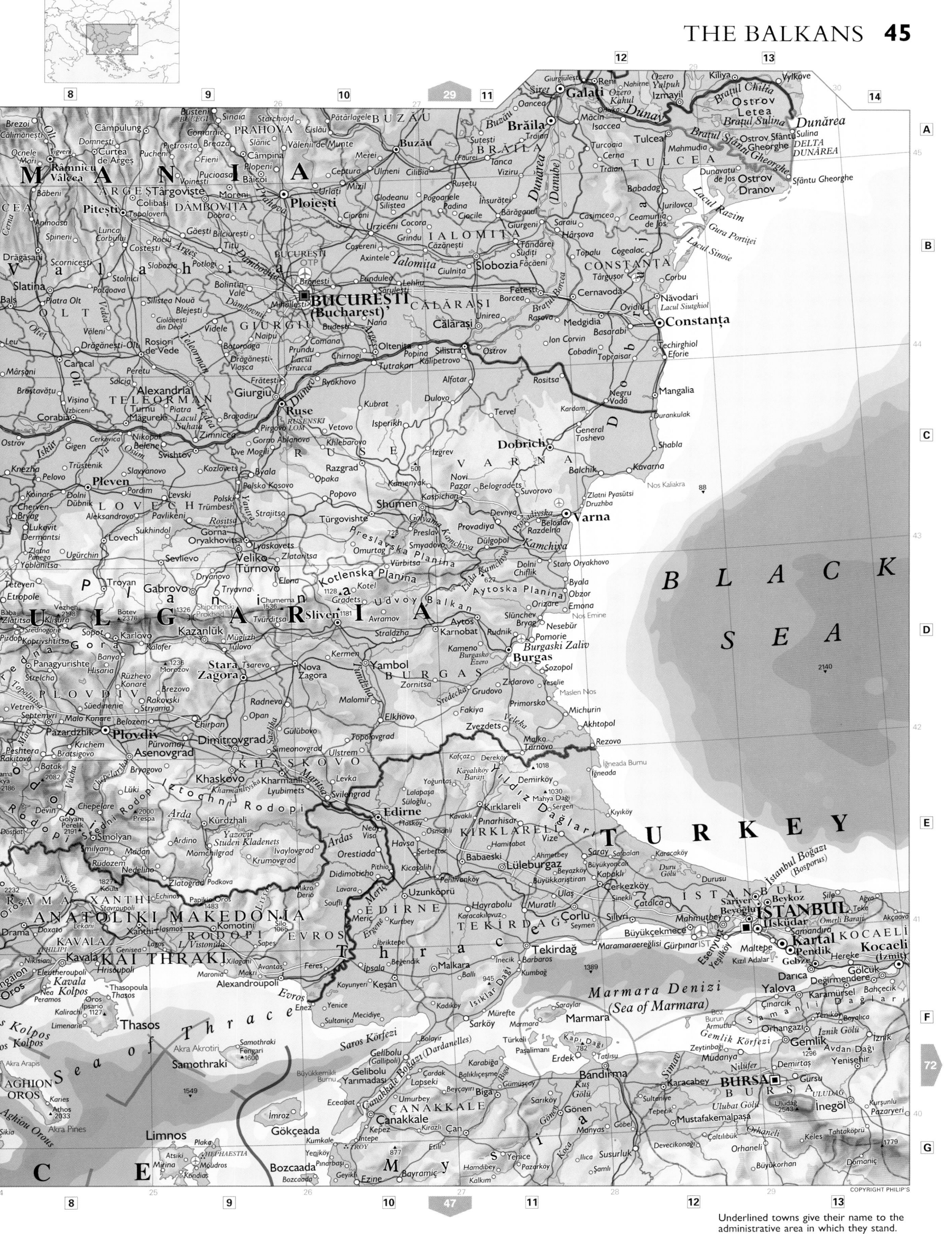

Underlined towns give their name to the
administrative area in which they stand.

1:2 200 000

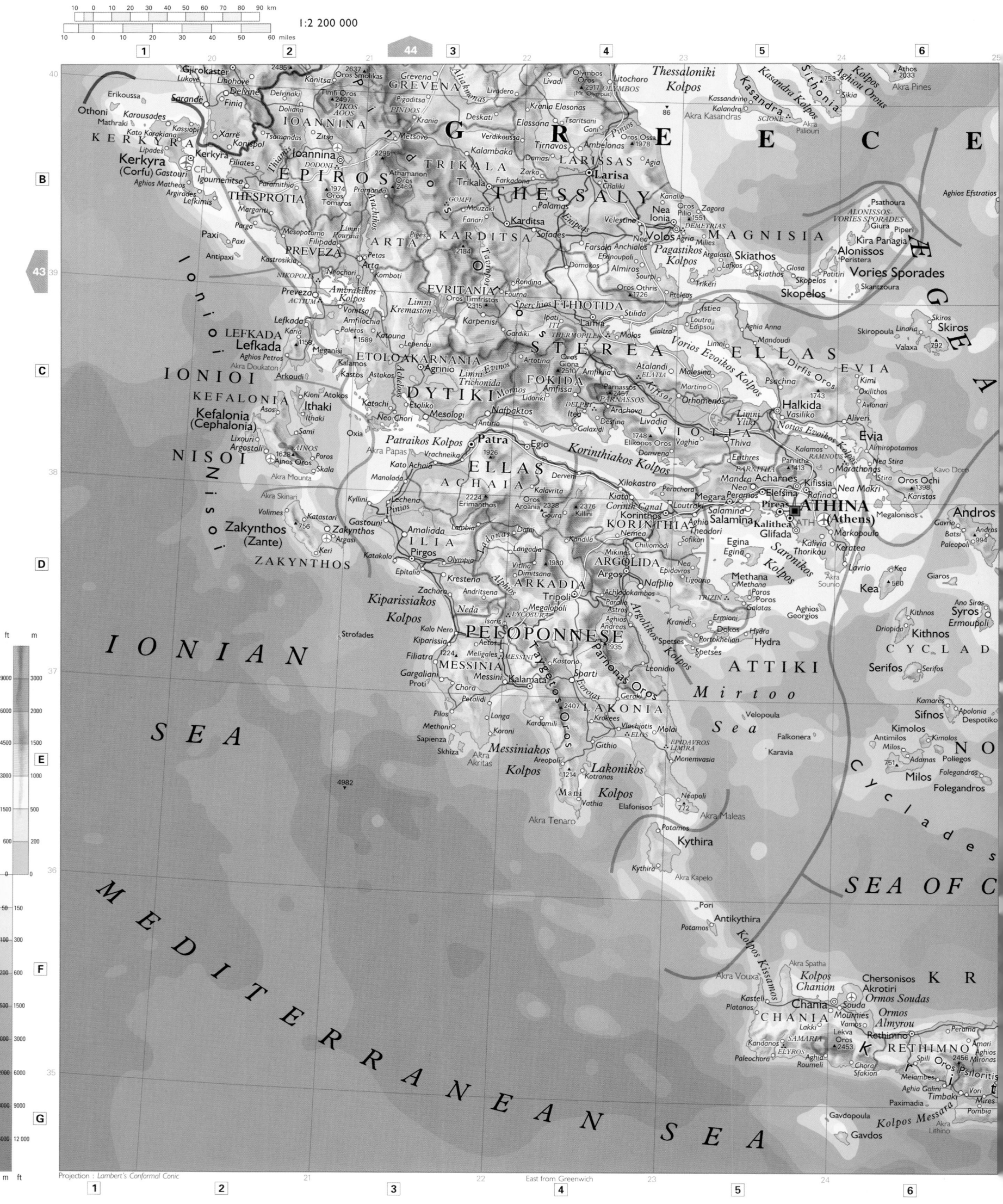

Projection : Lambert's Conformal Conic

East from Greenwich

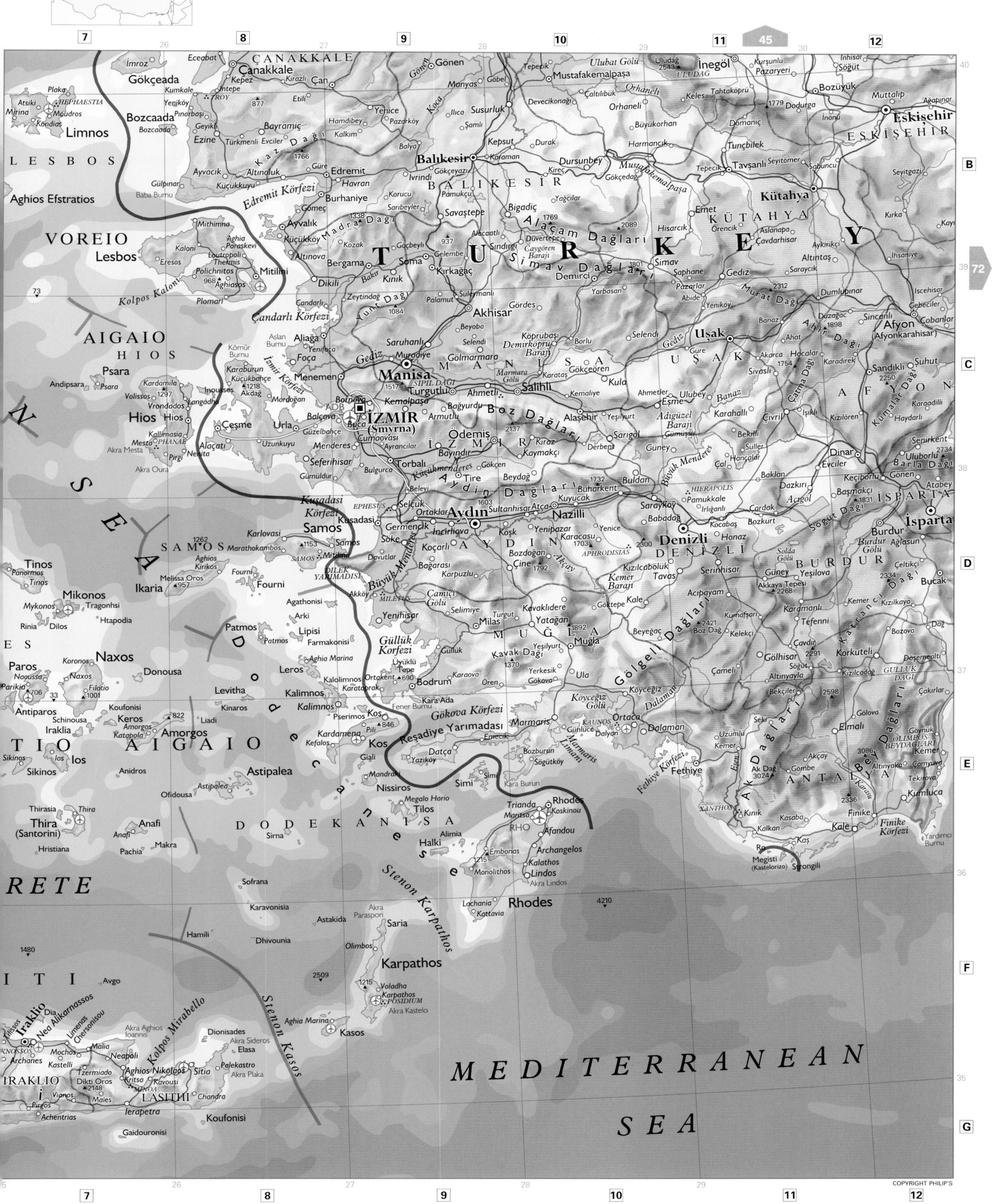

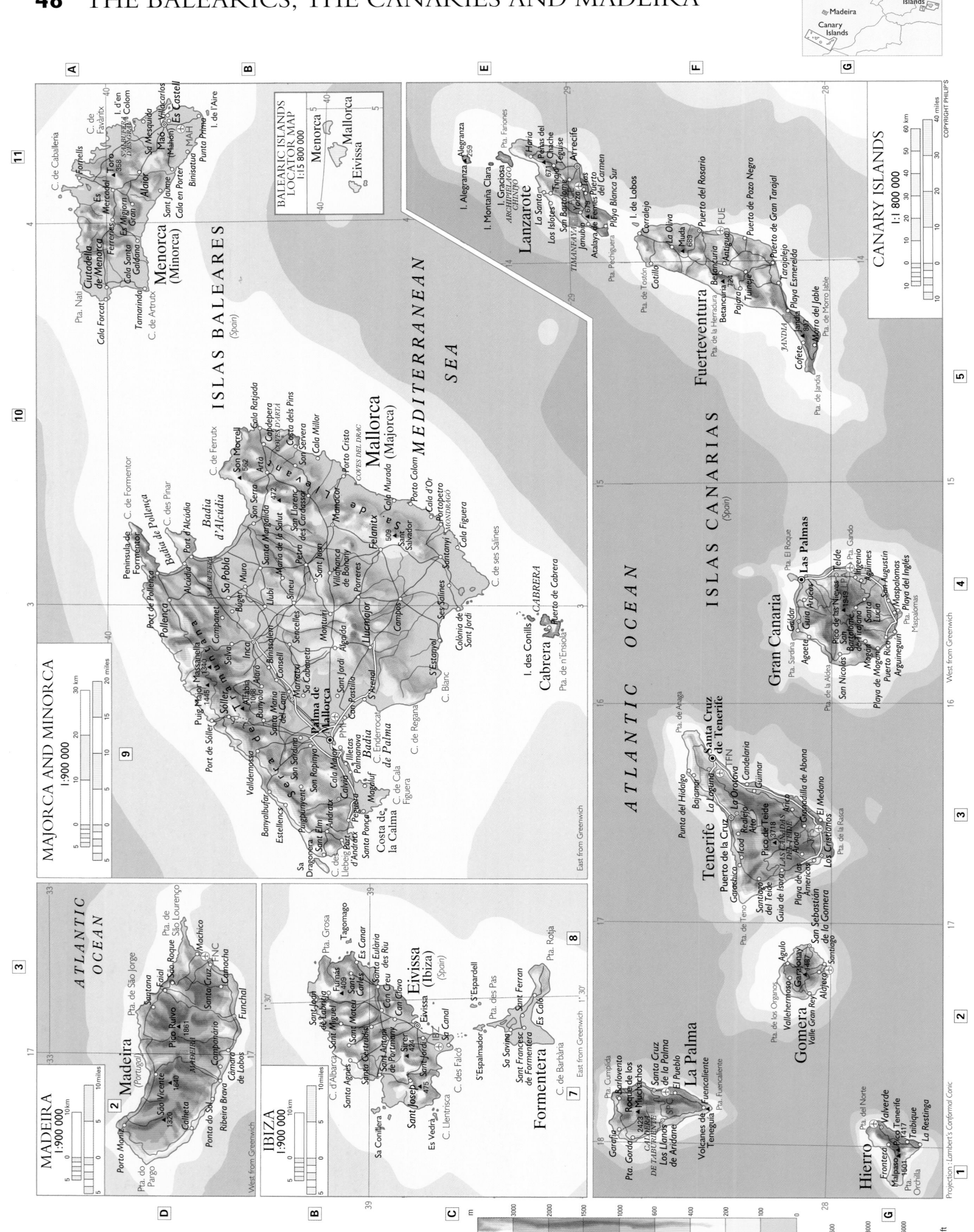

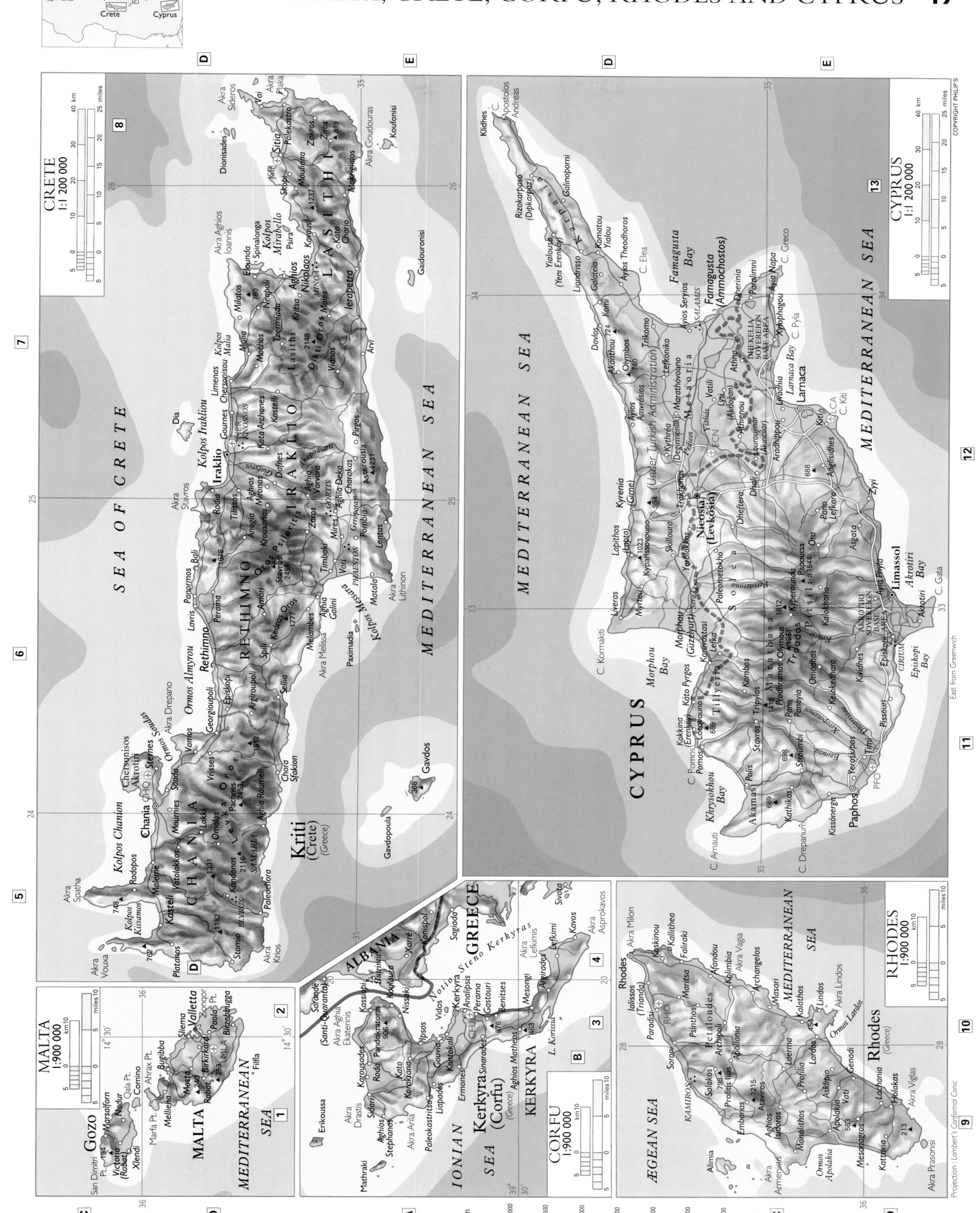

1:44 400 000

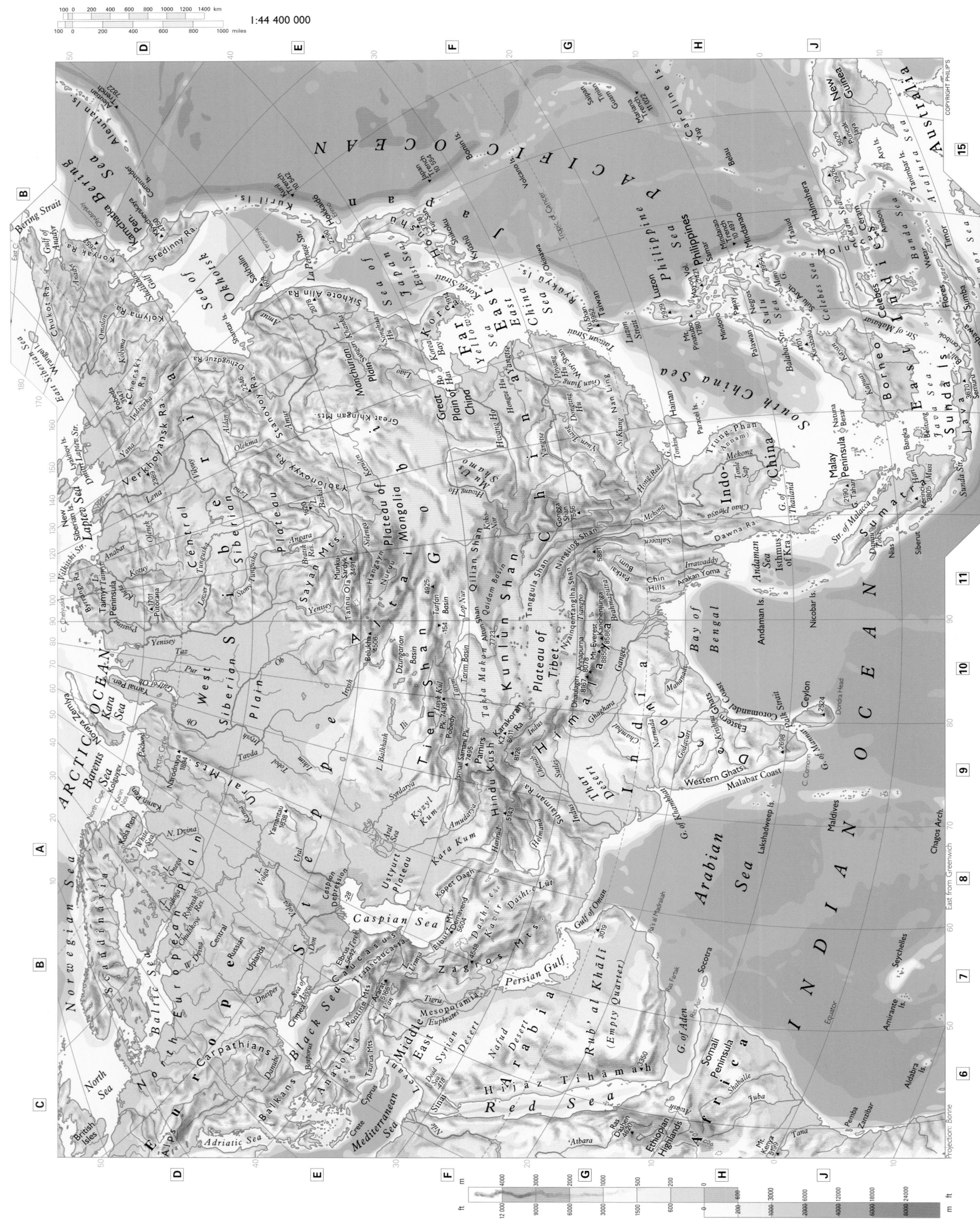

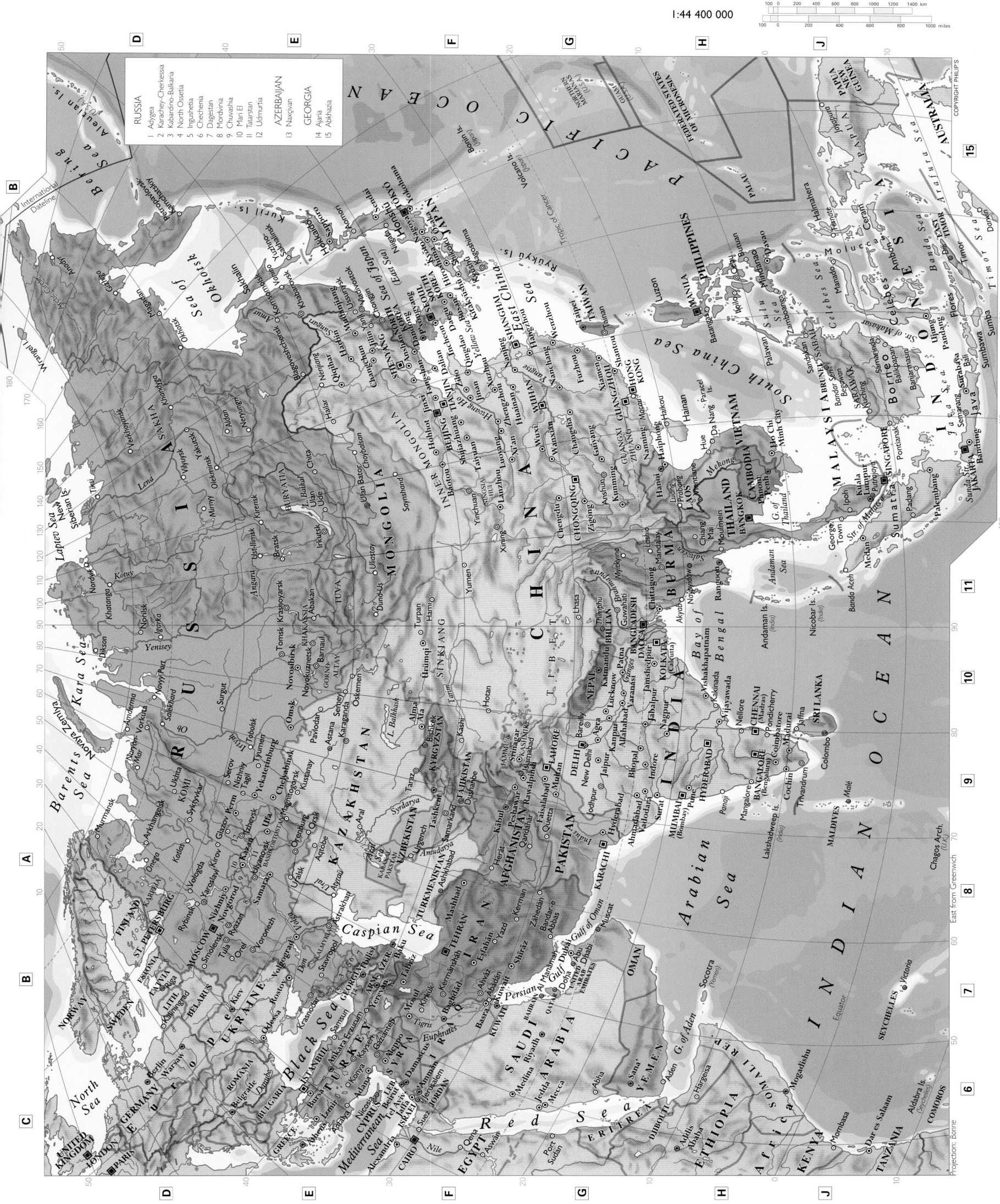

1:44 400 000

Projection: Bonne

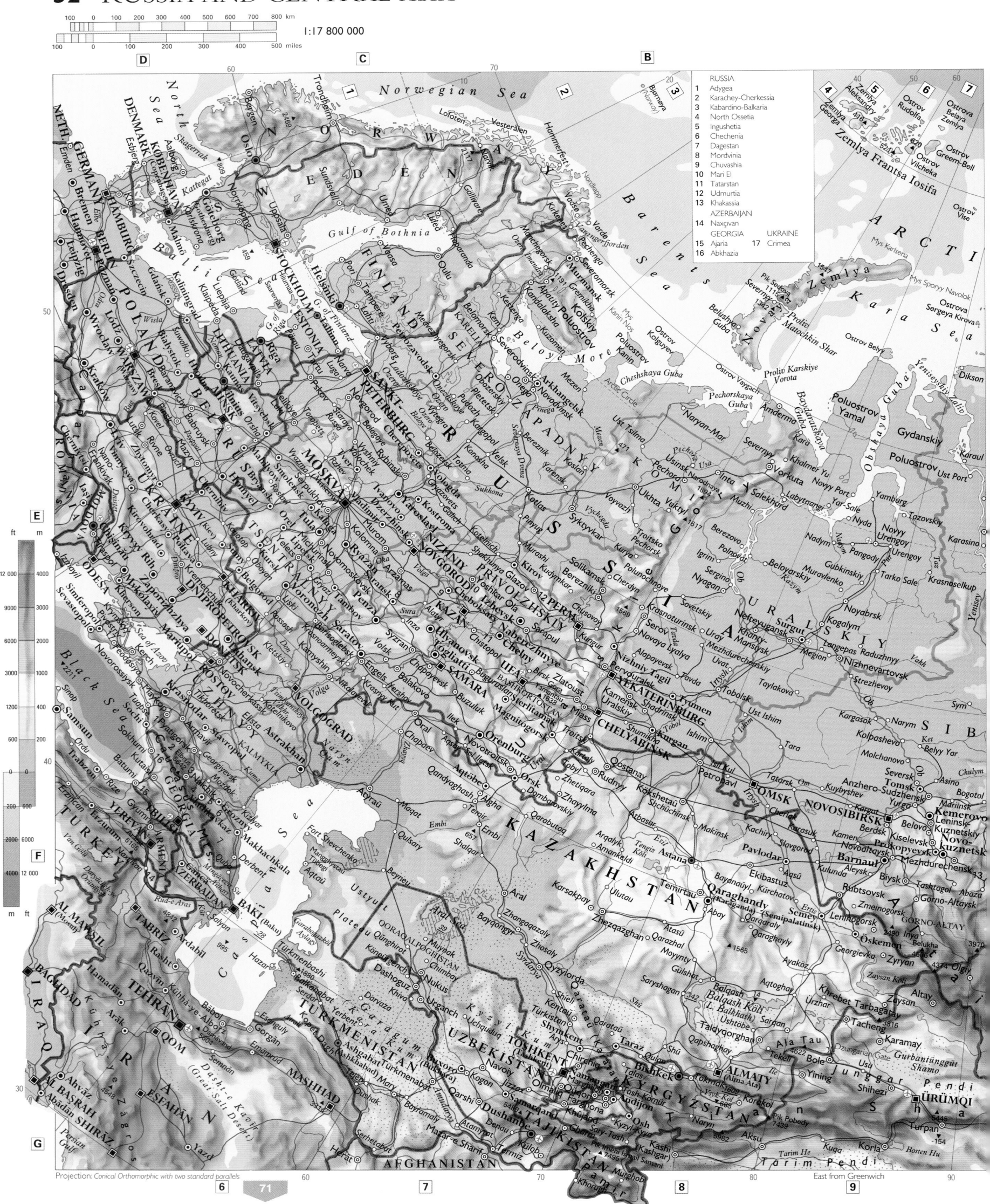

1:17 800 000

	RUSSIA
1	Adygea
2	Karachey-Cherkessia
3	Kabardino-Balkaria
4	North Ossetia
5	Ingushetia
6	Chechenia
7	Dagestan
8	Mordvinia
9	Chuvashia
10	Mari El
11	Tatarstan
12	Udmurtia
13	Khakassia
	AZERBAIJAN
14	Naxçivan
	GEORGIA
15	Ajaria
16	Abkhazia
	UKRAINE
17	Crimea

Projection: Conical Orthomorphic with two standard parallels

East from Greenwich

A 4 B C

8 9 10 11 12 13 14 15 16 17 18 19

70 80 70 180

OCEAN

Mys Dezhneva (East C.)
Bering Str.
Uelen
St. Lawrence I. (U.S.A.)
International Date Line

Mys Arkticheskiy
Ostrov Shmidta
Ostrov Ushakova
781 Ostrov Komsomolets
Ostrov Pioner
Ostrov Oktyabrskoy Revolyutsii
965
Severnaya Zemlya
Ostrova Sergeya Kirova
Proliv Vilkitskogo
Ostrov Bolshevik 935
Ostrov Malyy Taymyr
Mys Chelyuskin
Ostrova Petra
Ostrov Russkiy

3800

Ostrov Genriyetty
Ostrova Delonga
Ostrov Bennetta
Ostrova Zhokhova
Ostrov Faddeyevskiy
Novosibirskiye Ostrova
Ostrov Malyy Lyakhovskiy
Ostrov Bolshoy Lyakhovskiy
Ostrov Kotelnyy
Lyakhovskiye Ostrova
374
Ostrov Belkovskiy
Ostrov Stolbovoy
Proliv Dmitriya Lapteva

Ostrov Vrangelya
Proliv Longa
Chukchi Sea
Chaunskaya Guba
Pevek
Chukotskoye Nagorye
Nagorye
1194
1843
Anadyrskiy Zaliv
Provideniya
Beringovskiy
Egvekinot
Mys Navarin
Anadyr
1853

Lapte v Sea

Byrranga
Poluostrov Gory Taymyr
1146
621
Oz. Taymyr

East Siberian Sea

Ambarchik
Cherskiy
Bilibino
Omolon
1762
2453
Koryakskoye Nagorye
2562
Bering Sea

Poluostrov Kamchatka

Laptev Sea

Ostrov Bolshoy Begichev
Nordvik
Novorybnoye
Khatanga
Zhilinda
Ust Olenek
Tit-Ary
Tiksi
Saskylakh
Bulun
Kyusyur
Kazachye
Ust Kuyga
Druzhina
Srednekolymsk
Nizhne Kolymsk
Chokurdakh
Deputatskiy

Chernaya
Volochanka
Kheta
Pyasina
Dudinka 1591
Norilsk Talnakh Gory Putorana 1678
1341
Igarka
Turukhansk
Noginsk
Nizhnyaya Tunguska
Tura
Yukta
Yessey
962
Udachnyy
Arctic Circle
Aykhal
Chernyshevskiy
Mirnyy
Suntar
Nyurba
Vilyuysk
Verkhnevilyuysk
Yakutsk
Nizhniy Bestyakh
Pokrovsk
Sinsk
Olekminsk
Tommot
Aldan 2264

Verkhoyansk 2389
Batagay
Sangar
Batamay
Namtsy
Ytyk-Kyuyel
Borogontsy
Khandyga
Okhotskiy Perevoz
Ust Maya
Yugorenok
2185
Gora Chen 2562 Ust-Nera 3147
Artyk
Oymyakon 2959
Susuman
Yagodnoye
Ust-Omchug
Ola
Magadan
Arka
Ulya

Kolyma
Taskan
Omsukchan
Orotukan
Palatka
1586
1780

Sea of Okhotsk

Srednekolymsk

Ust-Kamchatsk
Petropavlovsk-Kamchatskiy
Gora Klyuchevskaya 4750
Yelizovo
Ozernovskiy

V E R K H O Y A N S K I Y   K H R E B E T
K H R E B E T   C H E R S K O G O
S A K H A   (Y A K U T I A)
D A L N E V O S T O C H N Y Y

Kamandorskiye Ostrova

Yeniseysk
Lesosibirsk
Kodinsk
Boguchany
Kezhma
Vanavara
Yerbogachen
Lensk 599
Vitim
Neryungri
Nagornyy
Chara 2999
Kodinsk
Bodaybo
Mama
Korshunova
Ust-Ilimsk
Makarovo
Zheleznogorsk-Ilimskiy
Kirensk
Severobaykalsk
Bagdarin
Taksimo
Ust-Nyukzha
Kalakan
Tynda
Zeya
Skovorodino
Magdagachi
Ushumun
Chegdomyn
1906
Ayan
Nelkan
Chagda
Ust-Mil
Aim
Maya
2246
2371
Udskaya Guba
Shantar Ostrov Bolshoy Shantar
Ostrov Feklistova
Nikolayevsk-na-Amure
Aleksandrovsk-Sakhalinskiy

S T A N O V O Y   K H R E B E T
Y A B L O N O V Y Y   K H R E B E T

Sakhalin

Achinsk
Nazarovo Kansk
Krasnoyarsk
Zelenogorsk Ilanskiy
Tayshet
Alzamay
Nizhneudinsk
Tulun
Zima
Zalari
Cheremkhovo
Usolye Sibirskoye
Angarsk
Irkutsk 1509
Bratsk
Artemovsk
Chernogorsk
Minusinsk 2922
Abakan
Sayanogorsk 2026
Zapadnyy Vostochnyy Sayan Sayan
Turan
Kyzyl
Toora-Khem
Ay-Dovurak
Samagaltay 3276
Erzin
Kyakhta
Petrovsk-Zabaykalskiy
Ulan-Ude
Shyudyanka
Gusinoozersk
Zakamensk
Khilok
Chita
Shilka
Nerchinsk
Sretensk
Aginskoye
Olovyannaya
Borzya
Zabaykalsk
Manzhouli
Hailar
2519

Munku-Sardyk 3491
Khovsgol Nuur
Hatgal
Darhan
Möron
Mörön
Hentiyn Nuruu
Choybalsan
Tamsagbulag
Baruun-Urt
Öndörhaan

Hangayn Nuruu 3905
Uliastay
Tsetserleg
3617
Dund-Us
Altay
Bayanhongor
Arvayheer
Mandalgovi
Buyant-Uhaa
Choyr
Xilinhot
Linxi 1949

ULAANBAATAR
M O N G O L I A
G o b i

Dalandzadgad
Dalanzadgad

Har Us Nuur
Hyargas Nuur
Uvs Nuur
T A N N U O L A
(Aerhtai Shan)

4266
4885
Hami
Gaxun Nur

C H I N A
D o n g b e i   (M a n c h u r i a)

Hohhot
Baotou
Zhangjiakou
BEIJING
Tangshan
Dalian
Chengde
Yingkou
CHIFENG
JINXI
SHENYANG
ANSHAN
FUSHUN
Dandong
NORTH KOREA
Hamhung
Wonsan
PYONGYANG
NAMP'O
Kimch'aek
Ch'ongjin
Hunjiang
Tonghua
Siping
CHANGCHUN
JILIN
Vladivostok
Yanji
FUYU
QIQIHAR
DAQING
Yichun
HARBIN
MUDANJIANG
JIAMUSI
JIXI
Hegang
Baicheng
Zalantun
Bei'an
Fuyu
Nenjiang
Songhua
2744
Taonan

Helhe
Blagoveshchensk
Raychikhinsk
Poyarkovo
Zavitinsk
Progress
Obluchye
Birobidzhan
Khabarovsk
Komsomolsk-na-Amure
2078
Svobodnyy
Belogorsk
Shimanovsk
2221
Dzhalinda
Mogocha
Gulian 1908
Karymskaye
Baley
Sherlovaya Gora
Krasnokamensk
Khapcheranga

Amur
Bikin
Dalnerechensk
Spassk-Dalniy
Arsenev
Dalnegorsk
Ussuriysk
Kavalerovo
Artem
Partizansk
Nakhodka
Kraskino
3669
Terney
Amgu
1763

SAPPORO
Hokkaido
Hakodate
Aomori
Hachinohe
Akita
Honshu
Sado
Niigata
Toyama 3190
Kanazawa
JAPAN
KYOTO
KOBE
OSAKA

Sea of Japan (East Sea)
Ulleungdo
SEOUL
INCHEON
SOUTH KOREA
DAEJEON
DAEGU
BUSAN
GWANGJU

Kurilskiye Ostrova
Ostrova
1819
1599
2339
2290
4428
1535
Tatarskiy Proliv
Sovetskaya Gavan
Vanino
Uglegorsk
Poronaysk
Dolinsk
Yuzhno-Sakhalinsk
Kholmsk
Nevelsk
Korsakov
Gora Lopatina 1609

COPYRIGHT PHILIP'S

10 11 12 60 13 14
100 110 120 130

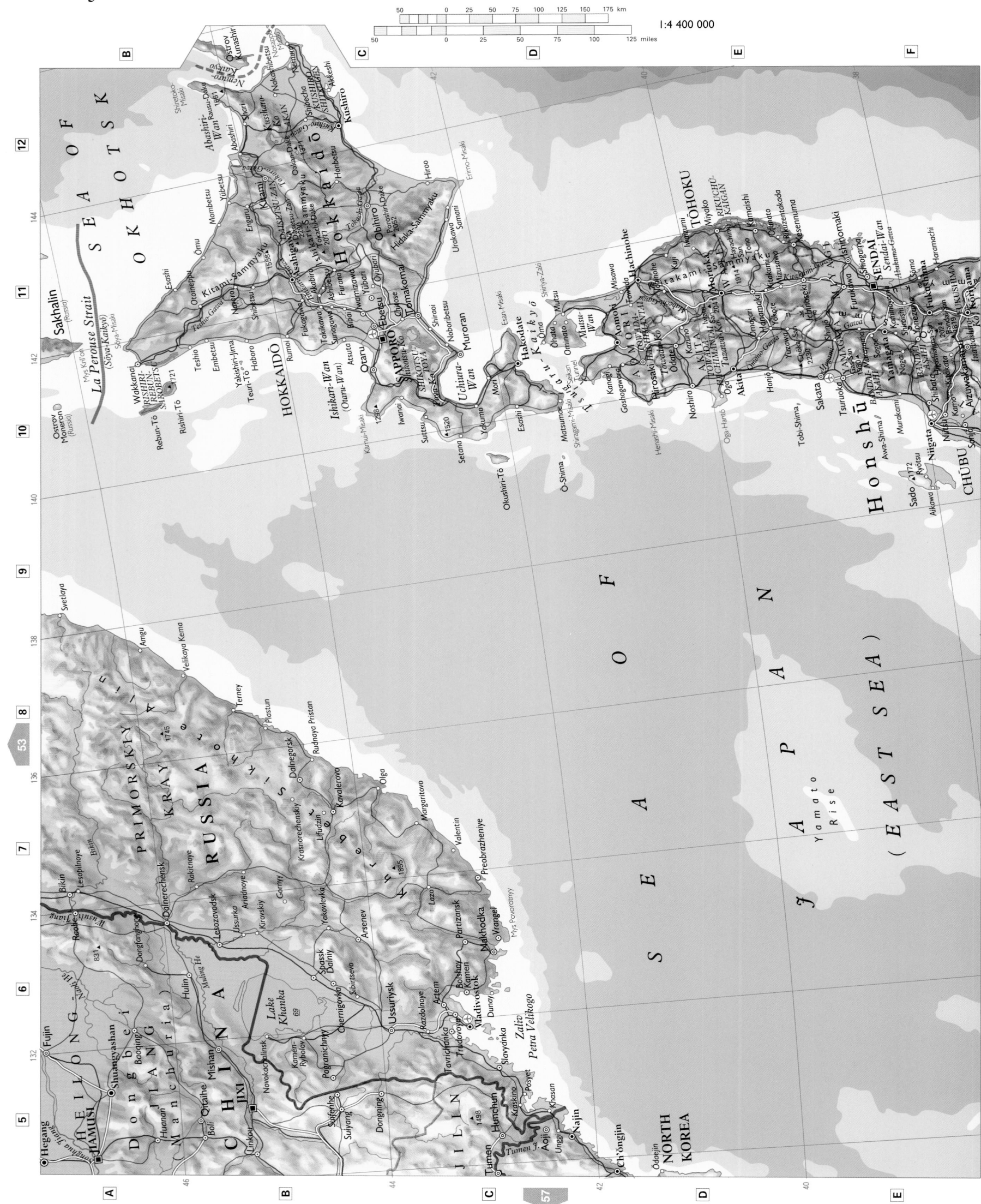

50 0 25 50 75 100 125 150 175 km

1:4 400 000

50 0 25 50 75 100 125 miles

SEA OF OKHOTSK

Sakhalin

La Perouse Strait
(Sōya-Kaikyō)

Ostrov Moneron
(Russia)

HOKKAIDŌ

Ostrov Kunashir

SHIRETOKO
KUSHIRO

Wakkanai
RISHIRI-
REBUN-
SAROBETSU

Rishiri-Tō
Rebun-Tō

SAPPORO

Ishikari-Wan
(Otaru-Wan)

SHIKOTSU-
TŌYA

Uchiura-
Wan

Mori

Hakodate

Tsugaru-Kaikyō

Okushiri-Tō

Ō-Shima

SEA OF

SVETLAYA

Amgu

Terney

RUSSIA

PRIMORSKY KRAY

Plastun

Rudnaya Pristan

Dalnegorsk

Olga

Margaritovo

Valentin

Preobrazheniye

Nakhodka

Vrangel

Mys Povorotnyy

Vladivostok

Zaliv
Petra Velikogo

HEILONGJIANG

Dongbei

Manchuria

CHINA

JILIN

NORTH
KOREA

Najin

JAPAN

(EAST SEA)

Yamato Rise

TŌHOKU

RIKUCHŪ-KAIGAN

Aomori

MORI

SENDAI

Sendai-Wan

Honshū

CHŪBU

Sado

Niigata

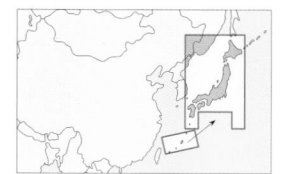

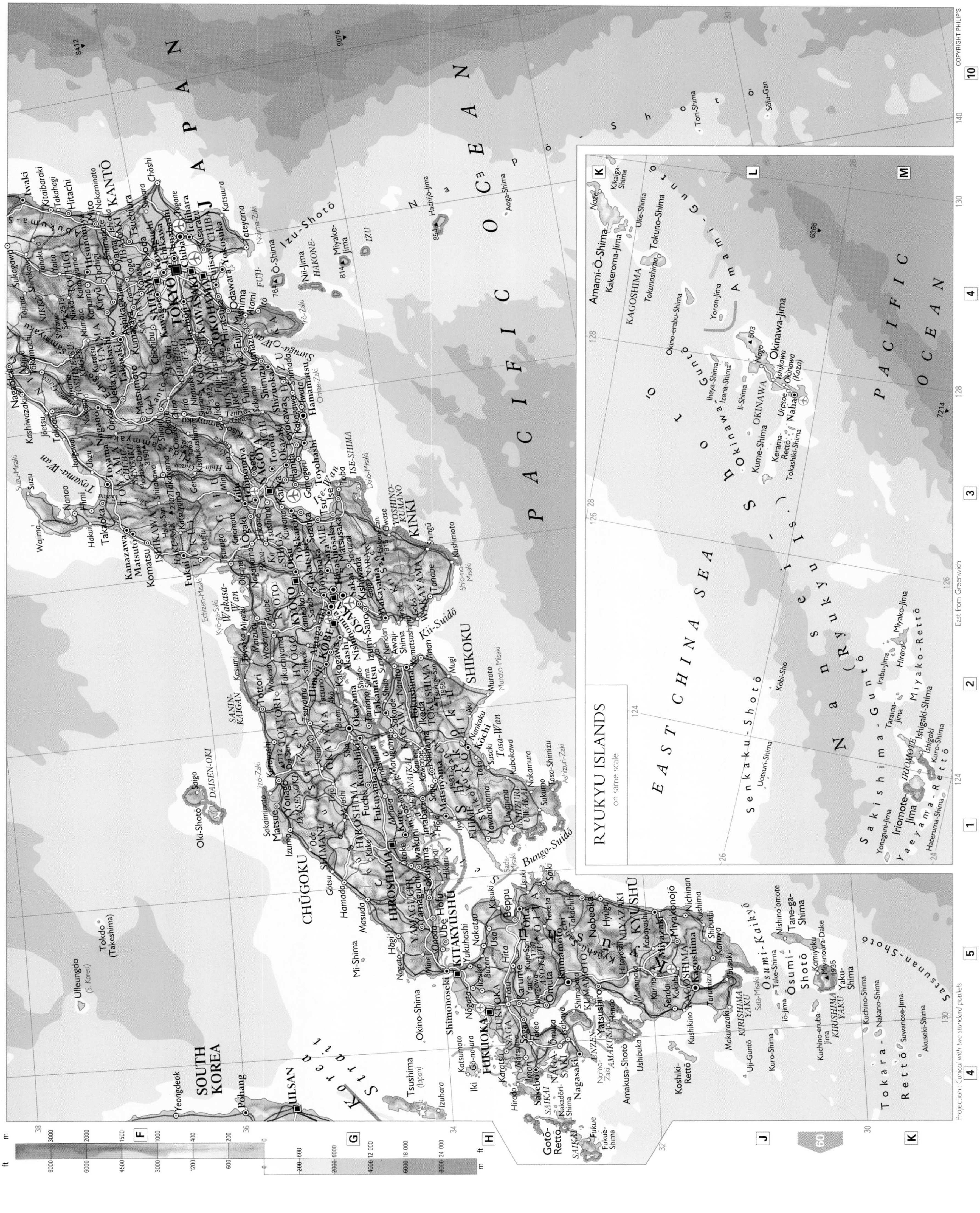

1:5 300 000

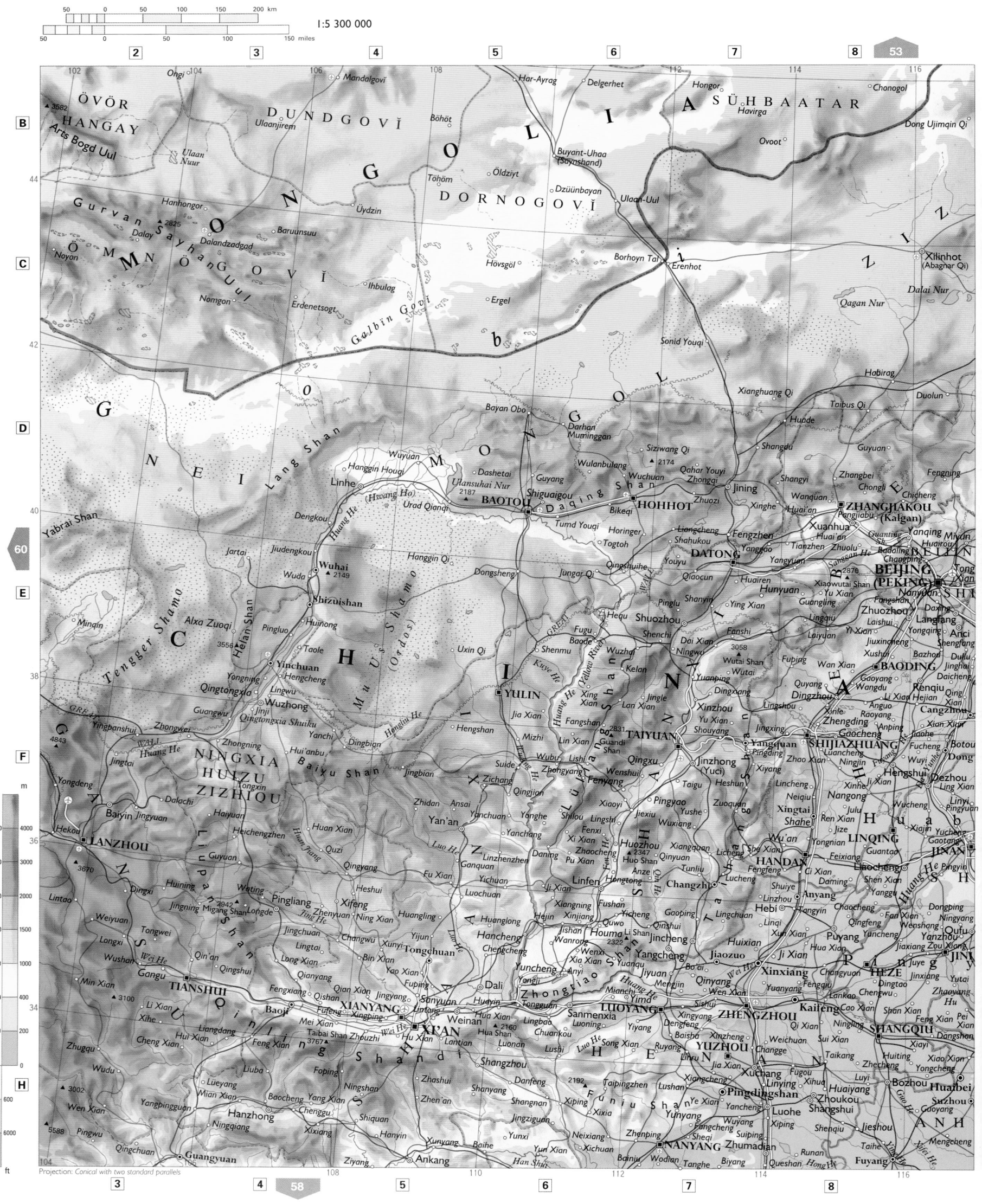

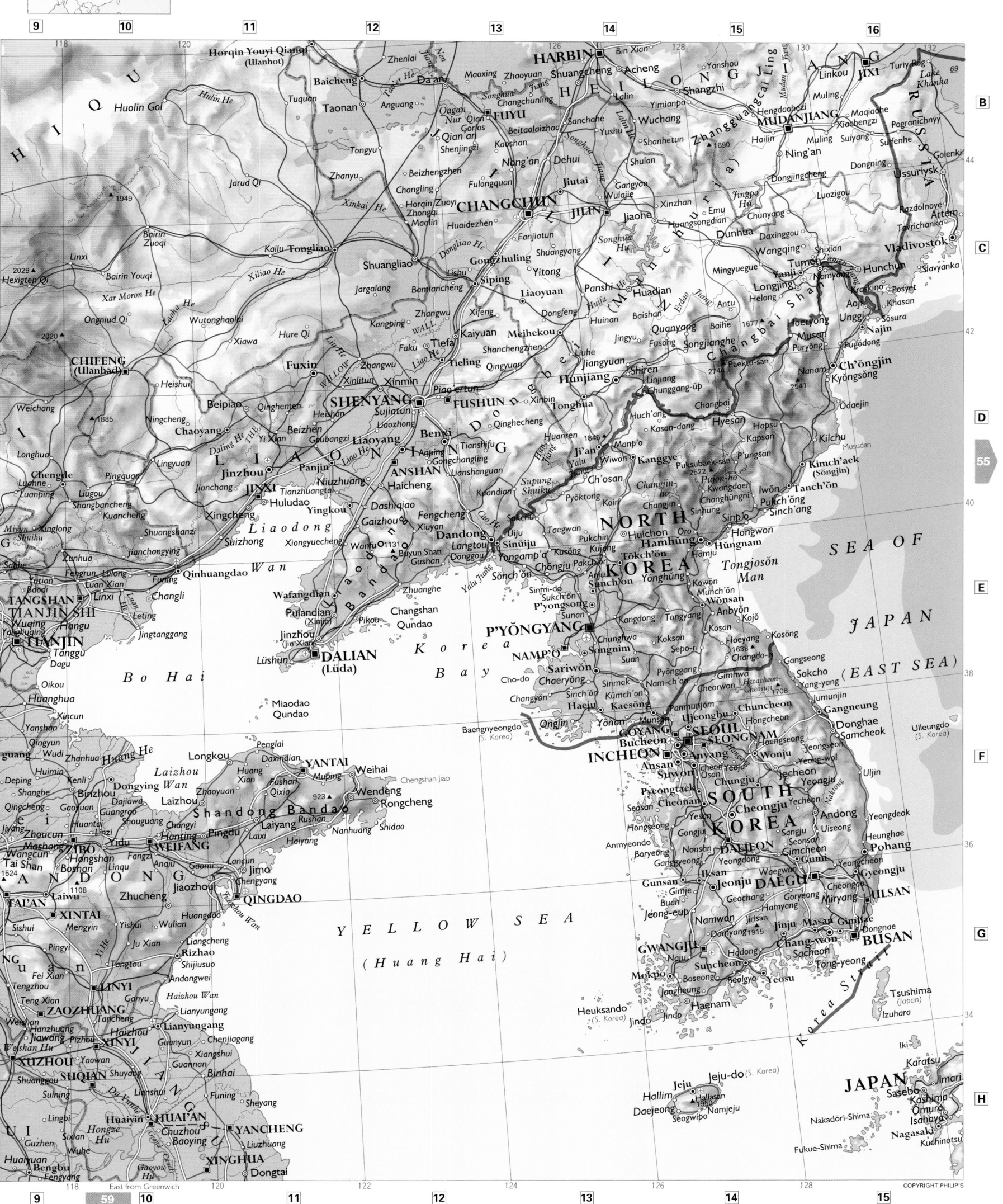

1:5 300 000

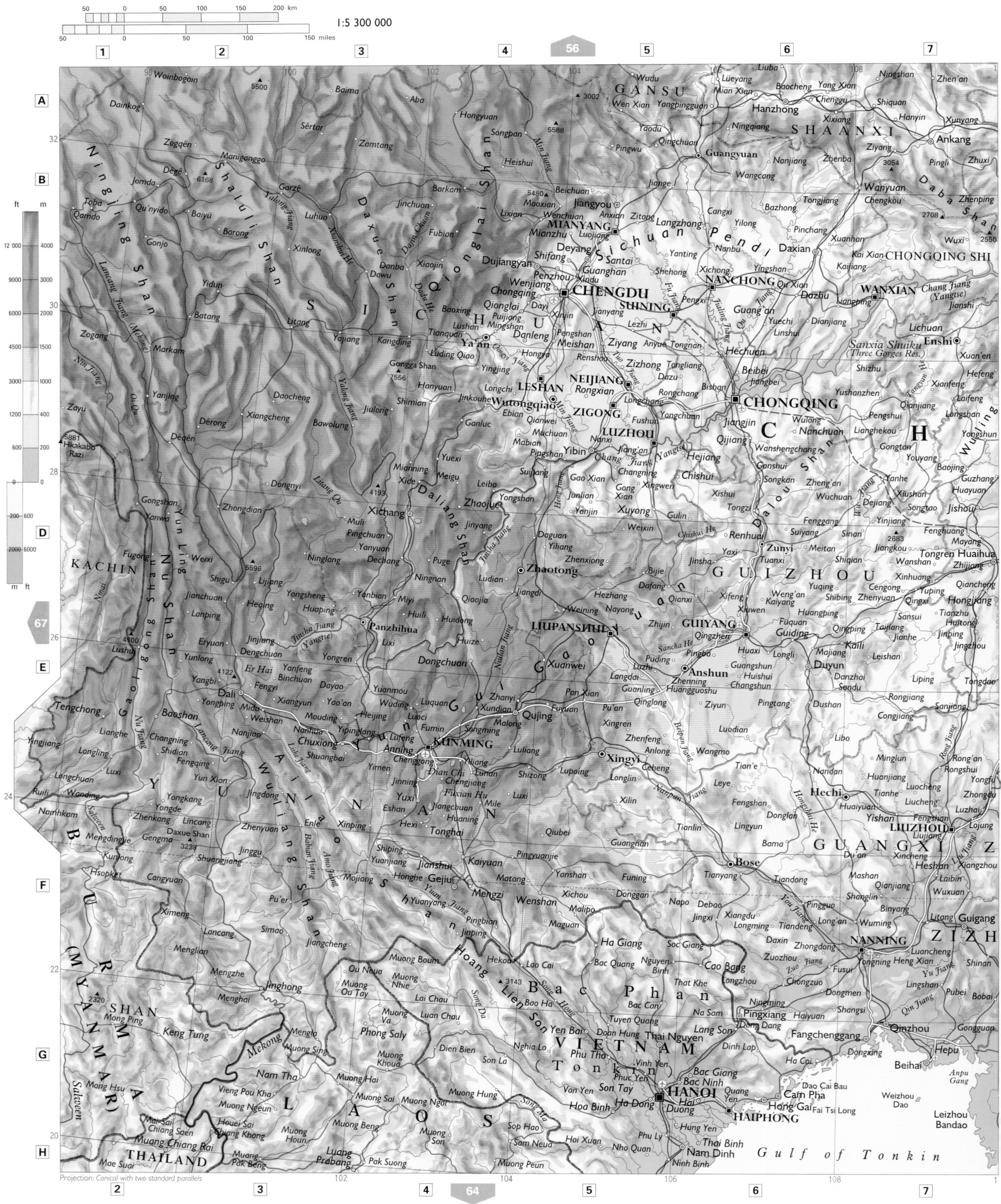

Projection: Conical with two standard parallels

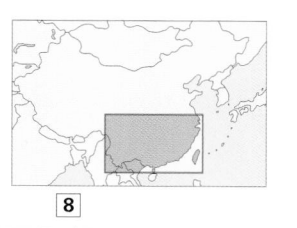

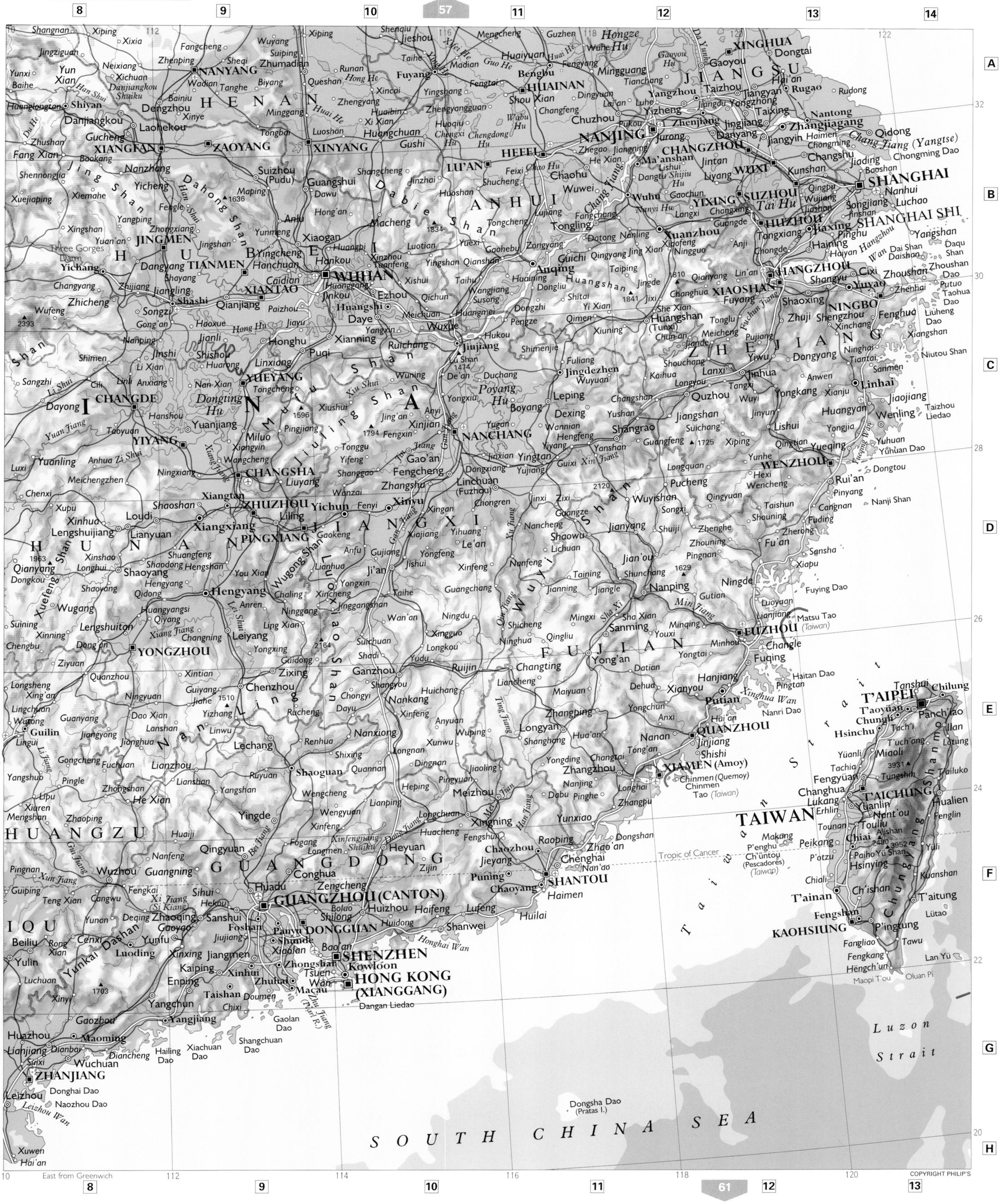

100 0 100 200 300 400 500 600 700 800 km
100 0 100 200 300 400 500 miles

1:17 800 000

COPYRIGHT PHILIP'S

RUSSIA

KAZAKHSTAN

MONGOLIA

NEI MONGOL ZIZHIQU (INNER MONGOLIA)

XINJIANG UYGUR ZIZHIQU (SINKIANG)

XIZANG ZIZHIQU (TIBET)

QINGHAI

GANSU

SICHUAN

YUNNAN

INDIA

NEPAL

BHUTAN

BANGLADESH

BURMA (MYANMAR)

THAILAND (SIAM)

LAOS

VIETNAM

NORTH KOREA

SOUTH KOREA

JAPAN

PHILIPPINES

TAIWAN (FORMOSA)

HONG KONG (Xianggang)

BEIJING
SHANGHAI
TIANJIN
SEOUL
PYONGYANG
FUKUOKA

YELLOW SEA
EAST CHINA SEA
SOUTH CHINA SEA
BAY OF BENGAL

Tarim Pendi
Taklimakan Shamo
Badain Jaran Shamo
Mu Us Shamo

Kunlun Shan
Qilian Shan
Tien Shan
Altai Shan

Huang He
Chang Jiang
Mekong
Irrawaddy

Tropic of Cancer

East from Greenwich

Projection: Bonne

m 6000 4000 3000 2000 1500 1000 400 200 0
ft 18 000 12 000 9000 6000 4500 3000 1200 600 0

1:17 800 000

1:6 700 000

50 0 100 150 200 250 300 km
50 0 50 100 150 200 miles

1 2 3 4 **59** 5 6 7 8

A **Dongsha Dao** (Pratas I.) **Luzon Strait** Itbayat I. Batanes Is. Batan I. A

P A C I F I C

20 20

Balintang Channel
Calayan I.

B Calayan I. Babuyan I. Camiguin I. B
Dalupiri I. Babuyan Islands Fuga I.
Mayraira Pt. **Babuyan Channel**
Bacarra Bangui Claveria Aparri Santa Ana Gonzaga
San Nicolas Laoag Kabugao Gattaran
18 Batac Tuao Tuguegarao Cagayan 18
Cabugao 2360 Tuao Mt. Cresta
Bangued Lubuagan △ 1685
C Vigan Santa Roxas Bontoc Ilagan Palanan Pt. C
Candon Maria Mt. Mateo Palanan
Tagudin Balaoan MT. DATA Santiago **Luzon**
San Fernando Mt. Pulog Cordon
Lingayen 2928 Solano
16 Bolinao HUNDRED **Baguio** Bayombong Casiguran 16
Alaminos ISLANDS Rosario Mt. Anacuao C. San Ildefonso
Lingayen Gulf Dagupan 1852
San Carlos San Manuel **P H I L I P P I N E**
D Santa Cruz Bayambang San Jose Baler Bay D
Masinloc Camiling Moncada Victoria Baler **S E A**
Iba 2037 Cuyapo La AURORA MEMORIAL
Tarlac Paz Gapan Dingalan
Concepcion Angeles **PHILIPPINES**
Mt. Pinatubo **San Fernando**
San Antonio 1780 Polillo Is.
Olongapo Oroni **Malabon** Patnanongan I.
BATAAN **Caloocan** Jomalig I.
Subic B. **Quezon City**
Bataan Manila **MANILA** Lamon Bay
14 Cavite Pasay Santa Cruz Paracale Pandan 14
Dasmariñas L. de Bay Lucban Labo
Tagaytay QUEZON Atimonan Daet **BICOL**
Nasugbu **San** Lucena Calauag Calabanga Viga Catanduanes
Balayan **Pablo** Lopez 1976 Naga San Andres
E Lemery **Lipa** Catanauan Mt. Isarog Iriga Virac E
Batangas Tayabas Bay Boac Nabua Ligao Rapu Rapu I.
Lubang 5245 C. Calavite Verde I. Pass Marin- Tabaco Mayon Vol.
Is. Mamburao duque Burias I. Legazpi Donsol Sorsogon
Calapan Victoria Pinamalayan Gubat
Mindoro LAKE NAUJAN Romblon Magallanes
Sablayan Mt. Baco Tablas Ticao I. Bulan San Bernardino Str.
Bongabong 2487 Sibuyan I. Irosin
12 APO REEF Roxas Odiongan SEA Aroroy Masbate Allen Mondragon Gamay 12
MARINE San Jose Masbate Mikagros Catarman Arteche
Busuanga I. Ilin I. Placer Calbayog Oras
Taft
F Culion I. Calamian Catbalogan **Samar** F
Group Pandan Kalibo VISAYAN Bilinan I. Borongan
Linapacan Str. Roxas SEA Caibiran Santa General MacArthur
Linapacan I. Tibiao Pilar Bantayan Carigara Rita Guiuan
Cuyo Is. 2117 Dao Ajuy Sara Calubian Palompon **Leyte** Basey
Bugasong Passi **Leyte** Tacloban
Cuyo Pototan **Panay** Silay Cadiz Bogo Ormoc Homonhon I.
San Jose **Iloilo** Victorias Sagay Tuburan Dulag Leyte Gulf
Dumaran I. Jordan San Carlos Danao Camotes Abuyog
Palawan Guimaras Binalbagan La 2450 Camotes Bato 10 497
10 ST. PAUL **Bacolod** Carlota CENTRAL CEBU Sea Baybay 10
1593 Hinigaran Himamaylan **Mandaue** San Juan Dinagat I.
Irahuan Honda Bay Kabankalan **Cebu** Maasin Surigao Str.
Puerto Princesa Sipalay Guihulngan Carcar Dinagat
1727 Cagayan Is. Hinoba-an Argao Bohol I. Siargao I.
Mt. Mantalingajan **Negros** Tanjay RATAH Panaon I. Placer
G 2085 Bais SIKATUNA Surigao Bucas Grande I. G
C. Buliluyan Bayawan Dumaguete **BOHOL** L. Mainit Carrascal
Bugsuk I. Siaton Siquijor I. Tagbilaran Cabadbaran Lanuza
Balabac I. Zamboanguita Camiguin I. 2012 **Butuan** Tandag
S U L U 5576 Talisayan Nasipit Tago
Balabac Strait Dipolog Dapitan SEA Balingasag Gingoog **Bayugan** Marihatag
8 Balambangan TUBBATAHA Manukan Oroquieta Opol Alubijid Lianga 8
Kudat Banggi Sindangan MT. Ozamiz **Cagayan de Oro** Talacogan Hinatuan
S E A Esperanza Bislig
H Langkon Cagayan Sulu Labason MALINDANG **Iligan** 2938 Malaybalay H
Kota Belud G. Kinabalu Liloy 2815 Tubod Marawi City Bunawan
Kota △ 4101 Siocon Kabasalan Pagadian L. Lanao Valencia Cateel
6 **Kinabalu** Senaja Jambongan Pilas Isabela Margosatubig Malabang Parang **M i n d a n a o** Baganga 6
Papar Telok Group Basilan I. Sibuco Illana Midsayap Panabo
62 Pangutaran Lamitan Bay Cotabato Pikit Mt. Apo **Davao** Tagum
Langkon Labuk Group Datu Piang 2954 Pantukan Manay
J Melalap SABAH Turtle Is. Jolo **Zamboanga** Talayan Kidapawan Digos Mati J
Keningau Samales Moro Gulf Kalamansig Davao
Kuamat MALAYSIA Jolo Group Lebak Koronadal Gulf C. San Agustin
Melalap Tawi-tawi Parang 2083 Malita
Borneo Group Talipao San Isidro
Teluk Darvel Tapul **General**
Pata I. 5824 **Santos** Tinaca Pt.
Sibutu Group Kiamba Sarangani Bay
Projection: Lambert's Conformal Conic Siasi Group Kumat Sarangani Is.
C E L E B E S **INDONESIA** Kep. Talaud

S O U T H

C H I N A

S E A

M i n d o r o Strait

Cagayan West Pass Cagayan East Pass

S U L U Archipelago

Sibutu Passage

Moro Gulf

S E A

East from Greenwich

1 2 3 4 **63** 5 6 7 8

Projection: Lambert's Conformal Conic

COPYRIGHT PHILIP'S

ft m
9000 3000
6000 2000
4500 1500
3000 1000
1200 400
600 200
0 0
200 600
4000 12 000
8000 24 000
m ft

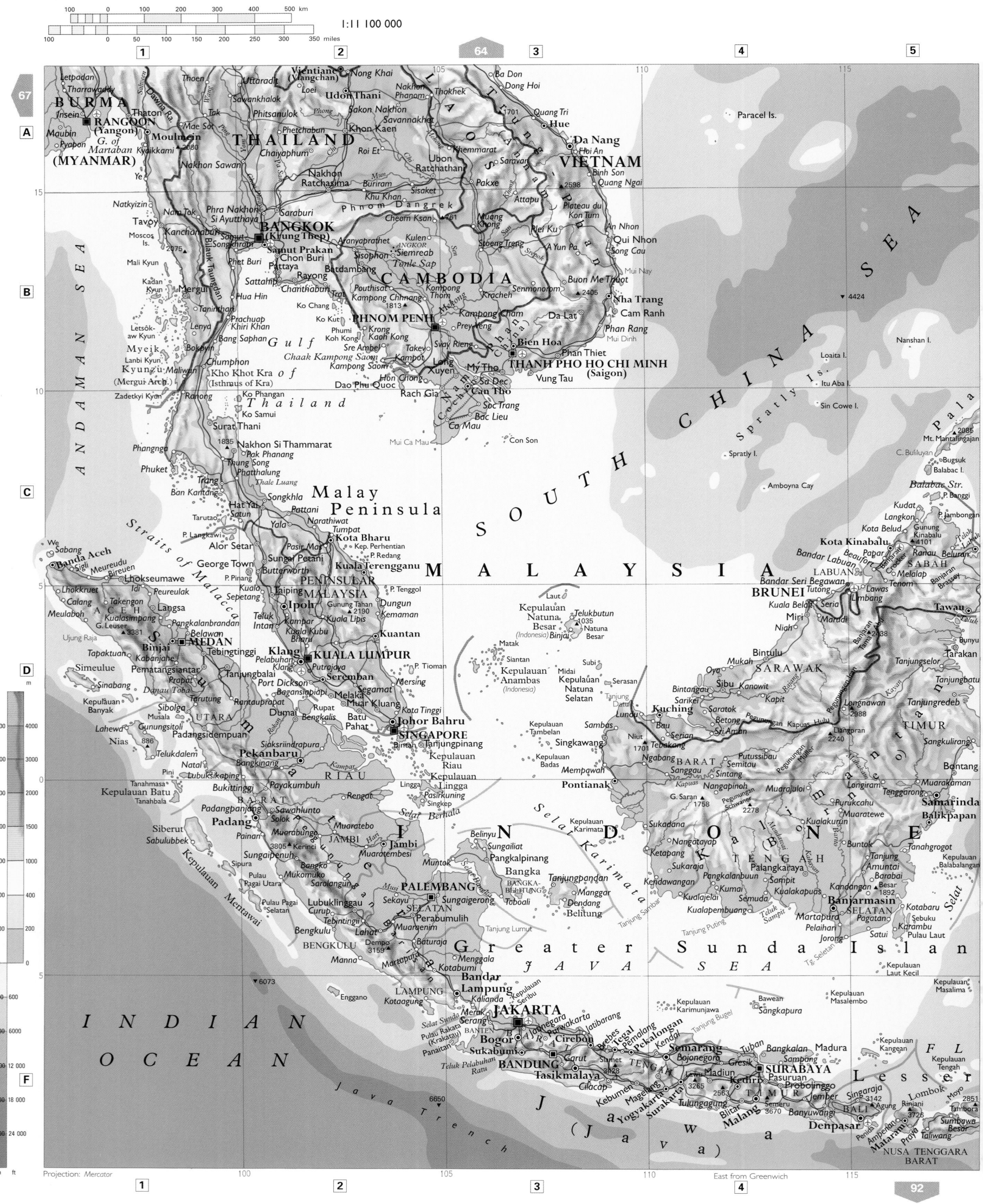

Projection: Mercator

East from Greenwich

PHILIPPINES

Claveria · Babuyan Chan. · C. Engaño
Bacarra · Laoag · Aparri · Tuguegarao · Palanan Pt. · Palanan
2048 · Tudo · Solano · Bayombong · Ilagan · Casiguran
Bangued · Vigan · Bontoc · Bolinao · Lingayen G. · Baguio · San Jose · C. San Ildefonso
San Fernando · Angeles · San Fernando · Cabanatuan
Dagupan · Tarlac · Polillo Is. · Luzon
Mt. Pinatubo 1759 · Olongapo · Malolos · Quezon City · Lamon Bay
Bataan · MANILA · Santa Cruz · Daet · Catanduanes
Manila B. · Cavite · Lipa · Lucena · Calauag · Virac
Lubang Is. · Batangas · 2188 · Naga · Mayon 2462 · Legazpi · Sorsogon
Calapan · Marinduque · Tabaco · Masbate · Bulan · San Bernardino Str.
5245 · Mamburao · Mindoro · Romblon · Tablas · Sibuyan · Masbate Sea · Catarman · Oras · Taft
Sablayan · Sibuyan · Masbate · Calbayog · Samar · General MacArthur
Calamian Group · Culion · San Jose · Pandan · Panay · Kalibo · Visayan · Borongan
2117 · Roxas · Sea · Catbalogan · Tacloban · Guiuan
Cuyo · Cuyo · Iloilo · Cadiz · Bogo · Leyte · Maasin · Dinagat 10 497
Taytay · Dumaran · San Carlos · Mandaue · Cebu · Siargao
Imuruan B. · Bacolod · Guimaras G. · 2435 · Talibon · Bohol · Surigao
Puerto Princesa · Negros · Tanjay · Siquijor · Camiguin · Tandag
5576 · Dumaguete · Bohol Sea · Butuan · L. 2012 · Ilanga
Dipolog · Oroquieta · Cagayan · Malaybalay · Cateela · Baganga
Sindangan · 2425 · Iligan · de Oro · 2938 · Tagum · 2804
Kabasalan · Ozamiz · Mindanao · 2954 · Mt. Apo · DAVAO · Mati
Siocon · Sibuco · Pagadian · Cotabato · Datu Piang · Digos
Zamboanga · Basilan B. · Moro G. · Illana B. · Lebak · Koronadal · 2083 · Malita · C. San Agustin
Parang · Isabela · Basilan · General Santos · Kiamba · 2954 · Tinaca Pt.
Jolo · Jolo · Samales Group · Sarangani Is. · Sarangani 5824

SULU SEA · Cagayan Is.
Pangutaran Group · Siasi · Tapul Group
Sandakan · Lahad Datu · Balimbing · Tawi-Tawi
Teluk Lahad · Semporna · Sipadan · Kepulauan Nanusa · Kepulauan Kawio
Karakelong · Beo · Kepulauan Talaud · Salibabu · Kaburuang

CELEBES SEA
Maratua · Tahuna · Pulau Sangihe · Tahulandang · Biaro
Bunaken · Manado · 2022 · Bangka · Doi · Galela · Tobelo · Akelamo
Amurang · Kema · Mayu · Jailolo · 1325 · Halmahera
Toli-Toli · Buol · Paleleh · Sumalata · Kuandang · Kotamobagu · Ternate · UTARA · Teluk Buli
Teluk Dondi · Malino · GORONTALO · 2490 · Tilamuta · Gorontalo · Tidore · Makian · Weda · Teluk Weda · Patani · Selat Gebe
Tanjung Mangkalihat · Tomini · Moutong · Kayoa · Wosi · Umera · Kepulauan Asia · Kepulauan Mapia
Donggala · Tomini · Teluk · Tomini · Kasiruta · Labuha · Gani · Tanjung Libobo
Palu · Toboli · Poh · 4970 · Obilatu · Bisa · Misool · Sailolof · Segat · Klamono
Pargi · Tojo · Tokala · Luwuk · Peleng · Mangole · Kawasi · Sesepe · Obi
2354 · Poso · 2630 · Banggai · Taliabu · Auponhia · Obi · Inanwatan · Teminabuan
Sulawesi (Celebes) · Kepulauan Banggai · Todeli · Kepulauan Sula · Fluk · Adua · Segun
BARAT · Danau Poso · Sanana · Lenmalu · Wahai
Mamuju · Malili · Kolonodale · Danau Towuti · TENGAH · Mondeodo · Manui · Namlea · Buru · Piru · Seram (Ceram) · Bula · Weri · Karufa
3074 · Masamba · Palopo · Kendari · Monse · 2736 · Kayeli · Amahai 3019 · Tehoru · Waru · Ibonma
Mamasa · 2799 · Malamala · Mekongga · Wowoni · Wamulan · Tifu · Namrole · Lima · Ambon · Saparua · Geser
Onang · Rantemario 3440 · Singkang · Pampanua · Kolaka · MALUKU · Gorong · Manggawitu
Majene · Piorang · Pangkajene · Buopinang · Raha · Muna · Lawele · Kepulauan Banda · Kepulauan Watubela
Teluk Mandar · Parepare · Watampone · Sinjai · Pising · Buton · Baubau · Wangiwangi · Bandanaira · Adi
Pangkajene · UJUNG PANDANG (Makasar) · 2871 · Bulukumba · Kabaena · Binongko · Tukangbesi · Har · Kai Besar · Kola · Gumzai
Bantaeng · Benteng · Binongko · Batuata · 7440 · Tual · Kai Kecil · Banda Elat · Dobo · Sewer · Wokam
Kepulauan Salayar · Bonerate · Kalaotoa · Gunungapi · Nila · Serua · Molu · Wangal · Rebi · Trangan · Gomogomo
Tanahjampea · Kalao · Damar · Teun · Daya · Tafermaar · Kepulauan Aru
Sumbawa · Sangeang 5123 · Komodo · Rinca · Pantar · Alor · Wetar · Wesiri · Romang · Barat · Tepa · Babar · Eliase · Selaru · Kepulauan Tanimbar
Bima · Raba · Ruteng · Flores · Larantuka · Lomblen · Kalabahi · Ataura · Baucau · Ilwaki · Kisar · Moa · Lakor · Sermata · Masela · Saumlaki · Tanjung Ngabordamlu
2850 · Aimere · Ende · Maumere · Solor · Selat Ombai · Dili · Tutuala Leti · Eliase
Parado · Selat Sape · Sumba · Membora · **NUSA TENGGARA TIMUR** · Pante Macassar (E. Timor) · 2963 · Viqueque · **EAST TIMOR**
Waikabubak · Melolo · Sawu Sea · Kupang · Kefamenanu · Nikiniki
Baing · Sawu · Baa · Roti
Raijua · Dana

PACIFIC OCEAN
Merir (Palau) · Tobi (Palau) · Helen Atoll (Palau) · 5798
Sopi · Berebere · Morotai · Kepulauan Raja Ampat · Selpele · Dampier · Waibeem · Kaironi · Manokwari · Supiori · Biak
Kepulauan Sangihe · Kepulauan Sangihe · Sorong · Jazirah Doberai · Kwoka · Numfoor · Warsa · Bosnik · Kepulauan Padaido
Karakitang · Siau · Waigeo · Kofiau · Batanta · Salawati · Warkapi · Yapen · Selat Yapen · 1496 · Biak
Equator
Ayu · Wakre · 2452 · Ransiki · Wasior · Yapen · Serui · Bonoi · Tanjung D'Urville · Kumamba
Dampier · Sonek · IRIAN JAYA · 2926 · Wasion · Wariap · Sarmi · Barapasi · Ansudu
Kepulauan Mapia · Salawati · Teminabuan · 2272 · Nuboi · Saberania · Genyem · Jayapura
IRIAN JAYA · BARAT · Babo · Wendesi · Cenderawasih · Pegunungan Van Rees · Sentani
Fakfak · Kokas · Wenut · Susunu · Kwatisore · Nabire · Woghote · Enarotali · Pegunungan · Tariku · Krau
Kaimana · Karufa · 5029 · Jaya · Maoke · Wamena · Krau · Jayawijaya
Teluk Berau · Teluk Fatagar · Adi · **PAPUA**
Manggawitu · Uta · Tembagapura · Puncak · 4730 · Wamena
Amamapare · Yapero · Puncak Mandala · Oksibil
Kepulauan Watubela · Agats · Mindiptana · Tanahmerah
Teluk Flamingo · Pulau · Pirimapun · Kepi · Bade
Kepulauan Aru · Wokam · Koba · Wangal · Muting · Okaba
Pulau Dolak · Kimaam · Pulau Komoran · Merauke
Tanjung Vals · Tanjung · Pangga · Tanjung Tampa
PAPUA NEW GUINEA

ARAFURA SEA
BANDA SEA
FLORES SEA
MOLUCCA SEA
CERAM SEA
SULU SEA
SUNDA IS.

JAVA AND MADURA
1:6 700 000

Scale: 50 · 0 · 50 · 100 · 150 · 200 · 250 · 300 km
50 · 0 · 50 · 100 · 150 · 200 miles

Selat Sunda · Merak · Tangerang · **JAKARTA** · Bawean · Sangkapura
Anyer · Bekasi · Karawang · Pamanukan · Kandanghaur · Kepulauan Karimunjawa
Pulau Pandeglang · Rangkasbitung · Bogor · Purwakarta · Subang · Indramayu · Tanjung Bugel
Rakata · Panaitan · Labuhan · Cianjur · Sumedang · Majalengka · Cirebon · Tegal · Pekalongan · Jepara · Rembang · Tuban · Tanjung Pangkah · Madura
Tanjung Guhakolak · **BANTEN** · Pelabuhanratu · Sukabumi · **BANDUNG** · 3078 · Ciremai · Kuningan · Pemalang · Kendal · Demak · Pati · Blora · Bangkalan · Tambuku · Sampang · Sumenep
Pelabuhan Ratu · Garut · Tasikmalaya · Purwakerto · Ciamis · Slamet · Wonosobo 3428 · **TENGAH** · Semarang · Purwodadi · Cepu · Gresik · Pamekasan
Pengalengan · Sindangbarang · Cijulang · Cilacap · Banyumas · Kebumen · Magelang · Boyolali · Surakarta · Ngawi · Jambang · **SURABAYA** · Selat Madura
Genteng · Nusa Kambangan · Karanganyar · 3265 · Yogyakarta · Madiun · Kediri · Pare · Sidoarjo · Pasuruan · Probolinggo · Situbondo
Wates · Bantul · **YOGY.** · 3339 · Ponorogo · 2563 · Limun · **TIMUR** · 3676 · **Malang** · 3332
Pacitan · Trenggalek · Blitar · 2565 · Semeru · Lumajang · Jember · Banyuwangi
Tulungagung · Wlingi · Pasirian · **Bali** · 3089 · Selat Bali
Nusa Barung

BALI
1:1 800 000
10 · 0 · 10 · 20 · 30 km
10 · 0 · 10 · 20 miles

3332 · Gunung Raung · Tanjung Batugondang · **BALI SEA** · Kubutambahan
Ketapang · Gilimanuk · Pulau Menjangan · Singaraja · Tejakula
Banyuwangi · Cekik · Gerokgak · Lovina · Bayun · Gunung · Tianyar
Glagah · Melaya · 1385 · Gunung Merbuk · Seririt · Kintamani · Batur · 1717 · Songan · Kubu
Jambewangi · Beluki · Busungbiu · Pupuan · Batukau · Bedugul · Penelokan · Gunung Culik
Genteng · Rogojampi · Negara · Mendoyo · Yehbuah · 2276 · Jatiluwih · Rendang · Agung 3142 · Saren · Amed
Srono · Muncar · Perancak · Pekutatan · Belimbing · Sembung · Tegallalang · Baturiti · Manggis · Tirtagangga
Tegalsari · Tjiuring · Pasar · Bojera · Blahkiuh · Ubud · Bangli · Candi Dasa · Karangasem (Amlapura)
Bajatrejo · Tabanan · Gianyar · Klungkung · Kusamba · Montongbuwoh · **Lombok**
Grajagan · **Bali** · Sukawati · Manggis · Ampenan · Lembuak
Jawa · Tanjung Kucur · **Denpasar** · Sanur · Selat Badung · Sampalan · **Mataram** · Teluk Terang
Tanjung Purwo · Semenanjung Blambangan · Danginpuri · Toyapakeh · 530 · Suwana · Lembar · Gerung
Teluk Jimbaran · Kuta · **Nusa Penida** · Tanjung Abah · Blongas
Uluwatu · DPS · Nusa Dua · Bukit Badung · Tanjung Bebera
Tanjung Mebulu · Tanjung Pangga · Tanjung Tampa

INDIAN OCEAN

COPYRIGHT PHILIP'S

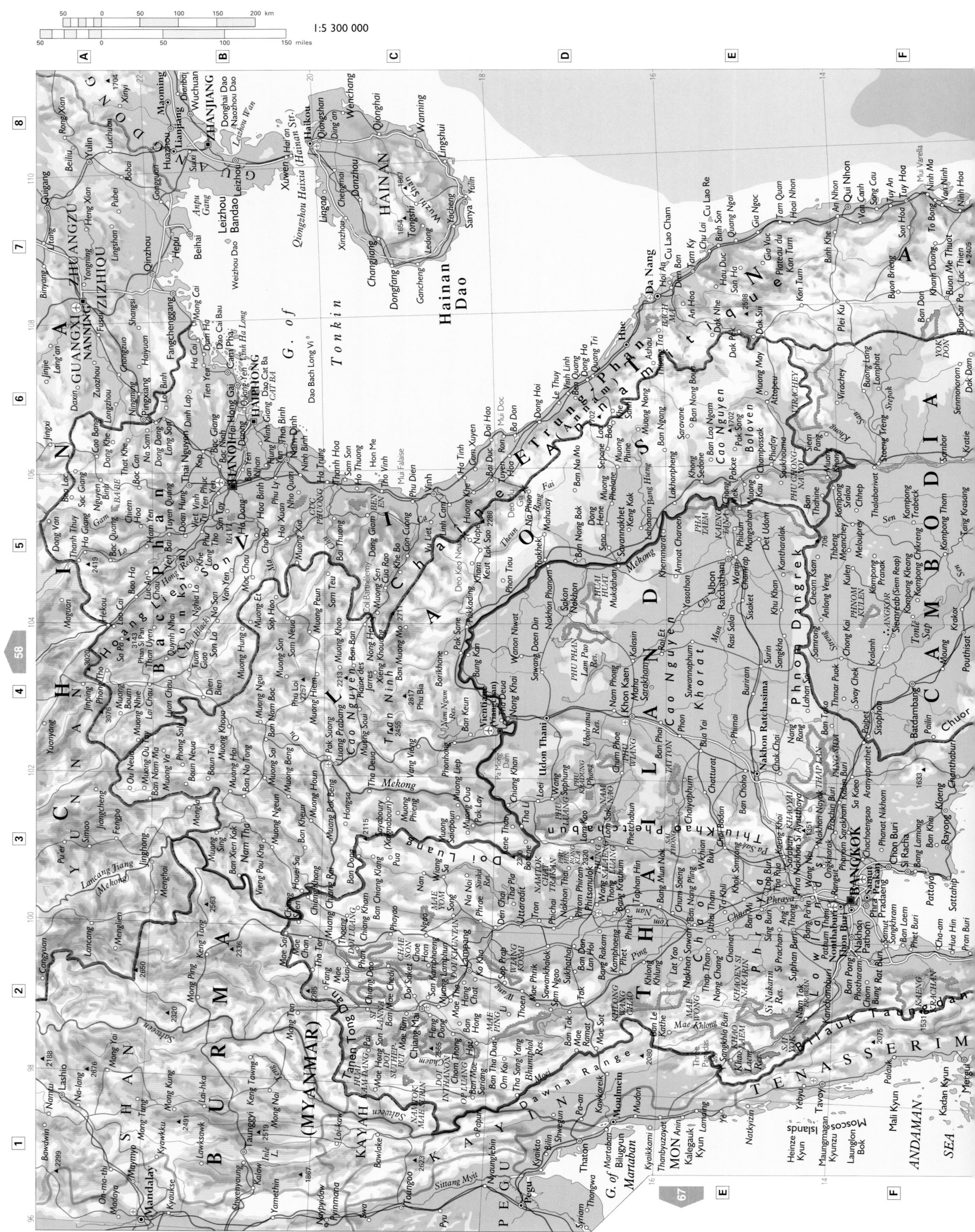

1:5 300 000

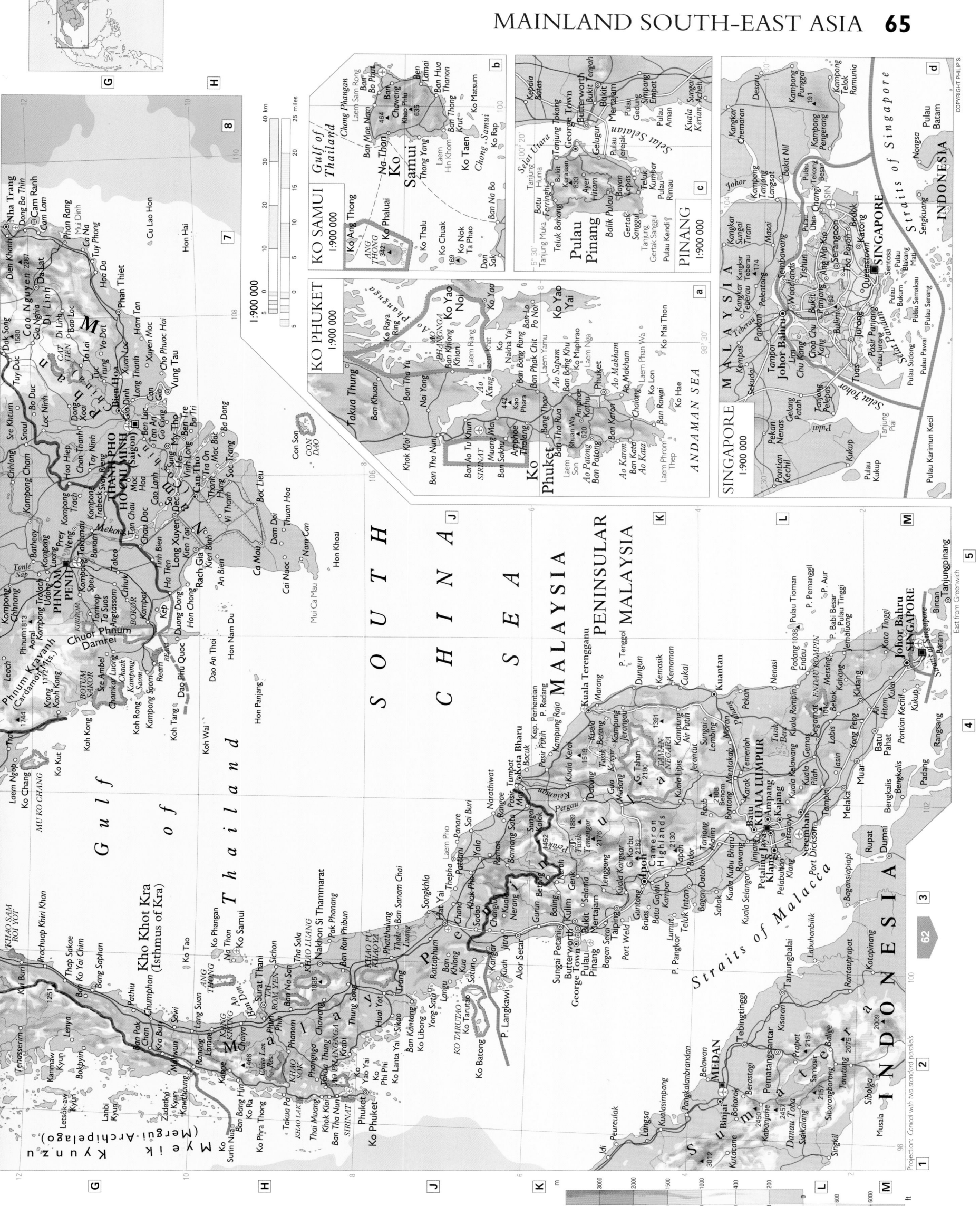

COPYRIGHT PHILIP'S

KO SAMUI
1:900 000

Gulf of Thailand

Chong Phangan
Ban Bo Phut
Ban Moe Nam
Ban Chaweng
Na-Thon
Ko Samui
Laem Sam Rong
Bari
Ben Lamai
Ban Hua Thanon
Khao Phu
Thong Yang
Laem Hin Khom
Ko Taen
Chong Samui
Ko Matsum
Ko Rap
Ko Ang Thong
ANG THONG
342 Ko Phaluai
Ko Thalu
Ko Chuak
Ko Nok Ta Phao
Ban Na Bo
Ko Phra

PINANG
1:900 000

Kepala Batas
Tanjung Tokong
Butterworth
George Town
Bukit Tengah
Simpang Empat
Pulau Jerejak
Bukit Mertajam
Kubang Semang
Tanjung Huma
Kenaian
464
Ayer Hitam
Bayan Lepas
833
Teluk Kumbar
Pulau Rimau
Balik Pulau
Gertak Sanggul
Pulau Kendi
5° 30'
100° 20'
Tanjung Muka
Batu Feringghi
169
Don Sak

SINGAPORE
1:900 000

Kangkar Chemaran
Desaru
Kampong Pungai
Telok Ramunia
Johor
Kampong Tanjung Langsat
Kota Tinggi
Ubin
Changi
Sembawang
Yishun
SIN
174
162
Singapore
Serangoon
Katong
Sentosa
Johor Bahru
Woodlands
Bukit Panjang
Chod Chu Kang
Bulim
Jurong
Pasir Panjang
Pulau Seletar
Kukup
Pontian Kechil
Pekan Nenas
Gelang Patah
Tanjung Pelepas
Tanjung Piai
Straits of Singapore
INDONESIA
Nongsa
Pulau Batam
East from Greenwich
104
Selat Johor
Selat Singapore

KO PHUKET
1:900 000

AO PHANGNGA
Ko Yao Noi
Ko Yao Yai
Ko Raya Ring
Ban Khlong Khian
Laem Kat
Nakha Yai
Ko Mai Thon
Ban Thong Wa
Ban Bang Rong
Phuket
Ban Phak Chit
Po Noi
Ao Po
Ao Sapam
Ban Bang Khu
Laem Nga
Ao Maprao
Takua Thung
Ko Khan
Nai Yong
442
Kao Phara
Ban Khuan
Ban Tha Yu
520
Muang Mai
Amphoe Thalang
Amphoe Kathu
Laem Son
Ao Patong
Ban Patong
Ao Karon
Ao Kata
Ban Karon
Ko Lon
Ko Hae
Ko Rawai
Laem Phrom Thep
Ao Makham
Ban Ao Tu Khun
SIRINAT
ANDAMAN SEA
99° 30'

Projection: Conical with two standard parallels

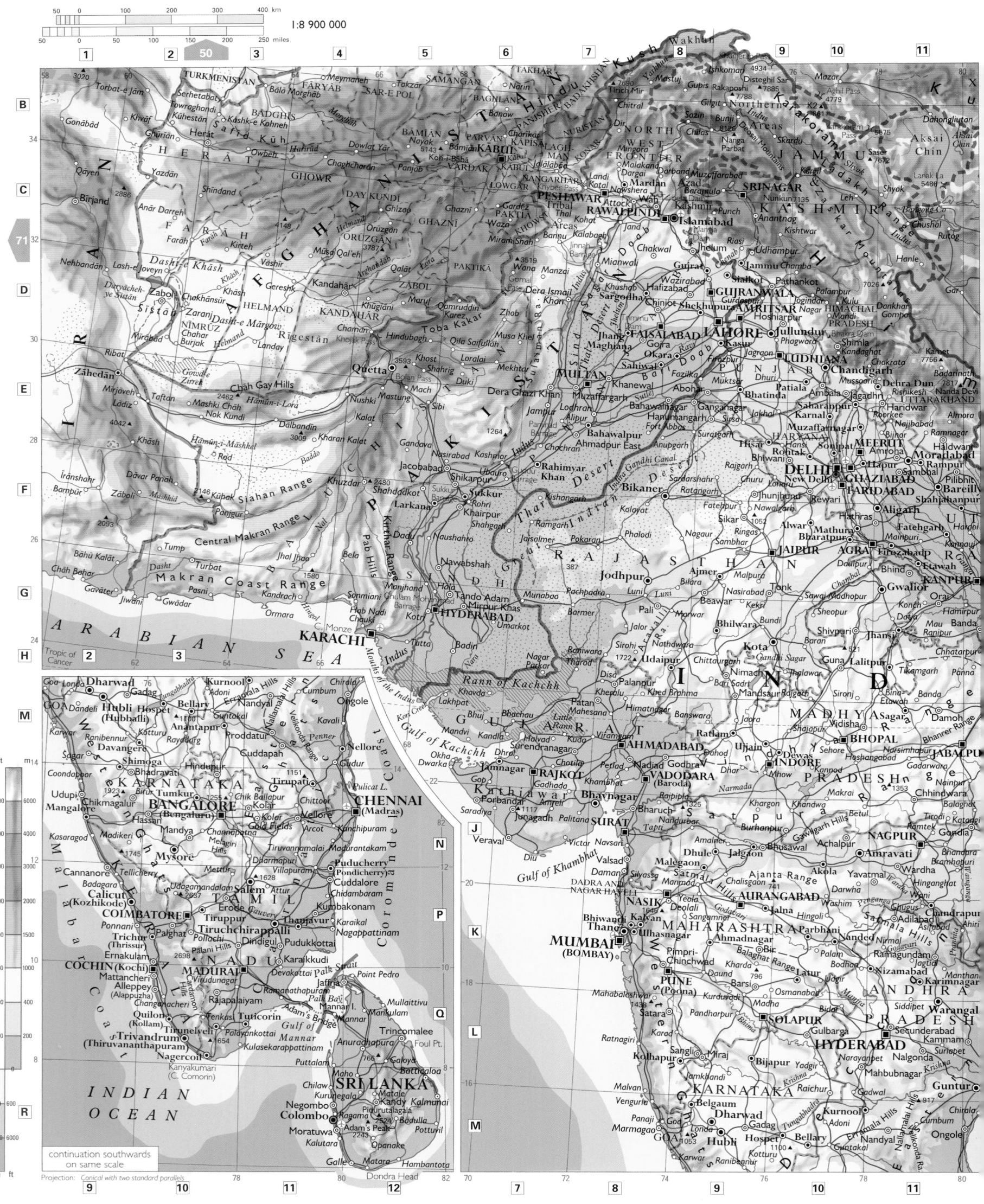

1:8 900 000

Projection: Conical with two standard parallels

continuation southwards on same scale

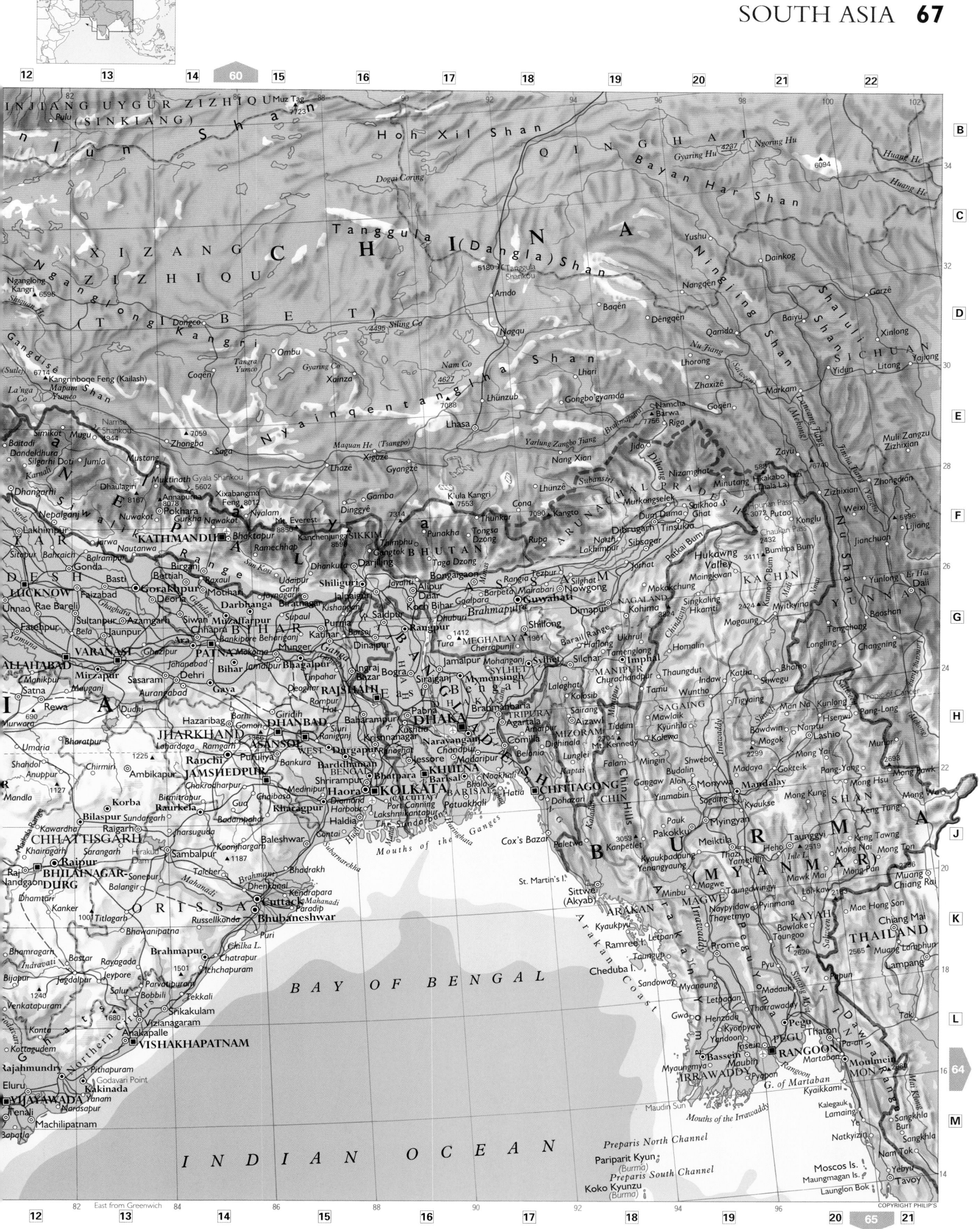

1:5 300 000

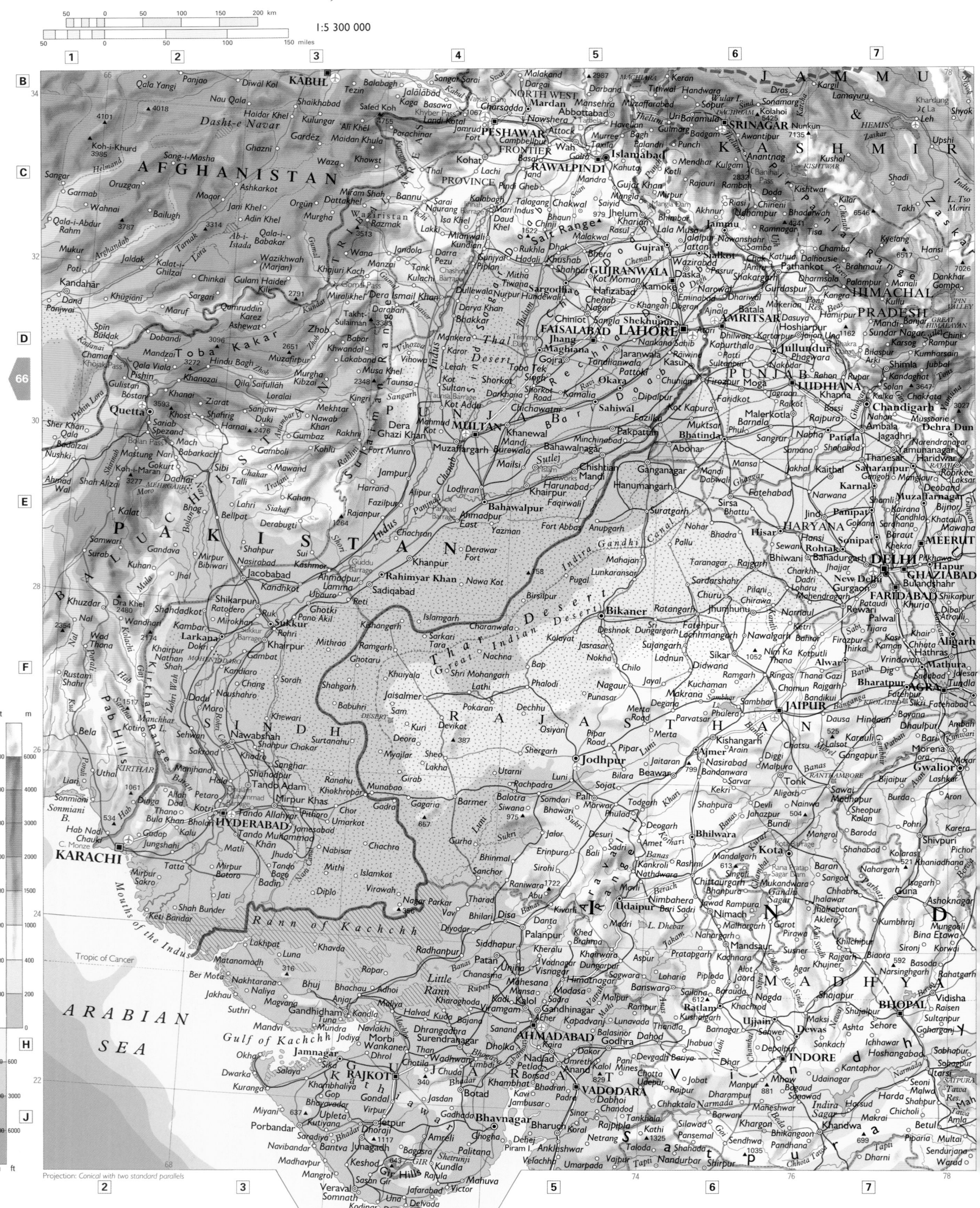

Projection: Conical with two standard parallels

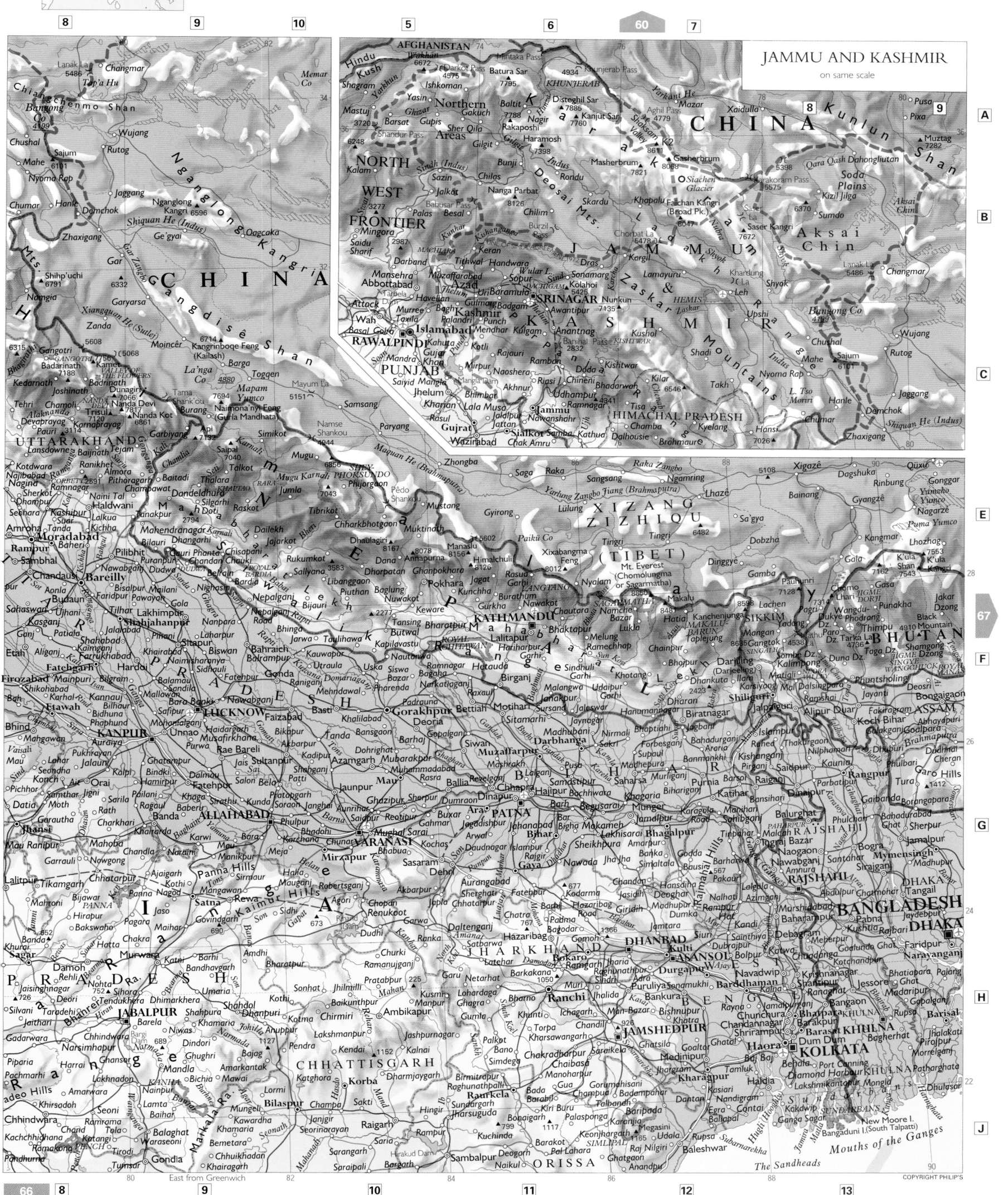

1:6 200 000

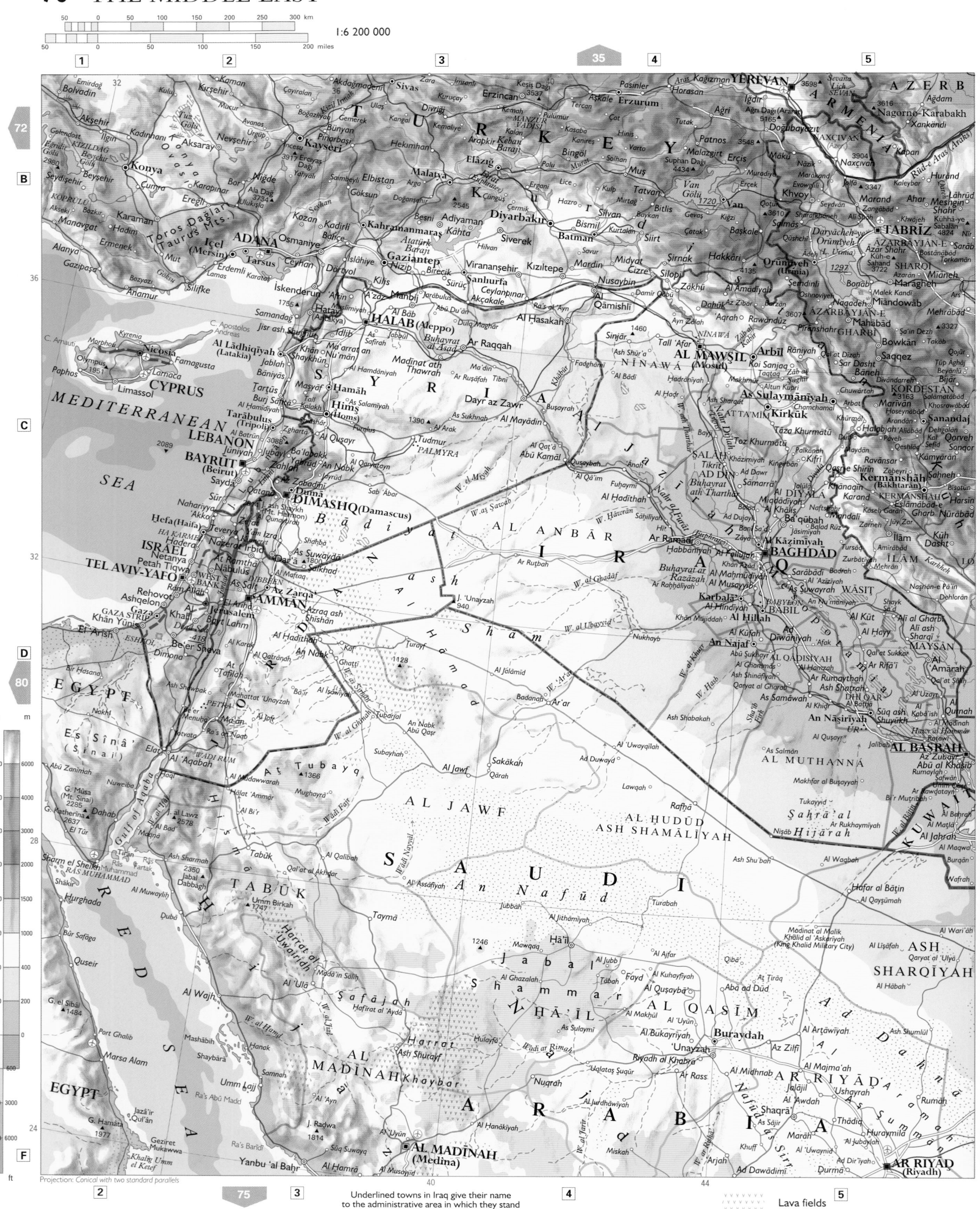

Projection: Conical with two standard parallels

Underlined towns in Iraq give their name
to the administrative area in which they stand

Lava fields

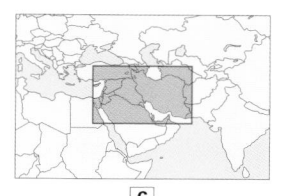

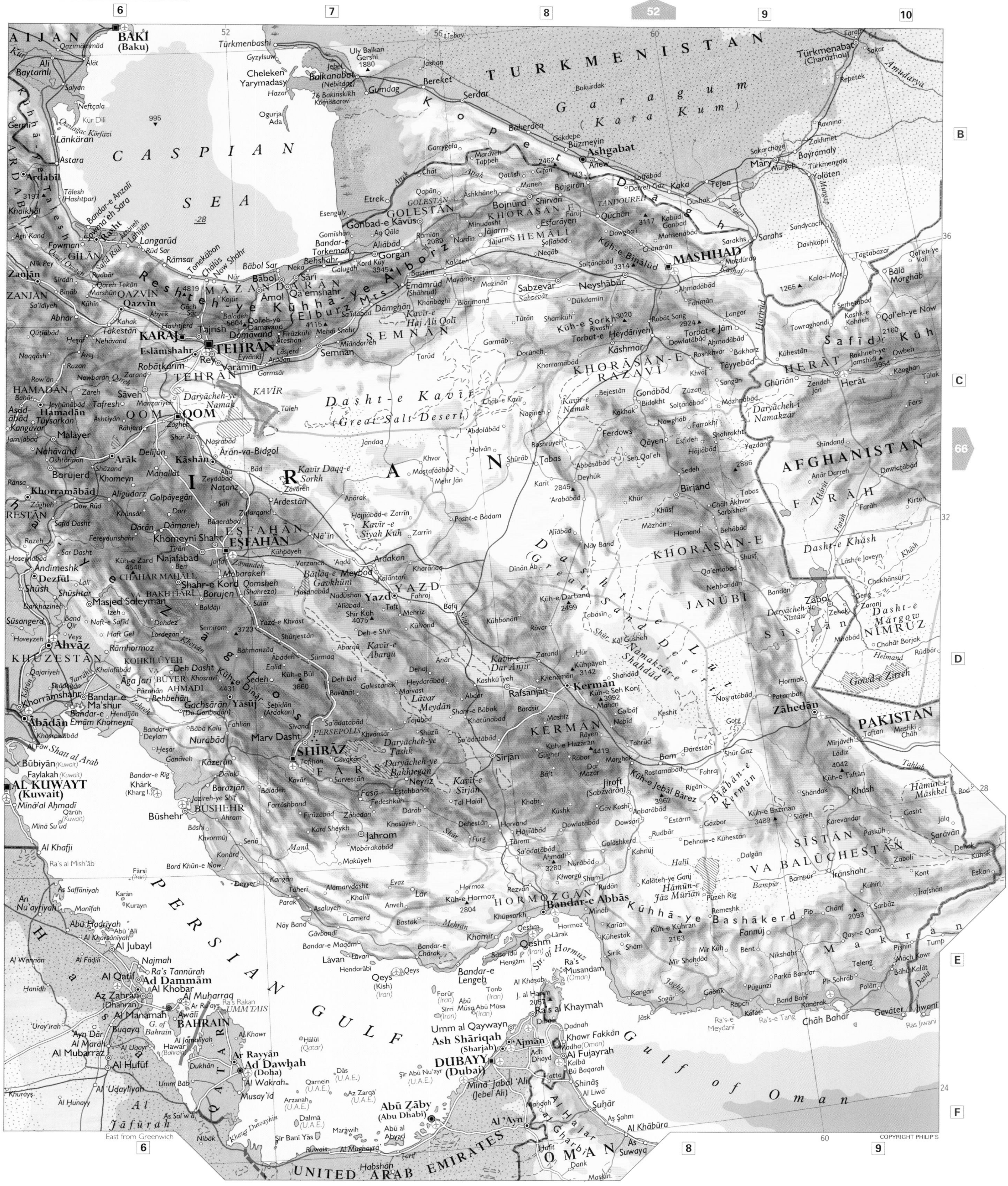

1 : 4 400 000

50   0   25 50 75 100 125 150 175 km
50   0   25 50 75 100 125 miles

| 1 | 2 | 3 | 4 | 33 | 5 | 6 | 7 |

A

BULGARIA

B L A C K   S E A

Stara Zagora
Yambol
Aytos
Burgas
Elkhovo
Michurin

45

B

Kırklareli
Edirne
Demirköy
İğneada
İğneada Burnu
Uzunköprü
Çorlu
Çerkezköy
Tekirdağ
İstanbul Boğazı (Bosporus)
Zonguldak
Bartın
Küre Dağları
SİNOP
Sinop
İnebolu
Abana
Ayancık
Erfelek
Kastamonu
Bafra
SAMSUN
Samsun
Terme
Ünye
Fatsa
Ordu

İSTANBUL
Kartal
Gebze
Kocaeli Sakarya (Adapazarı)
İzmit
Hendek
Düzce
Bolu
Gerede
Çerkeş
Çankırı
ILGAZ DAĞI
Tosya
Osmancık
Merzifon
Amasya
Çorum
Turhal
Tokat

Marmara Denizi
Sea of Marmara
Kapı Dağı
Erdek
Mudanya
Gemlik
İznik
Yalova

BURSA
Uludağ
İnegöl
Bilecik
Söğüt
Bozüyük
Eskişehir
Polatlı

C

Balıkesir
BALIKESİR
Dursunbey
Emet
Kütahya
Afyon (Afyonkarahisar)
ANKARA
Kırıkkale
Kırşehir
Yozgat
Sivas
SİVAS

İZMİR (Smyrna)
Manisa
Akhisar
Uşak
Nevşehir
Aksaray
Kayseri
KAYSERİ

D

Denizli
Isparta
Konya
KONYA
Karaman
NİĞDE
Niğde
ADANA
Kahramanmaraş
KAHRAMAN-MARAŞ

GREECE

Rhodes (Rhodes)

Antalya
ANTALYA
Manavgat
Alanya
İÇEL
İçel (Mersin)
Tarsus
ADANA
Gaziantep
HATAY
İskenderun

47

E

M E D I T E R R A N E A N

CYPRUS
Nicosia
Kyrenia
Famagusta
Morphou
Olympus
Larnaca
Limassol
Akrotiri
Paphos
Episkopi

Al Lādhiqīyah (Latakia)
Hamāh
Ḥimṣ (Homs)
SYRIA

F

S E A

Tarābulus (Tripoli)
LEBANON
BAYRŪT (Beirut)
Saydā
DIMASHQ (Damascus)
Ṣūr

G

ISRAEL
Hadera
Netanya
TEL AVIV-YAFO
Jerusalem
WEST BANK
AMMAN
JORDAN

32

| 80 | 3 | 4 | 5 | 74 | 7 |

Projection: Conical with two standard parallels

Division between Greeks and Turks
in Cyprus; Turks to the North.

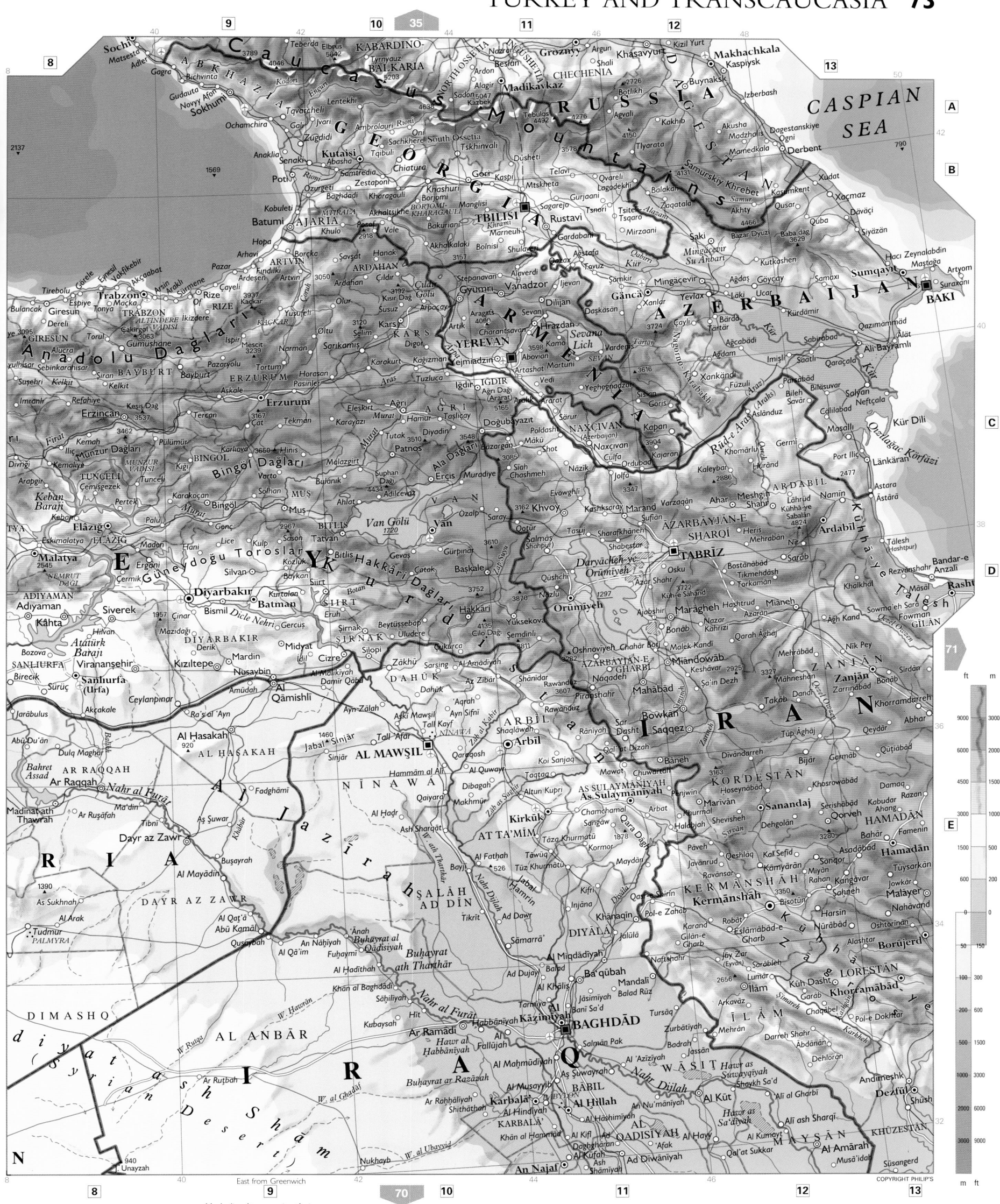

Underlined towns give their name
to the administrative area in which they stand

1:2 200 000

10 0 10 20 30 40 50 60 70 80 90 km
10 0 10 20 30 40 50 60 miles

| 1 | 2 | 3 | 4 | 72 | 5 | 6 |

CYPRUS
Paphos — Kividhes — Zyyi
Episkopi — Limassol — Akrotiri Bay — C. Gata
Episkopi Bay

2775

M E D I T E R R A N E A N

S E A

2089

Hims (Homs)
Furqlus
Shinshar
Al Hamidiyah
Tall Kalakh
Halba — ASH SHAMAL
Al Mina — Al Hirmil — Al Qusayr — HIMS
Tarabulus (Tripoli) — Zgharta — Qurnat as Sawda 3088
Al Batrun — Qartaba — Al Labwah — 2464 — Al Qaryatayn
Jubayl — Ibrahim — 2616 — Ba'labakk — An Nabk — Bi'r Ghadir
Juniyah — Bikfayya — Yabrud

BAYRUT (Beirut) — 2628 J. Sannin — **SYRIA**
Ash Shuwayfat — Alayh — Zahlah — Sirghaya — Al Qutayfah — Jayrud
Ad Damur — JABAL LUBNAN — Hawsh — An Nabk
LEBANON — Az Zabadani — Barada — Dumayr — Khan Abu Shamat
1942 J. al Barak — DIMASHB
Sayda (Sidon) — Jazzin — ash Shaykh (Mt. Hermon) 2814 — **DIMASHQ** (Damascus)
An Nabatiyah at Tahta — Marj 'Uyun — Qatana — Jaramanah — Al Hajanah
AL JANUB — Al Khiyam — Mas'ada — Al Kiswah — Buraq
Sur (Tyre) — Qiryat Shemona — Golan — DAR'A — As Sanamayn — Safa
1197 — Ar Qunaytirah — Shahba — Jabal
Nahariyya — Me'ona HAGALIL — Yam Kinneret (Sea of Galilee) — Izra — AS SUWAYDA
'Akko (Acre) 1208 — Zefat — Fiq — Shaykh Miskin — As Suwayda 1800
Qiryat Karmi'el — Yam HAZAFON — Teverya (Tiberias) 210 — Sahem al Jawlan — Salah
Mifraz Hefa — Yarmuk — Dar'a
Hefa (Haifa) — Qiryat Ata — Nazerat (Nazareth) — Tayibe — IRBID — Ar Ramtha
Daliyat el Karmel — HA KARMEL — Afula — Bet She'an — Busra ash Sham — Salkhad
Umm el Fahm — TEL MEGIDDO — AJLUN — J. Umm ad Daraj 1247 — Al Mafraq
CAESAREA — Jenin — Jarash — Umm al Qittayn
Hadera — Tulkarm — TUBAS — JARASH
ISRAEL — Shomron — SAMARIA — N. az Zarqa — AL MAFRAQ
Netanya — Nabulus — JIBBEEN — Az Zarqa
HAMERKAZ — Kefar Sava — AL BALQA
Herzliyya — Ra'anana — SHILO — As Salt — **AMMAN**
Bene Beraq — Petah Tiqwa — Wadi as Sir — Karama — AZ ZARQA
TEL AVIV-YAFO — Ramat Gan — WEST BANK — 243
Bat Yam — Lod — Ram Allah — 'AMMAN
Holon — Ramla — El Ariha (Jericho) — Na'ur
Rishon le Ziyyon — Yavne — Rehovot — At Tunayb — AMM
Ashdod — **Jerusalem** (Yerushalayim, Al Quds) — Ma'daba
Qiryat Mal'akhi — Bet Shemesh — Bayt Lahm (Bethlehem) — MA'DABA — AZ ZARQA
Ashqelon — Qiryat Gat — TEL LAKHISH — W. al Haydan — Dhiban
GAZA — Sederot — Al Khalil (Hebron) — Dead Sea — AL KARAK
GAZA STRIP — N. Shiqma — Az Zahiriyah — 'En Gedi — Al Karak
Khan Yunis — ESHKOL — JUDEA — Arad — MASADA 1305 — Al Mazar
Rafah — Bor Mashash — Sedom — W. al Hasa

Bur Sa'id (Port Said) — Bur Fu'ad
BUR SA'ID — Ras Burun — El Daheir — Be'er Sheva (Beersheba)
Khalig el Tina — Sabkhet el Bardawil — Dimona — 333 — AL KARAK — AT TAFILAH — W. al Ghadaf — W. al Makhruq
Ramani — Bir el 'Abd — El 'Arish — Bir el Gararat — Bir Lahfan — HADAROM — Sedom — Al Qatranah — Al Hadithah
El Qantara — Bir el Duweidar — Bir Kaseiba — W. el 'Arish — Qezi'ot — At Tafilah — Dana
Wahid — Bir Madkur — SHAMAL SINI — Abu Aweigila — 1305 — **JORDAN** — Ba'ir — W. Ba'ir
892 — Muweilih — Birein — Sede Boqer — Nijil — Ja'sh Shawmari 1072
Isma'iliya — Talata — Bir el Malhi — Mizpe Ramon — Mahattat 'Unayzah
Khamsa — **EGYPT** — Bir Hasana — 121 — PETRA — 1736
ISMA'ILIYA — El Buheirat el Murrat el Kubra (Great Bitter L.) — G. Yi 'Allaq 1094 — W. el Bruk — El 'Agrud — Hanegev (Negev Desert) — Wadi Musa — Ma'an
Gineifa — Bir el Thamada — W. el Mahlash — N. Paran — Al Jafr — Qa'el Jafr
El Suweis (Suez) — Mamarr Mitla — Bir Gebel Hisn — N. Hiyyon — MA'AN
'Adabiya — Uyun Musa — Nakhl — SINAI — El Kuntilla — Yotvata — Bi'r al Mari — Ra's an Naqb
Ain Sudr — W. Ruaq — El Thamad — Ras an Naqb — AL AQABAH 1435
Ras Sudr — G. el Kabrit 948 — W. Gidifi — 'En Avrona — Bi'r al Butayhat — Bi'r al Qattar — SAUDI
Gebel el Tih — WADI RUM — **ARABIA**
Ghubbet el Bus — EL SUWEIS — W. Abu Ga'da — JANUB SINI — Elat — 1592 Rum 1754 — Batn al Ghul
Bir Abu Sanduq 1272 — Ras Matarma — W. Abu'l Gifn — Bir el Biarat — Al 'Aqabah — Rum — At Tubayq
El Wabeira — 1165 — Bir el Heisi — Bir Taba — Gulf of Aqaba — 'Iz an Nuqaira — Haql — Al Mudawwarah

SAUDI ARABIA

--- 1974 Cease Fire Lines

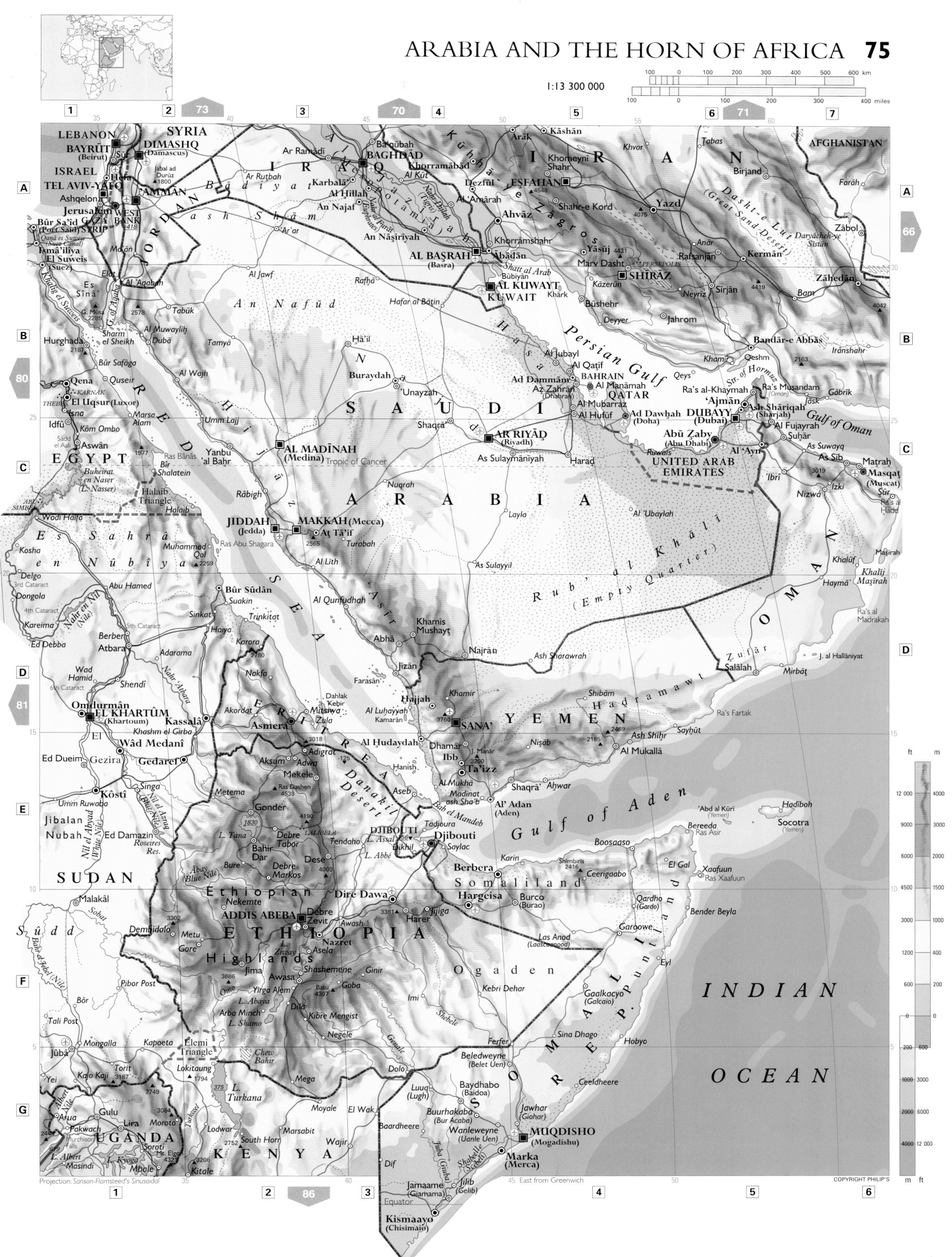

1:13 300 000

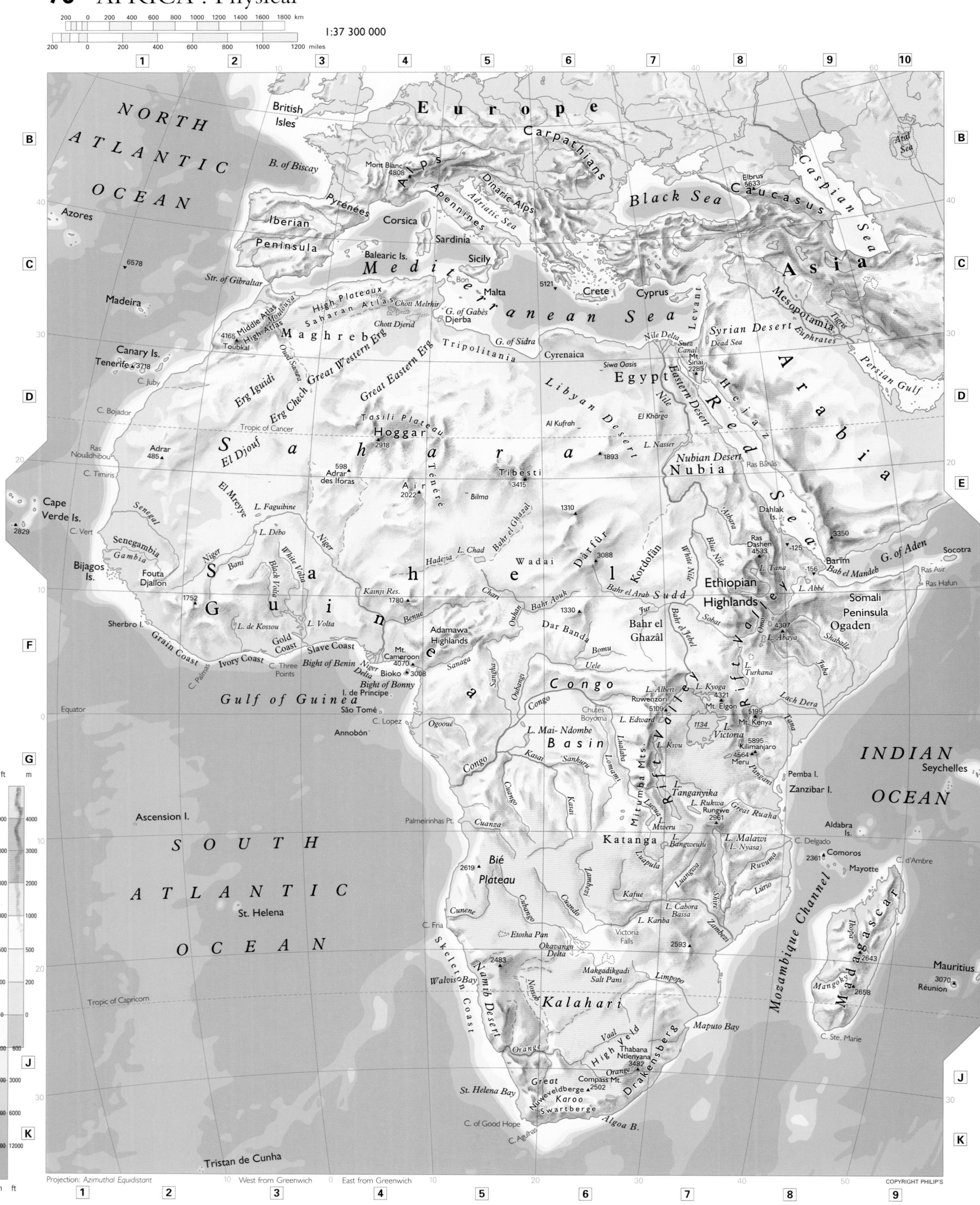

1:37 300 000

Projection: Azimuthal Equidistant

West from Greenwich 0 East from Greenwich

COPYRIGHT PHILIP'S

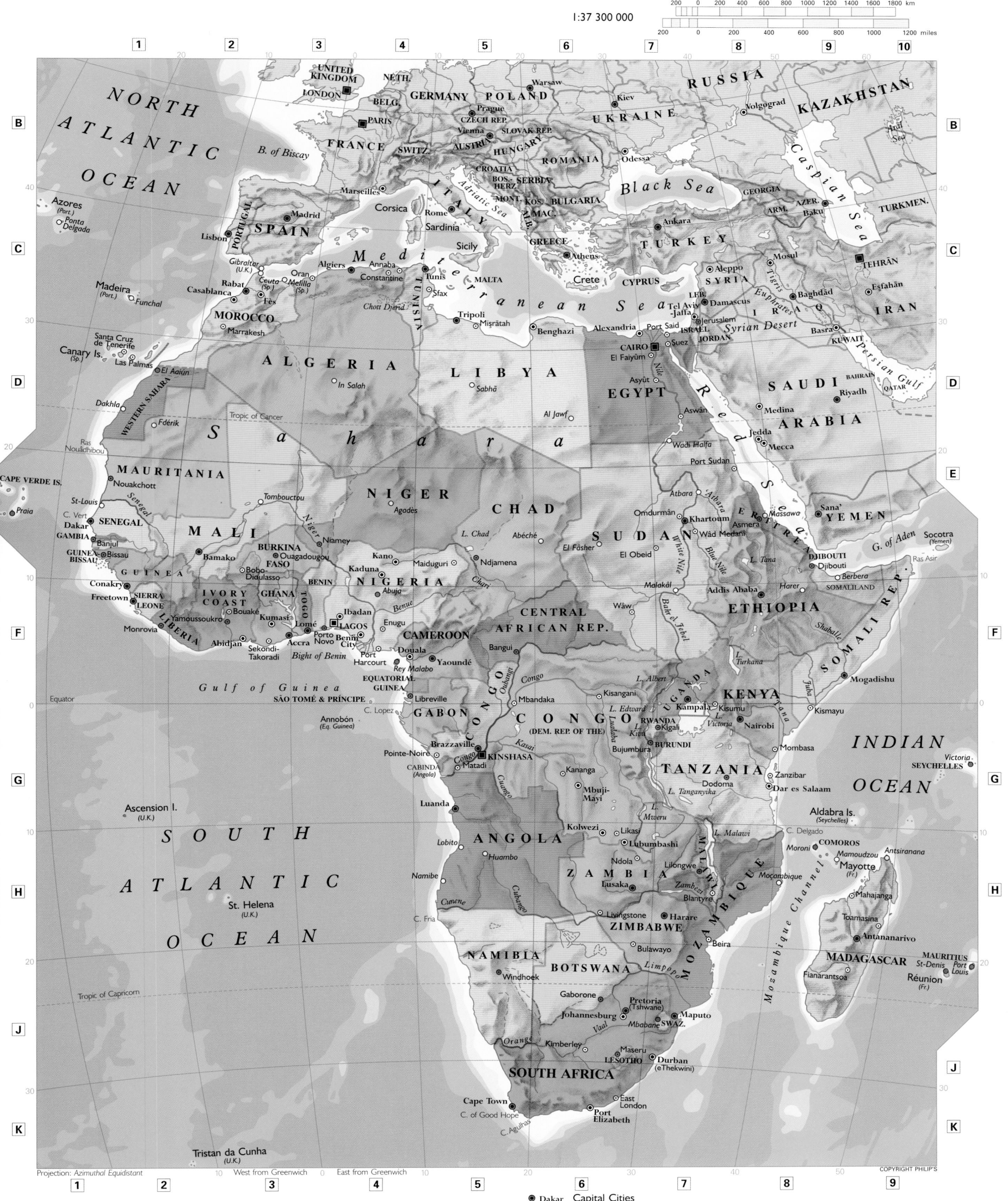

1:37 300 000

200 0 200 400 600 800 1000 1200 1400 1600 1800 km
200 0 200 400 600 800 1000 1200 miles

● Dakar Capital Cities

Projection: Azimuthal Equidistant

COPYRIGHT PHILIP'S

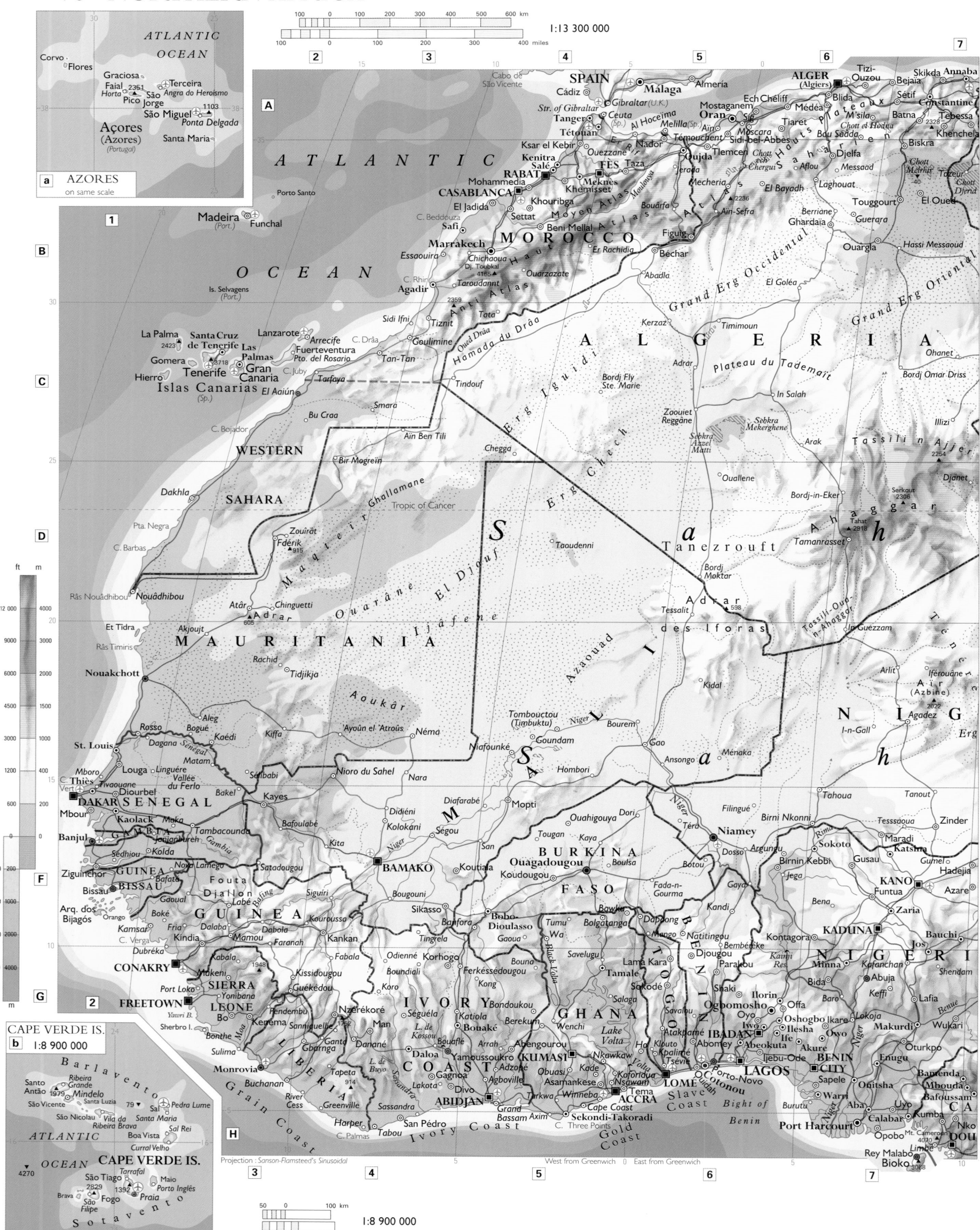

1:13 300 000

a AZORES
on same scale

ATLANTIC OCEAN

Corvo· °Flores
Graciosa
Faial 2351 °Terceira
Horta Pico °São Jorge Angra do Heroísmo
Pico São Miguel 1103
São Jorge
Ponta Delgada
Açores
(Azores)
(Portugal)
Santa Maria

b CAPE VERDE IS.
1:8 900 000

Barlavento
Santo
Antão 1979 Ribeira Grande
Mindelo
São Santa Luzia
Vicente São Nicolau 79
Vila da Ribeira Brava Sal
Santa Maria Pedra Lume
Sal Rei
Boa Vista
ATLANTIC Curral Velho
OCEAN
4270
CAPE VERDE IS.
São Tiago Tarrafal
2829 1392 Maio Porto Inglês
Brava Praia
São
Fogo Filipe
Sotavento

MOROCCO
ALGERIA
WESTERN SAHARA
MAURITANIA
SENEGAL
GAMBIA
GUINEA-BISSAU
GUINEA
SIERRA LEONE
LIBERIA
IVORY COAST
MALI
BURKINA FASO
GHANA
TOGO
BENIN
NIGER
NIGERIA
SPAIN

Projection : Sanson-Flamsteed's Sinusoidal

West from Greenwich / East from Greenwich

1:8 900 000

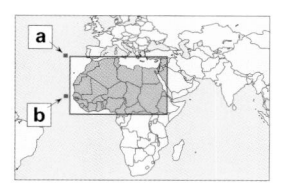

a
b

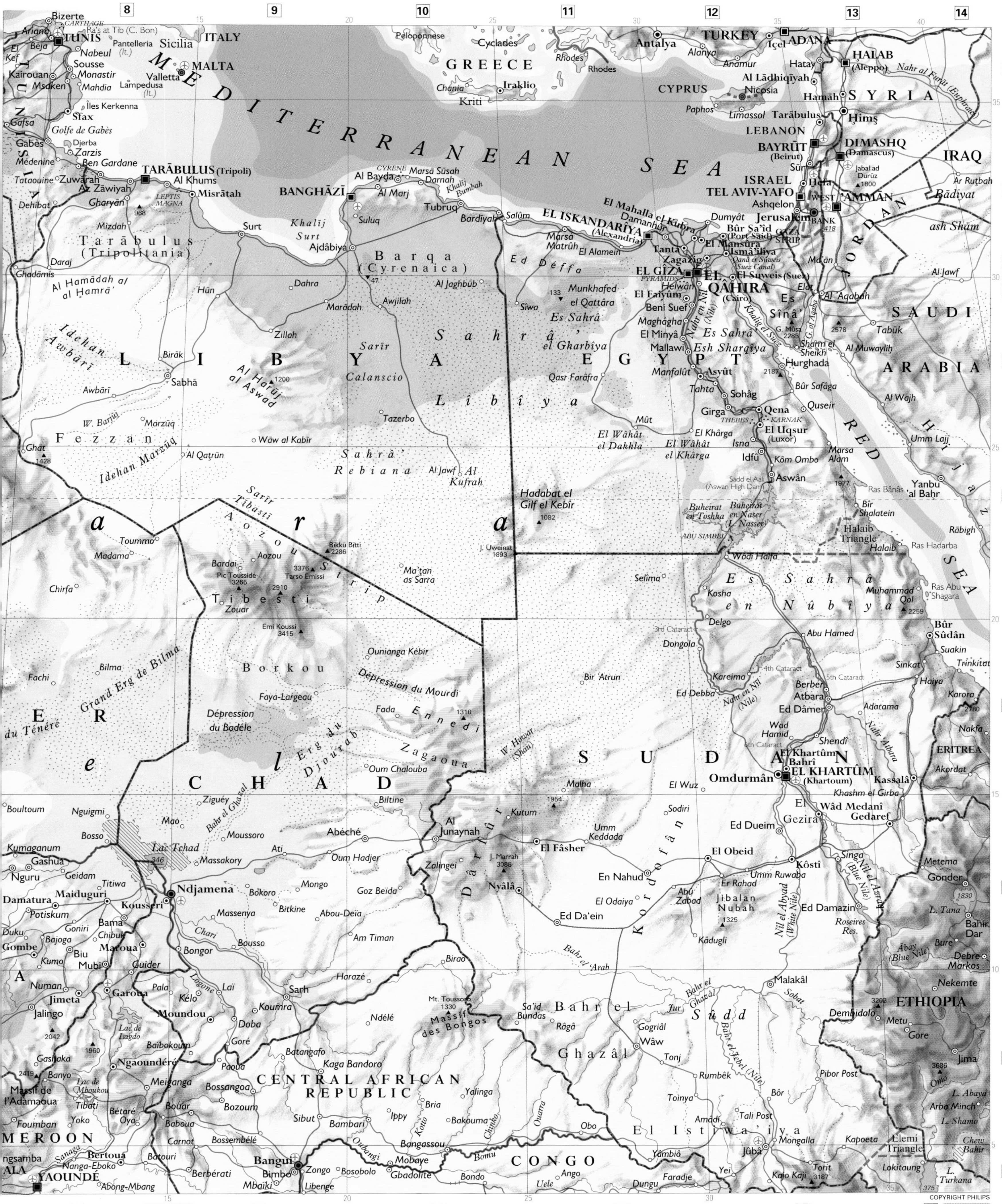

8 9 10 11 12 13 14

MEDITERRANEAN SEA

ITALY · Sicilia · MALTA · Valletta · Pantelleria · Lampedusa · GREECE · Peloponnese · Cyclades · Rhodes · Kriti · Chania · Iraklio · Rhodos · CYPRUS · Nicosia · Limassol · Paphos

TURKEY · Antalya · Alanya · Anamur · İçel · ADANA · Hatay · Al Lādhiqīya · HALAB (Aleppo) · Hamāh · Ḥimş · SYRIA · Tarābulus · BAYRŪT (Beirut) · LEBANON · DIMASHQ (Damascus) · IRAQ · Ar Ruṭba · Bādiyat ash Shām · Ṣūr · Haifa · ISRAEL · TEL AVIV-YAFO · Ashqelon · Jerusalem · WEST BANK · ʿAMMĀN · JORDAN · Maʿān · Al Jawf

TUNIS · CARTHAGE · Ariana · Bizerte · Nabeul · Sousse · Monastir · Mahdia · Kairouan · Msaken · Sfax · Îles Kerkenna · Sousse · El Kef · Béja · Gafsa · Gabès · Golfe de Gabès · Djerba · Zarzis · Médenine · Tataouine · Dehibat · Ben Gardane · Zuwārah · Az Zāwiyah · Gharyān · TARĀBULUS (Tripoli) · Al Khums · Misrātah · LEPTIS MAGNA · Mizdah · Ghadāmis · Daraj

LIBYA · Tarābulus (Tripolitania) · Al Hamādah al Hamrāʾ · Hūn · Surt · Dahra · Zillah · Marādah · Awjilah · Barqa (Cyrenaica) · BANGHĀZĪ · Al Marj · Al Bayda · CYRENE · Marsā Sūsah · Darnah · Tubruq · Bardiyah · Khalīj Surt · Suluq · Ajdābiya · Sirte

Fezzan · Idehan Awbārī · Birāk · Sabhā · Awbārī · Marzūq · Ghāt · Al Qaṭrūn · Idehan Marzūq · Sahrāʾ Rebiana · Al Harūj al Aswad · Tazerbo · Sarīr Calanscio · Sahrāʾ Lîbîya · Al Jawf · Al Kufrah · Hadabat el Gilf el Kebîr · J. Uweinat

EGYPT · EL ISKANDARÎYA (Alexandria) · Damanhûr · El Mahalla el Kubra · Tanta · Zagazig · EL QÂHIRA (Cairo) · EL GÎZA · PYRAMIDS · Helwân · Bûr Saʿîd (Port Said) · Dumyât · El Mansûra · Ismâʿîliya · El Suweis (Suez) · Suez Canal · Sînâʾ · SINAI · G. Mûsâ · Sharm el Sheikh · El Faiyûm · Beni Suef · Maghâgha · El Minyâ · Mallawi · Manfalût · Asyût · Tahta · Sohâg · Girga · Qena · KARNAK · THEBES · El Uqsur (Luxor) · Isna · Idfû · Kôm Ombo · Aswân · Aswan High Dam · Marsā Matrûh · El Alamein · Ed Déffa · Siwa · Munkhafed el Qaṭṭâra · Qaṭṭâra · Es Sahrâʾ el Gharbîya · Qasr Farâfra · El Wâhât el Dakhla · El Wâhât el Khârga · El Khârga · Mût · Esh Sharqîya

SAUDI ARABIA · Tabûk · Al Muwayliḥ · Al Wajh · Umm Lajj · Yanbuʿ al Bahr · Rābigh · Al ʿAqabah · G. of Aqaba · Elat · RED SEA · Hurghada · Bûr Safâga · Quseir · Marsa Alam · Ras Bânâs · Bîr Shalatein · Halaib Triangle · Halaib · Ras Hadarba · Wâdi Halfa · Selima · Es Sahrâʾ en Nûbîya · Kosha · Delgo · Dongola · Abu Hamed · Kareima · Ed Debba · 3rd Cataract · 4th Cataract · 5th Cataract · Berber · Atbara · Ed Dâmer · Wad Hamid · Shendî · El Khartûm Bahrî · KHARTOUM · EL KHARTÛM (Khartoum) · Omdurmân · Bûr Sûdân · Suakin · Sinkat · Trinkitat · Haiya · Karora · Nakfa · Akordat · ERITREA · Kassalâ · Khashm el Girba · Metema · Gonder · L. Tana · Bahir Dar · ʿAbay (Blue Nile) · Debre Markos · Nekemte · ETHIOPIA · Gore · Metu · Jima · Arba Minch · L. Abaya · L. Shamo · Chew Bahir · Elemi Triangle · L. Turkana

SUDAN · Dârfûr · J. Marrah · El Fâsher · Zalingei · Nyâlâ · En Nahud · Ed Daʿein · Kutum · Al Junaynah · Umm Keddada · Sodiri · Ed Dueim · Wâd Medanî · Gedaref · Gezira · El Obeid · Kôstî · Singa · Kordofân · Abû Zabad · Er Rahad · Umm Ruwaba · Jibalan Nubah · Kâdugli · Ed Damazin · Roseires Res. · Nil el Azraq (Blue Nile) · Nil el Abyad (White Nile) · Bahr el ʿArab · Bahr el Ghazâl · Ghazâl · Sudd · Râga · Wâw · Gogrîal · Tonj · Rumbêk · Bôr · Malakâl · Sobat · Pibor Post · Jûr · Toinya · Bahr el Jebel (Nile) · Amadi · Yâmbio · Jûba · El Istiwaʾîya · Torit · Kajo Kaji · Kapoeta · Mongalla

CHAD · Ndjamena · Lac Tchad · Mao · Moussoro · Ati · Abéché · Biltine · Oum Hadjer · Mongo · Bokoro · Massakory · Massaguet · Massenya · Bitkine · Am Timan · Abou-Deïa · Goz Beida · Zaguaoua · Ennedi · Fada · Oum Chalouba · Ounianga Kébir · Dépression du Mourdi · Dépression du Bodélé · Erg du Djourab · Borkou · Faya-Largeau · Bardai · Aozou · Aozou Strip · Pic Toussidé · Tibesti · Tarso Emissi · Zouar · Emi Koussi · Bikkū Bitti · Maʿtan as Sarra · Toummo · Madama · Chirfa · Sahara · Tibesti · Birao · Harazé · Sarh · Koumra · Doba · Goré · Moundou · Kélo · Laï · Bongor · Bousso · Massenya · Mt. Toussoro · Massif des Bongos

NIGER · Bilma · Fachi · Grand Erg de Bilma · Ténéré · du Ténéré · Nguigmi · Boultoum · Bosso · Kumaganum · Gashua · Nguru · Geidam · Titiwa · Damaturu · Maiduguri · Bama · Kousseri · Goniri · Potiskum · Chibuk · Mubi

CENTRAL AFRICAN REPUBLIC · Ngaoundéré · Meiganga · Bossangoa · Bouar · Bozoum · Batangafo · Kaga Bandoro · Sibut · Bambari · Bria · Bakouma · Ippy · Yalinga · Bangassou · Obo · Bondo · Uele · Dungu · Faradje · Yei

CAMEROON · YAOUNDÉ · Garoua · Maroua · Guider · Ngaoundéré · Bétaré Oya · Bertoua · Batouri · Berbérati · Carnot · Nola · Bangui · Zongo · Libenge · Mbaïki · Bimbo · Abong-Mbang · Yoko · Foumban

CONGO · Bangui · Gbadolite · Bosobolo · Mobaye · Ango · Bondo

Jos · Kano · Zaria · Gombe · Numan · Jimeta · Jalingo · Yola · Massif de l'Adamaoua · Lac de Lagdo · Gashaka · Banyo · Bafoussam

CONGO

COPYRIGHT PHILIPS

1:7 100 000

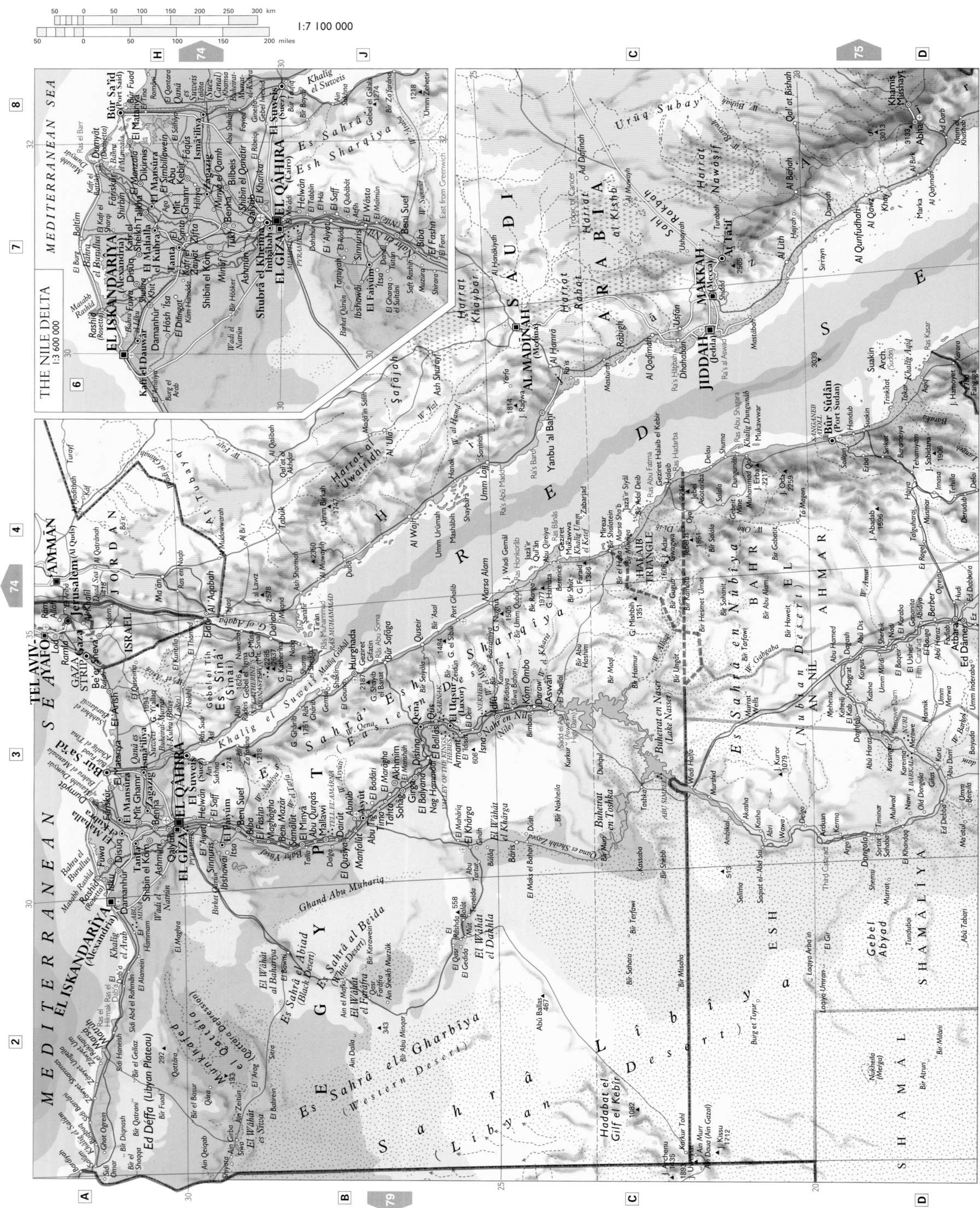

THE NILE DELTA
1:3 600 000

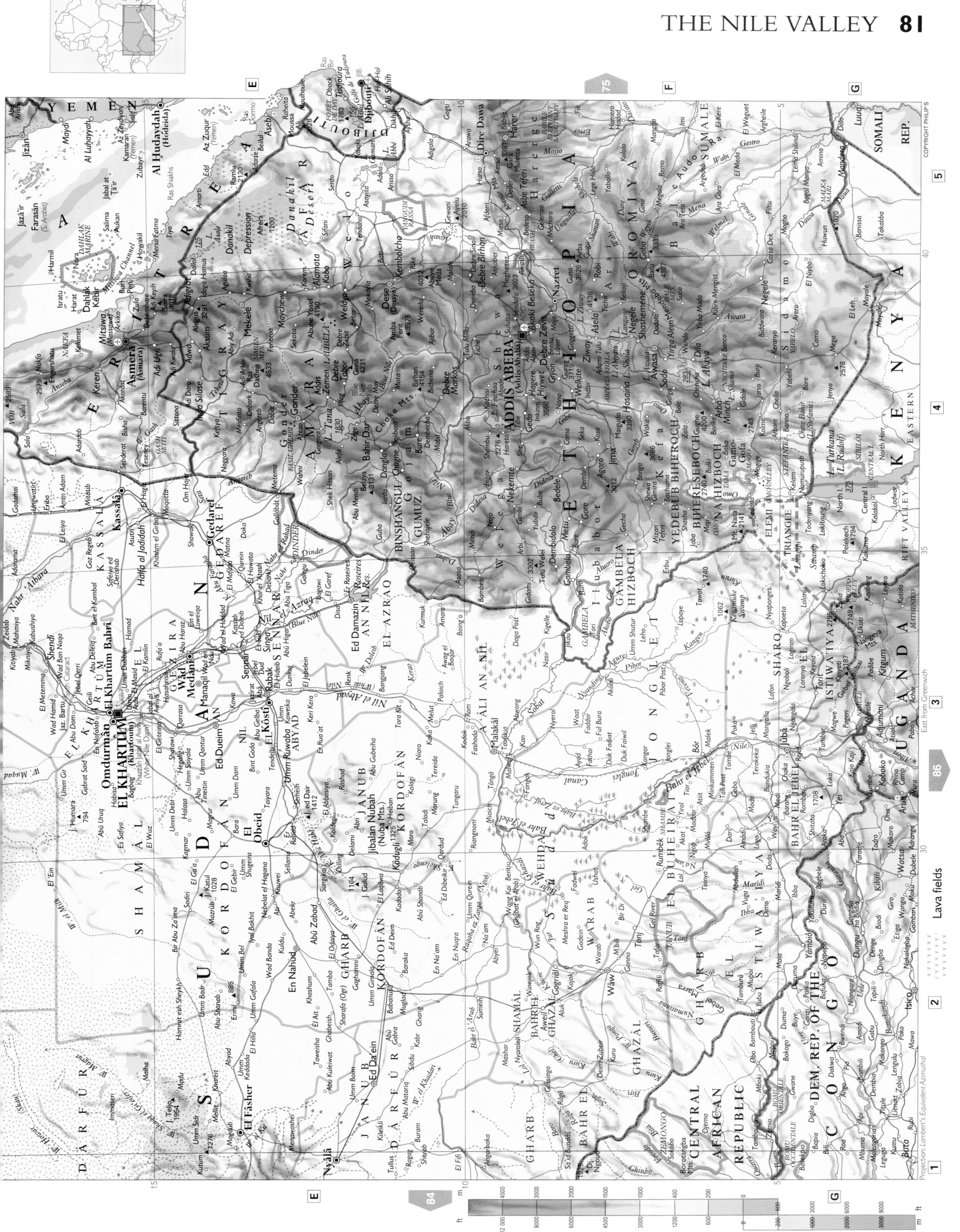

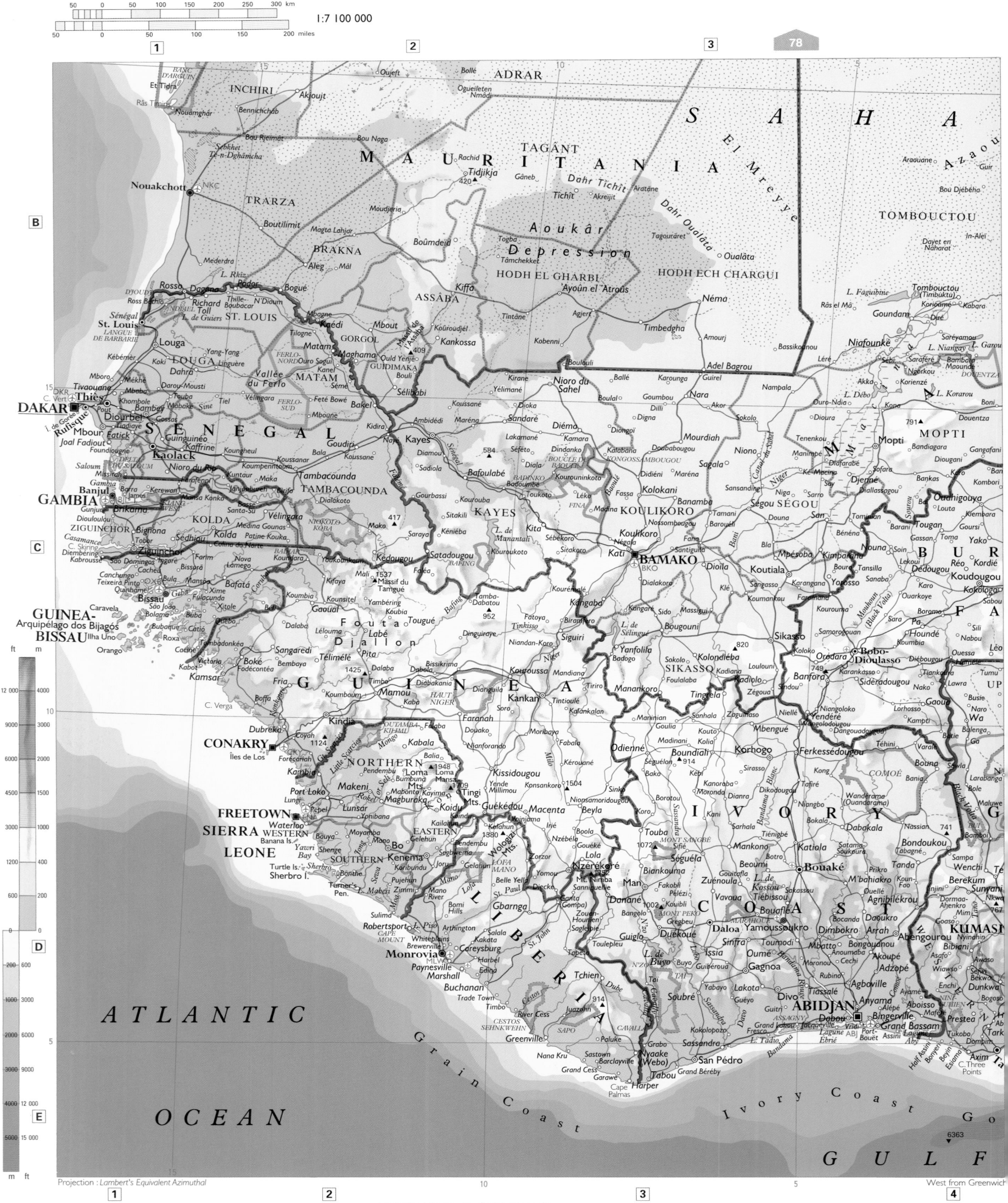

1:7 100 000

Projection : Lambert's Equivalent Azimuthal

Underlined towns give their name to the
administrative area in which they stand.

West from Greenwich

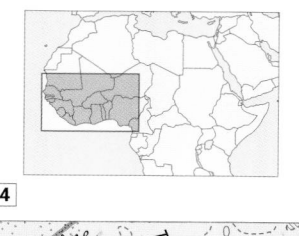

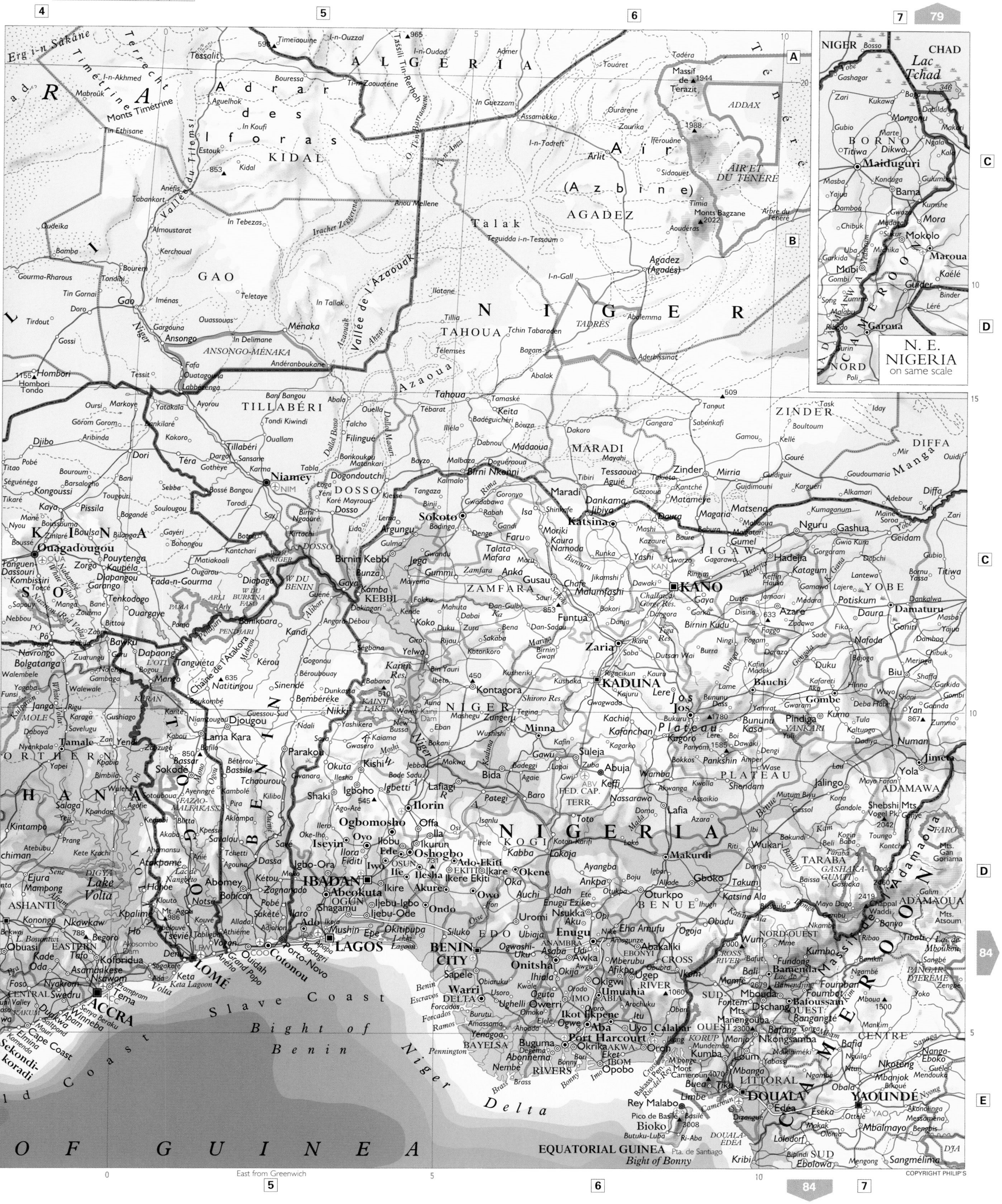

1:13 300 000

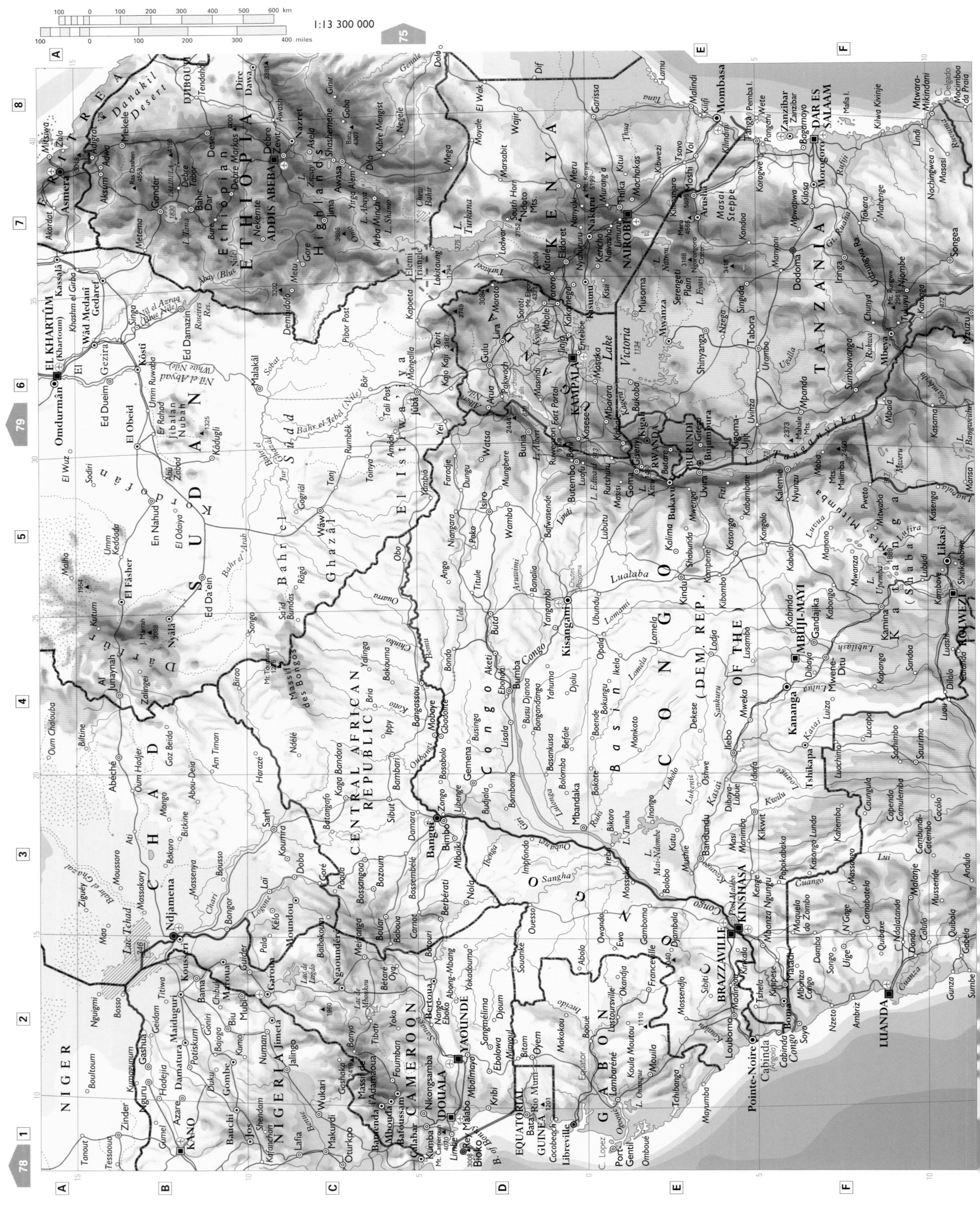

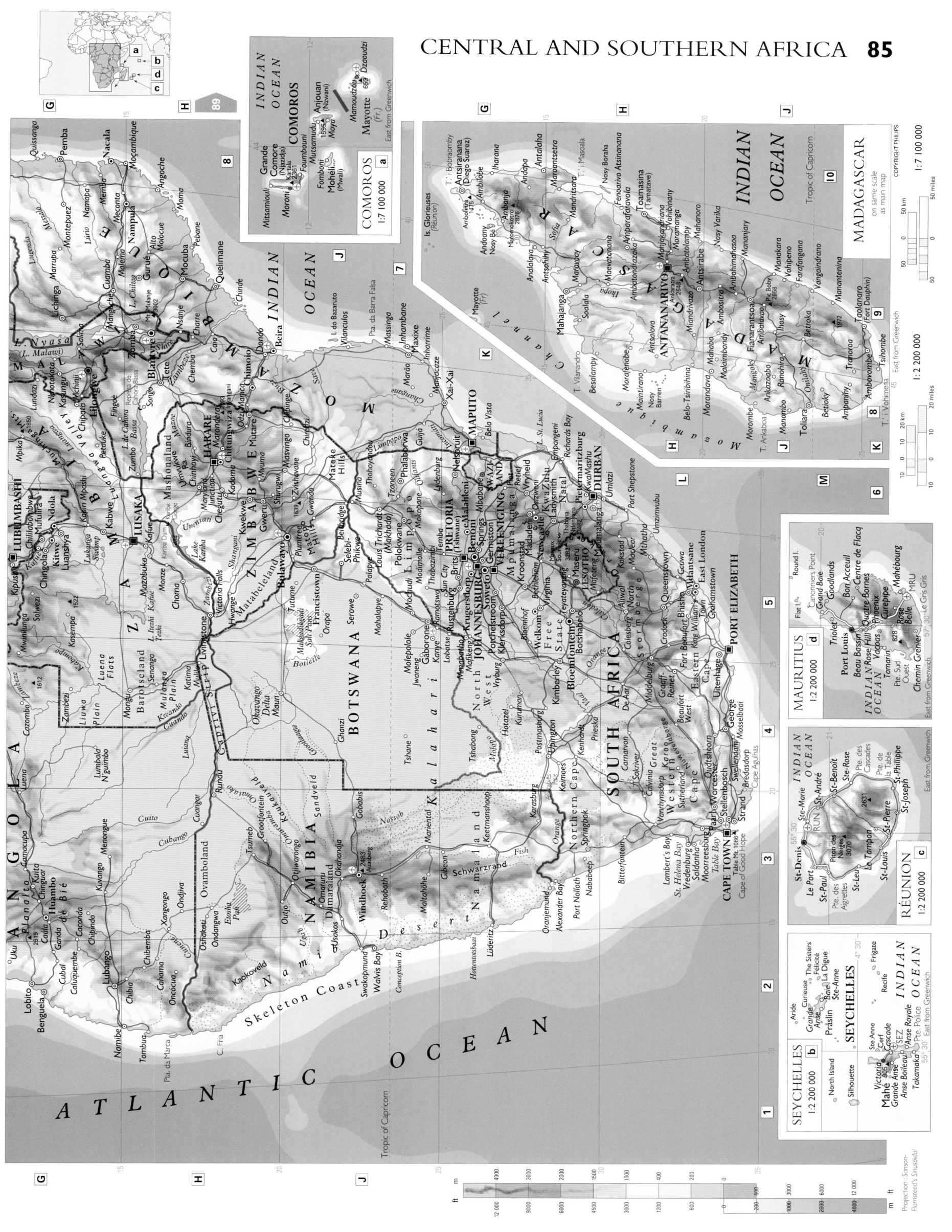

COMOROS

INDIAN OCEAN

Mitsamiouli
Grande
Comore
(Njazidja)
Moroni
Karthala
2361
Moya
Mohéli
(Mwali)
Foumbouni
Fomboni

Mutsamudu
1595▲
Anjouan
(Nzwani)

Mamoudzou ⊕ Dzaoudzi
652
Mayotte
(Fr.)

COMOROS
1:7 100 000
a

East from Greenwich

SEYCHELLES
1:2 200 000
b

North Island
Silhouette
Mahé
905
Victoria
Grande Anse
Anse Boileau
Takamaka

Aride
Grande
Praslin
Ste Anne
Cerf
Cascade
Anse Royale
Pte. Police

Curieuse
The Sisters
Félicité
Baie La Digue
Ste-Anne
Frigate
Recife

SEYCHELLES

INDIAN OCEAN

East from Greenwich

MADAGASCAR
on same scale
as main map
1:7 100 000

MAURITIUS
1:2 200 000
d

Flat I.
Round I.
Canonniers Point
Triolet
Goodlands
Bon Acceuil
Grand Baie
Centre de Flacq
Port Louis
Beau Bassin
Quatre Bornes
Vacoas
Phoenix
Curepipe
Rose Belle
Mahébourg
Chemin Grenier
677 30′ Le Gris Gris

INDIAN OCEAN

East from Greenwich

RÉUNION
1:2 200 000
c

St-Denis
Le Port
St-Paul
Pte. des
Aigrettes
Ste-Marie
St-André
Pte. de
la Table
St-Benoît
Ste-Rose
Piton des
Neiges
3070
Le Tampon
St-Louis
St-Pierre
St-Phillipe
St-Joseph

INDIAN OCEAN

East from Greenwich

MADAGASCAR

INDIAN OCEAN

ATLANTIC OCEAN

INDIAN OCEAN

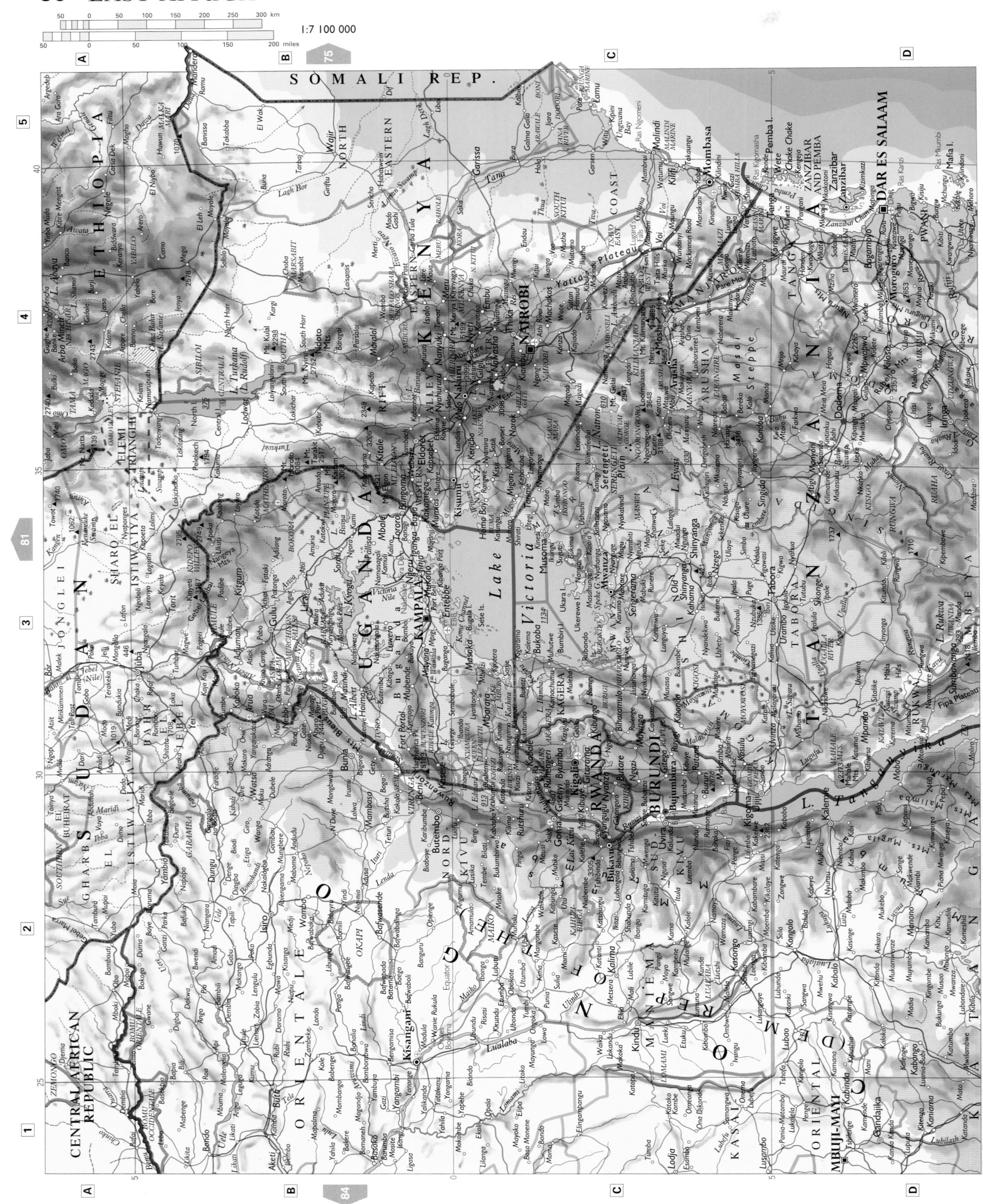

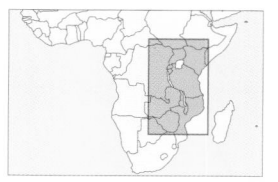

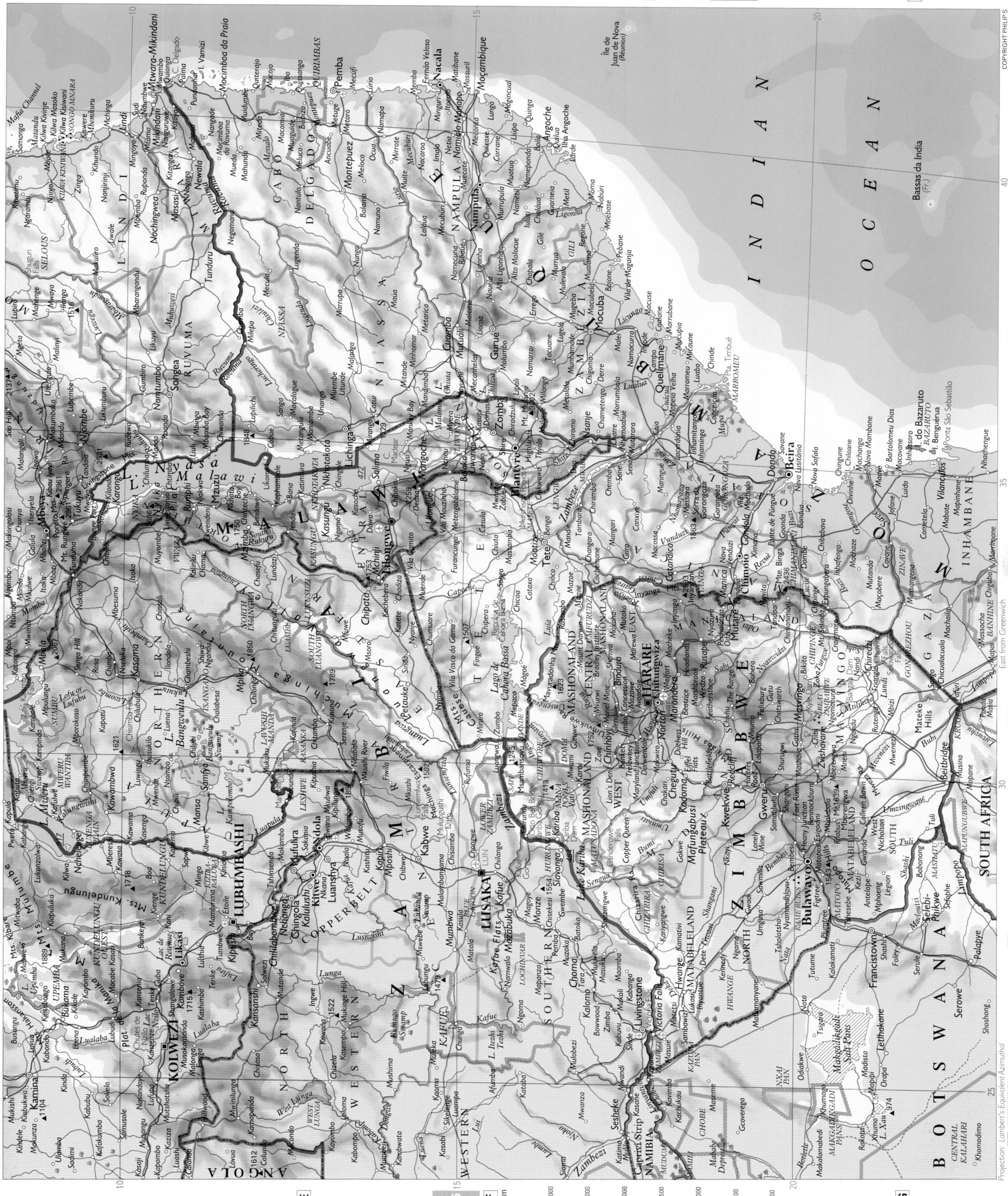

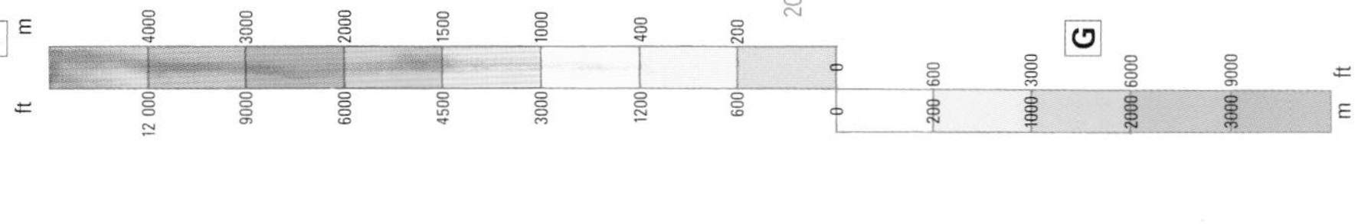

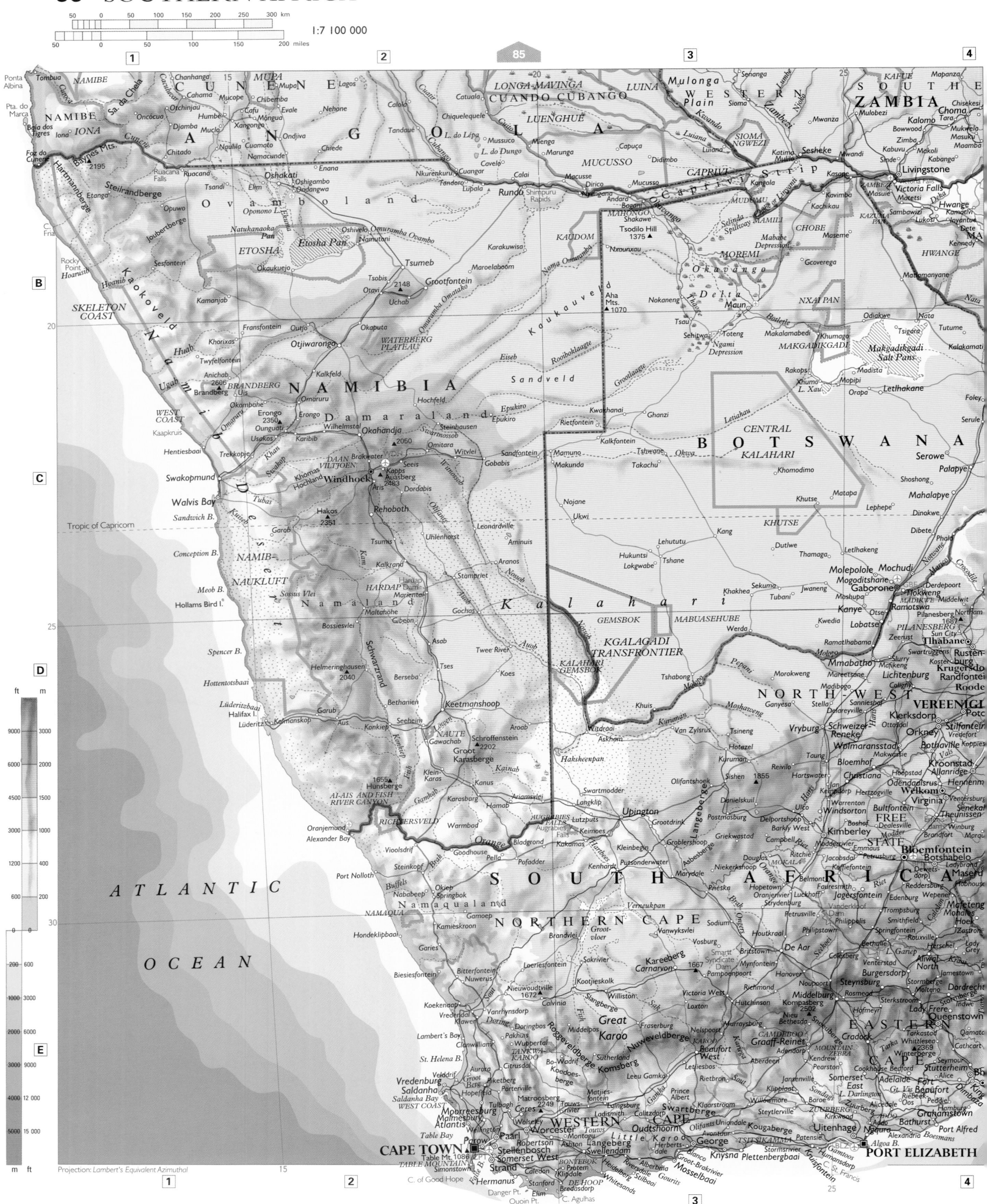

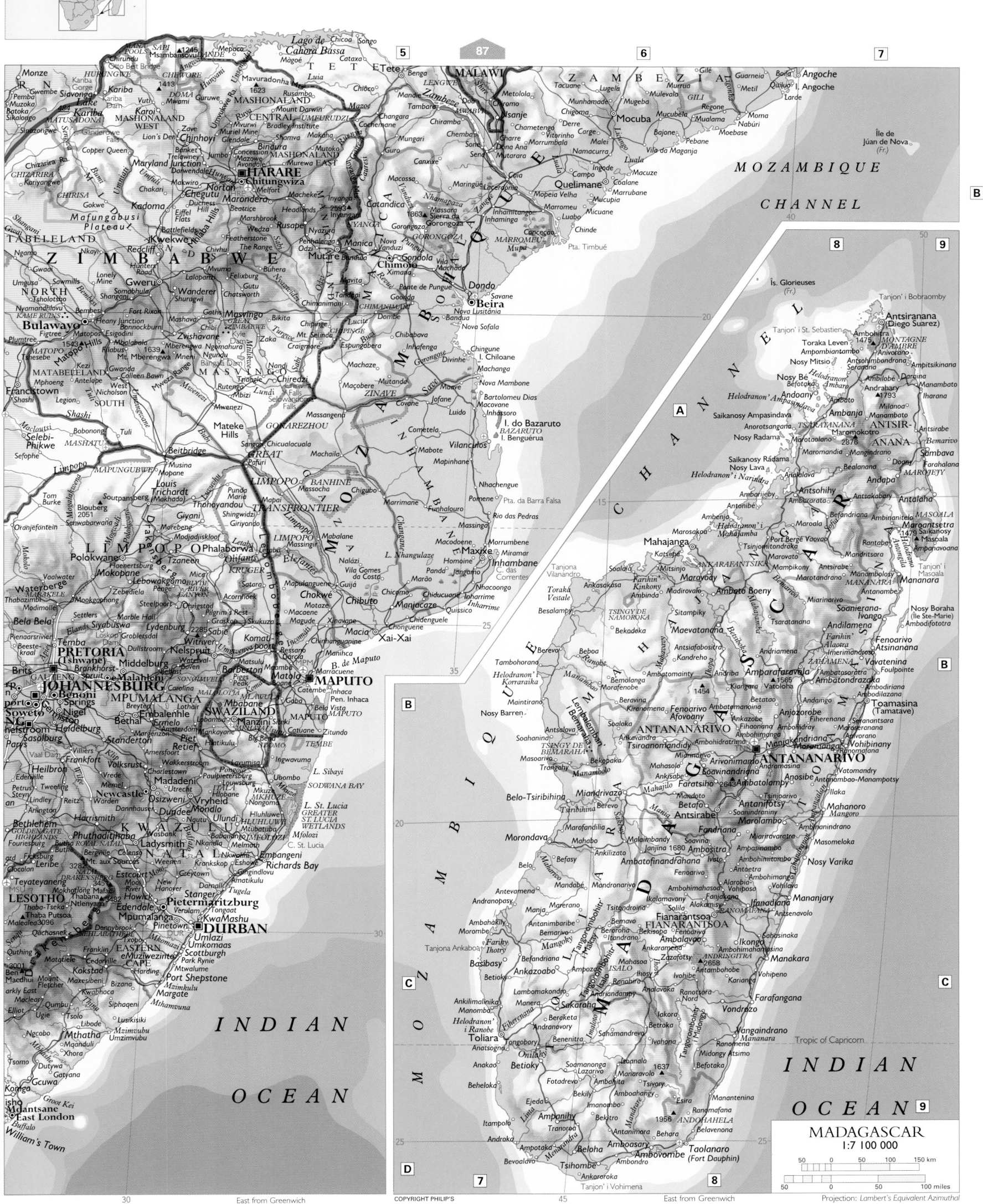

MOZAMBIQUE CHANNEL

MOZAMBIQUE

ZAMBIA

ZAMBEZIA

MALAWI

ZIMBABWE

HARARE
Chitungwiza

Bulawayo

Beira

Dondo

Savane

MATABELELAND

ZIMBABWE

GONAREZHOU

LIMPOPO

Polokwane

KRUGER

PRETORIA
(Tshwane)

JOHANNESBURG
Soweto

MPUMALANGA

SWAZILAND

MAPUTO

LESOTHO

KWAZULU
NATAL

Pietermaritzburg

DURBAN

EASTERN
CAPE

INDIAN

OCEAN

East London

MADAGASCAR

Antsiranana
(Diego Suarez)

MONTAGNE
D'AMBRE

ANTSIR-
ANANA

Nosy Be

Mahajanga

ANTANANARIVO

ANTANANARIVO

Antsirabe

Toamasina
(Tamatave)

Morondava

FIANARANTSOA

Toliara

Tropic of Capricorn

INDIAN

OCEAN

Taolanaro
(Fort Dauphin)

MADAGASCAR
1:7 100 000

50   0   50   100   150 km

50   0   50   100 miles

East from Greenwich

Projection: Lambert's Equivalent Azimuthal

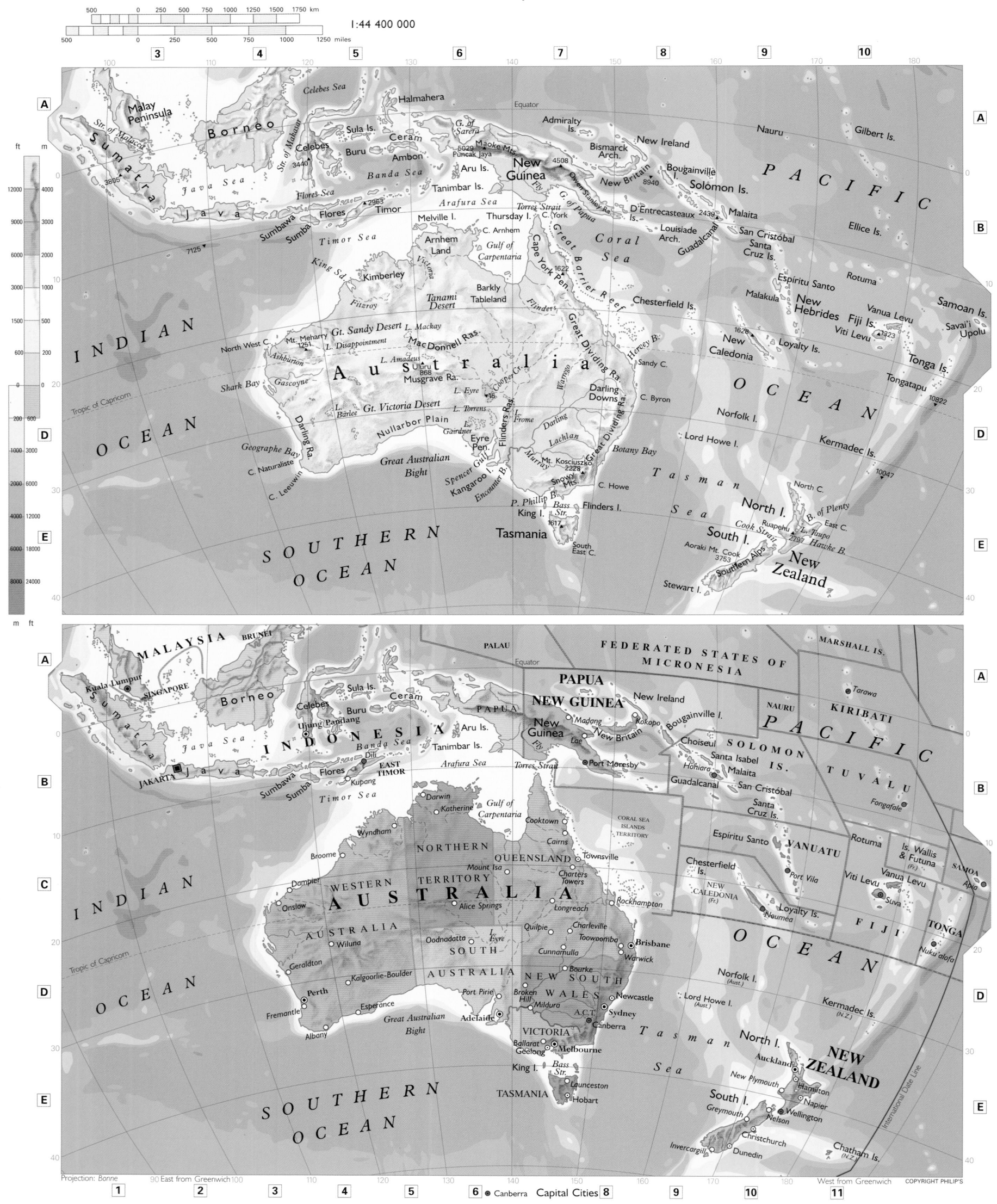

1:5 300 000

50 0 50 100 150 200 km
50 0 50 100 150 miles

FIJI a
on same scale

PACIFIC OCEAN

Great Sea Reef
Kia
Ringgold Is.
Udu Pt.
Labasa
Rabi
Vanua Levu
Yaqaga
Yasawa Group
Yadua
Bua
Savusavu Bay
Somosomo
Qamea
Taveuni
Nacula
Nabouwalu
Buca
Savusavu
Naitaba
Waya
Naviti
Bligh Water
Rakiraki
Nasau
Koro
Namenalala
Vanua Balavu
Mamanuca Group
Vomo
Tavua
Lautoka
Tomaniivi ▲1323
Lawaki
Levuka
Wakaya
Northern Lau Group
Vatu Vara
Mago
Cicia
Malolo
Nadi
KOROYANITU
Naval ▲1323
Korovou
Vunidawa
Nairai
Batiki
Sawaleke
Gau
Nayau
KORO SEA
Vanua Vatu
Lakeba Passage
Lakeba
Tubou
Viti Levu
Keiyasi
Sigatoka
Korolevu
Nausori
Suva
Beqa
Moala
Oneata
Moce
Namuka-i-Lau
Yagasa Cluster
FIJI
Vatulele
Yanuca
Matuku
Totoya
Fulaga
Ogea
Kadavu Passage
Ono
Kabara
Ogea Driki
Kadavu
Tavuki
Vunisea
Southern Lau Group
East from Greenwich
West from Greenwich

SAMOA
Asau
Safune
Falelima
Savai'i
1858 ▲
Satupa'itea
Saleloga
Taga
Manono
Mulifanua
Apia
Falefa
Falealili
Amaile
OLE PUPU PUE
Safata Bay
116 ▲
Siumu
'Upolu

PACIFIC OCEAN

AMERICAN SAMOA (U.S.A.)
Ofu Olosega
Ta'u
Tutuila Pago Pago
Leone Vaitogi
Aunu'u
AMERICAN SAMOA
Manu'a Is.
Luma

SAMOAN ISLANDS b
on same scale
West from Greenwich

TONGA c
on same scale

PACIFIC OCEAN

Fonualei
Toku
Vava'u
Neiafu
Late
Vava'u Group
Disney Reef
Home Reef
Ofolanga
Kao
Ha'ano
Foa Ha'apai Group
Tofua
Lifuka Uiha
Nomuka
Oto Tolu Group
Fonuafo'ou
Nomuka Group
Mango Group
Hunga Ha'apai
Tonumeia

TONGA
Nuku'alofa
Tongatapu
Tongatapu Group
Eua
West from Greenwich

TASMAN SEA

North Island

C. Reinga
C. Maria van Diemen
North C.
Houhora Heads
Rangaunu B.
Doubtless B.
Ahipara B.
Mangonui
Whangaroa Harb.
Kaitaia
Tauroa Pt.
Okaihau
Waitangi
C. Brett
Rawene
Opua
B. of Islands
Hokianga Harbour
Kaikohe
Hikurangi
Waipoua Forest
Whangarei
Dargaville
Whangarei Harb.
Bream Hd.
Bream B.
Waipu
Little Barrier I.
Warkworth
C. Rodney
Great Barrier I.
Helensville
C. Colville
Cuvier I.
Kaipara Harbour
Hauraki Gulf
Coromandel
Whitianga
Takapuna
AUCKLAND
Thames
Whangamata
Manukau
Papakura
Pukekohe
Whangamata
Mayor I.
Waiuku
Mercer
Waihi
Tauranga Harb.
Waikato
Paeroa
Mount Maunganui
Huntly
Te Aroha
Tauranga
Raglan
Morrinsville
Te Puke
Bay of Plenty
Whakaari (White I.)
Runaway
Hamilton
Cambridge
Whakatane
Kawhia Harbour
Te Awamutu
Putaruru
Rotorua
Matata
Opotiki
East C.
Kawhia
Otorohanga
Tokoroa
L. Rotorua
Murupara
Raukumara Ra.
Te Kuiti
Mangakino
Kinleith
L. Tarawera
UREWERA
Hikurangi ▲1753
Waitomo Caves
Mokai
Wairakei
Taneatua
Waikaremoana
Wapiro
North Taranaki Bight
Mokau
Mokau
Ongarue L.
Taupo
Tarawera
Motu
Tolaga Bay
New Plymouth
Waitara
Taumarunui
Turangi
Kaimanawa Mts.
Ormond
Gisborne
Inglewood
Whangamomona
L. Taupo
Waikaremoana
Nuhaka
Mt. Taranaki or Mt. Egmont ▲2518
WHANGANUI
Ruapehu ▲2797
TONGARIRO
Bay View
Poverty Bay
Opunake
C. Egmont
Stratford
Ohakune
Raetihi
Waiouru
Wairoa
Waikokopu
Kaponga
Eltham
Rangitaiki Ra.
Mahia Pen.
Hawera
Taihape
Napier
Hawke Bay
Patea
Waverley
Mangaweka
Ruahine Ra.
Hastings
C. Kidnappers
South Taranaki Bight
Wanganui
Marton
Hunterville
Waipawa
Bulls
Halcombe
Dannevirke
Waipukurau
Feilding
Woodville
Palmerston North
Foxton
Pahiatua
Shannon
Levin
Eketahuna
Otaki
Tararua Ra.
Masterton
Paraparaumu
Kapiti I.
Carterton
Greytown
C. Turnagain
Upper Hutt
Featherston
Martinborough
L. Wairarapa
Petone
Wellington
Lower Hutt
Eastbourne

South Island

C. Farewell
Golden B.
D'Urville I.
Collingwood
ABEL TASMAN
Takaka
Tasman B.
KAHURANGI
Tasman Mts.
Motueka
Pelorus
Karamea
Mapua
Havelock
Picton
Karamea Bight
Nelson
Richmond
Seddonville
Tadmor
Wakefield
Blenheim
Granity
Matiri
Seddon
Westport
Lyell
Murchison
L. Rotoiti
Renwick
Ward
Inangahua
NELSON LAKES
Cook Strait
PAPAROA
L. Rotoroa
Tapuae-o-Uenuku ▲2885
Punakaiki
Mt. Travers ▲2337
Blackball
Grey
Lewis Pass
Spenser Mts.
Runanga
Reefton
Hanmer Springs
Kaikoura
Greymouth
Stillwater
Clarence
Kumara
L. Brunner
Waiau
Hokitika
Jacksons
Culverden
Hurunui
Ross
ARTHUR'S PASS
Waikari
Amberley
Pegasus Bay
Arthur's Pass
Hawarden
Oxford
Waipara
Rangiora
Kaiapoi
Colridge
Springfield
Kaiapoi
New Brighton
Whitecliffs
Westland
Staveley
Riccarton
Christchurch
WESTLAND
Methven
Lincoln
Lyttelton
Abut Hd.
Banks Pen.
Mt. Cook
Aoraki Mt. Cook ▲3753
Tekapo
Southbridge
Little River
Akaroa
Mount Cook
Ellesmere
Rakaia
Jackson B.
Canterbury Plains
Okuru
Haast
Fairlie
Timaru
St. Andrews
MOUNT ASPIRING
Mt. Aspiring ▲3033
Ohau
L. Pukaki
Pleasant Point
Temuka
Milford Sd.
Mt. Earnslaw ▲2819
Tiritiri o te Moana
Canterbury Bight
Sutherland Falls
Milford Sound
L. Wanaka
Twizel
Bligh Sound
Wanaka
Omarama
Kurow
Waimate
George Sound
Arrowtown
Cromwell
Naseby
Oamaru
Secretary I.
Queenstown
Clyde
Maheno
Doubtful Sd.
L. Wakatipu
Alexandra
Dunstan Mts.
Hampden
Te Anau
Kingston
Roxburgh
Danaback
Palmerston
FIORDLAND
L. Te Anau
Eyre Mts.
Otago
Waikouaiti
Resolution I.
L. Manapouri
Garvie Mts.
Ettrick
Port Chalmers
Dusky Sd.
Manapouri
Mossburn
Umbrella Mts.
Kelso
Otago Harbour
Breaksea Sd.
Lumsden
Clutha
C. Saunders
Secretary I.
Southland
Nightcaps
Clinton
Dunedin
Clifden
Tuatapere
Ohai
Edievale
Lawrence
Milton
Mosgiel
L. Hauroko
Preservation Inlet
Winton
Gore
Balclutha
Orepuki
Riverton
Mataura
Kaitangata
Invercargill
Wyndham
Owaka
Bluff
Invercargill
Edendale
Tokanui
Tahakopa
South Invercargill
Ruapuke I.
Foveaux Str.
Halfmoon Bay
Solander I.
RAKIURA
Stewart I. (Rakiura)
Port Pegasus
South West C.

Projection: Conical with two standard parallels
East from Greenwich

PACIFIC OCEAN

TAHITI & MOOREA d
1:900 000

Pte. Aroa
B. de Matavai
Pte. Vénus
Papetoai
Paopao
Aruè
Mahina
Mt. Tohiea ▲1207
Papeete
Pirae
Pahenoo
Haapiti
Afareaitu
Faaa
Papenoo
Tiarei
Moorea (France)
Pte. Nuupere
Faaone
Hitiaa
Punaauia
Mt. Aorai ▲2060
Mt. Orohena ▲2241
Paea
Mt. Tetufera ▲1799
Lac Vaihiria
Faaone
Tahiti (France)
Maraa
Paea
Isthme de Taravao
Papara
Taravao
Afahiti
Pte. Tatatua
Atimaono
Mataiea
Vairao
Pueu
Tautira
Teahupoo
▲ Mt. Roonui 1332
Presqu'île de Taiarapu

West from Greenwich

COPYRIGHT PHILIP'S

10 0 10 km
10 0 10 miles
1:900 000

ft / m elevation scale:
9000 / 3000
6000 / 2000
3000 / 1000
1200 / 600
600 / 200
0
200 / 600
2000 / 6000
4000 / 12 000
6000 / 18 000
m / ft

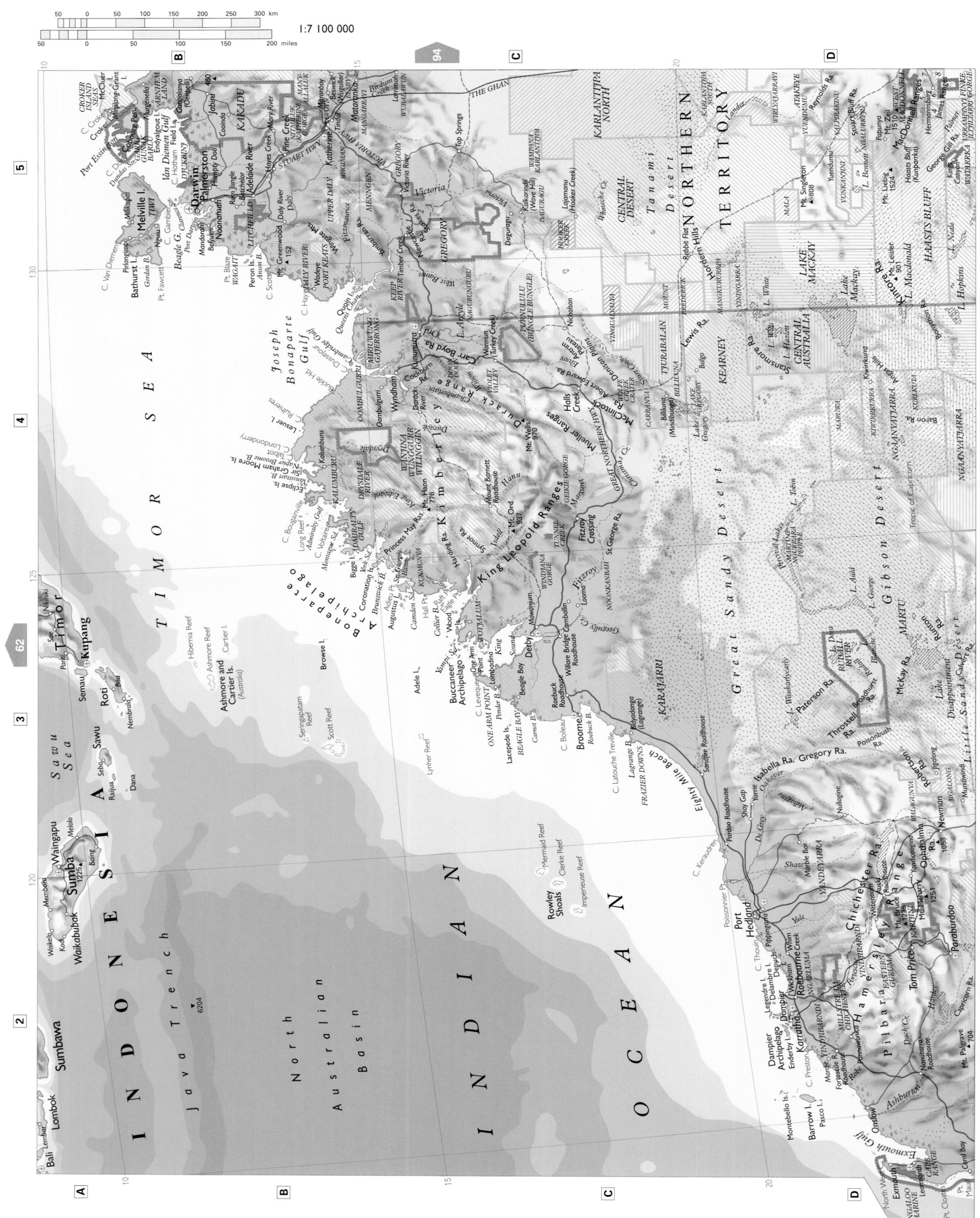

1:7 100 000

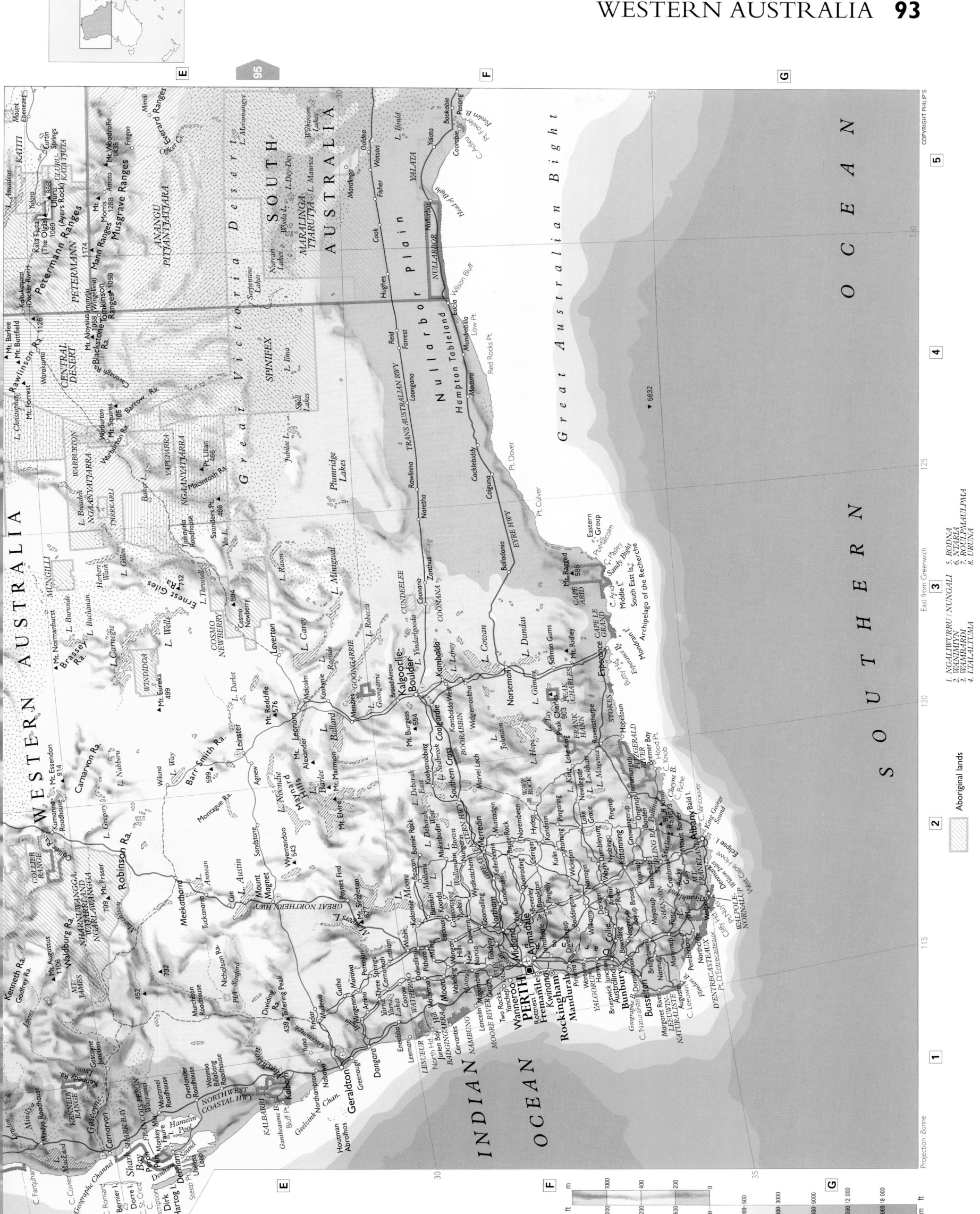

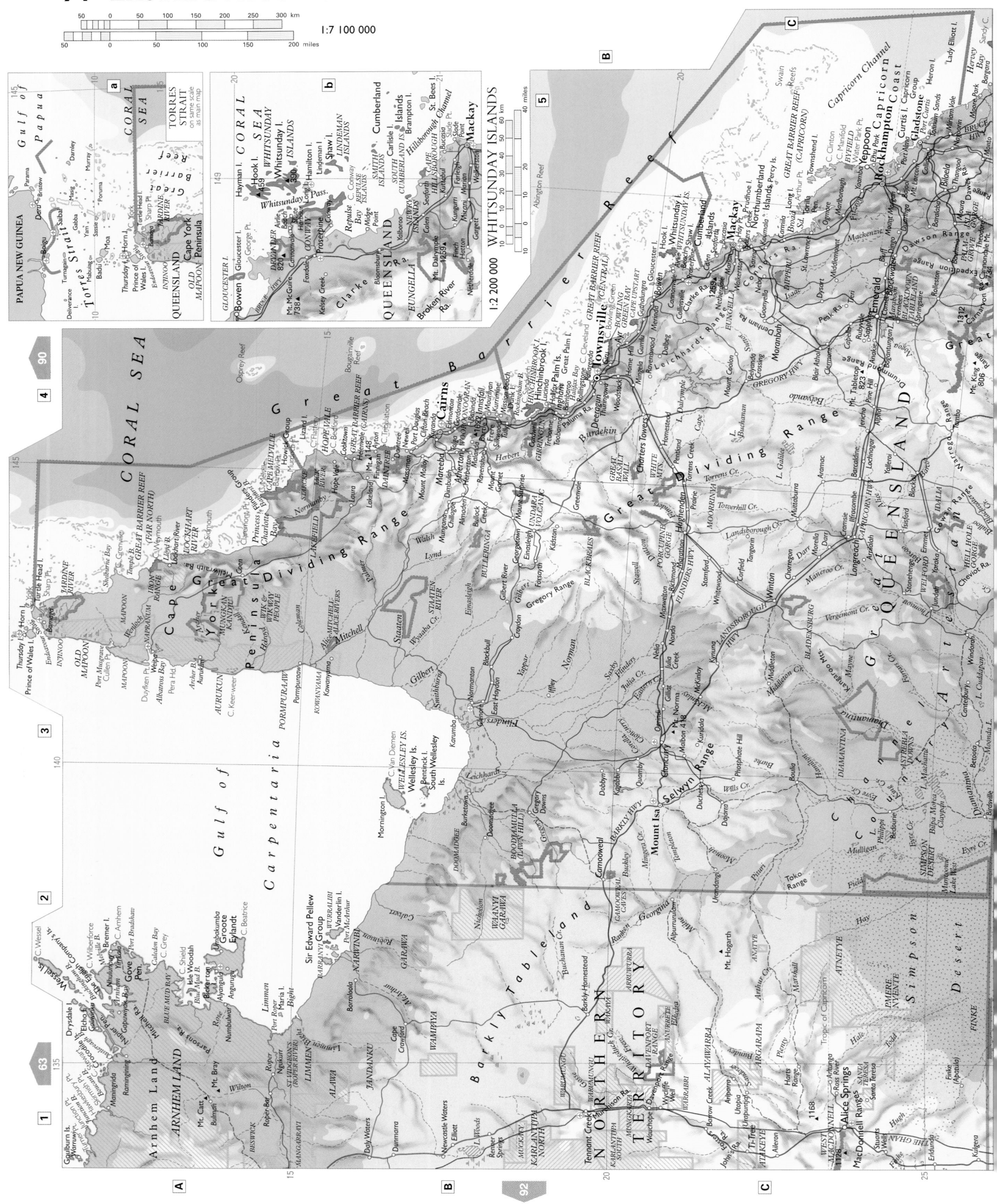

1:7 100 000

| 50 | 0 | 50 | 100 | 150 | 200 | 250 | 300 km |
| 50 | 0 | 50 | 100 | 150 | 200 miles |

PAPUA NEW GUINEA

Gulf of Papua

CORAL SEA

Torres Strait

QUEENSLAND

OLD MAPOON

Cape York Peninsula

TORRES STRAIT on same scale as main map

CORAL SEA

Cumberland Islands

WHITSUNDAY ISLANDS

QUEENSLAND

Mackay

1:2 200 000

Gulf of Carpentaria

CORAL SEA

Great Barrier Reef

Cairns

Townsville

Mackay

Rockhampton

Gladstone

GREAT DIVIDING RANGE

QUEENSLAND

NORTHERN TERRITORY

ARNHEM LAND

Alice Springs

MacDonnell Ranges

Simpson Desert

Tropic of Capricorn

TASMAN SEA

QUEENSLAND

Brisbane
Gold Coast
Sunshine Coast
Toowoomba
Ipswich
Bundaberg
Maryborough
Gympie
Nambour
Caloundra
Redcliffe
Beaudesert
Southport
Warwick
Dalby
Roma
Charleville
Cunnamulla

NEW SOUTH WALES

Sydney
Newcastle
Wollongong
Maitland
Gosford
Parramatta
Liverpool
Campbelltown
Penrith
Katoomba
Lithgow
Bathurst
Orange
Dubbo
Tamworth
Armidale
Grafton
Coffs Harbour
Port Macquarie
Taree
Forster
Nelson
Broken Hill
Wagga Wagga
Albury
Griffith
Bourke
Cobar
Nyngan
Narrabri
Moree
Inverell
Goulburn
Cooma
Nowra
Kiama
Queanbeyan

AUSTRALIAN CAPITAL TERRITORY

Canberra

VICTORIA

Melbourne
Geelong
Ballarat
Bendigo
Shepparton
Wodonga
Wangaratta
Traralgon
Morwell
Sale
Bairnsdale
Warrnambool
Horsham
Mildura
Swan Hill
Echuca
Colac
Portland
Dandenong
Frankston
Mornington
Sunbury
Werribee

SOUTH AUSTRALIA

Adelaide
Whyalla
Port Augusta
Port Pirie
Port Lincoln
Mount Gambier
Murray Bridge
Gawler
Naracoorte
Ceduna
Elizabeth
Salisbury

Lake Eyre
Lake Torrens
Lake Gairdner
Lake Frome
Lake Blanche

Eyre Peninsula
Yorke Peninsula
Kangaroo I.
Spencer Gulf
Gulf St Vincent
Flinders Ranges
Gawler Ranges

Sturt Stony Desert
Strzelecki Desert
Tirari Desert
Pedirka Desert

Great Dividing Range
Darling Downs
Grey Range
Barrier Range

Murray R.
Darling R.
Murrumbidgee R.
Lachlan R.
Macquarie R.
Cooper Cr.

TASMANIA

Hobart
Launceston
Devonport
Burnie
Glenorchy

Flinders Island
King Island
Cape Barren I.
Furneaux Group

Bass Strait

on same scale

Aboriginal lands

East from Greenwich

Projection: Bonne

ft m
15000 4500
10000 3000
6000 2000
4000 1200
2000 600
1000 400
0 200
0
-200

RUSSIA

Moskva
Volga
Yekaterinburg
Tomsk
Novosibirsk
Irkutsk
Oz. Baykal
Chita
Ob'
Lena
Okhotsk
Sea of Okhotsk
Poluostrov Kamchatka
Shirshov Ridge
Aleutian Basin
Bering Sea
Near Is. (U.S.A.)
Andreanof Is. (U.S.A.)
Aleutian
Astana (Aqmola)
Semey
KAZAKHSTAN
Aral Sea
Balqash Köl
Altai
MONGOLIA
Ulaanbaatar
Blagoveshchensk
Amur
Khabarovsk
Sakhalin
Kuril'skiye Ostrova (Russia)
Kurilskiye Ostrova
La Pérouse Str.
Kuril-Kamchatka Trench
10,542
Komandorskiye Ostrova (Russia)
Petropavlovsk-Kamchatskiy
7822
Aleutian Trench
Emperor Trough
Chinook Trough

Almaty
KYRGYZSTAN
Toshkent
Ürümqi
TAJIKISTAN
AFGHANISTAN
Kabul
Srinagar
PAKISTAN
Lahore
Delhi
Kanpur
Kunlun Shan
CHINA
Lanzhou
XIZANG
Lhasa
8850
Everest
NEPAL
Himalaya
Ganga
Brahmaputra
BANGLADESH
Kolkata (Calcutta)
Dhaka
Mandalay
BURMA
Irrawaddy
INDIA
Hyderabad
Bay of Bengal
Rangoon
Chennai (Madras)
Andaman Is. (India)
Beijing
Tianjin
Taiyuan
Xi'an
Nanjing
Wuhan
Chongqing
Changsha
Kunming
Guangzhou
Hong Kong
Macau
Hanoi
LAOS
VIETNAM
Mekong
Salween
THAILAND
Bangkok
CAMBODIA
Phnom Penh
Thanh Pho Ho Chi Minh
G. of Thailand
Nicobar Is. (India)
SRI LANKA
Colombo
Changchun
Shenyang
Dalian
Harbin
NORTH KOREA
SOUTH KOREA
Seoul
Qingdao
Kitakyūshū
Yellow Sea
Huang He
Chang Jiang
Hangzhou
Fuzhou
Shanghai
East China Sea
Taipei
TAIWAN
Hainan
C. Engano
Paracel Is.
Luzon
Mindoro
South China Sea
Palawan
Samar
Manila
PHILIPPINES
Mindanao
Davao
Sulu Sea
4101
Celebes Sea
Vladivostok
Hakodate
Sea of Japan
Sapporo
Sendai
Nagoya
Kyōto
Osaka
Ōsaka
Tōkyō
Yokohama
JAPAN
Fuji-San 3776
Shikoku
Kyūshū
10,554
Japan Trench
Okinawa
Ryūkyū-retto (Japan)
Philippine Sea
Kyushu-Palau Ridge
Iwo-Jima (Japan)
Ogasawara Gunto (Japan)
Kazan-Rettō (Japan)
Minami-Tori-Shima (Japan)
Shatsky Rise
Pacific
Northwest Pacific Basin
Emperor Seamount Chain
Midway Is. (U.S.A.)
Lisianski I. (U.S.A.)
Hawaii
International Date Line
West Mariana Basin
NORTHERN MARIANAS (U.S.A.)
Tinian
Saipan
East Mariana Basin
Challenger Deep 11,022
Mariana Trench
GUAM (U.S.A.)
10,497
Yap
Caroline Is.
Chuuk
PALAU
Melekeok
West Caroline Basin
Eauripik Rise
FED. STATES OF MICRONESIA
East Caroline Basin
Pohnpei
Palikir
Micronesia
MARSHALL IS.
Enewetak Atoll
Bikini Atoll
Kwajalein
Ralik Chain
Ratak Chain
Jaluit I.
Majuro
Wake I. (U.S.A.)
Mid-Pacific Mountains
PA
Mount
Central Pacific
Melanesia
Solomon Rise
Melanesian Basin
Butaritari
Tarawa
Banaba
Gilbert Is.
Nauru
NAURU
Phoenix Is.
Abariringa
Enderbury
Howland I. (U.S.A.)
Baker I. (U.S.A.)
KIR
O
Borneo
Ujung Pandang
Palembang
INDONESIA
Jakarta
Surabaya
Jawa
Java Sea
Sumatera
Sunda Islands
Kuala Lumpur
Singapore
PEN. MALAYSIA
MALAYSIA
BRUNEI
SABAH
SARAWAK
Sulawesi
Buru
Seram
Halmahera
Maluku
Banda Sea
7440
Flores Sea
Flores
Bali
Sumbawa
Sumba
Java Trench
Dili
EAST TIMOR
Timor
PAPUA
Puncak Jaya 5029
New Guinea
Admiralty Is.
New Ireland
Bismarck Arch.
New
Lae
Kokopo
8940
New Britain
Bougainville
PAPUA NEW GUINEA
Port Moresby
Arafura Sea
Torres Strait
C. York
Louisiade Arch.
Honiara
Guadalcanal
Santa Cruz Is.
9165
SOLOMON IS.
Fongafale
TUVALU
Tokelau (N.Z.)
SAMOA
Apia
Rotuma
Is. Wallis & Futuna (Fr.)
Vanua Levu
Viti Levu
Suva
FIJI
Nuku'alofa
TONGA
10,822
Tonga Trench
Espiritu Santo
VANUATU
Port Vila
Îs. Chesterfield
West Fiji Basin
7570
NEW CALEDONIA (Fr.)
Nouméa
Is. Loyauté
Indian Ocean scale bar:
ft m
12 000 4000
9000 3000
6000 2000
3000 1000
1500 500
600 200
0 0
200 600
1000 3000
2000 6000
4000 12 000
6000 18 000
8000 24 000
m ft

INDIAN
OCEAN
Ninety East Ridge
Cocos Is. (Austral.)
Christmas I. (Austral.)
Wharton Basin
Broken Ridge
Mid-Indian Ridge
Nouvelle Amsterdam (Fr.)
I. St. Paul (Fr.)
Is. Crozet (Fr.)
Kerguelen (Fr.)
Heard I. (Austral.)
North Australian Basin
C. Arnhem
Darwin
Gulf of Carpentaria
Broome
Exmouth Plateau
North West C.
Cairns
Townsville
AUSTRALIA
Mount Isa
Alice Springs
L. Eyre
Great Barrier Reef
Coral Sea Basin
Coral Sea
Great Dividing Ra.
Rockhampton
Brisbane
Middleton Basin
Lord Howe Rise
New Caledonia Trough
Norfolk Ridge
Norfolk I. (Austral.)
South Fiji Basin
Tonga Trench
Geraldton
Perth Basin
Perth
Naturaliste Plateau
Great Australian Bight
Albany
Adelaide
Murray
Darling
Sydney
Canberra
Mt. Kosciuszko 2228
Melbourne
Lord Howe I. (Austral.)
Kermadec Is. (N.Z.)
Kermadec Trench 10,047
Tasman Sea
Tasman Basin
Auckland
NEW ZEALAND
Wellington
Christchurch
Chatham Rise
Chatham Is. (N.Z.)
Bass Str.
Tasmania
Hobart
East Tasman Plateau
Aoraki Mt. Cook 3753
Dunedin
Bounty Trough
Bounty Is. (N.Z.)
Invercargill
Cook Strait
Louisville Ridge
South Tasman Rise
SOUTHERN
OCEAN
South Australian Basin
Auckland Is. (N.Z.)
Campbell Plateau
Campbell I. (N.Z.)
Antipodes Is. (N.Z.)
Macquarie Is. (Austral.)

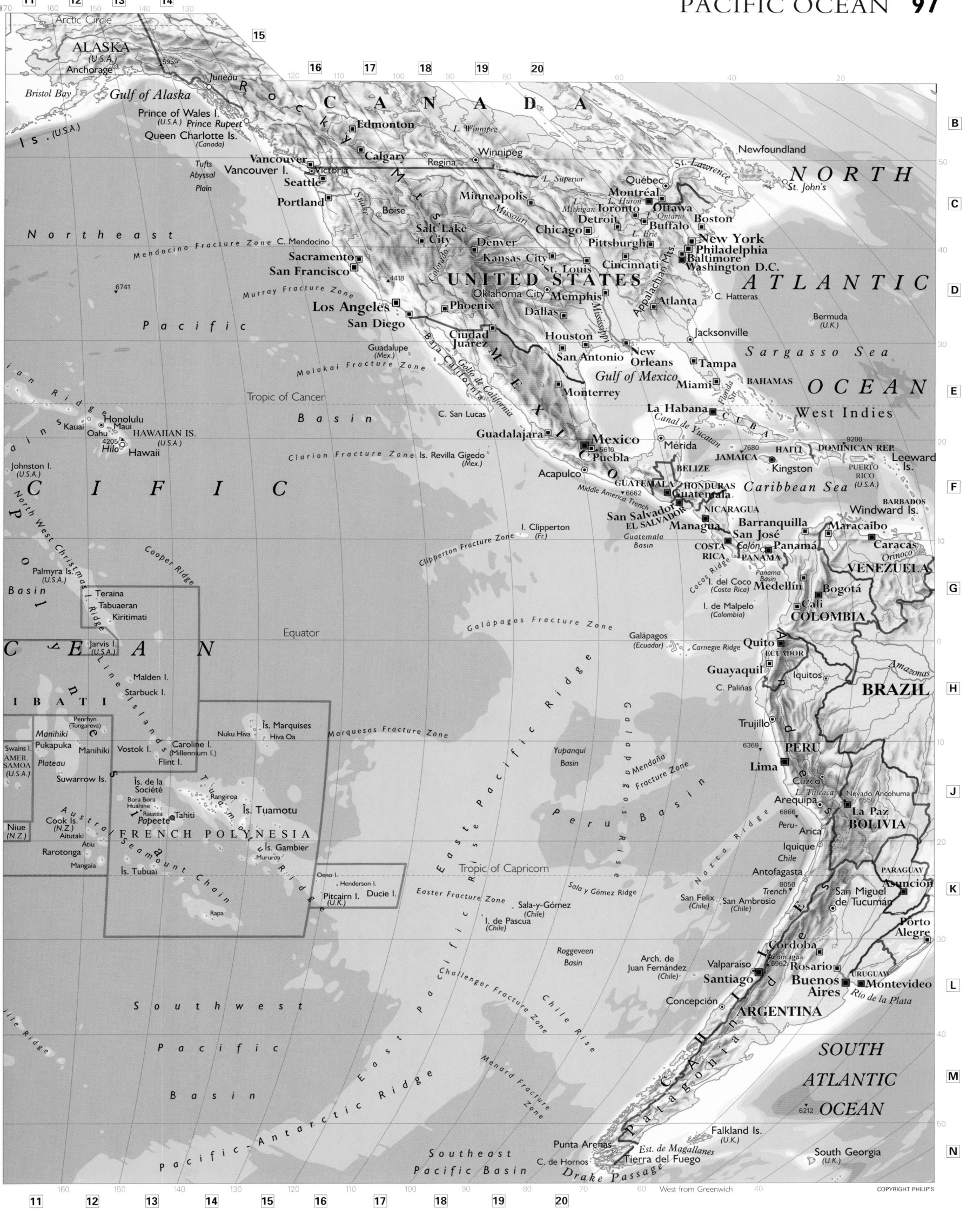

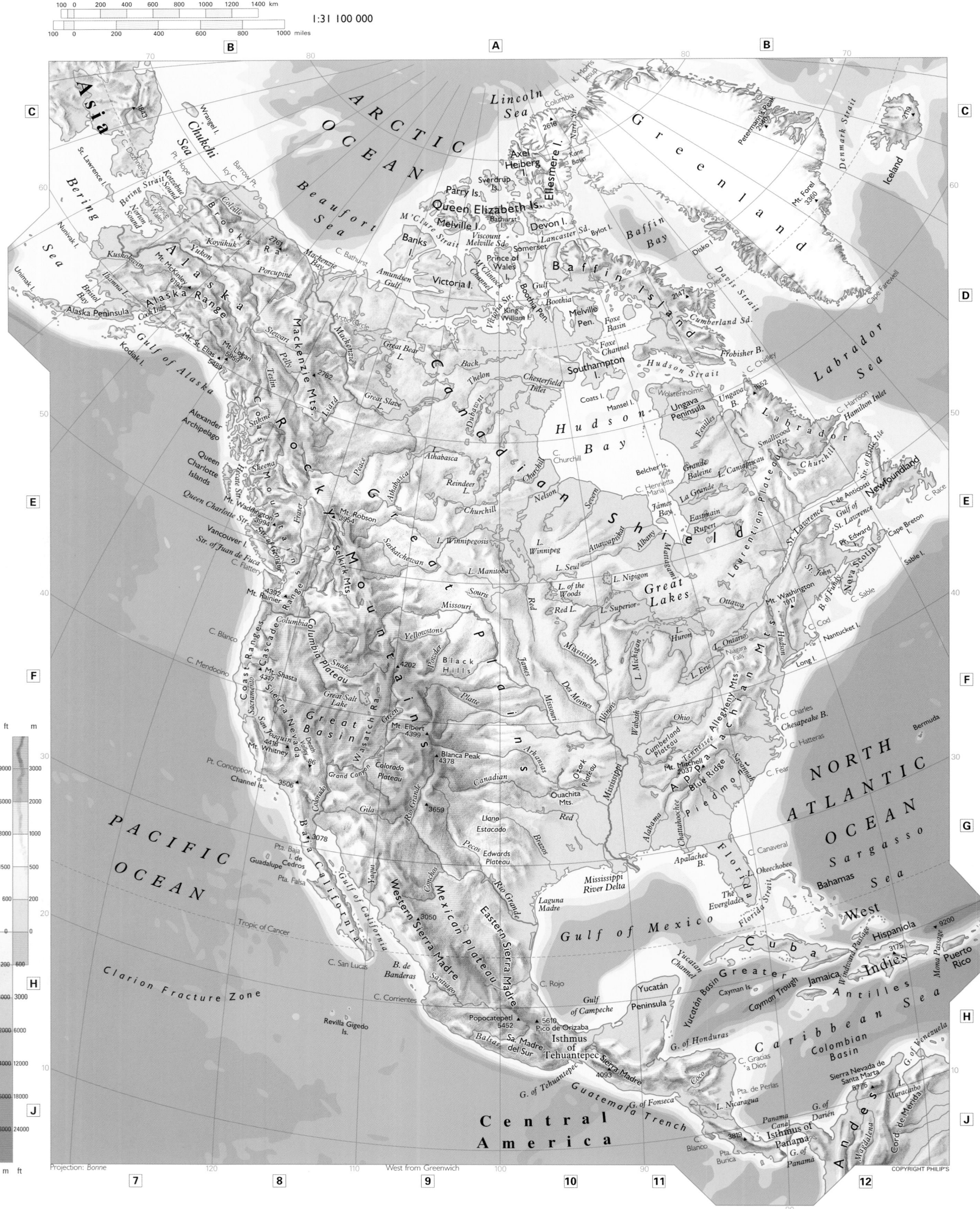

1:31 100 000

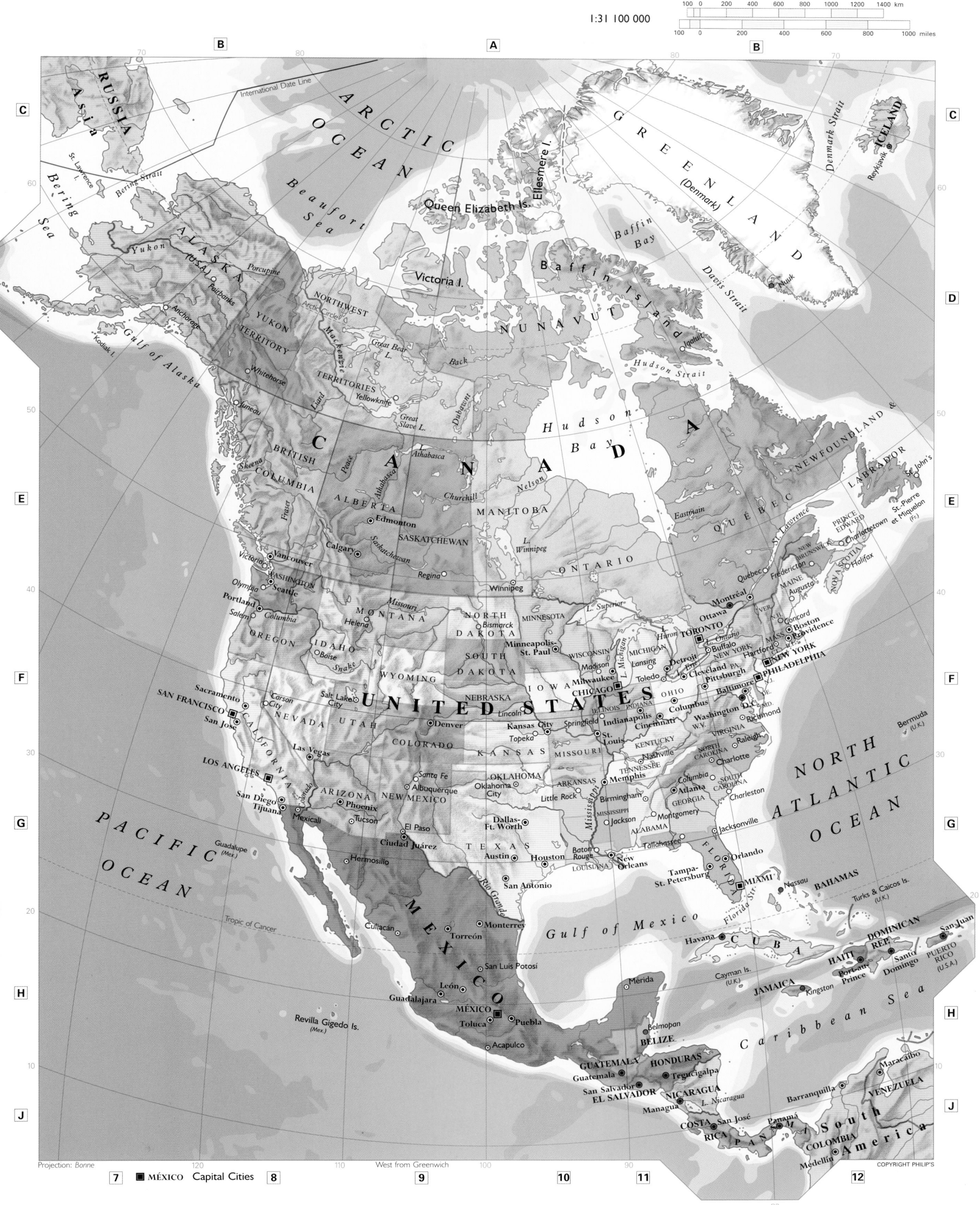

■ MÉXICO Capital Cities

100   0   100   200   300   400   500   600 km

100   0   100   200   300   400 miles

1:13 300 000

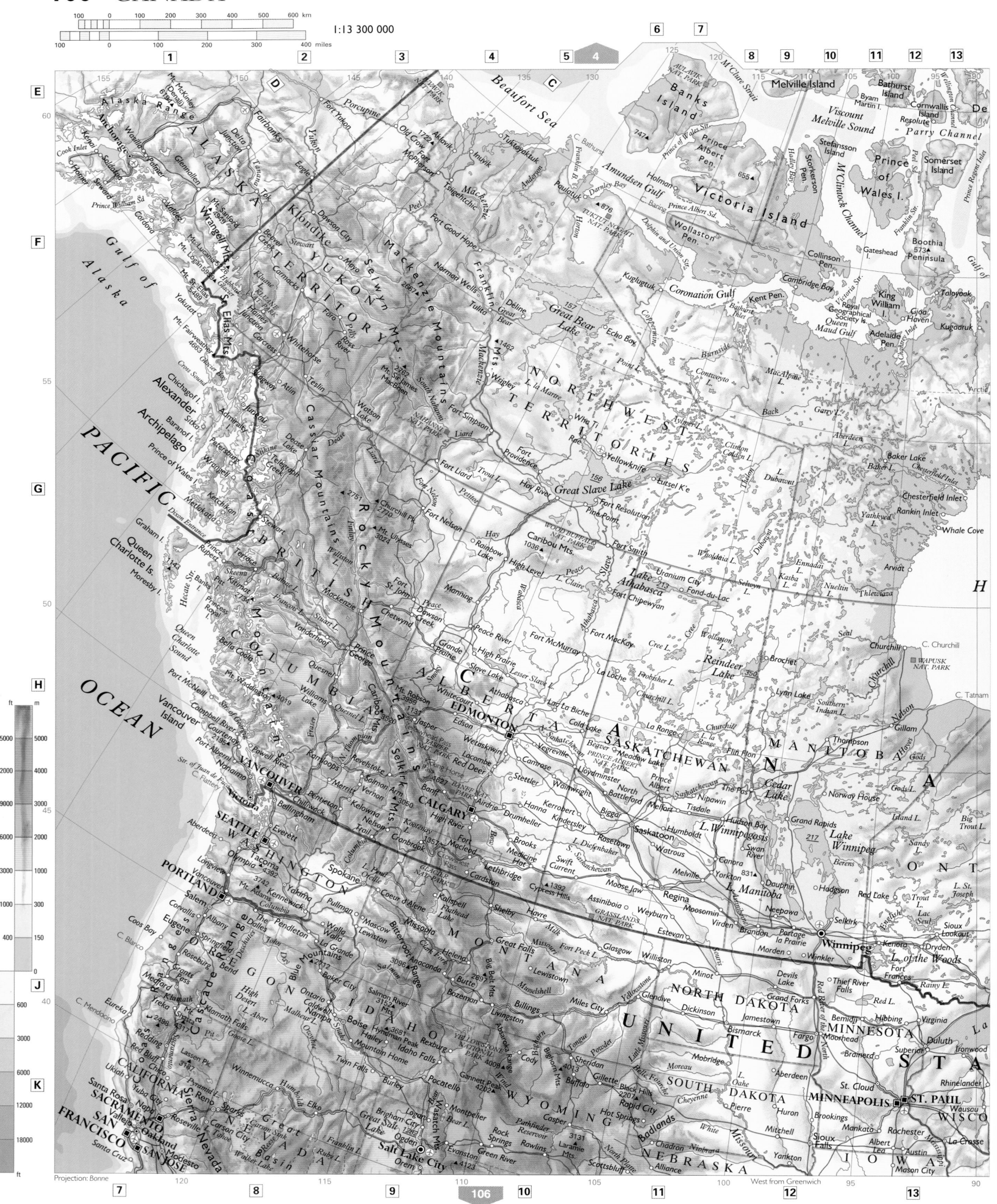

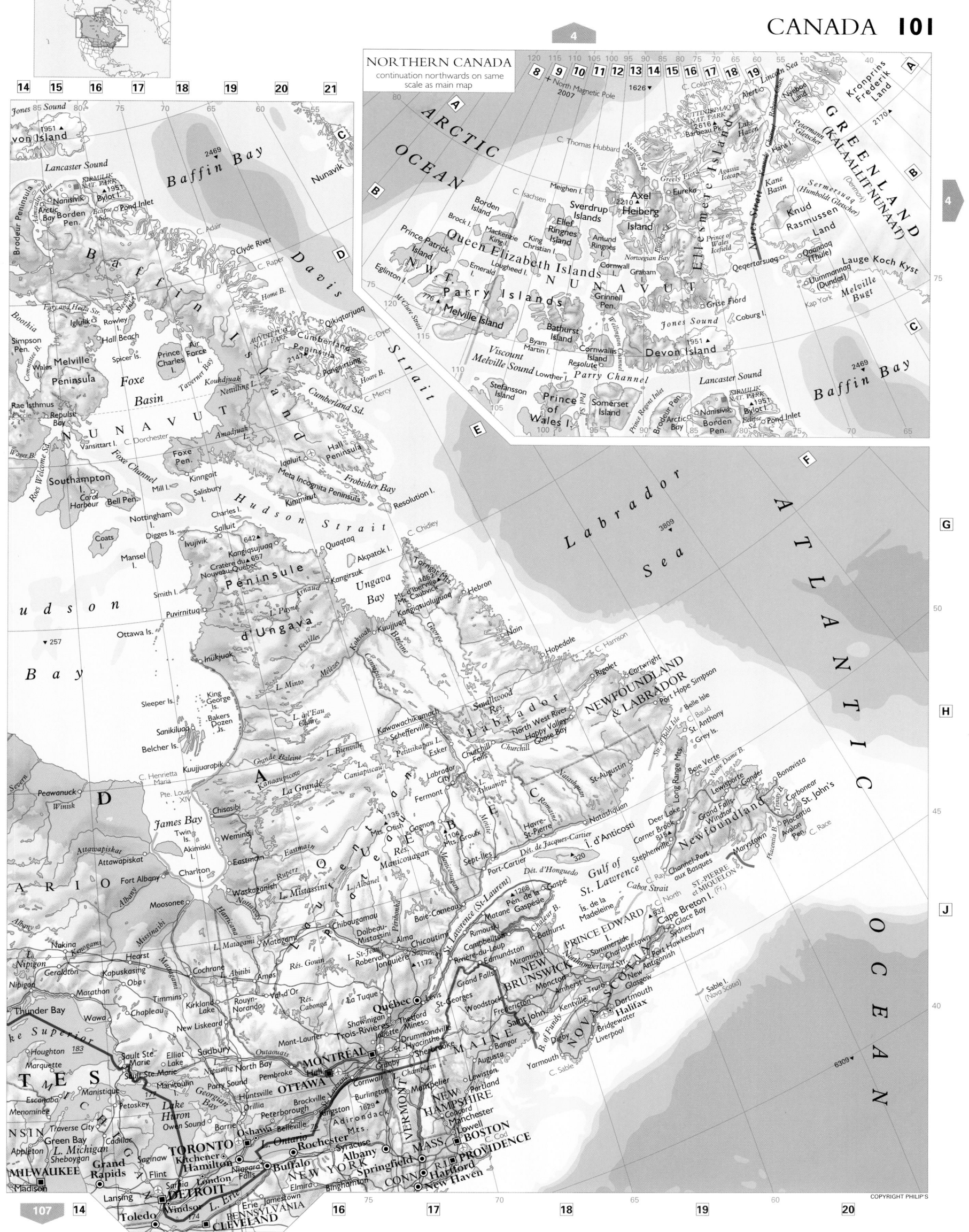

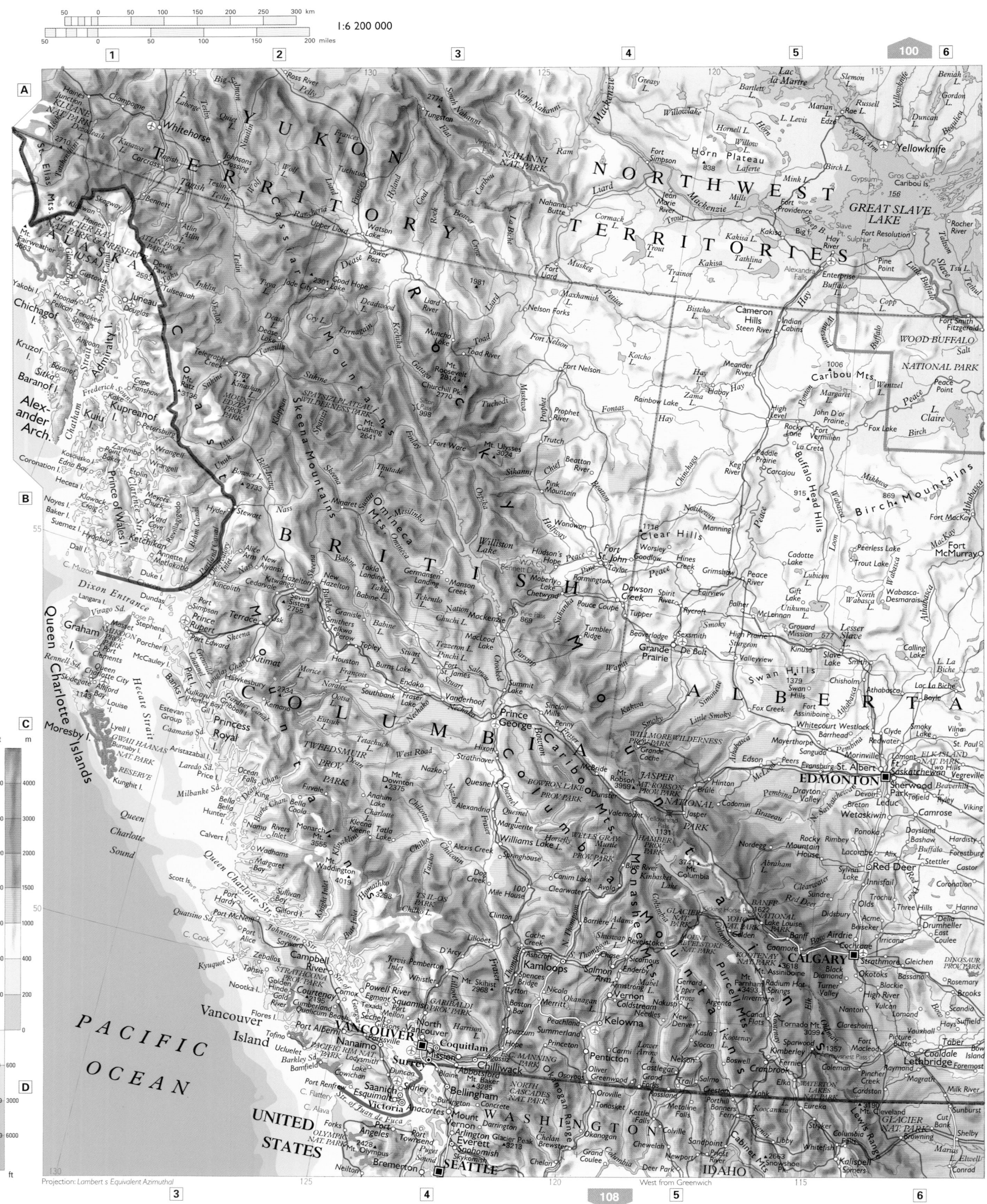

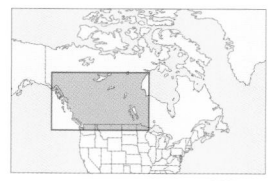

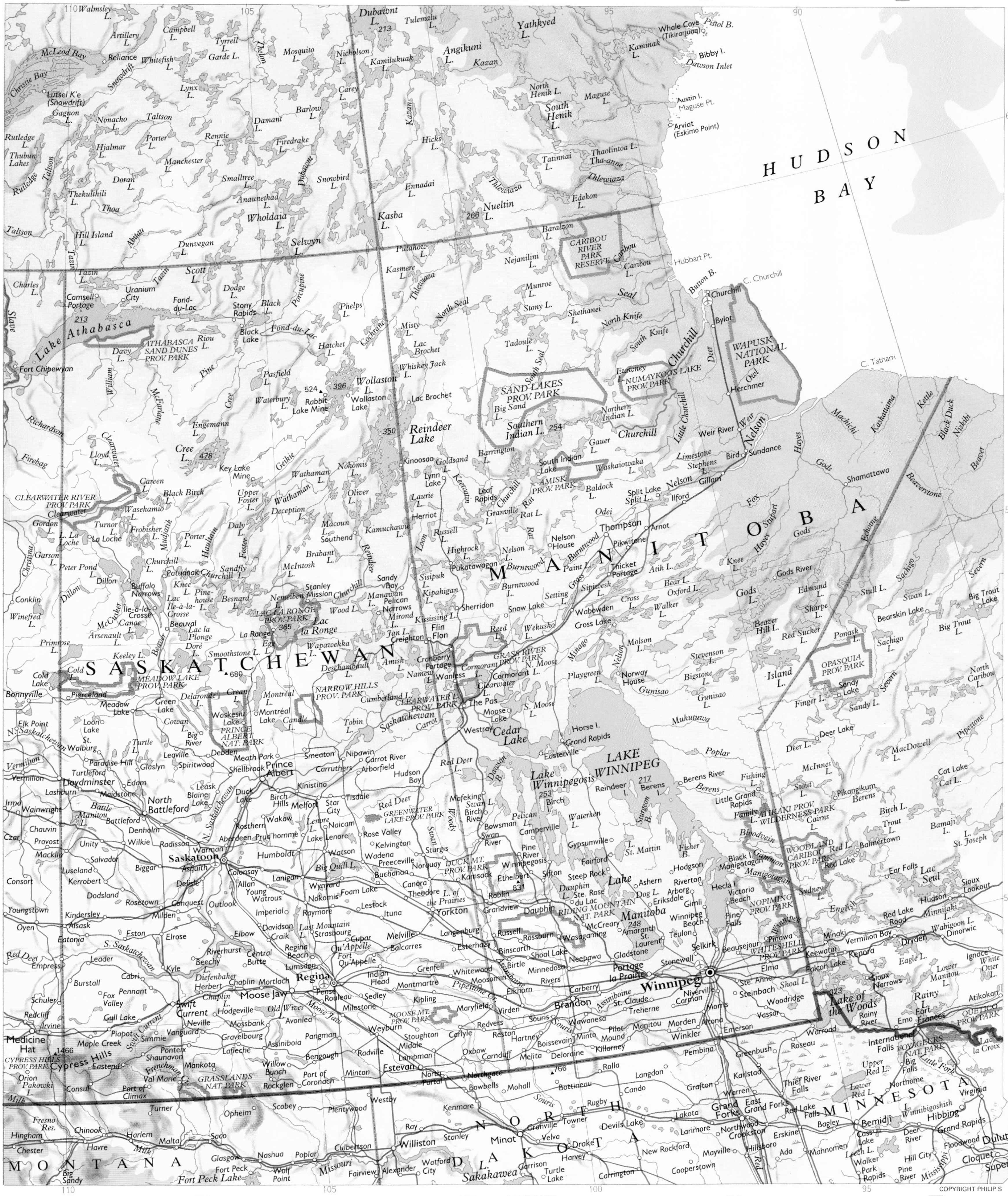

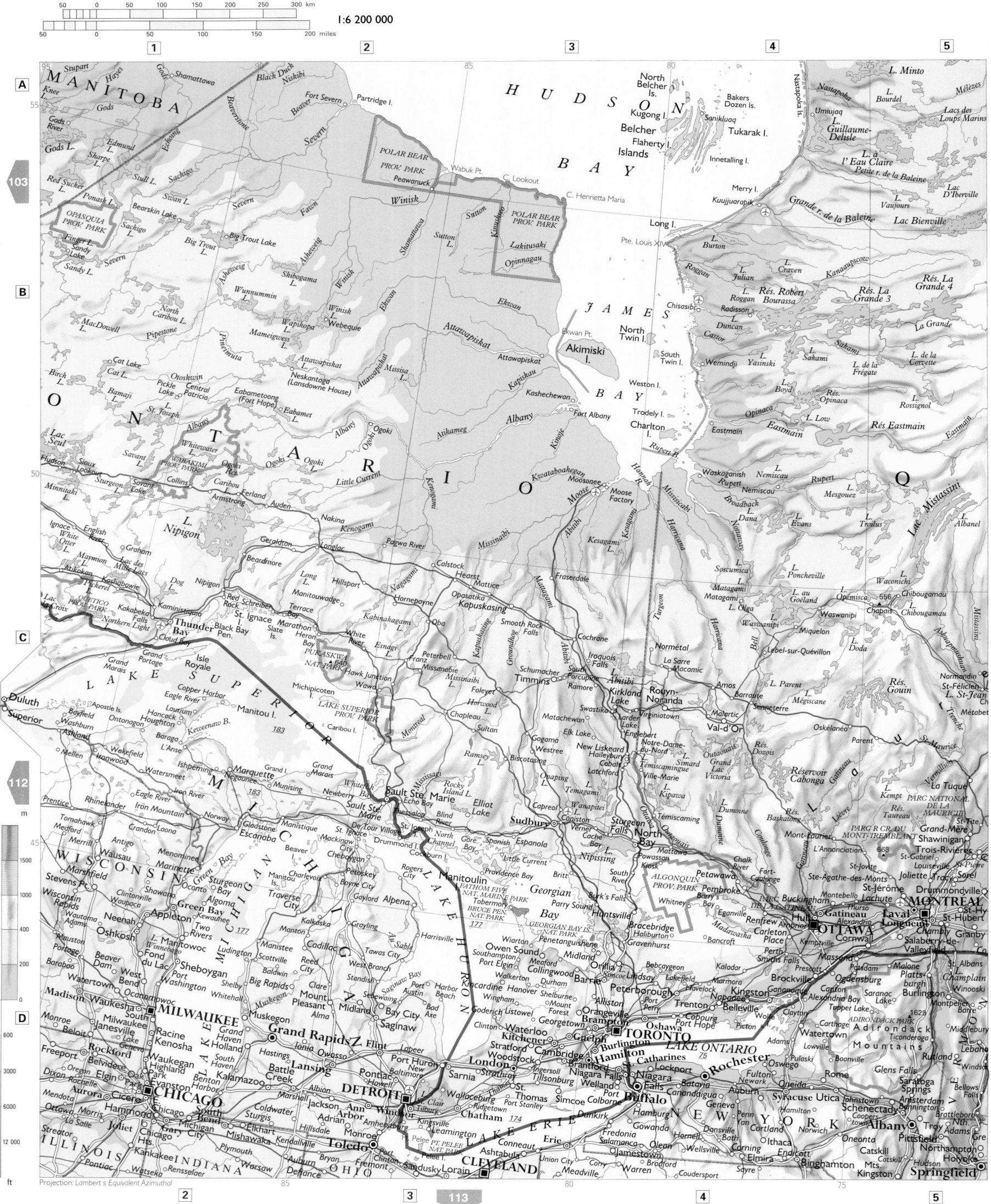

50 0 50 100 150 200 250 300 km
1:6 200 000
50 0 50 100 150 200 miles

Projection: Lambert's Equivalent Azimuthal

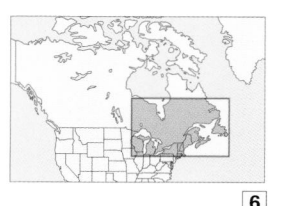

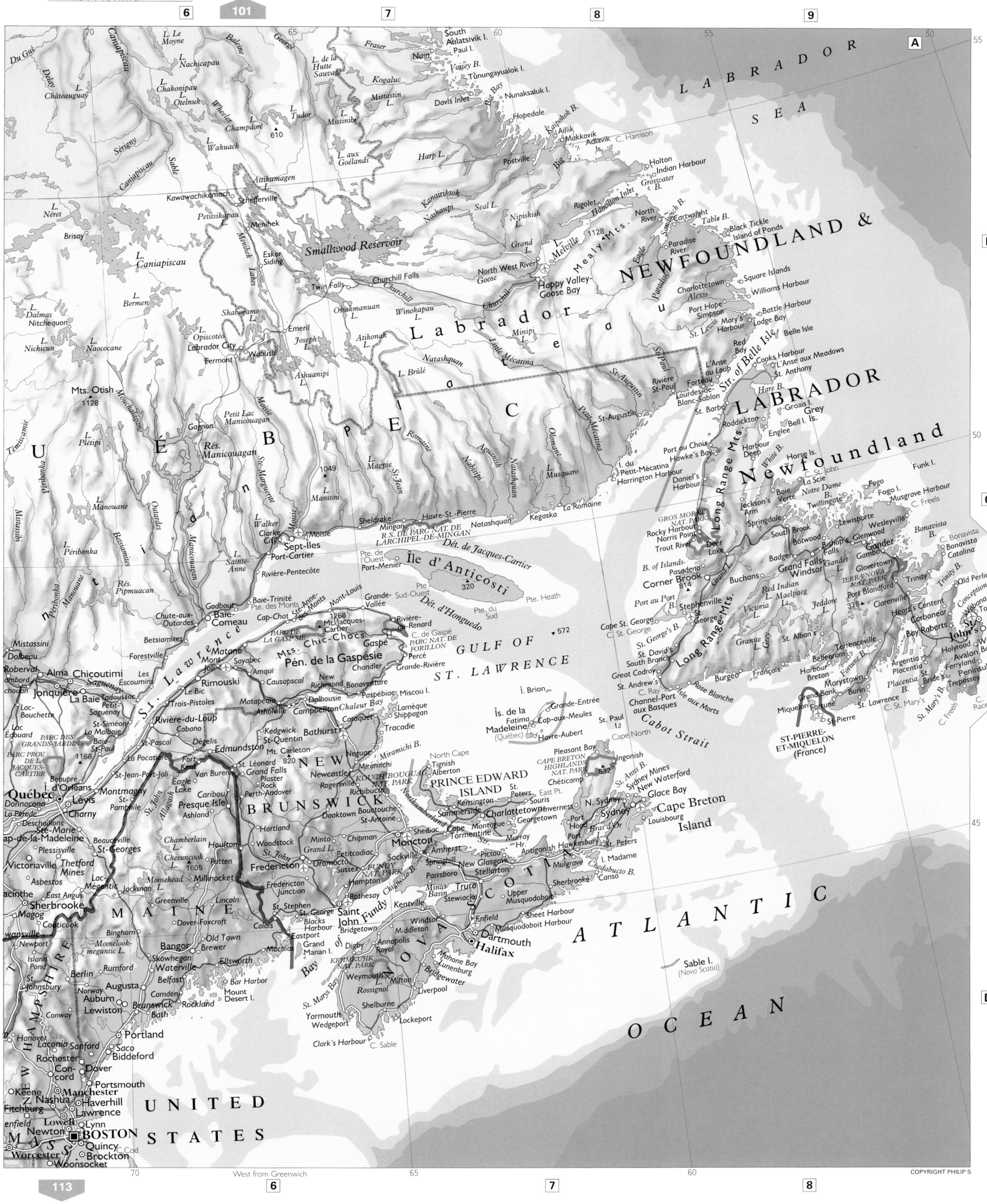

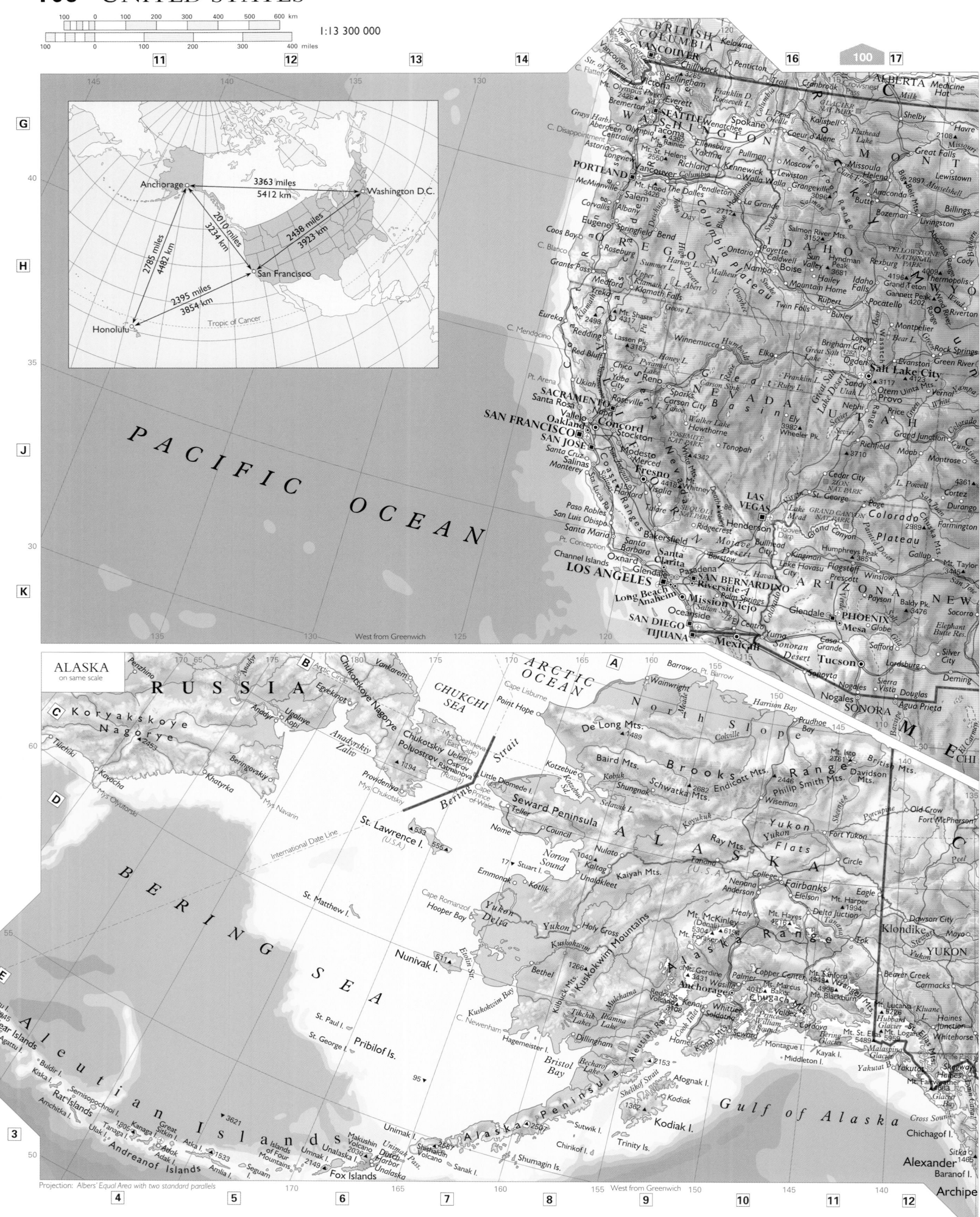

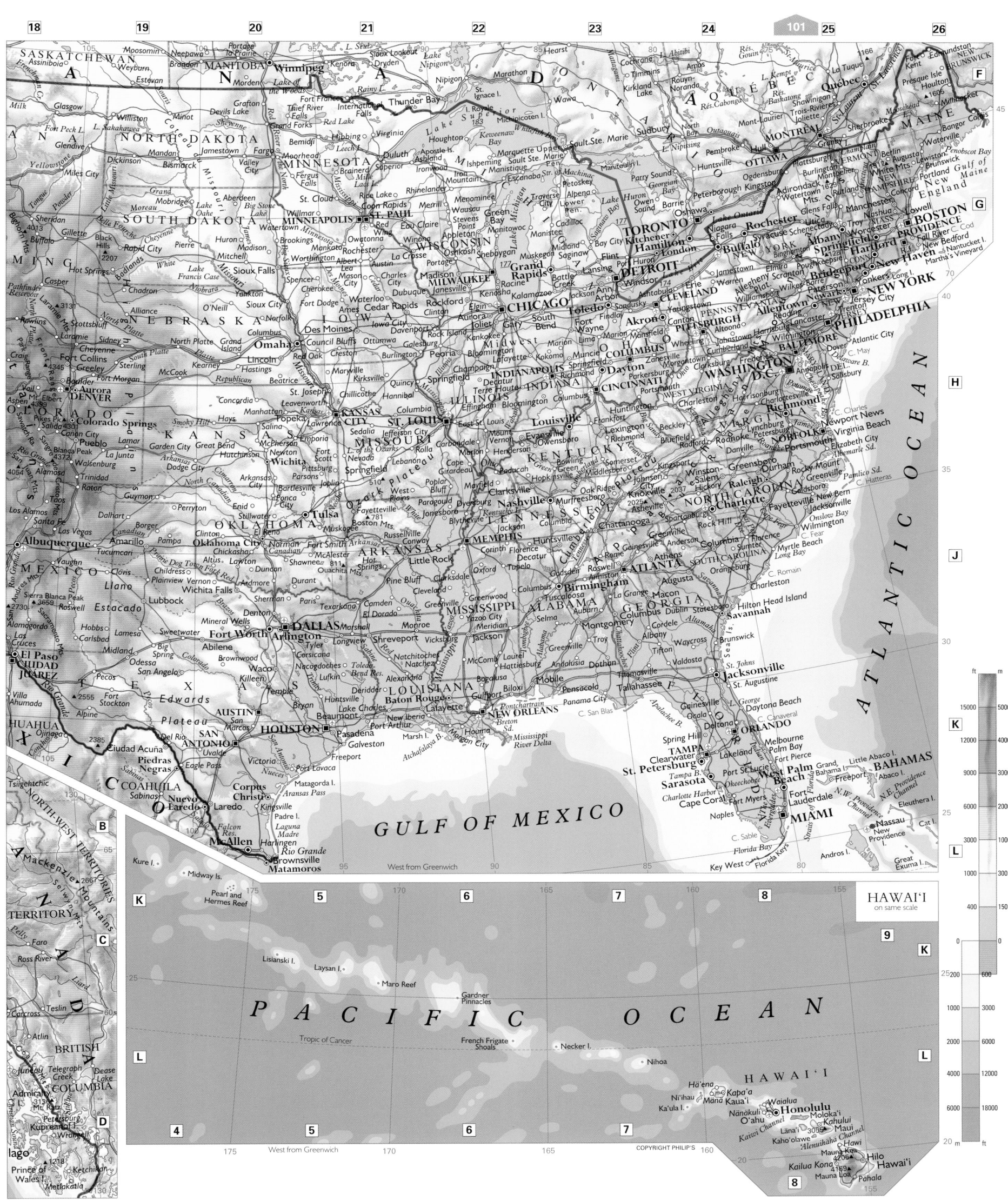

HAWAI'I
on same scale

COPYRIGHT PHILIP'S

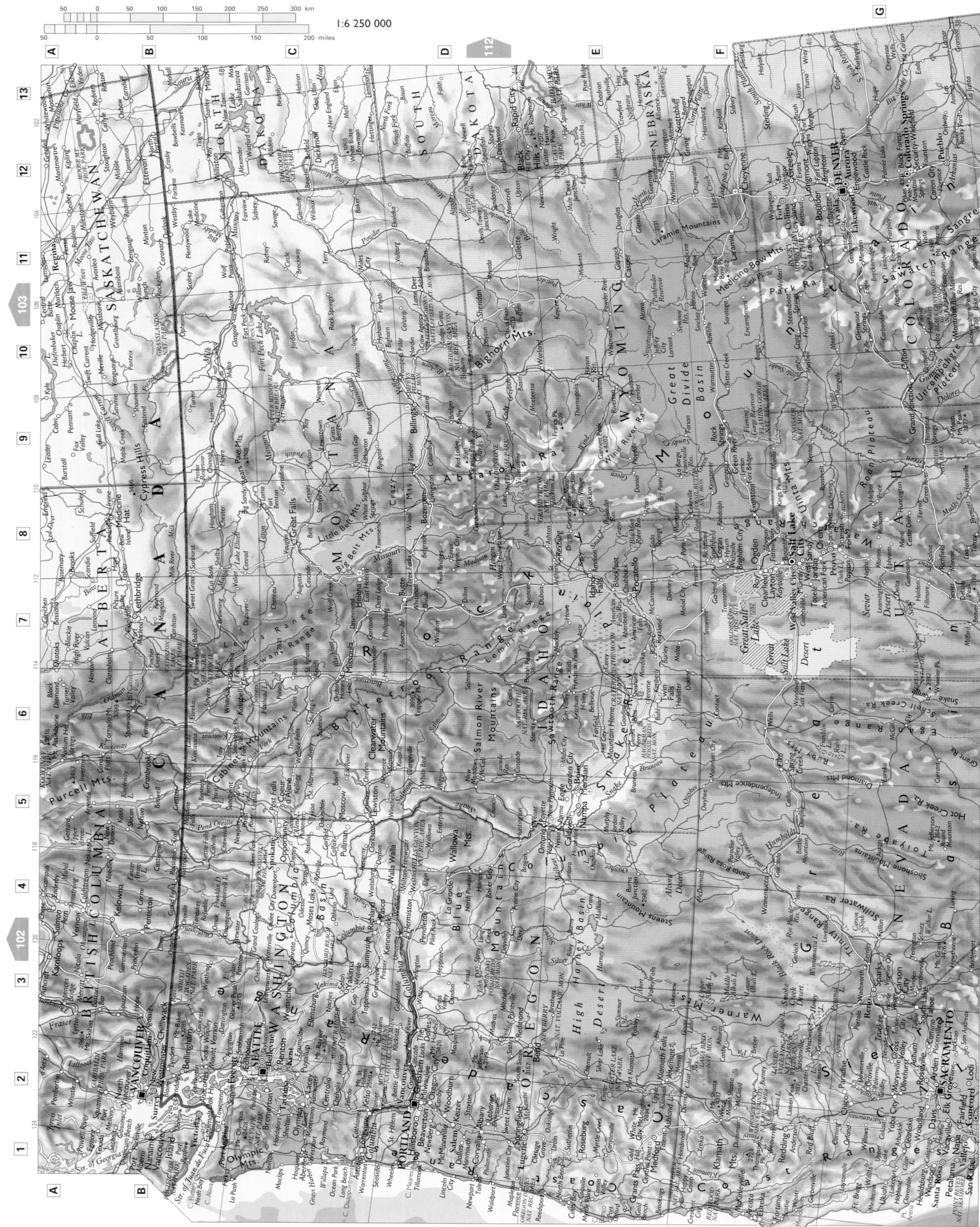

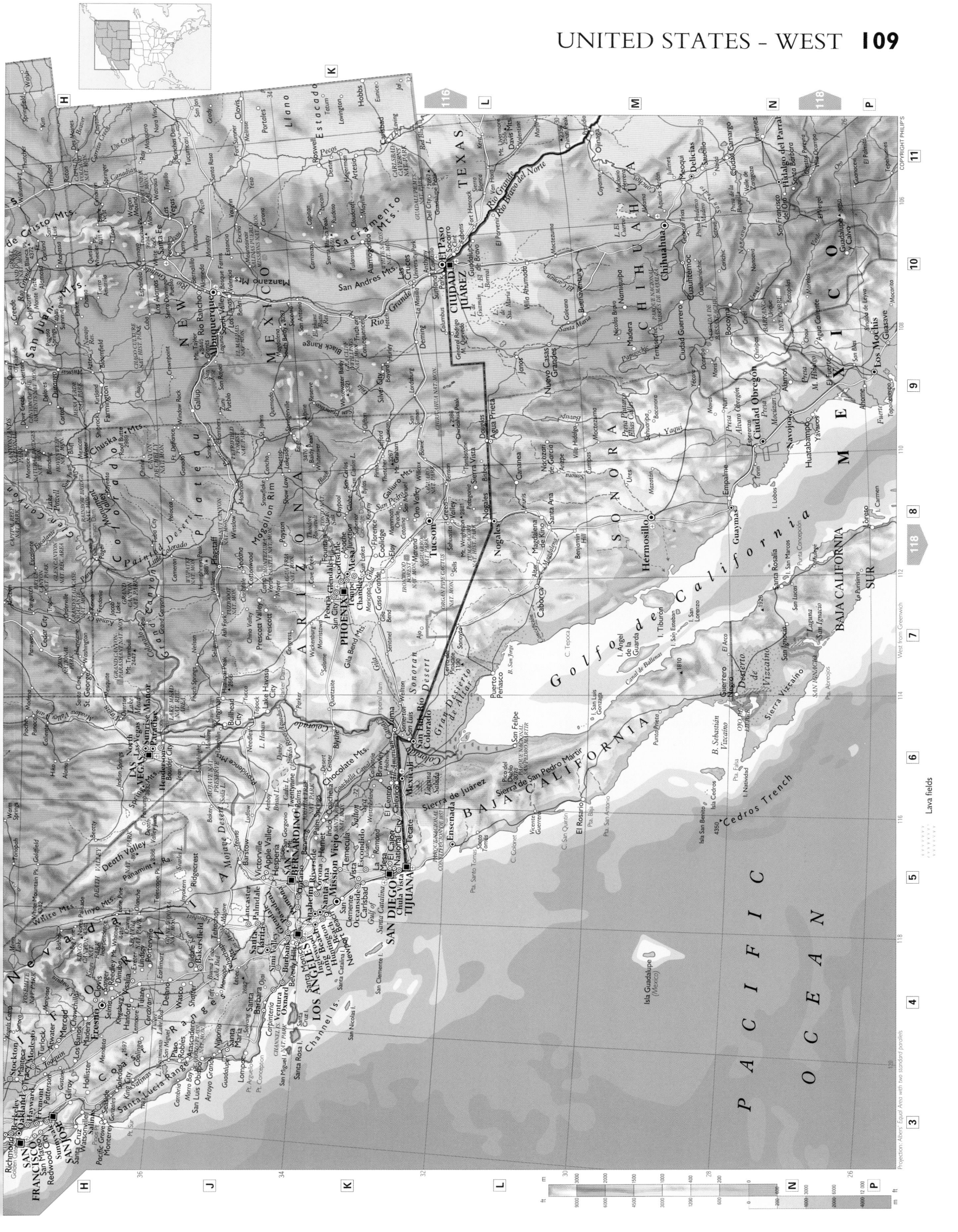

Projection: Albers Equal Area with two standard parallels

West from Greenwich

Lava fields

Scale 1:2 200 000

WESTERN WASHINGTON REGION
on same scale

PACIFIC OCEAN

BRITISH COLUMBIA

CANADA

Vancouver Island

Strait of Georgia

Strait of Juan de Fuca

OLYMPIC MOUNTAINS NATIONAL PARK

WASHINGTON

OREGON

SEATTLE

PORTLAND

Victoria

Sparks
Reno
Carson City
Lake Tahoe

SACRAMENTO

Sacramento Valley

San Joaquin Valley

SAN FRANCISCO
Oakland
SAN JOSE

Santa Clara Valley

Salinas Valley

Santa Lucia Range

Diablo Range

Fresno
Clovis
Visalia

YOSEMITE NATIONAL PARK

KINGS CANYON NATIONAL PARK

SEQUOIA NATIONAL PARK

Sierra Nevada

Inyo Mts.

White Mts.

Pahute Mesa

DEATH VALLEY

Monterey Bay

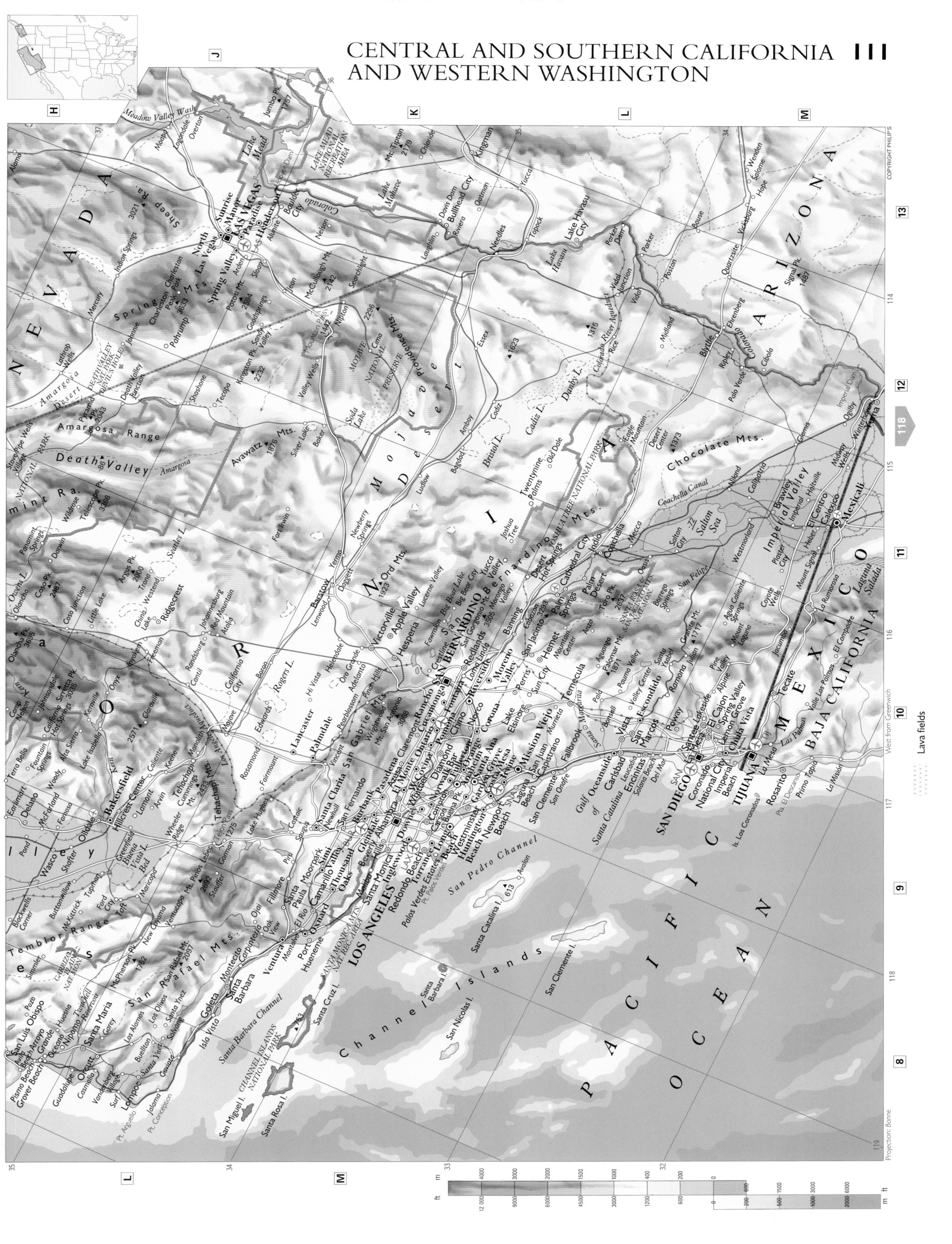

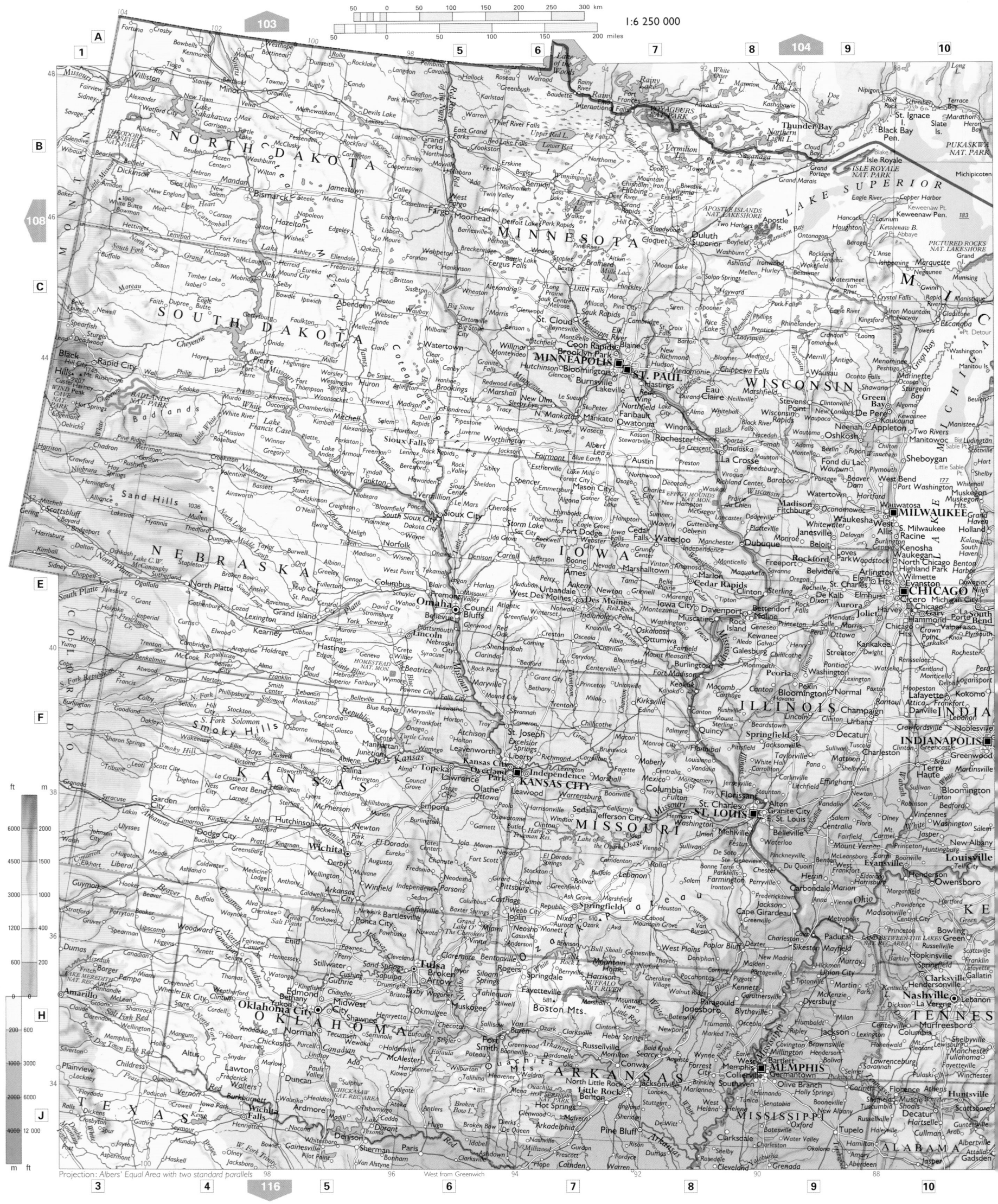

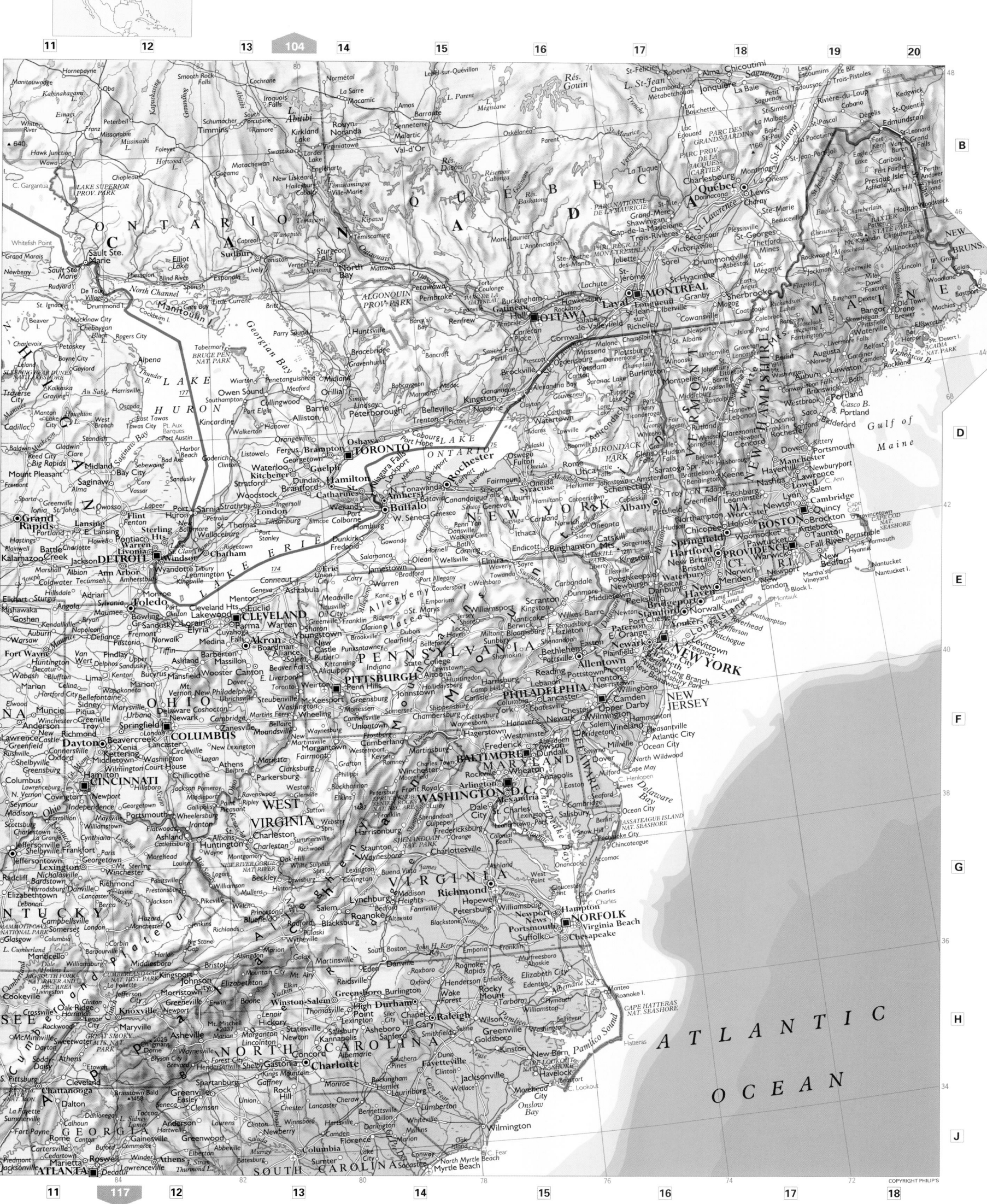

1:2 200 000

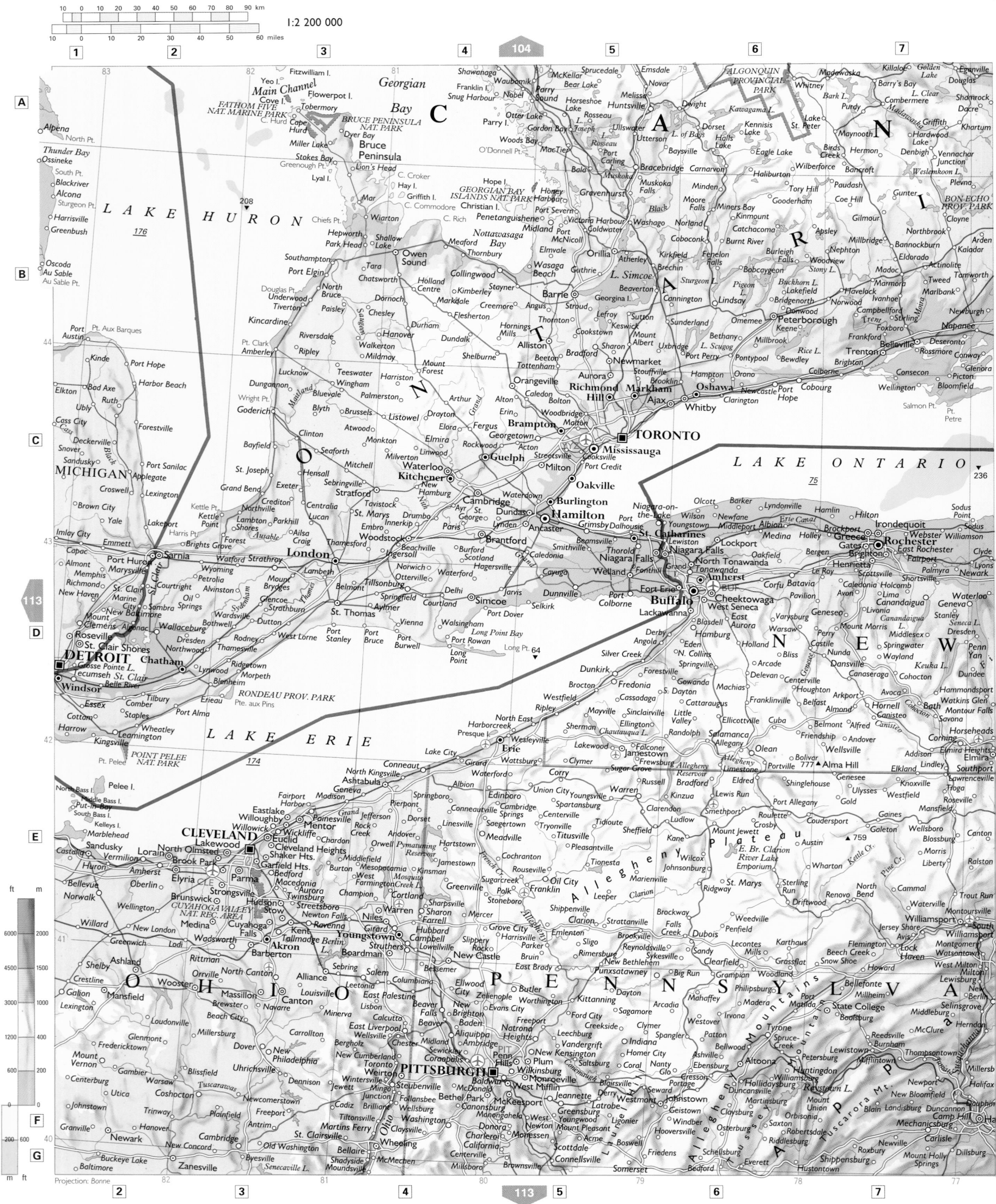

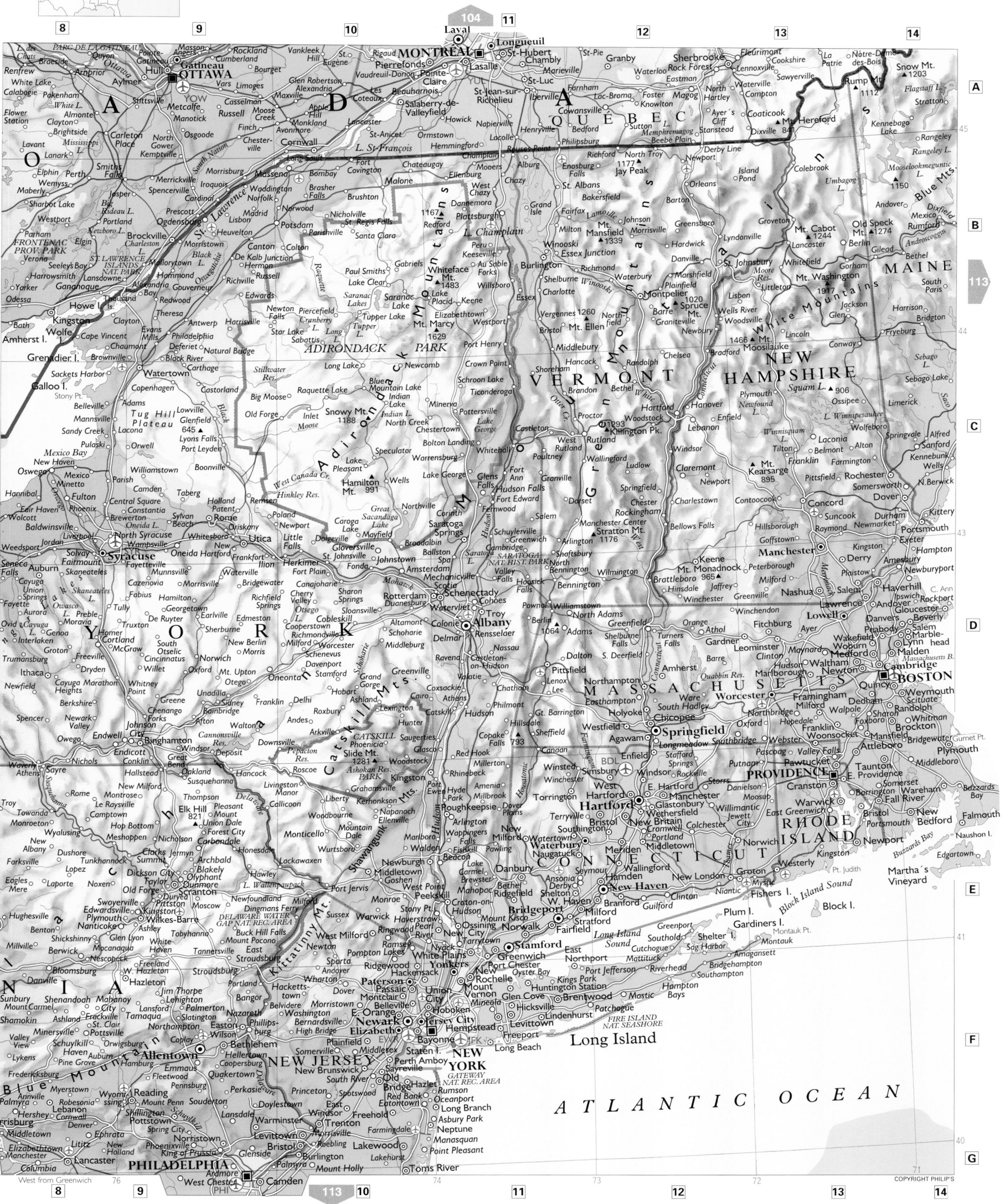

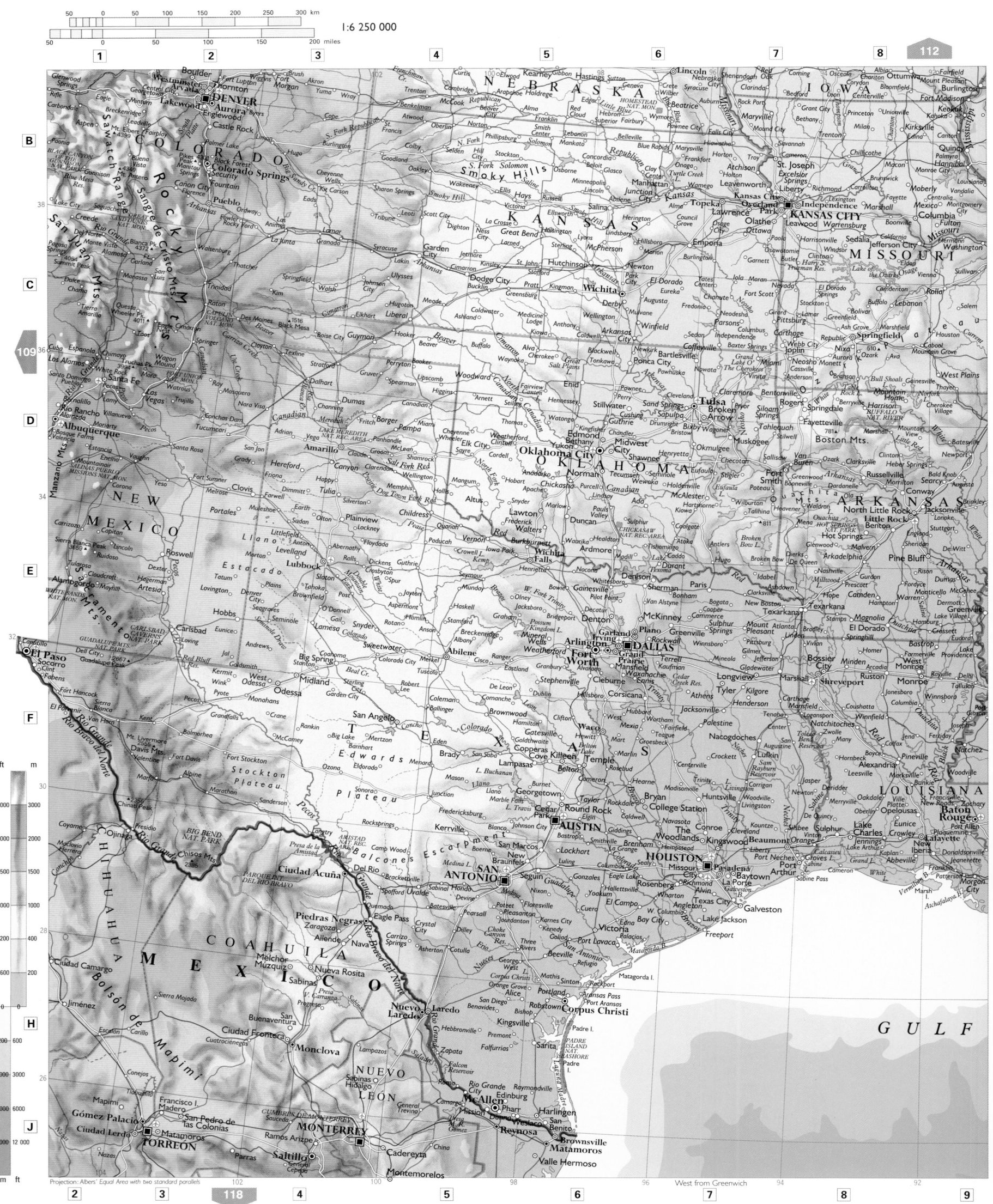

1:6 250 000

Projection: Albers' Equal Area with two standard parallels

West from Greenwich

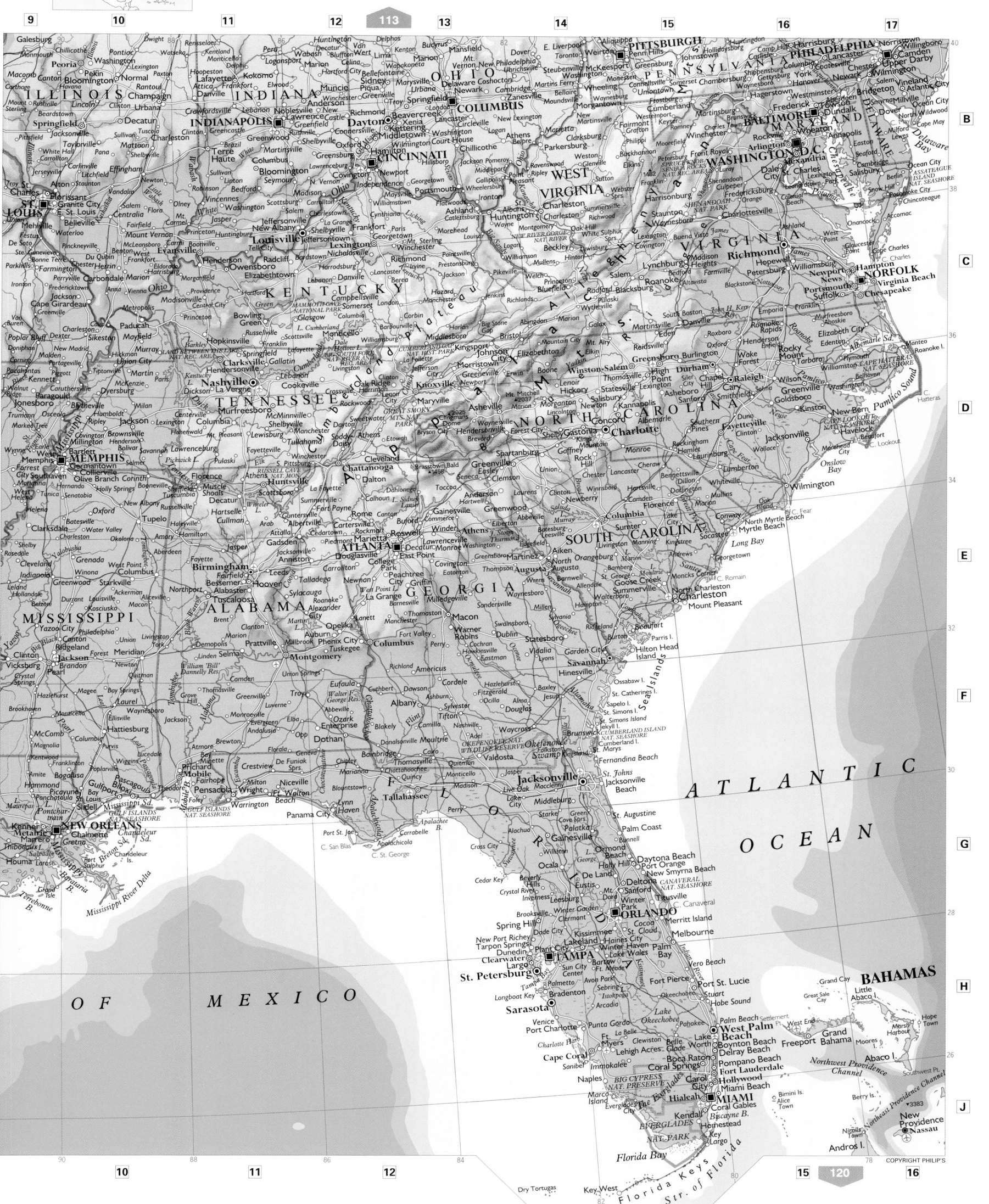

50 0   50   100   150   200   250   300 km

50 0   50   100   150   200 miles

1 : 7 100 000

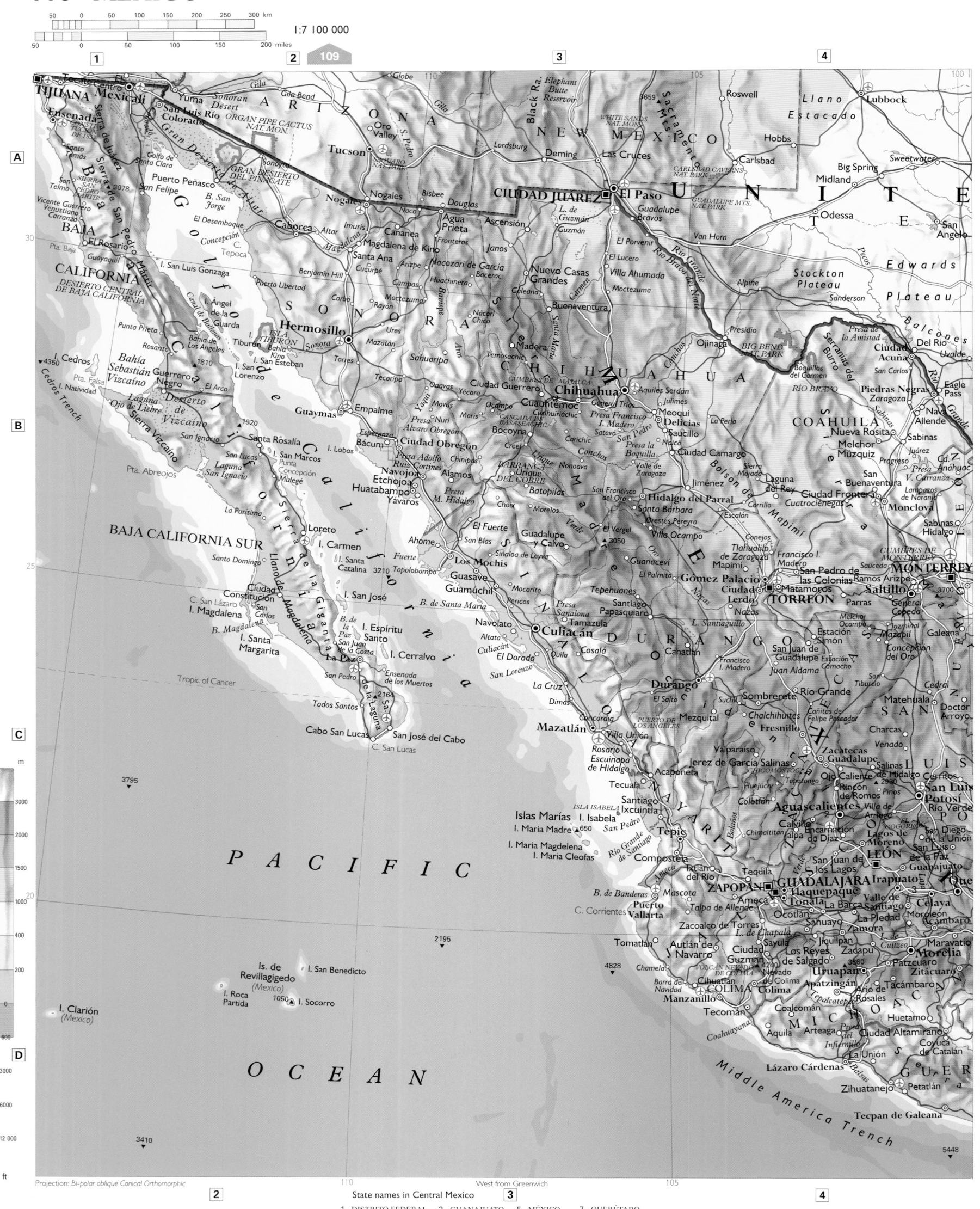

1

2

109

3

4

A

B

C

D

ft   m

9000 3000

6000 2000

4500 1500

3000 1000

1200   400

600   200

0   0

200   600

1000   3000

2000   6000

4000 12 000

m   ft

Projection: Bi-polar oblique Conical Orthomorphic

West from Greenwich

State names in Central Mexico

1 DISTRITO FEDERAL   3 GUANAJUATO   5 MÉXICO   7 QUERÉTARO
2 AGUASCALIENTES   4 HIDALGO   6 MORELOS   8 TLAXCALA

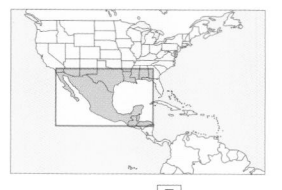

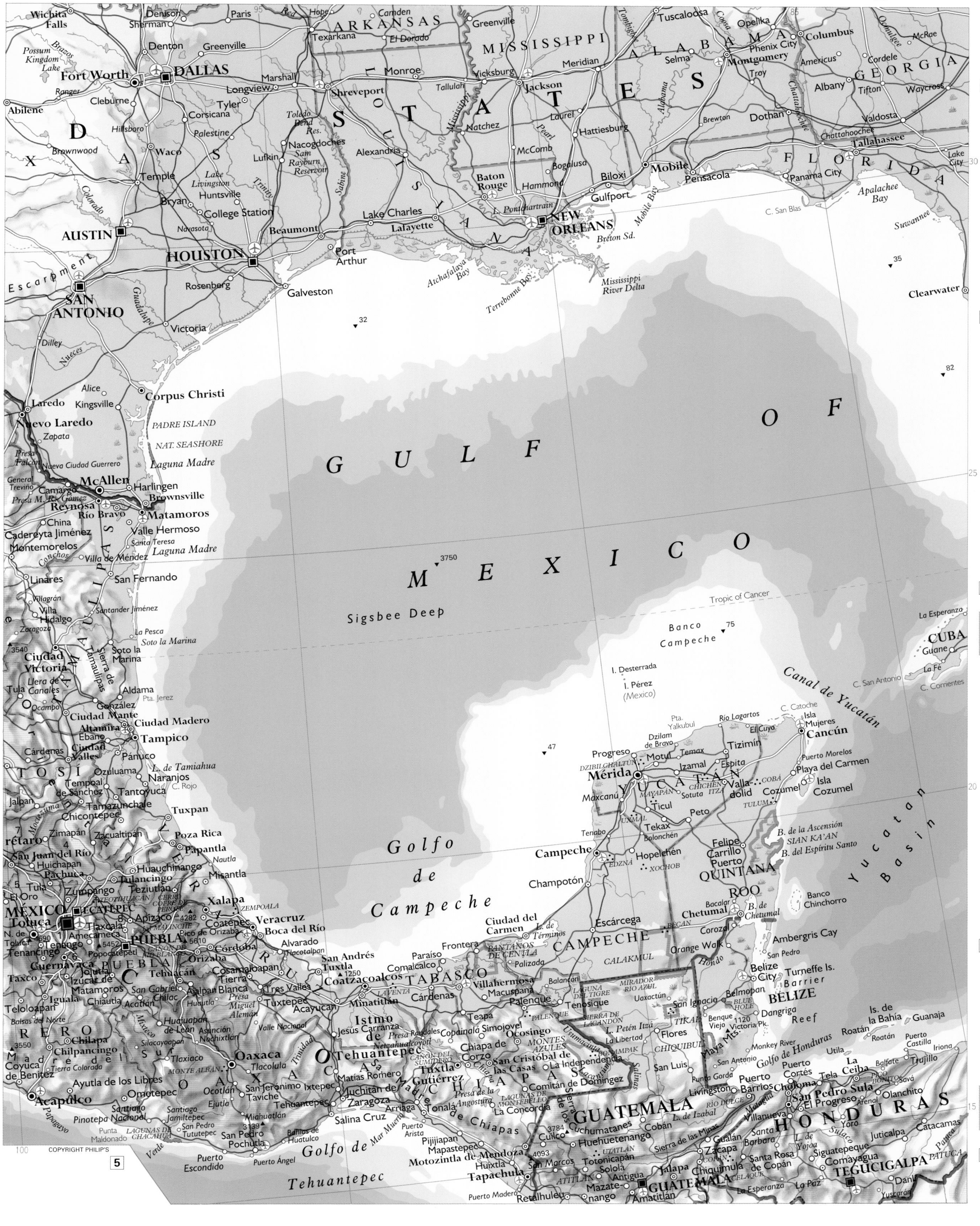

5 6 117 7 8

ARKANSAS
Wichita Falls
Denison
Paris
Camden
Greenville
Tuscaloosa
Opelika
Columbus
McRae
Cordele
Sherman
Texarkana
El Dorado
Greenville
MISSISSIPPI
Phenix City
Montgomery
Americus
Waco
Denton
Greenville
Monroe
Vicksburg
Meridian
Selma
Troy
Albany
Tifton
Waycross
GEORGIA
DALLAS
Fort Worth
Ranger
Longview
Marshall
Shreveport
Jackson
ALABAMA
Dothan
Valdosta
Abilene
Cleburne
Tyler
Corsicana
Toledo Bend Res.
Tallulah
Natchez
Laurel
Hattiesburg
Brewton
Chattahoochee
Tallahassee
Lake City
Hillsboro
Palestine
Lufkin
Nacogdoches
Sam Rayburn Reservoir
Alexandria
McComb
Bogalusa
Biloxi
Mobile
Pensacola
Panama City
FLORIDA
Brownwood
Temple
Bryan
Huntsville
LOUISIANA
Baton Rouge
Hammond
Gulfport
Apalachee Bay
Waco
Navasota
College Station
Lake Charles
Lafayette
NEW ORLEANS
Mobile Bay
C. San Blas
Suwannee
AUSTIN
HOUSTON
Beaumont
Port Arthur
Atchafalaya Bay
Terrebonne Bay
Breton Sd.
Mississippi River Delta
35
Clearwater
SAN ANTONIO
Rosenberg
Galveston
32
82
Dilley
Victoria
Alice
Kingsville
Corpus Christi
PADRE ISLAND
NAT. SEASHORE
Laredo
Nueces
GULF **OF**
Nuevo Laredo
Zapata
Laguna Madre
McAllen
Harlingen
Brownsville
MEXICO
General Trevino
Camargo
Presa M.R. Gomez
Reynosa
Río Bravo
Matamoros
3750
China
Valle Hermoso
Santa Teresa
Laguna Madre
Cadereyta Jiménez
Montemorelos
Villa de Méndez
Sigsbee Deep
Tropic of Cancer
La Esperanza
CUBA
Linares
San Fernando
Banco Campeche
75
Guane
La Fe
Villagrán
Santander Jiménez
La Pesca
Soto la Marina
Villa Hidalgo
Zaragoza
3540
I. Desterrada
I. Pérez (Mexico)
C. San Antonio
C. Corrientes
Ciudad Victoria
Llera de Canales
Tula
Ocampo
Sierra de Tamaulipas
Soto la Marina
Pta. Jerez
Canal de Yucatán
Jalpan
Ciudad Mante
Aldama
González
47
Pta. Yalkubul
Río Lagartos
El Cuyo
Isla Mujeres
Cancún
Ebano
Altamira
Ciudad Madero
Tampico
Progreso
Dzilam de Bravo
Temax
Tizimín
Puerto Morelos
Cárdenas
Ozuluama
Pánuco
L. de Tamiahua
DZIBILCHALTUN
Motul
Espita
Playa del Carmen
Temporal de Sánchez
Naranjos
C. Rojo
Mérida
Izamal
CHICHEN ITZA
Valladolid
Isla Cozumel
Tantoyuca
Maxcanú
MAYAPAN
Soluta
COBA
Cozumel
Jalpan
Tamazunchale
Chicontepec
Tuxpan
Ticul
Peto
TULUM
POTOSÍ
Zimapán
Zacualtipán
Poza Rica
Papantla
Nautla
UXMAL
Tekax
Tenabo
B. de la Ascensión
SIAN KA'AN
rétaro
San Juan del Río
Huichapan
Huauchinango
Misantla
Bolonchén
B. del Espíritu Santo
Pachuca
Tulancingo
Teziutlán
Campeche
Felipe Carrillo Puerto
Yucatan Basin
El Oro
Tula
Zumpango
EDZNA
Hopelchén
QUINTANA
Banco Chinchorro
MÉXICO
ECATEPEC
Xalapa
ZEMPOALA
Champotón
ROO
Toluca
Apizaco
Coatepec
Veracruz
Bacalar
Chetumal
B. de Chetumal
N. de Toluca
4690
Tlaxcala
Amecameca
MALINCHE 4282
Boca del Río
Golfo
Escárcega
BECAN
Corozal
Tenango
Popocatépetl
PUEBLA
Pico de Orizaba 5610
Alvarado
Orizaba
de
Ciudad del Carmen
L. de Términos
CALAKMUL
Orange Walk
Ambergris Cay
Cuernavaca
Iguala
Izúcar de Matamoros
Atlixco
San Gabriel Chilac
Córdoba
Tierra Blanca
San Andrés Tuxtla
Campeche
Frontera
Paraíso
Hondo
San Pedro
Belize City
Turneffe Is.
Taxco
Tlapa
Chiautla
Acatlán
Tehuacán
Presa Miguel Alemán
Cosamaloapan
Tuxtepec
Coatzacoalcos
Comalcalco
Palizada
BLUE HOLE
BELIZE
Barrier Reef
Telolopan
Huajuapan de León
Asunción Nochixtlán
Valle Nacional
Minatitlán
TABASCO
Villahermosa
Macuspana
Palenque
Balancán
MIRADOR-RÍO AZUL
Belmopan
Dangriga
RERO
Chilapa
Tlaxiaco
Acayucan
Cárdenas
Teapa
LA VENTA
Tenosique
CAMPECHE
San Ignacio
Benque Viejo
Is. de la Bahía
Guanaja
3550
Chilpancingo
Coyuca de Benitez
OAXACA
Tlacolula
MONTE ALBAN
Istmo de Tehuantepec
Jesús Carranza
Copainalá
Simojovel
Ocosingo
SIERRA DE LACANDON
LAGUNA DEL TIGRE
Uaxactún
CHIQUIBUL
Maya Mts.
Victoria Pk.
1120
Monkey River
Punta Gorda
Roatán
Utila
Golfo de Honduras
Puerto Cortés
Tela
La Ceiba
Roatán
Puerto Castilla
Iriona
Olanchito
Ayutla de los Libres
Ocotlán
Santiago Jamiltepec
San Pedro
Ejutla
Taviche
Tehuantepec
Zaragoza
Juchitán de Zaragoza
Arriaga
Tonalá
OAXACA
Tuxtla Gutiérrez
Chiapa de Corzo
San Cristóbal de las Casas
La Independencia
Comitán de Domínguez
CHIAPAS
LAGUNAS DE MONTEBELLO
3784
Cuchumatanes
GUATEMALA
Flores
L. Petén Itzá
TIKAL
San Antonio
San Luis
Livingston
RÍO DULCE
L. de Izabal
Puerto Barrios
Chixoy
San Pedro Sula
El Progreso
Arenal
Yoro
HONDURAS
Catacamas
Acapulco
Pinotepa Nacional
Punta Maldonado
PUNTA DE CHACAHUA
LAGUNAS
Tututepec
San Pedro Pochutla
Miahuatlán
Salina Cruz
CAÑON DEL SUMIDERO
CAÑON DEL RÍO LA VENTA
3550
Cintalapa
Suchiapa
Villaflores
Angostura
La Concordia
CHIQUIMULA
Río Dulce
Zacapa
Gualán
Santa Rosa de Copán
Santa Bárbara
L. de Yojoa
Siguatepeque
Comayagua
TEGUCIGALPA
Puerto Escondido
Puerto Ángel
Golfo de Tehuantepec
Mar Muerto
Pijijiapan
Mapastepec
Motozintla de Mendoza
Huixtla
Tapachula
San Marcos
Sololá
UTATLAN
Totonicapán
Quezaltenango
Retalhuleu
SIERRA DE LAS MINAS
4093
Coban
Huehuetenango
Jalapa
Chiquimula
Esquipulas
Jutiapa
Santa Rosa
La Esperanza
La Paz
Danli
Yuscarán
PATUCA
Tehuantepec
Puerto Madero
Mazatenango
GUATEMALA
Antigua
ATITLAN
Mazate-nango
Amatitlán

120
100
COPYRIGHT PHILIP'S

A
B
C
D
E

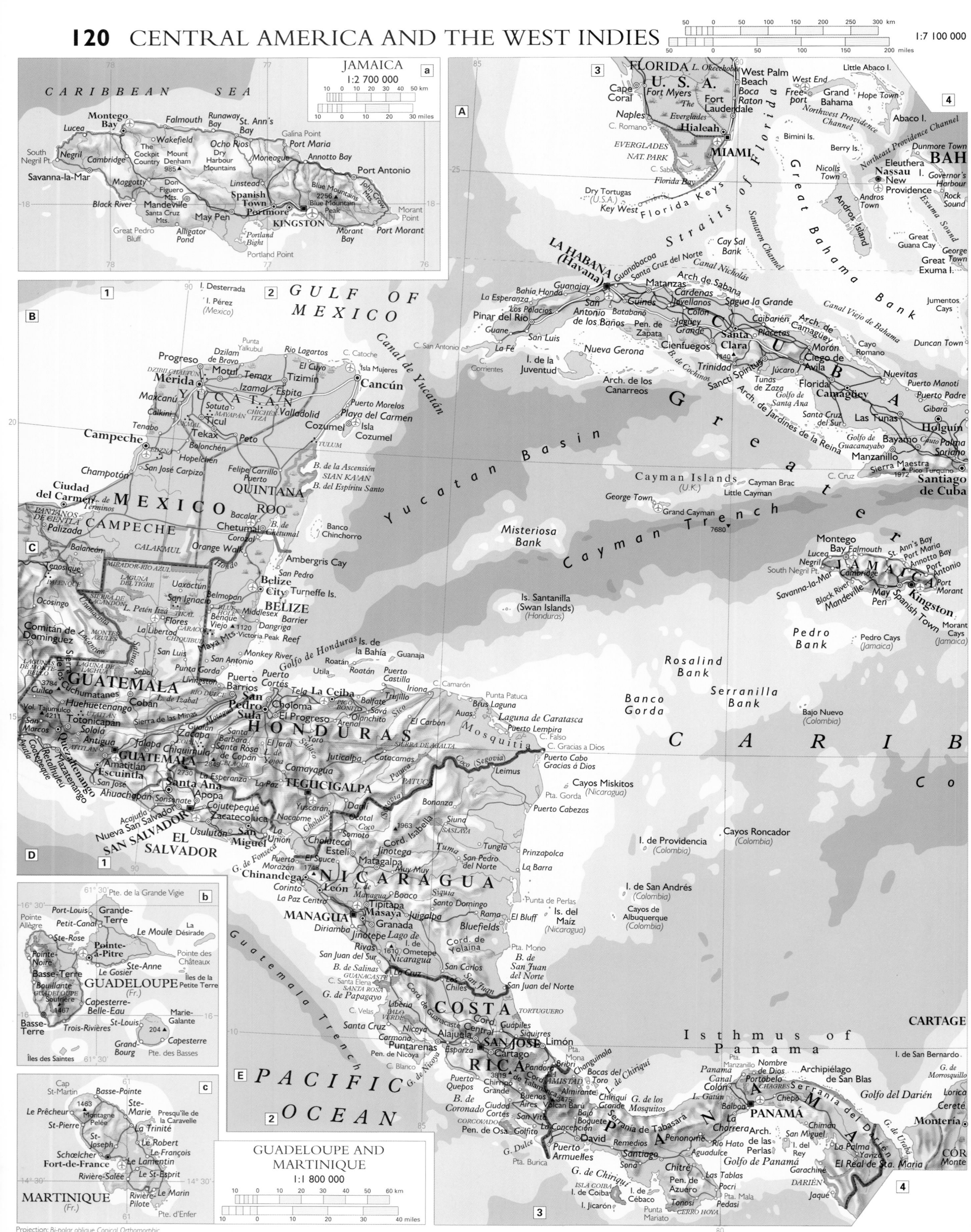

ATLANTIC OCEAN

PUERTO RICO (U.S.A.) 1:2 700 000 | d

Aguadilla, Isabela, Arecibo, Barceloneta, Manati, Vega Baja, Bayamón, SAN JUAN, Rio Grande, Carolina, Fajardo, Dewey, Culebra, Vieques, Esperanza, Mayagüez, San Sebastián, Adjuntas, Utuado, Cordillera Central, 1338 Cerro de Punta, Caguas, Sierra de Luquillo, Naguabo, Puerca, San German, Yauco, Mts. de Uroyan, Coamo, Cayey, Humacao, Yabucoa, Ponce, Guánica, Guayama, Pta. Aguila, I. Caja de Muertos

VIRGIN ISLANDS 1:1 800 000 | e

Virgin Islands (U.K.), Rufling Pt., Anegada, The Settlement, East Pt., Jost Van Dyke I., Guana I., Great Camanoe, Beef I., Virgin Gorda, Spanish Town, Virgin Is. (U.S.A.), Hans Lollik I., Tortola, Road Town, Peter I., Charlotte Amalie, Cruz Bay, St. John I., St. Thomas I., VIRGIN IS.

ST. LUCIA 1:890 000 | f

Cap Point, Pte. Hardy, Esperance Bay, Gros Islet, Castries, Girard, Marquis, Anse la Raye, Canaries, Millet, Dennery, Soufrière, Mt. Gimie 950, 750 Petit Piton, 796 Gros Piton, Trou Gras Pt., Micoud, Vierge Pt., Gros Piton Pt., Choiseul, Laborie, Vieux Fort, C. Moule à Chique, ST. LUCIA

BARBADOS 1:890 000 | g

Crab Hill, North Point, Spring Hall, Boscobelle, Fustic, Portland, 245 Belleplaine, Speightstown, Bathsheba, BARBADOS, Westmoreland, Hillcrest, Alleynes Bay, 340 Mt. Hillaby, Martin's Bay, Holetown, Massiah Street, Ragged Pt., Black Rock, Jackson, Bridgefield, Six Cross Roads, Bridgetown, Ellerton, Ivy, Edey, The Crane, Worthing, Oistins, St. Martins, Carlisle Bay, BGI, Chancery Lane, Oistins Bay, South Point

ATLANTIC OCEAN, AMAS, Arthur's Town, New Bight, Cat I., San Salvador I., Conception I., Rum Cay, Long I., Sandy Cay, Clarence Town, Crooked I. Passage, Samana Cay, Crooked I., Plana Cays, Albert Town, Snug Corner, Mayaguana I., Acklins I., Mira por vos Cay, Cay Verde, Hogsty Reef, Little Inagua I., Turks & Caicos Is. (U.K.), Caicos Is., Cockburn Town, Turks Is., Cay Santo Domingo, Lake Rose, INAGUA, Great Inagua I., Matthew Town, Mouchoir Bank, Silver Bank, Banes, Antilla, La Lucrecia, Moa, Mayari, Baracoa, Navidad Bank, Silver Bank Passage

Tropic of Cancer

Guantánamo, GUANTANAMO BAY (U.S.A.), Paso de los Vientos (Windward Passage), Cap-Haïtien, Monte Cristi, LA ISABELA, Santiago de los Caballeros, Puerto Plata, San Francisco de Macorís, Milwaukee Deep 9200, Puerto Rico Trench, Jean Rabel, Port-de-Paix, Fort Liberté, La Vega, Nagua, Samaná, Jamaica Channel, Jérémie, Gonaïves, Hinche, Pico Duarte 3175, HAÏTISES, Sánchez, Sabana de la Mar, Aguadilla, Arecibo, Bayamón, SAN JUAN, St-Marc, ARMANDO BERMUDEZ, Hato Mayor, C. Engaño, Carolina, St. Thomas, Anegada, Virgin Gorda, St. Croix, Île de la Gonâve, PORT-AU-PRINCE, DOMINICAN REP., San Pedro de Macorís, Higüey, Fajardo, Road Town, Tortola, Navassa I. (U.S.A.), Dame Marie, Massif de la Hotte, San Juan, 2880, L. Enriquillo, SIERRA DE BAHORUCO, Barahona, La Romana, Mayagüez, PUERTO RICO (U.S.A.), Ponce, Caguas, Vieques, Guayama, Charlotte Amalie, Virgin Is. (U.S.A.), Sombrero (U.K.), Anguilla (U.K.), St.-Martin (Fr.), Les Cayes, Aquin, Jacmel, Petit Goâve, Azua de Compostela, San Cristóbal, SANTO DOMINGO, ESTE, B. de Yuma, I. Saona, Isla Mona, Mona Passage, Frederiksted, Christiansted, St. Croix (U.S.A.), St. Eustatius (Neth.), Saba (Neth.), St. Maarten (Neth.), St.-Barthélemy (Fr.), Barbuda, Pointe-à-Gravois, Î. à Vache, Pedernales, I. Beata, C. Beata, Hispaniola, ANTIGUA & BARBUDA, Basseterre 1156, ST. KITTS & NEVIS, St. John's, Antigua, Nevis, Redonda, Montserrat (U.K.), Soufrière Hills 914, Guadeloupe Passage, Beata Ridge, Antilles, Ste-Rose, Le Moule, La Désirade, GUADELOUPE (Fr.) 1467, Pointe-à-Pitre, Basse-Terre, Marie-Galante (Fr.), Grand-Bourg, I. des Saintes (Fr.), Dominica Passage, Portsmouth, MORNE DIABLOTIN 1447, DOMINICA, MORNE TROIS PITONS, Roseau, Martinique Passage, I. de Aves (Venezuela), Mt. Pelée 1397, Ste-Marie, Le François, Fort-de-France, Rivière-Pilote, MARTINIQUE (Fr.), St. Lucia Channel, Castries, Soufrière, 950, ST. LUCIA, St. Vincent Passage, Soufrière 1234, St. Vincent, Speightstown 340, Kingstown, Bridgetown, BARBADOS, Bequia, ST. VINCENT & THE GRENADINES, Canouan, Carriacou, The Grenadines, St. George's, 840, GRENADA

Venezuelan Basin, CARIBBEAN SEA, Colombian Basin, Aves Ridge, Leeward Islands, Lesser Antilles, Windward Islands, Leeward Antilles

ABC Islands, Oranjestad, Aruba (Neth.), Curaçao, Bonaire, Willemstad, NETH. ANTILLES, Pta. Gallinas, MACUIRA, C. San Román, Pen. de Paraguaná, Punto Fijo, ARC. LOS ROQUES, Is. Las Aves (Ven.), Is. Los Roques (Ven.), I. Orchila (Ven.), I. Blanquilla (Ven.), Is. Los Hermanos (Ven.), Is. Los Testigos (Ven.), Tobago, Scarborough, Galera Point, Port of Spain, Trinidad, TRINIDAD & TOBAGO, Serpent's Mouth

COLOMBIA, Pta. Gallinas, Ríohacha, Uribia, GUAJIRA, Pen. de la Guajira, Santa Marta, Isla de Salamanca, Ciénaga, SA. NEVADA DE STA. MARTA, San Juan, Maicao, Golfo de Venezuela, Pta. Espada, Punta Cardón, Golfete de Coro, Coro, Puerto Cumarebo, La Vela, FALCÓN, Tucacas, Puerto Cabello, MARACAY, Maiquetía, La Guaira, CARACAS, MIRANDA, Cumaná, SUCRE, Carúpano, Güiria, G. de Paria, San Fernando, Río Claro, Arima, BARRAN-QUILLA, Soledad, Sabanalarga, Baranoa, Fundación, ATLÁNTICO, Calamar, MAGDALENA, Plato, Zambrano, El Carmen, Sincé, Mompós, Magangué, El Banco, Corozal, Sincelejo, San Marcos, Planeta Rica, Ayapel, Caucasia, Ciénaga, Valledupar, Agustín Codazzi, CÉSAR, Santa Marta, Sierra Nevada de Santa Marta 5775, La Concepción, Villa del Rosario, Machiques, Lago de Maracaibo, MARACAIBO, Santa Rita, Cabimas, Ciudad Ojeda, ZULIA, Mene Grande, Trujillo, LARA, Baragua, CERRO SAROCHE, YARACUY, BARQUISIMETO, San Felipe, Yaritagua, VALENCIA, Villa de Cura, Maracay, CARABOBO, La Victoria, San Juan de los Morros, Altagracia de Orituco, Los Teques, La Cruz, Barcelona, Maturín, MONAGAS, TRINIDAD & TOBAGO, Pariagúan, El Tigre, ANZOÁTEGUI, Ciudad Guayana, Soledad, Ciudad Bolívar, Upata, El Pao, Sierra Imataca, El Callao, Tumeremo, VENEZUELA, Orinoco, Embalse de Guri, AMACURO, DELTA, Tucupita

West from Greenwich, COPYRIGHT PHILIP'S

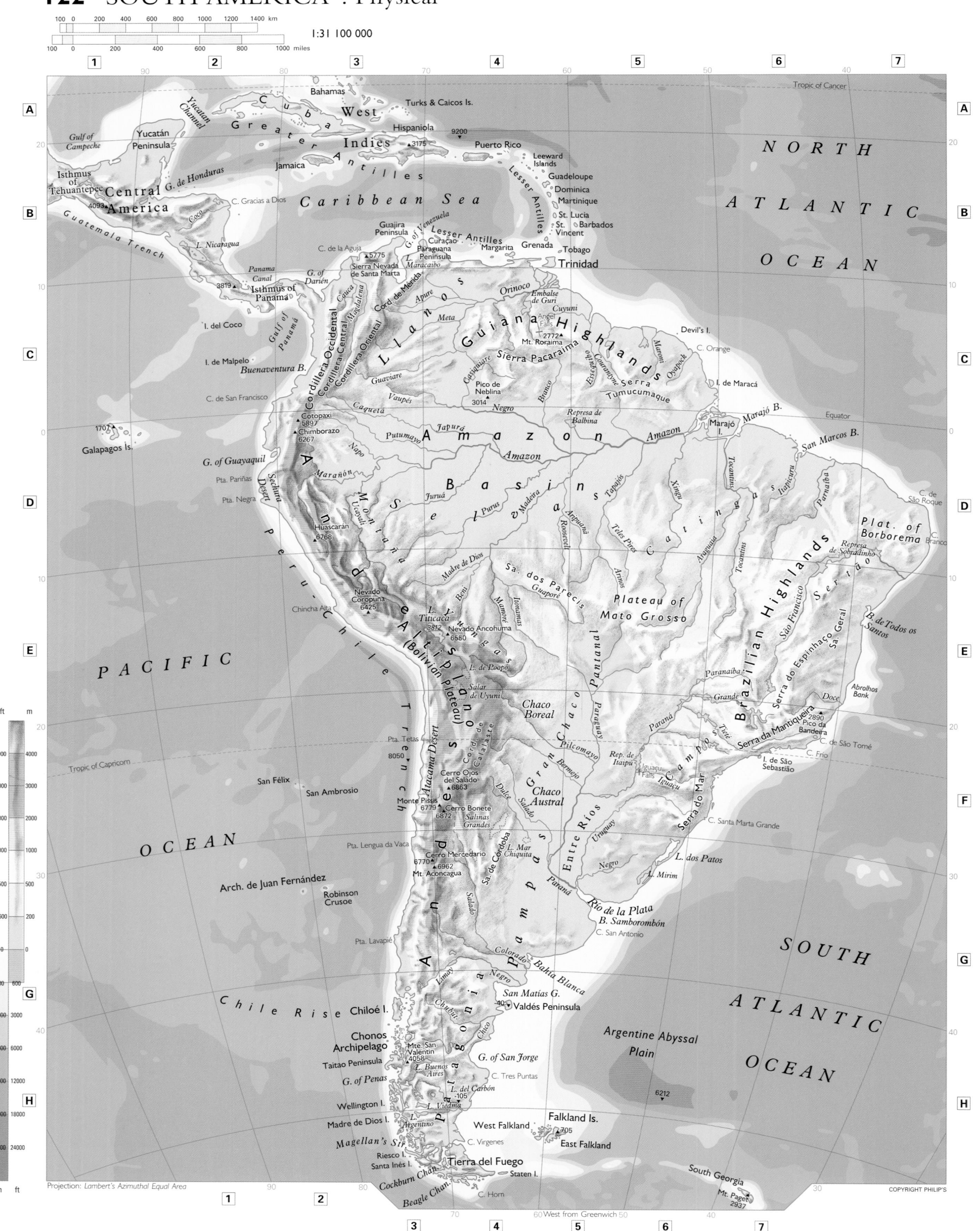

100 0 200 400 600 800 1000 1200 1400 km
100 0 200 400 600 800 1000 miles
1:31 100 000

Projection: Lambert's Azimuthal Equal Area

COPYRIGHT PHILIP'S

1:31 100 000

100 0 200 400 600 800 1000 1200 1400 km

100 0 200 400 600 800 1000 miles

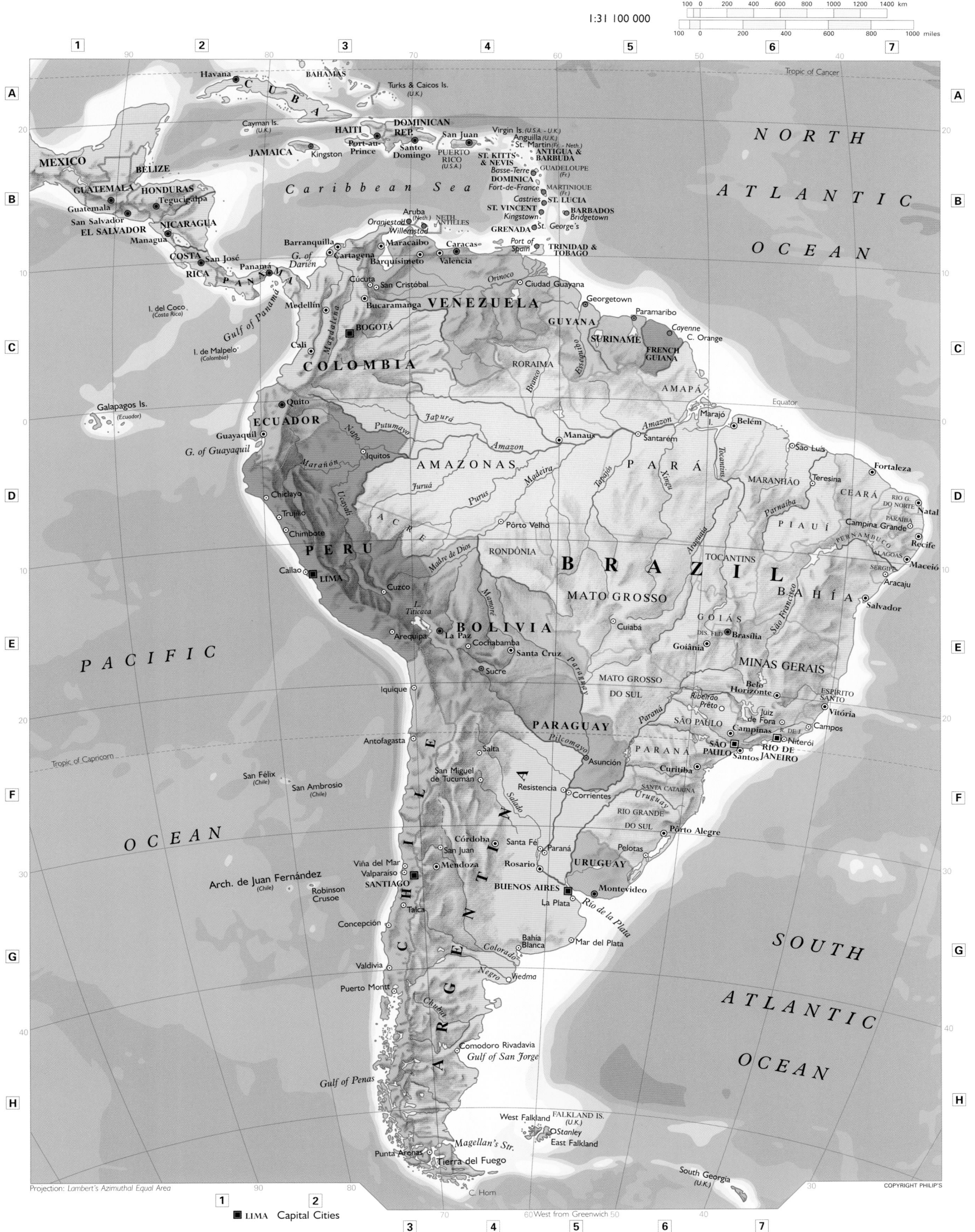

Tropic of Cancer

Havana
CUBA
BAHAMAS
Turks & Caicos Is.
(U.K.)

NORTH

Cayman Is.
(U.K.)
HAITI
DOMINICAN
REP.
San Juan
Virgin Is. (U.S.A. - U.K.)
Anguilla (U.K.)
St. Martin (Fr. - Neth.)
ANTIGUA &
BARBUDA

ATLANTIC

MEXICO
BELIZE
JAMAICA
Kingston
Port-au-
Prince
Santo
Domingo
PUERTO
RICO
(U.S.A.)
ST. KITTS
& NEVIS
Basse-Terre
DOMINICA
GUADELOUPE
(Fr.)

GUATEMALA
HONDURAS
Tegucigalpa
Caribbean Sea
Fort-de-France
MARTINIQUE
(Fr.)
Castries
ST. LUCIA

OCEAN

Guatemala
San Salvador
EL SALVADOR
NICARAGUA
Managua
ST. VINCENT
Kingstown
BARBADOS
Bridgetown

COSTA
RICA
San José
Panamá
PANAMA
Aruba
(Neth.)
Oranjestad
Willemstad
NETH.
ANTILLES
GRENADA
St. George's
Port of
Spain
TRINIDAD &
TOBAGO

I. del Coco
(Costa Rica)
G. of Darién
Barranquilla
Cartagena
Maracaibo
Caracas
Valencia
Orinoco

Gulf of Panamá
Medellín
Cúcuta
Bucaramanga
San Cristóbal
Barquisimeto
Ciudad Guayana

I. de Malpelo
(Colombia)
Cali
BOGOTÁ
VENEZUELA
GUYANA
Georgetown
Paramaribo
Cayenne
C. Orange

COLOMBIA
SURINAME
FRENCH
GUIANA
RORAIMA

Galapagos Is.
(Ecuador)
Quito
ECUADOR
Putumayo
Napo
Japurá
Branco
AMAPÁ
Equator

Guayaquil
G. of Guayaquil
Marañón
Iquitos
Amazon
AMAZONAS
Manaus
Amazon
Santarém
Belém
Marajó I.
São Luís

Chiclayo
Trujillo
Juruá
Ucayali
Purus
Madeira
PARÁ
Tocantins
MARANHÃO
Teresina
Fortaleza

Chimbote
ACRE
Pôrto Velho
RONDÔNIA
Xingu
Araguaia
PIAUÍ
CEARÁ
RIO G.
DO NORTE
Natal

PERU
Madre de Dios
BRAZIL
TOCANTINS
PARAÍBA
Campina
Grande
Recife

Callao
LIMA
Cuzco
Mamoré
MATO GROSSO
GOIÁS
São Francisco
PERNAMBUCO
ALAGOAS
SERGIPE
Maceió

Arequipa
L. Titicaca
La Paz
BOLIVIA
Cochabamba
Santa Cruz
Cuiabá
DIS. FED.
BRASÍLIA
Goiânia
BAHÍA
Aracaju
Salvador

Iquique
Sucre
MATO GROSSO
DO SUL
MINAS GERAIS
Belo
Horizonte
ESPÍRITO
SANTO

PACIFIC
Antofagasta
Salta
Paraguay
PARAGUAY
Paraná
Ribeirão
Prêto
SÃO PAULO
Juiz
de Fora
Vitória
Campos

San Félix
(Chile)
San Ambrosio
(Chile)
San Miguel
de Tucumán
Asunción
PARANÁ
SÃO
PAULO
Campinas
R. DE J.
Niterói
RIO DE
JANEIRO

OCEAN
Resistencia
Corrientes
Uruguay
SANTA CATARINA
Curitiba
Santos

Córdoba
San Juan
Santa Fé
Paraná
RIO GRANDE
DO SUL
Pôrto Alegre

Arch. de Juan Fernández
(Chile)
Robinson
Crusoe
Viña del Mar
Valparaíso
SANTIAGO
Mendoza
Rosario
Pelotas

Talca
CHILE
BUENOS AIRES
URUGUAY
Montevideo

Concepción
ARGENTINA
La Plata
Río de la Plata

Tropic of Capricorn
Pilcomayo
Salado
Bahía
Blanca
Mar del Plata

SOUTH

Valdivia
Colorado
Negro
Viedma

Puerto Montt

ATLANTIC

Comodoro Rivadavia
Gulf of San Jorge

Gulf of Penas

OCEAN

Magellan's Str.
West Falkland
FALKLAND IS.
(U.K.)
Stanley
East Falkland

Punta Arenas
Tierra del Fuego

C. Horn

South Georgia
(U.K.)

Projection: Lambert's Azimuthal Equal Area
COPYRIGHT PHILIP'S

60 West from Greenwich 50

LIMA Capital Cities

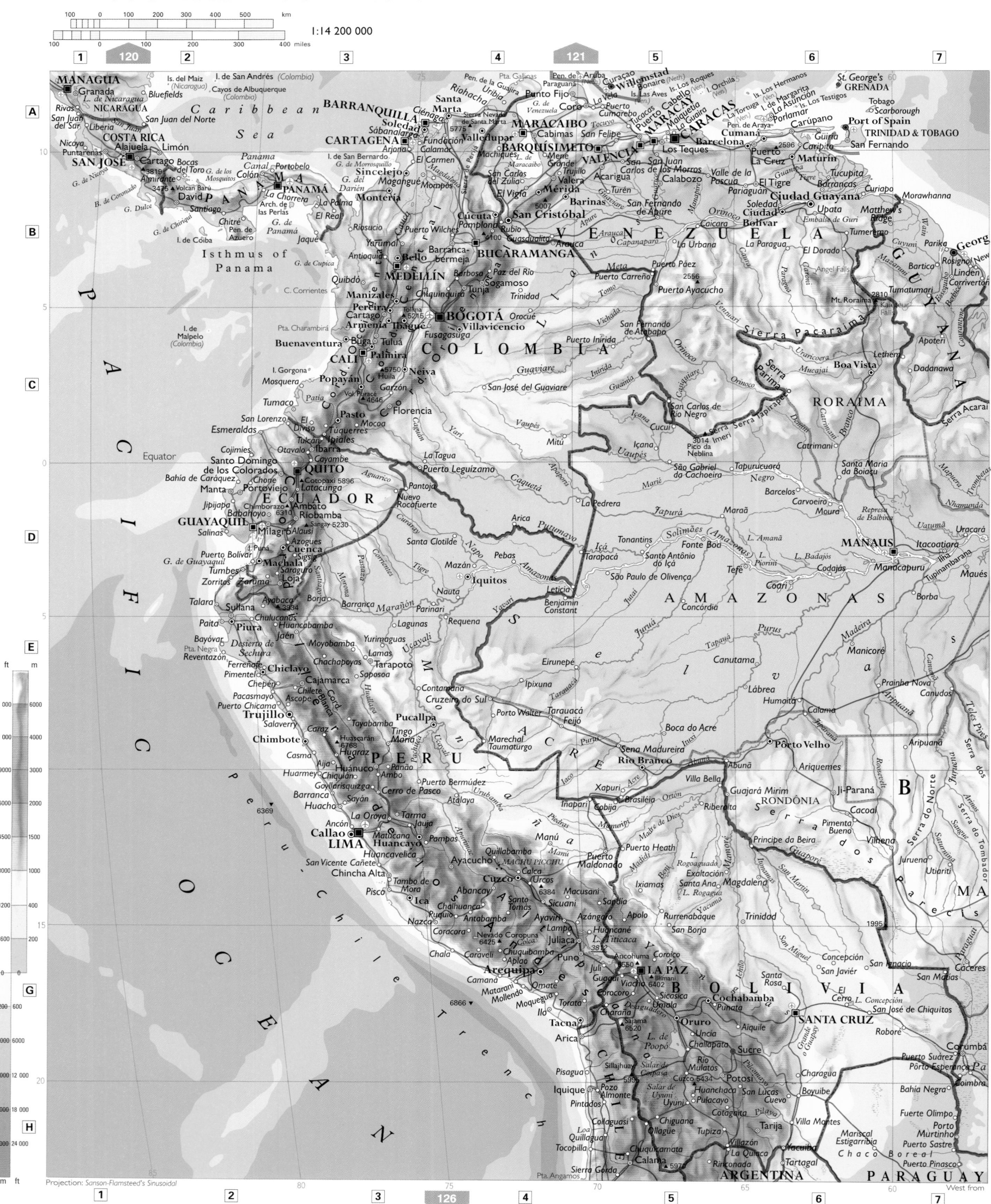

1:14 200 000

Projection: Sanson-Flamsteed's Sinusoidal

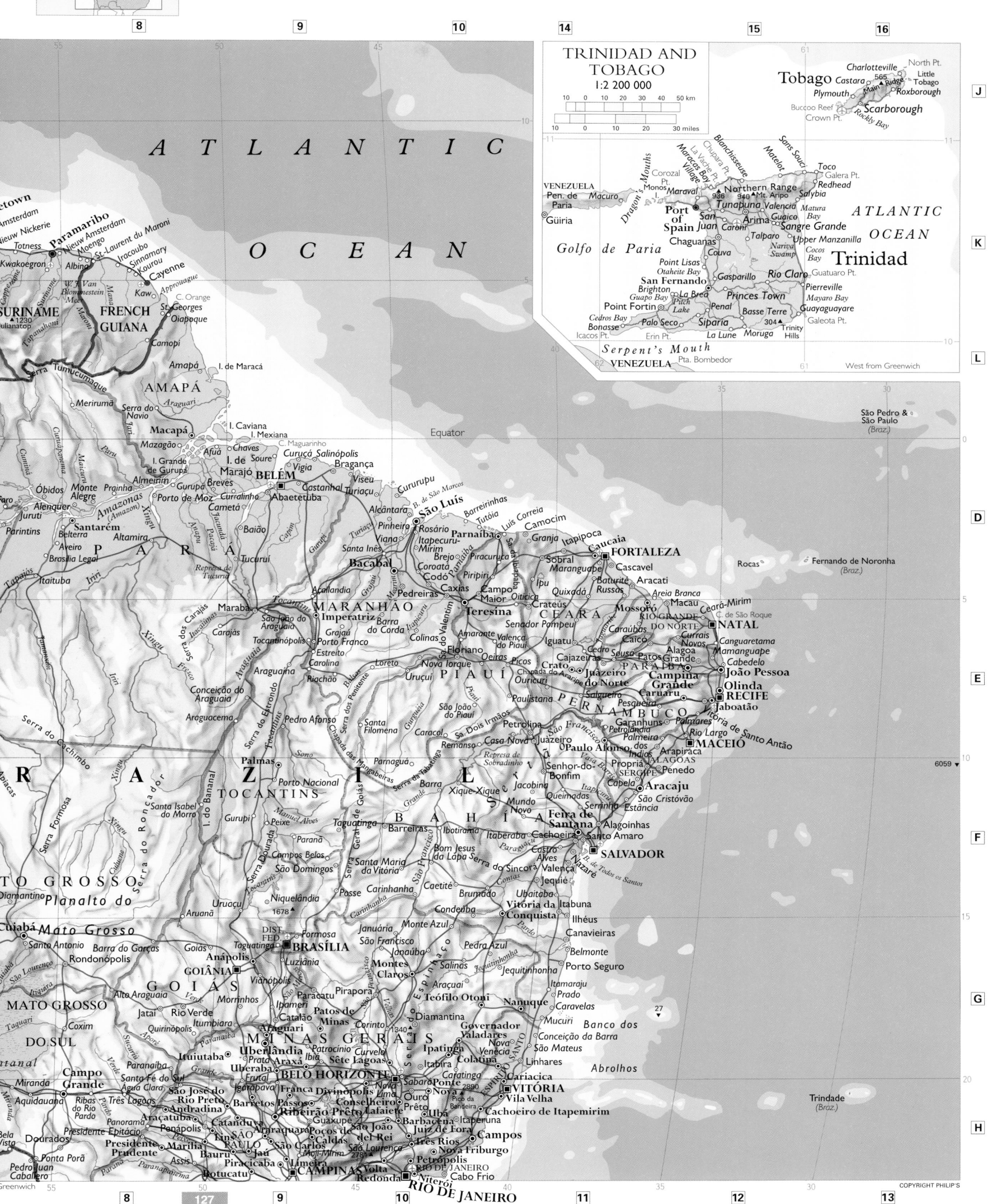

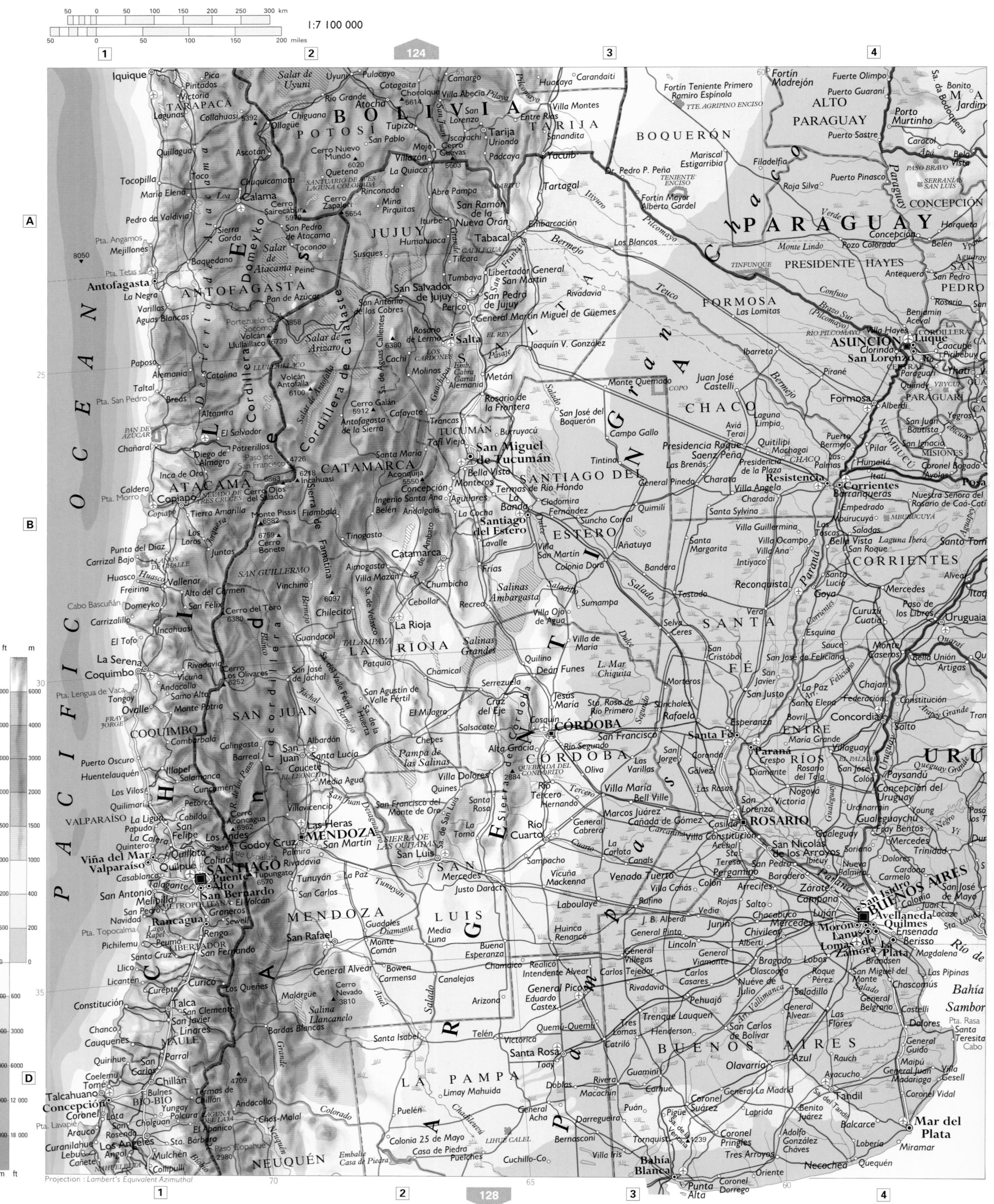

1:7 100 000

Projection : Lambert's Equivalent Azimuthal

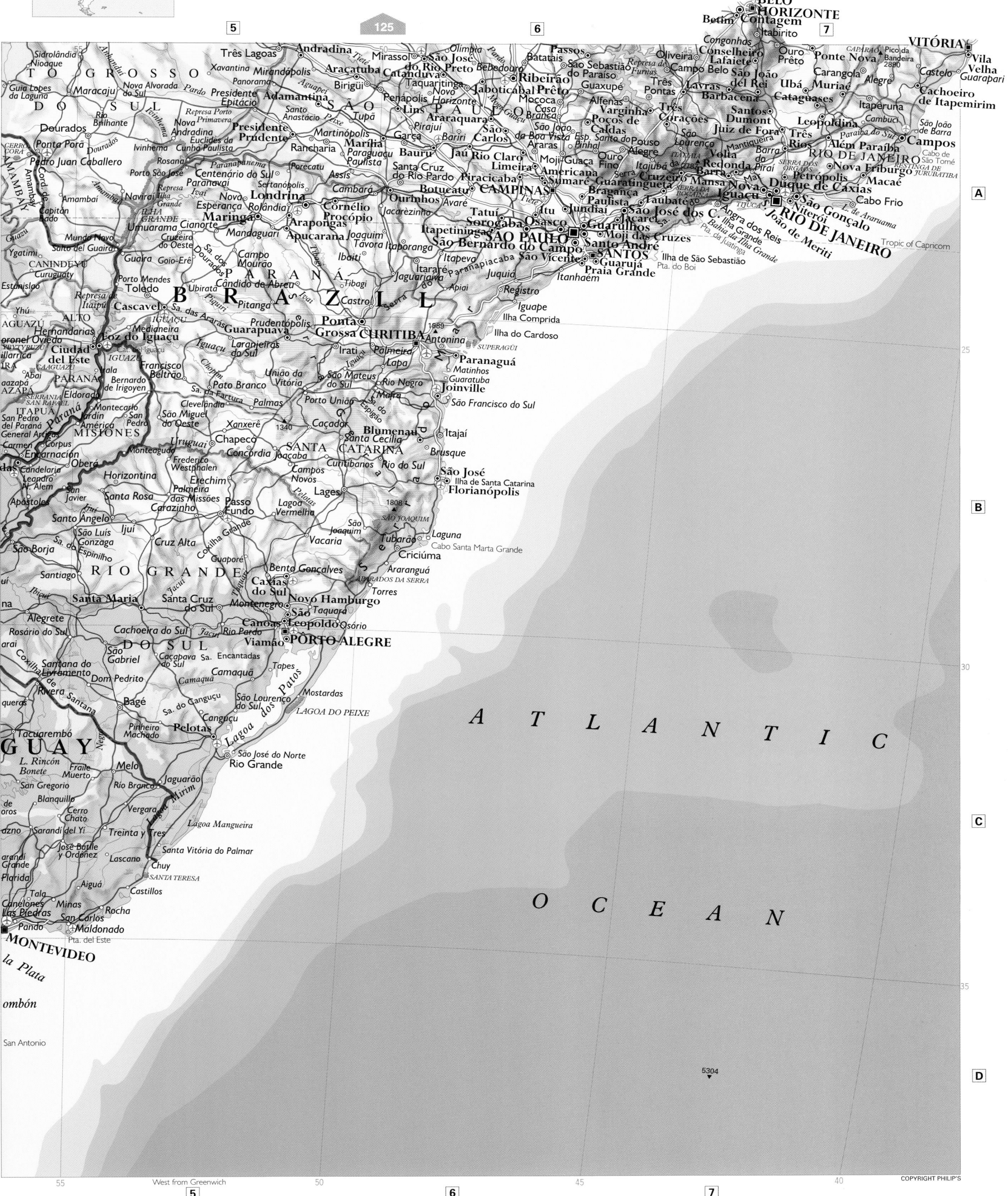

5   125   6   7

BELO
HORIZONTE
Betim Contagem Itabirito

Sidrolândia Nioaque   Olímpia   Passos   Batatais   Congonhas   Ouro   Ponte Nova   7   VITÓRIA
Guia Lopes   Três Lagoas   Andradina   Mirassol   São José   Oliveira   Conselheiro   Prêto   CAPARÃO Pico da   Vila
da Laguna   Xavantina Mirandópolis   Araçatuba Catanduva do Rio Prêto   Bebedouro   Ribeirão   Campo Belo São João   Carangola   Bandeira Velha
Maracaju   Panorama   Taquaritinga   Guaxupé   del Rei   Ubá   Muriaé   2890   Castelo   Guarapari
TO GROSSO   Nova Alvorada   Presidente   Biriguí   Taubaté   Jaboticabal Prêto   Lavras   Barbacena   Cataguases   de Itapemirim
Represa Porto   Epitácio   Lins   Araraquara   Alfenas Varginha   Três   Leopoldina   Cachoeiro
Santo   Adamantina   São João   Pouso   Corações   Juiz de Fora   Itaperuna   Cambuci
DO   Rio   Nova   Anastácio   Paixe   Tupã   Bauru   da Boa Vista   Esp. Santo do   Alegre   Volta   Três   Alem Paraíba   Campos

COPYRIGHT PHILIP'S

1:14 200 000

100 0 100 200 300 400 500 km
100 0 100 200 300 400 miles

Projection: Sanson-Flamsteed's Sinusoidal

West from Greenwich

COPYRIGHT PHILIP'S

ft m

12 000 4000
9000 3000
6000 2000
4500 1500
3000 1000
1200 400
600 200
0 0
200 600
2000 6000
4000 12 000
6000 18 000
8000 24 000
m ft

PARAGUAY

Chaco Boreal

Chaco Central

ASUNCIÓN

SÃO PAULO

RIO DE JANEIRO

NOVA IGUAÇU

CURITIBA

Ribeirão Prêto

Araraquara

Marília

Londrina

Maringá

Cascavel

Ponta Grossa

Florianópolis

Blumenau

Joinville

PÔRTO ALEGRE

Santa Maria

RIO GRANDE DO SUL

SANTA CATARINA

Pelotas

Rio Grande

URUGUAY

MONTEVIDEO

Salto

Paysandú

Durazno

Mercedes

Maldonado

BUENOS AIRES

La Plata

Rosario

Santa Fe

Paraná

CÓRDOBA

MENDOZA

SANTIAGO

Valparaíso

Viña del Mar

Rancagua

Talca

Concepción

Temuco

Valdivia

Puerto Montt

I. de Chiloé

San Miguel de Tucumán

Salta

Santiago del Estero

Catamarca

La Rioja

San Juan

San Luis

Río Cuarto

Bahía Blanca

Neuquén

Mar del Plata

Necochea

Tandil

Azul

Olavarría

Santa Rosa

General Roca

Viedma

Carmen de Patagones

Puerto Madryn

Trelew

Rawson

Pen. Valdés

Golfo San Matías

Comodoro Rivadavia

Golfo San Jorge

Puerto Deseado

Puerto San Julián

Puerto Santa Cruz

Río Gallegos

Punta Arenas

Ushuaia

Tierra del Fuego

Isla Grande de Tierra del Fuego

I. de Los Estados (Staten I.)

C. de Hornos (C. Horn)

Estrecho de Magallanes (Magellan's Str.)

Antofagasta

Calama

Tropic of Capricorn

Tarija

Villa Montes

Iquique (Peru-Chile Trench)

PACIFIC OCEAN

SOUTH ATLANTIC OCEAN

Argentine Abyssal Plain

FALKLAND ISLANDS (ISLAS MALVINAS) (U.K.)

West Falkland

East Falkland

Stanley

Port Darwin

South Georgia (U.K.)

Mt. Paget 2934

Grytviken

King Edward Pt.

Bird I.

Cerro Aconcagua 6960

Mt. San Valentín 4058

Cerro Fitz Roy 3405

INDEX TO WORLD MAPS

How to use the index

The index contains the names of all the principal places and features shown on the World Maps. Each name is followed by an additional entry in italics giving the country or region within which it is located. The alphabetical order of names composed of two or more words is governed primarily by the first word and then by the second. This is an example of the rule:

Miquelon *St-P. &M.* **105** C8
Mir *Niger* **83** C7
Mīr Kūh *Iran* **71** E8
Mīr Shahdād *Iran* **71** E8
Mira *Italy* **41** C9

Physical features composed of a proper name (Erie) and a description (Lake) are positioned alphabetically by the proper name. The description is positioned after the proper name and is usually abbreviated:

Erie, L. *N. Amer.* **114** D4

Where a description forms part of a settlement or administrative name however, it is always written in full and put in its true alphabetic position:

Mount Morris *U.S.A.* **114** D7

Names beginning with M' and Mc are indexed as if they were spelled Mac. Names beginning St. are alphabetised under Saint, but Sankt, Sint, Sant', Santa and San are all spelt in full and are alphabetised accordingly. If the same place name occurs two or more times in the index and all are in the same country, each is followed by the name of the administrative subdivision in which it is located. For example:

Jackson *Ky., U.S.A.* **113** G12
Jackson *Mich., U.S.A.* **113** D11
Jackson *Minn., U.S.A.* **112** D6

The number in bold type which follows each name in the index refers to the number of the map page where that feature or place will be found. This is usually the largest scale at which the place or feature appears.

The letter and figure which are in bold type immediately after the page number give the grid square on the map page, within which the feature is situated. The letter represents the latitude and the figure the longitude. A lower case letter immediately after the page number refers to an inset map on that page.

In some cases the feature itself may fall within the specified square, while the name is outside. This is usually the case only with features which are larger than a grid square.

Rivers are indexed to their mouths or confluences, and carry the symbol → after their names. The following symbols are also used in the index: ■ country, ▨ overseas territory or dependency, □ first order administrative area, △ national park, ⌓ other park (provincial park, nature reserve or game reserve), ✈ (LHR) principal airport (and location identifier), ❂ aboriginal land.

How to pronounce place names

English-speaking people usually have no difficulty in reading and pronouncing correctly English place names. However, foreign place name pronunciations may present many problems. Such problems can be minimised by following some simple rules. However, these rules cannot be applied to all situations, and there will be many exceptions.

1. In general, stress each syllable equally, unless your experience suggests otherwise.
2. Pronounce the letter 'a' as a broad 'a' as in 'arm'.
3. Pronounce the letter 'e' as a short 'e' as in 'elm'.
4. Pronounce the letter 'i' as a cross between a short 'i' and long 'e', as the two 'i's in 'California'.
5. Pronounce the letter 'o' as an intermediate 'o' as in 'soft'.
6. Pronounce the letter 'u' as an intermediate 'u' as in 'sure'.
7. Pronounce consonants hard, except in the Romance-language areas where 'g's are likely to be pronounced softly like 'j' in 'jam'; 'j' itself may be pronounced as 'y'; and 'x's may be pronounced as 'h'.
8. For names in mainland China, pronounce 'q' like the 'ch' in 'chin', 'x' like the 'sh' in 'she', 'zh' like the 'j' in 'jam', and 'z' as if it were spelled 'dz'. In general pronounce 'a' as in 'father', 'e' as in 'but', 'i' as in 'keep', 'o' as in 'or', and 'u' as in 'rule'.

Moreover, English has no diacritical marks (accent and pronunciation signs), although some languages do. The following is a brief and general guide to the pronunciation of those most frequently used in the principal Western European languages.

		Pronunciation as in
French	é	day and shows that the e is to be pronounced; e.g. Orléans.
	è	mare
	î	used over any vowel and does not affect pronunciation; shows contraction of the name, usually omission of 's' following a vowel.
	ç	's' before 'a', 'o' and 'u'.
	ë, ï, ü	over 'e', 'i' and 'u' when they are used with another vowel and shows that each is to be pronounced.
German	ä	fate
	ö	fur
	ü	no English equivalent; like French 'tu'
Italian	à, é	over vowels and indicates stress.
Portuguese	ã, õ	vowels pronounced nasally.
	ç	boss
	á	shows stress
	ô	shows that a vowel has an 'i' or 'u' sound combined with it.
Spanish	ñ	canyon
	ü	pronounced as w and separately from adjoining vowels.
	á	usually indicates that this is a stressed vowel.

Abbreviations

A.C.T. – Australian Capital Territory
A.R. – Autonomous Region
Afghan. – Afghanistan
Afr. – Africa
Ala. – Alabama
Alta. – Alberta
Amer. – America(n)
Arch. – Archipelago
Ariz. – Arizona
Ark. – Arkansas
Atl. Oc. – Atlantic Ocean
B. – Baie, Bahía, Bay, Bucht, Bugt
B.C. – British Columbia
Bangla. – Bangladesh
Barr. – Barrage
Bos.-H. – Bosnia-Herzegovina
C. – Cabo, Cap, Cape, Coast
C.A.R. – Central African Republic
C. Prov. – Cape Province
Calif. – California
Cat. – Catarata
Cent. – Central
Chan. – Channel
Colo. – Colorado
Conn. – Connecticut
Cord. – Cordillera
Cr. – Creek
Czech. – Czech Republic
D.C. – District of Columbia
Del. – Delaware
Dem. – Democratic
Dep. – Dependency
Des. – Desert
Dét. – Détroit
Dist. – District
Dj. – Djebel
Domin. – Dominica
Dom. Rep. – Dominican Republic
E. – East
E. Salv. – El Salvador
Eq. Guin. – Equatorial Guinea
Est. – Estrecho
Falk. Is. – Falkland Is.
Fd. – Fjord
Fla. – Florida
Fr. – French
G. – Golfe, Golfo, Gulf, Guba, Gebel
Ga. – Georgia
Gt. – Great, Greater
Guinea-Biss. – Guinea-Bissau
H.K. – Hong Kong
H.P. – Himachal Pradesh
Hants. – Hampshire
Harb. – Harbor, Harbour
Hd. – Head
Hts. – Heights
I.(s). – Île, Ilha, Insel, Isla, Island, Isle
Ill. – Illinois
Ind. – Indiana
Ind. Oc. – Indian Ocean
Ivory C. – Ivory Coast
J. – Jabal, Jebel
Jaz. – Jazīrah
Junc. – Junction
K. – Kap, Kapp
Kans. – Kansas
Kep. – Kepulauan
Ky. – Kentucky
L. – Lac, Lacul, Lago, Lagoa, Lake, Limni, Loch, Lough
La. – Louisiana
Ld. – Land
Liech. – Liechtenstein
Lux. – Luxembourg
Mad. P. – Madhya Pradesh
Madag. – Madagascar
Man. – Manitoba
Mass. – Massachusetts
Md. – Maryland
Me. – Maine
Medit. S. – Mediterranean Sea
Mich. – Michigan
Minn. – Minnesota
Miss. – Mississippi
Mo. – Missouri
Mont. – Montana
Mozam. – Mozambique
Mt.(s) – Mont, Montaña, Mountain
Mte. – Monte
Mti. – Monti
N. – Nord, Norte, North, Northern, Nouveau
N.B. – New Brunswick
N.C. – North Carolina
N. Cal. – New Caledonia
N. Dak. – North Dakota
N.H. – New Hampshire
N.I. – North Island
N.J. – New Jersey
N. Mex. – New Mexico
N.S. – Nova Scotia
N.S.W. – New South Wales
N.W.T. – North West Territory
N.Y. – New York
N.Z. – New Zealand
Nac. – Nacional
Nat. – National
Nebr. – Nebraska
Neths. – Netherlands
Nev. – Nevada
Nfld. & L. – Newfoundland and Labrador
Nic. – Nicaragua
O. – Oued, Ouadi
Occ. – Occidentale
Okla. – Oklahoma
Ont. – Ontario
Or. – Orientale
Oreg. – Oregon
Os. – Ostrov
Oz. – Ozero
P. – Pass, Passo, Pasul, Pulau
P.E.I. – Prince Edward Island
Pa. – Pennsylvania
Pac. Oc. – Pacific Ocean
Papua N.G. – Papua New Guinea
Pass. – Passage
Peg. – Pegunungan
Pen. – Peninsula, Péninsule
Phil. – Philippines
Pk. – Peak
Plat. – Plateau
Prov. – Province, Provincial
Pt. – Point
Pta. – Ponta, Punta
Pte. – Pointe
Qué. – Québec
Queens. – Queensland
R. – Rio, River
R.I. – Rhode Island
Ra. – Range
Raj. – Rajasthan
Recr. – Recreational, Récréatif
Reg. – Region
Rep. – Republic
Res. – Reserve, Reservoir
Rhld-Pfz. – Rheinland-Pfalz
S. – South, Southern, Sur
Si. Arabia – Saudi Arabia
S.C. – South Carolina
S. Dak. – South Dakota
S.I. – South Island
S. Leone – Sierra Leone
Sa. – Serra, Sierra
Sask. – Saskatchewan
Scot. – Scotland
Sd. – Sound
Sev. – Severnaya
Sib. – Siberia
Sprs. – Springs
St. – Saint
Sta. – Santa
Ste. – Sainte
Sto. – Santo
Str. – Strait, Stretto
Switz. – Switzerland
Tas. – Tasmania
Tenn. – Tennessee
Terr. – Territory, Territoire
Tex. – Texas
Tg. – Tanjung
Trin. & Tob. – Trinidad & Tobago
U.A.E. – United Arab Emirates
U.K. – United Kingdom
U.S.A. – United States of America
Ut. P. – Uttar Pradesh
Va. – Virginia
Vdkhr. – Vodokhranilishche
Vdskh. – Vodoskhovyshche
Vf. – Vírful
Vic. – Victoria
Vol. – Volcano
Vt. – Vermont
W. – Wadi, West
W. Va. – West Virginia
Wall. & F. Is. – Wallis and Futuna Is.
Wash. – Washington
Wis. – Wisconsin
Wlkp. – Wielkopolski
Wyo. – Wyoming
Yorks. – Yorkshire

A

A 'Âli an Nîl □ Sudan 81 F3
A Baña Spain 36 C2
A Cañiza Spain 36 C2
A Coruña Spain 36 B2
A Coruña □ Spain 36 B2
A Cruz do Incio Spain 36 C3
A Estrada Spain 36 C2
A Fonsagrada Spain 36 B3
A Guarda Spain 36 D2
A Gudiña Spain 36 C3
A Pobre Spain 36 C3
A Ramallosa Spain 36 C2
A Rúa Spain 36 C3
A Serra de Outes Spain 36 C2
Aabenraa Denmark 11 J3
Aabybro Denmark 11 G3
Aachen Germany 24 E2
Aalborg Denmark 11 G3
Aalborg Bugt Denmark 11 H4
Aalen Germany 25 G6
Aalestrup Denmark 11 H3
Aalst Belgium 17 D4
Aalten Neths. 17 C6
Aalter Belgium 17 C3
Äänekoski Finland 8 E21
Aarau Switz. 25 H4
Aarberg Switz. 25 H3
Aare → Switz. 25 H4
Aargau □ Switz. 25 H4
Aarhus = Århus Denmark 11 H4
Aars Denmark 11 H3
Aarschot Belgium 17 D4
Aba China 58 A3
Aba Dem. Rep. of the Congo 86 B3
Aba Nigeria 83 D6
Âbâ, Jazîrat Sudan 81 E3
Abaco I. Bahamas 120 A4
Abadab, J. Sudan 80 D4
Ābādān Iran 71 D6
Abade Ethiopia 81 F4
Ābādeh Iran 71 D7
Abadín Spain 36 B3
Abadla Algeria 78 B5
Abaetetuba Brazil 125 D9
Abagnar Qi = Xilinhot China 56 C9
Abah, Tanjung Indonesia 63 K18
Abai Paraguay 127 B4
Abak Nigeria 83 E6
Abakaliki Nigeria 83 D6
Abakan Russia 53 D10
Abala Niger 83 C5
Abalak Niger 83 B6
Abalemma Niger 83 B6
Abana Turkey 72 B6
Abancay Peru 124 F4
Abano Terme Italy 41 C8
Abarán Spain 39 G3
Abariringa Kiribati 96 H10
Abarqū Iran 71 D7
Abasha Georgia 35 J6
Abashiri Japan 54 B12
Abashiri-Wan Japan 54 C12
Abaújszántó Hungary 28 B6
Abava → Latvia 30 A8
Ābay = Nîl el Azraq → Sudan 81 D3
Abay Kazakhstan 52 E8
Abaya, L. Ethiopia 81 F4
Abaza Russia 52 D9
Abbadia di Fiastra ⌓ Italy 41 E10
Abbadia San Salvatore Italy 41 F8
'Abbāsābād Iran 71 C8
Abbay = Nîl el Azraq → Sudan 81 D3
Abbaye, Pt. U.S.A. 112 B9
Abbé, L. Ethiopia 81 E5
Abbeville France 19 B8
Abbeville Ala., U.S.A. 117 F12
Abbeville La., U.S.A. 116 G8
Abbeville S.C., U.S.A. 117 D13
Abbeyfeale Ireland 12 D2
Abbiategrasso Italy 40 C5
Abbot Ice Shelf Antarctica 5 D16
Abbotsford Canada 102 D4
Abbottabad Pakistan 68 B5
ABC Islands = Netherlands Antilles ☒ W. Indies 124 A5
Abd al Kūrī Yemen 75 E5
Ābdānān Iran 73 F12
Ābdar Iran 71 D7
'Abdolābād Iran 71 C8
Abdulpur Bangla. 69 G13
Abéché Chad 79 F10
Abejar Spain 38 D2
Abekr Sudan 81 E2
Abel Tasman △ N.Z. 91 D4
Abengourou Ivory C. 82 D4
Abenójar Spain 37 G6
Åbenrå = Aabenraa Denmark 11 J3
Abensberg Germany 25 G7
Abeokuta Nigeria 83 D5
Aberaeron U.K. 15 E3
Aberayron = Aberaeron U.K. 15 E3
Aberchirder U.K. 13 D6
Abercorn Australia 95 D5
Aberdare U.K. 15 F4
Aberdare △ Kenya 86 C4
Aberdare Ra. Kenya 86 C4
Aberdeen Australia 95 E5
Aberdeen Canada 103 C7
Aberdeen S. Africa 88 E3
Aberdeen U.K. 13 D6
Aberdeen Idaho, U.S.A. 108 E7
Aberdeen Md., U.S.A. 113 F15
Aberdeen Miss., U.S.A. 117 E10
Aberdeen S. Dak., U.S.A. 112 C4
Aberdeen Wash., U.S.A. 110 D3
Aberdeen, City of □ U.K. 13 D6
Aberdeen L. Canada 100 E12
Aberdeenshire □ U.K. 13 D6
Aberdovey = Aberdyfi U.K. 15 E3
Aberdyfi U.K. 15 E3
Aberfeldy U.K. 13 E5
Aberfoyle U.K. 13 E4
Abergavenny U.K. 15 F4
Abergele U.K. 14 D4
Abernathy U.S.A. 116 E4
Abert, L. U.S.A. 108 E3
Aberystwyth U.K. 15 E3
Abhā Si. Arabia 80 D5
Abhar Iran 73 D13
Abhayapuri India 69 F14
Abia □ Nigeria 83 D6
Abide Turkey 47 C11
Abidiya Sudan 80 D3
Abidjan Ivory C. 82 D4
Abilene Kans., U.S.A. 112 F5
Abilene Tex., U.S.A. 116 E5
Abingdon U.K. 15 F6
Abingdon U.S.A. 113 G13
Abington Reef Australia 94 B4
Abitau → Canada 103 B7
Abitibi → Canada 104 B3
Abitibi, L. Canada 104 C4
Abiy Adi Ethiopia 81 E4
Abiyata-Shala △ Ethiopia 81 F4
Abkhaz Republic = Abkhazia □ Georgia 35 J5
Abkhazia □ Georgia 35 J5
Abminga Australia 95 D1
Abnûb Egypt 80 B3
Åbo = Turku Finland 32 B2
Abohar India 68 D6
Aboisso Ivory C. 82 D4
Abomey Benin 83 D5
Abong-Mbang Cameroon 84 D2
Abonnema Nigeria 83 E6
Abony Hungary 28 C5
Aboso Ghana 82 D4
Abou-Deïa Chad 79 F9
Abovian Armenia 35 K7
Aboyne U.K. 13 D6
Abra Pampa Argentina 126 A2
Abraham L. Canada 102 C5
Abrantes Portugal 37 F2
Abreojos, Pta. Mexico 118 B2
Abri Esh Shamâliya, Sudan 80 C3
Abri Janub Kordofân, Sudan 81 E3
Abrolhos, Banco dos Brazil 125 F11
Abrud Romania 28 D8
Abruzzo □ Italy 41 F10
Absaroka Range U.S.A. 108 D9
Abtenau Austria 26 D6
Abu India 68 G5
Abū al Abyad U.A.E. 71 E7
Abū al Khaṣīb Iraq 70 D5
Abū 'Alī Si. Arabia 71 E6
Abū 'Alī → Lebanon 74 A4
Abu Ballas Egypt 80 C2
Abu Deleiq Sudan 81 D3
Abu Dhabi = Abū Ẓāby U.A.E. 71 E7
Abu Dis Sudan 80 D3
Abu Dom Sudan 81 D3
Abū Du'ān Syria 73 D8
Abu el Gaïn, W. → Egypt 74 F2
Abu Fatma, Ras Sudan 80 C4
Abû Gabra Sudan 81 E2
Abu Ga'da, W. → Egypt 74 F1
Abu Gelba Sudan 81 E3
Abu Gubeiha Sudan 81 E3
Abu Habl, Khawr → Sudan 81 E3
Abū Ḩadrīyah Si. Arabia 71 E6
Abu Hamed Sudan 80 D3
Abu Haraz An Nîl el Azraq, Sudan 80 D3
Abu Haraz El Gezira, Sudan 81 E3
Abu Haraz Esh Shamâliya, Sudan 80 D3
Abû Higar Sudan 81 E3
Abū Kamāl Syria 73 E9
Abu Kebîr Egypt 80 H7
Abu Kuleiwat Sudan 81 E2
Abū Madd, Ra's Si. Arabia 70 E3
Abu Matariq Sudan 81 E2
Abu Mendi Ethiopia 81 E4
Abū Mūsā U.A.E. 71 E7
Abū Qaṣr Si. Arabia 70 D3
Abu Qireiya Egypt 80 C4
Abu Qurqâs Egypt 80 B3
Abu Shagara, Ras Sudan 80 C4
Abu Shanab Sudan 81 E2
Abu Simbel Egypt 80 C3
Abū Şukhayr Iraq 73 G11
Abu Sultân Egypt 80 H8
Abu Tabari Sudan 80 D2
Abu Tig Egypt 80 B3
Abu Tiga Sudan 81 E3
Abu Tineitin Sudan 81 E3
Abû Uruq Sudan 81 D3
Abû Zabad Sudan 81 E2
Abū Ẓāby U.A.E. 71 E7
Abū Zeydābād Iran 71 C6
Abuja Nigeria 83 D6
Abukuma-Gawa → Japan 54 E10
Abukuma-Sammyaku Japan 54 F10
Abunã Brazil 124 E5
Abunã → Brazil 124 E5
Abune Yosef Ethiopia 81 E4
Aburo Dem. Rep. of the Congo 86 B3
Abut Hd. N.Z. 91 E3
Abuye Meda Ethiopia 81 E4
Abwong Sudan 81 F3
Åby Sweden 11 F10
Aby, Lagune Ivory C. 82 D4
Abyad Sudan 81 E2
Abyei Sudan 81 F2
Ābyek Iran 71 B6
Acadia △ U.S.A. 113 C19
Açailândia Brazil 125 D9
Acajutla El Salv. 120 D2
Acámbaro Mexico 118 D4
Acanthus Greece 44 F7
Acaponeta Mexico 118 C3
Acapulco Mexico 119 D5
Acaraí, Serra Brazil 124 C7
Acarigua Venezuela 124 B5
Acatlán Mexico 119 D5
Acayucán Mexico 119 D6
Accéglio Italy 40 D4
Accomac U.S.A. 113 G16
Accous France 20 E3
Accra Ghana 83 D4
Accrington U.K. 14 D5
Acebal Argentina 126 C3
Aceh □ Indonesia 62 D1
Acerra Italy 43 B7
Aceuchal Spain 37 G4
Achaia □ Greece 46 C3
Achalpur India 66 J10
Acharnes Greece 46 C5
Acheloos → Greece 46 C3
Acheng China 57 B14
Achenkirch Austria 26 D4
Achensee Austria 26 D4
Achentrias Greece 47 G7
Acher India 68 H5
Achern Germany 25 G4
Achill Hd. Ireland 12 C1
Achill I. Ireland 12 C1
Achim Germany 24 B5
Achinsk Russia 53 D10
Achladokambos Greece 46 D4
Acıgöl Turkey 47 D11
Acıpayam Turkey 47 D11
Acireale Italy 43 E8
Ackerman U.S.A. 117 E10
Acklins I. Bahamas 121 B5
Acme Canada 102 C6
Acme U.S.A. 114 F5
Aconcagua, Cerro Argentina 126 C2
Aconquija, Mt. Argentina 126 B2
Açores, Is. dos Atl. Oc. 78 a
Acornhoek S. Africa 89 C5
Acquapendente Italy 41 F8
Acquasanta Terme Italy 41 F10
Acquasparta Italy 41 F9
Acquaviva delle Fonti Italy 43 B9
Àcqui Terme Italy 40 D5
Acraman, L. Australia 95 E2
Acre = 'Akko Israel 74 C4
Acre □ Brazil 124 E4
Acre → Brazil 124 E5
Acri Italy 43 C9
Acs Hungary 28 C3
Actinolite Canada 114 B7
Actium Greece 46 C2
Acton Canada 114 C4
Ad Dafinah Si. Arabia 80 C5
Ad Daghghāran Iraq 73 G11
Ad Dammām Si. Arabia 71 E6
Ad Dāmūr Lebanon 74 B4
Ad Dawādimī Si. Arabia 70 E5
Ad Dawḩah Qatar 71 E6
Ad Dawr Iraq 73 E10
Ad Dir'īyah Si. Arabia 70 E5
Ad Dīwānīyah Iraq 73 F11
Ad Dujayl Iraq 73 F11
Ad Duwayd Si. Arabia 70 D4
Ada Ghana 83 D5
Ada Serbia 28 E5
Ada Minn., U.S.A. 112 B5
Ada Okla., U.S.A. 116 D6
Adabiya Egypt 74 F1
Adair, C. Canada 101 C17
Adaja → Spain 36 D6
Adak U.S.A. 106 E4
Adak I. U.S.A. 106 E4
Adamaoua □ Cameroon 83 D7
Adamaoua, Massif de l' Cameroon 83 D7
Adamawa □ Nigeria 83 D7
Adamawa Highlands = Adamaoua, Massif de l' Cameroon 83 D7
Adamello, Mte. Italy 40 B7
Adamello ⌓ Italy 40 B7
Adami Tulu Ethiopia 81 F4
Adaminaby Australia 95 F4
Adams Mass., U.S.A. 115 D11
Adams N.Y., U.S.A. 115 C8
Adams Wis., U.S.A. 112 D9
Adams, Mt. U.S.A. 110 D5
Adam's Bridge Sri Lanka 66 Q11
Adams L. Canada 102 C5
Adam's Peak Sri Lanka 66 R12
Adamuz Spain 37 G6
Adana Turkey 72 D6
Adana □ Turkey 72 D6
Adanero Spain 36 E6
Adapazarı = Sakarya Turkey 72 B4
Adar Gwagwa, J. Sudan 80 C4
Adarama Sudan 81 D3
Adare, C. Antarctica 5 D11
Adarte Eritrea 81 E5
Adaut Indonesia 63 F8
Adavale Australia 95 D3
Adda → Italy 40 C6
Addis Ababa = Addis Abeba Ethiopia 81 F4
Addis Abeba Ethiopia 81 F4
Addis Alem Ethiopia 81 F4
Addis Zemen Ethiopia 81 E4
Addison U.S.A. 114 D7
Addo S. Africa 88 E4
Addo △ S. Africa 88 E4
Adebour Niger 83 C7
Ādeh Iran 70 B5
Adel U.S.A. 117 F13
Adel Bagrou Mauritania 82 B3
Adelaide Australia 95 E2
Adelaide S. Africa 88 E4
Adelaide I. Antarctica 5 C17
Adelaide Pen. Canada 100 D12
Adelaide River Australia 92 B5
Adelaide Village Bahamas 120 A4
Adelanto U.S.A. 111 L9
Adele I. Australia 92 C3
Adélie, Terre Antarctica 5 C10
Adelie Land = Adélie, Terre Antarctica 5 C10
Adelsk Belarus 30 E10
Ademuz Spain 38 E3
Aden = Al 'Adan Yemen 75 E4
Aden, G. of Ind. Oc. 75 E4
Adendorp S. Africa 88 E3
Aderbissinat Niger 83 B6
Adh Dhayd U.A.E. 71 E7
Adhoi India 68 H4
Adi Indonesia 63 E8
Adi Arkai Ethiopia 81 E4
Adi Daro Ethiopia 81 E4
Adi Keyih Eritrea 81 E4
Adi Kwala Eritrea 81 E4
Adi Ugri Eritrea 81 E4
Adieu, C. Australia 93 F5
Adieu Pt. Australia 92 C3
Adigala Ethiopia 81 E5
Adige → Italy 41 C9
Adigrat Ethiopia 81 E4
Adıgüzel Barajı Turkey 47 C11
Adilabad India 66 K11
Adilcevaz Turkey 73 C10
Adirondack △ U.S.A. 115 C10
Adirondack Mts. U.S.A. 115 C10
Adis Abeba = Addis Abeba Ethiopia 81 F4
Adıyaman Turkey 73 D8
Adıyaman □ Turkey 73 D8
Adjohon Benin 83 D5
Adjud Romania 29 D12
Adjumani Uganda 86 B3
Adjuntas Puerto Rico 121 d
Adlavik Is. Canada 105 B8
Adler Russia 35 J4
Admer Algeria 83 A6
Admiralty G. Australia 92 B4
Admiralty Gulf ❂ Australia 92 B4
Admiralty I. U.S.A. 102 B2
Admiralty Inlet Canada 101 C14
Admiralty Is. Papua N. G. 90 B7
Adnan Menderes, İzmir ✈ (ADB) Turkey 47 C9
Ado Nigeria 83 D5
Ado-Ekiti Nigeria 83 D6
Adok Sudan 81 F3
Adola Ethiopia 81 E5
Adolfo González Chaves Argentina 126 D3
Adolfo Ruiz Cortines, Presa Mexico 118 B3
Adonara Indonesia 63 F6
Adoni India 66 M10
Adony Hungary 28 C3
Adour → France 20 E2
Adra India 69 H12
Adra Spain 37 J7
Adrano Italy 43 E7
Adrar Algeria 78 C6
Adrar Mauritania 78 D3
Adrar □ Mauritania 82 A3
Adrar des Iforas Africa 83 B5
Ádria Italy 41 C9
Adrian Mich., U.S.A. 113 E11
Adrian Tex., U.S.A. 116 D3
Adriatic Sea Medit. S. 6 G9
Adua Indonesia 63 E7
Adwa Ethiopia 81 E4
Adygea □ Russia 35 H5
Adzhar Republic = Ajaria □ Georgia 35 K6
Adzopé Ivory C. 82 D4
Ægean Sea Medit. S. 47 C7
Aerhtai Shan Mongolia 60 B4
Ærø Denmark 11 K4
Ærøskøbing Denmark 11 K4
Aetos Greece 46 D3
Afaahiti Tahiti 91 d
'Afak Iraq 73 F11
Afandou Greece 49 C10
Afar □ Ethiopia 81 E5
Afareaitu Moorea 91 d
Afdem Ethiopia 81 F5
Afghanistan ■ Asia 66 C4
Afikpo Nigeria 83 D6
Aflou Algeria 78 B6
Afognak I. U.S.A. 106 D9
Afragóla Italy 43 B7
Afram → Ghana 83 D4
Afrera Ethiopia 81 E5
Africa 76 E6
'Afrīn Syria 72 D7
Afşin Turkey 72 C7
Afton N.Y., U.S.A. 115 D9
Afton Wyo., U.S.A. 108 E8
Afuá Brazil 125 D8
'Afula Israel 74 C4
Afyon Turkey 47 C12
Afyon □ Turkey 47 C12
Afyonkarahisar = Afyon Turkey 47 C12
Aga Egypt 80 H7
Āgā Jarī Iran 71 D6
Agadés = Agadez Niger 83 B6
Agadez Niger 83 B6
Agadir Morocco 78 B4
Agaete Canary Is. 48 F4
Agaie Nigeria 83 D6
Agalega Is. Mauritius 3 E12
Ağapınar Turkey 47 B12
Agar India 68 H7
Agaro Ethiopia 81 F4
Agartala India 67 H17
Agăş Romania 29 D11
Agassiz Canada 102 D4
Agassiz Icecap Canada 101 A16
Agats Indonesia 63 F9
Agattu I. U.S.A. 106 E2
Agawam U.S.A. 115 D12
Agbélouvé Togo 83 D5
Agboville Ivory C. 82 D4
Ağcabädi Azerbaijan 35 K8
Ağdam Azerbaijan 35 L8
Ağdaş Azerbaijan 35 K8
Agde France 20 E7
Agde, C. d' France 20 E7
Agdzhabedi = Ağcabädi Azerbaijan 35 K8
Agen France 20 D4
Agerbæk Denmark 11 J2
Agersø Denmark 11 J5
Ageyevo Russia 32 E9
Aggteleki △ Hungary 28 B5
Āgh Kand Iran 73 D13
Aghathonisi Greece 47 D8
Aghia Anna Greece 46 C5
Aghia Deka Greece 49 D6
Aghia Ekaterinis, Akra Greece 49 A3
Aghia Galini Greece 49 D6
Aghia Marina Kasos, Greece 47 F8
Aghia Marina Leros, Greece 47 D8
Aghia Paraskevi Greece 47 B8
Aghia Roumeli Greece 46 F5
Aghia Varvara Greece 49 D7
Aghiasos Greece 47 B8
Aghio Theodori Greece 46 D5
Aghion Oros □ Greece 45 F8
Aghios Andreas Greece 46 D4
Aghios Efstratios Greece 46 B6
Aghios Georgios Greece 46 D5
Aghios Ioannis, Akra Greece 49 D7
Aghios Isidoros Greece 49 C9
Aghios Kirikos Greece 47 D8
Aghios Matheos Greece 49 B3
Aghios Mironas Greece 47 F7
Aghios Nikolaos Greece 49 D7
Aghios Petros Greece 46 C2
Aghios Stephanos Greece 49 A3
Aghiou Orous, Kolpos Greece 44 F7
Aghireşu Romania 29 D8
Agia Greece 46 B4
Aginskoye Russia 53 D12
Agjert Mauritania 82 B3
Ağlasun Turkey 47 D12
Agly → France 20 F7
Agnew Australia 93 E3
Agnibilékrou Ivory C. 82 D4
Agnita Romania 29 E9
Agnone Italy 41 G11
Ago-Are Nigeria 83 D5
Agofie Ghana 83 D5
Agogna → Italy 40 C5
Agoitz = Aoiz Spain 38 C3
Agön Sweden 10 C11
Agon Coutainville France 18 C5
Ágordo Italy 41 B9
Agori India 69 G10
Agouna Benin 83 D5
Agout → France 20 E5
Agra India 68 F7
Agrakhanskiy Poluostrov Russia 35 J8
Agramunt Spain 38 D6
Ágreda Spain 38 D3
Ağri Turkey 73 C10
Ağri □ Turkey 73 C10
Agri → Italy 43 B9
Ağri Daği Turkey 73 C11
Ağri Karakose = Ağri Turkey 73 C10
Agria Greece 46 B5
Agrigento Italy 42 E6
Agrinio Greece 46 C3
Agrópoli Italy 43 B7
Ağstafa Azerbaijan 35 K7
Agua Caliente Mexico 111 N10
Agua Caliente Springs U.S.A. 111 N10
Água Clara Brazil 125 H8
Agua Fria ⌓ U.S.A. 109 J8
Agua Hechicera Mexico 111 N10
Agua Prieta Mexico 118 A3
Aguadilla Puerto Rico 121 d
Aguadulce Panama 120 E3
Aguanga U.S.A. 111 M10
Aguanish Canada 105 B7
Aguanish → Canada 105 B7
Aguapey → Argentina 126 B4
Aguaray Guazú → Paraguay 126 A4
Aguarico → Ecuador 124 D3
Aguaro-Guariquito △ Venezuela 121 E6
Aguas → Spain 38 D4
Aguas Blancas Chile 126 A2
Aguas Calientes, Sierra de Argentina 126 B2
Aguascalientes Mexico 118 C4
Aguascalientes □ Mexico 118 C4
Agudo Spain 37 G6
Águeda Portugal 36 E2
Agueda → Spain 36 D4
Aguelhok Mali 83 B5
Aguié Niger 83 C6
Aguila, Punta Puerto Rico 121 d
Aguilafuente Spain 36 D6
Aguilar de Campóo Spain 36 C6
Aguilar de la Frontera Spain 37 H6
Aguilares Argentina 126 B2
Águilas Spain 39 H3
Agüimes Canary Is. 48 G4
Aguja, C. de la Colombia 122 B3
Agujereada, Pta. Puerto Rico 121 d
Agulaa Ethiopia 81 E4
Agulhas, C. S. Africa 88 E3
Agulo Canary Is. 48 F2
Agung, Gunung Indonesia 62 F5
Agur Uganda 86 B3
Agusan → Phil. 61 G6
Ağva Turkey 45 E13
Agvali Russia 35 J8
Aha Mts. Botswana 88 B3
Ahaggar Algeria 78 D7
Ahamansu Ghana 83 D5
Ahar Iran 73 C12
Ahat Turkey 47 C11
Ahaus Germany 24 C2
Ahipara B. N.Z. 91 A4
Ahir Dağı Turkey 47 C12
Ahiri India 66 K12
Ahlat Turkey 73 C10
Ahlen Germany 24 D3
Ahmad Wal Pakistan 68 E1
Ahmadabad India 68 H5
Aḩmadābād Khorāsān, Iran 71 C9
Aḩmadābād Khorāsān, Iran 71 C8
Aḩmadī Iran 71 E8
Ahmadnagar India 66 K9
Ahmadpur East Pakistan 68 E4
Ahmadpur Lamma Pakistan 68 E4
Ahmar, Mts. Ethiopia 81 F5
Ahmedabad = Ahmadabad India 68 H5
Ahmednagar = Ahmadnagar India 66 K9
Ahmetbey Turkey 45 E11
Ahmetler Turkey 47 C11
Ahmetli Turkey 47 C9
Ahoada Nigeria 83 D6
Ahome Mexico 118 B3
Ahoskie U.S.A. 117 C16
Ahr → Germany 24 E3
Ahram Iran 71 D6
Ahrax Pt. Malta 49 D1
Ahrensbök Germany 24 A6
Ahrensburg Germany 24 B6
Ahuachapán El Salv. 120 D2
Ahun France 19 F9
Åhus Sweden 11 J8
Ahvāz Iran 71 D6
Ahvenanmaa = Åland Finland 9 F19

Aḥwar Yemen 75 E4
Ahzar → Mali 83 B5
Ai → India 69 F14
Ai-Ais Namibia 88 D2
Ai-Ais and Fish River Canyon △ Namibia 88 C2
Aichach Germany 25 G7
Aichi □ Japan 55 G8
Aigle Switz. 25 J2
Aignay-le-Duc France 19 E11
Aigoual, Mt. France 20 D7
Aigre France 20 C4
Aigrettes, Pte. des Réunion 85 c
Aiguá Uruguay 127 C5
Aigueperse France 19 F10
Aigues → France 21 D8
Aigues-Mortes France 21 E8
Aigues-Mortes, G. d' France 21 E8
Aigües-Tortes i Estany de St. Maurici △ Spain 38 C4
Aiguilles France 21 D10
Aiguillon France 20 D4
Aigurande France 19 F8
Aihui = Heihe China 53 D13
Aija Peru 124 E3
Aikawa Japan 54 E9
Aiken U.S.A. 117 E14
Ailao Shan China 58 F3
Aileron Australia 94 C1
Aillant-sur-Tholon France 19 E10
Aillik Canada 105 A8
Ailsa Craig Canada 114 C3
Ailsa Craig U.K. 13 F3
Aim Russia 53 D14
Aimere Indonesia 63 F6
Aimogasta Argentina 126 B2
Ain □ France 19 F12
Ain → France 21 C9
Aïn Ben Tili Mauritania 78 C4
Ain Dalla Egypt 80 B2
Ain el Mafki Egypt 80 B2
Ain Girba Egypt 80 B2
Ain Murr Sudan 80 C2
Ain Qeiqab Egypt 80 B1
Aïn-Sefra Algeria 78 B5
Ain Sheikh Murzûk Egypt 80 B2
Ain Sudr Egypt 74 F2
Ain Sukhna Egypt 80 J8
Aïn Témouchent Algeria 78 A5
Ain Zeitûn Egypt 80 B2
Ainaži Latvia 32 D3
Ainos Oros Greece 46 C2
Ainsworth U.S.A. 112 D4
Aiquile Bolivia 124 G5
Aïr Niger 83 B6
Aïr et du Ténéré △ Niger 83 B6
Air Force I. Canada 101 D17
Air Hitam Malaysia 65 M4
Airaines France 19 C8
Airdrie Canada 102 C6
Airdrie U.K. 13 F5
Aire → France 19 C11
Aire → U.K. 14 D7
Aire, I. de l' Spain 48 B11
Aire-sur-la-Lys France 19 B9
Aire-sur-l'Adour France 20 E3
Airlie Beach Australia 94 b
Airvault France 18 F6
Aisch → Germany 25 F6
Aisne □ France 19 C10
Aisne → France 19 C9
Ait India 69 G8
Aitana, Sierra de Spain 39 G4
Aitkin U.S.A. 112 B7
Aitutaki Cook Is. 97 J12
Aiud Romania 29 D8
Aix-en-Provence France 21 E9
Aix-la-Chapelle = Aachen Germany 24 E2
Aix-les-Bains France 21 C9
Aixe-sur-Vienne France 20 C5
Aíyina = Egina Greece 46 D5
Aizawl India 67 H18
Aizenay France 18 F5
Aizkraukle Latvia 32 D3
Aizpute Latvia 30 B8
Aizuwakamatsu Japan 54 F9
Ajabshir Iran 73 D11
Ajaccio France 21 G12
Ajaccio, G. d' France 21 G12
Ajai △ Uganda 86 B3
Ajaigarh India 69 G9
Ajalpan Mexico 119 D5
Ajanta Ra. India 66 J9
Ajari Rep. = Ajaria □ Georgia 35 K6
Ajaria □ Georgia 35 K6
Ajax Canada 114 C5
Ajdābiyā Libya 79 B10
Ajdovščina Slovenia 41 C10
Ajibar Ethiopia 81 E4
Ajka Hungary 28 C2
'Ajlūn Jordan 74 C4
'Ajlūn □ Jordan 74 C4
'Ajmān U.A.E. 71 E7
Ajmer India 68 F6
Ajnala India 68 D6
Ajo U.S.A. 109 K7
Ajo, C. de Spain 36 B7
Ajuy Phil. 61 F5

Ak Dağ Turkey 47 E11
Ak Dağlar Turkey 72 C7
Ak Dağları Turkey 47 E11
Akaba Togo 83 D5
Akabira Japan 54 C11
Akagera △ Rwanda 86 C3
Akagera → Rwanda 86 C3
Akaki Beseka Ethiopia 81 F4
Akamas Cyprus 49 D11
Akan △ Japan 54 C12
Akanthou Cyprus 49 D12
Akaroa N.Z. 91 E4
Akasha Sudan 80 C3
Akashi Japan 55 G7
Akbarpur Bihar, India 69 G10
Akbarpur Ut. P., India 69 F10
Akçaabat Turkey 73 B8
Akçadağ Turkey 72 C7
Akçakale Turkey 73 D8
Akçakoca Turkey 72 B4
Akçaova Turkey 45 E13
Akçay Turkey 47 E11
Akçay → Turkey 47 D10
Akdağ Turkey 47 C9
Akdağmadeni Turkey 72 C6
Akdoğan = Lysi Cyprus 49 D12
Akelamo Indonesia 63 D7
Åkers styckebruk Sweden 10 E11
Åkersberga Sweden 10 E12
Aketi Dem. Rep. of the Congo 84 D4
Akhalkalaki Georgia 35 K6
Akhaltsikhe Georgia 35 K6
Akhisar Turkey 47 C9
Akhmīm Egypt 80 B3
Akhnur India 69 C6
Akhtopol Bulgaria 45 D11
Akhtuba → Russia 35 G8
Akhtubinsk Russia 35 F8
Akhty Russia 35 K8
Akhtyrka = Okhtyrka Ukraine 33 G8
Aki Japan 55 H6
Akimiski I. Canada 104 B3
Akimovka Ukraine 33 J8
Akıncı Burnu Turkey 72 D6
Akincilar = Louroujina Cyprus 49 E12
Åkirkeby Denmark 11 J8
Akita Japan 54 E10
Akita □ Japan 54 E10
Akjoujt Mauritania 82 B2
Akka Mali 82 B4
Akkaya Tepesi Turkey 47 D11
Akkeshi Japan 54 C12
'Akko Israel 74 C4
Akköy Turkey 47 D9
Akkuş Turkey 72 B7
Aklampa Benin 83 D5
Aklavik Canada 100 D4
Aklera India 68 G7
Akmenė Lithuania 30 B9
Akmenrags Latvia 30 B8
Akmonte = Almonte Spain 37 H4
Akō Japan 55 G7
Ako Nigeria 83 C7
Akôbô Sudan 81 F3
Akobo → Ethiopia 81 F3
Akola India 66 J10
Akonolinga Cameroon 83 E7
Akor Mali 82 B4
Akordat Eritrea 81 D4
Akosombo Dam Ghana 83 D5
Akot Sudan 81 F3
Akoupé Ivory C. 82 D4
Akpatok I. Canada 101 E18
Åkrahamn Norway 9 G11
Akranes Iceland 8 D2
Akreïjit Mauritania 82 B3
Akritas, Akra Greece 46 E3
Akron Colo., U.S.A. 108 F12
Akron Ohio, U.S.A. 114 E3
Akrotiri Cyprus 49 E11
Akrotiri, Akra Greece 45 F9
Akrotiri Bay Cyprus 49 E12
Aksai Chin China 69 B8
Aksaray Turkey 72 C6
Aksay = Aqsay Kazakhstan 52 D6
Akşehir Turkey 72 C4
Akşehir Gölü Turkey 72 C4
Akstafa = Ağstafa Azerbaijan 35 K7
Aksu China 60 B3
Aksu → Turkey 72 D4
Aksum Ethiopia 81 E4
Aktash Russia 34 C11
Aktsyabrski Belarus 23 B15
Aktyubinsk = Aqtöbe Kazakhstan 52 D6
Aku Nigeria 83 D6
Akure Nigeria 83 D6
Akureyri Iceland 8 D4
Akuseki-Shima Japan 55 K4
Akusha Russia 35 J8
Akwa-Ibom □ Nigeria 83 E6
Akwanga Nigeria 83 D6
Akyab = Sittwe Burma 67 J18
Akyazı Turkey 72 B4
Al 'Adan Yemen 75 E4
Al Aḥsā = Hasa Si. Arabia 71 E6

Al Ajfar Si. Arabia 70 E4
Al Amādīyah Iraq 73 D10
Al 'Amārah Iraq 73 G12
Al Anbār □ Iraq 70 C4
Al 'Aqabah Jordan 74 F4
Al 'Aqabah □ Jordan 74 F4
Al Arak Syria 73 E8
Al 'Aramah Si. Arabia 70 E5
Al 'Arṭāwīyah Si. Arabia 70 E5
Al 'Aṣimah = 'Ammān □ Jordan 74 D5
Al 'Assāfiyah Si. Arabia 70 D3
Al 'Awdah Si. Arabia 70 E5
Al 'Ayn Si. Arabia 70 E3
Al 'Ayn U.A.E. 71 E7
Al 'Azīzīyah Iraq 73 F11
Al Bāb Syria 72 D7
Al Bad' Si. Arabia 70 D2
Al Bādī Iraq 70 C4
Al Bāḥah Si. Arabia 80 C5
Al Baḥrah Kuwait 70 D5
Al Baḥral Mayyit = Dead Sea Asia 74 D4
Al Balqā' □ Jordan 74 C4
Al Bārūk, J. Lebanon 74 B4
Al Bāşah Si. Arabia 80 C5
Al Başrah Iraq 70 D5
Al Baṭḥā Iraq 70 D5
Al Batrūn Lebanon 74 A4
Al Baydā Libya 79 B10
Al Biqā Lebanon 74 A5
Al Bi'r Si. Arabia 70 D3
Al Bukayrīyah Si. Arabia 70 E4
Al Buraymī □ Oman 71 E8
Al Burayj Syria 74 A5
Al Faḍilī Si. Arabia 71 E6
Al Fallūjah Iraq 73 F10
Al Fatḥah Iraq 73 E10
Al Fāw Iraq 71 D6
Al Fujayrah U.A.E. 71 E8
Al Ghadaf, W. → Jordan 74 D5
Al Ghammās Iraq 70 D5
Al Ghazlān Si. Arabia 70 E4
Al Ḥadīthah Iraq 73 E10
Al Ḥadīthah Si. Arabia 74 D6
Al Ḥaḍr Iraq 73 E10
Al Ḥājānah Syria 74 B5
Al Ḥāmad Si. Arabia 70 D3
Al Ḥamdānīyah Syria 74 C3
Al Ḥamīdīyah Syria 74 A4
Al Ḥammār Iraq 70 D5
Al Ḥamrā' Si. Arabia 70 E3
Al Ḥamzah Iraq 70 D5
Al Ḥanākīyah Si. Arabia 70 E4
Al Ḥarūj al Aswad Libya 79 C9
Al Ḥasakah Syria 73 D9
Al Ḥaşakah Syria 73 D9
Al Ḥāshimīyah Iraq 73 G11
Al Ḥayy Iraq 73 F12
Al Ḥijarah Asia 70 D4
Al Ḥillah Iraq 73 F11
Al Ḥillah Si. Arabia 75 B4
Al Hindīyah Iraq 73 F11
Al Hirmil Lebanon 74 A5
Al Hoceïma Morocco 78 A5
Al Ḥudaydah Yemen 75 E3
Al Ḥudūd ash Shamālīyah □ Si. Arabia 70 D4
Al Hufūf Si. Arabia 71 E6
Al Ḥumaydah Si. Arabia 70 D2
Al Ḥunayy Si. Arabia 71 E6
Al Ḥisāwīyah Si. Arabia 70 D3
Al Jafr Jordan 74 E5
Al Jāfūrah Si. Arabia 71 E7
Al Jaghbūb Libya 79 C10
Al Jahrah Kuwait 70 D5
Al Jalāmīd Si. Arabia 70 D3
Al Jamalīyah Qatar 71 E6
Al Janūb □ Lebanon 74 B4
Al Jawf Libya 79 D10
Al Jawf Si. Arabia 70 D3
Al Jawf □ Si. Arabia 70 D3
Al Jazair = Algeria ■ Africa 78 C6
Al Jazirah Iraq 73 D9
Al Jithāmīyah Si. Arabia 70 E4
Al Jubayl Si. Arabia 71 E6
Al Jubaylah Si. Arabia 70 E5
Al Jubb Si. Arabia 70 E4
Al Junaynah Sudan 79 F10
Al Kabā'ish Iraq 70 D5
Al Karak Jordan 74 D4
Al Karak □ Jordan 74 E5
Al Kāẓimīyah Iraq 73 F11
Al Khābūrah Oman 71 F8
Al Khafji Si. Arabia 71 E6
Al Khalīl West Bank 74 D4
Al Khāliş Iraq 73 F11
Al Kharsānīyah Si. Arabia 71 E6
Al Khaşab Oman 71 D8
Al Khawr Qatar 71 E6
Al Khidr Iraq 70 D5
Al Khiyām Lebanon 74 B4
Al Khobar Si. Arabia 71 E6
Al Khums Libya 79 B8
Al Kifl Iraq 73 G11
Al Kiswah Syria 74 B5
Al Kūfah Iraq 73 F11
Al Kufrah Libya 79 D10
Al Kuhayfiyah Si. Arabia 70 E4

Al Kumayt Iraq 73 G12
Al Kūt Iraq 73 F11
Al Kuwayt Kuwait 70 D5
Al Labwah Lebanon 74 A5
Al Lādhiqīyah Syria 72 E6
Al Lādhiqīyah □ Syria 72 E6
Al Līth Si. Arabia 80 C5
Al Liwā' Oman 71 E8
Al Luḥayyah Yemen 75 D3
Al Madīnah Iraq 70 D5
Al Madīnah Si. Arabia 70 E3
Al Mafraq Jordan 74 C5
Al Mafraq □ Jordan 74 C5
Al Maghreb = Morocco ■ N. Afr. 78 B4
Al Maḥmūdīyah Iraq 73 F11
Al Majma'ah Si. Arabia 70 E5
Al Makhruq, W. → Jordan 74 D6
Al Makhūl Si. Arabia 70 E4
Al Mālikīyah Syria 73 D10
Al Manāmah Bahrain 71 E6
Al Maqwa' Kuwait 70 D5
Al Marāḥ Si. Arabia 71 E6
Al Marj Libya 79 B10
Al Maṭlā Kuwait 70 D5
Al Mawṣil Iraq 73 D10
Al Mayādin Syria 73 E9
Al Mazār Jordan 74 D4
Al Midhnab Si. Arabia 70 E5
Al Minā' Lebanon 74 A4
Al Miqdādīyah Iraq 73 E11
Al Mubarraz Si. Arabia 71 E6
Al Mudawwarah Jordan 74 F5
Al Mughayrā' U.A.E. 71 E7
Al Muḥarraq Bahrain 71 E6
Al Mukallā Yemen 75 E4
Al Mukhā Yemen 75 E3
Al Musayjīd Si. Arabia 70 E3
Al Musayyib Iraq 73 F11
Al Muthanná □ Iraq 70 D5
Al Muwayh Si. Arabia 80 C5
Al Muwaylih Si. Arabia 70 E3
Al Owuho = Otukpa Nigeria 83 D6
Al Qā'im Iraq 73 E9
Al Qādisīyah □ Iraq 70 D5
Al Qalībah Si. Arabia 70 D3
Al Qāmishlī Syria 73 D9
Al Qaryatayn Syria 74 A6
Al Qaṣīm □ Si. Arabia 70 E4
Al Qaṭ'ā Syria 73 E9
Al Qaṭīf Si. Arabia 71 E6
Al Qaṭrānah Jordan 74 D5
Al Qaṭrūn Libya 79 D9
Al Qawz Si. Arabia 80 D5
Al Qayṣūmah Si. Arabia 70 D5
Al Quds = Jerusalem Israel/West Bank 74 D4
Al Qunayṭirah Syria 74 C4
Al Qunfudhah Si. Arabia 80 D5
Al Qurnah Iraq 70 D5
Al Quṣayr Iraq 70 D5
Al Quṣayr Syria 74 A5
Al Qutayfah Syria 74 B5
Al Quwayr Iraq 73 D10
Al 'Ubaylah Si. Arabia 75 C5
Al 'Udayliyah Si. Arabia 71 E6
Al 'Ulā Si. Arabia 70 E3
Al 'Uqayr Si. Arabia 71 E6
Al 'Uwaynid Si. Arabia 70 E5
Al 'Uwayqīlah Si. Arabia 70 D4
Al 'Uyūn Ḥijāz, Si. Arabia 70 E3
Al 'Uyūn Najd, Si. Arabia 70 E4
Al 'Uzayr Iraq 70 D5
Al Wajh Si. Arabia 70 E3
Al Wakrah Qatar 71 E6
Al Waqbah Si. Arabia 70 D5
Al Wari'āh Si. Arabia 70 E5
Al Yaman = Yemen ■ Asia 75 E3
Ala Italy 40 C4
Ala Dağ Turkey 70 B2
Ala Dağları Turkey 73 C10
Ala Tau Asia 52 E9
Alabama □ U.S.A. 117 E11
Alabama → U.S.A. 117 E11
Alabaster U.S.A. 117 E11
Alaca Turkey 72 B6
Alaçam Turkey 72 B6
Alaçam Dağları Turkey 47 B10
Alacant = Alicante Spain 39 G4
Alaçatı Turkey 47 C8
Alachua U.S.A. 117 G13
Alaejos Spain 36 D5
Alagir Russia 35 J7
Alagna Valsésia Italy 40 C4
Alagoa Grande Brazil 125 E11
Alagoas □ Brazil 125 E11
Alagoinhas Brazil 125 F11
Alagón Spain 38 D3
Alagón → Spain 36 F4
Alaior Spain 48 B11
Alajero Canary Is. 48 F2
Alajuela Costa Rica 120 D3
Alakamisy Madag. 89 C8
Alaknanda → India 69 D8
Alakōl Kazakhstan 60 B3
Alakurtti Russia 8 C24
Alamarvdasht Iran 71 E7
Alamata Ethiopia 81 E4

Alameda Calif., U.S.A. 110 H4
Alameda N. Mex., U.S.A. 109 J10
Alaminos Phil. 61 C3
Alamo U.S.A. 111 H11
Alamogordo U.S.A. 109 K11
Alamos Mexico 118 B3
Alamosa U.S.A. 109 H11
Åland Finland 9 F19
Alandroal Portugal 37 G3
Ålands hav Europe 9 G18
Alange, Embalse d' Spain 37 G4
Alania = North Ossetia □ Russia 35 J7
Alanís Spain 37 G5
Alanya Turkey 72 D5
Alaotra, Farihin' Madag. 89 B8
Alapayevsk Russia 52 D7
Alappuzha = Alleppey India 66 Q10
Alar del Rey Spain 36 C6
Alaraz Spain 36 E5
Alarcón, Embalse de Spain 38 F2
Alaró Spain 48 B9
Alarobia-Vohiposa Madag. 89 C8
Alaşehir Turkey 47 C10
Alashtar Iran 73 F13
Alaska □ U.S.A. 106 C9
Alaska, G. of Pac. Oc. 100 F3
Alaska Peninsula U.S.A. 106 D8
Alaska Range U.S.A. 100 E1
Alássio Italy 40 D5
Älät Azerbaijan 35 L9
Alatau Shan = Ala Tau Asia 52 E9
Alatri Italy 41 G10
Alatyr Russia 34 C8
Alatyr → Russia 34 C8
Alausi Ecuador 124 D3
Álava □ Spain 38 C2
Alava, C. U.S.A. 108 B1
Alaverdi Armenia 35 K7
Alavo = Alavus Finland 8 E20
Alavus Finland 8 E20
Alawa ◇ Australia 94 B1
Alawoona Australia 95 E3
Alayawarra ◇ Australia 94 C1
'Alayh Lebanon 74 B4
Alazani → Azerbaijan 35 K8
Alba Italy 40 D5
Alba □ Romania 29 D8
Alba Adriática Italy 41 F10
Alba de Tormes Spain 36 E5
Alba-Iulia Romania 29 D8
Albac Romania 28 D7
Albacete Spain 39 F3
Albacete □ Spain 39 F3
Albacutya, L. Australia 95 F3
Albalate de las Nogueras Spain 38 E2
Albalate del Arzobispo Spain 38 D4
Alban France 20 E6
Albanel, L. Canada 104 B5
Albania ■ Europe 44 E4
Albano Laziale Italy 41 G9
Albany Australia 93 G2
Albany Ga., U.S.A. 117 F12
Albany N.Y., U.S.A. 115 D11
Albany Oreg., U.S.A. 108 D2
Albany Tex., U.S.A. 116 E5
Albany → Canada 104 B3
Albarca, C. d' Spain 48 B7
Albardón Argentina 126 C2
Albarracín Spain 38 E3
Albarracín, Sierra de Spain 38 E3
Albatera Spain 39 G4
Albatross B. Australia 94 A3
Albegna → Italy 41 F8
Albemarle U.S.A. 117 D14
Albemarle Sd. U.S.A. 117 C16
Albenga Italy 40 D5
Alberche → Spain 36 F6
Alberdi Paraguay 126 B4
Albères, Mts. France 20 F6
Ålberga Sweden 11 F10
Alberga → Australia 95 D2
Albersdorf Germany 24 A5
Albert France 19 C9
Albert, L. Africa 86 B3
Albert, L. Australia 95 F2
Albert Edward Ra. Australia 92 C4
Albert Lea U.S.A. 112 D7
Albert Nile → Uganda 86 B3
Albert Town Bahamas 121 B5
Alberta □ Canada 102 C6
Alberti Argentina 126 D3
Albertinia S. Africa 88 E3
Albertirsa Hungary 28 C4
Alberton Canada 105 C7
Albertville France 21 C10
Albertville U.S.A. 117 D11
Albi France 20 E6
Albia U.S.A. 112 E7
Albina Suriname 125 B8
Albina, Ponta Angola 88 B1
Albino Italy 40 C6
Albion Mich., U.S.A. 113 D11
Albion Nebr., U.S.A. 112 E4
Albion Pa., U.S.A. 114 E4

Albocàsser Spain 38 E5
Albolote Spain 37 H7
Alborán Medit. S. 37 K7
Alborea Spain 39 F3
Ålborg = Aalborg Denmark 11 G3
Ålborg Bugt = Aalborg Bugt Denmark 11 H4
Alborz, Reshteh-ye Kühhā-ye Iran 71 C7
Albox Spain 39 H2
Albufeira Portugal 37 H2
Albula → Switz. 25 J5
Albuñol Spain 37 J7
Albuquerque U.S.A. 109 J10
Albuquerque, Cayos de Caribbean 120 D3
Alburg U.S.A. 115 B11
Alburno, Mte. Italy 43 B8
Alburquerque Spain 37 F4
Albury Australia 95 F4
Alcácer do Sal Portugal 37 G2
Alcáçovas Portugal 37 G2
Alcalá de Guadaira Spain 37 H5
Alcalá de Henares Spain 36 E7
Alcalá de los Gazules Spain 37 J5
Alcalá de Xivert Spain 38 E5
Alcalá del Júcar Spain 39 F3
Alcalá del Río Spain 37 H5
Alcalá del Valle Spain 37 J5
Alcalá la Real Spain 37 H7
Álcamo Italy 42 E5
Alcanadre Spain 38 C2
Alcanadre → Spain 38 D4
Alcanar Spain 38 E5
Alcanede Portugal 37 F2
Alcanena Portugal 37 F2
Alcañices Spain 36 D4
Alcañiz Spain 38 D4
Alcântara Brazil 125 D10
Alcántara Spain 36 F4
Alcántara, Embalse de Spain 36 F4
Alcantarilla Spain 39 H3
Alcaracejos Spain 37 G6
Alcaraz Spain 39 G2
Alcaraz, Sierra de Spain 39 G2
Alcaudete Spain 37 H6
Alcázar de San Juan Spain 37 F7
Alchevsk Ukraine 33 H10
Alcira = Alzira Spain 39 F4
Alcobaça Portugal 37 F2
Alcobendas Spain 36 E7
Alcolea del Pinar Spain 38 D2
Alcorcón Spain 36 E7
Alcoutim Portugal 37 H3
Alcova U.S.A. 108 E10
Alcoy Spain 39 G4
Alcubierre, Sierra de Spain 38 D4
Alcublas Spain 38 F4
Alcúdia Spain 48 B10
Alcúdia, B. d' Spain 48 B10
Alcúdia, Sierra de la Spain 37 G6
Aldabra Is. Seychelles 77 G8
Aldama Mexico 119 C5
Aldan Russia 53 D13
Aldan → Russia 53 C13
Aldea, Pta. de la Canary Is. 48 G4
Aldeburgh U.K. 15 E9
Alder Pk. U.S.A. 110 K5
Alderney U.K. 15 H5
Aldershot U.K. 15 F7
Åled Sweden 11 H6
Aledo U.S.A. 112 E8
Alefa Ethiopia 81 E4
Aleg Mauritania 82 B2
Alegranza Canary Is. 48 E6
Alegranza, I. Canary Is. 48 E6
Alegre Brazil 127 A7
Alegrete Brazil 127 B4
Aleksandriya = Oleksandriya Kirovohrad, Ukraine 33 H7
Aleksandriya = Oleksandriya Rivne, Ukraine 23 C14
Aleksandrovskaya Russia 35 J8
Aleksandrov Russia 32 D10
Aleksandrov Gay Russia 34 E9
Aleksandrovac Serbia 44 C5
Aleksandrovac Serbia 44 B5
Aleksandrovka = Oleksandrovka Ukraine 33 H7
Aleksandrovo Bulgaria 45 C8
Aleksandrovsk-Sakhalinskiy Russia 53 D15
Aleksandrów Kujawski Poland 31 F5
Aleksandrów Łódzki Poland 31 G6
Aleksandry, Zemlya Russia 52 A5
Alekseyevka Samara, Russia 34 D10
Alekseyevka Voronezh, Russia 33 G10
Aleksin Russia 32 E9
Aleksinac Serbia 44 C5
Além Paraíba Brazil 127 A7
Alemania Argentina 126 B2
Alemania Chile 126 B2
Alençon France 18 D7
Alenquer Brazil 125 D8
'Alenuihāhā Channel U.S.A. 107 L8

Alépé *Ivory C.* **82** D4
Aleppo = Ḩalab *Syria* **72** D7
Aléria *France* **21** F13
Alert *Canada* **101** A20
Alès *France* **21** D8
Aleşd *Romania* **28** C7
Alessándria *Italy* **40** D5
Alet-les-Bains *France* **20** F6
Aletschhorn *Switz.* **25** J4
Aleutian Basin *Pac. Oc.* **96** B9
Aleutian Is. *Pac. Oc.* **106** E5
Aleutian Range *U.S.A.* **106** D9
Aleutian Trench *Pac. Oc.* **4** D17
Alexander *U.S.A.* **112** B2
Alexander, Mt. *Australia* **93** E3
Alexander Arch. *U.S.A.* **100** F4
Alexander Bay *S. Africa* **88** D2
Alexander City *U.S.A.* **117** E12
Alexander I. *Antarctica* **5** C17
Alexandra *Australia* **95** F4
Alexandra *N.Z.* **91** F2
Alexandra Falls *Canada* **102** A5
Alexandria = El
  Iskandarîya *Egypt* **80** H7
Alexandria *B.C., Canada* **102** C4
Alexandria *Ont., Canada* **115** A10
Alexandria *Romania* **29** G10
Alexandria *S. Africa* **88** E4
Alexandria *U.K.* **13** F4
Alexandria *La., U.S.A.* **116** F8
Alexandria *Minn., U.S.A.* **112** C6
Alexandria *S. Dak., U.S.A.* **112** D5
Alexandria *Va., U.S.A.* **113** F15
Alexandria Bay *U.S.A.* **115** B9
Alexandrina, L. *Australia* **95** F2
Alexandroúpoli *Greece* **45** F9
Alexis → *Canada* **105** B8
Alexis Creek *Canada* **102** C4
Aleysk *Russia* **52** D9
Alfabia *Spain* **48** B9
Alfambra *Spain* **38** E3
Alfândega da Fé *Portugal* **36** D4
Alfaro *Spain* **38** C3
Alfatar *Bulgaria* **45** C11
Alfeld *Germany* **24** D5
Alfenas *Brazil* **127** A6
Alföld *Hungary* **28** D5
Alfonsine *Italy* **41** D9
Alford *Aberds., U.K.* **13** D6
Alford *Lincs., U.K.* **14** D8
Alfred *Maine, U.S.A.* **115** C14
Alfred *N.Y., U.S.A.* **114** D7
Alfreton *U.K.* **14** D6
Alfta *Sweden* **10** C10
Algaida *Spain* **48** B9
Algar *Spain* **37** J5
Ålgård *Norway* **9** G11
Algarinejo *Spain* **37** H6
Algarve *Portugal* **37** J2
Algeciras *Spain* **37** J5
Algemesí *Spain* **39** F4
Alger *Algeria* **78** A6
Alger □ *Algeria* **39** J8
Alger ✈ (ALG) *Algeria* **39** J8
Algeria ■ *Africa* **78** C6
Algha *Kazakhstan* **52** E6
Alghero *Italy* **42** B1
Älghult *Sweden* **11** G9
Algiers = Alger *Algeria* **78** A6
Algoa B. *S. Africa* **88** E4
Algodonales *Spain* **37** J5
Algodor → *Spain* **36** F7
Algoma *U.S.A.* **112** C10
Algona *U.S.A.* **112** D6
Algonac *U.S.A.* **114** D2
Algonquin △ *Canada* **104** C4
Algorta *Uruguay* **128** C5
Alhama de Almería *Spain* **37** J8
Alhama de Aragón *Spain* **38** D3
Alhama de Granada *Spain* **37** H7
Alhama de Murcia *Spain* **39** H3
Alhambra *U.S.A.* **111** L8
Alhaurín el Grande *Spain* **37** J6
Alhucemas = Al Hoceïma
  Morocco **78** A5
'Alī al Gharbī *Iraq* **73** F12
'Alī ash Sharqī *Iraq* **73** F12
Äli Bayramlı *Azerbaijan* **35** L9
'Alī Khēl *Afghan.* **68** C3
Alī Sahîh *Djibouti* **81** E5
Alī Shāh *Iran* **70** B5
Ália *Italy* **42** E6
'Alīābād *Golestān, Iran* **71** B7
'Alīābād *Khorāsān, Iran* **71** C8
'Alīābād *Kordestān, Iran* **70** C5
'Alīābād *Yazd, Iran* **71** D7
Aliade *Nigeria* **83** D6
Aliaga *Spain* **38** E4
Aliağa *Turkey* **47** C8
Alibo *Ethiopia* **81** F4
Alibori → *Benin* **83** C5
Alicante *Spain* **39** G4
Alicante □ *Spain* **39** G4
Alicante ✈ (ALC) *Spain* **39** G4
Alice *S. Africa* **88** E4
Alice *U.S.A.* **116** H5

Alice → *Queens., Australia* **94** C3
Alice → *Queens., Australia* **94** B3
Alice, Punta *Italy* **43** C10
Alice Arm *Canada* **102** B3
Alice Springs *Australia* **94** C1
Alicedale *S. Africa* **88** E4
Aliceville *U.S.A.* **117** E10
Alicudi *Italy* **43** D7
Aliganj *India* **69** F8
Aligarh *Raj., India* **68** G7
Aligarh *Ut. P., India* **68** F8
Alīgūdarz *Iran* **71** C6
Alijó *Portugal* **36** D3
Alimia *Greece* **49** C9
Alingsås *Sweden* **11** G6
Alipur *Pakistan* **68** E4
Alipur Duar *India* **67** F16
Aliquippa *U.S.A.* **114** F4
Alishan *Taiwan* **59** F13
Aliste → *Spain* **36** D5
Alitus = Alytus *Lithuania* **32** E3
Aliveri *Greece* **46** C6
Aliwal North *S. Africa* **88** E4
Alix *Canada* **102** C6
Aljezur *Portugal* **37** H2
Aljustrel *Portugal* **37** H2
Alkamari *Niger* **83** C7
Alkmaar *Neths.* **17** B4
All American Canal *U.S.A.* **109** K6
Allada *Benin* **83** D5
Allagash → *U.S.A.* **113** B19
Allah Dad *Pakistan* **68** G2
Allahabad *India* **69** G9
Allan *Canada* **103** C7
Allanche *France* **20** C6
Allanridge *S. Africa* **88** D4
Allaqi, Wadi → *Egypt* **80** C3
Allariz *Spain* **36** C3
Allassac *France* **20** C5
Ålleberg *Sweden* **11** F7
Allegany *U.S.A.* **114** D6
Allegheny → *U.S.A.* **114** F5
Allegheny Mts. *U.S.A.* **113** F13
Allegheny Plateau *U.S.A.* **113** E14
Allegheny Res. *U.S.A.* **114** E6
Allègre *France* **20** C7
Allègre, Pte. *Guadeloupe* **120** b
Allen, Bog of *Ireland* **12** C5
Allen, L. *Ireland* **12** B3
Allendale *U.S.A.* **117** E14
Allende *Mexico* **118** B4
Allentown *U.S.A.* **115** F9
Allentsteig *Austria* **26** C8
Alleppey *India* **66** Q10
Allepuz *Spain* **38** E4
Aller → *Germany* **24** C5
Alleynes B. *Barbados* **121** g
Alliance *Nebr., U.S.A.* **112** D2
Alliance *Ohio, U.S.A.* **114** F3
Allier □ *France* **19** F9
Allier → *France* **19** F10
Alliford Bay *Canada* **102** C2
Alligator Pond *Jamaica* **120** a
Allinge *Denmark* **11** J8
Alliston *Canada* **114** B5
Alloa *U.K.* **13** E5
Allones *France* **18** D8
Allora *Australia* **95** D5
Allos *France* **21** D10
Alluitsup Paa *Greenland* **4** C5
Alma *Canada* **105** C5
Alma *Ga., U.S.A.* **117** F13
Alma *Kans., U.S.A.* **112** F5
Alma *Mich., U.S.A.* **113** D11
Alma *Nebr., U.S.A.* **112** E5
Alma *Wis., U.S.A.* **112** C8
Alma Ata = Almaty
  Kazakhstan **52** E8
Alma Hill *U.S.A.* **114** D7
Almacelles *Spain* **38** D5
Almada *Portugal* **37** G1
Almaden *Australia* **94** B3
Almadén *Spain* **37** G6
Almalyk = Olmaliq
  Uzbekistan **52** E7
Almanor, L. *U.S.A.* **108** F3
Almansa *Spain* **39** G3
Almanza *Spain* **36** C5
Almanzor, Pico *Spain* **36** E5
Almanzora → *Spain* **39** H3
Almaş, Munţii *Romania* **28** F7
Almassora *Spain* **38** F4
Almaty *Kazakhstan* **52** E8
Almazán *Spain* **38** D2
Almeirim *Brazil* **125** D8
Almeirim *Portugal* **37** F2
Almelo *Neths.* **17** B6
Almenar de Soria *Spain* **38** D2
Almenara *Spain* **38** F4
Almenara, Sierra de *Spain* **39** H3
Almendra, Embalse de *Spain* **36** D4
Almendralejo *Spain* **37** G4
Almere-Stad *Neths.* **17** B5
Almería *Spain* **37** J8
Almería □ *Spain* **39** H2
Almería, G. de *Spain* **39** J2
Almetyevsk *Russia* **34** C11
Älmhult *Sweden* **11** H8
Almirante *Panama* **120** E3

Almiropótamos *Greece* **46** C6
Almirós *Greece* **46** B4
Almodôvar *Portugal* **37** H2
Almodóvar del Campo *Spain* **37** G6
Almodóvar del Río *Spain* **37** H5
Almonte *Canada* **115** A8
Almonte *Spain* **37** H4
Almora *India* **69** E8
Almoradí *Spain* **39** G4
Almorox *Spain* **36** E6
Almoustarat *Mali* **83** B5
Älmsta *Sweden* **10** E12
Almudévar *Spain* **38** C4
Almuñécar *Spain* **37** J7
Almunge *Sweden* **10** E12
Almuradiel *Spain* **37** G7
Almus *Turkey* **72** B7
Almyrou, Ormos *Greece* **49** D6
Alness *U.K.* **13** D4
Alnmouth *U.K.* **14** B6
Alnwick *U.K.* **14** B6
Aloi *Uganda* **86** B3
Alon *Burma* **67** H19
Alonissos *Greece* **46** B5
Alónnisos-Northern
  Sporades △ *Greece* **46** B6
Alor *Indonesia* **63** F6
Alor Setar *Malaysia* **65** J3
Ålora *Spain* **37** J6
Alosno *Spain* **37** H3
Alot *India* **68** H6
Aloysius, Mt. *Australia* **93** E4
Alpaugh *U.S.A.* **110** K7
Alpe Apuane → *Italy* **40** D7
Alpedrinha *Portugal* **36** E3
Alpena *U.S.A.* **113** C12
Alpes-de-Haute-
  Provence □ *France* **21** D10
Alpes-Maritimes □ *France* **21** E11
Alpha *Australia* **94** C4
Alpha Ridge *Arctic* **4** A2
Alphen aan den Rijn *Neths.* **17** B4
Alphios → *Greece* **46** D3
Alpiarça *Portugal* **37** F2
Alpine *Ariz., U.S.A.* **109** K9
Alpine *Calif., U.S.A.* **111** N10
Alpine *Tex., U.S.A.* **116** F3
Alps *Europe* **22** E5
Alpu *Turkey* **72** C4
Alpurrurulam *Australia* **94** C2
Alqueta, Barragem do
  Portugal **37** G3
Alrø *Denmark* **11** J4
Als *Denmark* **11** K3
Alsace □ *France* **19** D14
Alsask *Canada* **103** C7
Alsasua *Spain* **38** C2
Alsek → *U.S.A.* **102** B1
Alsfeld *Germany* **24** E5
Alsta *Norway* **8** D15
Alstermo *Sweden* **11** H9
Alston *U.K.* **14** C5
Alta *Norway* **8** B20
Alta, Sierra *Spain* **38** E3
Alta Gracia *Argentina* **126** C3
Alta Sierra *U.S.A.* **111** K8
Altaelva → *Norway* **8** B20
Altafjorden *Norway* **8** A20
Altai = Aerhtai Shan
  Mongolia **60** B4
Altai = Gorno-Altay □
  Russia **52** D9
Altamaha → *U.S.A.* **117** F14
Altamira *Brazil* **125** D8
Altamira *Chile* **126** B2
Altamira *Mexico* **119** C5
Altamira, Cuevas de *Spain* **36** B6
Altamont *U.S.A.* **115** D10
Altamura *Italy* **43** B9
Altanbulag *Mongolia* **60** A5
Altar *Mexico* **118** A2
Altar, Gran Desierto de
  Mexico **118** B2
Altata *Mexico* **118** C3
Altavista *U.S.A.* **113** G14
Altay *China* **60** B3
Altdorf *Switz.* **25** J4
Alte Mellum *Germany* **24** B4
Altea *Spain* **39** G4
Altenberg *Germany* **24** E9
Altenbruch *Germany* **24** B4
Altenburg *Germany* **24** E8
Altenkirchen
  *Mecklenburg-Vorpommern,
  Germany* **24** A9
Altenkirchen *Rhld.-Pfz.,
  Germany* **24** E3
Altenmarkt *Austria* **26** D7
Alter do Chão *Portugal* **37** F3
Altınkaya Barajı *Turkey* **72** B6
Altınoluk *Turkey* **47** B8
Altınova *Turkey* **47** B8
Altıntaş *Turkey* **47** B12
Altınyaka *Turkey* **47** E12
Altınyayla *Turkey* **47** D11
Altiplano *Bolivia* **124** G5
Altkirch *France* **19** E14

Altmark *Germany* **24** C7
Altmühl → *Germany* **25** G7
Altmühltal △ *Germany* **25** G7
Altmunster *Austria* **26** D6
Alto Adige = Trentino-Alto
  Adige □ *Italy* **41** B8
Alto Araguaia *Brazil* **125** G8
Alto Cuchumatanes =
  Cuchumatanes, Sierra de
  los *Guatemala* **120** C1
Alto del Carmen *Chile* **126** B1
Alto Garda Bresciano △ *Italy* **40** C7
Alto Ligonha *Mozam.* **87** F4
Alto Molocue *Mozam.* **87** F4
Alto Paraguay □ *Paraguay* **126** A4
Alto Paraná □ *Paraguay* **127** B5
Alton *Canada* **114** C4
Alton *U.K.* **15** F7
Alton *Ill., U.S.A.* **112** F8
Alton *N.H., U.S.A.* **115** C13
Altona *Canada* **103** D9
Altoona *U.S.A.* **114** F6
Altötting *Germany* **25** G8
Altstätten *Switz.* **25** H5
Altun Kupri *Iraq* **73** E11
Altun Shan *China* **60** C3
Alturas *U.S.A.* **108** F3
Altus *U.S.A.* **116** D5
Alubijid *Phil.* **61** G6
Alucra *Turkey* **73** B8
Aluk *Sudan* **81** F2
Alūksne *Latvia* **32** D4
Alunda *Sweden* **10** D12
Alunite *U.S.A.* **111** K12
Aluoro → *Ethiopia* **81** F3
Alupka *Ukraine* **33** K8
Alushta *Ukraine* **33** K8
Alusi *Indonesia* **63** F8
Alustante *Spain* **38** E3
Alva *U.S.A.* **116** C5
Alvaiázere *Portugal* **36** F2
Älvängen *Sweden* **11** G6
Alvão △ *Portugal* **36** D3
Alvarado *Mexico* **119** D5
Alvarado *U.S.A.* **116** E6
Alvaro Obregón, Presa
  Mexico **118** B3
Älvdalen *Sweden* **10** C8
Alvear *Argentina* **126** B4
Alverca *Portugal* **37** G1
Alvesta *Sweden* **11** H8
Alvin *U.S.A.* **116** G7
Alvinston *Canada* **114** D3
Alvito *Portugal* **37** G3
Älvkarleby *Sweden* **10** D11
Alvord Desert *U.S.A.* **108** E4
Älvros *Sweden* **10** B8
Älvsbyn *Sweden* **8** D19
Alwar *India* **68** F7
Alxa Zuoqi *China* **56** E3
Alyangula *Australia* **94** A2
Alyata = Älät *Azerbaijan* **35** L9
Alyth *U.K.* **13** E5
Alzada *U.S.A.* **108** D11
Alzamay *Russia* **53** D11
Alzey *Germany* **25** F4
Alzira *Spain* **39** F4
Am Timan *Chad* **79** F10
Amadeus, L. *Australia* **93** D5
Amadi *Dem. Rep. of the Congo* **86** B2
Amâdi *Sudan* **81** F3
Amadjuak L. *Canada* **101** E17
Amadora *Portugal* **37** G1
Amagansett *U.S.A.* **115** F12
Amagasaki *Japan* **55** G7
Amager *Denmark* **11** J6
Amagunze *Nigeria* **83** D6
Amahai *Indonesia* **63** E7
Amaile *Samoa* **91** b
Amaiun-Maia *Spain* **38** B3
Amakusa-Shotō *Japan* **55** H5
Åmål *Sweden* **10** E6
Amalfi *Italy* **43** B7
Amaliáda *Greece* **46** D3
Amalner *India* **66** J9
Amamapare *Indonesia* **63** E9
Amambaí *Brazil* **127** A4
Amambaí → *Brazil* **127** A5
Amambay □ *Paraguay* **127** A4
Amambay, Cordillera de
  S. Amer. **127** A4
Amami-Guntō *Japan* **55** L4
Amami-Ō-Shima *Japan* **55** K4
Aman, Pulau *Malaysia* **65** c
Amaná, L. *Brazil* **124** D6
Amanat → *India* **69** G11
Amanda Park *U.S.A.* **110** C3
Amankeldi *Kazakhstan* **52** D7
Amantea *Italy* **43** C9
Amapá *Brazil* **125** C8
Amapá □ *Brazil* **125** C8
Amara *Sudan* **81** E3
Amara □ *Ethiopia* **81** E4
Amaranth *Canada* **103** C9
Amarante *Brazil* **125** E10
Amarante *Portugal* **36** D2
Amareleja *Portugal* **37** G3
Amargosa → *U.S.A.* **111** J10

Amargosa Desert *U.S.A.* **111** J10
Amargosa Range *U.S.A.* **111** J10
Amari *Greece* **49** D6
Amarillo *U.S.A.* **116** D4
Amârnâ, Tell el' *Egypt* **80** B3
Amaro, Mte. *Italy* **41** F11
Amarpur *India* **69** G12
Amarti *Eritrea* **81** E5
Amarwara *India* **69** H8
Amasra *Turkey* **72** B5
Amassama *Nigeria* **83** D6
Amasya *Turkey* **72** B6
Amasya □ *Turkey* **72** B6
Amata *Australia* **93** E5
Amatikulu *S. Africa* **89** D5
Amatitlán *Guatemala* **120** D1
Amatrice *Italy* **41** F10
Amay *Belgium* **17** D5
Amazon = Amazonas →
  S. Amer. **125** D8
Amazonas □ *Brazil* **124** E6
Amazonas → *S. Amer.* **125** D8
Amba Ferit *Ethiopia* **81** E4
Ambah *India* **68** F7
Ambahakily *Madag.* **89** C7
Ambahita *Madag.* **89** C8
Ambala *India* **68** D7
Ambalavao *Madag.* **89** C8
Ambanja *Madag.* **89** A8
Ambararata *Madag.* **89** B8
Ambarchik *Russia* **53** C17
Ambarijeby *Madag.* **89** A8
Ambaro, Helodranon'
  Madag. **89** A8
Ambato *Ecuador* **124** D3
Ambato *Madag.* **89** A8
Ambato, Sierra de *Argentina* **126** B2
Ambato Boeny *Madag.* **89** B8
Ambatofinandrahana
  Madag. **89** C8
Ambatolampy *Madag.* **89** B8
Ambatomainty *Madag.* **89** B8
Ambatomanoina *Madag.* **89** B8
Ambatondrazaka *Madag.* **89** B8
Ambatosoratra *Madag.* **89** B8
Ambelonas *Greece* **46** B4
Ambenja *Madag.* **89** B8
Amberg *Germany* **25** F7
Ambergris Cay *Belize* **119** D7
Ambérieu-en-Bugey *France* **21** C9
Amberley *Canada* **114** B3
Amberley *N.Z.* **91** E4
Ambert *France* **20** C7
Ambidédi *Mali* **82** C3
Ambikapur *India* **69** H10
Ambikol *Sudan* **80** C3
Ambilobé *Madag.* **89** A8
Ambinanindrano *Madag.* **89** C8
Ambinanitelo *Madag.* **89** B8
Ambinda *Madag.* **89** B8
Amble *U.K.* **14** B6
Ambleside *U.K.* **14** C5
Ambo *Peru* **124** F3
Amboahangy *Madag.* **89** C8
Ambodifototra *Madag.* **89** B8
Ambodilazana *Madag.* **89** B8
Ambodiriana *Madag.* **89** B8
Ambohidratrimo *Madag.* **89** B8
Ambohidray *Madag.* **89** B8
Ambohimahamasina *Madag.* **89** C8
Ambohimahasoa *Madag.* **89** C8
Ambohimanga *Madag.* **89** C8
Ambohimitombo *Madag.* **89** C8
Ambohitra *Madag.* **89** A8
Amboise *France* **18** E8
Ambon *Indonesia* **63** E7
Ambondro *Madag.* **89** D8
Amboseli, L. *Kenya* **86** C4
Amboseli △ *Kenya* **86** C4
Ambositra *Madag.* **89** C8
Ambovombe *Madag.* **89** D8
Amboy *U.S.A.* **111** L11
Amboyna Cay *S. China Sea* **62** C4
Ambridge *U.S.A.* **114** F4
Ambriz *Angola* **84** F2
Ambrolauri *Georgia* **73** A10
Amchitka I. *U.S.A.* **106** E3
Amderma *Russia* **52** C7
Amdhi *India* **69** H9
Amdo *China* **67** C17
Ameca *Mexico* **118** C4
Ameca → *Mexico* **118** C3
Amecameca de Juárez
  Mexico **119** D5
Ameland *Neths.* **17** A5
Amélia *Italy* **41** F9
America-Antarctica Ridge
  S. Ocean **5** B2
American Falls *U.S.A.* **108** E7
American Falls Res. *U.S.A.* **108** E7
American Fork *U.S.A.* **108** F8
American Highland *Antarctica* **5** D6
American Samoa ☑ *Pac. Oc.* **91** b
American Samoa △
  Amer. Samoa **91** b

Americus *U.S.A.* **117** E12
Amerigo Vespucci,
  Firenze ✈ (FLR) *Italy* **41** E8
Amersfoort *Neths.* **17** B5
Amersfoort *S. Africa* **89** D4
Amery Basin *S. Ocean* **5** C6
Amery Ice Shelf *Antarctica* **5** C6
Ames = Bertamirans *Spain* **36** C2
Ames *U.S.A.* **112** D7
Amesbury *U.S.A.* **115** D14
Amet *India* **68** G5
Amfíklia *Greece* **46** C4
Amfilochía *Greece* **46** C3
Amfípoli *Greece* **44** F7
Amfissa *Greece* **46** C4
Amga *Russia* **53** C14
Amga → *Russia* **53** C14
Amgu *Russia* **54** B8
Amgun → *Russia* **53** D14
Amherst *Canada* **105** C7
Amherst *Mass., U.S.A.* **115** D12
Amherst *N.Y., U.S.A.* **114** D6
Amherst *Ohio, U.S.A.* **114** E2
Amherst I. *Canada* **115** B8
Amherstburg *Canada* **104** D2
Amiata, Mte. *Italy* **41** F8
Amidon *U.S.A.* **112** B2
Amiens *France* **19** C9
Amindeo *Greece* **44** F5
Åminne *Sweden* **11** G7
Amino *Ethiopia* **81** G5
Aminuis *Namibia* **88** C2
Amīrābād *Iran* **70** C5
Amirante Is. *Seychelles* **50** J7
Amisk △ *Canada* **103** B9
Amisk L. *Canada* **103** C8
Amistad, Presa de la *Mexico* **118** B4
Amistad △ *U.S.A.* **116** G4
Amite *U.S.A.* **117** F9
Amla *India* **68** J8
Amlapura = Karangasem
  Indonesia **63** J18
Amlia I. *U.S.A.* **106** E5
Amlwch *U.K.* **14** D3
Amm Adam *Sudan* **81** D4
'Ammān *Jordan* **74** D4
'Ammān □ *Jordan* **74** D5
'Ammān ✈ (AMM) *Jordan* **74** D5
Ammanford *U.K.* **15** F4
Ammassalik = Tasiilaq
  Greenland **4** C6
Ammerån → *Sweden* **10** A10
Ammersee *Germany* **25** G7
Ammochostos =
  Famagusta *Cyprus* **49** D12
Ammon *U.S.A.* **108** E8
Amnat Charoen *Thailand* **64** E5
Amnura *Bangla.* **69** G13
Amo Jiang → *China* **58** F3
Åmol *Iran* **71** B7
Amorgós *Greece* **47** E7
Amory *U.S.A.* **117** E10
Amos *Canada* **104** C4
Åmot *Norway* **9** G13
Åmotfors *Sweden* **10** E6
Amoy = Xiamen *China* **59** E12
Ampanavoana *Madag.* **89** B9
Ampang *Malaysia* **65** L3
Ampanganela,
  Lakandranon' *Madag.* **89** C8
Ampanihy *Madag.* **89** C7
Amparafaravola *Madag.* **89** B8
Ampasinambo *Madag.* **89** C8
Ampasindava,
  Helodranon' *Madag.* **89** A8
Ampasindava, Saikanosy
  Madag. **89** A8
Ampenan *Indonesia* **62** F5
Amper *Nigeria* **83** D6
Amper → *Germany* **25** G7
Ampezzo *Italy* **41** B9
Amphoe Kathu *Thailand* **65** a
Amphoe Thalang *Thailand* **65** a
Ampitsikinana *Madag.* **89** A8
Ampombiantambo *Madag.* **89** A8
Amposta *Spain* **38** E5
Ampotaka *Madag.* **89** D7
Ampoza *Madag.* **89** C7
Amqui *Canada* **105** C6
Amravati *India* **66** J10
Amreli *India* **68** J4
Amritsar *India* **68** D6
Amroha *India* **69** E8
Amrum *Germany* **24** A4
Amsterdam *Neths.* **17** B4
Amsterdam ✈ (AMS) *Neths.* **17** B4
Amsterdam, I. = Nouvelle
  Amsterdam, Î. *Ind. Oc.* **3** F13
Amstetten *Austria* **26** C7
'Amūdah *Syria* **73** D9
Amudarya → *Uzbekistan* **52** E6
Amund Ringnes I. *Canada* **101** B12
Amundsen Abyssal Plain
  S. Ocean **5** C14
Amundsen Basin *Arctic* **4** A1
Amundsen Gulf *Canada* **100** C7
Amundsen Ridges *S. Ocean* **5** C14
Amundsen-Scott *Antarctica* **5** E

Amundsen Sea *Antarctica* **5** D15
Amungen *Sweden* **10** C9
Amuntai *Indonesia* **62** E5
Amur → *Russia* **53** D15
Amur, W. → *Sudan* **80** D3
Amurang *Indonesia* **63** D6
Amurrio *Spain* **38** B1
Amursk *Russia* **53** D14
Amusco *Spain* **36** C6
Amvrakikos Kolpos *Greece* **46** C2
Amvrosiyivka *Ukraine* **33** J10
Amyderya = Amudarya →
 Uzbekistan **52** E6
An Bien *Vietnam* **65** H5
An Cabhán = Cavan *Ireland* **12** B4
An Cóbh = Cóbh *Ireland* **12** E3
An Daingean = Dingle
 Ireland **12** D1
An Hoa *Vietnam* **64** E7
An Longfort = Longford
 Ireland **12** C4
An Muileann gCearr =
 Mullingar *Ireland* **12** C4
An Nabatiyah at Tahta
 Lebanon **74** B4
An Nabk *Si. Arabia* **70** D3
An Nabk *Syria* **74** A5
An Nafūd *Si. Arabia* **70** D4
An Nāḩīyah *Iraq* **73** E9
An Najaf *Iraq* **73** G11
An Nás = Naas *Ireland* **12** C5
An Nhon *Vietnam* **64** F7
An Nîl □ *Sudan* **80** D3
An Nîl el Abyad □ *Sudan* **81** E3
An Nîl el Azraq □ *Sudan* **81** E3
An Nu'ayrīyah *Si. Arabia* **71** E6
An Nu'mānīyah *Iraq* **73** F11
An Ros = Rush *Ireland* **12** C5
An tAonach = Nenagh
 Ireland **12** D3
An Thoi, Dao *Vietnam* **65** H5
An tInbhear Mór = Arklow
 Ireland **12** D5
An Uaimh *Ireland* **12** C5
Anabar → *Russia* **53** B12
'Anabtā *West Bank* **74** C4
Anaconda *U.S.A.* **108** C7
Anacortes *U.S.A.* **110** B4
Anacuao, Mt. *Phil.* **61** C4
Anadarko *U.S.A.* **116** D5
Anadia *Portugal* **36** E2
Anadolu *Turkey* **72** C5
Anadyr *Russia* **53** C18
Anadyr → *Russia* **53** C18
Anadyrskiy Zaliv *Russia* **53** C19
Anafi *Greece* **47** E7
Anaga, Pta. de *Canary Is.* **48** F3
Anagni *Italy* **41** G10
'Ānah *Iraq* **73** E10
Anaheim *U.S.A.* **111** M9
Anahim Lake *Canada* **102** C3
Anakapalle *India* **67** L13
Anakie *Australia* **94** C4
Anaklia *Georgia* **35** J5
Analalava *Madag.* **89** A8
Analavoka *Madag.* **89** C8
Analipsis *Greece* **49** A3
Anambar → *Pakistan* **68** D3
Anambas, Kepulauan
 Indonesia **62** D3
Anambas Is. = Anambas,
 Kepulauan *Indonesia* **62** D3
Anambra □ *Nigeria* **83** D6
Anamosa *U.S.A.* **112** D8
Anamur *Turkey* **72** D5
Anamur Burnu *Turkey* **72** D5
Anan *Japan* **55** H7
Anand *India* **68** H5
Ananes *Greece* **46** E6
Anangu Pitjantjatjara ◎
 Australia **93** E5
Anantapur *India* **66** M10
Anantnag *India* **69** C6
Ananyiv *Ukraine* **29** C14
Anapa *Russia* **33** K9
Anapodiaris → *Greece* **49** E7
Anápolis *Brazil* **125** G9
Anapu → *Brazil* **125** D8
Anār *Iran* **71** D7
Anārak *Iran* **71** C7
Anarisfjällen *Sweden* **10** A7
Anas → *India* **68** H5
Anatolia = Anadolu *Turkey* **72** C5
Anatsogno *Madag.* **89** C7
Añatuya *Argentina* **126** B3
Anatye ◎ *Australia* **94** C3
Anaunethad L. *Canada* **103** A8
Anbyŏn *N. Korea* **57** E14
Ancares, Sierra dos *Spain* **36** C4
Ancares △ *Spain* **36** C4
Ancaster *Canada* **114** C5
Ancenis *France* **18** E5
Anchor Bay *U.S.A.* **110** G3
Anchorage *U.S.A.* **100** E2
Anci *China* **56** E9
Ancohuma, Nevado *Bolivia* **124** G5
Ancón *Peru* **124** F3
Ancona *Italy* **41** E10

Ancud *Chile* **128** E2
Ancud, G. de *Chile* **128** E2
Ancy-le-Franc *France* **19** E11
Andacollo *Argentina* **126** D1
Andacollo *Chile* **126** C1
Andaingo *Madag.* **89** B8
Andalgalá *Argentina* **126** B2
Andalucía □ *Spain* **37** H6
Andalusia = Andalucía □
 Spain **37** H6
Andalusia *U.S.A.* **117** F11
Andaman Is. *Ind. Oc.* **51** G11
Andaman Sea *Ind. Oc.* **62** B1
Andamooka *Australia* **95** E2
Andapa *Madag.* **89** A8
Andara *Namibia* **88** B3
Andelot-Blancheville *France* **19** D12
Andenes *Norway* **8** B17
Andenne *Belgium* **17** D5
Andéranboukane *Mali* **83** B5
Andermatt *Switz.* **25** J4
Andernach *Germany* **24** E3
Andernos-les-Bains *France* **20** D2
Anderslöv *Sweden* **11** J7
Anderson *Alaska, U.S.A.* **106** C10
Anderson *Calif., U.S.A.* **108** F2
Anderson *Ind., U.S.A.* **113** E11
Anderson *Mo., U.S.A.* **112** G6
Anderson *S.C., U.S.A.* **117** D13
Anderson → *Canada* **100** D6
Anderstorp *Sweden* **11** G7
Andes *U.S.A.* **115** D10
Andes, Cord. de los *S. Amer.* **124** H5
Andfjorden *Norway* **8** B17
Andhra Pradesh □ *India* **66** L11
Andijon *Uzbekistan* **52** E8
Andikíthira = Antikythira
 Greece **46** F5
Andilamena *Madag.* **89** B8
Andīmeshk *Iran* **73** F13
Andímilos = Antimilos
 Greece **46** E6
Andíparos = Antiparos
 Greece **47** D7
Andipaxoi = Antipaxi *Greece* **46** B2
Andipsara *Greece* **47** C7
Andizhan = Andijon
 Uzbekistan **52** E8
Andoain *Spain* **38** B2
Andoany *Madag.* **89** A8
Andohahela △ *Madag.* **89** C8
Andong *S. Korea* **57** F15
Andongwei *China* **57** G10
Andorra *Spain* **38** E4
Andorra ■ *Europe* **20** F5
Andorra La Vella *Andorra* **20** F5
Andover *U.K.* **15** F6
Andover *Maine, U.S.A.* **115** B14
Andover *Mass., U.S.A.* **115** D13
Andover *N.J., U.S.A.* **115** F10
Andover *N.Y., U.S.A.* **114** D7
Andover *Ohio, U.S.A.* **114** E4
Andøya *Norway* **8** B16
Andradina *Brazil* **125** H8
Andrahary *Madag.* **89** A8
Andramasina *Madag.* **89** B8
Andranopasy *Madag.* **89** C7
Andranovory *Madag.* **89** C7
Andratx *Spain* **48** B9
Andreanof Is. *U.S.A.* **106** E4
Andreapol *Russia* **32** D7
Andrews *S.C., U.S.A.* **117** E15
Andrews *Tex., U.S.A.* **116** E3
Andreyevka *Russia* **34** D10
Ándria *Italy* **43** A9
Andriamena *Madag.* **89** B8
Andriandampy *Madag.* **89** C8
Andriba *Madag.* **89** B8
Andrijevica *Montenegro* **44** D3
Andringitra △ *Madag.* **89** C8
Andritsena *Greece* **46** D3
Androka *Madag.* **89** C7
Andros *Greece* **46** D6
Andros I. *Bahamas* **120** B4
Andros Town *Bahamas* **120** B4
Androscoggin → *U.S.A.* **115** C14
Andrychów *Poland* **31** J6
Andselv *Norway* **8** B18
Andújar *Spain* **37** G6
Andulo *Angola* **84** G3
Aneby *Sweden* **11** G8
Anéfis *Mali* **83** B5
Anegada *Br. Virgin Is.* **121** e
Anegada Passage *W. Indies* **121** C7
Aného *Togo* **83** D5
Anenni-Noi *Moldova* **29** D14
Anepmete *Papua N. G.* (?)
Aneto, Pico de *Spain* **38** C5
Anfu *China* **59** D10
Ang Mo Kio *Singapore* **65** d
Ang Thong *Thailand* **64** E3
Ang Thong, Ko *Thailand* **65** b
Ang Thong △ *Thailand* **65** b
Angamos, Punta *Chile* **126** A1
Angara → *Russia* **53** D10
Angara-Débou *Benin* **83** C5
Angarbka *Sudan* **81** F1
Angarsk *Russia* **53** D11
Angas Hills *Australia* **92** D4

Angaston *Australia* **95** E2
Ånge *Sweden* **10** B9
Ångel, Salto = Angel Falls
 Venezuela **124** B6
Ángel de la Guarda, I.
 Mexico **118** B2
Angel Falls *Venezuela* **124** B6
Angeles *Phil.* **61** D4
Ängelholm *Sweden* **11** H6
Angels Camp *U.S.A.* **110** G6
Anger → *Ethiopia* **81** F4
Angereb *Ethiopia* **81** E4
Angereb → *Ethiopia* **81** E4
Ängermanälven → *Sweden* **10** A11
Ångermanland *Sweden* **8** E17
Angermünde *Germany* **24** B9
Angers *Canada* **115** A9
Angers *France* **18** E6
Angerville *France* **19** D9
Ängesån → *Sweden* **8** C20
Angikuni L. *Canada* **103** A9
Angkor *Cambodia* **64** F4
Angledool *Australia* **95** D4
Anglès *Spain* **38** D7
Anglesey *U.K.* **14** D3
Anglesey, Isle of □ *U.K.* **14** D3
Anglet *France* **20** E2
Angleton *U.S.A.* **116** G7
Anglin → *France* **20** B4
Anglisidhes *Cyprus* **49** E12
Anglure *France* **19** D10
Angmagssalik = Tasiilaq
 Greenland **4** C6
Ango *Dem. Rep. of the Congo* **86** B2
Angoche *Mozam.* **87** F4
Angoche, I. *Mozam.* **87** F4
Angol *Chile* **126** D1
Angola *Ind., U.S.A.* **113** E11
Angola *N.Y., U.S.A.* **114** D5
Angola ■ *Africa* **85** G3
Angoulême *France* **20** C4
Angoumois *France* **20** C4
Angra do Heroísmo *Azores* **78** A1
Angra dos Reis *Brazil* **127** A7
Angrapa → *Russia* **30** D3
Angtassom *Cambodia* **65** G5
Angu *Dem. Rep. of the Congo* **86** B1
Anguang *China* **57** B12
Anguilla ☑ *W. Indies* **121** C7
Anguo *China* **56** E8
Angurugu *Australia* **94** A2
Angus *Canada* **114** B5
Angus □ *U.K.* **13** E6
Angwa → *Zimbabwe* **89** B5
Anhanduí → *Brazil* **127** A5
Anholt *Denmark* **11** H5
Anhua *China* **59** C8
Anhui □ *China* **59** B11
Anhwei = Anhui □ *China* **59** B11
Anichab *Namibia* **88** C1
Anidros *Greece* **47** E7
Anié *Togo* **83** D5
Animas → *U.S.A.* **109** H9
Anina *Romania* **28** E6
Aninoasa *Romania* **29** F9
Anivorano *Madag.* **89** B8
Anjalankoski *Finland* **32** B4
Anjar *India* **68** H4
Anji *China* **59** B12
Anjou *France* **18** E6
Anjouan *Comoros Is.* **85** a
Anjozorobe *Madag.* **89** B8
Anju *N. Korea* **57** E13
Anka *Nigeria* **83** C6
Ankaboa, Tanjona *Madag.* **89** C7
Ankang *China* **56** H5
Ankara *Turkey* **72** C5
Ankara → *Turkey* **72** C5
Ankarafantsika △ *Madag.* **89** B8
Ankaramena *Madag.* **89** C8
Ankaratra *Madag.* **89** B8
Ankarsrum *Sweden* **11** G10
Ankasakasa *Madag.* **89** B7
Ankavandra *Madag.* **89** B8
Ankazoabo *Madag.* **89** C7
Ankazobe *Madag.* **89** B8
Ankeny *U.S.A.* **112** E7
Ankilimalinika *Madag.* **89** C7
Ankilizato *Madag.* **89** C8
Ankisabe *Madag.* **89** B8
Anklam *Germany* **24** B9
Ankober *Ethiopia* **81** F4
Ankoro *Dem. Rep. of the Congo* **86** D2
Ankororoka *Madag.* **89** D8
Ankpa *Nigeria* **83** D6
Anlong *China* **58** E5
Anlong Veng *Cambodia* **64** E5
Anlu *China* **59** B9
Anmyeondo *S. Korea* **57** F14
Ånn *Sweden* **10** A6
Ann, C. *U.S.A.* **115** D14
Ann Arbor *U.S.A.* **113** D12
Anna *Russia* **34** E5
Anna *U.S.A.* **112** G9
Annaba *Algeria* **78** A7
Annaberg-Buchholz
 Germany **24** E9
Annalee → *Ireland* **12** B4

Annam *Vietnam* **64** E7
Annamitique, Chaîne *Asia* **64** D6
Annan *U.K.* **13** G5
Annan → *U.K.* **13** G5
Annapolis *U.S.A.* **113** F15
Annapolis Royal *Canada* **105** D6
Annapurna *Nepal* **69** E10
Annean, L. *Australia* **93** E2
Anneberg *Sweden* **11** G8
Annecy *France* **21** C10
Annecy, Lac d' *France* **21** C10
Annemasse *France* **19** F13
Annenskiy Most *Russia* **32** B9
Annette I. *U.S.A.* **102** B2
Anning *China* **58** E4
Anniston *U.S.A.* **117** E12
Annobón *Atl. Oc.* **77** G4
Annot *France* **21** E10
Annotto B. *Jamaica* **120** a
Annoville *U.S.A.* **115** F8
Annweiler *Germany* **25** F3
Ano Poroia *Greece* **44** E7
Ano Siros *Greece* **46** D6
Anogia *Greece* **49** D6
Anorotsangana *Madag.* **89** A8
Anosibe *Madag.* **89** B8
Anou Mellene *Mali* **83** B5
Anoumaba *Ivory C.* **82** D4
Anping *Hebei, China* **56** E8
Anping *Liaoning, China* **57** D12
Anpu Gang *China* **58** G7
Anqing *China* **59** B11
Anqiu *China* **57** F10
Anren *China* **59** D9
Ansager *Denmark* **11** J2
Ansai *China* **56** F5
Ansan *S. Korea* **57** F14
Ansbach *Germany* **25** F6
Anse Boileau *Seychelles* **85** b
Anse Royale *Seychelles* **85** b
Anseba → *Eritrea* **81** D4
Ansfelden *Austria* **26** C7
Anshan *China* **57** D12
Anshun *China* **58** D5
Ansião *Portugal* **36** F2
Ansley *U.S.A.* **112** E4
Ansó *Spain* **38** C4
Ansoáin *Spain* **38** C3
Anson *U.S.A.* **116** E5
Anson B. *Australia* **92** B5
Ansongo *Mali* **83** B5
Ansongo-Ménaka △ *Mali* **83** B5
Ansonia *U.S.A.* **115** E11
Anstruther *U.K.* **13** E6
Ansudu *Indonesia* **63** E9
Antabamba *Peru* **124** F4
Antakya = Hatay *Turkey* **72** D7
Antalaha *Madag.* **89** A9
Antalya *Turkey* **72** D4
Antalya □ *Turkey* **47** E12
Antalya Körfezi *Turkey* **72** D4
Antambohobe *Madag.* **89** C8
Antanambao-Manampotsy
 Madag. **89** B8
Antanambe *Madag.* **89** B8
Antananarivo *Madag.* **89** B8
Antananarivo □ *Madag.* **89** B8
Antanifotsy *Madag.* **89** B8
Antanimbaribe *Madag.* **89** C7
Antanimora *Madag.* **89** C8
Antarctic Pen. *Antarctica* **5** C18
Antarctica ■ *Antarctica* **5** E3
Antelope *Zimbabwe* **87** G2
Antequera *Paraguay* **126** A4
Antequera *Spain* **37** H6
Antero, Mt. *U.S.A.* **108** G10
Antevamena *Madag.* **89** C7
Anthony *Kans., U.S.A.* **112** G4
Anthony *N. Mex., U.S.A.* **109** K10
Anti Atlas *Morocco* **78** C4
Anti-Lebanon = Sharqi, Al
 Jabal ash *Lebanon* **74** B5
Antibes *France* **21** E11
Antibes, C. d' *France* **21** E11
Anticosti, Î. d' *Canada* **105** C7
Antifer, C. d' *France* **18** C7
Antigo *U.S.A.* **112** C9
Antigonish *Canada* **105** C7
Antigua *Canary Is.* **48** F5
Antigua *Guatemala* **120** D1
Antigua *W. Indies* **121** C7
Antigua & Barbuda ■
 W. Indies **121** C7
Antikythira *Greece* **46** F5
Antilla *Cuba* **120** B4
Antilles = West Indies
 Cent. Amer. **121** D7
Antimilos *Greece* **46** E6
Antioch *U.S.A.* **110** G5
Antioche, Pertuis d' *France* **20** B2
Antioquia *Colombia* **124** B3
Antiparos *Greece* **47** D7
Antipaxi *Greece* **46** B2
Antipodes Is. *Pac. Oc.* **96** M9
Antirio *Greece* **46** C3
Antlers *U.S.A.* **116** D7
Antoetra *Madag.* **89** C8

Antofagasta *Chile* **126** A1
Antofagasta □ *Chile* **126** A2
Antofagasta de la Sierra
 Argentina **126** B2
Antofalla *Argentina* **126** B2
Antofalla, Salar de *Argentina* **126** B2
Anton *U.S.A.* **116** E3
Antongila, Helodrano
 Madag. **89** B8
Antonibé *Madag.* **89** B8
Antonibé, Presqu'île d'
 Madag. **89** A8
Antonina *Brazil* **127** B6
Antrain *France* **18** D5
Antrim *U.K.* **12** B5
Antrim *U.S.A.* **114** F3
Antrim □ *U.K.* **12** B5
Antrim, Mts. of *U.K.* **12** A5
Antrim Plateau *Australia* **92** C4
Antrodoco *Italy* **41** F10
Antropovo *Russia* **34** A6
Antsakabary *Madag.* **89** B8
Antsalova *Madag.* **89** B7
Antsenavolo *Madag.* **89** C8
Antsiafabositra *Madag.* **89** B8
Antsirabe *Antananarivo,*
 Madag. **89** B8
Antsirabe *Antsiranana, Madag.* **89** A8
Antsirabe *Mahajanga, Madag.* **89** B8
Antsiranana *Madag.* **89** A8
Antsiranana □ *Madag.* **89** A8
Antsohihy *Madag.* **89** A8
Antsohimbondrona
 Seranana *Madag.* **89** A8
Antu *China* **57** C15
Antwerp = Antwerpen
 Belgium **17** C4
Antwerp *U.S.A.* **115** B9
Antwerpen *Belgium* **17** C4
Antwerpen □ *Belgium* **17** C4
Anupgarh *India* **68** E5
Anuppur *India* **69** H9
Anuradhapura *Sri Lanka* **66** Q12
Anurrete ◎ *Australia* **94** C2
Anveh *Iran* **71** E7
Anvers = Antwerpen
 Belgium **17** C4
Anvers I. *Antarctica* **5** C17
Anwen *China* **59** C13
Anxi *Fujian, China* **59** E12
Anxi *Gansu, China* **60** B4
Anxian *China* **58** B5
Anxiang *China* **59** C9
Anxious B. *Australia* **95** E1
Anyama *Ivory C.* **82** D4
Anyang *China* **56** F8
Anyang *S. Korea* **57** F14
Anyer *Indonesia* **63** G11
Anyi *Jiangxi, China* **59** C10
Anyi *Shanxi, China* **56** G6
Anyuan *China* **59** E10
Anyue *China* **58** B5
Anza *U.S.A.* **111** M10
Anze *China* **56** F7
Anzhero-Sudzhensk *Russia* **52** D9
Ánzio *Italy* **42** A5
Ao Makham *Thailand* **65** a
Ao Phangnga △ *Thailand* **65** a
Aoga-Shima *Japan* **55** H9
Aoiz *Spain* **38** C3
Aoji *N. Korea* **57** C16
Aomen = Macau *China* **59** F9
Aomori *Japan* **54** D10
Aomori □ *Japan* **54** D10
Aonla *India* **69** E8
Aorai, Mt. *Tahiti* **91** d
Aoraki Mount Cook *N.Z.* **91** E3
Aoral, Phnum *Cambodia* **65** G5
Aosta *Italy* **40** C4
Aotearoa = New Zealand ■
 Oceania **91** D6
Aoudéras *Niger* **83** B6
Aoukâr *Mauritania* **82** B3
Aozou Strip *Chad* **79** D9
Apá → *S. Amer.* **126** A4
Apache *U.S.A.* **116** D5
Apache Junction *U.S.A.* **109** K8
Apalachee B. *U.S.A.* **117** G13
Apalachicola *U.S.A.* **117** G12
Apalachicola → *U.S.A.* **117** G12
Apam *Ghana* **83** D4
Apapa *Nigeria* **83** D5
Apaporis → *Colombia* **124** D5
Aparados da Serra △ *Brazil* **127** B5
Aparri *Phil.* **61** B4
Apateu *Romania* **28** D6
Apatin *Serbia* **28** E4
Apatity *Russia* **8** C25
Apatula = Finke *Australia* **94** D1
Apatzingán *Mexico* **118** D4
Apeldoorn *Neths.* **17** B5
Apen *Germany* **24** B3
Apennines = Appennini
 Italy **40** D7
Aphrodisias *Turkey* **47** D10
Apia *Samoa* **91** b
Apiacás, Serra dos *Brazil* **124** E7
Apies → *S. Africa* **89** D4
Apizaco *Mexico* **119** D5

Aplao *Peru* **124** G4
Apo, Mt. *Phil.* **63** C7
Apolakia *Greece* **49** C9
Apolakia, Ormos *Greece* **49** C9
Apolda *Germany* **24** D7
Apollonia = Sūsah *Libya* **79** B10
Apollonia *Greece* **46** E6
Apolo *Bolivia* **124** F5
Apolonia *Greece* **46** E6
Apopa *El Salv.* **120** D2
Aporé → *Brazil* **125** G8
Apostle Is. *U.S.A.* **112** B8
Apostle Islands △ *U.S.A.* **112** B8
Apóstoles *Argentina* **127** B4
Apostolos Andreas, C.
 Cyprus **49** D13
Apostolovo *Ukraine* **33** J7
Apoteri *Guyana* **124** C7
Appalachian Mts. *U.S.A.* **113** G14
Äppelbo *Sweden* **10** D8
Appennini *Italy* **40** D7
Appennino Ligure *Italy* **40** D6
Appenzell-Ausser
 Rhoden □ *Switz.* **25** H5
Appenzell-Inner Rhoden □
 Switz. **25** H5
Appiano *Italy* **41** B8
Apple Hill *Canada* **115** A10
Apple Valley *U.S.A.* **111** L9
Appleby-in-Westmorland
 U.K. **14** C5
Appledore *U.K.* **15** F3
Appleton *U.S.A.* **112** C9
Approuague → *Fr. Guiana* **125** C8
Apricena *Italy* **41** G12
Aprília *Italy* **42** A5
Apsheronsk *Russia* **35** H4
Apsley *Canada* **114** B6
Apt *France* **21** E9
Apuane, Alpi *Italy* **40** D7
Apucarana *Brazil* **127** A5
Apulia = Púglia □ *Italy* **43** A9
Apure → *Venezuela* **124** B5
Apurimac → *Peru* **124** F4
Apuseni, Munții *Romania* **28** D7
Āq Qālā *Iran* **71** B7
Aqaba = Al 'Aqabah *Jordan* **74** F4
Aqaba, G. of *Red Sea* **70** D2
'Aqabah, Khalīj al =
 Aqaba, G. of *Red Sea* **70** D2
'Aqdā *Iran* **71** C7
Aqīq *Sudan* **80** D4
Aqiq, Khalîg *Sudan* **80** D4
Aqmola = Astana *Kazakhstan* **52** D8
Aqqikkol Hu *China* **60** C3
Aqrah *Iraq* **73** D10
Aqsay *Kazakhstan* **52** D6
Aqtaū *Kazakhstan* **52** E6
Aqtöbe *Kazakhstan* **52** D6
Aqtoghay *Kazakhstan* **52** E8
Aquidauana *Brazil* **125** H7
Aquila *Mexico* **118** D4
Aquiles Serdán *Mexico* **118** B3
Aquin *Haiti* **121** C5
Aquitaine □ *France* **20** D3
Ar Rafid *Syria* **74** C4
Ar Raḩḩālīyah *Iraq* **73** F10
Ar Ramādī *Iraq* **73** F10
Ar Ramtha *Jordan* **74** C5
Ar Raqqah *Syria* **73** E8
Ar Raqqah □ *Syria* **73** D8
Ar Rashidiya = Er Rachidia
 Morocco **78** B5
Ar Rass *Si. Arabia* **70** E4
Ar Rayyan *Qatar* **71** E6
Ar Rifā'ī *Iraq* **70** D5
Ar Riyāḑ *Si. Arabia* **70** E5
Ar Ru'ays *Qatar* **71** E6
Ar Rukhaymīyah *Iraq* **70** D5
Ar Rumaythah *Iraq* **70** D5
Ar Rumāfah *Syria* **73** E8
Ar Ruṣāfah *Syria* **73** E8
Ar Ruṭbah *Iraq* **73** F9
Ara *India* **69** G11
Ara Goro *Ethiopia* **81** F5
Ara Tera *Ethiopia* **81** F5
Arab *U.S.A.* **117** D11
'Arab, Bahr el → *Sudan* **81** F2
Arab, Khalîg el *Egypt* **80** A2
'Araba, W. → *Egypt* **80** J8
'Arabābād *Iran* **71** C8
Araban *Turkey* **72** D7
Arabatskaya Strelka *Ukraine* **33** K8
Arabba *Italy* **41** B8
Arabia *Asia* **50** F6
Arabian Desert = Es Sahrâ'
 Esh Sharqîya *Egypt* **80** B3
Arabian Gulf = Persian
 Gulf *Asia* **71** E6
Arabian Sea *Ind. Oc.* **50** G8
Araç *Turkey* **72** B5
Aracaju *Brazil* **125** F11
Aracati *Brazil* **125** D11
Araçatuba *Brazil* **127** A5
Aracena *Spain* **37** H4
Aracena, Sierra de *Spain* **37** H4
Arachova *Greece* **46** C4
Arachthos → *Greece* **46** B3
Aračinovo *Macedonia* **44** D5
Araçuaí *Brazil* **125** G10
'Arad *Israel* **74** D4

Arad *Romania* **28** D6
Arad □ *Romania* **28** D6
Arādān *Iran* **71** C7
Aradhippou *Cyprus* **49** E12
Arafura Sea *E. Indies* **90** B6
Aragats *Armenia* **35** K7
Aragón □ *Spain* **38** C3
Aragón → *Spain* **38** C3
Aragona *Italy* **42** E6
Araguacema *Brazil* **125** E9
Araguaia → *Brazil* **125** E9
Araguaína *Brazil* **125** E9
Araguari *Brazil* **125** G9
Araguari → *Brazil* **125** C9
Arahal *Spain* **37** H5
Arain *India* **68** F6
Arak *Algeria* **78** C6
Arāk *Iran* **71** C6
Araka *Sudan* **81** G3
Arakan Coast *Burma* **67** K19
Arakan Yoma *Burma* **67** K19
Araklı *Turkey* **73** B9
Araks = Aras, Rūd-e → *Asia* **35** K9
Aral *Kazakhstan* **52** E7
Aral Sea *Asia* **52** E7
Aral Tengizi = Aral Sea *Asia* **52** E7
Aralık *Turkey* **73** C11
Aralsk = Aral *Kazakhstan* **52** E7
Aralskoye More = Aral Sea *Asia* **52** E7
Aralsor, Ozero = Aralsor Köli *Kazakhstan* **35** F9
Aralsor Köli *Kazakhstan* **35** F9
Aramac *Australia* **94** C4
Aran I. *Ireland* **12** A3
Aran Is. *Ireland* **12** C2
Aranda de Duero *Spain* **36** D7
Arandān *Iran* **70** C5
Aranđelovac *Serbia* **44** B4
Aranjuez *Spain* **36** E7
Aranos *Namibia* **88** C2
Aranyaprathet *Thailand* **64** F4
Araouane *Mali* **82** B4
Arapahoe *U.S.A.* **112** E4
Arapey Grande → *Uruguay* **126** C4
Arapgir *Turkey* **73** C8
Arapiraca *Brazil* **125** E11
Arapis, Akra *Greece* **45** F8
Arapongas *Brazil* **127** A5
Ar'ar *Si. Arabia* **70** D4
Araranguá *Brazil* **127** B6
Araraquara *Brazil* **125** H9
Ararás, Serra das *Brazil* **127** B5
Ararat *Armenia* **73** C11
Ararat *Australia* **95** F3
Ararat, Mt. = Ağrı Dağı *Turkey* **73** C11
Araria *India* **69** F12
Araripe, Chapada do *Brazil* **125** E11
Araruama, L. de *Brazil* **127** A7
Aras = Aras, Rūd-e → *Asia* **35** K9
Aras, Rūd-e → *Asia* **35** K9
Aratāne *Mauritania* **82** B3
Arauca *Colombia* **124** B4
Arauca → *Venezuela* **124** B5
Arauco *Chile* **126** D1
Aravalli Range *India* **68** G5
Arawa *Ethiopia* **81** F5
Arawale → *Kenya* **86** C5
Araxá *Brazil* **125** G9
Araxes = Aras, Rūd-e → *Asia* **35** K9
Araya, Pen. de *Venezuela* **124** A6
Araz = Aras, Rūd-e → *Asia* **35** K9
Arba Gugu *Ethiopia* **81** F5
Arba Minch *Ethiopia* **81** F4
Arbat *Iraq* **73** E11
Árbatax *Italy* **42** C2
Arbi *Ethiopia* **81** F4
Arbīl *Iraq* **73** D11
Arbīl □ *Iraq* **73** D11
Arboga *Sweden* **10** E9
Arbois *France* **19** F12
Arbore *Ethiopia* **81** F4
Arboréa *Italy* **42** C1
Arborfield *Canada* **103** C8
Arborg *Canada* **103** C9
Arbre du Ténéré *Niger* **83** B7
Arbroath *U.K.* **13** E6
Arbuckle *U.S.A.* **110** F4
Arbus *Italy* **42** C1
Arc → *France* **21** C10
Arc-lès-Gray *France* **19** E12
Arcachon *France* **20** D2
Arcachon, Bassin d' *France* **20** D2
Arcade *U.S.A.* **114** D6
Arcadia *Fla., U.S.A.* **117** H14
Arcadia *La., U.S.A.* **116** E8
Arcadia *Pa., U.S.A.* **114** F6
Arcata *U.S.A.* **108** F1
Arcévia *Italy* **41** E9
Archanes *Greece* **47** F7
Archangel = Arkhangelsk *Russia* **52** C5
Archangelos *Greece* **49** C10
Archar *Bulgaria* **44** C6
Archbald *U.S.A.* **115** E9
Archena *Spain* **39** G3

Archer → *Australia* **94** A3
Archer B. *Australia* **94** A3
Archer Bend = Mungkan Kandju △ *Australia* **94** A3
Archers Post *Kenya* **86** B4
Arches △ *U.S.A.* **108** G9
Archidona *Spain* **37** H6
Archipel-de-Mingan △ *Canada* **105** B7
Archipiélago Chinijo △ *Canary Is.* **48** E6
Archipiélago Los Roques △ *Venezuela* **121** D6
Arci, Mte. *Italy* **42** C1
Arcidosso *Italy* **41** F8
Arcipelago de la Maddalena △ *Italy* **42** A2
Arcipelago Toscano △ *Italy* **40** F7
Arcis-sur-Aube *France* **19** D11
Arckaringa Cr. → *Australia* **95** D2
Arco *Italy* **40** C7
Arco *U.S.A.* **108** E7
Arcos de Jalón *Spain* **38** D2
Arcos de la Frontera *Spain* **37** J5
Arcos de Valdevez *Portugal* **36** D2
Arcot *India* **66** N11
Arcozelo *Portugal* **36** E3
Arctic Bay *Canada* **101** C14
Arctic Mid-Ocean Ridge *Arctic* **4** A
Arctic Ocean *Arctic* **4** B18
Arctic Red River = Tsiigehtchic *Canada* **100** D5
Arctowski *Antarctica* **5** C18
Arda → *Bulgaria* **45** E10
Arda → *Italy* **40** C7
Ardabīl *Iran* **73** C13
Ardabīl □ *Iran* **71** B6
Ardahan *Turkey* **73** B10
Ardahan □ *Turkey* **73** B10
Ardakān = Sepīdān *Iran* **71** D7
Ardakān *Iran* **71** C7
Ardala *Sweden* **11** F7
Ardales *Spain* **37** J6
Ardara *Ireland* **12** B3
Ardas → *Greece* **45** E10
Ardèche □ *France* **21** D8
Ardèche → *France* **21** D8
Ardee *Ireland* **12** C5
Arden *Canada* **114** B8
Arden *Denmark* **11** H3
Arden *Calif., U.S.A.* **110** G5
Arden *Nev., U.S.A.* **111** J11
Ardenne *Belgium* **17** E5
Ardennes = Ardenne *Belgium* **17** E5
Ardennes □ *France* **19** C11
Ardentes *France* **19** F8
Arderin *Ireland* **12** C4
Ardeşen *Turkey* **73** B9
Ardestān *Iran* **71** C7
Ardfert *Ireland* **12** D2
Ardglass *U.K.* **12** B6
Ardhéa = Aridea *Greece* **44** F6
Ardila → *Portugal* **37** G3
Ardino *Bulgaria* **45** E9
Ardivachar Pt. *U.K.* **13** D1
Ardlethan *Australia* **95** E4
Ardmore *Okla., U.S.A.* **116** D6
Ardmore *Pa., U.S.A.* **115** F9
Ardnamurchan, Pt. of *U.K.* **13** E2
Ardnave Pt. *U.K.* **13** F2
Ardon *Russia* **35** J7
Ardore *Italy* **43** D9
Ardres *France* **19** B8
Ardrossan *Australia* **95** E2
Ardrossan *U.K.* **13** F4
Ards Pen. *U.K.* **12** B6
Arduan *Sudan* **80** D3
Ardud *Romania* **28** C7
Åre *Sweden* **10** A7
Arecibo *Puerto Rico* **121** d
Areia Branca *Brazil* **125** E11
Arena, Pt. *U.S.A.* **110** G3
Arenal *Honduras* **120** C2
Arenas = Las Arenas *Spain* **36** B6
Arenas de San Pedro *Spain* **36** E5
Arenys de Mar *Spain* **38** D7
Arenzano *Italy* **40** D5
Areópoli *Greece* **46** E4
Arequipa *Peru* **124** G4
Arero *Ethiopia* **81** G4
Arès *France* **20** D2
Arévalo *Spain* **36** D6
Arezzo *Italy* **41** E8
Arga → *Spain* **38** C3
Arga *Turkey* **70** B3
Argalasti *Greece* **46** B5
Argamasilla de Alba *Spain* **37** F7
Argamasilla de Calatrava *Spain* **37** G6
Arganda del Rey *Spain* **36** E7
Arganil *Portugal* **36** E2
Argarapa ✪ *Australia* **94** C1
Argedeb *Ethiopia* **81** F5
Argelès-Gazost *France* **20** F3
Argelès-sur-Mer *France* **20** F7
Argens → *France* **21** E10
Argent-sur-Sauldre *France* **19** E9

Argenta *Canada* **102** C5
Argenta *Italy* **41** D8
Argentan *France* **18** D6
Argentário, Mte. *Italy* **41** F8
Argentat *France* **20** C5
Argenteuil *France* **19** D9
Argentia *Canada* **105** C9
Argentina ■ *S. Amer.* **128** D3
Argentine Basin *Atl. Oc.* **128** F6
Argentino, L. *Argentina* **128** G2
Argenton-Château *France* **18** F6
Argenton-sur-Creuse *France* **19** F8
Argeş □ *Romania* **29** F9
Argeş → *Romania* **29** F11
Arghandab → *Afghan.* **68** D1
Argheile *Ethiopia* **81** F5
Argirades *Greece* **49** B3
Argiroupoli *Greece* **49** D6
Argo *Sudan* **80** D3
Argolida □ *Greece* **46** D4
Argolikos Kolpos *Greece* **46** D4
Argonne *France* **19** C12
Argos *Greece* **46** D4
Argos Orestiko *Greece* **44** F5
Argostoli *Greece* **46** C2
Arguedas *Spain* **38** C3
Arguello, Pt. *U.S.A.* **111** L6
Arguineguín *Canary Is.* **48** G4
Argun *Russia* **35** J7
Argun → *Russia* **53** D13
Argungu *Nigeria* **83** C5
Argus Pk. *U.S.A.* **111** K9
Argyle, L. *Australia* **92** C4
Argyll △ *U.K.* **13** E4
Argyll & Bute □ *U.K.* **13** E3
Arhavi *Turkey* **73** B9
Århus *Denmark* **11** H4
Ariadnoye *Russia* **54** B7
Ariamsvlei *Namibia* **88** D2
Ariana *Tunisia* **79** A8
Ariano Irpino *Italy* **43** A8
Aribinda *Burkina Faso* **83** C4
Arica *Chile* **124** G4
Arica *Colombia* **124** D4
Arico *Canary Is.* **48** F3
Arid, C. *Australia* **93** F3
Arida *Japan* **55** G7
Aride *Seychelles* **85** b
Aridea *Greece* **44** F6
Ariège □ *France* **20** F5
Ariège → *France* **20** E5
Arienie *Israel* **80** A4
Arila, Akra *Greece* **49** A3
Arilje *Serbia* **44** C4
Arima *Trin. & Tob.* **121** D7
Arinos → *Brazil* **124** F7
Ario de Rosales *Mexico* **118** D4
Ariogala *Lithuania* **30** C11
Aripo, Mt. *Trin. & Tob.* **125** K15
Aripuanã *Brazil* **124** E6
Aripuanã → *Brazil* **124** E6
Ariquemes *Brazil* **124** E6
Arisaig *U.K.* **13** E3
Arish, W. el → *Egypt* **80** A3
Arissa *Ethiopia* **81** E5
Aristazabal I. *Canada* **102** C3
Arivonimamo *Madag.* **89** B8
Ariza *Spain* **38** D2
Arizaro, Salar de *Argentina* **126** A2
Arizona *Argentina* **126** D2
Arizona □ *U.S.A.* **109** J8
Arizpe *Mexico* **118** A2
'Arjah *Si. Arabia* **70** E5
Árjäng *Sweden* **10** E6
Arjeplog *Sweden* **8** C17
Arjepluovve = Arjeplog *Sweden* **8** C17
Arjona *Colombia* **124** A3
Arjona *Spain* **37** H6
Arjuna *Indonesia* **63** G15
Arka *Russia* **53** C15
Arkadak *Russia* **34** E6
Arkadelphia *U.S.A.* **116** D8
Arkadia □ *Greece* **46** D4
Arkaig, L. *U.K.* **13** E3
Arkalyk = Arqalyk *Kazakhstan* **52** D7
Arkansas □ *U.S.A.* **116** D8
Arkansas → *U.S.A.* **116** E9
Arkansas City *U.S.A.* **112** G5
Arkaroola *Australia* **95** E2
Arkavāz *Iran* **73** F12
Arkhángelos *Greece* **46** B5
Arki *Greece* **47** D8
Arki *India* **68** D7
Arkiko *Eritrea* **81** D4
Arklow *Ireland* **12** D5
Arkona, Kap *Germany* **24** A9
Arkösund *Sweden* **11** F10
Arkoudi *Greece* **46** C2
Arkport *U.S.A.* **114** D7
Arkticheskiy, Mys *Russia* **53** A10
Arkul *Russia* **34** B10
Arkville *U.S.A.* **115** D10
Arla *Sweden* **10** E10

Arlanda, Stockholm ✈ (ARN) *Sweden* **10** E11
Arlanza → *Spain* **36** C6
Arlanzón → *Spain* **36** C6
Arlbergpass *Austria* **26** D3
Arlbertunnel *Austria* **26** D3
Arles *France* **21** E8
Arli *Burkina Faso* **83** C5
Arli △ *Burkina Faso* **83** C5
Arlington *S. Africa* **89** D4
Arlington *N.Y., U.S.A.* **115** E11
Arlington *Oreg., U.S.A.* **108** D3
Arlington *S. Dak., U.S.A.* **112** C6
Arlington *Tex., U.S.A.* **116** E6
Arlington *Va., U.S.A.* **113** F15
Arlington *Vt., U.S.A.* **115** C11
Arlington *Wash., U.S.A.* **110** B4
Arlington Heights *U.S.A.* **112** D10
Arlit *Niger* **78** E7
Arlon *Belgium* **17** E5
Arltunga *Australia* **94** C1
Armadale *Australia* **93** F2
Armagh *U.K.* **12** B5
Armagh □ *U.K.* **12** B5
Armagnac *France* **20** E4
Armançon → *France* **19** E10
Armavir *Armenia* **35** H5
Armavir *Russia* **35** H5
Armenia *Colombia* **124** C3
Armenia ■ *Asia* **35** K7
Armeni *Romania* **28** E7
Armenistis, Akra *Greece* **49** C9
Armentières *France* **19** B9
Armidale *Australia* **95** E5
Armilla *Spain* **37** H7
Armories △ *France* **18** D3
Armour *U.S.A.* **112** D4
Armstrong *B.C., Canada* **102** C5
Armstrong *Ont., Canada* **104** B2
Armutlu *Bursa, Turkey* **45** F12
Armutlu *Izmir, Turkey* **47** C9
Arnarfjörður *Iceland* **8** D2
Arnaud → *Canada* **101** F18
Arnauti, C. *Cyprus* **49** D11
Arnay-le-Duc *France* **19** E11
Arnea *Greece* **44** F7
Arnedillo *Spain* **38** C2
Arnedo *Spain* **38** C2
Arnett *U.S.A.* **116** C5
Arnhem *Neths.* **17** C5
Arnhem, C. *Australia* **94** A2
Arnhem B. *Australia* **94** A2
Arnhem Land *Australia* **94** A1
Arnhem Land ✪ *Australia* **94** A1
Arnissa *Greece* **44** F5
Arno → *Italy* **40** E7
Arno Bay *Australia* **95** E2
Arnold *U.K.* **14** D6
Arnold *U.S.A.* **110** G6
Arnoldstein *Austria* **26** E6
Arnon → *France* **19** E9
Arnot *Canada* **103** B9
Arnøya *Norway* **8** A19
Arnprior *Canada* **115** A8
Arnsberg *Germany* **24** D4
Arnsberger Wald △ *Germany* **24** D4
Arnstadt *Germany* **24** E6
Aroa, Pte. *Moorea* **91** d
Aroab *Namibia* **88** D2
Aroania Oros *Greece* **46** D4
Aroche *Spain* **37** H4
Arochuku *Nigeria* **83** D6
Arolsen *Germany* **24** D5
Aron *India* **68** G6
Aron → *France* **19** F10
Arona *Canary Is.* **48** F3
Arona *Italy* **40** C5
Aroroy *Phil.* **61** E5
Aros → *Mexico* **118** B3
Arpa → *Asia* **73** C11
Arpaçay *Turkey* **73** B10
Arpajon *France* **19** D9
Arpajon-sur-Cère *France* **20** D6
Arpaşu de Sus *Romania* **29** E9
Arqalyk *Kazakhstan* **52** D7
Arrah = Ara *India* **69** G11
Arrah *Ivory C.* **82** D4
Arraiolos *Portugal* **37** G3
Arran *U.K.* **13** F3
Arras *France* **19** B9
Arrasate *Spain* **38** B2
Arrats → *France* **20** D4
Arreau *France* **20** F4
Arrecife *Canary Is.* **48** F6
Arrecifes *Argentina* **126** C3
Arrée, Mts. d' *France* **18** D3
Arrese *Denmark* **11** J6
Arriaga *Mexico* **119** D6
Arribes del Duero △ *Spain* **36** D4
Arrilalah *Australia* **94** C3
Arrino *Australia* **93** E2
Arriondas *Spain* **36** B5
Arromanches-les-Bains *France* **18** C6
Arronches *Portugal* **37** F3

Arros → *France* **20** E3
Arrow, L. *Ireland* **12** B3
Arrowtown *N.Z.* **91** F2
Arroyo de la Luz *Spain* **37** F4
Arroyo Grande *U.S.A.* **111** K6
Ars *Iran* **70** B5
Ars-sur-Moselle *France* **19** C13
Arsenault L. *Canada* **103** B7
Arsenev *Russia* **54** B6
Arsi *Ethiopia* **81** F4
Arsiero *Italy* **41** C8
Arsin *Turkey* **73** B8
Arsk *Russia* **34** B9
Årsunda *Sweden* **10** D10
Arta *Greece* **46** B3
Artà *Spain* **48** B10
Arta □ *Greece* **46** B3
Artà, Coves d *Spain* **48** B10
Artashat *Armenia* **73** B11
Arteaga *Mexico* **118** D4
Arteche *Phil.* **61** E6
Arteixo = Arteixo *Spain* **36** B2
Arteixo *Spain* **36** B2
Artem = Artyom *Azerbaijan* **35** K10
Artem *Russia* **54** C6
Artemovsk *Russia* **53** D10
Artemovsk *Ukraine* **33** H9
Artemovskiy *Russia* **35** G5
Artenay *France* **19** D8
Artern *Germany* **24** D7
Artesa de Segre *Spain* **38** D6
Artesia = Mosomane *Botswana* **88** C4
Artesia *U.S.A.* **109** K11
Arthington *Liberia* **82** D2
Arthur *Canada* **114** C4
Arthur → *Australia* **95** G3
Arthur Cr. → *Australia* **94** C2
Arthur Pt. *Australia* **94** C5
Arthur River *Australia* **93** F2
Arthur's Pass *N.Z.* **91** E3
Arthur's Pass △ *N.Z.* **91** E3
Arthur's Town *Bahamas* **121** B4
Artigas *Antarctica* **5** C18
Artigas *Uruguay* **126** C4
Artik *Armenia* **35** K6
Artillery L. *Canada* **103** A7
Artois *France* **19** B9
Artotina *Greece* **46** C4
Artova *Turkey* **72** B7
Artrutx, C. de *Spain* **48** B10
Artsyz *Ukraine* **29** D14
Artvin *Turkey* **73** B9
Artvin □ *Turkey* **73** B9
Artyk *Russia* **53** C15
Artyom *Azerbaijan* **35** K10
Aru, Kepulauan *Indonesia* **63** F8
Aru Is. = Aru, Kepulauan *Indonesia* **63** F8
Arua *Uganda* **86** B3
Aruanã *Brazil* **125** F8
Aruba ☑ *W. Indies* **121** D6
Arucas *Canary Is.* **48** F4
Arudy *France* **20** E3
Arué *Tahiti* **91** d
Arun → *Nepal* **69** F12
Arun → *U.K.* **15** G7
Arunachal Pradesh □ *India* **67** F19
Arusha *Tanzania* **86** C4
Arusha □ *Tanzania* **86** C4
Arusha △ *Tanzania* **86** C4
Arusha Chini *Tanzania* **86** C4
Aruwimi → *Dem. Rep. of the Congo* **86** B1
Arvada *Colo., U.S.A.* **108** G11
Arvada *Wyo., U.S.A.* **108** D10
Arvayheer *Mongolia* **53** E11
Arve → *France* **19** F13
Arvi *Greece* **49** E7
Arviat *Canada* **103** A10
Arvidsjaur *Sweden* **8** D18
Arvika *Sweden* **10** E6
Arvin *U.S.A.* **111** K8
Arwal *India* **69** G11
Arxan *China* **60** B6
Aryd *Sweden* **11** H8
Arys *Kazakhstan* **52** E7
Arzachena *Italy* **42** A2
Arzamas *Russia* **34** C6
Arzanah *U.A.E.* **71** E7
Arzgir *Russia* **35** H7
Arzignano *Italy* **41** C8
Arzúa *Spain* **36** C2
Aš *Czech Rep.* **26** A5
Ås *Sweden* **10** A8
As Pontes de García Rodríguez *Spain* **36** B3
Aş Şafā *Syria* **74** B6
As Saffānīyah *Si. Arabia* **71** E6
Aş Şahm *Oman* **71** E8
As Sājir *Si. Arabia* **70** E5
As Salamīyah *Syria* **72** D7
As Salmān *Iraq* **70** D5
As Salţ *Jordan* **74** C4
As Sal'w'a *Qatar* **71** E6
As Samāwah *Iraq* **70** D5
As Sanamayn *Syria* **74** B5
As Sohar = Şuḥār *Oman* **71** E8

As Sukhnah *Syria* **73** E8
As Sulaymānīyah *Iraq* **73** E11
As Sulaymānīyah □ *Iraq* **73** E11
As Sulaymī *Si. Arabia* **70** E4
As Sulayyil *Si. Arabia* **75** C4
As Summān *Si. Arabia* **70** E5
Aş Şuwar *Syria* **73** E9
Aş Suwaydā *Syria* **74** C5
Aş Suwaydā □ *Syria* **74** C5
As Suwayq *Oman* **71** F8
Aş Şuwayrah *Iraq* **73** F11
Åsa *Sweden* **11** G6
Asab *Namibia* **88** D2
Asaba *Nigeria* **83** D6
Asad, Buḥayrat al *Syria* **73** E8
Asadābād *Iran* **73** E13
Asafo *Ghana* **82** D4
Asahi-Gawa → *Japan* **55** G6
Asahigawa *Japan* **54** C11
Asale, L. *Ethiopia* **81** E5
Asaluyeh *Iran* **71** E7
Asamankese *Ghana* **83** D4
Asan → *India* **69** F8
Asansol *India* **69** H12
Åsarna *Sweden* **10** B8
Asau *Samoa* **91** b
Asayita *Ethiopia* **81** E5
Asbe Teferi *Ethiopia* **81** F5
Asbesberge *S. Africa* **88** D3
Asbestos *Canada* **105** C5
Asbury Park *U.S.A.* **115** F10
Ascea *Italy* **43** B8
Ascensión *Mexico* **118** A3
Ascensión, B. de la *Mexico* **119** D7
Ascension I. *Atl. Oc.* **77** G2
Aschach an der Donau *Austria* **26** C7
Aschaffenburg *Germany* **25** F5
Aschendorf *Germany* **24** B3
Aschersleben *Germany* **24** D7
Asciano *Italy* **41** E8
Áscoli Piceno *Italy* **41** F10
Áscoli Satriano *Italy* **43** A8
Ascope *Peru* **124** E3
Ascotán *Chile* **126** A2
Aseb *Eritrea* **81** E5
Åseda *Sweden* **11** G9
Asela *Ethiopia* **81** F4
Åsen *Sweden* **10** C7
Asenovgrad *Bulgaria* **45** D8
Asfeld *France* **19** C11
Asfûn el Matâ'na *Egypt* **80** B3
Aşgabat = Ashgabat *Turkmenistan* **71** B8
Asgata *Cyprus* **49** E12
Ash Fork *U.S.A.* **109** J7
Ash Grove *U.S.A.* **112** G7
Ash Shabakah *Iraq* **70** D4
Ash Shamāl □ *Lebanon* **74** A5
Ash Shāmīyah *Iraq* **73** G11
Ash Shāriqah *U.A.E.* **71** E7
Ash Sharmah *Si. Arabia* **70** D2
Ash Sharqāt *Iraq* **73** E10
Ash Shaţrah *Iraq* **70** D5
Ash Shawbak *Jordan* **70** D2
Ash Shihr *Yemen* **75** E4
Ash Shināfīyah *Iraq* **70** D5
Ash Shu'bah *Si. Arabia* **70** D5
Ash Shumlūl *Si. Arabia* **70** E5
Ash Shūr'a *Iraq* **70** D2
Ash Shurayf *Si. Arabia* **70** E3
Ash Shuwayfāt *Lebanon* **74** B4
Ashanti □ *Ghana* **83** D4
Ashau *Vietnam* **64** D6
Ashbourne *U.K.* **14** D6
Ashburn *U.S.A.* **117** F13
Ashburton *N.Z.* **91** E3
Ashburton → *Australia* **92** D1
Ashcroft *Canada* **102** C4
Ashdod *Israel* **74** D3
Ashdown *U.S.A.* **116** E7
Asheboro *U.S.A.* **117** D15
Ashern *Canada* **103** C9
Asherton *U.S.A.* **116** G5
Asheville *U.S.A.* **117** D13
Ashewat *Pakistan* **68** D3
Asheweig → *Canada* **104** B2
Ashford *Australia* **95** D5
Ashford *U.K.* **15** F8
Ashgabat *Turkmenistan* **71** B8
Ashibetsu *Japan* **54** C11
Ashikaga *Japan* **55** F9
Ashington *U.K.* **14** B6
Ashizuri-Uwakai △ *Japan* **55** H6
Ashizuri-Zaki *Japan* **55** H6
Ashkarkot *Afghan.* **68** C2
Ashkhabad = Ashgabat *Turkmenistan* **71** B8
Āshkhāneh *Iran* **71** B8
Ashland *Kans., U.S.A.* **112** G4
Ashland *Ky., U.S.A.* **113** F12
Ashland *Maine, U.S.A.* **113** B19
Ashland *Mont., U.S.A.* **108** D10
Ashland *Ohio, U.S.A.* **114** F2
Ashland *Oreg., U.S.A.* **108** E2
Ashland *Pa., U.S.A.* **115** F8
Ashland *Va., U.S.A.* **113** G15
Ashland *Wis., U.S.A.* **112** B8
Ashley *N. Dak., U.S.A.* **112** B4

Ashley *Pa., U.S.A.* **115** E9
Ashmore and Cartier Is.
　Ind. Oc. **92** B3
Ashmore Reef *Australia* **92** B3
Ashmûn *Egypt* **80** H7
Ashmyany *Belarus* **23** A13
Ashoknagar *India* **68** G7
Ashqelon *Israel* **74** D3
Ashta *India* **68** H7
Āshtiyān *Iran* **71** C6
Ashtabula *U.S.A.* **114** E4
Ashton *S. Africa* **88** E3
Ashton *U.S.A.* **108** D8
Ashuanipi, L. *Canada* **105** B6
Ashuapmushuan →
　Canada **104** C5
Ashville *U.S.A.* **114** F6
'Āṣī → *Asia* **72** D6
Asia **50** E9
Asia, Kepulauan *Indonesia* **63** D8
Asiago *Italy* **41** C8
Asifabad *India* **66** K11
Asinara *Italy* **42** A1
Asinara, G. dell' *Italy* **42** A1
Asino *Russia* **52** D9
Asipovichy *Belarus* **23** B15
'Asīr *Si. Arabia* **80** D5
Asir, Ras *Somali Rep.* **75** E5
Aşkale *Turkey* **73** C9
Askersund *Sweden* **11** F8
Askham *S. Africa* **88** D3
Askī Mawṣil *Iraq* **73** D10
Askim *Norway* **9** G14
Askio, Oros *Greece* **44** F5
Askja *Iceland* **8** D5
Asklipio *Greece* **49** C9
Askøyna *Norway* **8** F11
Asl *Egypt* **80** B3
Aslan Burnu *Turkey* **47** C8
Aslanapa *Turkey* **47** B11
Aslānduz *Iran* **73** C12
Asmara = Asmera *Eritrea* **81** D4
Asmera *Eritrea* **81** D4
Asnæs *Denmark* **11** J4
Åsnen *Sweden* **11** H8
Aso Kuju △ *Japan* **55** H5
Åsola *Italy* **40** C7
Asos *Greece* **46** C2
Asosa *Ethiopia* **81** E3
Asoteriba, Jebel *Sudan* **80** C4
Aspatria *U.K.* **14** C4
Aspe *Spain* **39** G4
Aspen *U.S.A.* **108** G10
Aspendos *Turkey* **72** D4
Aspermont *U.S.A.* **116** E4
Aspet *France* **20** E4
Aspiring, Mt. *N.Z.* **91** F2
Aspres-sur-Buëch *France* **21** D9
Asprokavos, Akra *Greece* **49** B4
Aspromonte △ *Italy* **43** D8
Aspur *India* **68** H6
Asquith *Canada* **103** C7
Assab = Aseb *Eritrea* **81** E5
Assâba □ *Mauritania* **82** B2
Assâba, Massif de l'
　Mauritania **82** B2
Assagny △ *Ivory C.* **82** D4
Assaikio *Nigeria* **83** D6
Assal, L. *Djibouti* **81** E5
Assam □ *India* **67** G18
Assamakka *Niger* **83** B6
Assateague Island △ *U.S.A.*
　113 F16
Asse *Belgium* **17** D4
Assémini *Italy* **42** C1
Assen *Neths.* **17** A6
Assens *Denmark* **11** J3
Assini *Ivory C.* **82** D4
Assiniboia *Canada* **103** D7
Assiniboine → *Canada* **103** D9
Assiniboine, Mt. *Canada* **102** C5
Assis *Brazil* **127** A5
Assisi *Italy* **41** E9
Assynt, L. *U.K.* **13** C3
Astaffort *France* **20** D4
Astakida *Greece* **47** F8
Astakos *Greece* **46** C3
Astana *Kazakhstan* **52** D8
Āstāneh *Iran* **71** B6
Astara *Azerbaijan* **73** C13
Āstārā *Iran* **73** C13
Astarabad = Gorgān *Iran* **71** B7
Asterousia *Greece* **49** E7
Asti *Italy* **40** D5
Astipalea *Greece* **47** E8
Astorga *Spain* **36** C4
Astoria *U.S.A.* **110** D3
Åstorp *Sweden* **11** H6
Astrakhan *Russia* **35** G9
Astrakhan □ *Russia* **35** G8
Astrebla Downs *Australia* **94** C3
Astudillo *Spain* **36** C6
Asturias □ *Spain* **36** B5
Asturias ✈ (OVD) *Spain* **36** B4
Asunción *Paraguay* **126** B4
Asunción Nochixtlán
　Mexico **119** D5
Åsunden *Sweden* **11** F9

Asutri *Sudan* **81** D4
Aswa → *Uganda* **86** B3
Aswa-Lolim △ *Uganda* **86** B3
Aswad, Ra's al *Si. Arabia* **80** C4
Aswân *Egypt* **80** C3
Aswan High Dam = Sadd
　el Aali *Egypt* **80** C3
Asyût *Egypt* **80** B3
Asyûti, Wadi → *Egypt* **80** B3
Aszód *Hungary* **28** C4
At Ṭafīlah *Jordan* **74** E4
At Ṭafīlah □ *Jordan* **74** E4
Aṭ Ṭā'if *Si. Arabia* **80** C5
At Ta'mīm □ *Iraq* **70** C5
Aṭ Ṭirāq *Si. Arabia* **70** E5
Aṭ Ṭubayq *Si. Arabia* **70** D3
Aṭ Ṭunayb *Jordan* **74** D4
Atabey *Turkey* **47** D12
Atacama □ *Chile* **126** B2
Atacama, Desierto de *Chile* **126** A2
Atacama, Salar de *Chile* **126** A2
Atakeye ⊚ *Australia* **92** D5
Atakpamé *Togo* **83** D5
Atalandi *Greece* **46** C4
Atalaya *Peru* **124** F4
Atalaya de Femes *Canary Is.* **48** F6
Atami *Japan* **55** G9
Atamyrat *Turkmenistan* **52** F7
Atâr *Mauritania* **78** D3
Atarfe *Spain* **37** H7
Atari *Pakistan* **68** D6
Atascadero *U.S.A.* **110** K6
Atasū *Kazakhstan* **52** E8
Atâr *Mauritania* **78** D3
Atari *Pakistan* **68** D6
Atascadero *U.S.A.* **110** K6
Atasū *Kazakhstan* **52** E8
Atatürk, İstanbul ✈ (IST)
　Turkey **45** F12
Atatürk Barajı *Turkey* **73** D8
Atauro *E. Timor* **63** F7
Ataviros *Greece* **49** C9
Atbara *Sudan* **80** D3
'Atbara, Nahr → *Sudan* **80** D3
Atbasar *Kazakhstan* **52** D7
Atça *Turkey* **47** D10
Atchafalaya B. *U.S.A.* **116** G9
Atchison *U.S.A.* **112** F6
Atebubu *Ghana* **83** D4
Ateca *Spain* **38** D3
Aterno → *Italy* **41** C7
Āteshān *Iran* **71** C7
Atessa *Italy* **41** F11
Atfih *Egypt* **80** J7
Ath *Belgium* **17** D3
Athabasca *Canada* **102** C6
Athabasca → *Canada* **103** B6
Athabasca, L. *Canada* **103** B7
Athabasca Sand Dunes △
　Canada **103** B7
Athamanon Oros *Greece* **46** B3
Athboy *Ireland* **12** C5
Athenry *Ireland* **12** C3
Athens = Athina *Greece* **46** D5
Athens *Ala., U.S.A.* **117** D11
Athens *Ga., U.S.A.* **117** E13
Athens *N.Y., U.S.A.* **115** D11
Athens *Ohio, U.S.A.* **113** F12
Athens *Pa., U.S.A.* **115** E8
Athens *Tenn., U.S.A.* **117** D12
Athens *Tex., U.S.A.* **116** E7
Atherley *Canada* **114** B5
Atherton *Australia* **94** B4
Athi River *Kenya* **86** C4
Athiéme *Benin* **83** D5
Athienou *Cyprus* **49** D12
Athina *Greece* **46** D5
Athina ✈ (ATH) *Greece* **46** D5
Athínai = Athina *Greece* **46** D5
Athlone *Ireland* **12** C4
Athna *Cyprus* **49** D12
Athol *U.S.A.* **115** D12
Atholl, Forest of *U.K.* **13** E5
Atholville *Canada* **105** C6
Athos *Greece* **45** F8
Athy *Ireland* **12** C5
Ati *Chad* **79** F9
Ati *Sudan* **81** E2
Atiak *Uganda* **86** B3
Atienza *Spain* **38** D2
Atiit *Sudan* **81** F3
Atik, L. *Canada* **103** B9
Atikaki △ *Canada* **103** C9
Atikameg → *Canada* **104** B3
Atikokan *Canada* **104** C1
Atikonak L. *Canada* **105** B7
Atimaono *Tahiti* **91** d
Atimonan *Phil.* **61** E4
Atitlán △ *Cent. Amer.* **119** E6
Atiu *Cook Is.* **97** J12
Atka *Russia* **53** C16
Atka I. *U.S.A.* **106** C5
Atkarsk *Russia* **34** E7
Atkinson *U.S.A.* **112** D14
Atlanta *Ga., U.S.A.* **117** E12
Atlanta *Tex., U.S.A.* **116** E7
Atlantic *U.S.A.* **112** E6
Atlantic City *U.S.A.* **113** F16
Atlantic-Indian Basin
　Antarctica **5** B4
Atlantic Ocean **2** D8

Atlas Mts. = Haut Atlas
　Morocco **78** B4
Atlin *Canada* **102** B2
Atlin, L. *Canada* **102** B2
Atlin □ *Canada* **102** B2
Atmore *U.S.A.* **117** F11
Atoka *U.S.A.* **116** D6
Atokos *Greece* **46** C2
Atolia *U.S.A.* **111** K9
Atqasuk *U.S.A.* **106** A8
Atrai → *Bangla.* **69** G13
Atrak = Atrek →
　Turkmenistan **71** B8
Ätran *Sweden* **11** G6
Ätran → *Sweden* **11** H6
Atrauli *India* **68** E8
Atrek → *Turkmenistan* **71** B8
Atri *Italy* **41** F10
Atsiki *Greece* **47** B7
Atsoum, Mts. *Cameroon* **83** D7
Atsuta *Japan* **54** C10
Attalla *U.S.A.* **117** D11
Attapu *Laos* **64** E6
Attawapiskat *Canada* **104** B3
Attawapiskat → *Canada* **104** B3
Attawapiskat L. *Canada* **104** B2
Attersee *Austria* **26** D6
Attica *Ind., U.S.A.* **112** E10
Attica *Ohio, U.S.A.* **114** E2
Attichy *France* **19** C10
Attigny *France* **19** C11
Attika = Attiki □ *Greece* **46** D5
Attikamagen L. *Canada* **105** B6
Attiki □ *Greece* **46** D5
Attleboro *U.S.A.* **115** E13
Attock *Pakistan* **68** C5
Attopeu = Attapu *Laos* **64** E6
Attu I. *U.S.A.* **106** C2
Attur *India* **66** P11
Atuel → *Argentina* **126** D2
Atura *Uganda* **86** B3
Atwater *U.S.A.* **110** H6
Atwood *Canada* **114** C3
Atwood *U.S.A.* **112** F3
Atyraū *Kazakhstan* **52** E6
Au Sable → *U.S.A.* **113** C12
Au Sable → *U.S.A.* **113** C12
Au Sable Forks *U.S.A.* **115** B11
Au Sable Pt. *U.S.A.* **114** B1
Auas *Honduras* **120** C3
Auasberg *Namibia* **88** C2
Aubagne *France* **21** E9
Aube □ *France* **19** D11
Aube → *France* **19** D10
Aubenas *France* **21** D8
Aubenton *France* **19** C11
Auberry *U.S.A.* **110** H7
Aubigny-sur-Nère *France* **19** E9
Aubin *France* **20** D6
Aubrac, Mts. d' *France* **20** D7
Auburn *Ala., U.S.A.* **117** E12
Auburn *Calif., U.S.A.* **110** G5
Auburn *Ind., U.S.A.* **113** E11
Auburn *Maine, U.S.A.* **113** C18
Auburn *N.Y., U.S.A.* **115** D8
Auburn *Nebr., U.S.A.* **112** E6
Auburn *Pa., U.S.A.* **115** F8
Auburn *Wash., U.S.A.* **110** C4
Auburn Ra. *Australia* **95** D5
Auburndale *U.S.A.* **117** G14
Aubusson *France* **20** C6
Auce *Latvia* **30** B9
Auch *France* **20** E4
Auchi *Nigeria* **83** D6
Auchterarder *U.K.* **13** E5
Auchtermuchty *U.K.* **13** E5
Auckland *N.Z.* **91** B5
Auckland Is. *Pac. Oc.* **96** N8
Aude □ *France* **20** E6
Aude → *France* **20** E7
Auden *Canada* **104** B2
Auderville *France* **18** C5
Audierne *France* **18** D2
Audincourt *France* **19** E13
Audo Ra. *Ethiopia* **81** F5
Audubon *U.S.A.* **112** E6
Auerbach *Germany* **24** E8
Augathella *Australia* **95** D4
Aughnacloy *U.K.* **12** B5
Aughrim *Ireland* **12** C5
Augrabies Falls *S. Africa* **88** D3
Augrabies Falls △ *S. Africa* **88** D3
Augsburg *Germany* **25** G6
Augsburg-Westliche
　Wälder △ *Germany* **25** G6
Augusta *Australia* **93** F2
Augusta *Italy* **43** E8
Augusta *Ark., U.S.A.* **116** D9
Augusta *Ga., U.S.A.* **117** E14
Augusta *Kans., U.S.A.* **112** G5
Augusta *Maine, U.S.A.* **113** C19
Augusta *Mont., U.S.A.* **108** C7
Augustenborg *Denmark* **11** K3
Augustów *Poland* **30** E9
Augustus, Mt. *Australia* **93** D2
Augustus I. *Australia* **92** C3
Aujuittuq = Grise Fiord
　Canada **101** B15

Aukan *Eritrea* **81** D5
Aukrug △ *Germany* **24** A5
Aukštaitija □ *Lithuania* **9** J22
Aukum *U.S.A.* **110** G6
Aulavik △ *Canada* **100** C8
Auld, L. *Australia* **93** D3
Aulla *Italy* **40** D6
Aulnay *France* **20** B3
Aulne → *France* **18** D2
Aulnoye-Aymeries *France* **19** B10
Ault *France* **18** B8
Ault *U.S.A.* **108** F11
Aulus-les-Bains *France* **20** F5
Aumale *France* **19** C8
Aumont-Aubrac *France* **20** D7
Auna *Nigeria* **83** C5
Auning *Denmark* **11** H4
Aunis *France* **20** B3
Aunu'u *Amer. Samoa* **91** b
Auponhia *Indonesia* **63** E7
Aur, Pulau *Malaysia* **65** L5
Auraiya *India* **69** F8
Aurangabad *Bihar, India* **69** G11
Aurangabad *Maharashtra,
　India* **66** K9
Auray *France* **18** E4
Aurich *Germany* **24** B3
Aurillac *France* **20** D6
Auronzo di Cadore *Italy* **41** B9
Aurora *Canada* **114** C5
Aurora *S. Africa* **88** E2
Aurora *Colo., U.S.A.* **108** G11
Aurora *Ill., U.S.A.* **112** E9
Aurora *Mo., U.S.A.* **112** G7
Aurora *N.Y., U.S.A.* **115** D8
Aurora *Nebr., U.S.A.* **112** E5
Aurora *Ohio, U.S.A.* **114** E3
Aurukun *Australia* **94** A3
Aurukun ⊚ *Australia* **94** A3
Aus *Namibia* **88** D2
Ausable → *Canada* **114** C3
Auschwitz = Oświęcim
　Poland **31** H6
Auski Roadhouse *Australia* **92** D2
Austerlitz = Slavkov u
　Brna *Czech Rep.* **27** B9
Austin *Minn., U.S.A.* **112** D7
Austin *Nev., U.S.A.* **108** G5
Austin *Pa., U.S.A.* **114** E6
Austin *Tex., U.S.A.* **116** F6
Austin, L. *Australia* **93** E2
Austin I. *Canada* **103** A10
Austra *Norway* **8** D14
Austral Is. = Tubuaï, Îs.
　French Polynesia **97** K13
Austral Seamount Chain
　Pac. Oc. **97** K13
Australia ■ *Oceania* **90** D6
Australian-Antarctic Basin
　S. Ocean **5** C9
Australian Capital
　Territory □ *Australia* **95** F4
Australind *Australia* **93** F2
Austria ■ *Europe* **26** E7
Austvågøya *Norway* **8** B16
Auterive *France* **20** E5
Authie → *France* **19** B8
Authon-du-Perche *France* **18** D7
Autlán de Navarro *Mexico* **118** D4
Autun *France* **19** F11
Auvergne □ *France* **20** C7
Auvergne, Mts. d' *France* **20** C6
Auvézère → *France* **20** C4
Auxerre *France* **19** E10
Auxi-le-Château *France* **19** B9
Auxonne *France* **19** E12
Auyán Tepui *Venezuela* **124** B6
Auyuittuq △ *Canada* **101** D18
Auzances *France* **19** F10
Av-Dovurak *Russia* **53** D10
Ava *U.S.A.* **112** G7
Avallon *France* **19** E10
Avalon *U.S.A.* **111** M8
Avalon Pen. *Canada* **105** C9
Avanos *Turkey* **72** C6
Avantas *Greece* **45** F9
Avaré *Brazil* **127** A6
Avawatz Mts. *U.S.A.* **111** K10
Avdan Dağı *Turkey* **45** F13
Aveiro *Brazil* **125** D7
Aveiro *Portugal* **36** E2
Aveiro □ *Portugal* **36** E2
Āvej *Iran* **71** C6
Avellaneda *Argentina* **126** C4
Avellino *Italy* **43** B7
Avenal *U.S.A.* **110** K6
Avenal *U.S.A.* **110** K6
Avery *U.S.A.* **108** C6
Aves, I. de *W. Indies* **121** C7
Aves, Is. las *Venezuela* **121** D6
Avesnes-sur-Helpe *France* **19** B10
Avesta *Sweden* **10** D10
Aveyron □ *France* **20** D6
Aveyron → *France* **20** D5
Avezzano *Italy* **41** F10
'Ayn, Wādī al *Oman* **71** F7
Ayn Dār *Si. Arabia* **71** E7

Aviano *Italy* **41** B9
Aviemore *U.K.* **13** D5
Avigliana *Italy* **40** C4
Avigliano *Italy* **43** B8
Avignon *France* **21** E8
Ávila *Spain* **36** E6
Ávila □ *Spain* **36** E6
Ávila, Sierra de *Spain* **36** E5
Avila Beach *U.S.A.* **111** K6
Avilés *Spain* **36** B5
Avintes *Portugal* **36** D2
Avis *Portugal* **37** F3
Avis *U.S.A.* **114** E7
Avísio → *Italy* **40** B8
Aviz *Portugal* **37** F3
Avize *France* **19** D11
Avlonari *Greece* **46** C6
Avlum *Denmark* **11** H2
Avoca *U.S.A.* **114** D7
Avoca → *Australia* **95** F3
Avoca → *Ireland* **12** C5
Avola *Canada* **102** C5
Avola *Italy* **43** F8
Avon *U.S.A.* **114** D7
Avon → *Australia* **93** F2
Avon → *Bristol, U.K.* **15** F5
Avon → *Dorset, U.K.* **15** G6
Avon → *Warks., U.K.* **15** E5
Avon Park *U.S.A.* **117** H14
Avondale *Zimbabwe* **87** F3
Avonlea *Canada* **103** D8
Avonmore *Canada* **115** A10
Avonmouth *U.K.* **15** F5
Avramov *Bulgaria* **45** D10
Avranches *France* **18** D5
Avre → *France* **18** D8
Avrig *Romania* **29** E9
Avrillé *France* **18** E6
Avtovac *Bos.-H.* **44** C2
Awa-Shima *Japan* **54** E9
Awag el Baqar *Sudan* **81** E3
A'waj → *Syria* **74** B5
Awaji-Shima *Japan* **55** G7
'Awālī *Bahrain* **71** E6
Awantipur *India* **69** C6
Awasa *Ethiopia* **81** F4
Awasa, L. *Ethiopia* **81** F4
Awash *Ethiopia* **81** F5
Awash → *Ethiopia* **81** E5
Awash △ *Ethiopia* **81** F5
Awaso *Ghana* **82** D4
Awatere → *N.Z.* **91** D5
Awbārī *Libya* **79** C8
Awbārī, Idehan *Libya* **79** C8
Awe, L. *U.K.* **13** E3
Aweil *Sudan* **81** F2
Awgu *Nigeria* **83** D6
Awjilah *Libya* **79** C10
Awka *Nigeria* **83** D6
Ax-les-Thermes *France* **20** F5
Axat *France* **20** F6
Axe → *U.K.* **15** F5
Axel Heiberg I. *Canada* **101** B14
Axim *Ghana* **82** E4
Axintele *Romania* **29** F11
Axios → *Greece* **44** F6
Axminster *U.K.* **15** G4
Axvall *Sweden* **11** F7
Ay *France* **19** C11
Ayabaca *Peru* **124** D3
Ayabe *Japan* **55** G7
Ayacucho *Argentina* **126** D4
Ayacucho *Peru* **124** F4
Ayaguz = Ayaköz *Kazakhstan* **52** E9
Ayaköz *Kazakhstan* **52** E9
Ayamé *Ivory C.* **82** D4
Ayamonte *Spain* **37** H3
Ayan *Russia* **53** D14
Ayancık *Turkey* **72** B6
Ayangba *Nigeria* **83** D6
Ayas *Turkey* **72** B5
Ayaviri *Peru* **124** F4
Aybastı *Turkey* **72** B7
Aydın *Turkey* **47** D9
Aydın □ *Turkey* **47** D9
Aydın Dağları *Turkey* **47** D10
Ayelu *Ethiopia* **81** E5
Ayenngré *Togo* **83** D5
Ayer *U.S.A.* **115** D13
Ayer Hitam *Malaysia* **65** c
Ayerbe *Spain* **38** C4
Ayer's Cliff *Canada* **115** A12
Ayers Rock = Uluru *Australia* **93** E5
Ayeyarwady =
　Irrawaddy → *Burma* **67** M19
Áyia Napa *Cyprus* **49** E13
Áyia Phyla *Cyprus* **49** E12
Áyios Amvrósios *Cyprus* **49** D12
Áyios Seryios *Cyprus* **49** D12
Áyios Theodhoros *Cyprus* **49** D13
Áyios Yeóryios = Aghios
　Georgios *Greece* **46** D5
Aykhal *Russia* **53** C12
Aykirikçi *Turkey* **47** B12
Aylesbury *U.K.* **15** F7
Aylmer *Canada* **114** D4
Aylmer, L. *Canada* **100** E10
'Ayn, Wādī al *Oman* **71** F7
Ayn Dār *Si. Arabia* **71** E7

Ayn Sifnī *Iraq* **73** D10
Ayn Zālah *Iraq* **73** D10
Ayna *Spain* **39** G2
Ayod *Sudan* **81** F3
Ayolas *Paraguay* **126** B4
Ayon, Ostrov *Russia* **53** C17
Ayora *Spain* **39** F3
Ayorou *Niger* **83** C5
'Ayoûn el 'Atroûs *Mauritania* **82** B3
Ayr *Australia* **94** B4
Ayr *Canada* **114** C4
Ayr *U.K.* **13** F4
Ayr → *U.K.* **13** F4
Ayrancı *Turkey* **72** D5
Ayrancılar *Turkey* **47** C9
Ayre, Pt. of *I. of Man* **14** C3
Aysha *Ethiopia* **81** E5
Ayton *Australia* **94** B4
Aytos *Bulgaria* **45** D11
Aytoska Planina *Bulgaria* **45** D11
Ayu, Kepulauan *Indonesia* **63** D8
Ayutla *Guatemala* **120** D1
Ayutla de los Libres *Mexico* **119** D5
Ayvacık *Turkey* **72** C2
Ayvalık *Turkey* **47** B8
Az Zabadānī *Syria* **74** B5
Aẓ Ẓāhirīyah *West Bank* **74** D3
Aẓ Ẓahrān *Si. Arabia* **71** E6
Az Zarqā *Jordan* **74** C5
Az Zarqā' *U.A.E.* **71** E7
Az Zarqā □ *Jordan* **74** C5
Az Zāwiyah *Libya* **79** B8
Az Zībār *Iraq* **73** D11
Az Zilfī *Si. Arabia* **70** E5
Az Zubayr *Iraq* **70** D5
Az Zuqur *Yemen* **81** E5
Azad Kashmir □ *Pakistan* **69** C5
Azambuja *Portugal* **37** F2
Azamgarh *India* **69** F10
Azángaro *Peru* **124** F4
Azar Shahr *Iran* **73** D11
Azara *Nigeria* **83** D6
Azarān *Iran* **73** D12
Azärbayjan =
　Azerbaijan ■ *Asia* **35** K9
Āzarbāyjān-e Gharbī □ *Iran* **70** B5
Āzarbāyjān-e Sharqī □ *Iran* **70** B5
Azare *Nigeria* **83** C7
Azay-le-Rideau *France* **18** E7
A'zāz *Syria* **72** D7
Azbine = Aïr *Niger* **83** B6
Azerbaijan ■ *Asia* **35** K9
Azezo *Ethiopia* **81** E4
Azimganj *India* **69** G13
Aznalcóllar *Spain* **37** H4
Azogues *Ecuador* **124** D3
Azores = Açores, Is. dos
　Atl. Oc. **78** a
Azov *Russia* **35** G4
Azov, Sea of *Europe* **33** J9
Azovskoye More = Azov,
　Sea of *Europe* **33** J9
Azpeitia *Spain* **38** B2
Azraq ash Shīshān *Jordan* **74** D5
Aztec *U.S.A.* **109** H10
Azúa de Compostela
　Dom. Rep. **121** C5
Azuaga *Spain* **37** G5
Azuara *Spain* **38** D4
Azuer → *Spain* **37** F7
Azuero, Pen. de *Panama* **120** E3
Azul *Argentina* **126** D4
Azusa *U.S.A.* **111** L9
Azzano Décimo *Italy* **41** C9
Azzel Matti, Sebkra *Algeria* **78** C6

B

Ba Be △ *Vietnam* **64** A5
Ba Don *Vietnam* **64** D6
Ba Dong *Vietnam* **65** H6
Ba Ngoi = Cam Lam *Vietnam* **65** G7
Ba Tri *Vietnam* **65** G6
Ba Vi △ *Vietnam* **64** B5
Ba Xian = Bazhou *China* **56** E9
Baa *Indonesia* **92** B3
Baamonde *Spain* **36** B3
Baardheere *Somali Rep.* **75** G3
Baarle-Nassau *Belgium* **17** C4
Bab el Mandeb *Red Sea* **75** E3
Baba *Bulgaria* **44** D7
Baba Burnu *Turkey* **47** B8
Babadag *Romania* **29** F13
Babadağ *Turkey* **47** D10
Babaeski *Turkey* **45** E11
Babahoyo *Ecuador* **124** D3
Babai = Sarju → *India* **69** F9
Babana *Nigeria* **83** C5
Babanusa *Sudan* **81** E2
Babar *Indonesia* **63** F7
Babar *Pakistan* **68** D3

Babarkach *Pakistan* **68** E3
Babayevo *Russia* **32** C8
Babb *U.S.A.* **108** B7
Babenhausen *Germany* **25** F4
Baberu *India* **69** G9
Babi Besar, Pulau *Malaysia* **65** L4
Babian Jiang → *China* **58** F3
Bābil □ *Iraq* **70** C5
Babile *Ethiopia* **81** F5
Babimost *Poland* **31** F2
Babinda *Australia* **94** B4
Babine *Canada* **102** B3
Babine → *Canada* **102** B3
Babine L. *Canada* **102** C3
Babiogórski △ *Poland* **31** J6
Babo *Indonesia* **63** E8
Babócsa *Hungary* **28** D2
Bābol *Iran* **71** B7
Bābol Sar *Iran* **71** B7
Baborów *Poland* **31** H5
Baboua *C.A.R.* **84** C2
Babruysk *Belarus* **23** B15
Babuhri *India* **68** F3
Babuna *Macedonia* **44** E5
Babura *Nigeria* **83** C6
Babusar Pass *Pakistan* **69** B5
Babušnica *Serbia* **44** C6
Babuyan Chan. *Phil.* **61** B4
Babylon *Iraq* **73** F11
Bač *Serbia* **28** E4
Bâc → *Moldova* **29** D14
Bac Can *Vietnam* **58** F5
Bac Giang *Vietnam* **58** G6
Bac Lieu *Vietnam* **65** H5
Bac Ninh *Vietnam* **58** G6
Bac Phan *Vietnam* **58** G5
Bac Quang *Vietnam* **58** F5
Bacabal *Brazil* **125** D10
Bacalar *Mexico* **119** D7
Bacan, Kepulauan *Indonesia* **63** E7
Bacarra *Phil.* **61** B4
Bacău *Romania* **29** D11
Bacău □ *Romania* **29** D11
Baccarat *France* **19** D13
Bacerac *Mexico* **118** A3
Băceşti *Romania* **29** D12
Bach Long Vi, Dao *Vietnam* **64** B6
Bach Ma △ *Vietnam* **64** D6
Bacharach *Germany* **25** E3
Bachhwara *India* **69** G11
Bachuma *Ethiopia* **81** F4
Bačina *Serbia* **44** C5
Back → *Canada* **100** D11
Bačka Palanka *Serbia* **28** E4
Bačka Topola *Serbia* **28** E4
Bäckebo *Sweden* **11** H10
Bäckefors *Sweden* **11** F6
Bäckhammar *Sweden* **10** E8
Bački Petrovac *Serbia* **28** E4
Backnang *Germany* **25** G5
Baco, Mt. *Phil.* **61** E4
Bacolod *Phil.* **61** F5
Bacqueville-en-Caux *France* **18** C8
Bács-Kiskun □ *Hungary* **28** D4
Bácsalmás *Hungary* **28** D4
Bacuag = Placer *Phil.* **61** G6
Bacuk *Malaysia* **65** J4
Bácum *Mexico* **118** B2
Bād *Iran* **71** C7
Bad → *U.S.A.* **112** C3
Bad Aussee *Austria* **26** D6
Bad Axe *U.S.A.* **114** C2
Bad Bergzabern *Germany* **25** F3
Bad Berleburg *Germany* **24** D4
Bad Bevensen *Germany* **24** B6
Bad Bramstedt *Germany* **24** B5
Bad Brückenau *Germany* **25** E5
Bad Doberan *Germany* **24** A7
Bad Driburg *Germany* **24** D5
Bad Ems *Germany* **25** E3
Bad Frankenhausen
  Germany **24** D7
Bad Freienwalde *Germany* **24** C10
Bad Goisern *Austria* **26** D6
Bad Harzburg *Germany* **24** D6
Bad Hersfeld *Germany* **24** E5
Bad Hofgastein *Austria* **26** D6
Bad Homburg *Germany* **25** E4
Bad Honnef *Germany* **24** E3
Bad Iburg *Germany* **24** C4
Bad Ischl *Austria* **26** D6
Bad Kissingen *Germany* **25** E6
Bad Königshofen *Germany* **25** E6
Bad Kreuznach *Germany* **25** F3
Bad Krozingen *Germany* **25** H3
Bad Laasphe *Germany* **24** E4
Bad Langensalza *Germany* **24** D6
Bad Lauterberg *Germany* **24** D6
Bad Leonfelden *Austria* **26** C7
Bad Liebenwerda *Germany* **24** D9
Bad Mergentheim *Germany* **25** F5
Bad Münstereifel *Germany* **24** E2
Bad Nauheim *Germany* **25** E4
Bad Neuenahr-Ahrweiler
  Germany **24** E3
Bad Neustadt *Germany* **25** E6
Bad Oeynhausen *Germany* **24** C4
Bad Oldesloe *Germany* **24** B6
Bad Orb *Germany* **25** E5
Bad Pyrmont *Germany* **24** D5
Bad Reichenhall *Germany* **25** H8
Bad Säckingen *Germany* **25** H3
Bad St. Leonhard *Austria* **26** E7
Bad Salzuflen *Germany* **24** C4
Bad Salzungen *Germany* **24** E6
Bad Schwartau *Germany* **24** B6
Bad Segeberg *Germany* **24** B6
Bad Tölz *Germany* **25** H7
Bad Urach *Germany* **25** G5
Bad Vöslau *Austria* **27** D9
Bad Waldsee *Germany* **25** H5
Bad Wildungen *Germany* **24** D5
Bad Wimpfen *Germany* **25** F5
Bad Windsheim *Germany* **25** F6
Bad Zwischenahn *Germany* **24** B4
Bada Barabil *India* **69** H11
Badagara *India* **66** P9
Badagri *Nigeria* **83** D5
Badajós, L. *Brazil* **124** D6
Badajoz *Spain* **37** G4
Badajoz □ *Spain* **37** G4
Badakhshān □ *Afghan.* **66** A7
Badalona *Spain* **38** D7
Badalzai *Afghan.* **68** C1
Badampahar *India* **67** H15
Badanah *Si. Arabia* **70** D4
Badarinath *India* **69** D8
Badas, Kepulauan *Indonesia* **62** D3
Baddam *India* **69** B6
Baddo → *Pakistan* **66** F4
Bade *Indonesia* **63** F9
Badeggi *Nigeria* **83** D6
Badéguichéri *Niger* **83** C6
Baden *Austria* **27** C9
Baden *Switz.* **25** H4
Baden *U.S.A.* **114** F4
Baden-Baden *Germany* **25** G4
Baden-Württemberg □
  Germany **25** G4
Badgam *India* **69** B6
Badgastein *Austria* **26** D6
Badger *Canada* **105** C8
Badger *U.S.A.* **110** J7
Bādghīs □ *Afghan.* **66** B3
Badgingarra △ *Australia* **93** F2
Badia Polésine *Italy* **41** C8
Badiar △ *Guinea* **82** C2
Badin *Pakistan* **68** G3
Badinka △ *Mali* **82** C3
Badlands *U.S.A.* **112** D2
Badlands △ *U.S.A.* **112** D2
Badogo *Mali* **82** C3
Badoumbé *Mali* **82** C2
Badrah *Iraq* **73** F11
Badrinath *India* **69** D8
Badu *Australia* **94** a
Badulla *Sri Lanka* **66** R12
Badung, Selat *Indonesia* **63** K18
Baena *Spain* **37** H6
Baengnyeongdo *S. Korea* **57** F13
Baeza *Spain* **37** H7
Bafang *Cameroon* **83** D7
Bafatá *Guinea-Biss.* **82** C2
Baffin B. *N. Amer.* **101** C19
Baffin I. *Canada* **101** D17
Bafia *Cameroon* **83** E7
Bafilo *Togo* **83** D5
Bafing → *Mali* **82** C2
Bafing △ *Mali* **82** C2
Bafliyūn *Syria* **70** B3
Bafoulabé *Mali* **82** C2
Bafoussam *Cameroon* **83** D7
Bāfq *Iran* **71** D7
Bafra *Turkey* **72** B6
Bafra Burnu *Turkey* **72** B7
Bāft *Iran* **71** D8
Bafut *Cameroon* **83** D7
Bafwasende
  Dem. Rep. of the Congo **86** B2
Bagaha *India* **69** F11
Bagam *Niger* **83** B6
Bagamoyo *Tanzania* **86** D4
Bagan Datoh *Malaysia* **65** L3
Bagan Serai *Malaysia* **65** K3
Baganga *Phil.* **61** H7
Bagani *Namibia* **88** B3
Bagansiapiapi *Indonesia* **62** D2
Bagasra *India* **68** J4
Bagaud *India* **68** H6
Bagawi *Sudan* **81** E3
Bagbag *Sudan* **81** D3
Bagdad *U.S.A.* **111** L11
Bagdarin *Russia* **53** D12
Bagé *Brazil* **127** C5
Bagenalstown = Muine
  Bheag *Ireland* **12** D5
Baggs *U.S.A.* **108** F10
Bagh *Pakistan* **69** C5
Baghain → *India* **69** G9
Baghdād *Iraq* **73** F11
Baghdadi *Georgia* **73** A10
Bagheria *Italy* **42** D6
Baghlān *Afghan.* **66** A6
Baghlān □ *Afghan.* **66** B6
Bagley *U.S.A.* **112** B6
Bagnara Cálabra *Italy* **43** D8
Bagnasco *Italy* **40** D5
Bagnères-de-Bigorre *France* **20** E4
Bagnères-de-Luchon *France* **20** F4
Bagni di Lucca *Italy* **40** D7
Bagno di Romagna *Italy* **41** E8
Bagnoles-de-l'Orne *France* **18** D6
Bagnols-sur-Cèze *France* **21** D8
Bagnorégio *Italy* **41** F9
Bago = Pegu *Burma* **67** L20
Bagodar *India* **69** G11
Bagoé → *Nigeria* **83** D7
Baguio *Phil.* **61** C4
Bāgyurdu *Turkey* **47** C9
Bagzane, Monts *Niger* **83** B6
Bah *India* **69** F8
Bahabón de Esgueva *Spain* **36** D7
Bahadurganj *India* **69** F12
Bahadurgarh *India* **68** E7
Bahama, Canal Viejo de
  W. Indies **120** B4
Bahamas ■ *N. Amer.* **121** B5
Bahār *Iran* **73** E13
Baharampur *India* **69** G13
Baharîya, El Wâhât al *Egypt* **80** B2
Baharu Pandan = Pandan
  Malaysia **65** d
Bahawalnagar *Pakistan* **68** E5
Bahawalpur *Pakistan* **68** E4
Bahçe *Turkey* **72** D7
Bahçecik *Turkey* **45** F13
Bäherden *Turkmenistan* **71** B8
Baheri *India* **69** E8
Bahgul → *India* **69** F8
Bahi *Tanzania* **86** D4
Bahi Swamp *Tanzania* **86** D4
Bahía = Salvador *Brazil* **125** F11
Bahía □ *Brazil* **125** F10
Bahía, Is. de la *Honduras* **120** C2
Bahía Blanca *Argentina* **126** D3
Bahía de Caráquez *Ecuador* **124** D2
Bahía Kino *Mexico* **118** B2
Bahía Laura *Argentina* **128** F3
Bahía Negra *Paraguay* **124** H7
Bahir Dar *Ethiopia* **81** E4
Bahmanzād *Iran* **71** D6
Bahr el Ahmar □ *Sudan* **80** D4
Bahr el Jabal □ *Sudan* **81** G3
Bahraich *India* **69** F9
Bahrain ■ *Asia* **71** E6
Bāhū Kalāt *Iran* **71** E9
Bai *Mali* **82** C4
Bai Bung, Mui = Ca Mau,
  Mui *Vietnam* **65** H5
Bai Duc *Vietnam* **64** C5
Bai Thuong *Vietnam* **64** C5
Baia de Aramă *Romania* **28** E7
Baia Mare *Romania* **29** C8
Baia-Sprie *Romania* **29** C8
Baião *Brazil* **125** D9
Baïbokoum *Chad* **79** G9
Baicheng *China* **57** B12
Băicoi *Romania* **29** E10
Baidoa = Baardheere
  Somali Rep. **75** G3
Baidoa = Baydhabo
  Somali Rep. **75** G3
Baie-Comeau *Canada* **105** C6
Baie-St-Paul *Canada* **105** C5
Baie Ste-Anne *Seychelles* **85** b
Baie-Trinité *Canada* **105** C6
Baie Verte *Canada* **105** C8
Baignes-Ste-Radegonde
  France **20** C3
Baigneux-les-Juifs *France* **19** E11
Baihar *India* **69** H9
Baihe *China* **56** H6
Ba'ījī *Iraq* **73** E10
Baijnath *India* **69** E8
Baikal, L. = Baykal, Oz.
  Russia **53** D11
Baikonur = Bayqongyr
  Kazakhstan **52** E7
Baikunthpur *India* **69** H10
Baile Átha Cliath = Dublin
  Ireland **12** C5
Baile Átha Fhirdhia =
  Ardee *Ireland* **12** C5
Baile Átha I = Athy *Ireland* **12** C5
Baile Átha Luain =
  Athlone *Ireland* **12** C4
Baile Átha Troim = Trim
  Ireland **12** C5
Baile Brigín = Balbriggan
  Ireland **12** C5
Báile Govora *Romania* **29** E9
Báile Herculane *Romania* **28** F7
Băile Olăneşti *Romania* **29** E9
Băile Tuşnad *Romania* **29** D10
Bailén *Spain* **37** G7
Băileşti *Romania* **29** F8
Baima *China* **58** A3
Bain-de-Bretagne *France* **18** E5
Bainbridge Ga., U.S.A. **117** F12
Bainbridge N.Y., U.S.A. **115** D9
Bainbridge Island *U.S.A.* **110** C4
Baing *Indonesia* **63** F6
Bainiu *China* **56** H7
Baiona *Spain* **36** C2
Bā'ir *Jordan* **74** E5
Bairiki = Tarawa *Kiribati* **96** G9
Bairin Youqi *China* **57** C10
Bairin Zuoqi *China* **57** C10
Bairnsdale *Australia* **95** F4
Bais *Phil.* **61** G5
Baisha *China* **56** G7
Baissa *Nigeria* **83** D7
Baitadi *Nepal* **69** E9
Baixa Limia-Sierra do
  Xurés △ *Spain* **36** D2
Baiyin *China* **56** F3
Baiyü *China* **58** B2
Baiyu Shan *China* **56** F4
Baiyuda *Sudan* **80** D3
Baj Baj *India* **69** H13
Baja *Hungary* **28** D3
Baja, Pta. *Mexico* **118** B1
Baja California *Mexico* **118** A1
Baja California □ *Mexico* **118** B2
Baja California Sur □
  Mexico **118** B2
Bajag *India* **69** H9
Bajamar *Canary Is.* **48** F3
Bajana *India* **68** H4
Bajatrejo *Indonesia* **63** J17
Bajera *Indonesia* **63** J18
Bājgīrān *Iran* **71** B8
Bajimba, Mt. *Australia* **95** D5
Bajina Bašta *Serbia* **44** C3
Bajmok *Serbia* **28** E4
Bajo Boquete *Panama* **120** E3
Bajo Nuevo *Caribbean* **120** C4
Bajoga *Nigeria* **83** C7
Bajool *Australia* **94** C5
Bak *Hungary* **28** D1
Bakar *Croatia* **41** C11
Bakassi Pen. *Cameroon* **83** E6
Bakel *Senegal* **82** C2
Baker Calif., U.S.A. **111** K10
Baker Mont., U.S.A. **108** C11
Baker, L. *Canada* **100** E12
Baker Bay *Phil.* **61** D4
Baker City *U.S.A.* **108** D5
Baker I. *Pac. Oc.* **96** G10
Baker I. *U.S.A.* **102** B2
Baker L. *Australia* **93** E5
Baker Lake *Canada* **100** E12
Bakers Creek *Australia* **94** C4
Bakers Dozen Is. *Canada* **104** A4
Bakersfield Calif., U.S.A. **111** K8
Bakersfield Vt., U.S.A. **115** B12
Bakharden = Bäherden
  Turkmenistan **71** B8
Bakhchysaray *Ukraine* **33** K7
Bakhmach *Ukraine* **33** G7
Bākhtarān = Kermānshāh
  Iran **73** E12
Bākhtarān □
  = Kermānshāh □ *Iran* **70** C5
Bakı *Azerbaijan* **35** K9
Bakır → *Turkey* **47** C9
Bakırdağı *Turkey* **72** C6
Bakkafjörður *Iceland* **8** C6
Bakkan *Turkey* **47** C11
Bako *Ethiopia* **81** F4
Bako *Ivory C.* **82** D3
Bakony *Hungary* **28** C2
Bakony Forest = Bakony
  Hungary **28** C2
Bakori *Nigeria* **83** C6
Bakouma *C.A.R.* **84** C4
Baksan *Russia* **35** J6
Bakswaho *India* **69** G8
Baku = Bakı *Azerbaijan* **35** K9
Bakundi *Nigeria* **83** D7
Bakuriani *Georgia* **73** B10
Bakutis Coast *Antarctica* **5** D15
Baky = Bakı *Azerbaijan* **35** K9
Bala *Canada* **114** A5
Bala *Senegal* **82** C2
Balâ *Turkey* **72** C5
Bala *U.K.* **14** E4
Bala, L. *U.K.* **14** E4
Balabac I. *Phil.* **62** C5
Balabac Str. *E. Indies* **62** C5
Balabagh *Afghan.* **68** B4
Ba'labakk *Lebanon* **74** B5
Balabalangan, Kepulauan
  Indonesia **62** E5
Bălăciţa *Romania* **29** F8
Balad *Iraq* **73** F11
Balad Rūz *Iraq* **73** F11
Bālādeh *Fārs, Iran* **71** D6
Bālādeh *Māzandaran, Iran* **71** B6
Balaghat *India* **69** J12
Balaghat Ra. *India* **66** K10
Balaguer *Spain* **38** D5
Balakän *Azerbaijan* **73** B12
Balakhna *Russia* **34** B6
Balakliya *Ukraine* **33** K7
Balakovo *Russia* **34** D8
Balamau *India* **69** F9
Bālan *Romania* **29** D10
Balancán *Mexico* **119** D6
Balanivka *Ukraine* **29** B14
Balashov *Russia* **34** E6
Balasinor *India* **68** H5
Balasore = Baleshwar *India* **67** J15
Balassagyarmat *Hungary* **28** B4
Balât *Egypt* **80** B2
Balaton *Hungary* **28** D2
Balaton-Felvidéki △ *Hungary* **28** D2
Balatonboglár *Hungary* **28** D2
Balatonfüred *Hungary* **28** D2
Balatonszentgyörgy *Hungary* **28** D2
Balayan *Phil.* **61** E4
Balazote *Spain* **39** G2
Balbieriškis *Lithuania* **30** D10
Balbigny *France* **21** C8
Balbina, Represa de *Brazil* **124** D7
Balboa *Panama* **120** E4
Balbriggan *Ireland* **12** C5
Balcarce *Argentina* **126** D4
Balcarres *Canada* **103** C8
Bălceşti *Romania* **29** F8
Balchik *Bulgaria* **45** C12
Balclutha *N.Z.* **91** G2
Balcones Escarpment *U.S.A.* **116** G5
Bald I. *Australia* **93** F2
Bald Knob *U.S.A.* **116** D9
Baldock L. *Canada* **103** B9
Baldwin Mich., U.S.A. **113** D11
Baldwin Pa., U.S.A. **114** F5
Baldwinsville *U.S.A.* **115** C8
Baldy Peak *U.S.A.* **109** K9
Bale *Croatia* **41** C10
Bale *Oromiya, Ethiopia* **81** F5
Bale *Oromiya, Ethiopia* **81** F5
Bale Mts. △ *Ethiopia* **81** F4
Baleares, Is. *Spain* **48** B10
Balearic Is. = Baleares, Is.
  Spain **48** B10
Baleine → *Canada* **105** A6
Baleine, Petite R. de la →
  Canada **104** A4
Băleni *Romania* **29** E12
Baler *Phil.* **61** D4
Baler Bay *Phil.* **61** D4
Baleshare *U.K.* **13** D1
Baleshwar *India* **67** J15
Baley *Russia* **53** D12
Balezino *Russia* **34** B11
Balfate *Honduras* **120** C2
Balgo *Australia* **92** D4
Bali *Cameroon* **83** D7
Bali *Greece* **49** D6
Bali *India* **68** G5
Bali □ *Indonesia* **62** F5
Bali, Selat *Indonesia* **63** J17
Bali, S. Leone **82** D2
Bali Sea *Indonesia* **63** J17
Balia *S. Leone* **82** D2
Baliapal *India* **69** J12
Balige *Indonesia* **65** L2
Baligród *Poland* **31** J9
Balik Pulau *Malaysia* **65** c
Balikesir *Turkey* **47** B9
Balıkesir □ *Turkey* **47** B9
Balīkh → *Syria* **73** E8
Balıklıçeşme *Turkey* **45** F11
Balikpapan *Indonesia* **62** E5
Balimbing *Phil.* **63** C5
Baling *Malaysia* **65** K3
Balingen *Germany* **25** G4
Balint *Romania* **28** E6
Balintang Channel *Phil.* **61** B4
Balkan Mts. = Stara
  Planina *Bulgaria* **44** C7
Balkanabat *Turkmenistan* **71** B7
Balkhash = Balqash
  Kazakhstan **52** E8
Balkhash, Ozero = Balqash
  Köli *Kazakhstan* **52** E8
Balladonia *Australia* **93** F3
Ballaghaderreen *Ireland* **12** C3
Ballarat *Australia* **95** F3
Ballard, L. *Australia* **93** E3
Ballater *U.K.* **13** D5
Ballé *Mali* **82** B3
Ballena, Canal de *Mexico* **118** B2
Balleny Is. *Antarctica* **5** C11
Balleroy *France* **18** C6
Ballerup *Denmark* **11** J6
Ballı *Turkey* **45** F11
Ballia *India* **69** G11
Ballina *Australia* **95** D5
Ballina *Ireland* **12** B2
Ballinasloe *Ireland* **12** C3
Ballinger *U.S.A.* **116** F5
Ballinrobe *Ireland* **12** C2
Ballinskelligs B. *Ireland* **12** E1
Ballon *France* **18** D7
Ballons des Vosges △ *France* **19** E14
Ballsh *Albania* **44** F3
Ballston Spa *U.S.A.* **115** D11
Ballyboghil *Ireland* **12** C5
Ballybunion *Ireland* **12** D2
Ballycanew *Ireland* **12** D5
Ballycastle *U.K.* **12** A5
Ballyclare *U.K.* **12** B5
Ballydehob *Ireland* **12** E2
Ballygawley *U.K.* **12** B4
Ballyhaunis *Ireland* **12** C3
Ballyheige *Ireland* **12** D2
Ballymena *U.K.* **12** B5
Ballymoney *U.K.* **12** A5
Ballymote *Ireland* **12** B3
Ballynahinch *U.K.* **12** B6
Ballyquintin Pt. *U.K.* **12** B6
Ballyshannon *Ireland* **12** B3
Balmaceda *Chile* **128** F2
Balmaseda *Spain* **38** B1
Balmazújváros *Hungary* **28** C6
Balmertown *Canada* **103** C10
Balmoral *Australia* **95** F3
Balmorhea *U.S.A.* **116** F3
Balochistan =
  Baluchistan □ *Pakistan* **66** F4
Balonne → *Australia* **95** D4
Balotra *India* **68** G5
Balqash *Kazakhstan* **52** E8
Balqash Köli *Kazakhstan* **52** E8
Balrampur *India* **69** F10
Balranald *Australia* **95** E3
Balş *Romania* **29** F9
Balsas → *Brazil* **125** E9
Balsas → *Mexico* **119** D5
Balsas del Norte *Mexico* **119** D5
Bålsta *Sweden* **10** E11
Balta *Romania* **28** F7
Balta *Ukraine* **29** B14
Baltanás *Spain* **36** D6
Baltasi *Moldova* **29** C12
Baltic Sea *Europe* **9** H18
Baltîm *Egypt* **80** H7
Baltimore *Ireland* **12** E2
Baltimore Md., U.S.A. **113** F15
Baltimore Ohio, U.S.A. **114** G2
Baltinglass *Ireland* **12** D5
Baltit *Pakistan* **69** A6
Baltiysk *Russia* **30** D6
Baltrum *Germany* **24** B3
Baluchistan □ *Pakistan* **66** F4
Baluqtybulaq *Kazakhstan* **34** E10
Balurghat *India* **69** G13
Balvi *Latvia* **32** D4
Balya *Turkey* **47** B9
Bam *Iran* **71** D8
Bama *China* **58** E6
Bama *Nigeria* **83** C7
Bamaga *Australia* **94** A3
Bamaji L. *Canada* **104** B1
Bamako *Mali* **82** C3
Bamba *Mali* **83** B4
Bambara Maoundé *Mali* **82** B4
Bambaroo *Australia* **94** B4
Bambaya *Guinea* **82** D2
Bamberg *Germany* **25** F6
Bamberg *U.S.A.* **117** E14
Bambesi *Ethiopia* **81** F3
Bambey *Senegal* **82** C1
Bambili *Dem. Rep. of the Congo* **86** B2
Bamboi *Ghana* **82** D4
Bamburgh *U.K.* **14** B6
Bamenda *Cameroon* **83** D7
Bamendjing, L. de *Cameroon* **83** D7
Bamfield *Canada* **102** D3
Bāmīān *Afghan.* **66** B5
Bamiancheng *China* **57** C13
Bamkin *Cameroon* **83** D7
Bampūr *Iran* **71** E8
Bampūr → *Iran* **71** E8
Ban *Burkina Faso* **82** C4
Ban Ao Tu Khun *Thailand* **65** a
Ban Ban *Laos* **64** C4
Ban Bang Hin *Thailand* **65** H2
Ban Bang Khu *Thailand* **65** a
Ban Bang Rong *Thailand* **65** a
Ban Bo Phut *Thailand* **65** b
Ban Chaweng *Thailand* **65** b
Ban Chiang Klang *Thailand* **64** C3
Ban Choho *Thailand* **64** E4
Ban Dan Lan Hoi *Thailand* **64** D2
Ban Don = Surat Thani
  Thailand **65** H2
Ban Don *Vietnam* **64** F6
Ban Don, Ao → *Thailand* **65** H2
Ban Dong *Thailand* **64** C3
Ban Hong *Thailand* **64** C2
Ban Hua Thanon *Thailand* **65** b
Ban Kantang *Thailand* **65** J2
Ban Karon *Thailand* **65** a
Ban Kata *Thailand* **65** a
Ban Keun *Laos* **64** C4
Ban Khai *Thailand* **64** F3
Ban Kheun *Laos* **64** B3
Ban Khlong Khian *Thailand* **65** a
Ban Khlong Kua *Thailand* **65** J3
Ban Khuan *Thailand* **65** J2
Ban Khuan Mao *Thailand* **65** J2
Ban Ko Yai Chim *Thailand* **65** G2
Ban Laem *Thailand* **64** F2
Ban Lamai *Thailand* **65** b
Ban Lao Ngam *Laos* **64** E6
Ban Le Kathe *Thailand* **64** E2
Ban Lo Po Noi *Thailand* **65** a
Ban Mae Chedi *Thailand* **64** C2
Ban Mae Nam *Thailand* **65** b
Ban Mae Sariang *Thailand* **64** C1
Ban Mê Thuôt = Buon Ma
  Thuot *Vietnam* **64** F7

Ban Mi *Thailand* **64** E3
Ban Muong Mo *Laos* **64** C4
Ban Na Bo *Thailand* **65** b
Ban Na Mo *Laos* **64** D5
Ban Na San *Thailand* **65** H2
Ban Na Tong *Laos* **64** B3
Ban Nam Bac *Laos* **64** B4
Ban Ngang *Laos* **64** E6
Ban Nong Bok *Laos* **64** D5
Ban Nong Boua *Laos* **64** E6
Ban Nong Pling *Thailand* **64** E3
Ban Pak Chan *Thailand* **65** G2
Ban Patong *Thailand* **65** a
Ban Phai *Thailand* **64** D4
Ban Phak Chit *Thailand* **65** a
Ban Pong *Thailand* **64** F2
Ban Rawai *Thailand* **65** a
Ban Ron Phibun *Thailand* **65** H2
Ban Sakhu *Thailand* **65** a
Ban Sanam Chai *Thailand* **65** J3
Ban Sangkha *Thailand* **64** E4
Ban Tak *Thailand* **64** D2
Ban Tako *Thailand* **64** E4
Ban Tha Dua *Thailand* **64** D2
Ban Tha Nun *Thailand* **65** a
Ban Tha Rua *Thailand* **65** a
Ban Tha Yu *Thailand* **65** a
Ban Thahine *Laos* **64** E5
Ban Thong Krut *Thailand* **65** b
Ban Xien Kok *Laos* **64** B3
Ban Yen Nhan *Vietnam* **64** B6
Banaba *Kiribati* **96** H8
Banalia *Dem. Rep. of the Congo* **86** B2
Banam *Cambodia* **65** G5
Banamba *Mali* **82** C3
Banana Is. *S. Leone* **82** D2
Bananal, I. do *Brazil* **125** F8
Banaras = Varanasi *India* **69** G10
Banas → *Gujarat, India* **68** H4
Banas → *Mad. P., India* **69** G9
Bânâs, Ras *Egypt* **80** C4
Banaz *Turkey* **47** C11
Banaz → *Turkey* **47** C11
Banbridge *U.K.* **12** B5
Banbury *U.K.* **15** E6
Banchory *U.K.* **13** D6
Banco *Ethiopia* **81** F4
Bancroft *Canada* **114** A7
Band *Romania* **29** D9
Band Boni *Iran* **71** E8
Band Qīr *Iran* **71** D6
Banda *Mad. P., India* **69** G8
Banda *Ut. P., India* **69** G9
Banda, Kepulauan *Indonesia* **63** E7
Banda Aceh *Indonesia* **62** C1
Banda Banda, Mt. *Australia* **95** E5
Banda Elat *Indonesia* **63** F8
Banda Is. = Banda, Kepulauan *Indonesia* **63** E7
Banda Sea *Indonesia* **63** F8
Bandai-Asahi △ *Japan* **54** F10
Bandama → *Ivory C.* **82** D4
Bandama Blanc → *Ivory C.* **82** D4
Bandama Rouge → *Ivory C.* **82** D4
Bandān *Iran* **71** D9
Bandanaira *Indonesia* **63** E7
Bandanwara *India* **68** F6
Bandar = Machilipatnam *India* **67** L12
Bandar-e Abbās *Iran* **71** E8
Bandar-e Anzalī *Iran* **73** D13
Bandar-e Bushehr = Būshehr *Iran* **71** D6
Bandar-e Chārak *Iran* **71** E7
Bandar-e Deylam *Iran* **71** D6
Bandar-e Emām Khomeynī *Iran* **71** D6
Bandar-e Lengeh *Iran* **71** E7
Bandar-e Maqām *Iran* **71** E7
Bandar-e Ma'shur *Iran* **71** D6
Bandar-e Rīg *Iran* **71** D6
Bandar-e Torkeman *Iran* **71** B7
Bandar Lampung *Indonesia* **62** F3
Bandar Maharani = Muar *Malaysia* **65** L4
Bandar Penggaram = Batu Pahat *Malaysia* **65** M4
Bandar Seri Begawan *Brunei* **62** D5
Bandar Sri Aman = Sri Aman *Malaysia* **62** D4
Bandawe *Malawi* **87** E3
Bande *Spain* **36** C3
Bandeira, Pico da *Brazil* **127** A7
Bandera *Argentina* **126** B3
Banderas, B. de *Mexico* **118** C3
Bandhavgarh *India* **69** H9
Bandi → *India* **68** F6
Bandiagara *Mali* **82** C4
Bandikui *India* **68** F7
Bandırma *Turkey* **45** F11
Bandjarmasin = Banjarmasin *Indonesia* **62** E4
Bandol *France* **21** E9
Bandon *Ireland* **12** E3
Bandon → *Ireland* **12** E3
Bandula *Mozam.* **87** F3
Bandundu *Dem. Rep. of the Congo* **84** E3

Bandung *Indonesia* **62** F3
Bané *Burkina Faso* **83** C4
Bâneasa *Romania* **29** E12
Bāneh *Iran* **73** E11
Banes *Cuba* **121** B4
Banff *Canada* **102** C5
Banff *U.K.* **13** D6
Banff △ *Canada* **102** C5
Banfora *Burkina Faso* **82** C4
Bang Fai → *Laos* **64** D5
Bang Hieng → *Laos* **64** D5
Bang Krathum *Thailand* **64** D3
Bang Lamung *Thailand* **64** F3
Bang Mun Nak *Thailand* **64** D3
Bang Pa In *Thailand* **64** E3
Bang Rakam *Thailand* **64** D3
Bang Saphan *Thailand* **65** G2
Bang Thao *Thailand* **65** a
Bangaduni I. *India* **69** J13
Bangala Dam *Zimbabwe* **87** G3
Bangalore *India* **66** N10
Banganga → *India* **68** F6
Bangangté *Cameroon* **83** D7
Bangaon *India* **69** H13
Bangassou *C.A.R.* **84** D4
Banggai *Indonesia* **63** E6
Banggai, Kepulauan *Indonesia* **63** E6
Banggai Arch. = Banggai, Kepulauan *Indonesia* **63** E6
Banggi, Pulau *Malaysia* **62** C5
Banghāzī *Libya* **79** B10
Bangjang *Sudan* **81** E3
Bangka *Sulawesi, Indonesia* **63** D7
Bangka *Sumatera, Indonesia* **62** E3
Bangka, Selat *Indonesia* **62** E3
Bangka-Belitung □ *Indonesia* **62** E3
Bangkalan *Indonesia* **63** G15
Bangkinang *Indonesia* **62** D2
Bangko *Indonesia* **62** E2
Bangkok *Thailand* **64** F3
Bangla = West Bengal □ *India* **69** H13
Bangladesh ■ *Asia* **67** H17
Bangli *Indonesia* **63** J18
Bangolo *Ivory C.* **82** D3
Bangong Co *China* **69** C8
Bangor *Down, U.K.* **12** B6
Bangor *Gwynedd, U.K.* **14** D3
Bangor *Maine, U.S.A.* **113** C19
Bangor *Pa., U.S.A.* **115** F9
Bangued *Phil.* **61** C4
Bangui *C.A.R.* **84** D3
Bangui *Phil.* **61** B4
Banguru *Dem. Rep. of the Congo* **86** B2
Bangweulu, L. *Zambia* **87** E3
Bangweulu Swamp *Zambia* **87** E3
Banhine △ *Mozam.* **89** C5
Bani *Burkina Faso* **83** C4
Baní *Dom. Rep.* **121** C5
Bani → *Mali* **82** C4
Bani Bangou *Niger* **83** B5
Banī Sa'd *Iraq* **73** F11
Bania *Ivory C.* **82** D4
Banihal Pass *India* **69** C6
Banikoara *Benin* **83** C5
Banissa *Kenya* **81** G5
Bāniyās *Syria* **72** E6
Banja Luka *Bos.-H.* **28** F2
Banjar *India* **68** D7
Banjar → *India* **69** H9
Banjarmasin *Indonesia* **62** E4
Banjul *Gambia* **82** C1
Banka *India* **69** G12
Bankas *Mali* **82** C4
Bankeryd *Sweden* **11** G8
Banket *Zimbabwe* **87** F3
Bankilaré *Niger* **83** C5
Bankipore *India* **67** G14
Banks I. = Moa *Australia* **94** a
Banks I. *B.C., Canada* **102** C3
Banks I. *N.W.T., Canada* **100** C7
Banks Pen. *N.Z.* **91** E4
Banks Str. *Australia* **95** G4
Bankura *India* **69** H12
Bankya *Bulgaria* **44** D7
Banmankhi *India* **69** G12
Bann → *Armagh, U.K.* **12** B5
Bann → *L'derry., U.K.* **12** A5
Bannalec *France* **18** E3
Bannang Sata *Thailand* **65** J3
Banning *U.S.A.* **111** M10
Banno *Ethiopia* **81** G4
Bannockburn *Canada* **114** B7
Bannockburn *U.K.* **13** E5
Bannockburn *Zimbabwe* **87** G2
Bannu *Pakistan* **66** C7
Bano *India* **69** H11
Bañolas = Banyoles *Spain* **38** C7
Banon *France* **21** D9
Baños de la Encina *Spain* **37** G7
Baños de Molgas *Spain* **36** C3
Bánovce nad Bebravou *Slovak Rep.* **27** C11
Banovići *Bos.-H.* **28** F3
Bansgaon *India* **69** F10
Banská Bystrica *Slovak Rep.* **27** C12
Banská Štiavnica *Slovak Rep.* **27** C11

Bansko *Bulgaria* **44** E7
Banskobystrický □ *Slovak Rep.* □
Banswara *India* **68** H6
Bantaeng *Indonesia* **63** F5
Bantaji *Nigeria* **83** D7
Bantayan *Phil.* **61** F5
Banten □ *Indonesia* **63** G11
Bantry *Ireland* **12** E2
Bantry B. *Ireland* **12** E2
Bantul *Indonesia* **63** G14
Bantva *India* **68** J4
Banya *Bulgaria* **45** D8
Banyak, Kepulauan *Indonesia* **62** D1
Banyalbufar *Spain* **48** B9
Banyeres de Mariola *Spain* **39** G4
Banyo *Cameroon* **83** D7
Banyoles *Spain* **38** C7
Banyuls-sur-Mer *France* **20** F7
Banyumas *Indonesia* **63** G13
Banyuwangi *Indonesia* **63** J17
Banzare Coast *Antarctica* **5** C9
Bao Ha *Vietnam* **58** F5
Bao Lac *Vietnam* **64** A5
Bao Loc *Vietnam* **65** G6
Bao'an = Shenzhen *China* **59** F10
Baocheng *China* **56** H4
Baode *China* **56** E6
Baodi *China* **57** E9
Baoding *China* **56** E8
Baoji *China* **56** G4
Baojing *China* **58** C7
Baokang *China* **59** B8
Baoshan *Shanghai, China* **59** B13
Baoshan *Yunnan, China* **58** E2
Baotou *China* **56** D6
Baoxing *China* **58** B4
Baoying *China* **57** H10
Baoyou = Ledong *China* **64** C7
Bap *India* **68** F5
Bapatla *India* **67** M12
Bapaume *France* **19** B9
Bāqerābād *Iran* **71** C6
Ba'qūbah *Iraq* **73** F11
Baquedano *Chile* **126** A2
Bar *Montenegro* **44** D3
Bar *Ukraine* **23** D14
Bar Bigha *India* **69** G11
Bar Harbor *U.S.A.* **113** C19
Bar-le-Duc *France* **19** D12
Bar-sur-Aube *France* **19** D11
Bar-sur-Seine *France* **19** D11
Bara *India* **69** G9
Bâra *Romania* **29** C12
Bara Banki *India* **69** F9
Barabai *Indonesia* **62** E5
Baraboo *U.S.A.* **112** D9
Baracoa *Cuba* **121** B5
Baradā → *Syria* **74** B5
Baradero *Argentina* **126** C4
Baraga *U.S.A.* **112** B9
Bărăganul *Romania* **29** F12
Baragoi *Kenya* **86** B4
Barah → *India* **68** F6
Barahona *Dom. Rep.* **121** C5
Barail Range *India* **67** G18
Barajas, Madrid ✈ (MAD) *Spain* **36** E7
Baraka *Sudan* **81** E2
Baraka → *Sudan* **80** D4
Barakar → *India* **69** G12
Barakot *India* **69** J11
Barakpur *India* **69** H13
Baralaba *Australia* **94** C4
Barameiya *Sudan* **80** D4
Baramula *India* **69** B6
Baran *India* **68** G7
Baran → *Pakistan* **68** G3
Barañain *Spain* **38** C3
Baranavichy *Belarus* **23** B14
Barani *Burkina Faso* **82** C4
Baranof *U.S.A.* **102** B2
Baranof I. *U.S.A.* **100** F4
Baranów Sandomierski *Poland* **31** H8
Baranya □ *Hungary* **28** E3
Baraolt *Romania* **29** D10
Baraona *Spain* **38** D2
Barapasi *Indonesia* **63** E9
Barasat *India* **69** H13
Barat Daya, Kepulauan *Indonesia* **63** F7
Barataria B. *U.S.A.* **117** G10
Barauda *India* **68** H6
Baraut *India* **68** E7
Barbacena *Brazil* **127** A7
Barbados ■ *W. Indies* **121** g
Barban *Croatia* **41** C11
Barbária, C. de *Spain* **48** C7
Barbaros *Turkey* **45** F11
Barbas, C. *W. Sahara* **78** D2
Barbàstro *Spain* **38** C5
Barbate *Spain* **37** J5
Barbate *France* **28** F7
Barbeau Pk. *Canada* **101** A16

Barberino di Mugello *Italy* **41** E8
Barberton *S. Africa* **89** D5
Barberton *U.S.A.* **114** E3
Barbezieux-St-Hilaire *France* **20** C3
Barbosa *Colombia* **124** B4
Barbourville *U.S.A.* **113** G12
Barbuda *W. Indies* **121** C7
Bârca *Romania* **29** G8
Barcaldine *Australia* **94** C4
Barcarrota *Spain* **37** G4
Barcellona Pozzo di Gotto *Italy* **43** D7
Barcelona *Spain* **38** D7
Barcelona *Venezuela* **124** A6
Barcelona □ *Spain* **38** D7
Barcelona-Prat ✈ (BCN) *Spain* **38** D7
Barceloneta *Puerto Rico* **121** d
Barcelonette *France* **21** D10
Barcelos *Brazil* **124** D6
Barcin *Poland* **31** F4
Barclayville *Liberia* **82** E3
Barcoo → *Australia* **94** D3
Barcs *Hungary* **28** E2
Barczewo *Poland* **30** E7
Bärdä *Azerbaijan* **35** K8
Bardaï *Chad* **79** D9
Bardas Blancas *Argentina* **126** D2
Barddhaman *India* **69** H12
Bardejov *Slovak Rep.* **27** B14
Bardera = Baardheere *Somali Rep.* ...
Bardi *Italy* **40** D6
Bardīyah *Libya* **79** B10
Bardolino *Italy* **40** C7
Bardonécchia *Italy* **40** C3
Bardsey I. *U.K.* **14** E3
Bardstown *U.S.A.* **113** G11
Bareilly *India* **69** E8
Barela *India* **69** H9
Barentin *France* **18** C7
Barenton *France* **18** D6
Barents Sea *Arctic* **4** B9
Barentu *Eritrea* **81** D4
Barfleur *France* **18** C5
Barfleur, Pte. de *France* **18** C5
Barga *Italy* **40** D7
Bargara *Australia* **94** C5
Bargas *Spain* **36** F6
Bârgăului Bistriţa → *Romania* **29** C9
Barge *Italy* **40** D4
Bargi Dam *India* **69** H9
Bargteheide *Germany* **24** B6
Barguzin *Russia* **53** D11
Barh *India* **69** G11
Barhaj *India* **69** F10
Barhi *India* **69** G11
Bari *India* **68** F7
Bari *Italy* **43** A9
Bari Doab *Pakistan* **68** D5
Bari Sadri *India* **68** G6
Bari Sardo *Italy* **42** C2
Barīdī, Ra's *Si. Arabia* **70** E3
Barīm *Yemen* **76** E8
Barinas *Venezuela* **124** B4
Baring, C. *Canada* **100** B8
Baringo, L. *Kenya* **86** B4
Bârîs *Egypt* **80** C3
Barisal *Bangla.* **67** H17
Barisal □ *Bangla.* **67** H17
Barisan, Pegunungan *Indonesia* **62** E2
Barito → *Indonesia* **62** E4
Baritú △ *Argentina* **126** A3
Barjac *France* **21** D8
Barjols *France* **21** E10
Barjūj, Wadi → *Libya* **79** C8
Bark L. *Canada* **114** A7
Barka = Baraka → *Sudan* **80** D4
Barkakana *India* **69** H11
Barkal, J. *Sudan* **80** D3
Barkam *China* **58** B4
Barker *U.S.A.* **114** C6
Barkley, L. *U.S.A.* **117** C10
Barkley Sound *Canada* **102** D3
Barkly East *S. Africa* **88** E4
Barkly Homestead *Australia* **94** B2
Barkly Tableland *Australia* **94** B2
Barkly West *S. Africa* **88** D3
Barkol, Wadi → *Sudan* **80** D3
Barla Dağı *Turkey* **47** C12
Bârlad *Romania* **29** D12
Bârlad → *Romania* **29** E12
Barlee, L. *Australia* **93** E2
Barlee, Mt. *Australia* **93** D4
Barletta *Italy* **43** A9
Barlinek *Poland* **31** F2
Barlovento *Canary Is.* **48** F2
Barlovento *C. Verde Is.* **78** b
Barlow L. *Canada* **103** A8
Barmedman *Australia* **95** E4
Barmer *India* **68** G4
Barmera *Australia* **95** E3
Barmouth *U.K.* **14** E3
Barmstedt *Germany* **24** B5
Barna → *India* **69** G10
Barnagar *India* **68** H6
Barnala *India* **68** D6
Barnard Castle *U.K.* **14** C6

Barnaul *Russia* **52** D9
Barnesville *Ga., U.S.A.* **117** E12
Barnesville *Minn., U.S.A.* **112** B5
Barnet □ *U.K.* **15** F7
Barneveld *Neths.* **17** B5
Barneville-Carteret *France* **18** C5
Barnhart *U.S.A.* **116** F4
Barnsley *U.K.* **14** D6
Barnstable *U.S.A.* **113** E18
Barnstaple *U.K.* **15** F3
Barnstaple Bay = Bideford Bay *U.K.* **15** F3
Barnwell *U.S.A.* **117** E14
Baro *Nigeria* **83** D6
Baro → *Ethiopia* **81** F3
Baroda = Vadodara *India* **68** H5
Baroda *India* **68** G7
Baroe *S. Africa* **88** E3
Barong *China* **58** B2
Barotseland *Zambia* **85** H4
Barouéli *Mali* **82** C3
Barpeta *India* **67** F17
Barqa *Libya* **79** C10
Barques, Pt. Aux *U.S.A.* **114** B2
Barquísimeto *Venezuela* **124** A5
Barr, Ras el *Egypt* **80** H7
Barr Smith Range *Australia* **93** E3
Barra *Brazil* **125** F10
Barra *Gambia* **82** C1
Barra *U.K.* **13** E1
Barra, Sd. of *U.K.* **13** D1
Barra de Navidad *Mexico* **118** D4
Barra do Corda *Brazil* **125** E9
Barra do Garças *Brazil* **125** G8
Barra do Piraí *Brazil* **127** A7
Barra Falsa, Pta. da *Mozam.* **89** C6
Barra Hd. *U.K.* **13** E1
Barra Mansa *Brazil* **127** A7
Barraba *Australia* **95** E5
Barrackpur = Barakpur *India* **69** H13
Barrafranca *Italy* **43** E7
Barraigh = Barra *U.K.* **13** E1
Barrāmīya *Egypt* **80** B3
Barranca *Lima, Peru* **124** F3
Barranca *Loreto, Peru* **124** D3
Barranca del Cobre △ *Mexico* **118** B3
Barrancabermeja *Colombia* **124** B4
Barrancas *Venezuela* **124** B6
Barrancos *Portugal* **37** G4
Barranqueras *Argentina* **126** B4
Barranquilla *Colombia* **124** A4
Barraute *Canada* **104** C4
Barre *Mass., U.S.A.* **115** D12
Barre *Vt., U.S.A.* **115** B12
Barreal *Argentina* **126** C2
Barreiras *Brazil* **125** F10
Barreirinhas *Brazil* **125** D10
Barreiro *Portugal* **37** G1
Barrême *France* **21** E10
Barren, Nosy *Madag.* **89** B7
Barretos *Brazil* **125** H9
Barrhead *Canada* **102** C6
Barrie *Canada* **114** B5
Barrier Ra. *Australia* **95** E3
Barrière *Canada* **102** C4
Barrington *U.S.A.* **115** E13
Barrington L. *Canada* **103** B8
Barrington Tops *Australia* **95** E5
Barringun *Australia* **95** D4
Barron *U.S.A.* **112** C8
Barrow *U.S.A.* **106** A8
Barrow → *Ireland* **12** D5
Barrow, Pt. *U.S.A.* **106** A8
Barrow Creek *Australia* **94** C1
Barrow I. *Australia* **92** D2
Barrow-in-Furness *U.K.* **14** C4
Barrow Pt. *Australia* **94** A3
Barrow Ra. *Australia* **93** E4
Barrow Str. *Canada* **4** B3
Barruecopardo *Spain* **36** D4
Barruelo de Santullán *Spain* **36** C6
Barry *U.K.* **15** F4
Barry's Bay *Canada* **114** A7
Barsalogho *Burkina Faso* **83** C4
Barsat *Pakistan* **69** A5
Barsham *Syria* **73** E9
Barsi *India* **66** K9
Barsinghausen *Germany* **24** C5
Barsoi *India* **67** G13
Barstow *U.S.A.* **111** L9
Barth *Germany* **24** A8
Barthélemy, Col *Vietnam* **64** C5
Bartica *Guyana* **124** B7
Bartın *Turkey* **72** B5
Bartle Frere *Australia* **94** B4
Bartlesville *U.S.A.* **116** C7
Bartlett *Calif., U.S.A.* **110** J8
Bartlett *Tenn., U.S.A.* **116** H10
Bartlett, L. *Canada* **102** A5
Bartolomeu Dias *Mozam.* **87** G4
Barton *U.S.A.* **115** B12
Barton upon Humber *U.K.* **14** D7
Bartoszyce *Poland* **30** D7
Bartow *U.S.A.* **117** H14
Barú, Volcan *Panama* **120** E3

Barumba *Dem. Rep. of the Congo* **86** B1
Baruth *Germany* **24** C9
Baruun Urt *Mongolia* **53** E12
Baruunsuu *Mongolia* **56** C3
Barvinkove *Ukraine* **33** H9
Barwani *India* **68** H6
Barwice *Poland* **30** E3
Barycz → *Poland* **31** G3
Barysaw *Belarus* **23** A15
Barysh *Russia* **34** D8
Barzân *Iraq* **70** B5
Bârzava *Romania* **28** D6
Bas-Rhin □ *France* **19** D14
Bašaid *Serbia* **28** E5
Bāsa'idū *Iran* **71** E7
Basal *Pakistan* **68** C5
Basankusa *Dem. Rep. of the Congo* **84** D3
Basarabeasca *Moldova* **29** D13
Basarabi *Romania* **29** F13
Basarabia = Bessarabiya *Moldova* **23** E15
Basauri *Spain* **38** B2
Basawa *Afghan.* **68** B4
Bascuñán, C. *Chile* **126** B1
Basel *Switz.* **25** H3
Basel, Euroairport ✈ (BSL) *Europe* **19** E14
Basel-Landschaft □ *Switz.* **25** H3
Basento → *Italy* **43** B9
Bashākerd, Kūhhā-ye *Iran* **71** E8
Bashaw *Canada* **102** C6
Bāshī *Iran* **71** D6
Bashkir Republic = Bashkortostan □ *Russia* **52** D6
Bashkortostan □ *Russia* **52** D6
Bashtanivka *Ukraine* **29** E14
Basibasy *Madag.* **89** C7
Basilan *Phil.* **61** H5
Basilan Str. *Phil.* **61** H5
Basildon *U.K.* **15** F8
Basilé *Eq. Guin.* **83** E6
Basilé, Pico de *Eq. Guin.* **83** E6
Basilicata □ *Italy* **43** B9
Basim = Washim *India* **66** J10
Basin *U.S.A.* **108** D9
Basingstoke *U.K.* **15** F6
Baška *Croatia* **41** D11
Başkale *Turkey* **73** C10
Baskatong, Rés. *Canada* **104** C4
Basle = Basel *Switz.* **25** H3
Başmakçı *Turkey* **47** D12
Basoda *India* **68** H7
Basoko *Dem. Rep. of the Congo* **86** B1
Basque, Pays *France* **20** E2
Basque Provinces = País Vasco □ *Spain* **38** C2
Basra = Al Başrah *Iraq* **70** D5
Bass Str. *Australia* **95** F4
Bassano *Canada* **102** C6
Bassano del Grappa *Italy* **41** C8
Bassar *Togo* **83** D5
Bassas da India *Ind. Oc.* **87** G4
Basse-Normandie □ *France* **18** D6
Basse-Pointe *Martinique* **120** c
Basse Santa-Su *Gambia* **82** C2
Basse-Terre *Guadeloupe* **120** b
Basse Terre *Trin. & Tob.* **125** K15
Bassein *Burma* **67** L19
Basses, Pte. des *Guadeloupe* **120** b
Basseterre *St. Kitts & Nevis* **121** C7
Bassett *U.S.A.* **112** D4
Bassi *India* **68** D7
Bassigny *France* **19** E12
Bassikounou *Mauritania* **82** B3
Bassila *Benin* **83** D5
Bassum *Germany* **24** C4
Båstad *Sweden* **11** H6
Bastak *Iran* **71** E7
Baştām *Iran* **71** B7
Bastar *India* **67** K12
Bastelica *France* **21** F13
Basti *India* **69** F10
Bastia *France* **21** F13
Bastogne *Belgium* **17** D5
Bastrop *La., U.S.A.* **116** E9
Bastrop *Tex., U.S.A.* **116** F6
Basuo = Dongfang *China* **64** C7
Bat Yam *Israel* **74** C3
Bata *Eq. Guin.* **84** D1
Bata *Romania* **28** D7
Bataan □ *Phil.* **61** D4
Batabanó *Cuba* **120** B3
Batabanó, G. de *Cuba* **120** B3
Batac *Phil.* **61** B4
Batagai *Russia* **53** C14
Batajnica *Serbia* **28** E5
Batak *Bulgaria* **45** E8
Batala *India* **68** D6
Batalha *Portugal* **36** F2
Batama *Dem. Rep. of the Congo* **86** B2
Batamay *Russia* **53** C13
Batang *China* **58** B2
Batang *Indonesia* **63** G13
Batangafo *C.A.R.* **84** C3
Batangas *Phil.* **61** E4
Batanta *Indonesia* **63** E8
Batatais *Brazil* **127** A6

Batavia *U.S.A.* **114** D6
Bataysk *Russia* **33** J10
Batchelor *Australia* **92** B5
Batdambang *Cambodia* **64** F4
Batemans B. *Australia* **95** F5
Batemans Bay *Australia* **95** F5
Batesburg-Leesville *U.S.A.* **117** E14
Batesville *Ark., U.S.A.* **116** D9
Batesville *Miss., U.S.A.* **117** D10
Batesville *Tex., U.S.A.* **116** G5
Bath *Canada* **115** B8
Bath *U.K.* **15** F5
Bath *Maine, U.S.A.* **113** D19
Bath *N.Y., U.S.A.* **114** D7
Bath & North East
  Somerset □ *U.K.* **15** F5
Batheay *Cambodia* **65** G5
Bathsheba *Barbados* **121** g
Bathurst *Australia* **95** E4
Bathurst *Canada* **105** C6
Bathurst *S. Africa* **88** E4
Bathurst, C. *Canada* **100** C6
Bathurst B. *Australia* **94** A3
Bathurst Harb. *Australia* **95** G4
Bathurst I. *Australia* **92** B5
Bathurst I. *Canada* **101** B11
Bathurst Inlet *Canada* **100** D10
Bati *Ethiopia* **81** E5
Batie *Burkina Faso* **82** D4
Batiki *Fiji* **91** a
Batlow *Australia* **95** F4
Batman *Turkey* **73** D9
Baṭn al Ghūl *Jordan* **74** F4
Batna *Algeria* **78** A7
Batobato = San Isidro *Phil.* **61** H7
Batočina *Serbia* **44** B5
Batoka *Zambia* **87** F2
Baton Rouge *U.S.A.* **116** F9
Batong, Ko *Thailand* **65** J2
Bátonyterenye *Hungary* **28** C4
Batopilas *Mexico* **118** B3
Batouri *Cameroon* **84** D2
Båtsfjord *Norway* **8** A23
Batsi *Greece* **46** D6
Battambang =
  Batdambang *Cambodia* **64** F4
Batticaloa *Sri Lanka* **66** R12
Battipáglia *Italy* **43** B7
Battle *U.K.* **15** G8
Battle → *Canada* **103** C7
Battle Creek *U.S.A.* **113** D11
Battle Ground *U.S.A.* **110** E4
Battle Harbour *Canada* **105** B8
Battle Lake *U.S.A.* **112** B6
Battle Mountain *U.S.A.* **108** F5
Battlefields *Zimbabwe* **87** F2
Battleford *Canada* **103** C7
Battonya *Hungary* **28** D6
Batu *Ethiopia* **81** F4
Batu *Malaysia* **65** L3
Batu, Kepulauan *Indonesia* **62** E1
Batu Ferringhi *Malaysia* **65** c
Batu Gajah *Malaysia* **65** K3
Batu Is. = Batu, Kepulauan
  Indonesia **62** E1
Batu Pahat *Malaysia* **65** M4
Batuata *Indonesia* **63** F6
Batugondang, Tanjung
  Indonesia **63** J17
Batukau, Gunung *Indonesia* **63** J18
Batumi *Georgia* **35** K5
Batur *Indonesia* **63** J18
Batur, Danau *Indonesia* **63** J18
Batur, Gunung *Indonesia* **63** J18
Batura Sar *Pakistan* **69** A6
Baturaja *Indonesia* **62** E2
Baturité *Brazil* **125** D11
Baturiti *Indonesia* **63** J18
Bau *Malaysia* **62** D4
Baubau *Indonesia* **63** F6
Baucau, E. *Timor* **63** F7
Bauchi *Nigeria* **83** C6
Bauchi □ *Nigeria* **83** C7
Baud *France* **18** E3
Baudette *U.S.A.* **112** A6
Bauer, C. *Australia* **95** E1
Bauhinia *Australia* **94** C4
Baukau = Baucau *E. Timor* **63** F7
Bauld, C. *Canada* **101** G20
Baume-les-Dames *France* **19** E13
Baunatal *Germany* **24** D5
Baunei *Italy* **42** B2
Baure *Nigeria* **83** C6
Bauru *Brazil* **127** A6
Bausi *India* **69** G12
Bauska *Latvia* **30** B11
Bautino *Kazakhstan* **35** H10
Bautzen *Germany* **24** D10
Bauya *S. Leone* **82** D2
Bavānāt *Iran* **71** D7
Bavanište *Serbia* **28** F5
Bavaria = Bayern □
  Germany **25** G7
Båven *Sweden* **10** E10
Bavispe → *Mexico* **118** B3
Bawdwin *Burma* **67** H20
Bawean *Indonesia* **62** F4
Bawku *Ghana* **83** C4
Bawlake *Burma* **67** K20

Bawolung *China* **58** C3
Baxley *U.S.A.* **117** F13
Baxoi *China* **58** B1
Baxter *U.S.A.* **112** B6
Baxter Springs *U.S.A.* **112** G6
Baxter State △ *U.S.A.* **113** B19
Bay, L. de *Phil.* **61** D4
Bay City *Mich., U.S.A.* **113** D12
Bay City *Tex., U.S.A.* **116** G7
Bay Minette *U.S.A.* **117** F11
Bay Roberts *Canada* **105** C9
Bay St. Louis *U.S.A.* **117** F10
Bay Springs *U.S.A.* **117** F10
Bay View *N.Z.* **91** C6
Baya *Dem. Rep. of the Congo* **87** E2
Bayamo *Cuba* **120** B4
Bayamón *Puerto Rico* **121** d
Bayan Har Shan *China* **60** C4
Bayan Hot = Alxa Zuoqi
  China **56** E3
Bayan Lepas *Malaysia* **65** c
Bayan Obo *China* **56** D5
Bayan-Ovoo = Erdenetsogt
  Mongolia **56** C4
Bayana *India* **68** F7
Bayanaūyl *Kazakhstan* **52** D8
Bayandalay *Mongolia* **56** C2
Bayanhongor *Mongolia* **53** E11
Bayard *N. Mex., U.S.A.* **109** K9
Bayard *Nebr., U.S.A.* **112** E2
Bayawan *Phil.* **61** G5
Baybay *Phil.* **61** F6
Bayburt *Turkey* **73** B9
Bayburt □ *Turkey* **73** B8
Baydaratskaya Guba *Russia* **52** C7
Baydhabo *Somali Rep.* **75** G3
Bayelsa □ *Nigeria* **83** E6
Bayerische Alpen *Germany* **25** H7
Bayerische Rhön *Germany* **25** E6
Bayerischer Spessart △
  Germany **25** F6
Bayerischer Wald *Germany* **25** G8
Bayern □ *Germany* **25** G7
Bayeux *France* **18** C6
Bayfield *Canada* **114** C3
Bayfield *U.S.A.* **112** B8
Bayındır *Turkey* **47** C9
Baykal, Oz. *Russia* **53** D11
Baykan *Turkey* **73** C9
Baynes Mts. *Namibia* **88** B1
Bayombong *Phil.* **61** C4
Bayon *France* **19** D13
Bayona = Baiona *Spain* **36** C2
Bayonne *France* **20** E2
Bayonne *U.S.A.* **115** F10
Bayovar *Peru* **124** E2
Bayqongyr *Kazakhstan* **52** E7
Bayram-Ali = Baýramaly
  Turkmenistan **71** B9
Baýramaly *Turkmenistan* **71** B9
Bayramiç *Turkey* **47** B8
Bayreuth *Germany* **25** F7
Bayrischzell *Germany* **25** H8
Bayrūt *Lebanon* **74** B4
Bays, L. of *Canada* **114** A5
Baysville *Canada* **114** A5
Bayt Laḥm *West Bank* **74** D4
Baytown *U.S.A.* **116** G7
Bayun *Indonesia* **63** J18
Bayzo *Niger* **83** C5
Baza *Spain* **37** H8
Bazar Dyuzu *Russia* **35** K8
Bazardüzü = Bazar Dyuzi
  Russia **35** K8
Bazarny Karabulak *Russia* **34** D8
Bazarnyy Syzgan *Russia* **34** D8
Bazaruto, I. do *Mozam.* **89** C6
Bazaruto △ *Mozam.* **89** C6
Bazas *France* **20** D3
Bazhong *China* **58** B6
Bazhou *China* **56** E9
Bazmān, Kūh-e *Iran* **71** D9
Baztan = Elizondo *Spain* **38** B3
Beach *U.S.A.* **112** B2
Beach City *U.S.A.* **114** F3
Beachport *Australia* **95** F3
Beachville *Canada* **114** C4
Beachy Hd. *U.K.* **15** G8
Beacon *Australia* **93** F2
Beacon *U.S.A.* **115** E11
Beaconsfield *Australia* **95** G4
Beagle, Canal *S. Amer.* **128** H3
Beagle Bay *Australia* **92** C3
Beagle Bay ◇ *Australia* **92** C3
Beagle G. *Australia* **92** B5
Béal an Átha = Ballina
  Ireland **12** B2
Béal Átha na Sluaighe =
  Ballinasloe *Ireland* **12** C3
Bealanana *Madag.* **89** A8
Beals Cr. → *U.S.A.* **116** E4
Beamsville *Canada* **114** C5
Bear → *Calif., U.S.A.* **110** G5
Bear → *Utah, U.S.A.* **106** G17
Béar, C. *France* **20** F7
Bear I. *Ireland* **12** E2
Bear L. *Canada* **103** B9
Bear L. *U.S.A.* **108** F8

Bear Lake *Canada* **114** A5
Beardmore *Canada* **104** C2
Beardmore Glacier *Antarctica* **5** E11
Beardstown *U.S.A.* **112** E8
Bearma → *India* **69** G8
Béarn *France* **20** E3
Bearpaw Mts. *U.S.A.* **108** B9
Bearskin Lake *Canada* **104** B1
Beas → *India* **68** D6
Beas de Segura *Spain* **37** G8
Beasain *Spain* **38** B2
Beata, C. *Dom. Rep.* **121** C5
Beata, I. *Dom. Rep.* **121** C5
Beatrice *U.S.A.* **112** E5
Beatrice *Zimbabwe* **87** F3
Beatrice, C. *Australia* **94** A2
Beatton → *Canada* **102** B4
Beatton River *Canada* **102** B4
Beatty *U.S.A.* **110** J10
Beattton → *Canada* **102** B4
Beaucaire *France* **21** E8
Beauce, Plaine de la *France* **19** D8
Beauceville *Canada* **105** C5
Beaudesert *Australia* **95** D5
Beaufort *France* **21** C10
Beaufort *Malaysia* **62** C5
Beaufort *N.C., U.S.A.* **117** D16
Beaufort *S.C., U.S.A.* **117** E14
Beaufort Sea *Arctic* **98** B5
Beaufort West *S. Africa* **88** E3
Beaugency *France* **19** E8
Beauharnois *Canada* **115** A11
Beaujeu *France* **19** F11
Beaujolais *France* **19** F11
Beaulieu → *Canada* **102** A6
Beaulieu-sur-Dordogne
  France **20** D5
Beaulieu-sur-Mer *France* **21** E11
Beauly *U.K.* **13** D4
Beauly → *U.K.* **13** D4
Beaumaris *U.K.* **14** D3
Beaumont *Belgium* **17** D4
Beaumont *France* **20** D4
Beaumont *U.S.A.* **116** F7
Beaumont-de-Lomagne
  France **20** E5
Beaumont-le-Roger *France* **18** C7
Beaumont-sur-Sarthe *France* **18** D7
Beaune *France* **19** E11
Beaune-la-Rolande *France* **19** D9
Beaupré *Canada* **105** C5
Beaupréau *France* **18** E6
Beauraing *Belgium* **17** D4
Beaurepaire *France* **21** C9
Beausejour *Canada* **103** C9
Beauvais *France* **19** C9
Beauval *Canada* **103** B7
Beauvoir-sur-Mer *France* **18** F4
Beauvoir-sur-Niort *France* **20** B3
Beaver *Okla., U.S.A.* **116** C4
Beaver *Pa., U.S.A.* **114** F4
Beaver *Utah, U.S.A.* **108** G7
Beaver → *B.C., Canada* **102** B4
Beaver → *Ont., Canada* **104** A2
Beaver → *Sask., Canada* **103** B7
Beaver → *U.S.A.* **116** C5
Beaver City *U.S.A.* **112** E4
Beaver Creek *Canada* **100** E3
Beaver Dam *U.S.A.* **112** D9
Beaver Falls *U.S.A.* **114** F4
Beaver Hill L. *Canada* **103** C10
Beaver I. *U.S.A.* **113** C11
Beavercreek *U.S.A.* **113** F11
Beaverhill L. *Canada* **102** C6
Beaverlodge *Canada* **102** B5
Beaverstone → *Canada* **104** B2
Beaverton *Canada* **114** B5
Beaverton *U.S.A.* **110** E4
Beawar *India* **68** F6
Bebedouro *Brazil* **127** A6
Bebera, Tanjung *Indonesia* **63** K18
Beboa *Madag.* **89** B7
Bebra *Germany* **24** E5
Becán *Mexico* **119** D7
Bécancour *Canada* **113** B17
Beccles *U.K.* **15** E9
Bečej *Serbia* **28** E5
Beceni *Romania* **29** E11
Becerreá *Spain* **36** C3
Béchar *Algeria* **78** B5
Becharof L. *U.S.A.* **106** D8
Bechyně *Czech Rep.* **26** B7
Beckley *U.S.A.* **113** G13
Beckum *Germany* **24** D4
Béclean *Romania* **29** C9
Bečov nad Teplou *Czech Rep.* **26** A5
Bečva → *Czech Rep.* **27** B10
Bédar *Spain* **39** H3
Bédarieux *France* **20** E7
Beddouza, C. *Morocco* **78** B4
Bedele *Ethiopia* **81** F4
Bederkesa *Germany* **24** B4
Bedeso *Ethiopia* **81** F5
Bedford *Canada* **115** A12
Bedford *S. Africa* **88** E4
Bedford *U.K.* **15** E7
Bedford *Ind., U.S.A.* **112** F10
Bedford *Iowa, U.S.A.* **112** E6
Bedford *Ohio, U.S.A.* **114** E3

Bear Lake *Canada* **114** A5
Bedford *Pa., U.S.A.* **114** F6
Bedford *Va., U.S.A.* **113** G14
Bedford, C. *Australia* **94** B4
Bedfordshire □ *U.K.* **15** E7
Będków *Poland* **31** G6
Bednja → *Croatia* **41** B13
Bednodemyanovsk *Russia* **34** D6
Bedok *Singapore* **65** d
Bedónia *Italy* **40** D6
Bedourie *Australia* **94** C2
Bedum *Neths.* **17** A6
Beebe Plain *Canada* **115** A12
Beech Creek *U.S.A.* **114** E7
Beechy *Canada* **103** C7
Beed = Bir *India* **66** K9
Beef I. *Br. Virgin Is.* **121** e
Beelitz *Germany* **24** C8
Beenleigh *Australia* **95** D5
Be'er Menuḥa *Israel* **70** D2
Be'er Sheva *Israel* **74** D3
Beersheba = Be'er Sheva
  Israel **74** D3
Beeskow *Germany* **24** C10
Beestekraal *S. Africa* **89** D4
Beeston *U.K.* **14** E6
Beeton *Canada* **114** B5
Beetzendorf *Germany* **24** C7
Beeville *U.S.A.* **116** G6
Befale *Dem. Rep. of the Congo* **84** D4
Befandriana *Mahajanga,
  Madag.* **89** B8
Befandriana *Toliara, Madag.* **89** C7
Befasy *Madag.* **89** C7
Befotaka *Antsiranana, Madag.* **89** A8
Befotaka *Fianarantsoa, Madag.* **89** C8
Bega *Australia* **95** F4
Bega, Canalul *Romania* **28** E5
Bégard *France* **18** D3
Beğendik *Turkey* **45** F10
Begoro *Ghana* **83** D4
Begusarai *India* **69** G12
Behābād *Iran* **71** C8
Behala *India* **69** H13
Behara *Madag.* **89** C8
Behbehān *Iran* **71** D6
Behm Canal *U.S.A.* **102** B2
Behshahr *Iran* **71** B7
Bei Jiang → *China* **59** F9
Bei'an *China* **60** B7
Beibei *China* **58** C6
Beichuan *China* **58** B5
Beihai *China* **58** G7
Beijing *China* **56** E9
Beijing □ *China* **56** E9
Beilen *Neths.* **17** B6
Beiliu *China* **59** F8
Beilngries *Germany* **25** F7
Beilpajah *Australia* **95** E3
Beilul *Eritrea* **81** E5
Beinn na Faoghla =
  Benbecula *U.K.* **13** D1
Beipan Jiang → *China* **58** E5
Beipiao *China* **57** D11
Beira *Mozam.* **87** F3
Beirut = Bayrūt *Lebanon* **74** B4
Beiseker *Canada* **102** C6
Beit Lekhem = Bayt Laḥm
  West Bank **74** D4
Beitaolaizhao *China* **57** B13
Beitbridge *Zimbabwe* **87** G3
Beiuș *Romania* **28** D7
Beizhen = Binzhou *China* **57** F10
Beizhen *China* **57** D11
Beizhengzhen *China* **57** B12
Beja *Portugal* **37** G3
Béja *Tunisia* **79** A7
Beja □ *Portugal* **37** H3
Bejaïa *Algeria* **78** A7
Béjar *Spain* **36** E5
Bejestān *Iran* **71** C8
Bekaa Valley = Al Biqâ
  Lebanon **74** A5
Bekçiler *Turkey* **47** E11
Békés *Hungary* **28** D6
Békés □ *Hungary* **28** D6
Békéscsaba *Hungary* **28** D6
Bekilli *Turkey* **47** C11
Bekily *Madag.* **89** C8
Bekisopa *Madag.* **89** C8
Bekitro *Madag.* **89** C8
Bekodoka *Madag.* **89** B8
Bekoji *Ethiopia* **81** F4
Bekok *Malaysia* **65** L4
Bekopaka *Madag.* **89** B7
Bekuli *Indonesia* **63** J17
Bekwai *Ghana* **83** D4
Bela *India* **69** G10
Bela *Pakistan* **68** F2
Bela Bela *S. Africa* **89** C4
Bela Crkva *Serbia* **28** F6
Bela Palanka *Serbia* **44** C6
Bela Vista *Brazil* **126** A4
Bela Vista *Mozam.* **89** D5
Bélábre *France* **20** B5
Belalcázar *Spain* **37** G5
Belan → *India* **69** G9
Belanovica *Serbia* **44** B4
Belarus ■ *Europe* **23** B14

Belau = Palau ■ *Palau* **90** A6
Belavenona *Madag.* **89** C8
Belawan *Indonesia* **62** D1
Belaya *Ethiopia* **81** E4
Belaya → *Russia* **33** J10
Belaya Glina *Russia* **35** G5
Belaya Kalitva *Russia* **35** F5
Belaya Tserkov = Bila
  Tserkva *Ukraine* **23** D16
Belaya Zemlya, Ostrova
  Russia **52** A7
Belcești *Romania* **29** C12
Belchatów *Poland* **31** G6
Belcher Is. *Canada* **104** A3
Belchite *Spain* **38** D4
Belden *U.S.A.* **110** F3
Beledweyne *Somali Rep.* **75** G4
Belém *Brazil* **125** D9
Belén *Argentina* **126** B2
Belén *Paraguay* **126** A4
Belen *Turkey* **72** D7
Belen *U.S.A.* **109** J10
Belene *Bulgaria* **45** C9
Bélesta *France* **20** F5
Belet Uen = Beledweyne
  Somali Rep. **75** G4
Belev *Russia* **32** F9
Belevi *Turkey* **47** C9
Belfair *U.S.A.* **110** C4
Belfast *S. Africa* **89** D5
Belfast *U.K.* **12** B6
Belfast *Maine, U.S.A.* **113** C19
Belfast *N.Y., U.S.A.* **114** D6
Belfast L. *U.K.* **12** B6
Belfield *U.S.A.* **112** B2
Belfort *France* **19** E13
Belfort, Territoire de □
  France **19** E13
Belfry *U.S.A.* **108** D9
Belgaum *India* **66** M9
Belgavi = Belgaum *India* **66** M9
Belgioioso *Italy* **40** C6
Belgium ■ *Europe* **17** D4
Belgodère *France* **21** F13
Belgorod *Russia* **33** G9
Belgorod □ *Russia* **33** G9
Belgrade = Beograd *Serbia* **44** B4
Belgrade *U.S.A.* **108** D8
Belgrano *Antarctica* **5** D1
Belhaven *U.S.A.* **117** D16
Béli *Guinea-Biss.* **82** C2
Beli *Nigeria* **83** D7
Beli Drim → *Europe* **44** D4
Beli Manastir *Croatia* **28** E3
Beli Timok → *Serbia* **44** C6
Beliu *Romania* **28** D6
Belize ■ *Cent. Amer.* **119** D7
Belize City *Belize* **119** D7
Beljakovci *Macedonia* **44** D5
Beljanica *Serbia* **44** B5
Belkovskiy, Ostrov *Russia* **53** B14
Bell → *Canada* **104** C4
Bell I. *Canada* **105** B8
Bell-Irving → *Canada* **102** B3
Bell Peninsula *Canada* **101** E15
Bell Ville *Argentina* **126** C3
Bella *Italy* **43** B8
Bella Bella *Canada* **102** C3
Bella Coola *Canada* **102** C3
Bella Unión *Uruguay* **126** C4
Bella Vista *Corrientes,
  Argentina* **126** B4
Bella Vista *Tucuman,
  Argentina* **126** B2
Bellac *France* **20** B5
Bellágio *Italy* **40** C6
Bellaire *U.S.A.* **114** F4
Bellária *Italy* **41** D9
Bellary *India* **66** M10
Bellata *Australia* **95** D4
Belle Fourche *U.S.A.* **112** C2
Belle Fourche → *U.S.A.* **107** G19
Belle Glade *U.S.A.* **117** H14
Belle-Île *France* **18** E3
Belle Isle *Canada* **105** B8
Belle Isle, Str. of *Canada* **105** B8
Belle Plaine *U.S.A.* **112** E8
Belle River *Canada* **114** D2
Belle Yella *Liberia* **82** D3
Belledonne *France* **21** C10
Bellefontaine *U.S.A.* **113** E12
Bellefonte *U.S.A.* **114** F7
Bellegarde *France* **19** E9
Bellegarde-en-Marche
  France **20** C6
Bellegarde-sur-Valserine
  France **19** F12
Bellême *France* **18** D7
Belleoram *Canada* **105** C8
Belleplaine *Barbados* **121** g

Belleville *Canada* **114** B7
Belleville *France* **19** F11
Belleville *Ill., U.S.A.* **112** F9
Belleville *Kans., U.S.A.* **112** F5
Belleville *N.J., U.S.A.* **115** F10
Belleville *N.Y., U.S.A.* **115** C8
Belleville-sur-Vie *France* **18** F5
Bellevue *Idaho, U.S.A.* **108** E6
Bellevue *Nebr., U.S.A.* **112** E6
Bellevue *Ohio, U.S.A.* **114** E2
Bellevue *Wash., U.S.A.* **110** C4
Belley *France* **21** C9
Bellin = Kangirsuk *Canada* **101** F18
Bellinge *Denmark* **11** J4
Bellingen *Australia* **95** E5
Bellingham *U.S.A.* **110** B4
Bellingshausen Abyssal
  Plain *S. Ocean* **5** C16
Bellingshausen Sea
  Antarctica **5** C17
Bellinzona *Switz.* **25** J5
Bello *Colombia* **124** B3
Bellows Falls *U.S.A.* **115** C12
Bellpat *Pakistan* **68** E3
Bellpuig *Spain* **38** D6
Belluno *Italy* **41** B9
Bellwood *U.S.A.* **114** F6
Bélmez *Spain* **37** G5
Belmont *Canada* **114** D3
Belmont *S. Africa* **88** D3
Belmont *U.S.A.* **114** D6
Belmonte *Brazil* **125** G11
Belmonte *Portugal* **36** E3
Belmonte *Spain* **39** F2
Belmopan *Belize* **119** D7
Belmullet *Ireland* **12** B2
Belo Horizonte *Brazil* **125** G10
Belo-sur-Mer *Madag.* **89** C7
Belo-Tsiribihina *Madag.* **89** B7
Belogorsk = Bilohirsk
  Ukraine **33** K8
Belogorsk *Russia* **53** D13
Belogradchik *Bulgaria* **44** C6
Belogradets *Bulgaria* **45** C11
Beloha *Madag.* **89** D8
Beloit *Kans., U.S.A.* **112** F4
Beloit *Wis., U.S.A.* **112** D9
Belokorovichi *Ukraine* **23** C15
Belomorsk *Russia* **52** C4
Belonia *India* **67** H17
Belopolye = Bilopillya
  Ukraine **33** G8
Belorechensk *Russia* **35** H4
Belorussia = Belarus ■
  Europe **23** B14
Beloslav *Bulgaria* **45** C11
Belovo *Bulgaria* **45** D8
Belovo *Russia* **52** D9
Belovodsk *Ukraine* **33** H10
Beloyarskiy *Russia* **52** C7
Beloye, Ozero *Russia* **32** B9
Beloye More *Russia* **8** C25
Belozem *Bulgaria* **45** D9
Belozersk *Russia* **32** B9
Belpasso *Italy* **43** E7
Belpre *U.S.A.* **113** F13
Belrain *India* **69** E9
Belt *U.S.A.* **108** C8
Beltana *Australia* **95** E2
Belterra *Brazil* **125** D8
Beltinci *Slovenia* **41** B13
Belton *U.S.A.* **116** F6
Belton L. *U.S.A.* **116** F6
Beltsy = Bălți *Moldova* **29** C12
Belturbet *Ireland* **12** B4
Belukha *Russia* **52** E9
Beluran *Malaysia* **62** C5
Belušiа *Slovak Rep.* **27** B11
Belushya Guba *Russia* **52** B6
Belušić *Serbia* **44** C5
Belvedere Maríttimo *Italy* **43** C8
Belvès *France* **20** D5
Belvidere *Ill., U.S.A.* **112** D9
Belvidere *N.J., U.S.A.* **115** F9
Belvís de la Jara *Spain* **36** F6
Belyando → *Australia* **94** C4
Belyando Crossing *Australia* **94** C4
Belyuen *Australia* **92** B5
Belyy *Russia* **32** E7
Belyy, Ostrov *Russia* **52** B8
Belyy Yar *Russia* **52** D9
Belz *Ukraine* **31** H11
Belżec *Poland* **31** H10
Belzig *Germany* **24** C8
Belzoni *U.S.A.* **117** E9
Belżyce *Poland* **31** G9
Bemaraha, Lembalemban' i
  Madag. **89** B7
Bemarivo *Madag.* **89** C7
Bemarivo → *Antsiranana,
  Madag.* **89** A9
Bemarivo → *Mahajanga,
  Madag.* **89** B8
Bemavo *Madag.* **89** C8
Bembéréke *Benin* **83** C5
Bembesi *Zimbabwe* **87** G2
Bembesi → *Zimbabwe* **87** F2
Bembézar → *Spain* **37** H5
Bembibre *Spain* **36** C4

Bemetara *India* **69** J9
Bemidji *U.S.A.* **112** B6
Bemolanga *Madag.* **89** B8
Ben *Iran* **71** C6
Ben Cruachan *U.K.* **13** E3
Ben Dearg *U.K.* **13** D4
Ben En △ *Vietnam* **64** C5
Ben Gardane *Tunisia* **79** B8
Ben Hope *U.K.* **13** C4
Ben Lawers *U.K.* **13** E4
Ben Lomond *N.S.W., Australia* **95** E5
Ben Lomond *Tas., Australia* **95** G4
Ben Lomond *U.K.* **13** E4
Ben Lomond △ *Australia* **95** G4
Ben Luc *Vietnam* **65** G6
Ben Macdhui *U.K.* **13** D5
Ben Mhor *U.K.* **13** D1
Ben More *Argyll & Bute, U.K.* **13** E2
Ben More *Stirling, U.K.* **13** E4
Ben More Assynt *U.K.* **13** C4
Ben Nevis *U.K.* **13** E3
Ben Quang *Vietnam* **64** D6
Ben Tre *Vietnam* **65** G6
Ben Vorlich *U.K.* **13** E4
Ben Wyvis *U.K.* **13** D4
Bena *Nigeria* **83** C6
Benalla *Australia* **95** F4
Benalmádena *Spain* **37** J6
Benares = Varanasi *India* **69** G10
Bénat, C. *France* **21** E10
Benavente *Portugal* **37** G2
Benavente *Spain* **36** C5
Benavides *U.S.A.* **116** H5
Benavides de Órbigo *Spain* **36** C5
Benbecula *U.K.* **13** D1
Benbonyathe Hill *Australia* **95** E2
Bend *U.S.A.* **108** D3
Bender Beyla *Somali Rep.* **75** F5
Bendery = Tighina *Moldova* **29** D14
Bendigo *Australia* **95** F3
Bendorf *Germany* **24** E3
Benē Beraq *Israel* **74** C3
Bénéna *Mali* **82** C4
Benenitra *Madag.* **89** C8
Benešov *Czech Rep.* **26** B7
Benevento *Italy* **43** A7
Benfeld *France* **19** D14
Benga *Mozam.* **87** E3
Bengal, Bay of *Ind. Oc.* **67** M17
Bengaluru = Bangalore
  India **66** N10
Bengbis *Cameroon* **83** E7
Bengbu *China* **57** H9
Benghazi = Banghāzī *Libya* **79** B10
Bengkalis *Indonesia* **65** M4
Bengkulu *Indonesia* **62** E2
Bengkulu □ *Indonesia* **62** E2
Bengough *Canada* **103** D7
Bengtsfors *Sweden* **10** E6
Benguela *Angola* **85** G2
Benguérua, I. *Mozam.* **89** C6
Benha *Egypt* **80** H7
Beni *Dem. Rep. of the Congo* **86** B2
Beni → *Bolivia* **124** F5
Beni Mazâr *Egypt* **80** B3
Beni Mellal *Morocco* **78** B4
Beni Suef *Egypt* **80** J7
Beniah L. *Canada* **102** A6
Benicarló *Spain* **38** E5
Benicássim *Spain* **38** E5
Benidorm *Spain* **39** G4
Benin ■ *Africa* **83** D5
Benin → *Nigeria* **83** D6
Benin, Bight of *W. Afr.* **83** E5
Benin City *Nigeria* **83** D6
Benissa *Spain* **39** G5
Benito Juárez *Argentina* **126** D4
Benitses *Greece* **49** A3
Benjamin Aceval *Paraguay* **126** A4
Benjamin Constant *Brazil* **124** D4
Benjamin Hill *Mexico* **118** A2
Benkelman *U.S.A.* **112** E3
Benkovac *Croatia* **41** D12
Bennett *Canada* **102** B2
Bennett, L. *Australia* **92** D5
Bennetta, Ostrov *Russia* **53** B15
Bennettsville *U.S.A.* **117** D15
Bennichchâb *Mauritania* **82** B1
Bennington *N.H., U.S.A.* **115** D11
Bennington *Vt., U.S.A.* **115** D11
Bénodet *France* **18** E2
Benom *Malaysia* **65** L4
Benoni *S. Africa* **89** D4
Benque Viejo *Belize* **119** D7
Bensheim *Germany* **25** F4
Benson *Ariz., U.S.A.* **109** L8
Benson *Minn., U.S.A.* **112** C6
Bent *Iran* **71** E8
Benteng *Indonesia* **63** F6
Bentinck I. *Australia* **94** B2
Bentiu *Sudan* **81** F2
Bentley Subglacial Trench
  Antarctica **5** E15
Bento Gonçalves *Brazil* **127** B5
Benton *Ark., U.S.A.* **116** D8
Benton *Calif., U.S.A.* **110** H8
Benton *Ill., U.S.A.* **112** F9
Benton *Pa., U.S.A.* **115** E8
Benton Harbor *U.S.A.* **112** D10

Bentong *Malaysia* **65** L3
Bentonville *U.S.A.* **116** C7
Bentu Liben *Ethiopia* **81** F4
Benue □ *Nigeria* **83** D6
Benue → *Nigeria* **83** D6
Benxi *China* **57** D12
Beo *Indonesia* **63** D7
Beograd *Serbia* **44** B4
Beograd ✈ (BEG) *Serbia* **44** C4
Beolgyo *S. Korea* **57** G14
Beoumi *Ivory C.* **82** D3
Bepan Jiang → *China* **58** E6
Beppu *Japan* **55** H5
Beqa *Fiji* **91** a
Beqaa Valley = Al Biqâ
  Lebanon **74** A5
Ber Mota *India* **68** H3
Bera, Tasik *Malaysia* **65** L4
Berach → *India* **68** G6
Beraketa *Madag.* **89** C7
Berane *Montenegro* **44** D3
Berastagi *Indonesia* **65** L2
Berat *Albania* **44** F3
Berau = Tanjungredeb
  Indonesia **62** D5
Berau, Teluk *Indonesia* **63** E8
Beravina *Madag.* **89** B8
Berber *Sudan* **80** D3
Berbera *Somali Rep.* **75** E4
Berbérati *C.A.R.* **84** D3
Berbice → *Guyana* **124** B7
Berceto *Italy* **40** D6
Berchidda *Italy* **42** B2
Berchtesgaden *Germany* **25** H8
Berchtesgaden △ *Germany* **25** H8
Berck *France* **19** B8
Berdichev = Berdychiv
  Ukraine **23** D15
Berdsk *Russia* **52** D9
Berdyansk *Ukraine* **33** J9
Berdychiv *Ukraine* **23** D15
Berea *U.S.A.* **113** G11
Berebere *Indonesia* **63** D7
Berehomet *Ukraine* **29** B10
Berehove *Ukraine* **28** B7
Bereket *Turkmenistan* **71** B7
Berekum *Ghana* **82** D4
Berenice *Egypt* **80** C4
Berens → *Canada* **103** C9
Berens I. *Canada* **103** C9
Berens River *Canada* **103** C9
Beresford *U.S.A.* **112** D5
Berestechko *Ukraine* **23** C13
Bereşti *Romania* **29** D12
Beretău → *Romania* **28** C6
Berettyó → *Hungary* **28** D6
Berettyóújfalu *Hungary* **28** C6
Berevo *Mahajanga, Madag.* **89** B7
Berevo *Toliara, Madag.* **89** B7
Bereza = Byaroza *Belarus* **33** F3
Berezhany *Ukraine* **23** D13
Berezina = Byarezina →
  Belarus **23** B16
Berezivka *Ukraine* **33** J6
Berezna *Ukraine* **33** G6
Bereznik *Russia* **52** C5
Berezniki *Russia* **52** D6
Berezovo *Russia* **52** C7
Berezyne *Ukraine* **29** D14
Berga *Spain* **38** C6
Berga *Sweden* **11** G10
Bergama *Turkey* **47** B9
Bérgamo *Italy* **40** C6
Bergara *Spain* **38** B2
Bergby *Sweden* **10** D11
Berge *Norway* **10** E2
Bergedorf *Germany* **24** B6
Bergeforsen *Sweden* **10** B11
Bergen
  Mecklenburg-Vorpommern,
  Germany **24** A9
Bergen *Niedersachsen,*
  Germany **24** C5
Bergen *Neths.* **17** B4
Bergen *Norway* **8** F11
Bergen *U.S.A.* **114** C7
Bergen op Zoom *Neths.* **17** C4
Bergerac *France* **20** D4
Bergheim *Germany* **24** E2
Bergholz *U.S.A.* **114** F4
Bergisch Gladbach *Germany* **17** D7
Bergisches Land △ *Germany* **24** E3
Bergkamen *Germany* **24** D3
Bergkvara *Sweden* **11** H10
Bergshamra *Sweden* **10** E12
Bergsjö *Sweden* **10** C11
Bergstrasse-Odenwald △
  Germany **25** F1
Bergues *France* **19** B9
Bergviken *Sweden* **10** C10
Bergville *S. Africa* **89** D4
Berhala, Selat *Indonesia* **62** E2
Berhampore =
  Baharampur *India* **69** G13
Berhampur = Brahmapur
  India **67** K14
Berheci → *Romania* **29** E12
Bering Glacier *U.S.A.* **106** C11

Bering Sea *Pac. Oc.* **98** D1
Bering Strait *Pac. Oc.* **106** B6
Beringovskiy *Russia* **53** C18
Berisso *Argentina* **126** C4
Berja *Spain* **37** J8
Berkeley *U.S.A.* **110** H4
Berkner I. *Antarctica* **5** D18
Berkovitsa *Bulgaria* **44** C7
Berkshire *U.S.A.* **115** D8
Berkshire Downs *U.K.* **15** F6
Berlanga *Spain* **37** G5
Berlenga, I. *Portugal* **37** F1
Berlin *Germany* **24** C9
Berlin *Md., U.S.A.* **113** F16
Berlin *N.H., U.S.A.* **115** B13
Berlin *N.Y., U.S.A.* **115** D11
Berlin *Wis., U.S.A.* **112** D9
Berlin □ *Germany* **24** C9
Berlin L. *U.S.A.* **114** E4
Berlin Tegel ✈ (TXL)
  Germany **24** C9
Bermeja, Sierra *Spain* **37** J5
Bermejo → *Formosa,*
  Argentina **126** B4
Bermejo → *San Juan,*
  Argentina **126** C2
Bermejo, Paso = Uspallata,
  P. de *Argentina* **126** C2
Bermen, L. *Canada* **105** B6
Bermeo *Spain* **38** B2
Bermillo de Sayago *Spain* **36** D4
Bermuda ☑ *Atl. Oc.* **99** F13
Bern *Switz.* **25** J3
Bern □ *Switz.* **25** J3
Bernalda *Italy* **43** B9
Bernalillo *U.S.A.* **109** J10
Bernardo de Irigoyen
  Argentina **127** B5
Bernardsville *U.S.A.* **115** F10
Bernasconi *Argentina* **126** D3
Bernau *Bayern, Germany* **25** H8
Bernau *Brandenburg, Germany* **24** C9
Bernay *France* **18** C7
Bernburg *Germany* **24** D7
Berndorf *Austria* **26** D9
Berne = Bern □ *Switz.* **25** J3
Berne = Bern □ *Switz.* **25** J3
Berner Alpen *Switz.* **25** J3
Berneray *U.K.* **13** D1
Bernier I. *Australia* **93** D1
Bernina, Piz *Switz.* **25** J5
Bernkastel-Kues *Germany* **25** F3
Beroroha *Madag.* **89** C8
Béroubouay *Benin* **83** C5
Beroun *Czech Rep.* **26** B7
Berounka → *Czech Rep.* **26** B7
Berovo *Macedonia* **44** E6
Berre, Étang de *France* **21** E9
Berre-l'Étang *France* **21** E9
Berri *Australia* **95** E3
Berriane *Algeria* **78** B6
Berry *Australia* **95** E5
Berry *France* **19** F8
Berry Is. *Bahamas* **120** A4
Berryessa, L. *U.S.A.* **110** G4
Berryville *U.S.A.* **116** C8
Berseba *Namibia* **88** D2
Bersenbrück *Germany* **24** C3
Bershad *Ukraine* **29** B14
Bertamirans *Spain* **36** C2
Berthold *U.S.A.* **112** A3
Berthoud *U.S.A.* **108** F11
Bertincourt *France* **19** B9
Bertoua *Cameroon* **84** D2
Bertraghboy B. *Ireland* **12** C2
Berwick *U.S.A.* **115** E8
Berwick-upon-Tweed *U.K.* **14** B6
Berwyn Mts. *U.K.* **14** E4
Beryslav *Ukraine* **33** J7
Berzasca *Romania* **28** F6
Berzence *Hungary* **28** D2
Besal *Pakistan* **69** B5
Besalampy *Madag.* **89** B7
Besançon *France* **19** E13
Besar *Indonesia* **62** E5
Beshenkovichi *Belarus* **32** E5
Beška *Serbia* **28** E5
Beslan *Russia* **35** J7
Besna Kobila *Serbia* **44** D6
Besnard L. *Canada* **103** B7
Besni *Turkey* **72** D7
Besor, N. → *Egypt* **74** D3
Bessarabia *Moldova* **23** E15
Bessarabka =
  Basarabeasca *Moldova* **29** D13
Bessèges *France* **21** D8
Bessemer *Ala., U.S.A.* **117** E11
Bessemer *Mich., U.S.A.* **112** B8
Bessemer *Pa., U.S.A.* **114** F4
Bessin *France* **18** C6
Bessines-sur-Gartempe
  France **20** B5
Beswick *Australia* **92** B5
Beswick ⦿ *Australia* **92** B5
Bet She'an *Israel* **74** C4
Bet Shemesh *Israel* **74** D4
Betafo *Madag.* **89** B8
Betancuria *Canary Is.* **48** F5
Betanzos *Spain* **36** B2

Bétaré Oya *Cameroon* **84** C2
Betatao *Madag.* **89** B8
Bétera *Spain* **39** F4
Bétérou *Benin* **83** D5
Bethal *S. Africa* **89** D4
Bethanien *Namibia* **88** D2
Bethany *Canada* **114** B6
Bethany *Mo., U.S.A.* **112** E6
Bethany *Okla., U.S.A.* **116** D6
Bethel *Alaska, U.S.A.* **106** C7
Bethel *Conn., U.S.A.* **115** E11
Bethel *Maine, U.S.A.* **115** B14
Bethel *Vt., U.S.A.* **115** C12
Bethel Park *U.S.A.* **114** F4
Béthenville *France* **19** C11
Bethlehem = Bayt Laḥm
  West Bank **74** D4
Bethlehem *S. Africa* **89** D4
Bethlehem *U.S.A.* **115** F9
Bethulie *S. Africa* **88** E4
Béthune *France* **19** B9
Béthune → *France* **18** C8
Betioky *Madag.* **89** C7
Betong *Malaysia* **65** J3
Betong *Thailand* **65** K3
Betoota *Australia* **94** D3
Betor *Ethiopia* **81** E4
Betpaqdala *Kazakhstan* **52** E8
Betroka *Madag.* **89** C8
Betsiamites *Canada* **105** C6
Betsiamites → *Canada* **105** C6
Betsiboka → *Madag.* **89** B8
Bettendorf *U.S.A.* **112** E8
Bettiah *India* **69** F11
Bettna *Sweden* **11** F10
Béttola *Italy* **40** D6
Betul *India* **66** J10
Betws-y-Coed *U.K.* **14** D4
Betxi *Spain* **38** F4
Betzdorf *Germany* **24** E3
Beuil *France* **21** D10
Beulah *Mich., U.S.A.* **112** C10
Beulah *N. Dak., U.S.A.* **112** B3
Beuvron → *France* **18** E8
Beveren *Belgium* **17** C4
Beverley *Australia* **93** F2
Beverley *U.K.* **14** D7
Beverly *U.S.A.* **115** D14
Beverly Hills *Calif., U.S.A.* **111** L8
Beverly Hills *Fla., U.S.A.* **117** G13
Beverungen *Germany* **24** D5
Bevoalavo *Madag.* **89** D7
Bewas → *India* **69** H8
Bewdley *Canada* **114** B6
Bex *Switz.* **25** J3
Bexhill *U.K.* **15** G8
Bey Dağları *Turkey* **47** E12
Beyānlū *Iran* **70** C5
Beyazköy *Turkey* **45** E11
Beyçayırı *Turkey* **45** F10
Beydağ *Turkey* **47** C10
Beyeğaç *Turkey* **47** D10
Beyin *Ghana* **82** D4
Beykoz *Turkey* **45** E13
Beyla *Guinea* **82** D3
Beynat *France* **20** C5
Beyneu *Kazakhstan* **52** E6
Beyoba *Turkey* **47** C9
Beyoğlu *Turkey* **45** E12
Beypazarı *Turkey* **72** B4
Beyşehir *Turkey* **72** D4
Beyşehir Gölü *Turkey* **72** D4
Beytüşşebap *Turkey* **73** D10
Bezdan *Serbia* **28** E3
Bezhetsk *Russia* **32** D9
Bezhta *Georgia* **35** J5
Béziers *France* **20** E7
Bezwada = Vijayawada
  India **67** L12
Bhabua *India* **69** G10
Bhachau *India* **66** H7
Bhadar → *Gujarat, India* **68** H5
Bhadar → *Gujarat, India* **68** J3
Bhadarwah *India* **69** C6
Bhadgaon = Bhaktapur
  Nepal **69** F11
Bhadohi *India* **69** G10
Bhadra *India* **68** E6
Bhadrakh *India* **67** J15
Bhadran *India* **68** H5
Bhadravati *India* **66** N9
Bhag *Pakistan* **68** E2
Bhagalpur *India* **69** G12
Bhagirathi → *Uttarakhand,*
  India **69** D8
Bhagirathi → *W. Bengal,*
  India **69** H13
Bhakkar *Pakistan* **68** D4
Bhakra Dam *India* **68** D7
Bhaktapur *Nepal* **69** F11
Bhamo *Burma* **67** G20
Bhandara *India* **66** J11
Bhanpura *India* **68** G6
Bhanrer Ra. *India* **69** H8
Bhaptiahi *India* **69** F12
Bharat = India ■ *Asia* **66** K11
Bharatpur *Chhattisgarh, India* **69** H9
Bharatpur *Raj., India* **68** F7
Bharatpur *Nepal* **69** F11
Bharno *India* **69** H11

Bharuch *India* **66** J8
Bhatinda *India* **68** D6
Bhatpara *India* **69** H13
Bhattu *India* **68** E6
Bhaun *Pakistan* **68** C5
Bhaunagar = Bhavnagar
  India **66** J8
Bhavnagar *India* **66** J8
Bhawari *India* **68** G5
Bhayavadar *India* **68** J4
Bhera *Pakistan* **68** C5
Bhikangaon *India* **68** J6
Bhilai = Bhilainagar-Durg
  India **67** J12
Bhilainagar-Durg *India* **67** J12
Bhilsa = Vidisha *India* **68** H7
Bhilwara *India* **68** G6
Bhima → *India* **66** L10
Bhimbar *Pakistan* **69** C6
Bhind *India* **69** F8
Bhinga *India* **69** F9
Bhinmal *India* **68** G5
Bhisho *S. Africa* **89** E4
Bhiwandi *India* **66** K8
Bhiwani *India* **68** E7
Bhogava → *India* **68** H5
Bhola *Bangla.* **67** H17
Bholari *Pakistan* **68** G3
Bhopal *India* **68** H7
Bhubaneshwar *India* **67** J14
Bhuj *India* **68** H3
Bhumiphol Res. *Thailand* **64** D2
Bhusawal *India* **66** J9
Bhutan ■ *Asia* **67** F17
Biafra, B. of = Bonny, Bight
  of *Africa* **83** E6
Biak *Indonesia* **63** E9
Biała *Poland* **31** H4
Biała → *Poland* **31** H7
Biała Piska *Poland* **30** E9
Biała Podlaska *Poland* **31** F10
Biała Rawska *Poland* **31** G7
Białobrzegi *Poland* **31** G7
Białogard *Poland* **30** D2
Białowieski △ *Poland* **31** F10
Białowieża *Poland* **31** F10
Biały Bór *Poland* **30** E3
Białystok *Poland* **31** E10
Biancavilla *Italy* **43** E7
Bianco *Italy* **43** D9
Biankouma *Ivory C.* **82** D3
Biaora *India* **68** H7
Biärjmand *Iran* **71** B7
Biaro *Indonesia* **63** D7
Biarritz *France* **20** E2
Bias *Indonesia* **63** J18
Biasca *Switz.* **25** J4
Biba *Egypt* **80** J7
Bibai *Japan* **54** C10
Bibbiena *Italy* **41** E8
Bibby I. *Canada* **103** A10
Bibei → *Spain* **36** C3
Biberach *Germany* **25** G5
Bibiani *Ghana* **82** D4
Bibungwa
  Dem. Rep. of the Congo **86** C2
Bicaj *Albania* **44** E4
Bicaz *Romania* **29** D11
Bicazu Ardelean *Romania* **29** D10
Bíccari *Italy* **43** A8
Bicester *U.K.* **15** F6
Bichena *Ethiopia* **81** E4
Bicheno *Australia* **95** G4
Bichia *India* **69** H9
Bichvinta *Georgia* **35** J5
Bickerton I. *Australia* **94** A2
Bicske *Hungary* **28** C3
Bid = Bir *India* **66** K9
Bida *Nigeria* **83** D6
Bidar *India* **66** L10
Biddeford *U.S.A.* **113** D18
Biddwara *Ethiopia* **81** F4
Bideford *U.K.* **15** F3
Bideford Bay *U.K.* **15** F3
Bidhuna *India* **69** F8
Bīdokht *Iran* **71** C8
Bidor *Malaysia* **65** K3
Bidyadanga *Australia* **92** C3
Bie *Sweden* **10** E10
Bié, Planalto de *Angola* **85** G3
Bieber *U.S.A.* **108** F3
Biebrza → *Poland* **31** E9
Biebrzański △ *Poland* **30** E9
Biecz *Poland* **31** J8
Biel *Switz.* **25** H3
Bielawa *Poland* **31** H3
Bielefeld *Germany* **24** C4
Bielersee *Switz.* **25** H3
Biella *Italy* **40** C5
Bielsk Podlaski *Poland* **31** F10
Bielsko-Biała *Poland* **31** J6
Bien Hoa *Vietnam* **65** G6
Bienne = Biel *Switz.* **25** H3
Bienvenida *Spain* **37** G4
Bienville, L. *Canada* **104** A5
Bierné *France* **18** E6
Bierun *Poland* **31** H6
Bierutów *Poland* **31** G4
Biescas *Spain* **38** C4

Biese → *Germany* **24** C7
Biesiesfontein *S. Africa* **88** E2
Bieszczadzki △ *Poland* **31** J9
Bietigheim-Bissingen
  Germany **25** G5
Bieżuń *Poland* **31** F6
Biferno → *Italy* **41** G12
Big → *Canada* **105** B8
Big B. *Canada* **105** A7
Big Bear City *U.S.A.* **111** L10
Big Bear Lake *U.S.A.* **111** L10
Big Belt Mts. *U.S.A.* **108** C8
Big Bend *Swaziland* **89** D5
Big Bend △ *U.S.A.* **116** G3
Big Black → *U.S.A.* **117** F10
Big Blue → *U.S.A.* **112** F5
Big Creek *U.S.A.* **110** H7
Big Cypress △ *U.S.A.* **117** H14
Big Desert *Australia* **95** F3
Big Falls *U.S.A.* **112** A7
Big Fork → *U.S.A.* **112** A7
Big Horn Mts. = Bighorn
  Mts. *U.S.A.* **108** D10
Big I. *Canada* **102** A5
Big Lake *U.S.A.* **116** F4
Big Moose *U.S.A.* **115** C10
Big Muddy Cr. → *U.S.A.* **108** B11
Big Pine *U.S.A.* **110** H8
Big Piney *U.S.A.* **108** E8
Big Quill L. *Canada* **103** C8
Big Rapids *U.S.A.* **113** D11
Big Rideau L. *Canada* **115** B8
Big River *Canada* **103** C7
Big Run *U.S.A.* **114** F6
Big Sable Pt. *U.S.A.* **112** C10
Big Salmon → *Canada* **102** A2
Big Sand L. *Canada* **103** B9
Big Sandy *U.S.A.* **108** B8
Big Sandy → *U.S.A.* **113** F12
Big Sandy Cr. = Sandy
  Cr. → *U.S.A.* **108** F9
Big Sandy Cr. → *U.S.A.* **108** G2
Big Sioux → *U.S.A.* **112** D5
Big South Fork △ *U.S.A.* **117** C12
Big Spring *U.S.A.* **116** E4
Big Stone City *U.S.A.* **112** C5
Big Stone Gap *U.S.A.* **113** G12
Big Stone L. *U.S.A.* **112** C5
Big Sur *U.S.A.* **110** J5
Big Timber *U.S.A.* **108** D9
Big Trout L. *Canada* **104** B2
Big Trout Lake *Canada* **104** B2
Biğa *Turkey* **45** F11
Biga → *Turkey* **45** F11
Bigadiç *Turkey* **47** B10
Biganos *France* **20** D3
Biggar *Canada* **103** C7
Biggar *U.K.* **13** F5
Bigge I. *Australia* **92** B4
Biggenden *Australia* **95** D5
Biggleswade *U.K.* **15** E7
Biggs *U.S.A.* **110** F5
Bighorn *U.S.A.* **108** C10
Bighorn → *U.S.A.* **108** C10
Bighorn Canyon △ *U.S.A.* **108** D10
Bighorn L. *U.S.A.* **108** D9
Bighorn Mts. *U.S.A.* **108** D10
Bignona *Senegal* **82** C1
Bigorre *France* **20** E4
Bigstone L. *Canada* **103** C9
Biguglia, Étang de *France* **21** F13
Bigwa *Tanzania* **86** D4
Bihać *Bos.-H.* **41** D12
Bihar *India* **69** G11
Bihar □ *India* **69** G12
Biharamulo *Tanzania* **86** C3
Biharamulo △ *Tanzania* **86** C3
Bihariganj *India* **69** G12
Biharkeresztes *Hungary* **28** C6
Bihor □ *Romania* **28** D7
Bihor, Munţii *Romania* **28** D7
Bijagós, Arquipélago dos
  Guinea-Biss. **82** C1
Bijaipur *India* **68** F7
Bijapur *Chhattisgarh, India* **67** K12
Bijapur *Karnataka, India* **66** L9
Bījār *Iran* **73** E12
Bijawar *India* **69** G8
Bijela *Montenegro* **44** D2
Bijeljina *Bos.-H.* **28** F4
Bijelo Polje *Montenegro* **44** C3
Bijie *China* **58** D5
Bijnor *India* **68** E8
Bikaner *India* **68** E5
Bikapur *India* **69** F10
Bikeqi *China* **56** D6
Bikfayyâ *Lebanon* **74** B4
Bikin *Russia* **54** A7
Bikin → *Russia* **54** A7
Bikini Atoll *Marshall Is.* **96** F8
Bikita *Zimbabwe* **89** C5
Bikkū Bīttī *Libya* **79** D9
Bikoué *Cameroon* **83** E7
Bila Tserkva *Ukraine* **23** D16
Bilanga *Burkina Faso* **83** C4
Bilara *India* **68** F5
Bilaspur *Chhattisgarh, India* **69** H10
Bilaspur *Punjab, India* **68** D7
Biläsuvar *Azerbaijan* **73** C13

Bilauk Taungdan *Thailand* 64 F2
Bilbao *Spain* 38 B2
Bilbao ✈ (BIO) *Spain* 38 B2
Bilbeis *Egypt* 80 H7
Bilbor *Romania* 29 C10
Bilche-Zolote *Ukraine* 29 B10
Bilciureşti *Romania* 29 F10
Bíldudalur *Iceland* 8 D2
Bílé Karpaty *Europe* 27 B11
Bileća *Bos.-H.* 44 D2
Bilecik *Turkey* 72 B4
Bilecik □ *Turkey* 72 B3
Bilećko Jezero *Bos.-H.* 44 D2
Bileh Savār *Iran* 73 C13
Bilgoraj *Poland* 31 H9
Bilgram *India* 69 F9
Bilhaur *India* 69 F9
Bilhorod-Dnistrovskyy
   Ukraine 33 J6
Bilibino *Russia* 53 C17
Bilibiza *Mozam.* 87 E5
Bilisht *Albania* 44 F5
Billdal *Sweden* 11 G5
Billiluna *Australia* 92 C4
Billings *U.S.A.* 108 D9
Billiton Is. = Belitung
   Indonesia 62 E3
Billsta *Sweden* 10 A12
Billund *Denmark* 11 J3
Bilma *Niger* 79 E8
Bilo Gora *Croatia* 28 E2
Biloela *Australia* 94 C5
Bilohirsk *Ukraine* 33 K8
Bilopillya *Ukraine* 33 G8
Biloxi *U.S.A.* 117 F10
Bilpa Morea Claypan
   Australia 94 D3
Biltine *Chad* 79 F10
Bilyarsk *Russia* 34 C10
Bima *Indonesia* 63 F5
Bimban *Egypt* 80 C3
Bimbila *Ghana* 83 D5
Bimbo *C.A.R.* 84 D3
Bimini Is. *Bahamas* 120 A4
Bin Xian *Heilongjiang, China* 57 B14
Bin Xian *Shaanxi, China* 56 G5
Bin Yauri *Nigeria* 83 C5
Bina-Etawah *India* 68 G8
Binalbagan *Phil.* 61 F5
Binalong *Australia* 95 E4
Bīnālūd, Kūh-e *Iran* 71 B8
Binatang = Bintangau
   Malaysia 62 D4
Binche *Belgium* 17 D4
Binchuan *China* 58 E3
Binder *Chad* 83 D7
Bindki *India* 69 F9
Bindslev *Denmark* 11 G4
Bindura *Zimbabwe* 87 F3
Binéfar *Spain* 38 D5
Bingara *Australia* 95 D5
Bingen *Germany* 25 F3
Bingerville *Ivory C.* 82 D4
Bingham *U.S.A.* 113 C19
Binghamton *U.S.A.* 115 D9
Bingöl *Turkey* 73 C9
Bingöl □ *Turkey* 73 C9
Bingöl Dağları *Turkey* 73 C9
Bingsjö *Sweden* 10 C9
Binh Dinh = An Nhon
   Vietnam 64 F7
Binh Khe *Vietnam* 64 F7
Binh Son *Vietnam* 64 E7
Binhai *China* 57 H10
Binic *France* 18 D4
Binisatua *Spain* 48 B11
Binissalem *Spain* 48 B9
Binjai *Indonesia* 62 D3
Binji *Nigeria* 83 C5
Binnaway *Australia* 95 E4
Binongko *Indonesia* 63 F6
Binscarth *Canada* 103 C8
Binshangul Gumuz □
   Ethiopia 81 E4
Bint Goda *Sudan* 81 E3
Bintan *Indonesia* 62 D2
Bintangau *Malaysia* 62 D4
Bintulu *Malaysia* 62 D4
Bintuni *Indonesia* 63 E8
Binyang *China* 58 F7
Binz *Germany* 24 A9
Binzert = Bizerte *Tunisia* 79 A7
Binzhou *China* 57 F10
Bío Bío □ *Chile* 126 D1
Bíobío → *Chile* 126 D1
Biograd na Moru *Croatia* 41 E12
Biogradska Gora △
   Montenegro 44 D3
Bioko *Eq. Guin.* 83 E6
Biokovo *Croatia* 41 E14
Bipindi *Cameroon* 83 E7
Bir *India* 66 K9
Bir, Ras *Djibouti* 81 E5
Bîr Abu Hashim *Egypt* 80 C3
Bîr Abu Minqar *Egypt* 80 B2
Bîr Abu Muḥammad *Egypt* 74 F3
Bi'r ad Dabbāghāt *Jordan* 74 E4
Bîr Adal Deib *Sudan* 80 C4

Bi'r al Butayyihāt *Jordan* 74 F4
Bi'r al Mārī *Jordan* 74 E4
Bi'r al Qattār *Jordan* 74 F4
Bîr 'Asal *Egypt* 80 B3
Bîr Atrun *Sudan* 80 D2
Bîr Beida *Egypt* 74 E3
Bîr Di *Sudan* 81 F2
Bîr Diqnash *Egypt* 80 A2
Bîr el 'Abd *Egypt* 74 D2
Bîr el Basur *Egypt* 80 B2
Bîr el Biarât *Egypt* 74 F3
Bîr el Duweidar *Egypt* 74 E1
Bîr el Garârât *Egypt* 74 D2
Bîr el Gellaz *Egypt* 80 A2
Bîr el Heisi *Egypt* 74 F2
Bîr el Jafir *Egypt* 74 E1
Bîr el Mâlḥi *Egypt* 74 E2
Bîr el Shaqqa *Egypt* 80 A2
Bîr el Thamâda *Egypt* 74 E2
Bîr Fuad *Egypt* 80 A2
Bîr Gebeil Ḥişn *Egypt* 74 E2
Bi'r Ghaḍir *Syria* 74 A6
Bîr Haimur *Egypt* 80 C3
Bîr Ḥasana *Egypt* 74 E2
Bîr Hōōker *Egypt* 80 H7
Bîr Kanayis *Egypt* 80 C3
Bîr Kaseiba *Egypt* 74 E2
Bîr Kerawein *Egypt* 80 B2
Bîr Lahfân *Egypt* 74 E2
Bîr Madkûr *Egypt* 74 E1
Bîr Maql *Egypt* 80 C3
Bîr Mîneiga *Sudan* 80 C4
Bîr Misaha *Egypt* 80 C2
Bîr Mogreïn *Mauritania* 78 C3
Bîr Murr *Egypt* 80 C3
Bi'r Muṭribah *Kuwait* 70 D5
Bîr Nakheila *Egypt* 80 C3
Bîr Qaṭia *Egypt* 74 E1
Bîr Qatrani *Egypt* 80 A2
Bîr Ranga *Egypt* 80 C4
Bîr Sahara *Egypt* 80 C2
Bîr Seiyâla *Egypt* 80 B3
Bîr Shalatein *Egypt* 80 C4
Bîr Shebb *Egypt* 80 C2
Bîr Shût *Egypt* 80 C4
Bîr Terfawi *Egypt* 80 C2
Bîr Umm Qubûr *Egypt* 80 C3
Bîr Ungât *Egypt* 80 C3
Bîr Za'farâna *Egypt* 80 J8
Bîr Zeidûn *Egypt* 80 B3
Birāk *Libya* 79 C8
Biramféro *Guinea* 82 C3
Biratnagar *Nepal* 69 F12
Birawa *Dem. Rep. of the Congo* 86 C2
Birch → *Canada* 102 B6
Birch Hills *Canada* 103 C7
Birch I. *Canada* 103 C9
Birch L. *N.W.T., Canada* 102 A5
Birch L. *Ont., Canada* 104 B1
Birch Mts. *Canada* 102 B6
Birch River *Canada* 103 C8
Birchip *Australia* 95 F3
Birchis *Romania* 28 E7
Bird *Canada* 103 B10
Bird I. = Aves, I. de *W. Indies* 121 C7
Bird I. *S. Georgia* 128 G13
Birds Creek *Canada* 114 A7
Birdsville *Australia* 94 D2
Birdum Cr. → *Australia* 92 C5
Birecik *Turkey* 73 D8
Birein *Israel* 74 E3
Bireuen *Indonesia* 62 C1
Birhan *Ethiopia* 81 E4
Biri → *Sudan* 81 F2
Birifo *Gambia* 82 C2
Birigüi *Brazil* 127 A5
Bîrjand *Iran* 71 C8
Birkenfeld *Germany* 25 F3
Birkenhead *U.K.* 14 D4
Birket Qârûn *Egypt* 80 J7
Birkfeld *Austria* 26 D8
Birkerød *Denmark* 11 J6
Bîrlad = Bârlad *Romania* 29 D12
Birmingham *U.K.* 15 E6
Birmingham *U.S.A.* 117 E11
Birmingham Int. ✈ (BHX)
   U.K. 15 E6
Birmitrapur *India* 67 H14
Birni Ngaouré *Niger* 83 C5
Birni Nkonni *Niger* 83 C6
Birnin Gwari *Nigeria* 83 C5
Birnin Kebbi *Nigeria* 83 C5
Birnin Kudu *Nigeria* 83 C6
Birobidzhan *Russia* 53 E14
Birr *Ireland* 12 C4
Birrie → *Australia* 95 D4
Birsilpur *India* 68 E5
Birsk *Russia* 52 D6
Birštonas *Lithuania* 30 D11
Birtle *Canada* 103 C8
Birur *India* 66 N9
Biržai *Lithuania* 30 D11
Birzebbuga *Malta* 49 D2
Bisa *Indonesia* 63 E7
Bisáccia *Italy* 43 A8
Bisacquino *Italy* 42 E6
Bisalpur *India* 69 E8
Bisbee *U.S.A.* 109 L9

Biscarrosse *France* 20 D2
Biscarrosse et de Parentis,
   Étang de *France* 20 D2
Biscay, B. of *Atl. Oc.* 6 F5
Biscayne B. *U.S.A.* 117 J14
Biscéglie *Italy* 43 A9
Bischheim *France* 19 D14
Bischofshofen *Austria* 26 D6
Bischofswerda *Germany* 24 D10
Bischwiller *France* 19 D14
Biscoe Is. *Antarctica* 5 C17
Biscostasing *Canada* 104 C3
Biševo *Croatia* 41 F13
Bisha *Eritrea* 81 D4
Bishah, W. → *Si. Arabia* 80 C5
Bishan *China* 58 C6
Bishkek *Kyrgyzstan* 52 E8
Bishnupur *India* 69 H12
Bisho = Bhisho *S. Africa* 89 E4
Bishop *Calif., U.S.A.* 110 H8
Bishop *Tex., U.S.A.* 116 M6
Bishop Auckland *U.K.* 14 C6
Bishop's Falls *Canada* 105 C8
Bishop's Stortford *U.K.* 15 F8
Bisignano *Italy* 43 C9
Bisina, L. *Uganda* 86 B3
Biskra *Algeria* 78 B7
Biskupiec *Poland* 30 E7
Bismarck *U.S.A.* 112 B3
Bismarck Arch. *Papua N. G.* 90 B7
Bismark *Germany* 24 C7
Bismil *Turkey* 73 D9
Biso *Uganda* 86 B3
Bison *U.S.A.* 112 C2
Bīsotūn *Iran* 73 E12
Bispgården *Sweden* 10 A10
Bissagos = Bijagós,
   Arquipélago dos
   Guinea-Biss. 82 C1
Bissau *Guinea-Biss.* 82 C1
Bissaula *Nigeria* 83 D7
Bissikrima *Guinea* 82 C2
Bissorã *Guinea-Biss.* 82 C1
Bistcho L. *Canada* 102 B5
Bistreţ *Romania* 29 G7
Bistrica = Ilirska-Bistrica
   Slovenia 41 C11
Bistriţa *Romania* 29 C9
Bistriţa → *Romania* 29 D11
Bistriţa Năsăud □ *Romania* 29 C9
Bistriţei, Munţii *Romania* 29 C10
Biswan *India* 69 F9
Bisztynek *Poland* 30 D7
Bitam *Gabon* 84 D2
Bitburg *Germany* 25 F2
Bitche *France* 19 C14
Bithynia *Turkey* 72 B4
Bitkine *Chad* 79 F9
Bitlis *Turkey* 73 C10
Bitlis □ *Turkey* 73 C10
Bitola *Macedonia* 44 E5
Bitolj = Bitola *Macedonia* 44 E5
Bitonto *Italy* 43 A9
Bitter Creek *U.S.A.* 108 F9
Bitter L. = Buheirat-
   Murrat-el-Kubra *Egypt* 80 H8
Bitterfeld *Germany* 24 D8
Bitterfontein *S. Africa* 88 E2
Bitterroot → *U.S.A.* 108 C6
Bitterroot Range *U.S.A.* 108 C6
Bitterwater *U.S.A.* 110 J6
Bitti *Italy* 42 B2
Bittou *Burkina Faso* 83 C4
Biu *Nigeria* 83 C7
Bivolari *Romania* 29 C12
Bivolu, Vf. *Romania* 29 C10
Biwa-Ko *Japan* 55 G8
Biwabik *U.S.A.* 112 B7
Bixad *Romania* 29 C8
Bixby *U.S.A.* 116 D7
Biyang *China* 56 H7
Biysk *Russia* 52 D9
Bizana *S. Africa* 89 E4
Bizen *Japan* 55 G7
Bizerte *Tunisia* 79 A7
Bjargtangar *Iceland* 8 D1
Bjärnum *Sweden* 11 H7
Bjästa *Sweden* 10 A12
Bjelasica *Montenegro* 44 D3
Bjelašnica *Bos.-H.* 28 G3
Bjelovar *Croatia* 41 C13
Bjerringbro *Denmark* 11 H3
Björbo *Sweden* 10 D8
Björklinge *Sweden* 10 D11
Björneborg = Pori *Finland* 32 B1
Björneborg *Sweden* 10 E8
Bjørnevatn *Norway* 8 B24
Bjørnøya *Arctic* 4 B8
Bjursås *Sweden* 10 D9
Bjuv *Sweden* 11 H6
Bla *Mali* 82 C3
Blace *Serbia* 44 C5
Blachownia *Poland* 31 H5
Black = Da → *Vietnam* 58 G5
Black → *Canada* 114 B5
Black → *Ariz., U.S.A.* 109 K8
Black → *Ark., U.S.A.* 116 D9
Black → *La., U.S.A.* 116 F9

Black → *Mich., U.S.A.* 114 D2
Black → *N.Y., U.S.A.* 115 C8
Black → *Wis., U.S.A.* 112 C8
Black Bay Pen. *Canada* 104 C2
Black Birch L. *Canada* 103 B7
Black Canyon of the
   Gunnison △ *U.S.A.* 108 G10
Black Diamond *Canada* 102 C6
Black Duck → *Canada* 104 A2
Black Forest =
   Schwarzwald *Germany* 25 G4
Black Forest *U.S.A.* 108 G11
Black Hd. *Ireland* 12 C2
Black Hills *U.S.A.* 112 D2
Black L. *Canada* 103 B7
Black L. *Mich., U.S.A.* 113 C11
Black L. *N.Y., U.S.A.* 115 B9
Black Lake *Canada* 103 B7
Black Mesa *U.S.A.* 116 C3
Black Mt. = Mynydd Du
   U.K. 15 F4
Black Mts. *U.K.* 15 F4
Black Range *U.S.A.* 109 K10
Black River *Jamaica* 120 a
Black River *U.S.A.* 115 C9
Black River Falls *U.S.A.* 112 C8
Black Rock *Barbados* 121 g
Black Rock Desert *U.S.A.* 108 F4
Black Sea *Eurasia* 6 G12
Black Tickle *Canada* 105 B8
Black Volta → *Africa* 82 D4
Black Warrior → *U.S.A.* 117 E11
Blackall *Australia* 94 C4
Blackball *N.Z.* 91 E3
Blackbraes △ *Australia* 94 B3
Blackbull *Australia* 94 B3
Blackburn *U.K.* 14 D5
Blackburn, Mt. *U.S.A.* 106 C11
Blackburn with Darwen □
   U.K. 14 D5
Blackdown Tableland △
   Australia 94 C4
Blackfoot *U.S.A.* 108 E7
Blackfoot → *U.S.A.* 108 C7
Blackfoot Res. *U.S.A.* 108 E8
Blackpool *U.K.* 14 D4
Blackpool □ *U.K.* 14 D4
Blackriver *U.S.A.* 114 B1
Blacks Harbour *Canada* 105 C6
Blacksburg *U.S.A.* 113 G13
Blacksod B. *Ireland* 12 B1
Blackstairs Mt. *Ireland* 12 D5
Blackstone *U.S.A.* 113 G14
Blackstone Ra. *Australia* 93 E4
Blackwater = West
   Road → *Canada* 102 C4
Blackwater *Australia* 94 C4
Blackwater → *Meath, Ireland* 12 C4
Blackwater → *Waterford,
   Ireland* 12 D4
Blackwater → *U.K.* 12 B5
Blackwell *U.S.A.* 116 C6
Blackwells *U.S.A.* 111 K7
Bladensburg △ *Australia* 94 C3
Blaenau Ffestiniog *U.K.* 14 E4
Blaenau Gwent □ *U.K.* 15 F4
Blagaj *Bos.-H.* 44 C1
Blagdon *France* 20 E5
Blagnac, Toulouse ✈ (TLS)
   France 20 E5
Blagodarnoye =
   Blagodarnyy *Russia* 35 H6
Blagodarnyy *Russia* 35 H6
Blagoevgrad *Bulgaria* 44 D7
Blagoveshchensk *Russia* 53 D13
Blahkiuh *Indonesia* 63 J18
Blain *France* 18 E5
Blain *U.S.A.* 114 F7
Blaine *Minn., U.S.A.* 112 C7
Blaine *Wash., U.S.A.* 110 B4
Blaine Lake *Canada* 103 C7
Blair *U.S.A.* 112 E5
Blair Athol *Australia* 94 C4
Blair Atholl *U.K.* 13 E5
Blairgowrie *U.K.* 13 E5
Blairsden *U.S.A.* 110 F6
Blairsville *U.S.A.* 114 F5
Blaj *Romania* 29 D8
Blakang Mati, Pulau *Singapore* 65 d
Blake Pt. *U.S.A.* 112 A9
Blakely *Ga., U.S.A.* 117 F12
Blakely *Pa., U.S.A.* 115 E9
Blâmont *France* 19 D13
Blanc, C. *Spain* 48 B9
Blanc, Mont *Europe* 21 C10
Blanca *S. Africa* 88 E4
Blanca, Cord. *Peru* 124 E3
Blanca Peak *U.S.A.* 109 H11
Blanche, L. *S. Austral.,
   Australia* 95 D2
Blanche, L. *W. Austral.,
   Australia* 92 D3
Blanchisseuse *Trin. & Tob.* 125 K15
Blanco *S. Africa* 88 E4
Blanco *U.S.A.* 116 F5
Blanco → *Argentina* 126 C2
Blanco, C. *Costa Rica* 120 E2

Blanco, C. *U.S.A.* 108 E1
Blanda → *Iceland* 8 D3
Blandford Forum *U.K.* 15 G5
Blanding *U.S.A.* 109 H9
Blanes *Spain* 38 D7
Blangy-sur-Bresle *France* 19 C9
Blanice → *Czech Rep.* 26 B7
Blankaholm *Sweden* 11 G10
Blankenberge *Belgium* 17 C3
Blankenburg *Germany* 24 D6
Blanquefort *France* 20 D3
Blanquilla *Venezuela* 121 D7
Blanquillo *Uruguay* 127 C4
Blansko *Czech Rep.* 27 B9
Blantyre *Malawi* 87 F4
Blarney *Ireland* 12 E3
Blasdell *U.S.A.* 114 D6
Blaszki *Poland* 31 G5
Blatná *Czech Rep.* 26 B6
Blato *Croatia* 41 F13
Blaubeuren *Germany* 25 G5
Blaustein *Germany* 25 G5
Blåvands Huk *Denmark* 11 J2
Blaydon *U.K.* 14 C6
Blaye *France* 20 C3
Blaye-les-Mines *France* 20 D6
Blayney *Australia* 95 E4
Blaze, Pt. *Australia* 92 B5
Błażowa *Poland* 31 J9
Bleckede *Germany* 24 B6
Bled *Slovenia* 41 B11
Blejeşti *Romania* 29 F10
Blekinge *Sweden* 9 H16
Blekinge län □ *Sweden* 11 H9
Blenheim *Canada* 114 D3
Blenheim *N.Z.* 91 D4
Bléone → *France* 21 D10
Blérancourt *France* 19 C10
Bletchley *U.K.* 15 F7
Bleus, Monts
   Dem. Rep. of the Congo 86 B3
Blida *Algeria* 78 A6
Blidö *Sweden* 10 E12
Blidsberg *Sweden* 11 G7
Blieskastel *Germany* 25 F3
Bligh Sound *N.Z.* 91 F1
Bligh Water *Fiji* 91 a
Blind River *Canada* 104 C3
Blinisht *Albania* 44 E3
Bliss *Idaho, U.S.A.* 108 E6
Bliss *N.Y., U.S.A.* 114 D6
Blissfield *U.S.A.* 114 F3
Blitar *Indonesia* 63 H15
Blitta *Togo* 83 D5
Block I. *U.S.A.* 115 E13
Block Island Sd. *U.S.A.* 115 E13
Bloemfontein *S. Africa* 88 D4
Bloemhof *S. Africa* 88 D4
Blois *France* 18 E8
Blomskog *Sweden* 10 E6
Blönduós *Iceland* 8 D3
Blongas *Indonesia* 63 K19
Bloodvein → *Canada* 103 C9
Bloody Foreland *Ireland* 12 A3
Bloomer *U.S.A.* 112 C8
Bloomfield *Canada* 114 C7
Bloomfield *Iowa, U.S.A.* 112 E7
Bloomfield *N. Mex., U.S.A.* 109 H10
Bloomfield *Nebr., U.S.A.* 112 D5
Bloomington *Ill., U.S.A.* 112 E9
Bloomington *Ind., U.S.A.* 112 F10
Bloomington *Minn., U.S.A.* 112 C7
Bloomsburg *U.S.A.* 115 F8
Bloomsbury *Australia* 94 b
Blora *Indonesia* 63 G14
Blossburg *U.S.A.* 114 E7
Blouberg *S. Africa* 89 C4
Blountstown *U.S.A.* 117 F12
Bludenz *Austria* 26 D2
Blue Earth *U.S.A.* 112 D6
Blue Hole △ *Belize* 120 C2
Blue Lagoon △ *Zambia* 87 F2
Blue Mesa Res. *U.S.A.* 108 G10
Blue Mountain Lake *U.S.A.*
   115 C10
Blue Mountain Pk. *Jamaica* 120 a
Blue Mt. *U.S.A.* 115 F8
Blue Mts. *Jamaica* 120 a
Blue Mts. *Maine, U.S.A.* 115 B14
Blue Mts. *Oreg., U.S.A.* 108 D4
Blue Mud B. *Australia* 94 A2
Blue Mud Bay ◎ *Australia* 94 A2
Blue Nile = Nîl el Azraq →
   Sudan 81 D3
Blue Nile Falls *Ethiopia* 81 E4
Blue Rapids *U.S.A.* 112 F5
Blue Ridge *U.S.A.* 113 G13
Blue River *Canada* 102 C5
Bluefield *U.S.A.* 113 G13
Bluefields *Nic.* 120 D3
Bluevale *Canada* 114 C3
Bluff *Australia* 94 C4
Bluff *N.Z.* 91 G2
Bluff *U.S.A.* 109 H9
Bluff Knoll *Australia* 93 F2
Bluff Pt. *Australia* 93 E1

Bluffton *U.S.A.* 113 E11
Blumenau *Brazil* 127 B6
Blunt *U.S.A.* 112 C4
Bly *U.S.A.* 108 E3
Blyde River Canyon ○
   S. Africa 89 C5
Blyth *Canada* 114 C3
Blyth *U.K.* 14 B6
Blythe *U.S.A.* 111 M12
Blytheville *U.S.A.* 117 D10
Bo *S. Leone* 82 D2
Bo Duc *Vietnam* 65 G6
Bo Hai *China* 57 E10
Bo Xian = Bozhou *China* 56 H8
Boa Vista *Brazil* 124 C6
Boa Vista *C. Verde Is.* 78 b
Boac *Phil.* 61 E4
Boaco *Nic.* 120 D2
Bo'ai *China* 56 G7
Boal *Spain* 36 B4
Boalsburg *U.S.A.* 114 F7
Boane *Mozam.* 89 D5
Boardman *U.S.A.* 114 E4
Bobadah *Australia* 95 E4
Bobai *China* 58 F7
Bobbili *India* 67 K13
Bóbbio *Italy* 40 D6
Bobcaygeon *Canada* 114 B6
Böblingen *Germany* 25 G5
Bobo-Dioulasso *Burkina Faso* 82 C4
Bobolice *Poland* 30 E3
Bobonong *Botswana* 87 G2
Boboshevo *Bulgaria* 44 D7
Bobov Dol *Bulgaria* 44 D7
Bóbr → *Poland* 31 F2
Bobraomby, Tanjon' i
   Madag. 89 A8
Bobrinets *Ukraine* 33 H7
Bobrov *Russia* 34 E5
Bobrovitsa *Ukraine* 33 G6
Bobruysk = Babruysk
   Belarus 23 B15
Boby, Pic *Madag.* 85 J9
Boca del Río *Mexico* 119 D5
Boca do Acre *Brazil* 124 E5
Boca Raton *U.S.A.* 117 H14
Bocanda *Ivory C.* 82 D4
Bocas del Dragón =
   Dragon's Mouths
   Venezuela 125 K15
Bocas del Toro *Panama* 120 E3
Boceguillas *Spain* 38 D7
Bochmanivka *Ukraine* 29 C14
Bochnia *Poland* 31 J7
Bocholt *Germany* 24 D2
Bochum *Germany* 24 D3
Bockenem *Germany* 24 C6
Boćki *Poland* 31 F10
Bocognano *France* 21 F13
Boconó *Mexico* 118 B3
Bocşa *Romania* 28 E6
Boda *Dalarna, Sweden* 10 C9
Böda *Kalmar, Sweden* 11 G11
Boda *Västernorrland, Sweden* 10 B10
Bodafors *Sweden* 11 G8
Bodaybo *Russia* 53 D12
Boddam *U.K.* 13 B7
Boddington *Australia* 93 F2
Bode Sadu *Nigeria* 83 D5
Bodega Bay *U.S.A.* 110 G3
Boden *Sweden* 8 D19
Bodensee *Europe* 25 H5
Bodenteich *Germany* 24 C6
Bodhan *India* 66 K10
Bodinga *Nigeria* 83 C6
Bodmin *U.K.* 15 G3
Bodmin Moor *U.K.* 15 G3
Bodø *Norway* 8 C16
Bodrog → *Hungary* 28 B5
Bodrum *Turkey* 47 D9
Bódva → *Hungary* 28 B5
Boën *France* 21 C8
Boende *Dem. Rep. of the Congo* 84 E4
Boerne *U.S.A.* 116 G5
Boesmans → *S. Africa* 88 E4
Boffa *Guinea* 82 C2
Bogalusa *U.S.A.* 117 F10
Bogan → *Australia* 95 D4
Bogan Gate *Australia* 95 E4
Bogandé *Burkina Faso* 83 C4
Bogantungan *Australia* 94 C4
Bogata *U.S.A.* 116 E7
Bogatić *Serbia* 44 B3
Boğazkale *Turkey* 72 B6
Boğazlıyan *Turkey* 72 C6
Bogen *Sweden* 10 D6
Bogense *Denmark* 11 J4
Bogetići *Montenegro* 44 D2
Boggabilla *Australia* 95 D5
Boggabri *Australia* 95 E5
Boggeragh Mts. *Ireland* 12 D3
Boglan = Solhan *Turkey* 73 C9
Bognor Regis *U.K.* 15 G7
Bogo *Phil.* 61 F6
Bogodukhov =
   Bohodukhiv *Ukraine* 33 G8
Bogol Manya *Ethiopia* 81 G5
Bogong, Mt. *Australia* 95 F4
Bogor *Indonesia* 62 F3

Bogoroditsk *Russia* 32 F10
Bogorodsk *Russia* 34 B6
Bogoso *Ghana* 82 D4
Bogotá *Colombia* 124 C4
Bogotol *Russia* 52 D9
Bogou *Togo* 83 C5
Bogra *Bangla.* 67 G16
Boguchany *Russia* 53 D10
Boguchar *Russia* 34 F5
Bogué *Mauritania* 82 B2
Boguszów-Gorce *Poland* 31 H3
Bohain-en-Vermandois
   France 19 C10
Bohdan *Ukraine* 29 B9
Bohemian Forest =
   Böhmerwald *Germany* 25 F9
Bohinjska Bistrica *Slovenia* 41 B11
Böhmerwald *Germany* 25 F9
Bohmte *Germany* 24 C4
Bohodukhiv *Ukraine* 33 G8
Bohol □ *Phil.* 61 G6
Bohol Sea *Phil.* 63 C6
Bohongou *Burkina Faso* 83 C5
Böhönye *Hungary* 28 D2
Bohorodchany *Ukraine* 29 B9
Bohorok *Indonesia* 65 L2
Bohuslän *Sweden* 11 F5
Bohuslev *Ukraine* 33 H6
Boi *Nigeria* 83 D6
Boi, Pta. do *Brazil* 127 A6
Boiaçu *Brazil* 124 D6
Boigu *Australia* 94 a
Boileau, C. *Australia* 92 C3
Boing'o *Sudan* 81 F3
Boiro *Spain* 36 C2
Boise *U.S.A.* 108 E5
Boise City *U.S.A.* 116 C3
Boissevain *Canada* 103 D8
Bóite → *Italy* 41 B9
Boitzenburg *Germany* 24 B9
Boizenburg *Germany* 24 B6
Bojador, C. *W. Sahara* 78 C3
Bojana → *Albania* 44 E3
Bojano *Italy* 43 A7
Bojanowo *Poland* 31 G3
Bøjden *Denmark* 11 J4
Bojnūrd *Iran* 71 B8
Bojonegoro *Indonesia* 63 G14
Boju *Nigeria* 83 D6
Boka *Serbia* 28 E5
Boka Kotorska *Montenegro* 44 D2
Bokala *Ivory C.* 82 D4
Bokani *Nigeria* 83 D6
Bokaro *India* 69 H11
Boké *Guinea* 82 C2
Bokhara → *Australia* 95 D4
Bokkos *Nigeria* 83 D6
Boknafjorden *Norway* 9 G11
Bokor △ *Cambodia* 65 G5
Bokora △ *Uganda* 86 B3
Bokoro *Chad* 79 F9
Bokpyin *Burma* 65 G2
Boksitogorsk *Russia* 32 C7
Bokungu
   Dem. Rep. of the Congo 84 E4
Bol *Croatia* 41 E13
Bolama *Guinea-Biss.* 82 C1
Bolan → *Pakistan* 68 E2
Bolan Pass *Pakistan* 66 E5
Bolaños → *Mexico* 118 C4
Bolaños de Calatrava *Spain* 37 G7
Bolayır *Turkey* 45 F10
Bolbec *France* 18 C7
Boldājī *Iran* 71 D6
Boldeşti-Scăeni *Romania* 29 E11
Bole *China* 60 B3
Bole *Ethiopia* 81 F4
Bole *Ghana* 82 D4
Bolekhiv *Ukraine* 23 D12
Bolesławiec *Poland* 31 G2
Bolgatanga *Ghana* 83 C4
Bolgrad = Bolhrad *Ukraine* 29 E13
Bolhrad *Ukraine* 29 E13
Bolinao *Phil.* 61 C3
Bolintin-Vale *Romania* 29 F10
Bolivar *Mo., U.S.A.* 112 G7
Bolivar *N.Y., U.S.A.* 114 D6
Bolivar *Tenn., U.S.A.* 117 D10
Bolivia ■ *S. Amer.* 124 G6
Bolivian Plateau =
   Altiplano *Bolivia* 124 G5
Boljevac *Serbia* 44 C5
Bolkhov *Russia* 32 F9
Bolków *Poland* 31 H3
Bollebygd *Sweden* 11 G6
Bollène *France* 21 D8
Bollnäs *Sweden* 10 C10
Bollon *Australia* 95 D4
Bollstabruk *Sweden* 10 B11
Bolmen *Sweden* 11 H7
Bolnisi *Georgia* 35 K7
Bolobo *Dem. Rep. of the Congo* 84 E3
Bologna *Italy* 41 D8
Bologna ✈ (BLQ) *Italy* 41 D8
Bologoye *Russia* 32 D8
Bolomba
   Dem. Rep. of the Congo 84 D3
Bolon, Ozero *Russia* 60 B8

Bolótana *Italy* 42 B1
Boloven, Cao Nguyen *Laos* 64 E6
Bolpur *India* 69 H12
Bolsena *Italy* 41 F8
Bolsena, L. di *Italy* 41 F8
Bolshakovo *Russia* 30 D8
Bolshaya Chernigovka
   Russia 34 D10
Bolshaya Glushitsa *Russia* 34 D10
Bolshaya Martynovka
   Russia 35 G5
Bolshaya Vradiyevka *Ukraine* 33 J6
Bolshevik, Ostrov *Russia* 53 B11
Bolshoy Anyuy → *Russia* 53 C17
Bolshoy Begichev, Ostrov
   Russia 53 B12
Bolshoy Kamen *Russia* 54 C6
Bolshoy Kavkas =
   Caucasus Mountains
   Eurasia 35 J7
Bolshoy Lyakhovskiy,
   Ostrov *Russia* 53 B15
Bolshoy Tyuters, Ostrov
   Russia 32 C4
Bolsward *Neths.* 17 A5
Bolt Head *U.K.* 15 G4
Boltaña *Spain* 38 C5
Boltigen *Switz.* 25 J3
Bolton *Canada* 114 C5
Bolton *U.K.* 14 D5
Bolton Landing *U.S.A.* 115 C11
Bolu *Turkey* 72 B4
Bolu □ *Turkey* 72 B4
Bolungavík *Iceland* 8 C2
Boluo *China* 59 F10
Bolvadin *Turkey* 72 C4
Bolzano *Italy* 41 B8
Bom Jesus da Lapa *Brazil* 125 F10
Boma *Dem. Rep. of the Congo* 84 F2
Bombala *Australia* 95 F4
Bombarral *Portugal* 37 F1
Bombay = Mumbai *India* 66 K8
Bombay *India* 66 K8
Bombay *U.S.A.* 115 B10
Bombedor, Pta. *Venezuela* 125 L15
Bomboma
   Dem. Rep. of the Congo 84 D3
Bombombwa
   Dem. Rep. of the Congo 86 B2
Bomi Hills *Liberia* 82 D2
Bomili *Dem. Rep. of the Congo* 86 B2
Bømlo *Norway* 9 G11
Bomokandi →
   Dem. Rep. of the Congo 86 B2
Bomu → *C.A.R.* 84 D4
Bon, C. = Ra's aţ Ţīb *Tunisia* 76 C5
Bon Acceuil *Mauritius* 85 d
Bon Echo △ *Canada* 114 B7
Bon Sar Pa *Vietnam* 64 F6
Bonāb *Āzarbāījān-e Sharqī,*
   Iran 73 D12
Bonāb *Zanjān, Iran* 73 D13
Bonaigarh *India* 69 J11
Bonaire *Neth. Ant.* 121 D6
Bonampak *Mexico* 119 D6
Bonang *Australia* 95 F4
Bonanza *Nic.* 120 D3
Bonaparte Arch. *Australia* 92 B3
Boñar *Spain* 36 C5
Bonar Bridge *U.K.* 13 D4
Bonasse *Trin. & Tob.* 125 K15
Bonaventure *Canada* 105 C6
Bonavista *Canada* 105 C9
Bonavista, C. *Canada* 105 C9
Bonavista B. *Canada* 105 C9
Bondeno *Italy* 41 D8
Bondo *Dem. Rep. of the Congo* 86 B1
Bondoukou *Ivory C.* 82 D4
Bondowoso *Indonesia* 63 G15
Bone, Teluk *Indonesia* 63 E6
Bonerate *Indonesia* 63 F6
Bonerate, Kepulauan
   Indonesia 63 F6
Bo'ness *U.K.* 13 E5
Bonete, Cerro *Argentina* 126 B2
Bong Son = Hoai Nhon
   Vietnam 64 E7
Bonga *Ethiopia* 81 F4
Bongabong *Phil.* 61 E4
Bongandanga
   Dem. Rep. of the Congo 84 D4
Bongor *Chad* 79 F9
Bongos, Massif des *C.A.R.* 84 C4
Bongouanou *Ivory C.* 82 D4
Bonham *U.S.A.* 116 E6
Boni *Mali* 82 B4
Boni △ *Kenya* 86 C5
Bonifacio *France* 21 G13
Bonifacio, Bouches de
   Medit. S. 42 A2
Bonin Is. = Ogasawara
   Gunto *Pac. Oc.* 51 F16
Bonke *Ethiopia* 81 F4
Bonkoukou *Niger* 83 C5
Bonn *Germany* 24 E3
Bonnat *France* 19 F8
Bonne Terre *U.S.A.* 112 G8
Bonners Ferry *U.S.A.* 108 B5
Bonnétable *France* 18 D7
Bonneval *France* 21 C11

Bonneval-sur-Arc *France* 18 D8
Bonneville *France* 19 F13
Bonney, L. *Australia* 95 F3
Bonnie Rock *Australia* 93 F2
Bonny *Nigeria* 83 E6
Bonny → *Nigeria* 83 E6
Bonny, Bight of *Africa* 83 E6
Bonny-sur-Loire *France* 19 E9
Bonnyrigg *U.K.* 13 F5
Bonnyville *Canada* 103 C6
Bono *Italy* 42 B2
Bonoi *Indonesia* 63 E9
Bonorva *Italy* 42 B1
Bonsall *U.S.A.* 111 M9
Bontang *Indonesia* 62 D5
Bontebok △ *S. Africa* 88 E3
Bonthe *S. Leone* 82 D2
Bontoc *Phil.* 61 C4
Bonyeri *Ghana* 82 D4
Bonyhád *Hungary* 28 D3
Bonython Ra. *Australia* 92 D4
Boodjamulla △ *Australia* 94 B2
Bookabie *Australia* 93 F5
Booker *U.S.A.* 116 C4
Boola *Guinea* 82 D3
Booligal *Australia* 95 E3
Boonah *Australia* 95 D5
Boone *Iowa, U.S.A.* 112 D7
Boone *N.C., U.S.A.* 117 C14
Booneville *Ark., U.S.A.* 116 D8
Booneville *Miss., U.S.A.* 117 D10
Boonville *Calif., U.S.A.* 110 F3
Boonville *Ind., U.S.A.* 112 F10
Boonville *Mo., U.S.A.* 112 F7
Boonville *N.Y., U.S.A.* 115 C9
Boorabbin △ *Australia* 93 F3
Boorindal *Australia* 95 E4
Boorowa *Australia* 95 E4
Boosaaso *Somali Rep.* 75 E4
Boothia, Gulf of *Canada* 100 C11
Boothia Pen. *Canada* 100 C13
Bootle *U.K.* 14 D4
Booué *Gabon* 84 E2
Boppard *Germany* 25 E3
Boquilla, Presa de la *Mexico* 118 B3
Boquillas del Carmen
   Mexico 118 B4
Bor *Czech Rep.* 26 B5
Bor *Russia* 34 B8
Bor *Serbia* 44 B6
Bôr *Sudan* 81 F3
Bor *Sweden* 11 G8
Bor *Turkey* 72 D6
Bor Mashash *Israel* 74 D3
Bora Bora *French Polynesia* 97 J12
Borah Peak *U.S.A.* 108 D7
Borang *Sudan* 81 G3
Borås *Sweden* 11 G6
Borāzjān *Iran* 71 D6
Borba *Brazil* 124 D7
Borba *Portugal* 37 G3
Borborema, Planalto da
   Brazil 122 D7
Borcea *Romania* 29 F12
Borçka *Turkey* 73 B9
Bord Khūn-e Now *Iran* 71 D6
Borda, C. *Australia* 95 F2
Bordeaux *France* 20 D3
Bordeaux ✈ (BOD) *France* 20 D3
Borden *Australia* 93 F2
Borden-Carleton *Canada* 105 C7
Borden I. *Canada* 101 B9
Borden Pen. *Canada* 101 C15
Border Ranges △ *Australia* 95 D5
Borders = Scottish
   Borders □ *U.K.* 13 F6
Bordertown *Australia* 95 F3
Borðeyri *Iceland* 8 D3
Bordighera *Italy* 40 E4
Bordj Fly Ste. Marie *Algeria* 78 C5
Bordj-in-Eker *Algeria* 78 D7
Bordj Mokhtar *Algeria* 78 D6
Bordj Omar Driss *Algeria* 78 C7
Bore *Ethiopia* 81 G4
Borehamwood *U.K.* 15 F7
Borek Wielkopolski *Poland* 31 G4
Borensberg *Sweden* 11 F9
Borgå = Porvoo *Finland* 32 B3
Borgarfjörður *Iceland* 8 D7
Borgarnes *Iceland* 8 D3
Børgefjellet *Norway* 8 D15
Borger *Neths.* 17 B6
Borger *U.S.A.* 116 D4
Borgholm *Sweden* 11 H10
Bórgia *Italy* 43 D9
Borgo San Dalmazzo *Italy* 40 D4
Borgo San Lorenzo *Italy* 41 E8
Borgo Val di Taro *Italy* 40 D6
Borgo Valsugana *Italy* 41 B8
Borgomanero *Italy* 40 C5
Borgorose *Italy* 41 F10
Borgosésia *Italy* 40 C5
Borhoyn Tal *Mongolia* 56 C6
Bori *Nigeria* 83 E6
Borikhane *Laos* 64 C4
Borisoglebsk *Russia* 34 E6
Borisov = Barysaw *Belarus* 23 A15
Borisovka *Russia* 33 G9
Borja *Peru* 124 D3

Borja *Spain* 38 D3
Borjas Blancas = Les
   Borges Blanques *Spain* 38 D5
Borjomi *Georgia* 35 K6
Børkop *Denmark* 11 J3
Borkou *Chad* 79 E9
Borkum *Germany* 24 B2
Borlänge *Sweden* 10 D9
Borley, C. *Antarctica* 5 C5
Borlu *Turkey* 47 C10
Bormida → *Italy* 40 D5
Bórmio *Italy* 40 B7
Borna *Germany* 24 D8
Borne Sulinowo *Poland* 30 E3
Borneo *E. Indies* 62 D5
Bornholm *Denmark* 11 J8
Bornholmsgattet *Europe* 11 J8
Borno □ *Nigeria* 83 C7
Bornos *Spain* 37 J5
Bornova *Turkey* 47 C9
Bornu Yassa *Nigeria* 83 C7
Boro → *Sudan* 81 F2
Borodino *Russia* 32 E8
Borodino *Ukraine* 29 D14
Borogontsy *Russia* 53 C14
Boromo *Burkina Faso* 82 C4
Boron *U.S.A.* 111 L9
Borongan *Phil.* 61 F6
Borotangba Mts. *C.A.R.* 81 F2
Borotou *Ivory C.* 82 D3
Borovan *Bulgaria* 44 C7
Borovichi *Russia* 32 C7
Borovsk *Russia* 32 E9
Borrby *Sweden* 11 J8
Borrego Springs *U.S.A.* 111 M10
Borriol *Spain* 38 E4
Borrisokane *Ireland* 12 D3
Borroloola *Australia* 94 B2
Borşa *Cluj, Romania* 29 D8
Borşa *Maramureş, Romania* 29 C9
Borsad *India* 68 H5
Borsec *Romania* 29 D10
Borshchiv *Ukraine* 29 B11
Borsod-Abaúj-Zemplén □
   Hungary 28 B6
Bort-les-Orgues *France* 20 C6
Borth *U.K.* 15 E3
Börtnan *Sweden* 10 B7
Borūjerd *Iran* 73 F13
Boryeong *S. Korea* 57 F14
Borynya *Ukraine* 31 J10
Boryslav *Ukraine* 31 J10
Boryspil *Ukraine* 33 G6
Borzhomi = Borjomi *Georgia* 35 K6
Borzna *Ukraine* 33 G7
Borzya *Russia* 53 D12
Bosa *Italy* 42 B1
Bosanska Dubica *Bos.-H.* 41 C13
Bosanska Gradiška *Bos.-H.* 28 E2
Bosanska Kostajnica
   Bos.-H. 41 C13
Bosanska Krupa *Bos.-H.* 41 D13
Bosanski Brod *Bos.-H.* 28 E2
Bosanski Novi *Bos.-H.* 41 C13
Bosanski Petrovac *Bos.-H.* 41 D13
Bosanski Šamac *Bos.-H.* 28 E3
Bosansko Grahovo *Bos.-H.* 41 D13
Boscastle *U.K.* 15 G3
Boscobelle *Barbados* 121 g
Bose *China* 58 F6
Boseong *S. Korea* 57 G14
Boshan *China* 57 F9
Boshof *S. Africa* 88 D4
Boshrūyeh *Iran* 71 C8
Bosilegrad *Serbia* 44 D6
Boskovice *Czech Rep.* 27 B9
Bosna → *Bos.-H.* 28 E3
Bosna i Hercegovina =
   Bosnia-Herzegovina ■
   Europe 28 G2
Bosnia-Herzegovina ■
   Europe 28 G2
Bosnik *Indonesia* 63 E9
Bosobolo
   Dem. Rep. of the Congo 84 D3
Bosporus = İstanbul Boğazı
   Turkey 45 E13
Bosque Farms *U.S.A.* 109 J10
Bossangoa *C.A.R.* 84 C3
Bossé Bangou *Niger* 83 C5
Bossier City *U.S.A.* 116 E8
Bosso *Niger* 83 C7
Bosso, Dallol → *Niger* 83 C5
Bostan *Pakistan* 68 D2
Bostānābād *Iran* 73 D12
Bosten Hu *China* 60 B3
Boston *U.K.* 14 E7
Boston *U.S.A.* 115 D13
Boston Bar *Canada* 102 D4
Boston Mts. *U.S.A.* 116 D8
Bosumtwi, L. *Ghana* 83 D4
Bosut → *Croatia* 28 E3
Boswell *Canada* 102 D5
Boswell *U.S.A.* 114 F5
Botad *India* 68 H4
Botan → *Turkey* 73 D10
Botany B. *Australia* 90 E8
Botene *Laos* 64 D3
Botev *Bulgaria* 45 D8

Botevgrad *Bulgaria* 44 D7
Bothaville *S. Africa* 88 D4
Bothnia, G. of *Europe* 8 F19
Bothwell *Australia* 95 G4
Bothwell *Canada* 114 D3
Boticas *Portugal* 36 D3
Botletle → *Botswana* 88 C3
Botlikh *Russia* 35 J8
Botna → *Moldova* 29 D14
Botoroaga *Romania* 29 F10
Botoşani *Romania* 29 C11
Botoşani □ *Romania* 29 C11
Botou *Burkina Faso* 83 C5
Botricello *Italy* 43 D9
Botro *Ivory C.* 82 D3
Botshabelo *S. Africa* 88 D4
Botswana ■ *Africa* 88 C3
Bottineau *U.S.A.* 112 A3
Bottnaryd *Sweden* 11 G7
Bottrop *Germany* 17 C6
Botucatu *Brazil* 127 A6
Botwood *Canada* 105 C8
Bou Djébéha *Mali* 82 B4
Bou Guema *Mauritania* 82 B2
Boromo *Burkina Faso* 82 C4
Boû Rjeïmât *Mauritania* 82 B1
Bou Saâda *Algeria* 78 A6
Bouaflé *Ivory C.* 82 D3
Bouaké *Ivory C.* 82 D3
Bouar *C.A.R.* 84 C3
Bouârfa *Morocco* 78 B5
Boucaut B. *Australia* 94 A1
Bouches-du-Rhône □ *France* 21 E9
Boucle de Baoulé △ *Mali* 82 C3
Boucles de la Seine
   Normande △ *France* 18 C7
Bouctouche *Canada* 105 C7
Bougainville, C. *Australia* 92 B4
Bougainville I. *Papua N. G.* 90 B8
Bougainville Reef *Australia* 94 B4
Bougie = Bejaïa *Algeria* 78 A7
Bougouni *Mali* 82 C3
Bouillon *Belgium* 17 E5
Boukombé *Benin* 83 C5
Boulal *Mali* 82 B3
Boulazac *France* 20 C4
Boulder *Colo., U.S.A.* 108 F11
Boulder *Mont., U.S.A.* 108 C7
Boulder City *U.S.A.* 111 K12
Boulder Creek *U.S.A.* 110 H4
Boulder Dam = Hoover
   Dam *U.S.A.* 111 K12
Bouli *Mauritania* 82 B2
Boulia *Australia* 94 C2
Bouligny *France* 19 C12
Boulogne → *France* 18 E5
Boulogne-sur-Gesse *France* 20 E4
Boulogne-sur-Mer *France* 19 B8
Bouloire *France* 18 E7
Boulouli *Mali* 82 B3
Boulsa *Burkina Faso* 83 C4
Boultoum *Niger* 83 C7
Bouma △ *Fiji* 91 a
Boûmdeïd *Mauritania* 82 B2
Boun Neua *Laos* 64 B3
Boun Tai *Laos* 64 B3
Bouna *Ivory C.* 82 D4
Boundary Peak *U.S.A.* 110 H8
Boundiali *Ivory C.* 82 D3
Bountiful *U.S.A.* 108 F8
Bounty Is. *Pac. Oc.* 96 M9
Bounty Trough *Pac. Oc.* 96 M9
Boura *Mali* 82 C4
Bourbon-Lancy *France* 19 F10
Bourbon-l'Archambault
   France 19 F10
Bourbonnais *France* 19 F10
Bourbonne-les-Bains *France* 19 E12
Bourbourg *France* 19 B9
Bourdel L. *Canada* 104 A5
Bourem *Mali* 83 B4
Bourg *France* 20 C3
Bourg-Argental *France* 21 C8
Bourg-de-Péage *France* 21 C9
Bourg-en-Bresse *France* 19 F12
Bourg-Lastic *France* 20 C6
Bourg-Madame *France* 20 F5
Bourg-St-Andéol *France* 21 D8
Bourg-St-Maurice *France* 21 C10
Bourganeuf *France* 20 C5
Bourgas = Burgas *Bulgaria* 45 D11
Bourges *France* 19 E9
Bourget *Canada* 115 A9
Bourget, Lac du *France* 21 C9
Bourgneuf, B. de *France* 18 E4
Bourgneuf-en-Retz *France* 18 E5
Bourgogne □ *France* 19 F11
Bourgoin-Jallieu *France* 21 C9
Bourgueil *France* 18 E7
Bourke *Australia* 95 E4
Bourne *U.K.* 14 E7
Bournemouth *U.K.* 15 G6
Bournemouth □ *U.K.* 15 G6
Bouroum *Burkina Faso* 83 C4
Bouse *U.S.A.* 111 M13
Boussac *France* 19 F9
Boussé *Burkina Faso* 83 C4
Bousso *Chad* 79 F9
Boussouma *Burkina Faso* 83 C4

Boutilimit *Mauritania* 82 B2
Boutonne → *France* 20 C3
Bouvet I. = Bouvetøya
   Antarctica 2 G10
Bouvetøya *Antarctica* 2 G10
Bouxwiller *France* 19 D14
Bouza *Niger* 83 C6
Bouzonville *France* 19 C13
Bova Marina *Italy* 43 E8
Bovalino Marina *Italy* 43 D9
Bovec *Slovenia* 41 B10
Bovill *U.S.A.* 108 C5
Bovino *Italy* 43 A8
Bovril *Argentina* 126 C4
Bow → *Canada* 102 C6
Bow Island *Canada* 108 B8
Bowbells *U.S.A.* 112 A2
Bowdle *U.S.A.* 112 C4
Bowelling *Australia* 93 F2
Bowen *Argentina* 126 D2
Bowen *Australia* 94 J6
Bowen Mts. *Australia* 95 F4
Bowers Basin *Pac. Oc.* 4 D16
Bowers Ridge *Pac. Oc.* 4 D17
Bowie *Ariz., U.S.A.* 109 K9
Bowie *Tex., U.S.A.* 116 E6
Bowkān *Iran* 73 D12
Bowland, Forest of *U.K.* 14 D5
Bowling Green *Ky., U.S.A.* 112 G10
Bowling Green *Ohio, U.S.A.* 113 E12
Bowling Green, C. *Australia* 94 B4
Bowling Green Bay △
   Australia 94 B4
Bowman *U.S.A.* 112 B2
Bowman I. *Antarctica* 5 C8
Bowmanville = Clarington
   Canada 114 C6
Bowmore *U.K.* 13 F2
Bowral *Australia* 95 E5
Bowraville *Australia* 95 E5
Bowron → *Canada* 102 C4
Bowron Lake △ *Canada* 102 C4
Bowser L. *Canada* 102 B3
Bowsman *Canada* 103 C8
Bowwood *Zambia* 87 F2
Box Cr. → *Australia* 95 E3
Boxholm *Sweden* 11 F9
Boxmeer *Neths.* 17 C5
Boxtel *Neths.* 17 C5
Boyabat *Turkey* 72 B6
Boyalıca *Turkey* 45 F13
Boyang *China* 59 C11
Boyany *Ukraine* 29 B11
Boyce *U.S.A.* 116 F8
Boyd L. *Canada* 104 B4
Boyle *Canada* 102 C6
Boyle *Ireland* 12 C3
Boyne → *Ireland* 12 C5
Boyne City *U.S.A.* 113 C11
Boynitsa *Bulgaria* 44 C6
Boynton Beach *U.S.A.* 117 H14
Boyolali *Indonesia* 63 G14
Boyoma, Chutes
   Dem. Rep. of the Congo 86 B2
Boysen Res. *U.S.A.* 108 E9
Boyuibe *Bolivia* 124 G6
Boyup Brook *Australia* 93 F2
Boz Burun *Turkey* 45 F12
Boz Dağı *Turkey* 47 D11
Boz Dağları *Turkey* 47 C10
Bozburun *Turkey* 47 E10
Bozcaada *Turkey* 72 C2
Bozdoğan *Turkey* 47 D10
Bozeman *U.S.A.* 108 D8
Bozen = Bolzano *Italy* 41 B8
Boževac *Serbia* 44 B5
Bozkır *Turkey* 72 D5
Bozkurt *Turkey* 47 D11
Bozouls *France* 20 D6
Bozoum *C.A.R.* 84 C3
Bozova *Antalya, Turkey* 47 D12
Bozova *Şanlıurfa, Turkey* 73 D8
Bozovici *Romania* 28 F7
Bozüyük *Turkey* 47 C11
Bozyazı *Turkey* 70 B2
Bra *Italy* 40 D4
Braås *Sweden* 11 G9
Brabant □ *Belgium* 17 D4
Brabant L. *Canada* 103 B8
Brabrand *Denmark* 11 H4
Brač *Croatia* 41 E13
Bracadale, L. *U.K.* 13 D2
Bracciano *Italy* 41 F9
Bracciano, L. di *Italy* 41 F9
Bracebridge *Canada* 114 A5
Bracieux *France* 18 E8
Bräcke *Sweden* 10 B9
Brackettville *U.S.A.* 116 G4
Brački Kanal *Croatia* 41 E13
Bracknell *U.K.* 15 F7
Bracknell Forest □ *U.K.* 15 F7
Brad *Romania* 28 D7
Brádano → *Italy* 43 B9
Bradenton *U.S.A.* 117 H13
Bradford *Canada* 114 B5
Bradford *U.K.* 14 D6
Bradford *Pa., U.S.A.* 114 E6
Bradford *Vt., U.S.A.* 115 C12

Bradley *Ark., U.S.A.* **116** E8
Bradley *Calif., U.S.A.* **110** K6
Bradley Institute *Zimbabwe* **87** F3
Brady *U.S.A.* **116** F5
Brædstrup *Denmark* **11** J3
Braeside *Canada* **115** A8
Braga *Portugal* **36** D2
Braga □ *Portugal* **36** D2
Bragadiru *Romania* **29** G10
Bragado *Argentina* **126** D3
Bragança *Brazil* **125** D9
Bragança *Portugal* **36** D4
Bragança □ *Portugal* **36** D4
Bragança Paulista *Brazil* **127** A6
Brahestad = Raahe *Finland* **8** D21
Brahmanbaria *Bangla.* **67** H17
Brahmani → *India* **67** J15
Brahmapur *India* **67** K14
Brahmaputra → *Asia* **69** H13
Braich-y-pwll *U.K.* **14** E3
Braidwood *Australia* **95** F4
Brăila *Romania* **29** E12
Brăila □ *Romania* **29** E12
Brainerd *U.S.A.* **112** B6
Braintree *U.K.* **15** F8
Braintree *U.S.A.* **115** D14
Brak → *S. Africa* **88** D3
Brake *Germany* **24** B4
Brakel *Germany* **24** D5
Brakna □ *Mauritania* **82** B2
Bräkne-Hoby *Sweden* **11** H9
Brakwater *Namibia* **88** C2
Brålanda *Sweden* **11** F6
Bramberg *Germany* **25** E6
Bramdrupdam *Denmark* **11** J3
Bramming *Denmark* **11** J2
Brämön *Sweden* **10** B11
Brampton *Canada* **114** C5
Brampton *U.K.* **14** C5
Brampton I. *Australia* **94** b
Bramsche *Germany* **24** C3
Branco → *Brazil* **124** D6
Brandberg *Namibia* **88** C1
Brandberg △ *Namibia* **88** C1
Brande *Denmark* **11** J3
Brandenburg =
  Neubrandenburg *Germany* **24** B9
Brandenburg *Germany* **24** C8
Brandenburg □ *Germany* **24** C9
Brandfort *S. Africa* **88** D4
Brando *France* **21** F13
Brandon *Canada* **103** D9
Brandon *U.S.A.* **115** C11
Brandon B. *Ireland* **12** D1
Brandon Mt. *Ireland* **12** D1
Brandsen *Argentina* **126** D4
Brandvlei *S. Africa* **88** E3
Brandýs nad Labem
  Czech Rep. **26** A7
Brănești *Romania* **29** F11
Branford *U.S.A.* **115** E12
Braniewo *Poland* **30** D6
Bransfield Str. *Antarctica* **5** C18
Brańsk *Poland* **31** F9
Branson *U.S.A.* **112** G7
Brantford *Canada* **114** C4
Brantôme *France* **20** C4
Branzi *Italy* **40** B6
Bras d'Or L. *Canada* **105** C7
Brasher Falls *U.S.A.* **115** B10
Brasil = Brazil ■ *S. Amer.* **125** F9
Brasil, Planalto *Brazil* **122** E6
Brasiléia *Brazil* **124** F5
Brasília *Brazil* **125** G9
Brasília Legal *Brazil* **125** D7
Braslaw *Belarus* **32** E4
Braslovče *Slovenia* **41** B12
Brașov *Romania* **29** E10
Brașov □ *Romania* **29** E10
Brass *Nigeria* **83** E6
Brass → *Nigeria* **83** E6
Brassac-les-Mines *France* **20** C7
Brasschaat *Belgium* **17** C4
Brassey, Banjaran *Malaysia* **62** D5
Brassey Ra. *Australia* **93** E3
Brasstown Bald *U.S.A.* **117** D13
Brastad *Sweden* **11** F5
Brastavățu *Romania* **29** G9
Bratan = Morozov *Bulgaria* **45** D9
Brateș *Romania* **29** E11
Bratislava *Slovak Rep.* **27** C10
Bratislava M.R. Štefánik ✈
  (BTS) *Slovak Rep.* **27** C10
Bratislavský □ *Slovak Rep.* **27** C10
Bratsigovo *Bulgaria* **45** D8
Bratsk *Russia* **53** D11
Brattleboro *U.S.A.* **115** D12
Bratunac *Bos.-H.* **28** F4
Braunau *Austria* **26** C6
Braunschweig *Germany* **24** C6
Braunton *U.K.* **15** F3
Brava *C. Verde Is.* **78** b
Bravicea *Moldova* **29** C13
Bråviken *Sweden* **11** F10
Bravo del Norte, Rio =
  Grande, Rio → *N. Amer.* **116** J6
Brawley *U.S.A.* **111** N11
Bray *Ireland* **12** C5
Bray, Mt. *Australia* **94** A1

Bray-sur-Seine *France* **19** D10
Brazeau → *Canada* **102** C5
Brazil *U.S.A.* **112** F10
Brazil ■ *S. Amer.* **125** F9
Brazilian Highlands =
  Brasil, Planalto *Brazil* **122** E6
Brazo Sur → *S. Amer.* **126** B4
Brazos → *U.S.A.* **116** G7
Brazzaville *Congo* **84** E3
Brčko *Bos.-H.* **28** F3
Brda → *Poland* **31** E5
Brdy *Czech Rep.* **26** B6
Bré = Bray *Ireland* **12** C5
Breaden, L. *Australia* **93** E4
Breaksea Sd. *N.Z.* **91** F1
Bream B. *N.Z.* **91** A5
Bream Hd. *N.Z.* **91** A5
Breas *Chile* **126** B1
Breaza *Romania* **29** E10
Brebes *Indonesia* **63** G13
Brechin *Canada* **114** B5
Brechin *U.K.* **13** E6
Brecht *Belgium* **17** C4
Břeclav *Czech Rep.* **27** C9
Brecon *U.K.* **15** F4
Brecon Beacons *U.K.* **15** F4
Brecon Beacons △ *U.K.* **15** F4
Breda *Neths.* **17** C4
Bredaryd *Sweden* **11** G7
Bredasdorp *S. Africa* **88** E3
Bredebro *Denmark* **11** J2
Bredstedt *Germany* **24** A4
Bree *Neths.* **17** C5
Bregalnica → *Macedonia* **44** E6
Bregenz *Austria* **26** D2
Bregovo *Bulgaria* **44** B6
Bréhal *France* **18** D5
Bréhat, Î. de *France* **18** D4
Breiðafjörður *Iceland* **8** D2
Breil-sur-Roya *France* **21** E11
Breisach *Germany* **25** G3
Brejo *Brazil* **125** D10
Bremen *Germany* **24** B4
Bremen □ *Germany* **24** B4
Bremer Bay *Australia* **93** F2
Bremer I. *Australia* **94** A2
Bremerhaven *Germany* **24** B4
Bremerton *U.S.A.* **110** C4
Bremervörde *Germany* **24** B5
Brenes *Spain* **37** H5
Brenham *U.S.A.* **116** F6
Brenne *France* **20** B5
Brenne △ *France* **20** B5
Brennerpass *Austria* **26** D4
Breno *Italy* **40** C7
Brent *U.S.A.* **117** E11
Brenta → *Italy* **41** C9
Brentwood *U.K.* **15** F8
Brentwood *Calif., U.S.A.* **110** H5
Brentwood *N.Y., U.S.A.* **115** F11
Bréscia *Italy* **40** C7
Breskens *Neths.* **17** C3
Breslau = Wrocław *Poland* **31** G4
Bresle → *France* **18** B8
Bressanone *Italy* **41** B8
Bressay *U.K.* **13** A7
Bresse *France* **19** F12
Bressuire *France* **18** F6
Brest *Belarus* **23** B12
Brest *France* **18** D2
Brest □ *Belarus* **33** F4
Brest-Litovsk = Brest
  Belarus **23** B12
Bretagne □ *France* **18** D3
Bretçu *Romania* **29** D11
Bretenoux *France* **20** D5
Breteuil *Eure, France* **18** D7
Breteuil *Oise, France* **19** C9
Breton *Canada* **102** C6
Breton, Pertuis *France* **20** B2
Breton Sd. *U.S.A.* **117** G10
Brett, C. *N.Z.* **91** A5
Bretten *Germany* **25** F4
Breuil-Cervínia *Italy* **40** C4
Brevard *U.S.A.* **117** D13
Breves *Brazil* **125** D8
Brewarrina *Australia* **95** E4
Brewer *U.S.A.* **113** C19
Brewer, Mt. *U.S.A.* **110** J8
Brewerville *Liberia* **82** D2
Brewster *N.Y., U.S.A.* **115** E11
Brewster *Ohio, U.S.A.* **114** F3
Brewster *Wash., U.S.A.* **108** B4
Brewster, Kap =
  Kangikajik *Greenland* **4** B6
Brewton *U.S.A.* **117** F11
Breyten *S. Africa* **89** D5
Breza *Bos.-H.* **28** F3
Brežice *Slovenia* **41** C12
Březnice *Czech Rep.* **26** B6
Breznik *Bulgaria* **44** D6
Brezno *Slovak Rep.* **27** C12
Brezoi *Romania* **29** E9
Brezovica *Kosovo* **44** D5
Brezovo *Bulgaria* **45** D9

Bria *C.A.R.* **84** C4
Briançon *France* **21** D10
Briare *France* **19** E9
Briático *Italy* **43** D9
Bribie I. *Australia* **95** D5
Bribri *Costa Rica* **120** E3
Briceni *Moldova* **29** B12
Bricquebec *France* **18** C5
Bridgefield *Barbados* **121** g
Bridgehampton *U.S.A.* **115** F12
Bridgend *U.K.* **15** F4
Bridgend □ *U.K.* **15** F4
Bridgenorth *Canada* **114** B6
Bridgeport *Calif., U.S.A.* **110** G7
Bridgeport *Conn., U.S.A.* **115** E11
Bridgeport *N.Y., U.S.A.* **115** C9
Bridgeport *Nebr., U.S.A.* **112** E2
Bridgeport *Tex., U.S.A.* **116** E6
Bridger *U.S.A.* **108** D9
Bridgeton *U.S.A.* **113** F16
Bridgetown *Australia* **93** F2
Bridgetown *Barbados* **121** g
Bridgetown *Canada* **105** D6
Bridgewater *Australia* **95** G4
Bridgewater *Canada* **105** D7
Bridgewater *Mass., U.S.A.* **115** E14
Bridgewater *N.Y., U.S.A.* **115** D9
Bridgewater, C. *Australia* **95** F3
Bridgnorth *U.K.* **15** E5
Bridgton *U.S.A.* **115** B14
Bridgwater *U.K.* **15** F4
Bridgwater B. *U.K.* **15** F4
Bridlington *U.K.* **14** C7
Bridlington B. *U.K.* **14** C7
Bridport *Australia* **95** G4
Bridport *U.K.* **15** G5
Briec *France* **18** D3
Brienne-le-Château *France* **19** D11
Brienon-sur-Armançon
  France **19** E10
Brienz *Switz.* **25** J4
Brienzersee *Switz.* **25** J3
Brière △ *France* **18** E4
Brig *Switz.* **25** J3
Brigg *U.K.* **14** D7
Brigham City *U.S.A.* **108** F7
Bright *Australia* **95** F4
Brighton *Australia* **95** F2
Brighton *Canada* **114** B7
Brighton *Trin. & Tob.* **125** K15
Brighton *U.K.* **15** G7
Brighton *U.S.A.* **114** C7
Brightside *Canada* **115** A8
Brignogan-Plage *France* **18** D2
Brignoles *France* **21** E10
Brihuega *Spain* **38** E2
Brikama *Gambia* **82** C1
Brilliant *U.S.A.* **114** F4
Brilon *Germany* **24** D4
Bríndisi *Italy* **43** B10
Brinje *Croatia* **41** D12
Brinkley *U.S.A.* **116** D9
Brinnon *U.S.A.* **110** C4
Brion, Î. *Canada* **105** C7
Brionne *France* **18** C7
Brionski *Croatia* **41** D10
Brioude *France* **20** C7
Briouze *France* **18** D6
Brisay *Canada* **105** B5
Brisbane *Australia* **95** D5
Brisbane → *Australia* **95** D5
Brisighella *Italy* **41** D8
Bristol *U.K.* **15** F5
Bristol *Conn., U.S.A.* **115** E12
Bristol *Pa., U.S.A.* **115** F10
Bristol *R.I., U.S.A.* **115** E13
Bristol *Tenn., U.S.A.* **117** C13
Bristol *Vt., U.S.A.* **115** B11
Bristol, City of □ *U.K.* **15** F5
Bristol B. *U.S.A.* **106** D8
Bristol Channel *U.K.* **15** F3
Bristol I. *Antarctica* **5** B1
Bristol L. *U.S.A.* **109** J6
Bristow *U.S.A.* **116** D6
Britain = Great Britain *Europe* **6** E5
British Columbia □ *Canada* **102** C3
British Indian Ocean Terr.
  = Chagos Arch. ☒ *Ind. Oc.* **50** J9
British Isles *Europe* **6** D6
British Mts. *N. Amer.* **106** B12
British Virgin Is. ☒ *W. Indies* **121** e
Brits *S. Africa* **89** D4
Britstown *S. Africa* **88** E3
Britt *Canada* **104** C3
Brittany = Bretagne □
  France **18** D3
Britton *U.S.A.* **112** C5
Brive-la-Gaillarde *France* **20** C5
Briviesca *Spain* **36** C7
Brixen = Bressanone *Italy* **41** B8
Brixham *U.K.* **15** G4
Brnaze *Croatia* **41** E13
Brnenský □ *Czech Rep.* **27** B9
Brno *Czech Rep.* **27** B9
Broach = Bharuch *India* **66** J8
Broad → *U.S.A.* **117** D14
Broad Arrow *Australia* **93** F3
Broad B. *U.K.* **13** C2
Broad Haven *Ireland* **12** B2

Broad Law *U.K.* **13** F5
Broad Pk. = Faichan
  Kangri *India* **69** B7
Broad Sd. *Australia* **94** C4
Broadalbin *U.S.A.* **115** C10
Broadback → *Canada* **104** B4
Broadhurst Ra. *Australia* **92** D3
Broads, The *U.K.* **14** E9
Broadus *U.S.A.* **108** D11
Broby *Sweden* **11** H8
Brocēni *Latvia* **30** B9
Brochet *Canada* **103** B8
Brochet, L. *Canada* **103** B8
Brock I. *Canada* **101** B9
Brocken *Germany* **24** D6
Brockport *U.S.A.* **114** C7
Brockton *U.S.A.* **115** D13
Brockville *Canada* **115** B9
Brockway *Mont., U.S.A.* **108** C11
Brockway *Pa., U.S.A.* **114** E6
Brocton *U.S.A.* **114** D5
Brod *Macedonia* **44** E5
Brodarevo *Serbia* **44** C3
Brodeur Pen. *Canada* **101** C14
Brodick *U.K.* **13** F3
Brodnica *Poland* **31** E6
Brody *Ukraine* **23** C13
Brogan *U.S.A.* **108** D5
Broglie *France* **18** C7
Brok *Poland* **31** F8
Broken Arrow *U.S.A.* **116** C7
Broken Bow *Nebr., U.S.A.* **112** E4
Broken Bow *Okla., U.S.A.* **116** D7
Broken Bow Lake *U.S.A.* **116** D7
Broken Hill *Australia* **95** E3
Broken Ridge *Ind. Oc.* **96** L1
Broken River Ra. *Australia* **94** b
Brokind *Sweden* **11** F9
Bromley *U.K.* **15** F8
Bromo *Indonesia* **63** G15
Bromölla *Sweden* **11** H8
Bromsgrove *U.K.* **15** E5
Brønderslev *Denmark* **11** G3
Brong-Ahafo □ *Ghana* **82** D4
Broni *Italy* **40** C6
Bronkhorstspruit *S. Africa* **89** D4
Brønnøysund *Norway* **8** D15
Bronte *Italy* **43** E7
Bronte Park *U.S.A.* **114** E4
Brook Park *U.S.A.* **114** E4
Brookhaven *U.S.A.* **117** F9
Brookings *Oreg., U.S.A.* **108** E1
Brookings *S. Dak., U.S.A.* **112** C5
Brooklin *Canada* **114** C6
Brooklyn Park *U.S.A.* **112** C7
Brooks *Canada* **102** C6
Brooks Range *U.S.A.* **106** B9
Brooksville *U.S.A.* **117** G13
Brookton *Australia* **93** F2
Brookville *Canada* **114** E5
Broom, L. *U.K.* **13** D3
Broome *Australia* **92** C3
Broons *France* **18** D4
Broora *U.K.* **13** C5
Brora → *U.K.* **13** C5
Brørup *Denmark* **11** J2
Brösarp *Sweden* **11** J8
Brosna → *Ireland* **12** C4
Broșteni *Mehedinți, Romania* **28** F7
Broșteni *Suceava, Romania* **29** C10
Brothers *U.S.A.* **108** E3
Brou *France* **18** D8
Brouage *France* **20** C2
Brough *U.K.* **14** C5
Brough Hd. *U.K.* **13** B5
Broughton Island =
  Qikiqtarjuaq *Canada* **101** D19
Broumov *Czech Rep.* **27** A9
Broup → *Ireland* **12** C4
Brovary *Ukraine* **33** G6
Brovst *Denmark* **11** G3
Brown, L. *Australia* **93** F2
Brown, Pt. *Australia* **95** E1
Brown City *U.S.A.* **114** C2
Brown Willy *U.K.* **15** G3
Brownfield *U.S.A.* **116** E3
Browning *U.S.A.* **108** B7
Brownsville *Oreg., U.S.A.* **108** D2
Brownsville *Pa., U.S.A.* **114** F5
Brownsville *Tenn., U.S.A.* **117** D10
Brownsville *Tex., U.S.A.* **116** J6
Brownville *U.S.A.* **115** C9
Brownwood *U.S.A.* **116** F5
Browse I. *Australia* **92** B3
Bruas *Malaysia* **65** K3
Bruay-la-Buissière *France* **19** B9
Bruce, Mt. *Australia* **92** D2
Bruce Pen. *Canada* **114** B3
Bruce Peninsula △ *Canada* **114** A3
Bruce Rock *Australia* **93** F2
Bruche → *France* **19** D14
Bruchsal *Germany* **25** F4
Bruck an der Leitha *Austria* **27** C9
Bruck an der Mur *Austria* **26** D8
Brue → *U.K.* **15** F5
Bruges = Brugge *Belgium* **17** C3
Brugg *Switz.* **25** H4
Brugge *Belgium* **17** C3
Bruin *U.S.A.* **114** E5
Brûk, W. el → *Egypt* **74** E2

Brûlé *Canada* **102** C5
Brûlé, L. *Canada* **105** B7
Brûlon *France* **18** E6
Brumado *Brazil* **125** F10
Brumath *France* **19** D14
Brumunddal *Norway* **8** F14
Bruneau *U.S.A.* **108** E6
Bruneau → *U.S.A.* **108** E6
Bruneck = Brunico *Italy* **41** B8
Brunei = Bandar Seri
  Begawan *Brunei* **62** D5
Brunei ■ *Asia* **62** D5
Brunflo *Sweden* **10** A8
Brunico *Italy* **41** B8
Brunna *Sweden* **10** E11
Brunnen *Switz.* **25** J4
Brunner, L. *N.Z.* **91** E3
Brunsbüttel *Germany* **24** B5
Brunssum *Neths.* **17** D5
Brunswick =
  Braunschweig *Germany* **24** C6
Brunswick *Ga., U.S.A.* **117** F14
Brunswick *Maine, U.S.A.* **113** D19
Brunswick *Md., U.S.A.* **113** F15
Brunswick *Mo., U.S.A.* **112** F7
Brunswick *Ohio, U.S.A.* **114** E3
Brunswick, Pen. de *Chile* **128** G2
Brunswick B. *Australia* **92** C3
Brunswick Junction *Australia* **93** F2
Brunt Ice Shelf *Antarctica* **5** D2
Bruntál *Czech Rep.* **27** B10
Brus Laguna *Honduras* **120** C3
Brusartsi *Bulgaria* **44** C7
Brush *U.S.A.* **108** F12
Brushton *U.S.A.* **115** B10
Brusio *Switz.* **25** J6
Brusque *Brazil* **127** B6
Brussel *Belgium* **17** D4
Brussel ✈ (BRU) *Belgium* **17** D5
Brussels = Brussel *Belgium* **17** D4
Brussels *Canada* **114** C3
Bruxelles = Brussel *Belgium* **17** D4
Bruyères *France* **19** D13
Bruz *France* **18** D5
Brwinów *Poland* **31** F7
Bryagovo *Bulgaria* **45** E9
Bryan *Ohio, U.S.A.* **113** E11
Bryan *Tex., U.S.A.* **116** F6
Bryan, Mt. *Australia* **95** E2
Bryanka *Ukraine* **33** H10
Bryansk *Bryansk, Russia* **33** F8
Bryansk *Dagestan, Russia* **35** H8
Bryansk □ *Russia* **33** F7
Bryanskoye = Bryansk
  Russia **35** H8
Bryce Canyon △ *U.S.A.* **109** H7
Bryne *Norway* **9** G11
Bryson City *U.S.A.* **117** D13
Bryukhovetskaya *Russia* **33** K10
Brza Palanka *Serbia* **44** B6
Brzeg *Poland* **31** H4
Brzeg Dolny *Poland* **31** G3
Brześć Kujawski *Poland* **31** F5
Brzesko *Poland* **31** J7
Brzeziny *Poland* **31** G6
Brzozów *Poland* **31** J9
Bsharri *Lebanon* **74** A5
Bū Baqarah *U.A.E.* **71** E8
Bu Craa *W. Sahara* **78** C3
Bū Ḥasā *U.A.E.* **71** F7
Bua *Fiji* **91** a
Bua *Sweden* **11** G6
Bua → *Malaysia* **87** E3
Bua Yai *Thailand* **64** E4
Buan *S. Korea* **57** G14
Buapinang *Indonesia* **63** E6
Buba *Guinea-Biss.* **82** C2
Bubanza *Burundi* **86** C2
Bubaque *Guinea-Biss.* **82** C1
Bube *Ethiopia* **81** F4
Bubi → *Zimbabwe* **87** G3
Būbiyān *Kuwait* **71** D6
Buca *Fiji* **91** a
Bucak *Turkey* **47** C9
Bucak *Turkey* **47** D12
Bucaramanga *Colombia* **124** B4
Bucas Grande I. *Phil.* **61** G6
Bucasia *Australia* **94** b
Buccaneer Arch. *Australia* **92** C3
Buccino *Italy* **43** B8
Buccoo Reef *Trin. & Tob.* **125** J16
Bucecea *Romania* **29** C11
Bucegi △ *Romania* **29** E10
Buchach *Ukraine* **23** D13
Buchan *U.K.* **13** D8
Buchan Ness *U.K.* **13** D7
Buchanan *Canada* **103** C8
Buchanan *Liberia* **82** D2
Buchanan, L. *Queens.,*
  Australia **94** C4
Buchanan, L. *W. Austral.,*
  Australia **93** E3
Buchanan, L. *U.S.A.* **116** F5
Buchanan Cr. → *Australia* **94** B2
Buchans *Canada* **105** C8
Bucharest = București
  Romania **29** F11
Bruin *U.S.A.* **114** E5
Brûk, W. el → *Egypt* **74** E2

Buchen *Germany* **25** F5
Bucheon *S. Korea* **57** F14
Buchholz *Germany* **24** B5
Buchloe *Germany* **25** G6
Buchon, Pt. *U.S.A.* **110** K6
Bück Hill Falls *U.S.A.* **115** E9
Bückeburg *Germany* **24** C5
Buckeye Lake *U.S.A.* **114** G2
Buckhannon *U.S.A.* **113** F13
Buckhaven *U.K.* **13** E5
Buckhorn L. *Canada* **114** B6
Buckie *U.K.* **13** D6
Buckingham *Canada* **104** C4
Buckingham *U.K.* **15** F7
Buckingham B. *Australia* **94** A2
Buckinghamshire □ *U.K.* **15** F7
Buckle Hd. *Australia* **92** B4
Buckleboo *Australia* **95** E2
Buckley *U.K.* **14** D4
Buckley → *Australia* **94** C2
Bucklin *U.S.A.* **112** G4
Bucks L. *U.S.A.* **110** F5
Bucquoy *France* **19** B9
București *Romania* **29** F11
București Otopeni ✈ (OTP)
  Romania **29** F11
Budacu, Vf. *Romania* **29** C10
Budalin *Burma* **67** H19
Budaörs *Hungary* **28** C3
Budapest *Hungary* **28** C4
Budapest □ *Hungary* **28** C4
Budapest ✈ (BUD) *Hungary* **28** C4
Budaun *India* **69** E8
Budd Coast *Antarctica* **5** C8
Buddusò *Italy* **42** B2
Bude *U.K.* **15** G3
Budennovsk *Russia* **35** H7
Budeşti *Romania* **29** F11
Budeyi *Ukraine* **29** B14
Budge Budge = Baj Baj
  India **69** H13
Budgewoi *Australia* **95** E5
Budia *Spain* **38** E2
Büdingen *Germany* **25** E5
Budjala *Dem. Rep. of the Congo* **84** D3
Budoni *Italy* **42** B2
Búdrio *Italy* **41** D8
Budva *Montenegro* **44** D2
Budzyń *Poland* **31** F3
Buea *Cameroon* **83** E6
Buellton *U.S.A.* **111** L6
Buena Esperanza *Argentina* **126** C2
Buena Park *U.S.A.* **111** M9
Buena Vista *Colo., U.S.A.* **108** G10
Buena Vista *Va., U.S.A.* **113** G14
Buena Vista Lake Bed
  U.S.A. **111** K7
Buenaventura *Colombia* **124** C3
Buenaventura *Mexico* **118** B3
Buendía, Embalse de *Spain* **38** E2
Buenos Aires *Argentina* **126** C4
Buenos Aires *Costa Rica* **120** E3
Buenos Aires □ *Argentina* **126** D4
Buenos Aires, L. *Argentina* **128** F2
Buffalo *Mo., U.S.A.* **112** G7
Buffalo *N.Y., U.S.A.* **114** D6
Buffalo *Okla., U.S.A.* **116** C5
Buffalo *S. Dak., U.S.A.* **112** C3
Buffalo *Wyo., U.S.A.* **108** D10
Buffalo → *Canada* **102** A5
Buffalo → *S. Africa* **89** D5
Buffalo → *U.S.A.* **116** C8
Buffalo Head Hills *Canada* **102** B5
Buffalo L. *Alta., Canada* **102** C6
Buffalo L. *N.W.T., Canada* **102** A5
Buffalo Narrows *Canada* **103** B7
Buffalo Springs *Kenya* **86** B4
Buffels → *S. Africa* **88** D2
Buford *U.S.A.* **117** D12
Bug → *Ukraine* **33** J6
Bug → *Poland* **31** F8
Buga *Colombia* **124** C3
Bugala I. *Uganda* **86** C3
Buganda *Uganda* **86** C3
Buganga *Uganda* **86** C3
Bugasong *Phil.* **61** F5
Bugeat *France* **20** C5
Bugel, Tanjung *Indonesia* **63** G14
Büger *Spain* **48** B9
Bugibba *Malta* **49** D1
Bugojno *Bos.-H.* **28** F2
Bugsuk I. *Phil.* **62** C5
Buguma *Nigeria* **83** E6
Bugun Shara *Mongolia* **60** B5
Bugungu □ *Uganda* **86** B3
Buguruslan *Russia* **52** D6
Buh → *Ukraine* **33** J6
Buharkent *Turkey* **47** D10
Buheirat-Murrat-el-Kubra
  Egypt **80** H8
Buhera *Zimbabwe* **89** B5
Bühl *Germany* **25** G4
Buhl *U.S.A.* **108** E6
Buhuşi *Romania* **29** C11
Bui △ *Ghana* **82** D4
Builth Wells *U.K.* **15** E4
Buinsk *Russia* **34** C9

Buir Nur *Mongolia* **60** B6
Buis-les-Baronnies *France* **21** D9
Buitrago del Lozoya *Spain* **36** E7
Bujalance *Spain* **37** H6
Bujanovac *Serbia* **44** D5
Bujaraloz *Spain* **38** D4
Buje *Croatia* **41** C10
Bujumbura *Burundi* **86** C2
Bük *Hungary* **28** C1
Buk *Poland* **31** F3
Bukachacha *Russia* **53** D12
Bukama
    Dem. Rep. of the Congo **87** D2
Bukavu *Dem. Rep. of the Congo* **86** C2
Bukene *Tanzania* **86** C3
Bukhara = Buxoro *Uzbekistan* **52** F7
Bukhoro = Buxoro *Uzbekistan* **52** F7
Bukima *Tanzania* **86** C3
Bukit Badung *Indonesia* **63** K18
Bukit Kerajaan *Malaysia* **65** c
Bukit Mertajam *Malaysia* **65** c
Bukit Ni *Malaysia* **65** d
Bukit Panjang *Singapore* **65** d
Bukit Tengah *Malaysia* **65** d
Bukittinggi *Indonesia* **62** E2
Bükk *Hungary* **28** B5
Bükki △ *Hungary* **28** B5
Bukoba *Tanzania* **86** C3
Bukum, Pulau *Singapore* **65** d
Bukuru *Nigeria* **83** D6
Bukuya *Uganda* **86** B3
Bül, Kuh-e *Iran* **71** D7
Bula *Guinea-Biss.* **82** C1
Bula *Indonesia* **63** E8
Bülach *Switz.* **25** H4
Bulahdelah *Australia* **95** E5
Bulan *Phil.* **61** E5
Bulancak *Turkey* **73** B8
Bulandshahr *India* **68** E7
Bulanık *Turkey* **73** C10
Bûlâq *Egypt* **80** B3
Bulawayo *Zimbabwe* **87** G2
Buldan *Turkey* **47** C10
Buldir I. *U.S.A.* **106** E3
Bulenga *Ghana* **82** D4
Bulgar *Russia* **34** C9
Bulgaria ■ *Europe* **45** D9
Bulgheria, Monte *Italy* **43** B8
Bulgurca *Turkey* **47** C9
Buli, Teluk *Indonesia* **63** D7
Buliluyan, C. *Phil.* **61** G2
Bulim *Singapore* **65** d
Bulki *Ethiopia* **81** F4
Bulkley → *Canada* **102** B3
Bull Shoals L. *U.S.A.* **116** C8
Bullaque → *Spain* **37** G6
Bullas *Spain* **39** G3
Bulle *Switz.* **25** J3
Bulleringa △ *Australia* **94** B3
Bullhead City *U.S.A.* **111** K12
Büllingen *Belgium* **17** D6
Bullock Creek *Australia* **94** B3
Bulloo → *Australia* **95** D3
Bulloo L. *Australia* **95** D3
Bulls *N.Z.* **91** D5
Bully-les-Mines *France* **19** B9
Bulman *Australia* **94** A1
Bulnes *Chile* **126** D1
Bulqizë *Albania* **44** E4
Bulsar = Valsad *India* **66** J8
Bultfontein *S. Africa* **88** D4
Bulukumba *Indonesia* **63** F6
Bulun *Russia* **53** B13
Bumba *Dem. Rep. of the Congo* **84** D4
Bumbah, Khalīj *Libya* **79** B10
Bumbeşti-Jiu *Romania* **29** E8
Bumbiri I. *Tanzania* **86** C3
Bumbuna *S. Leone* **82** D2
Bumhpa Bum *Burma* **67** F20
Bumi → *Zimbabwe* **87** F2
Buna *Kenya* **86** B4
Bunaken *Indonesia* **63** D6
Bunawan *Phil.* **61** G6
Bunazi *Tanzania* **86** C3
Bunbury *Australia* **93** F2
Bunclody *Ireland* **12** D5
Buncrana *Ireland* **12** A4
Bundaberg *Australia* **95** C5
Bünde *Germany* **24** C4
Bundey → *Australia* **94** C2
Bundi *India* **68** G6
Bundjalung △ *Australia* **95** D5
Bundoran *Ireland* **12** B3
Bundukia *Sudan* **81** F3
Bung Kan *Thailand* **64** C4
Bunga → *Nigeria* **83** C6
Bungay *U.K.* **15** E9
Bungil Cr. → *Australia* **95** D4
Bungle Bungle =
    Purnululu △ *Australia* **92** C4
Bungo-Suidō *Japan* **55** H6
Bungoma *Kenya* **86** B3
Bungotakada *Japan* **55** H5
Bungu *Tanzania* **86** D4
Bunia *Dem. Rep. of the Congo* **86** B3
Bunji *Pakistan* **69** B6
Bunkie *U.S.A.* **116** F8
Bunnell *U.S.A.* **117** G14
Buñol *Spain* **39** F4

Bunsuru *Nigeria* **83** C5
Buntok *Indonesia* **62** E4
Bununu Dass *Nigeria* **83** C6
Bununu Kasa *Nigeria* **83** D6
Bunya Mts. △ *Australia* **95** D5
Bünyan *Turkey* **72** C6
Bunyola *Spain* **48** B9
Bunyu *Indonesia* **62** D5
Bunza *Nigeria* **83** C5
Buol *Indonesia* **63** D6
Buon Brieng *Vietnam* **64** F7
Buon Ma Thuot *Vietnam* **64** F7
Buong Long *Cambodia* **64** F6
Buorkhaya, Mys *Russia* **53** B14
Buqayq *Si. Arabia* **71** E6
Buqbuq *Egypt* **80** A2
Bur Acaba = Buurhakaba
    Somali Rep. **75** G3
Bûr Fuad *Egypt* **80** H8
Bûr Safâga *Egypt* **70** E2
Bûr Sa'îd *Egypt* **80** H8
Bûr Sûdân *Sudan* **80** D4
Bûr Taufiq *Egypt* **80** J8
Bura *Kenya* **86** C5
Burakin *Australia* **93** F2
Buram *Sudan* **81** E2
Burao = Burco *Somali Rep.* **75** F4
Burâq *Syria* **74** B5
Buraydah *Si. Arabia* **70** E4
Burbank *U.S.A.* **111** L8
Burco *Somali Rep.* **75** F4
Burda *India* **68** G6
Burdekin → *Australia* **94** B4
Burdur *Turkey* **47** D12
Burdur □ *Turkey* **47** D12
Burdur Gölü *Turkey* **47** D12
Burdwan = Barddhaman
    India **69** H12
Bure *Gojam, Ethiopia* **81** E4
Bure *Ilubabor, Ethiopia* **81** F4
Bure → *U.K.* **14** E9
Büren *Germany* **24** D4
Bureya → *Russia* **53** E13
Burford *Canada* **114** C4
Burg *Germany* **24** C7
Burg auf Fehmarn *Germany* **24** A7
Burg el Arab *Egypt* **80** H6
Burg et Tuyur *Sudan* **80** C2
Burg Stargard *Germany* **24** B9
Burgas *Bulgaria* **45** D11
Burgas □ *Bulgaria* **45** D10
Burgaski Zaliv *Bulgaria* **45** D11
Burgdorf *Germany* **24** C6
Burgdorf *Switz.* **25** H3
Burgenland □ *Austria* **27** D9
Burgeo *Canada* **105** C8
Burgersdorp *S. Africa* **88** E4
Burgess, Mt. *Australia* **93** F3
Burghausen *Germany* **25** G8
Burghead *U.K.* **13** D5
Búrgio *Italy* **42** E6
Burglengenfeld *Germany* **25** F8
Burgohondo *Spain* **36** E6
Burgos *Spain* **36** C7
Burgos □ *Spain* **36** C7
Burgstädt *Germany* **24** E8
Burgsvik *Sweden* **11** G12
Burguillos del Cerro *Spain* **37** G4
Burgundy = Bourgogne □
    France **19** F11
Burhaniye *Turkey* **47** B8
Burhanpur *India* **66** J10
Burhi Gandak → *India* **69** G12
Burhner → *India* **69** H9
Buri Pen. *Eritrea* **81** D4
Burias I. *Phil.* **61** E5
Burica, Pta. *Costa Rica* **120** E3
Burien *U.S.A.* **110** C4
Burigi, L. *Tanzania* **86** C3
Burigi △ *Tanzania* **86** C3
Burin *Canada* **105** C8
Buriram *Thailand* **64** E4
Burji *Ethiopia* **81** F4
Burkburnett *U.S.A.* **116** D5
Burke → *Australia* **94** C2
Burke Chan. *Canada* **102** C3
Burketown *Australia* **94** B2
Burkina Faso ■ *Africa* **82** C4
Burk's Falls *Canada* **104** C4
Burlada *Spain* **38** C3
Burleigh Falls *Canada* **114** B6
Burley *U.S.A.* **108** E7
Burlingame *U.S.A.* **110** H4
Burlington *Canada* **114** C5
Burlington *Colo., U.S.A.* **108** G12
Burlington *Iowa, U.S.A.* **112** E9
Burlington *Kans., U.S.A.* **112** F6
Burlington *N.C., U.S.A.* **117** C15
Burlington *N.J., U.S.A.* **115** F10
Burlington *Vt., U.S.A.* **115** B11
Burlington *Wash., U.S.A.* **110** B4
Burlington *Wis., U.S.A.* **112** D9
Burma ■ *Asia* **67** J20
Burnaby I. *Canada* **102** C2
Burnet *U.S.A.* **116** F5
Burney *U.S.A.* **108** F3
Burnham *U.S.A.* **114** F7
Burnham-on-Sea *U.K.* **15** F5
Burnie *Australia* **95** G4

Burnley *U.K.* **14** D5
Burns *U.S.A.* **108** E4
Burns Junction *U.S.A.* **108** E5
Burns Lake *Canada* **102** C3
Burnside → *Canada* **100** D10
Burnside, L. *Australia* **93** E3
Burnsville *U.S.A.* **112** C7
Burnt River *Canada* **114** B6
Burntwood → *Canada* **103** B9
Burntwood L. *Canada* **103** B8
Burqân *Kuwait* **70** D5
Burra *Australia* **95** E2
Burra *Nigeria* **83** C6
Burray *U.K.* **13** C6
Burrel *Albania* **44** E4
Burren *Ireland* **12** C2
Burren △ *Ireland* **12** C3
Burren Junction *Australia* **95** E4
Burriana *Spain* **38** F4
Burrinjuck, L. *Australia* **95** F4
Burro, Serranías del *Mexico* **118** B4
Burrow Hd. *U.K.* **13** G4
Burrum Coast △ *Australia* **95** D5
Burruyacú *Argentina* **126** B3
Burry Port *U.K.* **15** F3
Bursa *Turkey* **45** F13
Bursa □ *Turkey* **72** B3
Burseryd *Sweden* **11** G7
Burstall *Canada* **103** C7
Burton *Ohio, U.S.A.* **114** E3
Burton *S.C., U.S.A.* **117** E14
Burton, L. *Canada* **104** B4
Burton upon Trent *U.K.* **14** E6
Buru *Indonesia* **63** E7
Burullus, Bahra el *Egypt* **80** H7
Burûn, Râs *Egypt* **74** D2
Burundi ■ *Africa* **86** C3
Bururi *Burundi* **86** C2
Burutu *Nigeria* **83** D6
Burwell *U.S.A.* **112** E4
Burwick *U.K.* **13** C5
Bury *U.K.* **14** D5
Bury St. Edmunds *U.K.* **15** E8
Buryatia □ *Russia* **53** D12
Buryn *Ukraine* **33** G7
Burzenin *Poland* **31** G5
Busalla *Italy* **40** D5
Busan = Pusan *S. Korea* **57** G15
Busango Swamp *Zambia* **87** E2
Busaso = Boosaaso
    Somali Rep. **75** E4
Buşayrah *Syria* **73** E9
Busca *Italy* **40** D4
Bushat *Albania* **44** E3
Büshehr *Iran* **71** D6
Büshehr □ *Iran* **71** D6
Bushenyi *Uganda* **86** C3
Bushire = Büshehr *Iran* **71** D6
Bushtyna *Ukraine* **29** B8
Busia *Ghana* **82** C4
Businga *Dem. Rep. of the Congo* **84** D4
Büsingen *Germany* **25** H4
Busko-Zdrój *Poland* **31** H7
Busovača *Bos.-H.* **28** F2
Buşra ash Shām *Syria* **74** C5
Busselton *Australia* **93** F2
Busseri → *Sudan* **81** F2
Busseto *Italy* **40** D7
Bussière-Badil *France* **20** C4
Bussolengo *Italy* **40** C7
Bussum *Neths.* **17** B5
Buşteni *Romania* **29** E10
Busto, C. *Spain* **36** B4
Busto Arsízio *Italy* **40** C5
Busu Djanoa
    Dem. Rep. of the Congo **84** D4
Busuanga I. *Phil.* **61** E4
Büsüm *Germany* **24** A5
Busungbiu *Indonesia* **63** J17
Buta *Dem. Rep. of the Congo* **86** B1
Butare *Rwanda* **86** C2
Butaritari *Kiribati* **96** G9
Bute *U.K.* **13** F3
Bute Inlet *Canada* **102** C4
Butemba *Uganda* **86** B3
Butembo
    Dem. Rep. of the Congo **86** B2
Buteni *Romania* **28** D7
Butera *Italy* **43** E7
Butere *Kenya* **86** B3
Butha Qi *China* **60** B7
Butiaba *Uganda* **86** B3
Butler *Mo., U.S.A.* **112** F6
Butler *Pa., U.S.A.* **114** F5
Buton *Indonesia* **63** F6
Butte *Mont., U.S.A.* **108** C7
Butte *Nebr., U.S.A.* **112** D4
Butte Creek → *U.S.A.* **110** F5
Butterworth = Gcuwa
    S. Africa **89** E4
Butterworth *Malaysia* **65** c
Buttevant *Ireland* **12** D3
Buttfield, Mt. *Australia* **93** D4
Button B. *Canada* **103** B10
Buttonwillow *U.S.A.* **111** K7
Butty Hd. *Australia* **93** F3
Butuan *Phil.* **61** G6
Butuku-Luba *Eq. Guin.* **83** E6
Butung = Buton *Indonesia* **63** F6

Buturlinovka *Russia* **34** E5
Butzbach *Germany* **25** E4
Bützow *Germany* **24** B7
Buurhakaba *Somali Rep.* **75** G3
Buxa Duar *India* **69** F13
Buxar *India* **69** G10
Buxoro *Uzbekistan* **52** F7
Buxtehude *Germany* **24** B5
Buxton *U.K.* **14** D6
Buxy *France* **19** F11
Buy *Russia* **34** A5
Buyant-Uhaa *Mongolia* **60** B6
Buynaksk *Russia* **35** J8
Buyo *Ivory C.* **82** D3
Buyo, L. de *Ivory C.* **82** D3
Büyük Menderes → *Turkey* **47** D9
Büyükçekmece *Turkey* **45** E12
Büyükkarıştıran *Turkey* **45** E11
Büyükkemikli Burnu
    Turkey **45** F10
Büyükorhan *Turkey* **47** B10
Büyükyoncalı *Turkey* **45** E11
Buzançais *France* **18** F8
Buzău *Romania* **29** E11
Buzău □ *Romania* **29** E11
Buzău → *Romania* **29** E12
Buzău, Pasul *Romania* **29** E11
Buzen *Japan* **55** H5
Buzet *Croatia* **41** C10
Buzi → *Mozam.* **87** F3
Büzmeyin *Turkmenistan* **71** B8
Buzuluk *Russia* **52** D6
Buzuluk → *Russia* **34** E6
Buzzards Bay *U.S.A.* **115** E14
Bwana Mkubwe
    Dem. Rep. of the Congo **87** E2
Bwindi △ *Uganda* **86** C2
Byala *Ruse, Bulgaria* **45** C9
Byala *Varna, Bulgaria* **45** D11
Byala Slatina *Bulgaria* **44** C7
Byam Martin I. *Canada* **101** B11
Byarezina → *Belarus* **23** B16
Byaroza *Belarus* **33** F3
Bychawa *Belarus* **31** G9
Byczyna *Poland* **31** G5
Bydgoszcz *Poland* **31** E5
Byelorussia = Belarus ■
    Europe **23** B14
Byers *U.S.A.* **108** G11
Byesville *U.S.A.* **114** G3
Byfield △ *Australia* **94** C5
Bykhaw *Belarus* **23** B16
Bykhov = Bykhaw *Belarus* **23** B16
Bykovo *Russia* **34** F7
Bylas *U.S.A.* **109** K8
Bylot *Canada* **103** B10
Bylot I. *Canada* **101** C16
Byrd, C. *Antarctica* **5** C17
Byrock *Australia* **95** E4
Byron, C. *Australia* **95** D5
Byron Bay *Australia* **95** D5
Byrranga, Gory *Russia* **53** B11
Byrranga Mts. = Byrranga,
    Gory *Russia* **53** B11
Byrum *Denmark* **11** G5
Byske *Sweden* **8** D19
Byskeälven → *Sweden* **8** D19
Bystrytsya *Ukraine* **29** B9
Bystrzyca → *Dolnośląskie,*
    Poland **31** G3
Bystrzyca → *Lubelskie, Poland* **31** G9
Bystrzyca Kłodzka *Poland* **31** H3
Bytča *Slovak Rep.* **27** B11
Bytkiv *Ukraine* **29** B9
Bytom *Poland* **31** H5
Bytom Odrzański *Poland* **31** G2
Bytów *Poland* **30** D4
Byumba *Rwanda* **86** C3
Bzenec *Czech Rep.* **27** C10
Bzura → *Poland* **31** F7

C

C.W. McConaughy, L.
    U.S.A. **112** E3
Ca → *Vietnam* **64** C5
Ca Mau *Vietnam* **65** H5
Ca Mau, Mui *Vietnam* **65** H5
Ca Na *Vietnam* **65** G7
Caacupé *Paraguay* **126** B4
Caaguazú △ *Paraguay* **127** B4
Caála *Angola* **85** G3
Caamaño Sd. *Canada* **102** C3
Caazapá *Paraguay* **126** B4
Caazapá □ *Paraguay* **127** B4
Cabadbaran *Phil.* **61** G6
Cabalian = San Juan *Phil.* **61** F6
Caballería, C. de *Spain* **48** A11
Cabana de Bergantiños *Spain* **36** B2
Cabanaquinta *Spain* **36** B5
Cabanatuan *Phil.* **61** D4
Cabañeros △ *Spain* **37** F6
Cabanes *Spain* **38** E5
Cabano *Canada* **105** C6
Čabar *Croatia* **41** C11
Cabazon *U.S.A.* **111** M10
Cabedelo *Brazil* **125** E12
Cabeza del Buey *Spain* **37** G5

Cabezón de la Sal *Spain* **36** B6
Cabildo *Chile* **126** C1
Cabimas *Venezuela* **124** A4
Cabinda *Angola* **84** F2
Cabinda □ *Angola* **84** F2
Cabinet Mts. *U.S.A.* **108** B6
Cabo Blanco *Argentina* **128** F3
Cabo de Gata-Níjar △ *Spain* **39** J2
Cabo Frio *Brazil* **127** A7
Cabo Pantoja *Peru* **124** D3
Cabo San Lucas *Mexico* **118** C3
Cabo Verde = Cape Verde
    Is. ■ *Atl. Oc.* **78** b
Cabonga, Réservoir *Canada* **104** C4
Caboolture *Australia* **95** D5
Caborca *Mexico* **118** A2
Cabora Bassa Dam =
    Cahora Bassa, Lago de
    Mozam. **87** F3
Cabot, Mt. *U.S.A.* **115** B13
Cabot Hd. *Canada* **114** A3
Cabot Str. *Canada* **105** C8
Cabra *Spain* **37** H6
Cabra del Santo Cristo *Spain* **37** H7
Cábras *Italy* **42** C1
Cabrera *Spain* **48** B9
Cabrera, Sierra *Spain* **36** C4
Cabrera △ *Spain* **39** F7
Cabri *Canada* **103** C7
Cabriel → *Spain* **39** F3
Cabugao *Phil.* **61** C4
Cacabelos *Spain* **36** C4
Caçador *Brazil* **127** B5
Čačak *Serbia* **44** C4
Caçapava do Sul *Brazil* **127** C5
Cáccamo *Italy* **42** E6
Cacém *Portugal* **37** G1
Cáceres *Brazil* **124** G7
Cáceres *Spain* **37** F4
Cáceres □ *Spain* **36** F5
Cache Bay *Canada* **104** C4
Cache Cr. → *U.S.A.* **110** G5
Cache Creek *Canada* **102** C4
Cacheu *Guinea-Biss.* **82** C1
Cachi *Argentina* **126** B2
Cachimbo, Serra do *Brazil* **125** E7
Cachinal de la Sierra *Chile* **126** A2
Cachoeira *Brazil* **125** F11
Cachoeira do Sul *Brazil* **127** C5
Cachoeiro de Itapemirim
    Brazil **127** A7
Cachopo *Portugal* **37** H3
Cacine *Guinea-Biss.* **82** C1
Cacoal *Brazil* **124** F6
Cacólo *Angola* **84** G3
Caconda *Angola* **85** G3
Caddo *U.S.A.* **116** D6
Cader Idris *U.K.* **14** E4
Cadereyta de Jiménez
    Mexico **118** B5
Cadí, Sierra del *Spain* **38** C6
Cadí-Moixeró △ *Spain* **38** C7
Cadibarrawirracanna, L.
    Australia **95** D2
Cadillac *France* **20** D3
Cadillac *U.S.A.* **113** C11
Cadiz *Phil.* **61** F5
Cádiz *Spain* **37** J4
Cadiz *Calif., U.S.A.* **111** L11
Cadiz *Ohio, U.S.A.* **114** F4
Cádiz □ *Spain* **37** J5
Cadiz L. *U.S.A.* **111** L11
Cádiz, G. de *Spain* **37** J3
Cadney Park *Australia* **95** D1
Cadomin *Canada* **102** C5
Cadotte Lake *Canada* **102** B5
Cadours *France* **20** E5
Cadoux *Australia* **93** F2
Caen *France* **18** C6
Caernarfon *U.K.* **14** D3
Caernarfon B. *U.K.* **14** D3
Caernarvon = Caernarfon
    U.K. **14** D3
Caerphilly *U.K.* **15** F4
Caerphilly □ *U.K.* **15** F4
Caesarea *Israel* **74** C3
Caetité *Brazil* **125** F10
Cafayate *Argentina* **126** B2
Cafu *Angola* **88** B2
Cagayan → *Phil.* **61** B4
Cagayan de Oro *Phil.* **61** G6
Cagayan Is. *Phil.* **61** G4
Cagayan Sulu I. *Phil.* **61** H3
Cagli *Italy* **41** E9
Cágliari *Italy* **42** C2
Cágliari, G. di *Italy* **42** C2
Cagnano Varano *Italy* **41** G12
Cagnes-sur-Mer *France* **21** E11
Caguán → *Colombia* **124** D4
Caguas *Puerto Rico* **121** d
Caha Mts. *Ireland* **12** E2
Cahama *Angola* **88** B1
Caher *Ireland* **12** D4
Cahersiveen *Ireland* **12** E1
Cahora Bassa, L. de *Mozam.* **87** F3
Cahora Bassa, Lago de
    Mozam. **87** F3

Cahore Pt. *Ireland* **12** D5
Cahors *France* **20** D5
Cahul *Moldova* **29** E13
Caì Du, Dao *Vietnam* **58** G6
Cai Nuoc *Vietnam* **65** H5
Caia *Mozam.* **87** F4
Caianda *Angola* **87** E1
Caibarién *Cuba* **120** B4
Caibiran *Phil.* **61** F6
Caicara *Venezuela* **124** B5
Caicó *Brazil* **125** E11
Caicos Is. *Turks & Caicos* **121** B5
Caicos Passage *W. Indies* **121** B5
Caidian *China* **59** B10
Caiguna *Australia* **93** F4
Căinari *Moldova* **29** E14
Caird Coast *Antarctica* **5** D1
Cairn Gorm *U.K.* **13** D5
Cairngorm Mts. *U.K.* **13** D5
Cairngorms △ *U.K.* **13** D5
Cairnryan *U.K.* **13** G3
Cairns *Australia* **94** B4
Cairns L. *Canada* **103** C10
Cairo = El Qâhira *Egypt* **80** H7
Cairo *Ga., U.S.A.* **117** F12
Cairo *Ill., U.S.A.* **112** G9
Cairo *N.Y., U.S.A.* **115** D11
Cairo Montenotte *Italy* **40** D5
Caiseal = Cashel *Ireland* **12** D4
Caisleán an Bharraigh =
    Castlebar *Ireland* **12** C2
Caithness *U.K.* **13** C5
Caithness, Ord of *U.K.* **13** C5
Caja de Muertos, I.
    Puerto Rico **121** d
Cajamarca *Peru* **124** E3
Cajarc *France* **20** D5
Cajazeiras *Brazil* **125** E11
Čajetina *Serbia* **44** C3
Çakırgol *Turkey* **73** B8
Çakırlar *Turkey* **47** E12
Čakovec *Croatia* **41** B13
Çal *Turkey* **47** C11
Cala *Spain* **37** H4
Cala → *Spain* **37** H4
Cala Cadolar, Punta de =
    Rotja, Pta. *Spain* **39** G6
Cala d'Or *Spain* **48** B10
Cala en Porter *Spain* **48** B11
Cala Figuera *Spain* **48** B10
Cala Figuera, C. de *Spain* **48** B9
Cala Forcat *Spain* **48** B10
Cala Major *Spain* **48** B9
Cala Mezquida = Sa
    Mesquida *Spain* **48** B11
Cala Millor *Spain* **48** B10
Cala Murada *Spain* **48** B10
Cala Ratjada *Spain* **48** B10
Cala Santa Galdana *Spain* **48** B10
Calabanga *Phil.* **61** E5
Calabar *Nigeria* **83** E6
Calabogie *Canada* **115** A8
Calabozo *Venezuela* **124** B5
Calábria □ *Italy* **43** C9
Calábria △ *Italy* **43** C9
Calaburras, Pta. de *Spain* **37** J6
Calaceite *Spain* **38** D5
Calacuccia *France* **21** F13
Calafat *Romania* **28** G7
Calafell *Spain* **38** D6
Calahorra *Spain* **38** C3
Calais *France* **19** B8
Calais *U.S.A.* **113** C20
Calakmul △ *Mexico* **119** D7
Calalaste, Cord. de *Argentina* **126** B2
Calama *Brazil* **124** E6
Calama *Chile* **126** A2
Calamar *Colombia* **124** A4
Calamian Group *Phil.* **61** F3
Calamocha *Spain* **38** E3
Calamonte *Spain* **37** G4
Călan *Romania* **28** E7
Calañas *Spain* **37** H4
Calanda *Spain* **38** D4
Calang *Indonesia* **62** D1
Calangiánus *Italy* **42** B2
Calanscio, Sarīr *Libya* **79** C10
Calapan *Phil.* **61** E4
Călărași *Moldova* **29** C13
Călărași *Romania* **29** F12
Călărași □ *Romania* **29** F12
Calasparra *Spain* **39** G3
Calatafimi *Italy* **42** E5
Calatayud *Spain* **38** D3
Călățele *Romania* **28** D8
Calato = Kalathos *Greece* **47** E10
Calauag *Phil.* **61** E5
Calavà, C. *Italy* **43** D7
Calavite, C. *Phil.* **61** E4
Calayan *Phil.* **61** B4
Calca *Peru* **124** F4
Calcasieu L. *U.S.A.* **116** G8
Calcium *U.S.A.* **115** B9
Calcutta = Kolkata *India* **69** H13
Calcutta *U.S.A.* **114** F4
Caldaro *Italy* **41** B8
Caldas da Rainha *Portugal* **37** F1
Caldas de Reis *Spain* **36** C2

Calder ➔ *U.K.* **14** D6
Caldera *Chile* **126** B1
Caldera de Taburiente △
  Canary Is. **48** F2
Caldwell *Idaho, U.S.A.* **108** E5
Caldwell *Kans., U.S.A.* **112** G5
Caldwell *Tex., U.S.A.* **116** F6
Caledon *Canada* **114** C5
Caledon *S. Africa* **88** E2
Caledon ➔ *S. Africa* **88** E4
Caledon B. *Australia* **94** A2
Caledonia *Canada* **114** C5
Caledonia *U.S.A.* **114** D7
Calella *Spain* **38** D7
Calemba *Angola* **88** B2
Calen *Australia* **94** b
Calenzana *France* **21** F12
Caletones *Chile* **126** B1
Calexico *U.S.A.* **111** N11
Calf of Man *I. of Man* **14** C3
Calgary *Canada* **102** C6
Calheta *Madeira* **48** D2
Calhoun *U.S.A.* **117** D12
Cali *Colombia* **124** C3
Calicut *India* **66** P9
Caliente *U.S.A.* **109** H6
California *Mo., U.S.A.* **112** F7
California *Pa., U.S.A.* **114** F5
California □ *U.S.A.* **110** H7
California, Baja, T.N. =
  Baja California □ *Mexico* **118** B2
California, Baja, T.S. = Baja
  California Sur □ *Mexico* **118** B2
California, G. de *Mexico* **118** B2
California City *U.S.A.* **111** K9
California Hot Springs
  U.S.A. **111** K8
Cälilabad *Azerbaijan* **73** C13
Calilegua △ *Argentina* **126** B3
Cälimäneşti *Romania* **29** E9
Cälimani, Munţii *Romania* **29** C10
Calingasta *Argentina* **126** C2
Calipatria *U.S.A.* **111** M11
Calistoga *U.S.A.* **110** G4
Calitri *Italy* **43** B8
Calitzdorp *S. Africa* **88** E3
Callabonna, L. *Australia* **95** D3
Callac *France* **18** D3
Callan *Ireland* **12** D4
Callander *U.K.* **13** E4
Callao *Peru* **124** F3
Callicoon *U.S.A.* **115** E9
Calling Lake *Canada* **102** B6
Calliope *Australia* **94** C5
Callosa de Segura *Spain* **39** G4
Callosa d'En Sarrià *Spain* **39** G4
Calma, Costa de la *Spain* **48** B9
Calne *U.K.* **15** F6
Calola *Angola* **88** B2
Calolbon = San Andres *Phil.* **61** E6
Calonge *Spain* **38** D8
Caloocan *Phil.* **61** D4
Calore ➔ *Italy* **43** A7
Caloundra *Australia* **95** D5
Calpe *Spain* **39** G5
Calpella *U.S.A.* **110** F3
Calpine *U.S.A.* **110** F3
Calstock *Canada* **104** C3
Caltabellotta *Italy* **42** E6
Caltagirone *Italy* **43** E7
Caltanissetta *Italy* **43** E7
Çaltılıbük *Turkey* **45** G12
Caluire-et-Cuire *France* **19** G11
Calulo *Angola* **84** G2
Caluso *Italy* **40** C4
Calvados □ *France* **18** C6
Calvert ➔ *Australia* **94** B2
Calvert I. *Canada* **102** C3
Calvert Ra. *Australia* **92** D3
Calvi *France* **21** F12
Calvià *Spain* **48** B9
Calvillo *Mexico* **118** C4
Calvinia *S. Africa* **88** E2
Calvo, Mte. *Italy* **41** G12
Calwa *U.S.A.* **110** J7
Calzada Almuradiel =
  Almuradiel *Spain* **37** G7
Calzada de Calatrava *Spain* **37** G7
Cam ➔ *U.K.* **15** E8
Cam Lam *Vietnam* **65** G7
Cam Pha *Vietnam* **58** G6
Cam Ranh *Vietnam* **65** G7
Cam Xuyen *Vietnam* **64** C6
Camabatela *Angola* **84** G3
Camacha *Madeira* **48** D3
Camacupa *Angola* **85** G3
Camagüey *Cuba* **120** B4
Camaiore *Italy* **40** E7
Camaná *Peru* **124** G4
Camanche Res. *U.S.A.* **110** G6
Camaquã *Brazil* **127** C5
Camaquã ➔ *Brazil* **127** C5
Câmara de Lobos *Madeira* **48** D3
Camararat, C. *France* **21** E10
Camarès *France* **20** E6
Camaret-sur-Mer *France* **18** D2
Camargo *Mexico* **119** B5
Camargue *France* **21** E8

Camargue △ *France* **21** E8
Camarillo *U.S.A.* **111** L7
Camariñas *Spain* **36** B1
Camarón, C. *Honduras* **120** C2
Camarones *Argentina* **128** E3
Camas *Spain* **37** H4
Camas *U.S.A.* **110** E4
Camas Valley *U.S.A.* **108** E2
Cambará *Australia* **92** C3
Cambará *Brazil* **127** A5
Cambay = Khambhat *India* **68** H5
Cambay, G. of =
  Khambhat, G. of *India* **66** J8
Cambil *Spain* **37** H7
Cambo-les-Bains *France* **20** E2
Cambodia ■ *Asia* **64** F5
Camborne *U.K.* **15** G2
Cambrai *France* **19** B10
Cambre *Spain* **36** B2
Cambria *U.S.A.* **110** K5
Cambrian Mts. *U.K.* **15** E4
Cambridge *Canada* **114** C4
Cambridge *Jamaica* **120** a
Cambridge *N.Z.* **91** B5
Cambridge *U.K.* **15** E8
Cambridge *Mass., U.S.A.* **115** D13
Cambridge *Minn., U.S.A.* **112** C7
Cambridge *N.Y., U.S.A.* **115** C11
Cambridge *Nebr., U.S.A.* **112** E4
Cambridge *Ohio, U.S.A.* **114** F3
Cambridge Bay *Canada* **100** D11
Cambridge G. *Australia* **92** B4
Cambridge Springs *U.S.A.* **114** E4
Cambridgeshire □ *U.K.* **15** E7
Cambrils *Spain* **38** D6
Cambuci *Brazil* **127** A7
Cambundi-Catembo *Angola* **84** G3
Camden *Australia* **95** B5
Camden *Ala., U.S.A.* **117** F11
Camden *Ark., U.S.A.* **116** E8
Camden *Maine, U.S.A.* **113** C19
Camden *N.J., U.S.A.* **115** G9
Camden *N.Y., U.S.A.* **115** C9
Camden *S.C., U.S.A.* **117** D14
Camden Sd. *Australia* **92** C3
Camdenton *U.S.A.* **112** F7
Camelford *U.K.* **15** G3
Çameli *Turkey* **47** D11
Camenca *Moldova* **29** B13
Camerino *Italy* **41** E10
Cameron *Ariz., U.S.A.* **109** J8
Cameron *La., U.S.A.* **116** G8
Cameron *Mo., U.S.A.* **112** F6
Cameron *Tex., U.S.A.* **116** F6
Cameron Highlands *Malaysia* **65** K3
Cameron Hills *Canada* **102** B5
Cameroon ■ *Africa* **79** G7
Cameroun ➔ *Cameroon* **83** E6
Cameroun, Mt. *Cameroon* **83** E6
Cametá *Brazil* **125** D9
Camerota *Italy* **43** B8
Camiçi Gölü *Turkey* **47** D9
Camiguin □ *Phil.* **61** G6
Camiguin I. *Phil.* **61** B4
Camiling *Phil.* **61** D4
Camilla *U.S.A.* **117** F12
Caminha *Portugal* **36** D2
Camino *U.S.A.* **110** G6
Cammal *U.S.A.* **114** E7
Cammarata *Italy* **42** E6
Camocim *Brazil* **125** D10
Camooweal *Australia* **94** B2
Camooweal Caves △
  Australia **94** C2
Camopi *Fr. Guiana* **125** C8
Camotes Is. *Phil.* **61** F6
Camotes Sea *Phil.* **61** F6
Camp Hill *U.S.A.* **114** F8
Camp Nelson *U.S.A.* **111** J8
Camp Pendleton *U.S.A.* **111** M9
Camp Verde *U.S.A.* **109** J8
Camp Wood *U.S.A.* **116** G4
Campagna *Italy* **43** B8
Campana *Argentina* **126** C4
Campana, I. *Chile* **128** F1
Campanário *Madeira* **48** D2
Campanario *Spain* **37** G5
Campanet *Spain* **48** B9
Campánia □ *Italy* **43** B7
Campbell *S. Africa* **88** D3
Campbell *Calif., U.S.A.* **110** H5
Campbell *Ohio, U.S.A.* **114** E4
Campbell I. *Pac. Oc.* **96** N8
Campbell L. *Canada* **103** A7
Campbell Plateau *S. Ocean* **5** A11
Campbell River *Canada* **102** C3
Campbellford *Canada* **114** B7
Campbellpur *Pakistan* **68** C5
Campbellsville *U.S.A.* **113** G11
Campbellton *Canada* **105** C6
Campbelltown *Australia* **95** E5
Campbeltown *U.K.* **13** F3
Campeche *Mexico* **119** D6
Campeche □ *Mexico* **119** D6
Campeche, Golfo de *Mexico* **119** D6
Câmpeni *Romania* **28** D8
Camperdown *Australia* **95** F3
Camperville *Canada* **103** C8

Câmpia Turzii *Romania* **29** D8
Campidano *Italy* **42** C1
Campíglia Maríttima *Italy* **40** E7
Campillo de Altobuey *Spain* **39** F3
Campillos *Spain* **37** H6
Câmpina *Romania* **29** E10
Campina Grande *Brazil* **125** E11
Campinas *Brazil* **127** A6
Campione *Italy* **21** C12
Campo *Spain* **38** C5
Campo de Criptana *Spain* **37** F7
Campo de Gibraltar *Spain* **37** J5
Campo Grande *Brazil* **125** H8
Campo Maior *Brazil* **125** D10
Campo Maior *Portugal* **37** F3
Campo Mourão *Brazil* **127** A5
Campo Túres *Italy* **41** B8
Campobasso *Italy* **41** G12
Campobello di Licata *Italy* **42** E6
Campobello di Mazara *Italy* **42** E5
Campofelice di Roccella *Italy* **42** E6
Campomarino *Italy* **41** G12
Camporeale *Italy* **42** E6
Camporrobles *Spain* **38** F3
Campos *Brazil* **127** A7
Campos *Spain* **48** B10
Campos Belos *Brazil* **125** F9
Campos del Paraíso =
  Carrascosa del Campo
  Spain **38** E2
Campos Novos *Brazil* **127** B5
Camprodon *Spain* **38** C7
Camptonville *U.S.A.* **110** F5
Camptown *U.S.A.* **115** E8
Câmpulung *Argeş, Romania* **29** E10
Câmpulung *Suceava,
  Romania* **29** C10
Câmpuri *Romania* **29** D11
Camrose *Canada* **102** C6
Camsell Portage *Canada* **103** B7
Cannóbio *Italy* **40** B5
Cannock *U.K.* **15** E5
Cannonball ➔ *U.S.A.* **112** B3
Cannondale Mt. *Australia* **94** D4
Cannonsville Res. *U.S.A.* **115** D9
Cannonvale *Australia* **94** b
Canoas *Brazil* **127** B5
Canoe L. *Canada* **103** B7
Canon City *U.S.A.* **108** G11
Cañon de Río Blanco △
  Mexico **119** D5
Cañón del Río Lobos △ *Spain* **36** D7
Cañón del Sumidero △
  Mexico **119** D5
Canonniers Pt. *Mauritius* **85** d
Canora *Canada* **103** C8
Canosa di Púglia *Italy* **43** A9
Canowindra *Australia* **95** E4
Canso *Canada* **105** C7
Cantabria □ *Spain* **36** B7
Cantabria, Sierra de *Spain* **38** C2
Cantabrian Mts. =
  Cantábrica, Cordillera
  Spain **36** C5
Cantábrica, Cordillera *Spain* **36** C5
Cantal □ *France* **20** C6
Cantal, Plomb du *France* **20** C6
Cantanhede *Portugal* **36** E2
Cantavieja *Spain* **38** E4
Čantavir *Serbia* **28** E4
Cantemir *Moldova* **29** D13
Canterbury *Australia* **94** D3
Canterbury *U.K.* **15** F9
Canterbury Bight *N.Z.* **91** F3
Canterbury Plains *N.Z.* **91** E3
Cantil *U.S.A.* **111** K9
Cantillana *Spain* **37** H5
Canton = Guangzhou *China* **59** F9
Canton *Ga., U.S.A.* **117** D12
Canton *Ill., U.S.A.* **112** E8
Canton *Miss., U.S.A.* **117** E9
Canton *Mo., U.S.A.* **112** E8
Canton *N.Y., U.S.A.* **115** B9
Canton *Ohio, U.S.A.* **114** F3
Canton *S. Dak., U.S.A.* **112** D5
Canton *L. U.S.A.* **116** C5
Cantù *Italy* **40** C6
Canudos *Brazil* **124** E7
Canumã ➔ *Brazil* **124** D7
Canutama *Brazil* **124** E6
Canutillo *U.S.A.* **116** F1
Canvey *U.K.* **15** F8
Canyon *U.S.A.* **116** D4
Canyon De Chelly △ *U.S.A.* **109** H9
Canyonlands △ *U.S.A.* **109** G9
Canyons of the Ancients △
  U.S.A. **109** H9
Canyonville *U.S.A.* **108** E2
Cao Bang *Vietnam* **58** F6
Cao He ➔ *China* **57** D13
Cao Lanh *Vietnam* **65** G5
Cao Xian *China* **56** G8
Cáorle *Italy* **41** C9
Cap-aux-Meules *Canada* **105** C7
Cap-Chat *Canada* **105** C6
Cap-de-la-Madeleine *Canada* **104** C5
Cap-Haïtien *Haiti* **121** C5
Cap Pt. *St. Lucia* **121** f

Canet-Plage *France* **20** F7
Cañete *Chile* **126** D1
Cañete *Spain* **38** E3
Cañete de las Torres *Spain* **37** H7
Cangas *Spain* **36** C2
Cangas de Onís *Spain* **36** B5
Cangas del Narcea *Spain* **36** B4
Cangnan *China* **59** D13
Canguaretama *Brazil* **125** E11
Canguçu *Brazil* **127** C5
Canguçu, Serra do *Brazil* **127** C5
Cangwu *China* **59** F8
Cangxi *China* **58** B5
Cangzhou *China* **56** E9
Caniapiscau ➔ *Canada* **105** A6
Caniapiscau, L. *Canada* **105** B6
Canicatti *Italy* **42** E6
Canicattini Bagni *Italy* **43** E8
Caniles *Spain* **37** H8
Canim Lake *Canada* **102** C4
Canindeyu □ *Paraguay* **127** A5
Canino *Italy* **41** F8
Canisteo *U.S.A.* **114** D7
Canisteo ➔ *U.S.A.* **114** D7
Cañitas de Felipe Pescador
  Mexico **119** C5
Cañizal *Spain* **36** D5
Canjáyar *Spain* **37** H8
Çankırı *Turkey* **72** B5
Çankırı □ *Turkey* **72** B5
Cankuzo *Burundi* **86** C3
Canmore *Canada* **102** C5
Cann River *Australia* **95** F4
Canna *U.K.* **13** D2
Cannanore *India* **66** P9
Cannes *France* **21** E11
Canning Town = Port
  Canning *India* **69** H13
Cannington *Canada* **114** B5

Capac *U.S.A.* **114** C2
Capáccio *Italy* **43** B8
Capaci *Italy* **42** D6
Capanaparo ➔ *Venezuela* **124** B5
Capánnori *Italy* **40** E7
Capbreton *France* **20** E2
Capdenac *France* **20** D6
Capdepera *Spain* **38** F8
Cape ➔ *Australia* **94** C4
Cape Arid △ *Australia* **93** F3
Cape Barren I. *Australia* **95** G4
Cape Breton Highlands △
  Canada **105** C7
Cape Breton I. *Canada* **105** C7
Cape Charles *U.S.A.* **113** G15
Cape Coast *Ghana* **83** D4
Cape Cod △ *U.S.A.* **113** E18
Cape Coral *U.S.A.* **117** H14
Cape Crawford *Australia* **94** B2
Cape Dorset = Kinngait
  Canada **101** E16
Cape Fear ➔ *U.S.A.* **117** E15
Cape Girardeau *U.S.A.* **112** G9
Cape Hatteras △ *U.S.A.* **117** D7
Cape Hillsborough △ *Australia* **94** b
Cape Le Grand △ *Australia* **93** F3
Cape Lookout △ *U.S.A.* **117** D16
Cape May *U.S.A.* **113** F16
Cape May Point *U.S.A.* **113** F16
Cape Melville △ *Australia* **94** A3
Cape Mount △ *Liberia* **82** D2
Cape Range △ *Australia* **92** D1
Cape St. George *Canada* **105** C8
Cape Tormentine *Canada* **105** C7
Cape Town *S. Africa* **88** E2
Cape Upstart △ *Australia* **94** B4
Cape Verde Is. ■ *Atl. Oc.* **78** b
Cape Vincent *U.S.A.* **115** B8
Cape York Peninsula
  Australia **94** A3
Capela *Brazil* **125** F11
Capella *Australia* **94** C4
Capendu *France* **20** E6
Capestang *France* **20** E7
Capesterre-Belle-Eau
  Guadeloupe **120** b
Capesterre-de-Marie-
  Galante *Guadeloupe* **120** b
Capim ➔ *Brazil* **125** D9
Capistrello *Italy* **41** G10
Capitan *U.S.A.* **109** K11
Capitán Arturo Prat
  Antarctica **5** C17
Capitol Reef △ *U.S.A.* **109** G8
Capitola *U.S.A.* **110** J5
Capizzi *Italy* **43** E7
Capo d'Orlando *Italy* **43** E7
Capodichino, Nápoli ✈
  (NAP) *Italy* **43** B7
Capoterra *Italy* **42** C1
Cappadocia *Turkey* **72** C6
Capraia *Italy* **40** E6
Caprara, Pta. *Italy* **42** A1
Caprarola *Italy* **41** F9
Capreol *Canada* **104** C3
Caprera *Italy* **42** A2
Capri *Italy* **43** B7
Capricorn Coast *Australia* **94** C5
Capricorn Group *Australia* **94** C5
Capricorn Ra. *Australia* **92** D2
Caprino Veronese *Italy* **40** C7
Caprivi Game △ *Namibia* **88** B3
Caprivi Strip *Namibia* **88** B3
Caps et Marais d'Opale △
  France **19** B9
Captains Flat *Australia* **95** F4
Captieux *France* **20** D3
Capulin Volcano △ *U.S.A.* **116** C3
Caquetá ➔ *Colombia* **124** D5
Caracal *Romania* **29** F9
Caracas *Venezuela* **124** A5
Caracol *Belize* **120** C2
Caracol *Mato Grosso do Sul,
  Brazil* **126** A4
Caracol *Piauí, Brazil* **125** E10
Carajas *Brazil* **125** E8
Carajás, Serra dos *Brazil* **125** E8
Carangola *Brazil* **127** A7
Caransebeş *Romania* **28** E7
Carantec *France* **18** D3
Caraquet *Canada* **105** C6
Caraş Severin □ *Romania* **28** E7
Caraşova *Romania* **28** E6
Caratasca, L. de *Honduras* **120** C3
Caratinga *Brazil* **125** G10
Caraúbas *Brazil* **125** E11
Caravaca de la Cruz *Spain* **39** G3
Caravággio *Italy* **40** C6
Caravela *Guinea-Biss.* **82** C1
Caravelas *Brazil* **125** G11
Caraveli *Peru* **124** G4
Caravelle, Presqu'île de la
  Martinique **120** c
Caraz *Peru* **124** E3
Carazinho *Brazil* **127** B5
Carballino = O Carballiño
  Spain **36** C2
Carballo *Spain* **36** B2

Carberry *Canada* **103** D9
Carbó *Mexico* **118** B2
Carbón, L. del *Argentina* **122** G3
Carbonara, C. *Italy* **42** C2
Carbondale *Colo., U.S.A.* **108** G10
Carbondale *Ill., U.S.A.* **112** G9
Carbondale *Pa., U.S.A.* **115** E9
Carbonear *Canada* **105** C9
Carboneras *Spain* **39** J3
Carboneras de Guadazaón
  Spain **38** F3
Carbónia *Italy* **42** C1
Carcabuey *Spain* **37** H6
Carcagente = Carcaixent
  Spain **39** F4
Carcaixent *Spain* **39** F4
Carcajou *Canada* **102** B5
Carcar *Phil.* **61** F5
Carcarana ➔ *Argentina* **126** C3
Carcasse, C. *Haiti* **121** C5
Carcassonne *France* **20** E6
Carcross *Canada* **102** A2
Çardak *Çanakkale, Turkey* **45** F10
Çardak *Denizli, Turkey* **47** D11
Cardamon Hills *India* **66** Q10
Cardamon Mts. =
  Kravanh, Chuor Phnum
  Cambodia **65** G4
Cardeña *Spain* **37** G6
Cárdenas *Cuba* **120** B3
Cárdenas *San Luis Potosí,
  Mexico* **119** C5
Cárdenas *Tabasco, Mexico* **119** D6
Cardener ➔ *Spain* **38** D6
Cardenete *Spain* **38** F3
Cardiff *U.K.* **15** F4
Cardiff □ *U.K.* **15** F4
Cardiff-by-the-Sea *U.S.A.* **111** M9
Cardigan *U.K.* **15** E3
Cardigan B. *U.K.* **15** E3
Cardinal *Canada* **115** B9
Cardona *Spain* **38** D6
Cardona *Uruguay* **126** C4
Cardoso, Ilha do *Brazil* **127** B5
Cardston *Canada* **102** D6
Cardwell *Australia* **94** B4
Careen L. *Canada* **103** B7
Carei *Romania* **28** C7
Careme = Ciremay *Indonesia* **63** G13
Carentan *France* **18** C5
Carey *U.S.A.* **108** E7
Carey, L. *Australia* **93** E3
Carey L. *Canada* **103** A8
Careysburg *Liberia* **82** D2
Cargèse *France* **21** F12
Carhaix-Plouguer *France* **18** D3
Carhué *Argentina* **126** D3
Caria *Turkey* **47** D10
Cariacica *Brazil* **125** H10
Cariati *Italy* **43** C9
Caribbean Sea *W. Indies* **121** D5
Cariboo Mts. *Canada* **102** C4
Caribou *U.S.A.* **113** B19
Caribou ➔ *Man., Canada* **103** B10
Caribou ➔ *N.W.T., Canada* **102** A3
Caribou I. *Canada* **104** C2
Caribou Is. *Canada* **102** A6
Caribou L. *Man., Canada* **103** B9
Caribou L. *Ont., Canada* **104** B2
Caribou Mts. *Canada* **102** B5
Caribou River △ *Canada* **103** B9
Caribrod = Dimitrovgrad
  Serbia **44** C6
Carichíc *Mexico* **118** B3
Carigara *Phil.* **61** F6
Carignan *France* **19** C12
Carignano *Italy* **40** D4
Carinda *Australia* **95** E4
Cariñena *Spain* **38** D3
Carinhanha *Brazil* **125** F10
Carinhanha ➔ *Brazil* **125** F10
Carini *Italy* **42** D6
Cariño *Spain* **36** B3
Carínola *Italy* **42** A6
Carinthia = Kärnten □
  Austria **26** E6
Caripito *Venezuela* **124** A6
Carlet *Spain* **39** F4
Carleton, Mt. *Canada* **105** C6
Carleton Place *Canada* **115** A8
Carletonville *S. Africa* **88** D4
Cârlibaba *Romania* **29** C10
Carlin *U.S.A.* **108** F5
Carlingford L. *U.K.* **12** B5
Carlinville *U.S.A.* **112** F9
Carlisle *U.K.* **14** C5
Carlisle *U.S.A.* **114** F7
Carlisle B. *Barbados* **121** g
Carlisle I. *Australia* **94** b
Carlit, Pic *France* **20** F5
Carloforte *Italy* **42** C1
Carlos Casares *Argentina* **126** D3
Carlos Tejedor *Argentina* **126** D3
Carlow *Ireland* **12** D5
Carlow □ *Ireland* **12** D5
Carlsbad *Calif., U.S.A.* **111** M9
Carlsbad *N. Mex., U.S.A.* **109** K11
Carlsbad Caverns △ *U.S.A.* **109** K11
Carluke *U.K.* **13** F5

Carlyle *Canada* **103** D8
Carmacks *Canada* **100** E4
Carmagnola *Italy* **40** D4
Carman *Canada* **103** D9
Carmarthen *U.K.* **15** F3
Carmarthen B. *U.K.* **15** F3
Carmarthenshire □ *U.K.* **15** F3
Carmaux *France* **20** D6
Carmel *U.S.A.* **115** E11
Carmel-by-the-Sea *U.S.A.* **110** J5
Carmel Valley *U.S.A.* **110** J5
Carmelo *Uruguay* **126** C4
Carmen *Paraguay* **127** B4
Carmen ➜ *Mexico* **118** A3
Carmen, I. *Mexico* **118** B2
Carmen de Patagones
  Argentina **128** E4
Cármenes *Spain* **36** C5
Carmensa *Argentina* **126** D2
Carmi *Canada* **102** D5
Carmi *U.S.A.* **112** F9
Carmichael *U.S.A.* **110** G5
Carmila *Australia* **94** C4
Carmona *Costa Rica* **120** E2
Carmona *Spain* **37** H5
Carn Ban *U.K.* **13** D4
Carn Eige *U.K.* **13** D3
Carnac *France* **18** E3
Carnamah *Australia* **93** E2
Carnarvon *Australia* **93** D1
Carnarvon *Canada* **114** A6
Carnarvon *S. Africa* **88** E3
Carnarvon ➜ *Australia* **94** C4
Carnarvon Ra. *Queens.,*
  Australia **94** D4
Carnarvon Ra. *W. Austral.,*
  Australia **93** E3
Carnation *U.S.A.* **110** C5
Carncastle *U.K.* **12** B6
Carndonagh *Ireland* **12** A4
Carnduff *Canada* **103** D8
Carnegie *U.S.A.* **114** F4
Carnegie, L. *Australia* **93** E3
Carnegie Ridge *Pac. Oc.* **97** H19
Carnic Alps = Karnische
  Alpen *Europe* **26** E6
Carniche Alpi = Karnische
  Alpen *Europe* **26** E6
Carnot *C.A.R.* **84** D3
Carnot, C. *Australia* **95** E2
Carnot B. *Australia* **92** C3
Carnoustie *U.K.* **13** E6
Carnsore Pt. *Ireland* **12** D5
Caro *U.S.A.* **113** D12
Caroga Lake *U.S.A.* **115** C10
Carol City *U.S.A.* **117** J14
Carolina *Brazil* **125** E9
Carolina *Puerto Rico* **121** d
Carolina *S. Africa* **89** D5
Caroline I. *Kiribati* **97** H12
Caroline Is. *Micronesia* **96** G6
Caroni *Trin. & Tob.* **125** K15
Caroní ➜ *Venezuela* **124** B6
Caronie = Nébrodi, Monti
  Italy **43** E7
Caroona *Australia* **95** E5
Carpathians *Europe* **23** D11
Carpaţii Meridionali *Romania* **29** E9
Carpentaria, G. of *Australia* **94** A2
Carpentras *France* **21** D9
Carpi *Italy* **40** D7
Cărpineni *Moldova* **29** D13
Carpinteria *U.S.A.* **111** L7
Carpio *Spain* **36** D5
Carr Boyd Ra. *Australia* **92** C4
Carra, L. *Ireland* **12** C2
Carrabelle *U.S.A.* **117** G12
Carraig Mhachdire Rois =
  Carrickmacross *Ireland* **12** C5
Carraig na Siúire =
  Carrick-on-Suir *Ireland* **12** D4
Carral *Spain* **36** B2
Carranya ◎ *Australia* **92** C4
Carranza, Presa V. *Mexico* **118** B4
Carrara *Italy* **40** D7
Carrascal *Phil.* **61** G6
Carrascosa del Campo *Spain* **38** E2
Carrauntoohill *Ireland* **12** D2
Carrick-on-Shannon *Ireland* **12** C3
Carrick-on-Suir *Ireland* **12** D4
Carrickfergus *U.K.* **12** B6
Carrieton *Australia* **95** E2
Carrillo *Mexico* **118** B4
Carrington *U.S.A.* **112** B4
Carrión ➜ *Spain* **36** D6
Carrión de los Condes *Spain* **36** C6
Carrizal Bajo *Chile* **126** B1
Carrizalillo *Chile* **126** B1
Carrizo Cr. ➜ *U.S.A.* **109** H12
Carrizo Plain △ *U.S.A.* **110** K7
Carrizo Springs *U.S.A.* **116** G5
Carrizozo *U.S.A.* **109** K11
Carroll *U.S.A.* **112** D6
Carrollton *Ga., U.S.A.* **117** E12
Carrollton *Ill., U.S.A.* **112** F8
Carrollton *Ky., U.S.A.* **113** F11
Carrollton *Mo., U.S.A.* **112** F7
Carrollton *Ohio, U.S.A.* **114** F3

Carron ➜ *U.K.* **13** D4
Carron, L. *U.K.* **13** D3
Carrot ➜ *Canada* **103** C8
Carrot River *Canada* **103** C8
Carrouges *France* **18** D6
Carrù *Italy* **40** D4
Carruthers *Canada* **103** C7
Carsa Dek *Ethiopia* **81** F4
Çarşamba *Turkey* **72** B7
Carsóli *Italy* **41** F10
Carson *Calif., U.S.A.* **111** M8
Carson *N. Dak., U.S.A.* **112** B3
Carson ➜ *U.S.A.* **110** F8
Carson City *U.S.A.* **110** F7
Carson Sink *U.S.A.* **108** G4
Cartagena *Colombia* **124** A3
Cartagena *Spain* **39** H4
Cartago *Colombia* **124** C3
Cartago *Costa Rica* **120** E3
Cártama *Spain* **37** J6
Cartaxo *Portugal* **37** F2
Cartaya *Spain* **37** H3
Cartersville *U.S.A.* **117** D12
Carterton *N.Z.* **91** D5
Carthage *Tunisia* **42** F3
Carthage *Ill., U.S.A.* **112** E8
Carthage *Mo., U.S.A.* **112** G6
Carthage *N.Y., U.S.A.* **113** D16
Carthage *Tex., U.S.A.* **116** E7
Cartier I. *Australia* **92** B3
Cartwright *Canada* **105** B8
Caruaru *Brazil* **125** E11
Carúpano *Venezuela* **124** A6
Caruthersville *U.S.A.* **112** G9
Carvin *France* **19** B9
Carvoeiro *Brazil* **124** D6
Carvoeiro, C. *Portugal* **37** F1
Cary *U.S.A.* **117** D15
Casa, Pas de la = Envalira,
  Port d' *Europe* **38** C6
Casa Branca *Portugal* **37** G2
Casa de Piedra *Argentina* **126** D2
Casa de Piedra, Embalse
  Argentina **126** D2
Casa Grande *U.S.A.* **109** K8
Casa Nova *Brazil* **125** E10
Casablanca *Chile* **126** C1
Casablanca *Morocco* **78** B4
Casacalenda *Italy* **41** G11
Casalbordino *Italy* **41** F11
Casale Monferrato *Italy* **40** C5
Casalmaggiore *Italy* **40** D7
Casalpusterlengo *Italy* **40** C6
Casamance ➜ *Senegal* **82** C1
Casarano *Italy* **43** B11
Casares *Spain* **37** J5
Casas Ibáñez *Spain* **39** F3
Casasimarro *Spain* **39** F2
Casatejada *Spain* **36** F5
Casavieja *Spain* **36** E6
Cascada de Basaseachic △
  Mexico **118** B3
Cascade *Seychelles* **85** b
Cascade *Idaho, U.S.A.* **108** D5
Cascade *Mont., U.S.A.* **108** C8
Cascade Locks *U.S.A.* **110** D5
Cascade Ra. *U.S.A.* **110** D5
Cascade Res. *U.S.A.* **108** D5
Cascades, Pte. des *Réunion* **85** c
Cascais *Portugal* **37** G1
Cascavel *Brazil* **127** A5
Cáscina *Italy* **40** E7
Casco B. *U.S.A.* **113** D19
Caselle Torinese *Italy* **40** C4
Caserta *Italy* **43** A7
Casey *Antarctica* **5** C8
Caseyr, Raas = Asir, Ras
  Somali Rep. **75** E5
Cashel *Ireland* **12** D4
Casiguran *Phil.* **61** C5
Casilda *Argentina* **126** C3
Casimcea *Romania* **29** F13
Casino *Australia* **95** D5
Casiquiare ➜ *Venezuela* **124** C5
Casma *Peru* **124** E3
Casmalia *U.S.A.* **111** L6
Cásola Valsénio *Italy* **41** D8
Cásoli *Italy* **41** F11
Caspe *Spain* **38** D4
Casper *U.S.A.* **108** E10
Caspian Depression *Eurasia* **35** G9
Caspian Sea *Eurasia* **35** G9
Cass City *U.S.A.* **114** C1
Cass Lake *U.S.A.* **112** B6
Cassà de la Selva *Spain* **38** D7
Cassadaga *U.S.A.* **114** D5
Cassel *France* **19** B9
Casselman *Canada* **115** A9
Casselton *U.S.A.* **112** B5
Cassiar Mts. *Canada* **102** B2
Cassino *Italy* **42** A6
Cassis *France* **21** E9
Castagneto Carducci *Italy* **40** E7
Castaic *U.S.A.* **111** L8
Castalia *U.S.A.* **114** E2
Castanhal *Brazil* **125** D9

Castara *Trin. & Tob.* **125** J16
Castéggio *Italy* **40** C6
Castejón de Monegros *Spain* **38** D4
Castèl di Sangro *Italy* **41** G11
Castèl San Giovanni *Italy* **40** C6
Castèl San Pietro Terme *Italy* **41** D8
Castelbuono *Italy* **43** E7
Castelfidardo *Italy* **41** E10
Castelfiorentino *Italy* **40** E7
Castelfranco Emília *Italy* **40** D8
Castelfranco Véneto *Italy* **41** C8
Casteljaloux *France* **20** D4
Castellabate *Italy* **43** B7
Castellammare, G. di *Italy* **42** D5
Castellammare del Golfo
  Italy **42** D5
Castellammare di Stábia
  Italy **43** B7
Castellamonte *Italy* **40** C4
Castellane *France* **21** E10
Castellaneta *Italy* **43** B9
Castelli *Argentina* **126** D4
Castelló de la Plana *Spain* **38** F4
Castellón de la Plana □ *Spain* **38** E4
Castellote *Spain* **38** E4
Castelmáuro *Italy* **41** G11
Castelnau-de-Médoc *France* **20** C3
Castelnau-Magnoac *France* **20** E4
Castelnaudary *France* **20** E5
Castelnovo ne' Monti *Italy* **40** D7
Castelnuovo di Val di
  Cécina *Italy* **40** E7
Castelo *Brazil* **127** A7
Castelo Branco *Portugal* **36** F3
Castelo Branco □ *Portugal* **36** F3
Castelo de Paiva *Portugal* **36** D2
Castelo de Vide *Portugal* **37** F3
Castelsardo *Italy* **42** B1
Castelsarrasin *France* **20** D5
Casteltérmini *Italy* **42** E6
Castelvetrano *Italy* **42** E5
Casterton *Australia* **95** F3
Castets *France* **20** E2
Castiglion Fiorentino *Italy* **41** E8
Castiglione del Lago *Italy* **41** E9
Castiglione della Pescáia
  Italy **40** F7
Castiglione delle Stiviere
  Italy **40** C7
Castilblanco *Spain* **37** F5
Castile *U.S.A.* **114** D6
Castilla, Playa de *Spain* **37** J4
Castilla-La Mancha □ *Spain* **37** F7
Castilla y León □ *Spain* **36** D6
Castillo de Locubín *Spain* **37** H7
Castillon-en-Couserans
  France **20** F5
Castillonès *France* **20** D4
Castillos *Uruguay* **127** C5
Castle Dale *U.S.A.* **108** G8
Castle Douglas *U.K.* **13** G5
Castle Rock *Colo., U.S.A.* **108** G11
Castle Rock *Wash., U.S.A.* **110** D4
Castlebar *Ireland* **12** C2
Castlebay *U.K.* **13** E1
Castleblaney *Ireland* **12** B5
Castlederg *U.K.* **12** B4
Castleford *U.K.* **14** D6
Castlegar *Canada* **102** D5
Castlemaine *Australia* **95** F3
Castlemaine *Ireland* **12** D2
Castlepollard *Ireland* **12** C4
Castlerea *Ireland* **12** C3
Castlereagh ➜ *Australia* **95** E4
Castlereagh B. *Australia* **94** A2
Castleton *U.S.A.* **115** C11
Castleton-on-Hudson
  U.S.A. **115** D11
Castletown *I. of Man* **14** C3
Castletown Bearhaven
  Ireland **12** E2
Castor *Canada* **102** C6
Castor ➜ *Canada* **104** B4
Castorland *U.S.A.* **115** C9
Castres *France* **20** E6
Castricum *Neths.* **17** B4
Castries *St. Lucia* **121** f
Castril *Spain* **37** H8
Castro *Brazil* **127** A6
Castro *Chile* **128** E2
Castro Alves *Brazil* **125** F11
Castro del Río *Spain* **37** H6
Castro-Urdiales *Spain* **36** B7
Castro Valley *U.S.A.* **110** H4
Castro Verde *Portugal* **37** H2
Castrojeriz *Spain* **36** C6
Castropol *Spain* **36** B4
Castroreale *Italy* **43** D8
Castrovíllari *Italy* **43** C9
Castroville *U.S.A.* **110** J5
Castuera *Spain* **37** G5
Çat *Turkey* **73** C9
Cat Ba, Dao *Vietnam* **64** B6
Cat Ba △ *Vietnam* **64** B6
Cat I. *Bahamas* **121** B4
Cat L. *Canada* **104** B1
Cat Lake *Canada* **104** B1
Cat Tien △ *Vietnam* **65** G6
Čata *Slovak Rep.* **27** D11

Catacamas *Honduras* **120** D2
Cataguases *Brazil* **127** A7
Çatak *Turkey* **73** C10
Çatalağzı *Turkey* **72** B4
Catalão *Brazil* **125** G9
Çatalca *Turkey* **45** C12
Catalina *Canada* **105** C9
Catalina *Chile* **126** B2
Catalina *U.S.A.* **109** K8
Catalonia = Cataluña □
  Spain **38** D6
Cataluña □ *Spain* **38** D6
Catamarca *Argentina* **126** B2
Catamarca □ *Argentina* **126** B2
Catanauan *Phil.* **61** E5
Catanduanes □ *Phil.* **61** E6
Catanduva *Brazil* **127** A6
Catánia *Italy* **43** E8
Catánia, G. di *Italy* **43** E8
Catanzaro *Italy* **43** D9
Catarman *Phil.* **61** E6
Catatumbo-Bari △ *Colombia* **121** E5
Catbalogan *Phil.* **61** F6
Catchacoma *Canada* **114** B6
Cateel *Phil.* **61** H7
Catembe *Mozam.* **89** D5
Caterham *U.K.* **15** F7
Cathair na Mart =
  Westport *Ireland* **12** C2
Cathair Saidhbhín =
  Cahersiveen *Ireland* **12** E1
Cathcart *S. Africa* **88** E4
Cathedral City *U.S.A.* **111** M10
Cathlamet *U.S.A.* **110** D3
Catió *Guinea-Biss.* **82** C1
Catlettsburg *U.S.A.* **113** F12
Catma Dağı *Turkey* **47** C11
Catoche, C. *Mexico* **119** C7
Catriló *Argentina* **126** D3
Catrimani *Brazil* **124** C6
Catrimani ➜ *Brazil* **124** C6
Catskill *U.S.A.* **115** D11
Catskill △ *U.S.A.* **115** D10
Catskill Mts. *U.S.A.* **115** D10
Catt, Mt. *Australia* **94** A1
Cattaraugus *U.S.A.* **114** D6
Catterick *U.K.* **14** C6
Cáttolica *Italy* **41** E9
Cáttolica Eraclea *Italy* **42** E6
Catuala *Angola* **88** B2
Catuane *Mozam.* **89** D5
Catur *Mozam.* **87** E4
Caubvick, Mt. = Iberville,
  Mt. d' *Canada* **101** F19
Cauca ➜ *Colombia* **124** B4
Caucaia *Brazil* **125** D11
Caucasus Mountains *Eurasia* **35** J7
Caucete *Argentina* **126** C2
Caudete *Spain* **39** G3
Caudry *France* **19** B10
Cauese Mts. *Mozam.* **87** F3
Caulnes *France* **18** D4
Caulónia *Italy* **43** D9
Caungula *Angola* **84** F3
Cauquenes *Chile* **126** D1
Caura ➜ *Venezuela* **124** B6
Cauresi ➜ *Mozam.* **87** F3
Căuşani *Moldova* **29** D14
Causapscal *Canada* **105** C6
Caussade *France* **20** D5
Causse-Méjean *France* **20** D7
Causses du Quercy △ *France* **20** D5
Cauterets *France* **20** F3
Cauvery ➜ *India* **66** P11
Caux, Pays de *France* **18** C7
Cava de' Tirreni *Italy* **43** B7
Cávado ➜ *Portugal* **36** D2
Cavagrande del Cassibile △
  Italy **43** F8
Cavaillon *France* **21** E9
Cavalaire-sur-Mer *France* **21** E10
Cavalese *Italy* **41** B8
Cavalier *U.S.A.* **112** A5
Cavalla = Cavally ➜ *Africa* **82** E3
Cavallà ➜ *Liberia* **82** D3
Cavallo, Î. de *France* **21** G13
Cavally ➜ *Africa* **82** E3
Cavan *Ireland* **12** B4
Cavan □ *Ireland* **12** C4
Cavárzere *Italy* **41** C9
Cave Creek *U.S.A.* **109** K8
Cavenagh Ra. *Australia* **93** E4
Cavendish *Australia* **95** F3
Caviana, I. *Brazil* **125** C8
Cavite *Phil.* **61** D4
Cavnic *Romania* **29** C8
Cavour *Italy* **40** D4
Cavtat *Croatia* **44** D2
Cawndilla L. *Australia* **95** E3
Cawnpore = Kanpur *India* **69** F9
Caxias *Brazil* **125** D10
Caxias do Sul *Brazil* **127** B5
Çay *Turkey* **72** C4
Cay Sal Bank *Bahamas* **120** B4
Cayambe *Ecuador* **124** C3

Çaycuma *Turkey* **72** B5
Çayeli *Turkey* **73** B9
Cayenne *Fr. Guiana* **125** B8
Cayey *Puerto Rico* **121** d
Caygören Barajı *Turkey* **47** B10
Çayıralan *Turkey* **72** C6
Çaylı *Azerbaijan* **73** B12
Caylus *France* **20** D5
Cayman Brac *Cayman Is.* **120** C4
Cayman Is. ☑ *W. Indies* **120** C3
Cayman Trough *Caribbean* **98** H11
Cayres *France* **20** D7
Cayuga *Canada* **114** D5
Cayuga *U.S.A.* **115** D8
Cayuga Heights *U.S.A.* **115** D8
Cayuga L. *U.S.A.* **115** D8
Cazalla de la Sierra *Spain* **37** H5
Căzăneşti *Romania* **29** F12
Cazaubon *France* **20** E3
Cazaux et de Sanguinet,
  Étang de *France* **20** D2
Cazenovia *U.S.A.* **115** D9
Cazères *France* **20** E5
Cazin *Bos.-H.* **41** D12
Čazma *Croatia* **41** C13
Cazombo *Angola* **85** G4
Cazorla *Spain* **37** H8
Cazorla, Sierra de *Spain* **37** G8
Cea ➜ *Spain* **36** C5
Ceamurlia de Jos *Romania* **29** F13
Ceanannus Mor *Ireland* **12** C5
Ceará = Fortaleza *Brazil* **125** D11
Ceará □ *Brazil* **125** E11
Ceará-Mirim *Brazil* **125** E11
Ceatharlach = Carlow
  Ireland **12** D5
Ceauru, L. *Romania* **29** F8
Cébaco, I. de *Panama* **120** E3
Cebollar *Argentina* **126** B2
Cebollera, Sierra de *Spain* **38** D2
Cebreros *Spain* **36** E6
Cebu *Phil.* **61** F5
Cebu □ *Phil.* **61** F5
Čečava *Bos.-H.* **28** F2
Ceccano *Italy* **42** A6
Cece *Hungary* **28** D3
Cechi *Ivory C.* **82** D4
Čechy = Bohemia *Czech Rep.* **26** A7
Cécina *Italy* **40** E7
Cécina ➜ *Italy* **40** E7
Ceclavín *Spain* **36** F4
Cedar ➜ *U.S.A.* **112** E8
Cedar City *U.S.A.* **109** H7
Cedar Creek Res. *U.S.A.* **116** E6
Cedar Falls *Iowa, U.S.A.* **112** D7
Cedar Falls *Wash., U.S.A.* **110** C5
Cedar Key *U.S.A.* **117** G13
Cedar L. *Canada* **103** C9
Cedar Park *U.S.A.* **116** F6
Cedartown *U.S.A.* **117** D12
Cedarvale *Canada* **102** B3
Cedarville *S. Africa* **89** E4
Cedeira *Spain* **36** B2
Cedral *Mexico* **118** C4
Cedrino ➜ *Italy* **42** B2
Cedro *Brazil* **125** E11
Cedros, I. *Mexico* **118** B1
Cedros B. *Trin. & Tob.* **125** K15
Ceduna *Australia* **95** E1
Ceel Gaal *Somali Rep.* **75** E5
Ceel Waaq *Kenya* **86** B5
Ceeldheere *Somali Rep.* **75** G4
Ceerigaabo *Somali Rep.* **75** E4
Cefalù *Italy* **43** D7
Cega ➜ *Spain* **36** D6
Ceglédi *Hungary* **28** C4
Céglie Messápico *Italy* **43** B10
Cehegín *Spain* **39** G3
Ceheng *China* **58** E5
Cehu-Silvaniei *Romania* **29** C8
Ceica *Romania* **28** D7
Ceira ➜ *Portugal* **36** E2
Celano *Italy* **41** F10
Celanova *Spain* **36** C3
Celaque △ *Honduras* **120** D2
Celaya *Mexico* **118** C4
Celebes = Sulawesi *Indonesia* **63** E6
Celebes Sea *Indonesia* **63** D6
Čelić *Bos.-H.* **28** F3
Celina *U.S.A.* **113** E11
Celinac *Bos.-H.* **28** F2
Celje *Slovenia* **41** B12
Celldömölk *Hungary* **28** C2
Celle *Germany* **24** C6
Celorico da Beira *Portugal* **36** E3
Celtic Sea *Atl. Oc.* **16** F2
Cenderwasih, Teluk *Indonesia* **63** E9
Cengong *China* **58** D7
Ceno ➜ *Italy* **40** D7
Centallo *Italy* **40** D4
Centelles *Spain* **38** D7
Center *N. Dak., U.S.A.* **112** B3

Center *Tex., U.S.A.* **116** F7
Centerburg *U.S.A.* **114** F2
Centerville *Calif., U.S.A.* **110** J7
Centerville *Iowa, U.S.A.* **112** E7
Centerville *Pa., U.S.A.* **114** F5
Centerville *Tenn., U.S.A.* **117** D11
Centerville *Tex., U.S.A.* **116** F7
Cento *Italy* **41** D8
Central = Tsentralnyy □
  Russia **74** C4
Central □ *Ghana* **83** D4
Central □ *Kenya* **86** C4
Central □ *Malawi* **87** E3
Central □ *Zambia* **87** E2
Central, Cordillera *Colombia* **124** C4
Central, Cordillera
  Costa Rica **120** D3
Central, Cordillera
  Dom. Rep. **121** C5
Central, Cordillera *Phil.* **61** C4
Central, Cordillera
  Puerto Rico **121** d
Central African Rep. ■
  Africa **79** G9
Central America *America* **98** H11
Central Australia ◎ *Australia* **92** D4
Central Butte *Canada* **103** C7
Central City *Colo., U.S.A.* **108** G11
Central City *Ky., U.S.A.* **112** G10
Central City *Nebr., U.S.A.* **112** E4
Central Desert ◎ *Australia* **92** C5
Central I. *Kenya* **86** B4
Central Island △ *Kenya* **86** B4
Central Kalahari △ *Botswana* **88** C3
Central Makran Range
  Pakistan **66** F4
Central Pacific Basin
  Pac. Oc. **96** G10
Central Patricia *Canada* **104** B1
Central Point *U.S.A.* **108** E2
Central Russian Uplands
  Europe **6** E13
Central Siberian Plateau
  Russia **50** B12
Central Square *U.S.A.* **115** C8
Centralia *Canada* **114** C3
Centralia *Ill., U.S.A.* **112** F9
Centralia *Mo., U.S.A.* **112** F7
Centralia *Wash., U.S.A.* **110** D4
Centre □ *Cameroon* **83** E7
Centre de Flacq *Mauritius* **85** d
Centreville *N.Y., U.S.A.* **114** D6
Centreville *Pa., U.S.A.* **114** E5
Cenxi *China* **59** F8
Čeotina ➜ *Bos.-H.* **44** C2
Cephalonia = Kefalonia
  Greece **46** C2
Čepin *Croatia* **28** E3
Ceprano *Italy* **42** A6
Ceptura *Romania* **29** E11
Cepu *Indonesia* **63** G14
Ceram = Seram *Indonesia* **63** E7
Ceram Sea = Seram Sea
  Indonesia **63** E7
Cerbère *France* **20** F7
Cerbicales, Îs. *France* **21** G13
Cercal *Portugal* **37** H2
Cerdaña *Spain* **38** C6
Cère ➜ *France* **20** D5
Cerea *Italy* **41** C8
Ceredigion □ *U.K.* **15** E3
Ceres *Argentina* **126** B3
Ceres *S. Africa* **88** E2
Ceres *U.S.A.* **110** H6
Céret *France* **20** F6
Cerf *Seychelles* **85** b
Cergy *France* **19** C9
Cerignola *Italy* **43** A8
Cerigo = Kythira *Greece* **46** E5
Cérilly *France* **19** F9
Cerisiers *France* **19** D10
Cerizay *France* **18** F6
Çerkeş *Turkey* **72** B5
Çerkezköy *Turkey* **45** E12
Cerknica *Slovenia* **41** C11
Cerkovica *Bulgaria* **45** C8
Cermerno *Serbia* **44** C4
Çermik *Turkey* **73** C8
Cerna *Romania* **29** E13
Cerna ➜ *Romania* **29** F8
Cernavodă *Romania* **29** F13
Cernay *France* **19** E14
Cernik *Croatia* **28** E2
Cerralvo, I. *Mexico* **118** C3
Cerralvo *Mexico* **118** B5
Cërrik *Albania* **44** E3
Cerritos *Mexico* **118** C4
Cerro Chato *Uruguay* **127** C4
Cerro Cofre de Perote △
  Mexico **119** D5
Cerro Corá △ *Paraguay* **127** A4
Cerro de Pasco *Peru* **124** F3
Cerro el Copey △ *Venezuela* **121** D7
Cerro Hoya △ *Panama* **120** E3
Cerro Saroche △ *Venezuela* **121** D6
Certaldo *Italy* **40** E8
Cervaro ➜ *Italy* **43** A8
Cervati, Monte *Italy* **43** B8
Cerventes = Australia *Australia* **93** F2
Cervera *Spain* **38** D6

Cervera de Pisuerga *Spain* 36 C6
Cervera del Río Alhama
  Spain 38 C3
Cervéteri *Italy* 41 F9
Cérvia *Italy* 41 D9
Cervignano del Friuli *Italy* 41 C10
Cervinara *Italy* 43 A7
Cervione *France* 21 F13
Cervo *Spain* 36 B3
Cesarò *Italy* 43 E7
Cesena *Italy* 41 D9
Cesenático *Italy* 41 D9
Cēsis *Latvia* 32 D3
Česká Lípa *Czech Rep.* 26 A7
Česká Rep. = Czech Rep. ■
  Europe 26 B8
Česká Třebová *Czech Rep.* 27 B9
České Budějovice *Czech Rep.* 26 C7
České Velenice *Czech Rep.* 26 C7
Českobudějovický □
  Czech Rep. 26 B7
Českomoravská Vrchovina
  Czech Rep. 26 B8
Český Brod *Czech Rep.* 26 A7
Český Krumlov *Czech Rep.* 26 C7
Český Těšín *Czech Rep.* 27 B11
Česma → *Croatia* 41 C13
Çeşme *Turkey* 47 C8
Cessnock *Australia* 95 E5
Cesson-Sévigné *France* 18 D5
Cestas *France* 20 D3
Cestos → *Liberia* 82 D3
Cestos Sehnkwehn △ *Liberia* 82 D3
Cetate *Romania* 28 F8
Cetin Grad *Croatia* 41 C12
Cetina → *Croatia* 41 E13
Cetinje *Montenegro* 44 D2
Cetraro *Italy* 43 C8
Ceuta *N. Afr.* 78 A4
Ceva *Italy* 40 D5
Cévennes *France* 20 D7
Cévennes △ *France* 20 D7
Ceyhan *Turkey* 72 D6
Ceyhan → *Turkey* 72 D6
Ceylanpınar *Turkey* 73 D9
Ceylon = Sri Lanka ■ *Asia* 66 R12
Cèze → *France* 21 D8
Cha-am *Thailand* 64 F2
Chabanais *France* 20 C4
Chabeuil *France* 21 D9
Chablais *France* 19 F13
Chablis *France* 19 E10
Chacabuco *Argentina* 126 C3
Chachapoyas *Peru* 124 E3
Chachoengsao *Thailand* 64 F3
Chachran *Pakistan* 68 E4
Chachro *Pakistan* 68 G4
Chaco □ *Argentina* 126 B3
Chaco □ *Paraguay* 126 B4
Chaco → *U.S.A.* 109 H9
Chaco △ *Argentina* 126 B4
Chaco Austral *S. Amer.* 128 B4
Chaco Boreal *S. Amer.* 124 H6
Chaco Central *S. Amer.* 128 A4
Chaco Culture △ *U.S.A.* 109 H10
Chacon, C. *U.S.A.* 102 C2
Chad ■ *Africa* 79 F8
Chad, L. = Tchad, L. *Chad* 79 F8
Chadileuvú → *Argentina* 126 D2
Chadron *U.S.A.* 112 D2
Chadyr-Lunga =
  Ciadâr-Lunga *Moldova* 29 D13
Chae Hom *Thailand* 64 C2
Chae Son △ *Thailand* 64 C2
Chaem → *Thailand* 64 C2
Chaeryŏng *N. Korea* 57 E13
Chafe *Nigeria* 83 C6
Chagai Hills = Chāh Gay
  Hills *Afghan.* 66 E3
Chagda *Russia* 53 D14
Chaghcharân *Afghan.* 66 B4
Chagne *Ethiopia* 81 E4
Chagny *France* 19 F11
Chagoda *Russia* 32 C8
Chagos Arch. ☑ *Ind. Oc.* 50 J9
Chagres △ *Panama* 120 E4
Chaguanas *Trin. & Tob.* 125 K15
Chāh Ākhvor *Iran* 71 C8
Chāh Bahar *Iran* 71 E9
Chāh-e Kavīr *Iran* 71 C8
Chāh Gay Hills *Afghan.* 66 E3
Chahār Borj *Iran* 73 D11
Chahār Borjak *Afghan.* 66 D3
Chahār Mahāll va
  Bakhtīarī □ *Iran* 71 C6
Chai Badan *Thailand* 64 E3
Chaibasa *India* 69 H11
Chaillé-les-Marais *France* 20 B2
Chainat *Thailand* 64 E3
Chaiya *Thailand* 65 H2
Chaiyaphum *Thailand* 64 E4
Chaj Doab *Pakistan* 68 C5
Chajari *Argentina* 126 C4
Chak Amru *Pakistan* 68 C6
Chaka *Sudan* 81 G3
Chakar → *Pakistan* 68 E3
Chakari *Zimbabwe* 89 B4
Chake Chake *Tanzania* 86 D4

Chakhānsūr *Afghan.* 66 D3
Chakonipau, L. *Canada* 105 A6
Chakradharpur *India* 69 H11
Chakrata *India* 68 D7
Chakwal *Pakistan* 68 C5
Chala *Peru* 124 G4
Chalais *France* 20 C4
Chalchihuites *Mexico* 118 C4
Chalcis = Halkida *Greece* 46 C5
Châlette-sur-Loing *France* 19 D9
Chaleur B. *Canada* 105 C6
Chalfant *U.S.A.* 110 H8
Chalhuanca *Peru* 124 F4
Chaliki *Greece* 46 B4
Chalindrey *France* 19 E12
Chaling *China* 59 D9
Chalisgaon *India* 66 J9
Chalk River *Canada* 104 C4
Chalkar, Ozero = Shalkar
  Köli *Kazakhstan* 34 E10
Chalky Inlet *N.Z.* 91 G1
Challans *France* 18 F5
Challapata *Bolivia* 124 G5
Challawa Gorge Res. *Nigeria* 83 C6
Challenger Deep *Pac. Oc.* 96 F6
Challenger Fracture Zone
  Pac. Oc. 97 L17
Challis *U.S.A.* 108 D6
Chalmette *U.S.A.* 117 G10
Chalon-sur-Saône *France* 19 F11
Chalong *Thailand* 65 a
Chalonnes-sur-Loire *France* 18 E6
Châlons-en-Champagne
  France 19 D11
Chálten, Cerro = Fitz Roy,
  Cerro *Argentina* 128 F2
Châlus *France* 20 C4
Chālūs *Iran* 71 B6
Cham *Germany* 25 F8
Cham, Cu Lao *Vietnam* 64 E7
Chama *U.S.A.* 109 H10
Chamaicó *Argentina* 126 D3
Chaman *Pakistan* 66 D5
Chamba *India* 68 C7
Chamba *Tanzania* 87 E4
Chambal → *India* 69 F8
Chamberlain *U.S.A.* 112 D4
Chamberlain → *Australia* 92 C4
Chamberlain L. *U.S.A.* 113 B19
Chambers *U.S.A.* 109 J9
Chambersburg *U.S.A.* 113 F15
Chambéry *France* 21 C9
Chambeshi → *Zambia* 84 G6
Chambly *Canada* 115 A11
Chambord *Canada* 105 C5
Chamboulive *France* 20 C5
Chamchamal *Iraq* 73 E11
Chamela *Mexico* 118 D3
Chamical *Argentina* 126 C2
Chamkar Luong *Cambodia* 65 G4
Chamoli *India* 69 D8
Chamonix-Mont Blanc
  France 21 C10
Chamouchouane =
  Ashuapmushuan →
  Canada 104 C5
Champa *India* 69 H10
Champagne *Canada* 102 A1
Champagne *France* 19 D11
Champagnole *France* 19 F12
Champaign *U.S.A.* 112 E9
Champassak *Laos* 64 E5
Champaubert *France* 19 D10
Champawat *India* 69 E9
Champdeniers-St-Denis
  France 20 B3
Champdoré, L. *Canada* 105 A6
Champeix *France* 20 C7
Champion *U.S.A.* 114 E4
Champlain *U.S.A.* 115 B11
Champlain, L. *U.S.A.* 115 B11
Champlitte *France* 19 E12
Champotón *Mexico* 119 D6
Champua *India* 69 H11
Chamusca *Portugal* 37 F2
Chana *Thailand* 65 J3
Chañaral *Chile* 126 B1
Chanārān *Iran* 71 B8
Chanasma *India* 68 H5
Chancery Lane *Barbados* 121 g
Chanco *Chile* 126 D1
Chand *India* 69 J8
Chandan *India* 69 G12
Chandan Chauki *India* 69 E9
Chandannagar *India* 69 H13
Chandausi *India* 69 E8
Chandeleur Is. *U.S.A.* 117 G10
Chandeleur Sd. *U.S.A.* 117 G10
Chandigarh *India* 68 D7
Chandil *India* 69 H12
Chandler *Australia* 95 D1
Chandler *Canada* 105 C7
Chandler *Ariz., U.S.A.* 109 K8
Chandler *Okla., U.S.A.* 116 D6
Chandod *India* 68 J5
Chandpur *Bangla.* 67 H17
Chandra *Greece* 49 D8
Chandrapur *India* 66 K11
Chânf *Iran* 71 E9

Chang *Pakistan* 68 F3
Chang, Ko *Thailand* 65 G4
Ch'ang Chiang = Chang
  Jiang → *China* 59 B13
Chang Jiang → *China* 59 B13
Chang-won *S. Korea* 57 G15
Changa *India* 69 C7
Changanacheri *India* 66 Q10
Changanassery =
  Changanacheri *India* 66 Q10
Changane → *Mozam.* 89 C5
Changbai *China* 57 D15
Changbai Shan *China* 57 C15
Changchiak'ou =
  Zhangjiakou *China* 56 D8
Ch'angchou = Changzhou
  China 59 B12
Changchun *China* 57 C13
Changchunling *China* 57 B13
Changde *China* 59 C8
Changdo-ri *N. Korea* 57 E14
Changfeng *China* 59 A11
Changhai = Shanghai
  China 59 B13
Changhua *China* 59 B12
Changhua *Taiwan* 59 E13
Changhŭngni *N. Korea* 57 D15
Changi *Singapore* 65 d
Changi, Singapore ✈ (SIN)
  Singapore 65 M4
Changjiang *China* 64 C7
Changjin *N. Korea* 57 D14
Changjin-ho *N. Korea* 57 D14
Changle *China* 59 E12
Changli *China* 57 E10
Changling *China* 57 B12
Changlun *Malaysia* 65 J3
Changning *Hunan, China* 59 D9
Changning *Sichuan, China* 58 C5
Changning *Yunnan, China* 58 E2
Changping *China* 56 D9
Changsha *China* 59 C9
Changshan *China* 59 C12
Changshan Qundao *China* 57 E12
Changshu *China* 59 B13
Changshun *China* 58 D6
Changtai *China* 59 E11
Changting *China* 59 E11
Changuinola *Panama* 120 E3
Changwu *China* 56 G4
Changxing *China* 59 B12
Changyang *China* 59 B8
Changyi *China* 57 F10
Changyŏn *N. Korea* 57 E13
Changyuan *China* 56 G8
Changzhi *China* 56 F7
Changzhou *China* 59 B12
Chanhanga *Angola* 88 B1
Chania *Greece* 49 D6
Chania □ *Greece* 49 D6
Chanion, Kolpos *Greece* 49 D5
Chanlar = Xanlar *Azerbaijan* 35 K8
Channapatna *India* 66 N10
Channel Is. *U.K.* 15 H5
Channel Is. *U.S.A.* 111 M7
Channel Islands △ *U.S.A.* 111 L7
Channel-Port aux Basques
  Canada 105 C8
Channel Tunnel *Europe* 15 F9
Channing *U.S.A.* 116 D3
Chantada *Spain* 36 C3
Chanthaburi *Thailand* 64 F4
Chantilly *France* 19 C9
Chantonnay *France* 18 F5
Chantrey Inlet *Canada* 100 D12
Chanute *U.S.A.* 112 G6
Chanza → *Spain* 37 H3
Chao Hu *China* 59 B11
Chao Phraya → *Thailand* 64 F3
Chao Phraya Lowlands
  Thailand 64 E3
Chaocheng *China* 56 F8
Chaohu *China* 59 B11
Chaoyang *Guangdong, China* 59 F11
Chaoyang *Liaoning, China* 57 D11
Chaozhou *China* 59 F11
Chapaev *Kazakhstan* 34 E10
Chapais *Canada* 104 C5
Chapala *Mozam.* 87 F4
Chapala, L. de *Mexico* 118 C4
Chapayevsk *Russia* 34 D9
Chapecó *Brazil* 127 B5
Chapel Hill *U.S.A.* 117 D15
Chapleau *Canada* 104 C3
Chaplin *Canada* 103 C7
Chaplin L. *Canada* 103 C7
Chaplino *Ukraine* 33 H9
Chaplygin *Russia* 32 F11
Chappell *U.S.A.* 112 E2
Chapra = Chhapra *India* 69 G11
Chaqâbal *Iran* 73 F12
Chara *Russia* 53 D12
Charadai *Argentina* 126 B4
Charagua *Bolivia* 124 G6
Charakas *Greece* 49 D7
Charambirá, Punta
  Colombia 124 C3
Charaña *Bolivia* 124 G5
Charantsavan *Armenia* 35 K7

Charanwala *India* 68 F5
Charata *Argentina* 126 B3
Charcas *Mexico* 118 C4
Charcot I. *Antarctica* 5 C17
Chard *U.K.* 15 G5
Chardon *U.S.A.* 114 E3
Chardzhou =
  Türkmenabat
  Turkmenistan 71 B9
Charente □ *France* 20 C4
Charente → *France* 20 C2
Charente-Maritime □ *France* 20 C3
Chari → *Chad* 79 F8
Chārīkār *Afghan.* 66 B6
Chariton *U.S.A.* 112 E7
Chariton → *U.S.A.* 112 F7
Chärjew = Türkmenabat
  Turkmenistan 71 B9
Charkhari *India* 69 G8
Charkhi Dadri *India* 68 E7
Charleroi *Belgium* 17 D4
Charleroi *U.S.A.* 114 F5
Charles, C. *U.S.A.* 113 G16
Charles, Peak *Australia* 93 F3
Charles City *U.S.A.* 112 D7
Charles de Gaulle, Paris ✈
  (CDG) *France* 19 D9
Charles I. *Canada* 101 E17
Charles L. *Canada* 103 B6
Charles Town *U.S.A.* 113 F15
Charlesbourg *Canada* 113 B18
Charleston *Ill., U.S.A.* 112 F9
Charleston *Miss., U.S.A.* 117 D9
Charleston *Mo., U.S.A.* 112 G9
Charleston *S.C., U.S.A.* 117 E15
Charleston *W. Va., U.S.A.* 113 F13
Charleston L. *Canada* 115 B9
Charleston Peak *U.S.A.* 111 J11
Charlestown *Ireland* 12 C3
Charlestown *S. Africa* 89 D4
Charlestown *Ind., U.S.A.* 113 F11
Charlestown *N.H., U.S.A.* 115 C12
Charlestown of Aberlour
  U.K. 13 D5
Charleville = Rath Luirc
  Ireland 12 D3
Charleville *Australia* 95 D4
Charleville-Mézières *France* 19 C11
Charlevoix *U.S.A.* 113 C11
Charlieu *France* 19 F11
Charlotte *Mich., U.S.A.* 113 D11
Charlotte *N.C., U.S.A.* 117 D14
Charlotte *Vt., U.S.A.* 115 B11
Charlotte Amalie
  U.S. Virgin Is. 121 e
Charlotte Harbor *U.S.A.* 117 H13
Charlotte L. *Canada* 102 C3
Charlottenberg *Sweden* 10 E6
Charlottesville *U.S.A.* 113 F14
Charlottetown *Nfld. & L.,
  Canada* 105 B8
Charlottetown *P.E.I., Canada* 105 C7
Charlotteville *Trin. & Tob.* 125 J16
Charlton *Australia* 95 F3
Charlton I. *Canada* 104 B4
Charmes *France* 19 D13
Charny *Canada* 105 C5
Charnyany *Belarus* 31 G11
Charolles *France* 19 F11
Chârost *France* 19 F9
Charre *Mozam.* 87 F4
Charroux *France* 20 B4
Charsadda *Pakistan* 68 B4
Charters Towers *Australia* 94 C4
Chartres *France* 18 D8
Chartre *France* 21 C9
Chascomús *Argentina* 126 D4
Chase *Canada* 102 C5
Chasefu *Zambia* 87 E3
Chashma Barrage *Pakistan* 68 C4
Chasseneuil-sur-Bonnieure
  France 20 C4
Chāt *Iran* 71 B7
Chatal Balkan = Udvoy
  Balkan *Bulgaria* 45 D10
Château-Arnoux-St-Auban
  France 21 D10
Château-Chinon *France* 19 E10
Château-d'Olonne *France* 20 B2
Château-du-Loir *France* 18 E7
Château-Gontier *France* 18 E6
Château-la-Vallière *France* 18 E7
Château-Landon *France* 19 D9
Château-Renard *France* 19 D9
Château-Renault *France* 18 E7
Château-Salins *France* 19 D13
Château-Thierry *France* 19 C10
Châteaubourg *France* 18 D5
Châteaubriant *France* 18 E5
Châteaudun *France* 18 D8
Chateaugay *U.S.A.* 115 B10
Châteaugiron *France* 18 D5
Châteauguay, L. *Canada* 105 A5
Châteaulin *France* 18 D2
Châteaumeillant *France* 19 F9
Châteauneuf-du-Faou *France* 18 D3
Châteauneuf-sur-Charente
  France 20 C3

Châteauneuf-sur-Cher
  France 19 F9
Châteauneuf-sur-Loire
  France 19 E9
Châteaurenard *France* 21 E8
Châteauroux *France* 19 F8
Châteauvillain *France* 19 D11
Châteaux, Pte. des *Guadeloupe* 120 b
Châtelaillon-Plage *France* 20 B2
Châtelguyon *France* 20 C7
Châtellerault *France* 18 F7
Châtelus-Malvaleix *France* 19 F9
Chatham = Miramichi
  Canada 105 C6
Chatham *Canada* 114 D2
Chatham *U.K.* 15 F8
Chatham *U.S.A.* 115 D11
Chatham Is. *Pac. Oc.* 96 M10
Chatham Rise *Pac. Oc.* 96 M10
Châtillon *Italy* 40 C4
Châtillon-Coligny *France* 19 E9
Châtillon-en-Diois *France* 21 D9
Châtillon-sur-Indre *France* 18 F8
Châtillon-sur-Loire *France* 19 E9
Châtillon-sur-Seine *France* 19 E11
Chatmohar *Bangla.* 69 G13
Chatra *India* 69 G11
Chatrapur *India* 67 K14
Chats, L. des *Canada* 115 A8
Chatsu *India* 68 F6
Chatsworth *Canada* 114 B4
Chatsworth *Zimbabwe* 87 F3
Châttagâm = Chittagong
  Bangla. 67 H17
Chattahoochee *U.S.A.* 117 F12
Chattahoochee → *U.S.A.* 117 F12
Chattanooga *U.S.A.* 117 D12
Chatteris *U.K.* 15 E8
Chatturat *Thailand* 64 E3
Chau Doc *Vietnam* 65 G5
Chaudes-Aigues *France* 20 D7
Chauffailles *France* 19 F11
Chaukan Pass *Burma* 67 F20
Chaumont *France* 19 D12
Chaumont *U.S.A.* 115 B8
Chaumont-en-Vexin *France* 19 C8
Chaumont-sur-Loire *France* 18 E8
Chaunay *France* 20 B4
Chaunskaya G. *Russia* 53 C17
Chauny *France* 19 C10
Chausey, Îs. *France* 18 D5
Chaussin *France* 19 F12
Chautauqua L. *U.S.A.* 114 D5
Chauvigny *France* 18 F7
Chauvin *Canada* 103 C6
Chavanges *France* 19 D11
Chaves *Brazil* 125 D9
Chaves *Portugal* 36 D3
Chawang *Thailand* 65 H2
Chazelles-sur-Lyon *France* 21 C8
Chazy *U.S.A.* 115 B11
Cheb *Czech Rep.* 26 A5
Cheboksarskoye Vdkhr.
  Russia 34 B8
Cheboksary *Russia* 34 B8
Cheboygan *U.S.A.* 113 C11
Chebsara *Russia* 32 C10
Chech, Erg *Africa* 78 D5
Chechelnyk *Ukraine* 29 B14
Chechen, Ostrov *Russia* 35 H8
Chechenia = Chechenia □
  Russia 35 J7
Checeno-Ingush Republic
  = Chechenia □ *Russia* 35 J7
Chechnya = Chechenia □
  Russia 35 J7
Checiny *Poland* 31 H7
Checotah *U.S.A.* 116 D7
Chedabucto B. *Canada* 105 C7
Cheduba I. *Burma* 67 K18
Cheektowaga *U.S.A.* 114 D6
Cheepie *Australia* 95 D4
Chef-Boutonne *France* 20 B3
Chegdomyn *Russia* 53 D14
Chegga *Mauritania* 78 C4
Chegutu *Zimbabwe* 87 F3
Chehalis *U.S.A.* 110 D4
Chehalis → *U.S.A.* 110 D3
Cheile Nerei-Beusnita △
  Romania 28 F6
Cheiron, Mt. *France* 21 E10
Cheju = Jeju *S. Korea* 57 H14
Cheju-do = Jeju-do *S. Korea* 57 H14
Chekalin *Russia* 32 E9
Chekhovo *Russia* 30 D7
Chekiang = Zhejiang □
  China 59 C13
Chel = Kuru, Bahr el →
  Sudan 81 F2
Chela, Sa. da *Angola* 88 B1
Chelan *U.S.A.* 108 C3
Chelan, L. *U.S.A.* 108 B3
Cheleken = Hazar
  Turkmenistan 52 F6
Cheleken Yarymadasy
  Turkmenistan 71 B7
Chelforó *Argentina* 128 D3
Chelkar = Shalqar
  Kazakhstan 52 E6
Chella *Ethiopia* 81 F4

Chelles *France* 19 D9
Chelm *Poland* 31 G10
Chelmno *Poland* 31 E5
Chelmsford *U.K.* 15 F8
Chelmża *Poland* 31 E5
Chelsea *Australia* 95 F4
Chelsea *U.S.A.* 115 C12
Cheltenham *U.K.* 15 F5
Chelva *Spain* 38 F4
Chelyabinsk *Russia* 52 D7
Chelyuskin, C. =
  Chelyuskin, Mys *Russia* 53 B11
Chelyuskin, Mys *Russia* 53 B11
Chemainus *Canada* 110 B3
Chemba *Mozam.* 85 H6
Chembar = Belinskiy *Russia* 34 D6
Chemillé *France* 18 E6
Chemin Grenier *Mauritius* 85 d
Chemnitz *Germany* 24 E8
Chemult *U.S.A.* 108 E3
Chen, Gora *Russia* 53 C15
Chenab → *Pakistan* 68 D4
Chenab Nagar *Pakistan* 68 D5
Chenango Forks *U.S.A.* 115 D9
Chencha *Ethiopia* 81 F4
Chenchiang = Zhenjiang
  China 59 A12
Cheney *U.S.A.* 108 C5
Cheng Xian *China* 56 H3
Chengbu *China* 59 D8
Chengcheng *China* 56 G5
Chengchou = Zhengzhou
  China 56 G7
Chengde *China* 57 D9
Chengdong Hu *China* 59 A11
Chengdu *China* 58 B5
Chenggong *China* 58 E4
Chenggu *China* 56 H4
Chenghai *China* 59 F11
Chengjiang *China* 58 E4
Chengkou *China* 58 B7
Chengmai *China* 64 C7
Ch'engtu = Chengdu *China* 58 B5
Chengwu *China* 56 G8
Chengxi Hu *China* 59 A11
Chengyang *China* 57 F11
Chenjiagang *China* 57 G10
Chennai *India* 66 N12
Chenôve *France* 19 E12
Chenxi *China* 59 C8
Chenzhou *China* 59 E9
Cheò, Eilean a' = Skye *U.K.* 13 D2
Cheom Ksan *Cambodia* 64 E5
Cheonan *S. Korea* 57 F14
Cheongdo *S. Korea* 57 G15
Cheongju *S. Korea* 57 F14
Cheorwon *S. Korea* 57 E14
Chepelare *Bulgaria* 45 E8
Chepén *Peru* 124 E3
Chepes *Argentina* 126 C2
Chepo *Panama* 120 E4
Chepstow *U.K.* 15 F5
Chequamegon B. *U.S.A.* 112 B8
Cher □ *France* 19 E9
Cher → *France* 18 E7
Chérádi *Italy* 43 B10
Cherasco *Italy* 40 D4
Cheraw *U.S.A.* 117 D15
Cherbourg *France* 18 C5
Cherdakly *Russia* 34 C9
Cherdyn *Russia* 52 C6
Cheremkhovo *Russia* 53 D11
Cherepovets *Russia* 32 C9
Chergui, Chott ech *Algeria* 78 B6
Cherikov = Cherykaw
  Belarus 23 B16
Cherkasy *Ukraine* 33 H7
Cherkasy □ *Ukraine* 33 H6
Cherkessk *Russia* 35 H6
Cherlak *Russia* 52 D8
Chernaya *Russia* 53 B9
Chernelytsya *Ukraine* 29 B10
Cherni *Bulgaria* 44 D7
Chernigov = Chernihiv
  Ukraine 33 G6
Chernigovka *Russia* 54 B6
Chernihiv *Ukraine* 33 G6
Chernihiv □ *Ukraine* 33 G7
Chernivtsi *Chernivtsi, Ukraine* 29 B10
Chernivtsi □ *Ukraine* 29 B10
Chernobyl = Chornobyl
  Ukraine 23 C16
Chernogorsk *Russia* 53 D10
Chernomorskoye =
  Chornomorske *Ukraine* 33 K7
Chernovtsy = Chernivtsi
  Ukraine 29 B10
Chernyakhovsk *Russia* 30 D8
Chernyanka *Russia* 33 G9
Chernysheyskiy *Russia* 53 C12
Chernyye Zemli *Russia* 35 H8
Cherokee *Iowa, U.S.A.* 112 D6
Cherokee *Okla., U.S.A.* 116 C5
Cherokee Village *U.S.A.* 116 C9
Cherokees, Grand Lake O'
  The *U.S.A.* 116 C7
Cherrapunji *India* 67 G17

Cherry Valley *U.S.A.* **115** D10
Cherskiy *Russia* **53** C17
Cherskogo Khrebet *Russia* **53** C15
Chersonisos *Greece* **49** D7
Chersonisos Akrotiri *Greece* **49** D6
Chertkovo *Russia* **33** H11
Cherven *Belarus* **23** B15
Cherven-Bryag *Bulgaria* **45** C8
Chervonoarmiyske *Ukraine* **29** E13
Chervonohrad *Ukraine* **23** C13
Cherwell → *U.K.* **15** F6
Cherykaw *Belarus* **23** B16
Chesapeake *U.S.A.* **113** G15
Chesapeake B. *U.S.A.* **113** F14
Cheshire □ *U.K.* **14** D5
Cheshskaya Guba *Russia* **52** C5
Cheshunt *U.K.* **15** F7
Chesil Beach *U.K.* **15** G5
Chesley *Canada* **114** B3
Cheste *Spain* **39** F4
Chester *U.K.* **14** D5
Chester *Calif., U.S.A.* **108** F3
Chester *Ill., U.S.A.* **112** G9
Chester *Mont., U.S.A.* **108** B8
Chester *Pa., U.S.A.* **113** F16
Chester *S.C., U.S.A.* **117** D14
Chester *Vt., U.S.A.* **115** C12
Chester *W. Va., U.S.A.* **114** F4
Chester-le-Street *U.K.* **14** C6
Chesterfield *U.K.* **14** D6
Chesterfield, Îs. *N. Cal.* **90** C8
Chesterfield Inlet *Canada* **100** E13
Chesterton Ra. *Australia* **95** D4
Chesterton Range △
    Australia **95** D4
Chestertown *U.S.A.* **115** C11
Chesterville *Canada* **115** A9
Chesuncook L. *U.S.A.* **113** C19
Chéticamp *Canada* **105** C7
Chetrosu *Moldova* **29** B12
Chetumal *Mexico* **119** D7
Chetumal, B. de *Cent. Amer.* **119** D7
Chetwynd *Canada* **102** B4
Chevanceaux *France* **20** C3
Cheviot, The *U.K.* **14** B5
Cheviot Hills *U.K.* **14** B5
Cheviot Ra. *Australia* **94** D3
Chew Bahir *Ethiopia* **81** G4
Chewelah *U.S.A.* **108** B5
Chewore △ *Zimbabwe* **87** F2
Cheyenne *Okla., U.S.A.* **116** D5
Cheyenne *Wyo., U.S.A.* **108** F11
Cheyenne → *U.S.A.* **112** C3
Cheyenne Wells *U.S.A.* **108** G12
Cheyne B. *Australia* **93** F2
Chhabra *India* **68** G7
Chhaktala *India* **68** H6
Chhapra *India* **69** G11
Chhata *India* **68** F7
Chhatarpur *Jharkhand, India* **69** G11
Chhatarpur *Mad. P., India* **69** G8
Chhattisgarh □ *India* **69** J10
Chhep *Cambodia* **64** F5
Chhindwara *Mad. P., India* **69** H8
Chhindwara *Mad. P., India* **69** H8
Chhlong *Cambodia* **65** F5
Chhota Tawa → *India* **68** H7
Chhoti Kali Sindh → *India* **68** G6
Chhuikhadan *India* **69** J9
Chhuk *Cambodia* **65** G5
Chi → *Thailand* **64** E5
Chiai *Taiwan* **59** F13
Chiali *Taiwan* **59** F13
Chiamboni *Somali Rep.* **84** E8
Chianciano Terme *Italy* **41** E8
Chiang Dao *Thailand* **64** C2
Chiang Kham *Thailand* **64** C3
Chiang Khan *Thailand* **64** D3
Chiang Khong *Thailand* **58** G3
Chiang Mai *Thailand* **64** C2
Chiang Rai *Thailand* **58** H2
Chiang Saen *Thailand* **58** G3
Chianti *Italy* **41** E8
Chiapa → *Mexico* **119** D6
Chiapa de Corzo *Mexico* **119** D6
Chiapas □ *Mexico* **119** D6
Chiapas, Sa. Madre de
    Mexico **119** D6
Chiaramonte Gulfi *Italy* **43** E7
Chiaravalle *Italy* **41** E10
Chiaravalle Centrale *Italy* **43** D9
Chiari *Italy* **40** C6
Chiatura *Georgia* **35** J6
Chiautla de Tapia *Mexico* **119** D5
Chiávari *Italy* **40** D6
Chiavenna *Italy* **40** B6
Chiba *Japan* **55** G10
Chiba □ *Japan* **55** G10
Chibabava *Mozam.* **89** C5
Chibemba *Cunene, Angola* **85** H2
Chibemba *Huíla, Angola* **88** B2
Chibi *Zimbabwe* **89** C5
Chibia *Angola* **85** H2
Chibougamau *Canada* **104** C5
Chibougamau, L. *Canada* **104** C5
Chibuk *Nigeria* **83** C7
Chibuto *Mozam.* **89** C5
Chic-Chocs, Mts. *Canada* **105** C6
Chicacole = Srikakulam
    India **67** K13

Chicago *U.S.A.* **112** E10
Chicago Heights *U.S.A.* **112** E10
Chicagof I. *U.S.A.* **100** F4
Chichaoua *Morocco* **78** B4
Chichawatni *Pakistan* **68** D5
Chichén-Itzá *Mexico* **119** C7
Chicheng *China* **56** D8
Chichester *U.K.* **15** G7
Chichester Ra. *Australia* **92** D2
Chichibu *Japan* **55** F9
Chichibu-Tama △ *Japan* **55** G9
Ch'ich'ihaerh = Qiqihar
    China **53** E13
Chicholi *India* **68** H8
Chickasaw △ *U.S.A.* **116** D6
Chickasha *U.S.A.* **116** D6
Chiclana de la Frontera *Spain* **37** J4
Chiclayo *Peru* **124** E3
Chico *U.S.A.* **110** F5
Chico → *Chubut, Argentina* **128** E3
Chico → *Santa Cruz,*
    Argentina **128** G3
Chicoa *Mozam.* **87** F3
Chicomo *Mozam.* **89** C5
Chicomostoc *Mexico* **118** C4
Chicontepec *Mexico* **119** C5
Chicopee *U.S.A.* **115** D12
Chicoutimi *Canada* **105** C5
Chicualacuala *Mozam.* **89** C5
Chidambaram *India* **66** P11
Chidenguele *Mozam.* **89** C5
Chidley, C. *Canada* **101** E19
Chiduacane *Mozam.* **89** C5
Chiede *Angola* **88** B2
Chiefs Pt. *Canada* **114** B3
Chiem Hoa *Vietnam* **64** A5
Chiemsee *Germany* **25** H8
Chiengi *Zambia* **87** D2
Chiengmai = Chiang Mai
    Thailand **64** C2
Chienti → *Italy* **41** E10
Chieri *Italy* **40** C4
Chiers → *France* **19** C11
Chiesa in Valmalenco *Italy* **40** B6
Chiese → *Italy* **40** C7
Chieti *Italy* **41** F11
Chifeng *China* **57** C10
Chigirin *Ukraine* **33** H7
Chignecto B. *Canada* **105** C7
Chiguana *Bolivia* **126** A2
Chigwell *U.K.* **15** F8
Chihli, G. of = Bo Hai *China* **57** E10
Chihuahua *Mexico* **118** B3
Chihuahua □ *Mexico* **118** B3
Chiili = Shīeli *Kazakhstan* **52** E7
Chik Bollapur *India* **66** N10
Chikmagalur *India* **66** N9
Chikwawa *Malawi* **87** F3
Chilanga *Zambia* **87** F2
Chilapa *Mexico* **119** D5
Chilas *Pakistan* **69** B6
Chilaw *Sri Lanka* **66** R11
Chilcotin → *Canada* **102** C4
Childers *Australia* **95** D5
Childress *U.S.A.* **116** D4
Chile ■ *S. Amer.* **128** D2
Chile Rise *Pac. Oc.* **97** L18
Chilecito *Argentina* **126** B2
Chilete *Peru* **124** E3
Chilia, Brațul → *Romania* **29** E14
Chililabombwe *Zambia* **87** E2
Chilim *Pakistan* **69** B6
Chilin = Jilin *China* **57** C14
Chiliomodi *Greece* **46** D4
Chilka L. *India* **67** K14
Chilko → *Canada* **102** C4
Chilko L. *Canada* **102** C4
Chillagoe *Australia* **94** B3
Chillán *Chile* **126** D1
Chillicothe *Ill., U.S.A.* **112** E9
Chillicothe *Mo., U.S.A.* **112** F7
Chillicothe *Ohio, U.S.A.* **113** F12
Chilliwack *Canada* **102** D4
Chilo *India* **68** F5
Chiloane, I. *Mozam.* **89** C5
Chiloé, I. de *Chile* **128** E2
Chilpancingo *Mexico* **119** D5
Chiltern Hills *U.K.* **15** F7
Chilton *U.S.A.* **112** C9
Chilubi *Zambia* **87** E2
Chilubula *Zambia* **87** E3
Chilumba *Malawi* **87** E3
Chilung *Taiwan* **59** E13
Chilwa, L. *Malawi* **87** F4
Chimaltitán *Mexico* **118** C4
Chimán *Panama* **120** E4
Chimanimani *Zimbabwe* **89** B5
Chimay *Belgium* **17** D4
Chimayo *U.S.A.* **109** J11
Chimba *Zambia* **87** D3
Chimbay *Uzbekistan* **52** E6
Chimborazo *Ecuador* **124** D3
Chimbote *Peru* **124** E3
Chimkent = Shymkent
    Kazakhstan **52** E7
Chimoio *Mozam.* **87** F3
Chimpembe *Zambia* **87** D2
Chin □ *Burma* **67** J18
Chin Hills *Burma* **67** H18

Chin Ling Shan = Qinling
    Shandi *China* **56** H5
China *Mexico* **119** B5
China ■ *Asia* **60** D6
China, Great Plain of *Asia* **50** E13
China Lake *U.S.A.* **111** K9
Chinan = Jinan *China* **56** F9
Chinandega *Nic.* **120** D2
Chinati Peak *U.S.A.* **116** G2
Chincha Alta *Peru* **124** F3
Chinchaga → *Canada* **102** B5
Chinchilla *Australia* **95** D5
Chinchilla de Monte
    Aragón *Spain* **39** G3
Chinchorro, Banco *Mexico* **119** D7
Chinchou = Jinzhou *China* **57** D11
Chincoteague *U.S.A.* **113** G16
Chinde *Mozam.* **87** F4
Chindwin → *Burma* **67** J19
Chineni *India* **69** C6
Chinga *Mozam.* **87** F4
Chingola *Zambia* **87** E2
Chingole *Malawi* **87** E3
Ch'ingtao = Qingdao *China* **57** F11
Chinguetti *Mauritania* **78** D3
Chingune *Mozam.* **89** C5
Chinhanguanine *Mozam.* **89** D5
Chinhoyi *Zimbabwe* **87** F3
Chini *India* **68** D8
Chiniot *Pakistan* **68** D5
Chínipas *Mexico* **118** B3
Chinji *Pakistan* **68** C5
Chinju = Jinju *S. Korea* **57** G15
Chinko → *C.A.R.* **84** D4
Chinle *U.S.A.* **109** H9
Chinmen *Taiwan* **59** E13
Chinmen Tao *Taiwan* **59** E12
Chinnampo = Namp'o
    N. Korea **57** E13
Chino *Japan* **55** G9
Chino *U.S.A.* **111** L9
Chino Valley *U.S.A.* **109** J7
Chinon *France* **18** E7
Chinook *U.S.A.* **108** B9
Chinook Trough *Pac. Oc.* **96** C10
Chinsali *Zambia* **87** E3
Chinsura = Chunchura
    India **69** H13
Chióggia *Italy* **41** C9
Chíos = Hios *Greece* **47** C8
Chipata *Zambia* **87** E3
Chiperceni *Moldova* **29** C13
Chipindo *Angola* **85** G3
Chipinge *Zimbabwe* **87** G3
Chipinge △ *Zimbabwe* **87** G3
Chipiona *Spain* **37** J4
Chipley *U.S.A.* **117** F12
Chipman *Canada* **105** C6
Chipoka *Malawi* **87** E3
Chippawa *U.K.* **15** F5
Chippewa → *U.S.A.* **112** C7
Chippewa Falls *U.S.A.* **112** C8
Chipping Norton *U.K.* **15** F6
Chiprovtsi *Bulgaria* **44** C6
Chiputneticook Lakes
    N. Amer. **113** C20
Chiquián *Peru* **124** F3
Chiquibul △ *Belize* **120** C2
Chiquimula *Guatemala* **120** D2
Chiquinquira *Colombia* **124** B4
Chir → *Russia* **35** F6
Chirala *India* **66** M12
Chiramba *Mozam.* **87** F3
Chirawa *India* **68** E6
Chirchiq *Uzbekistan* **52** E7
Chiredzi *Zimbabwe* **89** C5
Chiricahua △ *U.S.A.* **109** K9
Chiricahua Peak *U.S.A.* **109** L9
Chirikof I. *U.S.A.* **106** D8
Chiriquí, G. de *Panama* **120** E3
Chiriquí, L. de *Panama* **120** E3
Chirisa △ *Zimbabwe* **87** F2
Chirivira Falls *Zimbabwe* **87** G3
Chirmiri *India* **69** H10
Chirnogi *Romania* **29** F11
Chirpan *Bulgaria* **45** D9
Chirripó Grande, Cerro
    Costa Rica **120** E3
Chirundu *Zimbabwe* **89** B4
Chisamba *Zambia* **87** E2
Chisapani *Nepal* **69** E9
Chisasibi *Canada* **104** B4
Chisholm *Canada* **102** C6
Chisholm *U.S.A.* **112** B7
Chishtian Mandi *Pakistan* **68** E5
Chishui *China* **58** C5
Chishui He → *China* **58** C5
Chisimaio = Kismaayo
    Somali Rep. **75** H3
Chisimba Falls *Zambia* **87** E3
Chișinău *Moldova* **29** C13
Chișinău ✈ (KIV) *Moldova* **29** C13
Chișineu Criș *Romania* **28** D6
Chisone → *Italy* **40** D4
Chisos Mts. *U.S.A.* **116** G3
Chistopol *Russia* **34** C10
Chita *Russia* **53** D12
Chitipa *Malawi* **87** D3

Chitose *Japan* **54** C10
Chitral *Pakistan* **66** B7
Chitré *Panama* **120** E3
Chittagong *Bangla.* **67** H17
Chittagong □ *Bangla.* **67** G17
Chittaurgarh *India* **68** G6
Chittoor *India* **66** N11
Chitungwiza *Zimbabwe* **87** F3
Chiusi *Italy* **41** E8
Chiva *Spain* **39** F4
Chivasso *Italy* **40** C4
Chivhu *Zimbabwe* **87** F3
Chivilcoy *Argentina* **126** C4
Chiwanda *Tanzania* **87** E3
Chixi *China* **59** G9
Chizarira *Zimbabwe* **87** F2
Chizarira △ *Zimbabwe* **87** F2
Chizela *Zambia* **87** E2
Chkalov = Orenburg *Russia* **52** D6
Chkolovsk *Russia* **34** B6
Chloride *U.S.A.* **111** K12
Chlumec nad Cidlinou
    Czech Rep. **26** A8
Chmielnik *Poland* **31** H7
Cho Bo *Vietnam* **58** G5
Cho-do *N. Korea* **57** E13
Cho Phuoc Hai *Vietnam* **65** G6
Choa Chu Kang *Singapore* **65** d
Choba *Kenya* **86** B4
Chobe △ *Botswana* **88** B4
Chociwel *Poland* **30** E2
Chocianów *Poland* **31** G2
Chocolate Mts. *U.S.A.* **111** M11
Choctawhatchee → *U.S.A.* **117** F11
Choda *India* **68** H4
Chodecz *Poland* **31** F6
Chodov *Czech Rep.* **26** A5
Chodziez *Poland* **31** F3
Choele Choel *Argentina* **128** D3
Choiseul *St. Lucia* **121** f
Choiseul *Solomon Is.* **90** B8
Choix *Mexico* **118** B3
Chojna *Poland* **31** F1
Chojnice *Poland* **30** E4
Chojnów *Poland* **31** G2
Chok Chai *Thailand* **64** E4
Chōkai-San *Japan* **54** E10
Choke Canyon Res. *U.S.A.* **116** G5
Choke Mts. *Ethiopia* **81** E4
Chokurdakh *Russia* **53** B15
Cholame *U.S.A.* **110** K6
Cholet *France* **18** E6
Cholguan *Chile* **126** D1
Choloma *Honduras* **120** C2
Choluteca *Honduras* **120** D2
Choluteca → *Honduras* **120** D2
Chom Bung *Thailand* **64** F2
Chom Thong *Thailand* **64** C2
Choma *Zambia* **87** F2
Chomolungma = Everest,
    Mt. *Nepal* **69** E12
Chomun *India* **68** F6
Chomutov *Czech Rep.* **26** A6
Chon Buri *Thailand* **64** F3
Chon Thanh *Vietnam* **65** G6
Chone *Ecuador* **124** D3
Chong Kai *Cambodia* **64** F4
Chong Mek *Thailand* **64** E5
Chong Phangan *Thailand* **65** b
Chong Samui *Thailand* **65** b
Chongde *China* **59** B13
Chongjin *N. Korea* **57** D15
Chŏngju *N. Korea* **57** E13
Chongli *China* **56** D8
Chongming *China* **59** B13
Chongming Dao *China* **59** B13
Chongqing *Chongqing, China* **58** C6
Chongqing *Sichuan, China* **58** B4
Chongqing Shi □ *China* **58** C6
Chongren *China* **59** D11
Chonguene *Mozam.* **89** C5
Chongwe *Zambia* **87** F2
Chongyi *China* **59** E10
Chongzuo *China* **58** F6
Chonos, Arch. de los *Chile* **128** F2
Chop *Ukraine* **28** B7
Chopim → *Brazil* **127** B5
Chor *Pakistan* **68** G3
Chora *Greece* **46** D3
Chora Sfakion *Greece* **49** D6
Chorbat La *India* **69** B7
Chorley *U.K.* **14** D5
Chorna *Ukraine* **29** C14
Chornobyl *Ukraine* **23** C16
Chornomorske *Ukraine* **33** K7
Chorolque, Cerro *Bolivia* **126** A2
Choroszcz *Poland* **31** E9
Chorregon *Australia* **94** C3
Chorro el Indio △ *Venezuela* **121** E5
Chortkiv *Ukraine* **23** D13
Chorzele *Poland* **31** E7
Chorzów *Poland* **31** H5
Chos-Malal *Argentina* **126** D1
Ch'osan *N. Korea* **57** D13
Choszczno *Poland* **31** E2
Choteau *U.S.A.* **108** C7
Chotěboř *Czech Rep.* **26** B8
Chotila *India* **68** H4
Chotta Udepur *India* **68** H6
Chowchilla *U.S.A.* **110** H6

Choybalsan *Mongolia* **60** B6
Choyr *Mongolia* **53** E11
Christchurch *N.Z.* **91** E4
Christchurch *U.K.* **15** G6
Christian I. *Canada* **114** B4
Christian Sd. *U.S.A.* **107** D13
Christiana *S. Africa* **88** D4
Christiansfeld *Denmark* **11** J3
Christiansted *U.S. Virgin Is.* **121** C7
Christie B. *Canada* **103** A6
Christina → *Canada* **103** B6
Christmas Cr. → *Australia* **92** C4
Christmas I. = Kiritimati
    Kiribati **97** G12
Christmas I. *Ind. Oc.* **96** J2
Christopher, L. *Australia* **93** D4
Chrudim *Czech Rep.* **26** B8
Chrzanów *Poland* **31** H6
Chtimba *Malawi* **87** E3
Chū = Shū *Kazakhstan* **52** E8
Chu → *Vietnam* **64** C5
Chu Lai *Vietnam* **64** E7
Chuadanga *Bangla.* **69** H13
Chuak, Ko *Thailand* **65** b
Ch'uanchou = Quanzhou
    China **59** E12
Chuankou *China* **56** G6
Chubbuck *U.S.A.* **108** E7
Chūbu □ *Japan* **55** F8
Chubu-Sangaku △ *Japan* **55** F8
Chubut □ *Argentina* **128** E3
Chuchi L. *Canada* **102** B4
Chuda *India* **68** H4
Chudovo *Russia* **32** C6
Chudskoye, Ozero *Russia* **32** C4
Chugach Mts. *U.S.A.* **106** C10
Chugoku □ *Japan* **55** G6
Chūgoku-Sanchi *Japan* **55** G6
Chuguyev = Chuhuyiv
    Ukraine **33** H9
Chugwater *U.S.A.* **108** F11
Chuhuyiv *Ukraine* **33** H9
Chuka *Kenya* **86** C4
Chukchi Plateau *Arctic* **4** B17
Chukchi Sea *Russia* **53** C19
Chukotskiy Mys *Russia* **106** C5
Chukotskiy Poluostrov
    Russia **106** B5
Chukotskoye Nagorye
    Russia **53** C18
Chula Vista *U.S.A.* **111** N9
Chulucanas *Peru* **124** E2
Chulym → *Russia* **52** D9
Chum Phae *Thailand* **64** D4
Chum Saeng *Thailand* **64** E3
Chumar *India* **69** C8
Chumbicha *Argentina* **126** B2
Chumerna *Bulgaria* **45** D9
Chumikan *Russia* **53** D14
Chumphon *Thailand* **65** G2
Chumuare *Mozam.* **87** E3
Chuna → *Russia* **53** D10
Chun'an *China* **59** C12
Chuncheon *S. Korea* **57** F14
Chunchura *India* **69** H13
Chunga *Zambia* **87** F2
Chunggang-ŭp *N. Korea* **57** D14
Chunghwa *N. Korea* **57** E13
Chungju *S. Korea* **57** F14
Chungking = Chongqing
    China **58** C6
Chungli *Taiwan* **59** E13
Chungt'iaoshan =
    Zhongtiao Shan *China* **56** G6
Chungyang Shanmo *Taiwan* **59** F13
Chunian *Pakistan* **68** D6
Chunya *Tanzania* **87** D3
Chunyang *China* **57** C15
Chupara Pt. *Trin. & Tob.* **125** K15
Chuquibamba *Peru* **124** G4
Chuquicamata *Chile* **126** A2
Chur *Switz.* **25** J5
Churachandpur *India* **67** G18
Church Stretton *U.K.* **15** E5
Churchill *Canada* **103** B10
Churchill → *Man., Canada* **103** B10
Churchill → *Nfld. & L.,*
    Canada **105** B7
Churchill, C. *Canada* **103** B10
Churchill Falls *Canada* **105** B7
Churchill L. *Canada* **103** B7
Churchill Pk. *Canada* **102** B3
Churki *India* **69** H10
Churu *India* **68** E6
Churún Merú = Angel
    Falls *Venezuela* **124** B6
Chushal *India* **69** C8
Chuska Mts. *U.S.A.* **109** H9
Chusovoy *Russia* **52** D6
Chute-aux-Outardes *Canada* **105** C6
Chuuk = Truk *Micronesia* **96** G7
Chuvash Republic =
    Chuvashia □ *Russia* **34** C8
Chuvashia □ *Russia* **34** C8
Chuwārtah *Iraq* **73** E11
Chuxiong *China* **58** E3
Chuy *Uruguay* **127** C5
Chuzhou *China* **59** A12

Ci Xian *China* **56** F8
Ciacova *Romania* **28** E6
Ciadâr-Lunga *Moldova* **29** D13
Ciamis *Indonesia* **63** G13
Cianjur *Indonesia* **63** G12
Cianorte *Brazil* **127** A5
Cibola *U.S.A.* **111** M12
Çiçekdağı *Turkey* **72** C6
Cicero *U.S.A.* **112** E10
Cicia *Fiji* **91** a
Cidacos → *Spain* **38** C3
Cide *Turkey* **72** B5
Ciéagas del Cataumbo △
    Venezuela **121** E5
Ciechanów *Poland* **31** F7
Ciechanowiec *Poland* **31** E9
Ciechocinek *Poland* **31** F5
Ciego de Ávila *Cuba* **120** B4
Ciénaga *Colombia* **124** A4
Cienfuegos *Cuba* **120** B3
Cierp-Gaud *France* **20** F4
Cíes, Is. *Spain* **36** C2
Cieszanów *Poland* **31** H10
Cieszyn *Poland* **31** J5
Cieza *Spain* **39** G3
Çifteler *Turkey* **72** C4
Cifuentes *Spain* **38** E2
Cihanbeyli *Turkey* **72** C5
Cihuatlán *Mexico* **118** D4
Cijara, Embalse de *Spain* **37** F6
Cijulang *Indonesia* **63** G13
Cilacap *Indonesia* **63** G13
Çıldır *Turkey* **73** B10
Çıldır Gölü *Turkey* **73** B10
Cilento e Vallo di Diano △
    Italy **43** B8
Cili *China* **59** C8
Cilibia *Romania* **29** E12
Cilicia *Turkey* **72** D5
Cill Airne = Killarney *Ireland* **12** D2
Cill Chainnigh = Kilkenny
    Ireland **12** D4
Cill Dara = Kildare *Ireland* **12** C5
Cill Mhantáin = Wicklow
    Ireland **12** C5
Cilo Dağı *Turkey* **73** D10
Cima *U.S.A.* **111** K11
Cimarron *Kans., U.S.A.* **112** C5
Cimarron *N. Mex., U.S.A.* **109** H11
Cimarron → *U.S.A.* **116** C6
Cimişlia *Moldova* **29** C13
Cimone, Mte. *Italy* **40** D7
Çınar *Turkey* **73** D9
Çınarcık *Turkey* **45** F13
Cinca → *Spain* **38** D5
Cincar *Bos.-H.* **28** G2
Cincinnati *U.S.A.* **113** F11
Cincinnatus *U.S.A.* **115** D9
Çine *Turkey* **47** D10
Ciney *Belgium* **17** D5
Cíngoli *Italy* **41** E10
Cinigiano *Italy* **41** F8
Cinto, Mte. *France* **21** F12
Cintruénigo *Spain* **38** C3
Ciocile *Romania* **29** F12
Ciolănești din Deal *Romania* **29** F10
Ciorani *Romania* **29** F11
Čiovo *Croatia* **41** E13
Circeo, Mte. *Italy* **42** A6
Çırçır *Turkey* **72** C7
Circle *Alaska, U.S.A.* **106** B11
Circle *Mont., U.S.A.* **108** C11
Circleville *U.S.A.* **113** F12
Cirebon *Indonesia* **62** F3
Ciremay *Indonesia* **63** G13
Cirencester *U.K.* **15** F6
Cireşu *Romania* **28** F7
Cirey-sur-Vezouze *France* **19** D13
Ciriè *Italy* **40** C4
Cirium *Cyprus* **49** E11
Cirò *Italy* **43** C10
Cirò Marina *Italy* **43** C10
Ciron → *France* **20** D3
Cisco *U.S.A.* **116** E5
Cislău *Romania* **29** E11
Cisna *Poland* **31** J9
Cisnădie *Romania* **29** E9
Cisterna di Latina *Italy* **42** A5
Cisternino *Italy* **43** B10
Cistierna *Spain* **36** C5
Citeli-Ckaro =
    Tsiteli-Tsqaro *Georgia* **35** K8
Citlaltépetl = Orizaba, Pico
    de *Mexico* **119** D5
Citrus Heights *U.S.A.* **110** G5
Citrusdal *S. Africa* **88** E2
Città del Vaticano =
    Vatican City ■ *Europe* **41** G9
Città della Pieve *Italy* **41** F9
Città di Castello *Italy* **41** E9
Città Sant' Angelo *Italy* **41** F11
Cittadella *Italy* **41** C8
Cittaducale *Italy* **41** F9
Cittanova *Italy* **43** D9
Ciuc, Munții *Romania* **29** D11
Ciucaş, Vf. *Romania* **29** E10
Ciucea *Romania* **28** D7
Ciuciulea *Moldova* **29** C12

Ciuciuleni *Moldova* **29** C13
Ciudad Acuña *Mexico* **118** B4
Ciudad Altamirano *Mexico* **118** D4
Ciudad Anáhuac *Mexico* **118** B4
Ciudad Bolívar *Venezuela* **124** B6
Ciudad Camargo *Mexico* **118** B3
Ciudad Cortés *Costa Rica* **120** E3
Ciudad de México *Mexico* **119** D5
Ciudad de Valles *Mexico* **119** C5
Ciudad del Carmen *Mexico* **119** D6
Ciudad del Este *Paraguay* **127** B5
Ciudad Delicias = Delicias
  Mexico **118** B3
Ciudad Frontera *Mexico* **118** B4
Ciudad Guayana *Venezuela* **124** B6
Ciudad Guerrero *Mexico* **118** B3
Ciudad Guzmán *Mexico* **118** D4
Ciudad Juárez *Mexico* **118** A3
Ciudad Lerdo *Mexico* **118** B4
Ciudad Madero *Mexico* **119** C5
Ciudad Mante *Mexico* **119** C5
Ciudad Obregón *Mexico* **118** B3
Ciudad Real *Spain* **37** G7
Ciudad Real □ *Spain* **37** G7
Ciudad Rodrigo *Spain* **36** E4
Ciudad Victoria *Mexico* **119** C5
Ciudadela *Spain* **48** B10
Ciulniţa *Romania* **29** F12
Ciumeghiu *Romania* **28** D6
Ciuperceni *Romania* **28** F8
Civa Burnu *Turkey* **72** B7
Cividale del Friuli *Italy* **41** B10
Civita Castellana *Italy* **41** F9
Civitanova Marche *Italy* **41** E10
Civitavécchia *Italy* **41** F8
Civray *France* **20** B4
Çivril *Turkey* **47** C11
Cixerri → *Italy* **42** C1
Cixi *China* **59** B13
Cizre *Turkey* **73** D10
Clackmannanshire □ *U.K.* **13** E5
Clacton-on-Sea *U.K.* **15** F9
Clain → *France* **18** F7
Claire, L. *Canada* **102** B6
Clairton *U.S.A.* **114** F5
Clairvaux-les-Lacs *France* **19** F12
Claise → *France* **20** B5
Clallam Bay *U.S.A.* **110** B2
Clamecy *France* **19** E11
Clanton *U.S.A.* **117** E11
Clanwilliam *S. Africa* **88** E2
Clara *Ireland* **12** C4
Claraville *U.S.A.* **111** K8
Clare *Australia* **95** E2
Clare *U.S.A.* **113** D11
Clare □ *Ireland* **12** D3
Clare → *Ireland* **12** C2
Clare I. *Ireland* **12** C1
Claremont *Calif., U.S.A.* **111** L9
Claremont *N.H., U.S.A.* **115** C12
Claremont Pt. *Australia* **94** A3
Claremore *U.S.A.* **116** C7
Claremorris *Ireland* **12** C3
Clarence → *Australia* **95** D5
Clarence → *N.Z.* **91** E4
Clarence, I. *Chile* **128** G2
Clarence I. *Antarctica* **5** C18
Clarence Str. *Australia* **92** B5
Clarence Town *Bahamas* **121** B5
Clarendon *Pa., U.S.A.* **114** E5
Clarendon *Tex., U.S.A.* **116** D4
Clarenville *Canada* **105** C9
Claresholm *Canada* **102** D6
Clarie Coast *Antarctica* **5** C9
Clarinda *U.S.A.* **112** E6
Clarington *Canada* **114** C6
Clarion *Iowa, U.S.A.* **112** D7
Clarion *Pa., U.S.A.* **114** E5
Clarion → *U.S.A.* **114** E5
Clarion Fracture Zone
  Pac. Oc. **98** H7
Clark *U.S.A.* **112** C5
Clark, Pt. *Canada* **114** B3
Clark Fork *U.S.A.* **108** B5
Clark Fork → *U.S.A.* **108** B5
Clarkdale *U.S.A.* **109** J7
Clarke City *Canada* **105** B6
Clarke I. *Australia* **95** G4
Clarke Ra. *Australia* **94** b
Clarks Fork
  Yellowstone → *U.S.A.* **108** D9
Clark's Harbour *Canada* **105** D6
Clarks Hill L. = J. Strom
  Thurmond L. *U.S.A.* **117** E13
Clarks Summit *U.S.A.* **115** E9
Clarksburg *U.S.A.* **113** F13
Clarksdale *U.S.A.* **117** D9
Clarkston *U.S.A.* **108** C5
Clarksville *Ark., U.S.A.* **116** D8
Clarksville *Tenn., U.S.A.* **117** C11
Clarksville *Tex., U.S.A.* **116** E7
Clatskanie *U.S.A.* **110** D3
Claude *U.S.A.* **116** D4
Claveria *Phil.* **61** B4
Clay *U.S.A.* **110** G5
Clay Center *U.S.A.* **112** F5
Claypool *U.S.A.* **109** K8
Claysburg *U.S.A.* **114** F6
Claysville *U.S.A.* **114** F4

Clayton *Canada* **115** A8
Clayton *N. Mex., U.S.A.* **109** H12
Clayton *N.Y., U.S.A.* **115** B8
Clear, C. *Ireland* **12** E2
Clear, L. *Canada* **114** A7
Clear Hills *Canada* **102** B5
Clear I. *Ireland* **12** E2
Clear L. *U.S.A.* **110** F4
Clear Lake *Iowa, U.S.A.* **112** D7
Clear Lake *S. Dak., U.S.A.* **112** C5
Clear Lake Res. *U.S.A.* **108** F3
Clearfield *Pa., U.S.A.* **114** E6
Clearfield *Utah, U.S.A.* **108** F7
Clearlake *U.S.A.* **110** G4
Clearwater *Canada* **102** C4
Clearwater *U.S.A.* **117** H13
Clearwater → *Alta., Canada* **102** C6
Clearwater → *Alta., Canada* **103** B6
Clearwater L. *Canada* **103** C9
Clearwater Lake ○ *Canada* **103** C8
Clearwater Mts. *U.S.A.* **108** C6
Clearwater River ○ *Canada* **103** B7
Cleburne *U.S.A.* **116** E6
Clee Hills *U.K.* **15** E5
Cleethorpes *U.K.* **14** D7
Cleeve Cloud *U.K.* **15** F6
Clelles *France* **21** D9
Clemson *U.S.A.* **117** D13
Clerke Reef *Australia* **92** C2
Clermont *Australia* **94** C4
Clermont *France* **19** C9
Clermont *U.S.A.* **117** G14
Clermont-en-Argonne
  France **19** C12
Clermont-Ferrand *France* **20** C7
Clermont-l'Hérault *France* **20** E7
Clerval *France* **19** E13
Clervaux *Lux.* **17** D6
Cles *Italy* **40** B8
Clevedon *U.K.* **15** F5
Cleveland *Miss., U.S.A.* **117** E9
Cleveland *Ohio, U.S.A.* **114** E3
Cleveland *Okla., U.S.A.* **116** C6
Cleveland *Tenn., U.S.A.* **117** D12
Cleveland *Tex., U.S.A.* **116** F7
Cleveland, C. *Australia* **94** B4
Cleveland, Mt. *U.S.A.* **108** B7
Cleveland Heights *U.S.A.* **114** E3
Clevelândia *Brazil* **127** B5
Clew B. *Ireland* **12** C2
Clewiston *U.S.A.* **117** H14
Clifden *Ireland* **12** C1
Clifden *N.Z.* **91** G1
Cliffdell *U.S.A.* **110** D5
Cliffy Hd. *Australia* **93** G2
Clifton *Australia* **95** D5
Clifton *Ariz., U.S.A.* **109** K9
Clifton *Colo., U.S.A.* **108** G9
Clifton *Tex., U.S.A.* **116** F6
Clifton Beach *Australia* **94** B4
Clinch → *U.S.A.* **117** D12
Clingmans Dome *U.S.A.* **117** D13
Clint *U.S.A.* **116** F1
Clinton *B.C., Canada* **102** C4
Clinton *Ont., Canada* **114** C3
Clinton *N.Z.* **91** G2
Clinton *Ark., U.S.A.* **116** D8
Clinton *Conn., U.S.A.* **115** E12
Clinton *Ill., U.S.A.* **112** E9
Clinton *Ind., U.S.A.* **112** F10
Clinton *Iowa, U.S.A.* **112** E8
Clinton *Mass., U.S.A.* **115** D13
Clinton *Miss., U.S.A.* **117** E9
Clinton *Mo., U.S.A.* **112** F7
Clinton *N.C., U.S.A.* **117** D15
Clinton *Okla., U.S.A.* **116** D5
Clinton *S.C., U.S.A.* **117** D14
Clinton *Tenn., U.S.A.* **117** C12
Clinton *Wash., U.S.A.* **110** C4
Clinton, C. *Australia* **94** C5
Clinton Colden L. *Canada* **100** E10
Clintonville *U.S.A.* **112** C9
Clipperton, I. *Pac. Oc.* **97** F17
Clipperton Fracture Zone
  Pac. Oc. **97** G16
Clisham *U.K.* **13** D2
Clisson *France* **18** E5
Clitheroe *U.K.* **14** D5
Clo-oose *Canada* **110** B2
Cloates, Pt. *Australia* **92** D1
Clocolan *S. Africa* **89** D4
Clodomira *Argentina* **126** B3
Clogher Hd. *Ireland* **12** C5
Clonakilty *Ireland* **12** E3
Clonakilty B. *Ireland* **12** E3
Cloncurry *Australia* **94** C3
Cloncurry *Ireland* **12** C5
Cloncurry → *Australia* **94** B3
Clondalkin *Ireland* **12** C5
Clones *Ireland* **12** B4
Clonmel *Ireland* **12** D4
Cloppenburg *Germany* **24** C4
Cloquet *U.S.A.* **112** B7
Clorinda *Argentina* **126** B4
Cloud Bay *Canada* **104** C2
Cloud Peak *U.S.A.* **108** D10
Cloudcroft *U.S.A.* **109** K11
Cloverdale *U.S.A.* **110** G4
Clovis *Calif., U.S.A.* **110** J7

Clovis *N. Mex., U.S.A.* **109** J12
Cloyes-sur-le-Loir *France* **18** E8
Cloyne *Canada* **114** B7
Cluain Meala = Clonmel
  Ireland **12** D4
Cluj *Romania* **29** D8
Cluj-Napoca *Romania* **29** D8
Clunes *Australia* **95** F3
Cluny *France* **19** F11
Cluses *France* **19** F13
Clusone *Italy* **40** C6
Clutha → *N.Z.* **91** G2
Clwyd → *U.K.* **14** D4
Clyde *Canada* **102** C6
Clyde *N.Z.* **91** F2
Clyde *U.S.A.* **114** C8
Clyde, Firth of → *U.K.* **13** F3
Clyde → *U.K.* **13** F4
Clyde Muirshiel ○ *U.K.* **13** F4
Clyde River *Canada* **101** C18
Clydebank *U.K.* **13** F4
Clymer *N.Y., U.S.A.* **114** D5
Clymer *Pa., U.S.A.* **114** D5
Ćmielów *Poland* **31** H8
Côa → *Portugal* **36** D3
Coachella *U.S.A.* **111** M10
Coachella Canal *U.S.A.* **111** N12
Coahoma *U.S.A.* **116** E4
Coahuayana → *Mexico* **118** D4
Coahuila □ *Mexico* **118** B4
Coal → *Canada* **102** B3
Coalane *Mozam.* **87** F4
Coalcomán *Mexico* **118** D4
Coaldale *Canada* **102** D6
Coalgate *U.S.A.* **116** D6
Coalinga *U.S.A.* **110** J6
Coalisland *U.K.* **12** B5
Coalville *U.K.* **14** E6
Coalville *U.S.A.* **108** F8
Coamo *Puerto Rico* **121** d
Coari *Brazil* **124** D6
Coast □ *Kenya* **86** C4
Coast Mts. *Canada* **102** C3
Coast Ranges *U.S.A.* **110** G4
Coatbridge *U.K.* **13** F4
Coatepec *Mexico* **119** D5
Coatepeque *Guatemala* **120** D1
Coatesville *U.S.A.* **113** F16
Coaticook *Canada* **115** A13
Coats I. *Canada* **101** E15
Coats Land *Antarctica* **5** D1
Coatzacoalcos *Mexico* **119** D6
Cobá *Mexico* **119** C7
Cobadin *Romania* **29** F13
Cobalt *Canada* **104** C4
Cobán *Guatemala* **120** C1
Çobanlar *Turkey* **47** C12
Cobar *Australia* **95** E4
Cóbh *Ireland* **12** E3
Cobija *Bolivia* **124** F5
Cobleskill *U.S.A.* **115** D10
Coboconk *Canada* **114** B6
Cobourg *Canada* **114** C6
Cobourg Pen. *Australia* **92** B5
Cobram *Australia* **95** F4
Cóbué *Mozam.* **87** E3
Coburg *Germany* **25** E6
Coburg I. *Canada* **101** B16
Coca *Spain* **36** D6
Cocanada = Kakinada *India* **67** L13
Cocentaina *Spain* **39** G4
Cochabamba *Bolivia* **124** G5
Cochem *Germany* **25** E3
Cochemane *Mozam.* **87** F3
Cochin *India* **66** Q10
Cochin China = Nam-Phan
  Vietnam **65** G6
Cochran *U.S.A.* **117** E13
Cochrane *Alta., Canada* **102** C6
Cochrane *Ont., Canada* **104** C3
Cochrane *Chile* **128** F2
Cochrane → *Canada* **103** B8
Cochrane, L. *Chile* **128** F2
Cochranton *U.S.A.* **114** E4
Cockburn *Australia* **95** E3
Cockburn, Canal *Chile* **128** G2
Cockburn I. *Canada* **104** C3
Cockburn Ra. *Australia* **92** C4
Cockermouth *U.K.* **14** C4
Cocklebiddy *Australia* **93** F4
Cockpit Country, The *Jamaica* **120** a
Coco → *Cent. Amer.* **120** D3
Coco, I. del *Pac. Oc.* **97** G19
Cocoa *U.S.A.* **117** G14
Cocobeach *Gabon* **84** D1
Cocora *Romania* **29** F12
Cocos B. *Trin. & Tob.* **125** K15
Cocos Is. *Ind. Oc.* **96** J1
Cocos Ridge *Pac. Oc.* **97** G19
Cod, C. *U.S.A.* **113** D18
Codajás *Brazil* **124** D6
Codigoro *Italy* **41** D9
Codlea *Romania* **29** E10
Codó *Brazil* **125** D10
Codogno *Italy* **40** C6
Codróipo *Italy* **41** C10
Codru, Munţii *Romania* **28** D7
Cody *U.S.A.* **108** D9
Coe Hill *Canada* **114** B7

Coelemu *Chile* **126** D1
Coen *Australia* **94** A3
Coesfeld *Germany* **24** D3
Coeur d'Alene *U.S.A.* **108** C5
Coeur d'Alene L. *U.S.A.* **108** C5
Coevorden *Neths.* **17** B6
Cofete *Canary Is.* **48** F5
Coffeyville *U.S.A.* **112** G6
Coffin B. *Australia* **95** E2
Coffin Bay *Australia* **95** E2
Coffin Bay △ *Australia* **95** E2
Coffin Bay Peninsula
  Australia **95** E2
Coffs Harbour *Australia* **95** E5
Cofrentes *Spain* **39** F3
Cogalnic → *Moldova* **29** E14
Cogealac *Romania* **29** F13
Coghinas → *Italy* **42** B1
Coghinas, L. del *Italy* **42** B2
Cognac *France* **20** C3
Cogne *Italy* **40** C4
Cogolin *France* **21** E10
Cogolludo *Spain* **38** E1
Cohocton *U.S.A.* **114** D7
Cohocton → *U.S.A.* **114** D7
Cohoes *U.S.A.* **115** D11
Cohuna *Australia* **95** F3
Coiba, I. de *Panama* **120** E3
Coig → *Argentina* **128** G3
Coigeach, Rubha *U.K.* **13** C3
Coihaique *Chile* **128** F2
Coimbatore *India* **66** P10
Coimbra *Brazil* **124** G7
Coimbra *Portugal* **36** E2
Coimbra □ *Portugal* **36** E2
Coín *Spain* **37** J6
Coipasa, Salar de *Bolivia* **124** G5
Cojimies *Ecuador* **124** C3
Cojocna *Romania* **29** D8
Cojutepequé *El Salv.* **120** D2
Čoka *Serbia* **28** E5
Cokeville *U.S.A.* **108** E8
Colac *Australia* **95** F3
Colatina *Brazil* **125** G10
Colbeck, C. *Antarctica* **5** D13
Colborne *Canada* **114** C7
Colby *U.S.A.* **112** F3
Colchester *U.K.* **15** F8
Colchester *U.S.A.* **115** E12
Cold → *Canada* **103** C7
Cold Lake *Alta., Canada* **100** G9
Cold Lake *Alta., Canada* **103** C6
Coldstream *Canada* **102** C5
Coldstream *U.K.* **13** F6
Coldwater *Canada* **114** B5
Coldwater *Kans., U.S.A.* **112** G4
Coldwater *Mich., U.S.A.* **113** E11
Colebrook *U.S.A.* **115** B13
Coleman *Canada* **102** D6
Coleman *U.S.A.* **116** F5
Coleman → *Australia* **94** B3
Colenso *S. Africa* **89** D4
Coleraine *Australia* **95** F3
Coleraine *U.K.* **12** A5
Coleridge, L. *N.Z.* **91** E3
Colesberg *S. Africa* **88** E4
Coleville *U.S.A.* **110** G7
Colfax *Calif., U.S.A.* **110** F6
Colfax *La., U.S.A.* **116** F8
Colfax *Wash., U.S.A.* **108** C5
Colibaşi *Moldova* **29** E13
Colibaşi *Romania* **29** F9
Cólico *Italy* **40** B6
Colima *Mexico* **118** D4
Colima □ *Mexico* **118** D4
Colima, Nevado de *Mexico* **118** D4
Colina *Chile* **126** C1
Colina do Norte *Guinea-Biss.* **82** C2
Colinas *Brazil* **125** E10
Colindres *Spain* **36** B7
Coll *U.K.* **13** E2
Collahuasi *Chile* **126** A2
Collarada, Peña *Spain* **38** C4
Collarenebri *Australia* **95** D4
Colle di Val d'Elsa *Italy* **40** E8
Collécchio *Italy* **40** D7
Colleen Bawn *Zimbabwe* **87** G2
College *U.S.A.* **106** C10
College Park *U.S.A.* **117** E12
College Station *U.S.A.* **116** F6
Collesalvetti *Italy* **40** E7
Colli Euganei ○ *Italy* **41** C8
Collie *Australia* **93** F2
Collier B. *Australia* **92** C3
Collier Ra. *Australia* **93** D2
Collier Range △ *Australia* **93** D2
Collierville *U.S.A.* **117** D10
Collina, Passo di *Italy* **40** D7
Collingwood *Canada* **114** B4
Collingwood *N.Z.* **91** D4
Collins *U.S.A.* **104** B2
Collins Bay *Canada* **115** B8
Collinson Pen. *Canada* **100** D11
Collinsville *Australia* **94** C4
Collipulli *Chile* **126** D1

Collooney *Ireland* **12** B3
Colmar *France* **19** D14
Colmars *France* **21** D10
Colmenar *Spain* **37** J6
Colmenar de Oreja *Spain* **36** E7
Colmenar Viejo *Spain* **36** E7
Colo → *Australia* **95** E5
Cologne = Köln *Germany* **24** E2
Colom, I. d'en *Spain* **48** B11
Coloma *U.S.A.* **110** G6
Colomb-Béchar = Béchar
  Algeria **78** B5
Colombey-les-Belles *France* **19** D12
Colombey-les-Deux-Églises
  France **19** D11
Colombia ■ *S. Amer.* **124** C4
Colombian Basin *S. Amer.* **98** H12
Colombo *Sri Lanka* **66** R11
Colomiers *France* **20** E5
Colón *B. Aires, Argentina* **126** C3
Colón *Entre Ríos, Argentina* **126** C4
Colón *Cuba* **120** B3
Colón *Panama* **120** E4
Colón, Arch. de *Ecuador* **122** D1
Colonia del Sacramento
  Uruguay **126** C4
Colonia Dora *Argentina* **126** B3
Colonial Beach *U.S.A.* **113** F15
Colonie *U.S.A.* **115** D11
Colonna, C. *Italy* **43** C10
Colonsay *Canada* **103** C7
Colonsay *U.K.* **13** E2
Colorado □ *U.S.A.* **108** G11
Colorado → *Argentina* **128** D4
Colorado → *N. Amer.* **109** L6
Colorado → *U.S.A.* **116** G7
Colorado City *U.S.A.* **116** E4
Colorado Plateau *U.S.A.* **109** H8
Colorado River Aqueduct
  U.S.A. **111** L12
Colorado Springs *U.S.A.* **108** G11
Colorno *Italy* **40** D7
Colstrip *U.S.A.* **108** D10
Colton *U.S.A.* **115** B10
Columbia *Ky., U.S.A.* **113** G11
Columbia *La., U.S.A.* **116** E8
Columbia *Miss., U.S.A.* **117** F10
Columbia *Mo., U.S.A.* **112** F7
Columbia *Pa., U.S.A.* **115** F8
Columbia *S.C., U.S.A.* **117** D14
Columbia *Tenn., U.S.A.* **117** D11
Columbia → *N. Amer.* **110** D2
Columbia, C. *Canada* **101** A18
Columbia, District of □
  U.S.A. **113** F15
Columbia Basin *U.S.A.* **108** C4
Columbia Falls *U.S.A.* **108** B6
Columbia Mts. *Canada* **102** C5
Columbia Plateau *U.S.A.* **108** E5
Columbiana *U.S.A.* **114** F4
Columbretes, Is. *Spain* **38** F5
Columbus *Ga., U.S.A.* **117** E12
Columbus *Ind., U.S.A.* **113** F11
Columbus *Kans., U.S.A.* **112** G6
Columbus *Miss., U.S.A.* **117** E10
Columbus *Mont., U.S.A.* **108** D9
Columbus *N. Mex., U.S.A.* **109** L10
Columbus *Nebr., U.S.A.* **112** E5
Columbus *Ohio, U.S.A.* **113** F12
Columbus *Tex., U.S.A.* **116** G6
Colunga *Spain* **36** B5
Colusa *U.S.A.* **110** F4
Colville *U.S.A.* **108** B5
Colville → *U.S.A.* **106** A9
Colville, C. *N.Z.* **91** B5
Colwood *Canada* **110** B3
Colwyn Bay *U.K.* **14** D4
Coma *Ethiopia* **81** F4
Comácchio *Italy* **41** D9
Comalcalco *Mexico* **119** D6
Comallo *Argentina* **128** E2
Comana *Romania* **29** F11
Comanche *U.S.A.* **116** F5
Comandante Ferraz
  Antarctica **5** C18
Comăneşti *Romania* **29** D11
Comarnic *Romania* **29** E10
Comayagua *Honduras* **120** D2
Combahee → *U.S.A.* **117** E14
Combarbalá *Chile* **126** C1
Combe Martin *U.K.* **15** F3
Combeaufontaine *France* **19** E12
Comber *Canada* **114** D2
Comber *U.K.* **12** B6
Combermere *Canada* **114** A7
Comblain-au-Pont *Belgium* **17** D5
Combourg *France* **18** D5
Combrailles *France* **19** F9
Combronde *France* **20** C7
Comet *Australia* **94** C4
Comilla *Bangla.* **67** H17
Comino *Malta* **49** C1
Comino, C. *Italy* **42** B2
Cómiso *Italy* **43** F7
Comitán de Domínguez
  Mexico **119** D6

Commentry *France* **19** F9
Commerce *Ga., U.S.A.* **117** D13
Commerce *Tex., U.S.A.* **116** E7
Commercy *France* **19** D12
Committee B. *Canada* **101** D14
Commodore, C. *Canada* **114** B4
Commonwealth B. *Antarctica* **5** C10
Commoron Cr. → *Australia* **95** D5
Communism Pk. = imeni
  Ismail Samani, Pik
  Tajikistan **52** F8
Como *Italy* **40** C6
Como, Lago di *Italy* **40** B6
Comodoro Rivadavia
  Argentina **128** F3
Comoé → *Ivory C.* **82** D4
Comoé △ *Ivory C.* **82** D4
Comorâşte *Romania* **28** E6
Comorin, C. =
  Kannyakumari *India* **66** Q10
Comoros ■ *Ind. Oc.* **85** a
Comox *Canada* **102** D4
Compiègne *France* **19** C9
Comporta *Portugal* **37** G2
Compostela *Mexico* **118** C4
Comprida, I. *Brazil* **127** A6
Compton *Canada* **115** A13
Compton *U.S.A.* **111** M8
Comrat *Moldova* **29** D13
Con Cuong *Vietnam* **64** C5
Con Dao △ *Vietnam* **65** H6
Con Son *Vietnam* **65** H6
Conakry *Guinea* **82** D2
Conara *Australia* **95** G4
Concarneau *France* **18** E3
Conceição *Mozam.* **87** F4
Conceição da Barra *Brazil* **125** G11
Conceição do Araguaia
  Brazil **125** E9
Concepción *Argentina* **126** B2
Concepción *Bolivia* **124** G6
Concepción *Chile* **126** D1
Concepción *Mexico* **119** D6
Concepción *Paraguay* **126** A4
Concepción □ *Chile* **126** D1
Concepción → *Mexico* **118** A2
Concepción, Est. de *Chile* **128** G2
Concepción, L. *Bolivia* **124** G6
Concepción, Pta. *Mexico* **118** B2
Concepción del Oro *Mexico* **118** C4
Concepción del Uruguay
  Argentina **126** C4
Conception, Pt. *U.S.A.* **111** L6
Conception B. *Canada* **105** C9
Conception B. *Namibia* **88** C1
Conception I. *Bahamas* **121** B4
Concession *Zimbabwe* **87** F3
Conchas Dam *U.S.A.* **109** J11
Conches-en-Ouche *France* **18** D7
Concho *U.S.A.* **109** J9
Concho → *U.S.A.* **116** F5
Conchos → *Chihuahua,
  Mexico* **118** B4
Conchos → *Chihuahua,
  Mexico* **118** B3
Conchos → *Tamaulipas,
  Mexico* **119** B5
Concord *Calif., U.S.A.* **110** H4
Concord *N.C., U.S.A.* **117** D14
Concord *N.H., U.S.A.* **115** C13
Concordia *Antarctica* **5** D17
Concordia *Argentina* **126** C4
Concórdia *Amazonas, Brazil* **124** D5
Concórdia *Sta. Catarina,
  Brazil* **127** B5
Concordia *Mexico* **118** C3
Concordia *U.S.A.* **112** F5
Concrete *U.S.A.* **108** B3
Condamine *Australia* **95** D5
Condat *France* **20** C6
Conde *U.S.A.* **112** C4
Condé-sur-Noireau *France* **18** D6
Condeúba *Brazil* **125** F10
Condobolin *Australia* **95** E4
Condom *France* **20** E4
Condon *U.S.A.* **108** D3
Conegliano *Italy* **41** C9
Conejera, I. = Conills, I. des
  Spain **48** B9
Conejos *Mexico* **118** B4
Conemaugh → *U.S.A.* **114** F5
Conero △ *Italy* **41** E10
Confolens *France* **20** B4
Confuso → *Paraguay* **126** B4
Congaz *Moldova* **29** D13
Conghua *China* **59** F9
Congjiang *China* **58** E7
Congleton *U.K.* **14** D5
Congo (Brazzaville) =
  Congo ■ *Africa* **84** E3
Congo (Kinshasa) = Congo,
  Dem. Rep. of the ■ *Africa* **84** E4
Congo ■ *Africa* **84** E3
Congo → *Africa* **84** F2
Congo, Dem. Rep. of the ■
  Africa **84** E4
Congo Basin *Africa* **84** E4
Congonhas *Brazil* **127** A7
Congress *U.S.A.* **109** J7

Conil de la Frontera *Spain* **37** J4
Conills, I. des *Spain* **48** B9
Coniston *Canada* **104** C3
Conjeeveram =
    Kanchipuram *India* **66** N11
Conklin *Canada* **103** B6
Conklin *U.S.A.* **113** D9
Conn, L. *Ireland* **12** B2
Connacht □ *Ireland* **12** C2
Conneaut *U.S.A.* **114** E4
Conneautville *U.S.A.* **114** E4
Connecticut □ *U.S.A.* **115** E12
Connecticut → *U.S.A.* **115** E12
Connell *U.S.A.* **108** C4
Connellsville *U.S.A.* **114** F5
Connemara *Ireland* **12** C2
Connemara △ *Ireland* **12** C2
Connerré *France* **18** D7
Connersville *U.S.A.* **113** F11
Connors Ra. *Australia* **94** C4
Conoename → *Suriname* **125** B7
Conques *France* **20** D6
Conquest *Canada* **103** C7
Conrad *U.S.A.* **108** B8
Conrad Rise *S. Ocean* **5** B5
Conran, C. *Australia* **95** F4
Conroe *U.S.A.* **116** F7
Consecon *Canada* **114** C7
Conselheiro Lafaiete *Brazil* **127** A7
Consell *Spain* **48** B9
Conselve *Italy* **41** C8
Consett *U.K.* **14** C6
Consort *Canada* **103** C6
Constance = Konstanz
    Germany **25** H5
Constance, L. = Bodensee
    Europe **25** H5
Constanța *Romania* **29** F13
Constanța □ *Romania* **29** F13
Constantina *Spain* **37** H5
Constantine *Algeria* **78** A7
Constitución *Chile* **126** D1
Constitución *Uruguay* **126** C4
Constitución de 1857 △
    Mexico **118** A1
Consuegra *Spain* **37** F7
Consul *Canada* **103** D7
Contact *U.S.A.* **108** F6
Contai *India* **69** J12
Contamana *Peru* **124** E4
Contarina *Italy* **41** C9
Contas → *Brazil* **125** F11
Contes *France* **21** E11
Contoocook *U.S.A.* **115** C13
Contra Costa *Mozam.* **89** D5
Contres *France* **18** E8
Contrexéville *France* **19** D12
Contwoyto L. *Canada* **100** D9
Conversano *Italy* **43** B10
Conway = Conwy *U.K.* **14** D4
Conway → Conwy → *U.K.* **14** D4
Conway *Australia* **94** b
Conway *Canada* **114** B8
Conway *Ark., U.S.A.* **116** D8
Conway *N.H., U.S.A.* **115** C13
Conway *S.C., U.S.A.* **117** E15
Conway, C. *Australia* **94** b
Conway, L. *Australia* **95** D2
Conwy *U.K.* **14** D4
Conwy □ *U.K.* **14** D4
Conwy → *U.K.* **14** D4
Coober Pedy *Australia* **95** D1
Cooch Behar = Koch Bihar
    India **67** F16
Cooinda *Australia* **92** B5
Cook *Australia* **93** F5
Cook *U.S.A.* **112** B7
Cook, B. *Chile* **128** H3
Cook, C. *Canada* **102** C3
Cook, Mt. = Aoraki Mount
    Cook *N.Z.* **91** E3
Cook Inlet *U.S.A.* **100** F1
Cook Is. *Pac. Oc.* **97** J12
Cook Strait *N.Z.* **91** D5
Cookeville *U.S.A.* **117** C12
Cookhouse *S. Africa* **88** E4
Cooks Harbour *Canada* **105** B8
Cookshire *Canada* **115** A13
Cookstown *Canada* **114** B5
Cookstown *U.K.* **12** B5
Cooksville *Canada* **114** C4
Cooktown *Australia* **94** B4
Coolabah *Australia* **95** E4
Cooladdi *Australia* **95** D4
Coolah *Australia* **95** E4
Coolamon *Australia* **95** E4
Coolgardie *Australia* **93** F3
Coolidge *U.S.A.* **109** K8
Coolidge Dam *U.S.A.* **109** K8
Cooma *Australia* **95** F4
Coon Rapids *U.S.A.* **112** C7
Coonabarabran *Australia* **95** E4
Coonamble *Australia* **95** E4
Coonana ○ *Australia* **93** F3
Coonana *Australia* **93** F3
Coondapoor *India* **66** N9
Cooninnie, L. *Australia* **95** D2
Cooper *U.S.A.* **116** E7
Cooper Cr. → *Australia* **95** D2

Cooper Ridge *Pac. Oc.* **97** G12
Cooperstown *N. Dak., U.S.A.* **112** B4
Cooperstown *N.Y., U.S.A.* **115** D10
Coorabie *Australia* **93** F5
Coorow *Australia* **93** E2
Cooroy *Australia* **95** D5
Coos Bay *U.S.A.* **108** E1
Coosa → *U.S.A.* **117** E11
Cootamundra *Australia* **95** E4
Cootehill *Ireland* **12** B4
Copahue Paso *Argentina* **126** D1
Copainalá *Mexico* **119** D6
Copake *U.S.A.* **115** D11
Copalnic Mănăștur *Romania* **29** C8
Copán *Honduras* **120** D2
Cope *U.S.A.* **108** G12
Cope, C. *Spain* **39** H3
Copenhagen = København
    Denmark **11** J6
Copenhagen *U.S.A.* **115** C9
Copertino *Italy* **43** B11
Copiapó *Chile* **126** B1
Copiapó → *Chile* **126** B1
Coplay *U.S.A.* **115** F9
Copo △ *Argentina* **126** B3
Copp L. *Canada* **102** A6
Copparo *Italy* **41** D8
Copper Canyon = Barranca
    del Cobre △ *Mexico* **118** B3
Copper Center *U.S.A.* **106** C10
Copper Harbor *U.S.A.* **112** B10
Copper Queen *Zimbabwe* **87** F2
Copperas Cove *U.S.A.* **116** F6
Copperbelt □ *Zambia* **87** E2
Coppermine = Kugluktuk
    Canada **100** D8
Coppermine → *Canada* **100** D8
Copperopolis *U.S.A.* **110** H6
Copșa Mică *Romania* **29** D9
Coquet → *U.K.* **14** B6
Coquille *U.S.A.* **108** E1
Coquimbo *Chile* **126** C1
Coquimbo □ *Chile* **126** C1
Coquitlam *Canada* **102** D4
Corabia *Romania* **29** G9
Coracora *Peru* **124** G4
Coraki *Australia* **95** D5
Coral *U.S.A.* **114** F5
Coral Bay *Australia* **92** D1
Coral Gables *U.S.A.* **117** J14
Coral Harbour *Canada* **101** E15
Coral Sea *Pac. Oc.* **90** C8
Coral Sea Basin *Pac. Oc.* **96** J7
Coral Sea Islands Terr. □
    Australia **90** C8
Coral Springs *U.S.A.* **117** H14
Coraopolis *U.S.A.* **114** F4
Corato *Italy* **43** A9
Corbeil-Essonnes *France* **19** D9
Corbett △ *India* **69** E8
Corbie *France* **19** C9
Corbières *France* **20** F6
Corbigny *France* **19** E10
Corbin *U.S.A.* **113** G11
Corbones → *Spain* **37** H5
Corbu *Romania* **29** F13
Corby *U.K.* **15** E7
Corcaigh = Cork *Ireland* **12** E3
Corcoran *U.S.A.* **110** J7
Corcovado △ *Costa Rica* **120** E3
Cordele *U.S.A.* **117** F13
Cordell *U.S.A.* **116** D5
Cordenòns *Italy* **41** C9
Cordes-sur-Ciel *France* **20** D5
Córdoba *Argentina* **126** C3
Córdoba *Mexico* **119** D5
Córdoba *Spain* **37** H6
Córdoba □ *Argentina* **126** C3
Córdoba □ *Spain* **37** G6
Córdoba, Sierra de *Argentina* **126** C3
Cordon *Phil.* **61** C4
Cordova *U.S.A.* **100** E2
Corella *Spain* **38** C3
Corella → *Australia* **94** B3
Corfield *Australia* **94** C3
Corfu = Kerkyra *Greece* **49** A3
Corfu *U.S.A.* **114** D6
Corfu ✈ (CFU) *Greece* **46** B1
Corfu, Str. of = Kerkyras,
    Notio Steno *Greece* **49** A4
Corgo = O Corgo *Spain* **36** C3
Cori *Italy* **42** A5
Coria *Spain* **36** F4
Coria del Río *Spain* **37** H4
Corigliano Cálabro *Italy* **43** C9
Coringa Is. *Australia* **94** B4
Corinth = Korinthos *Greece* **46** D4
Corinth *Miss., U.S.A.* **117** D10
Corinth *N.Y., U.S.A.* **115** C11
Corinth, G. of =
    Korinthiakos Kolpos
    Greece **46** C4
Corinth Canal *Greece* **46** D4
Corinto *Brazil* **125** G10
Corinto *Nic.* **120** D2
Cork *Ireland* **12** E3
Cork □ *Ireland* **12** E3
Cork Harbour *Ireland* **12** E3

Corlay *France* **18** D3
Corleone *Italy* **42** E6
Corleto Perticara *Italy* **43** B9
Çorlu *Turkey* **45** E11
Cormack L. *Canada* **102** A4
Cormòns *Italy* **41** C10
Cormorant *Canada* **103** C8
Cormorant L. *Canada* **103** C8
Corn Is. = Maíz, Is. del *Nic.* **120** D3
Cornalvo △ *Spain* **37** F4
Cornélio Procópio *Brazil* **127** A5
Corner Brook *Canada* **105** C8
Cornești *Moldova* **29** C13
Corníglio *Italy* **40** D7
Corning *Ark., U.S.A.* **117** C9
Corning *Calif., U.S.A.* **108** G2
Corning *Iowa, U.S.A.* **112** E6
Corning *N.Y., U.S.A.* **114** D7
Corno Grande *Italy* **41** F10
Cornwall *Canada* **115** A10
Cornwall *U.S.A.* **115** F8
Cornwall □ *U.K.* **15** G3
Cornwall I. *Canada* **101** B13
Cornwallis I. *Canada* **101** B13
Corny Pt. *Australia* **95** E2
Coro *Venezuela* **124** A5
Coroatá *Brazil* **125** D10
Corocoro *Bolivia* **124** G5
Coroico *Bolivia* **124** G5
Coromandel *N.Z.* **91** B5
Coromandel Coast *India* **66** N12
Corona *Calif., U.S.A.* **111** M9
Corona *N. Mex., U.S.A.* **109** J11
Coronado *U.S.A.* **111** N9
Coronado, B. de *Costa Rica* **120** E3
Coronados, Is. Los *Mexico* **111** N9
Coronation *Canada* **102** C6
Coronation Gulf *Canada* **100** D10
Coronation I. *Antarctica* **5** C18
Coronation Is. *Australia* **92** B3
Coronda *Argentina* **126** C3
Coronel *Chile* **126** D1
Coronel Bogado *Paraguay* **126** B4
Coronel Dorrego *Argentina* **126** D3
Coronel Oviedo *Paraguay* **126** B4
Coronel Pringles *Argentina* **126** D3
Coronel Suárez *Argentina* **126** D3
Coronel Vidal *Argentina* **126** D4
Coropuna, Nevado *Peru* **124** G4
Corowa *Australia* **95** F4
Corozal *Belize* **119** D7
Corozal Pt. *Trin. & Tob.* **125** K15
Corps *France* **21** D9
Corpus *Argentina* **127** B4
Corpus Christi *U.S.A.* **116** H6
Corpus Christi, L. *U.S.A.* **116** G6
Corral de Almaguer *Spain* **37** F7
Corralejo *Canary Is.* **48** F6
Corraun Pen. *Ireland* **12** C2
Corréggio *Italy* **40** D7
Corrèze □ *France* **20** C5
Corrèze → *France* **20** C5
Corrib, L. *Ireland* **12** C2
Corridónia *Italy* **41** E10
Corrientes *Argentina* **126** B4
Corrientes □ *Argentina* **126** B4
Corrientes → *Argentina* **126** C4
Corrientes → *Peru* **124** D4
Corrientes, C. *Colombia* **124** B3
Corrientes, C. *Cuba* **120** B3
Corrientes, C. *Mexico* **118** C3
Corrigan *U.S.A.* **116** F7
Corrigin *Australia* **93** F2
Corriverton *Guyana* **124** B7
Corry *U.S.A.* **114** E5
Corse □ *France* **21** G13
Corse, C. *France* **21** E13
Corse △ *France* **21** F13
Corse-du-Sud □ *France* **21** G13
Corsica = Corse □ *France* **21** G13
Corsicana *U.S.A.* **116** E6
Corte *France* **21** F13
Corte Pinto *Portugal* **37** H3
Cortegana *Spain* **37** H4
Cortés, Mar de =
    California, G. de *Mexico* **118** B2
Cortez *U.S.A.* **109** H9
Cortina d'Ampezzo *Italy* **41** B9
Cortland *N.Y., U.S.A.* **115** D8
Cortland *Ohio, U.S.A.* **114** E4
Cortona *Italy* **41** E8
Corubal → *Guinea-Biss.* **82** C2
Coruche *Portugal* **37** G2
Çoruh → *Turkey* **35** K5
Çorum *Turkey* **72** B6
Çorum □ *Turkey* **72** B6
Corumbá *Brazil* **124** G7
Corund *Romania* **29** D10
Corunna = A Coruña *Spain* **36** B2
Corvallis *U.S.A.* **108** D2
Corvette, L. de la *Canada* **104** B5
Corvo *Azores* **78** a
Corydon *U.S.A.* **112** E7
Cosalá *Mexico* **118** C3
Cosamaloapan de Carpio
    Mexico **119** D5
Cosenza *Italy* **43** C9

Coșereni *Romania* **29** F11
Coshocton *U.S.A.* **114** F3
Cosmo Newberry *Australia* **93** E3
Cosmo Newberry ○ *Australia* **93** E3
Cosmonaut Sea *S. Ocean* **5** C5
Cosne-Cours-sur-Loire
    France **19** E9
Coso Junction *U.S.A.* **111** J9
Coso Pk. *U.S.A.* **111** J9
Cospeito *Spain* **36** B3
Cosquín *Argentina* **126** C3
Cossato *Italy* **40** C5
Cossé-le-Vivien *France* **18** E6
Cosson → *France* **18** E8
Costa Blanca *Spain* **39** G4
Costa Brava *Spain* **38** D8
Costa Cálida *Spain* **39** H3
Costa Daurada *Spain* **38** D6
Costa del Sol *Spain* **37** J6
Costa dels Pins *Spain* **48** B10
Costa Mesa *U.S.A.* **111** M9
Costa Rica ■ *Cent. Amer.* **120** E3
Costa Smeralda *Italy* **42** A2
Costești *Romania* **29** F9
Costigliole d'Asti *Italy* **40** D5
Cosumnes → *U.S.A.* **110** G5
Coswig *Sachsen, Germany* **24** D9
Coswig *Sachsen-Anhalt,
    Germany* **24** D8
Cotabato *Phil.* **61** H6
Cotagaita *Bolivia* **126** A2
Côte d'Azur *France* **21** E11
Côte-d'Ivoire = Ivory
    Coast ■ *Africa* **82** D4
Côte d'Or *France* **19** E11
Côte-d'Or □ *France* **19** E11
Coteau des Prairies *U.S.A.* **112** C5
Coteau du Missouri *U.S.A.* **112** B4
Cotentin *France* **18** C5
Côtes-d'Armor □ *France* **18** D4
Côtes de Meuse *France* **19** C12
Côtes-du-Nord =
    Côtes-d'Armor □ *France* **18** D4
Cotiella *Spain* **38** C5
Cotiujeni *Moldova* **29** C13
Cotonou *Benin* **83** D5
Cotopaxi *Ecuador* **124** D3
Cotronei *Italy* **43** C9
Cotswold Hills *U.K.* **15** F5
Cottage Grove *U.S.A.* **108** E2
Cottam *Canada* **114** D2
Cottbus *Germany* **24** D10
Cottonwood *U.S.A.* **109** J7
Cotulla *U.S.A.* **116** G5
Coubre, Pte. de la *France* **20** C2
Couches *France* **19** F11
Couço *Portugal* **37** G2
Coudersport *U.S.A.* **114** E6
Couedic, C. du *Australia* **95** F2
Couëron *France* **18** E5
Couesnon → *France* **18** D5
Couhé *France* **20** B4
Coulanges-sur-Yonne
    France **19** E10
Coulee City *U.S.A.* **108** C4
Coulee Dam Nat. Recr.
    Area = Lake Roosevelt △
    U.S.A. **108** B4
Coulman I. *Antarctica* **5** D11
Coulommiers *France* **19** D10
Coulon → *France* **21** E9
Coulonge → *Canada* **104** C4
Coulonges-sur-l'Autize
    France **20** B3
Coulounieix-Chamiers
    France **20** C4
Coulterville *U.S.A.* **110** H6
Council *Alaska, U.S.A.* **106** C7
Council *Idaho, U.S.A.* **108** D5
Council Bluffs *U.S.A.* **112** E6
Council Grove *U.S.A.* **112** F5
Coupeville *U.S.A.* **110** B4
Courantyne → *S. Amer.* **124** B7
Courcelles *Belgium* **17** D4
Courchevel *France* **21** C10
Courçon *France* **20** B3
Couronne, C. *France* **21** E9
Cours-la-Ville *France* **19** F11
Coursan *France* **20** E7
Courseulles-sur-Mer *France* **18** C6
Courtenay *Canada* **102** D4
Courtenay *U.S.A.* **119** D10
Courtland *Canada* **114** D4
Courtland *U.S.A.* **110** G5
Courtrai = Kortrijk *Belgium* **17** D3
Courtright *Canada* **114** D2
Coushatta *U.S.A.* **116** E8
Coutances *France* **18** C5
Coutras *France* **20** C3
Coutts Crossing *Australia* **95** D5
Couva *Trin. & Tob.* **125** K15
Couvin *Belgium* **17** D4
Covarrubias *Spain* **36** C7
Covasna *Romania* **29** E11
Covasna □ *Romania* **29** E10
Cove I. *Canada* **114** A3
Coventry *U.K.* **15** E6

Covilhã *Portugal* **36** E3
Covington *Ga., U.S.A.* **117** E13
Covington *Ky., U.S.A.* **113** F11
Covington *Tenn., U.S.A.* **117** D10
Covington *Va., U.S.A.* **113** G14
Cowal, L. *Australia* **95** E4
Cowan, L. *Australia* **93** F3
Cowan L. *Canada* **103** C7
Cowangie *Australia* **95** F3
Cowansville *Canada* **115** A12
Coward Springs *Australia* **95** D2
Cowcowing Lakes *Australia* **93** F2
Cowdenbeath *U.K.* **13** E5
Cowell *Australia* **95** E2
Cowes *U.K.* **15** G6
Cowichan L. *Canada* **110** B2
Cowlitz → *U.S.A.* **110** D4
Cowra *Australia* **95** E4
Cox → *Australia* **94** b
Coxilha Grande *Brazil* **127** B5
Coxim *Brazil* **125** G8
Cox's Bazar *Bangla.* **67** J17
Coyah *Guinea* **82** D2
Coyote Wells *U.S.A.* **111** N11
Coyuca de Benitez *Mexico* **119** D4
Coyuca de Catalán *Mexico* **118** D4
Cozad *U.S.A.* **112** E4
Cozes *France* **20** C3
Cozumel *Mexico* **119** C7
Cozumel, Isla *Mexico* **119** C7
Crab Hill *Barbados* **121** g
Cracow = Kraków *Poland* **31** H6
Cracow *Australia* **95** D5
Cradle Mt.-Lake St. Clair △
    Australia **95** G4
Cradock *Australia* **95** E2
Cradock *S. Africa* **88** E4
Craig *U.S.A.* **108** F10
Craigavon *U.K.* **12** B5
Craigmore *Zimbabwe* **87** G3
Craik *Canada* **103** C7
Crailsheim *Germany* **25** F6
Craiova *Romania* **29** F8
Cramsie *Australia* **94** C3
Cranberry L. *U.S.A.* **115** B10
Cranberry Portage *Canada* **103** C8
Cranbrook *Australia* **93** F2
Cranbrook *Canada* **102** D5
Crandon *U.S.A.* **112** C9
Crane *Oreg., U.S.A.* **108** E4
Crane *Tex., U.S.A.* **116** F3
Crane, The *Barbados* **121** g
Cranston *U.S.A.* **115** E13
Craon *France* **18** E6
Craonne *France* **19** C10
Craponne-sur-Arzon *France* **20** C7
Crasna *Romania* **29** D12
Crasna → *Romania* **28** C7
Crasnei, Munții *Romania* **29** C8
Crater L. *U.S.A.* **108** E2
Crater Lake △ *U.S.A.* **108** E2
Craters of the Moon △
    U.S.A. **108** E7
Crateús *Brazil* **125** E10
Crati → *Italy* **43** C9
Crato *Brazil* **125** E11
Crato *Portugal* **37** F3
Craven, L. *Canada* **104** B4
Crawford *U.S.A.* **112** D2
Crawfordsville *U.S.A.* **112** E10
Crawley *U.K.* **15** F7
Crazy Mts. *U.S.A.* **108** C8
Crean L. *Canada* **103** C7
Crécy-en-Ponthieu *France* **19** B8
Crediton *Canada* **114** C3
Crediton *U.K.* **15** G4
Cree → *Canada* **103** B7
Cree → *U.K.* **13** G4
Cree L. *Canada* **103** B7
Creede *U.S.A.* **109** H10
Creekside *U.S.A.* **114** F5
Creel *Mexico* **118** B3
Creemore *Canada* **114** B4
Creighton *Canada* **103** C8
Creighton *U.S.A.* **112** D5
Creil *France* **19** C9
Crema *Italy* **40** C6
Cremona *Italy* **40** C7
Crepaja *Serbia* **28** E5
Crépy *France* **19** C9
Crépy-en-Valois *France* **19** C9
Cres *Croatia* **41** D11
Crescent City *U.S.A.* **108** F1
Crescentino *Italy* **40** C5
Crespo *Argentina* **126** C3
Cresson *U.S.A.* **114** F6
Crest *France* **21** D9
Cresta, Mt. *Phil.* **61** C5
Crestline *Calif., U.S.A.* **111** L9
Crestline *Ohio, U.S.A.* **114** F2
Creston *Canada* **102** D5
Creston *Calif., U.S.A.* **110** K6
Creston *Iowa, U.S.A.* **112** E6
Crestview *Calif., U.S.A.* **110** H8
Crestview *Fla., U.S.A.* **117** F11
Crêt de la Neige *France* **19** F12
Crete = Kriti *Greece* **49** D7
Crete *U.S.A.* **112** E5
Crete, Sea of *Greece* **47** E7

Créteil *France* **19** D9
Creus, C. de *Spain* **38** C8
Creuse □ *France* **19** F9
Creuse → *France* **20** B4
Creutzwald *France* **19** C13
Creuzburg *Germany* **24** D6
Crèvecœur-le-Grand *France* **19** C9
Crevillent *Spain* **39** G4
Crewe *U.K.* **14** D5
Crewkerne *U.K.* **15** G5
Crianlarich *U.K.* **13** E4
Criciúma *Brazil* **127** B6
Cricova *Moldova* **29** C13
Crieff *U.K.* **13** E5
Crikvenica *Croatia* **41** C11
Crimea □ *Ukraine* **33** K8
Crimean Pen. = Krymskyy
    Pivostriv *Ukraine* **33** K8
Crimmitschau *Germany* **24** E8
Cristuru Secuiesc *Romania* **29** D10
Crișul Alb → *Romania* **28** D6
Crișul Negru → *Romania* **28** D6
Crișul Repede → *Romania* **28** D5
Criuleni *Moldova* **29** C14
Crivitz *Germany* **24** B7
Crna → *Macedonia* **44** E5
Crna Gora =
    Montenegro ■ *Europe* **44** D3
Crna Gora *Macedonia* **44** D5
Crna Reka = Crna →
    Macedonia **44** E5
Crna Trava *Serbia* **44** D6
Crni Drim → *Macedonia* **44** E4
Crni Timok → *Serbia* **44** C6
Crnoljeva Planina *Kosovo* **44** D5
Črnomelj *Slovenia* **41** C12
Croagh Patrick *Ireland* **12** C2
Croatia ■ *Europe* **41** C13
Crocker, Banjaran *Malaysia* **62** C5
Crockett *U.S.A.* **116** F7
Crocodile = Umgwenya →
    Mozam. **89** D5
Crocodile Is. *Australia* **94** A1
Crocq *France* **20** C6
Crodo *Italy* **40** B5
Crohy Hd. *Ireland* **12** B3
Croisette, C. *France* **21** E9
Croisic, Pte. du *France* **18** E4
Croix, L. la *Canada* **104** C1
Croker, C. *Australia* **92** B5
Croker, C. *Canada* **114** B4
Croker I. *Australia* **92** B5
Croker Islands Seas ○
    Australia **92** B5
Cromarty *U.K.* **13** D4
Cromer *U.K.* **14** E9
Cromwell *N.Z.* **91** F2
Cromwell *U.S.A.* **115** E12
Cronat *France* **19** F10
Crook *U.K.* **14** C6
Crooked → *Canada* **102** C4
Crooked → *U.S.A.* **108** D3
Crooked I. *Bahamas* **121** B5
Crooked Island Passage
    Bahamas **121** B5
Crookston *Minn., U.S.A.* **112** B5
Crookston *Nebr., U.S.A.* **112** D3
Crookwell *Australia* **95** E4
Cropane-Micone △ *Italy* **43** D9
Crosby *U.K.* **14** D4
Crosby *N. Dak., U.S.A.* **112** A2
Crosby *Pa., U.S.A.* **114** E6
Crosbyton *U.S.A.* **116** E4
Crosia *Italy* **43** C9
Cross → *Nigeria* **83** D6
Cross City *U.S.A.* **117** G13
Cross Fell *U.K.* **14** C5
Cross L. *Canada* **103** C9
Cross Lake *Canada* **103** C9
Cross River □ *Nigeria* **83** D6
Cross River △ *Nigeria* **83** D6
Cross Sound *U.S.A.* **100** F4
Crossett *U.S.A.* **116** E9
Crosshaven *Ireland* **12** E3
Crossmaglen *U.K.* **12** B5
Crossmolina *Ireland* **12** B2
Crossville *U.S.A.* **117** D12
Croswell *U.S.A.* **114** C2
Croton-on-Hudson *U.S.A.* **115** E11
Crotone *Italy* **43** C10
Crow → *Canada* **102** B4
Crow Agency *U.S.A.* **108** D10
Crow Hd. *Ireland* **12** E1
Crowell *U.S.A.* **116** E5
Crowley *U.S.A.* **116** F8
Crowley, L. *U.S.A.* **110** H8
Crown Point *Ind., U.S.A.* **112** E10
Crown Point *N.Y., U.S.A.* **115** C11
Crown Pt. *Trin. & Tob.* **125** J16
Crownpoint *U.S.A.* **109** J9
Crows Landing *U.S.A.* **110** H5
Crows Nest *Australia* **95** D5
Crowsnest Pass *Canada* **102** D6
Croydon *Australia* **94** B3
Croydon □ *U.K.* **15** F7
Crozet, Is. *Ind. Oc.* **3** G12
Crozon *France* **18** D2
Crusheen *Ireland* **12** D3
Cruz, C. *Cuba* **120** C4

Cruz Alta *Brazil* 127 B5
Cruz Bay *U.S. Virgin Is.* 121 e
Cruz del Eje *Argentina* 126 C3
Cruzeiro *Brazil* 127 A6
Cruzeiro do Oeste *Brazil* 127 A5
Cruzeiro do Sul *Brazil* 124 E4
Cry L. *Canada* 102 B3
Crystal Bay *U.S.A.* 110 F7
Crystal Brook *Australia* 95 E2
Crystal City *U.S.A.* 116 G5
Crystal Falls *U.S.A.* 112 B9
Crystal River *U.S.A.* 117 G13
Crystal Springs *U.S.A.* 117 F9
Csenger *Hungary* 28 C7
Csongrád *Hungary* 28 D5
Csongrád □ *Hungary* 28 D5
Csorna *Hungary* 28 C2
Csurgo *Hungary* 28 D2
Cu Lao Hon *Vietnam* 65 G7
Cua Rao *Vietnam* 64 C5
Cuácua → *Mozam.* 87 F4
Cuamato *Angola* 88 B2
Cuamba *Mozam.* 87 E4
Cuando → *Angola* 85 H4
Cuando Cubango □ *Angola* 88 B3
Cuangar *Angola* 88 B2
Cuango = Kwango →
  Dem. Rep. of the Congo 84 E3
Cuanza → *Angola* 84 F2
Cuarto → *Argentina* 126 C3
Cuatrociénegas *Mexico* 118 B4
Cuauhtémoc *Mexico* 118 B3
Cuba *Portugal* 37 G3
Cuba *N. Mex., U.S.A.* 109 H10
Cuba *N.Y., U.S.A.* 114 D6
Cuba ■ *W. Indies* 120 B4
Cubango → *Africa* 88 B3
Çubuk *Turkey* 72 B5
Cuc Phuong △ *Vietnam* 64 B5
Cuchumatanes, Sierra de
  los *Guatemala* 120 C1
Cuckfield *U.K.* 15 F7
Cucuí *Brazil* 124 C5
Cucurpé *Mexico* 118 A2
Cúcuta *Colombia* 124 B4
Cudalbi *Romania* 29 E12
Cuddalore *India* 66 P11
Cuddapah *India* 66 M11
Cuddapan, L. *Australia* 94 D3
Cudillero *Spain* 36 B4
Cue *Australia* 93 E2
Cuéllar *Spain* 36 D6
Cuenca *Ecuador* 124 D3
Cuenca *Spain* 38 E2
Cuenca □ *Spain* 38 F3
Cuenca, Serranía de *Spain* 38 F3
Cuenca Alta del
  Manzanares △ *Spain* 36 E7
Cuerda del Pozo, Embalse
  de la *Spain* 38 D2
Cuernavaca *Mexico* 119 D5
Cuero *U.S.A.* 116 G6
Cuers *France* 21 E10
Cueva de la Quebrada del
  Toro △ *Venezuela* 121 D6
Cuevas del Almanzora *Spain* 39 H3
Cuevo *Bolivia* 124 H6
Cugir *Romania* 29 E8
Cugnaux *France* 20 E5
Cuhai-Bakony → *Hungary* 28 C2
Cuiabá *Brazil* 125 G7
Cuiabá → *Brazil* 125 G7
Cuijk *Neths.* 17 C5
Cuilco *Guatemala* 120 C1
Cuillin Hills *U.K.* 13 D2
Cuillin Sd. *U.K.* 13 D2
Cuilo = Kwilu →
  Dem. Rep. of the Congo 84 E3
Cuiseaux *France* 19 F12
Cuito → *Angola* 88 B3
Cuitzeo, L. de *Mexico* 118 D4
Cujmir *Romania* 28 F7
Cukai *Malaysia* 65 K4
Çukurca *Turkey* 73 D10
Culbertson *U.S.A.* 108 B11
Culcairn *Australia* 95 F4
Culebra *Puerto Rico* 121 d
Culebra, Sierra de la *Spain* 36 C4
Culfa *Azerbaijan* 73 C11
Culgoa → *Australia* 95 D4
Culgoa Flood Plain △
  Australia 95 D4
Culiacán *Mexico* 118 C3
Culiacán → *Mexico* 118 C3
Culik *Indonesia* 63 J18
Culion *Phil.* 61 F3
Cúllar *Spain* 37 H8
Cullarin Ra. *Australia* 95 E4
Cullen *U.K.* 13 D6
Cullen Pt. *Australia* 94 A3
Cullera *Spain* 39 F4
Cullman *U.S.A.* 117 D11
Cullompton *U.K.* 15 G4
Culpeper *U.S.A.* 113 F7
Culuene → *Brazil* 125 F8
Culver, Pt. *Australia* 93 F3
Culverden *N.Z.* 91 E4
Cumaná *Venezuela* 124 A6

Cumaovası *Turkey* 47 C9
Cumberland *B.C., Canada* 102 D4
Cumberland *Ont., Canada* 115 A9
Cumberland *U.S.A.* 113 F14
Cumberland → *U.S.A.* 112 G9
Cumberland, L. *U.S.A.* 113 G11
Cumberland Gap △ *U.S.A.* 113 G12
Cumberland I. *U.S.A.* 117 F14
Cumberland Island △
  U.S.A. 117 F14
Cumberland Is. *Australia* 94 b
Cumberland L. *Canada* 103 C8
Cumberland Pen. *Canada* 101 D19
Cumberland Plateau *U.S.A.*
  117 D12
Cumberland Sd. *Canada* 101 D18
Cumbernauld *U.K.* 13 F5
Cumborah *Australia* 95 D4
Cumbres de Majalca △
  Mexico 118 B3
Cumbres de Monterrey △
  Mexico 118 B4
Cumbres Mayores *Spain* 37 G4
Cumbria □ *U.K.* 14 C5
Cumbrian Mts. *U.K.* 14 C5
Cumbum *India* 66 M11
Cuminá → *Brazil* 125 D7
Cummings Mt. *U.S.A.* 111 K8
Cummins *Australia* 95 E2
Cumnock *Australia* 95 E4
Cumnock *U.K.* 13 F4
Cumpas *Mexico* 118 B3
Çumra *Turkey* 72 D5
Cumplida, Pta. *Canary Is.* 48 F2
Cunco *Chile* 128 D2
Cuncumén *Chile* 126 C1
Cundeelee ۞ *Australia* 93 F3
Cunderdin *Australia* 93 F2
Cunene → *Angola* 88 B1
Cúneo *Italy* 40 D4
Çüngüş *Turkey* 70 B3
Cunillera, I. = Sa Conillera
  Spain 48 C7
Cunlhat *France* 20 C7
Cunnamulla *Australia* 95 D4
Cuorgnè *Italy* 40 C4
Cupar *Canada* 103 C8
Cupar *U.K.* 13 E5
Cupcini *Moldova* 29 B12
Cupertino *U.S.A.* 110 H4
Cupica, G. de *Colombia* 124 B3
Čuprija *Serbia* 44 C5
Curaçao *Neth. Ant.* 121 D6
Curanilahue *Chile* 126 D1
Curaray → *Peru* 124 D4
Cure → *France* 19 E10
Curepipe *Mauritius* 85 d
Curepto *Chile* 126 D1
Curiapo *Venezuela* 124 B6
Curicó *Chile* 126 C1
Curieuse *Seychelles* 85 b
Curinga *Italy* 43 D9
Curitiba *Brazil* 127 B6
Curitibanos *Brazil* 127 B5
Currabubula *Australia* 95 E5
Currais Novos *Brazil* 125 E11
Curral Velho *C. Verde Is.* 78 b
Curralinho *Brazil* 125 D9
Currane, L. *Ireland* 12 E1
Currant *U.S.A.* 108 G6
Currawinya △ *Australia* 95 D3
Current → *U.S.A.* 116 C9
Currie *Australia* 95 F3
Currie *U.S.A.* 108 F6
Curtea de Argeş *Romania* 29 E9
Curtici *Romania* 28 D6
Curtin Springs *Australia* 93 E5
Curtis *U.S.A.* 112 E3
Curtis Group *Australia* 95 F4
Curtis I. *Australia* 94 C5
Curuápanema → *Brazil* 125 D7
Curuçá *Brazil* 125 D9
Curuguaty *Paraguay* 127 A4
Curup *Indonesia* 62 E2
Cururupu *Brazil* 125 D10
Curuzú Cuatiá *Argentina* 126 B4
Curvelo *Brazil* 125 G10
Cusco = Cuzco *Peru* 124 F4
Cushendall *U.K.* 12 A5
Cushing *U.S.A.* 116 D6
Cushing, Mt. *Canada* 102 B3
Cusihuiriáchic *Mexico* 118 B3
Cusna, Mte. *Italy* 40 D7
Cusset *France* 19 F10
Custer *U.S.A.* 112 D2
Cut Bank *U.S.A.* 108 B7
Cutchogue *U.S.A.* 115 E12
Cuthbert *U.S.A.* 117 F12
Cutler *U.S.A.* 110 J7
Cutro *Italy* 43 C9
Cuttaburra → *Australia* 95 D3
Cuttack *India* 67 J14
Cuvier, C. *Australia* 93 D1
Cuvier I. *N.Z.* 91 B5
Cuxhaven *Germany* 24 B4
Cuyahoga Falls *U.S.A.* 114 E3
Cuyahoga Valley △ *U.S.A.* 114 E3
Cuyapo *Phil.* 61 D4
Cuyo *Phil.* 61 F4

Cuyo East Pass *Phil.* 61 F4
Cuyo West Pass *Phil.* 61 F4
Cuyuni → *Guyana* 124 B7
Cuzco *Bolivia* 124 H5
Cuzco *Peru* 124 F4
Čvrsnica *Bos.-H.* 28 G2
Cwmbran *U.K.* 15 F4
Cyangugu *Rwanda* 86 C2
Cyclades *Greece* 46 E6
Cyclades □ *Greece* 46 D6
Cygnet *Australia* 95 G4
Cynthiana *U.S.A.* 113 F11
Cypress Hills *Canada* 103 D7
Cypress Hills △ *Canada* 103 D7
Cyprus ■ *Asia* 49 E12
Cyrenaica = Barqa *Libya* 79 C10
Cyrene *Libya* 79 B10
Czaplinek *Poland* 30 E3
Czar *Canada* 103 C6
Czarna → *Łódzkie, Poland* 31 G6
Czarna → *Świętokrzyskie,*
  Poland 31 H8
Czarna Białostocka *Poland* 31 E10
Czarna Woda *Poland* 30 E5
Czarne *Poland* 30 E3
Czarnków *Poland* 31 F3
Czarnków *Poland* 31 F3
Czersk *Poland* 30 E4
Czerwieńsk *Poland* 31 F2
Czeremcha *Poland* 31 F10
Czerniejewo *Poland* 31 F4
Czech Rep. ■ *Europe* 26 B8
Czechowice-Dziedzice *Poland* 31 J5
Czempiń *Poland* 31 F3
Czerwionka-Leszczyny
  Poland 31 H5
Częstochowa *Poland* 31 H6
Członków *Poland* 31 E3
Człuchów *Poland* 30 E4
Czyżew-Osada *Poland* 31 F9

D

Da → *Vietnam* 58 G5
Da Hinggan Ling *China* 60 B7
Da Lat *Vietnam* 65 G7
Da Nang *Vietnam* 64 D7
Da Qaidam *China* 60 C4
Da Yunhe → *Hopei, China* 57 E9
Da Yunhe → *Jiangsu, China* 57 G11
Da'an *China* 57 B13
Daan Viljoen △ *Namibia* 88 C2
Dab'a, Ras el *Egypt* 80 H6
Daba Shan *China* 58 B7
Dabai *China* 56 F8
Dabakala *Ivory C.* 82 D4
Daba Shan *China* 58 B7
Dabas *Hungary* 28 C4
Dabat *Ethiopia* 81 E4
Dabbagh, Jabal *Si. Arabia* 70 E2
Dabhoi *India* 68 H5
Dabie *Poland* 31 F5
Dabie Shan *China* 59 B10
Dabilda *Cameroon* 83 C7
Dabnou *Niger* 83 C6
Dabo = Pasirkuning
  Indonesia 62 E2
Dabola *Guinea* 82 C2
Dabou *Ivory C.* 82 D4
Daboya *Ghana* 83 D4
Dabravolya *Belarus* 31 F10
Dąbrowa Białostocka
  Poland 30 E10
Dąbrowa Górnicza *Poland* 31 H6
Dąbrowa Tarnowska *Poland* 31 H7
Dabu *China* 59 E11
Dabung *Malaysia* 65 K4
Dabus → *Ethiopia* 81 E4
Dacato → *Ethiopia* 81 F5
Dacca = Dhaka *Bangla.* 69 H14
Dacca □ = Dhaka □ *Bangla.* 69 G14
Dachau *Germany* 25 G7
Dachigam △ *India* 68 B6
Dachstein, Hoher *Austria* 26 D6
Dačice *Czech Rep.* 26 B8
Dacre *Canada* 114 A8
Dadanawa *Guyana* 124 C7
Daday *Turkey* 72 B5
Dade City *U.S.A.* 117 G13
Dadhar *Pakistan* 68 E2
Dadiya *Nigeria* 83 D7
Dadra & Nagar Haveli □
  India 66 J8
Dadri = Charkhi Dadri *India* 68 E7
Dadu *Pakistan* 68 F2
Dadu He → *China* 58 C4
Daegu *S. Korea* 57 G15
Daejeon *S. Korea* 57 F14
Daejeong *S. Korea* 57 H14
Daet *Phil.* 61 D5
Dafang *China* 58 D5
Dafnes *Greece* 49 D7
Dafni *Greece* 46 D5
Dağ *Turkey* 47 D12
Dagana *Senegal* 82 B1
Dagash *Sudan* 80 D3
Dagestan □ *Russia* 35 J8
Dagestanskiye Ogni *Russia* 35 J9
Daggett *U.S.A.* 111 L10

Daghestan Republic =
  Dagestan □ *Russia* 35 J8
Daghfeli *Sudan* 80 D3
Dağlı U.K. 13 F4
Dağlıq Qarabağ =
  Nagorno-Karabakh □
  Azerbaijan 73 C12
Dağō = Hiiumaa *Estonia* 32 C2
Dagu *China* 57 E9
Daguan *China* 58 D4
Dagupan *Phil.* 61 C4
Daguragu *Australia* 92 C5
Daguragu ۞ *Australia* 92 C5
Dahab *Egypt* 70 D2
Dahlak Kebir *Eritrea* 81 D5
Dahlak Marine △ *Eritrea* 81 D5
Dahlenburg *Germany* 24 B6
Dahlonega *U.S.A.* 117 D13
Dahme *Germany* 24 D9
Dahod *India* 68 H6
Dahong Shan *China* 59 B9
Dahongliutan *China* 69 B8
Dahra *Libya* 79 C9
Dahra *Senegal* 82 B1
Dahshûr *Egypt* 80 J7
Dahûk *Iraq* 73 D10
Dahûk □ *Iraq* 73 D10
Dai Hao *Vietnam* 64 C6
Dai-Sen *Japan* 55 G6
Dai Shan *China* 59 B14
Dai Xian *China* 56 E7
Daicheng *China* 56 E9
Daikondi = Day Kundī □
  Afghan. 66 C5
Daimiel *Spain* 37 F7
Daingean *Ireland* 12 C4
Dainkog *China* 58 A1
Daintree *Australia* 94 B4
Daintree △ *Australia* 94 B4
Daiō-Misaki *Japan* 55 G8
Dair, J. ed *Sudan* 81 E3
Dairût *Egypt* 80 B3
Daisen-Oki △ *Japan* 55 G6
Daisetsu-Zan *Japan* 54 C11
Daisetsu-Zan △ *Japan* 54 C11
Dajarra *Australia* 94 C2
Dajiawa *China* 57 F10
Dajin Chuan → *China* 58 B3
Dak Dam *Cambodia* 64 F6
Dak Nhe *Vietnam* 64 E6
Dak Pek *Vietnam* 64 E6
Dak Song *Vietnam* 65 F6
Dak Sui *Vietnam* 64 E6
Dakar *Senegal* 82 C1
Dakar □ *Senegal* 82 C1
Dakhla *W. Sahara* 78 D2
Dakhla, El Wâhât el *Egypt* 80 B2
Dakingari *Nigeria* 83 C5
Dakor *India* 68 H5
Dakoro *Niger* 83 C6
Dakota City *U.S.A.* 112 D5
Đakovica *Kosovo* 44 D4
Đakovo *Croatia* 28 E3
Dalaba *Guinea* 82 C2
Dalachi *China* 56 F3
Dalai Nur *China* 56 C9
Dālakī *Iran* 71 D6
Dalälven → *Sweden* 10 D10
Dalaman *Turkey* 47 E10
Dalaman → *Turkey* 47 E10
Dalandzadgad *Mongolia* 56 C3
Dalap-Uliga-Darrit =
  Majuro *Marshall Is.* 96 G9
Dalarna *Sweden* 10 D8
Dalarnas län □ *Sweden* 10 C8
Dālbandīn *Pakistan* 66 E4
Dalbeattie *U.K.* 13 G5
Dalbeg *Australia* 94 C4
Dalbosjön *Sweden* 11 F6
Dalby *Australia* 95 D5
Dalby *Sweden* 11 J7
Dalby Söderskog △ *Sweden* 11 J7
Dale City *U.S.A.* 113 F15
Dale Hollow L. *U.S.A.* 117 C12
Dalga *Egypt* 80 B3
Dalgán *Iran* 71 E8
Dalhart *U.S.A.* 116 C3
Dalhousie *Canada* 105 C6
Dalhousie *India* 68 C7
Dali *Shaanxi, China* 56 G5
Dali *Yunnan, China* 58 E3
Dalian *China* 57 E11
Daliang Shan *China* 58 D4
Daling He → *China* 57 D11
Dāliyat el Karmel *Israel* 74 C4
Dalj *Croatia* 28 E3
Dalkeith *U.K.* 13 F5
Dalkey *Ireland* 12 C5
Dallas *Oreg., U.S.A.* 108 D2
Dallas *Tex., U.S.A.* 116 E6
Dalles, The *U.S.A.* 108 D3
Dallol *Ethiopia* 81 E5
Dalmā *U.A.E.* 71 E7
Dalmacija *Croatia* 41 E13
Dalmas, L. *Canada* 105 B5
Dalmatia = Dalmacija
  Croatia 41 E13
Dalmau *India* 69 F9
Dalmellington *U.K.* 13 F4
Dalnegorsk *Russia* 54 B7
Dalnerechensk *Russia* 54 B6

Dalnevostochnyy □ *Russia* 53 C14
Daloa *Ivory C.* 82 D3
Dalou Shan *China* 58 C6
Dalry *U.K.* 13 F4
Dalrymple, L. *Australia* 94 C4
Dalrymple, Mt. *Australia* 94 b
Dals Långed *Sweden* 11 F6
Dalsjöfors *Sweden* 11 G7
Dalsland *Sweden* 11 F6
Dalton *Ga., U.S.A.* 117 D12
Dalton *Mass., U.S.A.* 115 D11
Dalton *Nebr., U.S.A.* 112 E2
Dalton-in-Furness *U.K.* 14 C4
Dalupiri I. *Phil.* 61 B4
Dalvík *Iceland* 8 D4
Dálvvadis = Jokkmokk
  Sweden 8 C18
Dalwallinu *Australia* 93 F2
Daly → *Australia* 92 B5
Daly City *U.S.A.* 110 H4
Daly L. *Canada* 103 B7
Daly River *Australia* 92 B5
Daly River-Port Keats ۞
  Australia 92 B4
Daly Waters *Australia* 94 B1
Dalyan *Turkey* 47 E10
Dam Doi *Vietnam* 65 H5
Dam Ha *Vietnam* 64 B6
Damachova *Belarus* 31 G10
Daman *India* 66 J8
Dāmaneh *Iran* 71 C6
Damanhûr *Egypt* 80 H7
Damanzhuang *China* 56 E9
Damaq *Iran* 73 E13
Damar *Indonesia* 63 F7
Damara *C.A.R.* 84 D3
Damaraland *Namibia* 88 C2
Damascus = Dimashq *Syria* 74 B5
Damasi *Greece* 46 B4
Damaturu *Nigeria* 83 C7
Damāvand *Iran* 71 C7
Damāvand, Qolleh-ye *Iran* 71 C7
Damba *Angola* 84 F3
Dambaa *Nigeria* 83 C7
Dame Marie *Haiti* 121 C5
Dāmghān *Iran* 71 B7
Damiel *Spain* 37 F7
Damietta = Dumyât *Egypt* 80 H7
Daming *China* 56 F8
Damīr Qābū *Syria* 70 B4
Dammam = Ad Dammām
  Si. Arabia 71 E6
Dammarie-les-Lys *France* 19 D9
Dammartin-en-Goële *France* 19 C9
Damme *Germany* 24 C4
Damodar → *India* 69 H12
Damoh *India* 69 H8
Dampier *Australia* 92 D2
Dampier, Selat *Indonesia* 63 E8
Dampier Arch. *Australia* 92 D2
Damrei, Chuor Phnom
  Cambodia 65 G4
Damvillers *France* 19 C12
Damyang *S. Korea* 57 G14
Dan-Gulbi *Nigeria* 83 C6
Dan-Sadau *Nigeria* 83 C6
Dana *Indonesia* 63 F6
Dana *Jordan* 74 E4
Dana, L. *Canada* 104 B4
Dana, Mt. *U.S.A.* 110 H7
Danané *Ivory C.* 82 D3
Danao *Phil.* 61 F6
Danau Poso *Indonesia* 63 E6
Danba *China* 58 B3
Danbury *U.S.A.* 115 E11
Danby L. *U.S.A.* 109 J6
Dand *Afghan.* 68 D1
Dande △ *Zimbabwe* 87 F3
Dandeldhura *Nepal* 69 E9
Dandeli *India* 66 M9
Dandenong *Australia* 95 F4
Dandī *Iran* 73 D12
Dandī *Egypt* 80 J7
Dandong *China* 57 D13
Danfeng *China* 56 H6
Dangan Liedao *China* 59 F10
Dangé-St-Romain *France* 20 B4
Dăngeni *Romania* 29 C11
Danger Is. = Pukapuka
  Cook Is. 97 J11
Danger Pt. *S. Africa* 88 E2
Danginpuri *Indonesia* 63 K18
Dangla *Ethiopia* 81 E4
Dangla Shan = Tanggula
  Shan *China* 60 C4
Dangora *Nigeria* 83 C6
Dangrek, Mts. = Dangrek,
  Phnom *Thailand* 64 E5
Dangrek, Phnom *Thailand* 64 E5
Dangriga *Belize* 119 D7
Dangshan *China* 56 G9

Dangtu *China* 59 B12
Dangyang *China* 59 B8
Daniel *U.S.A.* 108 E8
Daniel's Harbour *Canada* 105 B8
Danielskuil *S. Africa* 88 D3
Danielson *U.S.A.* 115 E13
Danilov *Russia* 32 A11
Danilov Russia 34 E7
Danilovgrad *Montenegro* 44 D3
Danilovka *Russia* 34 E7
Daning *China* 56 F6
Danja *Nigeria* 83 C6
Danjiangkou *China* 59 A8
Danjiangkou Shuiku *China* 59 A8
Dank *Oman* 71 F8
Dankalwa *Nigeria* 83 C7
Dankama *Nigeria* 83 C7
Dankhar Gompa *India* 68 C8
Dankov *Russia* 32 F10
Danleng *China* 58 B4
Danlí *Honduras* 120 D2
Danmark = Denmark ■
  Europe 11 J3
Dannemora *U.S.A.* 115 B11
Dannenberg *Germany* 24 B7
Dannevirke *N.Z.* 91 D6
Dannhauser *S. Africa* 89 D5
Dansville *U.S.A.* 114 D7
Danta *India* 68 G5
Dantan *India* 69 J12
Dante = Xaafuun *Somali Rep.* 75 E5
Danube = Dunărea →
  Europe 29 E14
Danvers *U.S.A.* 115 D14
Danville *Ill., U.S.A.* 112 E10
Danville *Ky., U.S.A.* 113 G11
Danville *Pa., U.S.A.* 115 F8
Danville *Va., U.S.A.* 113 G14
Danville *Vt., U.S.A.* 115 B12
Danyang *China* 59 B12
Danzhai *China* 58 D6
Danzhou *China* 64 C7
Danzig = Gdańsk *Poland* 30 D5
Dão → *Portugal* 36 E2
Dao Xian *China* 59 E8
Daocheng *China* 58 C3
Daoukro *Ivory C.* 82 D4
Dapaong *Togo* 83 C5
Dapchi *Nigeria* 83 C7
Dapitan *Phil.* 61 G5
Daqing Shan *China* 56 D6
Daqq-e Sorkh, Kavīr *Iran* 71 C7
Daqu Shan *China* 59 B14
Dar Banda *Africa* 76 F6
Dar el Beida = Casablanca
  Morocco 78 B4
Dar es Salaam *Tanzania* 86 D4
Dar Mazār *Iran* 71 D8
Dar'ā *Syria* 74 C5
Dar'ā □ *Syria* 74 C5
Dārāb *Iran* 71 D7
Daraban *Pakistan* 68 D4
Darabani *Romania* 29 B11
Daraina *Madag.* 89 A8
Daraj *Libya* 79 B8
Dārān *Iran* 71 C6
Đaravica *Kosovo* 44 D4
Daraw *Egypt* 80 C3
Dārayyā *Syria* 74 B5
Darazo *Nigeria* 83 C7
Darband *Pakistan* 68 B5
Darband, Kūh-e *Iran* 71 D8
Darbhanga *India* 69 F11
D'Arcy *Canada* 102 C4
Darda *Croatia* 28 E3
Dardanelle *Ark., U.S.A.* 116 D8
Dardanelle *Calif., U.S.A.* 110 G7
Dardanelles = Çanakkale
  Boğazı *Turkey* 45 F10
Dare → *Ethiopia* 81 F5
Darende *Turkey* 72 C7
Dārestān *Iran* 71 D8
Darfo *Italy* 40 C7
Dârfûr *Sudan* 79 F10
Dargai *Pakistan* 68 B4
Dargaville *N.Z.* 91 A4
Dargol *Niger* 83 C5
Darhan *Mongolia* 60 B5
Darhan Muminggan
  Lianheqi *China* 56 D6
Dari *Sudan* 81 F3
Darıca *Turkey* 72 B3
Darién, G. del *Colombia* 124 B3
Darién △ *Panama* 120 E4
Dariganga = Ovoot *Mongolia* 56 B7
Darjeeling = Darjiling *India* 69 F13
Darjiling *India* 69 F13
Darkan *Australia* 93 F2
Darkhana *Pakistan* 68 D5
Darkhazīneh *Iran* 71 D6
Darkot Pass *Pakistan* 69 A5
Darling → *Australia* 95 E3
Darling Downs *Australia* 95 D5
Darling Ra. *Australia* 93 F2
Darlington *U.K.* 14 C6
Darlington *U.S.A.* 117 D15
Darlington □ *U.K.* 14 C6
Darlington, L. *S. Africa* 88 E4
Darlot, L. *Australia* 93 E3
Darłowo *Poland* 30 D3

Dărmănești *Bacău, Romania* **29** D11
Dărmănești *Suceava, Romania* **29** C11
Darmstadt *Germany* **25** F4
Darnah *Libya* **79** B10
Darnall *S. Africa* **89** D5
Darney *France* **19** D13
Darnley *Australia* **94** a
Darnley, C. *Antarctica* **5** C6
Darnley B. *Canada* **100** D7
Daroca *Spain* **38** D3
Darou-Mousti *Senegal* **82** B1
Darr → *Australia* **94** C3
Darra Pezu *Pakistan* **68** C4
Darreh Shahr *Iran* **73** F12
Darrequeira *Argentina* **126** D3
Darrington *U.S.A.* **108** B3
Darsser Ort *Germany* **24** A8
Dart → *U.K.* **15** G4
Dart, C. *Antarctica* **5** D14
Dartford *U.K.* **15** F8
Dartmoor *U.K.* **15** G4
Dartmoor △ *U.K.* **15** G4
Dartmouth *Canada* **105** D7
Dartmouth *U.K.* **15** G4
Dartmouth Res. *Australia* **95** D4
Dartuch, C. = Artrutx, C. de *Spain* **48** B10
Daruvar *Croatia* **28** E2
Darvaza *Turkmenistan* **52** E6
Darvel, Teluk = Lahad Datu, Telok *Malaysia* **63** D5
Darwen *U.K.* **14** D5
Darwendale *Zimbabwe* **89** B5
Darwha *India* **66** J10
Darwin *Australia* **92** B5
Darwin *U.S.A.* **111** J9
Darya Khan *Pakistan* **68** D4
Daryāchēh-ye Bakhtegān *Iran* **71** D7
Daryoi Amu = Amudarya → *Uzbekistan* **52** E6
Dās *U.A.E.* **71** E7
Dashen, Ras *Ethiopia* **81** E4
Dashetai *China* **56** D5
Dashkesan = Daşkäsän *Azerbaijan* **35** K7
Dashköpri *Turkmenistan* **71** B9
Dashoguz *Turkmenistan* **52** E6
Dasht → *Pakistan* **66** G2
Daska *Pakistan* **68** C6
Daşkäsän *Azerbaijan* **35** K7
Dassa *Benin* **83** D5
Dasuya *India* **68** D6
Datça *Turkey* **47** E9
Datia *India* **69** G8
Datian *China* **59** E11
Datong *Anhui, China* **59** B11
Datong *Shanxi, China* **56** D7
Dattakhel *Pakistan* **68** C3
Datteln *Germany* **24** D3
Datu, Tanjung *Indonesia* **62** D3
Datu Piang *Phil.* **61** H6
Datuk, Tanjong = Datu, Tanjung *Indonesia* **62** D3
Daua = Dawa → *Africa* **81** G5
Daud Khel *Pakistan* **68** C4
Daudnagar *India* **69** G11
Daugava → *Latvia* **32** D3
Daugavpils *Latvia* **32** E4
Daulpur *India* **68** F7
Daun *Germany* **25** E2
Dauphin *Canada* **103** C8
Dauphin *U.S.A.* **114** F8
Dauphin I. *U.S.A.* **103** D9
Dauphiné *France* **21** C9
Daura *Borno, Nigeria* **83** C7
Daura *Katsina, Nigeria* **83** C6
Dausa *India* **68** F7
Däväçi *Azerbaijan* **35** K9
Davangere *India* **66** M9
Davao *Phil.* **61** H6
Davao G. *Phil.* **61** H6
Dăvar Panāh = Sarāvān *Iran* **71** E9
Davenport *Calif., U.S.A.* **110** H4
Davenport *Iowa, U.S.A.* **112** E8
Davenport *Wash., U.S.A.* **108** C4
Davenport Ra. *Australia* **94** C1
Davenport Range △ *Australia* **94** C1
Daventry *U.K.* **15** E6
David *Panama* **120** E3
David City *U.S.A.* **112** E5
David Glacier *Antarctica* **5** D21
David Gorodok = Davyd Haradok *Belarus* **23** B14
Davidson *Canada* **103** C7
Davidson Mts. *U.S.A.* **106** B11
Davis *Antarctica* **5** C6
Davis *U.S.A.* **110** G5
Davis Dam *U.S.A.* **111** K12
Davis Inlet *Canada* **105** A7
Davis Mts. *U.S.A.* **116** F3
Davis Sea *Antarctica* **5** C7
Davis Str. *N. Amer.* **101** D19
Davlos *Cyprus* **49** D12
Davo → *Ivory C.* **82** D3
Davos *Switz.* **25** J5

Davy L. *Canada* **103** B7
Davyd Haradok *Belarus* **23** B14
Dawa → *Africa* **81** G5
Dawaki *Bauchi, Nigeria* **83** D6
Dawaki *Kano, Nigeria* **83** C6
Dawei = Tavoy *Burma* **64** E2
Dawes Ra. *Australia* **94** C5
Dawlish *U.K.* **15** G4
Dawna Ra. *Burma* **64** D2
Dawros Hd. *Ireland* **12** B3
Dawson *U.S.A.* **117** F12
Dawson, I. *Chile* **128** G2
Dawson B. *Canada* **103** C8
Dawson City *Canada* **100** E4
Dawson Creek *Canada* **102** B4
Dawson Inlet *Canada* **103** A10
Dawson Ra. *Australia* **94** C4
Dawu *Hubei, China* **59** B9
Dawu *Sichuan, China* **58** B3
Dax *France* **20** E2
Daxian *China* **58** B6
Daxin *China* **58** F6
Daxindian *China* **57** F11
Daxinggou *China* **57** C15
Daxue Shan *Sichuan, China* **58** B3
Daxue Shan *Yunnan, China* **58** F2
Day Kundī △ *Afghan.* **66** C5
Dayao *China* **58** E3
Daye *China* **59** B10
Dayet en Naharat *Mali* **82** B4
Dayi *China* **58** B4
Daylesford *Australia* **95** F3
Dayong *China* **59** C8
Dayr az Zawr *Syria* **73** E9
Dayr az Zawr □ *Syria* **73** E9
Daysland *Canada* **102** C6
Dayton *Nev., U.S.A.* **110** F7
Dayton *Ohio, U.S.A.* **113** F11
Dayton *Pa., U.S.A.* **114** F5
Dayton *Tenn., U.S.A.* **117** D12
Dayton *Wash., U.S.A.* **108** C5
Dayton *Wyo., U.S.A.* **108** D10
Daytona Beach *U.S.A.* **117** G14
Dayu *China* **59** E10
Dayville *U.S.A.* **108** D4
Dazhu *China* **58** B6
Dazu *China* **58** C5
De Aar *S. Africa* **88** E3
De Biesbosch △ *Neths.* **17** C4
De Funiak Springs *U.S.A.* **117** F11
De Grey → *Australia* **92** D2
De Haan *Belgium* **17** C3
De Hoge Veluwe △ *Neths.* **17** B5
De Hoop → *S. Africa* **88** E3
De Kalb Junction *U.S.A.* **115** B9
De Kennemerduinen △ *Neths.* **17** B4
De Land *U.S.A.* **117** G14
De Leon *U.S.A.* **116** E5
De Long Mts. *U.S.A.* **106** B7
De Panne *Belgium* **17** C2
De Pere *U.S.A.* **112** C9
De Queen *U.S.A.* **116** D7
De Quincy *U.S.A.* **116** F8
De Ruyters *U.S.A.* **115** D9
De Smet *U.S.A.* **112** C5
De Soto *U.S.A.* **112** F8
De Tour Village *U.S.A.* **113** B12
De Witt *U.S.A.* **116** D9
Dead Sea *Asia* **74** D4
Deadwood *U.S.A.* **112** C2
Deadwood L. *Canada* **102** B3
Deal *U.K.* **15** F9
Deal I. *Australia* **95** F4
Dealesville *S. Africa* **88** D4
De'an *China* **59** C10
Dean → *Canada* **102** C3
Dean, Forest of *U.K.* **15** F5
Dean Chan. *Canada* **102** C3
Deán Funes *Argentina* **126** C3
Dease → *Canada* **102** B3
Dease L. *Canada* **102** B2
Dease Lake *Canada* **102** B2
Death Valley *U.S.A.* **111** J10
Death Valley △ *U.S.A.* **111** J9
Death Valley Junction *U.S.A.* **111** J10
Deauville *France* **18** C7
Deba *Spain* **38** B2
Deba Habe *Nigeria* **83** C7
Debagram *India* **69** H14
Debaltsevo *Ukraine* **33** H10
Debao *China* **58** F6
Debar *Macedonia* **44** E4
Debark *Ethiopia* **81** E4
Debden *Canada* **103** C7
Dębica *Poland* **31** H8
Dęblin *Poland* **31** G8
Dębno *Poland* **31** F1
Débo, L. *Mali* **82** B4
DeBolt *Canada* **102** B5
Deborah East, L. *Australia* **93** F2
Deborah West, L. *Australia* **93** F2
Debre *Serbia* **44** B3
Debre Birhan *Ethiopia* **81** F4
Debre Markos *Ethiopia* **81** E4
Debre May *Ethiopia* **81** E4
Debre Sina *Ethiopia* **81** F4

Debre Tabor *Ethiopia* **81** E4
Debre Zebit *Ethiopia* **81** E4
Debre Zeyit *Ethiopia* **81** F4
Debrecen *Hungary* **28** C6
Debrzno *Poland* **30** E4
Dečani *Kosovo* **44** D4
Decatur *Ala., U.S.A.* **117** D11
Decatur *Ga., U.S.A.* **117** E12
Decatur *Ill., U.S.A.* **112** F9
Decatur *Ind., U.S.A.* **113** E11
Decatur *Tex., U.S.A.* **116** E6
Decazeville *France* **20** D6
Deccan *India* **66** L11
Deception Bay *Australia* **95** D5
Deception I. *Antarctica* **5** C17
Deception L. *Canada* **103** B8
Dechang *China* **58** D4
Dechhu *India* **68** F5
Děčín *Czech Rep.* **26** A7
Decize *France* **19** F10
Deckerville *U.S.A.* **114** C2
Decollatura *Italy* **43** C9
Decorah *U.S.A.* **112** D8
Deda *Romania* **29** D9
Dedéagach = Alexandroupoli *Greece* **45** F9
Deder *Ethiopia* **81** F5
Dedham *U.S.A.* **115** D13
Dedoplis Tskaro = Tsiteli-Tsqaro *Georgia* **35** K8
Dédougou *Burkina Faso* **82** C4
Dedovichi *Russia* **32** D5
Dedza *Malawi* **87** E3
Dee → *Aberds., U.K.* **13** D6
Dee → *Dumf. & Gall., U.K.* **13** G4
Dee → *Wales, U.K.* **14** D4
Deep B. *Canada* **102** A5
Deepwater *Australia* **95** D5
Deer → *Canada* **103** B10
Deer L. *Canada* **103** C10
Deer Lake *Nfld. & L., Canada* **105** C8
Deer Lake *Ont., Canada* **103** C10
Deer Lodge *U.S.A.* **108** C7
Deer Park *U.S.A.* **108** C5
Deer River *U.S.A.* **112** B7
Deeragun *Australia* **94** B4
Deerdepoort *S. Africa* **88** C4
Defiance *U.S.A.* **113** E11
Degana *India* **68** F6
Dêgê *China* **58** B2
Degebe → *Portugal* **37** G3
Degeberga *Sweden* **11** J8
Dégelis *Canada* **105** C6
Degema *Nigeria* **83** E6
Degerfors *Sweden* **10** E8
Degerhamn *Sweden* **11** H10
Deggendorf *Germany* **25** G8
Degh → *Pakistan* **68** D5
Değirmendere *Turkey* **45** F13
Degirmenlik = Kythréa *Cyprus* **49** D12
Deh Bīd *Iran* **71** D7
Deh Dasht *Iran* **71** D6
Deh-e Shīr *Iran* **71** D7
Dehaj *Iran* **71** D7
Dehak *Iran* **71** E9
Dehdez *Iran* **71** D6
Dehej *India* **68** J5
Dehestān *Iran* **71** D7
Dehgolān *Iran* **73** E12
Dehibat *Tunisia* **79** B8
Dehlorān *Iran* **73** F12
Dehnow-e Kūhestān *Iran* **71** E8
Dehra Dun *India* **68** D8
Dehri *India* **69** G11
Dehua *China* **59** E12
Dehui *China* **57** B13
Deim Zubeir *Sudan* **81** F2
Deinze *Belgium* **17** D3
Dej *Romania* **29** C8
Deje *Sweden* **10** E7
Dejiang *China* **58** C7
Deka → *Zimbabwe* **88** B4
DeKalb *U.S.A.* **112** E9
Dekemhare *Eritrea* **81** D4
Dekese *Dem. Rep. of the Congo* **84** E4
Del Mar *U.S.A.* **111** N9
Del Norte *U.S.A.* **109** H10
Del Rio *U.S.A.* **116** G4
Delai *Sudan* **80** D4
Delambre I. *Australia* **92** D2
Delami *Sudan* **81** E3
Delano *U.S.A.* **111** K7
Delano Peak *U.S.A.* **108** G7
Delareyville *S. Africa* **88** D4
Delaronde L. *Canada* **103** C7
Delavan *U.S.A.* **112** D9
Delaware *U.S.A.* **113** E12
Delaware □ *U.S.A.* **113** F16
Delaware → *U.S.A.* **115** G9
Delaware B. *U.S.A.* **113** F16
Delaware Water Gap △ *U.S.A.* **115** E10
Delay → *Canada* **105** A5
Delbrück *Germany* **24** D4
Delčevo *Macedonia* **44** E6
Delegate *Australia* **95** F4
Delémont *Switz.* **25** H3
Delevan *U.S.A.* **114** D6

Delft *Neths.* **17** B4
Delfzijl *Neths.* **17** A6
Delgado, C. *Mozam.* **87** E5
Delgerhet *Mongolia* **56** B6
Delgo *Sudan* **80** C3
Delhi *Canada* **114** D4
Delhi *India* **68** E7
Delhi *La., U.S.A.* **116** E9
Delhi *N.Y., U.S.A.* **115** D10
Deli Jovan *Serbia* **44** B6
Delia *Canada* **102** C6
Delice → *Turkey* **72** C6
Delicias *Mexico* **118** B3
Delījān *Iran* **71** C6
Déline *Canada* **100** D7
Delisle *Canada* **103** C7
Dell City *U.S.A.* **116** F2
Dell Rapids *U.S.A.* **112** D5
Delle *France* **19** E14
Delmar *U.S.A.* **115** D11
Delmenhorst *Germany* **24** B4
Delnice *Croatia* **41** C11
Delonga, Ostrova *Russia* **53** B15
Deloraine *Australia* **95** G4
Deloraine *Canada* **103** D8
Delphi *Greece* **46** C4
Delphi *U.S.A.* **112** E10
Delphos *U.S.A.* **113** E11
Delray Beach *U.S.A.* **117** H14
Delportshoop *S. Africa* **88** D3
Delsbo *Sweden* **10** C10
Delta *Colo., U.S.A.* **108** G9
Delta *Utah, U.S.A.* **108** G7
Delta □ *Nigeria* **83** D6
Delta del Ebre △ *Spain* **38** E5
Delta del Po △ *Italy* **41** D9
Delta du Saloum △ *Senegal* **82** C1
Delta Dunărea △ *Romania* **29** E14
Delta Junction *U.S.A.* **100** E2
Deltona *U.S.A.* **117** G14
Delungra *Australia* **95** D5
Delvada *India* **68** J4
Delvinaki *Greece* **46** B2
Delvinë *Albania* **44** G4
Delyatyn *Ukraine* **29** B9
Demak *Indonesia* **63** G14
Demanda, Sierra de la *Spain* **38** C2
Demavend = Damāvand, Qolleh-ye *Iran* **71** C7
Dembecha *Ethiopia* **81** E4
Dembi *Ethiopia* **81** F4
Dembia *C.A.R.* **86** B1
Dembia *Dem. Rep. of the Congo* **86** B2
Dembidolo *Ethiopia* **81** F3
Demchok *India* **69** C8
Demer → *Belgium* **17** D4
Demetrias *Greece* **46** B5
Demidov *Russia* **32** E6
Deming *N. Mex., U.S.A.* **109** K10
Deming *Wash., U.S.A.* **110** B4
Demini → *Brazil* **124** D6
Demirci *Turkey* **47** B10
Demirköprü Baraji *Turkey* **47** C10
Demirköy *Turkey* **45** E11
Demmin *Germany* **24** B9
Demonte *Italy* **40** D4
Demopolis *U.S.A.* **117** E11
Dempo *Indonesia* **62** E2
Demyansk *Russia* **32** D7
Den Bosch = 's-Hertogenbosch *Neths.* **17** C5
Den Burg *Neths.* **17** A4
Den Chai *Thailand* **64** D3
Den Haag = 's-Gravenhage *Neths.* **17** B4
Den Helder *Neths.* **17** B4
Den Oever *Neths.* **17** B5
Denain *France* **19** B10
Denair *U.S.A.* **110** H6
Denali = McKinley, Mt. *U.S.A.* **100** E1
Denau *Uzbekistan* **52** F7
Denbigh *Canada* **114** A7
Denbigh *U.K.* **14** D4
Denbighshire □ *U.K.* **14** D4
Dendang *Indonesia* **62** E3
Dendermonde *Belgium* **17** C4
Deneba *Ethiopia* **81** F4
Denge *Nigeria* **83** C6
Dengchuan *China* **58** E3
Dengfeng *China* **56** G7
Dengi *Nigeria* **83** D6
Dengkou *China* **56** D4
Dengzhou *China* **59** A9
Denham *Australia* **93** E1
Denham, Mt. *Jamaica* **120** a
Denham Ra. *Australia* **94** C4
Denham Sd. *Australia* **93** E1
Denholm *Canada* **103** C7
Denia *Spain* **39** G5
Denial B. *Australia* **95** E1
Deniliquin *Australia* **95** F3
Denison *Iowa, U.S.A.* **112** D7
Denison *Tex., U.S.A.* **116** E6
Denison Plains *Australia* **92** C4
Denizli *Turkey* **47** D11
Denizli □ *Turkey* **47** D11

Denman Glacier *Antarctica* **5** C7
Denmark *Australia* **93** F2
Denmark ■ *Europe* **11** J3
Denmark Str. *Atl. Oc.* **98** C17
Dennery *St. Lucia* **121** f
Dennison *U.S.A.* **114** F3
Denny *U.K.* **13** E5
Denpasar *Indonesia* **62** F5
Denpasar ✈ (DPS) *Indonesia* **63** K18
Denton *Mont., U.S.A.* **108** C9
Denton *Tex., U.S.A.* **116** E6
D'Entrecasteaux, Pt. *Australia* **93** F2
D'Entrecasteaux △ *Australia* **93** F2
D'Entrecasteaux Is. *Papua N. G.* **90** B8
Denu *Ghana* **83** D5
Denver *Colo., U.S.A.* **108** G11
Denver *Pa., U.S.A.* **115** F8
Denver City *U.S.A.* **116** E3
Deoband *India* **68** E7
Deogarh *India* **68** G5
Deoghar *India* **69** G12
Deolali *India* **66** K8
Deoli = Devli *India* **68** G6
Déols *France* **19** F8
Deora *India* **68** F4
Deori *India* **69** H8
Deoria *India* **69** F10
Deosai Mts. *Pakistan* **69** B6
Deosri *India* **69** F14
Depalpur *India* **68** H6
Deping *China* **57** F9
Deposit *U.S.A.* **115** D9
Depuch I. *Australia* **92** D2
Deputatskiy *Russia* **53** C14
Dêqên *China* **58** C2
Deqing *China* **59** F9
Dera Ghazi Khan *Pakistan* **68** D4
Dera Ismail Khan *Pakistan* **68** D4
Derabugti *Pakistan* **68** E3
Derawar Fort *Pakistan* **68** E4
Derbent *Russia* **35** J9
Derbent *Turkey* **47** C10
Derby *Australia* **92** C3
Derby *U.K.* **14** E6
Derby *Conn., U.S.A.* **115** E11
Derby *Kans., U.S.A.* **112** G5
Derby *N.Y., U.S.A.* **114** D6
Derby City □ *U.K.* **14** E6
Derby Line *U.S.A.* **115** B12
Derbyshire □ *U.K.* **14** D6
Đerdap △ *Serbia* **44** B6
Derdepoort *S. Africa* **88** C4
Dereham *U.K.* **15** E8
Dereköy *Turkey* **45** E11
Dereli *Turkey* **73** B8
Derg → *U.K.* **12** B4
Derg, L. *Ireland* **12** D3
Dergachi = Derhaci *Ukraine* **33** G9
Derhaci *Ukraine* **33** G9
Deridder *U.S.A.* **116** F8
Derik *Turkey* **73** D9
Derinkuyu *Turkey* **72** C6
Dermantsi *Bulgaria* **45** C8
Dermott *U.S.A.* **116** E9
Dêrong *China* **58** C2
Derry = Londonderry *U.K.* **12** B4
Derry = Londonderry □ *U.K.* **12** B4
Derry *N.H., U.S.A.* **115** D13
Derry *Pa., U.S.A.* **114** F5
Derryveagh Mts. *Ireland* **12** B3
Derudub *Sudan* **80** D4
Derval *France* **18** E5
Derveni *Greece* **46** C4
Derventa *Bos.-H.* **28** F2
Derwent → *Cumb., U.K.* **14** C4
Derwent → *Derby, U.K.* **14** E6
Derwent → *N. Yorks., U.K.* **14** D7
Derwent Water *U.K.* **14** C4
Des Moines *Iowa, U.S.A.* **112** E7
Des Moines *N. Mex., U.S.A.* **109** H12
Des Moines *Wash., U.S.A.* **110** C4
Des Moines → *U.S.A.* **112** E8
Desa *Romania* **28** G8
Desaguadero → *Argentina* **126** C2
Desaguadero → *Bolivia* **124** G5
Desantne *Ukraine* **29** E14
Desar *Malaysia* **65** d
Descanso, Pta. *Mexico* **111** N9
Descartes *France* **20** B4
Deschaillons-sur-St-Laurent *Canada* **105** C5
Deschambault L. *Canada* **103** C8
Deschutes → *U.S.A.* **108** D3
Dese *Ethiopia* **81** E4
Deseado → *Argentina* **128** F3
Desenzano del Garda *Italy* **40** C7
Deseronto *Canada* **114** B7
Desert Center *U.S.A.* **111** M11
Desert Hot Springs *U.S.A.* **111** M10
Desfina *Greece* **46** C4
Deshnok *India* **68** F5
Desierto Central de Baja California △ *Mexico* **118** B2
Deskati *Greece* **44** G5
Desna → *Ukraine* **23** C16
Desnățui → *Romania* **29** G8

Desolación, I. *Chile* **128** G2
Despeñaperros, Paso *Spain* **37** G7
Despeñaperros △ *Spain* **37** G7
Despotiko *Greece* **46** E6
Despotovac *Serbia* **44** B5
Dessau *Germany* **24** D8
Dessye = Dese *Ethiopia* **81** E4
D'Estrees B. *Australia* **95** F2
Desuri *India* **68** G5
Desvres *France* **19** B8
Det Udom *Thailand* **64** E5
Deta *Romania* **28** E6
Dete *Zimbabwe* **88** B4
Đetinja → *Serbia* **44** C4
Detmold *Germany* **24** D4
Detour, Pt. *U.S.A.* **112** C10
Detroit *U.S.A.* **114** D1
Detroit Lakes *U.S.A.* **112** B6
Detva *Slovak Rep.* **27** C12
Deua △ *Australia* **95** F4
Deurne *Neths.* **17** C5
Deutsch-Luxemburgischer △ *Germany* **25** F2
Deutsche Bucht *Germany* **24** A4
Deutschland = Germany ■ *Europe* **24** E6
Deutschlandsberg *Austria* **26** E8
Deux-Sèvres □ *France* **18** F6
Deva *Romania* **28** E7
Devakottai *India* **66** Q11
Devaprayag *India* **69** D8
Dévaványa *Hungary* **28** C5
Deveci Dağları *Turkey* **72** B7
Devecikonağı *Turkey* **45** G12
Devecser *Hungary* **28** C2
Develi *Turkey* **72** C6
Deventer *Neths.* **17** B6
Deveron → *U.K.* **13** D6
Devesel *Romania* **28** F7
Devgadh Bariya *India* **68** H5
Devikot *India* **68** F4
Devils Den *U.S.A.* **110** K7
Devils Hole = Death Valley → *U.S.A.* **111** J9
Devils Lake *U.S.A.* **112** A4
Devils Paw *Canada* **102** B2
Devils Postpile △ *U.S.A.* **110** H7
Devils Tower *U.S.A.* **108** D11
Devils Tower △ *U.S.A.* **108** D11
Devin *Bulgaria* **45** E8
Devine *U.S.A.* **116** G5
Devizes *U.K.* **15** F6
Devli *India* **68** G6
Devnya *Bulgaria* **45** C11
Devoll → *Albania* **44** F4
Devon *Canada* **102** C6
Devon □ *U.K.* **15** G4
Devon I. *Canada* **101** B15
Devonport *Australia* **95** G4
Devonport *N.Z.* **91** B5
Devrek *Turkey* **72** B4
Devrekâni *Turkey* **72** B5
Devrez → *Turkey* **72** B6
Dewas *India* **68** H7
Dewetsdorp *S. Africa* **88** D4
Dewey *Puerto Rico* **121** d
Dexing *China* **59** C11
Dexter *Maine, U.S.A.* **113** C19
Dexter *Mo., U.S.A.* **112** G9
Dexter *N. Mex., U.S.A.* **109** K11
Dey-Dey, L. *Australia* **93** E5
Deyang *China* **58** B5
Deyhūk *Iran* **71** C8
Deyyer *Iran* **71** E6
Dez → *Iran* **73** F13
Dezadeash L. *Canada* **102** A1
Dezfūl *Iran* **73** F13
Dezhneva, Mys *Russia* **53** C19
Dezhou *China* **56** F9
Dhadhar → *India* **69** G11
Dhahaban *Si. Arabia* **80** C4
Dhahiriya = Az̧ Z̧āhirīyah *West Bank* **74** D3
Dhahran = Az̧ Z̧ahrān *Si. Arabia* **71** E6
Dhak *Pakistan* **68** C5
Dhaka *Bangla.* **69** H14
Dhaka □ *Bangla.* **69** G14
Dhali *Cyprus* **49** D12
Dhamār *Yemen* **75** E3
Dhampur *India* **69** E8
Dhamtari *India* **69** J12
Dhanbad *India* **69** H12
Dhangarhi *Nepal* **69** E9
Dhankuta *Nepal* **69** F12
Dhanpuri *India* **69** H9
Dhar *India* **68** H6
Dharampur *India* **68** H6
Dharamsala = Dharmsala *India* **68** C7
Dharan *Nepal* **69** F12
Dhariwal *India* **68** D6
Dharla → *Bangla.* **69** G13
Dharmapuri *India* **66** N11
Dharmapuri *India* **69** H10
Dharmjaygarh *India* **69** H10
Dharmsala *India* **68** C7
Dharni *India* **68** J7
Dharwad *India* **66** M9

Dhasan → India 69 G8
Dhaulagiri Nepal 69 E10
Dhebar, L. India 68 G6
Dheftera Cyprus 49 D12
Dhenkanal India 67 J14
Dherinia Cyprus 49 D12
Dheskáti = Deskati Greece 44 G5
Dhī Qār □ Iraq 70 D5
Dhiarrizos Cyprus 49 E11
Dhībān Jordan 74 D4
Dhilwan India 68 D6
Dhimarkhera India 69 H9
Dhodhekánisos =
    Dodecanese Greece 47 E8
Dholka India 68 H5
Dhomokós = Domokos
    Greece 46 B4
Dhoraji India 68 J4
Dhragonísi = Tragonhsi
    Greece 47 D7
Dhrangadhra India 68 H4
Dhrol India 68 H4
Dhuburi India 67 F16
Dhule India 66 J9
Di-ib, W. → Sudan 80 C4
Di Linh Vietnam 65 G7
Di Linh, Cao Nguyen
    Vietnam 65 G7
Dia Greece 49 D7
Diabakania Guinea 82 C2
Diablo Range U.S.A. 110 J5
Diafarabé Mali 82 C4
Diala Mali 82 C3
Dialakoro Mali 82 C3
Dialakoto Senegal 82 C2
Diallassagou Mali 82 C4
Diamante Argentina 126 C3
Diamante Italy 43 C8
Diamante → Argentina 126 C2
Diamantina Brazil 125 G10
Diamantina → Australia 95 D2
Diamantina △ Australia 94 C3
Diamantino Brazil 125 F7
Diamond Bar U.S.A. 111 L9
Diamond Harbour India 69 H13
Diamond Is. Australia 94 B5
Diamond Mts. U.S.A. 108 G6
Diamond Springs U.S.A. 110 G6
Diamou Mali 82 C2
Dian Chi China 58 E4
Dianalund Denmark 11 J5
Dianbai China 59 G8
Diancheng China 59 G8
Dianjiang China 58 B6
Diano Marina Italy 40 E5
Dianra Ivory C. 82 D3
Diaoyu Tai = Senkaku-
    Shotō E. China Sea 55 M1
Diapaga Burkina Faso 83 C5
Diapangou Burkina Faso 83 C5
Diariguila Guinea 82 C2
Dībā U.A.E. 71 E8
Dibagah Iraq 73 E10
Dibai India 68 E8
Dibaya Dem. Rep. of the Congo 84 F4
Dibaya-Lubue
    Dem. Rep. of the Congo 84 E3
Dibbeen △ Jordan 74 C4
D'Iberville, Lac Canada 104 A5
Dibete Botswana 88 C4
Dibrugarh India 67 F19
Dickens U.S.A. 116 E4
Dickinson U.S.A. 112 B2
Dickson U.S.A. 117 C11
Dickson City U.S.A. 115 E9
Dicle Barajı Turkey 73 C9
Dicle Nehri → Turkey 73 D9
Dicomano Italy 41 E8
Didesa, W. → Ethiopia 81 E4
Didiéni Mali 82 C3
Didimoticho Greece 45 E10
Didsbury Canada 102 C6
Didwana India 68 F6
Die France 21 D9
Diébougou Burkina Faso 82 C4
Diecke Guinea 82 D3
Diefenbaker, L. Canada 103 C7
Diego de Almagro Chile 126 B1
Diego Suarez =
    Antsiranana Madag. 89 A8
Diekirch Lux. 17 E6
Diéma Mali 82 C3
Diembéring Senegal 82 C1
Diemelsee △ Germany 24 D4
Dien Ban Vietnam 64 E7
Dien Bien Vietnam 58 B4
Dien Khanh Vietnam 65 F7
Diepholz Germany 24 C4
Dieppe France 18 C8
Dierks U.S.A. 116 D7
Diest Belgium 17 D5
Dietikon Switz. 25 H4
Dieulefit France 21 D9
Dieuze France 19 D13
Dif Somali Rep. 75 G3
Diffa Niger 83 C7
Diffa □ Niger 83 B7
Differdange Lux. 17 E5
Dig India 68 F7

Digba Dem. Rep. of the Congo 86 B2
Digby Canada 105 D6
Digges Is. → Canada 101 E16
Diggi India 68 F6
Dighinala Bangla. 67 H18
Dighton U.S.A. 112 F3
Digna Mali 82 C3
Digne-les-Bains France 21 D10
Digoin France 19 F11
Digor Turkey 73 B10
Digos Phil. 61 H6
Digranes Iceland 8 C6
Digul → Indonesia 63 F9
Digya △ Ghana 83 D5
Dihang = Brahmaputra →
    Asia 69 H13
Dijlah, Nahr → Asia 70 D5
Dijon France 19 E12
Dikhil Djibouti 81 E5
Dikili Turkey 47 B8
Dikirnis Egypt 80 H7
Dikkil = Dikhil Djibouti 81 E5
Dikodougou Ivory C. 82 D3
Diksmuide Belgium 17 C2
Dikson Russia 52 B9
Dikti Oros Greece 49 D7
Dikwa Nigeria 83 C7
Dila Ethiopia 81 F4
Dilek Yarimadisi △ Turkey 47 D9
Dili E. Timor 63 F7
Dilijan Armenia 35 K7
Dilinata Greece 46 C2
Dilizhan = Dilijan Armenia 35 K7
Dilj Croatia 28 E3
Dillenburg Germany 24 E4
Dilley U.S.A. 116 G5
Dilli = Delhi India 68 E7
Dilli Mali 82 C3
Dilling Sudan 81 E2
Dillingen Bayern, Germany 25 G6
Dillingen Saarland, Germany 25 F2
Dillingham U.S.A. 106 D8
Dillon Canada 103 B7
Dillon Mont., U.S.A. 108 D7
Dillon S.C., U.S.A. 117 D15
Dillon → Canada 103 B7
Dillsburg U.S.A. 114 F7
Dilolo Dem. Rep. of the Congo 84 G4
Dilos Greece 47 D7
Dilove Ukraine 29 C9
Dimas Mexico 118 C3
Dimashq Syria 74 B5
Dimashq □ Syria 74 B5
Dimbaza S. Africa 89 E4
Dimbokro Ivory C. 82 D4
Dimboola Australia 95 F3
Dâmbovița =
    Dâmbovița → Romania 29 F11
Dimbulah Australia 94 B4
Dimitrovgrad Bulgaria 45 D9
Dimitrovgrad Russia 34 D9
Dimitrovgrad Serbia 44 C6
Dimitrovo = Pernik Bulgaria 44 D7
Dimitsana Greece 46 D4
Dimmitt U.S.A. 116 D3
Dimo Sudan 81 F2
Dimona Israel 74 D4
Dimovo Bulgaria 44 C6
Dinagat Phil. 61 F6
Dinajpur Bangla. 67 G16
Dinan France 18 D4
Dīnān Āb Iran 71 C8
Dinant Belgium 17 D4
Dinapur India 69 G11
Dinar Turkey 47 C12
Dīnār, Kūh-e Iran 71 D6
Dinara Planina Croatia 41 D13
Dinard France 18 D4
Dinaric Alps = Dinara
    Planina Croatia 41 D13
Dindanko Mali 82 C3
Dinder, Nahr ed → Sudan 81 E3
Dinder △ Sudan 81 E4
Dindigul India 66 P11
Dindori India 69 H9
Ding Xian = Dingzhou China 56 E8
Dinga Pakistan 68 C5
Dingalan Phil. 61 D4
Ding'an China 64 C8
Dingbian China 56 F4
Dingelstädt Germany 24 D6
Dingle Ireland 12 D1
Dingle Sweden 11 F5
Dingle B. Ireland 12 D1
Dingmans Ferry U.S.A. 115 E10
Dingnan China 59 E10
Dingo Australia 94 C4
Dingolfing Germany 25 G8
Dingtao China 56 G8
Dinguiraye Guinea 82 C2
Dingwall U.K. 13 D4
Dingxi China 56 G3
Dingxiang China 56 E7
Dingyuan China 59 A11
Dingzhou China 56 E8
Dinh, Mui Vietnam 65 G7
Dinh Lap Vietnam 58 G6
Dinin → Ireland 12 D4
Dinira △ Venezuela 121 E6

Dinokwe Botswana 88 C4
Dinorwic Canada 103 D10
Dinosaur → Canada 102 C6
Dinosaur △ U.S.A. 108 F9
Dinuba U.S.A. 110 J7
Diö Sweden 11 H8
Dioïla Mali 82 C3
Dioka Mali 82 C2
Diongoï Mali 82 C3
Dionisades Greece 49 D8
Diósgyör Hungary 28 B5
Diosig Romania 28 C7
Diougani Mali 82 C4
Diouloulou Senegal 82 C1
Dioura Mali 82 C3
Diourbel Senegal 82 C1
Diourbel □ Senegal 82 C1
Dipalpur Pakistan 68 D5
Dipkarpaz = Rizokarpaso
    Cyprus 49 D13
Diplo Pakistan 68 G3
Dipolog Phil. 61 G5
Dipperu △ Australia 94 C4
Dir Pakistan 68 B7
Diré Mali 82 B4
Dire Dawa Ethiopia 81 F5
Dirfis Oros Greece 46 C5
Diriamba Nic. 120 D2
Dirk Hartog I. Australia 93 E1
Dirranbandi Australia 95 D4
Disa India 68 G5
Disa Sudan 81 E3
Disappointment, C. U.S.A. 108 C1
Disappointment, L. Australia 92 D3
Disaster B. Australia 95 F4
Discovery B. Australia 95 F3
Disentis Muster Switz. 25 J4
Dishna Egypt 80 B3
Disina Nigeria 83 C6
Disko = Qeqertarsuaq
    Greenland 98 C14
Disna = Dzisna → Belarus 32 E5
Disney Reef Tonga 91 c
Diss U.K. 15 E9
Disteghil Sar Pakistan 69 A6
District of Columbia □
    U.S.A. 113 F15
Distrito Federal □ Brazil 125 G9
Distrito Federal □ Mexico 119 D5
Disûq Egypt 80 H7
Diu India 68 J4
Dīvāndarreh Iran 73 E12
Dives → France 18 C6
Dives-sur-Mer France 18 C6
Divichi = Däväçi Azerbaijan 35 K9
Divide U.S.A. 108 D7
Dividing Ra. Australia 93 E2
Divinópolis Brazil 125 H10
Divjake Albania 44 F3
Divnoye Russia 35 H6
Divo Ivory C. 82 D3
Divriği Turkey 73 C8
Dīwāl Kol Afghan. 68 B2
Dixie Mt. U.S.A. 110 F6
Dixon Calif., U.S.A. 110 G5
Dixon Ill., U.S.A. 112 E9
Dixon Entrance U.S.A. 100 G5
Dixville Canada 115 A13
Diyadin Turkey 73 C10
Diyālā □ Iraq 70 C5
Diyālā → Iraq 73 F11
Diyarbakır Turkey 73 D9
Diyarbakır □ Turkey 73 D9
Diyodar India 68 G4
Dizangué Cameroon 83 E6
Djakarta = Jakarta Indonesia 62 F3
Djamba Angola 88 B1
Djambala Congo 84 E2
Djanet Algeria 78 D7
Djawa = Jawa Indonesia 62 F3
Djelfa Algeria 78 B6
Djema C.A.R. 86 A2
Djenné Mali 82 C4
Djerba, Î. de Tunisia 79 B8
Djerid, Chott Tunisia 78 B7
Djibo Burkina Faso 83 C4
Djibouti Djibouti 81 E5
Djibouti ■ Africa 81 E5
Djolu Dem. Rep. of the Congo 84 D4
Djougou Benin 83 D5
Djoum Cameroon 84 D2
Djourab, Erg du Chad 79 E9
Djugu Dem. Rep. of the Congo 86 B3
Djukbinj △ Australia 92 B5
Djúpivogur Iceland 8 D6
Djurås Sweden 10 D9
Djurö △ Sweden 11 F7
Djursland Denmark 11 H4
Dmitriya Lapteva, Proliv
    Russia 53 B15
Dmitriyev Lgovskiy Russia 33 F8
Dmitrov Russia 32 D9
Dmitrovsk-Orlovskiy Russia 33 F8
Dnepr = Dnipro → Ukraine 33 J7
Dneprodzerzhinsk =
    Dniprodzerzhynsk Ukraine 33 H8
Dneprodzerzhinskoye
    Vdkhr. =
    Dniprodzerzhynske
    Vdskh. Ukraine 33 H8

Dnepropetrovsk =
    Dnipropetrovsk Ukraine 33 H8
Dneprorudnoye =
    Dniprorudne Ukraine 33 J8
Dnestr = Dnister → Europe 23 E16
Dnieper = Dnipro → Ukraine 33 J7
Dniester = Dnister →
    Europe 23 E16
Dnipro → Ukraine 33 J7
Dniprodzerzhynsk Ukraine 33 H8
Dniprodzerzhynske Vdskh.
    Ukraine 33 H8
Dnipropetrovsk Ukraine 33 H8
Dnipropetrovsk □ Ukraine 33 H8
Dniprorudne Ukraine 33 J8
Dnister → Europe 23 E16
Dnistrovskyy Lyman Ukraine 33 J6
Dno Russia 32 D5
Dnyapro = Dnipro →
    Ukraine 33 J7
Do Gonbadān = Gachsārān
    Iran 71 D6
Doaktown Canada 105 C6
Doan Hung Vietnam 58 G5
Doany Madag. 89 A8
Doba Chad 79 G9
Dobandi Pakistan 68 D2
Dobbiaco Italy 41 B9
Dobbyn Australia 94 B3
Dobczyce Poland 31 J7
Dobele Latvia 30 B10
Dobele □ Latvia 30 B10
Döbeln Germany 24 D9
Doberai, Jazirah Indonesia 63 E8
Doblas Argentina 126 D3
Dobo Indonesia 63 F8
Doboj Bos.-H. 28 F3
Dobra Wielkopolskie, Poland 31 G5
Dobra Zachodnio-Pomorskie,
    Poland 30 E2
Dobra Dâmbovița, Romania 29 F10
Dobra Hunedoara, Romania 28 E7
Dobre Miasto Poland 30 E7
Dobreşti Romania 28 D7
Dobrich Bulgaria 45 C11
Dobrinishta Bulgaria 44 E7
Dobříš Czech Rep. 26 B7
Dobrodzień Poland 31 H5
Dobromyl Ukraine 31 J9
Dobron Ukraine 28 B7
Dobropole Ukraine 33 H9
Dobrovolsk Russia 30 D9
Dobruja Romania 29 F13
Dobrush Belarus 23 B16
Dobrzany Poland 30 E2
Dobrzyń nad Wisłą Poland 31 F6
Doc, Mui Vietnam 64 D6
Docker River =
    Kaltukatjara Australia 93 D4
Docksta Sweden 10 A12
Doctor Arroyo Mexico 118 C4
Doctor Pedro P. Peña
    Paraguay 126 A3
Doda India 69 C6
Doda, L. Canada 104 C4
Dodecanese Greece 47 E8
Dodekanisa = Dodecanese
    Greece 47 E8
Dodekanisa □ Greece 47 E8
Dodge City U.S.A. 112 G3
Dodge L. Canada 103 B7
Dodgeville U.S.A. 112 D8
Dodo Cameroon 83 D7
Dodo Sudan 81 F2
Dodola Ethiopia 81 F4
Dodoma Tanzania 86 D4
Dodoma □ Tanzania 86 D4
Dodoni Greece 46 B2
Dodori △ Kenya 86 C5
Dodsland Canada 103 C7
Dodson U.S.A. 108 B9
Dodurga Turkey 47 B11
Doesburg Neths. 17 B6
Doetinchem Neths. 17 C6
Dog Creek Canada 102 C4
Dog L. Man., Canada 103 C9
Dog L. Ont., Canada 104 C2
Doğanşehir Turkey 72 C7
Dogliani Italy 40 D4
Dogondoutchi Niger 83 C5
Dogran Pakistan 68 D5
Doğubayazıt Turkey 73 C11
Doguéraoua Niger 83 C6
Doha = Ad Dawḥah Qatar 71 E6
Dohazari Bangla. 67 H18
Dohrighat India 69 F10
Doi Indonesia 63 D7
Doi Inthanon △ Thailand 64 C2
Doi Khuntan △ Thailand 64 C2
Doi Luang Thailand 64 C3
Doi Luang △ Thailand 64 C2
Doi Saket Thailand 64 C2
Doi Suthep △ Thailand 64 C2
Dois Irmãos, Sa. Brazil 125 E10
Dojransko Jezero Macedonia 44 E6
Doka Sudan 81 E4
Dokkum Neths. 17 A5
Dokos Greece 46 D5

Dokri Pakistan 68 F3
Dokuchayevsk Ukraine 33 J9
Dol-de-Bretagne France 18 D5
Dolac Kosovo 44 D4
Dolak, Pulau Indonesia 63 F9
Dolbeau-Mistassini Canada 105 C5
Dole France 19 E12
Doleib, Wadi → Sudan 81 E3
Dolenji Logatec Slovenia 41 C11
Dolgellau U.K. 14 E4
Dolgelley = Dolgellau U.K. 14 E4
Dolhasca Romania 29 C11
Doliana Greece 46 B2
Dolianova Italy 42 C2
Dolina = Dolyna Ukraine 29 D9
Dolinsk Russia 53 E15
Dolinskaya = Dolynska
    Ukraine 33 H7
Dolj □ Romania 29 F8
Dollard Neths. 17 A7
Dolo Ethiopia 81 G5
Dolo Italy 41 C9
Dolomites = Dolomiti Italy 41 B8
Dolomiti Italy 41 B8
Dolomiti Bellunesi △ Italy 41 B9
Dolores Argentina 126 D4
Dolores Uruguay 126 C4
Dolores U.S.A. 109 H9
Dolores → U.S.A. 108 G9
Dolovo Serbia 28 B5
Dolphin, C. Falk. Is. 128 G5
Dolphin and Union Str.
    Canada 100 B8
Dolsk Poland 31 G4
Dolyna Ukraine 29 D9
Dolynska Ukraine 33 H7
Dolynske Ukraine 29 C14
Dolzhanskaya Russia 33 J9
Dom Pedrito Brazil 127 C5
Doma Nigeria 83 D6
Doma = Zimbabwe 87 B5
Domaniç Turkey 47 B11
Domariaganj → India 69 F10
Domasi Malawi 87 F4
Domažlice Czech Rep. 26 B5
Dombarovskiy Russia 52 D6
Dombås Norway 8 E13
Dombasle-sur-Meurthe
    France 19 D13
Dombes France 21 C9
Dombóvár Hungary 28 D3
Dombrád Hungary 28 B6
Dome Argus Antarctica 5 E12
Dome C. Antarctica 5 D17
Dome Fuji Antarctica 5 D5
Domel I. = Letsôk-aw
    Kyun Burma 65 G2
Domérat France 19 F9
Domeyko Chile 126 B1
Domeyko, Cordillera Chile 126 A2
Domfront France 18 D6
Dominador Chile 126 A2
Dominica ■ W. Indies 121 C7
Dominica Passage W. Indies 121 C7
Dominican Rep. ■ W. Indies 121 C5
Dömitz Germany 24 B7
Domme France 20 D5
Dommel → Neths. 17 C5
Domodóssola Italy 40 B5
Domogled-Valea Cernei △
    Romania 28 F7
Domokos Greece 46 B4
Dompaire France 19 D13
Dompierre-sur-Besbre
    France 19 F10
Dompim Ghana 82 D4
Domrémy-la-Pucelle France 19 D12
Domvena Greece 46 C4
Domville, Mt. Australia 95 D5
Domžale Slovenia 41 B11
Don → Russia 33 J10
Don → Aberds., U.K. 13 D6
Don → S. Yorks., U.K. 14 D7
Don, C. Australia 92 B5
Don Benito Spain 37 G5
Don Figuerero Mts. Jamaica 120 a
Don Sak Thailand 65 b
Dona Ana = Nhamaabué
    Mozam. 87 F4
Doña Mencía Spain 37 H6
Donaghadee U.K. 12 B6
Donaghmore Ireland 12 B5
Donald Australia 95 F3
Donaldsonville U.S.A. 116 F9
Donalsonville U.S.A. 117 F12
Doñana △ Spain 37 J4
Donau = Dunărea →
    Europe 29 E14
Donau → Austria 27 C10
Donau Auen △ Austria 27 C9
Donaueschingen Germany 25 H4
Donauwörth Germany 25 G6
Doncaster U.K. 14 D6
Dondo Angola 84 F2
Dondo Mozam. 87 F3

Dondo, Teluk Indonesia 63 D6
Dondra Head Sri Lanka 66 S12
Dondușeni Moldova 29 B12
Donegal Ireland 12 B3
Donegal □ Ireland 12 B4
Donegal B. Ireland 12 B3
Donets → Russia 35 G5
Donets Basin Ukraine 6 F13
Donetsk Ukraine 33 J9
Donetsk □ Ukraine 33 J9
Dong Ba Thin Vietnam 65 F7
Dong Dang Vietnam 58 G6
Dong Giam Vietnam 64 C5
Dong Ha Vietnam 64 D6
Dong Hene Laos 64 D5
Dong Hoi Vietnam 64 D6
Dong Jiang → China 59 F10
Dong Khe Vietnam 58 F6
Dong Ujimqin Qi China 56 B9
Dong Van Vietnam 64 A5
Dong Xoai Vietnam 65 G6
Donga Nigeria 83 D7
Donga → Nigeria 83 D7
Dong'an China 59 D8
Dongara Australia 93 E1
Dongbei China 54 A5
Dongchuan China 58 D4
Dongco China 67 C14
Donges France 18 E4
Dongfang China 64 C7
Dongfeng China 57 C13
Donggala Indonesia 63 E5
Donggan China 58 F5
Donggang China 57 E13
Dongguan China 59 F9
Dongguang China 56 F9
Donghae S. Korea 57 F15
Donghai Dao China 59 G8
Dongjingcheng China 57 B15
Dongkou China 59 D8
Donglan China 58 E6
Dongliu China 59 B11
Dongmen China 58 F6
Dongnae S. Korea 57 G15
Dongning China 57 B16
Dongnyi China 58 C3
Dongola Sudan 80 D3
Dongping China 56 G9
Dongsha Dao S. China Sea 59 G11
Dongshan China 59 F11
Dongsheng China 56 E6
Dongtai China 57 H11
Dongting Hu China 59 C9
Dongtou China 59 D13
Dongxiang China 59 C11
Dongxing China 58 G7
Dongyang China 59 C13
Dongzhi China 59 B11
Donington, C. Australia 95 E2
Doniphan U.S.A. 112 G8
Donja Stubica Croatia 41 C12
Donji Dušnik Serbia 44 C6
Donji Miholjac Croatia 28 E3
Donji Milanovac Serbia 44 B8
Donji Vakuf Bos.-H. 28 F2
Dønna Norway 8 C15
Donna U.S.A. 116 H5
Donnacona Canada 105 C5
Donnelly's Crossing N.Z. 91 A4
Donnybrook Australia 93 F2
Donnybrook S. Africa 89 D4
Donora U.S.A. 114 F5
Donousa Greece 47 D7
Donskoy Russia 32 F10
Donsol Phil. 61 E5
Donwood Canada 114 B6
Donzère France 21 D8
Donzy France 19 E10
Doomadgee Australia 94 B2
Doomadgee △ Australia 94 B2
Doon → U.K. 13 F4
Doon Doon ○ Australia 92 C4
Dora, L. Australia 92 D3
Dora Báltea → Italy 40 C5
Dora Ripária → Italy 40 C4
Doran L. Canada 103 A7
Dorchester U.K. 15 G5
Dorchester, C. Canada 101 D16
Dordabis Namibia 88 C2
Dordogne □ France 20 C4
Dordogne → France 20 C3
Dordrecht Neths. 17 C4
Dordrecht S. Africa 88 E4
Dore → France 20 C7
Dore, Mts. France 20 C6
Doré L. Canada 103 C7
Dorfen Germany 25 G8
Dorgali Italy 42 B2
Dori Burkina Faso 83 C4
Doring → S. Africa 88 E2
Doringbos S. Africa 88 E2
Dorking U.K. 15 F7
Dormaa-Ahenkro Ghana 82 D4
Dormans France 19 C10
Dormo, Ras Eritrea 81 E5

Dornbirn *Austria* **26** D2
Dornes *France* **19** F10
Dorneşti *Romania* **29** C11
Dornie *U.K.* **13** D3
Dornoch *Canada* **114** B4
Dornoch *U.K.* **13** D4
Dornoch Firth *U.K.* **13** D4
Dornogovĭ □ *Mongolia* **56** C6
Doro *Mali* **83** B4
Doro, Kavo *Greece* **46** C6
Dorog *Hungary* **28** C3
Dorogobuzh *Russia* **32** E7
Dorohoi *Romania* **29** C11
Döröö Nuur *Mongolia* **60** B4
Dorr *Iran* **71** C6
Dorre I. *Australia* **93** E1
Dorrigo *Australia* **95** E5
Dorris *U.S.A.* **108** F3
Dorset *Canada* **114** A6
Dorset *Ohio, U.S.A.* **114** E4
Dorset *Vt., U.S.A.* **115** C11
Dorset □ *U.K.* **15** G5
Dorsten *Germany* **24** D2
Dortmund *Germany* **24** D3
Dortmund-Ems-Kanal ➤
    Germany **24** D3
Dörtyol *Turkey* **72** D7
Dorum *Germany* **24** B4
Doruma *Dem. Rep. of the Congo* **86** B2
Dorūneh *Iran* **71** C8
Dos Bahías, C. *Argentina* **128** E3
Dos Hermanas *Spain* **37** H5
Dos Palos *U.S.A.* **110** J6
Döşemealtı *Turkey* **47** D12
Dosso *Niger* **83** C5
Dosso □ *Niger* **83** C5
Dosso △ *Niger* **83** C5
Dothan *U.S.A.* **117** F12
Doty *U.S.A.* **110** D3
Douai *France* **19** B10
Douako *Guinea* **82** D2
Douala *Cameroon* **83** E6
Douarnenez *France* **18** D2
Doubabougou *Mali* **82** C3
Double Island Pt. *Australia* **95** D5
Double Mountain Fork ➤
    U.S.A. **116** E4
Doubrava ➤ *Czech Rep.* **26** A8
Doubs □ *France* **19** E13
Doubs ➤ *France* **19** F12
Doubtful Sd. *N.Z.* **91** F1
Doubtless B. *N.Z.* **91** A4
Doudeville *France* **18** C7
Doué-la-Fontaine *France* **18** E6
Douentza *Mali* **82** C4
Douentza △ *Mali* **82** B4
Douglas *Canada* **114** A8
Douglas *I. of Man* **14** C3
Douglas *S. Africa* **88** D3
Douglas *Ariz., U.S.A.* **109** L9
Douglas *Ga., U.S.A.* **117** F13
Douglas *Wyo., U.S.A.* **108** E11
Douglas Apsley △ *Australia* **95** G4
Douglas Chan. *Canada* **102** C3
Douglas Pt. *Canada* **114** B3
Douglasville *U.S.A.* **117** E12
Doukaton, Akra *Greece* **46** C2
Doulevant-le-Château
    France **19** D11
Doullens *France* **19** B9
Doumen *China* **59** F9
Douna *Mali* **82** C3
Dounreay *U.K.* **13** C5
Dourada, Serra *Brazil* **125** F9
Dourados *Brazil* **127** A5
Dourados ➤ *Brazil* **127** A5
Dourados, Serra dos *Brazil* **127** A5
Dourdan *France* **19** D9
Douro ➤ *Europe* **36** D2
Douvaine *France* **19** F13
Douvres-la-Délivrande
    France **18** C6
Douze ➤ *France* **20** E3
Dove ➤ *U.K.* **14** E6
Dove Creek *U.S.A.* **109** H9
Dover *Australia* **95** G4
Dover *U.K.* **15** F9
Dover *Del., U.S.A.* **113** F16
Dover *N.H., U.S.A.* **115** C14
Dover *N.J., U.S.A.* **115** F10
Dover *Ohio, U.S.A.* **114** F3
Dover, Pt. *Australia* **93** F4
Dover, Str. of *Europe* **15** G9
Dover-Foxcroft *U.S.A.* **113** C19
Dover Plains *U.S.A.* **115** E11
Dovey = Dyfi ➤ *U.K.* **15** E3
Dovhe *Ukraine* **29** B8
Dovrefjell *Norway* **8** E13
Dow Rūd *Iran* **71** C6
Dowa *Malawi* **87** E3
Dowagiac *U.S.A.* **112** E10
Dowerin *Australia* **93** F2
Dowgha'i *Iran* **71** B8
Dowlatābād *Kermān, Iran* **71** D8
Dowlatābād *Khorāsān, Iran* **71** C8
Down □ *U.K.* **12** B5
Downey *Calif., U.S.A.* **111** M8
Downey *Idaho, U.S.A.* **108** E7
Downham Market *U.K.* **15** E8

Downieville *U.S.A.* **110** F6
Downpatrick *U.K.* **12** B6
Downpatrick Hd. *Ireland* **12** B2
Downsville *U.S.A.* **115** D10
Downton, Mt. *Canada* **102** C4
Dowsārī *Iran* **71** D8
Doxato *Greece* **45** E8
Doyle *U.S.A.* **110** E6
Doylestown *U.S.A.* **115** F9
Dozois, Rés. *Canada* **104** C4
Dra Khel *Pakistan* **68** F2
Drâa, C. *Morocco* **78** C3
Drâa, Hamada du *Algeria* **78** C4
Drâa, Oued ➤ *Morocco* **78** C3
Drac ➤ *France* **21** C9
Drac, Coves del *Spain* **48** B10
Dračevo *Macedonia* **44** E5
Drachten Neths. **17** A6
Drăgăneşti *Moldova* **29** C13
Drăgăneşti-Olt *Romania* **29** F9
Drăgăneşti-Vlaşca *Romania* **29** F10
Dragaš *Kosovo* **44** D4
Drăgăşani *Romania* **29** F9
Dragichyn *Belarus* **23** B13
Dragocvet *Serbia* **44** C5
Dragon's Mouths *Venezuela* **125** K15
Dragovishtitsa *Bulgaria* **44** D6
Draguignan *France* **21** E10
Drahove *Ukraine* **29** B8
Drain *U.S.A.* **108** E2
Drake *U.S.A.* **112** B3
Drake Passage *S. Ocean* **5** B17
Drakensberg *S. Africa* **89** D4
Drama *Greece* **45** E8
Drama □ *Greece* **45** E8
Drammen *Norway* **9** G14
Drangajökull *Iceland* **8** C2
Dranov, Ostrov *Romania* **29** F14
Dras *India* **69** B6
Drastis, Akra *Greece* **49** A3
Drau = Drava ➤ *Croatia* **28** E3
Drava ➤ *Croatia* **28** E3
Dravograd *Slovenia* **41** B12
Drawa ➤ *Poland* **31** F2
Drawieński △ *Poland* **31** E2
Drawno *Poland* **31** E2
Drawsko Pomorskie *Poland* **30** E2
Drayton *Canada* **114** C4
Drayton Valley *Canada* **102** C6
Dreieich *Germany* **25** E4
Dren *Kosovo* **44** D5
Drenthe □ *Neths.* **17** B6
Drepano, Akra *Greece* **49** D6
Drepanum, C. *Cyprus* **49** E11
Dresden *Canada* **114** D2
Dresden *Germany* **24** D9
Dresden *U.S.A.* **114** D8
Dreux *France* **18** D8
Drezdenko *Poland* **31** F2
Driffield *U.K.* **14** C7
Driftwood *U.S.A.* **114** E6
Driggs *U.S.A.* **108** E8
Drin ➤ *Albania* **44** D3
Drin i Zi ➤ *Albania* **44** E4
Drina ➤ *Bos.-H.* **44** B3
Drîncea ➤ *Romania* **28** F7
Drinjača ➤ *Bos.-H.* **28** F4
Driopida *Greece* **46** D6
Drissa =
    Vyerkhnyadzvinsk *Belarus* **32** E4
Drniš *Croatia* **41** E13
Drøbak *Norway* **9** G14
Drobeta-Turnu Severin
    Romania **28** F7
Drobin *Poland* **31** F6
Drochia *Moldova* **29** B12
Drogheda *Ireland* **12** C5
Drogichin = Dragichyn
    Belarus **23** B13
Drogobych = Drohobych
    Ukraine **31** J10
Drohiczyn *Poland* **31** F9
Drohobych *Ukraine* **31** J10
Droichead Atha =
    Drogheda *Ireland* **12** C5
Droichead na Bandan =
    Bandon *Ireland* **12** E3
Droichead Nua *Ireland* **12** C5
Droitwich *U.K.* **15** E5
Drôme □ *France* **21** D9
Drôme ➤ *France* **21** D8
Dromedary, C. *Australia* **95** F5
Dromiling △ *Germany* **24** C7
Dromore *U.K.* **12** B4
Dromore West *Ireland* **12** B3
Dronero *Italy* **40** D4
Dronfield *U.K.* **14** D6
Dronne ➤ *France* **20** C3
Dronning Maud Land
    Antarctica **5** D3
Dronninglund *Denmark* **11** G4
Dronten *Neths.* **17** B5
Dropt ➤ *France* **20** D3
Drosendorf *Austria* **26** C8
Droué *France* **18** D8
Druk Yul = Bhutan ■ *Asia* **67** F17
Drumbo *Canada* **114** C4
Drumcliff *Ireland* **12** B3
Drumheller *Canada* **102** C6

Drummond *U.S.A.* **108** C7
Drummond I. *U.S.A.* **113** B12
Drummond Pt. *Australia* **95** E2
Drummond Ra. *Australia* **94** C4
Drummondville *Canada* **104** C5
Drumright *U.S.A.* **116** D6
Druskininkai *Lithuania* **32** E2
Drut ➤ *Belarus* **23** B16
Druya *Belarus* **32** E4
Druzhba *Bulgaria* **45** C12
Druzhina *Russia* **53** C15
Drvar *Bos.-H.* **41** D13
Drvenik *Croatia* **41** E13
Drwęca ➤ *Poland* **31** E5
Dry Harbour Mts. *Jamaica* **120** a
Dry Tortugas *U.S.A.* **117** F13
Dryander △ *Australia* **94** b
Dryanovo *Bulgaria* **45** D9
Dryden *Canada* **103** D10
Dryden *U.S.A.* **115** D8
Drygalski I. *Antarctica* **5** C7
Drygalski Ice Tongue
    Antarctica **5** D21
Drysdale ➤ *Australia* **92** B4
Drysdale I. *Australia* **94** A2
Drysdale River △ *Australia* **92** B4
Drzewica *Poland* **31** G7
Drzewiczka ➤ *Poland* **31** G7
Dschang *Cameroon* **83** D7
Du Gué ➤ *Canada* **104** A5
Du He *China* **59** A8
Du Quoin *U.S.A.* **112** F9
Du'an *China* **58** F7
Duanesburg *U.S.A.* **115** D10
Duaringa *Australia* **94** C4
Duarte, Pico *Dom. Rep.* **121** D5
Dubai = Dubayy *U.A.E.* **71** E7
Dubăsari *Moldova* **29** C14
Dubăsari Vdkhr. *Moldova* **29** C13
Dubawnt ➤ *Canada* **103** A8
Dubawnt L. *Canada* **103** A8
Dubayy *U.A.E.* **71** E7
Dubbo *Australia* **95** E4
Dube ➤ *Liberia* **82** D3
Dübele *Dem. Rep. of the Congo* **86** B2
Dübendorf *Switz.* **25** H4
Dubica *Croatia* **41** C13
Dublin *Ireland* **12** C5
Dublin *Ga., U.S.A.* **117** E13
Dublin *Tex., U.S.A.* **116** E5
Dublin □ *Ireland* **12** C5
Dublin ✈ (DUB) *Ireland* **12** C5
Dubna *Russia* **32** D9
Dubnica nad Váhom
    Slovak Rep. **27** C11
Dubno *Ukraine* **23** C13
Dubois *Idaho, U.S.A.* **108** D7
DuBois *Pa., U.S.A.* **114** E6
Dubossary = Dubăsari
    Moldova **29** C14
Dubossary Vdkhr. =
    Dubăsari Vdkhr. *Moldova* **29** C13
Dubove *Ukraine* **29** B8
Dubovka *Russia* **35** F7
Dubovskoye *Russia* **35** G6
Dubrajpur *India* **69** H12
Dubréka *Guinea* **82** D2
Dubrovitsa = Dubrovytsya
    Ukraine **23** C14
Dubrovnik *Croatia* **44** D2
Dubrovytsya *Ukraine* **23** C14
Dubuque *U.S.A.* **112** D8
Dubysa ➤ *Lithuania* **30** C10
Duchang *China* **59** C11
Duchesne *U.S.A.* **108** F8
Duchess *Australia* **94** C2
Ducie I. *Pac. Oc.* **97** K15
Duck ➤ *U.S.A.* **117** C11
Duck Cr. ➤ *Australia* **92** D2
Duck Lake *Canada* **103** C7
Duck Mountain △ *Canada* **103** C8
Duckwall, Mt. *U.S.A.* **110** H6
Duderstadt *Germany* **24** D6
Dudhi *India* **69** G10
Dudinka *Russia* **53** C9
Dudley *U.K.* **15** E5
Dudwa *India* **69** E9
Dudwa △ *India* **69** E9
Duékoué *Ivory C.* **82** D3
Dueñas *Spain* **36** D6
Duero = Douro ➤ *Europe* **36** D2
Dufftown *U.K.* **13** D5
Dufourspitz *Switz.* **25** K3
Dugi Otok *Croatia* **41** D11
Dugo Selo *Croatia* **41** C13
Dujiangyan *China* **58** B4
Duk Fadiat *Sudan* **81** F3
Duk Faiwil *Sudan* **81** F3
Dukat *Albania* **44** F3
Dūkdamīn *Iran* **71** C8
Dukhān *Qatar* **71** E6
Dukhovshchina *Russia* **32** E7
Duki *Pakistan* **66** D6
Dukla *Poland* **31** J8

Duku *Bauchi, Nigeria* **83** C7
Duku *Sokoto, Nigeria* **83** C5
Dulag *Phil.* **61** F6
Dulce *U.S.A.* **109** H10
Dulce ➤ *Argentina* **126** C3
Dulce, G. *Costa Rica* **120** E3
Dulf *Iraq* **70** C5
Duliu *China* **56** E9
Dullewala *Pakistan* **68** D4
Dullstroom *S. Africa* **89** D5
Duluth *U.S.A.* **112** B7
Dum Dum *India* **69** H13
Dum Duma *India* **67** F19
Dūmā *Syria* **74** B5
Dumaguete *Phil.* **61** G5
Dumai *Indonesia* **62** D2
Dumaran *Phil.* **61** F3
Dumas *Ark., U.S.A.* **116** E9
Dumas *Tex., U.S.A.* **116** D4
Dumayr *Syria* **74** B5
Dumbarton *U.K.* **13** F4
Dumbleyung *Australia* **93** F2
Dumbrăveni *Romania* **29** D9
Dumfries *U.K.* **13** F5
Dumfries & Galloway □ *U.K.* **13** F5
Dumitreşti *Romania* **29** E11
Dumka *India* **69** G12
Dumlupınar *Turkey* **47** C12
Dümmer *Germany* **24** C4
Dümmer △ *Germany* **24** C4
Dumoine ➤ *Canada* **104** C4
Dumoine, L. *Canada* **104** C4
Dumont d'Urville *Antarctica* **5** C10
Dumont d'Urville Sea *S. Ocean* **5** C9
Dumraon *India* **69** G11
Dumyât *Egypt* **80** H7
Dumyât, Masabb *Egypt* **80** H7
Dún Dealgan = Dundalk
    Ireland **12** B5
Dún Garbhán =
    Dungarvan *Ireland* **12** D4
Dún Laoghaire *Ireland* **12** C5
Dun-le-Palestel *France* **19** F8
Dun-sur-Auron *France* **19** F9
Dun-sur-Meuse *France* **19** C12
Duna = Dunărea ➤ *Europe* **29** E14
Duna-Drava △ *Hungary* **28** D3
Duna-völgyi-főcsatorna
    Hungary **28** D3
Dunaföldvár *Hungary* **28** D3
Dunagiri *India* **69** D8
Dunaj = Dunărea ➤
    Europe **29** E14
Dunajec ➤ *Poland* **31** H7
Dunajská Streda *Slovak Rep.* **27** C10
Dunakeszi *Hungary* **28** C4
Dunapataj *Hungary* **28** D3
Dunărea ➤ *Europe* **29** E14
Dunaszekcső *Hungary* **28** D3
Dunaújváros *Hungary* **28** D3
Dunav = Dunărea ➤
    Europe **29** E14
Dunavaţu de Jos *Romania* **29** F14
Dunavtsi *Bulgaria* **44** C6
Dunay *Russia* **54** C6
Dunayivtsi *Ukraine* **29** B11
Dunback *N.Z.* **91** F3
Dunbar *U.K.* **13** E6
Dunblane *U.K.* **13** E5
Duncan *Canada* **110** B3
Duncan *Ariz., U.S.A.* **109** K9
Duncan *Okla., U.S.A.* **116** D6
Duncan, L. *Canada* **102** A6
Duncan L. *Canada* **102** A6
Duncan Town *Bahamas* **120** B4
Duncannon *U.S.A.* **114** F8
Duncansby Head *U.K.* **13** C5
Duncansville *U.S.A.* **114** F6
Dundaga *Latvia* **30** A9
Dundalk *Canada* **114** B4
Dundalk *Ireland* **12** B5
Dundalk *U.S.A.* **113** F15
Dundalk Bay *Ireland* **12** C5
Dundas = Uummannaq
    Greenland **101** B18
Dundas *Canada* **114** C5
Dundas, L. *Australia* **93** F3
Dundas I. *Canada* **102** C2
Dundas Str. *Australia* **92** B5
Dundee *S. Africa* **89** D5
Dundee *U.K.* **13** E6
Dundee *U.S.A.* **114** D8
Dundee City □ *U.K.* **13** E6
Dundgovĭ □ *Mongolia* **56** B4
Dundrum *U.K.* **12** B6
Dundrum B. *U.K.* **12** B6
Dunedin *N.Z.* **91** F3
Dunedin *U.S.A.* **117** G13
Dunfanaghy *Ireland* **12** A4
Dunfermline *U.K.* **13** E5
Dungannon *Canada* **114** C3
Dungannon *U.K.* **12** B5
Dungarpur *India* **68** H5
Dungarvan *Ireland* **12** D4

Dungarvan Harbour *Ireland* **12** D4
Dungeness *U.K.* **15** G8
Dunglow *Ireland* **12** B3
Dungo, L. do *Angola* **88** B2
Dungog *Australia* **95** E5
Dungu *Dem. Rep. of the Congo* **86** B2
Dungun *Malaysia* **65** K4
Dunhua *China* **57** C15
Dunhuang *China* **60** B4
Dunk I. *Australia* **94** B4
Dunkassa *Benin* **83** C5
Dunkeld *Australia* **95** E4
Dunkeld *U.K.* **13** E5
Dunkerque *France* **19** A9
Dunkery Beacon *U.K.* **15** F4
Dunkirk = Dunkerque
    France **19** A9
Dunkirk *U.S.A.* **114** D5
Dunkuj *Sudan* **81** E3
Dunkwa *Central, Ghana* **82** D4
Dunkwa *Central, Ghana* **83** D4
Dúnleary = Dún Laoghaire
    Ireland **12** C5
Dunleer *Ireland* **12** C5
Dunmanus B. *Ireland* **12** E2
Dunmanway *Ireland* **12** E2
Dunmarra *Australia* **94** B1
Dunmore *U.S.A.* **115** E9
Dunmore East *Ireland* **12** D5
Dunmore Hd. *Ireland* **12** D1
Dunmore Town *Bahamas* **120** A4
Dunn *U.S.A.* **117** D15
Dunnellon *U.S.A.* **117** G13
Dunnet Hd. *U.K.* **13** C5
Dunning *U.S.A.* **112** E3
Dunnville *Canada* **114** D5
Dunolly *Australia* **95** F3
Dunoon *U.K.* **13** F4
Dunqul *Egypt* **80** C3
Duns *U.K.* **13** F6
Dunseith *U.S.A.* **112** A3
Dunshaughlin *Ireland* **12** C5
Dunsmuir *U.S.A.* **108** F2
Dunstable *U.K.* **15** F7
Dunstan Mts. *N.Z.* **91** F2
Dunster *Canada* **102** C5
Dunvegan *U.K.* **13** D2
Dunvegan L. *Canada* **103** A7
Duolun *China* **56** C9
Duong Dong *Vietnam* **65** G4
Dupree *U.S.A.* **112** C3
Dupuyer *U.S.A.* **108** B7
Duque de Caxias *Brazil* **127** A7
Durack ➤ *Australia* **92** C4
Durack Ra. *Australia* **92** C4
Durack River *Australia* **92** C4
Durağan *Turkey* **72** B6
Durak *Turkey* **47** B10
Đurakovac *Kosovo* **44** D4
Durance ➤ *France* **21** E8
Durand *U.S.A.* **112** C8
Durango *Mexico* **118** C4
Durango *U.S.A.* **109** H10
Durango □ *Mexico* **118** C4
Durankulak *Bulgaria* **45** C12
Durant *Miss., U.S.A.* **117** E10
Durant *Okla., U.S.A.* **116** E6
Duratón ➤ *Spain* **36** D6
Durazno *Uruguay* **126** C4
Durazzo = Durrës *Albania* **44** E3
Durban *France* **20** F6
Durban *S. Africa* **89** D5
Durbuy *Belgium* **17** D5
Dúrcal *Spain* **37** J7
Đurđevac *Croatia* **28** D2
Düren *Germany* **24** E2
Durg = Bhilainagar-Durg
    India **67** J12
Durgapur *India* **69** H12
Durham *Canada* **114** B4
Durham *U.K.* **14** C6
Durham *Calif., U.S.A.* **110** F5
Durham *N.C., U.S.A.* **117** D15
Durham *N.H., U.S.A.* **115** C14
Durham □ *U.K.* **14** C6
Durlas = Thurles *Ireland* **12** D4
Durleşti *Moldova* **29** C13
Durmă *Si. Arabia* **70** E5
Durmitor *Montenegro* **44** C2
Durmitor △ *Serbia* **44** C3
Durness *U.K.* **13** C4
Durrës *Albania* **44** E3
Durrow *Ireland* **12** D4
Dursey I. *Ireland* **12** E1
Dursley *U.K.* **15** F5
Dursunbey *Turkey* **47** B10
Durtal *France* **18** E6
Duru *Dem. Rep. of the Congo* **86** B2
Duru Gölü *Turkey* **45** E12
Durusu *Turkey* **45** E12
Durūz, Jabal ad *Jordan* **74** C5
D'Urville, Tanjung *Indonesia* **63** E9
D'Urville I. *N.Z.* **91** D4
Duryea *U.S.A.* **115** E9
Dūsh *Egypt* **80** C3
Dushak *Turkmenistan* **71** B9
Dushan *China* **58** E6

Dushanbe *Tajikistan* **52** F7
Dusheti *Georgia* **35** J7
Dushore *U.S.A.* **115** E8
Dusky Sd. *N.Z.* **91** F1
Dussejour, C. *Australia* **92** B4
Düsseldorf *Germany* **24** D2
Düsseldorf Rhein-Ruhr ✈
    (DUS) *Germany* **24** D2
Duszniki-Zdrój *Poland* **31** H3
Dutch Harbor *U.S.A.* **106** E6
Dutlwe *Botswana* **88** C3
Dutsan Wai *Nigeria* **83** C6
Dutse *Nigeria* **83** C6
Dutton *Canada* **114** D3
Dutton ➤ *Australia* **94** C3
Dutywa *S. Africa* **89** E4
Duved *Sweden* **10** A6
Düvertepe *Turkey* **47** B10
Duwayhin, Khawr *U.A.E.* **71** E6
Duyfken Pt. *Australia* **94** A3
Duyun *China* **58** D6
Düzağac *Turkey* **47** C12
Düzce *Turkey* **72** B4
Düzce □ *Turkey* **72** B4
Dve Mogili *Bulgaria* **45** C9
Dvina, Severnaya ➤ *Russia* **6** C14
Dvinsk = Daugavpils *Latvia* **32** E4
Dvor *Croatia* **41** C13
Dvůr Králové nad Labem
    Czech Rep. **26** A8
Dwarka *India* **68** H3
Dwellingup *Australia* **93** F2
Dwight *Canada* **114** A5
Dwight *U.S.A.* **112** E9
Dyakove *Ukraine* **28** B7
Dyatkovo *Russia* **32** F8
Dyatlovo = Dzyatlava
    Belarus **23** B13
Dyce *U.K.* **13** D6
Dyer, C. *Canada* **101** D19
Dyer Bay *Canada* **114** A3
Dyer Plateau *Antarctica* **5** D17
Dyersburg *U.S.A.* **117** C10
Dyfi ➤ *U.K.* **15** E3
Dyje ➤ *Czech Rep.* **27** C9
Dymer *Ukraine* **23** C16
Dynów *Poland* **31** J9
Dysart *Australia* **94** C4
Dyviziya *Ukraine* **29** E14
Dzaoudzi *Mayotte* **85** a
Dzerzhinsk *Russia* **34** B6
Dzhalinda *Russia* **53** D13
Dzhambul = Taraz
    Kazakhstan **52** E8
Dzhankoy *Ukraine* **33** K8
Dzhanybek = Zhänibek
    Kazakhstan **34** F8
Dzharylhach, Ostriv *Ukraine* **33** J7
Dzhezkazgan =
    Zhezqazghan *Kazakhstan* **52** E7
Dzhizak = Jizzax *Uzbekistan* **52** E7
Dzhugdzur, Khrebet *Russia* **53** D14
Dzhulynk *Ukraine* **29** B14
Dzhuryn *Ukraine* **29** B13
Dzhvari = Jvari *Georgia* **35** J6
Działdowo *Poland* **31** E7
Działoszyce *Poland* **31** H7
Działoszyn *Poland* **31** G5
Dzibilchaltún *Mexico* **119** C7
Dzierzgoń *Poland* **30** E6
Dzierżoniów *Poland* **31** H3
Dzilam de Bravo *Mexico* **119** C7
Dzisna *Belarus* **32** E5
Dzisna ➤ *Belarus* **32** E5
Dziwnów *Poland* **30** D1
Dzūkija △ *Lithuania* **9** J21
Dzungarian Basin =
    Junggar Pendi *China* **60** B3
Dzüünmod *Mongolia* **60** B5
Dzyarzhynsk *Belarus* **23** B14
Dzyatlava *Belarus* **23** B13

E

E.C. Manning △ *Canada* **102** D4
Eabamet L. *Canada* **104** B2
Eabametoong *Canada* **104** B2
Éadan Doire = Edenderry
    Ireland **12** C4
Eads *U.S.A.* **108** G12
Eagar *U.S.A.* **109** J9
Eagle *Alaska, U.S.A.* **100** E3
Eagle *Colo., U.S.A.* **108** G10
Eagle ➤ *Canada* **105** B8
Eagle Butte *U.S.A.* **112** C3
Eagle Grove *U.S.A.* **112** D7
Eagle L. *Canada* **103** D10
Eagle L. *Calif., U.S.A.* **108** F3
Eagle L. *Maine, U.S.A.* **113** B19
Eagle Lake *Canada* **114** A6
Eagle Lake *Maine, U.S.A.* **113** B19
Eagle Lake *Tex., U.S.A.* **116** G6
Eagle Mountain *U.S.A.* **111** M11
Eagle Nest *U.S.A.* **109** H11
Eagle Pass *U.S.A.* **116** G4
Eagle Pk. *U.S.A.* **110** G7
Eagle Pt. *Australia* **92** C3
Eagle River *Mich., U.S.A.* **112** B9
Eagle River *Wis., U.S.A.* **112** C9

Eaglehawk *Australia* **95** F3
Eagles Mere *U.S.A.* **115** E8
Ealing □ *U.K.* **15** F7
Ear Falls *Canada* **103** C10
Earle *U.S.A.* **117** D9
Earlimart *U.S.A.* **111** K7
Earlville *U.S.A.* **115** D9
Earn ⇒ *U.K.* **13** E5
Earn, L. *U.K.* **13** E4
Earnslaw, Mt. *N.Z.* **91** F2
Earth *U.S.A.* **116** D3
Easley *U.S.A.* **117** D13
East Anglia *U.K.* **14** E9
East Angus *Canada* **105** C5
East Antarctica *Antarctica* **5** D7
East Aurora *U.S.A.* **114** D6
East Ayrshire □ *U.K.* **13** F4
East Bengal *Bangla.* **67** G17
East Beskids = Východné
  Beskydy *Europe* **27** B15
East Brady *U.S.A.* **114** F5
East Branch Clarion River
  L. *U.S.A.* **114** E6
East C. = Dezhneva, Mys
  Russia **53** C19
East C. *N.Z.* **91** B7
East Caroline Basin *Pac. Oc.* **96** G6
East Chicago *U.S.A.* **112** E10
East China Sea *Asia* **60** C7
East Coulee *Canada* **102** C6
East Dereham = Dereham
  U.K. **15** E8
East Dunbartonshire □ *U.K.* **13** F4
East Falkland *Falk. Is.* **128** G5
East Grand Forks *U.S.A.* **112** B5
East Greenwich *U.S.A.* **115** E13
East Grinstead *U.K.* **15** F8
East Hartford *U.S.A.* **115** E12
East Haydon *Australia* **94** B3
East Helena *U.S.A.* **108** C8
East Indies *Asia* **50** J14
East Kilbride *U.K.* **13** F4
East Lansing *U.S.A.* **113** D11
East Liverpool *U.S.A.* **114** F4
East London *S. Africa* **89** E4
East Lothian □ *U.K.* **13** F6
East Main = Eastmain
  Canada **104** B4
East Mariana Basin *Pac. Oc.* **96** F7
East Northport *U.S.A.* **115** F11
East Orange *U.S.A.* **115** F10
East Pacific Rise *Pac. Oc.* **97** J17
East Palestine *U.S.A.* **114** F4
East Pine *Canada* **102** B4
East Point *U.S.A.* **117** E12
East Providence *U.S.A.* **115** E13
East Pt. *Br. Virgin Is.* **121** e
East Pt. *Canada* **105** C7
East Renfrewshire □ *U.K.* **13** F4
East Retford *U.K.* **14** D7
East Riding of Yorkshire □
  U.K. **14** D7
East Rochester *U.S.A.* **114** C7
East St. Louis *U.S.A.* **112** F8
East Schelde =
  Oosterschelde ⇒ *Neths.* **17** C4
East Sea = Japan, Sea of *Asia* **54** E7
East Siberian Sea *Russia* **53** B17
East Stroudsburg *U.S.A.* **115** E9
East Sussex □ *U.K.* **15** G8
East Tasman Plateau
  Pac. Oc. **96** M7
East Tawas *U.S.A.* **113** C12
East Timor ■ *Asia* **63** F7
East Toorale *Australia* **95** E4
East Walker ⇒ *U.S.A.* **110** G7
East Windsor *U.S.A.* **115** F10
Eastbourne *N.Z.* **91** D5
Eastbourne *U.K.* **15** G8
Eastend *Canada* **103** D7
Easter Fracture Zone
  Pac. Oc. **97** K16
Easter I. = Pascua, I. de
  Chile **97** K17
Eastern □ *Ghana* **83** D4
Eastern □ *Kenya* **86** C4
Eastern □ *S. Leone* **82** D2
Eastern Cape □ *S. Africa* **88** E4
Eastern Cr. ⇒ *Australia* **94** C3
Eastern Desert = Es Sahrâ'
  Esh Sharqîya *Egypt* **80** B3
Eastern Ghats *India* **66** N11
Eastern Group = Lau Group
  Fiji **91** a
Eastern Group *Australia* **93** F3
Eastern Guruma ⊚ *Australia* **92** D2
Eastern Transvaal =
  Mpumalanga □ *S. Africa* **89** D5
Easterville *Canada* **103** C9
Easthampton *U.S.A.* **115** D12
Eastlake *U.S.A.* **114** E3
Eastland *U.S.A.* **116** E5
Eastleigh *U.K.* **15** G6
Eastmain *Canada* **104** B4
Eastmain ⇒ *Canada* **104** B4
Eastman *Canada* **115** A12
Eastman *U.S.A.* **117** E13
Easton *Md., U.S.A.* **113** F15
Easton *Pa., U.S.A.* **115** F9

Easton *Wash., U.S.A.* **110** C5
Eastport *U.S.A.* **113** C20
Eastsound *U.S.A.* **110** B4
Eaton *U.S.A.* **108** F11
Eatonia *Canada* **103** C7
Eatonton *U.S.A.* **117** E13
Eatontown *U.S.A.* **115** F10
Eatonville *U.S.A.* **110** D4
Eau Claire *U.S.A.* **112** C8
Eau Claire, L. à l' *Canada* **104** A5
Eauripik Rise *Pac. Oc.* **96** G6
Eauze *France* **20** E4
Eban *Nigeria* **83** D5
Ebano *Mexico* **119** C5
Ebbegebirge △ *Germany* **24** D3
Ebbw Vale *U.K.* **15** F4
Ebeltoft *Denmark* **11** H4
Ebeltoft Vig *Denmark* **11** H4
Ebensburg *U.S.A.* **114** F6
Ebensee *Austria* **26** D6
Eber Gölü *Turkey* **72** C4
Eberbach *Germany* **25** F4
Eberswalde-Finow *Germany* **24** C9
Ebetsu *Japan* **54** C10
Ebian *China* **58** C4
Ebingen *Germany* **25** G5
Éboli *Italy* **43** B8
Ebolowa *Cameroon* **83** E7
Ebonda *Dem. Rep. of the Congo* **84** D4
Ebonyi □ *Nigeria* **83** D6
Ebrach *Germany* **25** F6
Ebre = Ebro ⇒ *Spain* **38** E5
Ébrié, Lagune *Ivory C.* **82** D4
Ebro ⇒ *Spain* **38** E5
Ebro, Embalse del *Spain* **36** C7
Ebstorf *Germany* **24** B6
Ecatepec de Morelos *Mexico* **119** D5
Ecbatana = Hamadān *Iran* **73** E13
Eceabat *Turkey* **45** F10
Ech Chéliff *Algeria* **78** A6
Echigo-Sammyaku *Japan* **55** F9
Echinos *Greece* **45** E9
Échirolles *France* **21** C9
Echizen-Misaki *Japan* **55** G7
Echmiadzin = Yejmiadzin
  Armenia **35** K7
Echo Bay *N.W.T., Canada* **100** D8
Echo Bay *Ont., Canada* **104** C3
Echoing ⇒ *Canada* **104** B1
Echternach *Lux.* **17** E6
Echuca *Australia* **95** F3
Écija *Spain* **37** H5
Eckental *Germany* **25** F7
Eckernförde *Germany* **24** A5
Eclipse I. *Australia* **93** G2
Eclipse Is. *Australia* **92** B4
Eclipse Sd. *Canada* **101** C16
Écommoy *France* **18** E7
Écouché *France* **18** D6
Ecrins △ *France* **21** D10
Ecuador ■ *S. Amer.* **124** D3
Écueillé *France* **18** E8
Ed *Sweden* **11** F5
Ed Dabbura *Sudan* **80** D3
Ed Da'ein *Sudan* **81** E2
Ed Damazin *Sudan* **79** F12
Ed Dâmer *Sudan* **80** D3
Ed Dar el Beida =
  Casablanca *Morocco* **78** B4
Ed Debba *Sudan* **80** D3
Ed Déffa *Egypt* **80** A2
Ed Deim *Sudan* **81** E2
Ed Dueim *Sudan* **81** E3
Edam *Canada* **103** C7
Edam *Neths.* **17** B5
Edane *Sweden* **10** E6
Édéa *Cameroon* **83** E7
Edebäck *Sweden* **10** D7
Edehon L. *Canada* **103** A9
Edelény *Hungary* **28** B5
Eden *Australia* **95** F4
Eden *N.C., U.S.A.* **117** C15
Eden *N.Y., U.S.A.* **114** D6
Eden *Tex., U.S.A.* **116** F5
Eden ⇒ *U.K.* **14** C4
Edenburg *S. Africa* **88** D4
Edendale *S. Africa* **89** D5
Edenderry *Ireland* **12** C4
Edenton *U.S.A.* **117** C16
Edenville *S. Africa* **89** D4
Eder ⇒ *Germany* **24** D5
Eder-Stausee *Germany* **24** D4
Edessa *Greece* **44** F6
Edewecht *Germany* **24** B3
Edfu = Idfû *Egypt* **80** C3
Edgar *U.S.A.* **112** E5
Edgartown *U.S.A.* **115** E14
Edge Hill *U.K.* **15** E6
Edgefield *U.S.A.* **117** E14

Edgeley *U.S.A.* **112** B4
Edgemont *U.S.A.* **112** D2
Edgeøya *Svalbard* **4** B9
Edgeworth *U.S.A.* **112** D2
Édhessa = Edessa *Greece* **44** F6
Edievale *N.Z.* **91** F2
Edina *Liberia* **82** D2
Edina *U.S.A.* **112** E7
Edinboro *U.S.A.* **114** E4
Edinburg *U.S.A.* **116** H5
Edinburgh *U.K.* **13** F5
Edinburgh ✈ (EDI) *U.K.* **13** F5
Edinburgh, City of □ *U.K.* **13** F5
Edineţ *Moldova* **29** B12
Edirne *Turkey* **45** E10
Edirne □ *Turkey* **45** E10
Edison *U.S.A.* **110** B4
Edithburgh *Australia* **95** F2
Edmeston *U.S.A.* **115** D9
Edmond *U.S.A.* **116** D6
Edmonds *U.S.A.* **110** C4
Edmonton *Australia* **94** B4
Edmonton *Canada* **102** C6
Edmund L. *Canada* **104** B1
Edmundston *Canada* **105** C6
Edna *U.S.A.* **116** G6
Edo □ *Nigeria* **83** D6
Edolo *Italy* **40** B7
Edremit *Turkey* **47** B9
Edremit Körfezi *Turkey* **47** B8
Edsbro *Sweden* **10** E12
Edsbyn *Sweden* **10** C9
Edson *Canada* **102** C5
Eduardo Castex *Argentina* **126** D3
Edward ⇒ *U.S.A.* **95** F3
Edward, L. *Africa* **86** C2
Edward VII Land *Antarctica* **5** E13
Edwards *Calif., U.S.A.* **111** L9
Edwards *N.Y., U.S.A.* **115** B9
Edwards Plateau *U.S.A.* **116** F4
Edwardsville *U.S.A.* **115** E9
Edzná *Mexico* **119** D6
Edzo *Canada* **102** A5
Eeklo *Belgium* **17** C3
Eesti = Estonia ■ *Europe* **32** C3
Eferding *Austria* **26** C7
Effigy Mounds △ *U.S.A.* **112** D8
Effingham *U.S.A.* **112** F9
Eforie *Romania* **29** F13
Efxinoupoli *Greece* **46** B4
Ega ⇒ *Spain* **38** C3
Égadi, Ísole *Italy* **42** E5
Egan Range *U.S.A.* **108** G6
Eganville *Canada* **114** A7
Eger = Cheb *Czech Rep.* **26** A5
Eger *Hungary* **28** C5
Eger ⇒ *Hungary* **28** C5
Egersund *Norway* **9** G12
Egg L. *Canada* **103** B7
Eggegebirge Südlicher
  Teutoburger Wald △
  Germany **24** D4
Eggenburg *Austria* **26** C8
Eggenfelden *Germany* **25** G8
Éghezée *Belgium* **17** D4
Egina *Greece* **46** D5
Eginio *Greece* **44** F6
Egio *Greece* **46** C4
Égletons *France* **20** C6
Eglinton I. *Canada* **101** B8
Egmont *Canada* **102** D4
Egmont, C. *N.Z.* **91** C4
Egmont, Mt. = Taranaki,
  Mt. *N.Z.* **91** C5
Egmont △ *N.Z.* **91** C5
Egra *India* **69** J12
Eğridir *Turkey* **72** D4
Eğridir Gölü *Turkey* **72** D4
Egtved *Denmark* **11** J3
Éguzon-Chantôme *France* **19** F8
Egvekinot *Russia* **53** C19
Egyek *Hungary* **28** C5
Egypt ■ *Africa* **80** B3
Eha Amufu *Nigeria* **83** D6
Ehime □ *Japan* **55** H6
Ehingen *Germany* **25** G5
Ehrenberg *U.S.A.* **111** M12
Ehrwald *Austria* **26** D3
Eibar *Spain* **38** B2
Eichstätt *Germany* **25** G7
Eider ⇒ *Germany* **24** A4
Eidsvold *Australia* **95** D5
Eidsvoll *Norway* **9** F14
Eifel *Germany* **25** E2
Eiffel Flats *Zimbabwe* **87** F3
Eiger *Switz.* **40** B5
Eigg *U.K.* **13** E2
Eighty Mile Beach *Australia* **92** C3
Eil, L. *U.K.* **13** E3
Eildon, L. *Australia* **95** F4
Eilean Sar = Western
  Isles □ *U.K.* **13** D1
Eilenburg *Germany* **24** D8
Eillenburg *Germany* **24** D8
Ein el Luweiqa *Sudan* **81** E3
Einasleigh *Australia* **94** B3
Einasleigh ⇒ *Australia* **94** B3
Einbeck *Germany* **24** D5
Eindhoven *Neths.* **17** C5
Einsiedeln *Switz.* **25** H4

Eire = Ireland ■ *Europe* **12** C4
Eiríksjökull *Iceland* **8** D3
Eirunepé *Brazil* **124** E5
Eiseb ⇒ *Namibia* **88** C2
Eisenach *Germany* **24** E6
Eisenberg *Germany* **24** E7
Eisenerz *Austria* **26** D7
Eisenhüttenstadt *Germany* **24** C10
Eisenkappel *Austria* **26** E7
Eisenstadt *Austria* **27** D9
Eisfeld *Germany* **25** E6
Eisleben *Germany* **24** D7
Eislingen *Germany* **25** G5
Eivissa *Spain* **48** C7
Eixe, Serra do *Spain* **36** C4
Ejea de los Caballeros *Spain* **38** C3
Ejeda *Madag.* **89** C7
Ejura *Ghana* **83** D4
Ejutla *Mexico* **119** D5
Ekalaka *U.S.A.* **108** D11
Ekaterinburg =
  Yekaterinburg *Russia* **52** D7
Ekenäs = Tammisaari
  Finland **32** B2
Ekenässjön *Sweden* **11** G9
Ekerö *Sweden* **10** E11
Eket *Nigeria* **83** E6
Eketahuna *N.Z.* **91** D5
Ekibastuz *Kazakhstan* **52** D8
Ekiti □ *Nigeria* **83** D6
Ekoli *Dem. Rep. of the Congo* **86** C1
Ekoln *Sweden* **10** E11
Ekshärad *Sweden* **10** D7
Eksjö *Sweden* **11** G8
Ekuma ⇒ *Namibia* **88** B2
Ekwan ⇒ *Canada* **104** B3
Ekwan Pt. *Canada* **104** B3
El Aaiún *W. Sahara* **78** C3
El Abanico *Chile* **126** D1
El Abbasiya *Sudan* **81** E3
El 'Agrûd *Egypt* **74** E3
El Ait *Sudan* **81** E2
El 'Aiyat *Egypt* **80** J7
El Alamein *Egypt* **80** A2
El 'Aqaba, W. ⇒ *Egypt* **74** E2
El 'Arag *Egypt* **80** A2
El Arīḥā *West Bank* **74** D4
El 'Arîsh *Egypt* **74** D2
El 'Arîsh, W. ⇒ *Egypt* **74** D2
El Asnam = Ech Chéliff
  Algeria **78** A6
El Astillero *Spain* **36** B7
El Badâri *Egypt* **80** B3
El Bahrein *Egypt* **80** B2
El Ballâs *Egypt* **80** B3
El Balyana *Egypt* **80** B3
El Baqeir *Sudan* **80** D3
El Barco de Ávila *Spain* **36** E5
El Barco de Valdeorras = O
  Barco *Spain* **36** C4
El Bauga *Sudan* **80** D3
El Bawiti *Egypt* **80** B2
El Bayadh *Algeria* **78** B6
El Bierzo *Spain* **36** C4
El Bluff *Nic.* **120** D3
El Bonillo *Spain* **39** G2
El Buheirat □ *Sudan* **81** F3
El Burgo de Osma *Spain* **38** D1
El Cajon *U.S.A.* **111** N10
El Calafate *Argentina* **128** G2
El Campello *Spain* **39** G4
El Campo *U.S.A.* **116** G6
El Capitan *U.S.A.* **110** H7
El Carbón *Honduras* **120** C2
El Carmen *Colombia* **124** B3
El Centro *U.S.A.* **111** N11
El Cerro *Bolivia* **124** G6
El Cerro de Andévalo *Spain* **37** H4
El Compadre *Mexico* **111** N10
El Coronil *Spain* **37** H5
El Cuy *Argentina* **128** B3
El Cuyo *Mexico* **119** C7
El Dab'a *Egypt* **80** H6
El Daheir *Egypt* **74** D3
El Deir *Egypt* **80** B3
El Descanso *Mexico* **111** N10
El Desemboque *Mexico* **118** A2
El Dilingat *Egypt* **80** H7
El Diviso *Colombia* **124** C3
El Djouf *Mauritania* **78** D4
El Dorado *Mexico* **118** C3
El Dorado *Ark., U.S.A.* **116** E8
El Dorado *Kans., U.S.A.* **112** G5
El Dorado *Venezuela* **124** B6
El Dorado Springs *U.S.A.* **112** G6
El 'Ein *Sudan* **81** D2
El Ejido *Spain* **37** J8
El Escorial *Spain* **36** E6
El Espinar *Spain* **36** D6
El Faiyûm *Egypt* **80** J7
El Fâsher *Sudan* **81** E2
El Ferrol = Ferrol *Spain* **36** B2
El Fifi *Sudan* **81** E2
El Fuerte *Mexico* **118** B3
El Ga'a *Sudan* **81** E2
El Garef *Sudan* **81** E3
El Gebir *Sudan* **81** E2
El Gedida *Egypt* **80** B2

El Geneina = Al Junaynah
  Sudan **79** F10
El Geteina *Sudan* **81** E3
El Gezira □ *Sudan* **81** E3
El Gir *Sudan* **80** D2
El Giza *Egypt* **80** J7
El Gogorrón △ *Mexico* **118** C4
El Goléa *Algeria* **78** B6
El Golfo de Santa Clara
  Mexico **118** A2
El Gouna *Egypt* **80** B3
El Grau *Spain* **39** G4
El Guácharo △ *Venezuela* **121** D7
El Guache △ *Venezuela* **121** E6
El Hagiz *Sudan* **81** D4
El Hâi *Egypt* **80** J7
El Hammam *Egypt* **80** A2
El Hawata *Sudan* **81** E3
El Heiz *Egypt* **80** B2
El Hideib *Sudan* **81** E3
El Hilla *Sudan* **81** E2
El 'Idisât *Egypt* **80** B3
El Iskandarîya *Egypt* **80** H7
El Istiwa'iya *Sudan* **79** G11
El Jadida *Morocco* **78** B4
El Jardal *Honduras* **120** D2
El Jebelein *Sudan* **81** E3
El Kab *Sudan* **80** D3
El Kafr el Sharqi *Egypt* **80** H7
El Kamlin *Sudan* **81** D3
El Karaba *Sudan* **80** D3
El Kef □ *Tunisia* **79** A7
El Kere *Ethiopia* **81** F5
El Khandaq *Sudan* **80** D3
El Khanka *Egypt* **80** H7
El Khârga *Egypt* **80** B3
El Khartûm ■ *Sudan* **81** D3
El Khartûm □ *Sudan* **81** D3
El Khartûm Bahrî *Sudan* **81** D3
El Kuntilla *Egypt* **74** E3
El Laqâwa *Sudan* **81** E2
El Leh *Ethiopia* **81** G4
El Leiya *Sudan* **81** D4
El Leoncito △ *Argentina* **126** C2
El Lucero *Mexico* **118** A3
El Maestrazgo *Spain* **38** E4
El Mafâza *Sudan* **81** E3
El Maghra *Egypt* **80** A2
El Mahalla el Kubra *Egypt* **80** H7
El Mahârîq *Egypt* **80** B3
El Maimûn *Egypt* **80** J7
El Maks el Bahari *Egypt* **80** C3
El Malpais △ *U.S.A.* **109** J10
El Manshâh *Egypt* **80** B3
El Mansûra *Egypt* **80** H7
El Manzala *Egypt* **80** H7
El Marâgha *Egypt* **80** B3
El Masid *Sudan* **81** D3
El Masnou *Spain* **38** D7
El Matarîya *Egypt* **80** H8
El Meda *Ethiopia* **81** F5
El Medano *Canary Is.* **48** F3
El Ménia = El Goléa *Algeria* **78** B6
El Metemma *Sudan* **81** E3
El Milagro *Argentina* **126** C2
El Minyâ *Egypt* **80** B3
El Monte *U.S.A.* **111** L8
El Montseny *Spain* **38** D7
El Mreyyé *Mauritania* **82** B3
El Niybo *Ethiopia* **81** G4
El Obeid *Sudan* **81** E3
El Odaiya *Sudan* **81** E2
El Oro *Mexico* **119** D4
El Oued *Algeria* **78** B7
El Palmar △ *Argentina* **126** C4
El Palmito, Presa *Mexico* **118** B3
El Paso *U.S.A.* **116** F1
El Pedernoso *Spain* **39** F2
El Pedroso *Spain* **37** H5
El Pinacate y Gran Desierto
  de Altar = Gran Desierto
  del Pinacate △ *Mexico* **118** A2
El Pobo de Dueñas *Spain* **38** E3
El Portal *U.S.A.* **110** H7
El Porvenir *Mexico* **118** A3
El Prat de Llobregat *Spain* **38** D7
El Progreso *Honduras* **120** C2
El Pueblito *Mexico* **118** B3
El Pueblo *Canary Is.* **48** F2
El Puente del Arzobispo *Spain* **36** F5
El Puerto de Santa María
  Spain **37** J4
El Qâhira *Egypt* **80** H7
El Qantara *Egypt* **74** E1
El Qasr *Egypt* **80** B2
El Qubâbât *Egypt* **80** J7
El Quseima *Egypt* **74** E3
El Qusîya *Egypt* **80** B3
El Râshda *Egypt* **80** B2
El Real de Santa María
  Panama **124** B3
El Reno *U.S.A.* **107** H20
El Rey △ *Argentina* **126** A3
El Ridisiya *Egypt* **80** C3
El Rio *U.S.A.* **111** L7
El Ronquillo *Spain* **37** H4
El Roque, Pta. *Canary Is.* **48** F4
El Rosarito *Mexico* **118** B2
El Rubio *Spain* **37** H5

El Saff *Egypt* **80** J7
El Salto *Mexico* **118** C3
El Salvador ■ *Cent. Amer.* **120** D2
El Sauce *Nic.* **120** D2
El Saucejo *Spain* **37** H5
El Shallal *Egypt* **80** J7
El Simbillawein *Egypt* **80** H7
El Sueco *Mexico* **118** B3
El Suweis *Egypt* **80** J8
El Tabbîn *Egypt* **80** J7
El Tamarâni, W. ⇒ *Egypt* **74** E3
El Thamad *Egypt* **74** F3
El Tigre *Venezuela* **124** B6
El Tîh, Gebel *Egypt* **74** F2
El Tîna *Egypt* **80** H8
El Tofo *Chile* **126** B1
El Tránsito *Chile* **126** B1
El Tûr *Egypt* **70** D2
El Turbio *Argentina* **128** G2
El Uqsur *Egypt* **80** B3
El Valle □ *Spain* **39** H3
El Vendrell *Spain* **38** D6
El Vergel *Mexico* **118** B3
El Vigía *Venezuela* **124** B4
El Viso del Alcor *Spain* **37** H5
El Wabeira *Egypt* **74** F2
El Waqf *Egypt* **80** B3
El Weguet *Ethiopia* **81** F5
El Wuz *Sudan* **81** D3
Elafonisos *Greece* **46** E4
Élancourt *France* **19** D8
Elasa *Greece* **47** D9
Elassona *Greece* **46** B4
Elat *Israel* **74** F3
Elatia *Greece* **46** C4
Elâzığ *Turkey* **73** C8
Elâzığ □ *Turkey* **73** C8
Elba *Italy* **40** F7
Elba *U.S.A.* **117** F11
Elbasan *Albania* **44** E4
Elbe *U.S.A.* **110** D4
Elbe ⇒ *Europe* **24** B4
Elbe-Seitenkanal *Germany* **24** C6
Elbert, Mt. *U.S.A.* **108** G10
Elberton *U.S.A.* **117** D13
Elbeuf *France* **18** C8
Elbing = Elbląg *Poland* **30** D6
Elbistan *Turkey* **72** C7
Elbląg *Poland* **30** D6
Elbow *Canada* **103** C7
Elbrus *Russia* **35** J6
Elbufer-Drawehn △ *Germany* **24** B6
Elburz Mts. = Alborz,
  Reshteh-ye Kūhhā-ye *Iran* **71** C7
Elche *Spain* **39** G4
Elche de la Sierra *Spain* **39** G2
Elcho I. *Australia* **94** A2
Elda *Spain* **39** G4
Eldama Ravine *Kenya* **86** B4
Elde ⇒ *Germany* **24** B7
Eldon *Mo., U.S.A.* **112** F7
Eldon *Wash., U.S.A.* **110** C3
Eldora *U.S.A.* **112** D7
Eldorado *Argentina* **127** B5
Eldorado *Canada* **114** B7
Eldorado *Ill., U.S.A.* **112** G9
Eldorado *Tex., U.S.A.* **116** F4
Eldoret *Kenya* **86** B4
Eldred *U.S.A.* **114** E6
Elea, C. *Cyprus* **49** D13
Eleanora, Pk. *Australia* **93** F3
Elefantes ⇒ *Africa* **89** C5
Elefsina *Greece* **46** C5
Eleftherios Venizelos ✈
  (ATH) *Greece* **46** D5
Elektrogorsk *Russia* **32** E10
Elektrostal *Russia* **32** E10
Elele *Nigeria* **83** D6
Elemi Triangle *Africa* **81** G4
Elena *Bulgaria* **45** D9
Elephant Butte Res. *U.S.A.* **109** K10
Elephant I. *Antarctica* **5** C18
Eleshnitsa *Bulgaria* **44** C7
Eleşkirt *Turkey* **73** C10
Eleuthera *Bahamas* **120** B4
Eleutheroupoli *Greece* **45** F8
Elgin *Canada* **115** B8
Elgin *U.K.* **13** D5
Elgin *Ill., U.S.A.* **112** D9
Elgin *N. Dak., U.S.A.* **112** B3
Elgin *Oreg., U.S.A.* **108** D5
Elgin *Tex., U.S.A.* **116** F6
Elgoibar *Spain* **38** B2
Elgon, Mt. *Africa* **86** B3
Eliase *Indonesia* **63** F8
Elikonos Oros *Greece* **46** C4
Elim *Namibia* **88** B2
Elim *S. Africa* **88** E2
Elin Pelin *Bulgaria* **44** D7
Elista *Russia* **35** G7
Elizabeth *Australia* **95** E2
Elizabeth *U.S.A.* **115** F10
Elizabeth City *U.S.A.* **117** C16
Elizabethton *U.S.A.* **117** C13
Elizabethtown *Ky., U.S.A.* **113** G11
Elizabethtown *N.Y., U.S.A.* **115** B11
Elizabethtown *Pa., U.S.A.* **115** F8
Elizondo *Spain* **38** B3
Elk *Poland* **30** E9

Elk ⇝ *Canada* **102** C5
Elk ⇝ *Poland* **30** E9
Elk ⇝ *U.S.A.* **117** D11
Elk City *U.S.A.* **116** D5
Elk Creek *U.S.A.* **110** F4
Elk Grove *U.S.A.* **110** G5
Elk Island △ *Canada* **102** C6
Elk Lake *Canada* **104** C3
Elk Point *Canada* **103** C6
Elk River *Idaho, U.S.A.* **108** C5
Elk River *Minn., U.S.A.* **112** C7
Elkedra ⇝ *Australia* **94** C2
Elkhart *Ind., U.S.A.* **113** E11
Elkhart *Kans., U.S.A.* **112** G3
Elkhorn *Canada* **103** D8
Elkhorn ⇝ *U.S.A.* **112** E5
Elkhovo *Bulgaria* **45** D10
Elkin *U.S.A.* **117** C14
Elkins *U.S.A.* **113** F14
Elkland *U.S.A.* **114** E7
Elko *Canada* **102** D5
Elko *U.S.A.* **108** F6
Elkton *U.S.A.* **114** C1
Ellas = Greece ■ *Europe* **46** B3
Ellef Ringnes I. *Canada* **101** B11
Ellen, Mt. *U.S.A.* **115** B12
Ellenburg *U.S.A.* **115** B11
Ellendale *U.S.A.* **112** B4
Ellensburg *U.S.A.* **108** C3
Ellenville *U.S.A.* **115** E10
Ellerton *Barbados* **121** g
Ellery, Mt. *Australia* **95** F4
Ellesmere, L. *N.Z.* **91** G4
Ellesmere I. *Canada* **101** B16
Ellesmere Island = Quttinirpaaq △ *Canada* **101** A17
Ellesmere Port *U.K.* **14** D5
Ellice Is. = Tuvalu ■ *Pac. Oc.* **90** B10
Ellicottville *U.S.A.* **114** D6
Ellington *U.S.A.* **114** D5
Elliot *Australia* **94** B1
Elliot *S. Africa* **89** E4
Elliot Lake *Canada* **104** C3
Elliotdale = Xhora *S. Africa* **89** E4
Ellis *U.S.A.* **112** F4
Elliston *Australia* **95** E1
Ellisville *U.S.A.* **117** F10
Ellon *U.K.* **13** D6
Ellore = Eluru *India* **67** L12
Ellsworth *Kans., U.S.A.* **112** F4
Ellsworth *Maine, U.S.A.* **113** C19
Ellsworth Land *Antarctica* **5** D16
Ellsworth Mts. *Antarctica* **5** D16
Ellwangen *Germany* **25** G6
Ellwood City *U.S.A.* **114** F4
Elm *Switz.* **25** J5
Elm-Lappwald △ *Germany* **24** C6
Elma *Canada* **103** D9
Elma *U.S.A.* **110** D3
Elmadağ *Turkey* **72** C5
Elmalı *Turkey* **47** E11
Elmhurst *U.S.A.* **112** E10
Elmina *Ghana* **83** D4
Elmira *Canada* **114** C4
Elmira *U.S.A.* **114** D8
Elmira Heights *U.S.A.* **114** D8
Elmore *Australia* **95** F3
Elmshorn *Germany* **24** B5
Elmvale *Canada* **114** B5
Elne *France* **20** F6
Elora *Canada* **114** C4
Elos *Greece* **46** E4
Elounda *Greece* **49** D7
Eloy *U.S.A.* **109** K8
Éloyes *France* **19** D13
Elphin *Canada* **115** B8
Elrose *Canada* **103** C7
Elsby △ *Australia* **92** B5
Elsdorf *Germany* **24** E2
Elsie *U.S.A.* **110** E3
Elsinore = Helsingør *Denmark* **11** H6
Elster ⇝ *Germany* **24** D7
Elsterwerda *Germany* **24** D9
Eltanin Fracture Zone System *S. Ocean* **5** B14
Eltham *N.Z.* **91** C5
Elton *Russia* **35** F8
Elton, Ozero *Russia* **35** F8
Eltville *Germany* **25** E4
Eluru *India* **67** L12
Elvas *Portugal* **37** G3
Elven *France* **18** E4
Elverum *Norway* **8** F14
Elvire ⇝ *Australia* **92** C4
Elvire, Mt. *Australia* **93** E2
Elvo ⇝ *Italy* **40** C5
Elwell, L. = Tiber Res. *U.S.A.* **108** B8
Elwood *Ind., U.S.A.* **113** E11
Elwood *Nebr., U.S.A.* **112** E4
Elx = Elche *Spain* **39** G4
Ely *U.K.* **15** E8
Ely *Minn., U.S.A.* **112** B8
Ely *Nev., U.S.A.* **108** G6
Elyria *U.S.A.* **114** E2
Elyros *Greece* **46** F5
Elz ⇝ *Germany* **25** G3

Emådalen *Sweden* **10** C8
eMalahleni *S. Africa* **89** D4
Emämrüd *Iran* **71** B7
Emån ⇝ *Sweden* **11** G10
Embarcación *Argentina* **126** A3
Embetsu *Japan* **54** B10
Embi *Kazakhstan* **52** E6
Embi ⇝ *Kazakhstan* **52** E6
Embonas *Greece* **49** C9
Embro *Canada* **114** C4
Embrun *France* **21** D10
Embu *Kenya* **86** C4
Emden *Germany* **24** B3
Emecik *Turkey* **47** E9
Emerald *Australia* **94** C4
Emerald I. *Canada* **101** B9
Emerson *Canada* **103** D9
Emet *Turkey* **47** B11
Emi Koussi *Chad* **79** E9
Emília-Romagna □ *Italy* **40** D8
Emilius, Mte. *Italy* **40** C4
Eminabad *Pakistan* **68** C6
Emine, Nos *Bulgaria* **45** D11
Emirdağ *Turkey* **72** C4
Emissi, Tarso *Chad* **79** D9
Emlenton *U.S.A.* **114** E5
Emlichheim *Germany* **24** C2
Emmaboda *Sweden* **11** H9
Emmaus *S. Africa* **88** D4
Emmaus *U.S.A.* **115** F9
Emme ⇝ *Switz.* **25** H3
Emmeloord *Neths.* **17** B5
Emmen *Neths.* **17** B6
Emmen *Switz.* **25** H4
Emmendingen *Germany* **25** G3
Emmental *Switz.* **25** J3
Emmerich *Germany* **24** D2
Emmet *Australia* **94** C3
Emmetsburg *U.S.A.* **112** D6
Emmett *Idaho, U.S.A.* **108** E5
Emmett *Mich., U.S.A.* **114** D2
Emmonak *U.S.A.* **106** C7
Emo *Canada* **103** D10
Emőd *Hungary* **28** C5
Emona *Bulgaria* **45** D11
Empalme *Mexico* **118** B2
Empangeni *S. Africa* **89** D5
Empedrado *Argentina* **126** B4
Emperor Seamount Chain *Pac. Oc.* **96** D9
Emperor Trough *Pac. Oc.* **96** C9
Empoli *Italy* **40** E7
Emporia *Kans., U.S.A.* **112** F5
Emporia *Va., U.S.A.* **113** G15
Emporium *U.S.A.* **114** E6
Empress *Canada* **103** C7
Empty Quarter = Rub' al Khālī *Si. Arabia* **75** D4
Ems ⇝ *Germany* **24** B3
Emsdale *Canada* **114** A5
Emsdetten *Germany* **24** C3
Emu *China* **57** C15
Emu Park *Australia* **94** C5
eMuziwezinto *S. Africa* **89** E5
'En 'Avrona *Israel* **74** F4
'En Boqeq *Israel* **71** D4
'En Gedi *Israel* **71** D4
En Nahud *Sudan* **81** E2
En Nofalab *Sudan* **81** D3
Ena *Japan* **55** G8
Enana *Namibia* **88** B2
Enånger *Sweden* **10** C11
Enard B. *U.K.* **13** C3
Enare = Inarijärvi *Finland* **8** B23
Enarotali *Indonesia* **63** E9
Encampment *U.S.A.* **108** F10
Encantadas, Serra *Brazil* **127** C5
Encarnación *Paraguay* **127** B4
Encarnación de Diaz *Mexico* **118** C4
Enchi *Ghana* **82** D4
Encinitas *U.S.A.* **111** M9
Encino *U.S.A.* **109** J11
Encounter B. *Australia* **95** F2
Encs *Hungary* **28** B6
Endako *Canada* **102** C3
Endau *Kenya* **86** C4
Endau Rompin △ *Malaysia* **65** L4
Ende *Indonesia* **63** F6
Endeavour Str. *Australia* **94** A3
Endelave *Denmark* **11** J4
Enderbury I. *Kiribati* **96** H10
Enderby *Canada* **102** C5
Enderby Abyssal Plain *S. Ocean* **5** C6
Enderby I. *Australia* **92** D2
Enderby Land *Antarctica* **5** C5
Enderlin *U.S.A.* **112** B5
Enderrocat, C. *Spain* **48** B9
Endicott *U.S.A.* **115** D8
Endicott Mts. *U.S.A.* **106** B4
Endwell *U.S.A.* **115** D8
Endyalgout I. *Australia* **92** B5
Eneabba *Australia* **93** E2
Enewetak Atoll *Marshall Is.* **96** F8
Enez *Turkey* **45** F10
Enfer, Pte. d' *Martinique* **120** c
Enfield *Canada* **105** D7
Enfield *Conn., U.S.A.* **115** E12
Enfield *N.C., U.S.A.* **117** C16

Enfield *N.H., U.S.A.* **115** C12
Engadin *Switz.* **25** J6
Engaño, C. *Dom. Rep.* **121** C6
Engaño, C. *Phil.* **63** A6
Engaru *Japan* **54** B11
Engcobo = Ngcobo *S. Africa* **89** E4
Engelberg *Switz.* **25** J4
Engels *Russia* **34** E8
England *U.S.A.* **116** D9
England □ *U.K.* **15** E5
Englee *Canada* **105** B8
Englehart *Canada* **104** C4
Englewood *U.S.A.* **108** G11
English ⇝ *Canada* **103** C10
English Bazar = Ingraj Bazar *India* **69** G13
English Channel *Europe* **15** G6
English Company's Is., The *Australia* **94** A2
English River *Canada* **104** C1
Engures ezers *Latvia* **30** A10
Enguri ⇝ *Georgia* **35** J5
Enid *U.S.A.* **116** C6
Enipeas ⇝ *Greece* **46** B4
Enkhuizen *Neths.* **17** B5
Enköping *Sweden* **10** E11
Enle *China* **58** F3
Enna *Italy* **43** E7
Ennadai L. *Canada* **103** A8
Ennedi *Chad* **79** E10
Enngonia *Australia* **95** D4
Ennigerloh *Germany* **24** D4
Ennis *Ireland* **12** D3
Ennis *Mont., U.S.A.* **108** D8
Ennis *Tex., U.S.A.* **116** E6
Enniscorthy *Ireland* **12** D5
Enniskillen *U.K.* **12** B4
Ennistimon *Ireland* **12** D2
Enns *Austria* **26** C7
Enns ⇝ *Austria* **26** C7
Eno *Finland* **8** E24
Enontekiö *Finland* **8** B20
Enosburg Falls *U.S.A.* **115** B12
Enping *China* **59** F9
Enriquillo, L. *Dom. Rep.* **121** C5
Enschede *Neths.* **17** B6
Ensenada *Argentina* **126** C4
Ensenada *Mexico* **118** A1
Ensenada de los Muertos *Mexico* **118** C2
Enshi *China* **58** B7
Ensisheim *France* **19** E14
Entebbe *Uganda* **86** B3
Enterprise *Canada* **102** A5
Enterprise *Ala., U.S.A.* **117** F12
Enterprise *Oreg., U.S.A.* **108** D5
Entorno de Doñana △ *Spain* **37** J4
Entraygues-sur-Truyère *France* **20** D6
Entre Ríos *Bolivia* **126** A3
Entre Ríos □ *Argentina* **126** C4
Entrepeñas, Embalse de *Spain* **38** E2
Entroncamento *Portugal* **37** F2
Enugu *Nigeria* **83** D6
Enugu □ *Nigeria* **83** D6
Enugu Ezike *Nigeria* **83** D6
Enumclaw *U.S.A.* **110** C5
Envalira, Port d' *Europe* **38** C6
Envermeu *France* **18** C8
Enviken *Sweden* **10** D9
Enying *Hungary* **28** D3
Enza ⇝ *Italy* **40** D7
Eochaill = Youghal *Ireland* **12** E4
Eólie, Ís. *Italy* **43** D7
Epanomi *Greece* **44** F6
Epe *Neths.* **17** B5
Epe *Nigeria* **83** D5
Épernay *France* **19** C10
Épernon *France* **19** D8
Ephesus *Turkey* **47** D9
Ephraim *U.S.A.* **108** G8
Ephrata *Pa., U.S.A.* **115** F8
Ephrata *Wash., U.S.A.* **108** C4
Epidavros Limira *Greece* **46** E5
Épila *Spain* **38** D3
Épinac *France* **19** F11
Épinal *France* **19** D13
Epiros □ *Greece* **46** B2
Episkopi *Cyprus* **49** E11
Episkopi *Greece* **49** D6
Episkopi Bay *Cyprus* **49** E11
Epitalio *Greece* **46** D3
Eppan = Appiano *Italy* **41** B8
Eppingen *Germany* **25** F4
Epsom *U.K.* **15** F7
Epukiro *Namibia* **88** C2
Equatoria = El Istiwa'iya *Sudan* **79** G11
Equatorial Guinea ■ *Africa* **84** D1
Er Hai *China* **58** E3
Er Rachidia *Morocco* **78** B5
Er Rahad *Sudan* **81** E3
Er Rif *Morocco* **78** A5
Er Rogel *Sudan* **80** D4
Er Roseires *Sudan* **81** E3

Er Rua'at *Sudan* **81** E3
Eraclea *Italy* **41** C9
Erāwadī Myit = Irrawaddy ⇝ *Burma* **67** M19
Erāwadī Myitwanya = Irrawaddy, Mouths of the *Burma* **67** M19
Erawan △ *Thailand* **64** E2
Erba *Italy* **40** C6
Erba *Sudan* **80** D4
Erba, J. *Sudan* **80** C4
Erbaa *Turkey* **72** B7
Erbeskopf *Germany* **25** F3
Erbil = Arbīl *Iraq* **73** D11
Erbu *Ethiopia* **81** E3
Erçek *Turkey* **70** B4
Erçiş *Turkey* **73** C10
Erciyaş Dağı *Turkey* **70** B2
Érd *Hungary* **28** C3
Erdao Jiang ⇝ *China* **57** C14
Erdek *Turkey* **45** F11
Erdemli *Turkey* **72** D6
Erdene = Ulaan-Uul *Mongolia* **56** B6
Erdenetsogt *Mongolia* **56** C4
Erding *Germany* **25** G7
Erdre ⇝ *France* **18** E5
Erebus, Mt. *Antarctica* **5** D11
Erechim *Brazil* **127** B5
Ereğli *Konya, Turkey* **72** D6
Ereğli *Zonguldak, Turkey* **72** B4
Erei, Monti *Italy* **43** E7
Erenhot *China* **56** C7
Eresma ⇝ *Spain* **36** D6
Eresos *Greece* **47** B9
Erfelek *Turkey* **72** B6
Erfenisdam *S. Africa* **88** D4
Erfstadt *Germany* **24** E2
Erft ⇝ *Germany* **24** D2
Erfurt *Germany* **24** E7
Ergani *Turkey* **73** C8
Ergel *Mongolia* **56** C5
Ergene ⇝ *Turkey* **45** E10
Ergeni Vozvyshennost *Russia* **35** G7
Érgli *Latvia* **32** D3
Erhlin *Taiwan* **59** F13
Eria ⇝ *Spain* **36** C5
Eriba *Sudan* **81** D4
Eriboll, L. *U.K.* **13** C4
Érice *Italy* **42** D5
Erie *U.S.A.* **114** D4
Erie, L. *N. Amer.* **114** D4
Erie Canal *U.S.A.* **114** D7
Erieau *Canada* **114** D3
Erigavo = Ceerigaabo *Somali Rep.* **75** E4
Erikoussa *Greece* **49** A3
Eriksdale *Canada* **103** C9
Erimanthos *Greece* **46** D3
Erimo-misaki *Japan* **54** D11
Erin *Canada* **114** C4
Erin Pt. *Trin. & Tob.* **125** K15
Erinpura *India* **68** G5
Eriskay *U.K.* **13** D1
Erithres *Greece* **46** C5
Eritrea ■ *Africa* **81** E4
Erjas ⇝ *Portugal* **36** F3
Erkelenz *Germany* **24** D1
Erkner *Germany* **24** C9
Erlangen *Germany* **25** F6
Erldunda *Australia* **94** D1
Ermelo *Neths.* **17** B5
Ermelo *S. Africa* **89** D4
Ermenek *Turkey* **72** D5
Ermil *Sudan* **81** E2
Ermioni *Greece* **46** D5
Ermones *Greece* **49** A3
Ermoupoli *Greece* **46** D6
Ernakulam *India* **66** Q10
Erne ⇝ *Ireland* **12** B3
Erne, Lower L. *U.K.* **12** B4
Erne, Upper L. *U.K.* **12** B4
Ernée *France* **18** D6
Ernest Giles Ra. *Australia* **93** E3
Ernstberg *Germany* **25** E2
Erode *India* **66** P10
Eromanga *Australia* **95** D3
Erongo *Namibia* **88** C2
Erquy *France* **18** D4
Erramala Hills *India* **66** M11
Errentería *Spain* **38** B3
Errer ⇝ *Ethiopia* **81** F5
Erri-Nundra △ *Australia* **95** F4
Errigal *Ireland* **12** A3
Erris Hd. *Ireland* **12** B1
Ersekë *Albania* **44** F4
Erskine *U.S.A.* **112** B6
Erstein *France* **19** D14
Ertholmene *Denmark* **11** J9
Ertil *Russia* **34** E5
Ertis = Irtysh ⇝ *Russia* **52** C7
Eruh *Turkey* **73** D10
Eruwa *Nigeria* **83** D5
Ervy-le-Châtel *France* **19** D10
Erwin *U.S.A.* **117** C13
Eryuan *China* **58** D2
Erzgebirge *Germany* **24** E8
Erzin *Russia* **53** D10
Erzincan *Turkey* **73** C8
Erzincan □ *Turkey* **73** C8

Erzurum *Turkey* **73** C9
Erzurum □ *Turkey* **73** C9
Es Caló *Spain* **48** C8
Es Canar *Spain* **48** B8
Es Mercadal *Spain* **48** B11
Es Migjorn Gran *Spain* **48** B11
Es Safiya *Sudan* **81** D3
Es Sahrâ al Beida *Egypt* **80** B2
Es Sahrâ' Esh Sharqîya *Egypt* **80** B3
Es Sînâ' *Egypt* **74** F2
Es Sûkî *Sudan* **81** E3
Es Vedrà *Spain* **48** C7
Esambo *Dem. Rep. of the Congo* **86** C1
Esan-Misaki *Japan* **54** D10
Esashi *Hokkaidō, Japan* **54** B11
Esashi *Hokkaidō, Japan* **54** D10
Esbjerg *Denmark* **11** J2
Esbo = Espoo *Finland* **32** B3
Escalante *U.S.A.* **109** H8
Escalante ⇝ *U.S.A.* **109** H8
Escalón *Mexico* **118** B4
Escambia ⇝ *U.S.A.* **117** F11
Escanaba *U.S.A.* **112** C10
Esch-sur-Alzette *Lux.* **17** E6
Eschede *Germany* **24** C6
Eschwege *Germany* **24** D6
Eschweiler *Germany* **24** E2
Escondido *U.S.A.* **111** M9
Escravos ⇝ *Nigeria* **83** D6
Escuinapa de Hidalgo *Mexico* **118** C3
Escuintla *Guatemala* **120** D1
Eséka *Cameroon* **83** E7
Eşen ⇝ *Turkey* **47** E11
Esenguly *Turkmenistan* **52** F6
Esens *Germany* **24** B3
Esenyurt *Turkey* **45** E12
Esera ⇝ *Spain* **38** C5
Eşfahān *Iran* **71** C6
Eşfahān □ *Iran* **71** C6
Esfarāyen *Iran* **71** B8
Esfideh *Iran* **71** C8
Esgueva ⇝ *Spain* **36** D6
Esh Sham = Dimashq *Syria* **74** B5
Esh Shamâlîya □ *Sudan* **80** D2
Esha Ness *U.K.* **13** A7
Eshan *China* **58** E4
Eshkol △ *Israel* **74** D3
Eshowe *S. Africa* **89** D5
Esiama *Ghana* **82** E4
Esigodini *Zimbabwe* **89** C4
Esil = Ishim ⇝ *Russia* **52** D8
Esino ⇝ *Italy* **41** E10
Esira *Madag.* **89** C8
Esk ⇝ *Dumf. & Gall., U.K.* **13** G5
Esk ⇝ *N. Yorks., U.K.* **14** C7
Eskān *Iran* **71** E9
Esker *Canada* **105** B6
Eskifjörður *Iceland* **8** D7
Eskilsäter *Sweden* **11** F7
Eskilstuna *Sweden* **10** E10
Eskimalatya *Turkey* **73** C8
Eskimo Point = Arviat *Canada* **103** A10
Eskişehir *Turkey* **47** B12
Eskişehir □ *Turkey* **47** B12
Esla ⇝ *Spain* **36** D4
Eslāmābād-e Gharb *Iran* **73** E12
Eslāmshahr *Iran* **71** C6
Eslöv *Sweden* **11** J7
Eşme *Turkey* **47** C10
Esme *Turkey* **72** B5
Esmeraldas *Ecuador* **124** C3
Esna = Isna *Egypt* **80** B3
Esnagi L. *Canada* **104** C3
Espalion *France* **20** D6
España = Spain ■ *Europe* **7** H5
Espanola *Canada* **104** C3
Espanola *U.S.A.* **109** J10
Esparreguera *Spain* **38** D6
Esparza *Costa Rica* **120** E3
Espelkamp *Germany* **24** C4
Esperança *Australia* **93** F3
Esperança B. *Australia* **93** F3
Esperance Harbour *St. Lucia* **121** f
Esperantina *Antarctica* **5** C18
Esperanza *Argentina* **126** C3
Esperanza *Phil.* **61** G6
Esperanza *Puerto Rico* **121** d
Espéraza *France* **20** F6
Espichel, C. *Portugal* **37** G1
Espiel *Spain* **37** G5
Espigão, Serra do *Brazil* **127** B5
Espinazo, Sierra del = Espinhaço, Serra do *Brazil* **125** G10
Espinhaço, Serra do *Brazil* **125** G10
Espinho *Portugal* **36** D2
Espinilho, Serra do *Brazil* **127** B5
Espinosa de los Monteros *Spain* **36** B7
Espírito Santo □ *Brazil* **125** H10
Espírito Santo do Pinhal *Brazil* **127** A6
Espíritu Santo *Vanuatu* **90** C9
Espíritu Santo, B. del *Mexico* **119** D7
Espíritu Santo, I. *Mexico* **118** C2
Espita *Mexico* **119** C7
Espiye *Turkey* **73** B8

Espoo *Finland* **32** B3
Espuña, Sierra de *Spain* **39** H3
Esquel *Argentina* **128** E2
Esquimalt *Canada* **110** B3
Esquina *Argentina* **126** C4
Essaouira *Morocco* **78** B4
Essebie *Dem. Rep. of the Congo* **86** B3
Essen *Belgium* **17** C4
Essen *Germany* **24** D3
Essendon, Mt. *Australia* **93** E3
Essequibo ⇝ *Guyana* **124** B7
Essex *Canada* **114** D2
Essex *Calif., U.S.A.* **111** L11
Essex *N.Y., U.S.A.* **115** B11
Essex □ *U.K.* **15** F8
Essex Junction *U.S.A.* **115** B11
Esslingen *Germany* **25** G5
Essonne □ *France* **19** D9
Estaca de Bares, C. de *Spain* **36** A3
Estagel *France* **20** F6
Estados, I. de Los *Argentina* **128** G4
Eştahbānāt *Iran* **71** D7
Estância *Brazil* **125** F11
Estancia *U.S.A.* **109** J10
Estärm *Iran* **71** D8
Estarreja *Portugal* **36** E2
Estats, Pic d' *Spain* **38** C6
Estcourt *S. Africa* **89** D4
Este *Italy* **41** C8
Este □ *Dom. Rep.* **121** C6
Estelí *Nic.* **120** D2
Estella *Spain* **38** C2
Estellencs *Spain* **48** B9
Estena ⇝ *Spain* **37** F6
Estepa *Spain* **37** H6
Estepona *Spain* **37** J5
Esterhazy *Canada* **103** C8
Esternay *France* **19** D10
Esterri d'Aneu *Spain* **38** C6
Estevan *Canada* **103** D8
Estevan Group *Canada* **102** C3
Estherville *U.S.A.* **112** D6
Estissac *France* **19** D10
Eston *Canada* **103** C7
Estonia ■ *Europe* **32** C3
Estoril *Portugal* **37** G1
Estouk *Mali* **83** B5
Estreito *Brazil* **125** E9
Estrela, Serra da *Portugal* **36** E3
Estrella *Spain* **37** G7
Estremoz *Portugal* **37** G3
Estrondo, Serra do *Brazil* **125** E9
Esztergom *Hungary* **28** C3
Et Tîdra *Mauritania* **82** B1
Etah *India* **69** F8
Étain *France* **19** C12
Étampes *France* **19** D9
Etanga *Namibia* **88** B1
Étaples *France* **19** B8
Etawah *India* **69** F8
Etawney L. *Canada* **103** B9
Etchojoa *Mexico* **118** B3
Ete *Nigeria* **83** D6
eThekwini = Durban *S. Africa* **89** D5
Ethel *U.S.A.* **110** D4
Ethelbert *Canada* **103** C8
Ethiopia ■ *Africa* **75** F3
Ethiopian Highlands *Ethiopia* **75** F2
Etili *Turkey* **45** G10
Etive, L. *U.K.* **13** E3
Etna *Italy* **43** E7
Etoile *Dem. Rep. of the Congo* **87** E2
Etoliko *Greece* **46** C3
Etolin Strait *U.S.A.* **106** C6
Etoloakarnania □ *Greece* **46** C3
Etosha △ *Namibia* **88** B2
Etosha Pan *Namibia* **88** B2
Etowah *U.S.A.* **117** D12
Étréchy *France* **19** D9
Étrek *Turkmenistan* **71** B7
Étrépagny *France* **19** C9
Étretat *France* **18** C7
Ettelbruck *Lux.* **17** E6
Ettlingen *Germany* **25** G4
Ettrick Water ⇝ *U.K.* **13** F6
Etuku *Dem. Rep. of the Congo* **86** C2
Etulia *Moldova* **29** E13
Etzná-Tixmucuy = Edzná *Mexico* **119** D6
Eu *France* **18** B8
Eua *Tonga* **91** c
Euboea = Evia *Greece* **46** C6
Eucla *Australia* **93** F4
Euclid *U.S.A.* **114** E3
Eucumbene, L. *Australia* **95** F4
Eudora *U.S.A.* **116** E9
Eufaula *Ala., U.S.A.* **117** F12
Eufaula *Okla., U.S.A.* **116** D7
Eufaula L. *U.S.A.* **116** D7
Eugene *U.S.A.* **108** D2
Eugowra *Australia* **95** E4
Eulo *Australia* **95** D4
Eungella △ *Australia* **94** b

Eunice *La., U.S.A.* **116** F8
Eunice *N. Mex., U.S.A.* **109** K12
Eupen *Belgium* **17** D6
Euphrates = Furāt, Nahr
　al → *Asia* **70** D5
Eure □ *France* **18** C8
Eure → *France* **18** C8
Eure-et-Loir □ *France* **18** D8
Eureka *Canada* **101** B14
Eureka *Calif., U.S.A.* **108** F1
Eureka *Kans., U.S.A.* **112** G5
Eureka *Mont., U.S.A.* **108** B6
Eureka *Nev., U.S.A.* **108** G6
Eureka *S. Dak., U.S.A.* **112** C4
Eureka, Mt. *Australia* **93** E3
Eureka Sd. *Canada* **101** B15
Euroa *Australia* **95** F4
Europa, Île *Ind. Oc.* **85** J8
Europa, Picos de *Spain* **36** B6
Europa, Pt. *Gib.* **37** J5
Europe **6** E10
Europoort *Neths.* **17** C4
Euskirchen *Germany* **24** E2
Eustis *U.S.A.* **117** G14
Eutin *Germany* **24** A6
Eutsuk L. *Canada* **102** C3
Evale *Angola* **88** B2
Evans *U.S.A.* **108** F11
Evans, L. *Canada* **104** B4
Evans City *U.S.A.* **114** F4
Evans Head *Australia* **95** D5
Evansburg *Canada* **102** C5
Evanston *Ill., U.S.A.* **112** D10
Evanston *Wyo., U.S.A.* **108** F8
Evansville *U.S.A.* **112** G10
Évaux-les-Bains *France* **19** F9
Evaz *Iran* **71** E7
Evciler *Afyon, Turkey* **47** C11
Evciler *Çanakkale, Turkey* **47** B8
Eveleth *U.S.A.* **112** B8
Evensk *Russia* **53** C16
Everard, L. *Australia* **95** E2
Everard Ranges *Australia* **93** E5
Everest, Mt. *Nepal* **69** E12
Everett *Pa., U.S.A.* **114** F6
Everett *Wash., U.S.A.* **110** C4
Everglades, The *U.S.A.* **117** J14
Everglades △ *U.S.A.* **117** J14
Everglades City *U.S.A.* **117** J14
Evergreen *Ala., U.S.A.* **117** F11
Evergreen *Mont., U.S.A.* **108** B6
Everöd *Sweden* **11** J8
Evertsberg *Sweden* **10** C7
Evesham *U.K.* **15** E6
Evia *Greece* **46** C6
Evia □ *Greece* **46** C5
Évian-les-Bains *France* **19** F13
Evinos → *Greece* **46** C3
Évisa *France* **21** F12
Evje *Norway* **9** G12
Évora *Portugal* **37** G3
Évora □ *Portugal* **37** G3
Evowghlī *Iran* **73** C11
Évreux *France* **18** C8
Evritania □ *Greece* **46** B3
Évron *France* **18** D6
Evros □ *Greece* **45** E10
Evros → *Greece* **72** B2
Evrotas → *Greece* **46** E4
Évry *France* **19** D9
Évvoia = Evia *Greece* **46** C6
Ewe, L. *U.K.* **13** D3
Ewing *U.S.A.* **112** D4
Ewo *Congo* **84** E2
Exaltación *Bolivia* **124** F5
Excelsior Springs *U.S.A.* **112** F6
Excideuil *France* **20** C5
Exe → *U.K.* **15** G4
Exeter *Canada* **114** C3
Exeter *U.K.* **15** G4
Exeter *Calif., U.S.A.* **110** J7
Exeter *N.H., U.S.A.* **115** D14
Exmoor *U.K.* **15** F4
Exmoor △ *U.K.* **15** F4
Exmouth *Australia* **92** D1
Exmouth *U.K.* **15** G4
Exmouth G. *Australia* **92** D1
Exmouth Plateau *Ind. Oc.* **96** J3
Expedition △ *Australia* **95** D4
Expedition Ra. *Australia* **94** C4
Extremadura □ *Spain* **37** G5
Exuma Sound *Bahamas* **120** B4
Eyasi, L. *Tanzania* **86** C4
Eye Pen. *U.K.* **13** C2
Eyemouth *U.K.* **13** F6
Eygues → = Aigues → *France* **21** D8
Eygurande *France* **19** G9
Eyjafjörður *Iceland* **8** C4
Eyl *Somali Rep.* **75** F4
Eymet *France* **20** D4
Eymoutiers *France* **20** C5
Eynesil *Turkey* **73** B8
Eyre (North), L. *Australia* **95** D2
Eyre (South), L. *Australia* **95** D2
Eyre, L. *Australia* **95** D2
Eyre Mts. *N.Z.* **91** F2
Eyre Pen. *Australia* **95** E2
Eysturoy *Færoe Is.* **8** E9
Eyvān = Jūy Zar *Iran* **73** F12

Eyvānkī *Iran* **71** C6
Ez Zeidab *Sudan* **80** D3
Ezcaray *Spain* **38** C1
Ežerėlis *Lithuania* **30** D10
Ezhou *China* **59** B10
Ezine *Turkey* **47** B8
Ezouza → *Cyprus* **49** E11

F

F.Y.R.O.M. = Macedonia ■
　Europe **44** E5
Faaa *Tahiti* **91** d
Faaborg *Denmark* **11** J4
Faaone *Tahiti* **91** d
Fabala *Guinea* **82** D3
Fabens *U.S.A.* **116** F1
Fabero *Spain* **36** C4
Fabius *U.S.A.* **115** D9
Fabriano *Italy* **41** E9
Făcăeni *Romania* **29** F12
Fachi *Niger* **79** E8
Fada *Chad* **79** E10
Fada-n-Gourma *Burkina Faso* **83** C5
Fadd *Hungary* **28** D3
Faddeyevskiy, Ostrov
　Russia **53** B15
Faddor *Sudan* **81** F3
Fadghāmī *Syria* **73** E9
Fadlab *Sudan* **80** D3
Faenza *Italy* **41** D8
Færoe Is. = Føroyar ☑ *Atl. Oc.* **8** F9
Fafa *Mali* **83** B5
Fafe *Portugal* **36** D2
Fagam *Nigeria* **83** C7
Făgăras *Romania* **29** E9
Făgăras, Munţii *Romania* **29** E9
Fågelfors *Sweden* **11** G9
Fågelmara *Sweden* **11** H9
Fagerhult *Sweden* **11** G9
Fagersta *Sweden* **10** D9
Făget *Romania* **28** E7
Făget, Munţii *Romania* **29** C8
Faggo *Nigeria* **83** C6
Fagnano, L. *Argentina* **128** G3
Fagnières *France* **19** D11
Faguibine, L. *Mali* **82** B4
Fahlīān *Iran* **71** D6
Fahraj *Kermān, Iran* **71** D8
Fahraj *Yazd, Iran* **71** D7
Fai Tsi Long *Vietnam* **58** G6
Faial *Azores* **78** a
Faial *Madeira* **48** D3
Faichan Kangri *India* **69** B7
Fair Haven *N.Y., U.S.A.* **115** C8
Fair Haven *Vt., U.S.A.* **113** D17
Fair Hd. *U.K.* **12** A5
Fair Isle *U.K.* **16** B6
Fair Oaks *U.S.A.* **110** G5
Fairbanks *U.S.A.* **100** E2
Fairbury *U.S.A.* **112** E6
Fairfax *U.S.A.* **115** B11
Fairfield *Ala., U.S.A.* **117** E11
Fairfield *Calif., U.S.A.* **110** G4
Fairfield *Conn., U.S.A.* **115** E11
Fairfield *Idaho, U.S.A.* **108** E6
Fairfield *Ill., U.S.A.* **112** F9
Fairfield *Iowa, U.S.A.* **112** E8
Fairfield *Tex., U.S.A.* **116** F6
Fairford *Canada* **103** C9
Fairhope *U.S.A.* **117** F11
Fairlie *N.Z.* **91** F3
Fairmead *U.S.A.* **110** H6
Fairmont *Minn., U.S.A.* **112** D6
Fairmont *W. Va., U.S.A.* **113** F13
Fairmount *Calif., U.S.A.* **111** L8
Fairmount *N.Y., U.S.A.* **115** C8
Fairplay *U.S.A.* **108** G10
Fairport *U.S.A.* **114** C7
Fairport Harbor *U.S.A.* **114** E3
Fairview *Canada* **102** B5
Fairview *Mont., U.S.A.* **108** C11
Fairview *Okla., U.S.A.* **116** C5
Fairweather, Mt. *U.S.A.* **102** B1
Faisalabad *Pakistan* **68** D5
Faith *U.S.A.* **112** C2
Faizabad *India* **69** F10
Fajardo *Puerto Rico* **121** d
Fajr, W. → *Si. Arabia* **70** D3
Fakenham *U.K.* **14** E8
Fåker *Sweden* **10** A8
Fakfak *Indonesia* **63** E8
Fakiya *Bulgaria* **45** D11
Fakobli *Ivory C.* **82** D3
Fakse *Denmark* **11** J6
Fakse Bugt *Denmark* **11** J6
Fakse Ladeplads *Denmark* **11** J6
Faku *China* **57** C12
Falaba *S. Leone* **82** D2
Falaise *France* **18** D6
Falaise, Mui *Vietnam* **64** C5
Falakro Oros *Greece* **44** E7
Falam *Burma* **67** H18
Falces *Spain* **38** C3
Fălciu *Romania* **29** D13
Falcó, C. des *Spain* **48** C7
Falcón, Presa *Mexico* **119** B5
Falcon Lake *Canada* **103** D9
Falcon Res. *U.S.A.* **116** H5

Falconara Maríttima *Italy* **41** E10
Falcone, C. del *Italy* **42** B1
Falconer *U.S.A.* **114** D5
Faléa *Mali* **82** C2
Falefa *Samoa* **91** b
Falelatai *Samoa* **91** b
Falelima *Samoa* **91** b
Falémé → *Senegal* **82** C2
Falerum *Sweden* **11** F10
Faleshty = Fălesti *Moldova* **29** C12
Fălesti *Moldova* **29** C12
Falfurrias *U.S.A.* **116** H5
Falher *Canada* **102** B5
Faliraki *Greece* **49** C10
Falkenberg *Germany* **24** D9
Falkenberg *Sweden* **11** H6
Falkensee *Germany* **24** C9
Falkirk *U.K.* **13** F5
Falkirk □ *U.K.* **13** F5
Falkland *U.K.* **13** E5
Falkland Is. ☑ *Atl. Oc.* **128** G5
Falkland Sd. *Falk. Is.* **128** G5
Falkonera *Greece* **46** E5
Falköping *Sweden* **11** F7
Fall River *U.S.A.* **115** E13
Fall River *U.S.A.* **116** E6
Fallbrook *U.S.A.* **111** M9
Fallon *U.S.A.* **108** G4
Falls City *U.S.A.* **112** E6
Falls Creek *U.S.A.* **114** E6
Falmouth *Jamaica* **120** a
Falmouth *U.K.* **15** G2
Falmouth *U.S.A.* **115** E14
Falsa, Pta. *Mexico* **118** B1
False B. *S. Africa* **88** E2
Falso, C. *Honduras* **120** C3
Falster *Denmark* **11** K5
Falsterbo *Sweden* **9** J15
Fălticeni *Romania* **29** C11
Falun *Sweden* **10** D9
Famagusta *Cyprus* **49** D12
Famagusta Bay *Cyprus* **49** D13
Famatina, Sierra de
　Argentina **126** B2
Famenin *Iran* **73** E13
Family L. *Canada* **103** C9
Famoso *U.S.A.* **111** K7
Fan Xian *China* **56** G8
Fana *Mali* **82** C3
Fanad Hd. *Ireland* **12** A4
Fanari *Greece* **46** B3
Fandriana *Madag.* **89** C8
Fánes-Sénnes e Braies △
　Italy **41** B9
Fang *Thailand* **58** H2
Fang Xian *China* **59** A8
Fangaga *Sudan* **80** D4
Fangak *Sudan* **81** F3
Fangchang *China* **59** B12
Fangcheng *China* **56** H7
Fangchenggang *China* **58** G7
Fangliao *Taiwan* **59** F13
Fangshan *China* **56** E6
Fangzi *China* **57** F10
Fannich, L. *U.K.* **13** D4
Fannūj *Iran* **71** E8
Fanø *Denmark* **11** J2
Fano *Italy* **41** E10
Fanshi *China* **56** E7
Fao = Al Fāw *Iraq* **71** D6
Faqirwali *Pakistan* **68** E5
Fâqûs *Egypt* **80** H7
Far East =
　Dalnevostochnyy □
　Russia **53** C14
Far East *Asia* **50** E14
Fara in Sabina *Italy* **41** F9
Faradje *Dem. Rep. of the Congo* **86** B2
Farafangana *Madag.* **89** C8
Farafenni *Gambia* **82** C1
Farâfra, El Wâhât el *Egypt* **80** B2
Farāh *Afghan.* **66** C3
Farāh □ *Afghan.* **66** C3
Farahalana *Madag.* **89** A9
Faraid, Gebel *Egypt* **80** C4
Farako *Ivory C.* **82** D4
Faramana *Burkina Faso* **82** C4
Faranah *Guinea* **82** C2
Farasān, Jazā'ir *Si. Arabia* **75** D3
Farasān Is. = Farasān,
　Jazā'ir *Si. Arabia* **75** D3
Faratsiho *Madag.* **89** C8
Fardes → *Spain* **37** H7
Fareham *U.K.* **15** G6
Farewell *U.S.A.* **114** D3
Farewell, C. *N.Z.* **91** D4
Farewell C. = Nunap Isua
　Greenland **98** D15
Färgelanda *Sweden* **11** F5
Farghona *Uzbekistan* **52** E8
Fargo *U.S.A.* **112** B5
Fār'iah, W. al → *West Bank* **74** C4
Faribault *U.S.A.* **112** C7
Faridabad *India* **68** E6
Faridkot *India* **68** D6
Faridpur *Bangla.* **69** H13
Faridpur *India* **69** E8

Farim *Guinea-Biss.* **82** C1
Farīmān *Iran* **71** C8
Fariones, Pta. *Canary Is.* **48** E6
Fâriskûr *Egypt* **80** H7
Farkadona *Greece* **46** B4
Farleigh *Australia* **94** b
Farmakonisi *Greece* **47** D9
Farmerville *U.S.A.* **116** E8
Farmingdale *U.S.A.* **115** F10
Farmington *Canada* **102** B4
Farmington *Calif., U.S.A.* **110** H6
Farmington *Maine, U.S.A.* **113** C18
Farmington *Mo., U.S.A.* **112** G9
Farmington *N.H., U.S.A.* **115** C13
Farmington *N. Mex., U.S.A.* **109** H9
Farmington *Utah, U.S.A.* **108** F8
Farmington → *U.S.A.* **115** E12
Farmville *U.S.A.* **113** G14
Färnäs *Sweden* **10** D8
Farne Is. *U.K.* **14** B6
Färnebofjärden △ *Sweden* **10** D10
Farnham *Canada* **115** A12
Farnham, Mt. *Canada* **102** C5
Faro *Brazil* **125** D7
Faro *Canada* **100** E5
Faro *Portugal* **37** H3
Faro *Sweden* **9** H18
Fårö *Sweden* **9** H18
Faro □ *Portugal* **37** H3
Fårösund *Sweden* **11** G13
Farquhar, C. *Australia* **93** D1
Farräshband *Iran* **71** D7
Farrell *U.S.A.* **114** E4
Farrokhī *Iran* **71** C8
Farruch, C. = Ferrutx, C. de
　Spain **48** B10
Farrukhabad *India* **69** F8
Fārs □ *Iran* **71** D7
Fārsala *Greece* **46** B4
Fārsī *Iran* **71** E6
Farsø *Denmark* **11** H3
Farson *U.S.A.* **108** E9
Farsund *Norway* **9** G12
Fartak, Râs *Si. Arabia* **70** D2
Fartak, Ra's *Yemen* **75** D5
Fârtănesti *Romania* **29** E12
Fartura, Serra da *Brazil* **127** B5
Faru *Nigeria* **83** C6
Fārūj *Iran* **71** B8
Fårup *Denmark* **11** H3
Farvel, Kap = Nunap Isua
　Greenland **98** D15
Farwell *U.S.A.* **116** D3
Fāryāb □ *Afghan.* **66** B4
Fasā *Iran* **71** D7
Fasano *Italy* **43** B10
Fashoda *Sudan* **81** F3
Fasil Ghebbi *Ethiopia* **81** E4
Fassa *Mali* **82** C1
Fastiv *Ukraine* **23** C15
Fastnet Rock *Ireland* **12** E2
Fastov = Fastiv *Ukraine* **23** C15
Fatagar, Tanjung *Indonesia* **63** E8
Fatehabad *Haryana, India* **68** E6
Fatehabad *Ut. P., India* **68** F8
Fatehgarh *India* **69** F8
Fatehpur *Bihar, India* **69** G11
Fatehpur *Raj., India* **68** F6
Fatehpur *Ut. P., India* **69** G9
Fatehpur *Ut. P., India* **69** F9
Fatehpur Sikri *India* **68** F6
Fatesh *Russia* **33** F8
Fathai *Sudan* **81** F3
Fathom Five △ *Canada* **114** A3
Fatick *Senegal* **82** C1
Fatick □ *Senegal* **82** C1
Fatima *Canada* **105** C7
Fátima *Portugal* **37** F2
Fatoya *Guinea* **82** C3
Fatsa *Turkey* **72** B7
Faucille, Col de la *France* **19** F13
Faulkton *U.S.A.* **112** C4
Faulquemont *France* **19** C13
Faure I. *Australia* **93** E1
Făurei *Romania* **29** E12
Fauresmith *S. Africa* **88** D4
Fauske *Norway* **8** C16
Favara *Italy* **42** E6
Favāritx, C. de *Spain* **48** B11
Faverges *France* **21** C10
Favignana *Italy* **42** E5
Favignana, I. *Italy* **42** E5
Fawcett, Pt. *Australia* **92** B5
Fawn → *Canada* **104** A2
Fawnskin *U.S.A.* **111** L10
Faxaflói *Iceland* **8** D2
Faxälven → *Sweden* **10** A10
Faya-Largeau *Chad* **79** E9
Fayd *Si. Arabia* **70** E4
Fayence *France* **21** E10
Fayette *Ala., U.S.A.* **117** E11
Fayette *Mo., U.S.A.* **112** F7
Fayette *N.Y., U.S.A.* **115** D8
Fayetteville *Ark., U.S.A.* **116** C7
Fayetteville *N.C., U.S.A.* **117** D15
Fayetteville *N.Y., U.S.A.* **115** C9
Fayetteville *Tenn., U.S.A.* **117** D11

Fayied *Egypt* **80** H8
Faylakah *Kuwait* **71** D6
Fayón *Spain* **38** D5
Fazao-Malfakassa △ *Togo* **83** D5
Fazilka *India* **68** D6
Fazilpur *Pakistan* **68** E4
Fdérik *Mauritania* **78** D3
Feakle *Ireland* **12** D3
Feale → *Ireland* **12** D2
Fear, C. *U.S.A.* **117** E16
Feather → *U.S.A.* **108** G3
Feather Falls *U.S.A.* **110** F5
Featherston *N.Z.* **91** D5
Featherstone *Zimbabwe* **87** F3
Fécamp *France* **18** C7
Fedala = Mohammedia
　Morocco **78** B4
Federación *Argentina* **126** C4
Féderal *Argentina* **126** C4
Federal Capital Terr. □
　Nigeria **83** D6
Federal Way *U.S.A.* **110** C4
Fedeshkūh *Iran* **71** D7
Fehérgyarmat *Hungary* **28** C7
Fehmarn *Germany* **24** A7
Fehmarn Bælt *Europe* **11** K5
Fehmarn Belt = Fehmarn
　Bælt *Europe* **11** K5
Fei Xian *China* **57** G9
Feijó *Brazil* **124** E4
Feilding *N.Z.* **91** D5
Feixi *China* **59** B11
Feixiang *China* **56** F8
Fejér □ *Hungary* **28** C3
Fejø *Denmark* **11** K5
Feke *Turkey* **72** D6
Fekete → *Hungary* **28** C3
Felanitx *Spain* **48** B10
Feldbach *Austria* **26** E8
Feldberg
　Mecklenburg-Vorpommern,
　Germany **24** B9
Feldberg
　Baden-W., Germany **25** H3
Feldkirch *Austria* **26** D2
Feldkirchen *Austria* **26** E7
Félicité *Seychelles* **85** b
Felipe Carrillo Puerto
　Mexico **119** D7
Felixburg *Zimbabwe* **89** B5
Felixstowe *U.K.* **15** F9
Felletin *France* **20** C6
Fellingsbro *Sweden* **10** E9
Felton *U.S.A.* **110** H4
Feltre *Italy* **41** B8
Femer Bælt = Fehmarn
　Bælt *Europe* **11** K5
Femø *Denmark* **11** K5
Femunden *Norway* **8** E14
Fen He → *China* **56** G6
Fenelon Falls *Canada* **114** B6
Fener Burnu *Turkey* **47** E9
Feneroa *Ethiopia* **81** E4
Feng Xian *Jiangsu, China* **56** G9
Feng Xian *Shaanxi, China* **56** H4
Fengari *Greece* **45** F9
Fengcheng *Jiangxi, China* **59** C10
Fengcheng *Liaoning, China* **57** D13
Fengfeng *China* **56** F8
Fenggang *China* **58** D6
Fenghua *China* **59** C13
Fenghuang *China* **58** D7
Fengkai *China* **59** F8
Fengkang *Taiwan* **59** F13
Fengle *China* **59** B9
Fenglin *Taiwan* **59** F13
Fengning *China* **56** D9
Fengqing *China* **58** E2
Fengqiu *China* **56** G8
Fengrun *China* **57** E10
Fengshan *Guangxi Zhuangzu,*
　China **58** E6
Fengshan *Guangxi Zhuangzu,*
　China **58** E6
Fengshan *Taiwan* **59** F13
Fengshun *China* **59** F11
Fengtai *Anhui, China* **59** A11
Fengtai *Beijing, China* **56** E9
Fengxian *China* **59** B13
Fengxiang *China* **56** G4
Fengxin *China* **59** C10
Fengyang *China* **57** H9
Fengyi *China* **58** D3
Fengyüan *Taiwan* **59** E13
Fengzhen *China* **56** D7
Feno, C. de *France* **21** G13
Fenoarivo *Fianarantsoa,*
　Madag. **89** C8
Fenoarivo *Fianarantsoa,*
　Madag. **89** C8
Fenoarivo Afovoany *Madag.* **89** B8
Fenoarivo Atsinanana
　Madag. **89** B8
Fens, The *U.K.* **14** E7
Fensmark *Denmark* **11** J5
Fenton *U.S.A.* **113** D12
Fenxi *China* **56** F6
Fenyang *China* **56** F6

Fenyi *China* **59** D10
Feodosiya *Ukraine* **33** K8
Ferbane *Ireland* **12** C4
Ferdows *Iran* **71** C8
Fère-Champenoise *France* **19** D10
Fère-en-Tardenois *France* **19** C10
Ferentino *Italy* **41** G10
Feres *Greece* **45** F10
Fergana = Farghona
　Uzbekistan **52** E8
Fergus *Canada* **114** C4
Fergus Falls *U.S.A.* **112** B5
Feričanci *Croatia* **28** E2
Ferihegy, Budapest ✈
　(BUD) *Hungary* **28** C3
Ferkéssédougou *Ivory C.* **82** D3
Ferlach *Austria* **26** E7
Ferland *Canada* **104** B2
Ferlo, Vallée du *Senegal* **82** B2
Ferlo-Nord △ *Senegal* **82** B2
Ferlo-Sud △ *Senegal* **82** B2
Fermanagh □ *U.K.* **12** B4
Fermo *Italy* **41** E10
Fermont *Canada* **105** B6
Fermoselle *Spain* **36** D4
Fermoy *Ireland* **12** D3
Fernán Núñez *Spain* **37** H6
Fernández *Argentina* **126** B3
Fernandina Beach *U.S.A.* **117** F14
Fernando de Noronha
　Brazil **125** D12
Fernando Póo = Bioko
　Eq. Guin. **83** E6
Ferndale *Canada* **114** B3
Ferndale *U.S.A.* **110** B4
Fernie *Canada* **102** D5
Fernlees *Australia* **94** C4
Fernley *U.S.A.* **108** G4
Fernwood *U.S.A.* **115** C11
Ferozepore = Firozpur *India* **68** D6
Ferrandina *Italy* **43** B9
Ferrara *Italy* **41** D8
Ferrato, C. *Italy* **42** C2
Ferreira do Alentejo *Portugal* **37** G2
Ferreñafe *Peru* **124** E3
Ferrerías *Spain* **48** B11
Ferret, C. *France* **20** D2
Ferrette *France* **19** E14
Ferriday *U.S.A.* **116** F9
Ferriere *Italy* **40** D6
Ferrières *France* **19** D9
Ferro, Capo *Italy* **42** A2
Ferrol *Spain* **36** B2
Ferron *U.S.A.* **108** G8
Ferrutx, C. de *Spain* **48** B10
Ferryland *Canada* **105** C9
Fertile *U.S.A.* **112** B6
Fertő-Hanság △ *Hungary* **28** C1
Fertőszentmiklós *Hungary* **28** C1
Fès *Morocco* **78** B5
Fessenden *U.S.A.* **112** B4
Festus *U.S.A.* **112** F8
Feté Bowé *Senegal* **82** C2
Fetesti *Romania* **29** F12
Fethiye *Turkey* **47** E11
Fethiye Körfezi *Turkey* **47** E10
Fetlar *U.K.* **13** A8
Feuilles → *Canada* **101** F17
Feurs *France* **21** C8
Fez = Fès *Morocco* **78** B5
Fezzan *Libya* **79** C8
Fiambalá *Argentina* **126** B2
Fianarantsoa *Madag.* **89** C8
Fianarantsoa □ *Madag.* **89** B8
Fiche *Ethiopia* **81** F4
Fichtelgebirge *Germany* **25** E7
Fichtelgebirge △ *Germany* **25** E8
Ficksburg *S. Africa* **89** D4
Fidenza *Italy* **40** D7
Fiditi *Nigeria* **83** D5
Field → *Australia* **94** C2
Field I. *Australia* **92** B5
Fieni *Romania* **29** E10
Fier *Albania* **44** F3
Fierzë *Albania* **44** E4
Fife □ *U.K.* **13** E5
Fife △ *U.K.* **13** E5
Fife Ness *U.K.* **13** E6
Fifth Cataract *Sudan* **80** D3
Figari *France* **21** G13
Figeac *France* **20** D6
Figeholm *Sweden* **11** G10
Figline Valdarno *Italy* **41** E8
Figtree *Zimbabwe* **87** G2
Figueira Castelo Rodrigo
　Portugal **36** E4
Figueira da Foz *Portugal* **36** E2
Figueiró dos Vinhos *Portugal* **36** F2
Figueres *Spain* **38** C7
Figuig *Morocco* **78** B5
Fihaonana *Madag.* **89** B8
Fiherenana *Madag.* **89** C8
Fiherenana → *Madag.* **89** C7
Fiji ■ *Pac. Oc.* **91** a
Fik *Ethiopia* **81** F5
Fika *Nigeria* **83** C7
Filabres, Sierra de los *Spain* **37** H8
Filabusi *Zimbabwe* **89** C4

Filadélfia *Italy* **43** D9
Filadélfia *Paraguay* **126** A3
Fil'akovo *Slovak Rep.* **27** C12
Filchner Ice Shelf *Antarctica* **5** D1
Filey *U.K.* **14** C7
Filey B. *U.K.* **14** C7
Filfla *Malta* **49** D1
Filiaşi *Romania* **29** F8
Filiates *Greece* **46** B2
Filiatra *Greece* **46** D3
Filicudi *Italy* **43** D7
Filingué *Niger* **83** C5
Filiourí = Lissos *Greece* **45** E9
Filipada *Greece* **46** B2
Filipstad *Sweden* **10** E8
Filisur *Switz.* **25** J5
Fillmore *Calif., U.S.A.* **111** L8
Fillmore *Utah, U.S.A.* **108** G7
Filotio *Greece* **47** D7
Filottrano *Italy* **41** E10
Filtu *Ethiopia* **81** F5
Fimbul Ice Shelf *S. Ocean* **5** C2
Fina △ *Mali* **82** C3
Finale Emília *Italy* **41** D8
Finale Lígure *Italy* **40** D5
Fiñana *Spain* **37** H8
Finch *Canada* **115** A9
Finch Hatton *Australia* **94** b
Finchaa, L. *Ethiopia* **81** F4
Findhorn → *U.K.* **13** D5
Findlay *U.S.A.* **113** E12
Fine *U.S.A.* **115** B9
Finger L. *Canada* **104** B1
Finger Lakes *U.S.A.* **115** D8
Fíngoè *Mozam.* **87** E3
Finike *Turkey* **47** E12
Finike Körfezi *Turkey* **47** E12
Finiq *Albania* **44** G4
Finistère □ *France* **18** D3
Finisterre = Fisterra *Spain* **36** C1
Finisterre, C. = Fisterra, C.
  Spain **36** C1
Finke *Australia* **94** D1
Finke Gorge △ *Australia* **92** D5
Finland ■ *Europe* **8** E22
Finland, G. of *Europe* **32** C3
Finlay → *Canada* **102** B3
Finley *Australia* **95** F4
Finley *U.S.A.* **112** B5
Finn → *Ireland* **12** B4
Finnerödja *Sweden* **11** F8
Finnigan, Mt. *Australia* **94** B4
Finniss, C. *Australia* **95** E1
Finnmark *Norway* **8** B20
Finnsnes *Norway* **8** B18
Finspång *Sweden* **11** F9
Finsteraarhorn *Switz.* **25** J4
Finsterwalde *Germany* **24** D9
Fiora → *Italy* **41** F8
Fiordland △ *N.Z.* **91** F1
Fiorenzuola d'Arda *Italy* **40** D6
Fiq *Syria* **74** C4
Firat = Furāt, Nahr al →
  Asia **70** D5
Fire Island △ *U.S.A.* **115** F11
Firebag → *Canada* **103** B6
Firebaugh *U.S.A.* **110** J6
Firedrake L. *Canada* **103** A8
Firenze *Italy* **41** E8
Firenze Amerigo
  Vespucci ✈ (FLR) *Italy* **41** E8
Firenze Pisa ✈ (PSA) *Italy* **40** E7
Firenzuola *Italy* **41** D8
Firk, Sha'ib → *Iraq* **70** D5
Firmi *France* **20** D6
Firminy *France* **21** C8
Firozabad *India* **69** F8
Firozpur *India* **68** D6
Firozpur-Jhirka *India* **68** F7
Fīrūzābād *Iran* **71** D7
Fīrūzkūh *Iran* **71** C7
Firvale *Canada* **102** C3
Fish → *Namibia* **88** D2
Fish → *S. Africa* **88** E3
Fish River Canyon *Namibia* **88** D2
Fisher B. *Canada* **103** C9
Fishers I. *U.S.A.* **115** E13
Fishguard *U.K.* **15** E3
Fishing L. *Canada* **103** C9
Fishkill *U.S.A.* **115** E11
Fismes *France* **19** C10
Fisterra *Spain* **36** C1
Fisterra, C. *Spain* **36** C1
Fitchburg *Mass., U.S.A.* **115** D13
Fitchburg *Wis., U.S.A.* **112** D9
Fitz Roy *Argentina* **128** F3
Fitz Roy, Cerro *Argentina* **128** F2
Fitzgerald *Canada* **102** B6
Fitzgerald *U.S.A.* **117** F13
Fitzgerald River △ *Australia* **93** F3
Fitzmaurice → *Australia* **92** B5
Fitzroy → *Queens., Australia* **94** C5
Fitzroy → *W. Austral.,
  Australia* **92** C3
Fitzroy Crossing *Australia* **92** C4
Fitzwilliam I. *Canada* **114** A3
Fiuggi *Italy* **41** G10
Fiume = Rijeka *Croatia* **41** C11

Fiumicino, Roma ✈ (FCO)
  Italy **41** G9
Five Points *U.S.A.* **110** J6
Fivizzano *Italy* **40** D7
Fizi *Dem. Rep. of the Congo* **86** C2
Fjällbacka *Sweden* **11** F5
Fjärdhundra *Sweden* **10** E10
Fjellerup *Denmark* **11** H4
Fjerritslev *Denmark* **11** G3
Fjugesta *Sweden* **10** E8
Flagstaff *U.S.A.* **109** J8
Flagstaff L. *U.S.A.* **115** A14
Flaherty I. *Canada* **104** A4
Flåm *Norway* **8** F12
Flambeau → *U.S.A.* **112** C8
Flamborough Hd. *U.K.* **14** C7
Fläming *Germany* **24** C8
Flaming Gorge △ *U.S.A.* **108** F9
Flaming Gorge Res. *U.S.A.* **108** F9
Flamingo, Teluk *Indonesia* **63** F9
Flanders = Flandre *Europe* **19** B9
Flandre *Europe* **19** B9
Flandre-Occidentale =
  West-Vlaanderen □
  Belgium **17** D2
Flandre-Orientale = Oost-
  Vlaanderen □ *Belgium* **17** C3
Flandreau *U.S.A.* **112** C5
Flanigan *U.S.A.* **110** E7
Flannan Is. *U.K.* **13** C1
Flåsjön *Sweden* **8** D16
Flat → *Canada* **102** A3
Flat I. *Mauritius* **85** d
Flathead L. *U.S.A.* **108** C6
Flattery, C. *Australia* **94** A4
Flattery, C. *U.S.A.* **110** B2
Flatwoods *U.S.A.* **113** F12
Fleetwood *U.K.* **14** D4
Fleetwood *U.S.A.* **115** F9
Flekkefjord *Norway* **9** G12
Flemington *U.S.A.* **114** E7
Flen *Sweden* **10** E10
Flensburg *Germany* **24** A5
Flers *France* **18** D6
Flesherton *Canada* **114** B4
Flesko, Tanjung *Indonesia* **63** D6
Fleurance *France* **20** E4
Fleurier *Switz.* **25** J2
Fleurieu Pen. *Australia* **95** F2
Flevoland □ *Neths.* **17** B5
Flin Flon *Canada* **103** C8
Flinders → *Australia* **94** B3
Flinders B. *Australia* **93** F2
Flinders Group *Australia* **94** A3
Flinders I. *S. Austral., Australia* **95** E1
Flinders I. *Tas., Australia* **95** G4
Flinders Ranges *Australia* **95** E2
Flinders Reefs *Australia* **94** B4
Flint *U.K.* **14** D4
Flint *U.S.A.* **113** D12
Flint → *U.S.A.* **117** F12
Flint I. *Kiribati* **97** J12
Flintshire □ *U.K.* **14** D4
Fliseryd *Sweden* **11** G10
Flix *Spain* **38** D5
Flixecourt *France* **19** B9
Floby *Sweden* **11** F7
Floda *Sweden* **11** G6
Flodden *U.K.* **14** B5
Flogny-la-Chapelle *France* **19** E10
Floodwood *U.S.A.* **112** B7
Flora *U.S.A.* **112** F1
Florac *France* **20** D7
Florala *U.S.A.* **117** F11
Florence = Firenze *Italy* **41** E8
Florence *Ala., U.S.A.* **117** D11
Florence *Ariz., U.S.A.* **109** K8
Florence *Colo., U.S.A.* **108** G11
Florence *Oreg., U.S.A.* **108** D1
Florence *S.C., U.S.A.* **117** D15
Florence, L. *Australia* **95** D2
Florencia *Colombia* **124** C3
Florennes *Belgium* **17** D4
Florensac *France* **20** E7
Florenville *Belgium* **17** E5
Flores *Azores* **78** a
Flores *Guatemala* **120** C2
Flores *Indonesia* **63** F6
Flores I. *Canada* **102** D3
Flores Sea *Indonesia* **63** F6
Floreşti *Moldova* **29** C13
Floresville *U.S.A.* **116** G5
Floriano *Brazil* **125** E10
Florianópolis *Brazil* **127** B6
Florida *Cuba* **120** B4
Florida *Uruguay* **127** C4
Florida □ *U.S.A.* **117** G14
Florida, Straits of *U.S.A.* **120** B4
Florida B. *U.S.A.* **120** B3
Florida Keys *U.S.A.* **117** J14
Floridia *Italy* **43** E8
Florin *U.S.A.* **110** G5
Florina *Greece* **44** F5
Flórina □ *Greece* **44** F5
Florissant *U.S.A.* **112** F8
Florø *Norway* **8** F11
Flower Station *Canada* **115** A8
Flowerpot I. *Canada* **114** A3
Floydada *U.S.A.* **116** E4

Fluk *Indonesia* **63** E7
Flúmen → *Spain* **38** D4
Flumendosa → *Italy* **42** C2
Fluminimaggiore *Italy* **42** C1
Flushing = Vlissingen *Neths.* **17** C3
Fluvià → *Spain* **38** C8
Fly → *Papua N. G.* **90** B7
Foa *Tonga* **91** c
Foam Lake *Canada* **103** C8
Foča *Bos.-H.* **44** C2
Focha bers *U.K.* **13** D5
Focşani *Romania* **29** E12
Fochabers *U.K.* **13** D5
Fochville *S. Africa* **89** D4
Focşani *Romania* **29** E12
Fodécontéa *Guinea* **82** C2
Fogang *China* **59** F9
Fóggia *Italy* **43** A8
Foglia → *Italy* **41** E9
Fogo *Canada* **105** C9
Fogo *C. Verde Is.* **78** b
Fogo I. *Canada* **105** C9
Fohnsdorf *Austria* **26** D7
Föhr *Germany* **24** A4
Foia *Portugal* **37** H2
Foix *France* **20** E5
Fojnica *Bos.-H.* **28** G2
Fokida □ *Greece* **46** C4
Fokino *Russia* **32** F3
Fokku *Nigeria* **83** C5
Folda *Nord-Trøndelag, Norway* **8** D14
Folda *Nordland, Norway* **8** C16
Földeák *Hungary* **28** D5
Folegandros *Greece* **46** E6
Foley *Botswana* **88** C4
Foley *U.S.A.* **117** F11
Foleyet *Canada* **104** C3
Folgefonna *Norway* **9** F12
Foligno *Italy* **41** F9
Folkestone *U.K.* **15** F9
Folkston *U.S.A.* **117** F13
Follansbee *U.S.A.* **114** F4
Follónica *Italy* **40** F7
Follónica, G. di *Italy* **40** F7
Folsom L. *U.S.A.* **110** G5
Folteşti *Romania* **29** E13
Fomboni *Comoros Is.* **85** a
Fond-du-Lac *Canada* **103** B7
Fond du Lac *U.S.A.* **112** D9
Fond-du-Lac → *Canada* **103** B7
Fonda *U.S.A.* **115** D10
Fondi *Italy* **42** A6
Fonfría *Spain* **36** D4
Fongafale *Tuvalu* **90** B10
Fonni *Italy* **42** B2
Fonsagrada = A
  Fonsagrada *Spain* **36** B3
Fonseca, G. de *Cent. Amer.* **120** D2
Font-Romeu-Odeillo-Via
  France **20** F5
Fontaine-Française *France* **19** E12
Fontainebleau *France* **19** D9
Fontana *U.S.A.* **111** L9
Fontas → *Canada* **102** B4
Fonte Boa *Brazil* **124** D5
Fontem *Cameroon* **83** D6
Fontenay-le-Comte *France* **20** B3
Fontenelle Res. *U.S.A.* **108** E8
Fontur *Iceland* **8** C6
Fonuafo'ou *Tonga* **91** c
Fonualei *Tonga* **91** c
Fonyód *Hungary* **28** D2
Foochow = Fuzhou *China* **59** D12
Foping *China* **56** H5
Foraker, Mt. *U.S.A.* **106** C9
Forbach *France* **19** C13
Forbes *Australia* **95** E4
Forbesganj *India* **69** F12
Forcados *Nigeria* **83** D6
Forcados → *Nigeria* **83** D6
Forcalquier *France* **21** E9
Forchheim *Germany* **25** F7
Ford City *Calif., U.S.A.* **111** K7
Ford City *Pa., U.S.A.* **114** F5
Førde *Norway* **8** F11
Fords Bridge *Australia* **95** D4
Fordyce *U.S.A.* **116** E8
Forécariah *Guinea* **82** D2
Forel, Mt. *Greenland* **98** C16
Foremost *Canada* **102** D6
Forest *Canada* **114** C3
Forest *U.S.A.* **117** E10
Forest City *Iowa, U.S.A.* **112** D7
Forest City *N.C., U.S.A.* **117** D14
Forest City *Pa., U.S.A.* **115** E9
Forest Grove *U.S.A.* **110** E3
Forestburg *Canada* **102** C6
Foreste Casentinesi-Monte
  Falterona-Campigna △
  Italy **41** E8
Foresthill *U.S.A.* **110** F6
Forestier Pen. *Australia* **95** G4
Forestville *Canada* **105** C6
Forestville *Calif., U.S.A.* **110** G4
Forestville *N.Y., U.S.A.* **114** D5
Forêt d'Orient △ *France* **19** D11
Forez, Mts. du *France* **20** C7
Forfar *U.K.* **13** E6
Forillon △ *Canada* **105** C7
Forks *U.S.A.* **110** C2

Forksville *U.S.A.* **115** E8
Forlì *Italy* **41** D9
Forman *U.S.A.* **112** B5
Formazza *Italy* **40** B5
Formby Pt. *U.K.* **14** D4
Formentera *Spain* **48** C7
Formentor, C. de *Spain* **48** B10
Formentor, Pen. de *Spain* **48** B10
Former Yugoslav Republic
  of Macedonia =
  Macedonia ■ *Europe* **44** E5
Fórmia *Italy* **42** A6
Formígine *Italy* **40** D7
Formosa = Taiwan ■ *Asia* **59** F13
Formosa *Argentina* **126** B4
Formosa *Brazil* **125** G9
Formosa □ *Argentina* **126** B4
Formosa, Serra *Brazil* **125** F8
Formosa B. = Ungwana B.
  Kenya **86** C5
Fornells *Spain* **48** A11
Fornos de Algodres *Portugal* **36** E3
Fornovo di Taro *Italy* **40** D7
Føroyar ☒ *Atl. Oc.* **8** F9
Forres *U.K.* **13** D5
Forrest *Australia* **93** F4
Forrest, Mt. *Australia* **93** D4
Forrest City *U.S.A.* **117** D9
Forsayth *Australia* **94** B3
Forshaga *Sweden* **10** E7
Förslöv *Sweden* **11** H6
Forsmo *Sweden* **10** A11
Forssa *Finland* **32** B2
Forst *Germany* **24** D10
Forster *Australia* **95** E5
Forsvik *Sweden* **11** F8
Forsyth *U.S.A.* **108** C10
Fort Abbas *Pakistan* **68** E5
Fort Albany *Canada* **104** B3
Fort Assiniboine *Canada* **102** C6
Fort Augustus *U.K.* **13** D4
Fort Beaufort *S. Africa* **88** E4
Fort Benton *U.S.A.* **108** C8
Fort Bragg *U.S.A.* **108** G2
Fort Bridger *U.S.A.* **108** F8
Fort Chipewyan *Canada* **103** B6
Fort Clatsop = Lewis and
  Clark △ *U.S.A.* **110** D3
Fort Collins *U.S.A.* **108** E11
Fort-Coulonge *Canada* **104** C4
Fort Covington *U.S.A.* **115** B10
Fort Dauphin = Taolanaro
  Madag. **89** D8
Fort Davis *U.S.A.* **116** F3
Fort-de-France *Martinique* **120** c
Fort Defiance *U.S.A.* **109** J9
Fort Dodge *U.S.A.* **112** D6
Fort Edward *U.S.A.* **115** C11
Fort Erie *Canada* **114** D6
Fort Fairfield *U.S.A.* **113** B20
Fort Frances *Canada* **103** D10
Fort Franklin = Déline
  Canada **100** D7
Fort Garland *U.S.A.* **109** H11
Fort George = Chisasibi
  Canada **104** B4
Fort Good Hope *Canada* **100** D6
Fort Hancock *U.S.A.* **116** F2
Fort Hope = Eabametoong
  Canada **104** B2
Fort Irwin *U.S.A.* **111** K10
Fort Kent *U.S.A.* **113** B19
Fort Klamath *U.S.A.* **108** D3
Fort Laramie *U.S.A.* **108** E11
Fort Lauderdale *U.S.A.* **117** H14
Fort Liard *Canada* **102** A4
Fort Liberté *Haiti* **121** C5
Fort Lupton *U.S.A.* **108** F11
Fort MacKay *Canada* **102** B6
Fort Macleod *Canada* **102** D6
Fort McMurray *Canada* **102** B6
Fort McPherson *Canada* **100** D5
Fort Madison *U.S.A.* **112** E9
Fort Meade *U.S.A.* **117** H14
Fort Morgan *U.S.A.* **108** F12
Fort Myers *U.S.A.* **117** H14
Fort Nelson *Canada* **102** B4
Fort Nelson → *Canada* **102** B4
Fort Norman = Tulita
  Canada **100** E6
Fort Payne *U.S.A.* **117** D12
Fort Peck *U.S.A.* **108** B10
Fort Peck Dam *U.S.A.* **108** C10
Fort Peck L. *U.S.A.* **108** C10
Fort Pierce *U.S.A.* **117** H14
Fort Pierre *U.S.A.* **112** C3
Fort Plain *U.S.A.* **115** D10
Fort Portal *Uganda* **86** B3
Fort Providence *Canada* **102** A5
Fort Qu'Appelle *Canada* **103** C8
Fort Resolution *Canada* **102** A6
Fort Rixon *Zimbabwe* **87** G2
Fort Ross *U.S.A.* **110** G3
Fort Rupert =
  Waskaganish *Canada* **104** B4
Fort St. James *Canada* **102** C4
Fort St. John *Canada* **102** B4
Fort Saskatchewan *Canada* **102** C6

Fort Scott *U.S.A.* **112** G6
Fort Severn *Canada* **104** A2
Fort Shevchenko *Kazakhstan* **35** H10
Fort Simpson *Canada* **102** A4
Fort Smith *Canada* **102** B6
Fort Smith *U.S.A.* **116** D7
Fort Stockton *U.S.A.* **116** F3
Fort Sumner *U.S.A.* **109** J11
Fort Thompson *U.S.A.* **112** C4
Fort Union △ *U.S.A.* **109** J11
Fort Valley *U.S.A.* **117** E13
Fort Vermilion *Canada* **102** B5
Fort Walton Beach *U.S.A.* **117** F11
Fort Ware *Canada* **102** B3
Fort Wayne *U.S.A.* **113** E11
Fort William *U.K.* **13** E3
Fort Worth *U.S.A.* **116** E6
Fort Yates *U.S.A.* **112** B3
Fort Yukon *U.S.A.* **100** D2
Fortaleza *Brazil* **125** D11
Forteau *Canada* **105** B8
Fortescue → *Australia* **92** D2
Fortescue River Roadhouse
  Australia **92** D2
Forth → *U.K.* **13** E5
Forth, Firth of *U.K.* **13** E6
Fortore → *Italy* **41** G12
Fortrose *U.K.* **13** D4
Fortuna *Spain* **39** G3
Fortuna *Calif., U.S.A.* **108** F1
Fortuna *N. Dak., U.S.A.* **112** A2
Fortune *Canada* **105** C8
Fortune B. *Canada* **105** C8
Forūr *Iran* **71** E7
Fos-sur-Mer *France* **21** E8
Fosen *Norway* **8** E14
Foshan *China* **59** F9
Fosnavåg *Norway* **8** E11
Foso *Ghana* **83** D4
Fossano *Italy* **40** D4
Fossil *U.S.A.* **108** D3
Fossil Butte △ *U.S.A.* **108** F8
Fossombrone *Italy* **41** E9
Foster *Canada* **115** A12
Foster → *Canada* **103** B7
Fosters Ra. *Australia* **94** C1
Fostoria *U.S.A.* **113** E12
Fotadrevo *Madag.* **89** C8
Fouesnant *France* **18** E2
Fougères *France* **18** D5
Foul Pt. *Sri Lanka* **66** Q12
Foulness I. *U.K.* **15** F8
Foulpointe *Madag.* **89** B8
Foula *U.K.* **13** A6
Foulalaba *Mali* **82** C3
Foumban *Cameroon* **83** D7
Foumbot *Cameroon* **83** D7
Foumbouni *Comoros Is.* **85** a
Foundiougne *Senegal* **82** C1
Fountain *U.S.A.* **108** G11
Fountain Hills *U.S.A.* **109** K8
Fountain Springs *U.S.A.* **111** K8
Four Mountains, Is. of
  U.S.A. **106** E5
Fourchambault *France* **19** E10
Fouriesburg *S. Africa* **88** D4
Fourmies *France* **19** B11
Fourna *Greece* **46** B3
Fourni *Greece* **47** D8
Fours *France* **19** F10
Fourth Cataract *Sudan* **79** E12
Fouta Djallon *Guinea* **82** C2
Foux, Cap-à- *Haiti* **121** C5
Foveaux Str. *N.Z.* **91** G2
Fowey *U.K.* **15** G3
Fowler *Calif., U.S.A.* **110** J7
Fowler *Colo., U.S.A.* **108** G11
Fowler, Pt. *Australia* **93** F5
Fowlers B. *Australia* **93** F5
Fowman *Iran* **73** D13
Fox → *Canada* **103** B10
Fox Creek *Canada* **102** C5
Fox Is. *U.S.A.* **106** E6
Fox Lake *Canada* **102** B6
Fox Valley *Canada* **103** C7
Foxboro *Canada* **114** B7
Foxboro *U.S.A.* **115** D13
Foxdale *Australia* **94** b
Foxe Basin *Canada* **101** D16
Foxe Chan. *Canada* **101** E16
Foxe Pen. *Canada* **101** E16
Foxen *Sweden* **10** E5
Foxford *Ireland* **12** C2
Foxton *N.Z.* **91** D5
Foyle, Lough *U.K.* **12** A4
Foynes *Ireland* **12** D2
Foz *Spain* **36** B3
Foz do Cunene *Angola* **88** B1
Foz do Iguaçu *Brazil* **127** B5
Frackville *U.S.A.* **115** F8
Fraga *Spain* **38** D5
Fraile Muerto *Uruguay* **127** C5
Framingham *U.S.A.* **115** D13
Frampol *Poland* **31** H9
Franca *Brazil* **125** H9
Francavilla al Mare *Italy* **41** F11
Francavilla Fontana *Italy* **43** B10
France ■ *Europe* **7** F6
Frances *Australia* **95** F3

Frances → *Canada* **102** A3
Frances L. *Canada* **102** A3
Franceville *Gabon* **84** E2
Franche-Comté □ *France* **19** F12
Francis Case, L. *U.S.A.* **112** D4
Francisco Beltrão *Brazil* **127** B5
Francisco Ignacio Madero
  Coahuila, Mexico **118** B4
Francisco Ignacio Madero
  Durango, Mexico **118** C4
Francisco Ignacio Madero,
  Presa *Mexico* **118** B3
Francistown *Botswana* **89** C4
Francofonte *Italy* **43** E7
François *Canada* **105** C8
François L. *Canada* **102** C3
Francois Peron △ *Australia* **93** E1
Francs Pk. *U.S.A.* **108** E9
Franeker *Neths.* **17** A5
Frank Hann △ *Australia* **93** F3
Frankenberg *Germany* **24** D4
Frankenhöhe △ *Germany* **25** F6
Frankenthal *Germany* **25** F7
Frankenwald *Germany* **25** E7
Frankenwald △ *Germany* **25** E7
Frankford *Canada* **114** B7
Frankfort *S. Africa* **89** D4
Frankfort *Ind., U.S.A.* **112** E10
Frankfort *Kans., U.S.A.* **112** F5
Frankfort *Ky., U.S.A.* **113** F11
Frankfort *N.Y., U.S.A.* **115** C9
Frankfurt *Brandenburg,
  Germany* **24** C10
Frankfurt *Hessen, Germany* **25** E4
Frankfurt ✈ (FRA) *Germany* **25** E4
Fränkische Alb *Germany* **25** F7
Fränkische Rezat →
  Germany **25** F7
Fränkische Saale →
  Germany **25** E5
Fränkische Schweiz *Germany* **25** F7
Fränkische
  Schweiz-Veldensteiner
  Forst △ *Germany* **25** F7
Frankland → *Australia* **93** G2
Franklin *Ky., U.S.A.* **112** G10
Franklin *La., U.S.A.* **116** G9
Franklin *Mass., U.S.A.* **115** D13
Franklin *N.H., U.S.A.* **115** C13
Franklin *N.Y., U.S.A.* **115** D9
Franklin *Nebr., U.S.A.* **112** E4
Franklin *Pa., U.S.A.* **114** E5
Franklin *Va., U.S.A.* **113** G15
Franklin *W. Va., U.S.A.* **113** F14
Franklin B. *Canada* **100** D6
Franklin D. Roosevelt L.
  U.S.A. **108** B4
Franklin-Gordon Wild
  Rivers △ *Australia* **95** G4
Franklin I. *Antarctica* **5** D11
Franklin I. *Canada* **114** A4
Franklin L. *U.S.A.* **108** F6
Franklin Mts. *Canada* **100** D6
Franklin Str. *Canada* **100** C12
Franklinton *U.S.A.* **117** F9
Franklinville *U.S.A.* **114** D6
Frankston *Australia* **95** F4
Frånö *Sweden* **10** B11
Fransfontein *Namibia* **88** C2
Fränsta *Sweden* **10** B10
Frantsa Iosifa, Zemlya *Russia* **52** A6
Franz *Canada* **104** C3
Franz Josef Land = Frantsa
  Iosifa, Zemlya *Russia* **52** A6
Franz Josef Strauss ✈
  (MUC) *Germany* **25** G7
Franzburg *Germany* **24** A8
Frascati *Italy* **41** G9
Fraser *U.S.A.* **114** D2
Fraser → *B.C., Canada* **110** A3
Fraser → *Nfld. & L., Canada* **105** A7
Fraser, Mt. *Australia* **93** E2
Fraser I. *Australia* **95** D5
Fraser Lake *Canada* **102** C4
Fraserburg *S. Africa* **88** E3
Fraserburgh *U.K.* **13** D6
Fraserdale *Canada* **104** C3
Frashër *Albania* **44** F4
Frasne *France* **19** F13
Frăteşti *Romania* **29** G10
Frauenfeld *Switz.* **25** H4
Fray Bentos *Uruguay* **126** C4
Fray Jorge △ *Chile* **126** C1
Frazier Downs ۞ *Australia* **92** C3
Frechilla *Spain* **36** C6
Fredericia *Denmark* **11** J3
Frederick *Md., U.S.A.* **113** F15
Frederick *Okla., U.S.A.* **116** D5
Frederick *S. Dak., U.S.A.* **112** C4
Fredericksburg *Pa., U.S.A.* **115** F8
Fredericksburg *Tex., U.S.A.* **116** G5
Fredericksburg *Va., U.S.A.* **113** F15
Fredericktown *Mo., U.S.A.* **112** G8
Fredericktown *Ohio, U.S.A.* **114** F2
Frederico Westphalen *Brazil* **127** B5
Fredericton *Canada* **105** C6
Fredericton Junction *Canada* **105** C6
Frederikshåb = Paamiut
  Greenland **4** C5
Frederikshamn = Hamina
  Finland **32** B4

Frederikshavn *Denmark* 11 G4
Frederikssund *Denmark* 11 J6
Frederiksted *U.S. Virgin Is.* 121 C7
Frederiksværk *Denmark* 11 J6
Fredonia *Ariz., U.S.A.* 109 H7
Fredonia *Kans., U.S.A.* 112 G6
Fredonia *N.Y., U.S.A.* 114 D5
Fredriksberg *Sweden* 10 D8
Fredrikstad *Norway* 9 G14
Free State □ *S. Africa* 88 D4
Freehold *U.S.A.* 115 F10
Freeland *U.S.A.* 115 E9
Freels, C. *Nfld. & L., Canada* 105 C9
Freels, C. *Nfld. & L., Canada* 105 C9
Freeman *Calif., U.S.A.* 111 K9
Freeman *S. Dak., U.S.A.* 112 D5
Freeport *Bahamas* 120 A4
Freeport *Ill., U.S.A.* 112 D9
Freeport *N.Y., U.S.A.* 115 F11
Freeport *Ohio, U.S.A.* 114 F3
Freeport *Pa., U.S.A.* 114 F5
Freeport *Tex., U.S.A.* 116 G7
Freetown *S. Leone* 82 D2
Freeville *U.S.A.* 115 D8
Frégate, L. de la *Canada* 104 B5
Fregenal de la Sierra *Spain* 37 G4
Fregene *Italy* 41 G9
Fregon *Australia* 93 E5
Fréhel, C. *France* 18 D4
Freiberg *Germany* 24 E9
Freibourg = Fribourg *Switz.* 25 J3
Freiburg *Baden-W., Germany* 25 H3
Freiburg *Niedersachsen,
    Germany* 24 B5
Freilassing *Germany* 25 H8
Freire *Chile* 128 D2
Freirina *Chile* 126 B1
Freising *Germany* 25 G7
Freistadt *Austria* 26 C7
Freital *Germany* 24 D9
Fréjus *France* 21 E10
Fremantle *Australia* 93 F2
Fremont *Calif., U.S.A.* 110 H4
Fremont *Mich., U.S.A.* 113 D11
Fremont *Nebr., U.S.A.* 112 E5
Fremont *Ohio, U.S.A.* 113 E12
Fremont → *U.S.A.* 108 G8
French Camp *U.S.A.* 110 H5
French Cays = Plana Cays
    Bahamas 121 B5
French Creek → *U.S.A.* 114 E5
French Frigate Shoals
    U.S.A. 107 L6
French Guiana ☑ *S. Amer.* 125 C8
French Polynesia ☑ *Pac. Oc.* 97 J13
Frenchman Cr. → *N. Amer.*
    108 B10
Frenchman Cr. → *U.S.A.* 112 E3
Frenštát pod Radhoštěm
    Czech Rep. 27 B11
Fresco *Ivory C.* 82 D3
Fresco → *Brazil* 125 E8
Freshfield, C. *Antarctica* 5 C10
Fresnay-sur-Sarthe *France* 18 D7
Fresno *U.S.A.* 110 J7
Fresno Alhándiga *Spain* 36 E5
Fresno Res. *U.S.A.* 108 B9
Freudenstadt *Germany* 25 G4
Frévent *France* 19 B9
Frew → *Australia* 94 C2
Frewsburg *U.S.A.* 114 D5
Freycinet △ *Australia* 95 G4
Freycinet Pen. *Australia* 95 G4
Freyming-Merlebach *France* 19 C13
Freyung *Germany* 25 G9
Fria *Guinea* 82 C2
Fria, C. *Namibia* 88 B1
Friant *U.S.A.* 110 J7
Frías *Argentina* 126 B2
Fribourg *Switz.* 25 J3
Fribourg □ *Switz.* 25 J3
Fridafors *Sweden* 11 H8
Friday Harbor *U.S.A.* 110 B3
Friedberg *Bayern, Germany* 25 G6
Friedberg *Hessen, Germany* 25 E4
Friedens *U.S.A.* 114 F6
Friedland *Germany* 24 B9
Friedrichshafen *Germany* 25 H5
Friedrichskoog *Germany* 24 A4
Friedrichstadt *Germany* 24 A5
Friendship *U.S.A.* 114 D6
Friesach *Austria* 26 E7
Friesack *Germany* 24 C8
Friesland □ *Neths.* 17 A5
Friesoythe *Germany* 24 B3
Frigate *Seychelles* 85 b
Friggesund *Sweden* 10 C10
Frillesås *Sweden* 11 G6
Frinnaryd *Sweden* 11 G8
Frio → *U.S.A.* 116 G5
Frio, C. *Brazil* 122 F6
Friol *Spain* 36 B3
Friona *U.S.A.* 116 D3
Fristad *Sweden* 11 G6
Fritch *U.S.A.* 116 D4
Fritsla *Sweden* 11 G6
Fritzlar *Germany* 24 D5
Friuli-Venézia Giulia □ *Italy* 41 B9

Frobisher B. *Canada* 101 E18
Frobisher Bay = Iqaluit
    Canada 101 E18
Frobisher L. *Canada* 103 B7
Frohavet *Norway* 8 E13
Frohnleiten *Austria* 26 D8
Frolovo *Russia* 34 F6
Frombork *Poland* 30 D6
Frome *U.K.* 15 F5
Frome → *U.K.* 15 G5
Frome, L. *Australia* 95 E2
Frómista *Spain* 36 C6
Front Range *U.S.A.* 107 G18
Front Royal *U.S.A.* 113 F14
Fronteira *Portugal* 37 F3
Frontenac △ *Canada* 115 B8
Frontera *Canary Is.* 48 G2
Frontera *Mexico* 119 D6
Fronteras *Mexico* 118 A3
Frontignan *France* 20 E7
Frosinone *Italy* 42 A6
Frostburg *U.S.A.* 113 F14
Frostisen *Norway* 8 B17
Frouard *France* 19 D13
Frövi *Sweden* 10 E9
Frøya *Norway* 8 E13
Frumoasa *Romania* 29 D10
Frunze = Bishkek *Kyrgyzstan* 52 E8
Frunzivka *Ukraine* 29 C14
Fruška Gora *Serbia* 28 F5
Fruška Gora △ *Serbia* 44 A3
Frutal *Brazil* 125 H9
Frutigen *Switz.* 25 J3
Frýdek-Místek *Czech Rep.* 27 B11
Frýdlant *Czech Rep.* 26 A8
Fryeburg *U.S.A.* 115 B14
Fryvaldov = Jeseník
    Czech Rep. 27 A10
Fthiótida □ *Greece* 46 C4
Fu Jiang → *China* 58 C6
Fu Xian = Wafangdian
    China 57 E11
Fu Xian *China* 56 G5
Fu'an *China* 59 D12
Fubian *China* 58 B4
Fucécchio *Italy* 40 E7
Fucheng *China* 56 F9
Fuchou = Fuzhou *China* 59 D12
Fuchuan *China* 59 E8
Fuchū *Japan* 55 G6
Fuchun Jiang → *China* 59 B13
Fúcino, Piana del *Italy* 41 F10
Fuding *China* 59 D13
Fuencaliente *Canary Is.* 48 F2
Fuencaliente *Spain* 37 G6
Fuencaliente, Pta. *Canary Is.* 48 F2
Fuengirola *Spain* 37 J6
Fuenlabrada *Spain* 36 E7
Fuensalida *Spain* 36 E6
Fuente-Álamo *Spain* 39 G3
Fuente Álamo de Murcia
    Spain 39 H3
Fuente de Cantos *Spain* 37 G4
Fuente del Maestre *Spain* 37 G4
Fuente el Fresno *Spain* 37 F7
Fuente Obejuna *Spain* 37 G5
Fuente Palmera *Spain* 37 H5
Fuentes de Andalucía *Spain* 37 H5
Fuentes de Ebro *Spain* 38 D4
Fuentes de León *Spain* 37 G4
Fuentes de Oñoro *Spain* 36 E4
Fuentesaúco *Spain* 36 D5
Fuerte → *Mexico* 118 B3
Fuerte Olimpo *Paraguay* 126 A4
Fuerteventura *Canary Is.* 48 F6
Fuerteventura ✈ (FUE)
    Canary Is. 48 F6
Fufeng *China* 56 G5
Fuga I. *Phil.* 61 B4
Fugong *China* 58 D2
Fugou *China* 56 G8
Fugu *China* 56 E6
Fuhai *China* 60 B3
Fuḥaymī *Iraq* 73 E10
Fuhlsbüttel, Hamburg ✈
    (HAM) *Germany* 24 B5
Fuji *Japan* 55 G9
Fuji-Hakone-Izu △ *Japan* 55 G9
Fuji-San *Japan* 55 G9
Fuji-Yoshida *Japan* 55 G9
Fujian □ *China* 59 E12
Fujinomiya *Japan* 55 G9
Fujisawa *Japan* 55 G9
Fujiyama, Mt. = Fuji-San
    Japan 55 G9
Fukagawa *Japan* 54 C11
Fukien = Fujian □ *China* 59 E12
Fukuchiyama *Japan* 55 G7
Fukue-Shima *Japan* 55 H4
Fukui *Japan* 55 F8
Fukui □ *Japan* 55 G8
Fukuoka *Japan* 55 H5
Fukuoka □ *Japan* 55 H5
Fukushima *Japan* 54 F10
Fukushima □ *Japan* 54 F10
Fukuyama *Japan* 55 G6
Fulacunda *Guinea-Biss.* 82 C1
Fulaga *Fiji* 91 a
Fulda *Germany* 24 E5

Fulda → *Germany* 24 D5
Fulford Harbour *Canada* 110 B3
Fuliang *China* 59 C11
Fullerton *Calif., U.S.A.* 111 M9
Fullerton *Nebr., U.S.A.* 112 E5
Fulongquan *China* 57 B13
Fulton *Mo., U.S.A.* 112 F8
Fulton *N.Y., U.S.A.* 115 C8
Fulufjället *Sweden* 10 C6
Fulun → *Sweden* 10 C7
Fumay *France* 19 C11
Fumel *France* 20 D4
Fumin *China* 58 E4
Funabashi *Japan* 55 G10
Funafuti = Fongafale *Tuvalu* 90 B10
Funäsdalen *Sweden* 10 B6
Funchal *Madeira* 48 D3
Funchal ✈ (FNC) *Madeira* 48 D3
Fundación *Colombia* 124 A4
Fundão *Portugal* 36 E3
Fundong *Cameroon* 83 D7
Fundu Moldovei *Romania* 29 C10
Fundulea *Romania* 29 F11
Fundy, B. of *Canada* 105 D6
Fundy △ *Canada* 105 C6
Funhalouro *Mozam.* 89 C5
Funing *Hebei, China* 57 E10
Funing *Jiangsu, China* 57 H10
Funing *Yunnan, China* 58 F5
Funiu Shan *China* 56 H7
Funsi *Ghana* 82 C4
Funtua *Nigeria* 83 C6
Fuping *Hebei, China* 56 E8
Fuping *Shaanxi, China* 56 G5
Fuqing *China* 59 E12
Fuquan *China* 58 D6
Furano *Japan* 54 C11
Furāt, Nahr al → *Asia* 70 D5
Furmanov *Russia* 34 B5
Furnas, Represa de *Brazil* 127 A6
Furneaux Group *Australia* 95 G4
Furnás *Spain* 48 B8
Fürstenau *Germany* 24 C3
Fürstenberg *Germany* 24 B9
Fürstenfeld *Austria* 26 D9
Fürstenfeldbruck *Germany* 25 G7
Fürstenwalde *Germany* 24 C10
Fürth *Germany* 25 F6
Fürth im Wald *Germany* 25 F8
Furtwangen *Germany* 25 G4
Furudal *Sweden* 10 C9
Furukawa *Japan* 54 E10
Furulund *Sweden* 11 J7
Fury and Hecla Str. *Canada* 101 D15
Fusagasugá *Colombia* 124 C4
Fuscaldo *Italy* 43 C9
Fushan *Shandong, China* 57 F11
Fushan *Shanxi, China* 56 G6
Fushë Arrëz *Albania* 44 D4
Fushë Krujë *Albania* 44 E3
Fushun *Liaoning, China* 57 D12
Fushun *Sichuan, China* 58 C5
Fusong *China* 57 C14
Füssen *Germany* 25 H6
Fustic *Barbados* 121 g
Fusui *China* 58 F6
Futog *Serbia* 28 E4
Futuna *Wall. & F. Is.* 90 C11
Fuwa *Egypt* 80 H7
Fuxian Hu *China* 58 E4
Fuxin *China* 57 C11
Fuyang *Anhui, China* 56 H8
Fuyang *Zhejiang, China* 59 B12
Fuyang He → *China* 56 E9
Fuying Dao *China* 59 D13
Fuyu *Heilongjiang, China* 53 E13
Fuyu *Jilin, China* 57 B13
Fuyuan *China* 58 E5
Füzesgyarmat *Hungary* 28 C6
Fuzhou = Linchuan *China* 59 D11
Fuzhou *China* 59 D12
Füzuli *Azerbaijan* 73 C12
Fylde *U.K.* 14 D5
Fyn *Denmark* 11 J4
Fyne, L. *U.K.* 13 F3
Fynshav *Denmark* 11 K3

G

Ga *Ghana* 82 D4
Gaalkacyo *Somali Rep.* 75 F4
Gaanda *Nigeria* 83 C7
Gabas → *France* 20 E3
Gabba *Australia* 94 a
Gabela *Angola* 84 G2
Gabès *Tunisia* 79 B8
Gabès, G. de *Tunisia* 79 B8
Gabgaba, W. → *Egypt* 80 C3
Gabia la Grande *Spain* 37 H7
Gabin *Poland* 31 F6
Gabon ■ *Africa* 84 E2
Gaborone *Botswana* 88 C4
Gabriels *U.S.A.* 115 B10
Gábrík *Iran* 71 E8
Gabrovo *Bulgaria* 45 D9
Gacé *France* 18 D7
Gäch Sär *Iran* 71 B6

Fulda → *Germany* 24 D5
Gacko *Bos.-H.* 44 C2
Gadag *India* 66 M9
Gadamai *Sudan* 81 D4
Gadap *Pakistan* 68 G2
Gadarwara *India* 69 H8
Gadebusch *Germany* 24 B7
Gadein *Sudan* 81 F2
Gadhada *India* 68 J4
Gadhada *India* 68 J4
Gadra *Pakistan* 68 G4
Gadsden *U.S.A.* 117 D11
Gadwal *India* 66 L10
Gadyach = Hadyach *Ukraine* 33 G8
Găeşti *Romania* 29 F10
Gaeta *Italy* 42 A6
Gaeta, G. di *Italy* 42 A6
Gaffney *U.S.A.* 117 D14
Gafsa *Tunisia* 78 B7
Gagarawa *Nigeria* 83 C6
Gagaria *India* 68 G4
Gagarin *Russia* 32 E8
Găgăuzia □ *Moldova* 29 D13
Gaggenau *Germany* 25 G4
Gaghamni *Sudan* 81 E2
Gagino *Russia* 34 C7
Gagliano del Capo *Italy* 43 C11
Gagnef *Sweden* 10 D9
Gagnoa *Ivory C.* 82 D3
Gagnon *Canada* 105 B6
Gagnon, L. *Canada* 103 A6
Gagra *Georgia* 35 J5
Gahini *Rwanda* 86 C3
Gahmar *India* 69 G10
Gai Xian = Gaizhou *China* 57 D12
Gaidouronisi *Greece* 49 E7
Gail *U.S.A.* 116 E4
Gail → *Austria* 26 E6
Gaillac *France* 20 E5
Gaillimh = Galway *Ireland* 12 C2
Gaillon *France* 18 C8
Gaines *U.S.A.* 114 E7
Gainesville *Fla., U.S.A.* 117 G13
Gainesville *Ga., U.S.A.* 117 D13
Gainesville *Mo., U.S.A.* 112 G7
Gainesville *Tex., U.S.A.* 116 E6
Gainsborough *U.K.* 14 D7
Gairdner, L. *Australia* 95 E2
Gairloch *U.K.* 13 D3
Gairloch, L. *U.K.* 13 D3
Gaizhou *China* 57 D12
Gaj *Croatia* 28 E2
Gaj → *Pakistan* 68 F2
Gakuch *Pakistan* 69 A5
Galâla, Gebel el *Egypt* 80 J8
Galán, Cerro *Argentina* 126 B2
Galana → *Kenya* 86 C5
Galanta *Slovak Rep.* 27 C10
Galápagar *Spain* 36 E7
Galápagos = Colón, Arch.
    de Ecuador *Ecuador* 122 D1
Galapagos Fracture Zone
    Pac. Oc. 97 G17
Galapagos Rise *Pac. Oc.* 97 J18
Galashiels *U.K.* 13 F6
Galatas *Greece* 46 D5
Galateia *Cyprus* 49 D13
Galați *Romania* 29 E13
Galați □ *Romania* 29 E12
Galatia *Turkey* 72 C5
Galatina *Italy* 43 B11
Galátone *Italy* 43 B11
Galax *U.S.A.* 113 G13
Galaxídi *Greece* 46 C4
Galcaio = Gaalkacyo
    Somali Rep. 75 F4
Galdhøpiggen *Norway* 8 F13
Galeana *Chihuahua, Mexico* 118 A3
Galeana *Nuevo León, Mexico* 118 A3
Galegu *Sudan* 81 E4
Galela *Indonesia* 63 D7
Galeota Pt. *Trin. & Tob.* 125 K16
Galera *Spain* 39 H2
Galera Pt. *Trin. & Tob.* 121 D7
Galesburg *U.S.A.* 112 E8
Galestan △ *Iran* 71 B8
Galeton *U.S.A.* 114 E7
Galga *Ethiopia* 81 F4
Gali *Georgia* 35 J5
Galicea Mare *Romania* 29 F8
Galich *Russia* 34 A6
Galiche *Bulgaria* 44 C7
Galicia □ *Spain* 36 C3
Galičica △ *Macedonia* 44 E4
Galilee = Hagalil *Israel* 74 C4
Galilee, L. *Australia* 94 C4
Galilee, Sea of = Yam
    Kinneret *Israel* 74 C4
Galim *Cameroon* 83 D7
Galina Pt. *Jamaica* 120 a
Galinoporni *Cyprus* 49 D13
Galion *U.S.A.* 114 F2
Galiuro Mts. *U.S.A.* 109 K8
Galiwinku *Australia* 94 A2
Gallâbat *Sudan* 81 E4
Gallan Hd. *U.K.* 13 C1
Gallarate *Italy* 40 C5
Gallatin *U.S.A.* 117 C11
Gallatin → *U.S.A.* 108 D8
Galle *Sri Lanka* 66 R12

Gállego → *Spain* 38 D4
Gallegos → *Argentina* 128 G3
Galletti → *Ethiopia* 81 F5
Galley Hd. *Ireland* 12 E3
Gallipoli = Gelibolu *Turkey* 45 F10
Gallípoli *Italy* 43 B10
Gallipolis *U.S.A.* 113 F12
Gällivare *Sweden* 8 C19
Gallneukirchen *Austria* 26 C7
Gällö *Sweden* 10 B9
Gallo, C. *Italy* 42 D6
Gallocanta, L. de *Spain* 38 E3
Galloo I. *U.S.A.* 115 C8
Galloway *U.K.* 13 F4
Galloway, Mull of *U.K.* 13 G4
Galloway △ *U.K.* 13 F4
Gallup *U.S.A.* 109 J9
Gallur *Spain* 38 D3
Galt *U.S.A.* 110 G5
Galten *Denmark* 11 H3
Galtür *Austria* 26 E3
Galty Mts. *Ireland* 12 D3
Galtymore *Ireland* 12 D3
Galugah *Iran* 71 B7
Galva *U.S.A.* 112 E9
Galve de Sorbe *Spain* 38 D1
Galveston *U.S.A.* 116 G7
Galveston B. *U.S.A.* 116 G7
Gálvez *Argentina* 126 C3
Galway *Ireland* 12 C2
Galway □ *Ireland* 12 C2
Galway B. *Ireland* 12 C2
Gam → *Vietnam* 64 B5
Gamagōri *Japan* 55 G8
Gamari, L. *Ethiopia* 81 E5
Gamawa *Nigeria* 83 C7
Gamay *Phil.* 61 E6
Gambaga *Ghana* 83 C4
Gambat *Pakistan* 68 F3
Gambela *Ethiopia* 81 F3
Gambela △ *Ethiopia* 81 F3
Gambela □ *Ethiopia* 81 F3
Gambhir → *India* 68 F6
Gambia ■ *W. Afr.* 82 C1
Gambia → *W. Afr.* 82 C1
Gambier *U.S.A.* 114 F2
Gambier, C. *Australia* 92 B5
Gambier, Îs. *French Polynesia* 97 K14
Gambier Is. *Australia* 95 F2
Gambo *Canada* 105 C9
Gamboli *Pakistan* 68 E3
Gamboma *Congo* 84 E3
Gamka → *S. Africa* 88 E3
Gamkab → *Namibia* 88 D2
Gamlakarleby = Kokkola
    Finland 8 E20
Gamleby *Sweden* 11 G10
Gammon → *Canada* 103 C9
Gammon Ranges △ *Australia* 95 E2
Gamo-Gofa *Ethiopia* 81 F4
Gamou *Niger* 83 C6
Gamtoos → *S. Africa* 88 E4
Gan *France* 20 E3
Gan Goriama, Mts. *Cameroon* 83 D7
Gan Jiang → *China* 59 C11
Ganado *U.S.A.* 109 J9
Gananita *Sudan* 80 D3
Gananoque *Canada* 115 B8
Ganāveh *Iran* 71 D6
Gäncä *Azerbaijan* 35 K8
Gancheng *China* 64 C7
Gand = Gent *Belgium* 17 C3
Ganda *Angola* 85 G2
Gandajika
    Dem. Rep. of the Congo 84 F4
Gandak → *India* 69 G11
Gandava *Pakistan* 68 E2
Gander *Canada* 105 C9
Gander L. *Canada* 105 C9
Ganderkesee *Germany* 24 B4
Ganderowe Falls *Zimbabwe* 87 F2
Gandesa *Spain* 38 D5
Gandhi Sagar *India* 68 G6
Gandhinagar *India* 68 H5
Gandi *Nigeria* 83 C6
Gandia *Spain* 39 G4
Gandino *Italy* 40 C6
Gando, Pta. *Canary Is.* 48 G4
Gandole *Nigeria* 83 D7
Gâneb *Mauritania* 82 B2
Ganedidalem = Gani
    Indonesia 63 E7
Ganga → *India* 69 H14
Ganga Sagar *India* 69 J13
Gangafani *Mali* 82 C4
Gangan → *India* 69 E8
Ganganagar *India* 68 E5
Gangapur *India* 68 F7
Gangara *Niger* 83 C6
Gangaw *Burma* 67 H19
Gangdisê Shan *China* 69 D9
Ganges = Ganga → *India* 69 H14
Ganges *Canada* 102 D4
Ganges *France* 20 E7
Ganges, Mouths of the *India* 69 J14

Ganggyeong *S. Korea* 57 F14
Gånghester *Sweden* 11 G7
Ganghwa *S. Korea* 57 F14
Gangi *Italy* 43 E7
Gângiova *Romania* 29 G8
Gangneung *S. Korea* 57 F15
Gangoh *India* 68 E7
Gangotri *India* 69 D8
Gangotri △ *India* 69 D8
Gangseong *S. Korea* 57 E15
Gangtok *India* 67 F16
Gangu *China* 56 G3
Gangyao *China* 57 B14
Gani *Indonesia* 63 E7
Ganj *India* 69 F8
Ganluc *China* 58 C4
Gannat *France* 19 F10
Gannett Peak *U.S.A.* 108 E9
Ganquan *China* 56 F5
Gänserdorf *Austria* 27 C9
Ganshui *China* 58 C6
Gansu □ *China* 56 G3
Ganta *Liberia* 82 D3
Gantheaume, C. *Australia* 95 F2
Gantheaume B. *Australia* 93 E1
Gantsevichi = Hantsavichy
    Belarus 23 B14
Ganye *Nigeria* 83 D7
Ganyem = Genyem
    Indonesia 63 E10
Ganyu *China* 57 G10
Ganyushkino *Kazakhstan* 35 G9
Ganzhou *China* 59 E10
Gao *Mali* 83 B4
Gao Xian *China* 58 C5
Gao'an *China* 59 C10
Gaochun *China* 59 B12
Gaohe *China* 59 F9
Gaohebu *China* 59 B11
Gaokeng *China* 59 D9
Gaolan Dao *China* 59 G9
Gaoligong Shan *China* 58 E2
Gaomi *China* 57 F10
Gaoping *China* 56 G7
Gaotang *China* 56 F9
Gaoua *Burkina Faso* 82 C4
Gaoual *Guinea* 82 C2
Gaoxiong = Kaohsiung
    Taiwan 59 F13
Gaoyang *China* 56 E8
Gaoyao *China* 59 F9
Gaoyou *China* 59 A12
Gaoyuan *China* 57 F9
Gaoyou Hu *China* 57 H10
Gaozhou *China* 59 G8
Gap *France* 21 D10
Gapan *Phil.* 61 D4
Gapat → *India* 69 G10
Gapuwiyak *Australia* 94 A2
Gar *China* 60 C2
Gara, L. *Ireland* 12 C3
Garáb *Iran* 73 F12
Garabogazköl Aylagy
    Turkmenistan 52 E6
Garachico *Canary Is.* 48 F3
Garachiné *Panama* 120 E4
Garafia *Canary Is.* 48 F2
Garagum *Turkmenistan* 71 B8
Garah *Australia* 95 D4
Garajonay *Canary Is.* 48 F2
Garamba △
    Dem. Rep. of the Congo 86 B2
Garango *Burkina Faso* 83 C4
Garautha *India* 69 G8
Garawa ☉ *Australia* 94 B2
Garawe *Liberia* 82 E3
Garba Tula *Kenya* 86 B4
Garberville *U.S.A.* 108 F2
Garbiyang *India* 69 D9
Garbsen *Germany* 24 C5
Gard □ *France* 21 D8
Gard → *France* 21 E8
Garda, L. di *Italy* 40 C7
Gardabani *Georgia* 35 K7
Gårdby *Sweden* 11 H10
Garde L. *Canada* 103 A7
Gardelegen *Germany* 24 C7
Garden City *Ga., U.S.A.* 117 E14
Garden City *Kans., U.S.A.* 112 G3
Garden City *Tex., U.S.A.* 116 F4
Garden Grove *U.S.A.* 111 M9
Gardēz *Afghan.* 68 C3
Gardiki *Greece* 46 C3
Gardiner *Maine, U.S.A.* 113 C19
Gardiner *Mont., U.S.A.* 108 D8
Gardiners I. *U.S.A.* 115 E12
Gardner *U.S.A.* 113 D12
Gardner Canal *Canada* 102 C3
Gardner Pinnacles *U.S.A.* 107 L6
Gardnerville *U.S.A.* 110 G7
Gardno, Jezioro *Poland* 30 D4
Gardo = Qardho *Somali Rep.* 75 F4
Gardone Val Trómpia *Italy* 40 C7
Gárdony *Hungary* 28 C3
Gares = Puente la Reina
    Spain 38 C3
Garešnica *Croatia* 41 C13

Garéssio *Italy* **40** D5
Garey *U.S.A.* **111** L6
Garfield *U.S.A.* **108** C5
Garforth *U.K.* **14** D6
Gargaliani *Greece* **46** D3
Gargan, Mt. *France* **20** C5
Gargano △ *Italy* **41** G12
Gargantua, C. *Canada* **113** B11
Gargett *Australia* **94** b
Gargouna *Mali* **83** B5
Gargždai *Lithuania* **30** C8
Garibaldi △ *Canada* **102** D4
Gariep, L. *S. Africa* **88** E4
Garies *S. Africa* **88** E2
Garig Gunak Barlu △
   Australia **92** B5
Garigliano ➤ *Italy* **42** A6
Garissa *Kenya* **86** C4
Garkida *Nigeria* **83** C7
Garko *Nigeria* **83** C6
Garland *Tex., U.S.A.* **116** E6
Garland *Utah, U.S.A.* **108** F7
Garlasco *Italy* **40** C5
Garliava *Lithuania* **30** D10
Garlin *France* **20** E3
Garmāb *Semnān, Iran* **71** C8
Garmāb *Zanjān, Iran* **73** E13
Garmisch-Partenkirchen
   Germany **25** H7
Garmsār *Iran* **71** C7
Garner *U.S.A.* **112** D7
Garnett *U.S.A.* **112** F6
Garo Hills *India* **69** G14
Garoe = Garoowe *Somali Rep.* **75** F4
Garonne ➤ *France* **20** C3
Garonne, Canal Latéral à la
   France **20** D4
Garoowe *Somali Rep.* **75** F4
Garot *India* **68** G6
Garou, L. *Mali* **82** B4
Garoua *Cameroon* **83** D7
Garpenberg *Sweden* **10** D10
Garphyttan *Sweden* **10** E8
Garrauli *India* **69** G8
Garrel *Germany* **24** C4
Garrigues *France* **20** E7
Garrison *Mont., U.S.A.* **108** C7
Garrison *N. Dak., U.S.A.* **112** B3
Garrison Res. =
   Sakakawea, L. *U.S.A.* **112** B3
Garron Pt. *U.K.* **12** A6
Garrovillas de Alconétar
   Spain **37** F4
Garrucha *Spain* **39** H3
Garry ➤ *U.K.* **13** E5
Garry, L. *Canada* **100** D11
Garrygala *Turkmenistan* **71** B8
Garsen *Kenya* **86** C5
Garson L. *Canada* **103** B6
Garstang *U.K.* **14** D5
Gartempe ➤ *France* **20** B4
Gartz *Germany* **24** B10
Garu *Ghana* **83** C4
Garu *India* **69** H11
Garub *Namibia* **88** D2
Garut *Indonesia* **63** G12
Garvão *Portugal* **37** H2
Garvie Mts. *N.Z.* **91** F2
Garw ➤ *Garoua Cameroon* **83** D7
Garwa *India* **69** G10
Garwolin *Poland* **31** G8
Gary *U.S.A.* **112** E10
Garz *Germany* **24** A9
Garzê *China* **58** B3
Garzón *Colombia* **124** C3
Gas-San *Japan* **54** E10
Gasan Kuli = Esenguly
   Turkmenistan **52** F6
Gascogne *France* **20** E4
Gascogne, G. de *Europe* **20** E2
Gascony = Gascogne *France* **20** E4
Gascoyne ➤ *Australia* **93** D1
Gascoyne Junction *Australia* **93** E2
Gascueña *Spain* **38** E2
Gash, Wadi ➤ *Africa* **81** D4
Gash Setit = *Eritrea* **81** D4
Gashagar *Nigeria* **83** C7
Gashaka *Nigeria* **83** D7
Gashaka-Gumti △ *Nigeria* **83** D7
Gasherbrum *Pakistan* **69** B7
Gashua *Nigeria* **83** C7
Gasparillo *Trin. & Tob.* **125** K15
Gaspé *Canada* **105** C7
Gaspé, C. de *Canada* **105** C7
Gaspé Pen. = Gaspésie,
   Pén. de la *Canada* **105** C6
Gaspésie, Pén. de la *Canada* **105** C6
Gaspésie △ *Canada* **105** C6
Gassan *Burkina Faso* **82** C4
Gassol *Nigeria* **83** D7
Gasteiz = Vitoria-Gasteiz
   Spain **38** C2
Gastonia *U.S.A.* **117** D14
Gastouni *Greece* **46** D3
Gastouri *Greece* **46** B1
Gastre *Argentina* **128** E3
Gästrikland *Sweden* **10** D10
Gata, C. *Cyprus* **49** E12

Gata, C. de *Spain* **39** J2
Gata, Sierra de *Spain* **36** E4
Gataga ➤ *Canada* **102** B3
Gătaia *Romania* **28** E6
Gatchina *Russia* **32** C6
Gatehouse of Fleet *U.K.* **13** G4
Gates *U.S.A.* **114** C7
Gateshead *U.K.* **14** C6
Gateshead I. *Canada* **100** C11
Gatesville *U.S.A.* **116** F6
Gateway △ *U.S.A.* **115** F11
Gaths *Zimbabwe* **87** G3
Gâtinais *France* **19** D9
Gâtine, Hauteurs de *France* **20** B3
Gatineau *Canada* **115** A9
Gatineau ➤ *Canada* **104** C4
Gatineau △ *Canada* **104** C4
Gattaran *Phil.* **61** B4
Gatton *Australia* **95** D5
Gatún, L. *Panama* **120** E4
Gatwick, London ✈ (LGW)
   U.K. **15** F7
Gatyana *S. Africa* **89** E4
Gau *Fiji* **91** a
Gaucín *Spain* **37** J5
Gauer L. *Canada* **103** B9
Gauhati = Guwahati *India* **67** F17
Gauja ➤ *Latvia* **30** A11
Gaujas △ *Latvia* **9** H21
Gaula ➤ *Norway* **8** E14
Gauri Phanta *India* **69** E9
Gaustatoppen *Norway* **9** G13
Gauteng □ *S. Africa* **89** D4
Gāv Koshī *Iran* **71** D8
Gāvakān *Iran* **71** D7
Gavarnie *France* **20** F3
Gavāter *Iran* **71** E9
Gāvbandī *Iran* **71** E7
Gavdopoula *Greece* **49** E6
Gavdos *Greece* **49** E6
Gavi *Italy* **40** D5
Gavião *Portugal* **37** F3
Gāvkhūnī, Bāţlāq-e *Iran* **71** C7
Gävle *Sweden* **10** D11
Gävleborgs län □ *Sweden* **10** C10
Gävlebukten *Sweden* **10** D11
Gavorrano *Italy* **40** F7
Gavray *France* **18** D5
Gavrilov Yam *Russia* **32** D10
Gavrio *Greece* **46** D6
Gawachab *Namibia* **88** D2
Gawilgarh Hills *India* **66** J10
Gawler *Australia* **95** E2
Gawler Ranges *Australia* **95** E2
Gawu *Nigeria* **83** D6
Gaxun Nur *China* **60** B5
Gaya *India* **69** G11
Gaya ➤ *Niger* **83** C5
Gaya *Nigeria* **83** C6
Gayéri *Burkina Faso* **83** C5
Gaylord *U.S.A.* **113** C11
Gayndah *Australia* **95** D5
Gaysin = Haysyn *Ukraine* **29** B14
Gayvoron = Hayvoron
   Ukraine **29** B14
Gaza *Gaza Strip* **74** D3
Gaza □ *Mozam.* **89** C5
Gaza Strip ■ *Asia* **74** D3
Gazanjyk = Bereket
   Turkmenistan **71** B7
Gazaoua *Niger* **83** C6
Gāzbor *Iran* **71** D8
Gazi *Dem. Rep. of the Congo* **86** B1
Gaziantep *Turkey* **72** D7
Gaziantep □ *Turkey* **72** D7
Gazimağusa = Famagusta
   Cyprus **49** D12
Gazipaşa *Turkey* **72** D5
Gbadolite
   Dem. Rep. of the Congo **84** D4
Gbarnga *Liberia* **82** D3
Gboko *Nigeria* **83** D6
Gbongan *Nigeria* **83** D5
Gcoverega *Botswana* **88** B3
Gcuwa *S. Africa* **89** E4
Gdańsk *Poland* **30** D5
Gdańsk ✈ (GDN) *Poland* **30** D5
Gdańska, Zatoka *Poland* **30** D6
Gdov *Russia* **32** C4
Gdynia *Poland* **30** D5
Geba ➤ *Guinea-Biss.* **82** C1
Gebe *Indonesia* **63** D7
Gebeciler *Turkey* **47** C12
Gebeit Mine *Sudan* **80** C4
Gebel Abyad *Sudan* **80** D2
Gebel Iweibid *Egypt* **80** H8
Gebze *Turkey* **45** F13
Gecha *Ethiopia* **81** F4
Gedaref *Sudan* **81** E4
Gedaref □ *Sudan* **81** E4
Gediz *Turkey* **47** B11
Gediz ➤ *Turkey* **47** C8
Gedo *Ethiopia* **81** F4
Gèdre *France* **20** F4
Gedser *Denmark* **11** K5
Gedung, Pulau *Malaysia* **65** c
Geegully Cr. ➤ *Australia* **92** C3

Geel *Belgium* **17** C4
Geelong *Australia* **95** F3
Geelvink B. =
   Cenderawasih, Teluk
   Indonesia **63** E9
Geelvink Chan. *Australia* **93** E1
Geesthacht *Germany* **24** B6
Geidam *Nigeria* **83** C7
Geikie ➤ *Canada* **103** B8
Geikie Gorge △ *Australia* **92** C4
Geilenkirchen *Germany* **24** E2
Geili *Sudan* **81** D3
Geisingen *Germany* **25** H4
Geislingen *Germany* **25** G5
Geistown *U.S.A.* **114** F6
Geita *Tanzania* **86** C3
Gejiu *China* **58** F4
Gel ➤ *Sudan* **81** F2
Gel, Meydān-e *Iran* **71** D7
Gel River *Sudan* **81** F2
Gela *Italy* **43** E7
Gela, G. di *Italy* **43** F7
Gelahun *Liberia* **82** D2
Gelang Patah *Malaysia* **65** d
Gelderland □ *Neths.* **17** B6
Geldern *Germany* **24** D2
Geldrop *Neths.* **17** C5
Geleen *Neths.* **17** D5
Gelehun *S. Leone* **82** D2
Gelembe *Turkey* **47** B9
Gelemso *Ethiopia* **81** F5
Gelendost *Turkey* **72** C4
Gelendzhik *Russia* **33** K10
Gelib = Jilib *Somali Rep.* **75** G3
Gelibolu *Turkey* **45** F10
Gelibolu Yarımadası *Turkey* **45** F10
Gelidonya Burnu *Turkey* **72** D4
Gelnhausen *Germany* **25** E5
Gelnica *Slovak Rep.* **27** C13
Gelsenkirchen *Germany* **24** D3
Gelting *Germany* **24** A5
Gelugur *Malaysia* **65** c
Gemas *Malaysia* **65** L4
Gembloux *Belgium* **17** D4
Gembu *Nigeria* **83** D7
Gemena *Dem. Rep. of the Congo* **84** D3
Gemerek *Turkey* **72** C7
Gemla *Sweden* **11** H8
Gemlik *Turkey* **45** F13
Gemlik Körfezi *Turkey* **45** F12
Gemona del Friuli *Italy* **41** B10
Gemsa *Egypt* **80** B3
Gemsbok △ *Botswana* **88** D3
Gemünden *Germany* **25** E5
Genadi *Greece* **49** C9
Genale ➤ *Ethiopia* **81** F4
Genç *Turkey* **73** C9
Gençay *France* **20** B4
Geneina, Gebel *Egypt* **80** B3
General Acha *Argentina* **126** D3
General Alvear *B. Aires,
   Argentina* **126** D4
General Alvear *Mendoza,
   Argentina* **126** D2
General Artigas *Paraguay* **126** B4
General Belgrano *Argentina* **126** D4
General Bernardo
   O'Higgins *Antarctica* **5** C18
General Cabrera *Argentina* **126** C3
General Cepeda *Mexico* **118** B4
General Guido *Argentina* **126** D4
General Juan Madariaga
   Argentina **126** D4
General La Madrid
   Argentina **126** D3
General MacArthur *Phil.* **61** F6
General Martin Miguel de
   Güemes *Argentina* **126** A3
General Pico *Argentina* **126** D3
General Pinedo *Argentina* **126** B3
General Pinto *Argentina* **126** C3
General Roca *Argentina* **128** D3
General Santos *Phil.* **61** H6
General Toshevo *Bulgaria* **45** C12
General Treviño *Mexico* **119** B5
General Trías *Mexico* **118** B3
General Viamonte *Argentina* **126** D3
General Villegas *Argentina* **126** D3
Genesee *Idaho, U.S.A.* **108** C5
Genesee *Pa., U.S.A.* **114** E7
Genesee ➤ *U.S.A.* **114** C7
Geneseo *Ill., U.S.A.* **112** E8
Geneseo *N.Y., U.S.A.* **114** D7
Geneva = Genève *Switz.* **25** J2
Geneva *Ala., U.S.A.* **117** F12
Geneva *N.Y., U.S.A.* **114** D7
Geneva *Nebr., U.S.A.* **112** E5
Geneva *Ohio, U.S.A.* **114** E4
Geneva, L. = Léman, L.
   Europe **19** F13
Genève *Switz.* **25** J2
Gengenbach *Germany* **25** G4
Gengma *China* **58** F2
Genichesk = Henichesk
   Ukraine **33** J8
Genil ➤ *Spain* **37** H5
Genisea *Greece* **45** E8
Genk *Belgium* **17** D5
Genlis *France* **19** E12

Gennargentu, Mti. del *Italy* **42** B2
Gennes *France* **18** E6
Génova = Génova *Italy* **40** D5
Genoa *Australia* **95** F4
Genoa *N.Y., U.S.A.* **115** D8
Genoa *Nebr., U.S.A.* **112** E5
Genoa *Nev., U.S.A.* **110** F7
Génova *Italy* **40** D5
Génova ✈ (GOA) *Italy* **40** D5
Génova, G. di *Italy* **40** E6
Genriyetty, Ostrov *Russia* **53** B16
Gent *Belgium* **17** C3
Genteng *Bali, Indonesia* **63** J17
Genteng *Jawa Barat,
   Indonesia* **63** G12
Genthin *Germany* **24** C8
Genyem *Indonesia* **63** E10
Genzano di Lucánia *Italy* **43** B9
Genzano di Roma *Italy* **41** G9
Geoagiu *Romania* **29** E8
Geochang *S. Korea* **57** G14
Geographe B. *Australia* **93** F2
Geographe Chan. *Australia* **93** D1
Geokchay = Göyçay
   Azerbaijan **35** K8
Georga, Zemlya *Russia* **52** A5
George *S. Africa* **88** E3
George ➤ *Canada* **105** A6
George, L. *N.S.W., Australia* **95** F4
George, L. *S. Austral., Australia* **95** F3
George, L. *W. Austral.,
   Australia* **92** D3
George, L. *Uganda* **86** B3
George, L. *Fla., U.S.A.* **117** G14
George, L. *N.Y., U.S.A.* **115** C11
George Gill Ra. *Australia* **92** D5
George Pt. *Australia* **94** b
George River =
   Kangiqsualujjuaq *Canada* **101** F18
George Sound *N.Z.* **91** F1
George Town *Australia* **95** G4
George Town *Bahamas* **120** B4
George Town *Cayman Is.* **120** C3
George Town *Malaysia* **65** c
George V Land *Antarctica* **5** C10
George VI Sound *Antarctica* **5** D17
George West *U.S.A.* **116** G5
Georgetown = Janjanbureh
   Gambia **82** C2
Georgetown *Australia* **94** B3
Georgetown *Ont., Canada* **114** C5
Georgetown *P.E.I., Canada* **105** C7
Georgetown *Guyana* **124** B7
Georgetown *Calif., U.S.A.* **110** G6
Georgetown *Colo., U.S.A.* **108** G11
Georgetown *Ky., U.S.A.* **113** F11
Georgetown *N.Y., U.S.A.* **115** D9
Georgetown *Ohio, U.S.A.* **113** F12
Georgetown *S.C., U.S.A.* **117** E15
Georgetown *Tex., U.S.A.* **116** F6
Georgia □ *U.S.A.* **117** E13
Georgia ■ *Asia* **35** J6
Georgia, Str. of *N. Amer.* **110** A3
Georgia Basin *S. Ocean* **5** B1
Georgian Bay Islands △
   Canada **114** B4
Georgīevka *Kazakhstan* **52** E9
Georgina ➤ *Australia* **94** C2
Georgina I. *Canada* **114** B5
Georgioupoli *Greece* **49** D6
Georgiyevsk *Russia* **35** H7
Georgsmarienhütte *Germany* **24** C4
Gera *Germany* **24** E8
Geraardsbergen *Belgium* **17** D3
Geraki *Greece* **46** D4
Geral, Serra *Brazil* **127** B6
Geral de Goiás, Serra *Brazil* **125** F9
Geraldine *U.S.A.* **108** C8
Geraldton *Australia* **93** E1
Geraldton *Canada* **104** C2
Gérardmer *France* **19** D13
Gercüş *Turkey* **73** D9
Gerdine, Mt. *U.S.A.* **106** C9
Gerede *Turkey* **72** B5
Gerês, Sierra do *Portugal* **36** D3
Gereshk *Afghan.* **66** D4
Gerik *Malaysia* **65** K3
Gering *U.S.A.* **112** E2
Gerlach *U.S.A.* **108** F4
Gerlachovský štit
   Slovak Rep. **27** B13
German Bight = Deutsche
   Bucht *Germany* **24** A4
German Planina *Macedonia* **44** D6
Germansen Landing *Canada* **102** B4
Germantown *U.S.A.* **117** D10
Germany ■ *Europe* **24** E6
Germencik *Turkey* **47** D9
Germering *Germany* **25** G7
Germersheim *Germany* **25** F4
Germī *Iran* **73** C13
Germiston *S. Africa* **89** D4
Gernika-Lumo *Spain* **38** B2
Gernsheim *Germany* **25** F4
Gero *Japan* **55** G8

Gerokgak *Indonesia* **63** J17
Gerolzhofen *Germany* **25** F6
Gerona = Girona *Spain* **38** D7
Geropotamos ➤ *Greece* **49** D6
Gerrard *Canada* **102** C5
Gers □ *France* **20** E4
Gers ➤ *France* **20** D4
Gersfeld *Germany* **24** E5
Gersthofen *Germany* **25** G6
Gertak Sanggul *Malaysia* **65** c
Gertak Sanggul, Tanjung
   Malaysia **65** c
Gerung *Indonesia* **63** K19
Gerzat *France* **20** C7
Gerze *Turkey* **72** B6
Geseke *Germany* **24** D4
Geser *Indonesia* **63** E8
Gesso ➤ *Italy* **40** D4
Gestro, Wabi ➤ *Ethiopia* **81** G5
Getafe *Spain* **36** E7
Getinge *Sweden* **11** H6
Gettysburg *Pa., U.S.A.* **113** F15
Gettysburg *S. Dak., U.S.A.* **112** C4
Getxo *Spain* **38** B2
Getz Ice Shelf *Antarctica* **5** D14
Gevaş *Turkey* **73** C10
Gévaudan *France* **20** D7
Gevgelija *Macedonia* **44** E6
Gévora ➤ *Spain* **37** G4
Gewani *Ethiopia* **81** E5
Gex *France* **19** F13
Geyikli *Turkey* **47** B8
Geyser *U.S.A.* **108** C8
Geyserville *U.S.A.* **110** G4
Geyve *Turkey* **72** B4
Ghâbat el Arab = Wang
   Kai *Sudan* **81** F2
Ghabeish *Sudan* **81** E2
Ghadaf, W. al ➤ *Iraq* **73** F10
Ghadāmis *Libya* **79** B8
Ghaggar ➤ *India* **68** E6
Ghaghara ➤ *India* **69** G11
Ghaghat ➤ *Bangla.* **69** G13
Ghagra *India* **69** H11
Ghagra ➤ *India* **69** F9
Ghalla, Wadi el ➤ *Sudan* **81** E2
Ghallamane *Mauritania* **78** D4
Ghana ■ *W. Afr.* **83** D4
Ghansor *India* **69** H9
Ghanzi *Botswana* **88** C3
Gharb Bahr el Ghazâl □
   Sudan **81** F2
Gharb el Istiwa'iya □ *Sudan* **81** G3
Gharb Kordofân □ *Sudan* **81** E2
Gharbîya, Es Sahrâ el *Egypt* **80** B2
Ghardaïa *Algeria* **78** B6
Ghârib, G. *Egypt* **80** B3
Gharig *Sudan* **81** E2
Gharm *Tajikistan* **52** F8
Gharyān *Libya* **79** B8
Ghat *Libya* **79** D8
Ghatal *India* **69** H12
Ghatampur *India* **69** F9
Ghats, Eastern *India* **66** N11
Ghats, Western *India* **66** N9
Ghatsila *India* **69** H12
Ghaţţī *Si. Arabia* **70** D3
Ghawdex = Gozo *Malta* **49** C1
Ghazal, Bahr el ➤ *Chad* **79** F9
Ghazâl, Bahr el ➤ *Sudan* **81** F2
Ghaziabad *India* **68** E7
Ghazipur *India* **69** G10
Ghaznī *Afghan.* **68** C3
Ghaznī □ *Afghan.* **66** C6
Ghedi *Italy* **40** C7
Ghelari *Romania* **28** E7
Ghent = Gent *Belgium* **17** C3
Gheorghe Gheorghiu-Dej =
   Oneşti *Romania* **29** D11
Gheorgheni *Romania* **29** D10
Gherla *Romania* **29** C8
Ghidigeni *Romania* **29** D12
Ghilarza *Italy* **42** B1
Ghīnah, Wādī al ➤
   Si. Arabia **70** D3
Ghizar ➤ *Pakistan* **69** A5
Ghot Ogrein *Egypt* **80** A2
Ghotaru *India* **68** F4
Ghotki *Pakistan* **68** E3
Ghowr □ *Afghan.* **66** C4
Ghughri *India* **69** H9
Ghugus *India* **66** K11
Ghulam Mohammad
   Barrage *Pakistan* **68** G3
Ghūrīān *Afghan.* **66** B2
Gia Dinh *Vietnam* **65** G6
Gia Lai = Plei Ku *Vietnam* **64** F7
Gia Nghia *Vietnam* **65** G6
Gia Ngoc *Vietnam* **64** E7
Gia Vuc *Vietnam* **64** E7
Giali *Greece* **47** E9
Gialtra *Greece* **46** C4
Giamama = Jamaame
   Somali Rep. **75** G3
Gianitsa *Greece* **44** F6
Giannutri *Italy* **40** F8

Giant Forest *U.S.A.* **110** J8
Giant Mts. = Krkonoše
   Czech Rep. **26** A8
Giant Sequoia △ *U.S.A.* **110** K8
Giants Causeway *U.K.* **12** A5
Gianyar *Indonesia* **63** K18
Giarabub = Al Jaghbūb
   Libya **79** C10
Giaros *Greece* **46** D6
Giarre *Italy* **43** E8
Giaveno *Italy* **40** C4
Gibara *Cuba* **120** B4
Gibb ➤ *U.S.A.* **112** E4
Gibbon *U.S.A.* **112** E5
Gibe ➤ *Ethiopia* **81** F4
Gibellina Nuova *Italy* **42** E5
Gibeon *Namibia* **88** D2
Gibraleón *Spain* **37** H4
Gibraltar ☑ *Europe* **37** J5
Gibraltar, Str. of *Medit. S.* **37** K5
Gibraltar Range △ *Australia* **95** D5
Gibson Desert *Australia* **92** D4
Gibsons *Canada* **102** D4
Gibsonville *U.S.A.* **110** F6
Giddings *U.S.A.* **116** F6
Gidole *Ethiopia* **81** F4
Giebnegáisi = Kebnekaise
   Sweden **8** C18
Gien *France* **19** E9
Giengen *Germany* **25** G6
Giessen *Germany* **24** E4
Gīfan *Iran* **71** B8
Gifatin, Geziret *Egypt* **80** B3
Gifhorn *Germany* **24** C6
Gift Lake *Canada* **102** B5
Gifu *Japan* **55** G8
Gifu □ *Japan* **55** G8
Gigant *Russia* **35** G5
Giganta, Sa. de la *Mexico* **118** B2
Gigen *Bulgaria* **45** C8
Gigha *U.K.* **13** F3
Gíglio *Italy* **40** F7
Gignac *France* **20** E7
Gigüela ➤ *Spain* **37** F7
Gijón *Spain* **36** B5
Gikongoro *Rwanda* **86** C2
Gil I. *Canada* **102** C3
Gila ➤ *U.S.A.* **109** K6
Gila Bend *U.S.A.* **109** K7
Gila Bend Mts. *U.S.A.* **109** K7
Gila Cliff Dwellings △
   U.S.A. **109** K9
Gīlān □ *Iran* **71** B6
Gīlān-e Gharb *Iran* **73** E11
Gilău *Romania* **29** D8
Gilbert ➤ *Australia* **94** B3
Gilbert Is. *Kiribati* **90** A10
Gilbert River *Australia* **94** B3
Gilbert Seamounts *Pac. Oc.* **4** D18
Gilead *U.S.A.* **115** B14
Gilf el Kebîr, Hadabat el
   Egypt **80** C2
Gilford I. *Canada* **102** C3
Gilgandra *Australia* **95** E4
Gilgil *Kenya* **86** C4
Gilgit *India* **69** B6
Gilgit ➤ *Pakistan* **69** B6
Gili △ *Mozam.* **87** F4
Gilimanuk *Indonesia* **63** J17
Giljeva Planina *Europe* **44** C3
Gillam *Canada* **103** B10
Gilleleje *Denmark* **11** H6
Gillen, L. *Australia* **93** E3
Gilles, L. *Australia* **95** E2
Gillette *U.S.A.* **108** D11
Gilliat *Australia* **94** C3
Gillingham *U.K.* **15** F8
Gilmer *U.S.A.* **116** E7
Gilmore, L. *Australia* **93** F3
Gilmour *Canada* **114** B7
Gilo ➤ *Ethiopia* **81** F3
Gilort ➤ *Romania* **29** F8
Gilroy *U.S.A.* **110** H5
Gimbi *Ethiopia* **81** F4
Gimcheon *S. Korea* **57** F15
Gimhae *S. Korea* **57** G15
Gimhwa *S. Korea* **57** E14
Gimie, Mt *St. Lucia* **121** f
Gimje *S. Korea* **57** G14
Gimli *Canada* **103** C9
Gimo *Sweden* **10** D12
Gimone ➤ *France* **20** E5
Gimont *France* **20** E4
Gin Gin *Australia* **95** D5
Gináh *Egypt* **80** B3
Gingin *Australia* **93** F2
Gingindlovu *S. Africa* **89** D5
Gingoog *Phil.* **61** G6
Ginir *Ethiopia* **81** F5
Ginosa *Italy* **43** B9
Ginzo de Limia = Xinzo de
   Limia *Spain* **36** C3
Giofyros ➤ *Greece* **49** D7
Giohar = Jawhar *Somali Rep.* **75** G4
Gióia, G. di *Italy* **43** D8
Gióia del Colle *Italy* **43** B9
Gióia Táuro *Italy* **43** D8
Gioiosa Iónica *Italy* **43** D9
Gioiosa Marea *Italy* **43** D7

Giona, Oros Greece 46 C4
Giovi, Passo dei Italy 40 D5
Giovinazzo Italy 43 A9
Gir △ India 68 J4
Gir Hills India 68 J4
Girab India 68 F4
Girâfi, W. → Egypt 74 F3
Giraltovce Slovak Rep. 27 B14
Girard St. Lucia 121 D7
Girard Kans., U.S.A. 112 G6
Girard Ohio, U.S.A. 114 E4
Girard Pa., U.S.A. 114 E4
Girdle Ness U.K. 13 D6
Giresun Turkey 73 B8
Giresun □ Turkey 73 B8
Girga Egypt 80 B3
Giri → India 68 D7
Giridih India 69 G12
Girifalco Italy 43 D9
Giriftu Kenya 86 B4
Giriyondo S. Africa 89 C5
Girne = Kyrenia Cyprus 49 D12
Giro Nigeria 83 C5
Giromagny France 19 E13
Giron = Kiruna Sweden 8 C19
Girona Spain 38 D7
Girona □ Spain 38 C7
Gironde □ France 20 D3
Gironde → France 20 C2
Gironella Spain 38 C6
Girraween △ Australia 95 D5
Girringun △ Australia 94 B4
Giru Australia 94 B4
Girvan U.K. 13 F4
Gisborne N.Z. 91 C7
Gisenyi Rwanda 86 C2
Gislaved Sweden 11 G7
Gisors France 19 C8
Gitarama Rwanda 86 C2
Gitega Burundi 86 C2
Githio Greece 46 E4
Giuba = Juba → Somali Rep. 75 G3
Giugliano in Campania Italy 43 B7
Giulianova Italy 41 F10
Giura Greece 46 B6
Giurgeni Romania 29 F12
Giurgiu Romania 29 G10
Giurgiu □ Romania 29 F10
Giurgiulești Moldova 29 E13
Give Denmark 11 J3
Givet France 19 B11
Givors France 21 C8
Givry France 19 F11
Giyon Ethiopia 81 F4
Giza = El Gîza Egypt 80 J7
Giza Pyramids Egypt 80 J7
Gizab Afghan. 68 C1
Gizhiga Russia 53 C17
Gizhiginskaya Guba Russia 53 C16
Giżycko Poland 30 D8
Gizzeria Italy 43 D9
Gjalicë e Lumës, Mal. Albania 44 D4
Gjegjan Albania 44 E4
Gjirokastër Albania 44 F4
Gjoa Haven Canada 100 D12
Gjøvik Norway 8 F14
Gjuhës, Kep i Albania 44 F3
Glace Bay Canada 105 C8
Glacier △ Canada 102 C5
Glacier △ U.S.A. 108 B7
Glacier Bay U.S.A. 100 F4
Glacier Bay ⌂ U.S.A. 102 B1
Glacier Peak U.S.A. 108 B3
Gladewater U.S.A. 116 E7
Gladstone Queens., Australia 94 C5
Gladstone S. Austral., Australia 95 E2
Gladstone Canada 103 C9
Gladstone U.S.A. 112 C10
Gladwin U.S.A. 113 D11
Glafsfjorden Sweden 10 E6
Glagah Indonesia 63 J17
Głagów Małapolski Poland 31 H8
Glåma = Glomma → Norway 9 G14
Gláma Iceland 8 D2
Glamis U.S.A. 111 N11
Glamoč Bos.-H. 41 D13
Glamorgan, Vale of □ U.K. 15 F4
Glamsbjerg Denmark 11 J4
Glarus Switz. 25 H5
Glarus □ Switz. 25 J5
Glasco Kans., U.S.A. 112 F5
Glasco N.Y., U.S.A. 115 D11
Glasgow U.K. 13 F4
Glasgow Ky., U.S.A. 113 G11
Glasgow Mont., U.S.A. 108 B10
Glasgow, City of □ U.K. 13 F4
Glasgow Int. ✕ (GLA) U.K. 13 F4
Glaslyn Canada 103 C7
Glastonbury U.K. 15 F5
Glastonbury U.S.A. 115 E12
Glauchau Germany 24 E8
Glava Sweden 10 E6
Glavice Croatia 41 E13
Glazov Russia 34 A11
Gleichen Canada 102 C6
Gleisdorf Austria 26 D8
Gleiwitz = Gliwice Poland 31 H5
Glen U.S.A. 115 B13
Glen Affric U.K. 13 D3
Glen Canyon U.S.A. 109 H8
Glen Canyon ⌂ U.S.A. 109 H8
Glen Canyon Dam U.S.A. 109 H8
Glen Coe U.K. 13 E3
Glen Cove U.S.A. 115 F11
Glen Garry U.K. 13 D3
Glen Innes Australia 95 D5
Glen Lyon U.S.A. 115 E8
Glen Mor U.K. 13 D4
Glen More ⌂ U.K. 13 D5
Glen Moriston U.K. 13 D4
Glen Robertson Canada 115 A10
Glen Spean U.K. 13 E4
Glen Ullin U.S.A. 112 B3
Glénan, Îs. de France 18 E3
Glenariff △ Ireland 12 A5
Glenbeigh Ireland 12 D2
Glencoe Canada 114 D3
Glencoe S. Africa 89 D5
Glencoe U.S.A. 112 C6
Glencolumbkille Ireland 12 B3
Glendale Ariz., U.S.A. 109 K7
Glendale Calif., U.S.A. 111 L8
Glendale Zimbabwe 87 F3
Glendive U.S.A. 108 C11
Glendo U.S.A. 108 E11
Glenelg → Australia 95 F3
Glenfield U.S.A. 115 C9
Glengad Hd. Ireland 12 A4
Glengarriff Ireland 12 E2
Glenmont U.S.A. 114 F2
Glenmorgan Australia 95 D4
Glenn U.S.A. 110 F4
Glennallen U.S.A. 100 E2
Glennamaddy Ireland 12 C3
Glenns Ferry U.S.A. 108 E6
Glenora Canada 114 B7
Glenorchy Australia 95 G4
Glenore Australia 94 B3
Glenreagh Australia 95 E5
Glenrock U.S.A. 108 E11
Glenrothes U.K. 13 E5
Glens Falls U.S.A. 115 C11
Glenside U.S.A. 115 F9
Glenties Ireland 12 B3
Glenveagh △ Ireland 12 A3
Glenville U.S.A. 113 F13
Glenwood Canada 105 C9
Glenwood Ark., U.S.A. 116 D8
Glenwood Iowa, U.S.A. 112 E6
Glenwood Minn., U.S.A. 112 C6
Glenwood Wash., U.S.A. 110 D5
Glenwood Springs U.S.A. 108 G10
Glettinganes Iceland 8 D7
Glifada Greece 46 D5
Glimåkra Sweden 11 H8
Glin Ireland 12 D2
Glina Croatia 41 C13
Glinojeck Poland 31 F7
Gliwice Poland 31 H5
Globe U.S.A. 109 K8
Glodeanu Siliștea Romania 29 F11
Glodeni Moldova 29 C12
Glödnitz Austria 26 E7
Gloggnitz Austria 26 D8
Głogów Poland 31 G3
Głogówek Poland 31 H4
Glomma → Norway 9 G14
Glorieuses, Îs. Ind. Oc. 89 A8
Glosa Greece 46 B5
Glossop U.K. 14 D6
Gloucester Australia 95 E5
Gloucester U.K. 15 F5
Gloucester U.S.A. 115 D14
Gloucester I. Australia 94 b
Gloucester Island △ Australia 94 b
Gloucester Point U.S.A. 113 G15
Gloucestershire □ U.K. 15 F5
Gloversville U.S.A. 115 C10
Glovertown Canada 105 C9
Głowno Poland 31 G6
Głubczyce Poland 31 H4
Glubokiy Russia 35 F5
Glubokoye = Hlybokaye Belarus 32 E4
Głuchołazy Poland 31 H4
Glücksburg Germany 24 A5
Glückstadt Germany 24 B5
Glukhov = Hlukhiv Ukraine 33 G7
Glusk Belarus 23 B15
Głuszyca Poland 31 H3
Glyngøre Denmark 11 H2
Gmünd Kärnten, Austria 26 E6
Gmünd Niederösterreich, Austria 26 C8
Gmunden Austria 26 D6
Gnarp Sweden 10 B11
Gnesta Sweden 10 E11
Gniew Poland 30 E5
Gniewkowo Poland 31 F5
Gniezno Poland 31 F4
Gnjilane Kosovo 44 D5
Gnoien Germany 24 B8
Gnosjö Sweden 11 G7
Gnowangerup Australia 93 F2
Go Cong Vietnam 65 G6
Gō-no-ura Japan 55 H4
Goa India 66 M8
Goa □ India 66 M8
Goalen Hd. Australia 95 F5
Goalpara India 67 F17
Goaltor India 69 H12
Goalundo Ghat Bangla. 69 H13
Goaso Ghana 82 D4
Goat Fell U.K. 13 F3
Goba Ethiopia 81 F4
Goba Mozam. 89 D5
Gobabis Namibia 88 C2
Göbel Turkey 45 F12
Gobi Asia 56 C6
Gobō Japan 55 H7
Gobo Sudan 81 F3
Göçbeyli Turkey 47 B9
Goch Germany 24 D2
Gochas Namibia 88 C2
Godalming U.K. 15 F7
Godavari → India 67 L13
Godavari Pt. India 67 L13
Godbout Canada 105 C6
Godda India 69 G12
Godech Bulgaria 44 C7
Goderich Canada 114 C3
Goderville France 18 C7
Godfrey Ra. Australia 93 D2
Godhavn = Qeqertarsuaq Greenland 4 C5
Godhra India 68 H5
Gödöllő Hungary 28 C4
Godoy Cruz Argentina 126 C2
Gods → Canada 104 A1
Gods L. Canada 104 B1
Gods River Canada 103 C10
Godthåb = Nuuk Greenland 99 C14
Goeie Hoop, Kaap die = Good Hope, C. of S. Africa 88 E2
Goéland, L. au Canada 104 C4
Goélands, L. aux Canada 105 A7
Goeree Neths. 17 C3
Goes Neths. 17 C3
Goffstown U.S.A. 115 C13
Gogama Canada 104 C3
Gogebic, L. U.S.A. 112 B9
Goggetti Ethiopia 81 F4
Gogolin Poland 31 H5
Gogonou Benin 83 C5
Gogra = Ghaghara → India 69 G11
Gogriâl Sudan 81 F2
Gogti Ethiopia 81 E5
Gohana India 68 E7
Goharganj India 68 H7
Goi → India 68 H6
Goiânia Brazil 125 G9
Goiás Brazil 125 G8
Goiás □ Brazil 125 F9
Goio-Erê Brazil 127 A5
Góis Portugal 36 E2
Gojam Ethiopia 81 E4
Gojeb, Wabi → Ethiopia 81 F4
Gojō Japan 55 G7
Gojra Pakistan 68 D5
Gökçeada Turkey 45 F9
Gökçedağ Turkey 47 B10
Gökçen Turkey 47 C9
Gökçeören Turkey 47 C10
Gökçeyazı Turkey 47 B9
Gökırmak → Turkey 72 B6
Gökova Turkey 47 D10
Gökova Körfezi Turkey 47 E9
Göksu → Turkey 72 D6
Göksun Turkey 72 C7
Gokteik Burma 67 H20
Göktepe Turkey 47 D10
Gokurt Pakistan 68 E2
Gokwe Zimbabwe 89 B4
Gola India 69 E9
Golakganj India 69 F13
Golan Heights = Hagolan Syria 74 C4
Gołańcz Poland 31 F4
Golāshkerd Iran 71 E8
Golaya Pristen = Hola Pristan Ukraine 33 J7
Gölbaşı Adiyaman, Turkey 72 D7
Gölbaşı Ankara, Turkey 72 C5
Golchikha Russia 4 B12
Golconda U.S.A. 108 F5
Gölcük Kocaeli, Turkey 45 F13
Gölcük Niğde, Turkey 72 C6
Gold U.S.A. 114 E7
Gold Beach U.S.A. 108 E1
Gold Coast W. Afr. 83 E4
Gold Hill U.S.A. 108 E2
Gold River Canada 102 D3
Goldap Poland 30 D9
Goldberg Germany 24 B8
Golden Canada 102 C5
Golden B. N.Z. 91 D4
Golden Gate U.S.A. 109 H2
Golden Gate Highlands △ S. Africa 89 D4
Golden Hinde Canada 102 D3
Golden Lake Canada 114 A7
Golden Spike ⌂ U.S.A. 108 F7
Golden Vale Ireland 12 D3
Goldendale U.S.A. 108 D3
Goldfield U.S.A. 109 H5
Goldsand L. Canada 103 B8
Goldsboro U.S.A. 117 D16
Goldsmith U.S.A. 116 F3
Goldthwaite U.S.A. 116 F5
Golegã Portugal 37 F2
Goleniów Poland 30 E1
Golestān □ Iran 71 B7
Golestānak Iran 71 D7
Goleta U.S.A. 111 L7
Golfito Costa Rica 120 E3
Golfo Aranci Italy 42 B2
Golfo di Orosei e del Gennargentu △ Italy 42 B2
Gölgeli Dağları Turkey 47 D10
Gölhisar Turkey 47 D11
Goliad U.S.A. 116 G6
Golija Montenegro 44 C2
Golija Serbia 44 C4
Golina Poland 31 F5
Gölköy Turkey 72 B7
Göllersdorf Austria 26 C9
Gölmarmara Turkey 47 C9
Golo → France 21 F13
Gölova Turkey 47 E12
Golpāyegān Iran 71 C6
Gölpazarı Turkey 72 B4
Golra Pakistan 68 C5
Golspie U.K. 13 D5
Golub-Dobrzyń Poland 31 E6
Golubac Serbia 44 B5
Golyam Perelik Bulgaria 45 E8
Golyama Kamchiya → Bulgaria 45 C11
Goma Dem. Rep. of the Congo 86 C2
Gomal Pass Pakistan 68 D3
Gomati → India 69 G10
Gombari Dem. Rep. of the Congo 86 B2
Gombe Nigeria 83 C7
Gömbe Turkey 47 E11
Gombe □ Nigeria 83 C7
Gombe → Tanzania 86 C3
Gombe Stream △ Tanzania 86 C2
Gombi Nigeria 83 C7
Gomel = Homyel Belarus 23 B16
Gomera Canary Is. 48 F2
Gómez Palacio Mexico 118 B4
Gomfi Greece 46 B3
Gomīshān Iran 71 B7
Gommern Germany 24 C7
Gomogomo Indonesia 63 F8
Gomoh India 69 H12
Gomotartsi Bulgaria 44 B6
Gompa = Ganta Liberia 82 D3
Gonābād Iran 71 C8
Gonaïves Haiti 121 C5
Gonarezhou △ Zimbabwe 87 G3
Gonâve, G. de la Haiti 121 C5
Gonâve, Île de la Haiti 121 C5
Gonbad-e Kāvūs Iran 71 B7
Gönc Hungary 28 B6
Gonda India 69 F9
Gondal India 68 J4
Gonder Ethiopia 81 E4
Gondia India 66 J12
Gondola Mozam. 87 F3
Gondomar Portugal 36 D2
Gondrecourt-le-Château France 19 D12
Gönen Balıkesir, Turkey 45 F11
Gönen İsparta, Turkey 47 D12
Gönen → Turkey 45 F11
Gong Xian China 58 C5
Gong'an China 59 B9
Gongcheng China 59 E8
Gongga Shan China 58 C3
Gongguan China 58 G7
Gonghe China 60 C5
Gongju S. Korea 57 F14
Gongola → Nigeria 83 D7
Gongolgon Australia 95 E4
Gongshan China 58 D2
Gongtan China 58 C7
Gongzhuling China 57 C13
Goni Greece 46 B4
Goniadz Poland 30 E9
Goniri Nigeria 83 C7
Gonjo China 58 B2
Gonnesa Italy 42 C1
Gonnosfanádiga Italy 42 C1
Gonzaga Phil. 61 B5
Gonzales Calif., U.S.A. 110 J5
Gonzales Tex., U.S.A. 116 G6
González Mexico 119 C5
Good Hope, C. of S. Africa 88 E2
Good Hope Lake Canada 102 B3
Gooderham Canada 114 B6
Goodhouse S. Africa 88 D2
Gooding U.S.A. 108 E6
Goodland U.S.A. 112 F3
Goodlands Mauritius 85 d
Goodlow Canada 102 B4
Goodooga Australia 95 D4
Goodsprings U.S.A. 111 K11
Goole U.K. 14 D7
Goolgowi Australia 95 E4
Goomalling Australia 93 F2
Goomeri Australia 95 D5
Goonda Mozam. 87 F3
Goondiwindi Australia 95 D5
Goongarrie, L. Australia 93 F3
Goongarrie △ Australia 93 F3
Goonyella Australia 94 C4
Goose → Canada 105 B7
Goose Creek U.S.A. 117 E14
Goose L. U.S.A. 108 F3
Gop India 68 H3
Gopalganj India 69 F11
Göppingen Germany 25 G5
Gor Spain 37 H8
Góra Dolnośląskie, Poland 31 G3
Góra Mazowieckie, Poland 31 F7
Góra Kalwaria Poland 31 G8
Gorakhpur India 69 F10
Goražde Bos.-H. 28 G3
Gorbatov Russia 34 B6
Gorbea, Peña Spain 38 B2
Gorczański △ Poland 31 J7
Gorda, Pta. Canary Is. 48 F2
Gorda, Pta. Nic. 120 D3
Gordan B. Australia 92 B5
Gördes Turkey 47 C10
Gordon U.S.A. 112 D2
Gordon → Australia 95 G4
Gordon Bay Canada 114 A5
Gordon L. Alta., Canada 103 B6
Gordon L. N.W.T., Canada 102 A6
Gordonvale Australia 94 B4
Goré Chad 79 G9
Gore Ethiopia 81 F4
Gore N.Z. 91 G2
Gore Bay Canada 104 C3
Gorée, Île de Senegal 82 C1
Görele Turkey 73 B8
Goreme Turkey 72 C6
Gorey Ireland 12 D5
Gorg Iran 71 D8
Gorgān Iran 71 B7
Gorgol □ Mauritania 82 B2
Gorgona Italy 40 E6
Gorgona, I. Colombia 124 C3
Gorgora Ethiopia 81 E4
Gorgoram Nigeria 83 C7
Gorham U.S.A. 115 B13
Gori Georgia 35 J7
Goriganga → India 69 E9
Gorinchem Neths. 17 C4
Goris Armenia 73 C12
Goritsy Russia 32 D9
Gorízia Italy 41 C10
Gorj □ Romania 29 E8
Gorki = Horki Belarus 32 E6
Gorkiy = Nizhniy Novgorod Russia 34 B7
Gorkovskoye Vdkhr. Russia 34 B6
Gorleston U.K. 15 E9
Gorlice Poland 31 J8
Görlitz Germany 24 D10
Gorlovka = Horlivka Ukraine 33 H10
Gorman U.S.A. 111 L8
Gorna Dzhumayo = Blagoevgrad Bulgaria 44 D7
Gorna Oryakhovitsa Bulgaria 45 C9
Gornja Radgona Slovenia 41 B13
Gornja Tuzla Bos.-H. 28 F3
Gornji Grad Slovenia 41 B11
Gornji Milanovac Serbia 44 B4
Gornji Vakuf Bos.-H. 28 G2
Gorno Ablanovo Bulgaria 45 C9
Gorno-Altay □ Russia 52 D9
Gorno-Altaysk Russia 52 D9
Gornozavodsk Russia 53 E15
Gornyatskiy Russia 35 F5
Gornyy Primorsk, Russia 54 B6
Gornyy Saratov, Russia 34 E9
Gorodenka = Horodenka Ukraine 29 B10
Gorodets Russia 34 B6
Gorodishche = Horodyshche Ukraine 33 H6
Gorodishche Russia 34 D7
Gorodnya = Horodnya Ukraine 33 G6
Gorodok = Haradok Belarus 32 E6
Gorodok = Horodok Ukraine 23 D12
Gorodovikovsk Russia 35 G5
Gorokhov = Horokhiv Ukraine 23 C13
Gorokhovets Russia 34 B6
Gorom Gorom Burkina Faso 83 C4
Goromonzi Zimbabwe 87 F3
Gorong, Kepulauan Indonesia 63 E8
Gorongosa △ Mozam. 89 B5
Gorongose → Mozam. 89 C5
Gorongoza Mozam. 87 F3
Gorongoza, Sa. da Mozam. 87 F3
Gorontalo Indonesia 63 D6
Gorontalo □ Indonesia 63 D6
Goronyo Nigeria 83 C6
Górowo Iławeckie Poland 30 D7
Gorron France 18 D6
Gorshechnoye Russia 33 G10
Gort Ireland 12 C3
Gortis Greece 49 D6
Góry Bystrzyckie Poland 31 H3
Goryachiy Klyuch Russia 35 H4
Goryeong S. Korea 57 G15
Gorzkowice Poland 31 G6
Górzno Poland 31 E6
Gorzów Śląski Poland 31 G5
Gorzów Wielkopolski Poland 31 F2
Gosford Australia 95 E5
Goshen Calif., U.S.A. 110 J7
Goshen Ind., U.S.A. 113 E11
Goshen N.Y., U.S.A. 115 E10
Goshogawara Japan 54 D10
Goslar Germany 24 D6
Gospič Croatia 41 D12
Gosport U.K. 15 G6
Gossas Senegal 82 C1
Gosse → Australia 94 B1
Gossi Mali 83 B4
Gossinga Sudan 81 F2
Gostivar Macedonia 44 E4
Gostyń Poland 31 G4
Gostynin Poland 31 F6
Göta älv → Sweden 11 G5
Göta kanal Sweden 11 F9
Götaland Sweden 11 G8
Göteborg Sweden 11 G5
Götene Sweden 11 F7
Goteşti Moldova 29 D13
Gotha Germany 24 E6
Gothenburg = Göteborg Sweden 11 G5
Gothenburg U.S.A. 112 E3
Gothèye Niger 83 C5
Gotland Sweden 11 G12
Gotlands län □ Sweden 11 G12
Gotō-Rettō Japan 55 H4
Gotse Delchev Bulgaria 44 E7
Gotska Sandön Sweden 9 G18
Gōtsu Japan 55 G6
Góttero, Monte Italy 40 D6
Göttingen Germany 24 D5
Gottwald = Zmiyev Ukraine 33 H9
Gottwaldov = Zlín Czech Rep. 27 B10
Goubangzi China 57 D11
Gouda Neths. 17 B4
Goudiri Senegal 82 C2
Goudoumaria Niger 83 C7
Goudouras, Akra Greece 49 E8
Gouéké Guinea 82 D3
Gouin, Rés. Canada 104 C5
Gouitafla Ivory C. 82 D3
Goulburn Australia 95 E4
Goulburn Is. Australia 94 A1
Goulia Ivory C. 82 C3
Goulimine Morocco 78 C3
Goumbou Mali 82 B3
Goumenissa Greece 44 F6
Goundam Mali 82 B4
Goura Greece 46 D4
Gourbassi Mali 82 C2
Gourdon France 20 D5
Gouré Niger 83 C7
Gourin France 18 D3
Gourits → S. Africa 88 E3
Gourma-Rharous Mali 83 B4
Gournay-en-Bray France 19 C8
Gournes Greece 49 D7
Gourock U.K. 13 F4
Goursi Burkina Faso 82 C4
Gouverneur U.S.A. 115 B9
Gouvia Greece 49 A3
Gouzon France 19 F9
Gove Peninsula Australia 94 A2
Governador Valadares Brazil 125 G10
Governor's Harbour Bahamas 120 A4
Govindgarh India 69 G9
Gowan Ra. Australia 94 D4
Gowanda U.S.A. 114 D6
Gower U.K. 15 F3
Gowna, L. Ireland 12 C4
Goya Argentina 126 B4
Göyçay Azerbaijan 35 K8
Goyder Lagoon Australia 95 D2
Goyllarisquizga Peru 124 F3
Göynük Antalya, Turkey 47 E12
Göynük Bolu, Turkey 72 B4
Goz Beïda Chad 79 F10
Goz Regeb Sudan 81 D4
Gozdnica Poland 31 G2
Gozo Malta 49 C1
Graaff-Reinet S. Africa 88 E3
Grabo Ivory C. 82 D3
Grabow Germany 24 B7
Grabów nad Prosną Poland 31 G5
Gračac Croatia 41 D12
Gračanica Bos.-H. 28 F3
Graçay France 19 E8
Gracias a Dios, C. Honduras 120 D3
Graciosa Azores 78 a
Graciosa, I. Canary Is. 48 E6
Grad Sofiya □ Bulgaria 44 D7
Gradac Montenegro 44 C3
Gradačac Bos.-H. 28 F3
Gradeška Planina Macedonia 44 E6
Gradets Bulgaria 45 D10
Gradišče Slovenia 41 B12
Grădiştea de Munte Romania 29 E8
Grado Italy 41 C10
Grado Spain 36 B4

Grady *U.S.A.* **109** J12
Graeca, Lacul *Romania* **29** F11
Grafenau *Germany* **25** G9
Gräfenberg *Germany* **25** F7
Grafham Water *U.K.* **15** E7
Grafton *Canada* **104** C1
Grafton *N. Dak., U.S.A.* **112** A5
Grafton *W. Va., U.S.A.* **113** F13
Graham *Canada* **104** C1
Graham *U.S.A.* **116** E5
Graham, Mt. *U.S.A.* **109** K9
Graham Bell, Ostrov =
  Greem-Bell, Ostrov *Russia* **52** A7
Graham I. *B.C., Canada* **102** C2
Graham I. *Nunavut, Canada* **101** B13
Graham Land *Antarctica* **5** C17
Grahamstown *S. Africa* **88** E4
Grahamsville *U.S.A.* **115** E10
Grahovo *Montenegro* **44** D2
Graie, Alpi *Europe* **21** C11
Grain Coast *W. Afr.* **82** E3
Grajagan *Indonesia* **63** K17
Grajagan, Teluk *Indonesia* **63** K17
Grajaú *Brazil* **125** E9
Grajaú → *Brazil* **125** D10
Grajewo *Poland* **30** E9
Gramada *Bulgaria* **44** C6
Gramat *France* **20** D5
Grammichele *Italy* **43** E7
Grámmos, Óros *Greece* **44** F4
Grampian *U.S.A.* **114** F6
Grampian Highlands =
  Grampian Mts. *U.K.* **13** E5
Grampian Mts. *U.K.* **13** E5
Grampians, The *Australia* **95** F3
Gramsh *Albania* **44** F4
Gran Canaria *Canary Is.* **48** G4
Gran Chaco *S. Amer.* **126** B3
Gran Desierto del
  Pinacate △ *Mexico* **118** A2
Gran Paradiso *Italy* **40** C4
Gran Sasso d'Itália *Italy* **41** F10
Gran Sasso e Monti Della
  Laga △ *Italy* **41** F10
Granada *Nic.* **120** D2
Granada *Spain* **37** H7
Granada *U.S.A.* **108** G12
Granada □ *Spain* **37** H7
Granadilla de Abona
  Canary Is. **48** F3
Granard *Ireland* **12** C4
Granbury *U.S.A.* **116** E6
Granby *Canada* **115** A12
Granby *U.S.A.* **108** F11
Grand → *Canada* **114** D5
Grand → *Mo., U.S.A.* **112** F7
Grand → *S. Dak., U.S.A.* **112** C4
Grand Bahama I. *Bahamas* **120** A4
Grand Baie *Mauritius* **85** d
Grand Bank *Canada* **105** C8
Grand Bassam *Ivory C.* **82** D4
Grand Bend *Canada* **114** C3
Grand Béréby *Ivory C.* **82** E3
Grand-Bourg *Guadeloupe* **120** b
Grand Canal = Da
  Yunhe → *China* **57** E9
Grand Canyon *U.S.A.* **109** H7
Grand Canyon △ *U.S.A.* **109** H7
Grand Canyon-
  Parashant △ *U.S.A.* **109** H7
Grand Cayman *Cayman Is.* **120** C3
Grand Cess *Liberia* **82** E3
Grand Coulee *U.S.A.* **108** C4
Grand Coulee Dam *U.S.A.* **108** C4
Grand Erg de Bilma *Niger* **79** E8
Grand Falls *Canada* **105** C6
Grand Falls-Windsor *Canada* **105** C8
Grand Forks *Canada* **102** D5
Grand Forks *U.S.A.* **112** B5
Grand Gorge *U.S.A.* **115** D10
Grand Haven *U.S.A.* **112** D10
Grand I. *Mich., U.S.A.* **112** B10
Grand I. *N.Y., U.S.A.* **114** D6
Grand Island *U.S.A.* **112** E4
Grand Isle *La., U.S.A.* **117** G9
Grand Isle *Vt., U.S.A.* **115** B11
Grand Junction *U.S.A.* **108** G9
Grand L. *N.B., Canada* **105** C6
Grand L. *Nfld. & L., Canada* **105** C8
Grand L. *Nfld. & L., Canada* **105** B7
Grand L. *U.S.A.* **116** G8
Grand Lahou *Ivory C.* **82** D3
Grand Lake *U.S.A.* **108** F11
Grand-Lieu, L. de *France* **18** E5
Grand Manan I. *Canada* **105** D6
Grand Marais *Mich., U.S.A.* **113** B11
Grand Marais *Minn., U.S.A.* **104** C1
Grand-Mère *Canada* **104** C5
Grand Popo *Benin* **83** D5
Grand Portage *U.S.A.* **112** B9
Grand Prairie *U.S.A.* **116** E6
Grand Rapids *Canada* **103** C9
Grand Rapids *Mich., U.S.A.* **113** D11
Grand Rapids *Minn., U.S.A.* **112** B7
Grand St-Bernard, Col du
  Europe **25** K3
Grand Staircase-
  Escalante △ *U.S.A.* **109** H8
Grand Teton *U.S.A.* **108** E8

Grand Teton △ *U.S.A.* **108** E8
Grand Union Canal *U.K.* **15** E7
Grandas de Salime *Spain* **36** B4
Grande → *Jujuy, Argentina* **126** A2
Grande →
  Mendoza, Argentina **126** D2
Grande → *Bolivia* **124** G6
Grande → *Bahia, Brazil* **125** F10
Grande →
  Minas Gerais, Brazil **125** H8
Grande, B. *Argentina* **128** G3
Grande, Rio → *N. Amer.* **116** J6
Grande Anse *Seychelles* **85** b
Grande Baleine → *Canada* **104** A4
Grande Cache *Canada* **102** C5
Grande-Rivière *Canada* **105** C7
Grande-Terre *Guadeloupe* **120** b
Grande-Vallée *Canada* **105** C6
Grande Vigie, Pte. de la
  Guadeloupe **120** b
Grandfalls *U.S.A.* **116** F3
Grândola *Portugal* **37** G2
Grandpré *France* **19** C11
Grands Causses △ *France* **20** D6
Grands-Jardins △ *Canada* **105** C5
Grandview *Canada* **103** C8
Grandview *U.S.A.* **108** C4
Grandvilliers *France* **19** C8
Graneros *Chile* **126** C1
Grangemouth *U.K.* **13** E5
Granger *U.S.A.* **108** F9
Grängesberg *Sweden* **10** D9
Grangeville *U.S.A.* **108** D5
Granisle *Canada* **102** C3
Granite City *U.S.A.* **112** F8
Granite Falls *U.S.A.* **112** C6
Granite L. *Canada* **105** C8
Granite Mt. *U.S.A.* **111** M10
Granite Pk. *U.S.A.* **108** D9
Graniteville *U.S.A.* **115** B12
Granitola, C. *Italy* **42** E5
Granity *N.Z.* **91** D3
Granja *Brazil* **125** D10
Granja de Moreruela *Spain* **36** D5
Granja de Torrehermosa
  Spain **37** G5
Gränna *Sweden* **11** F8
Granollers *Spain* **38** D7
Gransee *Germany* **24** B9
Grant *U.S.A.* **112** E3
Grant, Mt. *U.S.A.* **108** G4
Grant City *U.S.A.* **112** E7
Grant I. *Australia* **92** B5
Grant Range *U.S.A.* **108** G6
Grantham *U.K.* **14** E7
Grantown-on-Spey *U.K.* **13** D5
Grants *U.S.A.* **109** J10
Grants Pass *U.S.A.* **108** E2
Grantsville *U.S.A.* **108** F7
Granville *France* **18** D5
Granville *N. Dak., U.S.A.* **112** A3
Granville *N.Y., U.S.A.* **115** C11
Granville *Ohio, U.S.A.* **114** F2
Granville L. *Canada* **103** B8
Graskop *S. Africa* **89** D5
Gräsö *Sweden* **10** D12
Grass → *Canada* **103** B9
Grass Range *U.S.A.* **108** C9
Grass River △ *Canada* **103** C8
Grass Valley *Calif., U.S.A.* **110** F6
Grass Valley *Oreg., U.S.A.* **108** D3
Grassano *Italy* **43** B9
Grasse *France* **21** E10
Grassflat *U.S.A.* **114** E6
Grasslands △ *Canada* **103** D7
Grassy *Australia* **95** G3
Gråsten *Denmark* **11** K3
Grästorp *Sweden* **11** F6
Gratkorn *Austria* **26** D8
Graulhet *France* **20** E5
Graus *Spain* **38** C5
Grave, Pte. de *France* **20** C2
Gravelbourg *Canada* **103** D7
Gravelines *France* **19** A9
's-Gravenhage *Neths.* **17** B4
Gravenhurst *Canada* **114** B5
Gravesend *Australia* **95** D5
Gravesend *U.K.* **15** F8
Gravina in Púglia *Italy* **43** B9
Gravois, Pointe-à- *Haiti* **121** C5
Gravone → *France* **21** G12
Gray *France* **19** E12
Grayling *U.S.A.* **113** C11
Grays *U.K.* **15** F8
Grays Harbor *U.S.A.* **108** C1
Grays L. *U.S.A.* **108** E8
Grays River *U.S.A.* **110** D3
Grayvoron *Russia* **33** G8
Graz *Austria* **26** D8
Grdelica *Serbia* **44** D6
Greasy L. *Canada* **102** A4
Great Abaco I. = Abaco I.
  Bahamas **120** A4

Great Artesian Basin
  Australia **94** C3
Great Australian Bight
  Australia **93** F5
Great Bahama Bank
  Bahamas **120** B4
Great Barrier I. *N.Z.* **91** B5
Great Barrier Reef *Australia* **94** B4
Great Barrier Reef △
  Australia **94** B4
Great Barrington *U.S.A.* **115** D11
Great Basalt Wall △ *Australia* **94** B4
Great Basin *U.S.A.* **108** G5
Great Basin △ *U.S.A.* **108** G6
Great Bear → *Canada* **100** E7
Great Bear L. *Canada* **100** D8
Great Belt = Store Bælt
  Denmark **11** J4
Great Bend *Kans., U.S.A.* **112** F4
Great Bend *Pa., U.S.A.* **115** E9
Great Blasket I. *Ireland* **12** D1
Great Britain *Europe* **6** E5
Great Camanoe *Br. Virgin Is.* **121** e
Great Codroy *Canada* **105** C8
Great Divide, The = Great
  Dividing Ra. *Australia* **94** C4
Great Divide Basin *U.S.A.* **108** E9
Great Dividing Ra. *Australia* **94** C4
Great Driffield = Driffield
  U.K. **14** C7
Great Exuma I. *Bahamas* **120** B4
Great Falls *U.S.A.* **108** C8
Great Fish = Groot-Vis →
  S. Africa **88** E4
Great Guana Cay *Bahamas* **120** B4
Great Himalayan △ *India* **68** D7
Great Inagua I. *Bahamas* **121** B5
Great Indian Desert = Thar
  Desert *India* **68** F7
Great Karoo *S. Africa* **88** E3
Great Khingan Mts. = Da
  Hinggan Ling *China* **60** B7
Great Lake *Australia* **95** G4
Great Lakes *N. Amer.* **98** E11
Great Limpopo
  Transfrontier △ *Africa* **89** C5
Great Malvern *U.K.* **15** E5
Great Miami → *U.S.A.* **113** F11
Great Ormes Head *U.K.* **14** D4
Great Ouse → *U.K.* **14** E8
Great Palm I. *Australia* **94** B4
Great Pedro Bluff *Jamaica* **120** a
Great Pee Dee → *U.S.A.* **117** E15
Great Plains *N. Amer.* **98** E9
Great Ruaha → *Tanzania* **86** D4
Great Sacandaga L. *U.S.A.* **115** C10
Great Saint Bernard Pass =
  Grand St-Bernard, Col du
  Europe **25** K3
Great Salt Desert = Kavīr,
  Dasht-e *Iran* **71** C7
Great Salt Desert = Lūt,
  Dasht-e *Iran* **71** D8
Great Salt L. *U.S.A.* **108** F7
Great Salt Lake Desert
  U.S.A. **108** F7
Great Salt Plains L. *U.S.A.* **116** C5
Great Sand Dunes △ *U.S.A.*
  109 H11
Great Sandy △ *Australia* **95** D5
Great Sandy Desert *Australia* **92** D3
Great Sangi = Sangihe,
  Pulau *Indonesia* **63** D7
Great Scarcies → *S. Leone* **82** D2
Great Sea Reef *Fiji* **91** a
Great Sitkin I. *U.S.A.* **106** E4
Great Skellig *Ireland* **12** E1
Great Slave L. *Canada* **102** A5
Great Smoky Mts. △ *U.S.A.*
  117 D13
Great Stour = Stour → *U.K.* **15** F9
Great Victoria Desert
  Australia **93** E4
Great Wall *Antarctica* **5** C18
Great Wall *China* **56** E5
Great Whernside *U.K.* **14** C6
Great Yarmouth *U.K.* **15** E9
Great Zab = Zāb al
  Kabīr → *Iraq* **73** D10
Great Zimbabwe *Zimbabwe* **87** G3
Greater Antilles *W. Indies* **121** C5
Greater London □ *U.K.* **15** F7
Greater Manchester □ *U.K.* **14** D5
Greater St. Lucia
  Wetlands △ *S. Africa* **89** D5
Greater Sudbury =
  Sudbury *Canada* **104** C3
Greater Sunda Is. *Indonesia* **62** F4
Grebbestad *Sweden* **11** F5
Grebenka = Hrebinka
  Ukraine **33** G7
Greco, C. *Cyprus* **49** E13
Greco, Mte. *Italy* **41** G10
Gredos, Sierra de *Spain* **36** E6
Greece *U.S.A.* **114** C7
Greece ■ *Europe* **46** B3
Greeley *Colo., U.S.A.* **108** F11
Greeley *Nebr., U.S.A.* **112** E4
Greely Fd. *Canada* **101** A15

Greem-Bell, Ostrov *Russia* **52** A7
Green → *Ky., U.S.A.* **112** G10
Green → *Utah, U.S.A.* **108** G9
Green B. *U.S.A.* **112** C10
Green Bay *U.S.A.* **112** C9
Green C. = Australia **95** F5
Green Cove Springs *U.S.A.* **117** G14
Green I. = Lü Tao *Taiwan* **59** F13
Green Lake *Canada* **103** C7
Green Mts. *U.S.A.* **115** C12
Green River *Utah, U.S.A.* **108** G8
Green River *Wyo., U.S.A.* **108** F9
Green Valley *U.S.A.* **109** L8
Greenbank *U.S.A.* **110** B4
Greenbush *Mich., U.S.A.* **114** B1
Greenbush *Minn., U.S.A.* **112** A5
Greencastle *U.S.A.* **112** F10
Greene *U.S.A.* **115** D9
Greenfield *Calif., U.S.A.* **110** J5
Greenfield *Calif., U.S.A.* **111** K8
Greenfield *Ind., U.S.A.* **113** F11
Greenfield *Iowa, U.S.A.* **112** E6
Greenfield *Mass., U.S.A.* **115** D12
Greenfield *Mo., U.S.A.* **112** G7
Greenfield Park *Canada* **115** A11
Greenland ☒ *N. Amer.* **99** C15
Greenland Sea *Arctic* **4** B7
Greenock *U.K.* **13** F4
Greenore *Ireland* **12** B5
Greenore Pt. *Ireland* **12** D5
Greenough *Australia* **93** E1
Greenough → *Australia* **93** E1
Greenough Pt. *Canada* **114** B3
Greenport *U.S.A.* **115** E12
Greensboro *N.C., U.S.A.* **117** E13
Greensboro *N.C., U.S.A.* **117** C15
Greensboro *Vt., U.S.A.* **115** B12
Greensburg *Ind., U.S.A.* **113** F11
Greensburg *Kans., U.S.A.* **112** G4
Greensburg *Pa., U.S.A.* **114** F5
Greenstone Pt. *U.K.* **13** D3
Greenvale *Australia* **94** B4
Greenville *Liberia* **82** D3
Greenville *Ala., U.S.A.* **117** F11
Greenville *Calif., U.S.A.* **110** E6
Greenville *Maine, U.S.A.* **113** C19
Greenville *Mich., U.S.A.* **113** D11
Greenville *Miss., U.S.A.* **117** E9
Greenville *Mo., U.S.A.* **112** G8
Greenville *N.C., U.S.A.* **117** D16
Greenville *N.H., U.S.A.* **115** D13
Greenville *N.Y., U.S.A.* **115** D10
Greenville *Ohio, U.S.A.* **113** E12
Greenville *Pa., U.S.A.* **114** E4
Greenville *S.C., U.S.A.* **117** D13
Greenville *Tex., U.S.A.* **116** E6
Greenwater Lake △ *Canada* **103** C8
Greenwich *Conn., U.S.A.* **115** E11
Greenwich *N.Y., U.S.A.* **115** C11
Greenwich *Ohio, U.S.A.* **114** E2
Greenwich □ *U.K.* **15** F8
Greenwood *Canada* **102** D5
Greenwood *Ark., U.S.A.* **116** D7
Greenwood *Ind., U.S.A.* **112** F10
Greenwood *Miss., U.S.A.* **117** E9
Greenwood *S.C., U.S.A.* **117** D13
Greenwood, Mt. *Australia* **92** B5
Gregbe *Ivory C.* **82** D3
Gregory *U.S.A.* **112** D4
Gregory → *Australia* **94** B2
Gregory, L. *S. Austral.,
  Australia* **95** D2
Gregory, L. *W. Austral.,
  Australia* **92** D4
Gregory, L. *W. Austral.,
  Australia* **93** E2
Gregory △ *Australia* **92** C5
Gregory Downs *Australia* **94** B2
Gregory Ra. *Queens., Australia* **94** B3
Gregory Ra. *W. Austral.,
  Australia* **92** D3
Greiffenberg *Germany* **24** B9
Greifswald *Germany* **24** A9
Greifswalder Bodden
  Germany **24** A9
Grein *Austria* **26** C7
Greiz *Germany* **24** E8
Gremikha *Russia* **52** C4
Grenaa *Denmark* **11** H4
Grenada *U.S.A.* **117** E10
Grenada ■ *W. Indies* **121** D7
Grenade *France* **20** E5
Grenadier I. *U.S.A.* **115** B8
Grenadines, The *St. Vincent* **121** D7
Grenchen *Switz.* **25** H3
Grenen *Denmark* **11** G4
Grenfell *Australia* **95** E4
Grenfell *Canada* **103** C8
Grenoble *France* **21** C9
Grenville, C. *Australia* **94** A3
Grenville, Chan. *Canada* **102** C3
Gréoux-les-Bains *France* **21** E9
Gresham *U.S.A.* **110** E4
Gresik *Indonesia* **63** G15
Gretna *U.K.* **13** F5
Gretna *U.S.A.* **117** G9
Greve Strand *Denmark* **11** J6
Greven *Germany* **24** C3

Grevena *Greece* **44** F5
Grevena □ *Greece* **44** F5
Grevenbroich *Germany* **24** D2
Grevenmacher *Lux.* **17** E6
Grevesmühlen *Germany* **24** B7
Grey → *Australia* **95** C8
Grey → *N.Z.* **91** E3
Grey, C. *Australia* **94** A2
Grey Ra. *Australia* **95** D3
Greybull *U.S.A.* **108** D9
Greymouth *N.Z.* **91** E3
Greystones *Ireland* **12** C5
Greytown *N.Z.* **91** D5
Greytown *S. Africa* **89** D5
Gribanovskiy *Russia* **34** E5
Gribbell I. *Canada* **102** C3
Gribës, Mal i *Albania* **44** F3
Gridley *U.S.A.* **110** F5
Griekwastad *S. Africa* **88** D3
Griesheim *Germany* **25** F4
Grieskirchen *Austria* **26** C6
Griffin *U.S.A.* **117** E12
Griffith *Australia* **95** E4
Griffith *Canada* **114** A7
Griffith I. *Canada* **114** B4
Grignols *France* **20** D3
Grigoriopol *Moldova* **29** C14
Grigoryevka = Hrymayliv
  Ukraine **23** D14
Grimes *U.S.A.* **110** F5
Grimma *Germany* **24** D8
Grimmen *Germany* **24** A9
Grimsay *U.K.* **13** D1
Grimsby *Canada* **114** C5
Grimsby *U.K.* **14** D7
Grímsey *Iceland* **8** C5
Grimshaw *Canada* **102** B5
Grimslöv *Sweden* **11** H8
Grimstad *Norway* **9** G13
Grindelwald *Switz.* **25** J4
Grindsted *Denmark* **11** J2
Grindu *Romania* **29** F11
Grinnell *U.S.A.* **112** E7
Grinnell Pen. *Canada* **101** B13
Gris-Nez, C. *France* **19** B8
Grise Fiord *Canada* **101** B15
Grisolles *France* **20** E5
Grisons = Graubünden □
  Switz. **25** J5
Grisslehamn *Sweden* **10** D12
Grmeč Planina *Bos.-H.* **41** D13
Groais I. *Canada* **105** B8
Grobiņa *Latvia* **30** B8
Groblersdal *S. Africa* **89** D4
Grobming *Austria* **26** D6
Grocka *Serbia* **44** B4
Gródek *Poland* **31** E10
Grodków *Poland* **31** H4
Grodno = Hrodna *Belarus* **30** E10
Grodzisk Mazowiecki *Poland* **31** F7
Grodzisk Wielkopolski
  Poland **31** F3
Grodzyanka = Hrodzyanka
  Belarus **23** B15
Groesbeck *U.S.A.* **116** F6
Groix *France* **18** E3
Groix, Î. de *France* **18** E3
Grójec *Poland* **31** G7
Gronau *Niedersachsen,
  Germany* **24** C4
Gronau *Nordrhein-Westfalen,
  Germany* **24** C3
Grong *Norway* **8** D15
Grönhögen *Sweden* **11** H10
Groningen *Neths.* **17** A6
Groningen □ *Neths.* **17** A6
Groom *U.S.A.* **116** D4
Groot → *S. Africa* **88** E3
Groot-Berg → *S. Africa* **88** E2
Groot-Brakrivier *S. Africa* **88** E3
Groot Karasberge *Namibia* **88** D2
Groot-Kei → *S. Africa* **89** E4
Groot-Vis → *S. Africa* **88** E4
Grootdrink *S. Africa* **88** D3
Groote Eylandt *Australia* **94** A2
Grootfontein *Namibia* **88** B2
Grootlaagte → *Africa* **88** C3
Grootvloer → *S. Africa* **88** E3
Gros C. *Canada* **102** A6
Gros Islet *St. Lucia* **121** f
Gros Morne △ *Canada* **105** C8
Gros Piton *St. Lucia* **121** f
Gros Piton Pt. *St. Lucia* **121** f
Grósio *Italy* **40** B7
Grosne → *France* **19** F11
Grossa, Pta. *Spain* **48** B8
Grosse Point *U.S.A.* **114** D2
Grossenbrode *Germany* **24** A7
Grossenhain *Germany* **24** D9
Grosser Arber *Germany* **25** F8
Grosser Plöner See *Germany* **24** A6
Grosseto *Italy* **41** F8
Grossgerungs *Austria* **26** C7
Grossglockner *Austria* **26** D5
Groswater B. *Canada* **105** B8
Groton *Conn., U.S.A.* **115** E12
Groton *N.Y., U.S.A.* **115** D8

Groton *S. Dak., U.S.A.* **112** C4
Grottáglie *Italy* **43** B10
Grottaminarda *Italy* **43** A8
Grottammare *Italy* **41** F10
Grouard Mission *Canada* **102** B5
Grouin, Pte. du *France* **18** D5
Groundhog → *Canada* **104** C3
Grouw *Neths.* **17** A5
Grove City *U.S.A.* **114** E4
Grove Hill *U.S.A.* **117** F11
Groveland *U.S.A.* **110** H6
Grover Beach *U.S.A.* **111** K6
Groves *U.S.A.* **116** G8
Groveton *U.S.A.* **115** B13
Grožnjan *Croatia* **41** C10
Groznyy *Russia* **35** J7
Grubišno Polje *Croatia* **28** E2
Grudovo *Bulgaria* **45** D11
Grudusk *Poland* **31** E7
Grudziądz *Poland* **30** E5
Gruinard B. *U.K.* **13** D3
Gruissan *France* **20** E7
Grumo Áppula *Italy* **43** A9
Grums *Sweden* **10** E7
Grünberg *Germany* **24** E4
Gründau *Germany* **25** E5
Grundy Center *U.S.A.* **112** D7
Grünstadt *Germany* **25** F4
Gruppo di Tessa △ *Italy* **40** B8
Gruvberget *Sweden* **10** C10
Gruver *U.S.A.* **116** C4
Gruyères *Switz.* **25** J3
Gruža *Serbia* **44** C5
Gryazi *Russia* **33** F10
Gryazovets *Russia* **32** C11
Grybów *Poland* **31** J7
Grycksbo *Sweden* **10** D9
Gryfice *Poland* **30** E2
Gryfino *Poland* **31** E1
Gryfów Śląski *Poland* **31** G2
Grythyttan *Sweden* **10** E8
Grytviken *S. Georgia* **128** G9
Gstaad *Switz.* **25** J3
Gua *India* **69** H11
Gua Musang *Malaysia* **65** K3
Guacanayabo, G. de *Cuba* **120** B4
Guachípas → *Argentina* **126** B2
Guadajoz → *Spain* **37** H6
Guadalajara *Mexico* **118** C4
Guadalajara *Spain* **38** E1
Guadalajara □ *Spain* **38** E2
Guadalcanal *Solomon Is.* **90** B9
Guadalcanal *Spain* **37** G5
Guadalén → *Spain* **37** G7
Guadales *Argentina* **126** C2
Guadalete → *Spain* **37** J4
Guadalimar → *Spain* **37** G7
Guadalmena → *Spain* **37** G8
Guadalmez → *Spain* **37** G5
Guadalope → *Spain* **38** D4
Guadalquivir → *Spain* **37** J4
Guadalupe =
  Guadeloupe ☒ *W. Indies* **120** b
Guadalupe *Mexico* **118** C4
Guadalupe *Spain* **37** F5
Guadalupe *U.S.A.* **111** L6
Guadalupe → *U.S.A.* **116** G6
Guadalupe, Sierra de *Spain* **37** F5
Guadalupe Bravos *Mexico* **118** A3
Guadalupe I. *Pac. Oc.* **98** G8
Guadalupe Mts. △ *U.S.A.* **116** F2
Guadalupe Peak *U.S.A.* **116** F2
Guadalupe y Calvo *Mexico* **118** B3
Guadarrama, Sierra de *Spain* **36** E7
Guadeloupe ☒ *W. Indies* **120** b
Guadeloupe = Guadeloupe ☒ *Guadeloupe* **120** b
Guadeloupe Passage
  W. Indies **121** C7
Guadiamar → *Spain* **37** J4
Guadiana → *Portugal* **37** H3
Guadiana Menor → *Spain* **37** H7
Guadiaro → *Spain* **37** J5
Guadiato → *Spain* **37** H5
Guadiela → *Spain* **38** E2
Guadix *Spain* **37** H7
Guafo, Boca del *Chile* **128** E2
Guaico *Trin. & Tob.* **125** K15
Guainía → *Colombia* **124** C5
Guaíra *Brazil* **127** A5
Guaíra □ *Paraguay* **126** B4
Guaire = Gorey *Ireland* **12** D5
Guaitecas, Is. *Chile* **128** E2
Guajará-Mirim *Brazil* **124** F5
Guajira, Pen. de la *Colombia* **124** A4
Gualán *Guatemala* **120** C2
Gualdo Tadino *Italy* **41** E9
Gualeguay *Argentina* **126** C4
Gualeguaychú *Argentina* **126** C4
Gualequay → *Argentina* **126** C4
Guam ☒ *Pac. Oc.* **96** F6
Guamini *Argentina* **126** D3
Guamúchil *Mexico* **118** B3
Guana I. *Br. Virgin Is.* **121** e
Guanabacoa *Cuba* **120** B3
Guanacaste, Cordillera de
  Costa Rica **120** D2
Guanacaste △ *Costa Rica* **120** D2
Guanaceví *Mexico* **118** B3
Guanahani = San Salvador
  I. *Bahamas* **121** B5

Hälsingland *Sweden* 10 C10
Halstead *U.K.* 15 F8
Haltern *Germany* 24 D3
Haltiatunturi *Finland* 8 B19
Halton □ *U.K.* 14 D5
Haltwhistle *U.K.* 14 C5
Ḥālūl *Qatar* 71 E7
Halvad *India* 68 H4
Ḥalvān *Iran* 71 C8
Ham *France* 19 C10
Ham Tan *Vietnam* 65 G6
Ham Yen *Vietnam* 64 A5
Hamab *Namibia* 88 D2
Hamad *Sudan* 81 D3
Hamada *Japan* 55 G6
Hamadān *Iran* 73 E13
Hamadān □ *Iran* 71 C6
Ḥamāh *Syria* 72 E7
Ḥamāh □ *Syria* 72 E7
Hamamatsu *Japan* 55 G8
Hamar *Norway* 8 F14
Hamâta, Gebel *Egypt* 70 E2
Hambantota *Sri Lanka* 66 R12
Hamber △ *Canada* 102 C5
Hamburg *Germany* 24 B5
Hamburg *Ark., U.S.A.* 116 E9
Hamburg *N.Y., U.S.A.* 114 D6
Hamburg *Pa., U.S.A.* 115 F9
Hamburg □ *Germany* 24 B5
Hamburg Fuhlsbüttel ✈
  (HAM) *Germany* 24 B5
Ḥamḍ, W. al ➤ *Si. Arabia* 70 E3
Hamden *U.S.A.* 115 E12
Hamdibey *Turkey* 47 B9
Häme *Finland* 32 B2
Hämeenlinna *Finland* 32 B3
Hamélé *Ghana* 82 C4
Hamelin Pool *Australia* 93 E1
Hameln *Germany* 24 C5
Hamerkaz □ *Israel* 74 C3
Hamero Hadad *Ethiopia* 81 F5
Hamersley Ra. *Australia* 92 D2
Hamhŭng *N. Korea* 57 E14
Hami *China* 60 B4
Hamili *Greece* 47 F8
Hamilton *Australia* 95 F3
Hamilton *Canada* 114 C5
Hamilton *N.Z.* 91 B5
Hamilton *U.K.* 13 F4
Hamilton *Ala., U.S.A.* 117 D11
Hamilton *Mont., U.S.A.* 108 C6
Hamilton *N.Y., U.S.A.* 115 D9
Hamilton *Ohio, U.S.A.* 113 F11
Hamilton *Tex., U.S.A.* 116 F5
Hamilton ➤ *Queens.,*
  Australia 94 C2
Hamilton ➤ *S. Austral.,*
  Australia 95 D2
Hamilton City *U.S.A.* 110 F4
Hamilton I. *Australia* 94 b
Hamilton Inlet *Canada* 105 B8
Hamilton Mt. *U.S.A.* 115 C10
Hamina *Finland* 32 B4
Hamirpur *H.P., India* 68 D7
Hamirpur *Ut. P., India* 69 G9
Hamitabat *Turkey* 45 E11
Hamju *N. Korea* 57 E14
Hamlet *U.S.A.* 117 D15
Hamley Bridge *Australia* 95 E2
Hamlin = Hameln *Germany* 24 C5
Hamlin *N.Y., U.S.A.* 114 C7
Hamlin *Tex., U.S.A.* 116 E4
Hamm *Germany* 24 D3
Hammām al Alīl *Iraq* 73 D10
Ḥammār, Hawr al *Iraq* 70 D5
Hammarstrand *Sweden* 10 A10
Hammelburg *Germany* 25 E5
Hammeren *Denmark* 11 J8
Hammerfest *Norway* 8 A20
Hamminkeln *Germany* 24 D2
Hammond *Ind., U.S.A.* 112 E10
Hammond *La., U.S.A.* 117 F9
Hammond *N.Y., U.S.A.* 115 B9
Hammondsport *U.S.A.* 114 D7
Hammonton *U.S.A.* 113 F16
Hamneda *Sweden* 11 H7
Hamoyet, Jebel *Sudan* 80 D4
Hampden *N.Z.* 91 F3
Hampshire □ *U.K.* 15 F6
Hampshire Downs *U.K.* 15 F6
Hampton *N.B., Canada* 105 C6
Hampton *Ont., Canada* 114 C6
Hampton *Ark., U.S.A.* 116 E8
Hampton *Iowa, U.S.A.* 112 D7
Hampton *N.H., U.S.A.* 115 D14
Hampton *S.C., U.S.A.* 117 E14
Hampton *Va., U.S.A.* 113 G15
Hampton Bays *U.S.A.* 115 F12
Hampton Tableland *Australia* 93 F4
Hamra *Sweden* 10 C8
Hamrat esh Sheykh *Sudan* 81 E2
Ḥamrin, Jabal *Iraq* 73 E11
Hamur *Turkey* 73 C10
Hamyang *S. Korea* 57 G14
Han i Hotit *Albania* 44 D3
Han Jiang ➤ *China* 59 F11
Han Shui ➤ *China* 59 B10
Hanak *Si. Arabia* 70 E3

Hanak *Turkey* 73 B10
Hanamaki *Japan* 54 E10
Hanang *Tanzania* 86 C4
Hanau *Germany* 25 E4
Hanbogd = Ihbulag *Mongolia* 56 C4
Hançalar *Turkey* 47 C11
Hânceşti *Moldova* 29 D13
Hancheng *China* 56 G6
Hanchuan *China* 59 B9
Hancock *Mich., U.S.A.* 112 B9
Hancock *N.Y., U.S.A.* 115 E9
Hancock *Vt., U.S.A.* 115 C12
Handa *Japan* 55 G8
Handa I. *U.K.* 13 C3
Handan *China* 56 F8
Handeni *Tanzania* 86 D4
Handlová *Slovak Rep.* 27 C11
Handub *Sudan* 80 D4
Handwara *India* 69 B6
Hanegev *Israel* 74 E4
Hanford *U.S.A.* 110 J7
Hanford Reach △ *U.S.A.* 108 C4
Hang Chat *Thailand* 64 C2
Hang Dong *Thailand* 64 C2
Hangang ➤ *S. Korea* 57 F14
Hangayn Nuruu *Mongolia* 60 B4
Hangchou = Hangzhou
  China 59 B13
Hanggin Houqi *China* 56 D4
Hanggin Qi *China* 56 E5
Hangu *China* 57 E9
Hangzhou *China* 59 B13
Hangzhou Wan *China* 59 B13
Hanh *Mongolia* 53 D11
Hanhongor *Mongolia* 56 C3
Hani *Turkey* 73 C9
Hania = Chania *Greece* 49 D6
Ḥanīdh *Si. Arabia* 71 E6
Ḥanīsh *Yemen* 75 E3
Haniska *Slovak Rep.* 27 C14
Hanjiang *China* 59 E12
Hankinson *U.S.A.* 112 B5
Hankö *Finland* 32 C2
Hankou *China* 59 B10
Hanksville *U.S.A.* 108 G8
Hanle *India* 69 C8
Hanmer Springs *N.Z.* 91 E4
Hann ➤ *Australia* 92 C4
Hann, Mt. *Australia* 92 C4
Hanna *Canada* 102 C6
Hanna *U.S.A.* 108 F10
Hannah B. *Canada* 104 B4
Hannibal *Mo., U.S.A.* 112 F8
Hannibal *N.Y., U.S.A.* 115 C8
Hannik *Sudan* 80 D3
Hannover *Germany* 24 C5
Hanö *Sweden* 11 H8
Hanöbukten *Sweden* 11 J8
Hanoi *Vietnam* 58 G5
Hanover = Hannover
  Germany 24 C5
Hanover *Canada* 114 B3
Hanover *S. Africa* 88 E3
Hanover *N.H., U.S.A.* 115 C12
Hanover *Ohio, U.S.A.* 114 F2
Hanover *Pa., U.S.A.* 113 F15
Hanover, I. *Chile* 128 G2
Hans Lollik I. *U.S. Virgin Is.* 121 e
Hansdiha *India* 69 G12
Hanshou *China* 59 C8
Hansi *H.P., India* 68 C7
Hansi *Haryana, India* 68 E6
Hanson, L. *Australia* 95 E2
Hanstholm *Denmark* 11 G2
Hantsavichy *Belarus* 23 B14
Hanumangarh *India* 68 E6
Hanyin *China* 58 A7
Hanyuan *China* 58 C5
Hanzhong *China* 56 H4
Hanzhuang *China* 57 G9
Haora *India* 69 H13
Haoxue *China* 59 B9
Haparanda *Sweden* 8 D21
Happy *U.S.A.* 116 D4
Happy Camp *U.S.A.* 108 F2
Happy Valley-Goose Bay
  Canada 105 B7
Hapsu *N. Korea* 57 D15
Hapur *India* 68 E7
Ḥaql *Si. Arabia* 74 F3
Har *Indonesia* 63 F8
Har-Ayrag *Mongolia* 56 B5
Har Hu *China* 60 C4
Har Us Nuur *Mongolia* 60 B4
Har Yehuda *Israel* 74 D3
Ḥarad *Si. Arabia* 75 C4
Haradok *Belarus* 32 E6
Häradsbäck *Sweden* 11 H8
Haramosh *Pakistan* 69 B6
Haranomachi *Japan* 54 F10
Harare *Zimbabwe* 87 F3
Harat *Eritrea* 81 D4
Harazé *Chad* 79 F3
Harbel *Liberia* 82 D2
Harbin *China* 57 B14
Harbıye *Turkey* 72 D7
Harbo *Sweden* 10 D11
Harboøre *Denmark* 11 H2
Harbor Beach *U.S.A.* 114 C2

Harborcreek *U.S.A.* 114 D5
Harbour Breton *Canada* 105 C8
Harbour Deep *Canada* 105 B8
Harburg *Germany* 24 B5
Harburger Berge △ *Germany* 24 B5
Ḥarda *India* 68 H7
Hardangerfjorden *Norway* 9 F12
Hardangervidda *Norway* 8 F12
Hardap △ *Namibia* 88 C2
Hardap Dam *Namibia* 88 C2
Hardenberg *Neths.* 17 B6
Harderwijk *Neths.* 17 B5
Hardey ➤ *Australia* 92 D2
Hardin *U.S.A.* 108 D10
Harding *S. Africa* 89 E4
Harding Ra. *Australia* 92 C3
Hardisty *Canada* 102 C6
Hardoi *India* 69 F9
Hardwar = Haridwar *India* 68 E8
Hardwick *U.S.A.* 115 B12
Hardwood Lake *Canada* 114 A7
Hardy, Pen. *Chile* 128 H3
Hardy, Pte. *St. Lucia* 121 f
Hare B. *Canada* 105 B8
Hareid *Norway* 8 E12
Haren *Germany* 24 C3
Harer *Ethiopia* 81 F5
Harerge *Ethiopia* 81 F5
Hareto *Ethiopia* 81 F4
Harfleur *France* 18 C7
Hargeisa *Somali Rep.* 75 F3
Harghita □ *Romania* 29 D10
Harghita, Munţii *Romania* 29 D10
Hargshamn *Sweden* 10 D12
Hari ➤ *Indonesia* 62 E2
Haria *Canary Is.* 48 E6
Haridwar *India* 68 E8
Harim, Jabal al *Oman* 71 E8
Haringhata ➤ *Bangla.* 67 J16
Ḥarīr, W. al ➤ *Syria* 74 C4
Harīrūd ➤ *Asia* 71 B9
Härjedalen *Sweden* 10 B7
Harlan *Iowa, U.S.A.* 112 E6
Harlan *Ky., U.S.A.* 113 G12
Hârlău *Romania* 29 C11
Harlech *U.K.* 14 E3
Harlem *U.S.A.* 108 B9
Hårlev *Denmark* 11 J6
Harlingen *Neths.* 17 A5
Harlingen *U.S.A.* 116 H6
Harlow *U.K.* 15 F8
Harlowton *U.S.A.* 108 C9
Harmancık *Turkey* 47 B11
Harmånger *Sweden* 10 C11
Harmil *Eritrea* 81 D5
Harnai *Pakistan* 68 D2
Harney Basin *U.S.A.* 108 E4
Harney L. *U.S.A.* 108 E4
Harney Peak *U.S.A.* 112 D2
Härnön *Sweden* 10 B12
Härnösand *Sweden* 10 B11
Haro *Spain* 38 C2
Haroldswick *U.K.* 13 A8
Harp L. *Canada* 105 A7
Harper *Liberia* 82 E3
Harper, Mt. *U.S.A.* 106 C11
Harplinge *Sweden* 11 H6
Harrai *India* 69 H8
Harrand *Pakistan* 68 E4
Ḥarrat Khaybar *Si. Arabia* 80 B5
Ḥarrat Nawāṣif *Si. Arabia* 80 C5
Harricana ➤ *Canada* 104 B4
Harriman *U.S.A.* 117 D12
Harrington Harbour *Canada* 105 B8
Harris *U.K.* 13 D2
Harris, L. *Australia* 95 E2
Harris, Sd. of *U.K.* 13 D1
Harris Pt. *Canada* 114 C2
Harrisburg *Ill., U.S.A.* 112 G9
Harrisburg *Nebr., U.S.A.* 112 E2
Harrisburg *Pa., U.S.A.* 114 F8
Harrismith *S. Africa* 89 D4
Harrison *Ark., U.S.A.* 116 C8
Harrison *Maine, U.S.A.* 115 B14
Harrison *Nebr., U.S.A.* 112 D2
Harrison, C. *Canada* 105 B8
Harrison Bay *U.S.A.* 106 A9
Harrison L. *Canada* 102 D4
Harrisonburg *U.S.A.* 113 F14
Harrisonville *U.S.A.* 112 F6
Harriston *Canada* 114 C4
Harrisville *Mich., U.S.A.* 114 B1
Harrisville *N.Y., U.S.A.* 115 B9
Harrisville *Pa., U.S.A.* 114 E5
Harrodsburg *U.S.A.* 113 G11
Harrogate *U.K.* 14 C6
Harrow *Canada* 114 D2
Harrow □ *U.K.* 15 F7
Harrowsmith *Canada* 115 B8
Harry S. Truman Res.
  U.S.A. 112 F7
Harsefeld *Germany* 24 B5
Harsewinkel *Germany* 24 D4
Harsın *Iran* 73 E12
Hârşova *Romania* 29 F12
Harstad *Norway* 8 B17
Harsud *India* 68 H7
Hart *U.S.A.* 112 D10
Hart, L. *Australia* 95 E2

Hartbees ➤ *S. Africa* 88 D3
Hartberg *Austria* 26 D8
Hartford *Conn., U.S.A.* 115 E12
Hartford *Ky., U.S.A.* 112 G10
Hartford *S. Dak., U.S.A.* 112 D5
Hartford *Vt., U.S.A.* 115 C12
Hartford *Wis., U.S.A.* 112 D9
Hartford City *U.S.A.* 113 E11
Hartland *Canada* 105 C6
Hartland *U.K.* 15 F3
Hartlepool *U.K.* 14 C6
Hartlepool □ *U.K.* 14 C6
Hartley Bay *Canada* 102 C3
Hartmannberge *Namibia* 88 B1
Hartney *Canada* 103 D8
Hârtop *Moldova* 29 D13
Harts ➤ *S. Africa* 88 D3
Harts Range *Australia* 94 C1
Hartselle *U.S.A.* 117 D11
Hartshorne *U.S.A.* 116 D7
Hartstown *U.S.A.* 114 E4
Hartsville *U.S.A.* 117 D14
Hartswater *S. Africa* 88 D3
Hartwell *U.S.A.* 117 D13
Harunabad *Pakistan* 68 E5
Harvand *Iran* 71 D7
Harvey *Australia* 93 F2
Harvey *Ill., U.S.A.* 112 E10
Harvey *N. Dak., U.S.A.* 112 B4
Harwich *U.K.* 15 F9
Haryana □ *India* 68 E7
Haryn ➤ *Belarus* 23 B14
Harz *Germany* 24 D6
Harz △ *Germany* 24 D6
Harzgerode *Germany* 24 D7
Hasa *Si. Arabia* 71 E6
Ḥasā, W. al ➤ *Jordan* 74 D4
Hasaheisa *Sudan* 81 E3
Ḥasanābād *Iran* 71 C7
Hasankeyf *Turkey* 73 D9
Ḥasb, W. ➤ *Iraq* 70 D5
Hasdo ➤ *India* 69 J10
Haselünne *Germany* 24 C3
Hashimoto *Japan* 55 G7
Hashtjerd *Iran* 71 C6
Hashtpur = Tālesh *Iran* 73 D13
Hashtrud *Iran* 73 D12
Haskell *U.S.A.* 116 E5
Haskovo = Khaskovo
  Bulgaria 45 E9
Hasköy *Turkey* 45 E10
Haslach *U.S.A.* 25 G4
Hasle *Denmark* 11 J8
Haslemere *U.K.* 15 F7
Haslev *Denmark* 11 J5
Hasparren *France* 20 E2
Hassa *Turkey* 72 D7
Hassberge △ *Germany* 25 E6
Hassela *Sweden* 10 B10
Hasselt *Belgium* 17 D5
Hassfurt *Germany* 25 E6
Hassi Messaoud *Algeria* 78 B7
Hässleholm *Sweden* 11 H7
Hassloch *Germany* 25 F4
Hästholmen *Sweden* 11 F8
Hastings *N.Z.* 91 C6
Hastings *U.K.* 15 G8
Hastings *Mich., U.S.A.* 113 D11
Hastings *Minn., U.S.A.* 112 C8
Hastings *Nebr., U.S.A.* 112 E4
Hastings Ra. *Australia* 95 E5
Hästveda *Sweden* 11 H7
Hat *Ukraine* 28 B7
Hat Yai *Thailand* 65 J3
Hatanbulag = Ergel *Mongolia* 56 C5
Hatay *Turkey* 72 D7
Hatay □ *Turkey* 72 D7
Hatch *U.S.A.* 109 K10
Hatchet L. *Canada* 103 B8
Haṭeg *Romania* 28 E7
Hateruma-Shima *Japan* 55 M1
Hatfield *Australia* 95 E3
Hatgal *Mongolia* 60 A5
Hathras *India* 68 F8
Hatia *Bangla.* 67 H17
Hato Mayor *Dom. Rep.* 121 C6
Hatta *India* 69 G8
Hatta *U.A.E.* 71 E8
Hattah *Australia* 95 E3
Hattah Kulkyne △ *Australia* 95 E3
Hatteras, C. *U.S.A.* 117 D17
Hattiesburg *U.S.A.* 117 F10
Hatvan *Hungary* 28 C4
Hau Duc *Vietnam* 64 E7
Haugesund *Norway* 9 G11
Haukipudas *Finland* 8 D21
Haultain ➤ *Canada* 103 B7
Hauraki G. *N.Z.* 91 B5
Hausruck *Austria* 26 C6
Haut Atlas *Morocco* 78 B4
Haut-Jura △ *France* 19 F9
Haut-Niger △ *Guinea* 82 C2
Haut-Rhin □ *France* 19 E14
Haut-Zaïre = Orientale □
  Dem. Rep. of the Congo 86 B2
Haute-Corse □ *France* 21 F13
Haute-Garonne □ *France* 20 E5
Haute-Loire □ *France* 20 C7
Haute-Marne □ *France* 19 D12

Haute-Normandie □ *France* 18 C7
Haute-Saône □ *France* 19 E13
Haute-Savoie □ *France* 21 C10
Haute-Vienne □ *France* 20 C5
Hautes-Alpes □ *France* 21 D10
Hautes Fagnes = Hohes
  Venn *Belgium* 17 D6
Hautes-Pyrénées □ *France* 20 F4
Hauteville-Lompnès *France* 21 C9
Hautmont *France* 19 B10
Hauts-de-Seine □ *France* 19 D9
Hauts Plateaux *Algeria* 78 B6
Hauzenberg *Germany* 25 G9
Havana = La Habana *Cuba* 120 B3
Havana *U.S.A.* 112 E8
Havant *U.K.* 15 G7
Havârna *Romania* 29 B11
Havasor = Kığzı *Turkey* 70 B4
Havasu, L. *U.S.A.* 111 L12
Havdhem *Sweden* 11 G12
Havel ➤ *Germany* 24 C8
Havelian *Pakistan* 68 B5
Havelock *Canada* 114 B7
Havelock *N.Z.* 91 D4
Havelock *U.S.A.* 117 D16
Haverfordwest *U.K.* 15 F3
Haverhill *U.K.* 15 E8
Haverhill *U.S.A.* 115 D13
Haverstraw *U.S.A.* 115 E11
Håverud *Sweden* 11 F6
Havirga *Mongolia* 56 B7
Havířov *Czech Rep.* 27 B11
Havlíčkův Brod *Czech Rep.* 26 B8
Havneby *Denmark* 11 J2
Havran *Turkey* 47 B9
Havre *U.S.A.* 108 B9
Havre-Aubert *Canada* 105 C7
Havre-St.-Pierre *Canada* 105 B7
Havsa *Turkey* 45 E10
Havza *Turkey* 72 B6
Haw ➤ *U.S.A.* 117 D15
Hawai'i *U.S.A.* 107 M8
Hawai'i □ *U.S.A.* 107 M8
Hawaiian Is. *Pac. Oc.* 97 E12
Hawaiian Ridge *Pac. Oc.* 97 E11
Hawarden *Canada* 112 D5
Hawea, L. *N.Z.* 91 F2
Hawera *N.Z.* 91 C5
Hawi *U.S.A.* 107 L8
Hawick *U.K.* 13 F6
Hawk Junction *Canada* 104 C3
Hawke B. *N.Z.* 91 C6
Hawker *Australia* 95 E2
Hawke's Bay *Canada* 105 B8
Hawkesbury *Canada* 104 C5
Hawkesbury I. *Canada* 102 C3
Hawkesbury Pt. *Australia* 94 A1
Hawkinsville *U.S.A.* 117 E13
Hawley *Minn., U.S.A.* 112 B5
Hawley *Pa., U.S.A.* 115 E9
Hawrān, W. ➤ *Iraq* 73 F10
Hawsh Mūssá *Lebanon* 74 B4
Hawthorne *U.S.A.* 108 G4
Hay *Australia* 95 E3
Hay ➤ *Australia* 94 C2
Hay ➤ *Canada* 102 A5
Hay, C. *Australia* 92 B4
Hay I. *Canada* 114 B4
Hay L. *Canada* 102 B5
Hay-on-Wye *U.K.* 15 E4
Hay Point *Australia* 94 C4
Hay River *Canada* 102 A5
Hay Springs *U.S.A.* 112 D2
Haya = Tehoru *Indonesia* 63 E7
Hayachine-San *Japan* 54 E10
Hayange *France* 19 C13
Hayastan = Armenia ■ *Asia* 35 K7
Haydān, W. al ➤ *Jordan* 74 D4
Haydarlı *Turkey* 47 C12
Hayden *U.S.A.* 108 F10
Hayes *U.S.A.* 112 C3
Hayes ➤ *Canada* 104 A1
Hayes, Mt. *U.S.A.* 106 C10
Hayes Creek *Australia* 92 B5
Hayle *U.K.* 15 G2
Hayling I. *U.K.* 15 G7
Hayman I. *Australia* 94 b
Haymana *Turkey* 72 C5
Hayrabolu *Turkey* 45 E11
Hays *Canada* 102 C6
Hays *U.S.A.* 112 F4
Haysyn *Ukraine* 29 B14
Hayvoron *Ukraine* 29 B14
Hayward *Calif., U.S.A.* 110 H4
Hayward *Wis., U.S.A.* 112 B8
Haywards Heath *U.K.* 15 G7
Hazafon □ *Israel* 74 C4
Hazar *Turkmenistan* 52 F6
Hazārān, Kūh-e *Iran* 71 D8
Hazard *U.S.A.* 113 G12
Hazaribag *India* 69 H11
Hazaribag Road *India* 69 G11
Hazebrouck *France* 19 B9
Hazelton *Canada* 102 B3
Hazelton *U.S.A.* 112 B3
Hazen *U.S.A.* 112 B3
Hazen, L. *Canada* 101 A17
Hazenmore *Canada* 103 D7
Hazerswoude-Dorp *Neths.* 17 B4
Hazlehurst *Ga., U.S.A.* 117 F13
Hazlehurst *Miss., U.S.A.* 117 F9

Hazlet *U.S.A.* 115 F10
Hazleton *U.S.A.* 115 F9
Hazlett, L. *Australia* 92 D4
Hazro *Turkey* 70 B4
He Xian *Anhui, China* 59 B12
He Xian *Guangxi Zhuangzu,*
  China 59 E8
Head of Bight *Australia* 93 F5
Headlands *Zimbabwe* 87 F3
Healdsburg *U.S.A.* 110 G4
Healdton *U.S.A.* 116 D6
Healesville *Australia* 95 F4
Healy *U.S.A.* 106 C10
Heany Junction *Zimbabwe* 89 C4
Heard I. *Ind. Oc.* 3 G13
Hearne *U.S.A.* 116 F6
Hearst *Canada* 104 C3
Heart ➤ *U.S.A.* 112 B3
Heart's Content *Canada* 105 C9
Heath, Pte. *Canada* 105 C7
Heathrow, London ✈
  (LHR) *U.K.* 15 F7
Heavener *U.S.A.* 116 D7
Hebbronville *U.S.A.* 116 H5
Hebei □ *China* 56 E9
Hebel *Australia* 95 D4
Heber *U.S.A.* 111 N11
Heber Springs *U.S.A.* 116 D8
Hebgen L. *U.S.A.* 108 D8
Hebi *China* 56 G8
Hebrides *U.K.* 6 D4
Hebrides, Sea of the *U.K.* 13 D2
Hebron = Al Khalīl
  West Bank 74 D4
Hebron *Canada* 101 F19
Hebron *N. Dak., U.S.A.* 112 B2
Hebron *Nebr., U.S.A.* 112 E5
Heby *Sweden* 10 E10
Hecate Str. *Canada* 102 C2
Heceta I. *U.S.A.* 102 B2
Hechi *China* 58 E7
Hechingen *Germany* 25 G4
Hechuan *China* 58 B6
Hecla *U.S.A.* 112 C4
Hecla I. *Canada* 103 C9
Hedal *Norway* 10 D3
Hédé *France* 18 D5
Hede *Sweden* 10 B7
Hedemora *Sweden* 10 D9
Hedensted *Denmark* 11 J3
Hedesunda *Sweden* 10 D10
Heerde *Neths.* 17 B6
Heerenveen *Neths.* 17 B5
Heerhugowaard *Neths.* 17 B4
Heerlen *Neths.* 17 D5
Ḥefa *Israel* 74 C4
Ḥefa □ *Israel* 74 C4
Hefei *China* 59 B11
Hefeng *China* 59 C8
Hegalig *Sudan* 81 E3
Hegang *China* 60 B8
Heiban *Sudan* 81 E3
Heichengzhen *China* 56 F4
Heide *Germany* 24 A5
Heidelberg *Germany* 25 F4
Heidelberg *S. Africa* 88 E3
Heidenau *Germany* 24 E9
Heidenheim *Germany* 25 G6
Heihe *China* 53 D13
Heijing *China* 58 E3
Heilbad Heiligenstadt
  Germany 24 D6
Heilbron *S. Africa* 89 D4
Heilbronn *Germany* 25 F5
Heiligenblut *Austria* 26 D5
Heiligenhafen *Germany* 24 A6
Heilongjiang □ *China* 60 B7
Heilunkiang =
  Heilongjiang □ *China* 60 B7
Heimaey *Iceland* 8 E3
Heinola *Finland* 32 B4
Heinsberg *Germany* 24 D2
Heinze Kyun *Burma* 64 E1
Heishan *China* 57 D12
Heishui *Liaoning, China* 57 C10
Heishui *Sichuan, China* 58 A4
Hejaz = Ḥijāz *Si. Arabia* 70 E3
Hejian *China* 56 E9
Hejiang *China* 58 C5
Hejin *China* 56 G6
Hekimhan *Turkey* 72 C7
Hekla *Iceland* 8 E4
Hekou *Guangdong, China* 59 F9
Hekou *Yunnan, China* 58 F4
Hel *Poland* 30 D5
Helagsfjället *Sweden* 10 B6
Helan Shan *China* 56 E3
Helechosa de los Montes
  Spain 37 F6
Helen Atoll *Pac. Oc.* 63 D8
Helena *Ark., U.S.A.* 117 D9
Helena *Mont., U.S.A.* 108 C7
Helendale *U.S.A.* 111 L9
Helensburgh *U.K.* 13 E4
Helensville *N.Z.* 91 B5
Helenvale *Australia* 94 B4
Helgasjön *Sweden* 11 H8
Helgeland *Norway* 8 C15
Helgoland *Germany* 24 A3

Heligoland = Helgoland *Germany* **24** A3
Heligoland B. = Deutsche Bucht *Germany* **24** A4
Heliopolis = Masr el Gedida *Egypt* **80** H7
Hell Hole Gorge △ *Australia* **94** D3
Hella *Iceland* **8** E3
Hellas = Greece ■ *Europe* **46** B3
Hellertown *U.S.A.* **115** F9
Hellespont = Çanakkale Boğazı *Turkey* **45** F10
Hellevoetsluis *Neths.* **17** C4
Hellín *Spain* **39** G3
Hells Canyon △ *U.S.A.* **108** D5
Hell's Gate △ *Kenya* **86** C4
Helmand □ *Afghan.* **66** D4
Helmand ➤ *Afghan.* **66** D2
Helme ➤ *Germany* **24** D7
Helmeringhausen *Namibia* **88** D2
Helmond *Neths.* **17** C5
Helmsdale *U.K.* **13** C5
Helmsdale ➤ *U.K.* **13** C5
Helmstedt *Germany* **24** C7
Helong *China* **57** C15
Helper *U.S.A.* **108** G8
Helsingborg *Sweden* **11** H6
Helsinge *Denmark* **11** H6
Helsingfors = Helsinki *Finland* **32** B3
Helsingør *Denmark* **11** H6
Helsinki *Finland* **32** B3
Helska, Mierzeja *Poland* **30** D5
Helston *U.K.* **15** G2
Helvellyn *U.K.* **14** C4
Helwân *Egypt* **80** J7
Hemel Hempstead *U.K.* **15** F7
Hemet *U.S.A.* **111** M10
Hemingford *U.S.A.* **112** D2
Hemis △ *India* **68** B7
Hemmingford *Canada* **115** A11
Hempstead *N.Y., U.S.A.* **115** F11
Hempstead *Tex., U.S.A.* **116** F6
Hemse *Sweden* **11** G12
Hemsön *Sweden* **10** B12
Henán *Sweden* **11** F5
Henan □ *China* **56** H8
Henares ➤ *Spain* **36** E7
Henashi-Misaki *Japan* **54** D9
Hendaye *France* **20** E2
Hendek *Turkey* **72** B4
Henderson *Argentina* **126** D3
Henderson *Ky., U.S.A.* **112** G10
Henderson *N.C., U.S.A.* **117** C15
Henderson *N.Y., U.S.A.* **115** D10
Henderson *Nev., U.S.A.* **111** J12
Henderson *Tenn., U.S.A.* **117** D10
Henderson I. *Pac. Oc.* **97** K15
Hendersonville *N.C., U.S.A.* **117** D13
Hendersonville *Tenn., U.S.A.* **117** C11
Hendījān *Iran* **71** D6
Hendorābī *Iran* **71** E7
Heng Jiang *China* **58** C5
Heng Xian *China* **58** F7
Hengcheng *China* **56** E4
Hèngch'un *Taiwan* **59** F13
Hengdaohezi *China* **57** B15
Hengelo *Neths.* **17** B6
Hengfeng *China* **59** C10
Hengshan *Hunan, China* **59** D9
Hengshan *Shaanxi, China* **56** F5
Hengshui *China* **56** F8
Hengyang *China* **59** D9
Henichesk *Ukraine* **33** J8
Hénin-Beaumont *France* **19** B9
Henley-on-Thames *U.K.* **15** F7
Henlopen, C. *U.S.A.* **113** F16
Hennan *Sweden* **10** B9
Hennebont *France* **18** E3
Hennenman *S. Africa* **88** D4
Hennessey *U.S.A.* **116** C6
Hennigsdorf *Germany* **24** C9
Henri Pittier △ *Venezuela* **121** D6
Henrietta *N.Y., U.S.A.* **114** C7
Henrietta *Tex., U.S.A.* **116** E5
Henrietta, Ostrov = Genriyetty, Ostrov *Russia* **53** B16
Henrietta Maria, C. *Canada* **104** A3
Henry *U.S.A.* **112** E9
Henryetta *U.S.A.* **116** D7
Henryville *Canada* **115** A11
Hensall *Canada* **114** C3
Henstedt-Ulzburg *Germany* **24** B6
Hentiesbaai *Namibia* **88** C1
Hentiyn Nuruu *Mongolia* **60** B5
Henty *Australia* **95** F4
Henzada *Burma* **67** L19
Hephaestia *Greece* **47** B7
Heping *China* **59** E10
Heppner *U.S.A.* **108** D4
Hepu *China* **58** G7
Heqing *China* **58** D3
Hequ *China* **56** E6
Hérāðsflói *Iceland* **8** D6
Hérāðsvötn ➤ *Iceland* **8** D4
Heraklion = Iraklio *Greece* **49** D7

Herald Cays *Australia* **94** B4
Herāt *Afghan.* **66** B3
Herāt □ *Afghan.* **66** B3
Hérault □ *France* **20** E7
Hérault ➤ *France* **20** E7
Herbault *France* **18** E8
Herbert *Canada* **103** C7
Herberton *Australia* **94** B4
Herbert ➤ *Australia* **94** B4
Herbertsdale *S. Africa* **88** E3
Herbignac *France* **18** E4
Herborn *Germany* **24** E4
Herby *Poland* **31** H5
Herceg-Novi *Montenegro* **44** D2
Herchmer *Canada* **103** B10
Herðubreið *Iceland* **8** D5
Hereford *U.K.* **15** E5
Hereford *U.S.A.* **116** D3
Herefordshire □ *U.K.* **15** E5
Hereke *Turkey* **45** F13
Herentals *Belgium* **17** C4
Herford *Germany* **24** C4
Héricourt *France* **19** E13
Herington *U.S.A.* **112** F5
Heris *Iran* **73** C12
Herisau *Switz.* **25** H5
Hérisson *France* **19** F9
Herkimer *U.S.A.* **115** D10
Herlong *U.S.A.* **110** E6
Herm *U.K.* **15** H5
Hermakivka *Ukraine* **29** B11
Hermann *U.S.A.* **112** F8
Hermannsburg *Australia* **92** D5
Hermannsburg *Germany* **24** C6
Hermanus *S. Africa* **88** E2
Herment *France* **20** C6
Hermidale *Australia* **95** E4
Hermiston *U.S.A.* **108** D4
Hermon *Canada* **114** A7
Hermon *U.S.A.* **115** B9
Hermon, Mt. = Shaykh, J. ash *Lebanon* **74** B4
Hermosillo *Mexico* **118** B2
Hernád ➤ *Hungary* **28** C6
Hernandarias *Paraguay* **127** B5
Hernandez *U.S.A.* **110** J6
Hernando *Argentina* **126** C3
Hernando *U.S.A.* **117** D10
Hernani *Spain* **38** B3
Herndon *U.S.A.* **114** F8
Herne *Germany* **17** C7
Herne Bay *U.K.* **15** F9
Herning *Denmark* **11** H2
Heroica Caborca = Caborca *Mexico* **118** A2
Heroica Nogales = Nogales *Mexico* **118** A2
Heron Bay *Canada* **104** C2
Heron I. *Australia* **94** C5
Herradura, Pta. de la *Canary Is.* **48** F3
Herreid *U.S.A.* **112** C3
Herrenberg *Germany* **25** G4
Herrera *Spain* **37** H6
Herrera de Alcántara *Spain* **37** F3
Herrera de Pisuerga *Spain* **36** C6
Herrera del Duque *Spain* **37** F5
Herrestad *Sweden* **11** F5
Herrin *U.S.A.* **112** G9
Herriot *Canada* **103** B8
Herrljunga *Sweden* **11** F7
Herschel I. *Canada* **4** C1
Hershey *U.S.A.* **115** F8
Herso *Greece* **44** E6
Herstal *Belgium* **17** D5
Hertford *U.K.* **15** F7
Hertfordshire □ *U.K.* **15** F7
's-Hertogenbosch *Neths.* **17** C5
Hertsa *Ukraine* **29** B11
Hertzogville *S. Africa* **88** D4
Hervás *Spain* **36** E5
Hervey B. *Australia* **94** C5
Herzberg *Brandenburg, Germany* **24** D9
Herzberg *Niedersachsen, Germany* **24** D6
Herzliyya *Israel* **74** C3
Herzogenburg *Austria* **26** C8
Ḥeşār *Fārs, Iran* **71** D6
Ḥeşār *Markazī, Iran* **71** C6
Hesdin *France* **19** B9
Heshan *China* **58** F7
Heshui *China* **56** G5
Heshun *China* **56** F7
Hesperia *U.S.A.* **111** L9
Hesse = Hessen □ *Germany* **24** E4
Hessen □ *Germany* **24** E4
Hessenreuther und Manteler Wald △ *Germany* **25** F8
Hestra *Sweden* **11** G7
Hetauda *Nepal* **69** F11
Hetch Hetchy Aqueduct *U.S.A.* **110** H5
Hettinger *U.S.A.* **112** B2
Hettstedt *Germany* **24** D7
Heuksando *S. Korea* **57** G13
Heunghae *S. Korea* **57** F15

Heuvelton *U.S.A.* **115** B9
Heves *Hungary* **28** C5
Heves □ *Hungary* **28** C5
Hewitt *U.S.A.* **116** F6
Hexham *U.K.* **14** C5
Hexi *Yunnan, China* **58** E4
Hexi *Zhejiang, China* **59** D12
Hexigten Qi *China* **57** C9
Heydarābād *Iran* **71** D7
Heysham *U.K.* **14** C5
Heyuan *China* **59** F10
Heze *China* **56** G8
Hezhang *China* **58** D5
Hi Vista *U.S.A.* **111** L9
Hialeah *U.S.A.* **117** J14
Hiawatha *U.S.A.* **112** F6
Hibbing *U.S.A.* **112** B7
Hibernia Reef *Australia* **92** B3
Hickman *U.S.A.* **112** G9
Hickory *U.S.A.* **117** D14
Hicks, Pt. *Australia* **95** F4
Hicks L. *Canada* **103** A9
Hicksville *U.S.A.* **115** F11
Hida *Romania* **29** C8
Hida-Gawa ➤ *Japan* **55** G8
Hida-Sammyaku *Japan* **55** F8
Hidaka-Sammyaku *Japan* **54** C11
Hidalgo *Mexico* **119** C5
Hidalgo □ *Mexico* **119** C5
Hidalgo, Presa M. *Mexico* **118** B3
Hidalgo del Parral *Mexico* **118** B3
Hiddensee *Germany* **24** A9
Hieflau *Austria* **26** D7
Hiendelaencina *Spain* **38** D2
Hierro *Canary Is.* **48** G1
Higashiajima-San *Japan* **54** F10
Higashiōsaka *Japan* **55** G7
Higgins *U.S.A.* **116** C4
Higgins Corner *U.S.A.* **110** F5
High Bridge *U.S.A.* **115** F10
High Desert *U.S.A.* **106** G15
High Level *Canada* **102** B5
High Point *U.S.A.* **117** D15
High Prairie *Canada* **102** B5
High River *Canada* **102** C6
High Tatra = Tatry *Slovak Rep.* **27** B13
High Veld *Africa* **76** J6
High Wycombe *U.K.* **15** F7
Highland □ *U.K.* **13** D4
Highland Park *U.S.A.* **112** D10
Highmore *U.S.A.* **112** C4
Highrock L. *Canada* **103** B8
Higüey *Dom. Rep.* **121** C6
Hihya *Egypt* **80** H7
Hiiumaa *Estonia* **32** C2
Híjar *Spain* **38** D4
Ḥijāz *Si. Arabia* **70** E3
Hijo = Tagum *Phil.* **61** H6
Hikari *Japan* **55** H5
Hikmak, Ras el *Egypt* **80** A2
Hiko *U.S.A.* **110** H11
Hikone *Japan* **55** G8
Hikurangi *Gisborne, N.Z.* **91** C6
Hikurangi *Northland, N.Z.* **91** A5
Hildburghausen *Germany* **24** E6
Hildesheim *Germany* **24** C5
Hill ➤ *Australia* **93** F2
Hill City *Idaho, U.S.A.* **108** E6
Hill City *Kans., U.S.A.* **112** F4
Hill City *Minn., U.S.A.* **112** B7
Hill City *S. Dak., U.S.A.* **112** D2
Hill Island L. *Canada* **103** A7
Hillaby, Mt. *Barbados* **121** g
Hillared *Sweden* **11** G7
Hillcrest *Barbados* **121** g
Hillcrest Center *U.S.A.* **111** K8
Hillegom *Neths.* **17** B4
Hillerød *Denmark* **11** J6
Hillerstorp *Sweden* **11** G7
Hillsboro *Kans., U.S.A.* **112** F5
Hillsboro *N. Dak., U.S.A.* **112** B5
Hillsboro *Ohio, U.S.A.* **113** F12
Hillsboro *Oreg., U.S.A.* **108** D2
Hillsboro *Tex., U.S.A.* **116** E6
Hillsborough *Grenada* **121** D7
Hillsborough *U.S.A.* **115** C13
Hillsborough Channel *Australia* **94** b
Hillsdale *Mich., U.S.A.* **113** E11
Hillsdale *N.Y., U.S.A.* **115** D11
Hillsport *Canada* **104** C2
Hillston *Australia* **95** E4
Hilo *U.S.A.* **107** M8
Hilton *U.S.A.* **114** C7
Hilton Head Island *U.S.A.* **117** E14
Hilvan *Turkey* **73** D8
Hilversum *Neths.* **17** B5
Himachal Pradesh □ *India* **68** D7
Himalaya *Asia* **69** E11
Himalchuli *Nepal* **69** E11
Himamaylan *Phil.* **61** F5
Himarë *Albania* **44** F3
Himatnagar *India* **68** H5
Himeji *Japan* **55** G7
Himi *Japan* **55** F8
Himmerland *Denmark* **11** H3
Ḥimş *Syria* **74** A5
Ḥimş □ *Syria* **74** A6

Hinche *Haiti* **121** C5
Hinchinbrook I. *Australia* **94** B4
Hinchinbrook Island △ *Australia* **94** B4
Hinckley *U.K.* **15** E6
Hinckley *U.S.A.* **112** B7
Hindaun *India* **68** F7
Hindmarsh, L. *Australia* **95** F3
Hindsholm *Denmark* **11** J4
Hindu Bagh *Pakistan* **68** D2
Hindu Kush *Asia* **66** B7
Hindupur *India* **66** N10
Hines Creek *Canada* **102** B5
Hinesville *U.S.A.* **117** F14
Hinganghat *India* **66** J11
Hingham *U.S.A.* **108** B8
Hingir *India* **69** J10
Hingoli *India* **66** K10
Hinigaran *Phil.* **61** F5
Hinis *Turkey* **73** C9
Hinna = Imi *Ethiopia* **81** F5
Hinna *Nigeria* **83** C7
Hinnerup *Denmark* **11** H4
Hinnøya *Norway* **8** B16
Hinojosa del Duque *Spain* **37** G5
Hinsdale *U.S.A.* **115** D12
Hinterrhein ➤ *Switz.* **25** J5
Hinthada = Henzada *Burma* **67** L19
Hinton *Canada* **102** C5
Hinton *U.S.A.* **113** G13
Hios *Greece* **47** C8
Hios □ *Greece* **47** C8
Hirado *Japan* **55** H4
Hirakud Dam *India* **67** J13
Hiran ➤ *India* **69** H8
Hirapur *India* **69** G8
Hirara *Japan* **55** M2
Hiratsuka *Japan* **55** G9
Hiroo *Japan* **54** C11
Hirosaki *Japan* **54** D10
Hiroshima *Japan* **55** G6
Hiroshima □ *Japan* **55** G6
Hirson *France* **19** C11
Hirtshals *Denmark* **11** G3
Hisar *India* **68** E6
Hisarcık *Turkey* **47** B11
Hisaria *Bulgaria* **45** D8
Hisb, Sha'ib = Ḥasb, W. ➤ *Iraq* **70** D5
Ḥismá *Si. Arabia* **70** D3
Hispaniola *W. Indies* **121** C5
Ḥīt *Iraq* **73** F10
Hita *Japan* **55** H5
Hitachi *Japan* **55** F10
Hitchin *U.K.* **15** F7
Hitiaa *Tahiti* **91** d
Hitoyoshi *Japan* **55** H5
Hitra *Norway* **8** E13
Hitzacker *Germany* **24** B7
Hiva Oa *French Polynesia* **97** H14
Hixon *Canada* **102** C4
Ḥiyyon, N. ➤ *Israel* **74** E4
Hjalmar L. *Canada* **103** A7
Hjälmaren *Sweden* **10** E9
Hjältevad *Sweden* **11** G9
Hjo *Sweden* **11** F8
Hjørring *Denmark* **11** G3
Hjort Trench *S. Ocean* **5** B10
Hjortkvarn *Sweden* **11** F9
Hkakabo Razi *Burma* **67** E20
Hkamti = Singkaling Hkamti *Burma* **67** G19
Hlinsko *Czech Rep.* **26** B8
Hlobane *S. Africa* **89** D5
Hlohovec *Slovak Rep.* **27** C10
Hlučín *Czech Rep.* **27** B11
Hluhluwe *S. Africa* **89** D5
Hluhluwe △ *S. Africa* **89** C5
Hlukhiv *Ukraine* **33** G7
Hlyboka *Ukraine* **29** B10
Hlybokaye *Belarus* **32** E4
Hnúšťa *Slovak Rep.* **27** C12
Ho *Ghana* **83** D5
Ho Chi Minh City = Thanh Pho Ho Chi Minh *Vietnam* **65** G6
Ho Thuong *Vietnam* **64** C5
Hoa Binh *Vietnam* **58** G5
Hoa Da *Vietnam* **65** G7
Hoa Hiep *Vietnam* **65** G5
Hoai Nhon *Vietnam* **64** E7
Hoang Lien Son *Vietnam* **58** F4
Hoanib ➤ *Namibia* **88** B2
Hoare B. *Canada* **101** D19
Hoarusib ➤ *Namibia* **88** B2
Hobart *Australia* **95** G4
Hobart *U.S.A.* **116** D5
Hobbs *U.S.A.* **109** K12
Hobbs Coast *Antarctica* **5** D14
Hobe Sound *U.S.A.* **117** H14
Hoboken *U.S.A.* **115** F10
Hobro *Denmark* **11** H3
Hoburgen *Sweden* **11** H12
Hobyo *Somali Rep.* **75** F4
Hocalar *Turkey* **47** C11
Hochfeld *Namibia* **88** C2
Hochharz △ *Germany* **24** D6
Hochschwab *Austria* **26** D8
Höchstadt *Germany* **25** F6

Hinche *Haiti* **121** C5
Hochtaunus △ *Germany* **25** E4
Hockenheim *Germany* **25** F4
Hodaka-Dake *Japan* **55** F8
Hodeida = Al Ḥudaydah *Yemen* **75** E3
Hodgeville *Canada* **103** C7
Hodgson *Canada* **103** C9
Hodh El Gharbi □ *Mauritania* **82** B3
Hódmezővásárhely *Hungary* **28** D5
Hodna, Chott el *Algeria* **78** A6
Hodonín *Czech Rep.* **27** C10
Hœdic, Î. de *France* **18** E4
Hoek van Holland *Neths.* **17** C4
Hoengseong *S. Korea* **57** F14
Hoeryong *N. Korea* **57** C15
Hoeyang *N. Korea* **57** E14
Hof *Germany* **25** E7
Hofgeismar *Germany* **24** D5
Hofheim *Germany* **25** E4
Hofmeyr *S. Africa* **88** E4
Höfn *Iceland* **8** D6
Hofors *Sweden* **10** D10
Hofsjökull *Iceland* **8** D4
Hofu *Japan* **55** G5
Hogan Group *Australia* **95** F4
Höganäs *Sweden* **11** H6
Hogarth, Mt. *Australia* **94** C2
Hoge Kempen △ *Belgium* **17** C5
Hoggar = Ahaggar *Algeria* **78** D7
Högsäter *Sweden* **11** F6
Högsby *Sweden* **11** G10
Högsjö *Sweden* **10** E9
Hogsty Reef *Bahamas* **121** B5
Hoh ➤ *U.S.A.* **110** C2
Hohd ech Chargui □ *Mauritania* **82** B3
Hohe Acht *Germany* **25** E3
Hohe Tauern *Austria* **26** D5
Hohe Tauern △ *Austria* **26** D5
Hohenau *Austria* **27** C9
Hohenems *Austria* **26** D2
Hohenloher Ebene *Germany* **25** F5
Hohenwald *U.S.A.* **117** D11
Hohenwestedt *Germany* **24** A5
Hoher Rhön = Rhön *Germany* **24** E5
Hoher Vogelsberg △ *Germany* **24** E5
Hohes Venn *Belgium* **17** D6
Hohes Venn-Eifel △ *Europe* **24** E2
Hohhot *China* **56** D6
Hohoe *Ghana* **83** D5
Hoi An *Vietnam* **64** E7
Hoi Xuan *Vietnam* **58** G5
Hoisington *U.S.A.* **112** F4
Højer *Denmark* **11** K2
Hōjō *Japan* **55** H6
Hok *Sweden* **11** G8
Hökensås *Sweden* **11** G8
Hökerum *Sweden* **11** G7
Hokianga Harbour *N.Z.* **91** A4
Hokitika *N.Z.* **91** E3
Hokkaidō □ *Japan* **54** C11
Hol-Hol *Djibouti* **81** E5
Hola *Kenya* **86** B4
Hola Pristan *Ukraine* **33** J7
Holakas *Greece* **49** D9
Holbæk *Denmark* **11** J5
Holbrook *Australia* **95** F4
Holbrook *U.S.A.* **109** J8
Holcomb *U.S.A.* **114** D7
Holden *U.S.A.* **108** G7
Holdenville *U.S.A.* **116** D6
Holdrege *U.S.A.* **112** E4
Holešov *Czech Rep.* **27** B10
Holguín *Cuba* **120** B4
Holíč *Slovak Rep.* **27** C10
Holice *Czech Rep.* **26** A8
Höljes *Sweden* **10** D6
Hollabrunn *Austria* **26** C9
Hollams Bird I. *Namibia* **88** C1
Holland = Netherlands ■ *Europe* **17** C5
Holland *Mich., U.S.A.* **112** D10
Holland *N.Y., U.S.A.* **114** D6
Holland Centre *Canada* **114** B4
Holland Patent *U.S.A.* **115** C9
Hollandale *U.S.A.* **117** E9
Holley *U.S.A.* **114** C6
Hollfeld *Germany* **25** F7
Hollidaysburg *U.S.A.* **114** F6
Hollis *U.S.A.* **116** D5
Hollister *Calif., U.S.A.* **110** J5
Hollister *Idaho, U.S.A.* **108** E6
Höllviken = Höllviksnäs *Sweden* **11** J6
Höllviksnäs *Sweden* **11** J6
Holly Hill *U.S.A.* **117** G14
Holly Springs *U.S.A.* **117** D10
Hollywood *U.S.A.* **117** H14
Holman *Canada* **100** C8
Hólmavík *Iceland* **8** D3
Holmen *U.S.A.* **112** D8
Holmes Reefs *Australia* **94** B4
Holmsjö *Sweden* **11** H9
Holmsjön *Västernorrland, Sweden* **10** B10
Holmsjön *Västernorrland, Sweden* **10** B9

Holmsland Klit *Denmark* **11** J2
Holmsund *Sweden* **8** E19
Holod *Romania* **28** D7
Holovne *Ukraine* **31** G11
Holozubyntsi *Ukraine* **29** B11
Holroyd ➤ *Australia* **94** A3
Holstebro *Denmark* **11** H2
Holsteinische Schweiz △ *Germany* **24** A6
Holsworthy *U.K.* **15** G3
Holton *Canada* **105** B8
Holton *U.S.A.* **112** F6
Holtville *U.S.A.* **111** N11
Holwerd *Neths.* **17** A5
Holy Cross *U.S.A.* **106** C8
Holy I. *Anglesey, U.K.* **14** D3
Holy I. *Northumberland, U.K.* **14** B6
Holyhead *U.K.* **14** D3
Holyoke *Colo., U.S.A.* **108** F12
Holyoke *Mass., U.S.A.* **115** D12
Holyrood *Canada* **105** C9
Holzkirchen *Germany* **25** H7
Holzminden *Germany* **24** D5
Homa Bay *Kenya* **86** C3
Homalin *Burma* **67** G19
Homand *Iran* **71** C8
Homathko ➤ *Canada* **102** C4
Homberg *Germany* **24** D5
Hombori *Mali* **83** B4
Hombori Tondo *Mali* **83** B4
Homburg *Germany* **25** F3
Home B. *Canada* **101** D18
Home Hill *Australia* **94** B4
Home Reef *Tonga* **91** c
Homedale *U.S.A.* **108** E5
Homer *Alaska, U.S.A.* **100** F1
Homer *La., U.S.A.* **116** E8
Homer *N.Y., U.S.A.* **115** D8
Homer City *U.S.A.* **114** F5
Homert △ *Germany* **24** D4
Homestead *Australia* **94** C4
Homestead *U.S.A.* **117** J14
Homestead △ *U.S.A.* **112** E6
Homoine *Mozam.* **89** C6
Homoljske Planina *Serbia* **44** B5
Homorod *Romania* **29** D10
Homs = Ḥimş *Syria* **74** A5
Homyel *Belarus* **23** B16
Homyel □ *Belarus* **33** F6
Hon Chong *Vietnam* **65** G5
Hon Hai *Vietnam* **65** H7
Hon Me *Vietnam* **64** C5
Honan = Henan □ *China* **56** H8
Honaz *Turkey* **47** D11
Honbetsu *Japan* **54** C11
Honcut *U.S.A.* **110** F5
Honda, Bahía *Cuba* **120** B3
Honda Bay *Phil.* **61** G3
Hondarribia *Spain* **38** B3
Hondeklipbaai *S. Africa* **88** E2
Hondo *Japan* **55** H5
Hondo *U.S.A.* **116** G5
Hondo, Río ➤ *Belize* **119** D7
Honduras ■ *Cent. Amer.* **120** D2
Honduras, G. de *Caribbean* **120** C2
Hønefoss *Norway* **9** F14
Honesdale *U.S.A.* **115** E9
Honey Harbour *Canada* **114** B5
Honey L. *U.S.A.* **110** E6
Honfleur *France* **18** C7
Høng *Denmark* **11** J5
Hong Gai *Vietnam* **58** G6
Hong He ➤ *China* **56** H8
Hong Hu *China* **59** C9
Hong Kong □ *China* **59** F10
Hong'an *China* **59** B10
Hongcheon *S. Korea* **57** F14
Honghai Wan *China* **59** F10
Honghe *China* **58** F4
Honghu *China* **59** C9
Hongjiang *China* **58** D7
Hongliu He ➤ *China* **56** F5
Hongor *Mongolia* **56** B7
Hongsa *Laos* **64** C3
Hongseong *S. Korea* **57** F14
Hongshui He ➤ *China* **58** F7
Hongtong *China* **56** F6
Honguedo, Détroit d' *Canada* **105** C7
Hongwon *N. Korea* **57** E14
Hongya *China* **58** C4
Hongyuan *China* **58** A4
Hongze Hu *China* **57** H10
Honiara *Solomon Is.* **90** B8
Honiton *U.K.* **15** G4
Honjō *Japan* **54** E10
Honkorâb, Ras *Egypt* **80** C4
Honningsvåg *Norway* **8** A21
Hönö *Sweden* **11** G5
Honolulu *U.S.A.* **107** L8
Honshū *Japan* **54** F9
Hontoria del Pinar *Spain* **38** D1
Hood, Mt. *U.S.A.* **108** D3
Hood, Pt. *Australia* **93** F2
Hood River *U.S.A.* **108** D3
Hoodsport *U.S.A.* **110** C3
Hooge *Germany* **24** A4
Hoogeveen *Neths.* **17** B6
Hoogezand-Sappemeer *Neths.* **17** A6

Hooghly = Hugli → *India* **69** J13
Hooghly-Chinsura =
  Chunchura *India* **69** H13
Hook Hd. *Ireland* **12** D5
Hook I. *Australia* **94** b
Hook of Holland = Hoek
  van Holland *Neths.* **17** C4
Hooker *U.S.A.* **116** C4
Hooker Creek = Lajamanu
  Australia **92** C5
Hooker Creek ⊙ *Australia* **92** C5
Hoonah *U.S.A.* **102** B1
Hooper Bay *U.S.A.* **106** C6
Hoopeston *U.S.A.* **112** E10
Hoopstad *S. Africa* **88** D4
Höör *Sweden* **11** J7
Hoorn *Neths.* **17** B5
Hoover *U.S.A.* **117** E11
Hoover Dam *U.S.A.* **111** K12
Hooversville *U.S.A.* **114** F6
Hop Bottom *U.S.A.* **115** E9
Hopa *Turkey* **73** B9
Hope *Canada* **102** D4
Hope *Ariz., U.S.A.* **111** M13
Hope *Ark., U.S.A.* **116** E8
Hope, L. *S. Austral., Australia* **95** D2
Hope, L. *W. Austral., Australia* **93** F3
Hope, Pt. *U.S.A.* **98** C3
Hope I. *Canada* **114** B4
Hope Town *Bahamas* **120** A4
Hope Vale *Australia* **94** B4
Hope Vale ⊙ *Australia* **94** B4
Hopedale *Canada* **105** A7
Hopedale *U.S.A.* **115** D13
Hopefield *S. Africa* **88** E2
Hopei = Hebei □ *China* **56** E9
Hopelchén *Mexico* **119** D7
Hopetoun *Vic., Australia* **95** F3
Hopetoun *W. Austral., Australia* **93** F3
Hopetown *S. Africa* **88** D3
Hopewell *U.S.A.* **113** G15
Hopfgarten *Austria* **26** D5
Hopkins, L. *Australia* **92** D4
Hopkinsville *U.S.A.* **112** G10
Hopland *U.S.A.* **110** G3
Hoquiam *U.S.A.* **110** D3
Hora Hoverla *Ukraine* **29** B9
Horasan *Turkey* **73** B10
Horaždóvice *Czech Rep.* **26** B6
Horb *Germany* **25** G4
Hörby *Sweden* **11** J7
Horcajo de Santiago *Spain* **38** F1
Hordern Hills *Australia* **92** D5
Horezu *Romania* **29** E8
Horgen *Switz.* **25** H4
Horgoš *Serbia* **28** D4
Hořice *Czech Rep.* **26** A8
Horinchove *Ukraine* **29** B8
Horinger *China* **56** D6
Horizontina *Brazil* **127** B5
Horki *Belarus* **32** E6
Horlick Mts. *Antarctica* **5** E15
Horlivka *Ukraine* **33** H10
Hormak *Iran* **71** D9
Hormoz *Iran* **71** E7
Hormoz, Jaz.-ye *Iran* **71** E8
Hormozgān □ *Iran* **71** E8
Hormuz, Kūh-e *Iran* **71** E7
Hormuz, Str. of *The Gulf* **71** E8
Horn *Austria* **26** C8
Horn *Sweden* **11** G9
Horn → *Canada* **102** A5
Horn, Cape = Hornos, C. de *Chile* **128** H3
Horn Head *Ireland* **12** A3
Horn I. *Australia* **94** A3
Horn Plateau *Canada* **102** A5
Hornachuelos *Spain* **37** H5
Hornavan *Sweden* **8** C17
Hornbeck *U.S.A.* **116** F8
Hornbrook *U.S.A.* **108** F2
Hornburg *Germany* **24** C6
Horncastle *U.K.* **14** D7
Horndal *Sweden* **10** D10
Hornell *U.S.A.* **114** D7
Hornell L. *Canada* **102** A5
Hornepayne *Canada* **104** C3
Horní Planá *Czech Rep.* **26** C7
Hornings Mills *Canada* **114** B4
Hornitos *U.S.A.* **110** H6
Hornos, C. de *Chile* **128** H3
Hornoy-le-Bourg *France* **19** C8
Hornsby *Australia* **95** B5
Hornsea *U.K.* **14** D7
Hornslandet *Sweden* **10** C11
Hörnum *Germany* **24** A4
Horobetsu = Noboribetsu
  Japan **54** C10
Horodenka *Ukraine* **29** B10
Horodnya *Ukraine* **33** G6
Horodok *Khmelnytskyy, Ukraine* **23** D14
Horodok *Lviv, Ukraine* **23** D12
Horodyshche *Ukraine* **33** H6
Horokhiv *Ukraine* **23** C13
Horovice *Czech Rep.* **26** B6
Horqin Youyi Qianqi *China* **57** A12
Horqueta *Paraguay* **126** A4

Horred *Sweden* **11** G6
Horse Cr. → *U.S.A.* **108** F12
Horse I. *Canada* **103** C9
Horse Is. *Canada* **105** B8
Horsefly L. *Canada* **102** C4
Horseheads *U.S.A.* **114** D8
Horsens *Denmark* **11** J3
Horseshoe Lake *Canada* **114** A5
Horsham *Australia* **95** F3
Horsham *U.K.* **15** F7
Horšovský Týn *Czech Rep.* **26** B5
Horta *Azores* **78** a
Horten *Norway* **9** G14
Hortobágy → *Hungary* **28** C6
Hortobágyi △ *Hungary* **28** C6
Horton *U.S.A.* **112** F6
Horton → *Canada* **100** D6
Horwood L. *Canada* **104** C3
Hosaina *Ethiopia* **81** F4
Hosapete = Hospet *India* **66** M10
Hoseynābād *Khuzestān, Iran* **71** C6
Hoseynābād *Kordestān, Iran* **73** E12
Hôsh 'Īsa *Egypt* **80** H7
Hoshangabad *India* **68** H7
Hoshiarpur *India* **68** D6
Hospet *India* **66** M10
Hoste, I. *Chile* **128** H3
Hostens *France* **20** D3
Hot *Thailand* **64** C2
Hot Creek Range *U.S.A.* **108** G5
Hot Springs *Ark., U.S.A.* **116** D8
Hot Springs *S. Dak., U.S.A.* **112** D2
Hot Springs △ *U.S.A.* **116** D8
Hotagen *Sweden* **8** E16
Hotan *China* **60** C2
Hotazel *S. Africa* **88** D3
Hotchkiss *U.S.A.* **108** G10
Hotham, C. *Australia* **92** B5
Hoting *Sweden* **8** D17
Hotolisht *Albania* **44** E4
Hotte, Massif de la *Haiti* **121** C5
Houat, Î. de *France* **18** E4
Houdan *France* **19** D8
Houei Sai *Laos* **58** G3
Houeillès *France* **20** D4
Houffalize *Belgium* **17** D5
Houghton *Mich., U.S.A.* **112** B9
Houghton *N.Y., U.S.A.* **114** D6
Houghton L. *U.S.A.* **113** C11
Houghton-le-Spring *U.K.* **14** C6
Houhora Heads *N.Z.* **91** A4
Houlton *U.S.A.* **113** B20
Houma *U.S.A.* **117** G9
Houndé *Burkina Faso* **82** C4
Hourtin *France* **20** C2
Hourtin-Carcans, Étang d' *France* **20** C2
Housatonic → *U.S.A.* **115** E11
Houston *Canada* **102** C3
Houston *Mo., U.S.A.* **112** G8
Houston *Tex., U.S.A.* **116** G7
Hout = Mogwadi → *S. Africa* **89** C4
Houtkraal *S. Africa* **88** E3
Houtman Abrolhos *Australia* **93** E1
Hovd □ *Mongolia* **60** B4
Hove *U.K.* **15** G7
Hovedstaden □ *Denmark* **11** J6
Hovenweep △ *U.S.A.* **109** H9
Hoveyzeh *Iran* **71** D6
Hovmantorp *Sweden* **11** H9
Hövsgöl *Mongolia* **56** C5
Hövsgöl Nuur *Mongolia* **60** A5
Hovsta *Sweden* **10** E9
Howakil *Eritrea* **81** D5
Howar, Wadi → *Sudan* **81** D2
Howard *Australia* **95** D5
Howard *Pa., U.S.A.* **114** F7
Howard *S. Dak., U.S.A.* **112** C5
Howe *U.S.A.* **108** E7
Howe, C. *Australia* **95** F5
Howe, West Cape *Australia* **93** G2
Howe I. *Canada* **115** B8
Howell *U.S.A.* **113** D12
Howick *Canada* **115** A11
Howick *S. Africa* **89** D5
Howick Group *Australia* **94** A4
Howitt, L. *Australia* **95** D2
Howland I. *Pac. Oc.* **96** G10
Howrah = Haora *India* **69** H13
Howth *Ireland* **12** C5
Howth Hd. *Ireland* **12** C5
Höxter *Germany* **24** D5
Hoy *U.K.* **13** C5
Hoya *Germany* **24** C5
Hoyanger *Norway* **8** F12
Hoyerswerda *Germany* **24** D10
Hoylake *U.K.* **14** D4
Hoyos *Spain* **36** E4
Hpa-an = Pa-an *Burma* **67** L20
Hpauchinango *Mexico* **119** C5
Hpunan Pass *Burma* **67** F20
Hradec Králové *Czech Rep.* **26** A8
Hrádek *Czech Rep.* **27** C9
Hranice *Czech Rep.* **27** D10
Hrazdan *Armenia* **35** K7
Hrebenka *Ukraine* **33** G7
Hrisoupoli *Greece* **45** F8
Hristiana *Greece* **47** E7
Hrodna *Belarus* **30** E10

Hrodna □ *Belarus* **32** F3
Hrodzyanka *Belarus* **23** B15
Hron → *Slovak Rep.* **27** D11
Hrubieszów *Poland* **31** H10
Hrubý Jeseník *Czech Rep.* **27** A10
Hrvatska = Croatia ■ *Europe* **41** C13
Hrymayliv *Ukraine* **23** D14
Hrynyava *Ukraine* **29** C9
Hsenwi *Burma* **67** H20
Hsiamen = Xiamen *China* **59** E12
Hsian = Xi'an *China* **56** G5
Hsinchu *Taiwan* **59** E13
Hsinhailien =
  Lianyungang *China* **57** G10
Hsinying *Taiwan* **59** F13
Hsopket *Burma* **58** F2
Hsüchou = Xuzhou *China* **57** G9
Htapodia *Greece* **47** D7
Hu Xian *China* **56** G5
Hua Hin *Thailand* **64** F2
Hua Xian *Henan, China* **56** G8
Hua Xian *Shaanxi, China* **56** G5
Hua'an *China* **59** E11
Huab → *Namibia* **88** B2
Huacheng *China* **59** E10
Huachinera *Mexico* **118** A3
Huacho *Peru* **124** F3
Huade *China* **56** D7
Huadian *China* **57** C14
Huadu *China* **59** F9
Huahine, Î. *French Polynesia* **97** J12
Huai Hat △ *Thailand* **64** D5
Huai He → *China* **59** A12
Huai Nam Dang △ *Thailand* **64** C2
Huai Yot *Thailand* **65** J2
Huai'an *Hebei, China* **56** D8
Huai'an *Jiangsu, China* **57** H10
Huaibei *China* **56** G9
Huaibin *China* **59** A10
Huaide = Gongzhuling *China* **57** C13
Huaidezhen *China* **57** C13
Huaihua *China* **58** D7
Huaiji *China* **59** F9
Huainan *China* **59** A11
Huaining *China* **59** B11
Huairen *China* **56** E7
Huairou *China* **56** D9
Huaiyang *China* **56** H8
Huaiyin *China* **57** H10
Huaiyuan *Anhui, China* **57** H9
Huaiyuan *Guangxi Zhuangzu, China* **58** E7
Huajuapán de León *Mexico* **119** D5
Hualapai Peak *U.S.A.* **109** J7
Hualien *Taiwan* **59** E13
Huallaga → *Peru* **124** E3
Huambo *Angola* **85** G3
Huan Jiang → *China* **56** G5
Huan Xian *China* **56** G4
Huancabamba *Peru* **124** E3
Huancane *Peru* **124** G5
Huancavelica *Peru* **124** F3
Huancayo *Peru* **124** F3
Huanchaca *Bolivia* **124** H5
Huang Hai = Yellow Sea *China* **57** G12
Huang He → *China* **57** F10
Huang Xian *China* **57** F11
Huangchuan *China* **59** A10
Huanggang *China* **59** B10
Huangguoshu *China* **58** E5
Huangling *China* **56** G5
Huanglong *China* **56** G5
Huanglongtan *China* **59** A8
Huangmei *China* **59** B10
Huangpi *China* **59** B10
Huangping *China* **58** D6
Huangshan *Anhui, China* **59** B12
Huangshan *Anhui, China* **59** C12
Huangshi *China* **59** B10
Huangsongdian *China* **57** C14
Huangyan *China* **59** C13
Huangyangsi *China* **59** D8
Huaning *China* **58** E4
Huanjiang *China* **58** E7
Huanren *China* **57** D13
Huantai *China* **57** F9
Huánuco *Peru* **124** E3
Huaping *China* **58** D3
Huaraz *Peru* **124** E3
Huarmey *Peru* **124** F3
Huarong *China* **59** C9
Huascarán, Nevado *Peru* **124** E3
Huasco *Chile* **126** B1
Huasco → *Chile* **126** B1
Huasna *U.S.A.* **111** K6
Huatabampo *Mexico* **118** B3
Huauchinango *Mexico* **119** C5
Huautla de Jiménez *Mexico* **119** D5
Huaxi *China* **58** D6
Huayin *China* **56** G6
Huayuan *China* **58** C7
Huayun *China* **58** B6
Huazhou *China* **59** G8
Hubballi = Hubli *India* **66** M9
Hubbard *Ohio, U.S.A.* **114** E4
Hubbard *Tex., U.S.A.* **116** F6

Hubbard Glacier *Canada* **100** E4
Hubbart Pt. *Canada* **103** B10
Hubei □ *China* **59** B9
Hubli *India* **66** M9
Huch'ang *N. Korea* **57** D14
Hucknall *U.K.* **14** D6
Huddersfield *U.K.* **14** D6
Hude *Germany* **24** B4
Hudi *Sudan* **80** D3
Hudiksvall *Sweden* **10** C11
Hudson *Canada* **104** B1
Hudson *Mass., U.S.A.* **115** D13
Hudson *N.Y., U.S.A.* **115** D11
Hudson *Wis., U.S.A.* **112** C7
Hudson *Wyo., U.S.A.* **108** E9
Hudson → *U.S.A.* **115** F11
Hudson, C. *Antarctica* **5** C20
Hudson Bay *Nunavut, Canada* **101** D14
Hudson Bay *Sask., Canada* **103** C8
Hudson Falls *U.S.A.* **115** C11
Hudson Mts. *Antarctica* **5** D16
Hudson Str. *Canada* **101** E18
Hudson's Hope *Canada* **102** B4
Hue *Vietnam* **64** D6
Huebra → *Spain* **36** D4
Huedin *Romania* **28** D8
Huehuetenango *Guatemala* **120** C1
Huejúcar *Mexico* **118** C4
Huélamo *Spain* **38** E3
Huelgoat *France* **18** D3
Huelma *Spain* **37** H7
Huelva *Spain* **37** H4
Huelva □ *Spain* **37** H4
Huelva → *Spain* **37** H5
Huentelauquén *Chile* **126** C1
Huércal-Overa *Spain* **39** H3
Huerta, Sa. de la *Argentina* **126** C2
Huertas, C. de las *Spain* **39** G4
Huerva → *Spain* **38** D4
Huesca *Spain* **38** C4
Huesca □ *Spain* **38** C5
Huéscar *Spain* **39** H2
Huetamo *Mexico* **118** D4
Huete *Spain* **38** E2
Hugh → *Australia* **94** D1
Hughenden *Australia* **94** C3
Hughesville *U.S.A.* **115** E8
Hugli → *India* **69** J13
Hugo *Colo., U.S.A.* **108** G12
Hugo *Okla., U.S.A.* **116** D7
Hugoton *U.S.A.* **112** G3
Hui Xian = Huixian *China* **56** G7
Hui Xian *China* **56** H4
Hui'an *China* **59** E12
Hui'anbu *China* **56** F4
Huichang *China* **59** E10
Huichapan *Mexico* **119** C5
Huichon *N. Korea* **57** D14
Huidong *Guangdong, China* **59** F10
Huidong *Sichuan, China* **58** D4
Huifa He → *China* **57** C14
Huila, Nevado del *Colombia* **124** C3
Huilai *China* **59** F11
Huili *China* **58** D4
Huimin *China* **57** F9
Huinan *China* **57** C14
Huinca Renancó *Argentina* **126** C3
Huining *China* **56** G3
Huinong *China* **56** E4
Huishui *China* **58** D6
Huisne → *France* **18** E7
Huiting *China* **56** G9
Huitong *China* **58** D7
Huixian *China* **56** G7
Huixtla *Mexico* **119** D6
Huize *China* **58** D4
Huizhou *China* **59** F10
Hukawng Valley *Burma* **67** F20
Hukou *China* **59** C11
Hukuntsi *Botswana* **88** C3
Ḥulayfā' *Si. Arabia* **70** E4
Hulin He → *China* **57** B12
Hull = Kingston upon Hull *U.K.* **14** D7
Hull *Canada* **115** A9
Hull → *U.K.* **14** D7
Hulst *Neths.* **17** C4
Hultsfred *Sweden* **11** G9
Hulun Nur *China* **60** B6
Hulyaypole *Ukraine* **33** J9
Huma, Tanjung *Malaysia* **65** c
Humacao *Puerto Rico* **121** d
Humahuaca *Argentina* **126** A2
Humaitá *Brazil* **124** E6
Humaitá *Paraguay* **126** B4
Humansdorp *S. Africa* **88** E3
Humara, J. *Sudan* **81** D3
Humbe *Angola* **88** B1
Humber → *U.K.* **14** D7
Humboldt *Canada* **103** C7
Humboldt *Iowa, U.S.A.* **112** D6
Humboldt *Tenn., U.S.A.* **117** D10
Humboldt → *U.S.A.* **108** G4
Humboldt Gletscher =
  Sermersuaq *Greenland* **101** B19
Hume *U.S.A.* **110** J8
Hume, L. *Australia* **95** F4
Humenné *Slovak Rep.* **27** C14

Hummelsta *Sweden* **10** E10
Humphreys, Mt. *U.S.A.* **110** H8
Humphreys Peak *U.S.A.* **109** J8
Humpolec *Czech Rep.* **26** B8
Humptulips *U.S.A.* **110** C3
Hūn *Libya* **79** C9
Hun Jiang → *China* **57** D13
Húnaflói *Iceland* **8** C3
Hunan □ *China* **59** D9
Hunchun *China* **57** C16
Hundested *Denmark* **11** J5
Hundewali *Pakistan* **68** D5
Hundred Mile House *Canada* **102** C4
Hunedoara *Romania* **28** E7
Hunedoara □ *Romania* **28** E7
Hünfeld *Germany* **24** E5
Hung Yen *Vietnam* **58** G6
Hunga Ha'apai *Tonga* **91** c
Hungary ■ *Europe* **27** D12
Hungary, Plain of *Europe* **6** F10
Hungerford *Australia* **95** D3
Hŭngnam *N. Korea* **57** E14
Hungt'ou Hsü = Lan Yü *Taiwan* **59** F13
Huni Valley *Ghana* **82** D4
Hunjiang *China* **57** D14
Hunneberg *Sweden* **11** F6
Hunnebostrand *Sweden* **11** F5
Hunsberge *Namibia* **88** D2
Hunsrück *Germany* **25** F3
Hunstanton *U.K.* **14** E8
Hunte → *Germany* **24** B4
Hunter *U.S.A.* **115** D10
Hunter I. *Australia* **95** G3
Hunter I. *Canada* **102** C3
Hunter Ra. *Australia* **95** E5
Hunters Road *Zimbabwe* **87** F2
Hunterville *N.Z.* **91** C5
Huntingburg *U.S.A.* **112** F10
Huntingdon *U.K.* **15** E7
Huntingdon *U.S.A.* **114** F6
Huntington *Ind., U.S.A.* **113** E11
Huntington *N.Y., U.S.A.* **115** F11
Huntington *Oreg., U.S.A.* **108** D5
Huntington *Utah, U.S.A.* **108** G8
Huntington *W. Va., U.S.A.* **113** F12
Huntington Beach *U.S.A.* **111** M9
Huntly *N.Z.* **91** B5
Huntly *U.K.* **13** D6
Huntsville *Canada* **114** A5
Huntsville *Ala., U.S.A.* **117** D11
Huntsville *Tex., U.S.A.* **116** F7
Hunyani → *Zimbabwe* **87** F3
Hunyuan *China* **56** E7
Hunza → *India* **69** B6
Huo Xian = Huozhou *China* **56** F6
Huong Khe *Vietnam* **64** C5
Huonville *Australia* **95** G4
Huoqiu *China* **59** A11
Huoshan *Anhui, China* **59** A12
Huoshan *Anhui, China* **59** B11
Huoshao Dao = Lü Tao *Taiwan* **59** F13
Huozhou *China* **56** F6
Hupeh = Hubei □ *China* **59** B9
Ḥūr *Iran* **71** D8
Hurānd *Iran* **73** C12
Ḥuraymīla *Si. Arabia* **70** E5
Hurbanovo *Slovak Rep.* **27** D11
Hurd, C. *Canada* **114** A3
Hure Qi *China* **57** C11
Hurezani *Romania* **29** F8
Hurghada *Egypt* **80** B3
Hurley *N. Mex., U.S.A.* **109** K9
Hurley *Wis., U.S.A.* **112** B8
Huron *Calif., U.S.A.* **110** J6
Huron *Ohio, U.S.A.* **114** E2
Huron *S. Dak., U.S.A.* **112** C4
Huron, L. *U.S.A.* **114** B2
Huron East *Canada* **114** C3
Hurricane *U.S.A.* **109** H7
Hurso *Ethiopia* **81** F5
Hurungwe △ *Zimbabwe* **87** F2
Hurunui → *N.Z.* **91** E4
Hurup *Denmark* **11** H2
Húsavík *Iceland* **8** C5
Huşi *Romania* **29** D13
Huskvarna *Sweden* **11** G8
Hustadvika *Norway* **8** E12
Hustontown *U.S.A.* **114** F6
Hustopeče *Czech Rep.* **27** C9
Husum *Germany* **24** A5
Husum *Sweden* **10** A13
Hutchinson *Kans., U.S.A.* **112** F5
Hutchinson *Minn., U.S.A.* **112** C6
Hutte Sauvage, L. de la *Canada* **105** A7
Hüttenberg *Austria* **26** E7
Hutton, Mt. *Australia* **95** D4
Huwun *Ethiopia* **81** G5
Huy *Belgium* **17** D5
Huzhou *China* **59** B13
Hvalpsund *Denmark* **11** H3
Hvammstangi *Iceland* **8** D3
Hvar *Croatia* **41** E13
Hvarski Kanal *Croatia* **41** E13
Hvítá → *Iceland* **8** D3
Hvizdets *Ukraine* **29** B10

Hwacheon-Cheosuji *S. Korea* **57** E14
Hwang Ho = Huang He → *China* **57** F10
Hwange *Zimbabwe* **87** F2
Hwange △ *Zimbabwe* **88** B4
Hyannis *Mass., U.S.A.* **113** E18
Hyannis *Nebr., U.S.A.* **112** E3
Hyargas Nuur *Mongolia* **60** B4
Hybo *Sweden* **10** C10
Hydaburg *U.S.A.* **102** B2
Hyde Park *U.S.A.* **115** E11
Hyden *Australia* **93** F2
Hyder *U.S.A.* **102** B2
Hyderabad *India* **66** L11
Hyderabad *Pakistan* **68** G3
Hydra *Greece* **46** D5
Hyères *France* **21** E10
Hyères, Îs. d' *France* **21** F10
Hyesan *N. Korea* **57** D15
Hyland → *Canada* **102** B3
Hyltebruk *Sweden* **11** H7
Hymia *India* **69** C8
Hyndman Peak *U.S.A.* **108** E6
Hyōgo □ *Japan* **55** G7
Hyrum *U.S.A.* **108** F8
Hysham *U.S.A.* **108** C10
Hythe *U.K.* **15** F9
Hyūga *Japan* **55** H5
Hyvinge = Hyvinkää *Finland* **32** B3
Hyvinkää *Finland* **32** B3

I

I-n-Akhmed *Mali* **83** B4
I-n-Gall *Niger* **83** B6
I-n-Oudad *Algeria* **83** A5
I-n-Ouzzal *Algeria* **83** A5
I-n-Tadreft *Niger* **83** B6
Iablaniţa *Romania* **28** F7
Iaco → *Brazil* **124** E5
Iacobeni *Romania* **29** C10
Iakora *Madag.* **89** C8
Ialissos *Greece* **49** C10
Ialomiţa □ *Romania* **29** F12
Ialomiţa → *Romania* **29** F12
Ialoveni *Moldova* **29** D13
Ialpug → *Moldova* **29** E13
Ianca *Romania* **29** E12
Iara *Romania* **29** D8
Iarda *Ethiopia* **81** E4
Iargara *Moldova* **29** D13
Iaşi *Romania* **29** C12
Iaşi □ *Romania* **29** C12
Iasmos *Greece* **45** E9
Ib → *India* **69** J10
Iba *Phil.* **61** D4
Ibadan *Nigeria* **83** D5
Ibagué *Colombia* **124** C3
Iballë *Albania* **44** D4
Ibănești *Botoșani, Romania* **29** B11
Ibănești *Mureş, Romania* **29** D9
Ibar → *Serbia* **44** C4
Ibaraki □ *Japan* **55** F10
Ibarra *Ecuador* **124** C3
Ibb *Yemen* **75** E3
Ibba *Sudan* **81** G2
Ibba, Bahr el → *Sudan* **81** G2
Ibbenbüren *Germany* **24** C3
Ibembo *Dem. Rep. of the Congo* **86** B1
Ibenga → *Congo* **84** D3
Ibera, L. *Argentina* **126** B4
Iberian Peninsula *Europe* **6** H5
Iberville *Canada* **115** A11
Iberville, Mt. d' *Canada* **101** F19
Ibeto *Nigeria* **83** C6
Ibi *Nigeria* **83** D6
Ibi *Spain* **39** G4
Ibiá *Brazil* **125** G9
Ibiapaba, Sa. da *Brazil* **125** D10
Ibicuí → *Brazil* **127** B4
Ibicuy *Argentina* **126** C4
Ibiza = Eivissa *Spain* **48** C7
Ibiza ✈ (IBZ) *Spain* **39** G6
Íblei, Monti *Italy* **43** E7
Ibo *Mozam.* **87** E5
Ibonma *Indonesia* **63** E8
Ibotirama *Brazil* **125** F10
Ibrāhīm → *Lebanon* **74** A4
'Ibri *Oman* **71** F8
İbriktepe *Turkey* **45** E10
Ibshawâi *Egypt* **80** J7
Ibu *Indonesia* **63** D7
Ibusuki *Japan* **55** J5
Ica *Peru* **124** F3
Iça → *Brazil* **124** D5
Icacos Pt. *Trin. & Tob.* **125** K15
Içana *Brazil* **124** C5
Içana → *Brazil* **124** C5
İçel *Turkey* **72** D6
İçel □ *Turkey* **72** D5
Iceland ■ *Europe* **8** D4
Iceland Basin *Atl. Oc.* **4** C7
Icelandic Plateau *Arctic* **4** C7
İçeriçumra *Turkey* **72** D5
Ich'ang = Yichang *China* **59** B8
Ichchapuram *India* **67** K14
Icheon *S. Korea* **57** F14
Ichhawar *India* **68** H7

Ichihara *Japan* **55** G10
Ichikawa *Japan* **55** G9
Ichilo → *Bolivia* **124** G6
Ichinohe *Japan* **54** D10
Ichinomiya *Japan* **55** G8
Ichinoseki *Japan* **54** E10
Ichnya *Ukraine* **33** G7
Icod *Canary Is.* **48** F3
Icy C. *U.S.A.* **98** B3
Ida Grove *U.S.A.* **112** D6
Idabel *U.S.A.* **116** E7
Idaga Hamus *Ethiopia* **81** E4
Idah *Nigeria* **83** D6
Idaho □ *U.S.A.* **108** D6
Idaho City *U.S.A.* **108** E6
Idaho Falls *U.S.A.* **108** E7
Idalia △ *Australia* **94** C3
Idanha-a-Nova *Portugal* **36** F3
Idar-Oberstein *Germany* **25** F3
Idensalmi = Iisalmi *Finland* **8** E22
Idfû *Egypt* **80** C3
Ídhra = Hydra *Greece* **46** D5
Idi *Indonesia* **62** C1
Idi, Oros = Psiloritis, Oros
  Greece **49** D6
İdil *Turkey* **73** D9
Idiofa *Dem. Rep. of the Congo* **84** E3
Idkerberget *Sweden* **10** D9
Idku *Egypt* **80** H7
Idku, Bahra el *Egypt* **80** H7
Idlib *Syria* **72** E7
Idlib □ *Syria* **72** E7
Idre *Sweden* **10** C6
Idria *U.S.A.* **110** J6
Idrija *Slovenia* **41** C11
Idritsa *Russia* **32** D5
Idutywa = Dutywa *S. Africa* **89** E4
Ieper *Belgium* **17** D2
Ierapetra *Greece* **49** E7
Ierissos *Greece* **44** F7
Ierissos Kolpos *Greece* **44** F7
Iernut *Romania* **29** D9
Iesi *Italy* **41** E10
Iésolo *Italy* **41** C9
Ifac, Penyal d' *Spain* **39** G5
Ifakara *Tanzania* **84** F7
'Ifāl, W. al → *Si. Arabia* **70** D2
Ifanadiana *Madag.* **89** C8
Ife *Nigeria* **83** D5
Iférouâne *Niger* **83** B6
Iffley *Australia* **94** B3
Ifon *Nigeria* **83** D6
Iforas, Adrar des *Africa* **83** B5
Ifould, L. *Australia* **93** F5
Igalo *Montenegro* **44** D2
Iganga *Uganda* **86** B3
Igarapava *Brazil* **125** H9
Igarka *Russia* **52** C9
Igbetti *Nigeria* **83** D5
Igbo-Ora *Nigeria* **83** D5
Igboho *Nigeria* **83** D5
Igbor *Nigeria* **83** D6
Iğdır *Turkey* **73** C11
Igelfors *Sweden* **11** F9
Iggesund *Sweden* **10** C11
Iglésias *Italy* **42** C1
Igloolik = Iglulik *Canada* **101** D15
Igluligaarjuk = Chesterfield
  Inlet *Canada* **100** E13
Iglulik *Canada* **101** D15
'Igma, Gebel el *Egypt* **80** B3
Ignace *Canada* **104** C1
İğneada *Turkey* **45** E11
İğneada Burnu *Turkey* **45** E12
Igoumenitsa *Greece* **46** B2
Igrim *Russia* **52** C7
Iguaçu → *Brazil* **127** B5
Iguaçu, Cat. del *Brazil* **127** B5
Iguaçu △ *Brazil* **127** B5
Iguaçu Falls = Iguaçu, Cat.
  del *Brazil* **127** B5
Iguala *Mexico* **119** D5
Igualada *Spain* **38** D6
Iguassu = Iguaçu → *Brazil* **127** B5
Iguatu *Brazil* **125** E11
Iguazú △ *Argentina* **127** B5
Iguidi, Erg *Africa* **78** C4
Iharana *Madag.* **89** A9
Ihbulag *Mongolia* **56** C4
Iheya-Shima *Japan* **55** L3
Ihiala *Nigeria* **83** D6
Ihosy *Madag.* **89** C8
Ihotry, Farihy *Madag.* **89** C7
Ihugh *Nigeria* **83** D6
Ii *Finland* **8** D21
Ii-Shima *Japan* **55** L3
Iida *Japan* **55** G8
Iijoki → *Finland* **8** D21
Iisalmi *Finland* **8** E22
Iiyama *Japan* **55** F9
Iizuka *Japan* **55** H5
Ijâfene *Mauritania* **78** D4
Ijebu-Igbo *Nigeria* **83** D5
Ijebu-Ode *Nigeria* **83** D5
Ijevan *Armenia* **73** B11
IJmuiden *Neths.* **17** B4
Ijo älv = Iijoki → *Finland* **8** D21
IJssel → *Neths.* **17** B5
IJsselmeer *Neths.* **17** B5

Ijuí *Brazil* **127** B5
Ijuí → *Brazil* **127** B4
Ikalamavony *Madag.* **89** C8
Ikale *Nigeria* **83** D6
Ikaluktutiak = Cambridge
  Bay *Canada* **100** D11
Ikang *Nigeria* **83** E6
Ikanga *Kenya* **86** C4
Ikara *Nigeria* **83** C6
Ikare *Nigeria* **83** D6
Ikaria *Greece* **47** D8
Ikast *Denmark* **11** H3
Ikeda *Japan* **55** G6
Ikeja *Nigeria* **83** D5
Ikela *Dem. Rep. of the Congo* **84** E4
Ikere *Nigeria* **83** D6
Ikhtiman *Bulgaria* **44** D7
Iki *Japan* **55** H4
Ikimba L. *Tanzania* **86** C3
Ikire *Nigeria* **83** D5
İkizdere *Turkey* **73** B9
Ikom *Nigeria* **83** D6
Ikongo *Madag.* **89** C8
Ikopa → *Madag.* **89** B8
Ikorongo △ *Tanzania* **86** C3
Ikot Ekpene *Nigeria* **83** D6
Ikparjuk = Arctic Bay
  Canada **101** C14
Iksan *S. Korea* **57** G14
Ikungu *Tanzania* **86** C3
Ikuntji = Haasts Bluff
  Australia **92** D5
Ikurun *Nigeria* **83** D5
Ila *Nigeria* **83** D5
Ilagan *Phil.* **61** C4
Ilaka *Madag.* **89** B8
Ilām *Iran* **73** F12
Ilam *Nepal* **69** F12
Ilām □ *Iran* **70** C5
Ilan *Taiwan* **59** E13
Ilanskiy *Russia* **53** D10
Ilaro *Nigeria* **83** D5
Ilatane *Niger* **83** B6
Ilawa *Poland* **30** E6
Ile → *Kazakhstan* **52** E8
Île-à-la-Crosse *Canada* **103** B7
Île-à-la-Crosse, Lac *Canada* **103** B7
Île-de-France □ *France* **19** D9
Ileanda *Romania* **29** C8
Ilebo *Dem. Rep. of the Congo* **84** E4
Ilek *Russia* **52** D6
Ilero *Nigeria* **83** D5
Ilesha *Kwara, Nigeria* **83** D5
Ilesha *Oyo, Nigeria* **83** D5
Ilford *Canada* **103** B9
Ilfracombe *Australia* **94** C3
Ilfracombe *U.K.* **15** F3
Ilgaz *Turkey* **72** B5
Ilgaz Dağları *Turkey* **72** B5
Ilgın *Turkey* **72** C4
Ilha Grande, Represa *Brazil* **127** A5
Ilha Grande △ *Brazil* **127** A5
Ílhavo *Portugal* **36** E2
Ilhéus *Brazil* **125** F11
Ili = Ile → *Kazakhstan* **52** E8
Ilia *Romania* **28** E7
Ilia □ *Greece* **46** D3
Iliamna L. *U.S.A.* **106** D8
Ilias, Profitis *Greece* **49** C9
Iliç *Turkey* **73** C8
Ilıca *Turkey* **47** B9
Iligan *Phil.* **61** G6
Iligan Bay *Phil.* **61** G6
Ilin I. *Phil.* **61** E4
Ilion *U.S.A.* **115** D9
Ilirska-Bistrica *Slovenia* **41** C11
Ilkeston *U.K.* **14** E6
Ilkley *U.K.* **14** D6
Illampu = Ancohuma,
  Nevado *Bolivia* **124** G5
Illana B. *Phil.* **61** H5
Illapel *Chile* **126** C1
Ille-et-Vilaine □ *France* **18** D5
Ille-sur-Têt *France* **20** F6
Illéla *Niger* **83** C6
Iller → *Germany* **25** G5
Illertissen *Germany* **25** G6
Illescas *Spain* **36** E7
Illetas *Spain* **48** B9
Illichivsk *Ukraine* **33** J6
Illiers-Combray *France* **18** D8
Illimani, Nevado *Bolivia* **124** G5
Illinois □ *U.S.A.* **112** E9
Illinois → *U.S.A.* **112** F8
Illizi *Algeria* **78** C7
Illkirch-Graffenstaden
  France **19** D14
Íllora *Spain* **37** H7
Ilm → *Germany* **24** D7
Ilma, L. *Australia* **93** E4
Ilmajoki *Finland* **8** E20
Ilmen, Ozero *Russia* **32** C6
Ilmenau *Germany* **24** E6
Ilnytsya *Ukraine* **28** B8
Ilo *Peru* **124** G4
Ilobu *Nigeria* **83** D5
Iloilo *Phil.* **61** F5
Ilomantsi *Finland* **8** E24
Ilora *Nigeria* **83** D5

Ilorin *Nigeria* **83** D5
Ilovatka *Russia* **34** E7
Ilovlya *Russia* **35** F7
Ilovlya → *Russia* **35** F7
Iłowa *Poland* **31** G2
Ilubabor *Ethiopia* **81** F4
Ilva Micǎ *Romania* **29** C9
Ilwaco *U.S.A.* **110** D2
Ilwaki *Indonesia* **63** F7
Ilyichevsk = Illichivsk
  Ukraine **33** J6
Iłża *Poland* **31** G8
Izanka → *Poland* **31** G8
Imabari *Japan* **55** G6
Imaloto → *Madag.* **89** C8
İmamoğlu *Turkey* **72** D6
Imandra, Ozero *Russia* **8** C25
Imanombo *Madag.* **89** C8
Imari *Japan* **55** H4
Imasa *Sudan* **80** D4
Imathia □ *Greece* **44** F6
Imatra *Finland* **32** B5
Iménas *Mali* **83** B5
imeni 26 Bakinskikh
  Komissarov = Neftçala
  Azerbaijan **73** C13
imeni 26 Bakinskikh
  Komissarov *Turkmenistan* **71** B7
imeni Ismail Samani, Pik
  Tajikistan **52** F8
Imeri, Serra *Brazil* **124** C5
Imerimandroso *Madag.* **89** B8
Imfolozi △ *S. Africa* **89** D5
Imi *Ethiopia* **81** F5
Imishly = İmişli *Azerbaijan* **35** L9
İmişli *Azerbaijan* **35** L9
Imlay *U.S.A.* **108** F4
Imlay City *U.S.A.* **114** D1
Immaseri *Sudan* **81** D2
Immenstadt *Germany* **25** H6
Immingham *U.K.* **14** D7
Immokalee *U.S.A.* **117** H14
Imo □ *Nigeria* **83** D6
Imo → *Nigeria* **83** E6
Ímola *Italy* **41** D8
Imotski *Croatia* **41** E14
Imperatriz *Brazil* **125** E9
Impéria *Italy* **40** E5
Imperial *Canada* **103** C7
Imperial *Calif., U.S.A.* **111** N11
Imperial *Nebr., U.S.A.* **112** E3
Imperial Beach *U.S.A.* **111** N9
Imperial Dam *U.S.A.* **111** N12
Imperial Res. *U.S.A.* **111** N12
Imperial Valley *U.S.A.* **111** N11
Imperieuse Reef *Australia* **92** C2
Impfondo *Congo* **84** D3
Imphal *India* **67** G18
Imphy *France* **19** F10
İmranlı *Turkey* **73** C8
İmroz = Gökçeada *Turkey* **45** F9
İmroz → *Turkey* **45** F9
Imst *Austria* **26** D3
Imuris *Mexico* **118** A2
Imuruan B. *Phil.* **61** B5
In Aleï *Mali* **82** B4
In Delimane *Mali* **83** B5
In Guezzam *Algeria* **83** B6
In Koufi *Mali* **83** B5
In Salah *Algeria* **78** C6
In Tallak *Mali* **83** B5
In Tebezas *Mali* **83** B5
Ina *Japan* **55** G8
Inagua △ *Bahamas* **121** B5
Inangahua *N.Z.* **91** D3
Inanwatan *Indonesia* **63** E8
Iñapari *Peru* **124** F5
Inari *Finland* **8** B22
Inarijärvi *Finland* **8** B22
Inawashiro-Ko *Japan* **54** F10
Inca *Spain* **48** B9
Inca de Oro *Chile* **126** B2
Incahuasi *Argentina* **126** B2
Incahuasi *Chile* **126** B1
İnce Burun *Turkey* **72** A6
İncekum Burnu *Turkey* **72** D5
İncesu *Turkey* **72** C6
Incheon *S. Korea* **57** F14
Inchiri □ *Mauritania* **82** B2
Incio = A Cruz do Incio *Spain* **36** C3
İncirliova *Turkey* **47** D9
Incline Village *U.S.A.* **108** G4
Incomáti → *Mozam.* **89** D5
Incudine, Mte. *France* **21** G13
Inda Silase *Ethiopia* **81** E4
Indal *Sweden* **10** B11
Indalsälven → *Sweden* **10** B11
Indaw *Burma* **67** G20
Indbir *Ethiopia* **81** F4
Independence *Calif., U.S.A.* **110** J8
Independence *Iowa, U.S.A.* **112** D9
Independence *Kans., U.S.A.* **112** G6
Independence *Ky., U.S.A.* **113** F11
Independence *Mo., U.S.A.* **112** F6
Independence Fjord *Greenland* **4** A6
Independence Mts. *U.S.A.* **108** F5
Independența *Romania* **29** E12
Index *U.S.A.* **110** C5
India ■ *Asia* **66** K11

Indian → *U.S.A.* **117** H14
Indian Cabins *Canada* **102** B5
Indian Harbour *Canada* **105** B8
Indian Head *Canada* **103** C8
Indian L. *U.S.A.* **115** C10
Indian Lake *U.S.A.* **115** C10
Indian Springs *U.S.A.* **111** J11
Indiana *U.S.A.* **114** F5
Indiana □ *U.S.A.* **113** F11
Indianapolis *U.S.A.* **112** F10
Indianola *Iowa, U.S.A.* **112** E7
Indianola *Miss., U.S.A.* **117** E9
Indigirka → *Russia* **53** B15
Indija *Serbia* **28** E5
Indio *U.S.A.* **111** M10
Indira Gandhi Canal *India* **68** F5
Indira Sagar *India* **68** H7
Indo-China *Asia* **50** G12
Indonesia ■ *Asia* **62** F5
Indore *India* **68** H6
Indramayu *Indonesia* **63** G13
Indravati → *India* **67** K12
Indre □ *France* **19** F8
Indre → *France* **18** E7
Indre-et-Loire □ *France* **18** E7
Indulkana *Australia* **95** D1
Indura *Belarus* **30** E10
Indus → *Pakistan* **68** G2
Indus, Mouths of the
  Pakistan **68** H3
İnebolu *Turkey* **72** B5
İnecik *Turkey* **45** F11
İnegöl *Turkey* **45** F13
Ineu *Romania* **28** D6
Infantes = Villanueva de
  los Infantes *Spain* **37** G7
Infiernillo, Presa del *Mexico* **118** D4
Infiesto *Spain* **36** B5
Ingelstad *Sweden* **11** H8
Ingenio *Canary Is.* **48** G4
Ingenio Santa Ana
  Argentina **126** B2
Ingersoll *Canada* **114** C4
Ingham *Australia* **94** B4
Ingleborough *U.K.* **14** C5
Inglewood *Queens., Australia* **95** D5
Inglewood *Vic., Australia* **95** F3
Inglewood *N.Z.* **91** C5
Inglewood *U.S.A.* **111** M8
Ingólfshöfði *Iceland* **8** E5
Ingolstadt *Germany* **25** G7
Ingomar *U.S.A.* **108** C10
Ingonish *Canada* **105** C7
Ingore *Guinea-Biss.* **82** C1
Ingraj Bazar *India* **69** G13
Ingrid Christensen Coast
  Antarctica **5** C6
Ingul = Inhul → *Ukraine* **33** J7
Ingulec = Inhulec → *Ukraine* **33** J7
Ingulets = Inhulets →
  Ukraine **33** J7
Inguri = Enguri → *Georgia* **35** J5
Ingushetia □ *Russia* **35** J7
Ingwavuma *S. Africa* **89** D5
Inhaca *Mozam.* **89** D5
Inhafenga *Mozam.* **89** C5
Inhambane *Mozam.* **89** C6
Inhambane □ *Mozam.* **89** C5
Inhaminga *Mozam.* **87** F4
Inharrime *Mozam.* **89** C6
Inharrime → *Mozam.* **89** C6
Inhisar *Turkey* **47** A12
Inhul → *Ukraine* **33** J7
Inhulec → *Ukraine* **33** J7
Inhulets → *Ukraine* **33** J7
Iniesta *Spain* **39** F3
Iniirida → *Colombia* **124** C5
Inírida → *Colombia* **124** C5
Inis = Ennis *Ireland* **12** D3
Inis Córthaidh =
  Enniscorthy *Ireland* **12** D5
Inishbofin *Ireland* **12** C1
Inisheer *Ireland* **12** C2
Inishfree B. *Ireland* **12** A3
Inishkea North *Ireland* **12** B1
Inishkea South *Ireland* **12** B1
Inishmaan *Ireland* **12** C2
Inishmore *Ireland* **12** C2
Inishmurray I. *Ireland* **12** B3
Inishowen Pen. *Ireland* **12** A4
Inishshark *Ireland* **12** C1
Inishturk *Ireland* **12** C1
Inishvickillane *Ireland* **12** D1
Injāna *Iraq* **73** E11
Injibara *Ethiopia* **81** E4
Injinoo ۞ *Australia* **94** A3
Injune *Australia* **95** D4
Inklin → *N. Amer.* **102** B2
Inland Kaikoura Ra. *N.Z.* **91** D4
Inland Sea = Setonaikai
  Japan **55** G6
Inle L. *Burma* **67** J20
Inlet *U.S.A.* **115** C10
Inn → *Austria* **26** C6
Innamincka *Australia* **95** D3
Inner Hebrides *U.K.* **13** E2
Inner Mongolia = Nei
  Monggol Zizhiqu □ *China* **56** D7
Inner Sound *U.K.* **13** D3

Innerkip *Canada* **114** C4
Innetalling I. *Canada* **104** A4
Innisfail *Australia* **94** B4
Innisfail *Canada* **102** C6
In'noshima *Japan* **55** G6
Innsbruck *Austria* **26** D4
Innviertel *Austria* **26** C6
Inny → *Ireland* **12** C4
Inongo *Dem. Rep. of the Congo* **84** E3
İnönü *Turkey* **47** B12
Inoucdjouac = Inukjuak
  Canada **101** F16
Inowrocław *Poland* **31** F5
Inscription, C. *Australia* **93** E1
Insein *Burma* **67** L20
Insjön *Sweden* **10** D9
Ińsko *Poland* **30** E2
Însurăței *Romania* **29** F12
Inta *Russia* **52** C6
Intendente Alvear *Argentina* **126** D3
İntepe *Turkey* **47** A8
Interlaken *Switz.* **25** J3
Interlaken *U.S.A.* **115** D8
International Falls *U.S.A.* **112** A7
Intiyaco *Argentina* **126** B3
Întorsura Buzăului *Romania* **29** E11
Inukjuak *Canada* **101** F16
Inútil, B. *Chile* **128** G2
Inuvik *Canada* **100** D5
Inveraray *U.K.* **13** E3
Inverbervie *U.K.* **13** E6
Invercargill *N.Z.* **91** G2
Inverclyde □ *U.K.* **13** F4
Inverell *Australia* **95** D5
Invergordon *U.K.* **13** D4
Inverloch *Australia* **95** F4
Invermere *Canada* **102** C5
Inverness *Canada* **105** C7
Inverness *U.K.* **13** D4
Inverness *U.S.A.* **117** G13
Inverurie *U.K.* **13** D6
Investigator Group *Australia* **95** E1
Investigator Str. *Australia* **95** F2
Inya *Russia* **52** D9
Inyanga *Zimbabwe* **87** F3
Inyangani *Zimbabwe* **87** F3
Inyantue *Zimbabwe* **88** B4
Inyo Mts. *U.S.A.* **110** J9
Inyokern *U.S.A.* **111** K9
Inyonga *Tanzania* **86** D3
Inza *Russia* **34** D8
Inzhavino *Russia* **34** D6
Iō-Jima *Japan* **55** J5
Ioannina *Greece* **46** B2
Ioannina □ *Greece* **46** B2
Iola *U.S.A.* **112** G6
Ion Corvin *Romania* **29** F12
Iona *U.K.* **13** E2
Ione *U.S.A.* **110** G6
Ionia *U.S.A.* **113** D11
Ionian Is. = Ionioi Nisoi
  Greece **46** C2
Ionian Sea *Medit. S.* **6** H9
Ionioi Nisoi *Greece* **46** C2
Ionioi Nisoi □ *Greece* **46** C2
Ios *Greece* **47** E7
Iowa □ *U.S.A.* **112** D7
Iowa → *U.S.A.* **112** E8
Iowa City *U.S.A.* **112** E8
Iowa Falls *U.S.A.* **112** D7
Iowa Park *U.S.A.* **116** E5
Ipala *Tanzania* **86** C3
Ipameri *Brazil* **125** G9
Ipati *Greece* **46** C4
Ipatinga *Brazil* **125** G10
Ipatovo *Russia* **35** H6
Ipel' → *Europe* **27** D11
Ipiales *Colombia* **124** C3
Ipin = Yibin *China* **58** D5
Ipixuna *Brazil* **124** E4
Ipoh *Malaysia* **65** K3
Ippy *C.A.R.* **84** C4
İpsala *Turkey* **45** F10
Ipsario, Oros *Greece* **45** F8
Ipswich *Australia* **95** D5
Ipswich *U.K.* **15** E9
Ipswich *Mass., U.S.A.* **115** D14
Ipswich *S. Dak., U.S.A.* **112** C4
Ipu *Brazil* **125** D10
Iqaluit *Canada* **101** E18
Iqualit = Icana → *Brazil* **124** C5
Iquique *Chile* **124** H4
Iquitos *Peru* **124** D4
Irabu-Jima *Japan* **55** M2
Iracoubo *Fr. Guiana* **125** B8
Irahuan *Phil.* **61** G3
Irafshān *Iran* **71** E9
Irai *Brazil* **127** B5
Irala *Paraguay* **127** B5
Iran ■ *Asia* **71** C7
Iran, Pegunungan *Malaysia* **62** D4
Iran Ra. = Iran,
  Pegunungan *Malaysia* **62** D4
İranshahr *Iran* **71** E9

Irapuato *Mexico* **118** C4
Iraq ■ *Asia* **73** F10
Irati *Brazil* **127** B5
Irbes saurums *Latvia* **30** A9
Irbid *Jordan* **74** C4
Irbid □ *Jordan* **74** C5
Irebu *Dem. Rep. of the Congo* **84** E3
Iregua → *Spain* **38** C7
Ireland ■ *Europe* **12** C4
Irele *Nigeria* **83** D6
Irgiz, Bolshaya → *Russia* **34** D9
Iri = Iksan *S. Korea* **57** G14
Irian Jaya = Papua □
  Indonesia **63** E9
Irian Jaya Barat □ *Indonesia* **63** E8
Irié *Guinea* **82** D3
Iriga *Phil.* **61** E5
Iringa *Tanzania* **86** D4
Iringa □ *Tanzania* **86** D4
Iriomote → *Japan* **55** M1
Iriomote-Jima *Japan* **55** M1
Iriona *Honduras* **120** C2
Iriri → *Brazil* **125** D8
Irish Republic ■ *Europe* **12** C4
Irish Sea *Europe* **14** D3
Irkutsk *Russia* **53** D11
Irlığanlı *Turkey* **47** D11
Irma *Canada* **103** C6
Irō-Zaki *Japan* **55** G9
Iroise, Mer d' *France* **18** D2
Iron Baron *Australia* **95** E2
Iron Gate = Portile de Fier
  Europe **28** F7
Iron Knob *Australia* **95** E2
Iron Mountain *U.S.A.* **112** C9
Iron Range △ *Australia* **94** A3
Iron River *U.S.A.* **112** B9
Irondequoit *U.S.A.* **114** C7
Ironton *Mo., U.S.A.* **112** G8
Ironton *Ohio, U.S.A.* **113** F12
Ironwood *U.S.A.* **112** B8
Ironwood Forest △ *U.S.A.* **109** K8
Iroquois *Canada* **115** B9
Iroquois Falls *Canada* **104** C3
Irosin *Phil.* **61** E6
Irpin *Ukraine* **23** C16
Irrara Cr. → *Australia* **95** D4
Irrawaddy □ *Burma* **67** L19
Irrawaddy → *Burma* **67** M19
Irrawaddy, Mouths of the
  Burma **67** M19
Irricana *Canada* **102** C6
Irrunytju *Australia* **93** E4
Irshava *Ukraine* **28** B8
Irsina *Italy* **43** B9
Irtysh → *Russia* **52** C7
Irumu *Dem. Rep. of the Congo* **86** B2
Irún *Spain* **38** B3
Irunea = Pamplona-Iruña
  Spain **38** C3
Irurzun *Spain* **38** C3
Irvine *Canada* **103** D6
Irvine *U.K.* **13** F4
Irvine *Calif., U.S.A.* **111** M9
Irvine *Ky., U.S.A.* **113** G12
Irvinestown *U.K.* **12** B4
Irvona *U.S.A.* **114** F6
Irving *U.S.A.* **116** E6
Irwin → *Australia* **93** E1
Irymple *Australia* **95** E3
Is, Jebel *Sudan* **80** C4
Is-sur-Tille *France* **19** E12
Isa *Nigeria* **83** C6
Isa Khel *Pakistan* **68** C4
Isaac → *Australia* **94** C4
Isabel *U.S.A.* **112** C3
Isabel, I. *Mexico* **118** C3
Isabela *Phil.* **61** H5
Isabela *Puerto Rico* **121** d
Isabela, Cord. Nic. **120** D2
Isabella, Cord. *Nic.* **120** D2
Isabella Ra. *Australia* **92** D3
Isaccea *Romania* **29** E13
Isachsen, C. *Canada* **101** B10
Ísafjarðardjúp *Iceland* **8** C2
Ísafjörður *Iceland* **8** C2
Isagarh *India* **68** G7
Isahaya *Japan* **55** H5
Isaka *Tanzania* **86** C3
Işalnița *Romania* **29** F8
Isalo △ *Madag.* **89** C8
Isan → *India* **69** F9
Isana = Içana → *Brazil* **124** C5
Isangano △ *Zambia* **87** E3
Isanlu Makutu *Nigeria* **83** D6
Isar → *Germany* **25** G8
Isarco → *Italy* **41** B8
Isaris *Greece* **46** D3
Íscar *Spain* **36** D6
İscehisar *Turkey* **47** C12
 Íschia *Italy* **42** B6
Isdell → *Australia* **92** C3
Ise *Japan* **55** G8
Ise-Shima △ *Japan* **55** G8
Ise-Wan *Japan* **55** G8
Isefjord *Denmark* **11** J5
Isel → *Austria* **26** E5
Iseo *Italy* **40** C7
Iseo, L. d' *Italy* **40** C7
Iseramagazi *Tanzania* **86** C3

Isère □ *France* **21** C9
Isère ➤ *France* **21** D8
Iserlohn *Germany* **24** D3
Isérnia *Italy* **43** A7
Iseyin *Nigeria* **83** D5
Isfahan = Eşfahān *Iran* **71** C6
Ishëm *Albania* **44** E3
Ishigaki *Japan* **55** M2
Ishigaki-Shima *Japan* **55** M2
Ishikari-Gawa ➤ *Japan* **54** C10
Ishikari-Sammyaku *Japan* **54** C11
Ishikari-Wan *Japan* **54** C10
Ishikawa □ *Japan* **55** L3
Ishikawa □ *Japan* **55** F8
Ishim *Russia* **52** D7
Ishim ➤ *Russia* **52** D8
Ishinomaki *Japan* **54** E10
Ishioka *Japan* **55** F10
Ishkoman *Pakistan* **69** A5
Ishpeming *U.S.A.* **112** B10
Isigny-sur-Mer *France* **18** C5
Işıklar Dağı *Turkey* **45** F11
Işıklı *Turkey* **47** C11
Isil Kul *Russia* **52** D8
Ísili *Italy* **42** C2
Isiolo *Kenya* **86** B4
Isiro *Dem. Rep. of the Congo* **86** B2
Isisford *Australia* **94** C3
İskenderun *Turkey* **72** D7
İskenderun Körfezi *Turkey* **72** D6
İskilip *Turkey* **72** B6
Iskŭr ➤ *Bulgaria* **45** C8
Iskŭr, Yazovir *Bulgaria* **44** D7
Iskut ➤ *Canada* **102** B2
Isla ➤ *U.K.* **13** E5
Isla Coiba △ *Panama* **120** E3
Isla Cristina *Spain* **37** H3
Isla de Salamanca △
  Colombia **121** D5
Isla Gorge △ *Australia* **94** D4
Isla Isabel △ *Mexico* **118** C3
Isla Tiburón y San
  Esteban △ *Mexico* **118** B2
Isla Vista *U.S.A.* **111** L7
İslâhiye *Turkey* **72** D7
Islam Headworks *Pakistan* **68** E5
Islamabad *Pakistan* **68** C5
Islamgarh *Pakistan* **68** F4
Islamkot *Pakistan* **68** G4
Islampur *Bihar, India* **69** G11
Islampur *W. Bengal, India* **69** F13
Island = Iceland ■ *Europe* **8** D4
Island L. *Canada* **103** C10
Island Lagoon *Australia* **95** E2
Island Pond *U.S.A.* **115** B13
Islands, B. of *Canada* **105** C8
Islands, B. of *N.Z.* **91** A5
Islay *U.K.* **13** F2
Isle ➤ *France* **20** D3
Isle aux Morts *Canada* **105** C8
Isle of Wight □ *U.K.* **15** G6
Isle Royale △ *U.S.A.* **112** B9
Isleton *U.S.A.* **110** G5
Ismail = Izmayil *Ukraine* **29** E13
İsmâ'ilîya *Egypt* **80** H8
Ismaning *Germany* **25** G7
Isna *Egypt* **80** B3
Isoanala *Madag.* **89** C8
Isogstalo *India* **69** B8
Ísola del Liri *Italy* **41** G10
Ísola della Scala *Italy* **40** C7
Ísola di Capo Rizzuto *Italy* **43** D10
Isparta *Turkey* **47** D12
İsparta □ *Turkey* **72** D4
Isperikh *Bulgaria* **45** C10
Íspica *Italy* **43** F7
İspir *Turkey* **73** B9
Israel ■ *Asia* **74** D3
Isratu *Eritrea* **81** D4
Issakly *Russia* **34** C10
Issia *Ivory C.* **82** D3
Issoire *France* **20** C7
Issoudun *France* **19** F8
Issyk-Kul, Ozero =
  Ysyk-Köl *Kyrgyzstan* **52** E8
Ist *Croatia* **41** D11
Istállós-kő *Hungary* **28** B5
İstanbul *Turkey* **45** E12
İstanbul □ *Turkey* **45** E12
İstanbul ✈ (IST) *Turkey* **45** F12
İstanbul Boğazı *Turkey* **45** E13
Istiéa *Greece* **46** C5
Isto, Mt. *U.S.A.* **106** B11
Istok *Kosovo* **44** D4
Istokpoga, L. *U.S.A.* **117** H14
Istra *Croatia* **41** C10
Istra ➤ *Russia* **32** D9
Istres *France* **21** E8
Istria = Istra *Croatia* **41** C10
Itá *Paraguay* **126** B4
Itaberaba *Brazil* **125** F10
Itabira *Brazil* **125** G10
Itabirito *Brazil* **127** A7
Itabuna *Brazil* **125** F11
Itacaunas ➤ *Brazil* **125** E9
Itaituba *Brazil* **125** D7
Itajaí *Brazil* **127** B6
Itajubá *Brazil* **127** A6

Itaka *Tanzania* **87** D3
Itala △ *S. Africa* **89** D5
Italy ■ *Europe* **7** G8
Itamaraju *Brazil* **125** G11
Itampolo *Madag.* **89** C7
Itandrano *Madag.* **89** C8
Itapecuru Mirim *Brazil* **125** D10
Itaperuna *Brazil* **127** A7
Itapetininga *Brazil* **127** A6
Itapeva *Brazil* **127** A6
Itapicuru ➤ *Bahia, Brazil* **125** F11
Itapicuru ➤ *Maranhão,
  Brazil* **125** D10
Itapipoca *Brazil* **125** D11
Itaquí *Brazil* **126** B4
Itararé *Brazil* **127** A6
Itatí *Argentina* **126** B4
Itatiaia △ *Brazil* **127** A7
Itbayat *Phil.* **61** A4
Itchen ➤ *U.K.* **15** G6
Itea *Greece* **46** C4
Itezhi Tezhi, L. *Zambia* **87** F2
Ithaca = Ithaki *Greece* **46** C2
Ithaca *U.S.A.* **115** D8
Itháki *Greece* **46** C2
Iti △ *Greece* **46** C4
Itiquira ➤ *Brazil* **125** G7
Itiyuro ➤ *Argentina* **126** A3
Itō *Japan* **55** G9
Itoigawa *Japan* **55** F8
Iton ➤ *France* **18** C8
Itonamas ➤ *Bolivia* **124** F6
Itri *Italy* **42** A6
Itsa *Egypt* **80** J7
Íttiri *Italy* **42** B1
Ittoqqortoormiit *Greenland* **4** B6
Itu *Brazil* **127** A6
Itu *Nigeria* **83** D6
Itu Aba I. *S. China Sea* **62** B4
Ituiutaba *Brazil* **125** G9
Itumbiara *Brazil* **125** G9
Ituna *Canada* **103** C8
Itunge Port *Tanzania* **87** D3
Iturbe *Argentina* **126** A2
Ituri ➤ *Dem. Rep. of the Congo* **86** B2
Iturup, Ostrov *Russia* **53** E15
Ituxi ➤ *Brazil* **124** E6
Itzehoe *Germany* **24** B5
Ivahona *Madag.* **89** C8
Ivaí ➤ *Brazil* **127** A5
Ivalo *Finland* **8** B22
Ivalojoki ➤ *Finland* **8** B22
Ivanava *Belarus* **23** B13
Ivangorod *Russia* **32** C5
Ivanhoe *Australia* **95** E3
Ivanhoe *Canada* **114** B7
Ivanhoe *Calif., U.S.A.* **110** J7
Ivanhoe *Minn., U.S.A.* **112** C5
Ivanhorod *Ukraine* **29** B14
Ivanić Grad *Croatia* **41** C13
Ivanjica *Serbia* **44** C4
Ivanjska *Bos.-H.* **28** F2
Ivankoyskoye Vdkhr. *Russia* **32** D9
Ivano-Frankivsk *Ukraine* **29** B9
Ivano-Frankivsk □ *Ukraine* **29** B9
Ivanovo = Ivanava *Belarus* **23** B13
Ivanovo *Russia* **32** D11
Ivanovo □ *Russia* **34** B5
Ivanščica *Croatia* **41** B13
Ivato *Madag.* **89** C8
Ivatsevichy *Belarus* **23** B13
Ivaylovgrad *Bulgaria* **45** E10
Ivinheima ➤ *Brazil* **127** A5
Ivinhema *Brazil* **127** A5
Ivohibe *Madag.* **89** C8
Ivory Coast *W. Afr.* **82** E4
Ivory Coast ■ *Africa* **82** D4
Ivösjön *Sweden* **11** H8
Ivrea *Italy* **40** C4
İvrindi *Turkey* **47** B9
Ivujivik *Canada* **101** E16
Ivvavik △ *Canada* **100** D4
Ivybridge *U.K.* **15** G4
Iwaizumi *Japan* **54** E10
Iwaki *Japan* **55** F10
Iwakuni *Japan* **55** G6
Iwamizawa *Japan* **54** C10
Iwanai *Japan* **54** C10
Iwata *Japan* **55** G8
Iwate □ *Japan* **54** E10
Iwate-San *Japan* **54** E10
Iwo *Nigeria* **83** D5
Iwŏn *N. Korea* **57** D15
Iwonicz-Zdrój *Poland* **31** J8
Ixiamas *Bolivia* **124** F5
Ixopo *S. Africa* **89** E5
Ixtepec *Mexico* **119** D5
Ixtlán del Río *Mexico* **118** C4
Iyal Bakhit *Sudan* **81** E2
Iyo *Japan* **55** H6
Izabal, L. de *Guatemala* **120** C2
Izamal *Mexico* **119** C7
Izberbash *Russia* **35** J8
Izbica *Poland* **31** H10

Izbica Kujawska *Poland* **31** F5
Izbiceni *Romania* **29** G9
Izena-Shima *Japan* **55** L3
Izgrev *Bulgaria* **45** C10
Izhevsk *Russia* **52** D6
Izmayil *Ukraine* **29** E13
İzmir *Turkey* **47** C9
İzmir □ *Turkey* **47** C9
İzmir Adnan Menderes ✈
  (ADB) *Turkey* **47** C9
İzmir Körfezi *Turkey* **47** C8
İzmit = Kocaeli *Turkey* **45** F13
Iznájar *Spain* **37** H6
Iznalloz *Spain* **37** H7
İznik *Turkey* **72** B3
İznik Gölü *Turkey* **45** F13
Izobil'nyy *Russia* **35** H5
Izola *Slovenia* **41** C10
Izra *Syria* **74** C5
Iztochni Rodopi *Bulgaria* **45** E9
Izu-Shotō *Japan* **55** G10
Izúcar de Matamoros
  Mexico **119** D5
Izumi-Sano *Japan* **55** G7
Izumo *Japan* **55** G6
Izyaslav *Ukraine* **23** C14
Izyum *Ukraine* **33** H9

J

J.F.K. Int. ✈ (JFK) *U.S.A.* **115** F11
J. Strom Thurmond L.
  U.S.A. **117** E13
Jaba *Ethiopia* **81** F4
Jabal at Ţāʾir *Red Sea* **81** D5
Jabalón ➤ *Spain* **37** G6
Jabalpur *India* **69** H8
Jabbūl *Syria* **70** B3
Jabiru *Australia* **92** B5
Jablah *Syria* **72** E6
Jablanac *Croatia* **41** D11
Jablanica *Bos.-H.* **28** G2
Jablonec nad Nisou
  Czech Rep. **26** A8
Jablonica *Slovak Rep.* **27** C10
Jabłonowo Pomorskie *Poland* **30** E6
Jablunkov *Czech Rep.* **27** B11
Jaboatão *Brazil* **125** E11
Jaboticabal *Brazil* **127** A6
Jabukovac *Serbia* **44** B6
Jaca *Spain* **38** C4
Jacareí *Brazil* **127** A6
Jacarèzinho *Brazil* **127** A6
Jack River △ *Australia* **94** A3
Jackman *U.S.A.* **113** C18
Jacksboro *U.S.A.* **116** E5
Jackson *Barbados* **121** g
Jackson *Ala., U.S.A.* **117** F11
Jackson *Calif., U.S.A.* **110** G6
Jackson *Ky., U.S.A.* **113** G12
Jackson *Mich., U.S.A.* **113** D11
Jackson *Minn., U.S.A.* **112** D6
Jackson *Miss., U.S.A.* **117** E9
Jackson *Mo., U.S.A.* **112** G9
Jackson *N.H., U.S.A.* **115** B13
Jackson *Ohio, U.S.A.* **113** F12
Jackson *Tenn., U.S.A.* **117** D10
Jackson *Wyo., U.S.A.* **108** E8
Jackson B. *N.Z.* **91** E2
Jackson L. *U.S.A.* **108** E8
Jacksons *N.Z.* **91** E3
Jackson's Arm *Canada* **105** C8
Jacksonville *Ala., U.S.A.* **117** E12
Jacksonville *Ark., U.S.A.* **116** D8
Jacksonville *Calif., U.S.A.* **110** H6
Jacksonville *Fla., U.S.A.* **117** F14
Jacksonville *Ill., U.S.A.* **112** F8
Jacksonville *N.C., U.S.A.* **117** D16
Jacksonville *Tex., U.S.A.* **116** F7
Jacksonville Beach *U.S.A.* **117** F14
Jacmel *Haiti* **121** C5
Jacob Lake *U.S.A.* **109** H7
Jacobabad *Pakistan* **68** E3
Jacobina *Brazil* **125** F10
Jacques-Cartier, Dét. de
  Canada **105** C7
Jacques-Cartier, Mt. *Canada* **105** C6
Jacques-Cartier △ *Canada* **105** C5
Jacqueville *Ivory C.* **82** D4
Jacuí ➤ *Brazil* **127** C5
Jacundá ➤ *Brazil* **125** D8
Jacumba *U.S.A.* **111** N10
Jade *Germany* **24** B4
Jade City *Canada* **102** B3
Jade Mt. = Yü Shan *Taiwan* **59** F13
Jadebusen *Germany* **24** B4
Jadovnik *Serbia* **44** C3
Jadraque *Spain* **38** E16
Jaén *Peru* **124** E3
Jaén *Spain* **37** H7
Jaén □ *Spain* **37** H7
Jafarabad *India* **68** J4
Jaffa = Tel Aviv-Yafo *Israel* **74** C3
Jaffa, C. *Australia* **95** F2
Jaffna *Sri Lanka* **66** Q12
Jaffrey *U.S.A.* **115** D12
Jagadhri *India* **68** D7
Jagadishpur *India* **69** G11
Jagdalpur *India* **67** K13

Jagersfontein *S. Africa* **88** D4
Jaghīn ➤ *Iran* **71** E8
Jagodina *Serbia* **44** B5
Jagraon *India* **68** D6
Jagst ➤ *Germany* **25** F5
Jagtial *India* **66** K11
Jaguariaíva *Brazil* **127** A6
Jaguaribe ➤ *Brazil* **125** D11
Jagüey Grande *Cuba* **120** B3
Jahanabad *India* **69** G11
Jahazpur *India* **68** G6
Jahrom *Iran* **71** D7
Jaijon *India* **68** D7
Jailolo *Indonesia* **63** D7
Jailolo, Selat *Indonesia* **63** D7
Jaipur *India* **68** F6
Jais *India* **69** F9
Jaisalmer *India* **68** F4
Jaisinghnagar *India* **69** H8
Jaitaran *India* **68** F5
Jaithari *India* **69** H8
Jājarm *Iran* **71** B8
Jajce *Bos.-H.* **28** F2
Jakam ➤ *India* **68** H6
Jakarta *Indonesia* **62** F3
Jakhal *India* **68** E6
Jakhau *India* **68** H3
Jakobstad = Pietarsaari
  Finland **8** E20
Jakupica *Macedonia* **44** E5
Jal *U.S.A.* **109** K12
Jalājil *Si. Arabia* **70** E5
Jalālābād *Afghan.* **68** B4
Jalalabad *India* **69** F8
Jalalpur Jattan *Pakistan* **68** C6
Jalama *U.S.A.* **111** L6
Jalapa *Guatemala* **120** D2
Jalapa Enríquez = Xalapa
  Mexico **119** D5
Jalasjärvi *Finland* **8** E20
Jalaun *India* **69** F8
Jaldhaka ➤ *Bangla.* **69** F13
Jalesar *India* **68** F8
Jaleswar *Nepal* **69** F11
Jalgaon *India* **66** J9
Jalībah *Iraq* **70** D5
Jalingo *Nigeria* **83** D7
Jalisco □ *Mexico* **118** D4
Jalkot *Pakistan* **69** B5
Jalna *India* **66** K9
Jalón ➤ *Spain* **38** D3
Jalor *India* **68** G5
Jalpa *Mexico* **118** C4
Jalpaiguri *India* **67** F16
Jalpan *Mexico* **119** C5
Jaluit I. *Marshall Is.* **96** G8
Jalūlā *Iraq* **73** E11
Jamaame *Somali Rep.* **75** G3
Jamaari *Nigeria* **83** C6
Jamaica ■ *W. Indies* **120** a
Jamalpur *Bangla.* **67** G16
Jamalpur *India* **69** G12
Jamalpurganj *India* **69** H13
Jamanxim ➤ *Brazil* **125** D7
Jambewangi *Indonesia* **63** J17
Jambi *Indonesia* **62** E2
Jambi □ *Indonesia* **62** E2
Jambongan, Pulau *Malaysia* **62** C5
Jambongon *Phil.* **61** H2
Jambusar *India* **68** H5
James ➤ *S. Dak., U.S.A.* **112** D5
James ➤ *Va., U.S.A.* **113** G15
James B. *Canada* **104** B3
James I. *Gambia* **82** C1
James Ranges *Australia* **92** D5
James Ross I. *Antarctica* **5** C18
Jamesabad *Pakistan* **68** G3
Jamestown *Australia* **95** E2
Jamestown *S. Africa* **88** E4
Jamestown *N. Dak., U.S.A.* **112** B4
Jamestown *N.Y., U.S.A.* **114** D5
Jamestown *Tenn., U.S.A.* **114** E4
Jamīlābād *Iran* **71** C6
Jamira ➤ *India* **69** J13
Jāmjö *Sweden* **11** H9
Jamkhandi *India* **66** L9
Jammerbugten *Denmark* **11** G3
Jammu *India* **68** C6
Jammu & Kashmir □ *India* **69** B7
Jamnagar *India* **68** H4
Jamni ➤ *India* **69** G8
Jampur *Pakistan* **68** E4
Jamrud *Pakistan* **68** C4
Jämsä *Finland* **32** B3
Jamshedpur *India* **69** H12
Jamtara *India* **69** H12
Jämtland □ *Sweden* **8** E16
Jämtlands län □ *Sweden* **10** B7
Jan L. *Canada* **103** C8
Jan Mayen *Arctic* **4** B7
Janakkala *Finland* **32** B3
Janakpur *India* **69** F11
Janaúba *Brazil* **125** G10
Jand *Pakistan* **68** C5
Jandanku ◎ *Australia* **94** B2
Jandaq *Iran* **71** C7
Jandía *Canary Is.* **48** F5
Jandía, Pta. de *Canary Is.* **48** F5

Jandía △ *Canary Is.* **48** F5
Jandola *Pakistan* **68** C4
Jandowae *Australia* **95** D5
Jándula ➤ *Spain* **37** G6
Janesville *U.S.A.* **112** D9
Janga *Ghana* **83** C4
Jangamo *Mozam.* **89** C6
Janghai *India* **69** G10
Jangheung *S. Korea* **57** G14
Janikowo *Poland* **31** F5
Janin = Ioannina □ *Greece* **46** B2
Janja *Bos.-H.* **28** F3
Janjanbureh *Gambia* **82** C2
Janjevo *Kosovo* **44** D5
Janjgir *India* **69** J10
Janjina *Croatia* **41** F14
Janjina *Madag.* **89** C8
Janos *Mexico* **118** A3
Jánoshalma *Hungary* **28** D4
Jánosháza *Hungary* **28** C2
Jánossomorja *Hungary* **28** C2
Janów *Poland* **31** H6
Janów Lubelski *Poland* **31** H9
Janów Podlaski *Poland* **31** F10
Janowiec Wielkopolski
  Poland **31** F4
Januária *Brazil* **125** G10
Janub △ *Sudan* **81** F2
Janub Dârfûr □ *Sudan* **81** E2
Janub Kordofân □ *Sudan* **81** E3
Janūb Sīnī □ *Egypt* **74** F2
Janubio *Canary Is.* **48** F6
Janville *France* **19** D8
Janzé *France* **18** E5
Jaora *India* **68** H6
Japan ■ *Asia* **55** G8
Japan, Sea of *Asia* **54** E7
Japan Trench *Pac. Oc.* **96** D6
Japen = Yapen *Indonesia* **63** E9
Japla *India* **69** G11
Japurá ➤ *Brazil* **124** D5
Jaquarão *Brazil* **127** C5
Jaqué *Panama* **120** E4
Jarābulus *Syria* **73** D8
Jaraicejo *Spain* **37** F5
Jaraíz de la Vera *Spain* **36** E5
Jarama ➤ *Spain* **36** E7
Jaramānah *Syria* **72** F7
Jarandilla de la Vera *Spain* **36** E5
Jaranwala *Pakistan* **68** D5
Jarash *Jordan* **74** C4
Jarash □ *Jordan* **74** C4
Järbo *Sweden* **10** D10
Jardim *Brazil* **126** A4
Jardín ➤ *Spain* **39** G2
Jardín América *Argentina* **127** B4
Jardine River △ *Australia* **94** A3
Jardines de la Reina, Arch.
  de los *Cuba* **120** B4
Jargalang *China* **57** C12
Jari ➤ *Brazil* **125** D8
Jarīr, W. al ➤ *Si. Arabia* **70** E4
Jārlåsa *Sweden* **10** E11
Jarmen *Germany* **24** B9
Järna *Dalarna, Sweden* **10** D8
Järna *Stockholm, Sweden* **10** E11
Jarnac *France* **20** C3
Jarny *France* **19** C12
Jarocin *Poland* **31** G4
Jaroměř *Czech Rep.* **26** A8
Jarosław *Poland* **31** H9
Järpås *Sweden* **11** F6
Järpen *Sweden* **10** A7
Jarrahdale *Australia* **93** F2
Jarrahi ➤ *Iran* **71** D6
Jarres, Plaine des *Laos* **64** C4
Jarso *Ethiopia* **81** F4
Jartai *China* **56** E3
Jarud Qi *China* **57** B11
Jarvenpää *Finland* **32** B3
Jarvis *Canada* **114** D4
Jarvis I. *Pac. Oc.* **97** H12
Jarvornik *Czech Rep.* **27** A10
Järvsö *Sweden* **10** C10
Jasdan *India* **68** H4
Jashpurnagar *India* **69** H11
Jasidih *India* **69** G12
Jasień *Poland* **31** G2
Jasin *Malaysia* **65** L4
Jāsk *Iran* **71** E8
Jasło *Poland* **31** J8
Jason Is. *Falk. Is.* **128** G4
Jasper *Alta., Canada* **102** C5
Jasper *Ont., Canada* **115** B9
Jasper *Ala., U.S.A.* **117** E11
Jasper *Fla., U.S.A.* **117** F13
Jasper *Ind., U.S.A.* **112** F10
Jasper *Tex., U.S.A.* **116** F7
Jasper △ *Canada* **102** C5
Jasrasar *India* **68** F5
Jassān *Iraq* **73** G11
Jastarnia *Poland* **30** D5
Jastrebarsko *Croatia* **41** C12
Jastrowie *Poland* **30** E3

Jastrzębie Zdrój *Poland* **31** J5
Jász-Nagykun-Szolnok □
  Hungary **28** C5
Jászapáti *Hungary* **28** C5
Jászárokszállás *Hungary* **28** C5
Jászberény *Hungary* **28** C4
Jászkisér *Hungary* **28** C5
Jászladány *Hungary* **28** C5
Jataí *Brazil* **125** G8
Jati *Pakistan* **68** G3
Jatibarang *Indonesia* **63** G13
Jatiluwih *Indonesia* **63** J18
Jatinegara *Indonesia* **63** G12
Játiva = Xàtiva *Spain* **39** G4
Jättendal *Sweden* **10** C11
Jaú *Brazil* **127** A6
Jauja *Peru* **124** F3
Jaunpur *India* **69** G10
Java = Jawa *Indonesia* **62** F3
Java Sea *Indonesia* **62** F3
Java Trench *Ind. Oc.* **62** F3
Javalambre, Sa. de *Spain* **38** E4
Javānrūd *Iran* **73** E12
Jávea *Spain* **39** G5
Jawa *Indonesia* **62** F3
Jawa Barat □ *Indonesia* **63** G12
Jawa Tengah □ *Indonesia* **63** G14
Jawa Timur □ *Indonesia* **63** G15
Jawad *India* **68** G6
Jawhar *Somali Rep.* **75** G4
Jawor *Poland* **31** G3
Jaworzno *Poland* **31** H6
Jaworzyna Śląska *Poland* **31** H3
Jawoyn ◎ *Australia* **92** B5
Jay Peak *U.S.A.* **115** B12
Jaya, Puncak *Indonesia* **63** E9
Jayanti *India* **67** F16
Jayapura *Indonesia* **63** E10
Jayawijaya, Pegunungan
  Indonesia **63** F9
Jaynagar *India* **69** F12
Jaypur = Jeypore *India* **67** K13
Jayrūd *Syria* **72** F7
Jayton *U.S.A.* **116** E4
Jāz Mūriān, Hāmūn-e *Iran* **71** E8
Jazīreh-ye Shīf *Iran* **71** D6
Jazminal *Mexico* **118** C4
Jazzīn *Lebanon* **74** B4
Jean *U.S.A.* **111** K11
Jean Marie River *Canada* **102** A4
Jean-Rabel *Haiti* **121** C5
Jeanerette *U.S.A.* **116** G9
Jeanette, Ostrov =
  Zhannetty, Ostrov *Russia* **53** B16
Jeannette *U.S.A.* **114** F5
Jebäl Bärez, Kūh-e *Iran* **71** D8
Jebba *Nigeria* **83** D5
Jebel, Bahr el ➤ *Sudan* **81** F3
Jebel Ali = Minā' Jabal 'Alī
  U.A.E. **71** E7
Jebel Dud *Sudan* **81** E3
Jebel Qerri *Sudan* **81** D3
Jecheon *S. Korea* **57** F15
Jedburgh *U.K.* **13** F6
Jedda = Jiddah *Si. Arabia* **75** C2
Jeddore L. *Canada* **105** C8
Jedlicze *Poland* **31** J8
Jędrzejów *Poland* **31** H7
Jedwabne *Poland* **31** E9
Jeetzel ➤ *Germany* **24** B7
Jefferson *Iowa, U.S.A.* **112** D7
Jefferson *Ohio, U.S.A.* **114** E4
Jefferson *Tex., U.S.A.* **116** E7
Jefferson, Mt. *Nev., U.S.A.* **108** G5
Jefferson, Mt. *Oreg., U.S.A.* **108** D3
Jefferson City *Mo., U.S.A.* **112** F7
Jefferson City *Tenn., U.S.A.* **117** C13
Jeffersontown *U.S.A.* **113** F11
Jeffersonville *U.S.A.* **113** F11
Jeffrey City *U.S.A.* **108** E10
Jega *Nigeria* **83** C5
Jeju *S. Korea* **57** H14
Jeju-do *S. Korea* **57** H14
Jēkabpils *Latvia* **32** D3
Jekyll I. *U.S.A.* **117** F14
Jelcz-Laskowice *Poland* **31** G4
Jelenia Góra *Poland* **31** H2
Jelgava *Latvia* **30** B10
Jelgava □ *Latvia* **30** B10
Jelica *Serbia* **44** C4
Jelli *Sudan* **81** F3
Jelšava *Slovak Rep.* **27** C13
Jemaja *Indonesia* **65** L5
Jemaluang *Malaysia* **65** L4
Jember *Indonesia* **63** H15
Jena *Germany* **24** E7
Jena *U.S.A.* **116** F8
Jenbach *Austria* **26** D4
Jenīn *West Bank* **74** C4
Jenkins *U.S.A.* **113** G12
Jenner *U.S.A.* **110** G3
Jennings *U.S.A.* **116** F8
Jeong-eup *S. Korea* **57** G14
Jeonju *S. Korea* **57** G14
Jepara *Indonesia* **63** G14
Jeparit *Australia* **95** F3
Jequié *Brazil* **125** F10
Jequitinhonha *Brazil* **125** G10
Jequitinhonha ➤ *Brazil* **125** G11

Jerada *Morocco* **78** B5
Jerantut *Malaysia* **65** L4
Jerejak, Pulau *Malaysia* **65** c
Jérémie *Haiti* **121** C5
Jerez, Pta. *Mexico* **119** C5
Jerez de García Salinas
  Mexico **118** C4
Jerez de la Frontera *Spain* **37** J4
Jerez de los Caballeros *Spain* **37** G4
Jericho = El Arīḥā *West Bank* **74** D4
Jericho *Australia* **94** C4
Jerichow *Germany* **24** C8
Jerid, Chott el = Djerid,
  Chott *Tunisia* **78** B7
Jerilderie *Australia* **95** F4
Jermyn *U.S.A.* **115** E9
Jerome *U.S.A.* **108** E6
Jerramungup *Australia* **93** F2
Jersey *U.K.* **15** H5
Jersey City *U.S.A.* **115** F10
Jersey Shore *U.S.A.* **114** E7
Jerseyville *U.S.A.* **112** F8
Jerusalem *Israel/West Bank* **74** D4
Jervis B. *Australia* **95** F5
Jervis Inlet *Canada* **102** C4
Jerzu *Italy* **42** C2
Jesenice *Slovenia* **41** B11
Jeseník *Czech Rep.* **27** A10
Jesenké *Slovak Rep.* **27** C13
Jesi = Iesi *Italy* **41** E10
Jessnitz *Germany* **24** D8
Jessore *Bangla.* **67** H16
Jesup *U.S.A.* **117** F14
Jesús Carranza *Mexico* **119** D5
Jesús María *Argentina* **126** C3
Jetmore *U.S.A.* **112** F4
Jetpur *India* **68** J4
Jeumont *France* **19** B11
Jevnaker *Norway* **9** F14
Jewett *U.S.A.* **114** F3
Jewett City *U.S.A.* **115** E13
Jeyḥūnābād *Iran* **71** C6
Jeypore *India* **67** K13
Jeziorak, Jezioro *Poland* **30** E6
Jeziorany *Poland* **30** E7
Jeziorka → *Poland* **31** F8
Jha Jha *India* **69** G12
Jhaarkand = Jharkhand □
  India **69** H11
Jhabua *India* **68** H6
Jhajjar *India* **68** E7
Jhal *Pakistan* **68** E2
Jhal Jhao *Pakistan* **66** F4
Jhalawar *India* **68** G7
Jhalida *India* **69** H11
Jhalrapatan *India* **68** G7
Jhang Maghiana *Pakistan* **68** D5
Jhansi *India* **69** G8
Jhargram *India* **69** H12
Jharia *India* **69** H12
Jharkhand □ *India* **69** H11
Jharsuguda *India* **67** J14
Jhelum *Pakistan* **68** C5
Jhelum → *Pakistan* **68** D5
Jhilmilli *India* **69** H10
Jhudo *Pakistan* **68** G3
Jhunjhunu *India* **68** E6
Ji-Paraná *Brazil* **124** F6
Ji Xian *Hebei, China* **56** F8
Ji Xian *Henan, China* **56** G8
Ji Xian *Shanxi, China* **56** F6
Jia Xian *Henan, China* **56** H7
Jia Xian *Shaanxi, China* **56** E6
Jiading *China* **59** B13
Jiahe *China* **59** E9
Jiaji = Qionghai *China* **64** C8
Jialing Jiang → *China* **58** C6
Jiamusi *China* **60** B8
Ji'an *Jiangxi, China* **59** D10
Ji'an *Jilin, China* **57** D14
Jianchang *China* **57** D11
Jianchangying *China* **57** D10
Jianchuan *China* **58** D2
Jiande *China* **59** C12
Jiang'an *China* **58** C5
Jiangbei *China* **58** C6
Jiangcheng *China* **58** F3
Jiangchuan *China* **58** E4
Jiangdi *China* **58** D3
Jiangdu *China* **59** A12
Jiange *China* **58** A5
Jianghua *China* **59** E8
Jiangjin *China* **58** C6
Jiangkou *China* **58** D7
Jiangle *China* **59** D11
Jiangling *China* **59** B9
Jiangmen *China* **59** F9
Jiangshan *China* **59** C12
Jiangsu □ *China* **57** H11
Jiangxi □ *China* **59** D11
Jiangyan *China* **59** A13
Jiangyin *China* **59** B13
Jiangyong *China* **59** E8
Jiangyou *China* **58** B5
Jianhe *China* **58** D7
Jianli *China* **59** C9
Jianning *China* **59** D11
Jian'ou *China* **59** D12

Jianshi *China* **58** B7
Jianshui *China* **58** F4
Jianyang *Fujian, China* **59** D12
Jianyang *Sichuan, China* **58** B5
Jiao Xian = Jiaozhou *China* **57** F11
Jiaohe *Hebei, China* **56** E9
Jiaohe *Jilin, China* **57** C14
Jiaojiang *China* **59** C13
Jiaoling *China* **59** E11
Jiaozhou *China* **57** F11
Jiaozhou Wan *China* **57** F11
Jiaozuo *China* **56** G7
Jiashan *China* **59** B13
Jiawang *China* **57** G9
Jiaxiang *China* **56** G9
Jiaxing *China* **59** B13
Jiayi = Chiai *Taiwan* **59** F13
Jiayu *China* **59** C9
Jibiya *Nigeria* **83** C6
Jibou *Romania* **29** C8
Jibuti = Djibouti ■ *Africa* **81** E5
Jicarón, I. *Panama* **120** E3
Jičín *Czech Rep.* **26** A8
Jiddah *Si. Arabia* **75** C2
Jido *India* **67** E19
Jieshou *China* **56** H8
Jiexiu *China* **56** F6
Jieyang *China* **59** F11
Jigalong *Australia* **92** D3
Jigalong ○ *Australia* **92** D3
Jigawa □ *Nigeria* **83** C6
Jigni *India* **69** G8
Jihlava *Czech Rep.* **26** B8
Jihlava → *Czech Rep.* **27** C9
Jihlavský □ *Czech Rep.* **26** B8
Jihočeský □ *Czech Rep.* **26** B7
Jihomoravský □ *Czech Rep.* **27** B9
Jijiga *Ethiopia* **75** F3
Jikamshi *Nigeria* **83** C6
Jikau *Sudan* **81** F3
Jilib *Somali Rep.* **75** G3
Jilin *China* **57** C14
Jilin □ *China* **57** C14
Jiloca → *Spain* **38** D3
Jilong = Chilung *Taiwan* **59** E13
Jim Thorpe *U.S.A.* **115** F9
Jima *Ethiopia* **81** F4
Jimbaran, Teluk *Indonesia* **63** K18
Jimbolia *Romania* **28** E5
Jimena de la Frontera *Spain* **37** J5
Jiménez *Mexico* **118** B4
Jimeta *Nigeria* **83** D7
Jimo *China* **57** F11
Jin Jiang → *China* **59** C10
Jin Xian = Jinzhou *Hebei,*
  China **56** E8
Jin Xian = Jinzhou *Liaoning,*
  China **57** E11
Jinan *China* **56** F9
Jinchang *China* **60** C5
Jincheng *China* **56** G7
Jinchuan *China* **58** B4
Jind *India* **68** E7
Jindabyne *Australia* **95** F4
Jindo *S. Korea* **57** G15
Jindřichův Hradec *Czech Rep.* **26** B8
Jing He → *China* **56** G5
Jing Shan *China* **59** B8
Jing Xian *China* **59** B12
Jing'an *China* **59** C10
Jingbian *China* **56** F5
Jingchuan *China* **56** G4
Jingde *China* **59** B12
Jingdezhen *China* **59** C11
Jingdong *China* **58** E3
Jinggangshan *China* **59** D10
Jinggu *China* **58** F3
Jinghai *China* **56** E9
Jinghong *China* **58** G3
Jingjiang *China* **59** A13
Jingle *China* **56** E6
Jingmen *China* **59** B9
Jingning *China* **56** G4
Jingpo Hu *China* **57** C15
Jingshan *China* **59** B9
Jingtai *China* **58** F3
Jingxi *China* **58** F6
Jingxing *China* **56** E8
Jingyang *China* **56** G5
Jingyu *China* **57** C14
Jingyuan *China* **56** F3
Jingzhou *China* **58** D7
Jingziguan *China* **56** H6
Jinhua *China* **59** C12
Jining *Nei Monggol Zizhiqu,*
  China **56** D7
Jining *Shandong, China* **56** G9
Jinja *Uganda* **86** B3
Jinjang *Malaysia* **65** L3
Jinji *China* **56** F4
Jinjiang *Fujian, China* **59** E12
Jinjiang *Yunnan, China* **58** D3
Jinjini *Ghana* **82** D4
Jinju *S. Korea* **57** G15
Jinkou *China* **59** B10
Jinkouhe *China* **58** C4
Jinmen Dao *China* **59** E12
Jinnah Barrage *Pakistan* **68** C4
Jinning *China* **58** E4

Jinotega *Nic.* **120** D2
Jinotepe *Nic.* **120** D2
Jinping *Guizhou, China* **58** D7
Jinping *Yunnan, China* **58** F4
Jinsha *China* **58** D6
Jinsha Jiang → *China* **58** C5
Jinshan *China* **59** B13
Jinshi *China* **59** C8
Jintan *China* **59** B12
Jinxi *Jiangxi, China* **59** D11
Jinxi *Liaoning, China* **57** E11
Jinxian *China* **59** C11
Jinxiang *China* **56** G9
Jinyang *China* **58** D4
Jinyun *China* **59** C13
Jinzhai *China* **59** B10
Jinzhong *China* **56** F7
Jinzhou *Hebei, China* **56** E8
Jinzhou *Liaoning, China* **57** E11
Jinzhou *Liaoning, China* **57** D11
Jiparaná → *Brazil* **124** E6
Jipijapa *Ecuador* **124** D2
Jiquilpan *Mexico* **118** D4
Jirisan *S. Korea* **57** G14
Jiroft *Iran* **71** D8
Jishan *China* **56** G6
Jishou *China* **58** C7
Jishui *China* **59** D10
Jisr ash Shughūr *Syria* **72** E7
Jitarning *Australia* **93** F2
Jitra *Malaysia* **65** J3
Jiu → *Romania* **29** F10
Jiudengkou *China* **56** E4
Jiujiang *Guangdong, China* **59** F9
Jiujiang *Jiangxi, China* **59** C10
Jiuling Shan *China* **59** C10
Jiulong = Kowloon *China* **59** F10
Jiulong *China* **58** C5
Jiutai *China* **57** B13
Jiuxincheng *China* **56** E8
Jiuyuhang *China* **59** B12
Jiwani *Pakistan* **66** G2
Jixi *Anhui, China* **59** B12
Jixi *Heilongjiang, China* **57** B16
Jiyang *China* **57** F9
Jiyuan *China* **56** G7
Jīzān *Si. Arabia* **75** D3
Jize *China* **56** F8
Jizera → *Czech Rep.* **26** A7
Jizl, Wādī al → *Si. Arabia* **70** E3
Jizō-Zaki *Japan* **55** G6
Jizzax *Uzbekistan* **52** E7
Joaçaba *Brazil* **127** B5
Joal Fadiout *Senegal* **82** C1
João Pessoa *Brazil* **125** E12
Joaquín V. González
  Argentina **126** B3
Jobat *India* **68** H6
Jobourg, Nez de *France* **18** C5
Jódar *Spain* **37** H7
Jodhpur *India* **68** F5
Jodiya *India* **68** H4
Joensuu *Finland* **8** E23
Jõetsu *Japan* **55** F9
Jœuf *France* **19** C12
Jofane *Mozam.* **89** C5
Jogbani *India* **69** F12
Jõgeva *Estonia* **32** C4
Jogjakarta = Yogyakarta
  Indonesia **62** F4
Johannesburg *S. Africa* **89** D4
Johannesburg *U.S.A.* **111** K9
Johansfors *Sweden* **11** H9
Johilla → *India* **69** H9
John Crow Mts. *Jamaica* **120** a
John Day *U.S.A.* **108** D4
John Day → *U.S.A.* **108** D3
John Day Fossil Beds △
  U.S.A. **108** D4
John D'or Prairie *Canada* **102** B5
John H. Kerr Res. *U.S.A.* **117** C15
John o' Groats *U.K.* **13** C5
Johnnie *U.S.A.* **111** J10
John's Ra. *Australia* **94** C1
Johnson *U.S.A.* **115** B12
Johnson City *Kans., U.S.A.* **112** G3
Johnson City *N.Y., U.S.A.* **115** D9
Johnson City *Tenn., U.S.A.* **117** C13
Johnson City *Tex., U.S.A.* **116** F5
Johnsonburg *U.S.A.* **114** E6
Johnsondale *U.S.A.* **111** K8
Johnsons Crossing *Canada* **102** A2
Johnston, L. *Australia* **93** F3
Johnston Falls =
  Mambilima Falls *Zambia* **87** E2
Johnston I. *Pac. Oc.* **97** F11
Johnstone Str. *Canada* **102** C3
Johnstown *Ireland* **12** D4
Johnstown *N.Y., U.S.A.* **115** C10
Johnstown *Ohio, U.S.A.* **114** F2
Johnstown *Pa., U.S.A.* **114** F6
Johor □ *Malaysia* **65** d
Johor Bahru *Malaysia* **65** d
Joigny *France* **19** E10
Joinville *Brazil* **127** B6
Joinville *France* **19** D12
Joinville I. *Antarctica* **5** C18
Jojutla *Mexico* **119** D5

Jokkmokk *Sweden* **8** C18
Jökulsá á Bru → *Iceland* **8** D6
Jökulsá á Fjöllum → *Iceland* **8** C5
Jolfā *Āzarbāijān-e Sharqī, Iran* **73** C11
Jolfā *Eṣfahan, Iran* **71** C6
Joliet *U.S.A.* **112** E9
Joliette *Canada* **104** C5
Jolo *Phil.* **61** J4
Jolon *U.S.A.* **110** K5
Jomalig I. *Phil.* **61** D5
Jombang *Indonesia* **63** G15
Jomda *China* **58** B2
Jonava *Lithuania* **32** E3
Jones Sound *Canada* **101** B15
Jonesboro *Ark., U.S.A.* **117** D9
Jonesboro *La., U.S.A.* **116** E8
Jong → *S. Leone* **82** D2
Jonglei *Sudan* **81** F3
Jonglei □ *Sudan* **81** F3
Joniškis *Lithuania* **30** B10
Jönköping *Sweden* **11** G8
Jönköpings län □ *Sweden* **11** G8
Jonquière *Canada* **105** C5
Jonsered *Sweden* **11** G6
Jonzac *France* **20** C3
Joplin *U.S.A.* **112** G6
Jora *India* **68** F6
Jordan *Mont., U.S.A.* **108** C10
Jordan *N.Y., U.S.A.* **115** C8
Jordan ■ *Asia* **74** E5
Jordan → *Asia* **74** D4
Jordan Valley *U.S.A.* **108** E5
Jordanów *Poland* **31** J6
Jorhat *India* **67** F19
Jori → *Norway* **10** B3
Jörn *Sweden* **8** D19
Jorong *Indonesia* **62** E4
Jørpeland *Norway* **9** G12
Jorquera → *Chile* **126** B2
Jos *Nigeria* **83** D6
Jos Plateau *Nigeria* **83** D6
Jošanička Banja *Serbia* **44** C4
José Batlle y Ordóñez
  Uruguay **127** C4
José de San Martín
  Argentina **128** E2
Joseni *Romania* **29** D10
Joseph, L. *Canada* **114** A5
Joseph Bonaparte G.
  Australia **92** B4
Joseph L. *Canada* **105** B6
Joshinath *India* **69** D8
Joshinetsu-Kōgen △ *Japan* **55** F9
Joshua Tree *U.S.A.* **111** L10
Joshua Tree △ *U.S.A.* **111** M10
Josselin *France* **18** E4
Jost Van Dyke I. *Br. Virgin Is.* **121** e
Jostedalsbreen *Norway* **8** F12
Jotunheimen *Norway* **8** F13
Joubertberge *Namibia* **88** B1
Joué-lès-Tours *France* **18** E7
Jourdanton *U.S.A.* **116** G5
Joutseno *Finland* **32** B5
Jovellanos *Cuba* **120** B3
Jowkār *Iran* **73** E13
Joyeuse *France* **21** D8
Józefów *Lubelskie, Poland* **31** H10
Józefów *Mazowieckie, Poland* **31** F8
Ju Xian *China* **57** F10
Juan Aldama *Mexico* **118** C4
Juan Bautista Alberdi
  Argentina **126** C3
Juan de Fuca, Str of.
  N. Amer. **110** B3
Juán de Nova *Ind. Oc.* **89** B7
Juan Fernández, Arch. de
  Pac. Oc. **122** G2
Juan José Castelli *Argentina* **126** B3
Juan L. Lacaze *Uruguay* **126** C4
Juankoski *Finland* **8** E23
Juárez *Mexico* **118** B4
Juárez, Sierra de *Mexico* **118** A1
Juàzeiro *Brazil* **125** E10
Juàzeiro do Norte *Brazil* **125** E11
Juazohn *Liberia* **82** D3
Jûbâ *Sudan* **81** G3
Juba → *Somali Rep.* **75** G3
Jubany *Antarctica* **5** C18
Jubayl *Lebanon* **74** A4
Jubbah *Si. Arabia* **70** D4
Jubbal *India* **68** D7
Jubbulpore = Jabalpur *India* **69** H8
Jûbek *Germany* **24** A5
Jubga *Russia* **35** H4
Jubilee L. *Australia* **93** E4
Juby, C. *Morocco* **78** C3
Júcar = Xúquer → *Spain* **39** F4
Júcaro *Cuba* **120** B4
Juchitán de Zaragoza
  Mexico **119** D5
Judea = Har Yehuda *Israel* **74** D3
Judenburg *Austria* **26** D7
Judith → *U.S.A.* **108** C9
Judith, Pt. *U.S.A.* **115** E13
Judith Gap *U.S.A.* **108** C9
Juelsminde *Denmark* **11** J4
Juigalpa *Nic.* **120** D2
Juillac *France* **20** C5
Juist *Germany* **24** B2
Juiz de Fora *Brazil* **127** A7

Jujuy □ *Argentina* **126** A2
Julesburg *U.S.A.* **108** F12
Juli *Peru* **124** G5
Julia Cr. → *Australia* **94** C3
Julia Creek *Australia* **94** C3
Juliaca *Peru* **124** G4
Julian *U.S.A.* **111** M10
Julian, L. *Canada* **104** B4
Julian Alps = Julijske Alpe
  Slovenia **41** B11
Julianatop *Suriname* **125** C7
Julianehåb = Qaqortoq
  Greenland **4** C5
Jülich *Germany* **24** E2
Julijske Alpe *Slovenia* **41** B11
Julimes *Mexico* **118** B3
Jullundur *India* **68** D6
Julu *China* **56** F8
Jumbo *Zimbabwe* **87** F3
Jumbo Pk. *U.S.A.* **111** J12
Jumentos Cays *Bahamas* **120** B4
Jumilla *Spain* **39** G3
Jumla *Nepal* **69** E10
Jumna = Yamuna → *India* **69** G9
Jumunjin *S. Korea* **57** F15
Junagadh *India* **68** J4
Junction *Tex., U.S.A.* **116** F5
Junction *Utah, U.S.A.* **109** G7
Junction B. *Australia* **94** A1
Junction City *Kans., U.S.A.* **112** F5
Junction City *Oreg., U.S.A.* **108** D2
Junction Pt. *Australia* **94** A1
Jundah *Australia* **94** C3
Jundiaí *Brazil* **127** A6
Juneau *U.S.A.* **102** B2
Junee *Australia* **95** E4
Jungfrau *Switz.* **25** J3
Junggar Pendi *China* **60** B3
Jungshahi *Pakistan* **68** G2
Juniata → *U.S.A.* **114** F7
Junín *Argentina* **126** C3
Junín de los Andes *Argentina* **128** D2
Jūniyah *Lebanon* **74** B4
Junlian *China* **58** C5
Juntas *Chile* **126** B2
Juntura *U.S.A.* **108** E4
Jur, Nahr el → *Sudan* **81** F2
Jura = Jura, Mts. du *Europe* **19** F13
Jura = Schwäbische Alb
  Germany **25** G5
Jura *U.K.* **13** F3
Jura □ *France* **19** F12
Jura □ *Switz.* **25** H3
Jūra → *Lithuania* **30** C9
Jura, Mts. du *Europe* **19** F13
Jura, Sd. of *U.K.* **13** F3
Jurbarkas *Lithuania* **30** C9
Jurien Bay *Australia* **93** F2
Jurilovca *Romania* **29** F13
Jūrmala *Latvia* **30** B10
Jurong *China* **59** B12
Jurong *Singapore* **65** d
Juruá → *Brazil* **124** D5
Juruena *Brazil* **124** F7
Juruena → *Brazil* **124** E7
Juruti *Brazil* **125** D7
Jussey *France* **19** E12
Justo Daract *Argentina* **126** C2
Jutaí → *Brazil* **124** D5
Jüterbog *Germany* **24** D9
Juticalpa *Honduras* **120** D2
Jutland = Jylland *Denmark* **11** H3
Juuka *Finland* **8** E23
Juventud, I. de la *Cuba* **120** B3
Juvigny-sous-Andaine
  France **18** D6
Juvisy-sous-Andaine
Juy Zar *Iran* **73** F12
Juye *China* **56** G9
Juzennecourt *France* **19** D11
Jvari *Georgia* **35** J6
Jwaneng *Botswana* **85** J4
Jyderup *Denmark* **11** J5
Jylland *Denmark* **11** H3
Jyväskylä *Finland* **32** A3

K

K2 *Pakistan* **69** B7
Ka → *Nigeria* **83** C5
Kaakha = Kaka *Turkmenistan* **71** B8
Kaap Plateau *S. Africa* **88** D3
Kaapkruis *Namibia* **88** C1
Kaapstad = Cape Town
  S. Africa **88** E2
Kaba *Guinea* **82** C2
Kabaena *Indonesia* **63** F6
Kabala *S. Leone* **82** D2
Kabale *Uganda* **86** C3
Kabalo *Dem. Rep. of the Congo* **86** D2
Kabambare
  Dem. Rep. of the Congo **86** C2
Kabango
  Dem. Rep. of the Congo **87** D2
Kabanjahe *Indonesia* **62** D1
Kabankalan *Phil.* **61** G5
Kabara *Fiji* **91** a
Kabara *Mali* **82** B4
Kabardinka *Russia* **33** K10
Kabardino-Balkaria □
  Russia **35** J6

Kabarega Falls =
  Murchison Falls *Uganda* **86** B3
Kabarnet *Kenya* **86** B4
Kabasalan *Phil.* **61** H5
Kabat *Indonesia* **63** J17
Kabba *Nigeria* **83** D6
Kabi *Niger* **83** C7
Kabin Buri *Thailand* **64** F3
Kabinakagami L. *Canada* **104** C3
Kabinda *Dem. Rep. of the Congo* **84** F4
Kabna *Sudan* **80** D3
Kabompo *Zambia* **87** E1
Kabompo → *Zambia* **85** G4
Kabondo
  Dem. Rep. of the Congo **87** D2
Kabongo
  Dem. Rep. of the Congo **86** D2
Kabot *Guinea* **82** C2
Kabou *Togo* **83** D5
Kabr *Sudan* **81** E2
Kabrît, G. el *Egypt* **74** F2
Kabrousse *Senegal* **82** C1
Kabūd Gonbad *Iran* **71** B8
Kabudar Ahang *Iran* **73** E13
Kabugao *Phil.* **61** B4
Kābul *Afghan.* **68** B3
Kābul □ *Afghan.* **66** B6
Kābul → *Pakistan* **68** C5
Kabunga
  Dem. Rep. of the Congo **86** C2
Kaburuang *Indonesia* **63** D7
Kabushiya *Sudan* **81** D3
Kabwe *Zambia* **87** E2
Kačanik *Kosovo* **44** D5
Kačerginė *Lithuania* **30** D10
Kachchh, Gulf of *India* **68** H3
Kachchh, Rann of *India* **68** H4
Kachchhidhana *India* **69** J8
Kachebera *Zambia* **87** E3
Kachia *Nigeria* **83** D6
Kachikau *Botswana* **88** B3
Kachin □ *Burma* **58** D1
Kachira, L. *Uganda* **86** C3
Kachīry *Kazakhstan* **52** D8
Kachisi *Ethiopia* **81** F4
Kachnara *India* **68** H6
Kachot *Cambodia* **65** G4
Kaçkar *Turkey* **73** B9
Kadam, Mt. *Uganda* **86** B3
Kadan *Czech Rep.* **26** A6
Kadan Kyun *Burma* **64** F2
Kadanai → *Afghan.* **68** D1
Kadarkút *Hungary* **28** D2
Kadavu *Fiji* **91** a
Kadavu Passage *Fiji* **91** a
Kade *Ghana* **83** D4
Kadhimain = Al
  Kāẓimīyah *Iraq* **73** F11
Kadi *India* **68** H5
Kadiana *Mali* **82** C3
Kadina *Australia* **95** E2
Kadınhanı *Turkey* **72** C5
Kadiolo *Mali* **82** C3
Kadipur *India* **69** F10
Kadirli *Turkey* **72** D7
Kadiyevka = Stakhanov
  Ukraine **33** H10
Kadodo *Sudan* **81** E2
Kadoka *U.S.A.* **112** D3
Kadoma *Zimbabwe* **87** F2
Kâdugli *Sudan* **81** E2
Kaduna *Nigeria* **83** C6
Kaduna □ *Nigeria* **83** C6
Kaduna → *Nigeria* **83** D6
Kaduy *Russia* **32** C9
Kaédi *Mauritania* **82** B2
Kaélé *Cameroon* **83** C7
Kaeng Khoï *Thailand* **64** E3
Kaeng Krachan △ *Thailand* **64** F2
Kaeng Tana △ *Thailand* **64** E5
Kaesŏng *N. Korea* **57** F14
Kāf *Si. Arabia* **70** D3
Kafan = Kapan *Armenia* **73** C12
Kafanchan *Nigeria* **83** D6
Kafareti *Nigeria* **83** C7
Kaffrine *Senegal* **82** C1
Kafin *Nigeria* **83** D6
Kafin Madaki *Nigeria* **83** C6
Kafinda *Zambia* **87** E3
Kafr el Battikh *Egypt* **80** H7
Kafr el Dauwâr *Egypt* **80** H7
Kafr el Sheikh *Egypt* **80** H7
Kafr el Zaiyât *Egypt* **80** H7
Kafue *Zambia* **87** F2
Kafue → *Zambia* **85** H5
Kafue △ *Zambia* **87** F2
Kafue Flats *Zambia* **87** F2
Kafulwe *Zambia* **87** D2
Kaga *Afghan.* **68** B4
Kaga Bandoro *C.A.R.* **84** C3
Kagarko *Nigeria* **83** D6
Kagawa □ *Japan* **55** G7
Kagera □ *Tanzania* **86** C3
Kagera → *Uganda* **86** C3
Kağızman *Turkey* **73** B10
Kagmar *Sudan* **81** E3
Kagoro *Nigeria* **83** D6
Kagoshima *Japan* **55** J5

Kagoshima □ *Japan* 55 J5
Kagul = Cahul *Moldova* 29 E13
Kahak *Iran* 71 B6
Kahama *Tanzania* 86 C3
Kahan *Pakistan* 68 E3
Kahang *Malaysia* 65 L4
Kahayan → *Indonesia* 62 E4
Kahe *Tanzania* 86 C4
Kahemba
   Dem. Rep. of the Congo 84 F3
Kahnūj *Iran* 71 E8
Kahoka *U.S.A.* 112 E8
Kaho'olawe *U.S.A.* 107 L8
Kahramanmaraş *Turkey* 72 D7
Kahramanmaraş □ *Turkey* 72 D7
Kâhta *Turkey* 73 D8
Kahul, Ozero *Ukraine* 29 E13
Kahului *U.S.A.* 107 L8
Kahurangi △ *N.Z.* 91 D4
Kahuta *Pakistan* 68 C5
Kahuzi-Biega △
   Dem. Rep. of the Congo 86 C2
Kai, Kepulauan *Indonesia* 63 F8
Kai Besar *Indonesia* 63 F8
Kai Is. = Kai, Kepulauan
   Indonesia 63 F8
Kai Kecil *Indonesia* 63 F8
Kai Xian *China* 58 B7
Kaiama *Nigeria* 83 D5
Kaiapoi *N.Z.* 91 E4
Kaieteur Falls *Guyana* 124 B7
Kaifeng *China* 56 G8
Kaihua *China* 59 C12
Kaijiang *China* 58 B6
Kaikohe *N.Z.* 91 A4
Kaikoura *N.Z.* 91 E4
Kailahun *S. Leone* 82 D2
Kailash = Kangrinboqe
   Feng *China* 69 D9
Kaili *China* 58 D6
Kailu *China* 57 C11
Kailua Kona *U.S.A.* 107 M8
Kaimaktsalan Oros =
   Voras Oros *Greece* 44 F5
Kaimana *Indonesia* 63 E8
Kaimanawa Mts. *N.Z.* 91 C5
Kaimganj *India* 69 F8
Kaimur Hills *India* 69 G10
Kainab → *Namibia* 88 D2
Kainji Dam *Nigeria* 83 D5
Kainji Lake △ *Nigeria* 83 C5
Kainji Res. *Nigeria* 83 C5
Kainuu *Finland* 8 D23
Kaipara Harbour *N.Z.* 91 B5
Kaiping *China* 59 F9
Kaipokok B. *Canada* 105 B8
Kaira *India* 68 H5
Kairana *India* 68 E7
Kaironi *Indonesia* 63 E8
Kairouan *Tunisia* 79 A8
Kaiserslautern *Germany* 25 F3
Kaiserstuhl *Germany* 25 G3
Kaitaia *N.Z.* 91 A4
Kaitangata *N.Z.* 91 G2
Kaithal *India* 68 E7
Kaitu → *Pakistan* 68 C4
Kaiwi Channel *U.S.A.* 107 L8
Kaiyang *China* 58 D6
Kaiyuan *Liaoning, China* 57 C13
Kaiyuan *Yunnan, China* 58 F4
Kaiyuh Mts. *U.S.A.* 106 C8
Kajaani *Finland* 8 D22
Kajabbi *Australia* 94 C3
Kajana = Kajaani *Finland* 8 D22
Kajang *Malaysia* 65 L3
Kajaran *Armenia* 73 C12
Kajiado *Kenya* 86 C4
Kajo Kaji *Sudan* 81 G3
Kajok *Sudan* 81 F2
Kajuru *Nigeria* 83 C6
Kaka *Sudan* 81 E3
Kaka *Turkmenistan* 71 B8
Kakabeka Falls *Canada* 104 C2
Kakadu △ *Australia* 92 B5
Kakamas *S. Africa* 88 D3
Kakamega *Kenya* 86 B3
Kakanj *Bos.-H.* 28 F3
Kakanui Mts. *N.Z.* 91 F3
Kakata *Liberia* 82 D2
Kakdwip *India* 69 J13
Kake *Japan* 55 G6
Kake *U.S.A.* 102 B2
Kakegawa *Japan* 55 G9
Kakeroma-Jima *Japan* 55 K4
Kakhib *Russia* 35 J8
Kakhk *Iran* 71 C8
Kakhovka *Ukraine* 33 J7
Kakhovske Vdskh. *Ukraine* 33 J7
Kakinada *India* 67 L13
Kakisa *Canada* 102 A5
Kakisa → *Canada* 102 A5
Kakisa L. *Canada* 102 A5
Kakogawa *Japan* 55 G7
Kakum △ *Ghana* 83 D4
Kakuma *Kenya* 86 B3
Kakwa → *Canada* 102 C5
Kal Güsheh *Iran* 71 D8
Kāl Sefid *Iran* 73 E12
Kala *Nigeria* 83 C7

Kalaallit Nunaat =
   Greenland ☑ *N. Amer.* 99 C15
Kalabagh *Pakistan* 68 C4
Kalabahi *Indonesia* 63 F6
Kalabana *Mali* 82 C3
Kalach *Russia* 34 E5
Kalach na Donu *Russia* 35 F6
Kaladan → *Burma* 67 J18
Kaladar *Canada* 114 B7
Kalahari *Africa* 88 C3
Kalahari Gemsbok △
   S. Africa 88 D3
Kalajoki *Finland* 8 D21
Kalakamati *Botswana* 89 C4
Kalakan *Russia* 53 D12
K'alak'unlun Shank'ou =
   Karakoram Pass *Asia* 69 B7
Kalam *Pakistan* 69 B5
Kalama *Dem. Rep. of the Congo* 86 C2
Kalama *U.S.A.* 110 E4
Kalamaria *Greece* 44 F6
Kalamata *Greece* 46 D4
Kalamazoo *U.S.A.* 113 D11
Kalamazoo → *U.S.A.* 112 D10
Kalambaka *Greece* 46 B3
Kalambo Falls *Tanzania* 87 D3
Kalamos *Attiki, Greece* 46 C5
Kalamos *Lefkada, Greece* 46 C2
Kalan *Turkey* 70 B3
Kalankalan *Guinea* 82 C3
Kalannie *Australia* 93 F2
Kalao *Indonesia* 63 F6
Kalaotoa *Indonesia* 63 F6
Kälarne *Sweden* 10 B10
Kalasin *Thailand* 64 D4
Kālat *Iran* 71 B9
Kalat *Pakistan* 66 E5
Kalāteh *Iran* 71 B7
Kalāteh-ye Ganj *Iran* 71 E8
Kalathos *Greece* 47 E10
Kalaus → *Russia* 35 H7
Kalavrita *Greece* 46 C4
Kalbā *U.A.E.* 71 E8
Kalbarri *Australia* 93 E1
Kalbarri △ *Australia* 93 E1
Kalburgi = Gulbarga *India* 66 L10
Kalce *Slovenia* 22 F8
Kale *Antalya, Turkey* 47 E12
Kale *Denizli, Turkey* 47 D10
Kalecik *Turkey* 72 B5
Kalegauk Kyun *Burma* 64 E1
Kalehe *Dem. Rep. of the Congo* 86 C2
Kalema *Tanzania* 86 C3
Kalemie *Dem. Rep. of the Congo* 86 D2
Kalety *Poland* 31 H5
Kalewa *Burma* 67 H19
Kaleybar *Iran* 73 C12
Kalgoorlie-Boulder *Australia* 93 F3
Kali → *India* 69 F8
Kali Sindh → *India* 68 G6
Kaliakra, Nos *Bulgaria* 45 C12
Kalianda *Indonesia* 62 F3
Kalibo *Phil.* 61 F5
Kalima *Dem. Rep. of the Congo* 86 C2
Kalimantan *Indonesia* 62 E4
Kalimantan Barat □
   Indonesia 62 E4
Kalimantan Selatan □
   Indonesia 62 E5
Kalimantan Tengah □
   Indonesia 62 E4
Kalimantan Timur □
   Indonesia 62 D5
Kálimnos *Greece* 47 D8
Kalimpong *India* 69 F13
Kaliningrad *Russia* 30 D7
Kaliningrad ✈ (KGD) *Russia* 30 D7
Kalininsk *Russia* 34 E7
Kalinkavichy *Belarus* 23 B15
Kalinkovichi =
   Kalinkavichy *Belarus* 23 B15
Kalinovik *Bos.-H.* 44 C2
Kalipetrovo *Bulgaria* 45 B11
Kalirachi *Greece* 45 F8
Kaliro *Uganda* 86 B3
Kalispell *U.S.A.* 108 B6
Kalisz *Poland* 31 G5
Kalisz Pomorski *Poland* 31 E2
Kalithea *Greece* 46 D5
Kaliua *Tanzania* 86 D3
Kalivia Thorikou *Greece* 46 D5
Kalix = Kalixälven →
   Sweden 8 D20
Kalix *Sweden* 8 D20
Kalixälven → *Sweden* 8 D20
Kalka *India* 68 D7
Kalkan *Turkey* 47 E11
Kalkarindji *Australia* 92 C5
Kalkaska *U.S.A.* 113 C11
Kalkfeld *Namibia* 88 C2
Kalkfontein *Botswana* 88 C3
Kalkrand *Namibia* 88 C2
Kållandsö *Sweden* 11 F7
Kallavesi *Finland* 8 E22
Kållered *Sweden* 11 G6
Kallimasia *Greece* 47 C8

Kallinge *Sweden* 11 H9
Kallmet *Albania* 44 E3
Kallsjön *Sweden* 8 E15
Kalmalo *Nigeria* 83 C6
Kalmar *Sweden* 11 H10
Kalmar län □ *Sweden* 11 G10
Kalmar sund *Sweden* 11 H10
Kalmykia □ *Russia* 35 G8
Kalna *India* 69 H13
Kalnai *India* 69 H10
Kalo Nero *Greece* 46 D3
Kalocsa *Hungary* 28 D4
Kalofer *Bulgaria* 45 D8
Kalokhorio *Cyprus* 49 E12
Kaloko *Dem. Rep. of the Congo* 86 D2
Kalol *Gujarat, India* 68 H5
Kalol *Gujarat, India* 68 H5
Kalomo *Zambia* 87 F2
Kaloni *Greece* 47 B8
Kaloni, Kolpos *Greece* 47 B8
Kalookan = Caloocan *Phil.* 61 D4
Kalpi *India* 69 F8
Kaltag *U.S.A.* 106 C7
Kaltern = Caldaro *Italy* 41 B8
Kaltukatjara *Australia* 93 D4
Kaltungo *Nigeria* 83 D7
Kalu *Pakistan* 68 G2
Kaluga *Russia* 32 E9
Kaluga □ *Russia* 32 E8
Kalulushi *Zambia* 87 E2
Kalumburu *Australia* 92 B4
Kalumburu ◎ *Australia* 92 B4
Kalundborg *Denmark* 11 J5
Kalush *Ukraine* 23 D13
Kaluszyn *Poland* 31 F8
Kalutara *Sri Lanka* 66 R12
Kalvarija *Lithuania* 30 D10
Kalyan *India* 66 K8
Kalyazin *Russia* 32 D9
Kam *Albania* 44 E4
Kam → *Nigeria* 83 D7
Kama *Dem. Rep. of the Congo* 86 C2
Kama → *Russia* 6 D16
Kamachumu *Tanzania* 86 C3
Kamaishi *Japan* 54 E10
Kamalia *Pakistan* 68 D5
Kaman *India* 68 F6
Kaman *Turkey* 72 C5
Kamanjab *Namibia* 88 B2
Kamapanda *Zambia* 87 E1
Kamara *Mali* 82 C3
Kamarān *Yemen* 75 D3
Kamativi *Zimbabwe* 88 B4
Kamba *Nigeria* 83 C5
Kambalda West *Australia* 93 F3
Kambar *Pakistan* 68 F3
Kambia *S. Leone* 82 D2
Kambolé *Togo* 83 D5
Kambolé *Zambia* 87 D3
Kambos *Cyprus* 49 D11
Kambove
   Dem. Rep. of the Congo 87 E2
Kamchatka, Poluostrov
   Russia 53 D17
Kamchatka Pen. =
   Kamchatka, Poluostrov
   Russia 53 D17
Kamchiya → *Bulgaria* 45 C11
Kame Ruins *Zimbabwe* 87 G2
Kamen *Russia* 52 D9
Kamen-Rybolov *Russia* 54 B6
Kamenica *Serbia* 44 C6
Kamenica *Serbia* 44 B3
Kamenice nad Lipou
   Czech Rep. 26 B8
Kamenjak, Rt *Croatia* 41 D10
Kamenka = Kaminka
   Ukraine 33 H7
Kamenka *Kazakhstan* 34 E10
Kamenka *Penza, Russia* 34 D6
Kamenka *Voronezh, Russia* 33 G10
Kamenka Bugskaya =
   Kamyanka-Buzka
   Ukraine 23 C13
Kamenka Dneprovskaya =
   Kamyanka-Dniprovska
   Ukraine 33 J8
Kamennomostskiy *Russia* 35 H5
Kameno *Bulgaria* 45 D11
Kamenolomni *Russia* 35 G5
Kamensk-Shakhtinskiy
   Russia 35 F5
Kamensk Uralskiy *Russia* 52 D7
Kamenskiy *Russia* 34 E7
Kamenskoye *Russia* 53 C17
Kamenyak *Bulgaria* 45 C10
Kamenz *Germany* 24 D10
Kameoka *Japan* 55 G7
Kamet *India* 69 D8
Kamiah *U.S.A.* 108 C5
Kamień Krajeński *Poland* 30 E4
Kamień Pomorski *Poland* 30 E1
Kamienna → *Poland* 31 G8
Kamienna Góra *Poland* 31 H3
Kamieńsk *Poland* 31 G6
Kamieskroon *S. Africa* 88 E2
Kamilukuak L. *Canada* 103 A8
Kamin-Kashyrskyy *Ukraine* 23 C13

Kamina *Dem. Rep. of the Congo* 87 D2
Kaminak L. *Canada* 103 A10
Kaministiquia *Canada* 104 C1
Kaminka *Ukraine* 33 H7
Kaminoyama *Japan* 54 E10
Kamiros *Greece* 49 C9
Kamituga
   Dem. Rep. of the Congo 86 C2
Kamla → *India* 69 G12
Kamloops *Canada* 102 C4
Kamnik *Slovenia* 41 B11
Kamo *Armenia* 35 K7
Kamo *Japan* 54 F9
Kamoke *Pakistan* 68 C6
Kamp → *Austria* 26 C8
Kampala *Uganda* 86 B3
Kampar *Malaysia* 65 K3
Kampar → *Indonesia* 62 D2
Kampen *Neths.* 17 B5
Kampene
   Dem. Rep. of the Congo 84 E5
Kamphaeng Phet *Thailand* 64 D2
Kampinoski △ *Poland* 31 F7
Kampolombo, L. *Zambia* 87 E2
Kampong Chhnang *Cambodia* 65 F5
Kampong Pengerang
   Malaysia 65 d
Kampong Punggai *Malaysia* 65 d
Kampong Saom *Cambodia* 65 G4
Kampong Saom, Chaak
   Cambodia 65 G4
Kampong Tanjong Langsat
   Malaysia 65 d
Kampong Telok Ramunia
   Malaysia 65 d
Kampot *Cambodia* 65 G5
Kampti *Burkina Faso* 82 C4
Kampuchea = Cambodia ■
   Asia 64 F5
Kampung Air Putih *Malaysia* 65 K4
Kampung Jerangau *Malaysia* 65 K4
Kampung Raja *Malaysia* 65 K4
Kampungbaru = Tolitoli
   Indonesia 63 D6
Kamrau, Teluk *Indonesia* 63 E8
Kamsack *Canada* 103 C8
Kamsar *Guinea* 82 C2
Kamskoye Ustye *Russia* 34 C9
Kamuchawie L. *Canada* 103 B8
Kamui-Misaki *Japan* 54 C10
Kamyanets-Podilskyy
   Ukraine 29 B11
Kamyanka-Buzka *Ukraine* 23 C13
Kamyanka-Dniprovska
   Ukraine 33 J8
Kamyanka *Belarus* 31 F10
Kamyanyets *Belarus* 31 F10
Kamyanyuki *Belarus* 31 F10
Kämyārān *Iran* 73 E12
Kamyshin *Russia* 34 E7
Kamyzyak *Russia* 35 G9
Kan *Sudan* 81 F3
Kanaaupscow → *Canada* 104 B4
Kanab *U.S.A.* 109 H7
Kanab Cr. → *U.S.A.* 109 H7
Kanacea *Lau Group, Fiji* 91 a
Kanacea *Taveuni, Fiji* 91 a
Kanaga I. *U.S.A.* 106 E4
Kanagi *Japan* 54 D10
Kanairiktok → *Canada* 105 A7
Kanalia *Greece* 46 B4
Kananga
   Dem. Rep. of the Congo 84 F4
Kanash *Russia* 34 C8
Kanaskat *U.S.A.* 110 C5
Kanastraíon, Ákra =
   Paliouri, Akra *Greece* 44 G7
Kanawha → *U.S.A.* 113 F12
Kanazawa *Japan* 55 F8
Kanchanaburi *Thailand* 64 E2
Kanchenjunga *Nepal* 69 F13
Kanchipuram *India* 66 N11
Kańczuga *Poland* 31 J9
Kandaghat *India* 68 D7
Kandahār *Afghan.* 66 D4
Kandahār □ *Afghan.* 66 D4
Kandalaksha *Russia* 8 C25
Kandangan *Indonesia* 62 E5
Kandanghaur *Indonesia* 63 G13
Kandanos *Greece* 49 D5
Kandava *Latvia* 30 A9
Kandavu = Kadavu *Fiji* 91 a
Kandavu Passage =
   Kadavu Passage *Fiji* 91 a
Kandhkot *Pakistan* 68 E3
Kandhla *India* 68 E7
Kandi *Benin* 83 C5
Kandi *India* 69 H13
Kandiaro *Pakistan* 68 F3
Kandila *Greece* 46 D4
Kandra *Turkey* 72 B4
Kandla *India* 68 H4
Kandos *Australia* 95 E4
Kandreho *Madag.* 89 B8
Kandy *Sri Lanka* 66 R12
Kane *U.S.A.* 114 E6
Kane Basin *Greenland* 101 B18
Kanel *Senegal* 82 B2
Kanevskaya *Russia* 35 G4
Kanfanar *Croatia* 41 C10

Kang *Botswana* 88 C3
Kang Krung △ *Thailand* 65 H2
Kangaba *Mali* 82 C3
Kangal *Turkey* 72 C7
Kangān *Fārs, Iran* 71 E7
Kangān *Hormozgān, Iran* 71 E8
Kangar *Malaysia* 65 J3
Kangaré *Mali* 82 C3
Kangaroo I. *Australia* 95 F2
Kangaroo Mts. *Australia* 94 C3
Kangasala *Finland* 32 B3
Kangāvar *Iran* 73 E12
Kangding *China* 58 B3
Kangdong *N. Korea* 57 E14
Kangean, Kepulauan
   Indonesia 62 F5
Kangean Is. = Kangean,
   Kepulauan *Indonesia* 62 F5
Kangen → *Sudan* 81 F3
Kanggye *N. Korea* 57 D14
Kangikajik *Greenland* 4 B6
Kangiqliniq = Rankin Inlet
   Canada 100 E13
Kangiqsualujjuaq *Canada* 101 F18
Kangiqsujuaq *Canada* 101 E17
Kangiqtugaapik = Clyde
   River *Canada* 101 C18
Kangirsuk *Canada* 101 F18
Kangkar Chemaran *Malaysia* 65 d
Kangkar Sungai Tiram
   Malaysia 65 d
Kangkar Teberau *Malaysia* 65 d
Kangping *China* 57 C12
Kangra *India* 68 C7
Kangrinboqe Feng *China* 69 D9
Kangto *China* 67 F18
Kanha △ *India* 69 H9
Kanhar → *India* 69 G10
Kani *Ivory C.* 82 D3
Kaniama
   Dem. Rep. of the Congo 86 D1
Kaniapiskau =
   Caniapiscau → *Canada* 105 A6
Kaniapiskau, L. =
   Caniapiscau, L. *Canada* 105 B6
Kanin, Poluostrov *Russia* 6 B14
Kanin Nos, Mys *Russia* 52 C6
Kanin Pen. = Kanin,
   Poluostrov *Russia* 6 B14
Kaninë *Albania* 44 F3
Kaniva *Australia* 95 F3
Kanjiža *Serbia* 28 D5
Kankaanpää *Finland* 32 B2
Kankakee *U.S.A.* 112 E2
Kankakee → *U.S.A.* 112 E9
Kankan *Guinea* 82 C3
Kankendy = Xankändi
   Azerbaijan 73 C12
Kanker *India* 67 J12
Kankossa *Mauritania* 82 B2
Kankroli *India* 68 G5
Kannapolis *U.S.A.* 117 D14
Kannauj *India* 69 F8
Kannod *India* 66 H10
Kannur = Cannanore *India* 66 P9
Kannyakumari *India* 66 Q10
Kano *Nigeria* 83 C6
Kano □ *Nigeria* 83 C6
Kan'onji *Japan* 55 G6
Kanoroba *Ivory C.* 82 D3
Kanowit *Malaysia* 62 D4
Kanoya *Japan* 55 J5
Kanpetlet *Burma* 67 J18
Kanpur *India* 69 F9
Kansas □ *U.S.A.* 112 F4
Kansas → *U.S.A.* 112 F6
Kansas City *Kans., U.S.A.* 112 F6
Kansas City *Mo., U.S.A.* 112 F6
Kansenia
   Dem. Rep. of the Congo 87 E2
Kansk *Russia* 53 D10
Kansu = Gansu □ *China* 56 G3
Kantaphor *India* 68 H7
Kantchari *Burkina Faso* 83 C5
Kantché *Niger* 83 C6
Kanté *Togo* 83 D5
Kantemirovka *Russia* 33 H10
Kantharalak *Thailand* 64 E5
Kanthi = Contai *India* 69 J12
Kantli → *India* 68 E6
Kantō □ *Japan* 55 F9
Kantō-Sanchi *Japan* 55 G9
Kanturk *Ireland* 12 D3
Kanuma *Japan* 55 F9
Kanus *Namibia* 88 D2
Kanye *Botswana* 88 C4
Kanzenze
   Dem. Rep. of the Congo 87 E2
Kanzi, Ras *Tanzania* 86 D4
Kao *Tonga* 91 c
Kao Phara *Thailand* 65 a
Kaohsiung *Taiwan* 59 F13
Kaokoveld *Namibia* 88 B1
Kaolack *Senegal* 82 C1
Kaolack □ *Senegal* 82 C1
Kaoshan *China* 57 B13
Kapa'a *U.S.A.* 107 L8
Kapadvanj *India* 68 H5

Kapakli *Turkey* 45 E11
Kapan *Armenia* 73 C12
Kapanga
   Dem. Rep. of the Congo 84 F4
Kapchagai = Qapshaghay
   Kazakhstan 52 E8
Kapedo *Kenya* 86 B4
Kapela = Velika Kapela
   Croatia 41 C12
Kapelo, Akra *Greece* 46 E5
Kapema *Dem. Rep. of the Congo* 87 E2
Kapenguria *Kenya* 86 B4
Kapfenberg *Austria* 26 D8
Kapı Dağı *Turkey* 45 F11
Kapiri Mposhi *Zambia* 87 E2
Kāpīsā □ *Afghan.* 66 B6
Kapiskau → *Canada* 104 B3
Kapit *Malaysia* 62 D4
Kapiti I. *N.Z.* 91 D5
Kaplan *U.S.A.* 116 F4
Kaplice *Czech Rep.* 26 C7
Kapoe *Thailand* 65 H2
Kapoeta *Sudan* 81 G3
Kápolnásnyék *Hungary* 28 C3
Kapos → *Hungary* 28 D3
Kaposvár *Hungary* 28 D2
Kapowsin *U.S.A.* 110 D4
Kappeln *Germany* 24 A5
Kappelshamn *Sweden* 11 G12
Kapps *Namibia* 88 C2
Kaprije *Croatia* 41 E12
Kapsabet *Kenya* 86 B4
Kapsan *N. Korea* 57 D15
Kapsukas = Marijampolė
   Lithuania 30 D10
Kaptai L. *Bangla.* 67 H18
Kapuas → *Indonesia* 62 E3
Kapuas Hulu, Pegunungan
   Malaysia 62 D4
Kapuas Hulu Ra. = Kapuas
   Hulu, Pegunungan
   Malaysia 62 D4
Kapulo *Dem. Rep. of the Congo* 87 D2
Kapunda *Australia* 95 E2
Kapuni *N.Z.* 91 C5
Kapurthala *India* 68 D6
Kapuskasing *Canada* 104 C3
Kapuskasing → *Canada* 104 C3
Kapustin Yar *Russia* 35 F7
Kaputar, Mt. *Australia* 95 E5
Kapuvár *Hungary* 28 C2
Kara *Russia* 52 C7
Kara, W. → *Si. Arabia* 80 C5
Kara Ada *Turkey* 47 E9
Kara Bogaz Gol, Zaliv =
   Garabogazköl Aylagy
   Turkmenistan 52 E6
Kara Burun *Turkey* 47 E9
Kara-Kala = Garrygala
   Turkmenistan 71 B8
Kara Kalpak Republic =
   Qoraqalpoghistan □
   Uzbekistan 52 E6
Kara Kum = Garagum
   Turkmenistan 71 B8
Kara Sea *Russia* 52 B8
Kara Kum = Garagum
   Turkmenistan 71 B8
Karaadilli *Turkey* 47 C12
Karabiğa *Turkey* 45 F11
Karabük *Turkey* 72 B5
Karabük □ *Turkey* 72 B5
Karaburun *Albania* 44 F3
Karaburun *Turkey* 47 C8
Karabutak = Qarabutaq
   Kazakhstan 52 E7
Karacabey *Turkey* 45 F12
Karacakılavuz *Turkey* 45 E11
Karacaköy *Turkey* 45 E12
Karacasu *Turkey* 47 D10
Karachala = Qaraçala
   Azerbaijan 35 L9
Karachayevsk *Russia* 35 J5
Karachev *Russia* 33 F8
Karachey-Cherkessia □
   Russia 35 J5
Karachi *Pakistan* 68 G2
Karad *India* 66 L9
Karadirek *Turkey* 47 C12
Karaga *Ghana* 83 D4
Karaganda = Qaraghandy
   Kazakhstan 52 E8
Karagayly = Qaraghayly
   Kazakhstan 52 E8
Karaginskiy, Ostrov *Russia* 53 D17
Karagola Road *India* 69 G12
Karagüney Dağları *Turkey* 72 B6
Karahallı *Turkey* 47 C12
Karaikal *India* 66 P11
Karaikkudi *India* 66 P11
Karaisali *Turkey* 72 D6
Karaj *Iran* 71 C6
Karajarri ◎ *Australia* 92 C3
Karak *Malaysia* 65 L4
Karakalpakstan =
   Qoraqalpoghistan □
   Uzbekistan 52 E6
Karakaya Barajı *Turkey* 73 C8
Karakelong *Indonesia* 63 D7
Karakitang *Indonesia* 63 D7

Karakoçan *Turkey* **73** C9
Karakol *Kyrgyzstan* **52** E8
Karakoram Pass *Asia* **69** B7
Karakoram Ra. *Pakistan* **69** B7
Karakurt *Turkey* **73** B10
Karakuwisa *Namibia* **88** B2
Karalon *Russia* **53** D12
Karama *Jordan* **74** D4
Karaman *Balıkesir, Turkey* **47** B9
Karaman *Konya, Turkey* **72** D5
Karamanlı *Turkey* **47** D11
Karamay *China* **60** B3
Karambu *Indonesia* **62** E5
Karamea Bight *N.Z.* **91** D3
Karamnasa → *India* **69** G10
Karamürsel *Turkey* **45** F13
Karān *Si. Arabia* **71** E6
Karand *Iran* **73** E12
Karangana *Mali* **82** C3
Karanganyar *Indonesia* **63** G13
Karangasem *Indonesia* **63** J18
Karanjia *India* **69** J11
Karankasso *Burkina Faso* **82** C4
Karaova *Turkey* **47** D9
Karapınar *Turkey* **72** D5
Karasburg *Namibia* **88** D2
Karasino *Russia* **52** C9
Karasjok *Norway* **8** B21
Karasu *Turkey* **45** F13
Karasu → *Turkey* **47** E12
Karasuk *Russia* **52** D8
Karasuyama *Japan* **55** F10
Karataş *Adana, Turkey* **72** D6
Karataş *Manisa, Turkey* **47** C10
Karataş Burnu *Turkey* **72** D6
Karatau, Khrebet =
  Qarataū *Kazakhstan* **52** E7
Karatoprak *Turkey* **47** D9
Karatsu *Japan* **55** H5
Karaul *Russia* **52** B9
Karauli *India* **68** F7
Karavastasë, L. e *Albania* **44** F3
Karavia *Greece* **46** E5
Karavostasi *Cyprus* **49** D11
Karawang *Indonesia* **63** G12
Karawanken *Europe* **26** E7
Karayazı *Turkey* **73** C10
Karazhal = Qarazhal
  Kazakhstan **52** E8
Karbalā *Iraq* **73** F11
Karbalā □ *Iraq* **73** F10
Kårböle *Sweden* **10** C9
Karcag *Hungary* **28** C5
Karcha → *Pakistan* **69** B7
Karchana *India* **69** G9
Karczew *Poland* **31** F8
Kardam *Bulgaria* **45** C12
Kardamila *Greece* **47** C8
Kardamili *Greece* **46** E4
Kardeljevo = Ploče *Croatia* **41** E14
Karditsa *Greece* **46** B3
Karditsa □ *Greece* **46** B3
Kärdla *Estonia* **32** C2
Kareeberge *S. Africa* **88** E3
Kareha → *India* **69** G12
Karelia □ *Russia* **8** D25
Karelian Republic =
  Karelia □ *Russia* **8** D25
Karera *India* **68** G8
Kärevändar *Iran* **71** E9
Kargasok *Russia* **52** D9
Kargat *Russia* **52** D9
Kargi *Kenya* **86** B4
Kargı *Turkey* **72** B6
Kargil *India* **69** B7
Kargopol *Russia* **32** B10
Kargowa *Poland* **31** F2
Karguéri *Niger* **83** C7
Karhal *India* **69** F8
Karia *Greece* **46** C2
Kariān *Iran* **71** E8
Karianga *Madag.* **89** C8
Kariba *Zimbabwe* **87** F2
Kariba, L. *Zimbabwe* **87** F2
Kariba Dam *Zimbabwe* **87** F2
Kariba Gorge *Zambia* **87** F2
Karibib *Namibia* **88** C2
Karies *Greece* **45** F8
Karijini △ *Australia* **92** D2
Karimata, Kepulauan
  Indonesia **62** E3
Karimata, Selat *Indonesia* **62** E3
Karimata Is. = Karimata,
  Kepulauan *Indonesia* **62** E3
Karimnagar *India* **66** K11
Karimun Kecil, Pulau
  Indonesia **65** d
Karimunjawa, Kepulauan
  Indonesia **62** F4
Karin *Somali Rep.* **75** E4
Karīt *Iran* **71** C8
Kariya *Japan* **55** G8
Kariyangwe *Zimbabwe* **89** B4
Karjala *Finland* **32** A5
Karkaralinsk = Qarqaraly
  Kazakhstan **52** E8
Karkheh → *Iran* **70** D5

Karkinitska Zatoka
  Ukraine **33** K7
Karkinitskiy Zaliv =
  Karkinitska Zatoka
  Ukraine **33** K7
Karkuk = Kirkūk *Iraq* **73** E11
Karkur Tohl *Egypt* **80** C2
Karl Liebknecht *Russia* **53** G8
Karla, L. = Volvi, L. *Greece* **44** F7
Karlantijpa North ✪
  Australia **92** C5
Karlantijpa South ✪
  Australia **92** D5
Karleby = Kokkola *Finland* **8** E20
Karlino *Poland* **30** D2
Karlova *Turkey* **73** C9
Karlovac *Croatia* **41** C12
Karlovarský □ *Czech Rep.* **26** A5
Karlovasi *Greece* **47** D8
Karlovka = Karlivka *Ukraine* **33** H8
Karlovo *Bulgaria* **45** D8
Karlovy Vary *Czech Rep.* **26** A5
Karlsbad = Karlovy Vary
  Czech Rep. **26** A5
Karlsborg *Sweden* **11** F8
Karlsena, Mys *Russia* **52** B7
Karlshamn *Sweden* **11** H8
Karlskoga *Sweden* **10** E8
Karlskrona *Sweden* **11** H9
Karlsruhe *Germany* **25** F4
Karlstad *Sweden* **10** E7
Karlstad *U.S.A.* **112** A5
Karlstadt *Germany* **25** F5
Karma *Niger* **83** C5
Karmélava *Lithuania* **30** D11
Karmi'el *Israel* **74** C4
Karnak *Egypt* **80** B3
Karnal *India* **68** E7
Karnali → *Nepal* **69** E9
Karnaphuli Res. = Kaptai
  L. *Bangla.* **67** H18
Karnaprayag *India* **69** D8
Karnataka □ *India* **66** N10
Karnes City *U.S.A.* **116** G6
Karnische Alpen *Europe* **26** E6
Kärnten □ *Austria* **26** E6
Karo *Mali* **82** C4
Karoi *Zimbabwe* **87** F2
Karon, Ao *Thailand* **65** c
Karonga *Malawi* **87** D3
Karoo △ *S. Africa* **88** E3
Karoonda *Australia* **95** F2
Karor *Pakistan* **68** D4
Karora *Sudan* **80** D4
Karounga *Mali* **82** B3
Karousades *Greece* **46** B1
Karpacz *Poland* **31** H2
Karpasia *Cyprus* **49** D13
Karpathos *Greece* **47** F9
Karpathos, Stenon *Greece* **47** F9
Karpatsky △ *Ukraine* **29** B9
Karpenisi *Greece* **46** C3
Karpuzlu *Turkey* **47** D9
Karpuz Burnu = Apostolos
  Andreas, C. *Cyprus* **49** D13
Karratha *Australia* **92** D2
Kars *Turkey* **73** B10
Kars □ *Turkey* **73** B10
Karsakpay *Kazakhstan* **52** E7
Karsha = Qarshi *Uzbekistan* **52** F7
Karshi = Qarshi *Uzbekistan* **52** F7
Karsiyang *India* **69** F13
Karsog *India* **68** D7
Karst = Kras *Croatia* **41** C10
Kartal *Turkey* **45** F13
Kartala *Comoros Is.* **85** a
Kartaly *Russia* **52** D7
Kartapur *India* **68** D6
Karthaus *U.S.A.* **114** E6
Kartuzy *Poland* **30** D5
Karufa *Indonesia* **63** E8
Karuma △ *Uganda* **86** B3
Karumba *Australia* **94** B3
Karumo *Tanzania* **86** C3
Karumwa *Tanzania* **86** C3
Kārūn → *Iran* **71** D6
Karungu *Kenya* **86** C3
Karup *Denmark* **11** H3
Karviná *Czech Rep.* **27** B11
Karwan → *India* **68** F8
Karwar *India* **66** M9
Karwendel △ *Austria* **26** D4
Karwi *India* **69** G9
Karymskoye *Russia* **53** D12
Kaş *Turkey* **47** E11
Kasaba *Turkey* **47** E11
Kasache *Malawi* **87** E3
Kasai →
  Dem. Rep. of the Congo **84** E3
Kasai-Oriental □
  Dem. Rep. of the Congo **86** D1
Kasaji *Dem. Rep. of the Congo* **87** E1
Kasama *Zambia* **87** E3
Kasan *N. Korea* **57** D14
Kasandra *Greece* **44** F7
Kasandra Kolpos *Greece* **44** F7

Kasandras, Akra *Greece* **44** G7
Kasane *Namibia* **88** B3
Kasanga *Tanzania* **87** D3
Kasanka △ *Zambia* **87** E3
Kasar, Ras *Sudan* **80** D4
Kasaragod *India* **66** N9
Kasba L. *Canada* **103** A8
Kāseh Garān *Iran* **70** C5
Kasempa *Zambia* **87** E2
Kasenga
  Dem. Rep. of the Congo **87** E2
Kasese *Uganda* **86** B3
Kasewa *Zambia* **87** E2
Kasganj *India* **69** F8
Kashabowie *Canada* **104** C1
Kashaf → *Iran* **71** C9
Kashan → *Iran* **73** F12
Kāshān *Iran* **71** C6
Kashechewan *Canada* **104** B3
Kashgar = Kashi *China* **60** C2
Kashi *China* **60** C2
Kashimbo
  Dem. Rep. of the Congo **87** E2
Kashin *Russia* **32** D9
Kashipur *India* **69** E8
Kashira *Russia* **32** E10
Kashiwazaki *Japan* **55** F9
Kashk-e Kohneh *Afghan.* **66** B3
Kashksaray *Iran* **73** C11
Kashkū'īyeh *Iran* **71** D7
Kāshmar *Iran* **71** C8
Kashmir *Asia* **69** C7
Kashmor *Pakistan* **68** E3
Kashpirovka *Russia* **34** D9
Kashun Noerh = Gaxun
  Nur *China* **60** B5
Kasiari *India* **69** H12
Kasimov *Russia* **34** C5
Kasinge *Dem. Rep. of the Congo* **86** D2
Kasiruta *Indonesia* **63** E7
Kaskaskia → *U.S.A.* **112** G9
Kaskattama → *Canada* **103** B10
Kaskinen *Finland* **8** E19
Kaskö = Kaskinen *Finland* **8** E19
Kaslo *Canada* **102** D5
Kasmere L. *Canada* **103** B8
Kasongo
  Dem. Rep. of the Congo **86** C2
Kasongo Lunda
  Dem. Rep. of the Congo **84** F3
Kasos *Greece* **47** F8
Kasos, Stenon *Greece* **47** F8
Kaspi *Georgia* **35** K7
Kaspichan *Bulgaria* **45** C11
Kaspiysk *Russia* **35** J8
Kaspiyskiy *Russia* **35** H8
Kassab ed Doleib *Sudan* **81** E3
Kassaba *Egypt* **80** C2
Kassalâ *Sudan* **81** D4
Kassalâ □ *Sudan* **81** D4
Kassandrino *Greece* **44** F7
Kassel *Germany* **24** D5
Kassinger *Sudan* **80** D3
Kassiopi *Greece* **49** A3
Kasson *U.S.A.* **112** C7
Kastamonu *Turkey* **72** B5
Kastamonu □ *Turkey* **72** B5
Kastav *Croatia* **41** C11
Kasteli *Greece* **49** D5
Kastelli *Greece* **49** D7
Kastellórizon = Megisti
  Greece **47** E11
Kastelo, Akra *Greece* **47** F9
Kasterlee *Belgium* **17** C4
Kastlösa *Sweden* **11** H10
Kastoria *Greece* **44** F5
Kastoria □ *Greece* **44** F5
Kastorias, L. *Greece* **44** F5
Kastornoye *Russia* **33** G10
Kastos *Greece* **46** C2
Kastrosikia *Greece* **46** B2
Kastrup, København ✈
  (CPH) *Denmark* **11** J6
Kastsyukovichy *Belarus* **32** F7
Kasulu *Tanzania* **86** C3
Kasumi *Japan* **55** G7
Kasumkent *Russia* **35** K9
Kasungu *Malawi* **87** E3
Kasungu △ *Malawi* **87** E3
Kasur *Pakistan* **68** D6
Kata, Ao *Thailand* **65** J2
Kata Archanes *Greece* **49** D7
Kata Tjuta *Australia* **93** E5
Kataba *Zambia* **87** F2
Katagum *Nigeria* **83** C7
Katahdin, Mt. *U.S.A.* **113** C19
Kataka = Cuttack *India* **67** J14
Katako Kombe
  Dem. Rep. of the Congo **86** C1
Katakolo *Greece* **46** D3
Katale *Tanzania* **86** C3
Katanda *Katanga,*
  Dem. Rep. of the Congo **86** D1
Katanda *Nord-Kivu,*
  Dem. Rep. of the Congo **86** C2
Katanga □
  Dem. Rep. of the Congo **86** D2
Katangi *India* **69** J11

Katanning *Australia* **93** F2
Katastari *Greece* **46** D2
Katavi △ *Tanzania* **86** D3
Katavi Swamp *Tanzania* **86** D3
Katerini *Greece* **44** F6
Katghora *India* **69** H10
Katha *Burma* **67** G20
Katherîna, Gebel *Egypt* **70** D2
Katherine *Australia* **92** B5
Katherine Gorge =
  Nitmiluk △ *Australia* **92** B5
Kathi *India* **68** J6
Kathiawar *India* **68** H4
Kathikas *Cyprus* **49** E11
Kathmandu *Nepal* **69** F11
Kathua *India* **68** C6
Kati *Mali* **82** C3
Katihar *India* **69** G12
Katima Mulilo *Namibia* **88** B3
Katimbira *Malawi* **87** E3
Katingan = Mendawai →
  Indonesia **62** E4
Katiola *Ivory C.* **82** D3
Katiti ✪ *Australia* **93** E5
Katlabukh, Ozero *Ukraine* **29** E14
Katlanovo *Macedonia* **44** E5
Katmandu = Kathmandu
  Nepal **69** F11
Katni = Murwara *India* **69** H9
Katni *India* **69** H9
Kato Achaia *Greece* **46** C3
Kato Chorio *Greece* **49** D7
Kato Korakiana *Greece* **49** A3
Káto Pyrgos *Cyprus* **49** D11
Katochi *Greece* **46** C3
Katompe
  Dem. Rep. of the Congo **86** D2
Katong *Singapore* **65** d
Katonga → *Uganda* **86** B3
Katoomba *Australia* **95** E5
Katouna *Greece* **46** C2
Katowice *Poland* **31** H6
Katrancı Dağı *Turkey* **47** D12
Katrine, L. *U.K.* **13** E4
Katrineholm *Sweden* **10** E10
Katsepe *Madag.* **89** B8
Katsina □ *Nigeria* **83** C6
Katsina *Nigeria* **83** C6
Katsina Ala *Nigeria* **83** D6
Katsina Ala → *Nigeria* **83** D6
Katsumoto *Japan* **55** H4
Katsuura *Japan* **55** G10
Katsuyama *Japan* **55** F8
Kattavia *Greece* **49** D9
Kattegat *Denmark* **11** H5
Katthammarsvik *Sweden* **11** G12
Katul, J. *Sudan* **81** E2
Katumba
  Dem. Rep. of the Congo **86** D2
Katwa *India* **69** H13
Katwijk *Neths.* **17** B4
Kąty Wrocławskie *Poland* **31** G3
Kaua'i *U.S.A.* **107** L8
Kaub *Germany* **25** E3
Kaudom △ *Namibia* **88** B3
Kaufbeuren *Germany* **25** H6
Kaufman *U.S.A.* **116** E6
Kauhajoki *Finland* **8** E20
Kaukauna *U.S.A.* **112** C9
Kaukauveld *Namibia* **88** C3
Ka'ula I. *U.S.A.* **107** L7
Kaunas *Lithuania* **30** D10
Kaunas (KUN) ✈ *Lithuania* **30** D11
Kaunia *Bangla.* **69** G13
Kaunos *Turkey* **47** E10
Kaura Namoda *Nigeria* **83** C6
Kauru *Nigeria* **83** C6
Kautokeino *Norway* **8** B20
Kauwapur *India* **69** D8
Kavacha *Russia* **53** C17
Kavadarci *Macedonia* **44** E6
Kavajë *Albania* **44** E3
Kavak *Turkey* **72** B7
Kavak Dağı *Turkey* **47** D10
Kavaklı *Turkey* **47** D10
Kavaklıdere *Turkey* **47** D10
Kavala *Greece* **45** F8
Kavala □ *Greece* **45** F8
Kavala Kolpos *Greece* **45** F8
Kavalerovo *Russia* **54** B7
Kavali *India* **69** M12
Kavār *Iran* **71** D7
Kavarna *Bulgaria* **45** C12
Kavi *India* **68** H5
Kavimba *Botswana* **88** B3
Kavīr, Dasht-e *Iran* **71** C7
Kavīr △ *Iran* **71** C7
Kavkaz *Russia* **33** K9
Kävlinge *Sweden* **11** J7
Kavos *Greece* **49** B4
Kavousi *Greece* **47** F7
Kaw *Fr. Guiana* **125** C8
Kawa *Sudan* **81** E3
Kawagama L. *Canada* **114** A6
Kawagoe *Japan* **55** G9
Kawaguchi *Japan* **55** G9
Kawambwa *Zambia* **87** D2
Kawanoe *Japan* **55** G6
Kawardha *India* **69** J9

Kawasaki *Japan* **55** G9
Kawasi *Indonesia* **63** E7
Kawawachikamach *Canada* **105** B6
Kawerau *N.Z.* **91** C6
Kawhia *N.Z.* **91** C5
Kawhia Harbour *N.Z.* **91** C5
Kawio, Kepulauan *Indonesia* **63** D7
Kawthaung *Burma* **65** H2
Kawthoolei = Kayin □
  Burma **67** L20
Kawthule = Kayin □
  Burma **67** L20
Kaxholmen *Sweden* **11** G8
Kaya *Burkina Faso* **83** C4
Kayah □ *Burma* **67** K20
Kayak I. *U.S.A.* **100** D11
Kayalıköy Barajı *Turkey* **45** E11
Kayan → *Indonesia* **62** D5
Kaycee *U.S.A.* **108** E10
Kayeli *Indonesia* **63** E7
Kayenta *U.S.A.* **109** H8
Kayes *Mali* **82** C2
Kayes □ *Mali* **82** C2
Kayı *Turkey* **47** B12
Kayima *S. Leone* **82** D2
Kayin □ *Burma* **67** L20
Kayoa *Indonesia* **63** E7
Kayomba *Zambia* **87** E1
Kaysatskoye *Russia* **34** F8
Kayseri *Turkey* **72** C6
Kayseri □ *Turkey* **72** C7
Kaysville *U.S.A.* **108** F8
Kaz Dağı *Turkey* **47** B9
Kazachye *Russia* **53** B14
Kazakhstan ■ *Asia* **52** E8
Kazan *Russia* **34** C9
Kazan → *Canada* **103** A9
Kazan-Rettō *Pac. Oc.* **96** E6
Kazanlık *Bulgaria* **45** D9
Kazanskaya *Russia* **34** F5
Kazatin = Kozyatyn *Ukraine* **23** D15
Kazbek *Russia* **35** J7
Kāzerūn *Iran* **71** D6
Kazi Magomed =
  Qazımämmäd *Azerbaijan* **35** K9
Kazimierz Dolny *Poland* **31** G8
Kazimierza Wielka *Poland* **31** H7
Kazincbarcika *Hungary* **28** B5
Kazl Rūda *Lithuania* **30** D10
Kaztalovka *Kazakhstan* **34** F9
Kazuma Pan △ *Zimbabwe* **87** F2
Kazumba
  Dem. Rep. of the Congo **86** D2
Kazuno *Japan* **54** D10
Kazym → *Russia* **52** C7
Kcynia *Poland* **31** F4
Ké-Macina *Mali* **82** C3
Kea *Greece* **46** D6
Keady *U.K.* **12** B5
Kearney *U.S.A.* **112** E4
Kearney ✪ *Australia* **92** D4
Kearny *U.S.A.* **109** K8
Keban *Turkey* **73** C8
Keban Barajı *Turkey* **73** C8
Kebbi □ *Nigeria* **83** C5
Kébémèr *Senegal* **82** B1
Kébi *Ivory C.* **82** D3
Kebnekaise *Sweden* **8** C18
Kebri Dehar *Ethiopia* **75** F3
Kebumen *Indonesia* **63** G13
Kecel *Hungary* **28** D4
Kechika → *Canada* **102** B3
Keçiborlu *Turkey* **47** D12
Kecskemét *Hungary* **28** D4
Kedada *Ethiopia* **81** F4
Kedgwick *Canada* **105** C6
Kediri *Indonesia* **62** F4
Kedjebi *Ghana* **83** D5
Kédougou *Senegal* **82** C2
Kedros Oros *Greece* **49** D6
Kędzierzyn-Koźle *Poland* **31** H5
Keeler *U.S.A.* **110** J9
Keeley L. *Canada* **103** C7
Keeling Is. = Cocos Is.
  Ind. Oc. **96** J1
Keelung = Chilung *Taiwan* **59** E13
Keene *Canada* **114** B6
Keene *Calif., U.S.A.* **111** K8
Keene *N.H., U.S.A.* **115** D12
Keene *N.Y., U.S.A.* **115** B11
Keep River △ *Australia* **92** C4
Keeper Hill *Ireland* **12** D3
Keerweer, C. *Australia* **94** A3
Keeshmanshoop *Namibia* **88** D2
Keetmanshoop *Namibia* **88** D2
Keewatin *Canada* **103** D10
Keewatin → *Canada* **103** B8
Kefa *Ethiopia* **81** F4
Kefalonia *Greece* **46** C2
Kefalonia □ *Greece* **46** C2
Kefalos *Greece* **47** F8
Kefamenanu *Indonesia* **63** F6
Kefar Sava *Israel* **74** C3
Keffi *Nigeria* **83** D6
Keffin Hausa *Nigeria* **83** C6
Keflavík *Iceland* **8** D2

Keftya *Ethiopia* **81** E4
Keg River *Canada* **102** B5
Kegaska *Canada* **105** B7
Kehancha *Kenya* **86** C3
Keheili *Sudan* **80** D3
Kehl *Germany* **25** G3
Keighley *U.K.* **14** D6
Keila *Estonia* **32** C3
Keimoes *S. Africa* **88** D3
Keita *Niger* **83** C6
Keitele *Finland* **8** E22
Keith *Australia* **95** F3
Keith, C. *Australia* **92** B5
Keiyasi *Fiji* **91** a
Keizer *U.S.A.* **108** D2
Kejimkujik △ *Canada* **105** D6
Kejserr Franz Joseph Fd.
  Greenland **4** B6
Kekri *India* **68** G6
Kelam *Ethiopia* **81** G4
Kelamet *Eritrea* **81** D4
Kelan *China* **56** E6
Kelang = Klang *Malaysia* **65** L3
Kelantan → *Malaysia* **65** J4
Kélcyrë *Albania* **44** F4
Kelekçi *Turkey* **47** D11
Keles *Turkey* **45** G13
Keleti-főcsatorna *Hungary* **28** C6
Kelheim *Germany* **25** G7
Kelkit *Turkey* **73** B8
Kelkit → *Turkey* **72** B7
Kellé *Niger* **83** C7
Kellerberrin *Australia* **93** F2
Kellett, C. *Canada* **4** B1
Kelleys I. *U.S.A.* **114** E2
Kellogg *U.S.A.* **108** C5
Kells = Ceanannus Mor
  Ireland **12** C5
Kelmė *Lithuania* **30** C9
Kelmentsi *Ukraine* **29** B11
Kélo *Chad* **79** G9
Kelokedhara *Cyprus* **49** E11
Kelowna *Canada* **102** D5
Kelsey Creek *Australia* **94** b
Kelseyville *U.S.A.* **110** G4
Kelso *N.Z.* **91** F2
Kelso *U.K.* **13** F6
Kelso *U.S.A.* **110** D4
Keluang = Kluang *Malaysia* **65** L4
Kelvington *Canada* **103** C8
Kem *Russia* **52** C4
Kema *Indonesia* **63** D7
Kemah *Turkey* **73** C8
Kemaliye *Erzincan, Turkey* **73** C8
Kemaliye *Manisa, Turkey* **47** C10
Kemalpaşa *Turkey* **47** C9
Kemaman *Malaysia* **65** K4
Kemano *Canada* **102** C3
Kemasik *Malaysia* **65** K4
Kembolcha *Ethiopia* **81** E4
Kemer *Antalya, Turkey* **47** E12
Kemer *Burdur, Turkey* **47** D12
Kemer *Muğla, Turkey* **47** E11
Kemer Barajı *Turkey* **47** D10
Kemerovo *Russia* **52** D9
Kemeru △ *Latvia* **30** B10
Kemi *Finland* **8** D21
Kemi älv = Kemijoki →
  Finland **8** D21
Kemi träsk = Kemijärvi
  Finland **8** C22
Kemijärvi *Finland* **8** C22
Kemijoki → *Finland* **8** D21
Kemmerer *U.S.A.* **108** F8
Kemmuna = Comino *Malta* **49** C1
Kemp, L. *U.S.A.* **116** E5
Kemp Land *Antarctica* **5** C5
Kempas *Malaysia* **65** d
Kempsey *Australia* **95** E5
Kempt, L. *Canada* **104** C5
Kempten *Germany* **25** H6
Kempton *Australia* **95** G4
Kemptville *Canada* **115** B9
Ken → *India* **69** G9
Kenai *U.S.A.* **100** E1
Kenai Mts. *U.S.A.* **106** D9
Kenamuke Swamp *Sudan* **81** F3
Kendai *India* **69** H10
Kendal *Indonesia* **63** G14
Kendal *U.K.* **14** C5
Kendall *Australia* **95** E5
Kendall *U.S.A.* **117** J14
Kendall → *Australia* **94** A3
Kendallville *U.S.A.* **113** E11
Kendari *Indonesia* **63** E6
Kendawangan *Indonesia* **62** E4
Kende *Nigeria* **83** C5
Kendi, Pulau *Malaysia* **65** c
Kendrapara *India* **67** J15
Këndrevicës, Maja e *Albania* **44** F3
Kendrew *S. Africa* **88** E3
Kene Thao *Laos* **64** D3
Kenedy *U.S.A.* **116** G6
Kenema *S. Leone* **82** D2
Keng Kok *Laos* **64** D5
Keng Tawng *Burma* **67** J21
Keng Tung *Burma* **58** G2
Kengeja *Tanzania* **86** D4
Kenhardt *S. Africa* **88** D3

Kéniéba *Mali* **82** C2
Kenitra *Morocco* **78** B4
Kenli *China* **57** F10
Kenmare *Ireland* **12** E2
Kenmare *U.S.A.* **112** A2
Kenmare River *Ireland* **12** E2
Kennebago Lake *U.S.A.* **115** A14
Kennebec *U.S.A.* **112** D4
Kennebec → *U.S.A.* **113** D19
Kennebunk *U.S.A.* **115** C14
Kennedy *Zimbabwe* **88** B4
Kennedy Kanal *Arctic* **101** A18
Kennedy Ra. *Australia* **93** D2
Kennedy Range △ *Australia* **93** D2
Kenner *U.S.A.* **117** G9
Kennet → *U.K.* **15** F7
Kenneth Ra. *Australia* **93** D2
Kennett *U.S.A.* **112** G8
Kennewick *U.S.A.* **108** C4
Kennisis Lake *Canada* **114** A6
Kenogami → *Canada* **104** B3
Kenora *Canada* **103** D10
Kenosha *U.S.A.* **112** D10
Kensington *Canada* **105** C7
Kent *Ohio, U.S.A.* **114** E3
Kent *Tex., U.S.A.* **116** F2
Kent *Wash., U.S.A.* **110** C4
Kent □ *U.K.* **15** F8
Kent Group *Australia* **95** F4
Kent Pen. *Canada* **100** D10
Kentaū *Kazakhstan* **52** E7
Kentland *U.S.A.* **112** E10
Kenton *U.S.A.* **113** E12
Kentucky □ *U.S.A.* **113** G11
Kentucky → *U.S.A.* **113** F11
Kentucky L. *U.S.A.* **112** G9
Kentville *Canada* **105** C7
Kentwood *U.S.A.* **117** F9
Kenya ■ *Africa* **86** B4
Kenya, Mt. *Kenya* **86** C4
Kenyir, Tasik *Malaysia* **65** K4
Keo Neua, Deo *Vietnam* **64** C5
Keokuk *U.S.A.* **112** E8
Keoladeo △ *India* **68** F7
Keonjhargarh *India* **69** J11
Kep *Cambodia* **65** G5
Kep *Vietnam* **64** B6
Kepala Batas *Malaysia* **65** c
Kepez *Turkey* **45** F10
Kepi *Indonesia* **63** F9
Kępice *Poland* **30** D3
Kępno *Poland* **31** G4
Kepsut *Turkey* **47** B10
Kerala □ *India* **66** P10
Kerama-Rettō *Japan* **55** L3
Keran *Pakistan* **69** B5
Keran △ *Togo* **83** C5
Kerang *Australia* **95** F3
Keranyo *Ethiopia* **81** F4
Kerao → *Sudan* **81** E3
Keratea *Greece* **46** D5
Keraudren, C. *Australia* **92** C2
Kerava *Finland* **32** B3
Kerch *Ukraine* **33** K9
Kerchenskiy Proliv *Black Sea* **33** K9
Kerchoual *Mali* **83** B5
Kerempe Burnu *Turkey* **72** A5
Keren *Eritrea* **81** D4
Kerewan *Gambia* **82** C1
Kerguelen *Ind. Oc.* **3** G13
Keri *Greece* **46** D2
Keri Kera *Sudan* **81** E3
Kericho *Kenya* **86** C4
Kerinci *Indonesia* **62** E2
Kerki = Atamyrat
  Turkmenistan **52** F7
Kerkini, L. *Greece* **44** E7
Kerkouane *Tunisia* **42** F4
Kerkrade *Neths.* **17** D6
Kerkyra *Greece* **49** A3
Kerkyra □ *Greece* **46** B1
Kerkyra ✈ (CFU) *Greece* **46** B1
Kerkyras, Notio Steno *Greece* **49** A4
Kerma *Sudan* **80** D3
Kermadec Is. *Pac. Oc.* **90** E11
Kermadec Trench *Pac. Oc.* **96** L10
Kermān *Iran* **71** D8
Kerman *U.S.A.* **110** J6
Kermān □ *Iran* **71** D8
Kermān, Bīābān-e *Iran* **71** D8
Kermānshāh *Iran* **73** E12
Kermānshāh □ *Iran* **70** C5
Kermen *Bulgaria* **45** D10
Kermit *U.S.A.* **116** F3
Kern → *U.S.A.* **111** K7
Kernhof *Austria* **26** D8
Kernow = Cornwall □ *U.K.* **15** G3
Kernville *U.S.A.* **111** K8
Keroh *Malaysia* **65** K3
Keros *Greece* **47** E7
Kérou *Benin* **83** C5
Kérouane *Guinea* **82** D3
Kerpen *Germany* **24** E2
Kerrera *U.K.* **13** E3
Kerrobert *Canada* **103** C7
Kerrville *U.S.A.* **116** F5
Kerry □ *Ireland* **12** D2
Kerry Hd. *Ireland* **12** D2
Kersa *Ethiopia* **81** F5

Kerulen → *Asia* **60** B6
Kervo = Kerava *Finland* **32** B3
Kerzaz *Algeria* **78** C5
Kesagami *Canada* **104** B3
Kesagami L. *Canada* **104** B3
Keşan *Turkey* **45** F10
Kesennuma *Japan* **54** E10
Keshāvar *Iran* **73** D12
Keshit *Iran* **71** D8
Keşiş Dağ *Turkey* **73** C8
Keskin *Turkey* **72** C5
Kestell *S. Africa* **89** D4
Kestenga *Russia* **8** D24
Keswick *U.K.* **14** C4
Keszthely *Hungary* **28** D2
Ket → *Russia* **52** D9
Keta *Ghana* **83** D5
Keta Lagoon *Ghana* **83** D5
Ketapang *Bali, Indonesia* **63** J17
Ketapang *Kalimantan,
  Indonesia* **62** E4
Ketchenery *Russia* **35** G7
Ketchikan *U.S.A.* **102** B2
Ketchum *U.S.A.* **108** E6
Kete Krachi *Ghana* **83** D4
Ketef, Khalig umm el *Egypt* **70** F2
Keti Bandar *Pakistan* **68** G2
Kétou *Benin* **83** D5
Ketri *India* **68** E6
Kętrzyn *Poland* **30** D8
Kettering *U.K.* **15** E7
Kettering *U.S.A.* **113** F11
Kettle → *Canada* **103** B11
Kettle Falls *U.S.A.* **108** B4
Kettle Point *Canada* **114** C2
Kettle Pt. *Canada* **114** C2
Kettleman City *U.S.A.* **110** J7
Kęty *Poland* **31** J6
Keuka L. *U.S.A.* **114** D7
Keuruu *Finland* **32** A3
Kevelaer *Germany* **24** D2
Kewanee *U.S.A.* **112** E9
Kewaunee *U.S.A.* **112** C10
Keweenaw B. *U.S.A.* **112** B9
Keweenaw Pen. *U.S.A.* **112** B9
Keweenaw Pt. *U.S.A.* **112** B10
Key, L. *Ireland* **12** C3
Key Lake Mine *Canada* **103** B7
Key Largo *U.S.A.* **117** J14
Key West *U.S.A.* **120** B3
Keyala *Sudan* **81** F3
Keynsham *U.K.* **15** F5
Keyser *U.S.A.* **113** F14
Kezhma *Russia* **53** D11
Kezi *Zimbabwe* **89** C4
Kežmarok *Slovak Rep.* **27** B13
Kgalagadi Transfrontier △
  Africa **88** D3
Khabarovsk *Russia* **53** E14
Khabr *Iran* **71** D8
Khābūr → *Syria* **73** E9
Khachmas = Xaçmaz
  Azerbaijan **35** K9
Khachrod *India* **68** H6
Khadari, W. el → *Sudan* **81** E2
Khadro *Pakistan* **68** F3
Khadyzhensk *Russia* **35** H4
Khadzhilyangar =
  Dahongliutan *China* **69** B8
Khaga *India* **69** G9
Khagaria *India* **69** G12
Khaipur *Pakistan* **68** E5
Khair *India* **68** F7
Khairabad *India* **69** F9
Khairagarh *India* **69** J9
Khairpur *Pakistan* **68** F3
Khairpur Nathan Shah
  Pakistan **68** F2
Khairwara *India* **68** H5
Khaisor → *Pakistan* **68** D3
Khajuri Kach *Pakistan* **68** C3
Khakassia □ *Russia* **52** D9
Khakhea *Botswana* **88** C3
Khalafābād *Iran* **71** D6
Khalilabad *India* **69** F10
Khalīlī *Iran* **71** E7
Khalkhāl *Iran* **73** D13
Khalkís = Halkida *Greece* **46** C5
Khalmer Yu *Russia* **52** C7
Khalūf *Oman* **75** C6
Kham Keut *Laos* **64** C5
Khamaria *India* **69** H9
Khambhaliya *India* **68** H3
Khambhat *India* **68** H5
Khambhat, G. of *India* **66** J8
Khamīr *Iran* **71** E7
Khamir *Yemen* **75** D3
Khamis Mushayt *Si. Arabia* **75** D3
Khamsa *Egypt* **74** E1
Khan → *Namibia* **88** C2
Khān Abū Shāmat *Syria* **74** B5
Khān al Baghdādī *Iraq* **73** G10
Khān al Ḥammād *Iraq* **73** G11
Khān Azād *Iraq* **70** C5
Khān Mujiddah *Iraq* **70** C4
Khān Shaykhūn *Syria* **72** E7
Khān Yūnis *Gaza Strip* **74** D3
Khanai *Pakistan* **68** D2
Khānaqīn *Iraq* **73** E11

Khānbāghī *Iran* **71** B7
Khandwa *India* **66** J10
Khandyga *Russia* **53** C14
Khanewal *Pakistan* **68** D5
Khangah Dogran *Pakistan* **68** D5
Khanh Duong *Vietnam* **64** F7
Khaniá = Chania *Greece* **49** D6
Khaniadhana *India* **68** G8
Khanka, L. *Asia* **54** B6
Khankendy = Xankändi
  Azerbaijan **73** C12
Khanna *India* **68** D7
Khanozai *Pakistan* **68** D2
Khanpur *Pakistan* **68** E4
Khanty-Mansiysk *Russia* **52** C7
Khao Laem △ *Thailand* **64** E2
Khao Laem Res. *Thailand* **64** E2
Khao Lak △ *Malaysia* **65** H2
Khao Luang △ *Thailand* **65** H2
Khao Phlu *Thailand* **65** b
Khao Pu-Khao Ya △ *Thailand* **65** J2
Khao Sam Roi Yot △
  Thailand **64** F2
Khao Sok △ *Thailand* **65** H2
Khao Yai △ *Thailand* **64** E3
Khaoen Si Nakarin △
  Thailand **64** E2
Khapalu *Pakistan* **69** B7
Khapcheranga *Russia* **53** E12
Khaptao △ *Nepal* **69** E9
Kharabali *Russia* **35** G8
Kharagauli *Georgia* **35** J6
Kharaghoda *India* **68** H4
Kharagpur *India* **69** H12
Kharan Kalat *Pakistan* **68** E3
Kharānaq *Iran* **71** C7
Kharda *India* **66** K9
Khardung La *India* **69** B7
Kharg = Khārk, Jazīreh-ye
  Iran **71** D6
Kharga, El Wâhât el *Egypt* **80** B3
Khargon *India* **66** J9
Khari → *India* **68** G6
Kharian *Pakistan* **68** C5
Kharit, Wadi el → *Egypt* **80** C3
Khārk, Jazīreh-ye *Iran* **71** D6
Kharkiv *Ukraine* **33** H9
Kharkiv □ *Ukraine* **33** H9
Kharkov = Kharkiv *Ukraine* **33** H9
Kharmanli *Bulgaria* **45** E9
Kharovsk *Russia* **32** C11
Kharsawangarh *India* **69** H11
Kharta *Turkey* **72** B3
Khartoum = El Khartûm
  Sudan **81** D3
Khartum *Canada* **114** A7
Khasan *Russia* **54** C5
Khâsh *Iran* **71** D9
Khashm el Girba *Sudan* **81** E4
Khashum *Sudan* **81** E2
Khashuri *Georgia* **35** J6
Khaskovo *Bulgaria* **45** E9
Khaskovo □ *Bulgaria* **45** E9
Khatanga *Russia* **53** B11
Khatanga → *Russia* **53** B11
Khatauli *India* **68** E7
Khatra *India* **69** H12
Khātūnābād *Iran* **71** D7
Khatyrka *Russia* **53** C18
Khavda *India* **68** H3
Khawr Fakkān *U.A.E.* **71** E8
Khay' *Si. Arabia* **80** D5
Khaybar, Ḥarrat *Si. Arabia* **70** E4
Khāzimiyah *Iraq* **70** C4
Khazzān Jabal al Awliyâ
  Sudan **81** D3
Khe Bo *Vietnam* **64** C5
Khe Long *Vietnam* **64** B5
Khe Sanh *Vietnam* **64** D6
Khed Brahma *India* **68** G5
Khekra *India* **68** E7
Khemarak Phouminville =
  Krong Kaoh Kong
  Cambodia **65** G4
Khemisset *Morocco* **78** B4
Khemmarat *Thailand* **64** D5
Khenāmān *Iran* **71** D8
Khenchela *Algeria* **78** A7
Khersān → *Iran* **71** D6
Kherson *Ukraine* **33** J7
Kherson □ *Ukraine* **33** J7
Kheta → *Russia* **53** B11
Khewari *Pakistan* **68** F3
Khilchipur *India* **68** G7
Khilok *Russia* **53** D12
Khíos = Hios *Greece* **47** C6
Khirsadoh *India* **69** H8
Khiuma = Hiiumaa *Estonia* **32** C2
Khiva *Uzbekistan* **52** E6
Khiva *Ukraine* **23** D14
Khlebarovo *Bulgaria* **45** C10
Khlong Khlung *Thailand* **64** D2
Khmelnytskyy *Ukraine* **23** D14
Khmelnytskyy □ *Ukraine* **33** H4
Khmer Rep. = Cambodia ■
  Asia **64** F5
Khoai, Hon *Vietnam* **65** H5

Khodoriv *Ukraine* **23** D13
Khodzent = Khūjand
  Tajikistan **52** E7
Khojak Pass *Afghan.* **68** D2
Khok Kloi *Thailand* **65** a
Khok Pho *Thailand* **65** J3
Khok Samrong *Thailand* **64** E3
Kholm *Russia* **32** B6
Kholm *Russia* **32** D6
Kholmsk *Russia* **53** E15
Khomārlu *Iran* **73** C12
Khomas Hochland *Namibia* **88** C2
Khomeyn *Iran* **71** C6
Khomeynī Shahr *Iran* **71** C6
Khombole *Senegal* **82** C1
Khomodino *Botswana* **88** C3
Khon Kaen *Thailand* **64** D4
Khong → *Cambodia* **64** F5
Khong Sedone *Laos* **64** E5
Khonuu *Russia* **53** C15
Khoper → *Russia* **34** F6
Khor el 'Atash *Sudan* **81** E3
Khorāsān □ *Iran* **71** C8
Khorat = Nakhon
  Ratchasima *Thailand* **64** E4
Khorat, Cao Nguyen *Thailand* **64** E4
Khorixas *Namibia* **88** C1
Khorol *Ukraine* **33** H7
Khorramābād *Khorāsān, Iran* **71** C8
Khorramābād *Lorestān, Iran* **73** F13
Khorramdarreh *Iran* **73** D13
Khorrāmshahr *Iran* **71** D6
Khorugh *Tajikistan* **52** F8
Khosravī *Iran* **71** D6
Khosrowābād *Khuzestān, Iran* **71** D6
Khosrowābād *Kordestān,
  Iran* **73** E12
Khost *Pakistan* **68** D2
Khosūyeh *Iran* **71** D7
Khotyn *Ukraine* **29** B11
Khouribga *Morocco* **78** B4
Khowst *Afghan.* **68** C3
Khowst □ *Afghan.* **66** C6
Khoyniki *Belarus* **23** C15
Khrami → *Georgia* **35** K7
Khrenovoye *Russia* **34** E5
Khrysokhou B. *Cyprus* **49** D11
Khu Khan *Thailand* **64** E5
Khuan Wa *Thailand* **65** a
Khudzhand = Khūjand
  Tajikistan **52** E7
Khuff *Si. Arabia* **70** E5
Khūgīānī *Afghan.* **68** D2
Khuis *Botswana* **88** D3
Khuiyala *India* **68** F4
Khūjand *Tajikistan* **52** E7
Khujner *India* **68** H7
Khulna *Bangla.* **67** H16
Khulna □ *Bangla.* **67** H16
Khulo *Georgia* **35** K6
Khumago *Botswana* **88** C3
Khunjerab △ *Pakistan* **69** A6
Khunjerab Pass = Kinjirap
  Daban *Asia* **66** A9
Khūnsorkh *Iran* **71** E8
Khunti *India* **69** H11
Khūr *Iran* **71** C8
Khurai *India* **68** G8
Khurayş *Si. Arabia* **71** E6
Khureit *Sudan* **81** E2
Khurja *India* **68** E7
Khūrmāl *Iraq* **73** E12
Khurr, Wādī al *Iraq* **70** C4
Khūsf *Iran* **71** C8
Khush *Ukraine* **29** B8
Khushab *Pakistan* **68** C5
Khust *Ukraine* **29** B8
Khutse △ *Botswana* **88** C3
Khuwei *Sudan* **81** E2
Khuzdar *Pakistan* **68** F2
Khūzestān □ *Iran* **71** D6
Khvāf *Iran* **71** C9
Khvājeh *Iran* **70** B5
Khvānsār *Iran* **71** D7
Khvatovka *Russia* **34** D9
Khvor *Iran* **71** C7
Khvorgū *Iran* **71** E8
Khvormūj *Iran* **71** D6
Khvoy *Iran* **73** C11
Khvoynaya *Russia* **32** C8
Khyber Pass *Afghan.* **68** B4
Khyriv *Ukraine* **31** J9
Kia *Fiji* **91** a
Kiabukwa
  Dem. Rep. of the Congo **87** D1
Kiama *Australia* **95** E5
Kiamba *Phil.* **61** H6
Kiambu *Kenya* **86** C4
Kiang West △ *Gambia* **82** C1
Kiangara *Madag.* **89** B8
Kiangsi = Jiangxi □ *China* **59** D11
Kiangsu = Jiangsu □ *China* **57** H11
Kiato *Greece* **46** C4
Kibæk *Denmark* **11** H2
Kibale △ *Uganda* **86** B3
Kibanga Port *Uganda* **86** B3
Kibara *Tanzania* **86** C3
Kibare, Mts.
  Dem. Rep. of the Congo **86** D2

Kibira △ *Burundi* **86** C3
Kiboga *Uganda* **86** B3
Kibombo
  Dem. Rep. of the Congo **86** C2
Kibondo *Tanzania* **86** C3
Kibumbu *Burundi* **86** C2
Kibungu *Rwanda* **86** C3
Kibuye *Burundi* **86** C2
Kibuye *Rwanda* **86** C2
Kibwesa *Tanzania* **86** D2
Kibwezi *Kenya* **86** C4
Kicasalih *Turkey* **45** E10
Kichha *India* **69** E8
Kichha → *India* **69** E8
Kicking Horse Pass *Canada* **102** C5
Kidal *Mali* **83** B5
Kidal □ *Mali* **83** B5
Kidapawan *Phil.* **61** H6
Kidderminster *U.K.* **15** E5
Kidepo Valley △ *Uganda* **86** B3
Kidete *Tanzania* **86** D4
Kidira *Senegal* **82** C2
Kidnappers, C. *N.Z.* **91** C6
Kidsgrove *U.K.* **14** D5
Kidston *Australia* **94** B3
Kidugallo *Tanzania* **86** D4
Kiel *Germany* **24** A6
Kiel Canal = Nord-Ostsee-
  Kanal *Germany* **24** A5
Kielce *Poland* **31** H7
Kielder Water □ *U.K.* **14** B5
Kieler Bucht *Germany* **24** A6
Kiembara *Burkina Faso* **82** C4
Kien Binh *Vietnam* **65** H5
Kien Tan *Vietnam* **65** G5
Kienge *Dem. Rep. of the Congo* **87** E2
Kiessé *Niger* **83** C5
Kiev = Kyyiv *Ukraine* **23** C16
Kifaya *Guinea* **82** C2
Kiffa *Mauritania* **82** B2
Kifisós → *Greece* **46** C5
Kifissia *Greece* **46** C5
Kifrī *Iraq* **73** E11
Kigali *Rwanda* **86** C3
Kigarama *Tanzania* **86** C3
Kigelle *Sudan* **81** F3
Kigezi □ *Uganda* **86** C2
Kiği *Turkey* **73** C9
Kigoma □ *Tanzania* **86** D2
Kigoma-Ujiji *Tanzania* **86** C2
Kigomasha, Ras *Tanzania* **86** C4
Kigosi △ *Tanzania* **86** C3
Kiğzı *Turkey* **70** B4
Kihnu *Estonia* **32** C3
Kii-Sanchi *Japan* **55** G8
Kii-Suidō *Japan* **55** H7
Kiira Dam *Uganda* **86** B3
Kikaiga-Shima *Japan* **55** K4
Kikinda *Serbia* **28** E5
Kikládhes = Cyclades *Greece* **46** E6
Kikwit *Dem. Rep. of the Congo* **84** F3
Kil *Sweden* **10** E7
Kilafors *Sweden* **10** C10
Kilar *India* **68** C7
Kilbeggan *Ireland* **12** C4
Kilbrannan Sd. *U.K.* **13** F3
Kilbuck Mts. *U.S.A.* **106** C8
Kilchu *N. Korea* **57** D15
Kilcoy *Australia* **95** D5
Kildare *Ireland* **12** C5
Kildare □ *Ireland* **12** C5
Kildinstroy *Russia* **8** B25
Kileikli *Sudan* **81** E2
Kilfinnane *Ireland* **12** D3
Kilgarvan *Ireland* **12** E2
Kilgore *U.S.A.* **116** E7
Kilgoris *Kenya* **86** C3
Kilibo *Benin* **83** D5
Kilifi *Kenya* **86** C4
Kilimanjaro *Tanzania* **86** C4
Kilimanjaro □ *Tanzania* **86** C4
Kilimli *Turkey* **72** B4
Kilindini *Kenya* **86** C4
Kilis *Turkey* **72** D7
Kilis □ *Turkey* **72** D7
Kiliya *Ukraine* **29** E14
Kilkee *Ireland* **12** D2
Kilkeel *U.K.* **12** B5
Kilkenny *Ireland* **12** D4
Kilkenny □ *Ireland* **12** D4
Kilkieran B. *Ireland* **12** C2
Kilkis *Greece* **44** F6
Kilkis □ *Greece* **44** E6
Killala *Ireland* **12** B2
Killala B. *Ireland* **12** B2
Killaloe *Canada* **114** A7
Killaloe *Ireland* **12** D3
Killarney *Australia* **95** D5
Killarney *Canada* **103** D9
Killarney *Ireland* **12** D2
Killarney △ *Ireland* **12** D2
Killary Harbour *Ireland* **12** C2
Killdeer *U.S.A.* **112** B3
Killeberg *Sweden* **11** H8
Killeen *U.S.A.* **116** F6

Killin *U.K.* **13** E4
Killiney *Ireland* **12** C5
Killington Pk. *U.S.A.* **115** C12
Killíni = Kyllini *Greece* **46** D3
Killini *Greece* **46** D4
Killorglin *Ireland* **12** D2
Killybegs *Ireland* **12** B3
Kilmarnock *U.K.* **13** F4
Kilmez *Russia* **34** B10
Kilmez → *Russia* **34** B10
Kilmore *Australia* **95** F3
Kilmore Quay *Ireland* **12** D5
Kilondo *Tanzania* **87** D3
Kilosa *Tanzania* **86** D4
Kilrush *Ireland* **12** D2
Kilwa Kisiwani *Tanzania* **87** D4
Kilwa Kivinje *Tanzania* **87** D4
Kilwa Masoko *Tanzania* **87** D4
Kilwinning *U.K.* **13** F4
Kim *U.S.A.* **109** H12
Kim → *Cameroon* **83** D7
Kimaam *Indonesia* **63** F9
Kimamba *Tanzania* **86** D4
Kimba *Australia* **95** E2
Kimball *Nebr., U.S.A.* **112** E2
Kimball *S. Dak., U.S.A.* **112** D4
Kimberley *Australia* **92** C4
Kimberley *B.C., Canada* **102** D5
Kimberley *Ont., Canada* **114** B4
Kimberley *S. Africa* **88** D3
Kimberly *U.S.A.* **108** E6
Kimch'aek *N. Korea* **57** D15
Kimchŏn *S. Korea* **57** F15
Kimi *Greece* **46** C6
Kimmirut *Canada* **101** E18
Kimovsk *Moskva, Russia* **32** E9
Kimovsk *Tula, Russia* **32** E10
Kimparana *Mali* **82** C4
Kimpese *Dem. Rep. of the Congo* **84** F2
Kimry *Russia* **32** D9
Kimstad *Sweden* **11** F9
Kinabalu, Gunung *Malaysia* **62** C5
Kinango *Kenya* **86** C4
Kinaros *Greece* **47** E8
Kinaskan L. *Canada* **102** B2
Kinbasket L. *Canada* **102** C5
Kincardine *Canada* **114** B3
Kincolith *Canada* **102** C3
Kinda *Dem. Rep. of the Congo* **87** D2
Kindberg *Austria* **26** D8
Kinde *U.S.A.* **114** C2
Kinder Scout *U.K.* **14** D6
Kindersley *Canada* **103** C7
Kindia *Guinea* **82** D2
Kindu *Dem. Rep. of the Congo* **86** C2
Kinel *Russia* **34** D10
Kineshma *Russia* **34** B6
Kinesi *Tanzania* **86** C3
King, L. *Australia* **93** F2
King, Mt. *Australia* **94** D4
King Christian I. *Canada* **101** B11
King City *U.S.A.* **110** J5
King Cr. → *Australia* **94** C2
King Edward → *Australia* **92** B4
King Edward Point
  S. Georgia **128** G9
King Frederick VI Land =
  Kong Frederik VI Kyst
  Greenland **4** C5
King George B. *Falk. Is.* **128** G4
King George I. *Antarctica* **5** C18
King George Is. *Canada* **101** F15
King George Sd. *Australia* **93** G2
King I. = Kadan Kyun
  Burma **64** F2
King I. *Australia* **95** F3
King I. *Canada* **102** C3
King Khalid Military City =
  Madinat al Malik Khālid
  al Askarīyah *Si. Arabia* **70** E5
King Leopold Ranges
  Australia **92** C4
King of Prussia *U.S.A.* **115** F9
King Sd. *Australia* **92** C3
King Sejong *Antarctica* **5** C18
King William I. *Canada* **100** D12
King William's Town
  S. Africa **88** E4
Kingaok = Bathurst Inlet
  Canada **100** D10
Kingaroy *Australia* **95** D5
Kingfisher *U.S.A.* **116** D6
Kingirbān *Iraq* **70** C5
Kingisepp = Kuressaare
  Estonia **32** C2
Kingisepp *Russia* **32** C5
Kingman *Ariz., U.S.A.* **111** K12
Kingman *Kans., U.S.A.* **112** G4
Kingoonya *Australia* **95** E2
Kingri *Pakistan* **68** D3
Kings → *U.S.A.* **110** J7
Kings Canyon *Australia* **92** D5
Kings Canyon △ *U.S.A.* **110** J8
King's Lynn *U.K.* **14** E8
Kings Park *U.S.A.* **115** F11
Kings Peak *U.S.A.* **108** F8
Kingsbridge *U.K.* **15** G4
Kingsburg *U.S.A.* **110** J7

Kingscote *Australia* **95 F2**
Kingscourt *Ireland* **12 C5**
Kingsford *U.S.A.* **112 C9**
Kingsland *U.S.A.* **117 F14**
Kingsport *U.S.A.* **117 C13**
Kingston *Canada* **115 B8**
Kingston *Jamaica* **120 a**
Kingston *N.Z.* **91 F2**
Kingston *N.H., U.S.A.* **115 D13**
Kingston *N.Y., U.S.A.* **115 E11**
Kingston *Pa., U.S.A.* **115 E9**
Kingston *R.I., U.S.A.* **115 E13**
Kingston Pk. *U.S.A.* **111 K11**
Kingston South East
  Australia **95 F2**
Kingston upon Hull *U.K.* **14 D7**
Kingston upon Hull □ *U.K.* **14 D7**
Kingston-upon-Thames □
  U.K. **15 F7**
Kingstown *St. Vincent* **121 D7**
Kingstree *U.S.A.* **117 E15**
Kingsville *Canada* **114 D2**
Kingsville *U.S.A.* **116 H6**
Kingussie *U.K.* **13 D4**
Kingwood *U.S.A.* **116 F7**
Kınık *Antalya, Turkey* **47 E11**
Kınık *İzmir, Turkey* **47 B9**
Kinistino *Canada* **103 C7**
Kinjirap Daban *Asia* **66 A9**
Kinkala *Congo* **84 E2**
Kinki □ *Japan* **55 H8**
Kinleith *N.Z.* **91 C5**
Kinlochleven *U.K.* **13 E4**
Kinmount *Canada* **114 B6**
Kinna *Sweden* **11 G6**
Kinnairds Hd. *U.K.* **13 D6**
Kinnared *Sweden* **11 G7**
Kinnarp *Sweden* **11 F7**
Kinneviken *Sweden* **11 F7**
Kinngait *Canada* **101 E16**
Kino Nuevo *Mexico* **118 B2**
Kinoje → *Canada* **104 B3**
Kinomoto *Japan* **55 G8**
Kinoni *Uganda* **86 C3**
Kinoosao *Canada* **103 B8**
Kinross *U.K.* **13 E5**
Kinsale *Ireland* **12 E3**
Kinsale, Old Hd. of *Ireland* **12 E3**
Kinsha = Chang Jiang →
  China **59 B13**
Kinshasa
  Dem. Rep. of the Congo **84 E3**
Kinsley *U.S.A.* **112 G4**
Kinsman *U.S.A.* **114 E4**
Kinston *U.S.A.* **117 D16**
Kintamani *Indonesia* **63 J18**
Kintampo *Ghana* **83 D4**
Kintore *U.K.* **13 D6**
Kintore Ra. *Australia* **92 D4**
Kintyre *U.K.* **13 F3**
Kintyre, Mull of *U.K.* **13 F3**
Kinushseo → *Canada* **104 A3**
Kinuso *Canada* **102 B5**
Kinvarra *Ireland* **12 C3**
Kinyangiri *Tanzania* **86 C3**
Kinyeti *Sudan* **81 G3**
Kinzig → *Germany* **25 G3**
Kinzua *U.S.A.* **114 E6**
Kioni *Greece* **46 C2**
Kiosk *Canada* **104 C4**
Kiowa *Kans., U.S.A.* **112 G4**
Kiowa *Okla., U.S.A.* **116 D7**
Kipahigan L. *Canada* **103 B8**
Kipanga *Tanzania* **86 D4**
Kiparissia *Greece* **46 D3**
Kiparissiakos Kolpos *Greece* **46 D3**
Kipawa, L. *Canada* **104 C4**
Kipembawe *Tanzania* **86 D3**
Kipengere Ra. *Tanzania* **87 D3**
Kipili *Tanzania* **86 D3**
Kipini *Kenya* **86 C5**
Kipling *Canada* **103 C8**
Kippure *Ireland* **12 C5**
Kipushi *Dem. Rep. of the Congo* **87 E2**
Kira Panagia *Greece* **46 B6**
Kirane *Mali* **82 B2**
Kiranomena *Madag.* **89 B8**
Kiraz *Turkey* **47 C10**
Kırazlı *Turkey* **45 F10**
Kirchhain *Germany* **24 E4**
Kirchheim *Germany* **25 G5**
Kirchheimbolanden *Germany* **25 F3**
Kirchschlag *Austria* **27 D9**
Kireç *Turkey* **45 B10**
Kirensk *Russia* **53 D11**
Kirghizia = Kyrgyzstan ■
  Asia **52 E8**
Kiribati ■ *Pac. Oc.* **90 B10**
Kırıkhan *Turkey* **72 D7**
Kırıkkale *Turkey* **72 C5**
Kirillov *Russia* **32 C10**
Kirin = Jilin *China* **57 C14**
Kirinyaga = Kenya, Mt.
  Kenya **86 C4**
Kirirom △ *Cambodia* **65 G5**
Kirishi *Russia* **32 C7**
Kirishima Yaku △ *Japan* **55 J5**
Kiritimati *Kiribati* **97 G12**
Kırka *Turkey* **47 B12**

Kırkağaç *Turkey* **47 B9**
Kirkby *U.K.* **14 D5**
Kirkby-in-Ashfield *U.K.* **14 D6**
Kirkby Lonsdale *U.K.* **14 C5**
Kirkby Stephen *U.K.* **14 C5**
Kirkcaldy *U.K.* **13 E5**
Kirkcudbright *U.K.* **13 G4**
Kirkenes *Norway* **8 B24**
Kirkfield *Canada* **114 B6**
Kirkintilloch *U.K.* **13 F4**
Kirkjubæjarklaustur *Iceland* **8 E4**
Kirkland *Canada* **110 C4**
Kirkland Lake *Canada* **104 C3**
Kırklareli *Turkey* **45 E11**
Kırklareli □ *Turkey* **45 E11**
Kirksville *U.S.A.* **112 E7**
Kirkūk *Iraq* **73 E11**
Kirkwall *U.K.* **13 C6**
Kirkwood *S. Africa* **88 E4**
Kirn *Germany* **25 F3**
Kirov *Kaluga, Russia* **32 E8**
Kirov *Kirov, Russia* **52 D5**
Kirovabad = Gäncä
  Azerbaijan **35 K8**
Kirovograd = Kirovohrad
  Ukraine **33 H7**
Kirovohrad *Ukraine* **33 H7**
Kirovohrad □ *Ukraine* **33 H6**
Kirovskiy *Astrakhan, Russia* **35 H9**
Kirovskiy *Kamchatka, Russia* **53 D16**
Kirovskiy *Primorsk, Russia* **54 B6**
Kirriemuir *U.K.* **13 E5**
Kirsanov *Russia* **34 D5**
Kırşehir *Turkey* **72 C6**
Kirtachi *Niger* **83 C5**
Kirthar △ *Pakistan* **68 F2**
Kirthar Range *Pakistan* **68 F2**
Kirtland *U.S.A.* **109 H9**
Kiruna *Sweden* **8 C19**
Kirundu
  Dem. Rep. of the Congo **86 C2**
Kirya *Russia* **34 C8**
Kiryū *Japan* **55 F9**
Kisa *Sweden* **11 G9**
Kisaga *Tanzania* **86 C3**
Kisalföld *Hungary* **28 C2**
Kisanga *Dem. Rep. of the Congo* **86 B2**
Kisangani
  Dem. Rep. of the Congo **86 B2**
Kisar *Indonesia* **63 F7**
Kisarawe *Tanzania* **86 D4**
Kisarazu *Japan* **55 G9**
Kisbér *Hungary* **28 C3**
Kiselevsk *Russia* **52 D9**
Kish = Qeys *Iran* **71 E7**
Kishanganga → *Pakistan* **69 B5**
Kishanganj *India* **69 F13**
Kishangarh *Raj., India* **68 F6**
Kishangarh *Raj., India* **68 F4**
Kishi *Nigeria* **83 D5**
Kishinev = Chişinău
  Moldova **29 C13**
Kishiwada *Japan* **55 G7**
Kishtwar *India* **68 C6**
Kisielice *Poland* **30 E6**
Kisigo → *Tanzania* **86 D3**
Kisii *Kenya* **86 C3**
Kisiju *Tanzania* **86 D4**
Kisir *Turkey* **73 B10**
Kisizi *Uganda* **86 C2**
Kiska I. *U.S.A.* **106 E3**
Kiskomárom = Zalakomár
  Hungary **28 D2**
Kiskörei-víztároló *Hungary* **28 C5**
Kiskőrös *Hungary* **28 D4**
Kiskundorozsma *Hungary* **28 D5**
Kiskunfélegyháza *Hungary* **28 D4**
Kiskunhalas *Hungary* **28 D4**
Kiskunmajsa *Hungary* **28 D4**
Kiskunság □ *Hungary* **28 D4**
Kislovodsk *Russia* **35 J6**
Kismaayo *Somali Rep.* **75 H3**
Kiso-Gawa → *Japan* **55 G8**
Kiso-Sammyaku *Japan* **55 G8**
Kisofukushima *Japan* **55 G8**
Kisoro *Uganda* **86 C2**
Kissamos = Kasteli *Greece* **49 D5**
Kissamos, Kolpos *Greece* **49 D5**
Kissidougou *Guinea* **82 D2**
Kissimmee *U.S.A.* **117 G14**
Kissimmee → *U.S.A.* **117 H14**
Kississing L. *Canada* **103 B8**
Kissónerga *Cyprus* **49 E11**
Kissu, J. *Sudan* **80 C2**
Kistanje *Croatia* **41 E12**
Kisújszállás *Hungary* **28 C5**
Kisumu *Kenya* **86 C3**
Kisvárda *Hungary* **28 B6**
Kiswani *Tanzania* **86 C4**
Kiswere *Tanzania* **87 D4**
Kit Carson *U.S.A.* **108 G12**
Kita *Mali* **82 C3**
Kitaibaraki *Japan* **55 F10**
Kitakami *Japan* **54 E10**
Kitakami-Gawa → *Japan* **54 E10**
Kitakami-Sammyaku *Japan* **54 E10**
Kitakata *Japan* **54 F9**
Kitakyūshū *Japan* **55 H5**

Kitale *Kenya* **86 B4**
Kitami *Japan* **54 C11**
Kitami-Sammyaku *Japan* **54 B11**
Kitangiri, L. *Tanzania* **86 C3**
Kitaya *Tanzania* **87 E5**
Kitchener *Canada* **114 C4**
Kitee *Finland* **32 A6**
Kitega = Gitega *Burundi* **86 C2**
Kitgum *Uganda* **86 B3**
Kíthira = Kythira *Greece* **46 E5**
Kithnos *Greece* **46 D6**
Kiti *Cyprus* **49 E12**
Kiti, C. *Cyprus* **49 E12**
Kitimat *Canada* **102 C3**
Kitinen → *Finland* **8 C22**
Kitiyab *Sudan* **81 D3**
Kitros *Greece* **44 F6**
Kitsman *Ukraine* **29 B10**
Kitsuki *Japan* **55 H5**
Kittakittaooloo, L. *Australia* **95 D2**
Kittanning *U.S.A.* **114 F5**
Kittatinny Mt. *U.S.A.* **115 F10**
Kittery *U.S.A.* **115 C14**
Kittilä *Finland* **8 C21**
Kitui *Kenya* **86 C4**
Kitwanga *Canada* **102 B3**
Kitwe *Zambia* **87 E2**
Kitzbühel *Austria* **26 D5**
Kitzbühler Alpen *Austria* **26 D5**
Kitzingen *Germany* **25 F6**
Kivarli *India* **68 G5**
Kivertsi *Ukraine* **23 C13**
Kividhes *Cyprus* **49 E11**
Kivik *Sweden* **11 J8**
Kivotos *Greece* **44 F5**
Kivu, L. *Dem. Rep. of the Congo* **86 C2**
Kiwirrkurra *Australia* **92 D4**
Kiwirrkurra ✿ *Australia* **92 D4**
Kiyev = Kyyiv *Ukraine* **23 C16**
Kiyevskoye Vdkhr. =
  Kyyivske Vdskh. *Ukraine* **23 C16**
Kıyıköy *Turkey* **45 E12**
Kiziba-Baluba △ *Congo* **87 E2**
Kiziguru *Rwanda* **86 C3**
Kızıl Adalar *Turkey* **45 F13**
Kizil Jilga *China* **69 B8**
Kizil Yurt *Russia* **35 J8**
Kızılcabölük *Turkey* **47 D11**
Kızılcadağ *Turkey* **47 D11**
Kızılcahamam *Turkey* **72 B5**
Kızılhisar *Turkey* **72 D3**
Kızılırmak *Turkey* **72 B5**
Kızılkaya *Turkey* **47 D12**
Kızılören *Turkey* **47 C12**
Kızıltepe *Turkey* **73 D9**
Kizimkazi *Tanzania* **86 D4**
Kizlyar *Russia* **35 J8**
Kizyl-Arvat = Serdar
  Turkmenistan **71 B8**
Kjellerup *Denmark* **11 H3**
Kjölur *Iceland* **8 D4**
Kladanj *Bos.-H.* **28 F3**
Kladnica *Serbia* **44 C4**
Kladno *Czech Rep.* **26 A7**
Kladovo *Serbia* **44 B6**
Klaeng *Thailand* **64 F3**
Klagenfurt *Austria* **26 E7**
Klaipėda *Lithuania* **30 C8**
Klaipėda □ *Lithuania* **30 C8**
Klaksvík *Færoe Is.* **8 E9**
Klamath → *U.S.A.* **108 F11**
Klamath Falls *U.S.A.* **108 E3**
Klamath Mts. *U.S.A.* **108 F2**
Klamono *Indonesia* **63 E8**
Klang *Malaysia* **65 L3**
Klanjec *Croatia* **41 B12**
Klappan → *Canada* **102 B3**
Klarälven → *Sweden* **10 E12**
Klässbol *Sweden* **10 E6**
Klatovy *Czech Rep.* **26 B6**
Klawer *S. Africa* **88 E2**
Klazienaveen *Neths.* **17 B6**
Klé *Mali* **82 C3**
Klecko *Poland* **31 F4**
Kleczew *Poland* **31 F5**
Kleena Kleene *Canada* **102 C4**
Klein-Karas *Namibia* **88 D2**
Klekovača *Bos.-H.* **41 D13**
Klembivka *Ukraine* **29 B13**
Klenoec *Macedonia* **44 E4**
Klenovec *Slovak Rep.* **27 C12**
Klerksdorp *S. Africa* **88 D4**
Kleszczele *Poland* **31 F10**
Kletnya *Russia* **32 F7**
Kletsk = Klyetsk *Belarus* **23 B14**
Kletskiy *Russia* **35 F6**
Kleve *Germany* **24 D2**
Klickitat *U.S.A.* **108 D3**
Klickitat → *U.S.A.* **110 E5**
Klidhes *Cyprus* **49 D13**
Klimovichi *Belarus* **32 F6**
Klin *Russia* **32 D9**
Klina *Kosovo* **44 D4**
Klinaklini → *Canada* **102 C3**
Klintehamn *Sweden* **11 G12**

Klintsy *Russia* **33 F7**
Klip → *S. Africa* **89 D4**
Klipdale *S. Africa* **88 E2**
Klippan *Sweden* **11 H7**
Klipplaat *S. Africa* **88 E3**
Klishkivtsi *Ukraine* **29 B11**
Klisura *Bulgaria* **45 D8**
Kljajićevo *Serbia* **28 E4**
Ključ *Bos.-H.* **41 D13**
Klobuck *Poland* **31 H5**
Kłodawa *Poland* **31 F5**
Kłodzko *Poland* **31 H3**
Klondike *Canada* **100 E4**
Klong Wang Chao △
  Thailand **64 D2**
Klos *Albania* **44 E4**
Klosterneuburg *Austria* **27 C9**
Klosters *Switz.* **25 J5**
Klötze *Germany* **24 C7**
Klouto *Togo* **83 D5**
Kluane △ *Canada* **102 A1**
Kluane L. *Canada* **100 E4**
Kluang *Malaysia* **65 L4**
Kluczbork *Poland* **31 H5**
Klukwan *U.S.A.* **102 B1**
Klungkung *Indonesia* **63 K18**
Klyetsk *Belarus* **23 B14**
Klyuchevskaya, Gora
  Russia **53 D17**
Klyuchi *Russia* **53 D17**
Knäred *Sweden* **11 H7**
Knaresborough *U.K.* **14 C6**
Knee L. *Man., Canada* **104 A1**
Knee L. *Sask., Canada* **103 B7**
Knezha *Bulgaria* **45 C8**
Knight Inlet *Canada* **102 C3**
Knighton *U.K.* **15 E4**
Knights Ferry *U.S.A.* **110 H6**
Knights Landing *U.S.A.* **110 G5**
Knin *Croatia* **41 D13**
Knislinge *Sweden* **11 H8**
Knjaževac *Serbia* **44 C6**
Knob, C. *Australia* **93 F2**
Knock *Ireland* **12 C3**
Knockmealdown Mts.
  Ireland **12 D4**
Knokke-Heist *Belgium* **17 C3**
Knossos *Greece* **49 D7**
Knowlton *Canada* **115 A12**
Knox *U.S.A.* **112 E10**
Knox Coast *Antarctica* **5 C8**
Knoxville *Iowa, U.S.A.* **112 E8**
Knoxville *Pa., U.S.A.* **114 E7**
Knoxville *Tenn., U.S.A.* **117 D13**
Knud Rasmussen Land
  Greenland **101 B20**
Knysna *S. Africa* **88 E3**
Knyszyn *Poland* **30 E9**
Ko Kha *Thailand* **64 C2**
Ko Tarutao △ *Thailand* **65 J2**
Ko Yao *Thailand* **65 a**
Koartac = Quaqtaq *Canada* **101 E18**
Koba *Indonesia* **63 F8**
Kobarid *Slovenia* **41 B10**
Kobayashi *Japan* **55 J5**
Kōbe *Japan* **55 G7**
Kobelyaky *Ukraine* **33 H8**
København *Denmark* **11 J6**
København ✈ (CPH)
  Denmark **11 J6**
Kobenni *Mauritania* **82 B3**
Kōbi-Sho *Japan* **55 M1**
Koblenz *Germany* **25 H8**
Kobo *Ethiopia* **81 E4**
Kobryn *Belarus* **23 B13**
Kobuk → *U.S.A.* **106 B7**
Kobuleti *Georgia* **35 K5**
Kobyletska Polyana *Ukraine* **29 B9**
Kobylin *Poland* **31 G4**
Kobyłka *Poland* **31 F8**
Kobylkino *Russia* **34 C6**
Koca → *Turkey* **45 F11**
Kocabaş *Turkey* **47 D11**
Kocaeli *Turkey* **45 F13**
Kocaeli □ *Turkey* **45 C10**
Kočane *Serbia* **44 C5**
Kočani *Macedonia* **44 E6**
Koçarlı *Turkey* **47 D9**
Koceljevo *Serbia* **44 B3**
Kočevje *Slovenia* **41 C11**
Koch Bihar *India* **67 F16**
Kochas *India* **69 G10**
Kocher → *Germany* **25 F5**
Kōchi *Japan* **55 H6**
Kōchi □ *Japan* **55 H6**
Kochiu = Gejiu *China* **58 F4**
Kochubey *Russia* **35 H8**
Kock *Poland* **31 G9**
Kodarma *India* **69 G11**
Kode *Sweden* **11 G5**
Kodi *Indonesia* **92 A2**
Kodiak *U.S.A.* **106 D9**
Kodiak I. *U.S.A.* **106 D9**
Kodinar *India* **68 J4**
Kodinsk *Russia* **53 D10**

Kodok *Sudan* **81 F3**
Kodori → *Georgia* **35 J5**
Kodyma *Ukraine* **29 B14**
Koedoesberge *S. Africa* **88 E3**
Koes *Namibia* **88 D2**
Kofçaz *Turkey* **45 E11**
Koffiefontein *S. Africa* **88 D4**
Kofiau *Indonesia* **63 E7**
Köflach *Austria* **26 D8**
Koforidua *Ghana* **83 D4**
Kōfu *Japan* **55 G9**
Koga *Japan* **55 F9**
Kogaluc → *Canada* **105 A7**
Køge *Denmark* **11 J6**
Køge Bugt *Denmark* **11 J6**
Kogi □ *Nigeria* **83 D6**
Kogin Baba *Nigeria* **83 D7**
Kogon *Uzbekistan* **52 F7**
Koh-i-Khurd *Afghan.* **68 C1**
Koh-i-Maran *Pakistan* **68 E2**
Kohat *Pakistan* **68 C4**
Kohima *India* **67 G19**
Kohkīlūyeh va Būyer
  Aḥmadi □ *Iran* **71 D6**
Kohler Ra. *Antarctica* **5 D15**
Kohlu *Pakistan* **68 E3**
Kohtla-Järve *Estonia* **32 C4**
Kohylnyk → *Ukraine* **29 E14**
Koi Sanjaq *Iraq* **73 D11**
Koidu *S. Leone* **82 D2**
Koillismaa *Finland* **8 C23**
Koin *N. Korea* **57 D14**
Koinare *Bulgaria* **45 C8**
Koindu *S. Leone* **82 D2**
Kojetín *Czech Rep.* **27 B10**
Kojŏ *N. Korea* **57 E14**
Kojonup *Australia* **93 F2**
Kojūr *Iran* **71 B6**
Kokand = Qŭqon *Uzbekistan* **52 E8**
Kokas *Indonesia* **63 E8**
Kokava *Slovak Rep.* **27 C12**
Kokchetav = Kökshetaū
  Kazakhstan **52 D7**
Kokemäenjoki → *Finland* **32 B1**
Kokhma *Russia* **34 B5**
Koki *Senegal* **82 B1**
Kokkola *Finland* **8 E20**
Koko *Nigeria* **83 C5**
Koko Kyunzu *Burma* **67 M18**
Kokologo *Burkina Faso* **82 C4**
Kokolopozo *Ivory C.* **82 D3**
Kokomo *U.S.A.* **112 E10**
Kokoro *Niger* **83 C5**
Koksan *N. Korea* **57 E14**
Kökshetaū *Kazakhstan* **52 D7**
Koksoak → *Canada* **101 F18**
Kokstad *S. Africa* **89 E4**
Kokubu *Japan* **55 J5**
Kola *Indonesia* **63 F8**
Kola *Russia* **8 B25**
Kola Pen. = Kolskiy
  Poluostrov *Russia* **6 B13**
Kolachi → *Pakistan* **68 F2**
Kolahoi *India* **69 B6**
Kolahun *Liberia* **82 D2**
Kolaka *Indonesia* **63 E6**
Kolar *India* **66 N11**
Kolar Gold Fields *India* **66 N11**
Kolaras *India* **68 G6**
Kolari *Finland* **8 C20**
Kolárovo *Slovak Rep.* **27 D10**
Kolašin *Montenegro* **44 D3**
Kolayat *India* **68 F5**
Kolbäck *Sweden* **10 E10**
Kolbäcksån → *Sweden* **10 E10**
Kolbermoor *Germany* **25 H8**
Kolbuszowa *Poland* **31 H8**
Kolchugino *Russia* **32 D10**
Kolda *Senegal* **82 C2**
Kolda □ *Senegal* **82 C2**
Koldegi *Sudan* **81 E3**
Kolding *Denmark* **11 J3**
Kolepom = Dolak, Pulau
  Indonesia **63 F9**
Kolguyev, Ostrov *Russia* **52 C5**
Kolhapur *India* **66 L9**
Kolia *Ivory C.* **82 D3**
Kolimbia *Greece* **49 C10**
Kolín *Czech Rep.* **26 A8**
Kolind *Denmark* **11 H4**
Kolkas rags *Latvia* **30 A9**
Kolkata *India* **69 H13**
Kollam = Quilon *India* **66 Q10**
Kölleda *Germany* **24 D7**
Kollum *Neths.* **17 A6**
Kolmanskop *Namibia* **88 D2**
Kolno *Germany* **24 C2**
Kolno *Poland* **30 E8**
Koło *Poland* **31 F5**
Kołobrzeg *Poland* **30 D2**
Kolochava *Ukraine* **29 B8**
Kologi *Sudan* **81 E3**
Kolokani *Mali* **82 C3**
Koloko *Burkina Faso* **82 C3**
Kololo *Ethiopia* **81 F5**
Kolomna *Russia* **32 D10**
Kolomyya *Ukraine* **29 B9**
Kolondiéba *Mali* **82 C3**
Kolonodale *Indonesia* **63 E6**

Kolonowskie *Poland* **31 H5**
Kolosib *India* **67 G18**
Kolpashevo *Russia* **52 D9**
Kolpino *Russia* **32 C6**
Kolpny *Russia* **33 F9**
Kolskiy Poluostrov *Russia* **6 B13**
Kolskiy Zaliv *Russia* **8 B26**
Kolsva *Sweden* **10 E9**
Kolubara → *Serbia* **44 B4**
Koluszki *Poland* **31 G6**
Kolwezi *Dem. Rep. of the Congo* **87 E2**
Kolyma → *Russia* **53 C17**
Kolymskoye Nagorye
  Russia **53 C16**
Kôm Hamâda *Egypt* **80 H7**
Kôm Ombo *Egypt* **80 C3**
Komadugu Gana → *Nigeria* **83 C7**
Komandorskiye Is. =
  Komandorskiye Ostrova
  Russia **53 D17**
Komandorskiye Ostrova
  Russia **53 D17**
Komárno *Slovak Rep.* **27 D11**
Komarnyky *Ukraine* **28 B8**
Komárom *Hungary* **28 C3**
Komárom-Esztergom □
  Hungary **28 C3**
Komatipoort *S. Africa* **89 D5**
Komatou Yialou *Cyprus* **49 D13**
Komatsu *Japan* **55 F8**
Komatsushima *Japan* **55 H7**
Kombissiri *Burkina Faso* **83 C4**
Kombori *Burkina Faso* **82 C4**
Komboti *Greece* **46 B3**
Kome Channel *Uganda* **86 C3**
Komen *Slovenia* **41 C10**
Komenda *Ghana* **83 D4**
Komi *Cyprus* **49 D13**
Komi □ *Russia* **52 C6**
Komiža *Croatia* **41 E13**
Komló *Hungary* **28 D3**
Kommunarsk = Alchevsk
  Ukraine **33 H10**
Kommunizma, Pik = imeni
  Ismail Samani, Pik
  Tajikistan **52 F8**
Komodo *Indonesia* **63 F5**
Komoran, Pulau *Indonesia* **63 F9**
Komoro *Japan* **55 F9**
Komotini *Greece* **45 E9**
Komovi *Montenegro* **44 D3**
Kompasberg *S. Africa* **88 E3**
Kompong Cham *Cambodia* **65 G5**
Kompong Chhnang =
  Kampong Chhnang
  Cambodia **65 F5**
Kompong Chikreng *Cambodia* **64 F5**
Kompong Kleang *Cambodia* **64 F5**
Kompong Luong *Cambodia* **65 G5**
Kompong Pranak *Cambodia* **64 F5**
Kompong Som = Kampong
  Saom *Cambodia* **65 G4**
Kompong Som, Chhung =
  Kampong Saom, Chaak
  Cambodia **65 G4**
Kompong Speu *Cambodia* **65 G5**
Kompong Sralau *Cambodia* **64 E5**
Kompong Thom *Cambodia* **64 F5**
Kompong Trabeck *Cambodia* **64 F5**
Kompong Trabeck *Cambodia* **65 G5**
Kompong Trach *Cambodia* **65 G5**
Kompong Tralach *Cambodia* **65 G5**
Komrat = Comrat *Moldova* **29 D13**
Komsberg *S. Africa* **88 E3**
Komsomolets, Ostrov
  Russia **53 A10**
Komsomolsk *Russia* **32 D11**
Komsomolsk-na-Amur
  Russia **53 D14**
Komsomolskiy *Russia* **34 C7**
Kömür Burnu *Turkey* **47 C8**
Kon Tum *Vietnam* **64 E7**
Kon Tum, Plateau du
  Vietnam **64 E7**
Kona *Mali* **82 C4**
Kona *Nigeria* **83 D7**
Konakovo *Russia* **32 D9**
Konar □ *Afghan.* **66 B7**
Konārī *Iran* **71 D6**
Konch *India* **69 G8**
Konde *Tanzania* **86 C4**
Kondias *Greece* **47 B7**
Kondinin *Australia* **93 F2**
Kondoa *Tanzania* **86 C4**
Kondopoga *Russia* **32 A8**
Kondratyevo *Russia* **53 D10**
Kondrovo *Russia* **32 E9**
Konduga *Nigeria* **83 C7**
Köneürgench *Turkmenistan* **52 E6**
Konevo *Russia* **32 A10**
Kong = Khong → *Cambodia* **64 F5**
Kong *Ivory C.* **82 D4**
Kong, Koh *Cambodia* **65 G4**
Kong Christian IX Land
  Greenland **4 C6**
Kong Christian X Land
  Greenland **4 B6**
Kong Frederik IX Land
  Greenland **4 C5**

Kong Frederik VI Kyst
 Greenland 4 C5
Kong Frederik VIII Land
 Greenland 4 B6
Kong Oscar Fjord *Greenland* 4 B6
Kongeå → *Denmark* 11 J2
Kongerslev *Denmark* 11 H4
Konglu *Burma* 67 F20
Kongola *Namibia* 88 B3
Kongolo *Kasai-Or.,*
 Dem. Rep. of the Congo 86 D1
Kongolo *Katanga,*
 Dem. Rep. of the Congo 86 D2
Kongor *Sudan* 81 F3
Kongossambougou △ *Mali* 82 C3
Kongoussi *Burkina Faso* 83 C4
Kongsberg *Norway* 9 G13
Kongsvinger *Norway* 9 F15
Kongwa *Tanzania* 86 D4
Koni *Dem. Rep. of the Congo* 87 E2
Koni, Mts.
 Dem. Rep. of the Congo 87 E2
Koniakari *Mali* 82 C2
Koniecpol *Poland* 31 H6
Königs Wusterhausen
 Germany 24 C9
Königsbrunn *Germany* 25 G6
Königslutter *Germany* 24 C6
Konin *Poland* 31 F5
Konispol *Albania* 44 G4
Konitsa *Greece* 46 A2
Konjic *Bos.-H.* 28 G2
Konkiep *Namibia* 88 D2
Konkouré → *Guinea* 82 D2
Könnern *Germany* 24 D7
Kono *S. Leone* 82 D2
Konongo *Ghana* 83 D4
Konosha *Russia* 32 B11
Kōnosu *Japan* 55 F9
Konotop *Ukraine* 33 G7
Konsankoro *Guinea* 82 D3
Końskie *Poland* 31 G7
Konstancin-Jeziorna *Poland* 31 F8
Konstantinovka =
 Kostyantynivka *Ukraine* 33 H9
Konstantinovsk *Russia* 35 G5
Konstantynów Łódźki *Poland* 31 G6
Konstanz *Germany* 25 H5
Kont *Iran* 71 E9
Kontagora *Nigeria* 83 C6
Kontcha *Cameroon* 83 D7
Kontiolahti *Finland* 8 E23
Kontokali *Greece* 49 A3
Konya *Turkey* 72 D5
Konya □ *Turkey* 72 D5
Konya Ovası *Turkey* 72 C5
Konz *Germany* 25 F2
Konza *Kenya* 86 C4
Koocanusa, L. *Canada* 108 B6
Kookynie *Australia* 93 E3
Koolyanobbing *Australia* 93 F2
Koonibba *Australia* 95 E1
Koorawatha *Australia* 95 E4
Koorda *Australia* 93 F2
Kooskia *U.S.A.* 108 C6
Kootenay → *U.S.A.* 102 D5
Kootenay L. *Canada* 102 C5
Kootenay L. *Canada* 108 B5
Kootjieskolk *S. Africa* 88 E3
Kopanovka *Russia* 35 G8
Kopaonik *Serbia* 44 C4
Kopaonik △ *Serbia* 44 C4
Kópavogur *Iceland* 8 D3
Kopayhorod *Ukraine* 29 B12
Koper *Slovenia* 41 C10
Kopervik *Norway* 9 G11
Kopet Dagh *Asia* 71 B8
Kopi *Australia* 95 E2
Köping *Sweden* 10 E10
Köpingsvik *Sweden* 11 H10
Kopište *Croatia* 41 F13
Koplik *Albania* 44 D3
Köpmanholmen *Sweden* 10 A12
Kopparberg *Sweden* 10 E9
Koppeh Dāgh = Kopet
 Dagh *Asia* 71 B8
Koppies *S. Africa* 89 D4
Koppom *Sweden* 10 E6
Koprivlen *Bulgaria* 44 E7
Koprivnica *Croatia* 41 B13
Kopřivnice *Czech Rep.* 27 B11
Koprivshtitsa *Bulgaria* 45 D8
Köprübaşı *Turkey* 47 C10
Köprülü △ *Turkey* 70 B1
Kopychyntsi *Ukraine* 23 D13
Kora △ *Kenya* 86 C4
Korab *Macedonia* 44 E4
Koral *India* 68 J5
Korarou, L. *Mali* 82 B4
Korba *India* 69 H10
Korbach *Germany* 24 D4
Korbu, G. *Malaysia* 65 K3
Korçë *Albania* 44 F4
Korčula *Croatia* 41 F13
Korčulanski Kanal *Croatia* 41 E13
Kord Kūy *Iran* 71 B7
Kord Sheykh *Iran* 71 D7
Kordestān = Kurdistan *Asia*
 73 D10

Kordestān □ *Iran* 70 C5
Kordié *Burkina Faso* 82 C4
Kordofân *Sudan* 79 F11
Koré Mayroua *Niger* 83 C5
Korea, North ■ *Asia* 57 E14
Korea, South ■ *Asia* 57 G15
Korea Bay *Korea* 57 E13
Korea Strait *Asia* 57 H15
Korem *Ethiopia* 81 E4
Korenevo *Russia* 33 G8
Korenovsk *Russia* 35 H4
Korets *Ukraine* 23 C14
Korfantów *Poland* 31 H4
Korgan *Turkey* 72 B7
Korgus *Sudan* 80 D3
Korhogo *Ivory C.* 82 D3
Koribundu *S. Leone* 82 D2
Korienzé *Mali* 82 B4
Korinthia □ *Greece* 46 D4
Korinthiakos Kolpos *Greece* 46 C4
Korinthos *Greece* 46 D4
Korioumé *Mali* 82 B4
Korissia, L. *Greece* 49 B3
Kōriyama *Japan* 54 F10
Korkuteli *Turkey* 47 D12
Kormakiti, C. *Cyprus* 49 D11
Körmend *Hungary* 28 C1
Kormor *Iraq* 73 E11
Kornat *Croatia* 41 E12
Kornat △ *Croatia* 41 E12
Korneshty = Corneşti
 Moldova 29 C13
Korneuburg *Austria* 27 C9
Kórnik *Poland* 31 F4
Koro *Fiji* 91 a
Koro *Ivory C.* 82 D3
Koro *Mali* 82 C4
Koro Sea *Fiji* 91 a
Korocha *Russia* 33 G9
Köroğlu Dağları *Turkey* 72 B5
Korogwe *Tanzania* 86 D4
Koroleve *Ukraine* 29 B8
Korolevu *Fiji* 91 a
Koronadal *Phil.* 61 H6
Koroni *Greece* 46 E3
Koronia, L. *Greece* 44 F7
Koronos *Greece* 47 D7
Koronowo *Poland* 31 E4
Koropets *Ukraine* 29 B10
Koror *Palau* 96 G5
Körös → *Hungary* 28 D5
Körös Maros △ *Hungary* 28 C5
Köröstarcsa *Hungary* 28 D6
Korosten *Ukraine* 23 C15
Korostyshev *Ukraine* 23 C15
Korotoyak *Russia* 33 G10
Korovou *Fiji* 91 a
Koroyanitu △ *Fiji* 91 a
Korraraika, Helodranon' i
 Madag. 89 B7
Korsakov *Russia* 53 E15
Korsberga *Sweden* 11 G9
Korshiv *Ukraine* 29 B10
Korshunovo *Russia* 53 D12
Korsør *Denmark* 11 J5
Korsun Shevchenkovskiy
 Ukraine 33 H6
Korsze *Poland* 30 D8
Korti *Sudan* 80 D3
Kortrijk *Belgium* 17 D3
Korucu *Turkey* 47 B9
Korwai *India* 68 G8
Koryakskoye Nagorye
 Russia 53 C18
Koryukovka *Ukraine* 33 G7
Kos *Greece* 47 E9
Kosa *Ethiopia* 81 F4
Kosan *N. Korea* 57 E14
Kosaya Gora *Russia* 32 E9
Kościan *Poland* 31 F3
Kościerzyna *Poland* 30 D4
Kosciusko *U.S.A.* 117 E10
Kosciuszko, Mt. *Australia* 95 F4
Kösély → *Hungary* 28 C6
Kosha *Sudan* 80 C3
Koshava *Bulgaria* 44 B7
K'oshih = Kashi *China* 60 C2
Koshiki-Rettō *Japan* 55 J7
Koshim → *Kazakhstan* 34 F10
Kosi *India* 68 F7
Kosi → *India* 69 E8
Košice *Slovak Rep.* 27 C14
Košický □ *Slovak Rep.* 27 C14
Kosiv *Ukraine* 29 B9
Kosjerić *Serbia* 44 B3
Köşk *Turkey* 47 D10
Kouris → *Cyprus* 49 E11
Kourou *Fr. Guiana* 125 B8
Kourouba *Mali* 82 C2
Koŭroudjél *Mauritania* 82 B2
Kouroukoto *Mali* 82 C2
Kourouma *Burkina Faso* 82 C4
Kourouninkoto *Mali* 82 C3
Kouroussa *Guinea* 82 C3
Koussané *Senegal* 82 C2
Koussanar *Senegal* 82 C2
Koussane *Senegal* 82 C2
Koussané *Mali* 82 C2
Kousséri *Cameroon* 79 F8
Koutiala *Mali* 82 C3

Koster *S. Africa* 88 D4
Kôsti *Sudan* 81 E3
Kostinbrod *Bulgaria* 44 D7
Kostolac *Serbia* 44 B5
Kostopil *Ukraine* 23 C14
Kostroma *Russia* 32 D11
Kostromo □ *Russia* 34 A6
Kostromskoye Vdkhr.
 Russia 32 D11
Kostryzhivka *Ukraine* 29 B10
Kostrzyn *Lubuskie, Poland* 31 F1
Kostrzyn *Wielkopolskie, Poland* 31 F4
Kostyantynivka *Ukraine* 33 H9
Kostyukovichi =
 Kastsyukovichy *Belarus* 32 F7
Koszalin *Poland* 30 D3
Kőszeg *Hungary* 28 C1
Kot Addu *Pakistan* 68 D4
Kot Kapura *India* 68 D6
Kot Moman *Pakistan* 68 C5
Kot Sultan *Pakistan* 68 D4
Kota *India* 68 G6
Kota Barrage *India* 68 G6
Kota Belud *Malaysia* 62 C5
Kota Bharu *Malaysia* 65 J4
Kota Kinabalu *Malaysia* 62 C5
Kota Tinggi *Malaysia* 65 M4
Kotaagung *Indonesia* 62 F2
Kotabaru *Indonesia* 62 E5
Kotabumi *Indonesia* 62 E2
Kotamobagu *Indonesia* 63 D6
Kotapinang *Indonesia* 65 M3
Kotcho L. *Canada* 102 B4
Kotdwara *India* 69 E8
Kotel *Bulgaria* 45 D10
Kotelnich *Russia* 34 A9
Kotelnikovo *Russia* 35 G6
Kotelnyy, Ostrov *Russia* 53 B14
Kothari → *India* 68 G6
Köthen *Germany* 24 D7
Kothi *Chhattisgarh, India* 69 H10
Kothi *Mad. P., India* 69 G9
Kotiro *Pakistan* 68 F2
Kotka *Finland* 32 B4
Kotlas *Russia* 52 C5
Kotlenska Planina *Bulgaria* 45 D10
Kotli *Pakistan* 68 C5
Kotlik *U.S.A.* 106 C7
Kotma *India* 69 H9
Koton-Karifi *Nigeria* 83 D6
Kotonkoro *Nigeria* 83 C6
Kotor *Montenegro* 44 D2
Kotor Varoš *Bos.-H.* 28 F7
Kotoriba *Croatia* 41 B13
Kotovo *Russia* 34 E7
Kotovsk *Russia* 34 D5
Kotovsk *Ukraine* 23 E15
Kotputli *India* 68 F7
Kotri *Pakistan* 68 G3
Kotronas *Greece* 46 E4
Kötschach-Mauthen *Austria* 26 E6
Kotto → *C.A.R.* 84 D4
Kotturu *India* 66 M10
Kotu Group *Tonga* 91 c
Kotuy → *Russia* 53 B11
Kotyuzhany *Ukraine* 29 B12
Kotzebue *U.S.A.* 106 B7
Kotzebue Sound *U.S.A.* 106 B7
Kouchibouguac △ *Canada* 105 C6
Koudougou *Burkina Faso* 82 C4
Koufonisi *Iraklio, Greece* 49 E8
Koufonisi *Notio Aigaio, Greece* 47 E7
Kougaberge *S. Africa* 88 E3
Kouibli *Ivory C.* 82 D3
Kouilou → *Congo* 84 E2
Koukdjuak → *Canada* 101 D17
Koula *Greece* 45 E8
Koula Moutou *Gabon* 84 E2
Koulen = Kulen *Cambodia* 64 F5
Koulikoro *Mali* 82 C3
Koulikoro □ *Mali* 82 C3
Kouloura *Greece* 49 A3
Koumala *Australia* 94 C4
Koumankou *Mali* 82 C3
Koumbia *Burkina Faso* 82 C4
Koumbia *Guinea* 82 C2
Koumboum *Guinea* 82 C2
Koumpenntoum *Senegal* 82 C2
Koumra *Chad* 79 G9
Koun-Fao *Ivory C.* 82 D4
Koundara *Guinea* 82 C2
Koundian *Guinea* 82 C3
Koungheul *Senegal* 82 C2
Kountze *U.S.A.* 116 F7
Koupéla *Burkina Faso* 83 C4

Kouto *Ivory C.* 82 D3
Kouvé *Togo* 83 D5
Kouvola *Finland* 32 B4
Kovačica *Serbia* 44 B5
Kovdor *Russia* 8 C24
Kovel *Ukraine* 23 C13
Kovin *Serbia* 28 F5
Kovrov *Russia* 34 B5
Kowal *Poland* 31 F6
Kowalewo Pomorskie *Poland* 31 E5
Kowanyama *Australia* 94 B3
Kowanyama ۞ *Australia* 94 B3
Kowloon *China* 59 F10
Kowŏn *N. Korea* 57 E14
Koyampattur =
 Coimbatore *India* 66 P10
Köyceğiz *Turkey* 47 E10
Köyceğiz Gölü *Turkey* 47 E10
Koyukuk → *U.S.A.* 106 C8
Koyulhisar *Turkey* 72 B7
Koyunyeri *Turkey* 45 F10
Koza = Okinawa *Japan* 55 L3
Kozak *Turkey* 47 B9
Kozaklı *Turkey* 72 C6
Kozan *Turkey* 72 D6
Kozani *Greece* 44 F5
Kozani □ *Greece* 44 F5
Kozara *Bos.-H.* 41 D14
Kozara △ *Bos.-H.* 41 D13
Kozarac *Bos.-H.* 41 D13
Kozelets *Ukraine* 33 G6
Kozelsk *Russia* 32 E8
Kozhikode = Calicut *India* 66 P9
Koziegłowy *Poland* 31 H6
Kozienice *Poland* 31 G8
Kozje *Slovenia* 41 B12
Kozloduy *Bulgaria* 44 C7
Kozlovets *Bulgaria* 45 C9
Kozlovka *Russia* 34 C9
Kozlu *Turkey* 72 B4
Kozluk *Turkey* 73 C9
Koźmin *Poland* 31 G4
Kozmodemyansk *Russia* 34 B8
Kożuchów *Poland* 31 G2
Kozyatyn *Ukraine* 23 D15
Kozyrevsk *Russia* 53 D16
Kpabia *Ghana* 83 D4
Kpalimé *Togo* 83 D5
Kpandae *Ghana* 83 D4
Kpessi *Togo* 83 D5
Kra, Isthmus of = Kra, Kho
 Khot *Thailand* 65 G2
Kra, Kho Khot *Thailand* 65 G2
Kra Buri *Thailand* 65 G2
Kraai → *S. Africa* 88 E4
Krabi *Thailand* 65 H2
Kracheh *Cambodia* 64 F6
Kragan *Indonesia* 63 G14
Kragerø *Norway* 9 G13
Kragujevac *Serbia* 44 B4
Krajenka *Poland* 31 E3
Krakatau = Rakata, Pulau
 Indonesia 62 F3
Krakatoa = Rakata, Pulau
 Indonesia 62 F3
Krakor *Cambodia* 64 F5
Kraków *Poland* 31 H6
Kraków ✈ (KRK) *Poland* 31 H6
Kralanh *Cambodia* 64 F4
Králíky *Czech Rep.* 27 A9
Kraljevo *Serbia* 44 C4
Kralovéhradecký □
 Czech Rep. 26 A8
Královský Chlmec
 Slovak Rep. 27 C14
Kralupy nad Vltavou
 Czech Rep. 26 A7
Kramatorsk *Ukraine* 33 H9
Kramfors *Sweden* 10 B11
Krania *Greece* 44 G5
Krania Elasonas *Greece* 46 B4
Kranidi *Greece* 46 D5
Kranj *Slovenia* 41 B11
Kranjska Gora *Slovenia* 41 B10
Krankskop *S. Africa* 89 D5
Krapina *Croatia* 41 B12
Krapina → *Croatia* 41 C12
Krapkowice *Poland* 31 H4
Kras *Croatia* 41 C10
Kraskino *Russia* 54 C5
Krāslava *Latvia* 32 E2
Kraslice *Czech Rep.* 26 A5
Krasnaya Gorbatka *Russia* 34 C5
Krasnaya Polyana *Russia* 35 J5
Krasne *Ukraine* 29 D14
Krasni Okny *Ukraine* 29 C14
Krásník *Poland* 31 H10
Krasnoarmeisk *Ukraine* 33 H9
Krasnoarmeysk *Russia* 34 E7
Krasnoarmeyskiy *Russia* 35 G6
Krasnobrod *Poland* 31 H10
Krasnodar *Russia* 35 H4
Krasnodar □ *Russia* 35 J4
Krasnodarskoye Vdkhr.
 Russia 35 H4
Krasnodon *Ukraine* 33 H10
Krasnogorskiy *Russia* 34 B9
Krasnograd = Krasnohrad
 Ukraine 33 H8

Krasnogvardeysk *Ukraine* 33 K8
Krasnogvardeyskoye *Russia* 35 H5
Krasnohrad *Ukraine* 33 H8
Krasnokamensk *Russia* 53 D12
Krasnokutsk *Ukraine* 33 G8
Krasnolesnyy *Russia* 33 G10
Krasnoperekopsk *Ukraine* 33 J7
Krasnorechenskiy *Russia* 54 B7
Krasnoselkup *Russia* 52 C9
Krasnoslobodsk *Mordvinia,*
 Russia 34 C6
Krasnoslobodsk *Volgograd,*
 Russia 35 F7
Krasnoturinsk *Russia* 52 D7
Krasnovodsk *Russia* 53 D10
Krasnoyarsk *Russia* 53 D10
Krasnoye = Krasnyy *Russia* 32 E6
Krasnoyilsk *Russia* 29 C10
Krasnozavodsk *Russia* 32 D10
Krasnoznamensk *Russia* 30 D9
Krasny Sulin *Russia* 33 J11
Krasnystaw *Poland* 31 H10
Krasnyy *Russia* 32 E6
Krasnyy Kholm *Russia* 32 C9
Krasnyy Kut *Russia* 34 E8
Krasnyy Liman *Ukraine* 33 H9
Krasnyy Luch *Ukraine* 33 H10
Krasnyy Profintern *Russia* 32 D11
Krasnyy Yar *Astrakhan,*
 Russia 35 G9
Krasnyy Yar *Samara, Russia* 34 D10
Krasnyy Yar *Volgograd, Russia* 34 E7
Krasnyye Baki *Russia* 34 B7
Krasnyyoskolske Vdskh.
 Ukraine 33 H9
Kraszna → *Hungary* 28 B7
Kratie = Kracheh *Cambodia* 64 F6
Kratovo *Macedonia* 44 D6
Krau *Indonesia* 63 E10
Kravanh, Chuor Phnum
 Cambodia 65 G4
Krefeld *Germany* 24 D2
Kremaston, L. *Greece* 46 C3
Kremen *Croatia* 41 D12
Kremenchuk *Ukraine* 33 H7
Kremenchuksk Vdskh.
 Ukraine 33 H7
Kremenets *Ukraine* 23 C13
Kremennaya *Ukraine* 33 H10
Kremges = Svitlovodsk
 Ukraine 33 H7
Kremmen *Germany* 24 C9
Kremmling *U.S.A.* 108 F10
Kremnica *Slovak Rep.* 27 C11
Krems *Austria* 26 C8
Kremsmünster *Austria* 26 C7
Krestena *Greece* 46 D3
Kretinga *Lithuania* 30 C8
Krettsy *Russia* 32 C7
Kreuzberg *Germany* 25 E5
Kreuztal *Germany* 24 E4
Kria Vrisi *Greece* 44 F6
Kribi *Cameroon* 83 E6
Krichem *Bulgaria* 45 D8
Krichev = Krychaw *Belarus* 23 B16
Kril'on, Mys *Russia* 54 B11
Krim *Slovenia* 41 C11
Krios, Akra *Greece* 49 D5
Krishna → *India* 67 M12
Krishnanagar *India* 69 H13
Kristdala *Sweden* 11 G10
Kristiansand *Norway* 9 G13
Kristianstad *Sweden* 11 H8
Kristiansund *Norway* 8 E12
Kristiinankaupunki *Finland* 8 E19
Kristinehamn *Sweden* 10 E8
Kristinestad =
 Kristiinankaupunki
 Finland 8 E19
Kriti *Greece* 49 D7
Kritsa *Greece* 49 D7
Kriva → *Macedonia* 44 D5
Kriva Palanka *Macedonia* 44 D6
Krivaja → *Bos.-H.* 28 F3
Krivelj *Serbia* 44 B5
Křivoklátsko △ *Czech Rep.* 26 A6
Krivoy Rog = Kryvyy Rih
 Ukraine 33 J7
Križevci *Croatia* 41 B13
Krk *Croatia* 41 C11
Krka *Slovenia* 41 C12
Krka → *Slovenia* 41 C12
Krka △ *Croatia* 41 E12
Krkonoše *Czech Rep.* 26 A8
Krkonoše △ *Czech Rep.* 26 A8
Krnov *Czech Rep.* 27 A10
Krobia *Poland* 31 G3
Krokees *Greece* 46 E4
Krokodil = Umgwenya →
 Mozam. 89 D5
Krokom *Sweden* 10 A8
Krokowa *Poland* 30 D5
Krolevets *Ukraine* 33 G7
Kroměříž *Czech Rep.* 27 B10
Kromy *Russia* 33 F8
Kronach *Germany* 25 E7
Krong Kaoh Kong *Cambodia* 65 G4
Kronobergs län □ *Sweden* 11 H8

Kronprins Christian Land
 Greenland 101
Kronprins Frederik Land
 Greenland 4 B5
Kronprins Olav Kyst
 Antarctica 5 C5
Kronprinsesse Märtha Kyst
 Antarctica 5 D2
Kronshtadt *Russia* 32 C5
Kroonstad △ *S. Africa* 88 D4
Kröpelin *Germany* 24 A7
Kropotkin *Russia* 35 H5
Kropp *Germany* 24 A5
Krosna *Lithuania* 30 D10
Krośniewice *Poland* 31 F6
Krosno *Poland* 31 J8
Krosno Odrzańskie *Poland* 31 F2
Krotoszyn *Poland* 31 G4
Krotovka *Russia* 34 D10
Krousonas *Greece* 49 D6
Krrabë *Albania* 44 E3
Krško *Slovenia* 41 C12
Krstača *Serbia* 44 D4
Kruger △ *S. Africa* 89 C5
Krugersdorp *S. Africa* 89 D4
Kruisfontein *S. Africa* 88 E3
Krujë *Albania* 44 E3
Krulevshchina =
 Krulyewshchyna *Belarus* 32 E4
Krulyewshchyna *Belarus* 32 E4
Krumbach *Germany* 25 G6
Krumë *Albania* 44 D4
Krumovgrad *Bulgaria* 45 E9
Krung Thep = Bangkok
 Thailand 64 F3
Krupanj *Serbia* 44 B3
Krupina *Slovak Rep.* 27 C12
Krupinica → *Slovak Rep.* 27 C11
Krupki *Belarus* 23 A15
Kruševac *Serbia* 44 C5
Kruševo *Macedonia* 44 E5
Krushelnyksya *Ukraine* 31 J10
Kruszwica *Poland* 31 F5
Krychaw *Belarus* 23 B16
Krymsk *Russia* 33 K10
Krymsky Poluostrov =
 Krymskyy Pivostriv
 Ukraine 33 K8
Krymskyy Pivostriv *Ukraine* 33 K8
Krynica *Poland* 31 J7
Krynica Morska *Poland* 30 D6
Krynki *Poland* 31 E10
Krynychne *Ukraine* 29 E13
Kryvyy Rih *Ukraine* 33 J7
Kryzhopil *Ukraine* 29 B13
Krzepice *Poland* 31 H5
Krzna → *Poland* 31 F10
Krzywiń *Poland* 31 G3
Krzyż Wielkopolski *Poland* 31 F2
Ksar el Kebir *Morocco* 78 B4
Ksar es Souk = Er Rachidia
 Morocco 78 B5
Ksiąz Wielkopolski *Poland* 31 F4
Kstovo *Russia* 34 B7
Ku, W. el → *Sudan* 81 E2
Kuah *Malaysia* 65 J2
Kuala Belait *Malaysia* 62 D4
Kuala Berang *Malaysia* 65 K4
Kuala Dungun = Dungun
 Malaysia 65 K4
Kuala Kangsar *Malaysia* 65 K3
Kuala Kelawang *Malaysia* 65 L4
Kuala Kerai *Malaysia* 65 K4
Kuala Kerian *Malaysia* 65 c
Kuala Kubu Bharu *Malaysia* 65 L4
Kuala Lipis *Malaysia* 65 K4
Kuala Lumpur *Malaysia* 65 L3
Kuala Nerang *Malaysia* 65 J3
Kuala Pilah *Malaysia* 65 L4
Kuala Rompin *Malaysia* 65 L4
Kuala Selangor *Malaysia* 65 L3
Kuala Sepetang *Malaysia* 65 K3
Kuala Terengganu *Malaysia* 65 K4
Kualajelai *Indonesia* 62 E4
Kualakapuas *Indonesia* 62 E4
Kualakurun *Indonesia* 62 E4
Kualapembuang *Indonesia* 62 E4
Kualasimpang *Indonesia* 62 D1
Kuancheng *China* 57 D10
Kuandang *Indonesia* 63 D6
Kuandian *China* 57 D13
Kuangchou = Guangzhou
 China 59 F9
Kuanshan *Taiwan* 59 F13
Kuantan *Malaysia* 65 L4
Kuba = Quba *Azerbaijan* 35 K9
Kuban → *Russia* 33 K9
Kuban Depression =
 Prikubanskaya
 Nizmennost *Russia* 35 H4
Kubaysah *Iraq* 73 G10
Kubenskoye, Ozero *Russia* 32 C5
Kubokawa *Japan* 55 H6
Kubu *Indonesia* 63 J18
Kubutambahan *Indonesia* 63 J18
Kucar, Tanjung *Indonesia* 63 K18
Kučevo *Serbia* 44 B5

Kuchaman *India* 68 F6
Kuchenspitze *Austria* 26 D3
Kuchinda *India* 69 J11
Kuching *Malaysia* 62 D4
Kuchino-eruba-Jima *Japan* 55 J5
Kuchinotsu *Japan* 55 H5
Kuchl *Austria* 26 D6
Kuchurhan → *Ukraine* 29 D14
Kucing = Kuching *Malaysia* 62 D4
Kuçovë *Albania* 44 D1
Küçükbahçe *Turkey* 47 C8
Küçükköy *Turkey* 47 B8
Küçükkuyu *Turkey* 47 B8
Küçükmenderes → *Turkey* 47 D9
Kud → *Pakistan* 68 F2
Kuda *India* 68 H4
Kudat *Malaysia* 62 C5
Kudirkos Naumiestis
  Lithuania 30 D9
Kudowa-Zdrój *Poland* 31 H3
Kudus *Indonesia* 63 G14
Kudymkar *Russia* 52 D6
Kueiyang = Guiyang *China* 58 D6
Kufra Oasis = Al Kufrah
  Libya 79 D10
Kufstein *Austria* 26 D5
Kugaaruk = Pelly Bay
  Canada 101 D14
Kugluktuk *Canada* 100 D8
Kugong I. *Canada* 104 A4
Küh Dasht *Iran* 73 F12
Küh-e-Jebāl Bārez *Iran* 71 D8
Kühak *Iran* 71 E9
Kuhan *Pakistan* 68 E2
Kühbonān *Iran* 71 D8
Kühestak *Iran* 71 E8
Kuhin *Iran* 71 B6
Kühīrī *Iran* 71 E9
Kuhmo *Finland* 8 D23
Kuhnsdorf *Austria* 26 E7
Kui Buri *Thailand* 65 F2
Kuiseb → *Namibia* 88 C1
Kuito *Angola* 85 G3
Kuiu I. *U.S.A.* 102 B2
Kujang *N. Korea* 57 E14
Kujawsko-Pomorskie □
  Poland 30 E5
Kuji *Japan* 54 D10
Kujū-San *Japan* 55 H5
Kukava *Ukraine* 29 B12
Kukavica *Serbia* 44 D5
Kukawa *Nigeria* 83 C7
Kukës *Albania* 44 D4
Kukmor *Russia* 34 B10
Kukup *Malaysia* 65 d
Kukup, Pulau *Malaysia* 65 d
Kukvidze *Russia* 34 E6
Kula *Bulgaria* 44 C6
Kula *Serbia* 28 E4
Kula *Turkey* 47 C10
Kulachi *Pakistan* 68 D4
Kulai *Malaysia* 65 M4
Kulaly, Ostrov = Kulaly
  Aral *Kazakhstan* 35 H10
Kulaly Aral *Kazakhstan* 35 H10
Kulasekarappattinam *India* 66 Q11
Kulautuva *Lithuania* 30 D10
Kuldīga *Latvia* 30 B8
Kuldīga □ *Latvia* 30 B8
Kuldu *Sudan* 81 E2
Kulebaki *Russia* 34 C6
Kulen *Cambodia* 64 F5
Kulen Vakuf *Bos.-H.* 41 D13
Kulgam *India* 69 C6
Kulgera *Australia* 94 D1
Kulim *Malaysia* 65 K3
Kulin *Australia* 93 F2
Kulkayu = Hartley Bay
  Canada 102 C3
Kullen *Sweden* 11 H6
Kullu *India* 68 D7
Kulmbach *Germany* 25 E7
Kulp *Turkey* 73 C9
Kulpawn → *Ghana* 83 D4
Kulsary = Qulsary
  Kazakhstan 52 E6
Kulti *India* 69 H12
Kulu *Turkey* 72 C5
Kulunda *Russia* 52 D8
Kulungar *Afghan.* 68 C3
Külvand *Iran* 71 D7
Kulwin *Australia* 95 F3
Kulyab = Kŭlob *Tajikistan* 52 F7
Kuma → *Russia* 35 H8
Kumafşarı *Turkey* 47 D11
Kumaganum *Nigeria* 83 C7
Kumagaya *Japan* 55 F9
Kumai *Indonesia* 62 E4
Kumalar Dağı *Turkey* 47 C12
Kumamba, Kepulauan
  Indonesia 63 E9
Kumamoto *Japan* 55 H5
Kumamoto □ *Japan* 55 H5
Kumanovo *Macedonia* 44 D5

Kumara *N.Z.* 91 E3
Kumarina Roadhouse
  Australia 93 D2
Kumasi *Ghana* 82 D4
Kumba *Cameroon* 83 E6
Kumbağ *Turkey* 45 F11
Kumbakonam *India* 66 P11
Kumbarilla *Australia* 95 D5
Kumbhraj *India* 68 G7
Kumbia *Australia* 95 D5
Kumbo *Cameroon* 83 D7
Kŭmch'ŏn *N. Korea* 57 E14
Kumdok *India* 69 C8
Kume-Shima *Japan* 55 L3
Kumeny *Russia* 34 A9
Kumharsain *India* 68 D7
Kumi *Uganda* 86 B3
Kumkale *Turkey* 45 G10
Kumla *Sweden* 10 E9
Kumluca *Turkey* 47 E12
Kumo *Nigeria* 83 C7
Kumo älv =
  Kokemäenjoki → *Finland* 32 B1
Kumon Bum *Burma* 67 F20
Kumylzhenskaya *Russia* 34 F6
Kunágota *Hungary* 28 D6
Kunashir, Ostrov *Russia* 53 E15
Kunda *Estonia* 32 C4
Kunda *India* 69 G9
Kundar → *Pakistan* 68 D3
Kundelungu △
  Dem. Rep. of the Congo 87 E2
Kundelungu Ouest △
  Dem. Rep. of the Congo 87 D2
Kundian *Pakistan* 68 C4
Kundla *India* 68 J4
Kung, Ao *Thailand* 65 a
Kunga → *Bangla.* 69 J13
Kungälv *Sweden* 11 G5
Kunghit I. *Canada* 102 C2
Kungrad = Qŭnghirot
  Uzbekistan 52 E6
Kungsängen *Sweden* 10 E11
Kungsbacka *Sweden* 11 G6
Kungsgården *Sweden* 10 D10
Kungshamn *Sweden* 11 F5
Kungsör *Sweden* 10 E10
Kungur *Russia* 52 D6
Kungurri *Australia* 94 b
Kunhar → *Pakistan* 69 B5
Kunhegyes *Hungary* 28 C5
Kuningan *Indonesia* 63 G13
Kunlong *Burma* 58 F2
Kunlun Shan *Asia* 60 C3
Kunmadaras *Hungary* 28 C5
Kunming *China* 58 E4
Kunmunya ☼ *Australia* 92 C3
Kunów *Poland* 31 H8
Kunshan *China* 59 B13
Kunszentmárton *Hungary* 28 D5
Kunszentmiklós *Hungary* 28 C4
Kuntaur *Senegal* 82 C2
Kununurra *Australia* 92 C4
Kunwari → *India* 69 F8
Kunya-Urgench =
  Köneürgench *Turkmenistan* 52 E6
Künzelsau *Germany* 25 F5
Kuopio *Finland* 8 E22
Kupa → *Croatia* 41 C13
Kupang *Indonesia* 63 F6
Kupreanof I. *U.S.A.* 102 B2
Kupres *Bos.-H.* 28 G2
Kupyansk *Ukraine* 33 H9
Kupyansk-Uzlovoi *Ukraine* 33 H9
Kuqa *China* 60 B3
Kür → *Azerbaijan* 73 C13
Kür Dili *Azerbaijan* 73 C13
Kura = Kür → *Azerbaijan* 73 C13
Kuranda *Australia* 94 B4
Kuranga *India* 68 H3
Kurashiki *Japan* 55 G6
Kurayn *Si. Arabia* 71 E6
Kurayoshi *Japan* 55 G6
Kŭrchatov *Kazakhstan* 52 D8
Kürdämir *Azerbaijan* 35 K9
Kurdistan *Asia* 73 D10
Kŭrdzhali *Bulgaria* 45 E9
Kure *Japan* 55 G6
Küre *Turkey* 72 B5
Küre Dağları *Turkey* 72 B6
Kure I. *U.S.A.* 107 K4
Kuressaare *Estonia* 32 C2
Kurgan *Russia* 52 D7
Kurganinsk *Russia* 35 H5
Kurgannaya =
  Kurganinsk *Russia* 35 H5
Kuri *India* 68 F4
Kuria Maria Is. =
  Hallāniyat, Jazā'ir al *Oman* 75 D6
Kuridala *Australia* 94 C3
Kurigram *Bangla.* 67 G16
Kurikka *Finland* 32 B4
Kuril Basin *Pac. Oc.* 4 E15
Kuril Is. = Kurilskiye
  Ostrova *Russia* 53 E16
Kuril-Kamchatka Trench
  Pac. Oc. 96 C7
Kurilsk *Russia* 53 E15

Kurilskiye Ostrova *Russia* 53 E16
Kurino *Japan* 55 J5
Kurinskaya Kosa = Kür
  Dili *Azerbaijan* 73 C13
Kurkur *Egypt* 80 C3
Kurkuta ☼ *Australia* 92 D4
Kurlovskiy *Russia* 34 C5
Kurmuk *Sudan* 81 E3
Kurnool *India* 66 M11
Kuro-Kagoshima, *Japan* 55 J4
Kuro-Shima *Okinawa, Japan* 55 M2
Kuror, J. *Sudan* 80 C3
Kurow *N.Z.* 91 F3
Kurów *Poland* 31 G9
Kurram → *Pakistan* 68 C4
Kurri Kurri *Australia* 95 E5
Kurrimine *Australia* 94 B4
Kursavka *Russia* 35 H6
Kurseong = Karsiyang *India* 69 F13
Kurshskaya Kosa △ *Russia* 30 C7
Kuršių Nerijos △ *Lithuania* 30 C8
Kursk *Russia* 33 G9
Kursk □ *Russia* 33 G9
Kuršumlija *Serbia* 44 C5
Kuršumlijska Banja *Serbia* 44 C5
Kurşunlu *Bursa, Turkey* 45 F13
Kurşunlu *Çankırı, Turkey* 72 B5
Kurtalan *Turkey* 73 D9
Kurtbey *Turkey* 45 E10
Kurtistown *U.S.A.* 107 M8
Kuru *Japan* 55 H7
Kuru, Bahr el → *Sudan* 81 F2
Kurucaşile *Turkey* 72 B5
Kuruçay *Turkey* 73 C8
Kurukshetra = Thanesar
  India 68 D7
Kuruktag *China* 60 B3
Kuruman *S. Africa* 88 D3
Kuruman → *S. Africa* 88 D3
Kurume *Japan* 55 H5
Kurun → *Sudan* 81 F3
Kurunegala *Sri Lanka* 66 R12
Kurya *Russia* 52 C6
Kus Gölü *Turkey* 45 F11
Kuşadası *Turkey* 72 D2
Kuşadası Körfezi *Turkey* 47 D8
Kusamba *Indonesia* 63 K18
Kusatsu *Japan* 55 F9
Kusawa L. *Canada* 102 A1
Kusel *Germany* 25 F3
Kushaka *Nigeria* 83 C6
Kushalgarh *India* 68 H6
Kushchevskaya *Russia* 35 G4
Kusheriki *Nigeria* 83 C6
Kushikino *Japan* 55 J5
Kushima *Japan* 55 J5
Kushimoto *Japan* 55 H7
Kushiro *Japan* 54 C12
Kushiro-Gawa → *Japan* 54 C12
Kushiro Shitsugen △ *Japan* 54 C12
Kŭshk *Iran* 71 D8
Kushka = Serhetabat
  Turkmenistan 71 C9
Kushnytsya *Ukraine* 29 B8
Kushol *India* 69 C7
Kushtia *Bangla.* 67 H16
Kuskokwim → *U.S.A.* 106 C7
Kuskokwim B. *U.S.A.* 106 D7
Kuskokwim Mts. *U.S.A.* 106 C8
Kusmi *India* 69 H9
Kusŏng *N. Korea* 57 E13
Kussharo-Ko *Japan* 54 C12
Kustanay = Qostanay
  Kazakhstan 52 D7
Kut, Ko *Thailand* 65 G4
Kuta *Indonesia* 63 K18
Kütahya *Turkey* 47 B12
Kütahya □ *Turkey* 47 B11
Kutaisi *Georgia* 35 J6
Kutaraja = Banda Aceh
  Indonesia 62 C1
Kutch, Gulf of = Kachchh,
  Gulf of *India* 68 H3
Kutch, Rann of =
  Kachchh, Rann of *India* 68 H4
Kutina *Croatia* 41 C13
Kutiyana *India* 68 J4
Kutjevo *Croatia* 28 E2
Kutkashen *Azerbaijan* 35 K8
Kutná Hora *Czech Rep.* 26 B8
Kutno *Poland* 31 F6
Kutse *Botswana* 88 C3
Kuttabul *Australia* 94 b
Kutu *Dem. Rep. of the Congo* 84 E3
Kutum *Sudan* 81 E1
Kúty *Slovak Rep.* 27 C10
Kuty *Ukraine* 29 B10
Kuujjuaq *Canada* 101 F18
Kuujjuarapik *Canada* 104 A4
Kuusamo *Finland* 8 D23
Kuusankoski *Finland* 32 B4
Kuvshinovo *Russia* 32 D8
Kuwait = Al Kuwayt *Kuwait* 70 D5
Kuwait ■ *Asia* 70 D5
Kuwana *Japan* 55 G8
Kuwana → *Japan* 69 F10
Kuybyshev = Samara
  Russia 34 D10
Kuybyshev *Russia* 52 D8

Kuybyshevo *Ukraine* 33 J9
Kuybyshevskoye Vdkhr.
  Russia 34 C9
Kuye He → *China* 56 E6
Kūyeh *Iran* 70 B5
Kuyto, Ozero *Russia* 8 D24
Kuyucak *Turkey* 47 D10
Kuyumba *Russia* 53 C10
Kuzey Anadolu Dağları
  Turkey 72 B7
Kuzmin *Serbia* 28 E4
Kuznetsk *Russia* 34 D8
Kuzomen *Russia* 52 C4
Kvænangen *Norway* 8 A19
Kværndrup *Denmark* 11 J4
Kvaløya *Norway* 8 B18
Kvänum *Sweden* 11 F7
Kvareli = Qvareli *Georgia* 35 K7
Kvarner *Croatia* 41 D11
Kvarnerič *Croatia* 41 D11
Kvicksund *Sweden* 10 E10
Kvillsfors *Sweden* 11 G9
Kvinesdal *Sweden* 10 E10
Kvisgleby *Sweden* 10 B11
Kvismare kanal *Sweden* 10 E9
Kwabhaca *S. Africa* 89 E4
Kwahaca = Mount Frere
  S. Africa 89 E4
Kwajalein *Marshall Is.* 96 G8
Kwakhanai *Botswana* 88 C3
Kwakoegron *Suriname* 125 B7
Kwale *Kenya* 86 C4
Kwale *Nigeria* 83 D6
KwaMashu *S. Africa* 89 D5
Kwando → *Africa* 88 B3
Kwangchow = Guangzhou
  China 59 F9
Kwango →
  Dem. Rep. of the Congo 84 E3
Kwangsi-Chuang =
  Guangxi Zhuangzu
  Zizhiqu □ *China* 58 F7
Kwangtung =
  Guangdong □ *China* 59 F9
Kwara □ *Nigeria* 83 D6
Kwataboahegan → *Canada* 104 B3
Kwatisore *Indonesia* 63 E8
KwaZulu Natal □ *S. Africa* 89 D5
Kweichow = Guizhou □
  China 58 D6
Kwekwe *Zimbabwe* 87 F2
Kwidzyn *Poland* 31 B5
Kwiha *Ethiopia* 81 E4
Kwilu →
  Dem. Rep. of the Congo 84 E3
Kwinana *Australia* 93 F2
Kwisa → *Poland* 31 G2
Kwoka *Indonesia* 63 E8
Kwolla *Nigeria* 83 D6
Kyabra Cr. → *Australia* 95 D3
Kyabram *Australia* 95 F4
Kyaikto *Burma* 64 D1
Kyakhta *Russia* 53 D11
Kyambura → *Uganda* 86 C3
Kyancutta *Australia* 95 E2
Kyaukpadaung *Burma* 67 J19
Kyaukpyu *Burma* 67 K18
Kyaukse *Burma* 67 J20
Kybartai *Lithuania* 30 D9
Kyburz *U.S.A.* 110 G6
Kyelang *India* 68 C7
Kyenjojo *Uganda* 86 B3
Kyjov *Czech Rep.* 27 B10
Kyle *Canada* 103 C7
Kyle Dam *Zimbabwe* 87 G3
Kyle of Lochalsh *U.K.* 13 D3
Kyll → *Germany* 25 E2
Kyllburg *Germany* 25 E2
Kyllini *Greece* 46 D3
Kymijoki → *Finland* 32 B4
Kymmene älv =
  Kymijoki → *Finland* 32 B4
Kyneton *Australia* 95 F3
Kynuna *Australia* 94 C3
Kyō-ga-Saki *Japan* 55 G7
Kyoga, L. *Uganda* 86 B3
Kyogle *Australia* 95 D5
Kyom → *Sudan* 81 F2
Kyŏngju = Gyeongju
  S. Korea 57 G15
Kyŏngsŏng *N. Korea* 57 D15
Kyonpyaw *Burma* 67 L19
Kyōto *Japan* 55 G7
Kyōto □ *Japan* 55 G7
Kyparissovouno *Cyprus* 49 D12
Kyperounda *Cyprus* 49 E11
Kypros = Cyprus ■ *Asia* 49 E12
Kyrenia *Cyprus* 49 D12
Kyritz *Germany* 24 C8
Kyrgyzstan ■ *Asia* 52 E8
Kyrkhult *Sweden* 11 H8
Kyrnasivka *Ukraine* 29 B13
Kyrnychky *Ukraine* 29 E14
Kyro älv = Kyrönjoki →
  Finland 8 E19
Kyrönjoki → *Finland* 8 E19
Kystatyam *Russia* 53 C13
Kysucké Nové Mesto
  Slovak Rep. 27 B11
Kytay, Ozero *Ukraine* 29 E14
Kythira *Greece* 46 E5
Kythréa *Cyprus* 49 D12

Kyunhla *Burma* 67 H19
Kyuquot Sound *Canada* 102 D3
Kyurdamir = Kürdämir
  Azerbaijan 35 K9
Kyūshū *Japan* 55 H5
Kyūshū □ *Japan* 55 H5
Kyushu-Palau Ridge *Pac. Oc.* 96 E5
Kyūshū-Sanchi *Japan* 55 H5
Kyustendil *Bulgaria* 44 D6
Kyusyur *Russia* 53 B13
Kyyiv *Ukraine* 23 C16
Kyyiv □ *Ukraine* 33 G6
Kyyivske Vdskh. *Ukraine* 23 C16
Kyzyl *Russia* 53 D10
Kyzyl Kum *Uzbekistan* 52 E7
Kyzyl-Kyya *Kyrgyzstan* 52 E8
Kyzyl Orda = Qyzylorda
  Kazakhstan 52 E7

L

La Albuera *Spain* 37 G4
La Alcarria *Spain* 38 E2
La Almarcha *Spain* 38 F2
La Almunia de Doña
  Godina *Spain* 38 D3
La Amistad △ *Cent. Amer.* 120 E3
La Asunción *Venezuela* 124 A6
La Baie *Canada* 105 C5
La Banda *Argentina* 126 B3
La Bañeza *Spain* 36 C5
La Barca *Mexico* 118 C4
La Barge *U.S.A.* 108 E8
La Barra *Nic.* 120 D3
La Bastide-Puylaurent
  France 20 D7
La Baule *France* 18 E4
La Belle *U.S.A.* 117 H14
La Biche → *Canada* 102 B4
La Biche, L. *Canada* 102 B6
La Bisbal d'Empordà *Spain* 38 D8
La Brea *Trin. & Tob.* 125 K15
La Brède *France* 20 D3
La Bresse *France* 19 D13
La Bureba *Spain* 36 C7
La Calera *Chile* 126 C1
La Campana △ *Chile* 126 C1
La Campiña *Spain* 37 H6
La Canal = Sa Canal *Spain* 48 C7
La Cañiza = A Cañiza *Spain* 36 C2
La Canourgue *France* 20 D7
La Capelle *France* 19 C10
La Carlota *Argentina* 126 C3
La Carlota *Phil.* 61 F5
La Carlota *Spain* 37 H6
La Carolina *Spain* 37 G7
La Cavalerie *France* 20 D7
La Ceiba *Honduras* 120 C2
La Chaise-Dieu *France* 20 C7
La Chapelle d'Angillon
  France 19 E9
La Chapelle-St-Luc *France* 19 D11
La Chapelle-sur-Erdre *France* 18 E5
La Charité-sur-Loire *France* 19 E10
La Chartre-sur-le-Loir *France* 18 E7
La Châtaigneraie *France* 20 B3
La Châtre *France* 19 F9
La Chaux-de-Fonds *Switz.* 25 H2
La Chorrera *Panama* 120 E4
La Ciotat *France* 21 E9
La Clayette *France* 19 F11
La Cocha *Argentina* 126 B2
La Concepción *Panama* 120 E3
La Concordia *Mexico* 119 D6
La Coruña = A Coruña *Spain* 36 B2
La Côte-St-André *France* 21 C9
La Courtine *France* 20 C6
La Crau *Bouches-du-Rhône,*
  France 21 E8
La Crau *Var, France* 21 E10
La Crescent *U.S.A.* 112 D8
La Crete *Canada* 102 B5
La Crosse *Kans., U.S.A.* 112 F4
La Crosse *Wis., U.S.A.* 112 D8
La Cruz *Costa Rica* 120 D2
La Cruz *Mexico* 118 C3
La Désirade *Guadeloupe* 120 b
La Digue *Seychelles* 85 b
La Esperanza *Cuba* 120 B3
La Esperanza *Honduras* 120 D2
La Estrada = A Estrada *Spain* 36 C2
La Faouët *France* 18 D3
La Fayette *U.S.A.* 117 D12
La Fé *Cuba* 120 B3
La Fère *France* 19 C10
La Ferté-Bernard *France* 18 D7
La Ferté-Gaucher *France* 19 D10
La Ferté-Macé *France* 18 D6
La Ferté-St-Aubin *France* 19 E8
La Ferté-sous-Jouarre
  France 19 D10
La Ferté-Vidame *France* 18 D7
La Flèche *France* 18 E6
La Follette *U.S.A.* 117 C12
La Fregeneda *Spain* 36 E4
La Fuente de San Esteban
  Spain 36 E4
La Gacilly *France* 18 E4
La Gineta *Spain* 39 F2

La Grand'Combe *France* 21 D8
La Grande *U.S.A.* 108 D4
La Grande → *Canada* 104 B5
La Grande 3, Rés. *Canada* 104 B4
La Grande 4, Rés. *Canada* 104 B5
La Grande-Motte *France* 21 E8
La Grange *Calif., U.S.A.* 110 H6
La Grange *Ga., U.S.A.* 117 E12
La Grange *Ky., U.S.A.* 113 F11
La Grange *Tex., U.S.A.* 116 G6
La Grave *France* 21 C10
La Guaira *Venezuela* 124 A5
La Guardia = A Guarda
  Spain 36 D2
La Gudiña = A Gudiña *Spain* 36 C3
La Guerche-de-Bretagne
  France 18 E5
La Guerche-sur-l'Aubois
  France 19 F9
La Habana *Cuba* 120 B3
La Haute Vallée de
  Chevreuse △ *France* 19 D8
La Haye-du-Puits *France* 18 C5
La Horra *Spain* 36 D7
La Independencia *Mexico* 119 D6
La Isabela *Dom. Rep.* 121 C5
La Jonquera *Spain* 38 C7
La Junta *U.S.A.* 108 H12
La Laguna *Canary Is.* 48 F3
La Libertad = Puerto
  Libertad *Mexico* 118 B2
La Libertad *Guatemala* 120 C1
La Ligua *Chile* 126 C1
La Línea de la Concepción
  Spain 37 J5
La Loche *Canada* 103 B7
La Londe-les-Maures *France* 21 E10
La Lora *Spain* 36 C7
La Loupe *France* 18 D8
La Louvière *Belgium* 17 D4
La Lune *Trin. & Tob.* 125 K15
La Machine *France* 19 F10
La Maddalena *Italy* 42 A2
La Malbaie *Canada* 105 C5
La Malinche △ *Mexico* 119 D5
La Mancha *Spain* 39 F2
La Mariña *Spain* 36 B3
La Martre, L. *Canada* 102 A5
La Mesa *Mexico* 111 N10
La Mesa *U.S.A.* 111 N9
La Mesilla *U.S.A.* 109 K10
La Misión *Mexico* 118 A1
La Mothe-Achard *France* 18 F5
La Motte-Chalançon *France* 21 D9
La Motte-du-Caire *France* 21 D10
La Motte-Servolex *France* 21 C9
La Moure *U.S.A.* 112 B4
La Muela *Spain* 38 D3
La Mure *France* 21 D9
La Negra *Chile* 126 A1
La Oliva *Canary Is.* 48 F6
La Orotava *Canary Is.* 48 F3
La Oroya *Peru* 124 F3
La Pacaudière *France* 19 F10
La Palma *Canary Is.* 48 F2
La Palma *Panama* 120 E4
La Palma del Condado *Spain* 37 H4
La Paloma *Chile* 126 C1
La Pampa □ *Argentina* 126 D2
La Paragua *Venezuela* 124 B6
La Paz *Entre Ríos, Argentina* 126 C4
La Paz *San Luis, Argentina* 126 C2
La Paz *Bolivia* 124 G5
La Paz *Honduras* 120 D2
La Paz *Mexico* 118 C2
La Paz *Phil.* 61 D4
La Paz Centro *Nic.* 120 D2
La Pedrera *Colombia* 124 D5
La Pérade *Canada* 105 C5
La Perla *Mexico* 118 B4
La Perouse Str. *Asia* 54 B11
La Pesca *Mexico* 119 C5
La Piedad *Mexico* 118 C4
La Pine *U.S.A.* 108 E3
La Plata *Argentina* 126 C4
La Pobla de Lillet *Spain* 38 C6
La Pobla de Segur *Spain* 38 C5
La Pocatière *Canada* 105 C5
La Pola de Gordón *Spain* 36 C5
La Porta *France* 21 F13
La Porte *U.S.A.* 114 E2
La Presanella *Italy* 40 B7
La Puebla = Sa Pobla *Spain* 38 F8
La Puebla de Cazalla *Spain* 37 H5
La Puebla de los Infantes
  Spain 37 H5
La Puebla de Montalbán
  Spain 36 F6
La Puebla del Río *Spain* 37 H4
La Puerta de Segura *Spain* 37 G8
La Purísima *Mexico* 118 B2
La Push *U.S.A.* 110 C2
La Quiaca *Argentina* 126 A2
La Réole *France* 20 D3
La Restinga *Canary Is.* 48 G2
La Rioja *Argentina* 126 B2
La Rioja □ *Argentina* 126 B2
La Rioja □ *Spain* 38 C2
La Robla *Spain* 36 C5

La Roche-Bernard *France* 18 E4
La Roche-Canillac *France* 20 C5
La Roche-en-Ardenne
  Belgium 17 D5
La Roche-sur-Foron *France* 19 F13
La Roche-sur-Yon *France* 18 F5
La Rochefoucauld *France* 20 C4
La Rochelle *France* 20 B2
La Roda *Spain* 39 F2
La Roda de Andalucía *Spain* 37 H6
La Romaine *Canada* 105 B7
La Romana *Dom. Rep.* 121 C6
La Ronge *Canada* 103 B7
La Rumorosa *Mexico* 111 N10
La Sabina = Sa Savina *Spain* 48 C7
La Sagra *Spain* 39 H2
La Salle *U.S.A.* 112 E9
La Sanabria *Spain* 36 C4
La Santa *Canary Is.* 48 E6
La Sarre *Canada* 104 C4
La Scie *Canada* 105 C8
La Selva *Spain* 38 C7
La Selva Beach *U.S.A.* 110 J5
La Selva del Camp *Spain* 38 D6
La Serena *Chile* 126 B1
La Serena *Spain* 37 G5
La Seu d'Urgell *Spain* 38 C6
La Seyne-sur-Mer *France* 21 E9
La Sila *Italy* 43 C9
La Solana *Spain* 37 G7
La Soufrière *St. Vincent* 121 D7
La Souterraine *France* 19 F8
La Spézia *Italy* 40 D6
La Suze-sur-Sarthe *France* 18 E7
La Tagua *Colombia* 124 C4
La Teste-de-Buch *France* 20 D2
La Tortuga *Venezuela* 121 D6
La Tour-du-Pin *France* 21 C9
La Tranche-sur-Mer *France* 18 F5
La Tremblade *France* 20 C2
La Trinité *Martinique* 120 c
La Tuque *Canada* 104 C5
La Unión *Chile* 128 E2
La Unión *El Salv.* 120 D2
La Unión *Mexico* 118 D4
La Unión *Spain* 39 H4
La Urbana *Venezuela* 124 B5
La Vache Pt. *Trin. & Tob.* 125 K15
La Vall d'Uixó *Spain* 38 F4
La Vecilla *Spain* 36 C5
La Vega *Dom. Rep.* 121 C5
La Vela de Coro *Venezuela* 124 A5
La Veleta *Spain* 37 H7
La Venta *Mexico* 119 D6
La Vergne *U.S.A.* 117 C11
La Villa Joiosa =
  Villajoyosa *Spain* 39 G4
La Voulte-sur-Rhône *France* 21 D8
Laa an der Thaya *Austria* 27 C9
Laaber, Grosse → *Germany* 25 G8
Laage *Germany* 24 B8
Laascaanood = Las Anod
  Somali Rep. 75 F4
Laatzen *Germany* 24 C5
Laba → *Russia* 35 H4
Labasa *Fiji* 91 a
Labason *Phil.* 61 G5
Labastide-Murat *France* 20 D5
Labastide-Rouairoux *France* 20 E6
Labbézenga *Mali* 83 B5
Labdah = Leptis Magna
  Libya 79 B8
Labe = Elbe → *Europe* 24 B4
Labé *Guinea* 82 C2
Laberge, L. *Canada* 102 A1
Labin *Croatia* 41 C11
Labinsk *Russia* 35 H5
Labis *Malaysia* 65 L4
Labiszyn *Poland* 31 F4
Labo *Phil.* 61 D5
Laboe *Germany* 24 A6
Laborec → *Slovak Rep.* 27 C14
Laborie *St. Lucia* 121 f
Labouheyre *France* 20 D3
Laboulaye *Argentina* 126 C3
Labrador *Canada* 105 B7
Labrador City *Canada* 105 B6
Labrador Sea *Atl. Oc.* 101 F21
Lábrea *Brazil* 124 E6
Labruguière *France* 20 E6
Labuan *Malaysia* 62 C5
Labuan, Pulau *Malaysia* 62 C5
Labuha *Indonesia* 63 E7
Labuhan *Indonesia* 63 G11
Labuhanbajo *Indonesia* 63 F6
Labuhanbilik *Indonesia* 65 L3
Labuk, Telok *Malaysia* 62 C5
Labyrinth, L. *Australia* 95 E2
Labytnangi *Russia* 52 C7
Laç *Albania* 44 E3
Lac-Bouchette *Canada* 105 C5
Lac Édouard *Canada* 104 C5
Lac La Biche *Canada* 102 C6
Lac la Martre = Wha Ti
  Canada 100 E8
Lac La Ronge △ *Canada* 103 B7
Lac-Mégantic *Canada* 105 C5
Lac Thien *Vietnam* 64 F7
Lacanau *France* 20 D2

Lacanau, Étang de *France* 20 D2
Lacantún → *Mexico* 119 D6
Lácara → *Spain* 37 G4
Lacaune *France* 20 E6
Lacaune, Mts. de *France* 20 E6
Laccadive Is. =
  Lakshadweep Is. *India* 3 D13
Lacepede B. *Australia* 95 F2
Lacepede Is. *Australia* 92 C3
Lacerdónia *Mozam.* 87 F4
Lacey *U.S.A.* 110 C4
Lachania *Greece* 49 D9
Lachhmangarh *India* 68 F6
Lachi *Pakistan* 68 C4
Lachine *Canada* 104 C5
Lachlan → *Australia* 95 E3
Lachute *Canada* 104 C5
Lackagh Hills *Ireland* 12 B3
Lackawanna *U.S.A.* 114 D6
Lackawaxen *U.S.A.* 115 E10
Lacolle *Canada* 115 A11
Lacombe *Canada* 102 C6
Lacona *U.S.A.* 115 C8
Láconi *Italy* 42 C2
Laconia *U.S.A.* 115 C13
Lacq *France* 20 E3
Ladakh Ra. *India* 69 C8
Ladek-Zdrój *Poland* 31 H3
Lådik *Turkey* 72 B6
Ladismith *S. Africa* 88 E3
Ladíspoli *Italy* 41 G9
Ladíz *Iran* 71 D9
Ladnun *India* 68 F6
Ladoga, L. = Ladozhskoye
  Ozero *Russia* 32 B6
Ladonas → *Greece* 46 D3
Ladozhskoye Ozero *Russia* 32 B6
Ladushkin *Russia* 30 D7
Lady Elliott I. *Australia* 94 C5
Lady Grey *S. Africa* 88 E4
Ladybrand *S. Africa* 88 D4
Ladysmith *Canada* 110 B3
Ladysmith *S. Africa* 89 D4
Ladysmith *U.S.A.* 112 C8
Ladyzhyn *Ukraine* 29 B14
Lae *Papua N. G.* 90 B7
Laem Hin Khom *Thailand* 65 b
Laem Khat *Thailand* 65 a
Laem Nga *Thailand* 65 a
Laem Ngop *Thailand* 65 F4
Laem Phan Wa *Thailand* 65 a
Laem Pho *Thailand* 65 J3
Laem Phrom Thep *Thailand* 65 a
Laem Riang *Thailand* 65 a
Laem Sam Rong *Thailand* 65 b
Laem Son *Thailand* 65 a
Laem Yamu *Thailand* 65 a
Laerma *Greece* 49 C9
Læsø *Denmark* 11 G5
Læsø Rende *Denmark* 11 G4
Lafayette *Ind., U.S.A.* 112 E10
Lafayette *La., U.S.A.* 116 F8
Lafayette *Tenn., U.S.A.* 117 C11
Laferte → *Canada* 102 A5
Lafia *Nigeria* 83 D6
Lafiagi *Nigeria* 83 D6
Lafkos *Greece* 46 B5
Lafleche *Canada* 103 D7
Lafon *Sudan* 81 F3
Lagan *Sweden* 11 H7
Lagan → *Sweden* 11 H6
Lagan → *U.K.* 12 B6
Lagarfljót → *Iceland* 8 D6
Lagdo, L. de *Cameroon* 79 G8
Lage *Germany* 24 D4
Lågen → *Oppland, Norway* 8 F14
Lågen → *Vestfold, Norway* 9 G14
Lägerdorf *Germany* 24 B5
Lages *Brazil* 127 B5
Laghouat *Algeria* 78 B6
Lagnieu *France* 21 C9
Lagny-sur-Marne *France* 19 D9
Lago *Italy* 43 C9
Lago de Sanabria y
  Entorno △ *Spain* 36 C4
Lagôa *Portugal* 37 H2
Lagoa do Peixe △ *Brazil* 127 C5
Lagoa Vermelha *Brazil* 127 B5
Lagoaça *Portugal* 36 D4
Lagodekhi *Georgia* 35 K8
Lagónegro *Italy* 43 B8
Lagonoy G. *Phil.* 61 E5
Lagos *Greece* 45 E9
Lagos *Nigeria* 83 D5
Lagos *Portugal* 37 H2
Lagos □ *Nigeria* 83 D5
Lagos de Moreno *Mexico* 118 C4
Lagrange = Bidyadanga
  Australia 92 C3
Lagrange B. *Australia* 92 C3
Laguardia *Spain* 38 C2
Laguépie *France* 20 D5
Laguna *Brazil* 127 B6
Laguna *U.S.A.* 109 J10
Laguna, Sa. de la *Mexico* 118 C3
Laguna Beach *U.S.A.* 111 M9
Laguna de Duera *Spain* 36 D6
Laguna de la Restinga △
  Venezuela 121 D6

Laguna de Lachuá △
  Guatemala 120 C1
Laguna del Laja △ *Chile* 126 D1
Laguna del Tigre =
  Guatemala 120 C1
Laguna Limpia *Argentina* 126 B4
Lagunas *Chile* 126 A2
Lagunas *Peru* 124 E3
Lagunas de Chacahua △
  Mexico 119 D5
Lagunas de Montebello △
  Mexico 119 D6
Lagunas de Ruidera △ *Spain* 39 G2
Lahad Datu *Malaysia* 63 D5
Lahad Datu, Telok *Malaysia* 63 D5
Lahan Sai *Thailand* 64 E4
Lahanam *Laos* 64 D5
Lahar *India* 69 F8
Laharpur *India* 69 F9
Lahat *Indonesia* 62 E2
Lahewa *Indonesia* 62 D1
Lāhījān *Iran* 71 B6
Lahn → *Germany* 25 E3
Lahnstein *Germany* 25 E3
Laholm *Sweden* 11 H7
Laholmsbukten *Sweden* 11 H6
Lahore *Pakistan* 68 D6
Lahr *Germany* 25 G3
Lahri *Pakistan* 68 E3
Lāhrūd *Iran* 73 C12
Lahti *Finland* 32 B3
Lahtis = Lahti *Finland* 32 B3
Laï *Chad* 79 G9
Lai Chau *Vietnam* 58 F4
Lai'an *China* 59 A12
Laibin *China* 58 F7
Laifeng *China* 58 C7
L'Aigle *France* 18 D7
Laignes *France* 19 E11
L'Aiguillon-sur-Mer *France* 20 B2
Laila = Layla *Si. Arabia* 75 C4
Laingsburg *S. Africa* 88 E3
Lainioälven → *Sweden* 8 C20
Lairg *U.K.* 13 C4
Laisamis *Kenya* 86 B4
Laishui *China* 56 E8
Laissac *France* 20 D6
Laiwu *China* 57 F9
Laixi *China* 57 F11
Laiyang *China* 57 F11
Laiyuan *China* 56 E8
Laizhou *China* 57 F10
Laizhou Wan *China* 57 F10
Laja → *Mexico* 118 C4
Lajamanu *Australia* 92 C5
Lajere *Nigeria* 83 C7
Lajkovac *Serbia* 44 B4
Lajosmizse *Hungary* 28 C4
Lak Sao *Laos* 64 C5
Lakaband *Pakistan* 68 D3
Lakamané *Mali* 82 C3
Lake *U.S.A.* 108 D8
Lake Alpine *U.S.A.* 110 G7
Lake Andes *U.S.A.* 112 D4
Lake Arthur *U.S.A.* 116 F8
Lake Bindegolly △ *Australia* 95 D3
Lake Cargelligo *Australia* 95 E4
Lake Charles *U.S.A.* 116 F8
Lake City *Colo., U.S.A.* 108 G10
Lake City *Fla., U.S.A.* 117 F13
Lake City *Mich., U.S.A.* 113 C11
Lake City *Minn., U.S.A.* 112 C7
Lake City *Pa., U.S.A.* 114 D4
Lake City *S.C., U.S.A.* 117 E15
Lake Cowichan *Canada* 102 D4
Lake District △ *U.K.* 14 C4
Lake Elsinore *U.S.A.* 111 M9
Lake Eyre △ *Australia* 95 D2
Lake Gairdner △ *Australia* 95 E2
Lake George *U.S.A.* 115 C11
Lake Grace *Australia* 93 F2
Lake Gregory ◎ *Australia* 92 D4
Lake Harbour = Kimmirut
  Canada 101 E18
Lake Havasu City *U.S.A.* 111 L12
Lake Hughes *U.S.A.* 111 L8
Lake Isabella *U.S.A.* 111 K8
Lake Jackson *U.S.A.* 116 G7
Lake King *Australia* 93 F2
Lake Lenore *Canada* 103 C8
Lake Louise *Canada* 102 C5
Lake Mackay ◎ *Australia* 92 D4
Lake Mburo △ *Uganda* 86 C3
Lake Mead △ *U.S.A.* 111 K12
Lake Meredith △ *U.S.A.* 116 D4
Lake Mills *U.S.A.* 112 D7
Lake Nakuru △ *Kenya* 86 C4
Lake Placid *U.S.A.* 115 B11
Lake Pleasant *U.S.A.* 115 C10
Lake Providence *U.S.A.* 116 E9
Lake Roosevelt △ *U.S.A.* 108 B4
Lake St. Peter *Canada* 114 A6
Lake Superior △ *Canada* 104 C3
Lake Torrens △ *Australia* 95 E2
Lake Village *U.S.A.* 116 E9
Lake Wales *U.S.A.* 117 H14
Lake Worth *U.S.A.* 117 H14
Lakeba *Fiji* 91 a

Lakeba Passage *Fiji* 91 a
Lakefield *Canada* 114 B6
Lakefield △ *Australia* 94 B3
Lakehurst *U.S.A.* 115 F10
Lakeland *Australia* 94 B3
Lakeland *U.S.A.* 117 G14
Lakemba = Lakeba *Fiji* 91 a
Lakeport *Calif., U.S.A.* 110 F4
Lakeport *Mich., U.S.A.* 114 C2
Lakes Entrance *Australia* 95 F4
Lakeside *Calif., U.S.A.* 111 N10
Lakeside *Nebr., U.S.A.* 112 D2
Lakeview *U.S.A.* 108 E3
Lakeville *U.S.A.* 112 C7
Lakewood *Colo., U.S.A.* 108 G11
Lakewood *N.J., U.S.A.* 115 F10
Lakewood *N.Y., U.S.A.* 114 D5
Lakewood *Ohio, U.S.A.* 114 E3
Lakewood *Wash., U.S.A.* 110 C4
Lakha *India* 68 F4
Lakhimpur *India* 69 F9
Lakhisarai *India* 69 G12
Lakhnadon *India* 69 H8
Lakhnau = Lucknow *India* 69 F9
Lakhonpheng *Laos* 64 E5
Lakhpat *India* 68 H3
Läki *Azerbaijan* 35 K8
Lakin *U.S.A.* 112 G3
Lakitusaki → *Canada* 104 B3
Lakki *Greece* 49 D5
Lakki *Pakistan* 68 C4
Lakonia □ *Greece* 46 E4
Lakonikos Kolpos *Greece* 46 E4
Lakor *Indonesia* 63 F7
Lakota *Ivory C.* 82 D3
Lakota *U.S.A.* 112 A4
Laksefjorden *Norway* 8 A22
Lakselv *Norway* 8 A21
Lakshadweep Is. *India* 3 D13
Lakshmanpur *India* 69 H10
Lakshmikantapur *India* 69 H13
Lala Musa *Pakistan* 68 C5
Lalaghat *India* 67 G18
Lalago *Tanzania* 86 C3
Lalapanzi *Zimbabwe* 87 F3
Lalapaşa *Turkey* 45 E10
Lalbenque *France* 20 D5
L'Albufera *Spain* 39 F4
L'Alcora *Spain* 38 E4
L'Alfàs del Pi *Spain* 39 G4
Lalganj *India* 69 G11
Lalgola *India* 69 G13
Lālī *Iran* 71 C6
Lalibela *Ethiopia* 81 E4
Lalin *China* 57 B14
Lalín *Spain* 36 C2
Lalin He → *China* 57 B13
Lalinde *France* 20 D4
Lalitapur *Nepal* 69 F11
Lalitpur *India* 69 G8
Lalkua *India* 69 E8
Lalsot *India* 68 F7
Lam Pao Res. *Thailand* 64 D4
Lama Kara *Togo* 83 D5
Lamae *Thailand* 65 H2
Lamaing *Burma* 64 E1
Lamar *Colo., U.S.A.* 108 G12
Lamar *Mo., U.S.A.* 112 G6
Lamas *Peru* 124 E3
Lamastre *France* 21 D8
Lamayuru *India* 69 B7
Lambach *Austria* 26 C6
Lamballe *France* 18 D4
Lambaréné *Gabon* 84 E2
Lambasa = Labasa *Fiji* 91 a
Lambay I. *Ireland* 12 C5
Lambert's Bay *S. Africa* 88 E2
Lambesc *France* 21 E9
Lambeth *Canada* 114 D3
Lambia *Greece* 46 D3
Lambomakondro *Madag.* 89 C7
Lambro → *Italy* 40 C6
Lambton Shores *Canada* 114 C3
Lame *Nigeria* 83 C6
Lame Deer *U.S.A.* 108 D10
Lamego *Portugal* 36 D3
Lamèque *Canada* 105 C7
Lameroo *Australia* 95 F3
Lamesa *U.S.A.* 116 E4
Lamia *Greece* 46 C4
Lamington △ *Australia* 95 D5
Lamitan *Phil.* 61 H5
Lammermuir Hills *U.K.* 13 F6
Lammhult *Sweden* 11 G8
Lamoille → *U.S.A.* 115 B11
Lamon B. *Phil.* 61 D5
Lamont *Canada* 102 C6
Lamont *Calif., U.S.A.* 111 K8
Lamont *Wyo., U.S.A.* 108 E10
Lamotte-Beuvron *France* 19 E9
Lampa *Peru* 124 G4
Lampang *Thailand* 64 C2
Lampasas *U.S.A.* 116 F5
Lampazos de Naranjo
  Mexico 118 B4
Lampedusa *Italy* 48 G5
Lampeter *U.K.* 15 E3
Lampman *Canada* 103 D8

Lamprechtshausen *Austria* 26 D5
Lampung □ *Indonesia* 62 F2
Lamta *India* 69 H9
Lamu *Kenya* 86 C5
Lamy *U.S.A.* 109 J11
Lan Xian *China* 56 E6
Lan Yü *Taiwan* 59 F13
Läna'i *U.S.A.* 107 L8
Lanak La *China* 69 B8
Lanak'o Shank'ou =
  Lanak La *China* 69 B8
Lanao, L. *Phil.* 61 H6
Lanark *Canada* 115 A8
Lanark *U.K.* 13 F5
Lanbi Kyun *Burma* 65 G2
Lancang *China* 58 F2
Lancang Jiang → *China* 58 G3
Lancashire □ *U.K.* 14 D5
Lancaster *U.K.* 14 C5
Lancaster *Calif., U.S.A.* 111 L8
Lancaster *Ky., U.S.A.* 113 G11
Lancaster *N.H., U.S.A.* 115 B13
Lancaster *Ohio, U.S.A.* 113 F12
Lancaster *Pa., U.S.A.* 115 F8
Lancaster *S.C., U.S.A.* 117 D14
Lancaster *Wis., U.S.A.* 112 D8
Lancaster Sd. *Canada* 101 C15
Lancelin *Australia* 93 F2
Lanchow = Lanzhou *China* 56 F2
Lanchyn *Ukraine* 29 B9
Lanciano *Italy* 41 F11
Lancun *China* 57 F11
Lançut *Poland* 31 H9
Land Between the Lakes ◎
  U.S.A. 117 C11
Landau *Bayern, Germany* 25 G8
Landau *Rhld-Pfz., Germany* 25 F4
Landeck *Austria* 26 D3
Lander *U.S.A.* 108 E9
Lander → *Australia* 92 D5
Landerneau *France* 18 D2
Landeryd *Sweden* 11 G7
Landes □ *France* 20 D2
Landes de Gascogne ◎
  France 20 D3
Landete *Spain* 38 F3
Landi Kotal *Pakistan* 68 B4
Landisburg *U.S.A.* 114 F7
Landivisiau *France* 18 D2
Landmannalaugar *Iceland* 8 E4
Landquart *Switz.* 25 J5
Landrecies *France* 19 B10
Land's End ◎ *U.K.* 15 G2
Landsberg *Germany* 25 G6
Landsborough Cr. →
  Australia 94 C3
Landsbro *Sweden* 11 G8
Landshut *Germany* 25 G8
Landskrona *Sweden* 11 J6
Landstuhl *Germany* 25 F3
Landvetter *Sweden* 11 G6
Lanesboro *U.S.A.* 115 E9
Lanester *France* 18 E3
Lanett *U.S.A.* 117 E12
Lang Shan *China* 56 D4
Lang Son *Vietnam* 58 G6
Lang Suan *Thailand* 65 H2
Langå *Denmark* 11 H3
La'nga Co *China* 69 D9
Langadás *Greece* 44 F7
Langadia *Greece* 46 D4
Långan → *Sweden* 10 A8
Langano, L. *Ethiopia* 81 F4
Langar *Iran* 71 D9
Langara I. *Canada* 102 C2
Langarüd *Iran* 71 B6
Långås *Sweden* 11 H6
Langdai *China* 58 D5
Langdon *U.S.A.* 112 A4
Långe Jan = Ölands södra
  udde *Sweden* 11 H10
Langeac *France* 20 C7
Langeais *France* 18 E7
Langeb Baraka → *Sudan* 80 D4
Langeberg *S. Africa* 88 E3
Langeberge *S. Africa* 88 D3
Langeland *Denmark* 11 K4
Langen *Hessen, Germany* 25 F4
Langen *Niedersachsen,*
  Germany 24 B4
Langenburg *Canada* 103 C8
Langeneß *Germany* 24 A4
Langenlois *Austria* 26 C8
Langeoog *Germany* 24 B3
Langeskov *Denmark* 11 J4
Länghem *Sweden* 11 G7
Langhirano *Italy* 40 D7
Langholm *U.K.* 13 F5
Langjökull *Iceland* 8 D3
Langkawi, Pulau *Malaysia* 65 J2
Langklip *S. Africa* 88 D3
Langkon *Malaysia* 62 C5
Langley *Canada* 110 A4
Langnau *Switz.* 25 J3
Langogne *France* 20 D7
Langon *France* 20 D3

Langøya *Norway* 8 B16
Langreo *Spain* 36 B5
Langres *France* 19 E12
Langres, Plateau de *France* 19 E12
Langsa *Indonesia* 62 D1
Långsele *Sweden* 10 A11
Långshyttan *Sweden* 10 D10
Langtang △ *Nepal* 69 E11
Langtry *U.S.A.* 116 G4
Langu *Thailand* 65 J2
Langue de Barbarie △
  Senegal 82 C1
Languedoc *France* 20 E7
Languedoc-Roussillon □
  France 20 E6
Langxi *China* 59 B12
Langxiangzhen *China* 56 E9
Langzhong *China* 58 B5
Lanigan *Canada* 103 C7
Lankao *China* 56 G8
Länkäran *Azerbaijan* 73 C13
Lanmeur *France* 18 D3
Lannemezan *France* 20 E4
Lannilis *France* 18 D2
Lannion *France* 18 D3
L'Annonciation *Canada* 104 C5
Lanouaille *France* 20 C5
Lanping *China* 58 D2
Lansdale *U.S.A.* 115 F9
Lansdowne *Australia* 95 E5
Lansdowne *Canada* 115 B8
Lansdowne *India* 69 E8
Lansdowne House =
  Neskantaga *Canada* 104 B2
L'Anse *U.S.A.* 112 B9
L'Anse au Loup *Canada* 105 B8
L'Anse aux Meadows
  Canada 105 B8
L'Anse la Raye *St. Lucia* 121 f
Lansford *U.S.A.* 115 F9
Lanshan *China* 59 E9
Lansing *U.S.A.* 113 D11
Lanslebourg-Mont-Cenis
  France 21 C10
Lanta Yai, Ko *Thailand* 65 J2
Lantewa *Nigeria* 83 C7
Lantian *China* 56 G5
Lanus *Argentina* 126 C4
Lanusei *Italy* 42 C2
Lanuza *Phil.* 61 G7
Lanxi *China* 59 C12
Lanzarote *Canary Is.* 48 F6
Lanzarote ✈ (ACE) *Canary Is.* 48 F6
Lanzhou *China* 56 F2
Lanzo Torinese *Italy* 40 C4
Lao → *Italy* 43 C8
Lao Bao *Laos* 64 D6
Lao Cai *Vietnam* 58 F4
Laoag *Phil.* 61 B4
Laoang *Phil.* 61 E6
Laoha He → *China* 57 C11
Laohekou *China* 59 A8
Laois □ *Ireland* 12 D4
Laon *France* 19 C10
Laona *U.S.A.* 112 C9
Laos ■ *Asia* 64 D5
Lapa *Brazil* 127 B6
Lapalisse *France* 19 F10
Lapeer *U.S.A.* 113 D12
Lapeyrade *France* 20 D3
Lapithos *Cyprus* 49 D12
Lapland = Lappland *Europe* 8 B21
LaPorte *Ind., U.S.A.* 112 E10
Laporte *Pa., U.S.A.* 115 E8
Lapovo *Serbia* 44 B5
Lappeenranta *Finland* 32 B5
Lappland *Europe* 8 B21
Lappo = Lapua *Finland* 8 E20
Laprida *Argentina* 126 D3
Lâpseki *Turkey* 45 F10
Laptev Sea *Russia* 53 B13
Lapua *Finland* 8 E20
Lăpuş → *Romania* 29 C8
Lapuş, Munţii *Romania* 29 C8
Lăpuşna *Moldova* 29 D13
Łapy *Poland* 31 F9
Laqiya Arba'in *Sudan* 80 C2
Laqiya Umran *Sudan* 80 D2
L'Áquila *Italy* 41 F10
Lār *Iran* 71 E7
Larabanga *Ghana* 82 D4
Laragne-Montéglin *France* 21 D9
Laramie *U.S.A.* 108 F11
Laramie Mts. *U.S.A.* 108 F11
Laranjeiras do Sul *Brazil* 127 B5
Larantuka *Indonesia* 63 F6
Larat *Indonesia* 63 F8
L'Arbresle *France* 21 C8
Lärbro *Sweden* 11 G12
Larde *Mozam.* 87 F4
Larder Lake *Canada* 104 C4
Lardos *Greece* 49 C10
Lardos, Akra = Lindos,
  Akra *Greece* 49 C10
Lardos, Ormos *Greece* 49 C10
Laredo *Spain* 36 B7
Laredo *U.S.A.* 116 H5

Laredo Sd. *Canada* **102** C3
Largentière *France* **21** D8
L'Argentière-la-Bessée
  France **21** D10
Largo *U.S.A.* **117** H13
Largs *U.K.* **13** F4
Lari *Italy* **40** E7
Lariang *Indonesia* **63** E5
Larimore *U.S.A.* **112** B5
Larino *Italy* **41** G11
Larisa *Greece* **46** B4
Larissas □ *Greece* **46** B4
Larkana *Pakistan* **68** F3
Larnaca *Cyprus* **49** E12
Larnaca Bay *Cyprus* **49** E12
Larne *U.K.* **12** B6
Larned *U.S.A.* **112** F4
Laroquebrou *France* **20** D6
Larose *U.S.A.* **117** G9
Larrimah *Australia* **92** C5
Larsen Ice Shelf *Antarctica* **5** C17
Laruns *France* **20** E1
Larvik *Norway* **9** G14
Larzac, Causse du *France* **20** E7
Las Alpujarras *Spain* **39** J1
Las Animas *U.S.A.* **108** G12
Las Anod *Somali Rep.* **75** F4
Las Arenas *Spain* **36** B6
Las Batuecas △ *Spain* **36** E4
Las Breñas *Argentina* **126** B3
Las Cabezas de San Juan
  Spain **37** J5
Las Cañadas del Teide △
  Canary Is. **48** F3
Las Cejas *Argentina* **128** B4
Las Chimeneas *Mexico* **111** N10
Las Cruces *U.S.A.* **109** K10
Las Flores *Argentina* **126** D4
Las Gabias = Gabia la
  Grande *Spain* **37** H7
Las Heras *Argentina* **126** C2
Las Lajas *Argentina* **128** D2
Las Lomitas *Argentina* **126** A3
Las Marismas *Spain* **37** H4
Las Minas *Spain* **37** H4
Las Navas de la Concepción
  Spain **37** H5
Las Navas del Marqués *Spain* **36** E6
Las Palmas *Argentina* **126** B4
Las Palmas *Canary Is.* **48** F4
Las Palmas → *Mexico* **111** N10
Las Palmas ✈ (LPA)
  Canary Is. **48** G4
Las Pedroñas *Spain* **39** F2
Las Piedras *Uruguay* **127** C4
Las Pipinas *Argentina* **126** D4
Las Plumas *Argentina* **128** E3
Las Rosas *Argentina* **126** C3
Las Rozas *Spain* **36** E7
Las Tablas *Panama* **120** E3
Las Toscas *Argentina* **126** B4
Las Truchas *Mexico* **118** D4
Las Tunas *Cuba* **120** B4
Las Varillas *Argentina* **126** C3
Las Vegas *N. Mex., U.S.A.* **109** J11
Las Vegas *Nev., U.S.A.* **111** J11
Las Vegas McCarran Int. ✈
  (LAS) *U.S.A.* **111** J11
Lasarte-Oria *Spain* **38** B2
Lascano *Uruguay* **127** C5
Lash-e Joveyn *Afghan.* **66** D2
Lashburn *Canada* **103** C7
Lashio *Burma* **67** H20
Lashkar *India* **68** F8
Łasin *Poland* **30** E6
Lasithi *Greece* **49** D7
Lasithi □ *Greece* **49** D7
Lāsjerd *Iran* **71** C7
Lask *Poland* **31** G6
Łaskarzew *Poland* **31** G8
Laško *Slovenia* **41** B12
Lassay-les-Châteaux *France* **18** D6
Lassen Pk. *U.S.A.* **108** F3
Lassen Volcanic △ *U.S.A.* **108** F3
Last Mountain L. *Canada* **103** C7
Lastchance Cr. → *U.S.A.* **110** E5
Lastoursville *Gabon* **84** E2
Lastovo *Croatia* **41** F13
Lastovski Kanal *Croatia* **41** F14
Lat Yao *Thailand* **64** E2
Latacunga *Ecuador* **124** D3
Latakia = Al Lādhiqīyah
  Syria **72** E6
Latchford *Canada* **104** C4
Late *Tonga* **91** c
Latehar *India* **69** H11
Laterza *Italy* **43** B9
Latham *Australia* **93** E2
Lathen *Germany* **24** C3
Lathi *India* **68** F4
Lathrop Wells *U.S.A.* **111** J10
Latiano *Italy* **43** B10
Latina *Italy* **42** A5
Latium □ = Lazio □ *Italy* **41** F9
Laton *U.S.A.* **110** J7
Latorytsya → *Slovak Rep.* **27** C14
Latouche Treville, C.
  Australia **92** C3
Latrobe *Australia* **95** G4
Latrobe *U.S.A.* **114** F5
Latrónico *Italy* **43** B9
Latvia ■ *Europe* **32** D2
Lau *Nigeria* **83** D7
Lau Group *Fiji* **91** a
Lauchhammer *Germany* **24** D9
Lauda-Königshofen *Germany* **25** F5
Lauenburg *Germany* **24** B6
Lauenburgische Seen △
  Germany **24** B6
Lauf *Germany* **25** F7
Lauge Koch Kyst *Greenland* **101** B20
Laughlin *U.S.A.* **109** J6
Laujar de Andarax *Spain* **39** H2
Laukaa *Finland* **8** E21
Launceston *Australia* **95** G4
Launceston *U.K.* **15** G3
Laune → *Ireland* **12** D2
Launglon Bok *Burma* **64** F1
Laupheim *Germany* **25** G5
Laura *Australia* **94** B3
Laureana di Borrello *Italy* **43** D9
Laurel *Miss., U.S.A.* **117** F10
Laurel *Mont., U.S.A.* **108** D9
Laurel Hill *U.S.A.* **114** F5
Laurencekirk *U.K.* **13** E6
Laurens *U.S.A.* **117** D13
Lauria *Italy* **43** B8
Laurie L. *Canada* **103** B8
Laurinburg *U.S.A.* **117** D15
Laurium *U.S.A.* **112** B9
Lausanne *Switz.* **25** J2
Laut *Indonesia* **62** D3
Laut, Pulau *Indonesia* **62** E5
Laut Kecil, Kepulauan
  Indonesia **62** E5
Lauterbach *Germany* **24** E5
Lauterecken *Germany* **25** F3
Lautoka *Fiji* **91** a
Lauzès *France* **20** D5
Lava → *Russia* **30** D8
Lava Beds △ *U.S.A.* **108** F3
Lavagh More *Ireland* **12** B3
Lavagna *Italy* **40** D6
Laval *France* **18** D6
Laval-des-Rapides *Canada* **104** C5
Lavalle *Argentina* **126** B2
Lāvān *Iran* **71** E7
Lavant → *Canada* **115** A8
Lāvar Meydān *Iran* **71** D7
Lavara *Greece* **45** E10
Lavardac *France* **20** D4
Lavaur *France* **20** E5
Lavelanet *France* **20** F5
Lavello *Italy* **43** A8
Laverton *Australia* **93** E3
Lavis *Italy* **40** B8
Lavos *Portugal* **36** E2
Lavradio *Portugal* **37** G1
Lavras *Brazil* **127** A7
Lavre *Portugal* **37** G2
Lavrio *Greece* **46** D6
Lavris *Greece* **49** D6
Lavumisa *Swaziland* **89** D5
Lavushi Manda △ *Zambia* **87** E3
Lawaki *Fiji* **91** a
Lawas *Malaysia* **62** D5
Lawele *Indonesia* **63** F6
Lawn Hill =
  Boodjamulla △ *Australia* **94** B2
Lawqah *Si. Arabia* **70** D4
Lawra *Ghana* **82** C4
Lawrence *N.Z.* **91** F2
Lawrence *Ind., U.S.A.* **112** F10
Lawrence *Kans., U.S.A.* **112** F6
Lawrence *Mass., U.S.A.* **115** D13
Lawrenceburg *Ind., U.S.A.* **113** F11
Lawrenceburg *Tenn., U.S.A.*
  117 D11
Lawrenceville *Ga., U.S.A.* **117** E13
Lawrenceville *Pa., U.S.A.* **114** E7
Laws *Canada* **103** C7
Lawton *U.S.A.* **110** H8
Lawu *Indonesia* **63** G14
Lawz, J. al *Si. Arabia* **80** B4
Laxá *Sweden* **11** F8
Laxford, L. *U.K.* **13** C3
Laxou *France* **19** D13
Lay → *France* **20** B2
Layla *Si. Arabia* **75** C4
Laylān *Iraq* **70** C5
Layon → *France* **18** E6
Laysan I. *U.S.A.* **107** K5
Layton *U.S.A.* **108** F8
Laytonville *U.S.A.* **108** G2
Lazarev *Russia* **53** D15
Lazarev Sea *S. Ocean* **5** C2
Lazarevac *Serbia* **44** B4
Lazarevskoye *Russia* **35** J4
Lazarivo *Madag.* **89** C8
Lázaro Cárdenas *Mexico* **118** D4
Lazdijai *Lithuania* **30** D10
Lazio □ *Italy* **41** F9
Lazo *Moldova* **29** C13
Lazo *Russia* **54** C6
Le Beausset *France* **21** E9
Le Bic *Canada* **105** C6
Le Blanc *France* **20** B5
Le Bleymard *France* **20** D7
Le Bourgneuf-la-Fôret *France* **18** D6
Le Bugue *France* **20** D4
Le Cateau Cambrésis *France* **19** B10
Le Caylar *France* **20** E7
Le Chambon-Feugerolles
  France **21** C8
Le Châtelet *France* **19** F9
Le Chesne *France* **19** C11
Le Cheylard *France* **21** D8
Le Conquet *France* **18** D2
Le Creusot *France* **19** F11
Le Croisic *France* **18** E4
Le Donjon *France* **19** F10
Le Dorat *France* **20** B5
Le François *Martinique* **120** c
Le Gosier *Guadeloupe* **120** b
Le Grand-Lucé *France* **18** E7
Le Grand-Pressigny *France* **18** F7
Le Grand-Quevilly *France* **18** C8
Le Gris Gris *Mauritius* **85** d
Le Havre *France* **18** C7
Le Lamentin *Martinique* **120** c
Le Lavandou *France* **21** E10
Le Lion-d'Angers *France* **18** E6
Le Louroux-Béconnais
  France **18** E6
Le Luc *France* **21** E10
Le Lude *France* **18** E7
Le Mans *France* **18** E7
Le Marin *Martinique* **120** c
Le Mars *France* **112** B9
Le Mayet-de-Montagne
  France **19** F10
Le Mêle-sur-Sarthe *France* **18** D7
Le Monastier-sur-Gazeille
  France **20** D7
Le Monêtier-les-Bains
  France **21** D10
Le Mont-Dore *France* **20** C6
Le Mont-St-Michel *France* **18** D5
Le Moule *Guadeloupe* **120** b
Le Moyne, L. *Canada* **105** A6
Le Muy *France* **21** E10
Le Palais *France* **18** E3
Le Perthus *France* **20** F6
Le Port *Réunion* **85** c
Le Prêcheur *Martinique* **120** c
Le Puy-en-Velay *France* **20** C7
Le Raysville *U.S.A.* **115** E8
Le Robert *Martinique* **120** c
Le Roy *U.S.A.* **114** D7
Le St-Esprit *Martinique* **120** c
Le Sueur *U.S.A.* **112** C7
Le Tampon *Réunion* **85** c
Le Teil *France* **21** D8
Le Teilleul *France* **18** D6
Le Theil *France* **18** D7
Le Thillot *France* **19** E13
Le Thuy *Vietnam* **64** D6
Le Touquet-Paris-Plage
  France **19** B8
Le Tréport *France* **18** B8
Le Val-d'Ajol *France* **19** E13
Le Verdon-sur-Mer *France* **20** C2
Le Vigan *France* **20** E7
Lea → *U.K.* **15** F8
Leach *Cambodia* **65** F4
Lead *U.S.A.* **112** C2
Leader *Canada* **103** C7
Leadville *U.S.A.* **108** G10
Leaf → *U.S.A.* **117** F10
Leaf Rapids *Canada* **103** B9
Leamington *Canada* **114** D2
Leamington *U.S.A.* **108** G7
Leamington Spa = Royal
  Leamington Spa *U.K.* **15** E6
Le'an *China* **59** D10
Leandro Norte Alem
  Argentina **127** B4
Leane, L. *Ireland* **12** D2
Learmonth *Australia* **92** D1
Leask *Canada* **103** C7
Leatherhead *U.K.* **15** F7
Leavenworth *Kans., U.S.A.* **112** F6
Leavenworth *Wash., U.S.A.* **108** C3
Leawood *U.S.A.* **112** F6
Łeba *Poland* **30** D4
Łeba → *Poland* **30** D4
Lebach *Germany* **25** F2
Lebak *Phil.* **61** H6
Lebam *U.S.A.* **110** D3
Lebane *Serbia* **44** D5
Lebanon *Ind., U.S.A.* **112** E10
Lebanon *Kans., U.S.A.* **112** F4
Lebanon *Ky., U.S.A.* **113** G11
Lebanon *Mo., U.S.A.* **112** G7
Lebanon *N.H., U.S.A.* **115** C12
Lebanon *Oreg., U.S.A.* **108** D2
Lebanon *Pa., U.S.A.* **115** F8
Lebanon *Tenn., U.S.A.* **117** C11
Lebanon ■ *Asia* **74** B5
Lebedyan *Russia* **32** F11
Lebedyn *Ukraine* **33** G8
Lebel-sur-Quévillon *Canada* **104** C4
Lebomboberge *S. Africa* **89** C5
Łebork *Poland* **30** D4
Lebrija *Spain* **37** J4
Łebsko, Jezioro *Poland* **30** D4
Lebu *Chile* **126** D1
Leca da Palmeira *Portugal* **36** D2
Lecce *Italy* **43** B11
Lecco *Italy* **40** C6
Lecco, L. di *Italy* **40** C6
Lécera *Spain* **38** D4
Lech *Austria* **26** D3
Lech → *Germany* **25** G6
Lechang *China* **59** E9
Lechena *Greece* **46** D3
Lechtaler Alpen *Austria* **26** D3
Lecontes Mills *U.S.A.* **114** E6
Lectoure *France* **20** E4
Łęczna *Poland* **31** G9
Łęczyca *Poland* **31** F6
Ledesma *Spain* **36** D5
Ledong *China* **64** C7
Leduc *Canada* **102** C6
Lee *U.S.A.* **115** D11
Lee → *Ireland* **12** E3
Lee Vining *U.S.A.* **110** H7
Leech L. *U.S.A.* **112** B6
Leechburg *U.S.A.* **114** F5
Leeds *U.K.* **14** D6
Leeds *U.S.A.* **117** E11
Leek *Neths.* **17** A6
Leek *U.K.* **14** D5
Leeman *Australia* **93** E1
Leeper *U.S.A.* **114** E5
Leer *Germany* **24** B3
Leesburg *U.S.A.* **117** G14
Leesville *U.S.A.* **116** F8
Leeton *Australia* **95** E4
Leetonia *U.S.A.* **114** F4
Leeu Gamka *S. Africa* **88** E3
Leeuwarden *Neths.* **17** A5
Leeuwin, C. *Australia* **93** F2
Leeuwin Naturaliste △
  Australia **93** F2
Leeward Is. *Atl. Oc.* **121** C7
Lefka *Cyprus* **49** D11
Lefkada *Greece* **46** C2
Lefkimis, Akra *Greece* **49** B4
Lefkimmi *Greece* **49** B4
Lefkoniko *Cyprus* **49** D12
Lefroy *Canada* **114** B5
Lefroy, L. *Australia* **93** F3
Leg → *Poland* **31** H8
Leganés *Spain* **36** E7
Legazpi *Phil.* **61** E5
Lège-Cap-Ferret *France* **20** D2
Lege Hida *Ethiopia* **81** F5
Legendre I. *Australia* **92** D2
Leghorn = Livorno *Italy* **40** E7
Legionowo *Poland* **31** F7
Legnago *Italy* **41** C8
Legnano *Italy* **40** C5
Legnica *Poland* **31** G3
Legrad *Croatia* **41** B13
Leh *India* **69** B7
Lehigh Acres *U.S.A.* **117** H14
Lehighton *U.S.A.* **115** F9
Lehliu *Romania* **29** F11
Leho *Sudan* **81** F3
Lehrte *Germany* **24** C5
Lehututu *Botswana* **88** C3
Lei Shui → *China* **59** D9
Leiah *Pakistan* **68** D4
Leibnitz *Austria* **26** E8
Leibo *China* **58** C4
Leicester *U.K.* **15** E6
Leicester City □ *U.K.* **15** E6
Leicestershire □ *U.K.* **15** E6
Leichhardt → *Australia* **94** B2
Leichhardt Ra. *Australia* **94** C4
Leiden *Neths.* **17** B4
Leie → *Belgium* **17** C3
Leier *Ireland* **12** D2
Leimen *Germany* **25** F4
Leimus *Nic.* **120** D3
Leine → *Germany* **24** C5
Leinefelde *Germany* **24** D6
Leinster *Australia* **93** E3
Leinster □ *Ireland* **12** C4
Leinster, Mt. *Ireland* **12** D5
Leipalingis *Lithuania* **30** D10
Leipzig *Germany* **24** D8
Leiria *Portugal* **36** F2
Leiria □ *Portugal* **36** F2
Leirvik *Norway* **9** G11
Leishan *China* **58** D7
Leisler, Mt. *Australia* **92** D4
Leith *U.K.* **13** F5
Leith Hill *U.K.* **15** F7
Leitha → *Europe* **27** D10
Leitir Ceanainn =
  Letterkenny *Ireland* **12** B4
Leitrim *Ireland* **12** B3
Leitrim □ *Ireland* **12** B4
Leitza *Spain* **38** B3
Leiyang *China* **59** D9
Leizhou *China* **59** G8
Leizhou Bandao *China* **58** G7
Leizhou Wan *China* **59** G8
Lek → *Neths.* **17** C4
Leka *Norway* **8** D14
Lekani *Greece* **45** E8
Lekbibaj *Albania* **44** D3
Lekeitio *Spain* **38** B2
Lekki Lagoon *Nigeria* **83** D5
Léko *Mali* **82** C3
Lekoui *Burkina Faso* **82** C4
Lekoui *Burkina Faso* **82** C4
Lekoumou →
Léko *Mali* **82** C3
Lekoui *Burkina Faso* **82** C4
Leksand *Sweden* **10** D9
Leland *Mich., U.S.A.* **113** C11
Leland *Miss., U.S.A.* **117** E9
Lelång *Sweden* **10** E6
Leleque *Argentina* **128** E2
Lelystad *Neths.* **17** B5
Lem *Denmark* **11** H2
Lema *Nigeria* **83** C5
Lema Shilindi *Ethiopia* **81** G5
Léman, L. *Europe* **19** F13
Lembar *Indonesia* **92** R19
Lembuak *Indonesia* **63** K19
Lemera *Dem. Rep. of the Congo* **86** C2
Lemery *Phil.* **61** E4
Lemhi Ra. *U.S.A.* **108** D7
Lemmer *Neths.* **17** B5
Lemmon *U.S.A.* **112** C2
Lemon Grove *U.S.A.* **111** N9
Lemoore *U.S.A.* **110** J7
Lempdes *France* **20** C7
Lemvig *Denmark* **11** H2
Lena → *Russia* **53** B13
Lenadoon Pt. *Ireland* **12** B2
Lenart *Slovenia* **41** B12
Lenartovce *Slovak Rep.* **27** C13
Lencloître *France* **18** F7
Lendava *Slovenia* **41** B13
Lendinara *Italy* **41** C8
Lengerich *Germany* **24** C3
Lenggong *Malaysia* **65** K3
Lenggries *Germany* **25** H7
Lengshuijiang *China* **59** D8
Lengshuitan *China* **59** D8
Lengua de Vaca, Pta. *Chile* **126** C1
Lengwe △ *Malawi* **87** F3
Lengyeltóti *Hungary* **28** D2
Lenhovda *Sweden* **11** G9
Lenin, Kanal → *Russia* **35** J7
Lenina, Kanal → *Russia* **35** J7
Leningrad = Sankt-Peterburg →
Leningrad □ *Russia* **32** C7
Lenino *Ukraine* **33** K8
Leninogorsk *Kazakhstan* **52** D9
Leninsk *Russia* **35** F7
Leninsk-Kuznetskiy *Russia* **52** D9
Leninskoye *Russia* **34** A8
Lenk *Switz.* **25** J3
Lenkoran = Länkäran
  Azerbaijan **73** C13
Lenmalu *Indonesia* **63** E8
Lenne → *Germany* **24** D3
Lennestadt *Germany* **24** D4
Lennox *U.S.A.* **112** D5
Lennoxville *Canada* **115** A13
Leno *Italy* **40** C7
Lenoir *U.S.A.* **117** D14
Lenoir City *U.S.A.* **117** D12
Lenore L. *Canada* **103** C8
Lenox *U.S.A.* **115** D11
Lens *France* **19** B9
Lensahn *Germany* **24** A6
Lensk *Russia* **53** C12
Lentas *Greece* **49** E6
Lentekhi *Georgia* **35** J6
Lenti *Hungary* **28** D1
Lentini *Italy* **43** E8
Lenwood *U.S.A.* **111** L9
Lenya *Burma* **65** G2
Lenzen *Germany* **24** B7
Léo *Burkina Faso* **82** C4
Leoben *Austria* **26** D8
Leodhas = Lewis *U.K.* **13** C2
Leola *U.S.A.* **112** C4
Leominster *U.K.* **15** E5
Leominster *U.S.A.* **115** D13
Léon *France* **20** E2
León *Mexico* **118** C4
León *Nic.* **120** D2
León *Spain* **36** C5
Leon → *U.S.A.* **116** F6
León □ *Spain* **36** C5
León, Montes de *Spain* **36** C4
Leonardo da Vinci,
  Roma ✈ (FCO) *Italy* **41** G9
Leonardtown *U.S.A.* **113** F15
Leonardville *Namibia* **88** C2
Leonessa *Italy* **41** F9
Leonforte *Italy* **43** E7
Leongatha *Australia* **95** F4
Leonidio *Greece* **46** D4
Leonora *Australia* **93** E3
Leopoldina *Brazil* **127** A7
Leopoldsburg *Belgium* **17** C5
Leoti *U.S.A.* **112** F3
Leova *Moldova* **29** D13
Leoville *Canada* **103** C7
Lepe *Spain* **37** H3
Lepel = Lyepyel *Belarus* **32** E5
Lepenou *Greece* **46** C3
Leping *China* **59** C11
Lépo, L. do *Angola* **88** B2
Lepontine, Alpi *Italy* **40** B5
Leposavić *Kosovo* **44** C4
Leppävirta *Finland* **8** E22
Lepsény *Hungary* **28** D3
Leptis Magna *Libya* **79** B8
Lequeitio = Lekeitio *Spain* **38** B2
Lercara Friddi *Italy* **42** E6
Léré *Chad* **83** D7
Léré *Mali* **82** B4
Lere *Bauchi, Nigeria* **83** D6
Lere *Kaduna, Nigeria* **83** C6
Leribe *Lesotho* **89** D4
Lérici *Italy* **40** D7
Lérida = Lleida *Spain* **38** D5
Lérins, Îs. de *France* **21** E11
Lerma *Spain* **36** C7
Leros *Greece* **47** D8
Lérouville *France* **19** D12
Lerum *Sweden* **11** G6
Lerwick *U.K.* **13** A7
Leş *Romania* **28** D6
Les Abrets *France* **21** C9
Les Andelys *France* **18** C8
Les Borges Blanques *Spain* **38** D5
Les Cayes *Haiti* **121** C5
Les Coteaux *Canada* **115** A10
Les Escoumins *Canada* **105** C6
Les Essarts *France* **18** F5
Les Herbiers *France* **18** F5
Les Minquiers, Plateau des
  Chan. Is. **18** D4
Les Pieux *France* **18** C5
Les Ponts-de-Cé *France* **18** E6
Les Riceys *France* **19** E11
Les Sables-d'Olonne *France* **20** B2
Les Vans *France* **21** D8
Lesbos *Greece* **47** B8
L'Escala *Spain* **38** C8
Leshan *China* **58** C4
Leshwe △
  Dem. Rep. of the Congo **87** E2
Lésina *Italy* **41** G12
Lésina, L. di *Italy* **41** G12
Lesjöfors *Sweden* **10** E8
Lesko *Poland* **31** J9
Leskov I. *Antarctica* **5** B1
Leskovac *Serbia* **44** C5
Leskovik *Albania* **44** F4
Leśna *Poland* **31** G2
Lesneven *France* **18** D2
Leśnica *Poland* **31** H5
Lešnica *Serbia* **44** B3
Lesnoye *Russia* **32** C8
Lesopilnoye *Russia* **54** A7
Lesotho ■ *Africa* **89** D4
Lesozavodsk *Russia* **54** B6
Lesparre-Médoc *France* **20** C3
L'Espluga de Francolí *Spain* **38** D6
Lessay *France* **18** C5
Lesse → *Belgium* **17** D5
Lesse et Lomme △ *Belgium* **17** D5
Lessebo *Sweden* **11** H9
Lesser Antilles *W. Indies* **121** D7
Lesser Slave L. *Canada* **102** B5
Lesser Sunda Is. *Indonesia* **63** F6
Lessines *Belgium* **17** D3
Lester B. Pearson Int.,
  Toronto ✈ (YYZ) *Canada* **114** C5
Lestock *Canada* **103** C8
Lesueur I. *Australia* **92** B4
Lesueur △ *Australia* **93** F2
Lésvos = Lesbos *Greece* **47** B8
Leszno *Poland* **31** G3
Letaba *S. Africa* **89** C5
Letea, Ostrov *Romania* **29** E14
Lethbridge *Canada* **102** D6
Lethem *Guyana* **124** C7
Leti, Kepulauan *Indonesia* **63** F7
Leti Is. = Leti, Kepulauan
  Indonesia **63** F7
Letiahau → *Botswana* **88** C3
Leticia *Colombia* **124** D5
Leting *China* **57** E10
Letjiesbos *S. Africa* **88** E3
Letlhakane *Botswana* **88** C4
Letlhakeng *Botswana* **88** C3
Letpadan *Burma* **67** L19
Letpan *Burma* **67** K19
Letsôk-aw Kyun *Burma* **65** G2
Letterkenny *Ireland* **12** B4
Leu *Romania* **29** F9
Leucadia *U.S.A.* **111** M9
Leucate *France* **20** F7
Leucate, Étang de *France* **20** F7
Leuchars *U.K.* **13** E6
Leuk *Switz.* **25** J3
Leuşeni *Moldova* **29** D13
Leuser, G. *Indonesia* **62** D1
Leutkirch *Germany* **25** H6
Leuven *Belgium* **17** D4
Leuze-en-Hainaut *Belgium* **17** D3
Lev Tolstoy *Russia* **32** F10
Levan *Albania* **44** F3
Levanger *Norway* **8** E14
Levant, Î. du *France* **21** E10
Lévanto *Italy* **40** D6

Lévanzo *Italy* **42** D5
Levelland *U.S.A.* **116** E3
Leven *U.K.* **13** E6
Leven, L. *U.K.* **13** E5
Leven, Toraka *Madag.* **89** A8
Leveque C. *Australia* **92** C3
Leverano *Italy* **43** B10
Leverkusen *Germany* **24** D3
Levice *Slovak Rep.* **27** C11
Lévico Terme *Italy* **41** C8
Levie *France* **21** G13
Levier *France* **19** F13
Levin *N.Z.* **91** D5
Lévis *Canada* **105** C5
Levis, L. *Canada* **102** A5
Levitha *Greece* **47** D8
Levittown *N.Y., U.S.A.* **115** F11
Levittown *Pa., U.S.A.* **115** F10
Levka *Bulgaria* **45** D10
Levka Oros *Greece* **49** D6
Levkás = Lefkáda *Greece* **46** C2
Levkás □ *Greece* **46** C2
Levkôsia = Nicosia *Cyprus* **49** D12
Levoča *Slovak Rep.* **27** B13
Levroux *France* **19** F8
Levski *Bulgaria* **45** C9
Levskigrad = Karlovo
   Bulgaria **45** D8
Levuka *Fiji* **91** a
Lewes *U.K.* **15** G8
Lewes *U.S.A.* **113** F16
Lewin Brzeski *Poland* **31** H4
Lewis *U.K.* **13** C2
Lewis = *U.S.A.* **110** E4
Lewis, Butt of *U.K.* **13** C2
Lewis and Clark △ *U.S.A.* **110** D3
Lewis Ra. *Australia* **92** D4
Lewis Range *U.S.A.* **108** B7
Lewis Run *U.S.A.* **114** E6
Lewisburg *Pa., U.S.A.* **114** F8
Lewisburg *Tenn., U.S.A.* **117** D11
Lewisburg *W. Va., U.S.A.* **113** G13
Lewisporte *Canada* **105** C8
Lewiston *Idaho, U.S.A.* **108** C5
Lewiston *Maine, U.S.A.* **113** C18
Lewiston *N.Y., U.S.A.* **114** C5
Lewistown *Mont., U.S.A.* **108** C9
Lewistown *Pa., U.S.A.* **114** F7
Lexington *Ill., U.S.A.* **112** E9
Lexington *Ky., U.S.A.* **113** F11
Lexington *Mich., U.S.A.* **114** C2
Lexington *Mo., U.S.A.* **112** F7
Lexington *N.C., U.S.A.* **117** D14
Lexington *N.Y., U.S.A.* **115** D10
Lexington *Nebr., U.S.A.* **112** E5
Lexington *Ohio, U.S.A.* **114** F2
Lexington *Tenn., U.S.A.* **117** D10
Lexington *Va., U.S.A.* **113** G14
Lexington Park *U.S.A.* **113** F15
Leyburn *U.K.* **14** C6
Leye *China* **58** E6
Leyland *U.K.* **14** D5
Leyre → *France* **20** D2
Leyte □ *Phil.* **61** F6
Leyte Gulf *Phil.* **61** F6
Leżajsk *Poland* **31** H9
Lezay *France* **20** B3
Lezhë *Albania* **44** E3
Lezhi *China* **58** B5
Lézignan-Corbières *France* **20** E6
Lezoux *France* **20** C7
Lgov *Russia* **33** G8
Lhasa *China* **60** D4
Lhazê *China* **60** D3
L'Hermite, I. *Chile* **128** H3
Lhokkruet *Indonesia* **62** D1
Lhokseumawe *Indonesia* **62** C1
L'Hospitalet de Llobregat
   Spain **38** D7
Li *Thailand* **64** D2
Li Jiang → *China* **59** E8
Li Shui → *China* **59** E8
Li Xian *Gansu, China* **56** G3
Li Xian *Hebei, China* **56** E8
Li Xian *Hunan, China* **59** C8
Liadi *Greece* **47** E8
Liancheng *China* **59** E11
Liancourt Rocks = Tokdo
   Asia **55** F5
Lianga *Phil.* **61** G7
Liangcheng
   Nei Monggol Zizhiqu, China **56** D7
Liangcheng *Shandong, China* **57** G10
Liangdang *China* **56** H4
Lianghe *China* **58** E2
Lianghekou *China* **58** C7
Liangping *China* **58** B6
Liangpran *Indonesia* **62** D4
Lianhua *China* **59** D9
Lianjiang *Fujian, China* **59** D12
Lianjiang *Guangdong, China* **59** G8
Lianping *China* **59** E10
Lianshan *China* **59** E9
Lianshanguan *China* **57** D12
Lianshui *China* **57** H10
Lianyuan *China* **59** D8
Lianyungang *China* **57** G10
Lianzhou *China* **59** E9
Liao He → *China* **57** D11

Liaocheng *China* **56** F8
Liaodong Bandao *China* **57** E12
Liaodong Wan *China* **57** D11
Liaoning □ *China* **57** D12
Liaotung, G. of = Liaodong
   Wan *China* **57** D11
Liaoyang *China* **57** D12
Liaoyuan *China* **57** C13
Liaozhong *China* **57** D12
Liapades *Greece* **49** A3
Liard → *Canada* **102** A4
Liard River *Canada* **102** B3
Liari *Pakistan* **68** G2
Libau = Liepāja *Latvia* **30** B8
Libby *U.S.A.* **108** B6
Libenge *Dem. Rep. of the Congo* **84** D3
Liberal *U.S.A.* **112** G3
Liberec *Czech Rep.* **26** A8
Liberecký □ *Czech Rep.* **26** A8
Liberia *Costa Rica* **120** D2
Liberia ■ *W. Afr.* **82** D3
Libertador □ *Chile* **126** C1
Liberty *Mo., U.S.A.* **112** F6
Liberty *N.Y., U.S.A.* **115** E10
Liberty *Pa., U.S.A.* **114** E7
Liberty *Tex., U.S.A.* **116** F7
Liberty-Newark Int. ✈
   (EWR) *U.S.A.* **115** F10
Libiąż *Poland* **31** H6
Lîbîya, Sahrâ' *Africa* **79** C10
Libo *China* **58** E6
Libobo, Tanjung *Indonesia* **63** E7
Libode *S. Africa* **89** E4
Libohovë *Albania* **44** F4
Libong, Ko *Thailand* **65** J2
Libourne *France* **20** D3
Libramont *Belgium* **17** E5
Librazhd *Albania* **44** E4
Libreville *Gabon* **84** D1
Libya ■ *N. Afr.* **79** C9
Libyan Desert = Lîbîya,
   Sahrâ' *Africa* **79** C10
Libyan Plateau = Ed Déffa
   Egypt **80** A2
Licantén *Chile* **126** D1
Licata *Italy* **42** E6
Licheng *China* **56** F7
Lichfield *U.K.* **15** E6
Lichinga *Mozam.* **87** E4
Lichtenburg *S. Africa* **88** D4
Lichtenfels *Germany* **25** E7
Lichuan *Hubei, China* **58** B7
Lichuan *Jiangxi, China* **59** D11
Licking → *U.S.A.* **113** F11
Licosa, Punta *Italy* **43** B7
Licungo → *Mozam.* **87** F4
Lida *Belarus* **23** B13
Liden *Sweden* **10** B10
Lidhult *Sweden* **11** H7
Lidköping *Sweden* **11** F7
Lido *Italy* **41** C9
Lido *Niger* **83** C5
Lido di Roma = Óstia, Lido
   di *Italy* **41** G9
Lidoriki *Greece* **46** C4
Lidzbark *Poland* **31** E6
Lidzbark Warmiński *Poland* **30** D7
Liebenwalde *Germany* **24** C9
Lieberose *Germany* **24** D10
Liebig, Mt. *Australia* **92** D5
Liebling *Romania* **28** E6
Liechtenstein ■ *Europe* **25** H5
Liège *Belgium* **17** D5
Liège □ *Belgium* **17** D5
Liegnitz = Legnica *Poland* **31** G3
Lieksa *Finland* **8** E24
Lienart *Dem. Rep. of the Congo* **86** B2
Lienyunchiangshih =
   Lianyungang *China* **57** G10
Lienz *Austria* **26** E5
Liepāja *Latvia* **30** B8
Liepāja □ *Latvia* **30** B8
Liepājas ezers *Latvia* **30** B8
Lier *Belgium* **17** C4
Liernais *France* **19** E11
Liești *Romania* **29** E12
Lietuva = Lithuania ■
   Europe **32** E2
Liévin *France* **19** B9
Lièvre → *Canada* **104** C4
Liezen *Austria* **26** D7
Liffey → *Ireland* **12** C5
Lifford *Ireland* **12** B4
Liffré *France* **18** D5
Lifudzin *Russia* **54** B7
Ligao *Phil.* **61** E5
Lightning Ridge *Australia* **95** D4
Lignano Sabbiadoro *Italy* **41** C10
Ligny-en-Barrois *France* **19** D12
Ligonha → *Mozam.* **87** F4
Ligonier *U.S.A.* **114** F5
Ligouri *Greece* **46** D5
Liguell *France* **18** E7
Liguria □ *Italy* **40** D5
Ligurian Sea *Medit. S.* **40** E5
Lihou Reefs and Cays
   Australia **94** B5
Lihué Calel △ *Argentina* **126** D2

Lijiang *China* **58** D3
Likasi *Dem. Rep. of the Congo* **87** E2
Likenäs *Sweden* **10** D7
Likhoslavl *Russia* **32** D8
Likhovskoy *Russia* **33** H11
Likikoma I. *Malawi* **87** E3
Likumburu *Tanzania* **87** D4
L'Île-Bouchard *France* **18** E7
L'Île-Rousse *France* **21** F12
Liling *China* **59** D9
Lilla Edet *Sweden* **11** F6
Lille *France* **19** B10
Lille Bælt *Denmark* **11** J3
Lillebonne *France* **18** C7
Lillehammer *Norway* **8** F14
Lillesand *Norway* **9** G13
Lillhärdal *Sweden* **10** C8
Lillian Pt. *Australia* **93** E4
Lillo *Spain* **36** F7
Lillooet *Canada* **102** C4
Lillooet → *Canada* **102** D4
Lilongwe *Malawi* **87** E3
Liloy *Phil.* **63** C6
Lim → *Europe* **44** C3
Lim Chu Kang *Singapore* **65** d
Lima *Indonesia* **63** E7
Lima *Peru* **124** F3
Lima *Mont., U.S.A.* **108** D7
Lima *N.Y., U.S.A.* **114** D7
Lima *Ohio, U.S.A.* **113** E11
Lima → *Portugal* **36** D2
Limassol *Cyprus* **49** E12
Limay → *Argentina* **128** D3
Limay Mahuida *Argentina* **126** D2
Limbach-Oberfrohna
   Germany **24** E8
Limbang *Brunei* **62** D5
Limbara, Mte. *Italy* **42** B2
Limbaži *Latvia* **32** D3
Limbdi *India* **68** H4
Limbe *Cameroon* **83** E6
Limburg *Germany* **25** E4
Limburg □ *Belgium* **17** C5
Limburg □ *Neths.* **17** C5
Limedsforsen *Sweden* **10** D7
Limeira *Brazil* **127** A6
Limenaria *Greece* **45** F8
Limenas Chersonisou *Greece* **47** F7
Limerick *Ireland* **12** D3
Limerick *U.S.A.* **115** C14
Limerick □ *Ireland* **12** D3
Limestone *U.S.A.* **114** D6
Limestone → *Canada* **103** B10
Limfjorden *Denmark* **11** H3
Limia = Lima → *Portugal* **36** D2
Limingen *Norway* **8** D15
Limmared *Sweden* **11** G7
Limmen Bight *Australia* **94** A2
Limmen Bight → *Australia* **94** B2
Limmen ⊙ *Australia* **94** B2
Límni *Greece* **46** C5
Límnos *Greece* **47** B7
Limoges *Canada* **115** A9
Limoges *France* **20** C5
Limón *Costa Rica* **120** E3
Limon *U.S.A.* **108** G12
Limone Piemonte *Italy* **40** D4
Limousin □ *France* **20** C5
Limousin, Plateaux du
   France **20** C5
Limoux *France* **20** E6
Limpopo □ *S. Africa* **89** C4
Limpopo → *Africa* **89** D5
Limuru *Kenya* **86** C4
Lin Xian *China* **56** F6
Lin'an *China* **59** B12
Linapacan I. *Phil.* **61** F3
Linapacan Str. *Phil.* **61** F3
Linares *Chile* **126** D1
Linares *Mexico* **119** C5
Linares *Spain* **37** G7
Linaria *Greece* **46** C6
Linaro, Capo *Italy* **41** F8
Línas Mte. *Italy* **42** C1
Linate, Milano ✈ (LIN) *Italy* **40** C6
Lincang *China* **58** F3
Lincheng *China* **56** F8
Linchuan *China* **59** D11
Lincoln = Beamsville
   Canada **114** C5
Lincoln *Argentina* **126** C3
Lincoln *N.Z.* **91** E4
Lincoln *U.K.* **14** D7
Lincoln *Calif., U.S.A.* **110** G5
Lincoln *Ill., U.S.A.* **112** E9
Lincoln *Kans., U.S.A.* **112** F4
Lincoln *Maine, U.S.A.* **113** C19
Lincoln *N.H., U.S.A.* **115** B13
Lincoln *N. Mex., U.S.A.* **109** K11
Lincoln *Nebr., U.S.A.* **112** E5
Lincoln City *U.S.A.* **108** D1
Lincoln Hav = Lincoln Sea
   Arctic **101** A21
Lincoln Sea *Arctic* **101** A21
Lincolnshire □ *U.K.* **14** D7

Lincolnshire Wolds *U.K.* **14** D7
Lincolnton *U.S.A.* **117** D14
Lind *U.S.A.* **108** C4
Linda *U.S.A.* **110** F5
Lindau *Germany* **25** H5
Lindeman I. *Australia* **94** b
Lindeman Islands △ *Australia* **94** b
Linden *Guyana* **124** B7
Linden *Ala., U.S.A.* **117** E11
Linden *Calif., U.S.A.* **110** G5
Linden *Tex., U.S.A.* **116** E7
Lindenhurst *U.S.A.* **115** F11
Lindesberg *Sweden* **10** E9
Lindesnes *Norway* **9** H12
Lindi *Tanzania* **87** D4
Lindi □ *Tanzania* **87** D4
Lindi → *Dem. Rep. of the Congo* **86** B2
Lindley *U.S.A.* **114** D7
Lindö *Sweden* **11** F10
Lindome *Sweden* **11** G6
Líndos *Greece* **49** C10
Líndos, Ákra *Greece* **49** C10
Lindoso *Portugal* **36** D2
Lindow *Germany* **24** C8
Lindsay *Canada* **114** B6
Lindsay *Calif., U.S.A.* **110** J7
Lindsay *Okla., U.S.A.* **116** D6
Lindsborg *U.S.A.* **112** F5
Lindsdal *Sweden* **11** H10
Line Islands *Pac. Oc.* **97** H12
Linesville *U.S.A.* **114** E4
Linfen *China* **56** F6
Ling Xian *Hunan, China* **59** D9
Ling Xian *Shandong, China* **56** F9
Lingao *China* **64** C7
Lingayen *Phil.* **63** A6
Lingayen G. *Phil.* **61** C4
Lingbi *China* **57** H9
Lingbo *Sweden* **10** C10
Lingchuan
   Guangxi Zhuangzu, China **59** E8
Lingchuan *Shanxi, China* **56** G7
Lingen *Germany* **24** C3
Lingga *Indonesia* **62** E2
Lingga, Kepulauan *Indonesia* **62** E2
Lingga Arch. = Lingga,
   Kepulauan *Indonesia* **62** E2
Linghem *Sweden* **11** F9
Lingle *U.S.A.* **108** E2
Lingqiu *China* **56** E8
Lingshan *China* **58** F7
Lingshi *China* **56** F6
Lingshou *China* **56** E8
Lingshui *China* **64** C8
Lingtai *China* **56** G4
Linguère *Senegal* **82** B1
Lingui *China* **59** E8
Lingwu *China* **56** E4
Lingyuan *China* **57** D10
Lingyun *China* **58** E6
Linhai *China* **59** C13
Linhares *Brazil* **125** G10
Linhe *China* **56** D4
Linjiang *China* **57** D14
Linköping *Sweden* **11** F9
Linkou *China* **57** B16
Linli *China* **59** C8
Linnhe, L. *U.K.* **13** E3
Linqi *China* **56** G7
Linqing *China* **56** F8
Linqu *China* **57** F10
Linru *China* **56** G7
Lins *Brazil* **127** A6
Linshu *China* **57** G10
Linshui *China* **58** B6
Linstead *Jamaica* **120** a
Linta → *Madag.* **89** D7
Linth → *Switz.* **25** H5
Linthal *Switz.* **25** J5
Linton *Ind., U.S.A.* **112** F10
Linton *N. Dak., U.S.A.* **112** B3
Lintong *China* **56** G5
Linwood *Canada* **114** C4
Linwu *China* **59** E9
Linxi *China* **57** C10
Linxia *China* **60** C5
Linxiang *China* **59** C9
Linyanti → *Africa* **88** B4
Linyi *China* **57** G10
Linz *Austria* **26** C7
Linz *Germany* **24** E3
Linzhenzhen *China* **56** F5
Linzi *China* **57** F10
Lion, G. du *France* **20** E7
Lionárisso *Cyprus* **49** D13
Lioni *Italy* **43** B8
Lions, G. of = Lion, G. du
   France **20** E7
Lion's Den *Zimbabwe* **87** F3
Lion's Head *Canada* **114** B3
Liozno = Lyozna *Belarus* **32** E6
Lipa *Phil.* **61** E4
Lipali *Mozam.* **87** F4
Lípari *Italy* **43** D7
Lípari, I. *Italy* **43** D7
Lípari, Is. = Eólie, Ís. *Italy* **43** D7
Lipcani *Moldova* **29** B11
Liperi *Finland* **8** E23
Lipetsk *Russia* **33** F10

Lipetsk □ *Russia* **34** D4
Lipiany *Poland* **31** E1
Liping *China* **58** D7
Lipisi *Greece* **47** D8
Lipkany = Lipcani *Moldova* **29** B11
Lipník nad Bečvou
   Czech Rep. **27** B10
Lipno *Poland* **31** F6
Lipova *Romania* **28** D6
Lipovets *Ukraine* **23** D15
Lippe → *Germany* **24** D2
Lippstadt *Germany* **24** D4
Lipscomb *U.S.A.* **116** C4
Lipsk *Poland* **30** E10
Lipsko *Poland* **31** G8
Liptovský Hrádok
   Slovak Rep. **27** B12
Liptovský Milkuláš
   Slovak Rep. **27** B12
Liptrap, C. *Australia* **95** F4
Lipu *China* **59** E8
Lira *Uganda* **86** B3
Liri → *Italy* **42** A6
Liria = Llíria *Spain* **39** F4
Lisala *Dem. Rep. of the Congo* **84** D4
Lisboa *Portugal* **37** G1
Lisboa □ *Portugal* **37** F1
Lisboa ✈ (LIS) *Portugal* **37** G1
Lisbon = Lisboa *Portugal* **37** G1
Lisbon *N. Dak., U.S.A.* **112** B5
Lisbon *N.H., U.S.A.* **115** B13
Lisbon *N.Y., U.S.A.* **115** B9
Lisbon *Ohio, U.S.A.* **114** F4
Lisbon Falls *U.S.A.* **113** D18
Lisburn *U.K.* **12** B5
Lisburne, C. *U.S.A.* **106** B6
Liscannor B. *Ireland* **12** D2
Lisdoonvarna *Ireland* **12** C2
Lishe Jiang → *China* **58** E3
Lishi *China* **56** F6
Lishu *China* **57** C13
Lishui *Jiangsu, China* **59** B12
Lishui *Zhejiang, China* **59** C12
Lisianski I. *U.S.A.* **107** K5
Lisichansk = Lysychansk
   Ukraine **33** H10
Lisieux *France* **18** C7
Liski *Russia* **33** G10
L'Isle-Jourdain *Gers, France* **20** E5
L'Isle-Jourdain *Vienne, France* **20** B4
L'Isle-sur-la-Sorgue *France* **21** E9
Lisle-sur-Tarn *France* **20** E5
Lismore *Australia* **95** D5
Lismore *Ireland* **12** D4
Lissos → *Greece* **45** E9
Lista *Norway* **9** G12
Lister, Mt. *Antarctica* **5** D11
Liston *Australia* **95** D5
Listowel *Canada* **114** C4
Listowel *Ireland* **12** D2
Lit *Sweden* **10** A8
Lit-et-Mixe *France* **20** D2
Litang *Guangxi Zhuangzu,
   China* **58** F7
Litang *Sichuan, China* **58** B3
Litang Qu → *China* **58** C3
Litani → *Lebanon* **74** B4
Litchfield *Calif., U.S.A.* **110** E6
Litchfield *Conn., U.S.A.* **115** E11
Litchfield *Ill., U.S.A.* **112** F9
Litchfield *Minn., U.S.A.* **114** C6
Litchfield △ *Australia* **92** B5
Liteni *Romania* **29** C11
Lithgow *Australia* **95** E5
Lithino, Ákra *Greece* **49** E6
Lithuania ■ *Europe* **32** E2
Litija *Slovenia* **41** B11
Lititz *U.S.A.* **115** F8
Litochoro *Greece* **44** F6
Litoměřice *Czech Rep.* **26** A7
Litomyšl *Czech Rep.* **27** B9
Litschau *Austria* **26** C8
Little Abaco *Bahamas* **120** A4
Little Barrier I. *N.Z.* **91** B5
Little Belt Mts. *U.S.A.* **108** C8
Little Bighorn Battlefield △
   U.S.A. **108** D10
Little Blue → *U.S.A.* **112** F5
Little Buffalo → *Canada* **102** A6
Little Cayman *Cayman Is.* **120** C3
Little Churchill → *Canada* **103** B9
Little Colorado → *U.S.A.* **109** H8
Little Current *Canada* **104** C3
Little Current → *Canada* **104** B3
Little Diomede I. *U.S.A.* **106** B5
Little Falls *Minn., U.S.A.* **112** C6
Little Falls *N.Y., U.S.A.* **115** C10
Little Fork → *U.S.A.* **112** A7
Little Grand Rapids *Canada* **103** C9
Little Humboldt → *U.S.A.* **108** F5
Little Inagua I. *Bahamas* **121** B5
Little Karoo *S. Africa* **88** E3
Little Khingan Mts. = Xiao
   Hinggan Ling *China* **60** B7
Little Lake *U.S.A.* **111** K9
Little Laut Is. = Laut Kecil,
   Kepulauan *Indonesia* **62** E5

Little Mecatina =
   Petit-Mécatina → *Canada* **105** B8
Little Minch *U.K.* **13** D2
Little Missouri → *U.S.A.* **112** B2
Little Ouse → *U.K.* **15** E9
Little Rann *India* **68** H4
Little Red → *U.S.A.* **116** D9
Little River *N.Z.* **91** E4
Little Rock *U.S.A.* **116** D8
Little Ruaha → *Tanzania* **86** D4
Little Sable Pt. *U.S.A.* **112** D10
Little Scarcies → *S. Leone* **82** D2
Little Sioux → *U.S.A.* **112** E5
Little Smoky → *Canada* **102** C5
Little Snake → *U.S.A.* **108** F9
Little Tobago *Trin. & Tob.* **125** J16
Little Valley *U.S.A.* **114** D6
Little Wabash → *U.S.A.* **112** G9
Little White → *U.S.A.* **112** D3
Little Zab = Zāb aş
   Şaghîr → *Iraq* **73** E10
Littlefield *U.S.A.* **116** E3
Littlehampton *U.K.* **15** G8
Littleton *U.S.A.* **115** B13
Littoral □ *Cameroon* **83** E7
Litvinov *Czech Rep.* **26** A6
Liu He → *China* **57** D11
Liu Jiang → *China* **58** F7
Liuba *China* **56** H4
Liucheng *China* **58** E7
Liugou *China* **57** D10
Liuhe *China* **57** C13
Liuheng Dao *China* **59** C14
Liujiang *China* **58** E7
Liukang Tenggaja =
   Sabalana, Kepulauan
   Indonesia **63** F5
Liuli *Tanzania* **87** E3
Liupanshui *China* **58** D5
Liuwa Plain *Zambia* **85** G4
Liuyang *China* **59** C9
Liuzhuang *China* **57** H11
Liuzhou *China* **58** E7
Livada *Romania* **28** C7
Livadero *Greece* **44** F5
Livadhia *Cyprus* **49** E12
Livádi *Greece* **46** A4
Livadia *Greece* **46** C4
Livarot *France* **18** D7
Live Oak *Calif., U.S.A.* **110** F5
Live Oak *Fla., U.S.A.* **117** F13
Lively *Canada* **113** B13
Liveras *Cyprus* **49** D11
Livermore *U.S.A.* **110** H5
Livermore, Mt. *U.S.A.* **116** F2
Livermore Falls *U.S.A.* **113** C18
Liverpool *Australia* **95** B5
Liverpool *Canada* **105** D7
Liverpool *U.K.* **14** D4
Liverpool *U.S.A.* **115** C8
Liverpool Bay *U.K.* **14** D4
Liverpool Ra. *Australia* **95** E5
Livingston *Guatemala* **120** C2
Livingston *U.K.* **13** F5
Livingston *Ala., U.S.A.* **117** E10
Livingston *Calif., U.S.A.* **110** H6
Livingston *Mont., U.S.A.* **108** D8
Livingston *S.C., U.S.A.* **117** E14
Livingston *Tenn., U.S.A.* **117** C12
Livingston *Tex., U.S.A.* **116** F7
Livingston Manor *U.S.A.* **115** E10
Livingston, L. *U.S.A.* **116** F7
Livingstone *Zambia* **87** F2
Livingstone Mts. *Tanzania* **87** D3
Livingstonia *Malawi* **87** E3
Livno *Bos.-H.* **28** G2
Livny *Russia* **33** F9
Livonia *Mich., U.S.A.* **113** D12
Livonia *N.Y., U.S.A.* **114** D7
Livorno *Italy* **40** E7
Livradois-Forez △ *France* **20** E7
Livramento *Brazil* **127** C4
Livron-sur-Drôme *France* **21** D8
Livyntsi *Ukraine* **29** B11
Liwale *Tanzania* **87** D4
Liwiec → *Poland* **31** F8
Liwonde *Malawi* **87** F4
Liwonde △ *Malawi* **87** F4
Lixi *China* **58** D3
Lixian *China* **58** B6
Lixouri *Greece* **46** C2
Liyang *China* **59** B12
Lizard I. *Australia* **94** A4
Lizard Pt. *U.K.* **15** H2
Lizarra = Estella *Spain* **38** C2
Lizzano *Italy* **43** B10
Ljig *Serbia* **44** B4
Ljubija *Bos.-H.* **41** D13
Ljubinje *Bos.-H.* **44** D2
Ljubišnja *Europe* **44** C3
Ljubljana *Slovenia* **41** B11
Ljubljana ✈ (LJU) *Slovenia* **41** B11
Ljubno *Slovenia* **41** B11
Ljubovija *Serbia* **44** B3
Ljugarn *Sweden* **11** G12
Ljung *Sweden* **11** F7
Ljungan → *Sweden* **10** B11
Ljungaverk *Sweden* **10** B10

Ljungby *Sweden* **11** H7
Ljungbyholm *Sweden* **11** H10
Ljungdalen *Sweden* **10** B6
Ljungsbro *Sweden* **11** F9
Ljungskile *Sweden* **11** F5
Ljusdal *Sweden* **10** C10
Ljusfallshammar *Sweden* **11** F9
Ljusnan → *Sweden* **10** C11
Ljusne *Sweden* **10** C11
Ljutomer *Slovenia* **41** B13
Llagostera *Spain* **38** D7
Llancanelo, Salina *Argentina* **126** D2
Llandeilo *U.K.* **15** F4
Llandovery *U.K.* **15** F4
Llandrindod Wells *U.K.* **15** E4
Llandudno *U.K.* **14** D4
Llanelli *U.K.* **15** F3
Llangollen *U.K.* **14** E4
Llanidloes *U.K.* **15** E4
Llano *U.S.A.* **116** F5
Llano → *U.S.A.* **116** F5
Llano Estacado *U.S.A.* **116** E3
Llanos *S. Amer.* **124** C4
Llanos de Challe △ *Chile* **126** B1
Llanquihue, L. *Chile* **128** E1
Llanwrtyd Wells *U.K.* **15** E4
Llebeig, C. des *Spain* **48** B9
Lleida *Spain* **38** D5
Lleida □ *Spain* **38** C6
Llentrisca, C. *Spain* **48** C7
Llera de Canales *Mexico* **119** C5
Llerena *Spain* **37** G5
Lleyn Peninsula *U.K.* **14** E3
Llico *Chile* **126** C1
Lliria *Spain* **39** F4
Llívia *Spain* **38** C6
Llobregat → *Spain* **38** D7
Llodio *Spain* **38** B2
Lloret de Mar *Spain* **38** D7
Lloseta *Spain* **48** B9
Lloyd B. *Australia* **94** A3
Lloyd L. *Canada* **103** B7
Lloydminster *Canada* **103** C7
Llubí *Spain* **48** B10
Llucena del Cid *Spain* **38** E4
Llucmajor *Spain* **48** B9
Llullaillaco, Volcán *S. Amer.* **126** A2
Llullaillaco △ *Chile* **126** A2
Lo → *Vietnam* **64** B5
Loa *U.S.A.* **108** G8
Loa → *Chile* **126** A1
Loaita I. *S. China Sea* **62** B4
Loange →
Dem. Rep. of the Congo **84** E4
Loano *Italy* **40** D5
Lobatse *Botswana* **88** D4
Löbau *Germany* **24** D10
Lobenstein *Germany* **24** E7
Lobería *Argentina* **126** D4
Löberöd *Sweden* **11** J7
Lobito *Angola* **85** G2
Lobo → *Ivory C.* **82** D3
Lobos *Argentina* **126** D4
Lobos, I. *Mexico* **118** B3
Lobos, I. de *Canary Is.* **48** F6
Łobżenica *Poland* **31** E4
Loc Binh *Vietnam* **64** B6
Loc Ninh *Vietnam* **65** G6
Locarno *Switz.* **25** J4
Loch Baghasdail =
Lochboisdale *U.K.* **13** D1
Loch Garman = Wexford
Ireland **12** D5
Loch Lomond and the
Trossachs △ *U.K.* **13** E4
Loch Nam Madadh =
Lochmaddy *U.K.* **13** D1
Lochaber *U.K.* **13** E3
Locharbriggs *U.K.* **13** F5
Lochboisdale *U.K.* **13** D1
Loche, L. La *Canada* **103** B7
Lochem *Neths.* **17** B6
Loches *France* **18** E7
Lochgilphead *U.K.* **13** E3
Lochinvar △ *Zambia* **87** F2
Lochinver *U.K.* **13** C3
Lochmaddy *U.K.* **13** D1
Lochnagar *Australia* **94** C4
Lochnagar *U.K.* **13** E5
Łochów *Poland* **31** F8
Lochy, L. *U.K.* **13** E4
Lock *Australia* **95** E2
Lock Haven *U.S.A.* **114** E7
Lockeford *U.S.A.* **110** G5
Lockeport *Canada* **105** D6
Lockerbie *U.K.* **13** F5
Lockhart *U.S.A.* **116** G6
Lockhart, L. *Australia* **93** F2
Lockhart River *Australia* **94** A3
Lockhart River *Australia* **94** A3
Lockney *U.S.A.* **116** D4
Lockport *U.S.A.* **114** C6
Locminé *France* **18** E4
Locri *Italy* **43** D9
Locronan *France* **18** D2
Lod *Israel* **74** D3
Lodeinoye Pole *Russia* **32** B7

Lodève *France* **20** E7
Lodge Bay *Canada* **105** B8
Lodge Grass *U.S.A.* **108** D10
Lodhran *Pakistan* **68** E4
Lodi *Italy* **40** C6
Lodi *Calif., U.S.A.* **110** G5
Lodi *Ohio, U.S.A.* **114** E3
Lodja *Dem. Rep. of the Congo* **86** C1
Lodosa *Spain* **38** C2
Lödöse *Sweden* **11** F6
Lodwar *Kenya* **86** B4
Łódź *Poland* **31** G6
Łódzkie □ *Poland* **31** G6
Loei *Thailand* **64** D3
Loengo *Dem. Rep. of the Congo* **86** C2
Loeriesfontein *S. Africa* **88** E2
Lofa → *Liberia* **83** D2
Lofa Mano △ *Liberia* **82** D2
Lofer *Austria* **26** D5
Lofoten *Norway* **8** B16
Lofsdalen *Sweden* **10** B7
Lofsen → *Sweden* **10** B7
Loftahammar *Sweden* **11** G10
Loga *Niger* **83** C5
Logan *Iowa, U.S.A.* **112** E6
Logan *Ohio, U.S.A.* **113** F12
Logan *Utah, U.S.A.* **108** F8
Logan *W. Va., U.S.A.* **113** G13
Logan, Mt. *Canada* **100** E3
Logandale *U.S.A.* **111** J12
Logansport *Ind., U.S.A.* **112** E10
Logansport *La., U.S.A.* **116** F8
Logirim *Sudan* **81** G3
Logo *Sudan* **81** F3
Logone → *Chad* **79** F9
Logroño *Spain* **38** C2
Logrosán *Spain* **37** F5
Løgstør *Denmark* **11** H3
Løgumkloster *Denmark* **11** J2
Lohals *Denmark* **11** J4
Lohardaga *India* **69** H11
Loharia *India* **68** H6
Loharu *India* **68** E6
Lohja *Finland* **32** B3
Löhne *Germany* **24** C4
Lohr *Germany* **25** F5
Lohri Wah → *Pakistan* **68** F2
Loi-kaw *Burma* **67** K20
Loimaa *Finland* **32** B2
Loir → *France* **18** E6
Loir-et-Cher □ *France* **18** E8
Loire □ *France* **21** C8
Loire → *France* **18** E4
Loire Anjou Touraine ○
France **18** E6
Loire-Atlantique □ *France* **18** E5
Loiret □ *France* **19** E9
Loitz *Germany* **24** B9
Loja *Ecuador* **124** D3
Loja *Spain* **37** H6
Loji = Kawasi *Indonesia* **63** E7
Lojo = Lohja *Finland* **32** B3
Løjt Kirkeby *Denmark* **11** J3
Lojung *China* **58** E7
Loka *Sudan* **81** G3
Lokandu
Dem. Rep. of the Congo **86** C2
Lokeren *Belgium* **17** C3
Lokgwabe *Botswana* **88** C3
Lokhvitsa *Ukraine* **33** G7
Lokichar *Kenya* **86** B4
Lokichokio *Kenya* **86** B3
Lokitaung *Kenya* **86** B4
Lokkan tekojärvi *Finland* **8** C22
Løkken *Denmark* **11** G3
Loknya *Russia* **32** D6
Loko *Nigeria* **83** D6
Lokoja *Nigeria* **83** D6
Lokolo →
Dem. Rep. of the Congo **84** E3
Lokot *Russia* **33** F8
Lol *Sudan* **81** F2
Lol → *Sudan* **81** F2
Lola *Guinea* **82** D3
Lola, Mt. *U.S.A.* **110** F6
Lolgorien *Kenya* **86** C3
Lolibai, Gebel *Sudan* **81** G3
Lolimi *Sudan* **81** G3
Loliondo *Tanzania* **86** C4
Lolland *Denmark* **11** K5
Lollar *Germany* **24** E4
Lolo *U.S.A.* **108** C6
Lolodorf *Cameroon* **83** E7
Lom *Bulgaria* **44** C7
Lom → *Bulgaria* **44** C7
Lom Kao *Thailand* **64** D3
Lom Sak *Thailand* **64** D3
Loma *U.S.A.* **108** C8
Loma Linda *U.S.A.* **111** L9
Loma Mansa *S. Leone* **82** D2
Loma Mts. *S. Leone* **82** D2
Lomalóma *Fiji* **91** a
Lomami →
Dem. Rep. of the Congo **86** B1
Lomas de Zamora *Argentina* **126** C4
Lombadina *Australia* **92** C3
Lombárdia □ *Italy* **40** C6
Lombardy = Lombárdia □
Italy **40** C6

Lombez *France* **20** E4
Lomblen *Indonesia* **63** F6
Lombok *Indonesia* **62** F5
Lombok, Selat *Indonesia* **63** K18
Lomé *Togo* **83** D5
Lomela *Dem. Rep. of the Congo* **84** E4
Lomela →
Dem. Rep. of the Congo **84** E4
Lomianki *Poland* **31** F7
Lomma *Sweden* **11** J7
Lommel *Belgium* **17** C5
Lomond *Canada* **102** C6
Lomond, L. *U.K.* **13** E4
Lomonosov Ridge *Arctic* **4** A
Lomphat *Cambodia* **64** F6
Lompobatang *Indonesia* **63** F5
Lompoc *U.S.A.* **111** L6
Łomża *Poland* **31** E9
Lon, Ko *Thailand* **65** a
Loncoche *Chile* **128** D2
Londa *India* **66** M9
Londiani *Kenya* **86** C4
Londinières *France* **18** C8
London *Canada* **114** D3
London *U.K.* **15** F7
London *Ky., U.S.A.* **113** G11
London *Ohio, U.S.A.* **113** F12
London, Greater □ *U.K.* **15** F7
London Gatwick ✈ (LGW)
U.K. **15** F7
London Heathrow ✈ (LHR)
U.K. **15** F7
London Stansted ✈ (STN)
U.K. **15** F7
Londonderry *U.K.* **12** B4
Londonderry □ *U.K.* **12** B4
Londonderry, C. *Australia* **92** B4
Londonderry, I. *Chile* **128** H2
Londres *Argentina* **128** B3
Londrina *Brazil* **127** A5
Lone Pine *U.S.A.* **110** J8
Lonely Mine *Zimbabwe* **89** B4
Long B. *U.S.A.* **117** E15
Long Beach *Calif., U.S.A.* **111** M8
Long Beach *N.Y., U.S.A.* **115** F11
Long Beach *Wash., U.S.A.* **110** D2
Long Branch *U.S.A.* **115** F11
Long Creek *U.S.A.* **108** D4
Long Eaton *U.K.* **14** E6
Long I. *Australia* **94** b
Long I. *Bahamas* **121** B4
Long I. *Canada* **104** B4
Long I. *Ireland* **12** E2
Long I. *U.S.A.* **115** F11
Long Island Sd. *U.S.A.* **115** E12
Long L. *Canada* **104** C2
Long L. *U.S.A.* **115** C10
Long Lake *U.S.A.* **115** C10
Long Point *Canada* **114** D4
Long Point B. *Canada* **114** D4
Long Prairie *U.S.A.* **112** C6
Long Prairie → *U.S.A.* **112** B6
Long Pt. *Ont., Canada* **114** D4
Long Pt. *Ont., Canada* **115** C8
Long Range Mts. *Canada* **105** C8
Long Reef *Australia* **92** B4
Long Sault *Canada* **115** A10
Long Str. = Longa, Proliv
Russia **53** C18
Long Thanh *Vietnam* **65** G6
Long Xian *China* **56** G4
Long Xuyen *Vietnam* **65** G5
Longa *Greece* **46** E3
Longa, Proliv *Russia* **53** C18
Long'an *China* **58** F5
Longarone *Italy* **41** B9
Longbenton *U.K.* **14** B6
Longboat Key *U.S.A.* **117** H13
Longchang *China* **58** C5
Longchi *China* **58** C5
Longchuan *Guangdong, China* **59** E10
Longchuan *Yunnan, China* **58** E1
Longde *China* **56** G4
Longeau *France* **19** E12
Longford *Australia* **95** G4
Longford *Ireland* **12** C4
Longford □ *Ireland* **12** C4
Longhai *China* **59** E11
Longhua *China* **57** D9
Longhui *China* **59** D8
Longido *Tanzania* **86** C4
Longiram *Indonesia* **62** E5
Longkou *Jiangxi, China* **59** D10
Longkou *Shandong, China* **57** F11
Longlac *Canada* **104** C2
Longli *China* **58** D6
Longlin *China* **58** E5
Longling *China* **58** E2
Longmeadow *U.S.A.* **115** D12
Longmen *China* **59** F10
Longming *China* **58** F6
Longmont *U.S.A.* **108** F11
Longnan *China* **59** E10
Longnawan *Indonesia* **62** D4
Longobucco *Italy* **43** C9
Longquan *China* **59** C12
Longreach *Australia* **94** C3
Longshan *China* **58** C7
Longsheng *China* **59** E8

Longué-Jumelles *France* **18** E6
Longueau *France* **19** C9
Longueuil *Canada* **115** A11
Longuyon *France* **19** C12
Longvic *France* **19** E12
Longview *Tex., U.S.A.* **116** E7
Longview *Wash., U.S.A.* **110** D4
Longwy *France* **19** C12
Longxi *China* **56** G3
Longyan *China* **59** E11
Longyearbyen *Svalbard* **4** B8
Longyou *China* **59** C12
Longzhou *China* **58** F6
Lonigo *Italy* **41** C8
Löningen *Germany* **24** C3
Lonja → *Croatia* **41** C13
Lonoke *U.S.A.* **116** D9
Lonquimay *Chile* **128** D2
Lons-le-Saunier *France* **19** F12
Lönsboda *Sweden* **11** H8
Lookout, C. *Canada* **104** A3
Lookout, C. *U.S.A.* **117** D16
Loolmalasin *Tanzania* **86** C4
Loon → *Alta., Canada* **102** B5
Loon → *Man., Canada* **103** B8
Loon Lake *Canada* **103** C7
Loongana *Australia* **93** F4
Loop Hd. *Ireland* **12** D2
Lop Buri *Thailand* **64** E3
Lop Nor = Lop Nur *China* **60** B4
Lop Nur *China* **60** B4
Lopare *Bos.-H.* **28** F3
Lopatin *Russia* **35** J8
Lopatina, Gora *Russia* **53** D15
Lopatka *Russia* **53** D16
Lopaye *Sudan* **81** F3
Lopez *Phil.* **61** E5
Lopez *U.S.A.* **115** E8
Lopez, C. *Gabon* **84** E1
Lopphavet *Norway* **8** A19
Lora → *Afghan.* **66** D4
Lora, Hāmūn-i- *Pakistan* **66** E4
Lora Cr. → *Australia* **95** D2
Lora del Río *Spain* **37** H5
Lorain *U.S.A.* **114** E2
Loralai *Pakistan* **68** D3
Lorca *Spain* **39** H3
Lord Howe I. *Pac. Oc.* **90** E8
Lord Howe Rise *Pac. Oc.* **96** L8
Lordsburg *U.S.A.* **109** K9
Loreto *Brazil* **125** E9
Loreto *Italy* **41** E10
Loreto *Mexico* **118** B2
Lorgues *France* **21** E10
Lorient *France* **18** E3
Lorin, Firth of *U.K.* **13** E3
Lorne *Australia* **95** F3
Loronyo *Sudan* **81** G3
Lorovouno *Cyprus* **49** D11
Lörrach *Germany* **25** H3
Lorraine □ *France* **19** D13
Lorraine △ *France* **19** D12
Los *Sweden* **10** C9
Los, Îles de *Guinea* **82** D2
Los Alamos *Calif., U.S.A.* **111** L6
Los Alamos *N. Mex., U.S.A.* **109** J10
Los Alcornocales △ *Spain* **37** J5
Los Altos *U.S.A.* **110** H4
Los Andes *Chile* **126** C1
Los Angeles *Chile* **126** D1
Los Angeles *U.S.A.* **111** M8
Los Angeles, Bahia de
Mexico **118** B2
Los Angeles Aqueduct
U.S.A. **111** K9
Los Angeles Int. ✈ (LAX)
U.S.A. **111** M8
Los Banos *U.S.A.* **110** H6
Los Barrios *Spain* **37** J5
Los Blancos *Argentina* **126** A3
Los Cardones △ *Argentina* **126** B2
Los Chiles *Costa Rica* **120** D3
Los Corrales de Buelna *Spain* **36** B6
Los Cristianos *Canary Is.* **48** F3
Los Gallardos *Spain* **39** H3
Los Gatos *U.S.A.* **110** H5
Los Haïtises △ *Dom. Rep.* **121** C6
Los Hermanos Is. *Venezuela* **121** D7
Los Islotes *Canary Is.* **48** E6
Los Llanos de Aridane
Canary Is. **48** F2
Los Loros *Chile* **126** B1
Los Lunas *U.S.A.* **109** J10
Los Mochis *Mexico* **118** B3
Los Monegros *Spain* **38** D4
Los Nietos *Spain* **39** H4
Los Olivos *U.S.A.* **111** L6
Los Palacios *Cuba* **120** B3
Los Palacios y Villafranca
Spain **37** H5
Los Queñes *Chile* **126** D1
Los Reyes de Salgado
Mexico **118** D4

Los Roques Is. *Venezuela* **121** D6
Los Santos de Maimona
Spain **37** G4
Los Teques *Venezuela* **124** A5
Los Testigos, Is. *Venezuela* **124** A6
Los Vilos *Chile* **126** C1
Los Yébenes *Spain* **37** F7
Losice *Poland* **31** F9
Lošinj *Croatia* **41** D11
Loskop Dam *S. Africa* **89** D4
Løsning *Denmark* **11** J3
Lossiemouth *U.K.* **13** D5
Lossnen △ *Sweden* **10** B6
Lostwithiel *U.K.* **15** G3
Lot □ *France* **20** D5
Lot → *France* **20** D4
Lot-et-Garonne □ *France* **20** D4
Lota *Chile* **126** D1
Lotagipi Swamp *Sudan* **81** G3
Lotfābād *Iran* **71** B8
Lothair *S. Africa* **89** D5
Lotorp *Sweden* **11** F9
Lötschbergtunnel *Switz.* **25** J3
Lotta → *Europe* **8** B24
Lotung *Taiwan* **59** E13
Loubomo *Congo* **84** E2
Loudéac *France* **18** D4
Loudi *China* **59** D8
Loudonville *U.S.A.* **114** F2
Loudun *France* **18** E7
Loue → *France* **19** E12
Louga *Senegal* **82** B1
Louga □ *Senegal* **82** B1
Loughborough *U.K.* **14** E6
Lougheed I. *Canada* **101** B10
Loughrea *Ireland* **12** C3
Loughros More B. *Ireland* **12** B3
Louhans *France* **19** F12
Louis Trichardt *S. Africa* **89** C4
Louis XIV, Pte. *Canada* **104** B4
Louisa *U.S.A.* **113** F12
Louisbourg *Canada* **105** C8
Louisburgh *Ireland* **12** C2
Louise I. *Canada* **102** C2
Louiseville *Canada* **104** C5
Louisiade Arch. *Papua N. G.* **90** C8
Louisiana *U.S.A.* **112** F8
Louisiana □ *U.S.A.* **116** F9
Louisville *Ky., U.S.A.* **113** F11
Louisville *Miss., U.S.A.* **117** E10
Louisville *Ohio, U.S.A.* **114** F3
Louisville Ridge *Pac. Oc.* **96** L10
Loulay *France* **20** B3
Loulé *Portugal* **37** H3
Loulouni *Mali* **82** C3
Loum *Cameroon* **83** E6
Louny *Czech Rep.* **26** A6
Loup City *U.S.A.* **112** E4
Loups Marins, Lacs des
Canada **104** A5
Lourdes *France* **20** E3
Lourdes-de-Blanc-Sablon
Canada **105** B8
Lourinhã *Portugal* **37** F1
Louroujina *Cyprus* **49** E12
Lousã *Portugal* **36** E2
Louta *Burkina Faso* **82** C4
Louth *Australia* **95** E4
Louth *Ireland* **12** C5
Louth □ *Ireland* **12** C5
Louth *U.K.* **14** D7
Loutra Edipsou *Greece* **46** C5
Loutraki *Greece* **46** D4
Loutropoli Thermis *Greece* **47** B8
Louvain = Leuven *Belgium* **17** D4
Louviers *France* **18** C8
Louwsburg *S. Africa* **89** D5
Lovat → *Russia* **32** C6
Lovćen *Montenegro* **44** D2
Lovćen △ *Montenegro* **44** D2
Lovech *Bulgaria* **45** C8
Lovech □ *Bulgaria* **45** C8
Loveland *U.S.A.* **108** E2
Lovell *U.S.A.* **108** D9
Lovelock *U.S.A.* **108** F4
Lóvere *Italy* **40** C7
Lövestad *Sweden* **11** J7
Loviisa *Finland* **32** B4
Loving *U.S.A.* **109** K11
Lovington *U.S.A.* **109** K12
Lovisa = Loviisa *Finland* **32** B4
Lovosice *Czech Rep.* **26** A7
Lovran *Croatia* **41** C11
Lovrin *Romania* **28** E5
Lövstabruk *Sweden* **10** D11
Lövstabukten *Sweden* **10** D11
Low, L. *Canada* **104** B4
Low Pt. *Australia* **93** F4
Low Tatra = Nízké Tatry
Slovak Rep. **27** C12
Lowa *Dem. Rep. of the Congo* **86** C2
Lowa →
Dem. Rep. of the Congo **86** C2
Lowell *U.S.A.* **115** D13
Lowellville *U.S.A.* **114** E4
Löwen → *Namibia* **88** D2
Lower Alkali L. *U.S.A.* **108** F3
Lower Arrow L. *Canada* **102** D5

Lower Austria =
Niederösterreich □ *Austria* **26** C8
Lower California = Baja
California *Mexico* **118** A1
Lower Hutt *N.Z.* **91** D5
Lower Lake *U.S.A.* **110** G4
Lower Manitou L. *Canada* **103** D10
Lower Post *Canada* **102** B3
Lower Red L. *U.S.A.* **112** B6
Lower Saxony =
Niedersachsen □ *Germany* **24** C4
Lower Tunguska =
Tunguska,
Nizhnyaya → *Russia* **53** C9
Lower Zambezi △ *Zambia* **87** F3
Lowestoft *U.K.* **15** E9
Lowgar □ *Afghan.* **66** B6
Łowicz *Poland* **31** F6
Lowther I. *Canada* **101** C12
Lowville *U.S.A.* **115** C9
Loxton *Australia* **95** E3
Loxton *S. Africa* **88** E3
Loyalton *U.S.A.* **110** F6
Loyalty Is. = Loyauté, Îs.
N. Cal. **90** D9
Loyang = Luoyang *China* **56** G7
Loyauté, Îs. *N. Cal.* **90** D9
Loyev = Loyew *Belarus* **23** C16
Loyew *Belarus* **23** C16
Loyoro *Uganda* **86** B3
Lož *Slovenia* **41** C11
Lozère □ *France* **20** D7
Loznica *Serbia* **44** B3
Lozova *Ukraine* **33** H9
Ltalaltuma ○ *Australia* **92** D5
Lü Shan *China* **59** C11
Lü Tao *Taiwan* **59** F13
Luachimo *Angola* **84** F4
Luajan → *India* **69** G11
Lualaba →
Dem. Rep. of the Congo **86** B2
Luambe △ *Zambia* **87** E3
Luampa *Zambia* **87** F1
Lu'an *China* **59** B11
Luan Chau *Vietnam* **58** G4
Luan He → *China* **57** E10
Luan Xian *China* **57** E10
Luancheng
Guangxi Zhuangzu, China **58** F7
Luancheng *Hebei, China* **56** F8
Luanco *Spain* **36** B5
Luanda *Angola* **84** F2
Luang, Thale *Thailand* **65** J3
Luang Prabang *Laos* **58** H4
Luangwa *Zambia* **87** F3
Luangwa → *Zambia* **87** E3
Luangwa Valley *Zambia* **87** E3
Luangwe = Loange →
Dem. Rep. of the Congo **84** E4
Luanne *China* **57** D9
Luanping *China* **57** D9
Luanshya *Zambia* **87** E2
Luapula □ *Zambia* **87** E2
Luapula → *Africa* **87** D2
Luarca *Spain* **36** B4
Luashi *Dem. Rep. of the Congo* **87** E3
Luau *Angola* **84** G4
Lubaczów *Poland* **31** H10
Lubań *Poland* **31** G2
Lubana, Ozero = Lubānas
Ezers *Latvia* **32** D4
Lubānas Ezers *Latvia* **32** D4
Lubang *Phil.* **61** E4
Lubang Is. *Phil.* **63** B6
Lubango *Angola* **85** G2
Lubao *Dem. Rep. of the Congo* **86** D2
Lubartów *Poland* **31** G9
Lubawa *Poland* **30** E6
Lübbecke *Germany* **24** C4
Lübben *Germany* **24** D9
Lübbenau *Germany* **24** D9
Lubbock *U.S.A.* **116** E4
Lübeck *Germany* **24** B6
Lübecker Bucht *Germany* **24** A6
Lubefu *Dem. Rep. of the Congo* **86** C1
Lubefu →
Dem. Rep. of the Congo **86** C1
Lubelskie □ *Poland* **31** G9
Lubero = Luofu
Dem. Rep. of the Congo **86** C2
Luberon △ *France* **21** E9
Lubersac *France* **20** C5
Lubicon L. *Canada* **102** B5
Lubień Kujawski *Poland* **31** F6
Lubilash →
Dem. Rep. of the Congo **84** F4
Lubin *Poland* **31** G3
Lublin *Poland* **31** G9
Lubliniec *Poland* **31** H5
Lubnān = Lebanon ■ *Asia* **74** B5
Lubnān, Jabal *Lebanon* **74** B4
Lubniewice *Poland* **31** F2
Lubny *Ukraine* **33** G7
Lubomierz *Poland* **31** G2
Luboń *Poland* **31** F3
Lubongola
Dem. Rep. of the Congo **86** C2
L'ubotín *Slovak Rep.* **27** B13
Lubraniec *Poland* **31** F5

Lubsko *Poland* **31** G1
Lübtheen *Germany* **24** B7
Lubuagan *Phil.* **61** C4
Lubudi *Dem. Rep. of the Congo* **84** F5
Lubudi ➤
  Dem. Rep. of the Congo **87** D2
Lubuklinggau *Indonesia* **62** E2
Lubuksikaping *Indonesia* **62** D2
Lubumbashi
  Dem. Rep. of the Congo **87** E2
Lubunda
  Dem. Rep. of the Congo **86** D2
Lubungu *Zambia* **87** E2
Lubuskie □ *Poland* **31** F2
Lubutu *Dem. Rep. of the Congo* **86** C2
Luc An Chau *Vietnam* **64** A5
Luc-en-Diois *France* **21** D9
Lucan *Canada* **114** C3
Lucania, Mt. *Canada* **100** E3
Lucas Channel = Main
  Channel *Canada* **114** A3
Lucban *Phil.* **61** D4
Lucca *Italy* **40** E7
Lucé *France* **18** D8
Luce Bay *U.K.* **13** G4
Lucea *Jamaica* **120** a
Lucedale *U.S.A.* **117** F10
Lucena *Phil.* **61** E4
Lucena *Spain* **37** H6
Lučenec *Slovak Rep.* **27** C12
Lucera *Italy* **43** A8
Lucerne = Luzern *Switz.* **25** H4
Lucerne *U.S.A.* **110** F4
Lucerne Valley *U.S.A.* **111** L10
Lucero *Mexico* **118** A3
Luchena ➤ *Spain* **39** H3
Lucheng *China* **56** F7
Lucheringo ➤ *Mozam.* **87** E4
Lüchow *Germany* **24** C7
Luchuan *China* **59** F8
Lucia *U.S.A.* **110** J5
Lucinda *Australia* **94** B4
Luckau *Germany* **24** D9
Luckenwalde *Germany* **24** C9
Luckhoff *S. Africa* **88** D3
Lucknow *Canada* **114** C3
Lucknow *India* **69** F9
Luçon *France* **20** B2
Lüda = Dalian *China* **57** E11
Luda Kamchiya ➤ *Bulgaria* **45** C11
Ludbreg *Croatia* **41** B13
Lüdenscheid *Germany* **24** D3
Lüderitz *Namibia* **88** D2
Lüderitzbaai *Namibia* **88** D2
Ludhiana *India* **68** D6
Ludian *China* **58** D4
Luding Qiao *China* **58** C4
Lüdinghausen *Germany* **24** D3
Ludington *U.S.A.* **112** D10
Ludlow *U.K.* **15** E5
Ludlow *Calif., U.S.A.* **111** L10
Ludlow *Pa., U.S.A.* **114** E6
Ludlow *Vt., U.S.A.* **115** C12
Ludus *Romania* **29** D9
Ludvika *Sweden* **10** D9
Ludwigsburg *Germany* **25** G5
Ludwigsfelde *Germany* **24** C9
Ludwigshafen *Germany* **25** F4
Ludwigslust *Germany* **24** B7
Ludza *Latvia* **32** H3
Lueki *Dem. Rep. of the Congo* **86** C2
Luena *Dem. Rep. of the Congo* **87** D2
Luena *Zambia* **87** E3
Luena Flats *Zambia* **85** G4
Luenha = Ruenya ➤ *Africa* **87** F3
Lüeyang *China* **56** H4
Lufeng *Guangdong, China* **59** F10
Lufeng *Yunnan, China* **58** E4
Lufira ➤
  Dem. Rep. of the Congo **87** D2
Lufkin *U.S.A.* **116** F7
Lufupa *Dem. Rep. of the Congo* **87** E1
Luga *Russia* **32** C5
Luga ➤ *Russia* **32** C5
Lugano *Switz.* **25** J4
Lugano, L. di *Switz.* **40** C6
Lugansk = Luhansk
  Ukraine **33** H10
Lugard's Falls *Kenya* **86** C4
Lugela *Mozam.* **87** F4
Lugenda ➤ *Mozam.* **87** E4
Lugh Ganana = Luuq
  Somali Rep. **75** G3
Lugnaquillia *Ireland* **12** D5
Lugo *Italy* **41** D8
Lugo *Spain* **36** B3
Lugo □ *Spain* **36** C3
Lugoj *Romania* **28** E6
Lugovoy = Qulan *Kazakhstan* **52** E8
Luhansk *Ukraine* **33** H10
Luhansk □ *Ukraine* **33** H10
Luhe *China* **59** A12
Luhe ➤ *Germany* **24** B6
Luhuo *China* **58** B3
Lui ➤ *Angola* **84** F3
Luiana *Angola* **88** B3
Luiana ➤ *Angola* **85** H4
Luichow Pen. = Leizhou
  Bandao *China* **58** G7

Luimneach = Limerick
  Ireland **12** D3
Luing *U.K.* **13** E3
Luino *Italy* **40** C5
Luís Correia *Brazil* **125** D10
Luitpold Coast *Antarctica* **5** D1
Luiza *Dem. Rep. of the Congo* **84** F4
Luizi *Dem. Rep. of the Congo* **86** D2
Luján *Argentina* **126** C4
Lujiang *China* **59** B11
Lukang *Taiwan* **59** E13
Lukanga Swamp *Zambia* **87** E2
Lukavac *Bos.-H.* **28** F3
Lukenie ➤
  Dem. Rep. of the Congo **84** E3
Lukolela
  Dem. Rep. of the Congo **86** D1
Lukosi *Zimbabwe* **87** F2
Lukovë *Albania* **44** G3
Lukovit *Bulgaria* **45** C8
Luków *Poland* **31** G9
Lukoyanov *Russia* **34** C7
Lukusuzi △ *Zambia* **87** E3
Luleå *Sweden* **8** D20
Luleälven ➤ *Sweden* **8** D20
Lüleburgaz *Turkey* **45** E11
Luliang *China* **58** E4
Lulima *Dem. Rep. of the Congo* **86** C2
Luling *U.S.A.* **116** G6
Lulong *China* **57** E10
Lulonga ➤
  Dem. Rep. of the Congo **84** D3
Lulua ➤
  Dem. Rep. of the Congo **84** E4
Luma *Amer. Samoa* **91** b
Lumajang *Indonesia* **63** H15
Lumār *Iran* **73** F12
Lumbala N'guimbo *Angola* **85** G4
Lumberton *U.S.A.* **117** D15
Lumsden *Canada* **103** C8
Lumsden *N.Z.* **91** F2
Lumut *Malaysia* **65** K3
Lumut, Tanjung *Indonesia* **62** E3
Luna *India* **68** H3
Lunan *China* **58** E4
Lunavada *India* **68** H5
Lunca *Romania* **29** C10
Lunca Corbului *Romania* **29** F9
Lund *Sweden* **11** J7
Lundazi *Zambia* **87** E3
Lunderskov *Denmark* **11** J3
Lundi ➤ *Zimbabwe* **87** G3
Lundu *Malaysia* **62** D3
Lundy *U.K.* **15** F3
Lune ➤ *U.K.* **14** C5
Lüneburg *Germany* **24** B6
Lüneburg Heath =
  Lüneburger Heide
  Germany **24** B6
Lüneburger Heide *Germany* **24** B6
Lunel *France* **21** E8
Lünen *Germany* **24** D3
Lunenburg *Canada* **105** D7
Lunéville *France* **19** D13
Lunga ➤ *Zambia* **87** E2
Lunga Lunga *Kenya* **86** C4
Lungi *S. Leone* **82** D2
Lunglei *India* **67** H18
Luni *India* **68** G5
Luni ➤ *India* **68** G4
Luninets = Luninyets
  Belarus **23** B14
Luning *U.S.A.* **108** G4
Lunino *Russia* **34** D7
Luninyets *Belarus* **23** B14
Lunkaransar *India* **68** E5
Lunsar *S. Leone* **82** D2
Lunsemfwa ➤ *Zambia* **87** E3
Lunsemfwa Falls *Zambia* **87** E2
Luo He ➤ *China* **56** G6
Luocheng *China* **58** E7
Luochuan *China* **56** G5
Luoci *China* **58** E4
Luodian *China* **58** E6
Luoding *China* **59** F8
Luofu *Dem. Rep. of the Congo* **86** C2
Luohe *China* **56** H8
Luojiang *China* **58** B5
Luonan *China* **56** G6
Luoning *China* **56** G6
Luoshan *China* **59** A10
Luotian *China* **59** B10
Luoxiao Shan *China* **59** D10
Luoyang *China* **56** G7
Luoyuan *China* **59** D12
Luozigou *China* **57** C16
Lupeni *Romania* **29** E8
Lupilichi *Mozam.* **87** E4
Łupków *Poland* **31** J9
Lupoing *China* **58** E5
Luquan *China* **58** E4
Luque *Paraguay* **126** B4
Luquillo, Sierra de *Puerto Rico* **121** d
Lúras *Italy* **42** B2
Luray *U.S.A.* **113** F14
Lure *France* **19** E13
Lurgan *U.K.* **12** B5
Lúrio *Mozam.* **87** E5

Lusaka *Zambia* **87** F2
Lusaka □ *Zambia* **87** F2
Lusambo
  Dem. Rep. of the Congo **86** C1
Lusangaye
  Dem. Rep. of the Congo **86** C2
Luseland *Canada* **103** C7
Lusenga Plain △ *Zambia* **87** D2
Lushan *Henan, China* **56** H7
Lushan *Sichuan, China* **58** B4
Lushi *China* **56** G6
Lushnjë *Albania* **44** F3
Lushoto *Tanzania* **86** C4
Lushui *China* **58** E2
Lüshun *China* **57** E11
Lusignan *France* **20** B4
Lusigny-sur-Barse *France* **19** D11
Lusk *U.S.A.* **108** E11
Lussac-les-Châteaux *France* **20** B4
Lustenau *Austria* **26** D2
Lūt, Dasht-e *Iran* **71** D8
Luta = Dalian *China* **57** E11
Lutherstadt Wittenberg
  Germany **24** D8
Luton *U.K.* **15** F7
Luton □ *U.K.* **15** F7
Łutsel K'e *Canada* **103** A6
Lutsk *Ukraine* **23** C13
Lutto = Lotta ➤ *Europe* **8** B24
Lützow Holmbukta *Antarctica* **5** C4
Lutzputs *S. Africa* **88** D3
Luuq *Somali Rep.* **75** G3
Luverne *Ala., U.S.A.* **117** F11
Luverne *Minn., U.S.A.* **112** D5
Luvua *Dem. Rep. of the Congo* **87** D2
Luvua ➤
  Dem. Rep. of the Congo **86** D2
Luvuvhu ➤ *S. Africa* **89** C5
Luwegu ➤ *Tanzania* **87** D4
Luwero *Uganda* **86** B3
Luwuk *Indonesia* **63** E6
Luxembourg *Lux.* **17** E6
Luxembourg □ *Belgium* **17** E5
Luxembourg ■ *Europe* **17** E5
Luxembourg ✈ (LUX) *Lux.* **17** E6
Luxeuil-les-Bains *France* **19** E13
Luxi *Hunan, China* **59** C8
Luxi *Yunnan, China* **58** E4
Luxi *Yunnan, China* **58** E4
Luxor = El Uqsur *Egypt* **80** B3
Luy-de-Béarn ➤ *France* **20** E3
Luy-de-France ➤ *France* **20** E3
Luyi *China* **56** H8
Luz-St-Sauveur *France* **20** F4
Luzern *Switz.* **25** H4
Luzern □ *Switz.* **25** H3
Luzhai *China* **58** E7
Luzhany *Ukraine* **29** B10
Luzhi *China* **58** D5
Luzhou *China* **58** C5
Luziânia *Brazil* **125** G9
Lužnice ➤ *Czech Rep.* **26** B7
Luzon *Phil.* **61** D4
Luzon Strait *Asia* **59** G13
Luzy *France* **19** F10
Luzzi *Italy* **43** C9
Lviv *Ukraine* **23** D13
Lviv □ *Ukraine* **33** H2
Lvov = Lviv *Ukraine* **23** D13
Lwówek *Poland* **31** F3
Lwówek Śląski *Poland* **31** G2
Lyakhavichy *Belarus* **23** B14
Lyakhovskiye, Ostrova
  Russia **53** B15
Lyaki = Läki *Azerbaijan* **35** K8
Lyal I. *Canada* **114** A3
Lyaskovets *Bulgaria* **45** C9
Lyasnaya *Belarus* **31** F10
Lybster *U.K.* **13** C5
Lycaonia *Turkey* **72** D5
Lychen *Germany* **24** B9
Lychkova *Russia* **32** D7
Lycia *Turkey* **47** E11
Lyckeby ➤ *Sweden* **11** H9
Lycksele *Sweden* **8** D18
Lycosura *Greece* **46** D4
Lydda = Lod *Israel* **74** D3
Lyddan I. *Antarctica* **5** D2
Lydenburg *S. Africa* **89** D5
Lydia *Turkey* **47** C10
Łydynia ➤ *Poland* **31** F7
Lyell *N.Z.* **91** D4
Lyell I. *Canada* **102** C2
Lyepyel *Belarus* **32** E5
Lygnern *Sweden* **11** G6
Lykens *U.S.A.* **115** F8
Lyman *Ukraine* **29** E14
Lyman *U.S.A.* **108** F8
Lymanske *Ukraine* **29** D14
Lyme B. *U.K.* **15** G4
Lyme Regis *U.K.* **15** G5
Lymington *U.K.* **15** G6
Lynchburg *U.S.A.* **113** G14
Lynd ➤ *Australia* **94** B3
Lynd Ra. *Australia* **95** D4
Lynden *Canada* **114** C4
Lynden *U.S.A.* **110** B4
Lyndhurst *Australia* **95** E2

Lyndon ➤ *Australia* **93** D1
Lyndonville *N.Y., U.S.A.* **114** C6
Lyndonville *Vt., U.S.A.* **115** B12
Lyngen *Norway* **8** B19
Lynher Reef *Australia* **92** C3
Lynn *U.S.A.* **115** D14
Lynn Canal *U.S.A.* **106** D12
Lynn Haven *U.S.A.* **117** F12
Lynn Lake *Canada* **103** B8
Lynnwood *U.S.A.* **110** C4
Lynton *U.K.* **15** F4
Lyntupy *Belarus* **32** E4
Lynx L. *Canada* **103** A7
Lyon *France* **21** C8
Lyon St-Exupery ✈ (LYS)
  France **21** C8
Lyonnais *France* **21** C8
Lyons = Lyon *France* **21** C8
Lyons *Ga., U.S.A.* **117** E13
Lyons *Kans., U.S.A.* **112** F4
Lyons *N.Y., U.S.A.* **114** C8
Lyons ➤ *Australia* **93** E2
Lyons Falls *U.S.A.* **115** C9
Lyozna *Belarus* **32** E6
Lys = Leie ➤ *Belgium* **17** C3
Lysá nad Labem *Czech Rep.* **26** A7
Lysekil *Sweden* **11** F5
Lysi *Cyprus* **49** D12
Lyskovo *Russia* **34** B7
Lystrup *Denmark* **11** H4
Lysvik *Sweden* **10** D7
Lysychansk *Ukraine* **33** H10
Lytham St. Anne's *U.K.* **14** D4
Lyttelton *N.Z.* **91** E4
Lytton *Canada* **102** C4
Lyuban *Russia* **32** C6
Lyubertsy *Russia* **32** E9
Lyubim *Russia* **32** C11
Lyubimets *Bulgaria* **45** E10
Lyuboml *Ukraine* **31** G11
Lyubotyn *Ukraine* **33** H8
Lyubytino *Russia* **32** C7
Lyudinovo *Russia* **32** F8

M

M.R. Stefanik, Bratislava ✈
  (BTS) *Slovak Rep.* **27** C10
Ma ➤ *Vietnam* **58** H5
Ma'adaba *Jordan* **74** E4
Maamba *Zambia* **88** B4
Ma'ān *Jordan* **74** E4
Ma'ān □ *Jordan* **74** F5
Maanselkä *Finland* **8** E23
Ma'anshan *China* **59** B12
Maarianhamina =
  Mariehamn *Finland* **9** F18
Ma'arrat an Nu'mān *Syria* **72** E7
Maas ➤ *Neths.* **17** C5
Maaseik *Belgium* **17** C5
Maasin *Phil.* **63** B6
Maastricht *Neths.* **17** D5
Maave *Mozam.* **89** C5
Mababe Depression
  Botswana **88** B3
Mabalane *Mozam.* **89** C5
Mabel L. *Canada* **102** C5
Mabenge
  Dem. Rep. of the Congo **86** B1
Maberly *Canada* **115** B8
Mabesi, L. *S. Leone* **82** D2
Mabian *China* **58** C4
Mabil *Ethiopia* **81** E4
Mablethorpe *U.K.* **14** D8
Mably *France* **19** F11
Maboma
  Dem. Rep. of the Congo **86** B2
Mabonto *S. Leone* **82** D2
Mabrouk *Mali* **83** B4
Mabuasehube △ *Botswana* **88** D3
Mabuiag *Australia* **94** a
Mac Bac *Vietnam* **65** H6
Macachín *Argentina* **126** D3
Macaé *Brazil* **127** A7
Macael *Spain* **39** H2
McAlester *U.S.A.* **116** D7
McAllen *U.S.A.* **116** H5
MacAlpine L. *Canada* **100** D11
Macamic *Canada* **104** C4
Macao = Macau *China* **59** F9
Macão *Portugal* **37** F3
Macapá *Brazil* **125** C8
Macarao △ *Venezuela* **121** D6
McArthur ➤ *Australia* **94** B2
McArthur, Port *Australia* **94** B2
Macau *Brazil* **125** E11
Macau *China* **59** F9
McBride *Canada* **102** C4
McCall *U.S.A.* **108** D5
McCamey *U.S.A.* **116** F3
McCammon *U.S.A.* **108** E7
McCarran Int., Las
  Vegas ✈ (LAS) *U.S.A.* **111** J11
McCauley I. *Canada* **102** C2
McCleary *U.S.A.* **110** C3
Macclenny *U.S.A.* **117** F13
Macclesfield *U.K.* **14** D5
M'Clintock Chan. *Canada* **100** C11
McClintock Ra. *Australia* **92** C4

McCloud *U.S.A.* **108** F2
McCluer I. *Australia* **92** B5
McClure *U.S.A.* **114** F7
McClure, L. *U.S.A.* **110** H6
M'Clure Str. *Canada* **101** C8
McClusky *U.S.A.* **112** B3
McComb *U.S.A.* **117** F9
McCook *U.S.A.* **112** E3
McCreary *Canada* **103** C9
McCullough Mt. *U.S.A.* **111** K11
McDermitt *U.S.A.* **108** F5
McDonald *U.S.A.* **114** F4
McDonald Is. *Ind. Oc.* **3** G13
MacDonnell Ranges
  Australia **92** D5
MacDowell L. *Canada* **104** B1
Macduff *U.K.* **13** D6
Maceda *Spain* **36** C3
Macedonia *U.S.A.* **114** E3
Macedonia ■ *Europe* **44** E5
Maceió *Brazil* **125** E11
Macenta *Guinea* **82** D3
Macerata *Italy* **41** E10
McFarland *U.S.A.* **111** K7
McFarlane ➤ *Canada* **103** B7
Macfarlane, L. *Australia* **95** E2
McGehee *U.S.A.* **116** E9
McGill *U.S.A.* **108** G6
Macgillycuddy's Reeks
  Ireland **12** E2
McGraw *U.S.A.* **115** D8
McGregor *U.S.A.* **112** D8
McGregor Ra. *Australia* **95** D3
McGuire, Mt. *Australia* **94** b
Mach *Pakistan* **68** E2
Māch Kowr *Iran* **71** E9
Machado = Jiparaná ➤
  Brazil **124** E7
Machagai *Argentina* **126** B3
Machakos *Kenya* **86** C4
Machala *Ecuador* **124** D3
Machanga *Mozam.* **89** C6
Machattie, L. *Australia* **94** C2
Machault *France* **19** C11
Machava *Mozam.* **89** D5
Machece *Mozam.* **87** F4
Macheke *Zimbabwe* **89** B5
Macheng *China* **59** B10
Machero *Spain* **37** F6
Machhu ➤ *India* **68** H4
Machiara △ *Pakistan* **68** B5
Machias *Maine, U.S.A.* **113** C20
Machias *N.Y., U.S.A.* **114** D6
Machichi ➤ *Canada* **103** B10
Machico *Madeira* **48** D3
Machilipatnam *India* **67** L12
Machiques *Venezuela* **124** A4
Machu Pichu *Peru* **124** F4
Machynlleth *U.K.* **15** E4
Macia *Mozam.* **89** D5
Maciejowice *Poland* **31** G8
McIlwraith Ra. *Australia* **94** A3
Măcin *Romania* **29** E13
Macina *Mali* **82** C4
McInnes L. *Canada* **103** C10
McIntosh *U.S.A.* **112** C3
McIntosh L. *Canada* **103** B8
Macintyre ➤ *Australia* **95** D5
Macizo Galaico *Spain* **36** C3
Maçka *Turkey* **73** B8
Mackay *Australia* **94** K7
Mackay *U.S.A.* **108** E7
Mackay ➤ *Canada* **102** B6
Mackay, L. *Australia* **92** D4
McKay Ra. *Australia* **92** D3
McKeesport *U.S.A.* **114** F5
McKellar *Canada* **114** A5
McKenna *U.S.A.* **110** D4
Mackenzie *Canada* **102** B4
McKenzie *U.S.A.* **117** C10
Mackenzie ➤ *Australia* **94** C4
Mackenzie ➤ *Canada* **100** D5
McKenzie ➤ *U.S.A.* **108** D2
Mackenzie Bay *Canada* **98** C6
Mackenzie City = Linden
  Guyana **124** B7
Mackenzie King I. *Canada* **101** B9
Mackenzie Mts. *Canada* **100** E7
Mackinac, Straits of *U.S.A.* **107** F23
Mackinaw City *U.S.A.* **113** C11
McKinlay *Australia* **94** C3
McKinlay ➤ *Australia* **94** C3
McKinley, Mt. *U.S.A.* **100** E1
McKinley Sea *Arctic* **4** A7
McKinney *U.S.A.* **116** E6
Mackinnon Road *Kenya* **86** C4
McKittrick *U.S.A.* **111** K7
Macklin *Canada* **103** C7
Macksville *Australia* **95** E5
McLaughlin *U.S.A.* **112** C3
Maclean *Australia* **95** D5
McLean *U.S.A.* **116** D4
McLeansboro *U.S.A.* **112** F9
Maclear *S. Africa* **89** E4

Maclear, C. *Malawi* **87** E3
Macleay ➤ *Australia* **95** E5
McLennan *Canada* **102** B5
McLeod ➤ *Canada* **102** C5
MacLeod, L. *Australia* **93** D1
McLeod B. *Canada* **103** A7
McLeod Lake *Canada* **102** C4
McLoughlin, Mt. *U.S.A.* **108** E2
McMechen *U.S.A.* **114** G4
McMinnville *Oreg., U.S.A.* **108** D2
McMinnville *Tenn., U.S.A.* **117** D12
McMurdo *Antarctica* **5** D11
McMurdo Sd. *Antarctica* **5** D11
McMurray = Fort
  McMurray *Canada* **102** B6
McMurray *U.S.A.* **110** B4
Maçobere *Mozam.* **87** G3
Macodoene *Mozam.* **89** C6
Macomb *U.S.A.* **112** E8
Macomer *Italy* **42** B1
Mâcon *France* **19** F11
Macon *Ga., U.S.A.* **117** E13
Macon *Miss., U.S.A.* **117** E10
Macon *Mo., U.S.A.* **112** F7
Macossa *Mozam.* **87** F3
Macoun L. *Canada* **103** B8
Macovane *Mozam.* **89** C6
McPherson *U.S.A.* **112** F5
McPherson Pk. *U.S.A.* **111** L7
McPherson Ra. *Australia* **95** D5
Macquarie ➤ *Australia* **95** E4
Macquarie Harbour *Australia* **95** G4
Macquarie Is. *Pac. Oc.* **96** N7
Macquarie Ridge *S. Ocean* **5** B10
MacRobertson Land
  Antarctica **5** D6
Macroom *Ireland* **12** E3
MacTier *Canada* **114** A5
Macubela *Mozam.* **87** F4
Macugnaga *Italy* **40** C4
Macuira △ *Colombia* **121** D5
Macuiza *Mozam.* **87** F3
Macumba ➤ *Australia* **95** D2
Macuro *Venezuela* **125** K15
Macusani *Peru* **124** F4
Macuse *Mozam.* **87** F4
Macuspana *Mexico* **119** D6
Macusse *Angola* **88** B3
Mada ➤ *Nigeria* **83** D6
Ma'dabā *Jordan* **74** D4
Ma'dabā □ *Jordan* **74** D4
Madadeni *S. Africa* **89** D5
Madagali *Nigeria* **83** C7
Madagascar ■ *Africa* **89** C8
Madā'in Sālih *Si. Arabia* **70** E3
Madama *Niger* **79** D8
Madame, Î. *Canada* **105** C7
Madan *Bulgaria* **45** E8
Madang *Papua N. G.* **90** B7
Madara *Nigeria* **83** C7
Madaripur *Bangla.* **67** H17
Madauk *Burma* **67** L20
Madawaska *Canada* **114** A7
Madawaska ➤ *Canada* **114** A7
Madaya *Burma* **67** H20
Madbar *Sudan* **81** F3
Maddalena *Italy* **42** A2
Maddaloni *Italy* **43** A7
Madeira *Atl. Oc.* **48** D3
Madeira ➤ *Brazil* **124** D7
Madeleine, Îs. de la *Canada* **105** C7
Maden *Turkey* **73** C8
Madera *Mexico* **118** B3
Madera *Calif., U.S.A.* **110** J6
Madera *Pa., U.S.A.* **114** F6
Madha *India* **66** L9
Madhavpur *India* **68** J3
Madhepura *India* **69** F12
Madhubani *India* **69** F12
Madhupur *India* **69** G12
Madhya Pradesh □ *India* **68** J8
Madidi ➤ *Bolivia* **124** F5
Madikeri *India* **66** N9
Madikwe △ *S. Africa* **89** D5
Madill *U.S.A.* **116** D6
Madimba
  Dem. Rep. of the Congo **84** E3
Ma'din *Syria* **73** E8
Madina *Mali* **82** C3
Madinani *Ivory C.* **82** D3
Madinat al Malik Khālid al
  Askarīyah *Si. Arabia* **70** E5
Madīnat ath Thawrah *Syria* **73** E8
Madingou *Gabon* **84** E2
Madirovalo *Madag.* **89** B8
Madison *Calif., U.S.A.* **110** G5
Madison *Fla., U.S.A.* **117** F13
Madison *Ind., U.S.A.* **113** F11
Madison *Nebr., U.S.A.* **112** E5
Madison *Ohio, U.S.A.* **114** E3
Madison *S. Dak., U.S.A.* **112** C5
Madison *Wis., U.S.A.* **112** D9
Madison ➤ *U.S.A.* **108** D8
Madison Heights *U.S.A.* **113** G14
Madisonville *Ky., U.S.A.* **112** G10
Madisonville *Tex., U.S.A.* **116** F7
Madista *Botswana* **88** C4
Madiun *Indonesia* **62** F4
Mado Gashi *Kenya* **86** B4

Madoc *Canada* 114 B7
Madon → *France* 19 D13
Madona *Latvia* 32 D4
Madonie *Italy* 42 E6
Madonna di Campíglio *Italy* 40 B7
Madra Daği *Turkey* 47 B9
Madrakah, Ra's al *Oman* 75 D6
Madras = Chennai *India* 66 N12
Madras = Tamil Nadu □
India 66 P10
Madras *U.S.A.* 108 D3
Madre, L. *U.S.A.* 116 J6
Madre, Sierra *Phil.* 61 C5
Madre de Dios → *Bolivia* 124 F5
Madre de Dios, I. *Chile* 128 G1
Madre del Sur, Sierra
Mexico 119 D5
Madre Occidental, Sierra
Mexico 118 B3
Madre Oriental, Sierra
Mexico 118 C5
Madri *India* 68 G5
Madrid *Spain* 36 E7
Madrid *U.S.A.* 115 B9
Madrid □ *Spain* 36 E7
Madrid Barajas ✈ (MAD)
Spain 36 E7
Madridejos *Spain* 37 F7
Madrigal de las Altas
Torres *Spain* 36 D6
Madrona, Sierra *Spain* 37 G6
Madroñera *Spain* 37 F5
Madu *Sudan* 81 E2
Madula *Dem. Rep. of the Congo* 86 B2
Madura *Australia* 93 F4
Madura *Indonesia* 63 G15
Madura, Selat *Indonesia* 63 G15
Madurai *India* 66 Q11
Madurantakam *India* 66 N11
Madzhalis *Russia* 35 J8
Mae Chan *Thailand* 64 B2
Mae Hong Son *Thailand* 64 C2
Mae Khlong → *Thailand* 64 F3
Mae Phrik *Thailand* 64 D2
Mae Ping △ *Thailand* 64 D2
Mae Ramat *Thailand* 64 D2
Mae Rim *Thailand* 64 C2
Mae Sai *Thailand* 58 G2
Mae Sot *Thailand* 64 D2
Mae Suai *Thailand* 58 H2
Mae Tha *Thailand* 64 C2
Mae Wong △ *Thailand* 64 E2
Mae Yom △ *Thailand* 64 C3
Maebashi *Japan* 55 F9
Maella *Spain* 38 D5
Maestra, Sierra *Cuba* 120 B4
Maevatanana *Madag.* 89 B8
Mafeking = Mafikeng
S. Africa 88 D4
Mafeking *Canada* 103 C8
Maféré *Ivory C.* 82 D4
Mafeteng *Lesotho* 88 D4
Maffra *Australia* 95 F4
Mafia I. *Tanzania* 86 D4
Mafikeng *S. Africa* 88 D4
Mafra *Brazil* 127 B6
Mafra *Portugal* 37 G1
Mafungabusi Plateau
Zimbabwe 87 F2
Magadan *Russia* 53 D16
Magadi *Kenya* 86 C4
Magadi, L. *Kenya* 86 C4
Magaliesburg *S. Africa* 89 D4
Magallanes, Estrecho de
Chile 128 G2
Magaluf *Spain* 39 F7
Magangué *Colombia* 124 B4
Magaria *Niger* 83 C6
Magburaka *S. Leone* 82 D2
Magdagachi *Russia* 53 D13
Magdalen Is. = Madeleine,
Îs. de la *Canada* 105 C7
Magdalena *Argentina* 126 D4
Magdalena *Bolivia* 124 F6
Magdalena *U.S.A.* 109 J10
Magdalena → *Colombia* 124 A4
Magdalena → *Mexico* 118 A2
Magdalena, B. *Mexico* 118 C2
Magdalena, I. *Mexico* 118 C2
Magdalena, Llano de
Mexico 118 C2
Magdalena de Kino *Mexico* 118 A2
Magdeburg *Germany* 24 C7
Magdelaine Cays *Australia* 94 B5
Magdub *Sudan* 81 E2
Magee *U.S.A.* 117 F10
Magelang *Indonesia* 62 F4
Magellan's Str. =
Magallanes, Estrecho de
Chile 128 G2
Magenta *Italy* 40 C5
Magenta, L. *Australia* 93 F2
Magerøya *Norway* 8 A21
Maggia → *Switz.* 25 D4
Maggiorasca, Mte. *Italy* 40 D6
Maggiore, Lago *Italy* 40 B5
Maggotty *Jamaica* 120 a
Maghâgha *Egypt* 80 B3

Maghama *Mauritania* 82 B2
Magherafelt *U.K.* 12 B5
Maghreb *N. Afr.* 78 B5
Magione *Italy* 41 E9
Magistralnyy *Russia* 53 D11
Maglaj *Bos.-H.* 28 B7
Magliano in Toscana *Italy* 41 F8
Máglie *Italy* 43 B11
Magnac-Laval *France* 20 B5
Magnetic Pole (North) *Canada* 4 A2
Magnetic Pole (South)
Antarctica 5 C9
Magnisia □ *Greece* 46 B5
Magnitogorsk *Russia* 52 D6
Magnolia *Ark., U.S.A.* 116 E8
Magnolia *Miss., U.S.A.* 117 F9
Magny-en-Vexin *France* 19 C8
Mago *Fiji* 91 a
Mago △ *Ethiopia* 81 F4
Magog *Canada* 115 A12
Magoro *Uganda* 86 B3
Magosa = Famagusta
Cyprus 49 D12
Magoulades *Greece* 49 A3
Magoye *Zambia* 87 F2
Magpie, L. *Canada* 105 B7
Magrath *Canada* 102 D6
Magre → *Spain* 39 F4
Magrur *Sudan* 81 E3
Magrur, Wadi → *Sudan* 81 D2
Magta Lahjar *Mauritania* 82 B2
Magu *Tanzania* 86 C3
Maguan *China* 58 F5
Maguarinho, C. *Brazil* 125 D9
Magude *Mozam.* 89 D5
Magurski △ *Poland* 31 J8
Mağusa = Famagusta
Cyprus 49 D12
Maguse L. *Canada* 103 A9
Maguse Pt. *Canada* 103 A10
Magvana *India* 68 H3
Magwe *Burma* 67 J19
Magwe □ *Burma* 67 J18
Magwe *Sudan* 81 G3
Magyarország =
Hungary ■ *Europe* 27 D12
Maha Sarakham *Thailand* 64 D4
Mahābād *Iran* 73 D11
Mahabharat Lekh *Nepal* 69 E10
Mahabo *Madag.* 89 C7
Mahadeo Hills *India* 69 H8
Mahaffey *U.S.A.* 114 F6
Mahagi *Dem. Rep. of the Congo* 86 B3
Mahajamba → *Madag.* 89 B8
Mahajamba, Helodranon' i
Madag. 89 B8
Mahajan *India* 68 E5
Mahajanga *Madag.* 89 B8
Mahajanga □ *Madag.* 89 B8
Mahajilo → *Madag.* 89 B8
Mahakam → *Indonesia* 62 E5
Mahalapye *Botswana* 88 C4
Mahale Mts. *Tanzania* 86 D3
Mahale Mts. △ *Tanzania* 86 D2
Maḥallāt *Iran* 71 C6
Māhān *Iran* 71 D8
Mahan → *India* 69 H10
Mahanadi → *India* 67 J15
Mahananda → *India* 69 G12
Mahanoro *Madag.* 89 B8
Mahanoy City *U.S.A.* 115 F8
Maharashtra □ *India* 66 J9
Mahasham, W. → *Egypt* 74 E3
Mahasoa *Madag.* 89 C8
Mahasolo *Madag.* 89 B8
Mahattat ash Shīdīyah
Jordan 74 F4
Mahattat 'Unayzah *Jordan* 74 E4
Mahavavy → *Madag.* 89 B8
Mahaxay *Laos* 64 D5
Mahbubnagar *India* 66 L10
Mahda *U.A.E.* 71 E8
Mahdia *Tunisia* 79 A8
Mahe *India* 69 G8
Mahé *Seychelles* 85 b
Mahé ✈ (SEZ) *Seychelles* 85 b
Mahébourg *Mauritius* 85 d
Mahendragarh *India* 68 E7
Mahendranagar *Nepal* 69 E9
Mahenge *Tanzania* 87 D4
Maheno *N.Z.* 91 F3
Mahesana *India* 68 H5
Maheshwar *India* 68 H6
Mahgawan *India* 69 F8
Mahi → *India* 68 H5
Mahia Pen. *N.Z.* 91 C6
Mahilyow *Belarus* 23 B16
Mahilyow □ *Belarus* 32 E6
Mahina *Tahiti* 91 d
Mahinerangi, L. *N.Z.* 91 F2
Mahmiya *Sudan* 81 D3
Mahmud Kot *Pakistan* 68 D4
Mahmudia *Romania* 29 E14
Mahmudiye *Turkey* 47 B12
Mahmutbey *Turkey* 45 E12
Mähnsehän *Iran* 73 D12
Mahnomen *U.S.A.* 112 B6
Mahoba *India* 69 G8
Mahón = Maó *Spain* 48 B11

Mahon, Menorca ✈ (MAH)
Spain 38 F9
Mahone Bay *Canada* 105 D7
Mahopac *U.S.A.* 115 E11
Mahuta *Nigeria* 83 C5
Mahuva *India* 68 J4
Mahya Daği *Turkey* 45 E11
Mai-Ndombe, L.
Dem. Rep. of the Congo 84 E3
Mai Thon, Ko *Thailand* 65 a
Maia *Portugal* 36 D2
Maials *Spain* 38 D5
Maïche *France* 19 E13
Maicuru → *Brazil* 125 D8
Máida *Italy* 43 D9
Maidan Khula *Afghan.* 68 C3
Maidenhead *U.K.* 15 F7
Maidstone *Canada* 103 C7
Maidstone *U.K.* 15 F8
Maiduguri *Nigeria* 83 C7
Maiella △ *Italy* 41 F11
Maieru§ *Romania* 29 E10
Maigatari *Nigeria* 83 C6
Maigh Nuad = Maynooth
Ireland 12 C5
Maignelay Montigny *France* 19 C9
Maigo *Phil.* 61 G5
Maigudo △ *Ethiopia* 81 F4
Maihar *India* 69 G9
Maikala Ra. *India* 67 J12
Maiko △
Dem. Rep. of the Congo 86 C2
Mailani *India* 69 E9
Maillezais *France* 20 B3
Mailsi *Pakistan* 68 E5
Main → *Germany* 25 F4
Main → *U.K.* 12 B5
Main Channel *Canada* 114 A3
Main Range △ *Australia* 95 D5
Main Ridge *Trin. & Tob.* 125 J16
Mainburg *Germany* 25 G7
Maine *France* 18 D6
Maine □ *U.S.A.* 113 C19
Maine → *Ireland* 12 D2
Maine, G. of *U.S.A.* 113 D19
Maine-et-Loire □ *France* 18 E6
Maïne-Soroa *Niger* 83 C7
Maingkwan *Burma* 67 F20
Mainistir an Corann =
Midleton *Ireland* 12 E3
Mainit, L. *Phil.* 61 G6
Mainland *Orkney, U.K.* 13 C5
Mainland *Shet., U.K.* 13 A7
Mainpuri *India* 69 F8
Maintal *Germany* 25 E4
Maintenon *France* 19 D8
Maintirano *Madag.* 89 B7
Mainz *Germany* 25 E4
Maio *C. Verde Is.* 78 b
Maipú *Argentina* 126 D4
Maiquetía *Venezuela* 124 A5
Máira → *Italy* 40 D4
Mairabari *India* 67 F18
Maisí *Cuba* 121 B5
Maisi, Pta. de *Cuba* 121 B5
Maitland *N.S.W., Australia* 95 E5
Maitland *S. Austral., Australia* 95 E2
Maitland → *Canada* 114 C3
Maitri *Antarctica* 5 D3
Maiyema *Nigeria* 83 C5
Maíz, Is. del Nic. *120* D3
Maizuru *Japan* 55 G7
Majalengka *Indonesia* 63 G13
Majanji *Uganda* 86 B3
Majene *Indonesia* 63 E5
Majete △ *Malawi* 87 F3
Majevica *Bos.-H.* 28 F3
Maji *Ethiopia* 81 F4
Majiang *China* 58 D6
Majorca = Mallorca *Spain* 48 B10
Majuro *Marshall Is.* 96 G9
Maka *Senegal* 82 C2
Makaha *Zimbabwe* 89 B5
Makak *Cameroon* 83 E7
Makalamabedi *Botswana* 88 C3
Makale *Indonesia* 63 E5
Makalu-Barun △ *Nepal* 69 F12
Makamba *Burundi* 86 C2
Makari *Cameroon* 83 C7
Makarikari =
Makgadikgadi Salt Pans
Botswana 88 C4
Makarov Basin *Arctic* 4 A
Makarovo *Russia* 53 D11
Makarska *Croatia* 41 E14
Makaryev *Russia* 34 B6
Makasar = Ujung Pandang
Indonesia 63 F5
Makasar, Selat *Indonesia* 63 E5
Makasar, Str. of =
Makasar, Selat *Indonesia* 63 E5
Makat = Maqat *Kazakhstan* 52 E6
Makedonija =
Macedonia ■ *Europe* 44 E5
Makeni *S. Leone* 82 D2
Makeyevka = Makiyivka
Ukraine 33 H9
Makgadikgadi △ *Botswana* 88 C3

Makgadikgadi Salt Pans
Botswana 88 C4
Makhachkala *Russia* 35 J8
Makhado = Louis
Trichardt *S. Africa* 89 C4
Makham, Ao *Thailand* 65 a
Makharadze = Ozurgeti
Georgia 35 K5
Makhfar al Buşayyah *Iraq* 70 D5
Makhmür *Iraq* 73 E10
Makian *Indonesia* 63 D7
Makindu *Kenya* 86 C4
Makinsk *Kazakhstan* 52 D8
Makira = San Cristóbal
Solomon Is. 90 C9
Makiv *Ukraine* 29 B11
Makiyivka *Ukraine* 33 H9
Makkah *Si. Arabia* 80 C4
Makkovik *Canada* 105 A8
Makó *Hungary* 28 D5
Mako *Senegal* 82 C2
Makogai *Fiji* 91 a
Makokou *Gabon* 84 D2
Makongo
Dem. Rep. of the Congo 86 B2
Makoro *Dem. Rep. of the Congo* 86 B2
Maków Mazowiecki *Poland* 31 F8
Maków Podhalański *Poland* 31 J6
Makra *Greece* 47 E7
Makrai *India* 68 H7
Makran Coast Range
Pakistan 66 G4
Makrana *India* 68 F6
Makrany *Belarus* 31 G11
Makri *Greece* 45 F9
Makrigialos *Greece* 49 D7
Mākū *Iran* 73 C11
Makunda *Botswana* 88 C3
Makung *Taiwan* 59 F12
Makurazaki *Japan* 55 J5
Makurdi *Nigeria* 83 D6
Makushin Volcano *U.S.A.* 106 E6
Makūyeh *Iran* 71 D7
Makwassie *S. Africa* 88 D4
Makwiro *Zimbabwe* 89 B5
Mâl *Mauritania* 82 B2
Mal B. *Ireland* 12 D2
Mala = Mallow *Ireland* 12 D3
Mala, Pta. *Panama* 120 E3
Mala Belozërka *Ukraine* 33 J8
Malá Fatra △ *Slovak Rep.* 27 B12
Mala Kapela *Croatia* 41 D12
Mala Panew → *Poland* 31 H4
Mala Vyska *Ukraine* 33 H6
Malabang *Phil.* 61 H6
Malabar Coast *India* 66 P9
Malabon *Phil.* 61 D4
Malabu *Nigeria* 83 D7
Malacca, Straits of *Indonesia* 65 L3
Malacky *Slovak Rep.* 27 C10
Malad City *U.S.A.* 108 E7
Maladeta *Spain* 38 C5
Maladzyechna *Belarus* 23 A14
Málaga *Spain* 37 J6
Málaga □ *Spain* 37 J6
Malagarasi *Tanzania* 86 D3
Malagarasi → *Tanzania* 86 D2
Malagasy Rep. =
Madagascar ■ *Africa* 89 C8
Malagón *Spain* 37 F7
Malagón → *Spain* 37 H3
Malahide *Ireland* 12 C5
Malaimbandy *Madag.* 89 C8
Malaita *Solomon Is.* 90 B9
Malakal *Sudan* 81 F3
Malakand *Pakistan* 68 B4
Malakula *Vanuatu* 90 C9
Malakwal *Pakistan* 68 C5
Malamala *Indonesia* 63 E6
Malanda *Australia* 94 B4
Malang *Indonesia* 62 F4
Malanga *Mozam.* 87 E4
Malangen *Norway* 8 B18
Malanje *Angola* 84 F3
Mälaren *Sweden* 10 E11
Malargüe *Argentina* 126 D2
Malartic *Canada* 104 C4
Malaryta *Belarus* 31 G11
Malatya *Turkey* 73 C8
Malatya □ *Turkey* 72 C7
Malawi ■ *Africa* 87 E3
Malawi, L. *Africa* 87 E3
Malay Pen. *Asia* 65 J3
Malaya Belozërka = Mala
Belozërka *Ukraine* 33 J8
Malaya Vishera *Russia* 32 C7
Malaya Viska = Mala
Vyska *Ukraine* 33 H6
Malaybalay *Phil.* 61 G6
Malāyer *Iran* 73 E13
Malaysia ■ *Asia* 65 K4
Malazgirt *Turkey* 73 C10
Mala ◎ *Australia* 92 D5
Malbaza *Niger* 83 C6
Malbon *Australia* 94 C3
Malbooma *Australia* 95 E1
Malbork *Poland* 30 D6
Malcésine *Italy* 40 C7

Malchin *Germany* 24 B8
Malchow *Germany* 24 B8
Malcolm *Australia* 93 E3
Malcolm, Pt. *Australia* 93 F3
Maldah *India* 69 G13
Malden *Mass., U.S.A.* 115 D13
Malden *Mo., U.S.A.* 112 G9
Malden I. *Kiribati* 97 H12
Maldives ■ *Ind. Oc.* 50 H9
Maldon *U.K.* 15 F8
Maldonado *Uruguay* 127 C5
Maldonado, Pta. *Mexico* 119 D5
Malè *Italy* 40 B7
Malé Karpaty *Slovak Rep.* 27 C10
Maleas, Ákra *Greece* 46 E5
Malebo, Pool *Africa* 84 E3
Malegaon *India* 66 J9
Malei *Mozam.* 87 F4
Malek *Sudan* 81 F3
Malek Kandī *Iran* 73 D12
Malela *Dem. Rep. of the Congo* 86 C2
Malema *Mozam.* 87 E4
Maleme *Greece* 49 D5
Mălerås *Sweden* 11 H9
Malerkotla *India* 68 D6
Males *Greece* 49 D7
Malesherbes *France* 19 D9
Maleshevska Planina *Europe* 44 E7
Malesina *Greece* 46 C5
Malestroit *France* 18 E4
Malfa *Italy* 43 D7
Malgobek *Russia* 35 J7
Malgomaj *Sweden* 8 D17
Malgrat de Mar *Spain* 38 D7
Malha *Sudan* 81 E2
Malhargarh *India* 68 G6
Malheur → *U.S.A.* 108 D5
Malheur L. *U.S.A.* 108 E4
Mali *Guinea* 82 C2
Mali ■ *Africa* 82 B4
Mali → *Burma* 67 G20
Mali Kanal *Serbia* 28 E4
Mali Kyun *Burma* 64 F2
Malia, Kolpos *Greece* 49 D7
Malibu *U.S.A.* 111 L8
Maliku *Indonesia* 63 E6
Malili *Indonesia* 63 E6
Malimba, Mts.
Dem. Rep. of the Congo 86 D2
Malin Hd. *Ireland* 12 A4
Malin Pen. *Ireland* 12 A4
Malindi *Kenya* 86 C5
Malindi Marine △ *Kenya* 86 C5
Malines = Mechelen *Belgium* 17 C4
Malino *Indonesia* 63 E6
Malinyi *Tanzania* 87 D4
Malipo *China* 58 F5
Maliq *Albania* 44 F4
Malita *Phil.* 63 C7
Maliwun *Burma* 65 G2
Maliya *India* 68 H4
Maljenik *Serbia* 44 C5
Malka → *Russia* 35 J6
Malka Mari △ *Kenya* 86 B5
Malkara *Turkey* 45 F10
Małkinia Górna *Poland* 31 F9
Malko Tŭrnovo *Bulgaria* 45 E11
Mallacoota Inlet *Australia* 95 F4
Mallaig *U.K.* 13 D3
Mallawa *India* 69 F9
Mallawan *India* 69 F9
Mallawi *Egypt* 80 B3
Mallemort *France* 21 E9
Málles Venosta *Italy* 40 B7
Mallicolo = Malakula
Vanuatu 90 C9
Mallorca *Spain* 48 B10
Mallorytown *Canada* 115 B9
Mallow *Ireland* 12 D3
Malmbäck *Sweden* 11 G8
Malmberget *Sweden* 8 C19
Malmédy *Belgium* 17 D6
Malmesbury *S. Africa* 88 E2
Malmivaara = Malmberget
Sweden 8 C19
Malmköping *Sweden* 10 E10
Malmö *Sweden* 11 J7
Malmslätt *Sweden* 11 F9
Malmyzh *Russia* 34 B10
Malnaş *Romania* 29 D10
Malo Konare *Bulgaria* 45 D8
Maloarkhangelsk *Russia* 33 F9
Malolo *Fiji* 91 a
Malolos *Phil.* 61 D4
Malolotja △ *Swaziland* 89 D5
Malombe L. *Malawi* 87 E4
Malomice *Poland* 31 G2
Malomir *Bulgaria* 45 D10
Malone *U.S.A.* 115 B10
Malong *China* 58 E5
Małopolskie □ *Poland* 31 J7
Malorad *Bulgaria* 44 C7
Måløy *Norway* 8 F11
Maloyaroslovets *Russia* 32 E9
Malpartida de Cáceres *Spain* 37 F4
Malpaso *Canary Is.* 48 G1

Malpaso, Presa =
Netzahualcóyotl, Presa
Mexico 119 D6
Malpelo, I. de *Colombia* 124 C2
Malpica de Bergantiños
Spain 36 B2
Malpur *India* 68 H5
Malpura *India* 68 F6
Mals = Málles Venosta *Italy* 40 B7
Malta *Idaho, U.S.A.* 108 E7
Malta *Mont., U.S.A.* 108 B10
Malta ■ *Europe* 49 D2
Maltahöhe *Namibia* 88 C2
Malton *Canada* 114 C5
Malton *U.K.* 14 C7
Maluku *Indonesia* 63 E7
Maluku □ *Indonesia* 63 E7
Maluku Sea = Molucca Sea
Indonesia 63 E6
Malumfashi *Nigeria* 83 C6
Malung *Sweden* 10 D7
Malungsfors *Sweden* 10 D7
Maluwe *Ghana* 82 D4
Malvan *India* 66 L8
Malvern *U.S.A.* 116 D8
Malvern Hills *U.K.* 15 E5
Malvinas, Is. = Falkland
Is. ☑ *Atl. Oc.* 128 G5
Malwal *Sudan* 81 F3
Malý Dunaj → *Slovak Rep.* 27 D11
Malya *Tanzania* 86 C3
Malye Derbety *Russia* 35 G7
Malyn *Ukraine* 23 C15
Malyy Lyakhovskiy,
Ostrov *Russia* 53 B15
Malyy Taymyr, Ostrov
Russia 53 B11
Mama *Russia* 53 D12
Mamadysh *Russia* 34 C10
Mamanguape *Brazil* 125 E11
Mamanuca Group *Fiji* 91 a
Mamarr Mitlā *Egypt* 74 E1
Mamasa *Indonesia* 63 E5
Mambasa
Dem. Rep. of the Congo 86 B2
Mamberamo → *Indonesia* 63 E9
Mambilima Falls *Zambia* 87 E2
Mambirima
Dem. Rep. of the Congo 87 E2
Mambo *Tanzania* 86 C4
Mambrui *Kenya* 86 C5
Mamburao *Phil.* 61 E4
Mamedkala *Russia* 73 A13
Mameigwess L. *Canada* 104 B2
Mamers *France* 18 D7
Mamfé *Cameroon* 83 D6
Mammoth *U.S.A.* 109 K8
Mammoth Cave △ *U.S.A.* 112 G10
Mamonovo *Russia* 30 D6
Mamoré → *Bolivia* 124 F5
Mamou *Guinea* 82 C2
Mamoudzou *Mayotte* 85 a
Mampikony *Madag.* 89 B8
Mampong *Ghana* 83 D4
Mamry, Jezioro *Poland* 30 D8
Mamuju *Indonesia* 63 E5
Mamuno *Botswana* 88 C3
Mamuras *Albania* 44 E3
Man *Ivory C.* 82 D3
Man, I. of *U.K.* 14 C3
Man-Bazar *India* 69 H12
Man Na *Burma* 67 H20
Mänä *U.S.A.* 107 J14
Mana → *Fr. Guiana* 125 B8
Mana Pools △ *Zimbabwe* 87 F2
Manaar, G. of = Mannar,
G. of *Asia* 66 Q11
Manacapuru *Brazil* 124 D6
Manacor *Spain* 48 B10
Manado *Indonesia* 63 D6
Managua *Nic.* 120 D2
Managua, L. de *Nic.* 120 D2
Manakara *Madag.* 89 C8
Manali *India* 68 C7
Manama = Al Manāmah
Bahrain 71 E6
Manambao → *Madag.* 89 B7
Manambato *Madag.* 89 A8
Manambolo → *Madag.* 89 B7
Manambolosy *Madag.* 89 B8
Mananara *Madag.* 89 B8
Mananara → *Madag.* 89 C8
Mananara △ *Madag.* 89 B8
Mananjary *Madag.* 89 C8
Manankoro *Mali* 82 C3
Manantali, L. de *Mali* 82 C2
Manantenina *Madag.* 89 C8
Manaos = Manaus *Brazil* 124 D7
Manapire → *Venezuela* 124 B5
Manapouri *N.Z.* 91 F1
Manapouri, L. *N.Z.* 91 F1
Manaqil *Sudan* 81 E3
Manār, Jabal *Yemen* 75 E3
Manaravolo *Madag.* 89 C8
Manas *China* 60 B3
Manas → *India* 67 F17
Manaslu *Nepal* 69 E11
Manasquan *U.S.A.* 115 F10

Manassa *U.S.A.* **109** H11
Manatí *Puerto Rico* **121** d
Manaung *Burma* **67** K18
Manaus *Brazil* **124** D7
Manavgat *Turkey* **72** D4
Manawan L. *Canada* **103** B8
Manay *Phil.* **61** H7
Manbij *Syria* **72** D7
Mancha Real *Spain* **37** H7
Manche □ *France* **18** C5
Manchegorsk *Russia* **52** C4
Manchester *U.K.* **14** D5
Manchester *Calif., U.S.A.* **110** G3
Manchester *Conn., U.S.A.* **115** E12
Manchester *Ga., U.S.A.* **117** E12
Manchester *Iowa, U.S.A.* **112** D8
Manchester *Ky., U.S.A.* **113** G12
Manchester *N.H., U.S.A.* **115** D13
Manchester *N.Y., U.S.A.* **114** D7
Manchester *Pa., U.S.A.* **115** F8
Manchester *Tenn., U.S.A.* **117** D11
Manchester *Vt., U.S.A.* **115** C11
Manchester Int. ✈ (MAN)
    U.K. **14** D5
Manchester L. *Canada* **103** A7
Manchhar L. *Pakistan* **68** F2
Manchuria = Dongbei *China* **54** A5
Manchurian Plain *China* **50** D14
Manciano *Italy* **41** F8
Mancifa *Ethiopia* **81** F5
Mand → *India* **69** J10
Mand → *Iran* **71** D7
Manda *Ludewe, Tanzania* **87** E3
Manda *Mbeya, Tanzania* **86** D3
Manda *Mbeya, Tanzania* **87** D3
Mandabé *Madag.* **89** C7
Mandaguari *Brazil* **127** A5
Mandah = Töhöm *Mongolia* **56** B5
Mandal *Norway* **9** G12
Mandala, Puncak *Indonesia* **63** E10
Mandalay *Burma* **67** J20
Mandale = Mandalay
    Burma **67** J20
Mandalgarh *India* **68** G6
Mandalgovĭ *Mongolia* **56** B4
Mandalī *Iraq* **73** F11
Mandan *U.S.A.* **112** B3
Mandaon *Phil.* **61** E5
Mandar, Teluk *Indonesia* **63** E5
Mándas *Italy* **42** C2
Mandaue *Phil.* **61** F5
Mandelieu-la-Napoule
    France **21** E10
Mandera *Kenya* **86** B5
Mandeville *Jamaica* **120** a
Mandi *India* **68** D7
Mandi Burewala *Pakistan* **68** D5
Mandi Dabwali *India* **68** E6
Mandiana *Guinea* **82** C3
Mandimba *Mozam.* **87** E4
Mandioli *Indonesia* **63** E7
Mandla *India* **69** H9
Mandø *Denmark* **11** J2
Mandorah *Australia* **92** B5
Mandoto *Madag.* **89** B8
Mandoudi *Greece* **46** C5
Mandra *Greece* **46** C5
Mandra *Pakistan* **68** C5
Mandraki *Greece* **47** E9
Mandrare → *Madag.* **89** D8
Mandritsara *Madag.* **89** B8
Mandronarivo *Madag.* **89** C8
Mandsaur *India* **68** G6
Mandurah *Australia* **93** F2
Mandúria *Italy* **43** B10
Mandvi *India* **68** H3
Mandya *India* **66** N10
Mandzai *Pakistan* **68** D2
Mané *Burkina Faso* **83** C4
Maneh *Iran* **71** B8
Manengouba, Mts. *Cameroon* **83** E6
Manera *Madag.* **89** C7
Manérbio *Italy* **40** C7
Maneroo Cr. → *Australia* **94** C3
Manfalût *Egypt* **80** B3
Manfredónia *Italy* **41** G12
Manfredónia, G. di *Italy* **41** G13
Manga *Burkina Faso* **83** C4
Manga *Niger* **83** C7
Mangabeiras, Chapada das
    Brazil **125** F9
Mangaia *Cook Is.* **97** K12
Mangalia *Romania* **29** G13
Mangalore *India* **66** N9
Mangaluru = Mangalore
    India **66** N9
Mangan *India* **69** F13
Mangawan *India* **69** G9
Mangaweka *N.Z.* **91** C5
Manggar *Indonesia* **62** E4
Manggawitu *Indonesia* **63** E8
Mangghystaū Tübegi
    Kazakhstan **52** E6
Manggis *Indonesia* **63** J18
Mangindrano *Madag.* **89** A8
Mangkalihat, Tanjung
    Indonesia **63** D5
Mangkururpa ⊗ *Australia* **92** D4
Mangla *Pakistan* **68** C5

Mangla Dam *Pakistan* **69** C5
Manglaur *India* **68** E7
Manglisi *Georgia* **35** K7
Mangnai *China* **60** C4
Mango *Togo* **83** C5
Mango *Tonga* **91** c
Mangoche *Malawi* **87** E4
Mangoky → *Madag.* **89** C7
Mangole *Indonesia* **63** E6
Mangombe
    Dem. Rep. of the Congo **86** C2
Mangonui *N.Z.* **91** A4
Mangoro → *Madag.* **89** B8
Mangrol *Mad. P., India* **68** J4
Mangrol *Raj., India* **68** G6
Mangualde *Portugal* **36** E3
Mangum *U.S.A.* **116** D5
Manguri *Australia* **95** A1
Mangyshlak, Poluostrov =
    Mangghystaū Tübegi
    Kazakhstan **52** E6
Manhattan *U.S.A.* **112** F5
Manhiça *Mozam.* **89** D5
Mania → *Madag.* **89** B8
Maniago *Italy* **41** B9
Manica *Mozam.* **89** B5
Manica □ *Mozam.* **89** B5
Manicaland □ *Zimbabwe* **87** F3
Manicoré *Brazil* **124** E6
Manicouagan → *Canada* **105** C6
Manicouagan, Rés. *Canada* **105** B6
Maniema □
    Dem. Rep. of the Congo **86** C2
Manīfah *Si. Arabia* **71** E6
Manifold, C. *Australia* **94** C5
Maniganggo *China* **58** B2
Manigotagan *Canada* **103** C9
Manigotagan → *Canada* **103** C9
Manihari *India* **69** G12
Manihiki *Cook Is.* **97** J11
Manihiki Plateau *Pac. Oc.* **97** J11
Manika, Plateau de la
    Dem. Rep. of the Congo **87** E2
Manikpur *India* **69** G9
Manila *Phil.* **61** D4
Manila *U.S.A.* **108** F9
Manila B. *Phil.* **61** D4
Manilla *Australia* **95** E5
Manimpé *Mali* **82** C3
Maningrida *Australia* **94** A1
Maninian *Ivory C.* **82** C3
Manipur □ *India* **67** G19
Manipur → *Burma* **67** H19
Manisa *Turkey* **47** C9
Manisa □ *Turkey* **47** C9
Manistee *U.S.A.* **112** C10
Manistee → *U.S.A.* **112** C10
Manistique *U.S.A.* **112** C10
Manitoba □ *Canada* **103** B9
Manitoba, L. *Canada* **103** C9
Manitou *Canada* **103** D9
Manitou, L. *Canada* **105** B6
Manitou Is. *U.S.A.* **113** C10
Manitou L. *Canada* **103** C7
Manitou Springs *U.S.A.* **108** G11
Manitoulin I. *Canada* **104** C3
Manitouwadge *Canada* **104** C2
Manitowoc *U.S.A.* **112** C10
Manizales *Colombia* **124** B3
Manja *Madag.* **89** C7
Manjacaze *Mozam.* **89** C5
Manjakandriana *Madag.* **89** B8
Manjhand *Pakistan* **68** G3
Manjimup *Australia* **93** F2
Manjo *Cameroon* **83** E6
Manjra → *India* **66** K10
Mankato *Kans., U.S.A.* **112** F4
Mankato *Minn., U.S.A.* **112** C6
Mankayane *Swaziland* **89** D5
Mankera *Pakistan* **68** D4
Mankim *Cameroon* **83** D7
Mankono *Ivory C.* **82** D3
Mankota *Canada* **103** D7
Manlay = Üydzin *Mongolia* **56** B4
Manlleu *Spain* **38** C7
Manmad *India* **66** J9
Mann Ranges *Australia* **93** E5
Manna *Indonesia* **62** E2
Mannahill *Australia* **95** E3
Mannar *Sri Lanka* **66** Q11
Mannar, G. of *Asia* **66** Q11
Mannar I. *Sri Lanka* **66** Q11
Mannheim *Germany* **25** F4
Manning *Canada* **102** B5
Manning *Oreg., U.S.A.* **110** E3
Manning *S.C., U.S.A.* **117** E14
Mannu → *Italy* **42** C2
Mannu, C. *Italy* **42** B1
Mannum *Australia* **95** E2
Mano *S. Leone* **82** D2
Mano → *Liberia* **82** D2
Mano River *Liberia* **82** D2
Manohar pur *India* **69** H11
Manokwari *Indonesia* **63** E8
Manolada *Greece* **46** C3
Manombo *Madag.* **89** C7
Manono
    Dem. Rep. of the Congo **86** D2

Manono *Samoa* **91** b
Manoppello *Italy* **41** F11
Manorhamilton *Ireland* **12** B3
Manosque *France* **21** E9
Manotick *Canada* **115** A9
Manouane → *Canada* **105** C5
Manouane, L. *Canada* **105** B5
Manp'o *N. Korea* **57** D14
Manpojin = Manp'o
    N. Korea **57** D14
Manpur *Chhattisgarh, India* **69** H10
Manpur *Mad. P., India* **68** H6
Manresa *Spain* **38** D6
Mansa *Gujarat, India* **68** H5
Mansa *Punjab, India* **68** E6
Mansa *Zambia* **87** E2
Mansa Konko *Gambia* **82** C1
Månsåsen *Sweden* **10** A8
Mansehra *Pakistan* **68** B5
Mansel I. *Canada* **101** E15
Mansfield *Australia* **95** F4
Mansfield *U.K.* **14** D6
Mansfield *La., U.S.A.* **116** E8
Mansfield *Mass., U.S.A.* **115** D13
Mansfield *Ohio, U.S.A.* **114** F2
Mansfield *Pa., U.S.A.* **114** E7
Mansfield *Tex., U.S.A.* **116** E6
Mansfield, Mt. *U.S.A.* **115** B12
Mansilla de las Mulas *Spain* **36** C5
Mansle *France* **20** C4
Mansôa *Guinea-Biss.* **82** C1
Manson Creek *Canada* **102** B4
Manta *Ecuador* **124** D2
Mantadia △ *Madag.* **89** B8
Mantalingajan, Mt. *Phil.* **61** G2
Mantare *Tanzania* **86** C3
Manteca *U.S.A.* **110** H5
Manteo *U.S.A.* **117** D17
Mantes-la-Jolie *France* **19** D8
Manthani *India* **66** K11
Manti *U.S.A.* **108** G8
Mantiqueira, Serra da
    Brazil **127** A7
Manton *U.S.A.* **113** C11
Mantorp *Sweden* **11** F9
Mántova *Italy* **40** C7
Mänttä *Finland* **32** A3
Mantua = Mántova *Italy* **40** C7
Manturovo *Russia* **34** A7
Manú *Peru* **124** F4
Manú → *Peru* **124** F4
Manu'a Is. *Amer. Samoa* **91** b
Manuel Alves → *Brazil* **125** F9
Manui *Indonesia* **63** E6
Manukau *N.Z.* **91** B5
Manuripi → *Bolivia* **124** F5
Many *U.S.A.* **116** F8
Manyallaluk ⊙ *Australia* **92** B5
Manyani *Kenya* **86** C4
Manyara, L. *Tanzania* **86** C4
Manyara △ *Tanzania* **86** C4
Manyas *Turkey* **45** F11
Manyava *Ukraine* **29** B9
Manych → *Russia* **35** G5
Manych-Gudilo, Ozero
    Russia **35** G6
Manyonga → *Tanzania* **86** C3
Manyoni *Tanzania* **86** D3
Manzai *Pakistan* **68** C4
Manzala, Bahra el *Egypt* **80** H7
Manzanar △ *U.S.A.* **110** J7
Manzanares *Spain* **37** F7
Manzaneda *Spain* **36** C3
Manzanillo *Cuba* **120** B4
Manzanillo *Mexico* **118** D4
Manzanillo, Pta. *Panama* **120** E4
Manzano Mts. *U.S.A.* **109** J10
Manzarīyeh *Iran* **71** C6
Manzhouli *China* **60** B6
Manzini *Swaziland* **89** D5
Manzur Vadisi △ *Turkey* **70** B3
Mao *Chad* **79** F9
Maó *Spain* **48** B11
Maoke, Pegunungan
    Indonesia **63** E9
Maolin *China* **57** C12
Maoming *China* **59** G8
Maopi T'ou *China* **59** G13
Maouri, Dallol → *Niger* **83** C5
Maoxian *China* **58** B4
Maoxing *China* **57** B13
Mapam Yumco *China* **69** D9
Mapastepec *Mexico* **119** D6
Mapia, Kepulauan *Indonesia* **63** D8
Mapimí *Mexico* **118** B4
Mapimí, Bolsón de *Mexico* **118** B4
Maping *China* **59** B9
Mapinga *Tanzania* **86** D4
Mapinhane *Mozam.* **89** C6
Maple Creek *Canada* **103** D7
Maple Valley *U.S.A.* **110** C4
Mapleton *U.S.A.* **108** D2
Mapoon ⊙ *Australia* **94** A3
Mapuera → *Brazil* **124** D7
Mapulanguene *Mozam.* **89** C5
Maputo *Mozam.* **89** D5
Maputo □ *Mozam.* **89** D5

Maputo, B. de *Mozam.* **89** D5
Maputo ○ *Mozam.* **89** D5
Maqat *Kazakhstan* **52** E6
Maqiaohe *China* **57** B16
Maqnā *Si. Arabia* **70** D2
Maqteïr *Mauritania* **78** D3
Maquan He =
    Brahmaputra → *Asia* **69** H13
Maqueda *Spain* **36** E6
Maquela do Zombo *Angola* **84** F3
Maquinchao *Argentina* **128** E3
Maquoketa *U.S.A.* **112** D8
Mar → *Canada* **114** B3
Mar, Serra do *Brazil* **127** B6
Mar Chiquita, L. *Argentina* **126** C3
Mar del Plata *Argentina* **126** D4
Mar Menor *Spain* **39** H4
Mara *Tanzania* **86** C3
Mara □ *Tanzania* **86** C3
Maraã *Brazil* **124** D5
Marabá *Brazil* **125** E9
Maraboon, L. *Australia* **94** C4
Maracá, I. de *Brazil* **125** C8
Maracaibo *Venezuela* **124** A4
Maracaibo, L. de *Venezuela* **124** B4
Maracaju *Brazil* **127** A4
Maracas Bay *Trin. & Tob.* **125** K15
Maracay *Venezuela* **124** A5
Maracena *Spain* **37** H7
Marādah *Libya* **79** C9
Maradi *Niger* **83** C6
Maradi □ *Niger* **83** C6
Marāgheh *Iran* **73** D12
Marāh *Si. Arabia* **70** E5
Marahuue △ *Ivory C.* **82** D3
Marajo, I. de *Brazil* **125** D9
Marākand *Iran* **70** B5
Marakele △ *S. Africa* **89** E4
Maralal *Kenya* **86** B4
Maralinga *Australia* **93** F5
Maralinga Tjarutja ⊙
    Australia **93** E5
Maramaereğlisi *Turkey* **45** F11
Marambio *Antarctica* **5** C18
Maramureş □ *Romania* **29** C9
Maran *Malaysia* **65** L4
Marana *U.S.A.* **109** K8
Maranboy *Australia* **92** B5
Maranchón *Spain* **38** D2
Marand *Iran* **73** C11
Marang *Malaysia* **65** K4
Maranguape *Brazil* **125** D11
Maranhão = São Luís *Brazil*
    125 D10
Maranhão □ *Brazil* **125** E9
Marano, L. di *Italy* **41** C10
Maranoa → *Australia* **95** D4
Marañón → *Peru* **124** D4
Marão *Mozam.* **89** C5
Maraş = Kahramanmaraş
    Turkey **72** D7
Mărăşeşti *Romania* **29** E12
Maratea *Italy* **43** C8
Marateca *Portugal* **37** G2
Marathasa *Cyprus* **49** E11
Marathokambos *Greece* **47** D8
Marathon *Australia* **94** C3
Marathon *Canada* **104** C2
Marathon *N.Y., U.S.A.* **115** D8
Marathon *Tex., U.S.A.* **116** F3
Marathonas *Greece* **46** C5
Marathóvouno *Cyprus* **49** D12
Maratua *Indonesia* **63** D5
Maraval *Trin. & Tob.* **125** K15
Maravatío *Mexico* **118** D4
Marawi City *Phil.* **61** G6
Marāwih *U.A.E.* **71** E7
Marāyia △ *Sudan* **81** G2
Marāyit, Wadi → *Sudan* **81** F2
Marié → *Brazil* **124** D5
Marie Byrd Land *Antarctica* **5** D14
Marie-Galante *Guadeloupe* **120** b
Mariecourt =
    Kangiqsujuaq *Canada* **101** E17
Mariefred *Sweden* **10** E11
Mariehamn *Finland* **9** F18
Marieholm *Sweden* **11** J7
Mariembourg *Belgium* **17** D4
Marienbad = Mariánské
    Lázně *Czech Rep.* **26** B5
Marienberg *Germany* **24** E5
Mariental *Namibia* **88** C2
Marienville *U.S.A.* **114** E5
Mariestad *Sweden* **11** F7
Marietta *Ga., U.S.A.* **117** E12
Marietta *Ohio, U.S.A.* **113** F13
Marieville *Canada* **115** A11
Mariga → *Nigeria* **83** C6
Marignane *France* **21** E9
Marihatag *Phil.* **61** G7
Mariinsk *Russia* **52** D9
Mariinskiy Posad *Russia* **34** B8
Marijampolė *Lithuania* **30** D10
Marijampolė □ *Lithuania* **30** D10
Marília *Brazil* **127** A6

Marckolsheim *France* **19** D14
Marco Island *U.S.A.* **117** J14
Marcos Juárez *Argentina* **126** C3
Mărculeşti *Moldova* **29** C13
Marcus Baker, Mt. *U.S.A.* **106** C10
Marcus I. = Minami-Tori-
    Shima *Pac. Oc.* **96** E7
Marcy, Mt. *U.S.A.* **115** B11
Mardan *Pakistan* **68** B5
Mardarivka *Ukraine* **29** C14
Mardie *Australia* **92** D2
Mardin *Turkey* **73** D9
Mårdsjö *Sweden* **10** A9
Marécchia → *Italy* **41** D9
Maree, L. *U.K.* **13** D3
Mareeba *Australia* **94** B4
Mareetsane *S. Africa* **88** D4
Maremma *Italy* **41** F8
Maremma ○ *Italy* **40** F8
Maréna *Kayes, Mali* **82** C2
Maréna *Koulikouro, Mali* **82** C3
Marengo *U.S.A.* **112** E7
Marennes *France* **20** C2
Marerano *Madag.* **89** C7
Marettimo *Italy* **42** F5
Mareuil *France* **20** C4
Marfa *U.S.A.* **116** F2
Marfa Pt. *Malta* **49** D1
Marganets = Marhanets
    Ukraine **33** J8
Margaret → *Australia* **92** C4
Margaret Bay *Canada* **102** C3
Margaret L. *Canada* **102** B5
Margaret River *Australia* **93** F2
Margarita, I. de *Venezuela* **124** A6
Margariti *Greece* **46** B2
Margaritovo *Russia* **54** C7
Margate *S. Africa* **89** E5
Margate *U.K.* **15** F9
Margeride, Mts. de la *France* **20** D7
Marghera, di Savóia *Italy* **43** A9
Marghilon *Uzbekistan* **52** E8
Marghita *Romania* **28** C7
Margonin *Poland* **31** F4
Margosatubig *Phil.* **61** H5
Marguerite *Canada* **102** C4
Marhanets *Ukraine* **33** J8
Mari El □ *Russia* **34** B8
Mari Indus *Pakistan* **68** C4
Mari Republic = Mari El □
    Russia **34** B8
María, Sa. de *Spain* **39** H2
María de la Salut *Spain* **48** B10
María Elena *Chile* **126** A2
María Grande *Argentina* **126** C4
Maria I. *N. Terr., Australia* **94** A2
Maria I. *Tas., Australia* **95** G4
Maria Island △ *Australia* **95** G4
Maria van Diemen, C. *N.Z.* **91** A4
Mariager *Denmark* **11** H3
Mariager Fjord *Denmark* **11** H4
Mariakani *Kenya* **86** C4
Mariala △ *Australia* **95** D4
Marian *Australia* **94** b
Marian L. *Canada* **102** A5
Mariana Trench *Pac. Oc.* **96** F6
Marianna *Ark., U.S.A.* **117** D9
Marianna *Fla., U.S.A.* **117** F12
Mariannelund *Sweden* **11** G9
Marias → *U.S.A.* **108** C8
Marías, Islas *Mexico* **118** C3
Mariato, Punta *Panama* **120** E3
Mariazell *Austria* **26** D8
Maribo *Denmark* **11** K5
Maribor *Slovenia* **41** B12
Marico → *Africa* **88** C4
Maricopa *Ariz., U.S.A.* **109** K7
Maricopa *Calif., U.S.A.* **111** K7
Marīdī *Sudan* **81** G2
Marīdī, Wadi → *Sudan* **81** F2
Marié → *Brazil* **124** D5
Marie Byrd Land *Antarctica* **5** D14

Marín *Spain* **36** C2
Marina *U.S.A.* **110** J5
Marinduque *Phil.* **63** B6
Marine City *U.S.A.* **114** D2
Marineo *Italy* **42** E6
Marinette *U.S.A.* **112** C10
Maringá *Brazil* **127** A5
Marinha Grande *Portugal* **36** F2
Marino *Italy* **41** G9
Marion *Ala., U.S.A.* **117** E11
Marion *Ill., U.S.A.* **112** G9
Marion *Ind., U.S.A.* **113** E11
Marion *Iowa, U.S.A.* **112** D8
Marion *Kans., U.S.A.* **112** F5
Marion *N.C., U.S.A.* **117** D13
Marion *Ohio, U.S.A.* **113** E12
Marion *S.C., U.S.A.* **117** D15
Marion *Va., U.S.A.* **113** G13
Marion, L. *U.S.A.* **117** E14
Mariposa *U.S.A.* **110** H7
Mariscal Estigarribia
    Paraguay **126** A3
Maritime Alps =
    Maritimes, Alpes *Europe* **21** D11
Maritimes, Alpes *Europe* **21** D11
Maritsa = Evros → *Greece* **72** B2
Maritsa *Greece* **49** C10
Mariupol *Ukraine* **33** J9
Mariusa △ *Venezuela* **121** E7
Marīvān *Iran* **73** E12
Marj 'Uyūn *Lebanon* **74** B4
Marka *Si. Arabia* **80** D5
Marka *Somali Rep.* **75** G3
Markam *China* **58** C3
Markaryd *Sweden* **11** H7
Markdale *Canada* **114** B4
Marked Tree *U.S.A.* **117** D9
Markelsdorfer Huk *Germany* **24** A7
Market Drayton *U.K.* **14** E5
Market Harborough *U.K.* **15** E7
Market Rasen *U.K.* **14** D7
Markham *Canada* **114** C5
Markham, Mt. *Antarctica* **5** E11
Marki *Poland* **31** F8
Märkische Schweiz ○
    Germany **24** C10
Markkleeberg *Germany* **24** D8
Markleeville *U.S.A.* **110** G7
Markopoulo *Greece* **21** D11
Markovac *Serbia* **44** B5
Markovo *Russia* **53** C17
Markoye *Burkina Faso* **83** C5
Marks *Russia* **34** E8
Marksville *U.S.A.* **116** F8
Markt Schwaben *Germany* **25** G7
Marktoberdorf *Germany* **25** H6
Marktredwitz *Germany* **25** E8
Marl *Germany* **24** D3
Marla *Australia* **95** D1
Marlbank *Canada* **114** B7
Marlboro *U.S.A.* **115** E11
Marlborough *Australia* **94** C4
Marlborough *U.K.* **15** F6
Marlborough □ *N.Z.* **115** D13
Marlborough Downs *U.K.* **15** F6
Marle *France* **19** C10
Marlin *U.S.A.* **116** F6
Marlow *Germany* **24** A8
Marlow *U.K.* **15** F7
Marlow *U.S.A.* **116** D6
Marmagao *India* **66** M8
Marmande *France* **20** D4
Marmara *Turkey* **45** F11
Marmara, Sea of =
    Marmara Denizi *Turkey* **45** F12
Marmara Denizi *Turkey* **45** F12
Marmara Gölü *Turkey* **47** C10
Marmaris *Turkey* **47** E10
Marmaris Limanı *Turkey* **47** E10
Marmion, Mt. *Australia* **93** E2
Marmion L. *Canada* **104** C1
Marmolada, Mte. *Italy* **41** B8
Marmolejo *Spain* **37** G6
Marmora *Canada* **114** B7
Mármora, La *Italy* **42** C2
Marmugao = Marmagao
    India **66** M8
Marnay *France* **19** E12
Marne *Germany* **24** B5
Marne □ *France* **19** D11
Marne → *France* **19** D10
Marneuli *Georgia* **35** K7
Maro Reef *U.S.A.* **107** K5
Maroala *Madag.* **89** B8
Maroantsetra *Madag.* **89** B8
Maroelaboom *Namibia* **88** B2
Marofandilia *Madag.* **89** C7
Marojejy △ *Madag.* **89** A8
Marolambo *Madag.* **89** C8
Maromandia *Madag.* **89** A8
Maromokotro *Madag.* **89** A8
Marondera *Zimbabwe* **87** F3
Maroni → *Fr. Guiana* **125** B8
Maronia *Greece* **45** F9
Maronne → *France* **20** C5
Maroochydore *Australia* **95** D5
Maroona *Australia* **95** F3
Maros → *Hungary* **28** D5
Marosakoa *Madag.* **89** B8

Maroseranana *Madag.* **89** B8
Maróstica *Italy* **41** C8
Marotandrano *Madag.* **89** B8
Marotaolano *Madag.* **89** A8
Maroua *Cameroon* **83** C7
Marovato *Madag.* **89** B8
Marovoay *Madag.* **89** B8
Marquard *S. Africa* **88** D4
Marquesas Fracture Zone
  Pac. Oc. **97** H15
Marquesas Is. = Marquises,
  Îs. *French Polynesia* **97** H14
Marquette *U.S.A.* **112** B10
Marquis *St. Lucia* **121** f
Marquise *France* **19** B8
Marquises, Îs.
  French Polynesia **97** H14
Marra, Djebel *Sudan* **79** F10
Marra, Gebel *Sudan* **81** F2
Marracuene *Mozam.* **89** D5
Marradi *Italy* **41** D8
Marrakech *Morocco* **78** B4
Marratxí *Spain* **38** F7
Marrawah *Australia* **95** G3
Marree *Australia* **95** D2
Marrero *U.S.A.* **117** G9
Marrimane *Mozam.* **89** C5
Marromeu *Mozam.* **89** B6
Marromeu △ *Mozam.* **89** B6
Marroquí, Punta *Spain* **37** K5
Marrowie Cr. → *Australia* **95** E4
Marrubane *Mozam.* **87** F4
Marrúbiu *Italy* **42** C1
Marrupa *Mozam.* **87** E4
Mars Hill *U.S.A.* **113** B20
Marsá 'Alam *Egypt* **80** B3
Marsá Matrûh *Egypt* **80** A2
Marsá Sha'b *Sudan* **80** C4
Marsabit *Kenya* **86** B4
Marsabit △ *Kenya* **86** B4
Marsala *Italy* **42** E5
Marsalforn *Malta* **49** C1
Mârşani *Romania* **29** F9
Marsberg *Germany* **24** C4
Marsciano *Italy* **41** F9
Marsden *Australia* **95** E4
Marseillan *France* **20** E7
Marseille *France* **21** E9
Marseille-Marignane ✕
  (MRS) *France* **21** E9
Marseilles = Marseille *France* **21** E9
Marsh I. *U.S.A.* **116** G9
Marshall *Liberia* **82** D2
Marshall *Ark., U.S.A.* **116** D8
Marshall *Mich., U.S.A.* **113** D11
Marshall *Minn., U.S.A.* **112** C6
Marshall *Mo., U.S.A.* **112** F7
Marshall *Tex., U.S.A.* **116** E7
Marshall → *Australia* **94** C2
Marshall Is. ■ *Pac. Oc.* **90** A10
Marshalltown *U.S.A.* **112** D7
Marshbrook *Zimbabwe* **89** B5
Marshfield *Mo., U.S.A.* **112** G7
Marshfield *Vt., U.S.A.* **115** B12
Marshfield *Wis., U.S.A.* **112** C8
Marshūn *Iran* **71** B6
Mársico Nuovo *Italy* **43** B8
Märsta *Sweden* **10** E11
Marstal *Denmark* **11** K4
Marstrand *Sweden* **11** G5
Mart *U.S.A.* **116** F6
Marta → *Italy* **41** F8
Martaban *Burma* **67** L20
Martaban, G. of *Burma* **67** L20
Martano *Italy* **43** B11
Martapura *Kalimantan,
  Indonesia* **62** E4
Martapura *Sumatera,
  Indonesia* **62** E2
Marte *Nigeria* **83** C7
Marte R. Gómez, Presa
  Mexico **119** B5
Martel *France* **20** D5
Martelange *Belgium* **17** E5
Martellago *Italy* **41** C9
Martés, Sierra *Spain* **39** F4
Martfű *Hungary* **28** C5
Martha's Vineyard *U.S.A.* **115** E14
Martigné-Ferchaud *France* **18** E5
Martigny *Switz.* **25** J3
Martigues *France* **21** E9
Martin *Slovak Rep.* **27** B11
Martin *S. Dak., U.S.A.* **112** D3
Martin *Tenn., U.S.A.* **117** C10
Martin → *Spain* **38** D4
Martin L. *U.S.A.* **117** E12
Martina Franca *Italy* **43** B10
Martinborough *N.Z.* **91** D5
Martinez *Calif., U.S.A.* **110** G4
Martinez *Ga., U.S.A.* **117** E13
Martinique ☑ *W. Indies* **120** c
Martinique Passage
  W. Indies **121** C7
Martino *Greece* **46** C5
Martinópolis *Brazil* **127** A5
Martin's Bay *Barbados* **121** g
Martins Ferry *U.S.A.* **114** F4
Martinsberg *Austria* **26** C8
Martinsburg *Pa., U.S.A.* **114** F6

Martinsburg *W. Va., U.S.A.* **113** F15
Martinsicuro *Italy* **41** F10
Martinsville *Ind., U.S.A.* **112** F10
Martinsville *Va., U.S.A.* **113** G14
Marton *N.Z.* **91** D5
Martorell *Spain* **38** D6
Martos *Spain* **37** H7
Martu ◎ *Australia* **92** D3
Maru *Nigeria* **83** C6
Marudi *Malaysia* **62** D4
Maruf *Afghan.* **66** D5
Marugame *Japan* **55** G6
Marunga *Angola* **88** B3
Marungu, Mts.
  Dem. Rep. of the Congo **86** D3
Maruwa ◎ *Australia* **92** D4
Marv Dasht *Iran* **71** D7
Marvast *Iran* **71** D7
Marvejols *France* **20** D7
Marvel Loch *Australia* **93** F2
Marwar *India* **68** G5
Mary *Turkmenistan* **71** B9
Maryborough = Port
  Laoise *Ireland* **12** C4
Maryborough *Queens.,
  Australia* **95** D5
Maryborough *Vic., Australia* **95** F3
Maryfield *Canada* **103** D8
Maryland ☐ *U.S.A.* **113** F15
Maryland Junction *Zimbabwe* **87** F3
Maryport *U.K.* **14** C4
Mary's Harbour *Canada* **105** B8
Marystown *Canada* **105** C8
Marysville *Calif., U.S.A.* **110** F5
Marysville *Kans., U.S.A.* **112** F5
Marysville *Mich., U.S.A.* **114** D2
Marysville *Ohio, U.S.A.* **113** E12
Marysville *Wash., U.S.A.* **110** B4
Maryville *Mo., U.S.A.* **112** E6
Maryville *Tenn., U.S.A.* **117** D13
Marzūq *Libya* **79** C8
Marzūq, Idehān *Libya* **79** D8
Masada *Israel* **74** D4
Masahunga *Tanzania* **86** C3
Masai *Malaysia* **65** d
Masai Mara △ *Kenya* **86** C4
Masai Steppe *Tanzania* **86** C4
Masaka *Uganda* **86** C3
Mäsäl *Iran* **73** D12
Masalembo, Kepulauan
  Indonesia **62** F4
Masalima, Kepulauan
  Indonesia **62** F5
Masallı *Azerbaijan* **73** C13
Masamba *Indonesia* **63** E6
Masan *S. Korea* **57** G15
Masandam, Ra's *Oman* **71** E8
Masasi *Tanzania* **87** E4
Masaya *Nic.* **120** D2
Masba *Nigeria* **83** C7
Masbate *Phil.* **61** E5
Máscali *Italy* **43** E8
Mascara *Algeria* **78** A6
Mascota *Mexico* **118** C4
Masela *Indonesia* **63** F7
Maseru *Lesotho* **88** D4
Mashaba *Zimbabwe* **87** G3
Mashābih *Si. Arabia* **70** E3
Mashan *China* **58** F7
Mashar *Sudan* **81** F2
Mashatu △ *Botswana* **89** C4
Mashegu *Nigeria* **83** D6
Masherbrum *Pakistan* **69** B7
Mashhad *Iran* **71** B8
Mashi *Nigeria* **83** C6
Mashīz *Iran* **71** D8
Mashkel, Hāmūn-i- *Pakistan* **71** D9
Mashki Chāh *Pakistan* **66** E3
Mashonaland *Zimbabwe* **85** H6
Mashonaland Central ☐
  Zimbabwe **89** B5
Mashonaland East ☐
  Zimbabwe **89** B5
Mashonaland West ☐
  Zimbabwe **89** B4
Mashrakh *India* **69** F11
Mashtaga = Maştağa
  Azerbaijan **35** K10
Masi Manimba
  Dem. Rep. of the Congo **84** E3
Masig *Australia* **94** a
Masindi *Uganda* **86** B3
Masindi Port *Uganda* **86** B3
Masinga Res. *Kenya* **86** C4
Maşīrah, Jazīrat *Oman* **75** C6
Maşīrah, Khalīj *Oman* **75** C6
Masisi *Dem. Rep. of the Congo* **86** C2
Masjed Soleyman *Iran* **71** D6
Mask, L. *Ireland* **12** C2
Maskin *Oman* **71** F8
Maslen Nos *Bulgaria* **45** D11
Maslinica *Croatia* **41** E13
Masnou = El Masnou *Spain* **38** D7
Masoala, Tanjon' i *Madag.* **89** B9
Masoala △ *Madag.* **89** B9
Masoarivo *Madag.* **89** B7
Masohi = Amahai *Indonesia* **63** E7
Masomeloka *Madag.* **89** C8

Mason *Nev., U.S.A.* **110** G7
Mason *Tex., U.S.A.* **116** F5
Mason City *U.S.A.* **112** D7
Maspalomas *Canary Is.* **48** G4
Maspalomas, Pta. *Canary Is.* **48** G4
Masqat *Oman* **75** C6
Masr el Gedida *Egypt* **80** H7
Massa *Italy* **40** D7
Massa Maríttima *Italy* **40** E7
Massachusetts ☐ *U.S.A.* **115** D13
Massachusetts B. *U.S.A.* **115** D14
Massafra *Italy* **43** B10
Massakory *Chad* **79** F9
Massamba *Mozam.* **87** F3
Massanella *Spain* **48** B9
Massangena *Mozam.* **89** C5
Massango *Angola* **84** F3
Massat *France* **20** F5
Massena *U.S.A.* **115** B10
Massenya *Chad* **79** F9
Masset *Canada* **102** C2
Masseube *France* **20** E4
Massiac *France* **20** C7
Massif Central *France* **20** D7
Massif des Bauges △ *France* **19** G13
Massigui *Mali* **82** C3
Massillon *U.S.A.* **114** F3
Massinga *Mozam.* **89** C6
Massingir *Mozam.* **89** C5
Masson-Angers *Canada* **115** A9
Masson I. *Antarctica* **5** C7
Maştağa *Azerbaijan* **35** K10
Mastanli = Momchilgrad
  Bulgaria **45** E9
Masterton *N.Z.* **91** D5
Masterton, Ko *Thailand* **65** b
Mastic *U.S.A.* **115** F12
Mastuj *Pakistan* **69** A5
Mastung *Pakistan* **66** E5
Mastūrah *Si. Arabia* **80** C3
Masty *Belarus* **23** B13
Masuda *Japan* **55** G5
Masuku = Franceville *Gabon* **84** E2
Masurian Lakes =
  Mazurski, Pojezierze
  Poland **30** E7
Masvingo *Zimbabwe* **87** G3
Masvingo ☐ *Zimbabwe* **87** G3
Maswa △ *Tanzania* **86** C3
Maşyāf *Syria* **72** E7
Mat → *Albania* **44** E3
Matabeleland *Zimbabwe* **85** H5
Matabeleland North ☐
  Zimbabwe **87** F2
Matabeleland South ☐
  Zimbabwe **87** G2
Matachel → *Spain* **37** G4
Matachewan *Canada* **104** C3
Matadi *Dem. Rep. of the Congo* **84** F2
Matagalpa *Nic.* **120** D2
Matagami *Canada* **104** C4
Matagami, L. *Canada* **104** C4
Matagorda B. *U.S.A.* **116** G6
Matagorda I. *U.S.A.* **116** G6
Mataiea *Tahiti* **91** d
Matak *Indonesia* **62** D3
Matala *Greece* **49** E6
Matam *Senegal* **82** B2
Matam ☐ *Senegal* **82** B2
Matameye *Niger* **83** C6
Matamoros *Campeche,
  Mexico* **119** D6
Matamoros *Coahuila, Mexico* **118** B4
Matamoros *Tamaulipas,
  Mexico* **119** B5
Matandu → *Tanzania* **87** D3
Matane *Canada* **105** C6
Matang *China* **58** F5
Matankari *Niger* **83** C5
Matanomadh *India* **68** H3
Matanzas *Cuba* **120** B3
Matapa *Botswana* **88** C3
Matapan, C. = Tenaro,
  Ákra *Greece* **46** E5
Matapédia *Canada* **105** C6
Matapo △ *Zimbabwe* **87** G2
Matara *Sri Lanka* **66** S12
Mataram *Indonesia* **62** F5
Matarani *Peru* **124** G4
Mataranka *Australia* **92** B5
Matarma, Râs *Egypt* **74** E1
Mataró *Spain* **38** D7
Matarraña → *Spain* **38** D5
Mataruška Banja *Serbia* **44** C4
Matatiele *S. Africa* **89** E4
Mataura *N.Z.* **91** G2
Matavai, B. de *Tahiti* **91** d
Matehuala *Mexico* **118** C4
Mateke Hills *Zimbabwe* **87** G3
Matelot *Trin. & Tob.* **125** K15
Matera *Italy* **43** B9
Matese, Monti del *Italy* **43** A7
Matese → *Italy* **43** A7
Mátészalka *Hungary* **28** C7
Matetsi *Zimbabwe* **87** F2

Matfors *Sweden* **10** B11
Matha *France* **20** C3
Matheniko △ *Uganda* **86** B3
Mathis *U.S.A.* **116** G6
Mathraki *Greece* **49** A3
Mathura *India* **68** F7
Mati *Phil.* **61** H7
Matiakoali *Burkina Faso* **83** C5
Matiali *India* **69** F13
Matías Romero *Mexico* **119** D5
Matibane *Mozam.* **87** E5
Matiri Ra. *N.Z.* **91** D4
Matjiesfontein *S. Africa* **88** E3
Matla → *India* **69** J13
Matlamanyane *Botswana* **88** B4
Matli *Pakistan* **68** G3
Matlock *U.K.* **14** D6
Matna *Sudan* **81** E4
Mato Grosso ☐ *Brazil* **125** F8
Mato Grosso, Planalto do
  Brazil **125** G8
Mato Grosso do Sul ☐ *Brazil* **125** G8
Matobo = Matapo △
  Zimbabwe **87** G2
Matochkin Shar, Proliv
  Russia **52** B6
Matopo Hills *Zimbabwe* **87** G2
Matopos *Zimbabwe* **87** G2
Matosinhos *Portugal* **36** D2
Matour *France* **19** F11
Matroosberg *S. Africa* **88** E2
Maţruḥ *Oman* **75** C6
Matsena *Nigeria* **83** C7
Matsesta *Russia* **35** J4
Matsu Tao *Taiwan* **59** E13
Matsue *Japan* **55** G6
Matsum, Ko *Thailand* **65** b
Matsumae *Japan* **54** D10
Matsumoto *Japan* **55** F9
Matsusaka *Japan* **55** G8
Matsuura *Japan* **55** H4
Matsuyama *Japan* **55** H6
Mattagami → *Canada* **104** B3
Mattancheri *India* **66** Q10
Mattawa *Canada* **104** C4
Matterhorn *Switz.* **25** K3
Mattersburg *Austria* **27** D9
Matthew Town *Bahamas* **121** B5
Matthews Ridge *Guyana* **124** B6
Mattice *Canada* **104** C3
Mattituck *U.S.A.* **115** F12
Mattō *Japan* **55** F8
Mattoon *U.S.A.* **112** F9
Matuba *Mozam.* **89** C5
Matucana *Peru* **124** F3
Matuku *Fiji* **91** a
Matūn = Khowst *Afghan.* **68** C3
Matura *Trin. & Tob.* **125** K15
Maturín *Venezuela* **124** B6
Matusadona △ *Zimbabwe* **87** F2
Matveyev Kurgan *Russia* **33** J10
Matxitxako, C. *Spain* **38** B2
Mau *Mad. P., India* **69** F8
Mau *Ut. P., India* **69** G10
Mau *Ut. P., India* **69** G9
Mau Escarpment *Kenya* **86** C4
Mau Ranipur *India* **69** G8
Maua *Kenya* **86** C4
Maua *Mozam.* **87** E4
Maubeuge *France* **19** B10
Maubin *Burma* **67** L19
Maubourguet *France* **20** E4
Maud, Pt. *Australia* **92** D1
Maud Rise *S. Ocean* **5** C3
Maude *Australia* **95** E3
Maudin Sun *Burma* **67** M19
Maués *Brazil* **124** D7
Mauganj *India* **69** G9
Maughold Hd. *I. of Man* **14** C3
Mauguio *France* **20** E7
Maui *U.S.A.* **107** L8
Maulamyaing = Moulmein
  Burma **67** L20
Maule ☐ *Chile* **126** D1
Mauléon-Licharre *France* **20** E3
Maumee *U.S.A.* **113** E12
Maumee → *U.S.A.* **113** E12
Maumere *Indonesia* **63** F6
Maumusson, Pertuis de
  France **20** C2
Maun *Botswana* **88** C3
Mauna Kea *U.S.A.* **107** M8
Mauna Loa *U.S.A.* **107** M8
Maunath Bhanjan = Mau
  India **69** G10
Maungmagan Kyunzu
  Burma **64** F1
Maungu *Kenya* **86** C4
Maupin *U.S.A.* **108** D3
Maure-de-Bretagne *France* **18** E5
Maurepas, L. *U.S.A.* **117** F9
Maures *France* **21** E10
Mauriac *France* **20** C6
Maurice, L. *Australia* **93** E5
Mauricie △ *Canada* **104** C5
Maurienne *France* **21** C10
Mauritania ■ *Africa* **78** D3
Mauritius ■ *Ind. Oc.* **85** d
Mauron *France* **18** D4

Maurs *France* **20** D6
Mauston *U.S.A.* **112** D8
Mauterndorf *Austria* **26** D6
Mauthen *Austria* **26** E6
Mauvezin *France* **20** E4
Mauzé-sur-le-Mignon *France* **20** B3
Mavli *India* **68** G5
Mavrovë *Albania* **44** F3
Mavrovo △ *Macedonia* **44** E4
Mavuradonha Mts. *Zimbabwe* **87** F3
Mawa *Dem. Rep. of the Congo* **86** B2
Mawai *India* **69** H9
Mawana *India* **68** E7
Mawand *Pakistan* **68** E3
Mawat *Iraq* **73** E11
Mawjib, W. al → *Jordan* **74** D4
Mawk Mai *Burma* **67** J20
Mawlaik *Burma* **67** H19
Mawlamyine = Moulmein
  Burma **67** L20
Mawqaq *Si. Arabia* **70** E4
Mawson Base *Antarctica* **5** C6
Mawson Coast *Antarctica* **5** C6
Max *U.S.A.* **112** B3
Maxcanú *Mexico* **119** C6
Maxesibeni *S. Africa* **89** E4
Maxhamish L. *Canada* **102** B4
Maxixe *Mozam.* **89** C6
Maxville *Canada* **115** A10
Maxwell *U.S.A.* **110** F4
Maxwelton *Australia* **94** C3
May, C. *U.S.A.* **113** F16
May Pen *Jamaica* **120** a
Maya *Spain* **38** B3
Maya → *Russia* **53** D14
Maya Mts. *Belize* **119** D7
Mayaguana *Bahamas* **121** B5
Mayagüez *Puerto Rico* **121** d
Mayahi *Niger* **83** C6
Mayaky *Ukraine* **29** C14
Mayals = Maials *Spain* **38** D5
Mayāmey *Iran* **71** B7
Mayang *China* **58** D7
Mayanup *Australia* **93** F2
Mayapán *Mexico* **119** C7
Mayarí *Cuba* **121** B4
Mayaro B. *Trin. & Tob.* **125** K16
Maybell *U.S.A.* **108** F9
Maybole *U.K.* **13** F4
Maychew *Ethiopia* **81** E4
Maydän *Iraq* **73** E11
Maydan *Ukraine* **29** B8
Maydī *Yemen* **81** D5
Mayen *Germany* **25** E3
Mayenne *France* **18** D6
Mayenne ☐ *France* **18** D6
Mayenne → *France* **18** E6
Mayer *U.S.A.* **109** J7
Mayerthorpe *Canada* **102** C5
Mayfield *Ky., U.S.A.* **112** G9
Mayfield *N.Y., U.S.A.* **115** C10
Mayhill *U.S.A.* **109** K11
Maykop *Russia* **35** H5
Maymyo *Burma* **64** A1
Maynard *Mass., U.S.A.* **115** D13
Maynard *Wash., U.S.A.* **110** C4
Maynard Hills *Australia* **93** E2
Mayne → *Australia* **94** C3
Maynooth *Canada* **114** A7
Maynooth *Ireland* **12** C5
Mayo *Canada* **100** E4
Mayo ☐ *Ireland* **12** C2
Mayo Daga *Nigeria* **83** D7
Mayo Faran *Nigeria* **83** D7
Mayon Volcano *Phil.* **61** E5
Mayor I. *N.Z.* **91** B6
Mayorga *Spain* **36** C5
Mayotte ☑ *Ind. Oc.* **85** a
Mayraira Pt. *Phil.* **61** B4
Maysán *Iraq* **70** D5
Mayskiy *Russia* **35** J7
Maysville *U.S.A.* **113** F12
Mayu *Indonesia* **63** D7
Mayville *N. Dak., U.S.A.* **112** B5
Mayville *N.Y., U.S.A.* **114** D5
Mazabuka *Zambia* **87** F2
Mazagán = El Jadida *Morocco* **78** B4
Mazagão *Brazil* **125** D8
Mazamet *France* **20** E6
Mazán *Peru* **124** D4
Māzandarān ☐ *Iran* **71** B7
Mazapil *Mexico* **118** C4
Mazara del Vallo *Italy* **42** E5
Mazarrón *Spain* **39** H3
Mazarrón, G. de *Spain* **39** H3
Mazaruni → *Guyana* **124** B7
Mazatán *Mexico* **118** B2
Mazatenango *Guatemala* **120** D1
Mazatlán *Mexico* **118** C3
Mažeikiai *Lithuania* **30** B9
Māzhān *Iran* **71** D8
Mazıdağı *Turkey* **73** D9
Mazīnān *Iran* **71** B8
Mazoe *Mozam.* **87** F3
Mazoe → *Mozam.* **87** F3
Mazowe *Zimbabwe* **87** F3
Mazowiecki = Poland **31** F8
Mazrûb *Sudan* **81** E2
Mazu Dao *China* **59** D12
Mazurski, Pojezierze *Poland* **30** E7

Mazyr *Belarus* **23** B15
Mba *Fiji* **91** a
Mbaba *Senegal* **82** C1
Mbabane *Swaziland* **89** D5
Mbagne *Mauritania* **82** B2
M'bahiakro *Ivory C.* **82** D4
Mbaïki *C.A.R.* **84** D3
Mbala *Zambia* **87** D3
Mbalabala *Zimbabwe* **89** C4
Mbale *Uganda* **86** B3
Mbalmayo *Cameroon* **83** E7
Mbam → *Cameroon* **83** E7
Mbamba Bay *Tanzania* **87** E3
Mbandaka
  Dem. Rep. of the Congo **84** D3
Mbanga *Cameroon* **83** E6
Mbanza Congo *Angola* **84** F2
Mbanza Ngungu
  Dem. Rep. of the Congo **84** F2
Mbarangandu *Tanzania* **87** D4
Mbarara *Uganda* **86** C3
Mbatto *Ivory C.* **82** D4
Mbengga = Beqa *Fiji* **91** a
Mbenkuru → *Tanzania* **87** D4
Mberengwa *Zimbabwe* **87** G2
Mberengwa, Mt. *Zimbabwe* **87** G2
Mberubu *Nigeria* **83** D6
Mbesuma *Zambia* **87** E3
Mbeya *Tanzania* **87** D3
Mbeya ☐ *Tanzania* **86** D3
Mbhashe → *S. Africa* **89** E4
M'bili *Sudan* **81** F2
Mbinga *Tanzania* **87** E4
Mbini = Río Muni ☐
  Eq. Guin. **84** D2
Mbizi *Zimbabwe* **87** G3
Mboki *C.A.R.* **81** F2
M'bonge *Cameroon* **83** E6
Mboro *Senegal* **82** B1
Mbouda *Cameroon* **83** D7
M'boukou, L. de *Cameroon* **83** D7
Mboune *Senegal* **82** C2
Mbour *Senegal* **82** C1
Mbout *Mauritania* **82** B2
Mbuji-Mayi
  Dem. Rep. of the Congo **86** D1
Mbulu *Tanzania* **86** C4
Mburucuyá *Argentina* **126** B4
Mburucuyá △ *Argentina* **126** B4
Mchinja *Tanzania* **87** D4
Mchinji *Malawi* **87** E3
Mdantsane *S. Africa* **89** E4
Mead, L. *U.S.A.* **111** J12
Meade *U.S.A.* **112** G3
Meade River = Atqasuk
  U.S.A. **106** A8
Meadow Lake *Canada* **103** C7
Meadow Lake △ *Canada* **103** C7
Meadow Valley Wash →
  U.S.A. **111** J12
Meadville *U.S.A.* **114** E4
Meaford *Canada* **114** B4
Mealhada *Portugal* **36** E2
Mealpaeg L. *Canada* **105** C8
Mealy Mts. *Canada* **105** B8
Meander River *Canada* **102** B5
Meares, C. *U.S.A.* **108** D1
Mearim → *Brazil* **125** D10
Meath ☐ *Ireland* **12** C5
Meath Park *Canada* **103** C7
Meaulne *France* **19** F9
Meaux *France* **19** D9
Mebechi-Gawa → *Japan* **54** D10
Mebulu, Tanjung *Indonesia* **63** K18
Mecanhelas *Mozam.* **87** F4
Mecca = Makkah *Si. Arabia* **80** C4
Mecca *U.S.A.* **111** M10
Mechanicsburg *U.S.A.* **114** F8
Mechanicville *U.S.A.* **115** D11
Mechara *Ethiopia* **81** F5
Mechelen *Belgium* **17** C4
Mecheria *Algeria* **78** B5
Mechernich *Germany* **24** E2
Mechetinskaya *Russia* **35** G5
Mecidiye *Turkey* **45** F10
Mecitözü *Turkey* **72** B6
Mecklenburg *Germany* **22** B7
Mecklenburg-
  Vorpommern ☐ *Germany* **24** B7
Mecklenburger Bucht
  Germany **24** A7
Meconta *Mozam.* **87** E4
Mecsek *Hungary* **28** D3
Mecubúri *Mozam.* **87** E4
Mecubúri → *Mozam.* **87** E5
Mecúfi *Mozam.* **87** E5
Meda *Portugal* **36** E3
Medan *Indonesia* **62** D1
Médanos de Coro △
  Venezuela **121** D6
Medanosa, Pta. *Argentina* **128** F3
Mede *Italy* **40** C5
Médéa *Algeria* **78** A6
Mededa *Bos.-H.* **28** G4
Medellín *Colombia* **124** B3
Medelpad *Sweden* **10** B10
Medemblik *Neths.* **17** B5
Mederdra *Mauritania* **82** B1
Medford *Mass., U.S.A.* **115** D13

Medford *Oreg., U.S.A.* **108** E2
Medford *Wis., U.S.A.* **112** C8
Medgidia *Romania* **29** F13
Medi *Sudan* **81** F3
Media Agua *Argentina* **126** C2
Media Luna *Argentina* **126** C2
Medianeira *Brazil* **127** B5
Medicina *Italy* **41** D8
Medicine Bow *U.S.A.* **108** F10
Medicine Bow Mts. *U.S.A.* **108** F10
Medicine Bow Pk. *U.S.A.* **108** F10
Medicine Hat *Canada* **103** D6
Medicine Lake *U.S.A.* **108** B11
Medicine Lodge *U.S.A.* **112** G4
Medina = Al Madīnah
    Si. Arabia **70** E3
Medina *N. Dak., U.S.A.* **112** B4
Medina *N.Y., U.S.A.* **114** C6
Medina *Ohio, U.S.A.* **114** E3
Medina → *U.S.A.* **116** G5
Medina de Pomar *Spain* **36** C7
Medina de Rioseco *Spain* **36** D5
Medina del Campo *Spain* **36** D6
Médina Gounas *Senegal* **82** C2
Medina L. *U.S.A.* **116** G5
Medina Sidonia *Spain* **37** J5
Medinaceli *Spain* **38** D2
Medinipur *India* **69** H12
Mediterranean Sea *Europe* **6** H7
Médoc *France* **20** C3
Medulin *Croatia* **41** D10
Medveđa *Serbia* **44** D5
Medvedevo *Russia* **34** B8
Medveditsa → *Tver, Russia* **32** D9
Medveditsa → *Volgograd, Russia* **34** F6
Medvedok *Russia* **34** B10
Medvezhi, Ostrava *Russia* **53** B17
Medvezhyegorsk *Russia* **52** C4
Medway □ *U.K.* **15** F8
Medway → *U.K.* **15** F8
Medzev *Slovak Rep.* **27** C13
Medzilaborce *Slovak Rep.* **27** B14
Medžitlija *Macedonia* **44** F5
Meekatharra *Australia* **93** E2
Meeker *U.S.A.* **108** F10
Meersburg *Germany* **25** H5
Meerut *India* **68** E7
Meeteetse *U.S.A.* **108** D9
Mega *Ethiopia* **81** G4
Megalo *Ethiopia* **81** F5
Megalo Horio *Greece* **47** E9
Megalonisos *Greece* **46** D4
Megalopoli *Greece* **46** D4
Meganisi *Greece* **46** C2
Megara *Greece* **46** D5
Megasini *India* **69** J12
Megdovas = Tavropos →
    Greece **46** B3
Megève *France* **21** C10
Meghalaya □ *India* **67** G17
Meghezez *Ethiopia* **81** F4
Meghna → *Bangla.* **67** H17
Megion *Russia* **52** C8
Mégiscane, L. *Canada* **104** C4
Megiste *Greece* **47** E11
Megisti *Greece* **47** E11
Megra *Russia* **32** B9
Mehadia *Romania* **28** F7
Meharry, Mt. *Australia* **92** D2
Mehedeby *Sweden* **10** D11
Mehedinți □ *Romania* **28** F7
Meheisa *Sudan* **80** D3
Mehlville *U.S.A.* **112** F8
Mehndawal *India* **69** F10
Mehr Jān *Iran* **71** C7
Mehrābād *Iran* **73** D12
Mehrābān *Iran* **73** C12
Mehrān *Iran* **73** F12
Mehrān → *Iran* **71** E7
Mehrgarh *Pakistan* **68** E2
Mehrīz *Iran* **71** D7
Mehun-sur-Yèvre *France* **19** E9
Mei Jiang → *China* **59** E11
Mei Xian *China* **56** G4
Meicheng *China* **59** C12
Meichengzhen *China* **59** C8
Meichuan *China* **59** B10
Meighen I. *Canada* **101** B12
Meigu *China* **58** C4
Meihekou *China* **57** C13
Meiktila *Burma* **67** J19
Meira, Serra de *Spain* **36** B3
Meiringen *Switz.* **25** J4
Meishan *China* **58** B4
Meissen *Germany* **24** D9
Meissner *Germany* **24** D5
Meissner-Kaufunger
    Wald △ *Germany* **24** D5
Meitan *China* **58** D6
Meizhou *China* **59** E11
Meja *India* **69** G10
Mejillones *Chile* **126** A1
Mekdela *Ethiopia* **81** E4
Mekele *Ethiopia* **81** E4
Mekerghene, Sebkra *Algeria* **78** C6

Mékhé *Senegal* **82** B1
Mekhtar *Pakistan* **66** D6
Meknès *Morocco* **78** B4
Meko *Nigeria* **83** D5
Mekong → *Asia* **65** H6
Mekongga *Indonesia* **63** E6
Mekrou → *Benin* **83** C5
Mekvari = Kür →
    Azerbaijan **73** C13
Mel *Italy* **41** B9
Melagiri Hills *India* **66** N10
Melaka *Malaysia* **65** L4
Melalap *Malaysia* **62** C5
Melambes *Greece* **49** D6
Melanesia *Pac. Oc.* **96** H7
Melanesian Basin *Pac. Oc.* **96** G8
Melaya *Indonesia* **63** J17
Melbourne *Australia* **95** F4
Melbourne *U.S.A.* **117** G14
Melchor Múzquiz *Mexico* **118** B4
Melchor Ocampo *Mexico* **118** C4
Méldola *Italy* **41** D9
Meldorf *Germany* **24** A5
Melegnano *Italy* **40** C6
Melenci *Serbia* **28** E5
Melenki *Russia* **34** C5
Mélèzes → *Canada* **104** A5
Melfi *Italy* **43** B8
Melfort *Canada* **103** C8
Melfort *Zimbabwe* **87** F3
Melgaço *Portugal* **36** C2
Melgar de Fernamental
    Spain **36** C6
Melhus *Norway* **8** E14
Melide *Spain* **36** C2
Meligales *Greece* **46** D3
Melilla *N. Afr.* **78** A5
Melilli *Italy* **43** E8
Melipilla *Chile* **126** C1
Melissa *Canada* **114** A5
Melissa, Akra *Greece* **49** D6
Melissa Oros *Greece* **47** D8
Melita *Canada* **103** D8
Mélito di Porto Salvo *Italy* **43** E8
Melitopol *Ukraine* **33** J8
Melk *Austria* **26** C8
Mellan Fryken *Sweden* **10** E7
Mellansel *Sweden* **8** E18
Mellbystrand *Sweden* **11** H6
Melle *France* **20** B3
Melle *Germany* **24** C4
Mellen *U.S.A.* **112** B8
Mellerud *Sweden* **11** F6
Mellette *U.S.A.* **112** C5
Mellid = Melide *Spain* **36** C2
Mellieha *Malta* **49** D1
Mellit *Sudan* **81** E2
Mellrichstadt *Germany* **24** E6
Melnik *Bulgaria* **44** E7
Mělník *Czech Rep.* **26** A7
Melnytsya Podilska *Ukraine* **29** B11
Melo *Uruguay* **127** C5
Melolo *Indonesia* **63** F6
Melouprey *Cambodia* **64** F5
Melrhir, Chott *Algeria* **78** B7
Melrose *Australia* **95** E4
Melrose *U.K.* **13** F6
Melrose *Minn., U.S.A.* **112** C6
Melrose *N. Mex., U.S.A.* **109** J12
Melstone *U.S.A.* **108** C10
Melsungen *Germany* **24** D5
Melton Mowbray *U.K.* **14** E7
Melun *France* **19** D9
Melut *Sudan* **81** E3
Melville *Canada* **103** C8
Melville, C. *Australia* **94** A3
Melville B. *Australia* **94** A2
Melville B. *Greenland* **101** B19
Melville I. *Australia* **92** B5
Melville I. *Canada* **101** B9
Melville Pen. *Canada* **101** D15
Melvin, Lough *Ireland* **12** B3
Mélykút *Hungary* **28** D4
Memaliaj *Albania* **44** F3
Memba *Mozam.* **87** E5
Memboro *Indonesia* **92** A2
Membrilla *Spain* **37** G7
Memel = Klaipėda *Lithuania* **30** C8
Memel *S. Africa* **89** D4
Memmingen *Germany* **25** H6
Mempawah *Indonesia* **62** D3
Memphis *Egypt* **80** J7
Memphis *Mich., U.S.A.* **114** D2
Memphis *Tenn., U.S.A.* **117** D9
Memphis *Tex., U.S.A.* **116** D4
Memphrémagog, L.
    N. Amer. **115** B12
Mena *Ukraine* **33** G7
Mena *U.S.A.* **116** D7
Mena → *Ethiopia* **81** F5
Menai Strait → *U.K.* **14** D3
Ménaka *Mali* **83** B5
Menan = Chao Phraya →
    Thailand **64** F3
Menarandra → *Madag.* **89** D7
Menard *U.S.A.* **116** F5
Menard Fracture Zone
    Pac. Oc. **97** M18

Menawashei *Sudan* **81** E1
Mendaña Fracture Zone
    Pac. Oc. **97** J18
Mendawai → *Indonesia* **62** E4
Mende *France* **20** D7
Mendebo Mts. *Ethiopia* **81** F4
Mendeleyev Ridge *Arctic* **4** B17
Menden *Germany* **24** D3
Menderes *Turkey* **47** C9
Mendhar *India* **69** C6
Mendi *Ethiopia* **81** F4
Mendip Hills *U.K.* **15** F5
Mendocino *U.S.A.* **108** G2
Mendocino, C. *U.S.A.* **108** F1
Mendocino Fracture Zone
    Pac. Oc. **97** D13
Mendota *Calif., U.S.A.* **110** J6
Mendota *Ill., U.S.A.* **112** E9
Mendoyo *Indonesia* **63** J17
Mendoza *Argentina* **126** C2
Mendoza □ *Argentina* **126** C2
Mene Grande *Venezuela* **124** B4
Menemen *Turkey* **47** C9
Menen *Belgium* **17** D3
Menfi *Italy* **42** E5
Mengdingjie *China* **58** F2
Mengeš *Slovenia* **41** B11
Menggala *Indonesia* **62** E3
Menghai *China* **58** G3
Mengibar *Spain* **37** H7
Mengjin *China* **56** G7
Mengla *China* **58** G3
Menglian *China* **58** F2
Mengshan *China* **59** E8
Mengyin *China* **57** G9
Mengzhe *China* **58** F3
Mengzi *China* **58** F4
Menihek *Canada* **105** B6
Menihek L. *Canada* **105** B6
Menin = Menen *Belgium* **17** D3
Menindee *Australia* **95** E3
Menindee L. *Australia* **95** E3
Meningie *Australia* **95** F2
Menjangan, Pulau *Indonesia* **63** J17
Menlo Park *U.S.A.* **110** H4
Menminee *U.S.A.* **112** C10
Menominee → *U.S.A.* **112** C10
Menomonie *U.S.A.* **112** C8
Menongue *Angola* **85** G3
Menorca *Spain* **48** B11
Menorca ✈ (MAH) *Spain* **38** F9
Mentakab *Malaysia* **65** L4
Mentawai, Kepulauan
    Indonesia **62** E1
Menton *France* **21** E11
Mentor *U.S.A.* **114** E3
Menzies *Australia* **93** E3
Meob B. *Namibia* **88** C1
Me'ona *Israel* **74** B4
Meoqui *Mexico* **118** B3
Mepaco *Mozam.* **87** F3
Meppel *Neths.* **17** B6
Meppen *Germany* **24** C3
Mequinenza *Spain* **38** D5
Mequinenza, Embalse de
    Spain **38** D5
Mer *France* **18** E8
Merak *Indonesia* **63** F12
Meramangye, L. *Australia* **93** E5
Meran = Merano *Italy* **41** B8
Merano *Italy* **41** B8
Merate *Italy* **40** C6
Merauke *Indonesia* **63** F10
Merbein *Australia* **95** E3
Merbuk, Gunung *Indonesia* **63** J17
Merca = Marka *Somali Rep.* **75** G3
Mercantour △ *France* **21** D10
Mercato Saraceno *Italy* **41** E9
Merced *U.S.A.* **110** H6
Merced → *U.S.A.* **110** H6
Merced Pk. *U.S.A.* **110** H7
Mercedes *B. Aires, Argentina* **126** C4
Mercedes *Corrientes,
    Argentina* **126** B4
Mercedes *San Luis, Argentina* **126** C2
Mercedes *Uruguay* **126** C4
Merceditas *Chile* **126** B1
Mercer *N.Z.* **91** B5
Mercer *U.S.A.* **114** E4
Mercer Island *U.S.A.* **110** C4
Mercury *U.S.A.* **111** J11
Mercy, C. *Canada* **101** D10
Merdrignac *France* **18** D4
Mere *U.K.* **15** F5
Meredith, C. *Falk. Is.* **128** G4
Meredith, L. *U.S.A.* **116** D4
Merefa *Ukraine* **33** H9
Merei *Romania* **29** E11
Merga = Nukheila *Sudan* **80** D2
Mergui *Burma* **64** F2
Mergui Arch. = Myeik
    Kyunzu *Burma* **65** G1
Méribel-les-Allues *France* **21** C10
Meriç *Turkey* **45** E10
Meriç → *Turkey* **45** F10
Mérida *Mexico* **119** C7
Mérida *Spain* **37** G4
Mérida *Venezuela* **124** B4

Mérida, Cord. de *Venezuela* **124** B4
Meriden *U.K.* **15** E6
Meriden *U.S.A.* **115** E12
Meridian *Calif., U.S.A.* **110** F5
Meridian *Idaho, U.S.A.* **108** E5
Meridian *Miss., U.S.A.* **117** E10
Mérignac *France* **20** D3
Merinda *Australia* **94** C4
Mering *Germany* **25** G6
Meringa *Nigeria* **83** C7
Merir *Pac. Oc.* **63** D8
Merirumã *Brazil* **125** C8
Merkel *U.S.A.* **116** E4
Mermaid Reef *Australia* **92** C2
Merowe *Sudan* **80** D3
Merowe Dam *Sudan* **80** D3
Merredin *Australia* **93** F2
Merrick *U.K.* **13** F4
Merrickville *Canada* **115** B9
Merrill *Oreg., U.S.A.* **108** E3
Merrill *Wis., U.S.A.* **112** C9
Merrimack → *U.S.A.* **115** D14
Merriman *U.S.A.* **112** D3
Merritt *Canada* **102** C4
Merritt Island *U.S.A.* **117** G14
Merriwa *Australia* **95** E5
Merry I. *Canada* **104** A4
Merryville *U.S.A.* **116** F8
Mersa Fatma *Eritrea* **81** E5
Mersch *Lux.* **17** E6
Merse → *Italy* **41** E8
Mersea I. *U.K.* **15** F8
Merseburg *Germany* **24** D7
Mersey → *U.K.* **14** D4
Merseyside □ *U.K.* **14** D4
Mersin = İçel *Turkey* **72** D6
Mersing *Malaysia* **65** L4
Merta *India* **68** F6
Merta Road *India* **68** F5
Merthyr Tydfil *U.K.* **15** F4
Merthyr Tydfil □ *U.K.* **15** F4
Merti *Kenya* **86** B4
Mértola *Portugal* **37** H3
Mertzon *U.S.A.* **116** F4
Méru *France* **20** C6
Meru *Kenya* **86** B4
Meru *Tanzania* **86** C4
Meru △ *Kenya* **86** B4
Merville *France* **19** B9
Méry-sur-Seine *France* **19** D10
Merzifon *Turkey* **72** B6
Merzig *Germany* **25** F2
Mesa *U.S.A.* **109** K8
Mesa Verde △ *U.S.A.* **109** H9
Mesagne *Italy* **43** B10
Mesanagros *Greece* **49** C9
Mesaoría *Cyprus* **49** D12
Meschede *Germany* **24** D4
Mescit *Turkey* **73** B9
Mesfinto *Ethiopia* **81** E4
Mesgouez, L. *Canada* **104** B5
Meshchovsk *Russia* **32** E8
Meshed = Mashhad *Iran* **71** B8
Meshgīn Shahr *Iran* **73** C12
Meshoppen *U.S.A.* **115** E8
Meshra er Req *Sudan* **81** F2
Mesilinka → *Canada* **102** B4
Meslay-du-Maine *France* **18** E6
Mesocco *Switz.* **25** J5
Mesologi *Greece* **46** C3
Mesongi *Greece* **49** B3
Mesopotamia = Al Jazirah
    Iraq **73** E10
Mesopotamia *U.S.A.* **114** E4
Mesopotamo *Greece* **46** B2
Mesoraca *Italy* **43** C9
Mésou Volímais = Volimes
    Greece **46** D2
Mesquite *U.S.A.* **109** H6
Messaad *Algeria* **78** B6
Messac *France* **18** E5
Messalo → *Mozam.* **87** E4
Messaména *Cameroon* **83** E7
Messara, Kolpos *Greece* **49** D6
Messina = Musina *S. Africa* **89** C5
Messina *Italy* **43** D8
Messina, Str. di *Italy* **43** D8
Messini *Greece* **46** D4
Messinia □ *Greece* **46** D3
Messiniakos Kolpos *Greece* **46** E4
Messkirch *Germany* **25** H5
Messlingen *Sweden* **10** B6
Mesta = Nestos → *Europe* **45** E8
Mesta, Akra *Greece* **47** C7
Mestanza *Spain* **37** G6
Mestre *Italy* **41** C9
Mesudiye *Turkey* **72** B7
Meta → *S. Amer.* **124** B5
Meta Incognita Pen. *Canada*
    101 E14
Metabetchouan *Canada* **105** C5
Mica *Greece* **49** C5
Micăsasa *Romania* **29** D9
Metaire *U.S.A.* **117** G9
Metalici, Munții *Romania* **28** D7
Metaline Falls *U.S.A.* **108** B5
Metallifere, Colline *Italy* **40** E8
Metán *Argentina* **126** B3
Metangula *Mozam.* **87** E3
Metauro → *Italy* **41** E10
Metcalfe *Canada* **115** A9

Metema *Ethiopia* **81** E4
Metengobalame *Mozam.* **87** E3
Methana *Greece* **46** D5
Methoni *Greece* **46** E3
Methven *N.Z.* **91** E3
Metil *Mozam.* **87** F4
Metković *Croatia* **41** E14
Metković *Croatia* **41** E14
Metlakatla *U.S.A.* **100** F5
Metlika *Slovenia* **41** C12
Metropolis *U.S.A.* **112** G9
Metropolitana □ *Chile* **126** C1
Metsovo *Greece* **46** B3
Metu *Ethiopia* **81** F4
Metz *France* **19** C13
Metzingen *Germany* **25** G5
Meulaboh *Indonesia* **62** D1
Meung-sur-Loire *France* **19** E8
Meureudu *Indonesia* **62** C1
Meurthe → *France* **19** D13
Meurthe-et-Moselle □
    France **19** D13
Meuse □ *France* **19** C12
Meuse → *Europe* **17** D5
Meuselwitz *Germany* **24** D8
Mexia *U.S.A.* **116** F6
Mexiana, I. *Brazil* **125** C9
Mexicali *Mexico* **111** N11
Mexican Plateau *Mexico* **98** G9
Mexican Water *U.S.A.* **109** H9
México *Mexico* **119** D5
Mexico *Maine, U.S.A.* **115** B14
Mexico *Mo., U.S.A.* **112** F9
Mexico *N.Y., U.S.A.* **115** C8
México □ *Mexico* **119** D5
Mexico ■ *Cent. Amer.* **118** C4
México, Ciudad de *Mexico* **119** D5
Mexico, G. of *Cent. Amer.* **119** C7
Mexico B. *U.S.A.* **115** A9
Meydān-e Naftūn *Iran* **71** D6
Meydani, Ra's-e *Iran* **71** E8
Meyenburg *Germany* **24** B8
Meyers Chuck *U.S.A.* **102** B2
Meymac *France* **20** C6
Meymaneh *Afghan.* **66** B4
Meyrueis *France* **20** D7
Meyssac *France* **20** C5
Meyzieu *France* **21** C8
Mezdra *Bulgaria* **44** C7
Mezen *Russia* **6** B14
Mezen → *Russia* **6** B14
Mézenc, Mt. *France* **21** D8
Mezeş, Munții *Romania* **28** C8
Mezha → *Russia* **32** E6
Mezhdurechensk *Russia* **52** D9
Mezhdurechenskiy *Russia* **52** D7
Mézidon-Canon *France* **18** C6
Mézières-en-Brenne *France* **20** B5
Mézilhac *France* **21** D8
Mézin *France* **20** D4
Mezőberény *Hungary* **28** D6
Mezőfalva *Hungary* **28** D3
Mezőhegyes *Hungary* **28** D5
Mezőkövácsháza *Hungary* **28** D5
Mezőkövesd *Hungary* **28** C5
Mézos *France* **20** D2
Mezőtúr *Hungary* **28** C5
Mezquital *Mexico* **118** C4
Mezzolombardo *Italy* **40** B8

Michoacán □ *Mexico* **118** D4
Michurin *Bulgaria* **45** D11
Michurinsk *Russia* **34** D5
Micoud *St. Lucia* **121** f
Micronesia *Pac. Oc.* **96** G7
Micronesia, Federated
    States of ■ *Pac. Oc.* **90** A8
Mid-Pacific Seamounts
    Pac. Oc. **96** F10
Midai *Indonesia* **62** D3
Midale *Canada* **103** D8
Middelburg *Neths.* **17** C3
Middelburg *Eastern Cape,
    S. Africa* **88** E4
Middelburg *Mpumalanga,
    S. Africa* **89** D4
Middelfart *Denmark* **11** J3
Middelpos *S. Africa* **88** E3
Middelwit *S. Africa* **88** C4
Middle Alkali L. *U.S.A.* **108** F3
Middle America Trench =
    Guatemala Trench
    Pac. Oc. **98** H10
Middle Bass I. *U.S.A.* **114** E2
Middle East *Asia* **50** E5
Middle Fork Feather →
    U.S.A. **110** F5
Middle I. *Australia* **93** F3
Middle Loup → *U.S.A.* **112** E4
Middleboro *U.S.A.* **115** E14
Middleburg *Fla., U.S.A.* **117** F14
Middleburg *Pa., U.S.A.* **114** F7
Middleburgh *U.S.A.* **115** D10
Middlebury *U.S.A.* **115** B11
Middlefield *U.S.A.* **114** E3
Middlemount *Australia* **94** C4
Middleport *N.Y., U.S.A.* **114** C6
Middleport *Ohio, U.S.A.* **113** F12
Middlesboro *U.S.A.* **113** G12
Middlesbrough *U.K.* **14** C6
Middlesbrough □ *U.K.* **14** C6
Middlesex *Belize* **120** C2
Middlesex *N.J., U.S.A.* **115** F10
Middlesex *N.Y., U.S.A.* **114** D7
Middleton *Australia* **94** C3
Middleton *Canada* **105** D6
Middleton Cr. → *Australia* **94** C3
Middleton I. *U.S.A.* **106** D10
Middletown *U.K.* **12** B5
Middletown *Calif., U.S.A.* **110** G4
Middletown *Conn., U.S.A.* **115** E12
Middletown *N.Y., U.S.A.* **115** E10
Middletown *Ohio, U.S.A.* **113** F11
Middletown *Pa., U.S.A.* **115** F8
Midge Point *Australia* **94** b
Midhurst *Canada* **114** B5
Midhurst *U.K.* **15** G7
Midi, Canal du → *France* **20** E5
Midi d'Ossau, Pic du *France* **20** F3
Midi-Pyrénées □ *France* **20** E5
Midland *Australia* **93** F2
Midland *Canada* **114** B5
Midland *Calif., U.S.A.* **111** M12
Midland *Mich., U.S.A.* **113** D11
Midland *Pa., U.S.A.* **114** F4
Midland *Tex., U.S.A.* **116** F3
Midlands □ *Zimbabwe* **87** F2
Midleton *Ireland* **12** E3
Midlothian *U.K.* **13** F5
Midnapore = Medinipur
    India **69** H12
Midongy, Tangorombohitr'
    i *Madag.* **89** C8
Midongy Atsimo *Madag.* **89** C8
Midou → *France* **20** E3
Midouze → *France* **20** E3
Midsayap *Phil.* **61** H6
Midtjylland □ *Denmark* **11** H2
Midu *China* **58** E3
Midway Is. *Pac. Oc.* **107** K4
Midway Wells *U.S.A.* **111** N11
Midwest *U.S.A.* **107** G22
Midwest *Wyo., U.S.A.* **108** E10
Midwest City *U.S.A.* **116** D6
Midyat *Turkey* **73** D9
Midzŏr *Bulgaria* **44** C7
Mie □ *Japan* **55** G8
Miechów *Poland* **31** H7
Miedwie, Jezioro *Poland* **31** E1
Międzybórz *Poland* **31** G4
Międzychód *Poland* **31** F2
Międzylesie *Poland* **31** H3
Międzyrzec Podlaski *Poland* **31** G9
Międzyrzecz *Poland* **31** F2
Międzyzdroje *Poland* **31** E1
Miejska Górka *Poland* **31** G3
Miélan *France* **20** E4
Mielec *Poland* **31** H8
Mienga *Angola* **88** B2
Miercurea-Ciuc *Romania* **29** D10
Miercurea Sibiului *Romania* **29** E8
Mieres *Spain* **36** B5
Mieroszów *Poland* **31** H3
Mieso *Ethiopia* **81** F5
Mieszkowice *Poland* **31** F1
Mifflintown *U.S.A.* **114** F7
Mifraz Hefa *Israel* **74** C4
Migennes *France* **19** E10
Migliarino *Italy* **41** D8

Migliarino-San Rossore-
Massaciuccoli △ *Italy* **40** E7
Migori *Kenya* **86** C3
Miguel Alemán, Presa
Mexico **119** D5
Miguelturra *Spain* **37** G7
Mihăileni *Romania* **29** C11
Mihăilești *Romania* **29** F11
Mihailovca *Moldova* **29** D13
Mihalgazi *Turkey* **47** A12
Mihalıççık *Turkey* **72** C4
Mihara *Japan* **55** G6
Miheșu de Cîmpie *Romania* **29** D9
Mijas *Spain* **37** J6
Mikese *Tanzania* **86** D4
Mikha-Tskhakaya =
Senaki *Georgia* **35** J6
Mikhailovka =
Mykhaylivka *Ukraine* **33** J8
Mikhaylov *Russia* **32** E10
Mikhaylovgrad =
Montana *Bulgaria* **44** C7
Mikhaylovka *Russia* **34** E6
Mikhnevo *Russia* **32** E9
Mikines *Greece* **46** D4
Mikkeli *Finland* **32** B4
Mikkwa → *Canada* **102** B6
Mikniya *Sudan* **81** D3
Mikołajki *Poland* **30** E8
Míkonos = Mykonos *Greece* **47** D7
Mikri Prespa, L. *Greece* **44** F5
Mikro Derio *Greece* **45** E10
Mikstat *Poland* **31** G4
Mikulov *Czech Rep.* **27** C9
Mikumi *Tanzania* **86** D4
Mikumi △ *Tanzania* **86** D4
Milaca *U.S.A.* **112** C7
Milagro *Ecuador* **124** D3
Milagros *Phil.* **61** E5
Milan = Milano *Italy* **40** C6
Milan *Mo., U.S.A.* **112** E7
Milan *Tenn., U.S.A.* **117** D10
Milange *Mozam.* **87** F4
Milano *Italy* **40** C6
Milano Linate ✈ (LIN) *Italy* **40** C6
Milanoa *Madag.* **89** A8
Milâs *Turkey* **47** D9
Milatos *Greece* **49** D7
Milazzo *Italy* **43** D8
Milbank *U.S.A.* **112** C5
Milbanke Sd. *Canada* **102** C3
Milden *Canada* **103** C7
Mildenhall *U.K.* **15** E8
Mildmay *Canada* **114** B3
Mildura *Australia* **95** E3
Mile *China* **58** E4
Miles *Australia* **95** D5
Miles City *U.S.A.* **108** C11
Milești *Moldova* **29** C13
Milestone *Canada* **103** D8
Mileto *Italy* **43** D9
Miletto, Mte. *Italy* **43** A7
Miletus *Turkey* **47** D9
Milevsko *Czech Rep.* **26** B7
Milford *Calif., U.S.A.* **110** F5
Milford *Conn., U.S.A.* **115** E11
Milford *Del., U.S.A.* **113** F16
Milford *Mass., U.S.A.* **115** D13
Milford *N.H., U.S.A.* **115** D13
Milford *N.Y., U.S.A.* **115** D10
Milford *Pa., U.S.A.* **115** E10
Milford *Utah, U.S.A.* **108** G7
Milford Haven *U.K.* **15** F2
Milford Sd. *N.Z.* **91** F1
Milford Sound *N.Z.* **91** F1
Milḥ, Baḥr al = Razzāzah,
Buḥayrat ar *Iraq* **73** D11
Milicz *Poland* **31** G4
Milies *Greece* **46** B5
Milikapiti *Australia* **92** B5
Miling *Australia* **93** F2
Militello in Val di Catánia
Italy **43** E7
Milk, Wadi el → *Sudan* **80** D3
Milk River *Canada* **102** D6
Mill → *U.S.A.* **114** D1
Mill I. *Antarctica* **5** C8
Mill I. *Canada* **101** E16
Mill Valley *U.S.A.* **110** H4
Millárs → *Spain* **38** F4
Millau *France* **20** D7
Millbridge *Canada* **114** B7
Millbrook *Canada* **114** B6
Millbrook *Ala., U.S.A.* **117** E11
Millbrook *N.Y., U.S.A.* **115** E11
Mille Lacs, L. des *Canada* **104** C1
Mille Lacs L. *U.S.A.* **112** B7
Milledgeville *U.S.A.* **117** E13
Millen *U.S.A.* **117** E14
Millennium I. = Caroline I.
Kiribati **97** H12
Miller *U.S.A.* **112** C4
Miller Lake *Canada* **114** A3
Millerovo *Russia* **35** F5
Millersburg *Ohio, U.S.A.* **114** F3
Millersburg *Pa., U.S.A.* **114** F8
Millerton *U.S.A.* **115** E11
Millerton L. *U.S.A.* **110** J7
Millet *St. Lucia* **121** f

Millevaches, Plateau de
France **20** C6
Millheim *U.S.A.* **114** F7
Millicent *Australia* **95** F3
Millington *U.S.A.* **117** D10
Millinocket *U.S.A.* **113** C19
Millmerran *Australia* **95** D5
Millom *U.K.* **14** C4
Mills L. *Canada* **102** A5
Millsboro *U.S.A.* **114** G5
Millstream Chichester △
Australia **92** D2
Millstreet *Ireland* **12** D2
Milltown Malbay *Ireland* **12** D2
Millville *N.J., U.S.A.* **113** F16
Millville *Pa., U.S.A.* **115** E8
Millwood L. *U.S.A.* **116** E8
Milna *Croatia* **41** E13
Milo *U.S.A.* **113** C19
Milo → *Guinea* **82** D3
Milon, Akra *Greece* **49** C10
Milos *Greece* **46** E6
Miłosław *Poland* **31** F4
Milot *Albania* **44** E3
Milparinka *Australia* **95** D3
Milpitas *U.S.A.* **110** H5
Miltenberg *Germany* **25** F5
Milton *N.S., Canada* **105** D7
Milton *Ont., Canada* **114** C5
Milton *N.Z.* **91** G2
Milton *Calif., U.S.A.* **110** G6
Milton *Fla., U.S.A.* **117** F11
Milton *Pa., U.S.A.* **114** F8
Milton *Vt., U.S.A.* **115** B11
Milton-Freewater *U.S.A.* **108** D4
Milton Keynes *U.K.* **15** E7
Milton Keynes □ *U.K.* **15** E7
Miluo *China* **59** C9
Milverton *Canada* **114** C4
Milwaukee *U.S.A.* **112** D10
Milwaukee Deep *Atl. Oc.* **121** C6
Milwaukie *U.S.A.* **110** E4
Mim *Ghana* **82** D4
Mimili *Australia* **93** E5
Mimizan *France* **20** D2
Mimoň *Czech Rep.* **26** A7
Min Jiang → *Fujian, China* **59** E12
Min Jiang → *Sichuan, China* **58** C5
Min Xian *China* **56** H3
Mina' Jabal 'Alī *U.A.E.* **71** E7
Mina Pirquitas *Argentina* **126** A2
Mīnā Su'ud *Si. Arabia* **71** D6
Mīnā'al Aḥmadī *Kuwait* **71** D6
Minago → *Canada* **103** C9
Minaki *Canada* **103** D10
Minamata *Japan* **55** H5
Minami-Arapusa △ *Japan* **55** G9
Minami-Tori-Shima *Pac. Oc.* **96** E7
Minas *Uruguay* **127** C4
Minas, Sierra de las
Guatemala **120** C2
Minas Basin *Canada* **105** C7
Minas de Riotinto *Spain* **37** H4
Minas Gerais □ *Brazil* **125** G9
Minatitlán *Mexico* **119** D6
Minbu *Burma* **67** J19
Minchinabad *Pakistan* **68** D5
Mincio → *Italy* **40** C7
Minčol *Slovak Rep.* **27** B13
Mindanao *Phil.* **61** H6
Mindanao Sea = Bohol Sea
Phil. **63** C6
Mindanao Trench *Pac. Oc.* **61** F7
Mindel → *Germany* **25** G6
Mindelheim *Germany* **25** G6
Mindelo *C. Verde Is.* **78** b
Minden *Canada* **114** B6
Minden *Germany* **24** C4
Minden *La., U.S.A.* **116** E8
Minden *Nev., U.S.A.* **110** G7
Mindiptana *Indonesia* **63** F10
Mindoro *Phil.* **61** E4
Mindoro Str. *Phil.* **61** E4
Mine *Japan* **55** G5
Minehead *U.K.* **15** F4
Mineola *N.Y., U.S.A.* **115** F11
Mineola *Tex., U.S.A.* **116** E7
Mineral King *U.S.A.* **110** J8
Mineral Wells *U.S.A.* **116** E5
Mineralnyye Vody *Russia* **35** H6
Miners Bay *Canada* **114** B6
Minersville *U.S.A.* **115** F8
Minerva *N.Y., U.S.A.* **115** C11
Minerva *Ohio, U.S.A.* **114** F3
Minervino Murge *Italy* **43** A9
Minetto *U.S.A.* **115** C8
Mingäçevir *Azerbaijan* **35** K8
Mingäçevir Su Anbarı
Azerbaijan **35** K8
Mingan *Canada* **105** B7
Mingechaur = Mingäçevir
Azerbaijan **35** K8
Mingechaurskoye
Vdkhr. = Mingäçevir Su
Anbarı *Azerbaijan* **35** K8
Mingela *Australia* **94** B4

Mingenew *Australia* **93** E2
Mingera Cr. → *Australia* **94** C2
Minggang *China* **59** A10
Mingguang *China* **59** A11
Mingin *Burma* **67** H19
Mingir *Moldova* **29** D13
Minglanilla *Spain* **39** F3
Minglun *China* **58** E7
Mingo Junction *U.S.A.* **114** F4
Mingora *Pakistan* **69** B5
Mingorría *Spain* **36** E6
Mingshan *China* **58** B4
Mingteke Daban =
Mintaka Pass *Pakistan* **69** A6
Mingxi *China* **59** D11
Mingyuegue *China* **57** C15
Minho = Miño → *Spain* **36** D2
Minhou *China* **59** E12
Minidoka *U.S.A.* **108** E7
Minigwal, L. *Australia* **93** E3
Minilya → *Australia* **93** D1
Minilya Roadhouse *Australia* **93** D1
Minipi L. *Canada* **105** B7
Minjilang *Australia* **92** B5
Mink L. *Canada* **102** A5
Minkammen *Sudan* **81** F3
Minna *Nigeria* **83** D6
Minneapolis *Kans., U.S.A.* **112** F5
Minneapolis *Minn., U.S.A.* **112** C7
Minnedosa *Canada* **103** C9
Minnesota □ *U.S.A.* **112** B6
Minnesota → *U.S.A.* **112** C7
Minnewaukan *U.S.A.* **112** A4
Minnipa *Australia* **95** E2
Minnitaki L. *Canada* **104** C1
Mino *Japan* **55** G8
Miño *Spain* **36** B2
Miño → *Spain* **36** D2
Minoa *Greece* **47** F7
Minorca = Menorca *Spain* **48** B11
Minot *U.S.A.* **112** A3
Minqin *China* **56** C2
Minqing *China* **59** D12
Minsen *Germany* **24** B3
Minsk *Belarus* **23** B14
Minsk □ *Belarus* **32** F4
Mińsk Mazowiecki *Poland* **31** F8
Mintabie *Australia* **95** D1
Mintaka Pass *Pakistan* **69** A6
Minto *Canada* **105** C6
Minto, L. *Canada* **104** A5
Minton *Canada* **103** D8
Minturn *U.S.A.* **108** G10
Minturno *Italy* **42** A6
Minudasht *Iran* **71** B8
Minûf *Egypt* **80** H7
Minusinsk *Russia* **53** D10
Minutang *India* **67** E20
Minvoul *Gabon* **84** D2
Minya el Qamh *Egypt* **80** H7
Minya Konka = Gongga
Shan *China* **58** C3
Mionica *Bos.-H.* **28** F3
Mionica *Serbia* **44** B4
Miquelon *Canada* **104** C4
Miquelon *St-P. & M.* **105** C8
Mir *Niger* **83** C7
Mīr Kūh *Iran* **71** E8
Mīr Shahdād *Iran* **71** E8
Mira *Italy* **41** C9
Mira *Portugal* **36** E2
Mira → *Portugal* **37** H2
Mira por vos Cay *Bahamas* **121** B5
Mirabela Eclano *Italy* **43** A7
Mirabello, Kolpos *Greece* **49** D7
Mirador-Río Azul △
Guatemala **120** C2
Miraj *India* **66** L9
Miram Shah *Pakistan* **68** C4
Miramar *Argentina* **126** D4
Miramar *Mozam.* **89** C6
Miramas *France* **21** E8
Mirambeau *France* **20** C3
Miramichi *Canada* **105** C6
Miramichi B. *Canada* **105** C7
Miramont-de-Guyenne
France **20** D4
Miranda *Brazil* **125** H7
Miranda → *Brazil* **124** G7
Miranda de Ebro *Spain* **38** C2
Miranda do Corvo *Portugal* **36** E2
Miranda do Douro *Portugal* **36** D4
Mirande *France* **20** E4
Mirandela *Portugal* **36** D3
Mirándola *Italy* **40** D8
Mirandópolis *Brazil* **127** A5
Mirango *Malawi* **87** E3
Mirani *Australia* **94** b
Mirano *Italy* **41** C9
Miras *Albania* **44** F4
Mirassol *Brazil* **127** A6
Mirbāṭ *Oman* **75** D5
Mirear *Egypt* **80** C4
Mirebeau *France* **18** F7
Mirebeau-sur-Bèze *France* **19** E12
Mirecourt *France* **19** D13
Mires *Greece* **49** D6
Mirgorod = Myrhorod
Ukraine **33** H7

Miri *Malaysia* **62** D4
Miriam Vale *Australia* **94** C5
Miribel *France* **19** G11
Mirim, L. *S. Amer.* **127** C5
Mirnyy *Antarctica* **5** C14
Mirnyy *Russia* **53** C12
Miroč *Serbia* **44** B6
Mirokhan *Pakistan* **68** F3
Mirond L. *Canada* **103** B8
Mirosławiec *Poland* **30** E3
Mirpur *Pakistan* **69** C5
Mirpur Batoro *Pakistan* **68** G3
Mirpur Bibiwari *Pakistan* **68** E2
Mirpur Khas *Pakistan* **68** G3
Mirpur Sakro *Pakistan* **68** G2
Mirria *Niger* **83** C6
Mirtağ *Turkey* **70** B4
Mirtoo Sea *Greece* **46** D5
Miryang *S. Korea* **57** G15
Mirzaani *Georgia* **35** K8
Mirzapur *India* **69** G10
Mirzapur-cum-
Vindhyachal = Mirzapur
India **69** G10
Misantla *Mexico* **119** D5
Misawa *Japan* **54** D10
Miscou I. *Canada* **105** C7
Mish'āb, Ra's al *Si. Arabia* **71** D6
Mishamo *Tanzania* **86** D3
Mishan *China* **54** B5
Mishawaka *U.S.A.* **112** E10
Mishbih, Gebel *Egypt* **80** C3
Mishima *Japan* **55** G9
Misión *Mexico* **111** N10
Misiones □ *Argentina* **127** B5
Misiones □ *Paraguay* **126** B4
Miskah *Si. Arabia* **70** E4
Miskitos, Cayos *Nic.* **120** D3
Miskolc *Hungary* **28** B5
Misool *Indonesia* **63** E8
Misr = Egypt ■ *Africa* **80** B3
Miṣrātah *Libya* **79** B9
Miṣrātah *Libya* **79** B9
Missanabie *Canada* **104** C3
Missinaibi → *Canada* **104** B3
Missinaibi L. *Canada* **104** C3
Mission *Canada* **102** D4
Mission *S. Dak., U.S.A.* **112** D3
Mission *Tex., U.S.A.* **116** H5
Mission Beach *Australia* **94** B4
Mission Viejo *U.S.A.* **111** M9
Missirah *Senegal* **82** C1
Missisa L. *Canada* **104** B2
Mississagi → *Canada* **104** C3
Mississauga *Canada* **114** C5
Mississippi □ *U.S.A.* **117** E10
Mississippi → *U.S.A.* **117** G10
Mississippi L. *U.S.A.* **115** A8
Mississippi River Delta
U.S.A. **117** G10
Mississippi Sd. *U.S.A.* **117** F10
Missoula *U.S.A.* **108** C6
Missouri □ *U.S.A.* **112** F7
Missouri → *U.S.A.* **112** F8
Missouri City *U.S.A.* **116** G7
Missouri Valley *U.S.A.* **112** E6
Mist *U.S.A.* **110** E3
Mistassibi → *Canada* **105** B5
Mistassini *Canada* **105** B5
Mistassini → *Canada* **105** C5
Mistassini, L. *Canada* **104** B5
Mistastin L. *Canada* **105** A7
Mistelbach *Austria* **27** C9
Misterbianco *Italy* **43** E8
Mistinibi, L. *Canada* **105** A7
Mistissini *Canada* **105** C5
Mistretta *Italy* **43** E7
Misty L. *Canada* **103** B8
Misurata = Miṣrātah *Libya* **79** B9
Mît Ghamr *Egypt* **80** H7
Mitande *Mozam.* **87** E4
Mitatib *Sudan* **81** D7
Mitchell *Australia* **95** D4
Mitchell *Canada* **114** C3
Mitchell *Nebr., U.S.A.* **112** E2
Mitchell *Oreg., U.S.A.* **108** D3
Mitchell *S. Dak., U.S.A.* **112** D4
Mitchell → *Australia* **94** B3
Mitchell, Mt. *U.S.A.* **117** D13
Mitchell-Alice Rivers △
Australia **94** B3
Mitchell Ra. *Australia* **94** A2
Mitchelstown *Ireland* **12** D3
Mitha Tiwana *Pakistan* **68** C5
Mithi *Pakistan* **68** G3
Mithimna *Greece* **47** B8
Mithrao *Pakistan* **68** F3
Mitilini *Greece* **47** B8
Mitilinii *Greece* **47** D8
Mitla Pass = Mamarr Mitlā
Egypt **74** E1
Mito *Japan* **55** F10
Mitrofanovka *Russia* **33** H10
Mitrovica = Kosovska
Mitrovica *Kosovo* **44** D4

Mitsamiouli *Comoros Is.* **85** a
Mitsinjo *Madag.* **89** B8
Mitsiwa *Eritrea* **81** D4
Mitsiwa Channel *Eritrea* **81** D5
Mitsukaidō *Japan* **55** F9
Mittagong *Australia* **95** E5
Mittelberg *Austria* **26** D3
Mittelfranken □ *Germany* **25** F6
Mittellandkanal → *Germany* **24** C4
Mittenwalde *Germany* **24** C9
Mittersill *Austria* **26** D5
Mitterteich *Germany* **25** F8
Mittimatalik = Pond Inlet
Canada **101** C16
Mittweida *Germany* **24** E8
Mitú *Colombia* **124** C4
Mitumba *Tanzania* **86** D3
Mitumba, Mts.
Dem. Rep. of the Congo **86** D2
Mitwaba
Dem. Rep. of the Congo **87** D2
Mityana *Uganda* **86** B3
Mixteco → *Mexico* **119** D5
Miyagi □ *Japan* **54** E10
Miyah, W. el → *Egypt* **80** C3
Miyah, W. el → *Syria* **70** C3
Miyake-Jima *Japan* **55** G9
Miyako *Japan* **54** E10
Miyako-Jima *Japan* **55** M2
Miyako-Rettō *Japan* **55** M2
Miyakonojō *Japan* **55** J5
Miyān Rahan *Iran* **73** E12
Miyani *India* **68** J3
Miyanoura-Dake *Japan* **55** J5
Miyazaki *Japan* **55** H5
Miyazaki □ *Japan* **55** H5
Miyazu *Japan* **55** G7
Miyet, Bahr el = Dead Sea
Asia **74** D3
Miyi *China* **58** D4
Miyoshi *Japan* **55** G6
Miyun *China* **56** D9
Miyun Shuiku *China* **57** D9
Mizan Teferi *Ethiopia* **81** F4
Mizdah *Libya* **79** B8
Mizen Hd. *Cork, Ireland* **12** E2
Mizen Hd. *Wicklow, Ireland* **12** D5
Mizhhirya *Ukraine* **29** B8
Mizhi *China* **56** F6
Mizil *Romania* **29** F11
Mizoram □ *India* **67** H18
Mizpe Ramon *Israel* **74** E3
Mizuho *Antarctica* **5** D5
Mizusawa *Japan* **54** E10
Mjällby *Sweden* **11** H8
Mjöbäck *Sweden* **11** G6
Mjölby *Sweden* **11** F9
Mjörn *Sweden* **11** G6
Mjøsa *Norway* **8** F14
Mkata *Tanzania* **86** D4
Mkhaya △ *Swaziland* **89** D5
Mkhuze △ *S. Africa* **89** D5
Mkokotoni *Tanzania* **86** D4
Mkomazi *Tanzania* **86** C4
Mkomazi → *S. Africa* **89** E5
Mkomazi △ *Tanzania* **86** C4
Mkulwe *Tanzania* **87** D3
Mkumbi, Ras *Tanzania* **86** D4
Mkushi *Zambia* **87** E2
Mkushi River *Zambia* **87** E2
Mkuze *S. Africa* **89** D5
Mladá Boleslav *Czech Rep.* **26** A7
Mladenovac *Serbia* **44** B4
Mlala Hills *Tanzania* **86** D3
Mlange = Mulanje, Mt.
Malawi **87** F4
Mlava → *Serbia* **44** B5
Mława *Poland* **31** E7
Mlawula △ *Swaziland* **89** D5
Mlinište *Bos.-H.* **41** D13
Mljet *Croatia* **41** F14
Mljet △ *Croatia* **41** F14
Mljetski Kanal *Croatia* **41** F14
Młynary *Poland* **30** D6
Mmabatho *S. Africa* **88** D4
Mme *Cameroon* **83** D7
Mnichovo Hradiště
Czech Rep. **26** A7
Mo i Rana *Norway* **8** C16
Moa *Australia* **94** a
Moa *Cuba* **121** B4
Moa *Indonesia* **63** F7
Moa → *S. Leone* **82** D2
Moab *U.S.A.* **108** G9
Moala *Fiji* **91** a
Moama *Australia* **95** F3
Moamba *Mozam.* **89** D5
Moapa *U.S.A.* **111** J12
Moate *Ireland* **12** C4
Moba *Dem. Rep. of the Congo* **86** D2
Mobārakābād *Iran* **71** D7
Mobaye *C.A.R.* **84** D4
Moberly *U.S.A.* **112** F7
Moberly Lake *Canada* **102** B4
Mobile *U.S.A.* **117** F10
Mobile B. *U.S.A.* **117** F11
Mobridge *U.S.A.* **112** C4
Moc Chau *Vietnam* **64** B5
Moc Hoa *Vietnam* **65** G5

Mocabe Kasari
Dem. Rep. of the Congo **87** D2
Moçambique =
Mozambique ■ *Africa* **87** F4
Moçambique *Mozam.* **87** F5
Mocanaqua *U.S.A.* **115** E8
Moce *Fiji* **91** a
Mochima △ *Venezuela* **121** D7
Mochos *Greece* **49** D7
Mochudi *Botswana* **88** C4
Mocimboa da Praia *Mozam.* **87** E5
Mociu *Romania* **29** D9
Möckeln *Sweden* **11** H8
Mockfjärd *Sweden* **10** D8
Moclips *U.S.A.* **110** C2
Mocoa *Colombia* **124** C3
Mococa *Brazil* **127** A6
Mocorito *Mexico* **118** B3
Moctezuma *Mexico* **118** B3
Moctezuma → *Mexico* **119** C5
Mocuba *Mozam.* **87** F4
Modane *France* **21** C10
Modasa *India* **68** H5
Modder → *S. Africa* **88** D3
Modderrivier *S. Africa* **88** D3
Módena *Italy* **40** D7
Modena *U.S.A.* **109** H7
Modesto *U.S.A.* **110** H6
Módica *Italy* **43** F7
Modimolle *S. Africa* **89** C4
Mödling *Austria* **27** C9
Modo *Sudan* **81** F3
Modra *Slovak Rep.* **27** C10
Modriča *Bos.-H.* **28** F3
Moe *Australia* **95** F4
Moebase *Mozam.* **87** F4
Moëlan-sur-Mer *France* **18** E3
Moengo *Suriname* **125** B8
Moffat *U.K.* **13** F5
Moga *India* **68** D6
Mogadishu = Muqdisho
Somali Rep. **75** G4
Mogador = Essaouira
Morocco **78** B4
Mogadouro *Portugal* **36** D4
Mogalakwena → *S. Africa* **89** C4
Mogami-Gawa → *Japan* **54** E10
Mogán *Canary Is.* **48** G4
Mogaung *Burma* **67** G20
Mogente = Moixent *Spain* **39** G4
Mogho *Ethiopia* **81** G5
Mogi das Cruzes *Brazil* **127** A6
Mogi-Guaçu → *Brazil* **127** A6
Mogi-Mirim *Brazil* **125** H9
Mogielnica *Poland* **31** G7
Mogige *Ethiopia* **81** F4
Mogilev = Mahilyow
Belarus **23** B16
Mogilev-Podolskiy =
Mohyliv-Podilskyy
Ukraine **29** B12
Mogilno *Poland* **31** F4
Mogincual *Mozam.* **87** F5
Mogliano Véneto *Italy* **41** C9
Mogocha *Russia* **53** D12
Mogok *Burma* **67** H20
Mogollon Rim *U.S.A.* **109** J8
Mógoro *Italy* **42** C1
Moguer *Spain* **37** H4
Mogumber *Australia* **93** F2
Mogwadi → *S. Africa* **89** C4
Mohács *Hungary* **28** E3
Mohales Hoek *Lesotho* **88** E4
Mohall *U.S.A.* **112** A3
Moḥammadābād *Iran* **71** B8
Mohammedia *Morocco* **78** B4
Mohana → *India* **69** G11
Mohanlalganj *India* **69** F9
Mohave, L. *U.S.A.* **111** K12
Mohawk → *U.S.A.* **115** D11
Moheda *Sweden* **11** G8
Mohéli *Comoros Is.* **85** a
Moher, Cliffs of *Ireland* **12** D2
Mohicanville Res. *U.S.A.* **114** F2
Möhne → *Germany* **24** D3
Mohns Ridge *Arctic* **4** B7
Mohoro *Tanzania* **86** D4
Mohsenābād *Iran* **71** B8
Mohyliv-Podilskyy *Ukraine* **29** B12
Moia *Sudan* **81** F2
Moidart, L. *U.K.* **13** E3
Moinești *Romania* **29** D11
Moira → *Canada* **114** B7
Moirans *France* **21** C9
Moirans-en-Montagne
France **19** F12
Moisaküla *Estonia* **32** C3
Moisie *Canada* **105** B6
Moisie → *Canada* **105** B6
Moissac *France* **20** D5
Moita *Portugal* **37** G2
Moixent *Spain* **39** G4
Mojácar *Spain* **39** H3
Mojados *Spain* **36** D6
Mojave *U.S.A.* **111** K8

Mojave △ *U.S.A.* **111** K11
Mojave Desert *U.S.A.* **111** L10
Mojiang *China* **58** F3
Mojjo → *Ethiopia* **81** F5
Mojkovac *Montenegro* **44** D3
Mojo *Bolivia* **126** A2
Mojo *Ethiopia* **81** F4
Mojokerto *Indonesia* **63** G15
Mokai *N.Z.* **91** C5
Mokambo
    Dem. Rep. of the Congo **87** E2
Mokameh *India* **69** G11
Mokau *N.Z.* **91** C5
Mokelumne → *U.S.A.* **110** G5
Mokelumne Hill *U.S.A.* **110** G6
Mokhotlong *Lesotho* **89** D4
Mŏklinta *Sweden* **10** D10
Mokoan, L. *Australia* **95** C4
Mokokchung *India* **67** F19
Mokolo *Cameroon* **83** C7
Mokolo → *S. Africa* **89** C4
Mokopane *S. Africa* **89** C4
Mokpo *S. Korea* **57** G14
Mokra Gora *Europe* **44** D4
Mokronog *Slovenia* **41** C12
Moksha → *Russia* **34** C6
Mokshan *Russia* **34** D7
Mokwa *Nigeria* **83** D6
Mol *Belgium* **17** C5
Mola di Bari *Italy* **43** A10
Molai *Greece* **46** E4
Molale *Ethiopia* **81** E4
Molara *Italy* **42** B2
Molat *Croatia* **41** D11
Molchanovo *Russia* **52** D9
Mold *U.K.* **14** D4
Moldava nad Bodvou
    Slovak Rep. **27** C14
Moldavia = Moldova ■
    Europe **29** C13
Molde *Norway* **8** E12
Moldova ■ *Europe* **29** C13
Moldova Nouă *Romania* **28** F6
Moldoveanu, Vf. *Romania* **29** E9
Moldoviţa *Romania* **29** C10
Mole → *U.K.* **15** F7
Mole △ *Ghana* **83** D4
Molepolole *Botswana* **88** C4
Molfetta *Italy* **43** A9
Molina de Aragón *Spain* **38** E3
Molina de Segura *Spain* **39** G3
Moline *U.S.A.* **112** E8
Molinella *Italy* **41** D8
Molinos *Argentina* **126** B2
Moliro *Dem. Rep. of the Congo* **86** D3
Moliterno *Italy* **43** B8
Molkom *Sweden* **10** E7
Mölle *Sweden* **11** H6
Molledo *Spain* **36** B6
Mollendo *Peru* **124** G4
Mollerin, L. *Australia* **93** F2
Mollerussa *Spain* **38** D5
Mollina *Spain* **37** H6
Mölln *Germany* **24** B6
Mölltorp *Sweden* **11** F8
Mölnlycke *Sweden* **11** G6
Molo *Kenya* **86** C4
Molochansk *Ukraine* **33** J8
Molochnoye, Ozero *Ukraine* **33** J8
Molodechno =
    Maladzyechna *Belarus* **23** A14
Molodezhnaya *Antarctica* **5** C9
Molodove *Ukraine* **29** D14
Moloka'i *U.S.A.* **107** L8
Molokai Fracture Zone
    Pac. Oc. **97** E15
Molong *Australia* **95** E4
Molopo → *Africa* **88** D3
Molos *Greece* **46** C4
Molsheim *France* **19** D14
Molson L. *Canada* **103** C9
Molteno *S. Africa* **88** E4
Molu *Indonesia* **63** F8
Molucca Sea *Indonesia* **63** E6
Moluccas = Maluku
    Indonesia **63** E7
Moma *Dem. Rep. of the Congo* **86** C1
Moma *Mozam.* **87** F4
Mombasa *Kenya* **86** C4
Mombetsu *Japan* **54** B11
Mombuey *Spain* **36** C4
Momchilgrad *Bulgaria* **45** E9
Momi *Dem. Rep. of the Congo* **86** C2
Mompós *Colombia* **124** B4
Møn *Denmark* **11** K6
Mon □ *Burma* **67** L20
Mona, Canal de la = Mona
    Passage *W. Indies* **121** C6
Mona, Isla *Puerto Rico* **121** C6
Mona, Pta. *Costa Rica* **120** E3
Mona Passage *W. Indies* **121** C6
Monaca *U.S.A.* **114** F4
Monaco ■ *Europe* **21** E11
Monadhliath Mts. *U.K.* **13** D4
Monadnock, Mt. *U.S.A.* **115** D12
Monaghan *Ireland* **12** B5
Monaghan □ *Ireland* **12** B5
Monahans *U.S.A.* **116** F3

Monapo *Mozam.* **87** E5
Monar, L. *U.K.* **13** D3
Monarch Mt. *Canada* **102** C3
Monashee Mts. *Canada* **102** C5
Monasterevin *Ireland* **12** C4
Monastir = Bitola *Macedonia* **44** E5
Monastir *Tunisia* **79** A8
Moncada *Phil.* **61** D4
Moncalieri *Italy* **40** D4
Moncalvo *Italy* **40** C5
Moncão *Portugal* **36** C2
Moncarapacho *Portugal* **37** H3
Moncayo, Sierra del *Spain* **38** D3
Monchegorsk *Russia* **8** C25
Mönchengladbach *Germany* **24** D2
Monchique *Portugal* **37** H2
Moncks Corner *U.S.A.* **117** E14
Monclova *Mexico* **118** B4
Moncontour *France* **18** D4
Moncton *Canada* **105** C7
Mondariz *Spain* **36** C2
Mondego → *Portugal* **36** E2
Mondego, C. *Portugal* **36** E2
Mondeodo *Indonesia* **63** E6
Mondeville *France* **18** C6
Mondolfo *Italy* **41** E10
Mondoñedo *Spain* **36** B3
Mondoví *Italy* **40** D4
Mondragon = Arrasate *Spain* **38** B2
Mondragon *Phil.* **61** E6
Mondragone *Italy* **42** A6
Mondrain I. *Australia* **93** F3
Moneague *Jamaica* **120** a
Monemvasia *Greece* **46** E5
Moneron, Ostrov *Russia* **54** A10
Monessen *U.S.A.* **114** F5
Monesterio *Spain* **37** G4
Monestier-de-Clermont
    France **21** D9
Monett *U.S.A.* **112** G7
Moneymore *U.K.* **12** B5
Monfalcone *Italy* **41** C10
Monflanquin *France* **20** D4
Monforte *Portugal* **37** F3
Monforte de Lemos *Spain* **36** C3
Mong Cai *Vietnam* **64** B6
Mong Hsu *Burma* **58** G2
Mong Kung *Burma* **67** J20
Mong Nai *Burma* **67** J20
Mong Pawk *Burma* **67** H21
Mong Ping *Burma* **58** G2
Mong Ton *Burma* **67** J21
Mong Wa *Burma* **67** J22
Mong Yai *Burma* **67** H21
Mongalla *Sudan* **81** F3
Mongers, L. *Australia* **93** E2
Monghyr = Munger *India* **69** G12
Mongibello = Etna *Italy* **43** E7
Mongo *Chad* **79** F9
Mongo → *S. Leone* **82** D2
Mongolia ■ *Asia* **53** E10
Mongolia, Plateau of *Asia* **50** D12
Mongonu *Nigeria* **83** C7
Mongu *Zambia* **85** H4
Mŏngua *Angola* **88** B2
Monifieth *U.K.* **13** E6
Monistrol-sur-Loire *France* **21** C8
Monkey Bay *Malawi* **87** E4
Monkey Mia *Australia* **93** E1
Monkey River *Belize* **119** D7
Mońki *Poland* **30** E9
Monkland *Canada* **115** A10
Monkoto
    Dem. Rep. of the Congo **84** E4
Monkton *Canada* **114** C3
Monmouth *U.K.* **15** F5
Monmouth *Ill., U.S.A.* **112** E8
Monmouth *Oreg., U.S.A.* **108** D2
Monmouthshire □ *U.K.* **15** F5
Mono → *Togo* **83** D5
Mono, Pta. *Nic.* **120** D3
Mono L. *U.S.A.* **110** H7
Monolith *U.S.A.* **111** K8
Monolithos *Greece* **49** C9
Monongahela *U.S.A.* **114** F5
Monópoli *Italy* **43** B10
Monor *Hungary* **28** C4
Monos I. *Trin. & Tob.* **125** K15
Monóvar *Spain* **39** G4
Monreal del Campo *Spain* **38** E3
Monreale *Italy* **42** D6
Monroe *Ga., U.S.A.* **117** E13
Monroe *La., U.S.A.* **116** E8
Monroe *Mich., U.S.A.* **113** E12
Monroe *N.C., U.S.A.* **117** D14
Monroe *N.Y., U.S.A.* **115** E10
Monroe *Utah, U.S.A.* **108** G7
Monroe *Wash., U.S.A.* **110** C5
Monroe *Wis., U.S.A.* **112** D9
Monroe City *U.S.A.* **112** F9
Monroeton *U.S.A.* **115** E8
Monroeville *Ala., U.S.A.* **117** F11
Monroeville *Pa., U.S.A.* **114** F5
Monrovia *Liberia* **82** D2
Mons *Belgium* **17** D3
Møns Klint *Denmark* **11** K6
Monsaraz *Portugal* **37** G3
Monse *Indonesia* **63** E6
Monségur *France* **20** D4

Monsélice *Italy* **41** C8
Mönsterås *Sweden* **11** G10
Mont Cenis, Col du *France* **21** C10
Montagne, Brazil **127** B5
Mont-de-Marsan *France* **20** E3
Mont-Joli *Canada* **105** C6
Mont-Laurier *Canada* **104** C4
Mont-Louis *Canada* **105** C6
Mont Peko △ *Ivory C.* **82** D3
Mont-roig del Camp *Spain* **38** D5
Mont-St-Michel, Le *France* **18** D5
Mont Sangbé △ *Ivory C.* **82** D3
Mont-Tremblant △ *Canada* **104** C5
Montabaur *Germany* **24** E3
Montagnac *France* **20** E7
Montagnana *Italy* **41** C8
Montagne d'Ambre △
    Madag. **89** A8
Montagne de Reims △
    France **19** C11
Montagu *S. Africa* **88** E3
Montagu I. *Antarctica* **5** B1
Montague *Canada* **105** C7
Montague, I. *Mexico* **118** A2
Montague I. *U.S.A.* **106** C10
Montague Ra. *Australia* **93** E2
Montague Sd. *Australia* **92** B4
Montaigu *France* **18** F5
Montalbán *Spain* **38** E4
Montalbano Iónico *Italy* **43** B9
Montalbo *Spain* **38** F2
Montalcino *Italy* **41** E8
Montalegre *Portugal* **36** D3
Montalto *Italy* **43** D8
Montalto di Castro *Italy* **41** F8
Montalto Uffugo *Italy* **43** C9
Montalvo *U.S.A.* **111** L7
Montamarta *Spain* **36** D5
Montana *Peru* **124** E4
Montana *Bulgaria* **44** C7
Montana □ *Bulgaria* **44** C7
Montana □ *U.S.A.* **108** C9
Montaña Clara, I. *Canary Is.* **48** E6
Montañas de Malaga △
    Spain **37** J6
Montánchez *Spain* **37** F4
Montargil *Portugal* **37** F2
Montargis *France* **19** E9
Montauban *France* **20** D5
Montauk *U.S.A.* **115** E13
Montauk Pt. *U.S.A.* **115** E13
Montbard *France* **19** E11
Montbarrey *France* **19** E12
Montbéliard *France* **19** E13
Montblanc *Spain* **38** D6
Montbrison *France* **21** C8
Montcalm, Pic de *France* **20** F5
Montceau-les-Mines *France* **19** F11
Montcenis *France* **21** B8
Montclair *U.S.A.* **115** F10
Montcornet *France* **19** C11
Montcuq *France* **20** D5
Montdidier *France* **19** C9
Monte Albán *Mexico* **119** D5
Monte Alegre *Brazil* **125** D8
Monte Azul *Brazil* **125** G10
Monte-Carlo *Monaco* **21** E11
Monte Caseros *Argentina* **126** C4
Monte Comán *Argentina* **126** C2
Monte Crísti *Dom. Rep.* **121** C5
Monte Cucco △ *Italy* **41** E9
Monte Lindo → *Paraguay* **126** A4
Monte Patria *Chile* **126** C1
Monte Quemado *Argentina* **126** B3
Monte Redondo *Portugal* **36** F2
Monte Rio *U.S.A.* **110** G4
Monte San Giovanni
    Campano *Italy* **42** A6
Monte San Savino *Italy* **41** E8
Monte Sant' Ángelo *Italy* **41** G12
Monte Santu, C. di *Italy* **42** B2
Monte Sibillini △ *Italy* **41** F10
Monte Subasio △ *Italy* **41** E9
Monte Vista *U.S.A.* **109** H10
Monteagudo *Argentina* **127** B5
Montealegre del Castillo
    Spain **39** G3
Montebello *Canada* **104** C5
Montebello Iónico *Italy* **43** E8
Montebello Is. *Australia* **92** D2
Montebelluna *Italy* **41** C9
Montebourg *France* **18** C5
Montecarlo *Argentina* **127** B5
Montecastrilli *Italy* **41** F9
Montecatini Terme *Italy* **40** E7
Montecito *U.S.A.* **111** L7
Montecristo *Italy* **40** F7
Montefalco *Italy* **41** F9
Montefiascone *Italy* **41** F9
Montefrío *Spain* **37** H7
Montegiórgio *Italy* **41** E10
Montego Bay *Jamaica* **120** a
Montehermoso *Spain* **36** E4
Montejícar *Spain* **37** H7
Montélimar *France* **21** D8
Montella *Italy* **43** B8
Montellano *Spain* **37** J5
Montello *U.S.A.* **112** D9
Montemor-o-Novo *Portugal* **37** G2
Montemor-o-Velho *Portugal* **36** E2

Montemorelos *Mexico* **119** B5
Montendre *France* **20** C3
Montenegro *Brazil* **127** B5
Montenegro ■ *Europe* **44** D3
Montenero di Bisáccia *Italy* **41** G11
Montepuez *Mozam.* **87** E4
Montepuez → *Mozam.* **87** E5
Montepulciano *Italy* **41** E8
Montereale *Italy* **41** F10
Montereau-Faut-Yonne
    France **19** D9
Monterey *U.S.A.* **110** J5
Monterey B. *U.S.A.* **110** J5
Montería *Colombia* **124** B3
Monteros *Argentina* **126** B2
Monterotondo *Italy* **41** F9
Monterrey *Mexico* **118** B4
Montes Azules △ *Mexico* **119** D6
Montes Claros *Brazil* **125** G10
Montesano *U.S.A.* **110** D3
Montesano sulla
    Marcellana *Italy* **43** B8
Montesárchio *Italy* **43** A7
Montescaglioso *Italy* **43** B9
Montesilvano *Italy* **41** F11
Montesinho △ *Portugal* **36** D4
Montevarchi *Italy* **41** E8
Montevideo *Uruguay* **127** C4
Montevideo *U.S.A.* **112** C6
Montezuma *U.S.A.* **112** E7
Montezuma Castle △ *U.S.A.* **109** J8
Montfaucon *France* **18** E5
Montfaucon-d'Argonne
    France **19** C12
Montfaucon-en-Velay *France* **21** C8
Montfort-le-Gesnois *France* **18** D7
Montfort-sur-Meu *France* **18** D5
Montfragüe △ *Spain* **36** F5
Montgenèvre *France* **21** D10
Montgomery *U.K.* **15** E4
Montgomery *Ala., U.S.A.* **117** E11
Montgomery *Pa., U.S.A.* **114** E8
Montgomery *W. Va., U.S.A.* **113** F13
Montgomery City *U.S.A.* **112** F8
Montguyon *France* **20** C3
Monthermé *France* **19** C11
Monthey *Switz.* **25** J2
Monthois *France* **19** C11
Monti *Italy* **42** B2
Monti Lucrétili △ *Italy* **41** F9
Monti Picentini △ *Italy* **43** B8
Monti Simbruini △ *Italy* **41** G10
Monticelli d'Ongina *Italy* **40** C6
Monticello *Ark., U.S.A.* **116** E9
Monticello *Fla., U.S.A.* **117** F13
Monticello *Ind., U.S.A.* **112** E10
Monticello *Iowa, U.S.A.* **112** D8
Monticello *Ky., U.S.A.* **113** G11
Monticello *Minn., U.S.A.* **112** C7
Monticello *Miss., U.S.A.* **117** F9
Monticello *N.Y., U.S.A.* **115** E10
Monticello *Utah, U.S.A.* **109** H9
Montichiari *Italy* **40** C7
Montier-en-Der *France* **19** D11
Montignac *France* **20** C5
Montigny-lès-Metz *France* **19** C13
Montigny-sur-Aube *France* **19** E11
Montijo *Portugal* **37** G2
Montijo *Spain* **37** G4
Montilla *Spain* **37** H6
Montivilliers *France* **18** C7
Montluçon *France* **19** F9
Montmagny *Canada* **105** C5
Montmarault *France* **19** F9
Montmartre *Canada* **103** C8
Montmédy *France* **19** C12
Montmélian *France* **21** C10
Montmirail *France* **19** D10
Montmoreau-St-Cybard
    France **20** C4
Montmorillon *France* **20** B4
Montmort-Lucy *France* **19** D10
Montoire-sur-le-Loir *France* **18** E7
Montongbuwoh *Indonesia* **63** K19
Montoro *Spain* **37** G6
Montour Falls *U.S.A.* **114** D8
Montoursville *U.S.A.* **114** E8
Montpelier *Idaho, U.S.A.* **108** E8
Montpelier *Vt., U.S.A.* **115** B12
Montpellier *France* **20** E7
Montpezat-de-Quercy *France* **20** D5
Montpon-Ménestérol *France* **20** D4
Montréal *Canada* **115** A11
Montréal *Aude, France* **20** E6
Montréal *Gers, France* **20** E4
Montreal → *Canada* **104** C3
Montreal L. *Canada* **103** C7
Montreal Lake *Canada* **103** C7
Montredon-Labessonnié
    France **20** E6
Montrésor *France* **18** E8
Montret *France* **19** F12
Montreuil *Pas-de-Calais,*
    France **19** B8
Montreuil *Seine-St-Denis,*
    France **19** D9
Montreuil-Bellay *France* **18** E6

Montreux *Switz.* **25** J2
Montrevel-en-Bresse *France* **19** F12
Montrichard *France* **18** E8
Montrose *U.K.* **13** E6
Montrose *Colo., U.S.A.* **108** G10
Montrose *Pa., U.S.A.* **115** E9
Monts, Pte. des *Canada* **105** C6
Montsalvy *France* **20** D6
Montsant, Serra de *Spain* **38** D6
Montsauche-les-Settons
    France **19** E11
Montsec, Serra del *Spain* **38** C5
Montseny △ *Spain* **38** D2
Montserrat *Spain* **38** D6
Montserrat ☑ *W. Indies* **121** C7
Montuenga *Spain* **36** D6
Montuiri *Spain* **48** B9
Monywa *Burma* **67** H19
Monza *Italy* **40** C6
Monze *Zambia* **87** F2
Monze, C. *Pakistan* **68** G2
Monzón *Spain* **38** D5
Mooers *U.S.A.* **115** B11
Mooi → *S. Africa* **89** D5
Mooi River *S. Africa* **89** D4
Moomba *Australia* **95** A3
Moonah → *Australia* **94** C2
Moonda, L. *Australia* **94** D3
Moonie *Australia* **95** D5
Moonie → *Australia* **95** D4
Moonta *Australia* **95** E2
Moora *Australia* **93** F2
Moorcroft *U.S.A.* **108** D11
Moore → *Australia* **93** F2
Moore, L. *Australia* **93** E2
Moore Falls *Canada* **114** B6
Moore Park *Australia* **94** C5
Moore Res. *U.S.A.* **115** B13
Moore River △ *Australia* **93** F2
Moorea *French Polynesia* **91** d
Moorefield *U.S.A.* **113** F14
Moorfoot Hills *U.K.* **13** F5
Moorhead *U.S.A.* **112** B5
Moormerland *Germany* **24** B3
Moorpark *U.S.A.* **111** L8
Moorreesburg *S. Africa* **88** E2
Moorrinya △ *Australia* **94** C3
Moosburg *Germany* **25** G7
Moose → *Canada* **104** B3
Moose → *U.S.A.* **115** C9
Moose Creek *Canada* **115** A10
Moose Factory *Canada* **104** B3
Moose Jaw *Canada* **103** C7
Moose Jaw → *Canada* **103** C7
Moose Lake *Canada* **103** C8
Moose Lake *U.S.A.* **112** B7
Moose Mountain △ *Canada* **103** D8
Moosehead L. *U.S.A.* **113** C19
Mooselookmeguntic L.
    U.S.A. **115** B14
Moosilauke, Mt. *U.S.A.* **115** B13
Moosomin *Canada* **103** C8
Moosonee *Canada* **104** B3
Moosup *U.S.A.* **115** E13
Mopane *S. Africa* **89** C4
Mopeia Velha *Mozam.* **87** F4
Mopipi *Botswana* **88** C3
Mopoi *C.A.R.* **86** A2
Mopti *Mali* **82** C4
Mopti □ *Mali* **82** C4
Moqatta *Sudan* **81** E4
Moqor *Afghan.* **68** C2
Moquegua *Peru* **124** G4
Mór *Hungary* **28** C3
Mora *Cameroon* **83** C7
Móra *Portugal* **37** G2
Mora *Spain* **37** F7
Mora *Sweden* **10** C8
Mora *Minn., U.S.A.* **112** C7
Mora *N. Mex., U.S.A.* **109** J11
Mora de Rubielos *Spain* **38** E4
Móra d'Ebre *Spain* **38** D5
Móra la Nova *Spain* **38** D5
Morača → *Montenegro* **44** D3
Moradabad *India* **69** E8
Morafenobe *Madag.* **89** B7
Morąg *Poland* **30** E6
Moral de Calatrava *Spain* **37** G7
Moraleja *Spain* **36** E4
Moramanga *Madag.* **89** B8
Moran *Kans., U.S.A.* **112** G6
Moran *Wyo., U.S.A.* **108** E8
Moranbah *Australia* **94** C4
Morang = Biratnagar *Nepal* **69** F12
Morano Cálabro *Italy* **43** C9
Morant Bay *Jamaica* **120** a
Morant Cays *Jamaica* **120** C4
Morant Pt. *Jamaica* **120** a
Morar *India* **68** F8
Morar, L. *U.K.* **13** E3
Moratalla *Spain* **39** G3
Moratuwa *Sri Lanka* **66** R11
Morava → *Slovak Rep.* **27** C9
Moravia *U.S.A.* **115** D8
Moravian Hts. =
    Českomoravská
    Vrchovina *Czech Rep.* **26** B8
Moravica → *Serbia* **44** C4
Moraviţa *Romania* **28** E6

Moravská Třebová
    Czech Rep. **27** B9
Moravské Budějovice
    Czech Rep. **26** B8
Morawa *Australia* **93** E2
Morawhanna *Guyana* **124** B7
Moray □ *U.K.* **13** D5
Moray Firth *U.K.* **13** D5
Morbach *Germany* **25** F3
Morbegno *Italy* **40** B6
Morbi *India* **68** H4
Morbihan □ *France* **18** E4
Mörbylånga *Sweden* **11** H10
Morcenx *France* **20** D3
Morcone *Italy* **43** A7
Mordelles *France* **18** D5
Morden *Canada* **103** D9
Mordoğan *Turkey* **47** C8
Mordovian Republic =
    Mordvinia □ *Russia* **34** C7
Mordovo *Russia* **34** D5
Mordvinia □ *Russia* **34** C7
Mordy *Poland* **31** F9
Moreau → *U.S.A.* **112** C3
Morebeng *S. Africa* **89** C4
Morecambe *U.K.* **14** C5
Morecambe B. *U.K.* **14** C5
Moree *Australia* **95** D4
Morehead *U.S.A.* **113** F12
Morehead City *U.S.A.* **117** D16
Morel → *India* **68** F7
Morelia *Mexico* **118** D4
Morella *Australia* **94** C3
Morella *Spain* **38** E4
Morelos *Mexico* **118** B3
Morelos □ *Mexico* **119** D5
Moremi △ *Botswana* **88** B3
Morena *India* **68** F8
Morena, Sierra *Spain* **37** G5
Moreni *Romania* **29** F10
Moreno Valley *U.S.A.* **111** M10
Moresby I. *Canada* **102** C2
Morestel *France* **21** C9
Moreton I. *Australia* **95** D5
Moreton Island △ *Australia* **95** D5
Moreuil *France* **19** C9
Morez *France* **19** F13
Morgan *U.S.A.* **108** F8
Morgan City *U.S.A.* **116** G9
Morgan Hill *U.S.A.* **110** H5
Morganfield *U.S.A.* **112** G10
Morganton *U.S.A.* **117** D14
Morgantown *U.S.A.* **113** F14
Morgenzon *S. Africa* **89** D4
Morges *Switz.* **25** J2
Morghak *Iran* **71** D8
Morgongåva *Sweden* **10** E10
Morhange *France* **19** D13
Morhar → *India* **69** G11
Mori *Italy* **40** C7
Mori *Japan* **54** C10
Moriarty *U.S.A.* **109** J10
Moribaya *Guinea* **82** D3
Morice L. *Canada* **102** C3
Moriki *Nigeria* **83** C6
Morinville *Canada* **102** C6
Morioka *Japan* **54** E10
Moris *Mexico* **118** B3
Morlaàs *France* **20** E3
Morlaix *France* **18** D3
Mörlunda *Sweden* **11** G9
Mormanno *Italy* **43** C8
Mormant *France* **19** D9
Mornington *Australia* **95** F4
Mornington, I. *Chile* **128** F1
Mornington I. *Australia* **94** B2
Mornos → *Greece* **46** C3
Moro *Pakistan* **68** F2
Moro *Sudan* **81** E3
Moro → *Pakistan* **68** E2
Moro G. *Phil.* **61** H5
Morocco ■ *N. Afr.* **78** B4
Morogoro *Tanzania* **86** D4
Morogoro □ *Tanzania* **86** D4
Moroleón *Mexico* **118** C4
Moron *Argentina* **126** C4
Morón *Cuba* **120** B4
Mörön *Mongolia* **53** E11
Morón de Almazán *Spain* **38** D2
Morón de la Frontera *Spain* **37** H5
Morona → *Peru* **124** D3
Morondava *Madag.* **89** C7
Morondo *Ivory C.* **82** D3
Morongo Valley *U.S.A.* **111** L10
Moroni *Comoros Is.* **85** a
Moroni *U.S.A.* **108** G8
Moronou *Ivory C.* **82** D4
Morotai *Indonesia* **63** D7
Moroto *Uganda* **86** B3
Moroto, Mt. *Uganda* **86** B3
Morozov *Bulgaria* **45** D9
Morozovsk *Russia* **35** F5
Morpeth *Canada* **114** D3
Morpeth *U.K.* **14** B6
Morphou *Cyprus* **49** D11
Morphou Bay *Cyprus* **49** D11
Morrilton *U.S.A.* **116** D8
Morrinhos *Brazil* **125** G9

Morrinsville *N.Z.* **91** B5
Morris *Canada* **103** D9
Morris *Ill., U.S.A.* **112** E9
Morris *Minn., U.S.A.* **112** C6
Morris *N.Y., U.S.A.* **115** D9
Morris *Pa., U.S.A.* **114** E7
Morris, Mt. *Australia* **93** E5
Morris Jesup, Kap *Greenland* **98** A16
Morrisburg *Canada* **115** B9
Morristown *Ariz., U.S.A.* **109** K7
Morristown *N.J., U.S.A.* **115** F10
Morristown *N.Y., U.S.A.* **115** D9
Morristown *Tenn., U.S.A.* **117** C13
Morrisville *N.Y., U.S.A.* **115** D9
Morrisville *Pa., U.S.A.* **115** F10
Morrisville *Vt., U.S.A.* **115** B12
Morro, Pta. *Chile* **126** B1
Morro Bay *U.S.A.* **110** K6
Morro del Jable *Canary Is.* **48** F5
Morro Jable, Pta. de
  Canary Is. **48** F5
Morrocoy △ *Venezuela* **121** D6
Morrosquillo, G. de *Colombia* **120** E4
Mörrum *Sweden* **11** H8
Morrumbene *Mozam.* **89** C6
Mörrumsån → *Sweden* **11** H8
Mors *Denmark* **11** H2
Morshansk *Russia* **34** D5
Mörsil *Sweden* **10** A7
Mortagne → *France* **19** D13
Mortagne-au-Perche *France* **18** D7
Mortagne-sur-Gironde
  France **20** C3
Mortagne-sur-Sèvre *France* **18** F6
Mortain *France* **18** D6
Mortara *Italy* **40** C5
Morteau *France* **19** E13
Morteros *Argentina* **126** C3
Mortlach *Canada* **103** C7
Mortlake *Australia* **95** F3
Morton *Tex., U.S.A.* **116** E3
Morton *Wash., U.S.A.* **110** D4
Moruga *Trin. & Tob.* **125** K15
Morundah *Australia* **95** E4
Moruya *Australia* **95** F5
Morvan *France* **19** E11
Morven *Australia* **95** D4
Morvern *U.K.* **13** E3
Morwell *Australia* **95** F4
Moryń *Poland* **31** F1
Morzine *France* **19** F13
Mosalsk *Russia* **32** E8
Mosbach *Germany* **25** F5
Mošćenice *Croatia* **41** C11
Mosciano Sant' Ángelo
  Italy **41** F10
Moscos Is. *Burma* **64** F1
Moscow = Moskva *Russia* **32** E9
Moscow *Idaho, U.S.A.* **108** C5
Moscow *Pa., U.S.A.* **115** E9
Mosel → *Europe* **19** B14
Moselle = Mosel → *Europe* **19** B14
Moselle □ *France* **19** D13
Moses Lake *U.S.A.* **108** C4
Mosgiel *N.Z.* **91** F3
Moshaweng → *S. Africa* **88** D3
Moshi *Tanzania* **86** C4
Moshi → *Nigeria* **83** D5
Moshupa *Botswana* **88** C4
Mosina *Poland* **31** F3
Mosjøen *Norway* **8** D15
Moskenesøya *Norway* **8** C15
Moskenstraumen *Norway* **8** C15
Moskva *Russia* **32** E9
Moskva □ *Russia* **32** D9
Moskva → *Russia* **32** E10
Moslavačka Gora *Croatia* **41** C13
Mosomane *Botswana* **88** C4
Mosonmagyaróvár *Hungary* **28** C2
Mošorin *Serbia* **28** E5
Mospino *Ukraine* **33** J9
Mosquera *Colombia* **124** C3
Mosquero *U.S.A.* **109** J12
Mosqueruela *Spain* **38** E4
Mosquitia *Honduras* **120** C3
Mosquito Coast =
  Mosquitia *Honduras* **120** C3
Mosquito Creek L. *U.S.A.* **114** E4
Mosquito L. *Canada* **103** A8
Mosquitos, G. de los *Panama* **120** E3
Moss *Norway* **9** G14
Moss Vale *Australia* **95** E5
Mossaka *Congo* **84** E3
Mossbank *Canada* **103** D7
Mossburn *N.Z.* **91** F2
Mosselbaai *S. Africa* **88** E4
Mossendjo *Congo* **84** E2
Mossgiel *Australia* **95** E3
Mossman *Australia* **94** B4
Mossingen *Germany* **25** G5
Mossman *Australia* **94** B4
Mossoró *Brazil* **125** E11
Mossuril *Mozam.* **87** E5
Most *Czech Rep.* **26** A6
Mosta *Malta* **49** D1
Mostaganem *Algeria* **78** A6
Mostar *Bos.-H.* **28** G2
Mostardas *Brazil* **127** C5

Mostiska = Mostyska
  Ukraine **31** J10
Móstoles *Spain* **36** E7
Mosty = Masty *Belarus* **23** B13
Mostyska *Ukraine* **31** J10
Mosul = Al Mawşil *Iraq* **73** D10
Mota *Ethiopia* **81** E4
Mota del Cuervo *Spain* **39** F2
Mota del Marqués *Spain* **36** D5
Motagua → *Guatemala* **120** C2
Motala *Sweden* **11** F9
Motaze *Mozam.* **89** C5
Moţca *Romania* **29** C11
Moth *India* **69** G8
Motherwell *U.K.* **13** F5
Motihari *India* **69** F11
Motilla del Palancar *Spain* **39** F3
Motnik *Slovenia* **41** B11
Motovun *Croatia* **41** C10
Motozintla de Mendoza
  Mexico **119** D6
Motril *Spain* **37** J7
Motru *Romania* **28** F7
Motru → *Romania* **29** F8
Mott *U.S.A.* **112** B2
Móttola *Italy* **43** B10
Motueka *N.Z.* **91** D4
Motueka → *N.Z.* **91** D4
Motul *Mexico* **119** C7
Mouchalagane → *Canada* **105** B6
Mouding *China* **58** E3
Moudjeria *Mauritania* **82** B2
Moudon *Switz.* **25** J2
Moudros *Greece* **47** B7
Mouhoun = Black
  Volta → *Africa* **82** D4
Mouila *Gabon* **84** E2
Moulamein *Australia* **95** F3
Moule à Chique, C. *St. Lucia* **121** f
Mouliana *Greece* **49** D7
Moulins *France* **19** F10
Moulmein *Burma* **67** L20
Moulouya, O. → *Morocco* **78** B5
Moultrie *U.S.A.* **117** F13
Moultrie, L. *U.S.A.* **117** E14
Mound City *Mo., U.S.A.* **112** E6
Mound City *S. Dak., U.S.A.* **112** C3
Moundou *Chad* **79** G9
Moundsville *U.S.A.* **114** G4
Moung *Cambodia* **64** F4
Mount Airy *U.S.A.* **117** C14
Mount Albert *Canada* **114** B5
Mount Aspiring △ *N.Z.* **91** F2
Mount Barker *S. Austral.,
  Australia* **95** F2
Mount Barker *W. Austral.,
  Australia* **93** F2
Mount Barnett Roadhouse
  Australia **92** C4
Mount Bellew Bridge *Ireland* **12** C3
Mount Brydges *Canada* **114** D3
Mount Burr *Australia* **95** F3
Mount Carmel = Ha
  Karmel △ *Israel* **74** C4
Mount Carmel *Ill., U.S.A.* **112** F10
Mount Carmel *Pa., U.S.A.* **115** F8
Mount Clemens *U.S.A.* **114** D2
Mount Coolon *Australia* **94** C4
Mount Darwin *Zimbabwe* **87** F3
Mount Desert I. *U.S.A.* **113** C19
Mount Dora *U.S.A.* **117** G14
Mount Ebenezer *Australia* **93** E5
Mount Edziza △ *Canada* **102** B2
Mount Elgon △ *E. Afr.* **86** B3
Mount Field △ *Australia* **95** G4
Mount Fletcher *S. Africa* **89** E4
Mount Forest *Canada* **114** C4
Mount Frankland △
  Australia **93** F2
Mount Frederick ☼ *Australia* **92** C4
Mount Gambier *Australia* **95** F3
Mount Garnet *Australia* **94** B4
Mount Holly *U.S.A.* **115** G10
Mount Holly Springs *U.S.A.* **114** F7
Mount Hope *N.S.W., Australia* **95** E4
Mount Hope *S. Austral.,
  Australia* **95** E2
Mount Isa *Australia* **94** C2
Mount James ☼ *Australia* **93** D2
Mount Jewett *U.S.A.* **114** E6
Mount Kaputar △ *Australia* **95** E5
Mount Kenya △ *Kenya* **86** C4
Mount Kisco *U.S.A.* **115** E11
Mount Laguna *U.S.A.* **111** N10
Mount Larcom *Australia* **94** C5
Mount Lofty Ranges
  Australia **95** E2
Mount Magnet *Australia* **93** E2
Mount Maunganui *N.Z.* **91** B6
Mount Molloy *Australia* **94** B4
Mount Morgan *Australia* **94** C5
Mount Morris *U.S.A.* **114** D7
Mount Pearl *Canada* **105** C9
Mount Penn *U.S.A.* **115** F9
Mount Perry *Australia* **95** D5
Mount Pleasant *Iowa, U.S.A.* **112** E8
Mount Pleasant *Mich.,
  U.S.A.* **113** D11
Mount Pleasant *Pa., U.S.A.* **114** F5

Mount Pleasant *S.C., U.S.A.*
  117 E15
Mount Pleasant *Tenn.,
  U.S.A.* **117** D11
Mount Pleasant *Tex., U.S.A.* **116** E7
Mount Pleasant *Utah,
  U.S.A.* **108** G8
Mount Pocono *U.S.A.* **115** E9
Mount Rainier △ *U.S.A.* **110** D5
Mount Revelstoke △
  Canada **102** C5
Mount Robson → *Canada* **102** C5
Mount St. Helens △ *U.S.A.* **110** D4
Mount Selinda *Zimbabwe* **89** C5
Mount Shasta *U.S.A.* **108** F2
Mount Signal *U.S.A.* **111** N11
Mount Sterling *Ill., U.S.A.* **112** F8
Mount Sterling *Ky., U.S.A.* **113** F12
Mount Surprise *Australia* **94** B3
Mount Union *U.S.A.* **114** F7
Mount Upton *U.S.A.* **115** D9
Mount Vernon *Ill., U.S.A.* **112** F9
Mount Vernon *Ind., U.S.A.* **112** G10
Mount Vernon *N.Y., U.S.A.* **115** F11
Mount Vernon *Ohio, U.S.A.* **114** F2
Mount Vernon *Wash.,
  U.S.A.* **110** B4
Mount William △ *Australia* **95** G4
Mounta, Akra *Greece* **46** C2
Mountain Ash *U.K.* **15** F4
Mountain Center *U.S.A.* **111** M10
Mountain City *Nev., U.S.A.* **108** F6
Mountain City *Tenn., U.S.A.*
  117 C14
Mountain Dale *U.S.A.* **115** E10
Mountain Grove *U.S.A.* **112** G7
Mountain Home *Ark.,
  U.S.A.* **116** C8
Mountain Home *Idaho,
  U.S.A.* **108** E6
Mountain Iron *U.S.A.* **112** B7
Mountain Pass *U.S.A.* **111** K11
Mountain View *Ark., U.S.A.* **116** D8
Mountain View *Calif.,
  U.S.A.* **110** H4
Mountain Zebra △ *S. Africa* **88** E4
Mountainair *U.S.A.* **109** J10
Mountlake Terrace *U.S.A.* **110** C4
Mountmellick *Ireland* **12** C4
Mountrath *Ireland* **12** D4
Moura *Australia* **94** C4
Moura *Brazil* **124** D6
Moura *Portugal* **37** G3
Mourão *Portugal* **37** G3
Mourdi, Dépression du *Chad* **79** E10
Mourdiah *Mali* **82** C3
Mourenx *France* **20** E3
Mouri *Ghana* **83** D4
Mourilyan *Australia* **94** B4
Mourmelon-le-Grand
  France **19** C11
Mourne → *U.K.* **12** B4
Mourne Mts. *U.K.* **12** B5
Mournies *Greece* **49** D6
Mouscron *Belgium* **17** D3
Moussa 'Ali *Djibouti* **81** E5
Moussoro *Chad* **79** F9
Mouthe *France* **19** F13
Moutier *Switz.* **25** H3
Moûtiers *France* **21** C10
Moutong *Indonesia* **63** D6
Mouy *France* **19** C9
Mouzaki *Greece* **46** B3
Mouzon *France* **19** C12
Movas *Mexico* **118** B3
Moville *Ireland* **12** A4
Mowandjum *Australia* **92** C3
Moy → *Ireland* **12** B2
Moya *Comoros Is.* **85** a
Moyale *Ethiopia* **86** B4
Moyale *Kenya* **81** G4
Moyamba *S. Leone* **82** D2
Moyen Atlas *Morocco* **78** B4
Moyo *Indonesia* **62** F5
Moyobamba *Peru* **124** E3
Moyowosi △ *Tanzania* **86** C3
Moyyero → *Russia* **53** C11
Moyynqum *Kazakhstan* **52** E8
Moyynty *Kazakhstan* **52** E8
Mozambique =
  Moçambique *Mozam.* **87** F5
Mozambique ■ *Africa* **87** F4
Mozambique Chan. *Africa* **89** B7
Mozdok *Russia* **35** J7
Mozdūrān *Iran* **71** B9
Mozhaysk *Russia* **32** E9
Mozhga *Russia* **34** B11
Mozhnābād *Iran* **71** C9
Mozirje *Slovenia* **41** B11
Mozyr = Mazyr *Belarus* **23** B15
Mpanda *Tanzania* **86** D3
Mpésoba *Mali* **82** C3
Mphoeng *Zimbabwe* **87** G2
Mpika *Zambia* **87** E3
Mpulungu *Zambia* **87** D3
Mpumalanga *S. Africa* **89** D5
Mpumalanga □ *S. Africa* **89** D5
Mpwapwa *Tanzania* **86** D4
Mqanduli *S. Africa* **89** E4

Mqinvartsveri = Kazbek
  Russia **35** J7
Mrągowo *Poland* **30** E8
Mramor *Serbia* **44** C5
Mrkonjić Grad *Bos.-H.* **28** F2
Mrkopalj *Croatia* **41** C11
Mrocza *Poland* **31** E4
Msaken *Tunisia* **79** A8
Msambansovu *Zimbabwe* **87** F3
M'sila → *Algeria* **78** A6
Msoro *Zambia* **87** E3
Msta → *Russia* **32** C6
Mstislavl = Mstsislaw
  Belarus **23** A16
Mstsislaw *Belarus* **23** A16
Mszana Dolna *Poland* **31** J7
Mszczonów *Poland* **31** G7
Mtama *Tanzania* **87** E4
Mtamvuna =
  Mthamvuna → *S. Africa* **89** E5
Mthamvuna → *S. Africa* **89** E5
Mthatha *S. Africa* **89** E4
Mtilikwe → *Zimbabwe* **87** G3
Mtirala △ *Georgia* **35** K6
Mtito Andei *Kenya* **86** C4
Mtsensk *Russia* **32** F9
Mtskheta *Georgia* **35** K7
Mtubatuba *S. Africa* **89** D5
Mtwalume *S. Africa* **89** E5
Mtwara-Mikindani *Tanzania* **87** E5
Mu Gia, Deo *Vietnam* **64** D5
Mu Ko Chang △ *Thailand* **65** G4
Mu Us Shamo *China* **56** E5
Muang Chiang Rai =
  Chiang Rai *Thailand* **58** H2
Muang Khong *Laos* **64** E5
Muang Lamphun *Thailand* **64** C2
Muang Mai *Thailand* **65** a
Muang Pak Beng *Laos* **58** H3
Muar *Malaysia* **65** L4
Muarabungo *Indonesia* **62** E2
Muaraenim *Indonesia* **62** E2
Muarajuloi *Indonesia* **62** E4
Muarakaman *Indonesia* **62** E5
Muaratebo *Indonesia* **62** E2
Muaratembesi *Indonesia* **62** E2
Muaratewe *Indonesia* **62** E4
Mubarakpur *India* **69** F10
Mubarraz = Al Mubarraz
  Si. Arabia **71** E6
Mubende *Uganda* **86** B3
Mubi *Nigeria* **83** C7
Mucajaí → *Brazil* **124** C6
Muchachos, Roque de los
  Canary Is. **48** F2
Muchinga Mts. *Zambia* **87** E3
Muchkapskiy *Russia* **34** E6
Muchuan *China* **58** C5
Muck *U.K.* **13** E2
Muckadilla *Australia* **95** D4
Muckaty ☼ *Australia* **94** B1
Muckle Flugga *U.K.* **13** A8
Mucur *Turkey* **72** C6
Mucuri *Brazil* **125** G11
Mucusso *Angola* **88** B3
Muda → *Canary Is.* **48** F6
Mudanjiang *China* **57** B15
Mudanya *Turkey* **45** F12
Muddy Cr. → *U.S.A.* **108** G8
Mudgee *Australia* **95** E4
Mudjatik → *Canada* **103** B7
Mudurnu *Turkey* **72** B4
Muecate *Mozam.* **87** E4
Mueda *Mozam.* **87** E4
Mueller Ranges *Australia* **92** C4
Muende *Mozam.* **87** E3
Muerto, Mar *Mexico* **119** D6
Mufu Shan *China* **59** C10
Mufulira *Zambia* **87** E2
Mufumbiro Range *Africa* **86** C2
Mugardos *Spain* **36** B2
Muge → *Portugal* **37** F2
Múggia *Italy* **41** C10
Mughal Sarai *India* **69** G10
Mughayrā' *Si. Arabia* **70** D3
Mugi *Japan* **55** H7
Mugia = Muxía *Spain* **36** B1
Mugila, Mts.
  Dem. Rep. of the Congo **86** D2
Muğla *Turkey* **47** D10
Muğla □ *Turkey* **47** D10
Muglad *Sudan* **81** E2
Müglizh *Bulgaria* **45** D9
Mugu *Nepal* **69** E10
Muhala *Congo* **86** D2
Muhammad, Râs *Egypt* **70** E2
Muhammad Qol *Sudan* **80** C4
Muhammadabad *India* **69** F10
Muhesi → *Tanzania* **86** D4
Mühlacker *Germany* **25** G4
Mühldorf *Germany* **25** G8
Mühlhausen *Germany* **24** D6
Mühlig Hofmann fjell
  Antarctica **5** D3
Mühlviertel *Austria* **26** C7
Muhos *Finland* **8** D21
Muhu *Estonia* **32** C2
Muhutwe *Tanzania* **86** C3

Muine Bheag *Ireland* **12** D5
Muineachán = Monaghan
  Ireland **12** B5
Muir, L. *Australia* **93** F2
Muir of Ord *U.K.* **13** D4
Mujeres, I. *Mexico* **120** B2
Mujnak = Muynak
  Uzbekistan **52** E6
Muka, Tanjung *Malaysia* **65** c
Mukacheve *Ukraine* **28** B7
Mukachevo = Mukacheve
  Ukraine **28** B7
Mukah *Malaysia* **62** D4
Mukandwara *India* **68** G6
Mukawwa, Geziret *Egypt* **70** F2
Mukawwar *Sudan* **80** C4
Mukdahan *Thailand* **64** D5
Mukden = Shenyang *China* **57** D12
Mukerian *India* **68** D6
Mukhavyets *Belarus* **31** F10
Mukhtolovo *Russia* **34** C6
Mukinbudin *Australia* **93** F2
Mukishi *Dem. Rep. of the Congo* **87** D1
Mukomuko *Indonesia* **62** E2
Mukomwenze
  Dem. Rep. of the Congo **86** D2
Mukono *Uganda* **86** B3
Muktsar *India* **68** D6
Mukur = Moqor *Afghan.* **68** C2
Mukutuwa → *Canada* **103** C9
Mukwela *Zambia* **87** F2
Mula *Spain* **39** G3
Mula → *Pakistan* **68** F2
Mulange
  Dem. Rep. of the Congo **86** C2
Mulanje, Mt. *Malawi* **87** F4
Mulchatna → *U.S.A.* **106** D8
Mulchén *Chile* **126** D1
Mulde → *Germany* **24** D8
Mule Creek Junction *U.S.A.*
  108 E11
Muleba *Tanzania* **86** C3
Mulegé *Mexico* **118** B2
Muleshoe *U.S.A.* **116** D3
Muletta, Gara *Ethiopia* **81** F5
Mulgrave *Canada* **105** C7
Mulgrave I. = Badu *Australia* **94** a
Mulhacén *Spain* **37** H7
Mülheim *Germany* **24** D2
Mulhouse *France* **19** E14
Muli *China* **58** D3
Mulifanua *Samoa* **91** b
Muling *China* **57** B16
Mull *U.K.* **13** E3
Mull, Sound of *U.K.* **13** E3
Mullach Íde = Malahide
  Ireland **12** C5
Mullaittivu *Sri Lanka* **66** Q12
Mullen *U.S.A.* **112** D3
Mullengudgery *Australia* **95** B4
Mullens *U.S.A.* **113** G13
Muller, Pegunungan
  Indonesia **62** D4
Mullet Pen. *Ireland* **12** B1
Mullewa *Australia* **93** E2
Müllheim *Germany* **25** H3
Mulligan → *Australia* **94** D2
Mullingar *Ireland* **12** C4
Mullins *U.S.A.* **117** D15
Mullsjö *Sweden* **11** G7
Mullumbimby *Australia* **95** D5
Mulobezi *Zambia* **87** F2
Mulonga Plain *Zambia* **85** H4
Mulroy B. *Ireland* **12** A4
Multan *Pakistan* **68** D4
Mulumbe, Mts.
  Dem. Rep. of the Congo **87** D2
Mulungushi Dam *Zambia* **87** E2
Mulvane *U.S.A.* **112** G5
Mulwad *Sudan* **80** D3
Mulwala, L. *Australia* **95** C4
Mumbai *India* **66** K8
Mumbwa *Zambia* **87** F2
Mumias *Kenya* **86** C4
Mumra *Russia* **35** H8
Mun → *Thailand* **64** E5
Muna *Indonesia* **63** F6
Munabao *India* **68** G4
Munamagi *Estonia* **32** D4
Muncan *Indonesia* **63** K18
Muncar *Indonesia* **63** J17
Münchberg *Germany* **25** E7
Müncheberg *Germany* **24** C10
München *Germany* **25** G7
München Franz Josef
  Strauss Int. ✈ (MUC)
  Germany **25** G7
Munchen-Gladbach =
  Mönchengladbach
  Germany **24** D2
Muncho Lake *Canada* **102** B3
Munch'ŏn *N. Korea* **57** E14
Muncie *U.S.A.* **113** E11
Muncoonie L. West *Australia* **94** D2
Mundabbera *Australia* **95** D5
Munday *U.S.A.* **116** E5
Mundemba *Cameroon* **83** E6
Münden *Germany* **24** D5
Münden → *Germany* **24** D5

Mundiwindi *Australia* **92** D3
Mundo → *Spain* **39** G2
Mundo Novo *Brazil* **125** F10
Mundra *India* **68** H3
Mundrabilla *Australia* **93** F4
Munera *Spain* **39** F2
Mungallala *Australia* **95** D4
Mungallala Cr. → *Australia* **95** D4
Mungana *Australia* **94** B3
Mungaoli *India* **68** G8
Mungari *Mozam.* **87** F3
Mungbere
  Dem. Rep. of the Congo **86** B2
Mungeli *India* **69** H9
Munger *India* **69** G12
Mungerannie *Australia* **95** A2
Mungilli ☼ *Australia* **93** E3
Mungkan Kandju △
  Australia **94** A3
Munich = München
  Germany **25** G7
Munising *U.S.A.* **112** B10
Munka-Ljungby *Sweden* **11** H6
Munkebo *Denmark* **11** J4
Munkedal *Sweden* **11** F5
Munkfors *Sweden* **10** E7
Munku-Sardyk *Russia* **53** D11
Münnerstadt *Germany* **25** E6
Munnsville *U.S.A.* **115** D9
Muñoz Gamero, Pen. *Chile* **128** G2
Munroe L. *Canada* **103** B9
Munsan *S. Korea* **57** F14
Munster *France* **19** D14
Münster *Niedersachsen,
  Germany* **24** C6
Münster
  *Nordrhein-Westfalen,
  Germany* **24** D3
Munster □ *Ireland* **12** D3
Muntadgin *Australia* **93** F2
Muntele Mare, Vf. *Romania* **29** D8
Muntok *Indonesia* **62** E3
Munzur Dağları *Turkey* **73** C8
Muong Beng *Laos* **58** G3
Muong Boum *Vietnam* **58** F4
Muong Et *Laos* **64** B5
Muong Hai *Laos* **58** G3
Muong Hiem *Laos* **64** B4
Muong Houn *Laos* **58** G3
Muong Hung *Vietnam* **58** G4
Muong Kau *Laos* **64** E5
Muong Khao *Laos* **64** C4
Muong Khoua *Laos* **58** G4
Muong Liep *Laos* **64** C4
Muong May *Laos* **64** E6
Muong Ngeun *Laos* **58** G3
Muong Ngoi *Laos* **58** G4
Muong Nong *Laos* **64** D6
Muong Nhie *Vietnam* **58** F4
Muong Ou Tay *Laos* **58** F3
Muong Oua *Laos* **58** G4
Muong Peun *Laos* **58** G4
Muong Phalane *Laos* **64** D5
Muong Phieng *Laos* **64** C3
Muong Phine *Laos* **64** D6
Muong Sai *Laos* **58** G3
Muong Saiapoun *Laos* **64** C3
Muong Sen *Vietnam* **64** C5
Muong Sing *Laos* **58** G3
Muong Son *Laos* **58** G4
Muong Soui *Laos* **64** C4
Muong Va *Laos* **58** G4
Muong Xia *Vietnam* **64** B5
Muonio *Finland* **8** C20
Muonio älv =
  Muonionjoki → *Finland* **8** C20
Muonioälven =
  Muonionjoki → *Finland* **8** C20
Muonionjoki → *Finland* **8** C20
Mupa → *Mozam.* **87** F4
Muping *China* **57** F11
Mupoi *Sudan* **81** F2
Muqaddam, Wadi → *Sudan* **80** D3
Muqdisho *Somali Rep.* **75** G4
Mur → *Austria* **27** E9
Mûr-de-Bretagne *France* **18** D4
Muradiye *Manisa, Turkey* **47** C9
Muradiye *Van, Turkey* **73** C10
Murakami *Japan* **54** E9
Muralag = Prince of Wales
  I. *Australia* **94** A3
Murallón, Cerro *Chile* **128** F2
Muranda *Rwanda* **86** C2
Murang'a *Kenya* **86** C4
Murashi *Russia* **52** D5
Murat *France* **20** C6
Murat → *Turkey* **73** C9
Murat Dağı *Turkey* **47** C11
Muratlı *Turkey* **45** E11
Murato *France* **21** F13
Murau *Austria* **26** D7
Murava *Belarus* **31** F11
Muravera *Italy* **42** C2
Murayama *Japan* **54** E10
Murça *Portugal* **36** D3
Murchison → *Australia* **93** E1
Murchison, Mt. *Antarctica* **5** D11
Murchison Falls *Uganda* **86** B3

Murchison Falls △ *Uganda* **86** B3
Murchison Ra. *Australia* **94** C1
Murchison Rapids *Malawi* **87** F3
Murchison Roadhouse
 Australia **93** E1
Murcia *Spain* **39** G3
Murcia □ *Spain* **39** H3
Murdo *U.S.A.* **112** D3
Murdoch Pt. *Australia* **94** A3
Mürefte *Turkey* **45** F11
Mureş □ *Romania* **29** D9
Mureş ➤ *Romania* **28** D5
Mureşul = Mureş ➤
 Romania **28** D5
Muret *France* **20** E5
Murewa *Zimbabwe* **89** B5
Murfreesboro *N.C., U.S.A.* **117** C16
Murfreesboro *Tenn., U.S.A.* **117** D11
Murgap = Murghob
 Tajikistan **52** F8
Murgap ➤ *Turkmenistan* **71** B9
Murgenella *Australia* **92** B5
Murgeni *Romania* **29** D13
Murgha Kibzai *Pakistan* **68** D3
Murghob *Tajikistan* **52** F8
Murgon *Australia* **95** D5
Muri *India* **69** H11
Muria *Indonesia* **63** G14
Muriaé *Brazil* **127** A7
Murias de Paredes *Spain* **36** C4
Muriel Mine *Zimbabwe* **87** F3
Müritz *Germany* **24** B8
Müritz △ *Germany* **24** B8
Murliganj *India* **69** G12
Murmansk *Russia* **8** B25
Murmashi *Russia* **8** B25
Murnau *Germany* **25** H7
Muro *France* **21** F12
Muro *Spain* **48** B10
Muro, C. de *France* **21** G12
Muro de Alcoy *Spain* **39** G4
Muro Lucano *Italy* **43** B8
Murom *Russia* **34** C5
Muroran *Japan* **54** C10
Muros *Spain* **36** C1
Muros e Noya, Ría de ➤
 Spain **36** C1
Muroto *Japan* **55** H7
Muroto-Misaki *Japan* **55** H7
Murovani Kurylivtsi
 Ukraine **29** B12
Murowana Goślina *Poland* **31** F3
Murphy *U.S.A.* **108** E5
Murphys *U.S.A.* **110** G6
Murrat *Sudan* **80** D2
Murrat Wells *Sudan* **80** C3
Murray *Australia* **94** a
Murray *Ky., U.S.A.* **112** G9
Murray *Utah, U.S.A.* **108** F8
Murray ➤ *Australia* **95** F2
Murray, L. *U.S.A.* **117** D14
Murray Bridge *Australia* **95** F2
Murray Fracture Zone
 Pac. Oc. **97** D14
Murray Harbour *Canada* **105** C7
Murray River △ *Australia* **95** E3
Murraysburg *S. Africa* **88** E3
Murree *Pakistan* **68** C5
Murrieta *U.S.A.* **111** M9
Murro di Porco, Capo *Italy* **43** F8
Murrumbidgee ➤ *Australia* **95** E3
Murrumburrah *Australia* **95** E4
Murrurundi *Australia* **95** E5
Murshid *Sudan* **80** C3
Murshidabad *India* **69** G13
Murska Sobota *Slovenia* **41** B13
Murtle L. *Canada* **102** C5
Murtoa *Australia* **95** F3
Murtosa *Portugal* **36** E2
Murungu *Tanzania* **86** C3
Mururoa *French Polynesia* **97** K14
Murwara *India* **69** H9
Murwillumbah *Australia* **95** D5
Mürz ➤ *Austria* **26** D8
Mürzzuschlag *Austria* **26** D8
Muş *Turkey* **73** C9
Muş □ *Turkey* **73** C9
Mûsa, Gebel *Egypt* **70** D2
Musa Khel *Pakistan* **68** D3
Mūsá Qal'eh *Afghan.* **66** C4
Musafirkhana *India* **69** F9
Musä'idah *Iraq* **73** H12
Musala *Bulgaria* **44** D7
Musala *Indonesia* **62** E1
Musan *N. Korea* **57** C15
Musangu
 Dem. Rep. of the Congo **87** E1
Musasa *Tanzania* **86** C3
Musay'īd *Qatar* **71** E6
Muscat = Masqat *Oman* **75** C6
Muscatine *U.S.A.* **112** E8
Muscle Shoals *U.S.A.* **117** D11
Musgedi =
 Unsengedsi ➤ *Zimbabwe* **87** F3
Musgrave Harbour *Canada* **105** C9
Musgrave Ranges *Australia* **93** E5
Mushie *Dem. Rep. of the Congo* **84** E3
Mushin *Nigeria* **83** D5
Musi ➤ *Indonesia* **62** E2

Musina *S. Africa* **89** C5
Muskeg ➤ *Canada* **102** A4
Muskegon *U.S.A.* **112** D10
Muskegon ➤ *U.S.A.* **112** D10
Muskegon Heights *U.S.A.* **112** D10
Muskogee *U.S.A.* **116** D7
Muskoka, L. *Canada* **114** B5
Muskoka Falls *Canada* **114** B5
Muskwa ➤ *Canada* **102** B4
Muslīmiyah *Syria* **70** B3
Musmar *Sudan* **80** D4
Musofu *Zambia* **87** E2
Musoma *Tanzania* **86** C3
Musquaro, L. *Canada* **105** B7
Musquodoboit Harbour
 Canada **105** D7
Musselburgh *U.K.* **13** F5
Musselshell ➤ *U.S.A.* **108** C10
Mussende *Angola* **84** G3
Mussidan *France* **20** C4
Mussomeli *Italy* **42** E6
Mussoorie *India* **68** D8
Mussuco *Angola* **88** B2
Mustafakemalpaşa *Turkey* **45** F12
Mustang *Nepal* **69** E10
Musters, L. *Argentina* **128** F3
Musudan *N. Korea* **57** D15
Muswellbrook *Australia* **95** E5
Muszyna *Poland* **31** J7
Mût *Egypt* **80** B2
Mut *Turkey* **72** D5
Mutanda *Mozam.* **89** C5
Mutanda *Zambia* **87** E2
Mutare *Zimbabwe* **87** F3
Mutawintji △ *Australia* **95** E3
Mutha *Kenya* **86** C4
Muting *Indonesia* **63** F10
Mutki = Mirtağ *Turkey* **70** B4
Mutoko *Zimbabwe* **89** B5
Mutomo *Kenya* **86** C4
Mutoray *Russia* **53** C11
Mutsamudu *Comoros Is.* **85** a
Mutshatsha
 Dem. Rep. of the Congo **87** E1
Mutsu *Japan* **54** D10
Mutsu-Wan *Japan* **54** D10
Muttaburra *Australia* **94** C3
Muttalip *Turkey* **47** B12
Mutton I. *Ireland* **12** D2
Mutuáli *Mozam.* **87** E4
Mutum Biyu *Nigeria* **83** D7
Mutumba *Burundi* **86** C2
Muweilih *Egypt* **74** E3
Muxía *Spain* **36** B1
Muy Muy *Nic.* **120** D2
Muyinga *Burundi* **86** C3
Muynak = Moʻynoq
 Uzbekistan **52** E6
Muyunkum, Peski =
 Moyynqum *Kazakhstan* **52** E8
Muzaffarabad *Pakistan* **69** B5
Muzaffargarh *Pakistan* **68** D4
Muzaffarnagar *India* **68** E7
Muzaffarpur *India* **69** F11
Muzafirpur *Pakistan* **68** D3
Muzhi *Russia* **52** C7
Muzillac *France* **18** E4
Muzūra *Egypt* **80** J7
Mvôlô *Sudan* **81** F2
Mvuma *Zimbabwe* **87** F3
Mvurwi *Zimbabwe* **87** F3
Mwabvi ◯ *Malawi* **87** F3
Mwadui *Tanzania* **86** C3
Mwali = Mohéli *Comoros Is.* **85** a
Mwambo *Tanzania* **87** E5
Mwandi *Zambia* **87** F1
Mwanza
 Dem. Rep. of the Congo **86** D2
Mwanza *Tanzania* **86** C3
Mwanza *Zambia* **87** F1
Mwanza □ *Tanzania* **86** C3
Mwaya *Tanzania* **87** D3
Mweelrea *Ireland* **12** C2
Mweka *Dem. Rep. of the Congo* **84** E4
Mwene-Ditu
 Dem. Rep. of the Congo **84** F4
Mwenezi *Zimbabwe* **87** G3
Mwenezi ➤ *Mozam.* **87** G3
Mwenga
 Dem. Rep. of the Congo **86** C2
Mweru, L. *Zambia* **87** D2
Mweru Wantipa △ *Zambia* **87** D2
Mweza Range *Zimbabwe* **87** G3
Mwilambwe
 Dem. Rep. of the Congo **86** D2
Mwimbi *Tanzania* **87** D3
Mwingi *Kenya* **86** C4
Mwinilunga *Zambia* **87** E1
My Tho *Vietnam* **65** G6
Myajlar *India* **68** F4
Myanaung *Burma* **67** K19
Myanmar = Burma ■ *Asia* **67** J20
Myaungmya *Burma* **67** L19
Mycenæ = Mikines *Greece* **46** D4
Myedna *Belarus* **31** G10
Myeik Kyunzu *Burma* **65** G1
Myerstown *U.S.A.* **115** F8
Myingyan *Burma* **67** J19
Myitkyina *Burma* **67** G20
Myjava *Slovak Rep.* **27** C10

Mykhaylivka *Ukraine* **33** J8
Mykines *Færoe Is.* **8** E9
Mykolayiv *Ukraine* **33** J7
Mykolayiv ➤ *Ukraine* **33** J6
Mykolayiv □ *Ukraine* **33** J6
Mykonos *Greece* **47** D7
Mymensingh *Bangla.* **67** G17
Mynydd Du *U.K.* **15** F4
Mýrdalsjökull *Iceland* **8** E4
Myrhorod *Ukraine* **33** H7
Myrtle Beach *U.S.A.* **117** E15
Myrtle Creek *U.S.A.* **108** E2
Myrtle Point *U.S.A.* **108** E1
Myrtou *Cyprus* **49** D12
Mysia *Turkey* **45** G11
Myślenice *Poland* **31** J6
Myślibórz *Poland* **31** F1
Mysłowice *Poland* **31** H6
Mysore = Karnataka □
 India **66** N10
Mysore *India* **66** N10
Mystic *U.S.A.* **115** E13
Mysuru = Mysore *India* **66** N10
Myszków *Poland* **31** H6
Myszyniec *Poland* **30** E8
Mytishchi *Russia* **32** E9
Mývatn *Iceland* **8** D5

N

Na Clocha Liatha =
 Greystones *Ireland* **12** C5
Na Hearadh = Harris *U.K.* **13** D2
Na Noi *Thailand* **64** C3
Na Phao *Laos* **64** D5
Na Sam *Vietnam* **58** F6
Na San *Vietnam* **64** B5
Na Thon *Thailand* **65** b
Naab ➤ *Germany* **25** F8
Na'am *Sudan* **81** F2
Na'am ➤ *Sudan* **81** F2
Naantali *Finland* **32** B1
Naas *Ireland* **12** C5
Nababeep *S. Africa* **88** D2
Nabadwip = Navadwip
 India **69** H13
Nabawa *Australia* **93** E1
Nabberu, L. *Australia* **93** E3
Nabburg *Germany* **25** F8
Naberezhnyye Chelny
 Russia **34** C11
Nabeul *Tunisia* **79** A8
Nabha *India* **68** D7
Nabīd *Iran* **71** D8
Nabire *Indonesia* **63** E9
Nabisar *Pakistan* **68** G3
Nabisipi ➤ *Canada* **105** B7
Nabiswera *Uganda* **86** B3
Nāblus = Nābulus *West Bank* **74** C4
Naboomspruit *S. Africa* **89** C4
Nabou *Burkina Faso* **82** C4
Nabouwalu *Fiji* **91** a
Nabua *Phil.* **61** E5
Nābulus *West Bank* **74** C4
Nacala *Mozam.* **87** E5
Nacaome *Honduras* **120** D2
Nacaroa *Mozam.* **87** E4
Naches *U.S.A.* **108** C3
Naches ➤ *U.S.A.* **110** D6
Nachicapau, L. *Canada* **105** A6
Nachingwea *Tanzania* **87** E4
Nachna *India* **68** F4
Náchod *Czech Rep.* **26** A9
Nacimiento, L. *U.S.A.* **110** K6
Naco *Mexico* **118** A3
Nacogdoches *U.S.A.* **116** F7
Nácori Chico *Mexico* **118** B3
Nacozari de García *Mexico* **118** A3
Nacula *Fiji* **91** a
Nådendal = Naantali *Finland* **32** B1
Nadi *Fiji* **91** a
Nadi *Sudan* **80** D3
Nadiad *India* **68** H5
Nădlac *Romania* **28** D5
Nador *Morocco* **78** B5
Nadur *Malta* **49** C1
Nadüshan *Iran* **71** C7
Nadvirna *Ukraine* **29** B9
Nadvornaya = Nadvirna
 Ukraine **29** B9
Nadym *Russia* **52** C8
Nadym ➤ *Russia* **52** C8
Nærbø *Norway* **9** G11
Næstved *Denmark* **11** J5
Nafada *Nigeria* **83** C7
Nafpaktos *Greece* **46** C3
Nafplio *Greece* **46** D4
Naft-e Safid *Iran* **71** D6
Naftshahr *Iran* **73** E11
Nafud Desert = An Nafūd
 Si. Arabia **70** D4
Nag Hammâdi *Egypt* **80** B3
Naga *Phil.* **61** E5
Nagagami ➤ *Canada* **104** B3
Nagahama *Japan* **55** G8

Nagai *Japan* **54** E10
Nagaland □ *India* **67** G19
Nagano *Japan* **55** F9
Nagano □ *Japan* **55** F9
Nagaoka *Japan* **55** F9
Nagaon = Nowgong *India* **67** F18
Nagappattinam *India* **66** P11
Nagar ➤ *Bangla.* **69** G13
Nagar Parkar *Pakistan* **68** G4
Nagasaki *Japan* **55** H4
Nagasaki □ *Japan* **55** H4
Nagato *Japan* **55** G5
Nagaur *India* **68** F5
Nagda *India* **68** H6
Nagercoil *India* **66** Q10
Nagina *India* **69** E8
Nagīneh *Iran* **71** C8
Nagir *Pakistan* **69** B5
Nagod *India* **69** G9
Nagold *Germany* **25** G4
Nagold ➤ *Germany* **25** G4
Nagoorin *Australia* **94** C5
Nagorno-Karabakh □
 Azerbaijan **73** C12
Nagornyy *Russia* **53** D13
Nagoya *Japan* **55** G8
Nagpur *India* **66** J11
Nagua *Dom. Rep.* **121** C6
Naguabo *Puerto Rico* **121** d
Nagurunguru ◉ *Australia* **92** C4
Nagyatád *Hungary* **28** D2
Nagyecsed *Hungary* **28** C7
Nagykálló *Hungary* **28** C6
Nagykanizsa *Hungary* **28** D2
Nagykáta *Hungary* **28** C4
Nagykőrös *Hungary* **28** C4
Naha *Japan* **55** L3
Nahan *India* **68** D7
Nahanni △ *Canada* **102** A4
Nahanni Butte *Canada* **102** A4
Nahargarh *Mad. P., India* **68** G6
Nahargarh *Raj., India* **68** G7
Nahariyya *Israel* **72** F6
Nahāvand *Iran* **73** E13
Nahe ➤ *Germany* **25** F3
Nahhne *Ukraine* **29** E13
Nahīya, W. ➤ *Egypt* **80** B3
Nahuel Huapi, L. *Argentina* **128** E2
Nahuelbuta △ *Chile* **126** D1
Nai Yong *Thailand* **65** a
Naicá *Mexico* **118** B3
Naicam *Canada* **103** C8
Naikoon △ *Canada* **102** C2
Naila *Germany* **25** E7
Naimisharanya *India* **69** F9
Naimona'nyi Feng *Nepal* **69** D9
Nain *Canada* **105** A7
Nā'īn *Iran* **71** C7
Naini Tal *India* **69** E8
Nainpur *India* **69** H9
Naintré *France* **18** F7
Nainwa *India* **68** G6
Naipu *Romania* **29** F10
Nairai *Fiji* **91** a
Nairn *U.K.* **13** D5
Nairobi *Kenya* **86** C4
Nairobi □ *Kenya* **86** C4
Naissaar *Estonia* **32** C3
Naita, Mt. *Ethiopia* **81** F4
Naitaba *Fiji* **91** a
Naivasha *Kenya* **86** C4
Naivasha, L. *Kenya* **86** C4
Najac *France* **20** D5
Najaf = An Najaf *Iraq* **73** G11
Najafābād *Iran* **71** C6
Najd *Si. Arabia* **75** B3
Nájera *Spain* **38** C2
Najerilla ➤ *Spain* **38** C2
Najibabad *India* **69** E8
Najin *N. Korea* **57** C16
Najmah *Si. Arabia* **71** E6
Najrān *Si. Arabia* **75** D3
Naju *S. Korea* **57** G14
Nakadōri-Shima *Japan* **55** H4
Nakalagba
 Dem. Rep. of the Congo **86** B2
Nakambé = White
 Volta ➤ *Ghana* **83** D4
Nakaminato *Japan* **55** F10
Nakamura *Japan* **55** H6
Nakano *Japan* **55** F9
Nakano-Shima *Japan* **55** K4
Nakashibetsu *Japan* **54** C12
Nakfa *Eritrea* **81** D4
Nakfa ◯ *Eritrea* **81** D4
Nakha Yai, Ko *Thailand* **65** a
Nakhichevan = Naxçıvan
 Azerbaijan **73** C11
Nakhichevan Rep. =
 Naxçıvan □ *Azerbaijan* **73** C11
Nakhl *Egypt* **74** F2
Nakhl-e Taqī *Iran* **71** E7
Nakhodka *Russia* **54** C6
Nakhon Nayok *Thailand* **64** E3
Nakhon Pathom *Thailand* **64** F3
Nakhon Phanom *Thailand* **64** D5
Nakhon Ratchasima *Thailand* **64** E4

Nakhon Sawan *Thailand* **64** E3
Nakhon Si Thammarat
 Thailand **65** H3
Nakhon Thai *Thailand* **64** D3
Nakhtarana *India* **68** H3
Nakina *Canada* **104** B2
Nakło nad Notecią *Poland* **31** E4
Nako *Burkina Faso* **82** C4
Nakodar *India* **68** D6
Nakskov *Denmark* **11** K5
Naktong ➤ *S. Korea* **57** G15
Nakuru *Kenya* **86** C4
Nakuru, L. *Kenya* **86** C4
Nakusp *Canada* **102** C5
Nal *Pakistan* **68** F2
Nal ➤ *Pakistan* **68** G1
Nalázi *Mozam.* **89** C5
Nalchik *Russia* **35** J6
Nalęczów *Poland* **31** G9
Nalerigu *Ghana* **83** C4
Nalgonda *India* **66** L11
Nalhati *India* **69** G12
Naliya *India* **68** H3
Nallamalai Hills *India* **66** M11
Nallıhan *Turkey* **72** B4
Nalón ➤ *Spain* **36** B4
Nalubaale Dam *Uganda* **86** B3
Nam Can *Vietnam* **65** H5
Nam-ch'on *N. Korea* **57** E14
Nam Co *China* **60** C4
Nam Dinh *Vietnam* **58** G6
Nam Du, Hon *Vietnam* **65** H5
Nam Nao △ *Thailand* **64** D3
Nam Ngum Res. *Laos* **64** C4
Nam-Phan *Vietnam* **65** G6
Nam Phong *Thailand* **64** D4
Nam Tha *Laos* **58** G3
Nam Tok *Thailand* **64** E2
Namacunde *Angola* **88** B2
Namacurra *Mozam.* **89** B6
Namak, Daryācheh-ye *Iran* **71** C7
Namak, Kavir-e *Iran* **71** C8
Namakzār, Daryācheh-ye
 Iran **71** C9
Namaland *Namibia* **88** C2
Namanga *Kenya* **86** C4
Namangan *Uzbekistan* **52** E8
Namapa *Mozam.* **87** E4
Namaqualand *S. Africa* **88** C2
Namasagali *Uganda* **86** B3
Namber *Indonesia* **63** E8
Nambour *Australia* **95** D5
Nambouwalu =
 Nabouwalu *Fiji* **91** a
Nambucca Heads *Australia* **95** E5
Nambung △ *Australia* **93** F2
Namche Bazar *Nepal* **69** F12
Namchonjŏm =
 Nam-ch'on *N. Korea* **57** E14
Namecunda *Mozam.* **87** E4
Namenalala *Fiji* **91** a
Nameponda *Mozam.* **87** F4
Náměšt' nad Oslavou
 Czech Rep. **27** B9
Námestovo *Slovak Rep.* **27** B12
Nametil *Mozam.* **87** F4
Namew L. *Canada* **103** C8
Namgia *India* **68** D8
Namhkam *Burma* **58** E1
Namialo *Mozam.* **87** E4
Namib Desert *Namibia* **88** C2
Namib-Naukluft △ *Namibia* **88** C2
Namibe *Angola* **85** H2
Namibe □ *Angola* **88** B1
Namibia ■ *Africa* **88** C2
Namibwoestyn = Namib
 Desert *Namibia* **88** C2
Namīn *Iran* **73** C13
Namlea *Indonesia* **63** E7
Namoi ➤ *Australia* **95** E4
Nampa *U.S.A.* **108** E5
Nampala *Mali* **82** B3
Nampo *N. Korea* **57** E13
Nampō-Shotō *Japan* **55** J10
Nampula *Mozam.* **87** F4
Namrole *Indonesia* **63** E7
Namse Shankou *China* **69** E10
Namsen ➤ *Norway* **8** D14
Namsos *Norway* **8** D14
Namtok Chat Trakan △
 Thailand **64** D3
Namtok Mae Surin △
 Thailand **64** C2
Namtsy *Russia* **53** C13
Namtu *Burma* **67** H20
Namtumbo *Tanzania* **87** E4
Namu *Canada* **102** C3
Namuka-i-Lau *Fiji* **91** a
Namur *Belgium* **17** D4
Namur □ *Belgium* **17** D4
Namuruputh *Kenya* **86** B4
Namutoni *Namibia* **88** B2
Namwala *Zambia* **87** F2
Namwon *S. Korea* **57** G14
Namyang *N. Korea* **57** C15
Namysłów *Poland* **31** G4
Nao, C. de la *Spain* **39** G5
Naococane, L. *Canada* **105** B5
Naoussa *Cyclades, Greece* **47** D7
Naoussa *Imathia, Greece* **44** F6
Naozhou Dao *China* **59** G8

Nan-ch'ang = Nanchang
 China **59** C10
Nan Ling *China* **59** E8
Nan Xian *China* **59** C9
Nana *Romania* **29** F11
Nana Kru *Liberia* **82** E4
Nanaimo *Canada* **102** D4
Nänäkuli *U.S.A.* **107** L8
Nanam *N. Korea* **57** D15
Nanan *China* **59** E12
Nanango *Australia* **95** D5
Nan'ao *China* **59** E8
Nanao *Japan* **55** F8
Nanbu *China* **58** B6
Nanchang *China* **59** C10
Nancheng *China* **59** D11
Nanching = Nanjing *China* **59** A12
Nanchong *China* **58** B6
Nanchuan *China* **58** C6
Nancy *France* **19** D13
Nanda Devi *India* **69** D8
Nanda Devi △ *India* **69** D8
Nanda Kot *India* **69** D9
Nandan *China* **58** E6
Nandan *Japan* **55** G7
Nanded *India* **66** K10
Nandewar Ra. *Australia* **95** E5
Nandi = Nadi *Fiji* **91** a
Nandigram *India* **69** H12
Nandurbar *India* **66** J9
Nandyal *India* **66** M11
Nanfeng *Guangdong, China* **59** F8
Nanfeng *Jiangxi, China* **59** D11
Nang Rong *Thailand* **64** E4
Nanga-Eboko *Cameroon* **83** E7
Nanga Parbat *Pakistan* **69** B6
Nangade *Mozam.* **87** E4
Nangapinoh *Indonesia* **62** E4
Nangarhär □ *Afghan.* **66** B7
Nangatayap *Indonesia* **62** E4
Nangbéto, L. de *Togo* **82** D5
Nangeya Mts. *Uganda* **86** B3
Nangis *France* **19** D10
Nangong *China* **56** F8
Nanhua *China* **58** E3
Nanhuang *China* **57** F11
Nanhui *China* **59** B13
Nanisivik *Canada* **101** C15
Nanjeko *Zambia* **87** F1
Nanji Shan *China* **59** D13
Nanjian *China* **58** E3
Nanjiang *China* **58** A6
Nanjing *Fujian, China* **59** E11
Nanjing *Jiangsu, China* **59** A12
Nanjirinji *Tanzania* **87** D4
Nankana Sahib *Pakistan* **68** D5
Nankang *China* **59** E10
Nanking = Nanjing *China* **59** A12
Nankoku *Japan* **55** H6
Nanling *China* **59** B12
Nanning *China* **58** F7
Nannup *Australia* **93** F2
Nanpan Jiang ➤ *China* **58** E6
Nanpara *India* **69** F9
Nanpi *China* **56** E9
Nanping *Fujian, China* **59** D12
Nanping *Henan, China* **59** C9
Nanri Dao *China* **59** E12
Nanripe *Mozam.* **87** E4
Nansei-Shotō =
 Ryūkyū-rettō *Japan* **55** M3
Nansen Basin *Arctic* **4** A10
Nansen Sd. *Canada* **101** A13
Nanshan I. *S. China Sea* **62** B5
Nansio *Tanzania* **86** C3
Nantawarrinna ◉ *Australia* **95** B2
Nanterre *France* **19** D9
Nantes *France* **18** E5
Nantiat *France* **20** B5
Nanticoke *U.S.A.* **115** E8
Nanton *Canada* **102** C6
Nantong *China* **59** A13
Nant'ou *Taiwan* **59** F13
Nantua *France* **19** F12
Nantucket I. *U.S.A.* **113** E18
Nantucket I. *U.S.A.* **113** E18
Nantulo *Mozam.* **87** E4
Nantwich *U.K.* **14** D5
Nanty Glo *U.S.A.* **114** F6
Nanuku Passage *Fiji* **91** a
Nanuque *Brazil* **125** G10
Nanusa, Kepulauan
 Indonesia **63** D7
Nanutarra Roadhouse
 Australia **92** D2
Nanxi *China* **58** C5
Nanxiong *China* **59** E10
Nanyang *China* **56** H7
Nanyi Hu *China* **59** B12
Nanyuki *Kenya* **86** B4
Nanzhang *China* **59** B8

Napa ➤ *U.S.A.* **110** G4
Napanee *Canada* **114** B8
Napanoch *U.S.A.* **115** E10
Nape *Laos* **64** C5
Nape Pass = Keo Neua,
  Deo *Vietnam* **64** C5
Napier *N.Z.* **91** C6
Napier Broome B. *Australia* **92** B4
Napier Pen. *Australia* **94** A2
Napierville *Canada* **115** A11
Naples = Nápoli *Italy* **43** B7
Naples *U.S.A.* **117** H14
Napo *China* **58** F5
Napo ➤ *Peru* **124** D4
Napoleon *N. Dak., U.S.A.* **112** B4
Napoleon *Ohio, U.S.A.* **113** E11
Nápoli *Italy* **43** B7
Nápoli, G. di *Italy* **43** B7
Nápoli Capodichino ✈
  (NAP) *Italy* **43** B7
Napopo *Dem. Rep. of the Congo* **86** B2
Naqâda *Egypt* **80** B3
Naqadeh *Iran* **73** D11
Naqb, Ra's an *Jordan* **74** F4
Naqqâsh *Iran* **71** C6
Nara *Japan* **55** G7
Nara *Mali* **82** B3
Nara □ *Japan* **55** G8
Nara Canal *Pakistan* **68** G3
Nara Visa *U.S.A.* **109** J12
Naracoorte *Australia* **95** F3
Naradhan *Australia* **95** E4
Naraini *India* **69** G9
Naranjos *Mexico* **119** C5
Narasapur *India* **67** L12
Narayangadh = Bharatpur
  Nepal **69** F11
Narayanganj *Bangla.* **67** H17
Narayanpet *India* **66** L10
Narberth *U.K.* **15** F3
Narbonne *France* **20** E7
Narcea ➤ *Spain* **36** B4
Nardin *Iran* **71** B7
Nardò *Italy* **43** B11
Narembeen *Australia* **93** F2
Narendranagar *India* **68** D8
Nares Str. *Arctic* **101** B18
Naretha *Australia* **93** F3
Narew ➤ *Poland* **31** F7
Nari ➤ *Pakistan* **68** F2
Narin *Afghan.* **66** A6
Narindra, Helodranon' i
  Madag. **89** A8
Narita *Japan* **55** G10
Nariva Swamp *Trin. & Tob.* **125** K15
Närke *Sweden* **10** E8
Narmada ➤ *India* **68** J5
Narman *Turkey* **73** B9
Narnaul *India* **68** E7
Narni *Italy* **41** F9
Naro *Ghana* **82** C4
Naro Fominsk *Russia* **32** E9
Narodnaya *Russia* **6** B17
Narok *Kenya* **86** C4
Narón *Spain* **36** B2
Narooma *Australia* **95** F5
Narrabri *Australia* **95** E4
Narran ➤ *Australia* **95** D4
Narrandera *Australia* **95** E4
Narrogin *Australia* **93** F2
Narromine *Australia* **95** E4
Narrow Hills △ *Canada* **103** C8
Narsimhapur *India* **69** H8
Narsinghgarh *India* **68** H7
Nartes, L. e *Albania* **44** F3
Nartkala *Russia* **35** J6
Naruto *Japan* **55** G7
Narva *Estonia* **32** C4
Narva ➤ *Russia* **32** C4
Narva Bay = Narva Laht
  Estonia **9** G22
Narva Laht *Estonia* **9** G22
Narvik *Norway* **8** B17
Narvskoye Vdkhr. *Russia* **32** C5
Narwana *India* **68** E7
Narwiański △ *Poland* **31** F9
Narwinbi ◎ *Australia* **94** B2
Naryan-Mar *Russia* **52** C6
Narym *Russia* **52** D9
Naryn *Kyrgyzstan* **52** E8
Naryn Qum *Kazakhstan* **35** G9
Nasa *Norway* **8** C16
Nasau *Fiji* **91** a
Năsăud *Romania* **29** C9
Nasca = Nazca *Peru* **124** F4
Naseby *N.Z.* **91** F3
Naselle *U.S.A.* **110** D3
Naser, Buheirat en *Egypt* **80** C3
Nashik = Nasik *India* **66** K8
Nashua *Mont., U.S.A.* **110** B10
Nashua *N.H., U.S.A.* **115** D13
Nashville *Ark., U.S.A.* **116** E8
Nashville *Ga., U.S.A.* **117** F13
Nashville *Tenn., U.S.A.* **117** C11
Našice *Croatia* **28** E3
Nasielsk *Poland* **31** F7
Nasik *India* **66** K8

Nasipit *Phil.* **61** G6
Nasir *Sudan* **81** F3
Nasirabad *India* **68** F6
Nasirabad *Pakistan* **68** E3
Nasiri = Ahvāz *Iran* **71** D6
Nasiriyah = An Nāşiriyah
  Iraq **70** D5
Naskaupi ➤ *Canada* **105** B7
Naso *Italy* **43** D7
Naşrābād *Iran* **71** C6
Nass ➤ *Canada* **102** C3
Nassarawa *Nigeria* **83** D6
Nassarawa □ *Nigeria* **83** D6
Nassau *Bahamas* **120** A4
Nassau *U.S.A.* **115** D11
Nassau, B. *Chile* **128** H3
Nasser, L. = Naser,
  Buheirat en *Egypt* **80** C3
Nassian *Ivory C.* **82** D4
Nässjö *Sweden* **11** G8
Nastapoka ➤ *Canada* **104** A4
Nastapoka, Is. *Canada* **104** A4
Nasugbu *Phil.* **61** D4
Näsum *Sweden* **11** H8
Näsviken *Sweden* **10** C10
Nata *Botswana* **88** C4
Nata ➤ *Botswana* **88** C4
Natal *Brazil* **125** E11
Natal *Indonesia* **62** D1
Natal Drakensberg △
  S. Africa **89** D4
Natalinci *Serbia* **28** B5
Naţanz *Iran* **71** C6
Natashquan *Canada* **105** B7
Natashquan ➤ *Canada* **105** B7
Natchez *U.S.A.* **116** F9
Natchitoches *U.S.A.* **116** F8
Natewa B. *Fiji* **91** a
Nathalia *Australia* **95** F4
Nathdwara *India* **68** G5
Nati, Pta. *Spain* **48** A10
Natimuk *Australia* **95** F3
Nation ➤ *Canada* **102** B4
National City *U.S.A.* **111** N9
Natitingou *Benin* **83** C5
Natividad, I. *Mexico* **118** B1
Natkyizin *Burma* **64** E1
Natron, L. *Tanzania* **86** C4
Natrona Heights *U.S.A.* **114** F5
Natrûn, W. el ➤ *Egypt* **80** H7
Natukanaoka Pan *Namibia* **88** B2
Natuna Besar, Kepulauan
  Indonesia **62** D3
Natuna Is. = Natuna Besar,
  Kepulauan *Indonesia* **62** D3
Natuna Selatan,
  Kepulauan *Indonesia* **62** D3
Natural Bridge *U.S.A.* **115** B9
Natural Bridges △ *U.S.A.* **109** H9
Naturaliste, C. *Tas., Australia* **95** G4
Naturaliste, C. *W. Austral.,
  Australia* **93** F2
Naturaliste Plateau *Ind. Oc.* **96** L3
Nau Qala *Afghan.* **68** B3
Naucelle *France* **20** D6
Nauders *Austria* **26** E3
Nauen *Germany* **24** C8
Naugatuck *U.S.A.* **115** E11
Naujaat = Repulse Bay
  Canada **101** D14
Naujoji Akmenė *Lithuania* **30** B9
Naumburg *Germany* **24** D7
Nauru ■ *Pac. Oc.* **90** B9
Naushahra = Nowshera
  Pakistan **68** B4
Naushahro *Pakistan* **68** F3
Naushon I. *U.S.A.* **115** E14
Nausori *Fiji* **91** a
Nauta *Peru* **124** D4
Nautanwa *India* **69** F10
Naute △ *Namibia* **88** D2
Nautla *Mexico* **119** C5
Nava *Mexico* **118** B4
Nava *Spain* **36** B5
Nava del Rey *Spain* **36** D5
Navadwip *India* **69** H13
Navahermosa *Spain* **37** F6
Navahrudak *Belarus* **23** B13
Navajo Res. *U.S.A.* **109** H10
Navalcarnero *Spain* **36** E6
Navalmoral de la Mata *Spain* **36** F5
Navalvillar de Pela *Spain* **37** F5
Navan = An Uaimh *Ireland* **12** C5
Navarin, Mys *Russia* **53** C17
Navarino, I. *Chile* **128** H3
Navarra □ *Spain* **38** C3
Navarre *U.S.A.* **114** F3
Navarro ➤ *U.S.A.* **110** F3
Navas de San Juan *Spain* **37** G7
Navasota *U.S.A.* **116** F6
Navassa I. *W. Indies* **121** C5
Nävekvarn *Sweden* **11** F10
Naver ➤ *U.K.* **13** C4
Navia *Spain* **36** B4
Navia ➤ *Spain* **36** B4
Navia de Suarna = A Pobre
  Spain **36** C3

Navibandar *India* **68** J3
Navidad *Chile* **126** C1
Naviraí *Brazil* **127** A5
Naviti *Fiji* **91** a
Navlakhi *India* **68** H4
Navlya *Russia* **33** F3
Năvodari *Romania* **29** F13
Navoiy *Uzbekistan* **52** E7
Navojoa *Mexico* **118** B3
Navolato *Mexico* **118** C3
Navrongo *Ghana* **83** C4
Navsari *India* **66** J8
Nawa Kot *Pakistan* **68** E4
Nawab Khan *Pakistan* **68** D3
Nawabganj *Ut. P., India* **69** F9
Nawabganj *Ut. P., India* **69** E8
Nawabshah *Pakistan* **68** F3
Nawada *India* **69** G11
Nawakot *Nepal* **69** F11
Nawalgarh *India* **68** F6
Nawanshahr *India* **69** C6
Nawar, Dasht-i- *Afghan.* **68** C3
Nawi *Sudan* **80** D3
Nawoiy = Navoiy *Uzbekistan* **52** E7
Naxçıvan *Azerbaijan* **73** C11
Naxçıvan □ *Azerbaijan* **73** C11
Naxos *Greece* **47** D7
Nay *France* **20** E3
Nay, Mui *Vietnam* **62** B3
Nāy Band *Būshehr, Iran* **71** E7
Nāy Band *Khorāsān, Iran* **71** C8
Nayakhan *Russia* **53** C16
Nayarit □ *Mexico* **118** C4
Nayau *Fiji* **91** a
Nayé *Senegal* **82** C2
Nayong *China* **58** D5
Nayoro *Japan* **54** B11
Naypyidaw *Burma* **64** C1
Nayyāl, W. ➤ *Si. Arabia* **70** D3
Nazar Kahrizi *Iran* **73** D12
Nazaré *Brazil* **125** F11
Nazaré *Portugal* **37** F1
Nazareth = Nazerat *Israel* **74** C4
Nazareth *U.S.A.* **115** F9
Nazarovo *Russia* **53** D10
Nazas *Mexico* **118** B4
Nazas ➤ *Mexico* **118** B4
Nazca *Peru* **124** F4
Nazca Ridge *Pac. Oc.* **97** K19
Naze *Japan* **55** K4
Naze, The *U.K.* **15** F9
Nazerat *Israel* **74** C4
Nāzik *Iran* **73** C11
Nazilli *Turkey* **47** D10
Nazinon = Red Volta ➤
  Africa **83** C4
Nazko *Canada* **102** C4
Nazko ➤ *Canada* **102** C4
Nāzlū *Iran* **73** D11
Nazret *Ethiopia* **81** F4
Nchanga *Zambia* **87** E2
Ncheu *Malawi* **87** E3
Ndala *Tanzania* **86** C3
Ndalatando *Angola* **84** F2
Ndali *Benin* **83** D5
Ndareda *Tanzania* **86** C4
Ndélé *C.A.R.* **84** C4
Ndiael △ *Senegal* **82** B1
Ndikinimeki *Cameroon* **83** E7
N'Dioum *Senegal* **82** B2
Ndjamena *Chad* **79** F8
Ndola *Zambia* **87** E2
Ndomo △ *S. Africa* **89** D5
Ndoto Mts. *Kenya* **86** B4
Nduguti *Tanzania* **86** C3
Nea Alikarnassos *Greece* **47** F7
Nea Anchialos *Greece* **46** B4
Nea Epidavros *Greece* **46** D5
Nea Ionia *Greece* **46** B4
Nea Kalikratia *Greece* **44** F7
Nea Makri *Greece* **46** C5
Nea Moudania *Greece* **44** F7
Nea Peramos *Attiki, Greece* **46** C5
Nea Peramos *Kavala, Greece* **45** F8
Nea Visa *Greece* **45** E10
Nea Zichni *Greece* **44** E7
Neagh, Lough *U.K.* **12** B5
Neah Bay *U.S.A.* **110** B2
Neale, L. *Australia* **92** D5
Neales ➤ *Australia* **95** D2
Neamţ □ *Romania* **29** C11
Neapoli *Kozani, Greece* **44** F5
Neapoli *Kriti, Greece* **49** D7
Neapoli *Lakonia, Greece* **46** E5
Near Is. *U.S.A.* **106** E2
Neath *U.K.* **15** F4
Neath Port Talbot □ *U.K.* **15** F4
Nebbi *Uganda* **86** B3
Nebbou *Burkina Faso* **83** C4
Nebelat el Hagana *Sudan* **81** E2
Nebine Cr. ➤ *Australia* **95** D4
Nebitdag = Balkanabat
  Turkmenistan **71** B7
Nebo *Australia* **94** C4
Nebolchy *Russia* **32** C7
Nebraska □ *U.S.A.* **112** E4
Nebraska City *U.S.A.* **112** E6
Nébrodi, Monti *Italy* **43** E7

Necedah *U.S.A.* **112** C8
Nechako ➤ *Canada* **102** C4
Neches ➤ *U.S.A.* **116** G8
Nechisar *Ethiopia* **81** F4
Neckar ➤ *Germany* **25** F4
Neckartal-Odenwald △
  Germany **25** F5
Necker I. *U.S.A.* **107** L7
Necochea *Argentina* **126** D4
Neda *Spain* **36** B2
Neda ➤ *Greece* **46** D3
Nedelino *Bulgaria* **45** E9
Nedelišće *Croatia* **41** B13
Nederland =
  Netherlands ■ *Europe* **17** C5
Nedoboyivtsi *Ukraine* **29** B11
Needles *Canada* **102** D5
Needles *U.S.A.* **111** L12
Needles, The *U.K.* **15** G6
Neembucú □ *Paraguay* **126** B4
Neemuch = Nimach *India* **68** G6
Neenah *U.S.A.* **112** C9
Neepawa *Canada* **103** C9
Neftçala *Azerbaijan* **73** C13
Neftegorsk *Krasnodar, Russia* **35** H4
Neftegorsk *Sakhalin, Russia* **53** D15
Neftekumsk *Russia* **35** H7
Nefteyugansk *Russia* **52** C8
Nefyn *U.K.* **14** E3
Négala *Mali* **82** C3
Negapatam =
  Nagappattinam *India* **66** P11
Negara *Indonesia* **63** J17
Negaunee *U.S.A.* **112** B10
Negele *Oromiya, Ethiopia* **81** F4
Negele *Oromiya, Ethiopia* **81** F4
Negev Desert = Hanegev
  Israel **74** E4
Negoiul, Vf. *Romania* **29** E9
Negombo *Sri Lanka* **66** R11
Negotin *Serbia* **44** B6
Negotino *Macedonia* **44** E6
Negra, Peña *Spain* **36** C4
Negra, Pta. *Mauritania* **78** D2
Negra, Pta. *Peru* **124** E2
Negrais, C. = Maudin Sun
  Burma **67** M19
Negreşti *Romania* **29** D12
Negreşti-Oaş *Romania* **29** C8
Negril *Jamaica* **120** a
Negro ➤ *Argentina* **128** E4
Negro ➤ *Brazil* **124** D7
Negro ➤ *Uruguay* **126** C4
Negros *Phil.* **61** G5
Negru Vodă *Romania* **29** G13
Neguac *Canada* **105** C6
Nehalem ➤ *U.S.A.* **110** E3
Nehāvand *Iran* **71** C6
Nehbandān *Iran* **71** D9
Nehoiu *Romania* **29** E11
Nei Monggol Zizhiqu □
  China **56** D7
Neiafu *Tonga* **91** c
Neiges, Piton des *Réunion* **85** c
Neijiang *China* **58** C5
Neillsville *U.S.A.* **112** C8
Neilton *U.S.A.* **108** C2
Neiqiu *China* **56** F8
Neiva *Colombia* **124** C3
Neixiang *China* **56** H6
Nejanilini L. *Canada* **103** B9
Nejd = Najd *Si. Arabia* **75** B3
Nejo *Ethiopia* **81** F4
Nekā *Iran* **71** B7
Nekemte *Ethiopia* **81** F4
Nêkheb *Egypt* **80** B3
Neksø *Denmark* **11** J9
Nelas *Portugal* **36** E3
Nelia *Australia* **94** C3
Nelidovo *Russia* **32** D7
Neligh *U.S.A.* **112** D4
Nelkan *Russia* **53** D14
Nellore *India* **66** M11
Nelson *Canada* **102** D5
Nelson *N.Z.* **91** D4
Nelson *U.K.* **14** D5
Nelson *Ariz., U.S.A.* **109** J7
Nelson *Nev., U.S.A.* **111** K12
Nelson ➤ *Canada* **103** C9
Nelson, C. *Australia* **95** F3
Nelson, Estrecho *Chile* **128** G2
Nelson Forks *Canada* **102** B4
Nelson House *Canada* **103** B9
Nelson L. *Canada* **103** B8
Nelson Lakes △ *N.Z.* **91** D4
Nelspoort *S. Africa* **88** E3
Nelspruit *S. Africa* **89** D5
Néma *Mauritania* **82** B3
Neman = Nemunas ➤
  Lithuania **30** C8
Neman *Russia* **30** C9
Nembe *Nigeria* **83** E6
Nembrala *Indonesia* **92** B3
Nemea *Greece* **46** D4
Nemeiben L. *Canada* **103** B7
Nemërçkë, Mal *Albania* **44** F4
Nemira, Vf. *Romania* **29** D11
Nemiscau *Canada* **104** B4
Nemiscau, L. *Canada* **104** B4

Nemours *France* **19** D9
Nemrut Dağı △ *Turkey* **73** C8
Nemšová *Slovak Rep.* **27** C11
Nemunas ➤ *Lithuania* **30** C8
Nemuro *Japan* **54** C12
Nemuro-Kaikyō *Japan* **54** C12
Nemyriv *Ukraine* **31** H10
Nen Jiang ➤ *China* **57** B13
Nenagh *Ireland* **12** D3
Nenana *U.S.A.* **106** C10
Nenasi *Malaysia* **65** L4
Nene ➤ *U.K.* **15** E8
Nenita *Greece* **47** C8
Nenjiang *China* **60** B7
Neno *Malawi* **87** F3
Neo Chori *Greece* **46** C3
Neochori *Greece* **46** B2
Neodesha *U.S.A.* **112** G6
Neon Petritsi *Greece* **44** E7
Neora Valley △ *India* **69** F13
Neosho *U.S.A.* **112** G6
Neosho ➤ *U.S.A.* **116** C7
Nepal ■ *Asia* **69** F11
Nepalganj *Nepal* **69** E9
Nepalganj Road *India* **69** E9
Nephi *U.S.A.* **108** G8
Nephin *Ireland* **12** B2
Nephin Beg Range *Ireland* **12** C2
Nepi *Italy* **41** F9
Nepomuk *Czech Rep.* **26** B6
Neptune *U.S.A.* **115** F10
Neqāb *Iran* **71** B8
Nera ➤ *Italy* **41** F9
Nera ➤ *Romania* **28** F6
Nérac *France* **20** D4
Nerang *Australia* **95** D5
Nerastro, Sarīr *Libya* **79** D10
Neratovice *Czech Rep.* **26** A7
Nerchinsk *Russia* **53** D12
Nereju *Romania* **29** E11
Nerekhta *Russia* **32** D11
Neresnytsya *Ukraine* **29** B8
Néret, L. *Canada* **105** B5
Neretvanski Kanal *Croatia* **41** E14
Neringa *Lithuania* **30** C8
Neris ➤ *Lithuania* **32** E3
Nerja *Spain* **37** J7
Nerl ➤ *Russia* **32** D11
Nerpio *Spain* **39** G2
Nerva *Spain* **37** H4
Nervi *Italy* **40** D6
Neryungri *Russia* **53** D13
Nescopeck *U.S.A.* **115** E8
Neshūr *Bulgaria* **45** D11
Neskantaga *Canada* **104** B2
Ness, L. *U.K.* **13** D4
Ness City *U.S.A.* **112** F4
Nesterov *Russia* **30** D9
Nesterov *Ukraine* **23** C12
Nestório *Greece* **44** F5
Nestos ➤ *Europe* **45** E8
Nesvady *Slovak Rep.* **27** D11
Nesvizh = Nyasvizh *Belarus* **23** B14
Netanya *Israel* **74** C3
Netarhat *India* **69** H11
Nete ➤ *Belgium* **17** C4
Netherdale *Australia* **94** b
Netherlands ■ *Europe* **17** C5
Netherlands Antilles ☑
  W. Indies **124** A5
Neto ➤ *Italy* **43** C10
Netrang *India* **68** J5
Nettancourt *France* **19** D11
Nettetal *Germany* **24** D2
Nettilling L. *Canada* **101** D17
Nettuno *Italy* **42** A5
Netzahualcóyotl, Presa
  Mexico **119** D6
Neu-Isenburg *Germany* **25** E4
Neu-Ulm *Germany* **25** G6
Neubrandenburg *Germany* **24** B9
Neubukow *Germany* **24** A7
Neuburg *Germany* **25** G7
Neuchâtel *Switz.* **25** J2
Neuchâtel □ *Switz.* **25** J2
Neuchâtel, Lac de *Switz.* **25** J2
Neudau *Austria* **26** D9
Neuenhagen *Germany* **24** C9
Neuenhaus *Germany* **24** C2
Neuf-Brisach *France* **19** D14
Neufahrn *Bayern, Germany* **25** G8
Neufahrn *Bayern, Germany* **25** G7
Neufchâteau *Belgium* **17** E5
Neufchâteau *France* **19** D12
Neufchâtel-en-Bray *France* **18** C8
Neufchâtel-sur-Aisne
  France **19** C11
Neuhaus *Germany* **24** B6
Neuillé-Pont-Pierre *France* **18** E7
Neuilly-St-Front *France* **19** C10
Neukalen *Germany* **24** B8
Neumarkt *Germany* **25** F7
Neumayer *Antarctica* **5** D17
Neumünster *Germany* **24** A5
Neung-sur-Beuvron *France* **19** E8
Neunkirchen *Austria* **26** D9
Neunkirchen *Germany* **25** F3
Neuquén *Argentina* **128** D3
Neuquén □ *Argentina* **126** D2

Neuruppin *Germany* **24** C8
Neusäss *Germany* **25** G6
Neuse ➤ *U.S.A.* **117** D16
Neusiedl *Austria* **27** D9
Neusiedler See *Austria* **27** D9
Neusiedler
  See-Seewinkel △ *Austria* **27** D9
Neuss *Germany* **24** D2
Neussargues-Moissac *France* **20** C7
Neustadt *Bayern, Germany* **25** G7
Neustadt *Bayern, Germany* **25** G7
Neustadt *Bayern, Germany* **25** F6
Neustadt *Bayern, Germany* **25** F7
Neustadt *Brandenburg,
  Germany* **24** C8
Neustadt *Hessen, Germany* **24** E5
Neustadt *Niedersachsen,
  Germany* **24** C5
Neustadt *Rhld-Pfz., Germany* **25** F4
Neustadt *Sachsen, Germany* **24** D10
Neustadt *Schleswig-Holstein,
  Germany* **24** A6
Neustadt *Thüringen, Germany* **24** E7
Neustrelitz *Germany* **24** B9
Neuvic *France* **20** C6
Neuville-sur-Saône *France* **21** C8
Neuvy-le-Roi *France* **18** E7
Neuvy-St-Sépulchre *France* **19** F8
Neuvy-sur-Barangeon
  France **19** E9
Neuwerk *Germany* **24** B4
Neuwied *Germany* **24** E3
Neva ➤ *Russia* **32** C6
Nevada *Iowa, U.S.A.* **112** D7
Nevada *Mo., U.S.A.* **112** G6
Nevada □ *U.S.A.* **108** G5
Nevada City *U.S.A.* **110** F6
Nevado, Cerro *Argentina* **126** D2
Nevado de Colima =
  Volcán de Colima △
  Mexico **118** D4
Nevado de Tres Cruces △
  Chile **126** B2
Nevel *Russia* **32** D5
Nevelsk *Russia* **53** E15
Nevers *France* **19** F10
Nevertire *Australia* **95** E4
Nevesinje *Bos.-H.* **44** C2
Neville *Canada* **103** D7
Nevinnomyssk *Russia* **35** H6
Nevis *St. Kitts & Nevis* **121** C7
Nevrokop = Gotse Delchev
  Bulgaria **44** E7
Nevşehir *Turkey* **72** C6
Nevşehir □ *Turkey* **72** C6
Nevskoye *Russia* **30** D9
New ➤ *U.S.A.* **113** G5
New Aiyansh *Canada* **102** B3
New Albany *Ind., U.S.A.* **113** F11
New Albany *Miss., U.S.A.* **117** D10
New Albany *Pa., U.S.A.* **115** E8
New Amsterdam *Guyana* **124** B7
New Baltimore *U.S.A.* **114** D2
New Bedford *U.S.A.* **115** E14
New Berlin *N.Y., U.S.A.* **115** D9
New Berlin *Pa., U.S.A.* **114** F8
New Bern *U.S.A.* **117** D16
New Bethlehem *U.S.A.* **114** F5
New Bight *Bahamas* **121** B4
New Bloomfield *U.S.A.* **114** F7
New Boston *U.S.A.* **116** E7
New Braunfels *U.S.A.* **116** G5
New Brighton *N.Z.* **91** E4
New Brighton *U.S.A.* **114** F4
New Britain *Papua N. G.* **90** B8
New Britain *U.S.A.* **115** E12
New Brunswick *U.S.A.* **115** F10
New Brunswick □ *Canada* **105** C6
New Bussa *Nigeria* **83** D6
New Caledonia ☑ *Pac. Oc.* **90** D9
New Caledonia Trough
  Pac. Oc. **96** L8
New Castile = Castilla-La
  Mancha □ *Spain* **37** F7
New Castle *Ind., U.S.A.* **113** F11
New Castle *Pa., U.S.A.* **114** F4
New City *U.S.A.* **115** E11
New Concord *U.S.A.* **114** G3
New Cumberland *U.S.A.* **114** F4
New Cuyama *U.S.A.* **111** L7
New Delhi *India* **68** E7
New Denver *Canada* **102** D5
New Don Pedro Res. *U.S.A.* **110** H6
New England *U.S.A.* **107** G25
New England *N. Dak., U.S.A.* **112** B2
New England Ra. *Australia* **95** E5
New Forest △ *U.K.* **15** G6
New Galloway *U.K.* **13** F4
New Glasgow *Canada* **105** C7
New Guinea *Oceania* **90** B6
New Halfa = Halfa al
  Jadidah *Sudan* **81** D4
New Hamburg *Canada* **114** C4
New Hampshire □ *U.S.A.* **115** C13
New Hampton *U.S.A.* **112** D7
New Hanover *S. Africa* **89** D5
New Hartford *U.S.A.* **115** C9
New Haven *Conn., U.S.A.* **115** E12
New Haven *Mich., U.S.A.* **114** D2

New Haven *N.Y., U.S.A.* **115** C8
New Hazelton *Canada* **102** B3
New Hebrides =
    Vanuatu ■ *Pac. Oc.* **90** C9
New Holland *U.S.A.* **115** F8
New Iberia *U.S.A.* **110** F9
New Ireland *Papua N. G.* **90** B8
New Jersey □ *U.S.A.* **113** F16
New Kensington *U.S.A.* **114** F5
New Lexington *U.S.A.* **113** F12
New Liskeard *Canada* **104** C4
New London *Conn., U.S.A.* **115** E12
New London *Ohio, U.S.A.* **114** E2
New London *Wis., U.S.A.* **112** C9
New Madrid *U.S.A.* **112** G9
New Martinsville *U.S.A.* **113** F13
New Meadows *U.S.A.* **108** D5
New Melones L. *U.S.A.* **110** H6
New Mexico □ *U.S.A.* **109** J11
New Milford *Conn., U.S.A.* **115** E11
New Milford *Pa., U.S.A.* **115** E9
New Moore I. *Ind. Oc.* **69** J13
New Norcia *Australia* **93** F2
New Norfolk *Australia* **95** G4
New Orleans *U.S.A.* **117** G9
New Philadelphia *U.S.A.* **114** F3
New Plymouth *N.Z.* **91** C5
New Plymouth *U.S.A.* **108** E5
New Port Richey *U.S.A.* **117** G13
New Providence *Bahamas* **120** A4
New Quay *U.K.* **15** E3
New Radnor *U.K.* **15** E4
New Richmond *Canada* **105** C6
New Richmond *U.S.A.* **112** C7
New River Gorge ⌒ *U.S.A.* **113** G13
New Roads *U.S.A.* **116** F9
New Rochelle *U.S.A.* **115** F11
New Rockford *U.S.A.* **112** B4
New Romney *U.K.* **15** G8
New Ross *Ireland* **12** D5
New Salem *U.S.A.* **112** B3
New Scone = Scone *U.K.* **13** E5
New Siberian I. = Novaya
    Sibir, Ostrov *Russia* **53** B16
New Siberian Is. =
    Novosibirskiye Ostrova
    Russia **53** B15
New Smyrna Beach *U.S.A.* **117** G14
New South Wales □
    Australia **95** E4
New Tecumseth = Alliston
    Canada **114** B5
New Town *U.S.A.* **112** B2
New Tredegar *U.K.* **15** F4
New Ulm *U.S.A.* **112** C7
New Waterford *Canada* **105** C7
New Westminster *Canada* **110** A4
New York *U.S.A.* **115** F11
New York □ *U.S.A.* **115** D9
New York J.F. Kennedy
    Int. ✈ (JFK) *U.S.A.* **115** F11
New Zealand ■ *Oceania* **91** D6
Newaj → *India* **68** G7
Newala *Tanzania* **87** E4
Newark *Del., U.S.A.* **113** F16
Newark *N.J., U.S.A.* **115** F10
Newark *N.Y., U.S.A.* **114** C7
Newark *Ohio, U.S.A.* **114** F2
Newark Liberty Int. ✈
    (EWR) *U.S.A.* **115** F10
Newark-on-Trent *U.K.* **14** D7
Newark Valley *U.S.A.* **115** D8
Newberg *U.S.A.* **108** D2
Newberry *Mich., U.S.A.* **113** B11
Newberry *S.C., U.S.A.* **117** D14
Newberry Springs *U.S.A.* **111** L10
Newboro L. *Canada* **115** B8
Newbridge = Droichead
    Nua *Ireland* **12** C5
Newburgh *Canada* **114** B8
Newburgh *U.S.A.* **115** E10
Newbury *U.K.* **15** F6
Newbury *N.H., U.S.A.* **115** B12
Newbury *Vt., U.S.A.* **115** B12
Newburyport *U.S.A.* **115** D14
Newcastle *Australia* **95** E5
Newcastle *N.B., Canada* **105** C6
Newcastle *Ont., Canada* **104** D4
Newcastle *S. Africa* **89** D4
Newcastle *U.K.* **12** B6
Newcastle *Calif., U.S.A.* **110** G5
Newcastle *Wyo., U.S.A.* **108** E11
Newcastle Emlyn *U.K.* **15** E3
Newcastle Ra. *Australia* **94** B1
Newcastle Waters *Australia* **94** B1
Newcastle-under-Lyme *U.K.* **14** D5
Newcastle-upon-Tyne *U.K.* **14** C6
Newcastle West *Ireland* **12** D2
Newcomb *U.S.A.* **115** C10
Newcomerstown *U.S.A.* **114** F3
Newdegate *Australia* **93** F2
Newell *Australia* **94** B4
Newell *U.S.A.* **112** C12
Newenham, C. *U.S.A.* **106** D7
Newfane *U.S.A.* **114** C6
Newfield *U.S.A.* **115** D8
Newfound L. *Canada* **115** C13
Newfoundland *Canada* **105** C8
Newfoundland *U.S.A.* **115** E9

Newfoundland &
    Labrador □ *Canada* **105** B8
Newhaven *U.K.* **15** G8
Newkirk *U.S.A.* **116** C6
Newlyn *U.K.* **15** G2
Newman *Australia* **92** D2
Newman *U.S.A.* **110** H5
Newmarket *Canada* **114** B5
Newmarket *Ireland* **12** D2
Newmarket *U.K.* **15** E8
Newmarket *U.S.A.* **115** C14
Newnan *U.S.A.* **117** E12
Newport *Ireland* **12** C2
Newport *I. of W., U.K.* **15** G6
Newport *Newport, U.K.* **15** F5
Newport *Ark., U.S.A.* **116** D9
Newport *Ky., U.S.A.* **113** F11
Newport *N.H., U.S.A.* **115** C12
Newport *N.Y., U.S.A.* **115** C9
Newport *Oreg., U.S.A.* **108** D1
Newport *Pa., U.S.A.* **114** F7
Newport *R.I., U.S.A.* **115** E13
Newport *Tenn., U.S.A.* **117** D13
Newport *Vt., U.S.A.* **115** B12
Newport *Wash., U.S.A.* **108** B5
Newport □ *U.K.* **15** F4
Newport Beach *U.S.A.* **111** M9
Newport News *U.S.A.* **113** G15
Newport Pagnell *U.K.* **15** E7
Newquay *U.K.* **15** G2
Newry *U.K.* **12** B5
Newry Islands △ *Australia* **94** b
Newton *Ill., U.S.A.* **112** F9
Newton *Iowa, U.S.A.* **112** E8
Newton *Kans., U.S.A.* **112** F5
Newton *Mass., U.S.A.* **115** D13
Newton *Miss., U.S.A.* **117** E10
Newton *N.C., U.S.A.* **117** D14
Newton *N.J., U.S.A.* **115** E10
Newton *Tex., U.S.A.* **116** F8
Newton Abbot *U.K.* **15** G4
Newton Aycliffe *U.K.* **14** C6
Newton Falls *N.Y., U.S.A.* **115** B10
Newton Falls *Ohio, U.S.A.* **114** E4
Newton Stewart *U.K.* **13** G4
Newtonmore *U.K.* **13** D4
Newtown *U.K.* **15** E4
Newtownabbey *U.K.* **12** B6
Newtownards *U.K.* **12** B6
Newtownbarry = Bunclody
    Ireland **12** D5
Newtownstewart *U.K.* **12** B4
Newville *U.S.A.* **114** F7
Nexon *France* **20** C5
Neya *Russia* **34** A6
Neyrīz *Iran* **71** D7
Neyshābūr *Iran* **71** B8
Nezhin = Nizhyn *Ukraine* **33** G6
Nezperce *U.S.A.* **108** C5
Nezvysko *Ukraine* **29** B10
Ngaanyatjarra ⊚ *Australia* **92** D4
Ngabang *Indonesia* **62** D3
Ngabordamlu, Tanjung
    Indonesia **63** F8
N'Gage *Angola* **84** F3
Ngala *Nigeria* **83** C7
Ngaliwurru Nungali ⊚
    Australia **92** D5
Ngalurrtju ⊚ *Australia* **92** D5
Ngambé *Centre, Cameroon* **83** D7
Ngambé *Littoral, Cameroon* **83** E7
Ngami Depression *Botswana* **88** C3
Ngamo *Zimbabwe* **87** F2
Nganbéto, L. de *Togo* **83** D5
Ngangala *Sudan* **81** G3
Nganglong Kangri *China* **69** C9
Ngao *Thailand* **64** C2
Ngaoundéré *Cameroon* **84** C2
Ngapara *N.Z.* **91** F3
Ngara *Tanzania* **86** C3
Ngaruma ⊚ *Australia* **92** D2
Ngawi *Indonesia* **63** G14
Ngcobo *S. Africa* **89** E4
Ngeru *Uganda* **86** B3
Ngha Lo *Vietnam* **58** G5
Ngoboli *Sudan* **81** G3
Ngoma *Malawi* **87** E3
Ngomahura *Zimbabwe* **87** G3
Ngomba *Tanzania* **87** D3
Ngomeni, Ras *Kenya* **86** C5
Ngong *Kenya* **86** C4
Ngop *Sudan* **81** F3
Ngordou *Mali* **82** B4
Ngoring Hu *China* **60** C4
Ngorkou *Mali* **82** B4
Ngorongoro *Tanzania* **86** C4
Ngorongoro ⌒ *Tanzania* **86** C4
Ngozi *Burundi* **86** C2
Ngudu *Tanzania* **86** C3
Nguigmi *Niger* **79** F8
Nguila *Cameroon* **83** D7
Nguiu *Australia* **92** B5
Ngukurr *Australia* **94** A1
Ngundu *Zimbabwe* **87** F3
Ngunga *Tanzania* **86** C3
Nguru *Nigeria* **83** C7
Nguru Mts. *Tanzania* **86** D4
Nguyen Binh *Vietnam* **58** F5

Nhacoongo *Mozam.* **89** C6
Nhamaabué *Mozam.* **87** F4
Nhamundá → *Brazil* **125** D7
Nhangulaze, L. *Mozam.* **89** C5
Nharnuwangga, Wajarri
    and Ngarlawangga ⊚
    Australia **93** D2
Nhill *Australia* **95** F3
Nho Quan *Vietnam* **58** G5
Nhulunbuy *Australia* **94** A2
Nia-nia *Dem. Rep. of the Congo* **86** B2
Niafounké *Mali* **82** B4
Niagara Falls *Canada* **114** C5
Niagara Falls *U.S.A.* **114** C6
Niagara-on-the-Lake
    Canada **114** C5
Niah *Malaysia* **62** D4
Niamey *Niger* **83** C5
Niamtougou *Togo* **83** D5
Niandan-Koro *Guinea* **82** C3
Nianforando *Guinea* **82** D2
Niangara
    Dem. Rep. of the Congo **86** B2
Niangay, L. *Mali* **82** B4
Niangbo *Ivory C.* **82** D3
Niangoloko *Burkina Faso* **82** C4
Niantic *U.S.A.* **115** E12
Niaro *Sudan* **81** E3
Nias *Indonesia* **62** D1
Niassa □ *Mozam.* **87** E4
Niassa △ *Mozam.* **87** E4
Nibāk *Si. Arabia* **71** E7
Nibe *Denmark* **11** H3
Nicaragua ■ *Cent. Amer.* **120** D2
Nicaragua, L. de *Nic.* **120** D2
Nicastro *Italy* **43** D9
Nice *France* **21** E11
Nice-Côte-d'Azur ✈ (NCE)
    France **21** E11
Niceville *U.S.A.* **117** F11
Nichicun, L. *Canada* **105** B5
Nichinan *Japan* **55** J5
Nicholás, Canal *W. Indies* **120** B3
Nicholasville *U.S.A.* **113** G11
Nichols *U.S.A.* **115** D8
Nicholson *Australia* **92** C4
Nicholson *U.S.A.* **115** E9
Nicholson → *Australia* **94** B2
Nicholson L. *Canada* **103** A8
Nicholson Ra. *Australia* **93** E2
Nicholville *U.S.A.* **115** B10
Nicola *Canada* **102** C3
Nicolls Town *Bahamas* **120** A4
Nicosia *Cyprus* **49** D12
Nicosia *Italy* **43** E7
Nicótera *Italy* **43** D8
Nicoya *Costa Rica* **120** D2
Nicoya, G. de *Costa Rica* **120** E3
Nicoya, Pen. de *Costa Rica* **120** E2
Nida *Lithuania* **30** C8
Nidd → *U.K.* **14** D6
Nidda *Germany* **25** E5
Nidda → *Germany* **25** E4
Nidwalden □ *Switz.* **25** J4
Nidzica *Poland* **31** E7
Niebüll *Germany* **24** A4
Nied → *Germany* **19** C13
Niederaula *Germany* **24** E5
Niederbayern □ *Germany* **25** G8
Niederbronn-les-Bains
    France **19** D14
Niedere Tauern *Austria* **26** D7
Niederlausitz *Germany* **24** D9
Niederösterreich □ *Austria* **26** C8
Niedersachsen □ *Germany* **24** C4
Niedersächsisches
    Wattenmeer △ *Germany* **24** B3
Niekerkshoop *S. Africa* **88** D3
Niellé *Ivory C.* **82** C3
Niemba *Dem. Rep. of the Congo* **86** D2
Niemen = Nemunas →
    Lithuania **30** C8
Niemodlin *Poland* **31** H4
Nienburg *Germany* **24** C5
Niepołomice *Poland* **31** H7
Niers → *Germany* **24** D1
Niesky *Germany* **24** D10
Nieszawa *Poland* **31** F5
Nieu Bethesda *S. Africa* **88** E3
Nieu Nickerie *Suriname* **125** B7
Nieuwoudtville *S. Africa* **88** E2
Nieuwpoort *Belgium* **17** C2
Nieuw Amsterdam
    Suriname **125** B7
Nieves, Pico de las *Canary Is.* **48** G4
Nièvre □ *France* **19** E10
Niga *Mali* **82** C3
Niğde *Turkey* **72** D6
Niğde □ *Turkey* **72** D6
Nigel *S. Africa* **89** D4
Niger □ *Nigeria* **83** D6
Niger ■ *W. Afr.* **83** E7
Niger → *W. Afr.* **83** D6
Niger Delta *Africa* **83** E6
Nigeria ■ *W. Afr.* **83** D6
Nighasin *India* **69** E9
Nightcaps *N.Z.* **91** F2
Nigrita *Greece* **44** F7
Nha Trang *Vietnam* **65** F7

Nihoa *U.S.A.* **107** L7
Nihon = Japan ■ *Asia* **55** G8
Nii-Jima *Japan* **55** G9
Niigata *Japan* **54** F9
Niigata □ *Japan* **55** F9
Niihama *Japan* **55** H6
Ni'ihau *U.S.A.* **107** L7
Niimi *Japan* **55** G6
Niitsu *Japan* **54** F9
Níjar *Spain* **39** J2
Nijkerk *Neths.* **17** B5
Nijmegen *Neths.* **17** C5
Nijverdal *Neths.* **17** B6
Nīk Pey *Iran* **73** D13
Nike *Nigeria* **83** D6
Nikel *Russia* **8** B24
Nikiniki *Indonesia* **92** A3
Nikisiani *Greece* **45** F8
Nikki *Benin* **83** D5
Nikkō *Japan* **55** F9
Nikkō △ *Japan* **55** F9
Nikolayev = Mykolayiv
    Ukraine **33** J7
Nikolayevsk *Russia* **34** E7
Nikolayevsk-na-Amur
    Russia **53** D15
Nikolsk *Russia* **34** D8
Nikolskoye *Russia* **53** D17
Nikopol *Bulgaria* **45** C8
Nikopol *Ukraine* **33** J8
Nikopolis *Greece* **46** B2
Niksar *Turkey* **72** B7
Nikšić *Montenegro* **44** D2
Nīl, Nahr en → *Africa* **80** H7
Nīl el Abyad → *Sudan* **81** D3
Nīl el Azraq → *Sudan* **81** D3
Nila *Indonesia* **63** F7
Niland *U.S.A.* **111** M11
Nile = Nīl, Nahr en → *Africa* **80** H7
Nile Delta *Egypt* **80** H7
Niles *Mich., U.S.A.* **112** E10
Niles *Ohio, U.S.A.* **114** E4
Nilüfer → *Turkey* **45** F12
Nim Ka Thana *India* **68** F6
Nimach *India* **68** G6
Nimba, Mts. *Africa* **82** D3
Nimbahera *India* **68** G6
Nîmes *France* **21** E8
Nimfaíon, Ákra = Pines,
    Akra *Greece* **45** F8
Nimmitabel *Australia* **95** F4
Nimule *Sudan* **81** G3
Nimule △ *Sudan* **81** G3
Nin *Croatia* **41** D12
Nīnawá *Iraq* **73** D10
Nīnawá □ *Iraq* **70** B4
Nindigully *Australia* **95** D4
Nineveh = Nīnawá *Iraq* **73** D10
Ning Xian *China* **56** G4
Ningaloo Marine ⌒ *Australia* **92** D1
Ning'an *China* **57** B15
Ningbo *China* **59** C13
Ningcheng *China* **57** D10
Ningde *China* **59** D12
Ningdu *China* **59** D10
Ningguang *China* **59** D9
Ningguo *China* **59** B12
Ninghai *China* **59** C13
Ninghua *China* **59** D11
Ningi *Nigeria* **83** C6
Ningjin *China* **56** F8
Ningjing Shan *China* **58** C2
Ninglang *China* **58** D3
Ningling *China* **56** G8
Ningming *China* **58** F6
Ningnan *China* **58** D4
Ningpo = Ningbo *China* **59** C13
Ningqiang *China* **56** H4
Ningshan *China* **56** H5
Ningsia Hui A.R. = Ningxia
    Huizu Zizhiqu □ *China* **56** F4
Ningwu *China* **56** E7
Ningxia Huizu Zizhiqu □
    China **56** F4
Ningxiang *China* **59** C9
Ningyang *China* **56** G9
Ningyuan *China* **59** E8
Ninh Binh *Vietnam* **58** G5
Ninh Giang *Vietnam* **64** B6
Ninh Hoa *Vietnam* **64** F7
Ninh Ma *Vietnam* **64** F7
Nini-Suhien △ *Ghana* **82** D4
Ninove *Belgium* **17** D4
Nioaque *Brazil* **127** A5
Niobrara *U.S.A.* **112** D4
Niobrara → *U.S.A.* **112** D4
Niokolo-Koba △ *Senegal* **82** C2
Niono *Mali* **82** C3
Nionsamoridougou *Guinea* **82** D3
Nioro du Rip *Senegal* **82** C1
Nioro du Sahel *Mali* **82** B3
Niort *France* **20** B3
Nipawin *Canada* **103** C8
Nipigon *Canada* **104** C2
Nipigon, L. *Canada* **104** C2

Nipishish L. *Canada* **105** B7
Nipissing, L. *Canada* **104** C4
Nipomo *U.S.A.* **111** K6
Nippon = Japan ■ *Asia* **55** G8
Nipton *U.S.A.* **111** K11
Niquelândia *Brazil* **125** F9
Nīr *Iran* **73** C12
Nirasaki *Japan* **55** G9
Nirmal *India* **66** K11
Nirmali *India* **69** F12
Niš *Serbia* **44** C5
Nisa *Portugal* **37** F3
Nišava → *Serbia* **44** C5
Niscemi *Italy* **43** F7
Nishinomiya *Japan* **55** G7
Nishino'omote *Japan* **55** J5
Nishiwaki *Japan* **55** G7
Niška Banja *Serbia* **44** C6
Niskibi → *Canada* **104** A2
Nisko *Poland* **31** H9
Nisporeni *Moldova* **29** C13
Nisqually → *U.S.A.* **110** C4
Nissaki *Greece* **49** A3
Nissan → *Sweden* **11** H6
Nissiros *Greece* **47** E9
Nissum Bredning *Denmark* **11** H2
Nissum Fjord *Denmark* **11** H2
Nistru = Dnister → *Europe* **23** E16
Nisutlin → *Canada* **102** A2
Nitchequon *Canada* **105** B5
Niterói *Brazil* **127** A7
Nith → *Canada* **114** C4
Nith → *U.K.* **13** F5
Nitmiluk △ *Australia* **92** B5
Nitra *Slovak Rep.* **27** C11
Nitra → *Slovak Rep.* **27** D11
Nitriansky □ *Slovak Rep.* **27** C11
Nittenau *Germany* **25** F8
Niue *Pac. Oc.* **97** J11
Niulan Jiang → *China* **58** D4
Niut *Indonesia* **62** D4
Niutou Shan *China* **59** C13
Niuzhuang *China* **57** D12
Nivala *Finland* **8** E21
Nivelles *Belgium* **17** D4
Nivernais *France* **19** E10
Niverville *Canada* **103** D9
Niwas *India* **69** H9
Nixa *U.S.A.* **112** G7
Nixon *U.S.A.* **116** G6
Nizamabad *India* **66** K11
Nizamghat *India* **67** E19
Nizhne Kolymsk *Russia* **53** C17
Nizhnekamsk *Russia* **34** C10
Nizhneudinsk *Russia* **53** D10
Nizhnevartovsk *Russia* **52** C8
Nizhniy Bestyakh *Russia* **53** C13
Nizhniy Chir *Russia* **35** F6
Nizhniy Lomov *Russia* **34** D6
Nizhniy Novgorod *Russia* **34** B7
Nizhniy Novgorod □ *Russia* **34** B7
Nizhniy Tagil *Russia* **52** D6
Nizhyn *Ukraine* **33** G6
Nizina Mazowiecka *Poland* **31** F8
Nizip *Turkey* **72** D7
Nízké Tatry *Slovak Rep.* **27** C12
Nízké Tatry △ *Slovak Rep.* **27** C12
Nízký Jeseník *Czech Rep.* **27** B10
Nizwá *Oman* **75** C6
Nizza Monferrato *Italy* **40** D5
Njakwa *Malawi* **87** E3
Njanji *Zambia* **87** E3
Njazidja = Grande Comore
    Comoros Is. **85** a
Njegoš *Montenegro* **44** D2
Njinjo *Tanzania* **87** D4
Njombe *Tanzania* **87** D3
Njombe → *Tanzania* **86** D3
Njurundabommen *Sweden* **10** B11
Nkambe *Cameroon* **83** D7
Nkana *Zambia* **87** E2
Nkandla *S. Africa* **89** D5
Nkawkaw *Ghana* **83** D4
Nkayi *Zimbabwe* **87** F2
Nkhotakota *Malawi* **87** E3
Nkhotakota △ *Malawi* **87** E3
Nkondwe *Tanzania* **86** D3
Nkongsamba *Cameroon* **83** E6
Nkoteng *Cameroon* **83** D7
Nkurenkuru *Namibia* **88** B2
Nkwanta *Ghana* **82** D4
Nmai → *Burma* **58** F2
Noakhali = Maijdi *Bangla.* **67** H17
Nobel *Canada* **114** A4
Nobeoka *Japan* **55** H5
Noblejas *Spain* **36** F7
Noblesville *U.S.A.* **112** E10
Noboribetsu *Japan* **54** C10
Noccundra *Australia* **95** D3
Noce → *Italy* **40** B8
Nocera Inferiore *Italy* **43** B7
Nocera Umbra *Italy* **41** E9
Noci *Italy* **43** B10
Nocona *U.S.A.* **116** E6
Nocrich *Romania* **29** E9

Noda *Japan* **55** G9
Nogales *Mexico* **118** A2
Nogales *U.S.A.* **109** L8
Nogaro *France* **20** E3
Nogat → *Poland* **30** D6
Nōgata *Japan* **55** H5
Nogent *France* **19** D12
Nogent-le-Rotrou *France* **18** D7
Nogent-sur-Seine *France* **19** D10
Noggara *Ethiopia* **81** E4
Noggerup *Australia* **93** F2
Noginsk *Moskva, Russia* **32** E10
Noginsk *Tunguska, Russia* **53** C10
Nogliki *Russia* **53** D15
Nogoa → *Australia* **94** C4
Nogoyá *Argentina* **126** C4
Nógrád □ *Hungary* **28** C4
Noguera Pallaresa → *Spain* **38** D5
Noguera Ribagorçana →
    Spain **38** D5
Nohar *India* **68** E6
Nohfelden *Germany* **25** F3
Nohta *India* **69** H8
Noia *Spain* **36** C2
Noire, Montagne *France* **20** E6
Noires, Mts. *France* **18** D3
Noirétable *France* **20** C7
Noirmoutier, Î. de *France* **18** F4
Noirmoutier-en-l'Île *France* **18** F4
Nojane *Botswana* **88** C3
Nojima-Zaki *Japan* **55** G9
Nok Kundi *Pakistan* **66** E3
Nok Ta Phao, Ko *Thailand* **65** b
Nokaneng *Botswana* **88** B3
Nokia *Finland* **32** B2
Nokomis *Canada* **103** C8
Nokomis L. *Canada* **103** B8
Nola *C.A.R.* **84** D3
Nola *Italy* **43** B7
Nolay *France* **19** F11
Noli, C. di *Italy* **40** D5
Nolinsk *Russia* **34** B9
Noma Omuramba →
    Namibia **88** B3
Nombre de Dios *Panama* **120** E4
Nome *U.S.A.* **106** C6
Nomo-Zaki *Japan* **55** H4
Nomuka *Tonga* **91** c
Nomuka Group *Tonga* **91** c
Nonacho L. *Canada* **103** A7
Nonancourt *France* **18** D8
Nonda *Australia* **94** C3
None *Italy* **40** D4
Nong Chang *Thailand* **64** E2
Nong Het *Laos* **64** C4
Nong Khai *Thailand* **64** D4
Nong'an *China* **57** B13
Nongoma *S. Africa* **89** D5
Nongsa *Indonesia* **65** d
Nonoava *Mexico* **118** B3
Nonsan *S. Korea* **57** F14
Nonthaburi *Thailand* **64** F3
Nontron *France* **20** C4
Nonza *France* **21** F13
Noonamah *Australia* **92** B5
Noondie, L. *Australia* **93** E2
Noonkanbah ⊚ *Australia* **92** C3
Noord Brabant □ *Neths.* **17** C5
Noord Holland □ *Neths.* **17** B4
Noordbeveland *Neths.* **17** C3
Noordoostpolder *Neths.* **17** B5
Noordwijk *Neths.* **17** B4
Noosa Heads *Australia* **95** D5
Nootka I. *Canada* **102** D3
Nopiming ⌒ *Canada* **103** C9
Nora *Eritrea* **81** D5
Nora *Sweden* **10** E9
Noralee *Canada* **102** C3
Noranda =
    Rouyn-Noranda *Canada* **104** C4
Norberg *Sweden* **10** D9
Nórcia *Italy* **41** F10
Norco *U.S.A.* **111** M9
Nord □ *Cameroon* **83** D7
Nord □ *France* **19** B10
Nord-Kivu □
    Dem. Rep. of the Congo **86** C2
Nord-Ostsee-Kanal *Germany* **24** A5
Nord-Ouest □ *Cameroon* **83** D7
Nord-Pas-de-Calais □ *France* **19** B9
Nordaustlandet *Svalbard* **4** B9
Nordborg *Denmark* **11** J3
Nordby *Denmark* **11** J2
Norddeich *Germany* **24** B3
Nordegg *Canada* **102** C5
Norden *Germany* **24** B3
Nordenham *Germany* **24** B4
Norderney *Germany* **24** B3
Norderstedt *Germany* **24** B5
Nordfjord *Norway* **8** F11
Nordfriesische Inseln
    Germany **24** A4
Nordhausen *Germany* **24** D6
Nordhorn *Germany* **24** C3
Norðoyar *Færoe Is.* **8** E9
Nördinge-Nol *Sweden* **11** G6
Nordingrå *Sweden* **10** B12
Nordjylland □ *Denmark* **11** G3
Nordkapp *Norway* **8** A21

Nordkapp *Svalbard* **4** A9
Nordkinnhalvøya *Norway* **8** A22
Nördlicher Teutoburger
  Wald-Wiehengebirge △
  Germany **24** C4
Nördlingen *Germany* **25** G6
Nordrhein-Westfalen □
  Germany **24** D3
Nordstrand *Germany* **24** A4
Nordvik *Russia* **53** B12
Nore ➤ *Ireland* **12** D4
Noreland *Canada* **114** B6
Norfolk = Simcoe *Canada* **114** D4
Norfolk *N.Y., U.S.A.* **115** B10
Norfolk *Nebr., U.S.A.* **112** D5
Norfolk *Va., U.S.A.* **113** G15
Norfolk □ *U.K.* **15** E8
Norfolk Broads △ *U.K.* **15** E9
Norfolk I. *Pac. Oc.* **90** D9
Norfolk Ridge *Pac. Oc.* **96** K8
Norfork L. *U.S.A.* **116** C8
Norge = Norway ■ *Europe* **8** E14
Norilsk *Russia* **53** C9
Norma, Mt. *Australia* **94** C3
Normal *U.S.A.* **112** E9
Norman *U.S.A.* **116** D6
Norman ➤ *Australia* **94** B3
Norman Wells *Canada* **100** D6
Normanby ➤ *Australia* **94** A3
Normandie-Maine △ *France* **18** D6
Normandin *Canada* **104** C5
Normanhurst, Mt. *Australia* **93** E3
Normanton *Australia* **94** B3
Normétal *Canada* **104** C4
Norquay *Canada* **103** C8
Norquinco *Argentina* **128** E2
Norra Dellen *Sweden* **10** C10
Norra Kvill △ *Sweden* **11** G9
Norra Ulvön *Sweden* **10** A12
Norrahammar *Sweden* **11** G8
Norrbottens län □ *Sweden* **8** C19
Nørre Åby *Denmark* **11** J3
Nørre Alslev *Denmark* **11** K5
Nørresundby *Denmark* **11** G3
Norrhult-Klavreström
  Sweden **11** G9
Norris Point *Canada* **105** C8
Norristown *U.S.A.* **115** F9
Norrköping *Sweden* **11** F10
Norrland *Sweden* **8** E16
Norrsundet *Sweden* **10** D11
Norrtälje *Sweden* **10** E12
Norseman *Australia* **93** F3
Norsk *Russia* **53** D14
Norte, Pta. del *Canary Is.* **48** G2
Norte, Serra do *Brazil* **124** F7
North, C. *Canada* **105** C7
North Adams *U.S.A.* **115** D11
North America **98** F10
North Arm *Canada* **102** A5
North Augusta *U.S.A.* **117** E14
North Australian Basin
  Ind. Oc. **92** B2
North Ayrshire □ *U.K.* **13** F4
North Bass I. *U.S.A.* **114** E2
North Battleford *Canada* **103** C7
North Bay *Canada* **104** C4
North Belcher Is. *Canada* **104** A4
North Bend *Oreg., U.S.A.* **108** E1
North Bend *Pa., U.S.A.* **114** E7
North Bend *Wash., U.S.A.* **110** C5
North Bennington *U.S.A.* **115** D11
North Berwick *U.K.* **13** E6
North Berwick *U.S.A.* **115** C14
North Bruce *Canada* **114** B3
North C. *Canada* **105** C7
North C. *N.Z.* **91** A4
North Canadian ➤ *U.S.A.* **116** D7
North Canton *U.S.A.* **114** F3
North Cape = Nordkapp
  Norway **8** A21
North Caribou L. *Canada* **104** B1
North Carolina □ *U.S.A.* **117** D15
North Cascades △ *U.S.A.* **108** B3
North Channel *Canada* **104** C3
North Channel *U.K.* **13** F3
North Charleston *U.S.A.* **117** E15
North Chicago *U.S.A.* **112** D10
North Collins *U.S.A.* **114** D6
North Creek *U.S.A.* **115** C11
North Dakota □ *U.S.A.* **112** B3
North Downs *U.K.* **15** F8
North East *U.S.A.* **114** D5
North East Frontier
  Agency = Arunachal
  Pradesh □ *India* **67** F19
North East Lincolnshire □
  U.K. **14** D7
North Eastern □ *Kenya* **86** B5
North Esk ➤ *U.K.* **13** E6
North European Plain *Europe* **6** E10
North Foreland *U.K.* **15** F9
North Fork *U.S.A.* **110** H7
North Fork American ➤
  U.S.A. **110** G5
North Fork Feather ➤
  U.S.A. **110** F5
North Fork Grand ➤
  U.S.A. **112** C2
North Fork Red ➤ *U.S.A.* **116** D5

North Frisian Is. =
  Nordfriesische Inseln
  Germany **24** A4
North Gower *Canada* **115** A9
North Hd. *Australia* **93** F1
North Henik L. *Canada* **103** A9
North Highlands *U.S.A.* **110** G5
North Horr *Kenya* **86** B4
North I. *Kenya* **86** B4
North I. *N.Z.* **91** C5
North I. *Seychelles* **85** b
North Kingsville *U.S.A.* **114** E4
North Kitui △ *Kenya* **86** C4
North Knife ➤ *Canada* **103** B10
North Koel ➤ *India* **69** G10
North Korea ■ *Asia* **57** E14
North Lakhimpur *India* **67** F19
North Lanarkshire □ *U.K.* **13** F5
North Las Vegas *U.S.A.* **111** J11
North Lincolnshire □ *U.K.* **14** D7
North Little Rock *U.S.A.* **116** D8
North Loup ➤ *U.S.A.* **112** E4
North Luangwa △ *Zambia* **87** E3
North Magnetic Pole *Canada* **4** A2
North Mankato *U.S.A.* **112** C6
North Minch *U.K.* **13** C3
North Moose L. *Canada* **103** C8
North Myrtle Beach *U.S.A.* **117** E15
North Nahanni ➤ *Canada* **102** A4
North Olmsted *U.S.A.* **114** E3
North Ossetia □ *Russia* **35** J7
North Pagai, I. = Pagai
  Utara, Pulau *Indonesia* **62** E2
North Palisade *U.S.A.* **110** H8
North Platte *U.S.A.* **112** E3
North Platte ➤ *U.S.A.* **112** E3
North Pole *Arctic* **4** A
North Portal *Canada* **103** D8
North Powder *U.S.A.* **108** D5
North Pt. *Barbados* **121** g
North Pt. *Trin. & Tob.* **125** J16
North Pt. *U.S.A.* **114** A1
North Rhine Westphalia =
  Nordrhein-Westfalen □
  Germany **24** D3
North River *Canada* **105** B8
North Ronaldsay *U.K.* **13** B6
North Saskatchewan ➤
  Canada **103** C7
North Sea *Europe* **6** D6
North Seal ➤ *Canada* **103** B9
North Slope *U.S.A.* **106** B9
North Somerset □ *U.K.* **15** F5
North Sydney *Canada* **105** C7
North Syracuse *U.S.A.* **115** C8
North Taranaki Bight *N.Z.* **91** C5
North Thompson ➤ *Canada* **102** C4
North Tonawanda *U.S.A.* **114** D6
North Troy *U.S.A.* **115** B12
North Twin I. *Canada* **104** B4
North Tyne ➤ *U.K.* **14** B5
North Uist *U.K.* **13** D1
North Vancouver *Canada* **110** A3
North Vernon *U.S.A.* **113** F11
North Wabasca L. *Canada* **102** B6
North Walsham *U.K.* **14** E9
North West =
  Severo-Zapadnyy □ *Russia* **52** C4
North-West □ *S. Africa* **88** D4
North West C. *Australia* **92** D1
North West Frontier □
  Pakistan **68** C4
North West Highlands *U.K.* **13** D4
North West River *Canada* **105** B7
North Western □ *Zambia* **87** E2
North Wildwood *U.S.A.* **113** F16
North York Moors *U.K.* **14** C7
North York Moors △ *U.K.* **14** C7
North Yorkshire □ *U.K.* **14** C6
Northallerton *U.K.* **14** C6
Northam *Australia* **93** F2
Northam *S. Africa* **88** C4
Northampton *Australia* **93** E1
Northampton *U.K.* **15** E7
Northampton *Mass., U.S.A.* **115** D12
Northampton *Pa., U.S.A.* **115** F9
Northamptonshire □ *U.K.* **15** E7
Northbridge *U.S.A.* **115** D13
Northbrook *Canada* **114** B7
Northcliffe *Australia* **93** F2
Northeast Pacific Basin
  Pac. Oc. **97** D13
Northeast Providence
  Chan. *W. Indies* **120** A4
Northeim *Germany* **24** D6
Northern □ *Limpopo □
  S. Africa* **89** C4
Northern □ *Malawi* **87** E3
Northern □ *S. Leone* **82** D2
Northern □ *Zambia* **87** E3
Northern Areas □ *Pakistan* **69** A5
Northern Cape □ *S. Africa* **88** D3
Northern Circars *India* **67** L13
Northern Indian L. *Canada* **103** B9
Northern Ireland □ *U.K.* **12** B5
Northern Lau Group *Fiji* **91** a
Northern Light L. *Canada* **104** c1
Northern Marianas ☑
  Pac. Oc. **96** F6

Northern Province □
  S. Africa **89** C4
Northern Range *Trin. & Tob.*
  125 K15
Northern Sporades *Greece* **46** B5
Northern Territory □
  Australia **92** D5
Northfield *Minn., U.S.A.* **112** C7
Northfield *Vt., U.S.A.* **115** B12
Northgate *Canada* **103** D8
Northland □ *N.Z.* **91** A4
Northome *U.S.A.* **112** B6
Northport *Ala., U.S.A.* **117** E11
Northport *Wash., U.S.A.* **108** B5
Northumberland, C. *Australia* **95** F3
Northumberland Is. *Australia* **94** C4
Northumberland Str.
  Canada **105** C7
Northville *U.S.A.* **115** C10
Northwest Pacific Basin
  Pac. Oc. **96** D8
Northwest Providence
  Channel *W. Indies* **120** A4
Northwest Territories □
  Canada **100** E8
Northwich *U.K.* **14** D5
Northwood *Iowa, U.S.A.* **112** D7
Northwood *N. Dak., U.S.A.* **112** B5
Norton *U.S.A.* **112** F4
Norton *Zimbabwe* **87** F3
Norton Sd. *U.S.A.* **106** C7
Nortorf *Germany* **24** A5
Norwalk *Calif., U.S.A.* **111** M8
Norwalk *Conn., U.S.A.* **115** E11
Norwalk *Iowa, U.S.A.* **112** E7
Norwalk *Ohio, U.S.A.* **114** E2
Norway *Maine, U.S.A.* **113** C18
Norway *Mich., U.S.A.* **112** C10
Norway ■ *Europe* **8** E14
Norway House *Canada* **103** C9
Norwegian B. *Canada* **101** B9
Norwegian Basin *Atl. Oc.* **4** C7
Norwegian Sea *Atl. Oc.* **6** B6
Norwich *Canada* **114** D4
Norwich *U.K.* **15** E9
Norwich *Conn., U.S.A.* **115** E12
Norwich *N.Y., U.S.A.* **115** D9
Norwood *Canada* **114** B7
Norwood *U.S.A.* **115** B10
Nosappu-Misaki *Japan* **54** C12
Noshiro *Japan* **54** D10
Nosivka *Ukraine* **33** G6
Nosovka = Nosivka *Ukraine* **33** G6
Noşratābād *Iran* **71** D8
Noss Hd. *U.K.* **13** C5
Nossebro *Sweden* **11** F6
Nossob ➤ *S. Africa* **88** D3
Nossombougou *Mali* **82** C3
Nosy Barren *Madag.* **85** H8
Nosy Bé *Madag.* **85** G9
Nosy Boraha *Madag.* **89** B8
Nosy Lava *Madag.* **89** A8
Nosy Varika *Madag.* **89** C8
Noteć ➤ *Poland* **31** F2
Notikewin ➤ *Canada* **102** B5
Notio Aigaio □ *47* E7
Notios Aiyaíon = Notio
  Aigaio □ *47* E7
Notios Evvoikos Kolpos
  Greece **46** C5
Noto *Italy* **43** F8
Noto, G. di *Italy* **43** F8
Notodden *Norway* **9** G13
Notre Dame B. *Canada* **105** C8
Notre-Dame-de-Koartac =
  Quaqtaq *Canada* **101** E18
Notre-Dame-des-Bois
  Canada **115** A13
Notre-Dame-d'Ivugivic =
  Ivujivik *Canada* **101** E16
Notre-Dame-du-Nord
  Canada **104** C4
Notsé *Togo* **83** D5
Nottawasaga B. *Canada* **114** B4
Nottaway ➤ *Canada* **104** B4
Nottingham *U.K.* **14** E6
Nottingham, City of □ *U.K.* **14** E6
Nottingham I. *Canada* **101** E16
Nottinghamshire □ *U.K.* **14** D6
Nottoway ➤ *U.S.A.* **113** G15
Notwane ➤ *Botswana* **88** C4
Nouâdhibou *Mauritania* **78** D2
Nouâdhibou, Râs *Mauritania* **78** D2
Nouakchott *Mauritania* **82** B1
Nouâmghâr *Mauritania* **82** B1
Nouméa *N. Cal.* **90** D9
Nouna *Burkina Faso* **82** C4
Noupoort *S. Africa* **88** E3
Nouveau Comptoir =
  Wemindji *Canada* **104** B4
Nouvelle Amsterdam, Î.
  Ind. Oc. **3** F13
Nouvelle-Calédonie = New
  Caledonia ☑ *Pac. Oc.* **90** D9
Nouzonville *France* **19** C11
Nová Baňa *Slovak Rep.* **27** C11
Nová Bystřice *Czech Rep.* **26** B8
Nova Esperança *Brazil* **127** A5
Nova Friburgo *Brazil* **127** A7

Nova Gorica *Slovenia* **41** C10
Nova Gradiška *Croatia* **28** E2
Nova Iguaçu *Brazil* **127** A7
Nova Iorque *Brazil* **125** E10
Nova Kakhovka *Ukraine* **33** J7
Nova Lamego = Gabú
  Guinea-Biss. **82** C2
Nova Lusitânia *Mozam.* **87** F3
Nova Mambone *Mozam.* **89** C6
Nova Odesa *Ukraine* **33** J6
Nová Paka *Czech Rep.* **26** A8
Nova Pavova *Serbia* **28** F5
Nova Scotia □ *Canada* **105** C7
Nova Siri *Italy* **43** B9
Nova Sofala *Mozam.* **89** C5
Nova Ushytsya *Ukraine* **29** B12
Nova Varoš *Serbia* **44** C3
Nova Venécia *Brazil* **125** G10
Nova Zagora *Bulgaria* **45** D10
Novaci *Macedonia* **44** E3
Novaci *Romania* **29** E8
Novafeltria *Italy* **41** E9
Novannenskiy =
  Novoannenskiy *Russia* **34** E6
Novar *Canada* **114** A5
Novara *Italy* **40** C5
Novato *U.S.A.* **110** G4
Novaya Kazanka =
  Zhangqala *Kazakhstan* **35** F9
Novaya Ladoga *Russia* **32** B7
Novaya Lyalya *Russia* **52** D7
Novaya Sibir, Ostrov *Russia* **53** B16
Novaya Zemlya *Russia* **52** B6
Nové Město *Slovak Rep.* **27** C10
Nové Město na Moravě
  Czech Rep. **26** B9
Nové Město nad Metují
  Czech Rep. **26** A9
Nové Zámky *Slovak Rep.* **27** C11
Novelda *Spain* **39** G4
Novellara *Italy* **40** D7
Noventa Vicentina *Italy* **41** C8
Novgorod *Russia* **32** C6
Novgorod □ *Russia* **32** C7
Novgorod-Severskiy =
  Novhorod-Siverskyy
  Ukraine **33** G7
Novhorod-Siverskyy *Ukraine* **33** G7
Novi Bečej *Serbia* **28** E5
Novi Knezevac *Serbia* **28** D5
Novi Lígure *Italy* **40** D5
Novi Pazar *Bulgaria* **45** C11
Novi Pazar *Serbia* **44** C4
Novi Sad *Serbia* **28** E4
Novi Slankamen *Serbia* **28** E5
Novi Travnik *Bos.-H.* **28** F2
Novi Vinodolski *Croatia* **41** C11
Novigrad *Istra, Croatia* **41** C10
Novigrad *Zadar, Croatia* **41** D12
Novigradsko More *Croatia* **41** D12
Novo Hamburgo *Brazil* **127** B5
Novo Mesto *Slovenia* **41** C12
Novo Miloševo *Serbia* **28** E5
Novoaleksandrovsk *Russia* **35** H5
Novoaleksandrovskaya =
  Novoaleksandrovsk
  Russia **35** H5
Novoaltaysk *Russia* **52** D9
Novoannenskiy *Russia* **34** E6
Novoazovsk *Ukraine* **33** J10
Novocheboksarsk *Russia* **34** B8
Novocherkassk *Russia* **35** G5
Novodevichye *Russia* **34** D9
Novodvinsk *Russia* **52** C5
Novogrudok =
  Navahrudak *Belarus* **23** B13
Novohrad-Volynskyy
  Ukraine **23** C14
Novokachalinsk *Russia* **54** B5
Novokhopersk *Russia* **34** E5
Novokuybyshevsk *Russia* **34** D9
Novokuznetsk *Russia* **52** D9
Novolazarevskaya *Antarctica* **5** D3
Novomirgorod *Ukraine* **33** H6
Novomoskovsk *Russia* **32** E10
Novomoskovsk *Ukraine* **33** H8
Novopolotsk =
  Navapolatsk *Belarus* **32** E5
Novorossiysk *Russia* **35** K9
Novorybnoye *Russia* **53** B11
Novorzhev *Russia* **32** D5
Novosej *Albania* **44** E4
Novoselytsya *Ukraine* **29** B11
Novoshakhtinsk *Russia* **33** J10
Novosibirsk *Russia* **52** D9
Novosibirskiye Ostrova
  Russia **53** B15
Novosil *Russia* **33** F9
Novosokolniki *Russia* **32** D6
Novotitarovskaya *Russia* **35** H4
Novotroitsk *Russia* **52** D6
Novoukrayinka *Ukraine* **33** H6
Novouljanovsk *Russia* **34** C9
Novouzensk *Russia* **34** E9
Novovolynsk *Ukraine* **31** H11
Novovoronezhskiy *Russia* **33** G10
Novoyavoriske *Ukraine* **31** J10

Novozybkov *Russia* **33** F6
Novska *Croatia* **41** C14
Nový Bor *Czech Rep.* **26** A7
Nový Bydžov *Czech Rep.* **26** A8
Novy Dvor *Belarus* **31** F11
Nový Jičín *Czech Rep.* **27** B11
Novy Dwór Mazowiecki
  Poland **31** F7
Novyy Afon *Georgia* **35** J5
Novyy Buh *Ukraine* **33** J7
Novyy Oskol *Russia* **33** G9
Novyy Port *Russia* **52** C8
Novyy Urengoy *Russia* **52** C8
Nowa Deba *Poland* **31** H8
Nowa Ruda *Poland* **31** H3
Nowa Sarzyna *Poland* **31** H9
Nowa Sól *Poland* **31** G2
Nowata *U.S.A.* **116** C7
Nowbarān *Iran* **71** C6
Nowe *Poland* **30** E5
Nowe Miasteczko *Poland* **31** G2
Nowe Miasto *Poland* **31** G7
Nowe Miasto Lubawskie
  Poland **30** E6
Nowe Skalmierzyce *Poland* **31** G4
Nowe Warpno *Poland* **30** E1
Nowghāb *Iran* **71** C8
Nowgong *Assam, India* **67** F18
Nowgong *Mad. P., India* **69** G8
Nowogard *Poland* **30** E2
Nowogród *Poland* **31** E8
Nowogród Bobrzanski
  Poland **31** G2
Nowogrodziec *Poland* **31** G2
Nowra *Australia* **95** E5
Nowshera *Pakistan* **66** C8
Nowy Dwór Gdański *Poland* **30** D6
Nowy Sącz *Poland* **31** J7
Nowy Staw *Poland* **30** D6
Nowy Targ *Poland* **31** J6
Nowy Tomyśl *Poland* **31** F3
Nowy Wiśnicz *Poland* **31** J7
Noxen *U.S.A.* **115** E9
Noyabr'sk *Russia* **52** C8
Noyant *France* **18** E7
Noyers *France* **19** E10
Noyon *France* **19** C9
Noyon *Mongolia* **56** C2
Nozay *France* **18** E5
Nqutu *S. Africa* **89** D5
Nsanje *Malawi* **87** F4
Nsawam *Ghana* **83** D4
Nseluka *Zambia* **87** D3
Nsomba *Zambia* **87** E2
Nsukka *Nigeria* **83** D6
Ntaria ✿ *Australia* **92** D5
Ntui *Cameroon* **83** E7
Ntungamo *Uganda* **86** C3
Nu Jiang ➤ *China* **58** E2
Nu Shan *China* **58** E2
Nuba Mts. = Nubah,
  Jibalan *Sudan* **81** E3
Nubah, Jibalan *Sudan* **81** E3
Nubia *Africa* **76** D7
Nubian Desert = Nûbîya,
  Es Sahrâ en *Sudan* **80** C3
Nûbîya, Es Sahrâ en *Sudan* **80** C3
Nubledo *Spain* **36** B5
Nuboai *Indonesia* **63** E9
Nubra ➤ *India* **69** B7
Nucet *Romania* **28** D7
Nueces ➤ *U.S.A.* **116** H6
Nueltin L. *Canada* **103** A9
Nuestra Señora del Rosario
  de Caá-Catí *Argentina* **126** B4
Nueva Carteya *Spain* **37** H6
Nueva Ciudad Guerrero
  Mexico **119** B5
Nueva Gerona *Cuba* **120** B3
Nueva Palmira *Uruguay* **126** C4
Nueva Rosita *Mexico* **118** B4
Nueva San Salvador *El Salv.* **120** D2
Nueva Tabarca *Spain* **39** G4
Nuéve de Julio *Argentina* **126** D3
Nuevitas *Cuba* **120** B4
Nuevo, G. *Argentina* **128** E4
Nuevo Casas Grandes
  Mexico **118** A3
Nuevo Laredo *Mexico* **119** B5
Nuevo León □ *Mexico* **118** C5
Nuevo Rocafuerte *Ecuador* **124** D3
Nugget Pt. *N.Z.* **91** G2
Nugrus, Gebel *Egypt* **80** C3
Nuhaka *N.Z.* **91** C6
Nuits-St-Georges *France* **19** E11
Nukey Bluff *Australia* **95** E2
Nukhayb *Iraq* **73** F10
Nuku Hiva *French Polynesia* **97** H13
Nuku'alofa *Tonga* **91** c
Nukus *Uzbekistan* **52** E6
Nulato *U.S.A.* **106** C8
Nules *Spain* **38** F4
Nullagine *Australia* **92** D3
Nullagine ➤ *Australia* **92** D3
Nullarbor *Australia* **93** F5
Nullarbor △ *Australia* **93** F2
Nullarbor Plain *Australia* **93** F4

Numalla, L. *Australia* **95** D3
Numan *Nigeria* **83** D7
Numata *Japan* **55** F9
Numatinna ➤ *Sudan* **81** F2
Numaykoos Lake △ *Canada* **103** B9
Numazu *Japan* **55** G9
Numbulwar *Australia* **94** A2
Numfoor *Indonesia* **63** E8
Numurkah *Australia* **95** F4
Nunaksaluk I. *Canada* **105** A7
Nunap Isua *Greenland* **98** D15
Nunavik *Greenland* **101** C21
Nunavut □ *Canada* **101** D15
Nunda *U.S.A.* **114** D7
Nuneaton *U.K.* **15** E6
Nungarin *Australia* **93** F2
Nungo *Mozam.* **87** E4
Nungwe *Tanzania* **86** C3
Nunivak I. *U.S.A.* **106** C6
Nunkun *India* **69** C7
Núoro *Italy* **42** B2
Nūr *Iran* **71** B7
Nūrābād *Hormozgān, Iran* **71** E8
Nūrābād *Lorestān, Iran* **73** E12
Nure ➤ *Italy* **40** C6
Nuremberg = Nürnberg
  Germany **25** F7
Nuri *Mexico* **118** B3
Nuri *Sudan* **80** D3
Nuriootpa *Australia* **95** E2
Nuristān □ *Afghan.* **66** B7
Nurlat *Russia* **34** C10
Nurmes *Finland* **8** E23
Nürnberg *Germany* **25** F7
Nurpur *Pakistan* **68** D4
Nurra, L = Terewah, L.
  Australia **95** D4
Nurrari Lakes *Australia* **93** E5
Nurri *Italy* **42** C2
Nürtingen *Germany* **25** G5
Nurzec ➤ *Poland* **31** F9
Nus *Italy* **40** C4
Nusa Barung *Indonesia* **63** H15
Nusa Dua *Indonesia* **63** K18
Nusa Kambangan *Indonesia* **63** G13
Nusa Tenggara Barat □
  Indonesia **62** F5
Nusa Tenggara Timur □
  Indonesia **63** F6
Nusaybin *Turkey* **73** D9
Nushki *Pakistan* **68** E2
Nuuk *Greenland* **99** C14
Nuupere, Pte. *Moorea* **91** d
Nuwakot *Nepal* **69** E10
Nuwayb'ī, W. an ➤
  Si. Arabia **74** F3
Nuweiba' *Egypt* **70** D2
Nuwerus *S. Africa* **88** E2
Nuweveldberge *S. Africa* **88** E3
Nuyts, Pt. *Australia* **93** G2
Nuyts Arch. *Australia* **95** E1
Nxai Pan △ *Botswana* **88** B3
Nxaunxau *Botswana* **88** B3
Nyaake *Liberia* **82** E3
Nyabing *Australia* **93** F2
Nyack *U.S.A.* **115** E11
Nyagan *Russia* **52** C7
Nyahanga *Tanzania* **86** C3
Nyahua *Tanzania* **86** D3
Nyahururu *Kenya* **86** B4
Nyaingêntanglha Shan
  China **60** C4
Nyakanazi *Tanzania* **86** C3
Nyakrom *Ghana* **83** D4
Nyâlâ *Sudan* **81** E1
Nyamandhlovu *Zimbabwe* **87** F2
Nyambiti *Tanzania* **86** C3
Nyamira *Kenya* **86** C3
Nyamlell *Sudan* **81** F2
Nyamwaga *Tanzania* **86** C3
Nyandekwa *Tanzania* **86** C3
Nyanding ➤ *Sudan* **81** F3
Nyandoma *Russia* **32** B11
Nyanga △ *Zimbabwe* **87** F3
Nyangana *Namibia* **88** B3
Nyanguge *Tanzania* **86** C3
Nyankpala *Ghana* **83** D4
Nyanza *Rwanda* **86** C2
Nyanza □ *Kenya* **86** C3
Nyanza-Lac *Burundi* **86** C2
Nyaponges *Sudan* **81** F3
Nyasa, L. = Malawi, L. *Africa* **87** E3
Nyasvizh *Belarus* **23** B14
Nyazura *Zimbabwe* **87** F3
Nyazwidzi ➤ *Zimbabwe* **87** G3
Nyborg *Denmark* **11** J4
Nybro *Sweden* **11** H9
Nyda *Russia* **52** C8
Nyeboe Land *Greenland* **101** A20
Nyeri *Kenya* **86** C4
Nyerol *Sudan* **81** F3
Nyhammar *Sweden* **10** D8
Nyika △ *Malawi* **87** E3
Nyimba *Zambia* **87** E3
Nyinahin *Ghana* **82** D4
Nyíradony *Hungary* **28** C6
Nyírbátor *Hungary* **28** C7
Nyíregyháza *Hungary* **28** C6
Nyiru, Mt. *Kenya* **86** B4

Nykarleby =
  Uusikaarlepyy *Finland* **8** E20
Nykøbing *Nordjylland,*
  Denmark **11** H2
Nykøbing *Sjælland, Denmark* **11** K5
Nykøbing *Sjælland, Denmark* **11** J5
Nyköping *Sweden* **11** F11
Nykroppa *Sweden* **10** E8
Nykvarn *Sweden* **10** E11
Nyland *Sweden* **10** A11
Nylstroom = Modimolle
  S. Africa **89** C4
Nymagee *Australia* **95** E4
Nymboida △ *Australia* **95** D5
Nymburk *Czech Rep.* **26** A8
Nynäshamn *Sweden* **11** F11
Nyngan *Australia* **95** E4
Nyoma Rap *India* **69** C8
Nyoman = Nemunas ➤
  Lithuania **30** C8
Nyon *Switz.* **25** J2
Nyong ➤ *Cameroon* **83** E6
Nyons *France* **21** D9
Nyou *Burkina Faso* **83** C4
Nýrsko *Czech Rep.* **26** B6
Nysa *Poland* **31** H4
Nysa ➤ *Europe* **24** C10
Nysa Kłodzka ➤ *Poland* **31** H4
Nysäter *Sweden* **10** E6
Nyslott = Savonlinna *Finland* **32** B5
Nyssa *U.S.A.* **108** E5
Nystad = Uusikaupunki
  Finland **32** B7
Nysted *Denmark* **11** K5
Nyunzu *Dem. Rep. of the Congo* **86** D2
Nyurba *Russia* **53** C12
Nyzhankovychi *Ukraine* **31** J9
Nyzhnohirskyy *Ukraine* **33** K8
Nyzhny Vorota *Ukraine* **28** B8
Nzébéla *Guinea* **82** D3
Nzega *Tanzania* **86** C3
Nzérékoré *Guinea* **82** D3
Nzeto *Angola* **84** F2
Nzilo, Chutes de
  Dem. Rep. of the Congo **87** E2
N'zo ➤ *Ivory C.* **82** D3
N'zo △ *Ivory C.* **82** D3
Nzubuka *Tanzania* **86** C3
Nzwani = Anjouan
  Comoros Is. **85** a

O

O Barco *Spain* **36** C4
O Carballiño *Spain* **36** C2
O Corgo *Spain* **36** C3
O Le Pupū Pu'e △ *Samoa* **91** b
O Pino *Spain* **36** C2
O Porriño *Spain* **36** C2
Ō-Shima *Hokkaidō, Japan* **54** D9
Ō-Shima *Shizuoka, Japan* **55** G9
Oa, Mull of *U.K.* **13** F2
Oacoma *U.S.A.* **112** D4
Oahe, L. *U.S.A.* **112** C3
Oahe Dam *U.S.A.* **112** C3
O'ahu *U.S.A.* **107** L8
Oak Harbor *U.S.A.* **110** B4
Oak Hill *U.S.A.* **113** G13
Oak Island *U.S.A.* **117** E15
Oak Ridge *U.S.A.* **117** C12
Oak View *U.S.A.* **111** L7
Oakan-Dake *Japan* **54** C12
Oakdale *Calif., U.S.A.* **110** H6
Oakdale *La., U.S.A.* **116** F8
Oakes *U.S.A.* **112** B4
Oakesdale *U.S.A.* **108** C5
Oakey *Australia* **95** D5
Oakfield *U.S.A.* **114** C6
Oakham *U.K.* **15** E7
Oakhurst *U.S.A.* **110** H7
Oakland *Calif., U.S.A.* **110** H4
Oakland *Pa., U.S.A.* **115** E9
Oakley *Idaho, U.S.A.* **108** E7
Oakley *Kans., U.S.A.* **112** F3
Oakover ➤ *Australia* **92** D3
Oakridge *U.S.A.* **108** E2
Oakville *Canada* **114** C5
Oakville *U.S.A.* **110** D3
Oamaru *N.Z.* **91** F3
Oancea *Romania* **29** E12
Oasi Faunistica di
  Vendicari △ *Italy* **43** F8
Oasis *Calif., U.S.A.* **110** H9
Oasis *Calif., U.S.A.* **111** M10
Oates Land *Antarctica* **5** C11
Oatman *U.S.A.* **111** K12
Oaxaca *Mexico* **119** D5
Oaxaca □ *Mexico* **119** D5
Ob ➤ *Russia* **52** C7
Oba *Canada* **104** C3
Obala *Cameroon* **83** E7
Obama *Japan* **55** G7
Oban *Nigeria* **83** D6
Oban *U.K.* **13** E3
Obbia = Hobyo *Somali Rep.* **75** F4
Oberá *Argentina* **127** B4
Oberammergau *Germany* **25** H7
Oberasbach *Germany* **25** F6
Oberbayern □ *Germany* **25** G7
Oberdrauburg *Austria* **26** E5

Obere Donau △ *Germany* **25** G5
Oberer Bayerischer
  Wald △ *Germany* **25** F8
Oberfranken □ *Germany* **25** E7
Oberhausen *Germany* **24** D2
Oberkirch *Germany* **25** G4
Oberlausitz *Germany* **24** D10
Oberlin *Kans., U.S.A.* **112** F3
Oberlin *La., U.S.A.* **116** F8
Oberlin *Ohio, U.S.A.* **114** E2
Obernai *France* **19** D14
Oberndorf *Germany* **25** G4
Oberon *Australia* **95** E4
Oberösterreich □ *Austria* **26** C7
Oberpfalz □ *Germany* **25** F8
Oberpfälzer Wald *Germany* **25** F8
Oberpfälzer Wald △ *Germany* **25** F8
Oberstdorf *Germany* **25** H6
Obertyn *Ukraine* **29** B10
Oberursel *Germany* **25** E4
Oberwart *Austria* **27** D9
Obi, Kepulauan *Indonesia* **63** E7
Obiaruku *Nigeria* **83** D6
Óbidos *Brazil* **125** D7
Óbidos *Portugal* **37** F1
Obihiro *Japan* **54** C11
Obilatu *Indonesia* **63** E7
Obilnoye *Russia* **35** G7
Obing *Germany* **25** G8
Objat *France* **20** C5
Obluchye *Russia* **53** E14
Obninsk *Russia* **32** E9
Obo *C.A.R.* **86** A2
Obock *Djibouti* **81** E5
Obodivka *Ukraine* **29** B14
Oborniki *Poland* **31** F3
Oborniki Śląskie *Poland* **31** G3
Oboyan *Russia* **33** G9
Obozerskaya = Obozerskiy
  Russia **52** C5
Obozerskiy *Russia* **52** C5
Obrenovac *Serbia* **44** B4
Obrovac *Croatia* **41** D12
Obruk *Turkey* **72** C5
Obrzycko *Poland* **31** F3
Observatory Inlet *Canada* **102** B3
Obshchi Syrt *Russia* **6** E16
Obskaya Guba *Russia* **52** C8
Obuasi *Ghana* **83** D4
Obubra *Nigeria* **83** D6
Obudu *Nigeria* **83** D6
Obwalden □ *Switz.* **25** J4
Obzor *Bulgaria* **45** D11
Ocala *U.S.A.* **117** G13
Ocampo *Chihuahua, Mexico* **118** B3
Ocampo *Tamaulipas, Mexico* **119** C5
Ocaña *Spain* **36** F7
Occidental, Cordillera
  Colombia **124** C3
Occidental, Grand Erg
  Algeria **78** B6
Ocean City *Md., U.S.A.* **113** F16
Ocean City *N.J., U.S.A.* **113** F16
Ocean City *Wash., U.S.A.* **110** C2
Ocean Falls *Canada* **102** C3
Ocean I. = Banaba *Kiribati* **96** H8
Ocean Park *U.S.A.* **110** D2
Oceano *U.S.A.* **111** K6
Oceanport *U.S.A.* **115** F10
Oceanside *U.S.A.* **111** M9
Ochagavía *Spain* **38** C3
Ochakiv *Ukraine* **33** J6
Ochamchira *Georgia* **35** J5
Ochi, Oros *Greece* **46** D6
Ochil Hills *U.K.* **13** E5
Ocho Rios *Jamaica* **120** a
Ochsenfurt *Germany* **25** F6
Ochsenhausen *Germany* **25** G5
Ocilla *U.S.A.* **117** F13
Ockelbo *Sweden* **10** D10
Ocmulgee ➤ *U.S.A.* **117** F13
Ocna Mureş *Romania* **29** D8
Ocna Sibiului *Romania* **29** E9
Ocnele Mari *Romania* **29** E9
Ocniţa *Moldova* **29** B12
Oconee ➤ *U.S.A.* **117** F13
Oconomowoc *U.S.A.* **112** D9
Oconto *U.S.A.* **112** C10
Oconto Falls *U.S.A.* **112** C10
Ocosingo *Mexico* **119** D6
Ocotal *Nic.* **120** D2
Ocotlán *Jalisco, Mexico* **118** C4
Ocotlán *Oaxaca, Mexico* **119** D5
Ocreza ➤ *Portugal* **37** F3
Ócsa *Hungary* **28** C4
Octeville *France* **18** C5
Oda *Ghana* **83** D4
Ōda *Japan* **55** G6
Oda, J. *Sudan* **80** C4
Ódáðahraun *Iceland* **8** D5
Ōdaejin *N. Korea* **57** D15
Ödåkra *Sweden* **11** H6
Odate *Japan* **54** D10
Odawara *Japan* **55** G9
Odda *Norway* **9** F12
Odder *Denmark* **11** J4
Odei ➤ *Canada* **103** B9
Odemira *Portugal* **37** H2
Ödemiş *Turkey* **47** C9
Odendaalsrus *S. Africa* **88** D4

Odensbacken *Sweden* **10** E9
Odense *Denmark* **11** J4
Odenwald = Neckartal-
  Odenwald *Germany* **25** F5
Odenwald *Germany* **25** F5
Oder ➤ *Europe* **24** B10
Oder-Havel Kanal *Germany* **24** C10
Oderzo *Italy* **41** C9
Odesa *Ukraine* **33** J5
Odesa □ *Ukraine* **33** J5
Ödeshög *Sweden* **11** F8
Odessa = Odesa *Ukraine* **33** J6
Odessa *Canada* **115** B8
Odessa *Tex., U.S.A.* **116** F3
Odessa *Wash., U.S.A.* **108** C4
Odiakwe *Botswana* **88** C4
Odiel ➤ *Spain* **37** H4
Odienné *Ivory C.* **82** D3
Odintsovo *Russia* **32** E9
Odiongan *Phil.* **61** E4
Odobești *Romania* **29** E12
Odolanów *Poland* **31** G4
O'Donnell *U.S.A.* **116** E4
O'Donnell Pt. *Canada* **114** A4
Odorheiu Secuiesc *Romania* **29** D10
Odoyevo *Russia* **32** F9
Odra = Oder ➤ *Europe* **24** B10
Odra ➤ *Spain* **36** C6
Odžaci *Serbia* **28** E4
Odžak *Bos.-H.* **28** E3
Odzi *Zimbabwe* **89** B5
Odzi ➤ *Zimbabwe* **89** B5
Oebisfelde *Germany* **24** C6
Oeiras *Brazil* **125** E10
Oeiras *Portugal* **37** G1
Oelrichs *U.S.A.* **112** D2
Oelsnitz *Germany* **25** E8
Oelwein *U.S.A.* **112** D8
Oeno □ *Pac. Oc.* **97** K14
Oenpelli = Gunbalanya
  Australia **92** B5
Oetz *Austria* **26** D3
Of *Turkey* **73** B9
Ofanto ➤ *Italy* **43** A9
Offa *Nigeria* **83** D5
Offaly □ *Ireland* **12** C4
Offenbach *Germany* **25** E4
Offenburg *Germany* **25** G3
Officer Cr. ➤ *Australia* **93** E5
Offida *Italy* **41** F10
Ofidousa *Greece* **47** E8
Ofolanga *Tonga* **91** c
Ofotfjorden *Norway* **8** B17
Ofu *Amer. Samoa* **91** b
Ōfunato *Japan* **54** E10
Oga *Japan* **54** E9
Oga-Hantō *Japan* **54** E9
Ogaden *Ethiopia* **75** F3
Ōgaki *Japan* **55** G8
Ogallala *U.S.A.* **112** E3
Ogasawara Gunto *Pac. Oc.* **51** F16
Ogbomosho *Nigeria* **83** D5
Ogden *U.S.A.* **108** F8
Ogdensburg *U.S.A.* **115** B9
Ogea Driki *Fiji* **91** a
Ogea Levu *Fiji* **91** a
Ogeechee ➤ *U.S.A.* **117** F14
Ogilby *U.S.A.* **111** N12
Oglio ➤ *Italy* **40** C7
Óglio Nord △ *Italy* **40** C6
Óglio Sud △ *Italy* **40** C7
Ogmore *Australia* **94** C4
Ognon ➤ *France* **19** E12
Ogoja *Nigeria* **83** D6
Ogoki *Canada* **104** B2
Ogoki ➤ *Canada* **104** B2
Ogoki L. *Canada* **104** B2
Ogoki Res. *Canada* **104** B2
Ogooué ➤ *Gabon* **84** E1
Ogowe = Ogooué ➤ *Gabon* **84** E1
Ogr = Sharafa *Sudan* **81** E2
Ográzden *Macedonia* **44** E6
Ogre *Latvia* **32** D3
Ogrein *Sudan* **80** D3
Ogulin *Croatia* **41** C12
Ogun □ *Nigeria* **83** D5
Ogurchinskiy, Ostrov
  Turkmenistan **71** B7
Oguta *Nigeria* **83** D6
Oğuzeli *Turkey* **72** D7
Ogwashi-Uku *Nigeria* **83** D6
Ogwe *Nigeria* **83** E6
Ohai *N.Z.* **91** F2
Ohakune *N.Z.* **91** C5
Ohata *Japan* **54** D10
Ohau, L. *N.Z.* **91** F2
Ohio □ *U.S.A.* **114** F2
Ohio ➤ *U.S.A.* **112** G9
Ohře ➤ *Czech Rep.* **26** A7
Ohre ➤ *Germany* **24** C7
Ohrid *Macedonia* **44** E4
Ohridsko Jezero *Macedonia* **44** E4
Ohrigstad *S. Africa* **89** C5
Oi Qu *China* **58** C2
Oiapoque *Brazil* **125**
Oikou *China* **57** E9
Oil City *U.S.A.* **114** E5

Oil Springs *Canada* **114** D2
Oildale *U.S.A.* **111** K7
Oinousa = Inousses *Greece* **47** C8
Oise □ *France* **19** C9
Oise ➤ *France* **19** C9
Oiseaux du Djoudj △ *Senegal* **82** B1
Oistins *Barbados* **121** g
Oistins B. *Barbados* **121** g
Ōita *Japan* **55** H5
Ōita □ *Japan* **55** H5
Oiticica *Brazil* **125** E10
Ojai *U.S.A.* **111** L7
Ojcowski △ *Poland* **31** H6
Ojinaga *Mexico* **118** B4
Ojiya *Japan* **55** F9
Ojo Caliente *Mexico* **118** C4
Ojo de Liebre, L. *Mexico* **118** B2
Ojos del Salado, Cerro
  Argentina **126** B2
Oka *Nigeria* **83** D5
Oka ➤ *Russia* **34** B7
Okaba *Indonesia* **63** F9
Okahandja *Namibia* **88** C2
Okanagan L. *Canada* **102** D5
Okandja *Gabon* **84** E2
Okanogan *U.S.A.* **108** B4
Okanogan ➤ *U.S.A.* **108** B4
Okanogan Range *N. Amer.* **102** D5
Okány *Hungary* **28** D6
Okapi △
  Dem. Rep. of the Congo **86** B2
Okaputa *Namibia* **88** C2
Okara *Pakistan* **68** D5
Okaukuejo *Namibia* **88** B2
Okavango Delta *Botswana* **88** B3
Okavango Swamp =
  Okavango Delta *Botswana* **88** B3
Okaya *Japan* **55** F9
Okayama *Japan* **55** G6
Okayama □ *Japan* **55** G6
Okazaki *Japan* **55** G8
Oke-Iho *Nigeria* **83** D5
Okecie, Warszawa ✈
  (WAW) *Poland* **31** F7
Okeechobee *U.S.A.* **117** H14
Okeechobee, L. *U.S.A.* **117** H14
Okefenokee △ *U.S.A.* **117** F13
Okefenokee Swamp △ *U.S.A.* **117** F13
Okehampton *U.K.* **15** G4
Okene *Nigeria* **83** D6
Okha *India* **68** H3
Okha *Russia* **53** D15
Okhotsk *Russia* **53** D15
Okhotsk, Sea of *Asia* **53** D15
Okhotskiy Perevoz *Russia* **53** C14
Okhtyrka *Ukraine* **33** G8
Oki-Shotō *Japan* **55** F6
Okiep *S. Africa* **88** D2
Okigwi *Nigeria* **83** D6
Okija *Nigeria* **83** D6
Okinawa *Japan* **55** L3
Okinawa □ *Japan* **55** L4
Okinawa-Guntō *Japan* **55** L4
Okinawa-Jima *Japan* **55** L4
Okino-erabu-Shima *Japan* **55** L4
Okitipupa *Nigeria* **83** D5
Oklahoma □ *U.S.A.* **116** D6
Oklahoma City *U.S.A.* **116** D6
Okmulgee *U.S.A.* **116** D7
Oknitsa = Ocniţa *Moldova* **29** B12
Oko, W. ➤ *Sudan* **80** C4
Okolo *Uganda* **86** B3
Okolona *U.S.A.* **117** E10
Okombahe *Namibia* **88** C2
Okonek *Poland* **30** E3
Okotoks *Canada* **102** C6
Okrika *Nigeria* **83** E6
Oksibil *Indonesia* **63** E10
Oktyabrsk = Qandyaghash
  Kazakhstan **52** E6
Oktyabrsk *Russia* **34** D9
Oktyabrskiy = Aktsyabrski
  Belarus **23** B15
Oktyabrskiy *Kamchatka,*
  Russia **53** D16
Oktyabrskiy *Rostov, Russia* **35** G5
Oktyabrskoy Revolyutsii,
  Ostrov *Russia* **53** B10
Oktyabrskoye = Zhovtneve
  Ukraine **33** J7
Okulovka *Russia* **32** C7
Okuru *N.Z.* **91** E2
Okushiri-Tō *Japan* **54** C9
Okuta *Nigeria* **83** D5
Okwa ➤ *Botswana* **88** C3
Ola *Russia* **53** D16
Ólafsfjörður *Iceland* **8** C4
Ólafsvík *Iceland* **8** D2
Olaine *Latvia* **30** D3
Olancha *U.S.A.* **111** J8
Olancha Pk. *U.S.A.* **111** J8
Olanchito *Honduras* **120** C2
Öland *Sweden* **11** H10
Ölands norra udde *Sweden* **11** G11
Ölands södra udde *Sweden* **11** H10
Olargues *France* **20** E6
Olary *Australia* **95** E3
Olascoaga *Argentina* **126** D3

Olathe *U.S.A.* **112** F6
Olavarría *Argentina* **126** D3
Oława *Poland* **31** H4
Olbernhau *Germany* **24** E9
Ólbia *Italy* **42** B2
Ólbia, G. di *Italy* **42** B2
Olching *Germany* **25** G7
Olcott *U.S.A.* **114** C6
Old Bahama Chan. =
  Bahama, Canal Viejo de
  W. Indies **120** B4
Old Baldy Pk. = San
  Antonio, Mt. *U.S.A.* **111** L9
Old Bridge *U.S.A.* **115** F10
Old Castile = Castilla y
  Leon □ *Spain* **36** D6
Old Crow *Canada* **100** D4
Old Dale *U.S.A.* **111** L11
Old Forge *N.Y., U.S.A.* **115** C10
Old Forge *Pa., U.S.A.* **115** E9
Old Mapoon ☼ *Australia* **94** A3
Old Perlican *Canada* **105** C9
Old Shinyanga *Tanzania* **86** C3
Old Speck Mt. *U.S.A.* **115** B14
Old Town *U.S.A.* **113** C19
Old Washington *U.S.A.* **114** F3
Old Wives L. *Canada* **103** C7
Oldbury *U.K.* **15** F5
Oldcastle *Ireland* **12** C4
Oldeani *Tanzania* **86** C4
Oldenburg *Niedersachsen,*
  Germany **24** B4
Oldenburg
  Schleswig-Holstein, Germany **24** A6
Oldenzaal *Neths.* **17** B6
Oldham *U.K.* **14** D5
Oldman ➤ *Canada* **102** D6
Oldmeldrum *U.K.* **13** D6
Olds *Canada* **102** C6
Olduvai Gorge *Tanzania* **86** C4
Oldziyt *Mongolia* **56** B5
Olean *U.S.A.* **114** D6
Olecko *Poland* **30** D9
Oléggio *Italy* **40** C5
Oleiros *Portugal* **36** F3
Oleiros *Spain* **36** B2
Olekma ➤ *Russia* **53** C13
Olekminsk *Russia* **53** C13
Oleksandriya *Kirovohrad,*
  Ukraine **33** H7
Oleksandriya *Rivne, Ukraine* **23** C14
Oleksandrovka *Ukraine* **33** H7
Olema *U.S.A.* **110** G4
Olenegorsk *Russia* **8** B25
Olenek *Russia* **53** C12
Olenek ➤ *Russia* **53** B13
Olenino *Russia* **32** D7
Oléron, Î. d' *France* **20** C2
Olesk *Ukraine* **31** G11
Oleśnica *Poland* **31** G4
Olesno *Poland* **31** H5
Olevsk *Ukraine* **23** C14
Olga, L. *Canada* **104** C4
Olgas, The = Kata Tjuta
  Australia **93** E5
Ölgiy *Mongolia* **52** E9
Ølgod *Denmark* **11** J2
Olhão *Portugal* **37** H3
Olhopil *Ukraine* **29** B14
Olhovatka *Russia* **30** D9
Olib *Croatia* **41** D11
Oliena *Italy* **42** B2
Oliete *Spain* **38** D4
Olifants = Elefantes ➤ *Africa* **89** C5
Olifants ➤ *Namibia* **88** C2
Olifantshoek *S. Africa* **88** D3
Olimbos *Greece* **47** F9
Olímpia *Brazil* **127** A6
Olimpos-Beydaglari △
  Turkey **47** E12
Olinda *Brazil* **125** E12
Olite *Spain* **38** C3
Oliva *Argentina* **126** C3
Oliva *Spain* **39** G4
Oliva, Punta del *Spain* **36** B5
Oliva de la Frontera *Spain* **37** G4
Olivares, Cerro los *Argentina* **126** C2
Olivares de Júcar *Spain* **38** F2
Olive Branch *U.S.A.* **117** D10
Olivehurst *U.S.A.* **110** G5
Oliveira de Azeméis *Portugal* **36** E2
Oliveira do Douro *Portugal* **36** D2
Olivenza *Spain* **37** G3
Oliver *Canada* **102** D5
Oliver L. *Canada* **103** B8
Olivet *France* **19** E8
Olkhovka *Russia* **34** F7
Olkusz *Poland* **31** H6
Ollagüe *Chile* **126** A2
Olmaliq *Uzbekistan* **52** E7
Olmedo *Spain* **36** D6
Olmeto *France* **21** G12
Olney *Ill., U.S.A.* **112** F9
Olney *Tex., U.S.A.* **116** E5
Olofström *Sweden* **11** H8
Oloitokitok *Kenya* **86** C4
Oloma *Cameroon* **83** E7
Olomane ➤ *Canada* **105** B7

Olomouc *Czech Rep.* **27** B10
Olomoucký □ *Czech Rep.* **27** B10
Olonets *Russia* **32** B7
Olongapo *Phil.* **61** D4
Olonne-sur-Mer *France* **20** B2
Oloron, Gave d' ➤ *France* **20** E3
Oloron-Ste-Marie *France* **20** E3
Olosega *Amer. Samoa* **91** b
Olosenga = Swains I.
  Amer. Samoa **97** J11
Olot *Spain* **38** C7
Olovo *Bos.-H.* **28** F3
Olovyannaya *Russia* **53** D12
Oloy ➤ *Russia* **53** C16
Olsberg *Germany* **24** D4
Olshammar *Sweden* **11** F8
Olshanka *Ukraine* **33** H6
Olshany *Ukraine* **33** G8
Olsztyn *Poland* **30** E7
Olsztynek *Poland* **30** E7
Olt □ *Romania* **29** F9
Olt ➤ *Romania* **29** G9
Olten *Switz.* **25** H3
Olteniţa *Romania* **29** F11
Olton *U.S.A.* **116** D3
Oltu *Turkey* **73** B10
Oluan Pi *Taiwan* **59** G13
Olula del Rio *Spain* **39** H2
Olur *Turkey* **73** B10
Olutanga *Phil.* **61** H5
Olvega *Spain* **38** D2
Olvera *Spain* **37** J5
Olymbos *Cyprus* **49** D12
Olymbos Oros *Greece* **44** F6
Olympia *Greece* **46** D3
Olympia *U.S.A.* **110** D4
Olympic △ *U.S.A.* **110** C3
Olympic Dam *Australia* **95** E2
Olympic Mts. *U.S.A.* **110** C3
Olympus *Cyprus* **49** E11
Olympus, Mt. = Olymbos
  Oros *Greece* **44** F6
Olympus, Mt. = Uludağ
  Turkey **45** F13
Olympus, Mt. *U.S.A.* **110** C3
Olyphant *U.S.A.* **115** E9
Olyutorskiy, Mys *Russia* **53** D18
Om ➤ *Russia* **52** D8
Om Hajer *Eritrea* **81** E4
Om Koi *Thailand* **64** D2
Ōma *Japan* **54** D10
Ōmachi *Japan* **55** F8
Omae-Zaki *Japan* **55** G9
Ōmagari *Japan* **54** E10
Omagh *U.K.* **12** B4
Omagh □ *U.K.* **12** B4
Omaha *U.S.A.* **112** E6
Omak *U.S.A.* **108** B4
Omalos *Greece* **49** D5
Oman ■ *Asia* **75** C6
Oman, G. of *Asia* **71** E8
Omaruru *Namibia* **88** C2
Omaruru ➤ *Namibia* **88** C1
Omate *Peru* **124** G4
Ombai, Selat *Indonesia* **63** F6
Omboué *Gabon* **84** E1
Ombrone ➤ *Italy* **40** F8
Omdurmân *Sudan* **81** D3
Omegna *Italy* **40** C5
Omemee *Canada* **114** B6
Omeonga
  Dem. Rep. of the Congo **86** C1
Ometepe, I. de *Nic.* **120** D2
Ometepec *Mexico* **119** D5
Ominato *Japan* **54** D10
Omineca ➤ *Canada* **102** B4
Omineca Mts. *Canada* **102** B3
Omiš *Croatia* **41** E13
Omišalj *Croatia* **41** C11
Omitara *Namibia* **88** C2
Ōmiya = Saitama *Japan* **55** G9
Omme Å ➤ *Denmark* **11** J2
Ommen *Neths.* **17** B6
Ömnögovi □ *Mongolia* **56** C3
Omo ➤ *Ethiopia* **81** F4
Omo △ *Ethiopia* **81** F4
Omo Valley *Ethiopia* **81** F4
Omodeo, L. *Italy* **42** B1
Omodhos *Cyprus* **49** E11
Omoko *Nigeria* **83** D6
Omolon ➤ *Russia* **53** C16
Omono-Gawa ➤ *Japan* **54** E10
Ompha *Canada* **115** B8
Omsk *Russia* **52** D8
Omsukchan *Russia* **53** C16
Ōmu *Japan* **54** B11
Omul, Vf. *Romania* **29** E10
Omulew ➤ *Poland* **31** E8
Ōmura *Japan* **55** H4
Omuramba Omatako ➤
  Namibia **88** B2
Omuramba Ovambo ➤
  Namibia **88** B2
Omurtag *Bulgaria* **45** C10
Ōmuta *Japan* **55** H5
Oña *Spain* **36** C7
Onaga *U.S.A.* **112** F6
Onalaska *U.S.A.* **112** D8
Onancock *U.S.A.* **113** G16
Onang *Indonesia* **63** E5

Onangue, L. *Gabon* **84** E2
Onaping L. *Canada* **104** C3
Oñati *Spain* **38** B2
Onavas *Mexico* **118** B3
Onawa *U.S.A.* **112** D5
Oncócua *Angola* **88** B1
Onda *Spain* **38** F4
Ondangwa *Namibia* **88** B2
Ondarroa *Spain* **38** B2
Ondava → *Slovak Rep.* **27** C14
Ondjiva *Angola* **88** B2
Ondo *Nigeria* **83** D5
Ondo □ *Nigeria* **83** D6
Öndörshil *Mongolia* **56** B5
Öndverðarnes *Iceland* **8** D2
One Arm Point *Australia* **92** C3
One Arm Point ○ *Australia* **92** C3
One Tree *Australia* **95** E3
Oneata *Fiji* **91** a
Onega *Russia* **52** C4
Onega → *Russia* **6** C13
Onega, L. = Onezhskoye
  Ozero *Russia* **32** B8
Oneida *U.S.A.* **115** C9
Oneida L. *U.S.A.* **115** C9
O'Neill *U.S.A.* **112** D4
Onekotan, Ostrov *Russia* **53** E16
Onema *Dem. Rep. of the Congo* **86** C1
Oneonta *U.S.A.* **115** D9
Oneşti *Romania* **29** D11
Onezhskoye Ozero *Russia* **32** B8
Ongarue *N.Z.* **91** C5
Ongea Levu = Ogea Levu *Fiji* **91** a
Ongers → *S. Africa* **88** E3
Ongerup *Australia* **93** F2
Ongjin *N. Korea* **57** F13
Ongkharak *Thailand* **64** E3
Ongniud Qi *China* **57** C10
Ongoka *Dem. Rep. of the Congo* **86** C2
Ongole *India* **66** M12
Ongon = Havirga *Mongolia* **56** B7
Oni *Georgia* **35** J6
Onida *U.S.A.* **112** C3
Onilahy → *Madag.* **89** C7
Onitsha *Nigeria* **83** D6
Ono *Fiji* **91** a
Onoda *Japan* **55** G5
Ons, I. de *Spain* **36** C2
Onsala *Sweden* **11** G6
Onslow *Australia* **92** D2
Onslow B. *U.S.A.* **117** D16
Ontake-San *Japan* **55** G8
Ontario *Calif., U.S.A.* **111** L9
Ontario *Oreg., U.S.A.* **108** D5
Ontario □ *Canada* **104** B2
Ontario, L. *N. Amer.* **114** C7
Ontinyent *Spain* **39** G4
Ontonagon *U.S.A.* **112** B9
Ontur *Spain* **39** G3
Onyx *U.S.A.* **111** K8
Oodnadatta *Australia* **95** D2
Ooldea *Australia* **93** F5
Oombulgurri *Australia* **92** C4
Oombulgurri ○ *Australia* **92** C4
Oorindi *Australia* **94** C3
Oost-Vlaanderen □ *Belgium* **17** C3
Oostende *Belgium* **17** C2
Oosterhout *Neths.* **17** C4
Oosterschelde → *Neths.* **17** C4
Oosterwolde *Neths.* **17** B6
Ootacamund =
  Udagamandalam *India* **66** P10
Ootsa L. *Canada* **102** C3
Ooty = Udagamandalam
  India **66** P10
Op Luang △ *Thailand* **64** C2
Opaka *Bulgaria* **45** C10
Opala *Dem. Rep. of the Congo* **86** C1
Opalenica *Poland* **31** F3
Opan *Bulgaria* **45** D9
Opanake *Sri Lanka* **66** R12
Opasatika *Canada* **104** C3
Opasquia △ *Canada* **104** B1
Opatija *Croatia* **41** C11
Opatów *Poland* **31** H8
Opava *Czech Rep.* **27** B10
Opelika *U.S.A.* **117** E12
Opelousas *U.S.A.* **116** F8
Opémisca, L. *Canada* **104** C5
Opheim *U.S.A.* **108** B10
Ophthalmia Ra. *Australia* **92** D2
Opi *Nigeria* **83** D6
Opinaca → *Canada* **104** B4
Opinaca, Rés. *Canada* **104** B4
Opinnagau → *Canada* **104** B3
Opiscotéo, L. *Canada* **105** B6
Opobo *Nigeria* **83** E6
Opochka *Russia* **32** D5
Opoczno *Poland* **31** G7
Opol *Phil.* **61** G6
Opole *Poland* **31** H4
Opole Lubelskie *Poland* **31** G8
Opolskie □ *Poland* **31** H5
Oponono L. *Namibia* **88** B2
Oporto = Porto *Portugal* **36** D2
Opotiki *N.Z.* **91** C6
Opp *U.S.A.* **117** F11
Oppdal *Norway* **8** E13
Óppido Mamertina *Italy* **43** D8
Opportunity *U.S.A.* **108** C5

Oprişor *Romania* **28** F8
Oprtalj *Croatia* **41** C10
Opua *N.Z.* **91** A5
Opunake *N.Z.* **91** C4
Opuwo *Namibia* **88** B1
Opuzen *Croatia* **41** E14
Ora *Cyprus* **49** E12
Oracle *U.S.A.* **109** K8
Oradea *Romania* **28** D6
Öræfajökull *Iceland* **8** D5
Orahovac *Kosovo* **44** D4
Orahovica *Croatia* **28** E2
Orai *India* **69** G8
Oraison *France* **21** E9
Oral = Zhayyq → *Kazakhstan* **6** F16
Oral *Kazakhstan* **34** E10
Oran *Algeria* **78** A5
Orange *Australia* **95** E4
Orange *France* **21** D8
Orange *Calif., U.S.A.* **111** M9
Orange *Mass., U.S.A.* **115** D12
Orange *Tex., U.S.A.* **116** F8
Orange *Va., U.S.A.* **113** F14
Orange → *S. Africa* **88** D2
Orange, C. *Brazil* **125** C8
Orange Cove *U.S.A.* **110** J7
Orange Free State = Free
  State □ *S. Africa* **88** D4
Orange Grove *U.S.A.* **116** H6
Orange Walk *Belize* **119** D7
Orangeburg *U.S.A.* **117** E14
Orangeville *Canada* **114** C4
Orango *Guinea-Biss.* **82** C1
Orani *Phil.* **61** D4
Oranienburg *Germany* **24** C9
Oranje = Orange → *S. Africa* **88** D2
Oranjemund *Namibia* **88** D2
Oranjerivier *S. Africa* **88** D3
Oranjestad *Aruba* **121** D5
Orapa *Botswana* **85** J5
Oras *Phil.* **61** E6
Orašje *Bos.-H.* **28** E3
Orăştie *Romania* **29** E8
Orava → *Slovak Rep.* **27** B12
Orava, Vodna nádrž
  Slovak Rep. **27** B12
Oraviţa *Romania* **28** E6
Orb → *France* **20** E7
Orba → *Italy* **40** D5
Ørbæk *Denmark* **11** J4
Orbe *Switz.* **25** J2
Orbec *France* **18** C7
Orbetello *Italy* **41** F8
Órbigo → *Spain* **36** C5
Orbisonia *U.S.A.* **114** F7
Orbost *Australia* **95** F4
Örbyhus *Sweden* **10** D11
Orcadas *Antarctica* **5** C18
Orcas I. *U.S.A.* **110** B4
Orce *Spain* **39** H2
Orce → *Spain* **39** H2
Orchard City *U.S.A.* **108** G10
Orchard Homes *U.S.A.* **108** C6
Orchid I. = Lan Yü *Taiwan* **59** F13
Orchies *France* **19** B10
Orchila, I. *Venezuela* **121** D6
Orchilla, Pta. *Canary Is.* **48** G1
Órcia → *Italy* **41** F8
Orco → *Italy* **40** C4
Orcutt *U.S.A.* **111** L6
Ord *U.S.A.* **112** E4
Ord → *Australia* **92** C4
Ord, Mt. *Australia* **92** C4
Ord Mts. *U.S.A.* **111** L10
Ordenes = Ordes *Spain* **36** B2
Orderville *U.S.A.* **109** H7
Ordes *Spain* **36** B2
Ordesa y Monte Perido △
  Spain **38** C4
Ording = St-Peter-Ording
  Germany **24** A4
Ordos = Mu Us Shamo *China* **56** E5
Ordu *Turkey* **72** B7
Ordu □ *Turkey* **72** B7
Ordubad *Azerbaijan* **73** C12
Orduña *Álava, Spain* **38** C2
Orduña *Granada, Spain* **37** H7
Ordway *U.S.A.* **108** G12
Ordzhonīkīdze *Ukraine* **33** J8
Ore *Dem. Rep. of the Congo* **86** B2
Ore Mts. = Erzgebirge
  Germany **24** E8
Orebić *Croatia* **41** F14
Örebro *Sweden* **10** E9
Örebro län □ *Sweden* **10** E8
Orecchiella △ *Italy* **40** D7
Oregon *U.S.A.* **112** D9
Oregon □ *U.S.A.* **108** E3
Oregon City *U.S.A.* **110** E4
Oregon Dunes △ *U.S.A.* **108** E1
Öregrund *Sweden* **10** D12
Öregrundsgrepen *Sweden* **10** D12
Orekhov = Orikhiv *Ukraine* **33** J8
Orekhovo-Zuyevo *Russia* **32** B10
Orel *Russia* **33** F9
Orel □ *Russia* **33** F9
Orel → *Ukraine* **33** H8
Orellana, Canal de *Spain* **37** F5
Orellana, Embalse de *Spain* **37** F5
Orellana la Vieja *Spain* **37** F5

Orem *U.S.A.* **108** F8
Ören *Turkey* **47** D9
Örencik *Turkey* **47** B11
Orenburg *Russia* **52** D6
Orense = Ourense *Spain* **36** C3
Orepuki *N.Z.* **91** G1
Orestes Pereyra *Mexico* **118** B3
Orestiada *Greece* **45** E10
Øresund *Europe* **11** J6
Orfanos Kolpos *Greece* **44** F7
Orford Ness *U.K.* **15** E9
Organ Pipe Cactus △ *U.S.A.* **109** K7
Organos, Pta. de los
  Canary Is. **48** F2
Organyà *Spain* **38** C6
Orgaz *Spain* **37** F7
Orgeyev = Orhei *Moldova* **29** C13
Orhaneli *Turkey* **45** G12
Orhaneli → *Turkey* **45** G12
Orhangazi *Turkey* **45** F13
Orhei *Moldova* **29** C13
Orhon Gol → *Mongolia* **53** D11
Ória *Italy* **43** B10
Oriental, Cordillera
  Colombia **124** B4
Oriental, Grand Erg *Algeria* **78** B7
Orientale □
  Dem. Rep. of the Congo **86** B2
Oriente *Argentina* **126** D3
Orihuela *Spain* **39** G4
Orihuela del Tremedal *Spain* **38** E3
Orikhiv *Ukraine* **33** J8
Orikum *Albania* **44** F3
Orillia *Canada* **114** B5
Orinoco → *Venezuela* **124** B6
Orion *Canada* **103** D6
Oriskany *U.S.A.* **115** C9
Orissa □ *India* **67** K14
Orissaare *Estonia* **32** C2
Oristano *Italy* **42** C1
Oristano, G. di *Italy* **42** C1
Orizaba *Mexico* **119** D5
Orizare *Bulgaria* **45** D11
Orjen *Bos.-H.* **44** D2
Orjiva *Spain* **37** J7
Orkanger *Norway* **8** E13
Örkelljunga *Sweden* **11** H7
Örken *Sweden* **11** G9
Örkény *Hungary* **28** C4
Orkla → *Norway* **8** E13
Orkney *S. Africa* **88** D4
Orkney □ *U.K.* **13** B5
Orkney Is. *U.K.* **13** B6
Orland *U.S.A.* **110** F4
Orlando *U.S.A.* **117** G14
Orlando, C. d' *Italy* **43** D7
Orléanais *France* **19** E9
Orléans *France* **19** E8
Orleans *U.S.A.* **115** B12
Orléans, Î. d' *Canada* **105** C5
Orlice → *Czech Rep.* **26** A8
Orlivka *Ukraine* **29** E13
Orlov *Slovak Rep.* **27** B13
Orlov Gay *Russia* **34** E9
Orlová *Czech Rep.* **27** B11
Orlovat *Serbia* **28** E5
Ormara *Pakistan* **66** G4
Ormea *Italy* **40** D4
Ormília *Greece* **44** F7
Ormoc *Phil.* **61** F6
Ormond *N.Z.* **91** C6
Ormond Beach *U.S.A.* **117** G14
Ormož *Slovenia* **41** B13
Ormskirk *U.K.* **14** D5
Ormstown *Canada* **115** A11
Ornans *France* **19** E13
Orne □ *France* **18** D7
Orne → *France* **18** C6
Orneta *Poland* **30** D7
Ornö *Sweden* **10** E12
Örnsköldsvik *Sweden* **10** A12
Oro *N. Korea* **57** D14
Oro → *Mexico* **118** B3
Oro Grande *U.S.A.* **111** L9
Oro Valley *U.S.A.* **109** K8
Orobie, Alpi *Italy* **40** B6
Orobie Bergamasche △ *Italy* **40** B6
Orobie Valtellinesi △ *Italy* **40** B6
Orocué *Colombia* **124** C4
Orodara *Burkina Faso* **82** C4
Orodo *Nigeria* **83** D6
Orofino *U.S.A.* **108** C5
Orohena, Mt. *Tahiti* **91** d
Orol Dengizi = Aral Sea *Asia* **52** E7
Oromíya □ *Ethiopia* **81** F5
Oromocto *Canada* **105** C6
Oron *Nigeria* **83** E6
Orono *Canada* **114** C6
Orono *U.S.A.* **113** C19
Oronsay *U.K.* **13** E2
Oropesa *Spain* **36** F5
Oroquieta *Phil.* **61** G5
Orosei *Italy* **42** B2
Orosei, G. di *Italy* **42** B2
Orosháza *Hungary* **28** D5
Oroszlány *Hungary* **28** C3
Orotukan *Russia* **53** C16
Oroville *Calif., U.S.A.* **110** F5

Oroville *Wash., U.S.A.* **108** B4
Oroville, L. *U.S.A.* **110** F5
Orrefors *Sweden* **11** H9
Orroroo *Australia* **95** E2
Orrviken *Sweden* **10** A8
Orrville *U.S.A.* **114** F3
Orsa *Sweden* **10** C8
Orsara di Púglia *Italy* **43** A8
Orsasjön *Sweden* **10** C8
Orsha *Belarus* **32** E6
Orsk *Russia* **52** D6
Orşova *Romania* **28** F7
Ørsted *Denmark* **11** H4
Örsundsbro *Sweden* **10** E11
Orta *Turkey* **72** B5
Orta, L. d' *Italy* **40** C5
Orta Nova *Italy* **43** A8
Ortaca *Turkey* **47** E10
Ortakent *Turkey* **47** D9
Ortaklar *Turkey* **47** D9
Ortaköy *Çorum, Turkey* **72** B6
Ortaköy *Niğde, Turkey* **72** C6
Orte *Italy* **41** F9
Ortegal, C. *Spain* **36** B3
Orthez *France* **20** E3
Ortigueira *Spain* **36** B3
Orting *U.S.A.* **110** C4
Ortisei *Italy* **41** B8
Ortles *Italy* **40** B7
Ortón → *Bolivia* **124** F5
Ortona *Italy* **41** F11
Ortonville *U.S.A.* **112** C5
Orūmīyeh *Iran* **73** D11
Orūmīyeh, Daryācheh-ye
  Iran **73** D11
Orune *Italy* **42** B2
Oruro *Bolivia* **124** G5
Orust *Sweden* **11** F5
Oruzgān □ *Afghan.* **66** C5
Orvault *France* **18** E5
Orvieto *Italy* **41** F9
Orwell *N.Y., U.S.A.* **115** C9
Orwell *Ohio, U.S.A.* **114** E4
Orwell → *U.K.* **15** F9
Orwigsburg *U.S.A.* **115** F8
Oryakhovo *Bulgaria* **44** C7
Orynyn *Ukraine* **29** B11
Oryol = Orel *Russia* **33** F9
Orzinuovi *Italy* **40** C6
Orzyc → *Poland* **31** F8
Orzysz *Poland* **30** E8
Osa *Poland* **30** E5
Osa, Pen. de *Costa Rica* **120** E3
Osage *U.S.A.* **112** D7
Osage → *U.S.A.* **112** F8
Osage City *U.S.A.* **112** F6
Ōsaka *Japan* **55** G7
Osan *S. Korea* **57** F14
Osawatomie *U.S.A.* **112** F6
Osborne *U.S.A.* **112** F4
Osby *Sweden* **11** H7
Osceola *Ark., U.S.A.* **117** D10
Osceola *Iowa, U.S.A.* **112** E7
Oschatz *Germany* **24** D9
Oschersleben *Germany* **24** C7
Óschiri *Italy* **42** B2
Oscoda *U.S.A.* **114** B1
Osečina *Serbia* **44** B3
Ösel = Saaremaa *Estonia* **32** C2
Osery *Russia* **32** D10
Osgoode *Canada* **115** A9
Osh *Kyrgyzstan* **52** E8
Oshakati *Namibia* **85** H3
Oshawa *Canada* **114** C6
Oshigambo *Namibia* **88** B2
Oshkosh *Nebr., U.S.A.* **112** E2
Oshkosh *Wis., U.S.A.* **112** C9
Oshmyany = Ashmyany
  Belarus **23** A13
Oshnovīyeh *Iran* **73** D11
Oshogbo *Nigeria* **83** D5
Oshtorīnān *Iran* **73** E13
Oshwe *Dem. Rep. of the Congo* **84** E3
Osi *Nigeria* **83** D6
Osieczna *Poland* **31** G3
Osijek *Croatia* **28** E3
Ósilo *Italy* **42** B1
Ósimo *Italy* **41** E10
Osin □ *Nigeria* **83** D5
Osipovichi = Asipovichy
  Belarus **23** B15
Osiyan *India* **68** F5
Osizweni *S. Africa* **89** D5
Oskaloosa *U.S.A.* **112** E7
Oskarshamn *Sweden* **11** G10
Oskarström *Sweden* **11** H6
Oskélanéo *Canada* **104** C4
Öskemen *Kazakhstan* **52** E9
Oskol → *Ukraine* **33** H9
Osku *Iran* **73** D12
Oslo *Norway* **9** G14
Oslob *Phil.* **61** G5
Oslofjorden *Norway* **9** G14
Osmanabad *India* **66** K10
Osmancık *Turkey* **72** B6
Osmaniye *Turkey* **72** D7
Osmanlı *Turkey* **45** E10
Ösmo *Sweden* **10** F11
Osnabrück *Germany* **24** C4

Ośno Lubuskie *Poland* **31** F1
Osogovska Planina
  Macedonia **44** D6
Osor *Italy* **41** D11
Osório *Brazil* **127** B5
Osorno *Chile* **128** E2
Osorno *Spain* **36** C6
Osorno, Vol. *Chile* **128** D2
Osoyoos *Canada* **102** D5
Ospika → *Canada* **102** B4
Osprey Reef *Australia* **94** A4
Oss *Neths.* **17** C5
Ossa, Mt. *Australia* **95** G4
Ossa, Oros *Greece* **46** B4
Ossa de Montiel *Spain* **39** G2
Ossabaw I. *U.S.A.* **117** F14
Osse → *France* **20** D4
Osse → *Nigeria* **83** D6
Ossi *Italy* **42** B1
Ossining *U.S.A.* **115** E11
Ossipee *U.S.A.* **115** C13
Ossokmanuan L. *Canada* **105** B7
Ossora *Russia* **53** D17
Ostashkov *Russia* **32** D7
Østavall *Sweden* **10** B9
Oste → *Germany* **24** B5
Ostend = Oostende *Belgium* **17** C2
Oster *Ukraine* **23** C16
Österbotten = Pohjanmaa
  Finland **8** E20
Osterburg *Germany* **24** C7
Osterburken *Germany* **25** F5
Österbybruk *Sweden* **10** D11
Österbymo *Sweden* **11** G9
Österdalälven → *Sweden* **10** C7
Österdalen *Norway* **10** C4
Osterforse *Sweden* **10** A11
Östergötlands län □ *Sweden* **11** F9
Osterholz-Scharmbeck
  Germany **24** B4
Østerild *Denmark* **11** G2
Östermyra = Seinäjoki
  Finland **8** E20
Osterode *Germany* **24** D6
Östersund *Sweden* **10** A8
Östervåla *Sweden* **10** D11
Osterwieck *Germany* **24** C6
Østfold □ *Norway* **9** G14
Ostfriesische Inseln *Germany* **24** B3
Ostfriesland *Germany* **24** B3
Osthammar *Sweden* **10** D12
Óstia, Lido di *Italy* **41** G9
Ostíglia *Italy* **41** C8
Östmark *Sweden* **10** D6
Östra Husby *Sweden* **11** F10
Ostrava *Czech Rep.* **27** B11
Ostravský □ *Czech Rep.* **27** B10
Ostróda *Poland* **30** E6
Ostrogozhsk *Russia* **33** G10
Ostroh *Ukraine* **23** C14
Ostrołęka *Poland* **31** E8
Ostrov *Bulgaria* **45** D9
Ostrov *Czech Rep.* **26** A5
Ostrov *Romania* **29** F12
Ostrov *Russia* **32** D5
Ostrów Lubelski *Poland* **31** G9
Ostrów Mazowiecka *Poland* **31** F8
Ostrów Wielkopolski *Poland* **31** G4
Ostrowiec-Świętokrzyski
  Poland **31** H8
Ostrožac *Bos.-H.* **28** G2
Ostrzeszów *Poland* **31** G4
Ostuni *Italy* **43** B10
Osum → *Albania* **44** F4
Osûm → *Bulgaria* **45** C8
Ōsumi-Kaikyō *Japan* **55** J5
Ōsumi-Shotō *Japan* **55** J5
Osun □ *Nigeria* **83** D5
Osuna *Spain* **37** H5
Oswegatchie → *U.S.A.* **115** B9
Oswego *U.S.A.* **115** C8
Oswego → *U.S.A.* **115** C8
Oswestry *U.K.* **14** E4
Oświęcim *Poland* **31** H6
Otaci *Moldova* **29** B12
Otago □ *N.Z.* **91** F2
Otago Harbour *N.Z.* **91** F3
Otah.eite B. *Trin. & Tob.* **125** K15
Ōtake *Japan* **55** G6
Otaki *N.Z.* **91** D5
Otaru *Japan* **54** C10
Otaru-Wan =
  Ishikari-Wan *Japan* **54** C10
Otava → *Czech Rep.* **26** B7
Otavalo *Ecuador* **124** C3
Otavi *Namibia* **88** B2
Otchinjau *Angola* **88** B1
Otego *U.S.A.* **115** D9
Otelec *Romania* **28** E5
Otelnuk, L. *Canada* **105** A6
Oţelu Roşu *Romania* **28** E7
Otero de Rey = Outeiro de
  Rei *Spain* **36** B3

Othello *U.S.A.* **108** C4
Othoni *Greece* **46** B1
Othris, Oros *Greece* **46** B4
Oti → *Africa* **83** D5
Oti □ *Togo* **83** C5
Otish, Mts. *Canada* **105** B5
Otjiwarongo *Namibia* **88** C2
Otmuchów *Poland* **31** H4
Oto Tolu Group *Tonga* **91** c
Otočac *Croatia* **41** D12
Otoineppu *Japan* **54** B11
Otok *Croatia* **41** E13
Otopeni, Bucureşti ✈
  (OTP) *Romania* **29** F11
Otorohanga *N.Z.* **91** C5
Otoskwin → *Canada* **104** B2
Otra → *Norway* **9** G13
Otradnyy *Russia* **34** D10
Otranto *Italy* **43** B11
Otranto, C. d' *Italy* **43** B11
Otranto, Str. of *Italy* **43** B11
Otrokovice *Czech Rep.* **27** B10
Otse *S. Africa* **88** D4
Ötsego L. *U.S.A.* **115** D10
Ōtsu *Japan* **55** G7
Ōtsuki *Japan* **55** G9
Ottawa *Canada* **115** A9
Ottawa *Ill., U.S.A.* **112** E9
Ottawa *Kans., U.S.A.* **112** F6
Ottawa Is. *Canada* **101** F15
Ottélé *Cameroon* **83** E7
Ottensheim *Austria* **26** C7
Otter Cr. → *U.S.A.* **115** B11
Otter Lake *Canada* **114** A5
Otterndorf *Germany* **24** B4
Otterup *Denmark* **11** J4
Otterville *Canada* **114** D4
Ottery St. Mary *U.K.* **15** G4
Otto Beit Bridge *Zimbabwe* **87** F2
Ottosdal *S. Africa* **88** D4
Ottumwa *U.S.A.* **112** E7
Otu *Nigeria* **83** D5
Otukpa *Nigeria* **83** D6
Oturkpo *Nigeria* **83** D6
Otway, B. *Chile* **128** G2
Otway, C. *Australia* **95** F3
Otwock *Poland* **31** F8
Otyniya *Ukraine* **29** B9
Ötztaler Ache → *Austria* **26** D3
Ötztaler Alpen *Austria* **26** E3
Ou → *Laos* **64** B4
Ou Neua *Laos* **58** F3
Ou-Sammyaku *Japan* **54** E10
Ouachita → *U.S.A.* **116** F9
Ouachita, L. *U.S.A.* **116** D8
Ouachita Mts. *U.S.A.* **116** D7
Ouagadougou *Burkina Faso* **83** C4
Ouahigouya *Burkina Faso* **82** C4
Ouahran = Oran *Algeria* **78** A5
Oualâta *Mauritania* **82** B3
Ouallam *Niger* **83** C5
Ouallene *Algeria* **78** D6
Ouarâne *Mauritania* **78** D3
Ouargaye *Burkina Faso* **83** C5
Ouargla *Algeria* **78** B7
Ouarkoye *Burkina Faso* **82** C4
Ouarra → *C.A.R.* **84** C4
Ouarzazate *Morocco* **78** B4
Ouassouas *Mali* **83** B5
Ouatagouna *Mali* **83** B5
Oubangi →
  Dem. Rep. of the Congo **84** E3
Ouche → *France* **19** E12
Ouddorp *Neths.* **17** C3
Oude Rijn → *Neths.* **17** B4
Oudenaarde *Belgium* **17** D3
Oudon → *France* **18** E5
Oudtshoorn *S. Africa* **88** E3
Ouella *Niger* **83** C5
Ouellé *Ivory C.* **82** D4
Ouémé → *Benin* **83** D5
Ouessa *Burkina Faso* **82** C4
Ouessant, Î. d' *France* **18** D1
Ouesso *Congo* **84** D3
Ouest □ *Cameroon* **83** D7
Ouest, Pte. de l' *Canada* **105** C7
Ouezzane *Morocco* **78** B4
Ougarou *Burkina Faso* **83** C5
Oughter, L. *Ireland* **12** B4
Oughterard *Ireland* **12** C2
Ouidah *Benin* **83** D5
Ouidi *Niger* **83** C7
Ouistreham *France* **18** C6
Oujda *Morocco* **78** B5
Oujeft *Mauritania* **82** A2
Oulainen *Finland* **8** D21
Ould Yenjé *Mauritania* **82** B2
Oullins *France* **21** C8
Oulu *Finland* **8** D21
Oulujärvi *Finland* **8** D22
Oulujoki → *Finland* **8** D21
Oulx *Italy* **40** C3
Oum Chalouba *Chad* **79** E10
Oum Hadjer *Chad* **79** F9
Oumé *Ivory C.* **82** D3
Ounasjoki → *Finland* **8** C21
Ounguati *Namibia* **88** C2

Ounianga Kébir *Chad* **79** E10
Our → *Lux.* **17** E6
Oura, Akra *Greece* **47** C8
Ouranoupoli *Greece* **44** F7
Ourârene *Niger* **83** B6
Ourcq → *France* **19** C10
Ourense *Spain* **36** C3
Ourense □ *Spain* **36** C3
Ouricuri *Brazil* **125** E10
Ourinhos *Brazil* **127** A6
Ouro Fino *Brazil* **127** A6
Ouro Prêto *Brazil* **127** A7
Ouro Sogui *Senegal* **82** B2
Oursi *Burkina Faso* **83** C4
Ourthe → *Belgium* **17** D5
Ouse → *E. Sussex, U.K.* **15** G8
Ouse → *N. Yorks., U.K.* **14** D7
Oust *France* **18** E4
Oust → *France* **20** F5
Outamba-Kilimi △ *S. Leone* **82** D2
Outaouais → *Canada* **104** C5
Outardes → *Canada* **105** C6
Outeiro de Rei *Spain* **36** B3
Outer Hebrides *U.K.* **13** D1
Outes = A Serra de Outes
   Spain **36** C2
Outjo *Namibia* **88** C2
Outlook *Canada* **103** C7
Outokumpu *Finland* **8** E23
Outreau *France* **19** B8
Ouvèze → *France* **21** E8
Ouyen *Australia* **95** F3
Ouzouer-le-Marché *France* **19** E8
Ovada *Italy* **40** D5
Ovalau *Fiji* **91** a
Ovalle *Chile* **126** C1
Ovamboland *Namibia* **88** B2
Ovanåker *Sweden* **10** C9
Ovar *Portugal* **36** E2
Overath *Germany* **24** E3
Overflakkee *Neths.* **17** C4
Overijssel □ *Neths.* **17** B6
Overland Park *U.S.A.* **112** F6
Overlander Roadhouse
   Australia **93** E1
Overton *U.S.A.* **111** J12
Övertorneå *Sweden* **8** C20
Överum *Sweden* **11** F10
Ovid *U.S.A.* **115** D8
Ovidiopol *Ukraine* **33** J6
Ovidiu *Romania* **29** F13
Oviedo *Spain* **36** B5
Ovišrags *Latvia* **30** A8
Ovoot *Mongolia* **56** B7
Övör Hangay □ *Mongolia* **56** B2
Ovoro *Nigeria* **83** D6
Øvre Årdal *Norway* **8** F12
Övre Fryken *Sweden* **10** E7
Ovruch *Ukraine* **23** C15
Owaka *N.Z.* **91** G2
Owambo = Ovamboland
   Namibia **88** B2
Owasco L. *U.S.A.* **115** D8
Owase *Japan* **55** G8
Owatonna *U.S.A.* **112** C7
Owbeh *Afghan.* **66** B3
Owego *U.S.A.* **115** D8
Owen Falls Dam =
   Nalubaale Dam *Uganda* **86** B3
Owen Sound *Canada* **114** B4
Owen Stanley Ra.
   Papua N. G. **90** B7
Oweniny → *Ireland* **12** B2
Owens → *U.S.A.* **110** J9
Owens L. *U.S.A.* **111** J9
Owensboro *U.S.A.* **112** G10
Owerri *Nigeria* **83** D6
Owl → *Canada* **103** B10
Owo *Nigeria* **83** D6
Owosso *U.S.A.* **113** D11
Owyhee *U.S.A.* **108** F5
Owyhee → *U.S.A.* **108** E5
Owyhee, L. *U.S.A.* **108** E5
Ox Mts. = Slieve Gamph
   Ireland **12** B3
Öxarfjörður *Iceland* **8** C5
Oxbow *Canada* **103** D8
Oxelösund *Sweden* **11** F11
Oxford *N.Z.* **91** E4
Oxford *U.K.* **15** F6
Oxford *Mass., U.S.A.* **115** D13
Oxford *Miss., U.S.A.* **117** D10
Oxford *N.C., U.S.A.* **117** C15
Oxford *N.Y., U.S.A.* **115** D9
Oxford *Ohio, U.S.A.* **113** F11
Oxford L. *Canada* **103** C9
Oxfordshire □ *U.K.* **15** F6
Oxia *Greece* **46** C2
Oxie *Sweden* **11** J7
Oxnard *U.S.A.* **111** L7
Oxsjövålen *Sweden* **10** B7
Oxus = Amudarya →
   Uzbekistan **52** E6
Oya *Malaysia* **62** D4
Oyama *Japan* **55** F9

Oyambre △ *Spain* **36** B6
Oyem *Gabon* **84** D2
Oyen *Canada* **103** C6
Oykel → *U.K.* **13** D4
Oymyakon *Russia* **53** C15
Oyo *Nigeria* **83** D5
Oyo *Sudan* **80** C4
Oyo □ *Nigeria* **83** D5
Oyonnax *France* **19** F12
Oyster Bay *U.S.A.* **115** F11
Ōyūbari *Japan* **54** C11
Özalp *Turkey* **73** C10
Ozamiz *Phil.* **61** G5
Ozark *Ala., U.S.A.* **117** F12
Ozark *Ark., U.S.A.* **116** D8
Ozark *Mo., U.S.A.* **112** G7
Ozark Plateau *U.S.A.* **112** G8
Ozarks, L. of the *U.S.A.* **112** F7
Ożarów *Poland* **31** H8
Ózd *Hungary* **28** B5
Ozernovskiy *Russia* **53** D16
Ozernoye *Russia* **34** E10
Ozero Svityaz *Ukraine* **31** G10
Ozersk *Russia* **30** D8
Ozette, L. *U.S.A.* **110** B2
Ozieri *Italy* **42** B2
Ozimek *Poland* **31** H5
Ozinki *Russia* **34** E9
Ozona *U.S.A.* **116** F4
Ozorków *Poland* **31** G6
Ozren *Bos.-H.* **28** G3
Ozuluama *Mexico* **119** C5
Ozun *Romania* **29** E10
Ozurgeti *Georgia* **35** K5

P

Pa *Burkina Faso* **82** C4
Pa-an *Burma* **67** L20
Pa Mong Dam *Thailand* **64** D4
Pa Sak → *Thailand* **64** E3
Paamiut *Greenland* **4** C5
Paar → *Germany* **25** G7
Paarl *S. Africa* **88** E2
Pab Hills *Pakistan* **68** F2
Pabbay *U.K.* **13** D1
Pabianice *Poland* **31** G6
Pabna *Bangla.* **67** G16
Pabo *Uganda* **86** B3
Pacaja → *Brazil* **125** D8
Pacaraima, Sa. *S. Amer.* **124** C6
Pacasmayo *Peru* **124** E3
Paceco *Italy* **42** E5
Pachia *Greece* **47** E7
Pachino *Italy* **43** F8
Pachitea → *Peru* **124** E4
Pachmarhi *India* **69** H8
Pachnes *Greece* **49** D6
Pachpadra *India* **68** G5
Pachuca *Mexico* **119** C5
Pacific Antarctic Ridge
   Pac. Oc. **5** B13
Pacific Grove *U.S.A.* **110** J5
Pacific Ocean **97** G14
Pacific Rim △ *Canada* **110** B2
Pacifica *U.S.A.* **110** H4
Pacitan *Indonesia* **63** H14
Packwood *U.S.A.* **110** D5
Pacov *Czech Rep.* **26** B8
Pacy-sur-Eure *France* **18** C8
Padaido, Kepulauan
   Indonesia **63** E9
Padang *Riau, Indonesia* **65** M4
Padang *Sumatera Barat,
   Indonesia* **62** E2
Padang Endau *Malaysia* **65** L4
Padangpanjang *Indonesia* **62** E2
Padangsidempuan *Indonesia* **62** D1
Padborg *Denmark* **11** K3
Paddle Prairie *Canada* **102** B5
Paderborn *Germany* **24** D4
Padeş, Vf. *Romania* **28** E7
Padma → *India* **69** G11
Pádova *Italy* **41** C8
Padra *India* **68** H5
Padrauna *India* **69** F10
Padre I. *U.S.A.* **116** H6
Padre Island △ *U.S.A.* **116** H6
Padrón *Spain* **36** C2
Padstow *U.K.* **15** G3
Padua = Pádova *Italy* **41** C8
Paducah *Ky., U.S.A.* **112** G9
Paducah *Tex., U.S.A.* **116** D4
Padul *Spain* **37** H7
Paea *Tahiti* **91** d
Paeroa *N.Z.* **91** B5
Paesana *Italy* **40** D4
Pafúri *Mozam.* **89** C5
Pag *Croatia* **41** D12
Paga *Ghana* **83** C4
Pagadian *Phil.* **61** H5
Pagai Selatan, Pulau
   Indonesia **62** E2
Pagai Utara, Pulau *Indonesia* **62** E2
Pagalu = Annobón *Atl. Oc.* **77** G4
Pagara *India* **69** G9
Pagastikós Kolpos *Greece* **46** B4
Pagatan *Indonesia* **62** E5
Page *U.S.A.* **109** H8

Pagégiai *Lithuania* **30** C8
Paget, Mt. *S. Georgia* **128** G9
Pago Pago *Amer. Samoa* **91** b
Pagosa Springs *U.S.A.* **109** H10
Pagwa River *Canada* **104** B2
Pāhala *U.S.A.* **107** M8
Pahang → *Malaysia* **65** L4
Pahang □ *Malaysia* **65** L4
Pahiatua *N.Z.* **91** D5
Pahokee *U.S.A.* **117** H14
Pahrump *U.S.A.* **111** J11
Pahute Mesa *U.S.A.* **110** H10
Pai *Thailand* **64** C2
Paicines *U.S.A.* **110** J5
Paide *Estonia* **32** C3
Paignton *U.K.* **15** G4
Paiho *Taiwan* **59** F13
Päijänne *Finland* **32** B3
Pailani *India* **69** G9
Pailin *Cambodia* **64** F4
Paimpol *France* **18** D3
Painan *Indonesia* **62** E2
Painesville *U.S.A.* **114** E3
Paint Hills = Wemindji
   Canada **104** B4
Paint L. *Canada* **103** B9
Painted Desert *U.S.A.* **109** H8
Paintsville *U.S.A.* **113** G12
Paisley *Canada* **114** B3
Paisley *U.K.* **13** F4
Paisley *U.S.A.* **108** E3
Paita *Peru* **124** E2
Paiva → *Portugal* **36** D2
Paizhou *China* **59** B9
Pajares *Spain* **36** B5
Pajares, Puerto de *Spain* **36** C5
Pajęczno *Poland* **31** G5
Pak Lay *Laos* **64** C3
Pak Phanang *Thailand* **65** H3
Pak Sane *Laos* **64** C4
Pak Song *Laos* **64** E6
Pak Suong *Laos* **58** H4
Pakaur *India* **69** G12
Pakch'ŏn *N. Korea* **57** E13
Pakenham *Canada* **115** A8
Pakhuis *S. Africa* **88** E2
Pakistan ■ *Asia* **68** E4
Pakkading *Laos* **64** C4
Pakokku *Burma* **67** J19
Pakowki L. *Canada* **103** D6
Pakpattan *Pakistan* **68** D5
Pakrac *Croatia* **28** E2
Pakruojis *Lithuania* **30** C10
Paks *Hungary* **28** D3
Paktīā □ *Afghan.* **66** C6
Paktīkā □ *Afghan.* **66** C6
Pakwach *Uganda* **86** B3
Pakxe *Laos* **64** E5
Pal Lahara *India* **69** J11
Pala *Chad* **79** G9
Pala *Dem. Rep. of the Congo* **86** D2
Pala *U.S.A.* **111** M9
Palabek *Uganda* **86** B3
Palacios *U.S.A.* **116** G6
Palafrugell *Spain* **38** C8
Palagiano *Italy* **43** B10
Palagonia *Italy* **43** E7
Palagruža *Croatia* **41** F13
Palaiseau *France* **19** D9
Palakkad = Palghat *India* **66** P10
Palam *India* **66** K10
Palamás *Greece* **46** B4
Palamós *Spain* **38** D8
Palampur *India* **68** C7
Palamut *Turkey* **47** C9
Palana *Australia* **95** F4
Palana *Russia* **53** D16
Palanan *Phil.* **61** C5
Palanan Pt. *Phil.* **61** C5
Palandri *Pakistan* **69** C5
Palanga *Lithuania* **30** C8
Palangkaraya *Indonesia* **62** E4
Palani Hills *India* **66** P10
Palanpur *India* **68** G5
Palapye *Botswana* **88** C4
Palas *Pakistan* **69** B5
Palas de Rei *Spain* **36** C3
Palasponga *India* **69** J11
Palatka *Russia* **53** C16
Palatka *U.S.A.* **117** G14
Palau *Italy* **42** A2
Palau ■ *Palau* **90** A6
Palauk *Burma* **64** F2
Palawan *Phil.* **61** G3
Palayankottai *India* **66** Q10
Palazzo, Pte. *France* **21** F12
Palazzo San Gervásio *Italy* **43** B8
Palazzolo Acréide *Italy* **43** E7
Paldiski *Estonia* **32** C3
Pale *Bos.-H.* **28** G3
Palekastro *Greece* **49** D8
Paleleh *Indonesia* **63** D6
Palembang *Indonesia* **62** E2
Palencia *Spain* **36** C6
Palencia □ *Spain* **36** C6
Palenque *Mexico* **119** D6
Paleochora *Greece* **49** D5
Paleokastritsa *Greece* **49** A3

Paleometokho *Cyprus* **49** D12
Paleopoli *Greece* **46** D6
Palermo *Italy* **42** D6
Palermo *Chile* **124** A3
Palermo ✈ (PMO) *Italy* **42** D6
Paleros *Greece* **46** C2
Palestina *Chile* **126** A2
Palestine *Asia* **74** D4
Palestine *U.S.A.* **116** F7
Palestrina *Italy* **41** G9
Paletwa *Burma* **67** J18
Palghat *India* **66** P10
Palgrave, Mt. *Australia* **92** D2
Pali *India* **68** G5
Palikir *Micronesia* **96** G7
Palinuro *Italy* **43** B8
Palinuro, C. *Italy* **43** B8
Palisades Res. *U.S.A.* **108** E8
Paliseul *Belgium* **17** E5
Palitana *India* **68** J4
Palizada *Mexico* **119** D6
Palk Bay *Asia* **66** Q11
Palk Strait *Asia* **66** Q11
Palkānah *Iraq* **70** C5
Palkhed *India* **68** K5
Palkonda *India* **69** H11
Palkot *India* **69** H11
Pallanza = Verbánia *Italy* **40** C5
Pallarenda *Australia* **94** B4
Pallasovka *Russia* **34** E8
Pallës, Bishti i *Albania* **44** E3
Pallinup → *Australia* **93** F2
Pallisa *Uganda* **86** B3
Pallu *India* **68** E6
Palm Bay *U.S.A.* **117** G14
Palm Beach *U.S.A.* **117** H14
Palm Coast *U.S.A.* **117** G14
Palm Desert *U.S.A.* **111** M10
Palm Is. *Australia* **94** B4
Palm Springs *U.S.A.* **111** M10
Palm-Grove △ *Australia* **94** C4
Palma *Mozam.* **87** E5
Palma, B. de *Spain* **48** B9
Palma de Mallorca *Spain* **48** B9
Palma de Mallorca ✈
   (PMI) *Spain* **39** F7
Palma del Río *Spain* **37** H5
Palma di Montechiaro *Italy* **42** E6
Palma Nova = Palmanova
   Spain **48** B9
Palma Soriano *Cuba* **120** B4
Palmanova *Spain* **48** B9
Palmares *Brazil* **125** E11
Palmarola *Italy* **42** B5
Palmas *Brazil* **127** B5
Palmas *C. Liberia* **82** E3
Pálmas, G. di *Italy* **42** D1
Palmdale *U.S.A.* **111** L8
Palmeira das Missões *Brazil* **127** B5
Palmeira dos Índios *Brazil* **125** E11
Palmela *Portugal* **37** G2
Palmer *Antarctica* **5** C17
Palmer *U.S.A.* **100** E2
Palmer → *Australia* **94** B3
Palmer Arch. *Antarctica* **5** C17
Palmer Land *Antarctica* **5** D18
Palmerston *Australia* **92** B5
Palmerston *Canada* **114** C4
Palmerston *N.Z.* **91** F3
Palmerston North *N.Z.* **91** D5
Palmerton *U.S.A.* **115** F9
Palmetto *U.S.A.* **117** H13
Palmi *Italy* **43** D8
Palmira *Argentina* **126** C2
Palmira *Colombia* **124** C3
Palmyra = Tudmur *Syria* **73** E8
Palmyra *Mo., U.S.A.* **112** F8
Palmyra *N.J., U.S.A.* **115** F9
Palmyra *N.Y., U.S.A.* **114** C7
Palmyra *Pa., U.S.A.* **115** F8
Palmyra Is. *Pac. Oc.* **97** G11
Palo Alto *U.S.A.* **110** H4
Palo Seco *Trin. & Tob.* **125** K15
Palo Verde *U.S.A.* **111** M12
Palo Verde △ *Costa Rica* **120** D2
Paloich *Sudan* **81** E3
Palomar Mt. *U.S.A.* **111** M10
Palompon *Phil.* **61** F6
Palopo *Indonesia* **63** E6
Palos, C. de *Spain* **39** H4
Palos de la Frontera *Spain* **37** H4
Palos Verdes, Pt. *U.S.A.* **111** M8
Palos Verdes Estates *U.S.A.* **111** M8
Pålsboda *Sweden* **10** E9
Palu *Indonesia* **63** E5
Palu *Turkey* **73** C9
Paluke *Liberia* **82** D3
Paluma Ra. *Australia* **94** B4
Paluzza *Italy* **41** B10
Palwal *India* **68** E7
Pama *Burkina Faso* **83** C5
Pama △ *Burkina Faso* **83** C5
Pamanukan *Indonesia* **63** G12
Pamekasan *Indonesia* **63** G15
Pamenang *Indonesia* **63** J19
Pamiers *France* **20** E5
Pamir *Tajikistan* **52** F8
Pamlico → *U.S.A.* **117** D16
Pamlico Sd. *U.S.A.* **117** D17
Pampa *U.S.A.* **116** D4

Pampa de las Salinas
   Argentina **126** C2
Pampanua *Indonesia* **63** E6
Pampas *Argentina* **126** D3
Pampas *Peru* **124** F3
Pamphylia *Turkey* **72** D4
Pamplona *Colombia* **124** B4
Pamplona-Iruña *Spain* **38** C3
Pampoenpoort *S. Africa* **88** E3
Pamukçu *Turkey* **47** B9
Pamukkale *Turkey* **47** D11
Pan de Azúcar *Chile* **126** A2
Pan de Azúcar △ *Chile* **126** B1
Pan Xian *China* **58** E5
Pana *U.S.A.* **112** F9
Panabo *Phil.* **61** H6
Panaca *U.S.A.* **109** H6
Panagyurishte *Bulgaria* **45** D8
Panaitan *Indonesia* **63** G11
Panaji *India* **66** M8
Panamá *Panama* **120** E4
Panama ■ *Cent. Amer.* **120** E4
Panamá, G. de *Panama* **120** E4
Panama, Isthmus of
   Cent. Amer. **98** J12
Panama Basin *Pac. Oc.* **97** G19
Panama Canal *Panama* **120** E4
Panama City *U.S.A.* **117** F12
Panamint Range *U.S.A.* **111** J9
Panamint Springs *U.S.A.* **111** J9
Panão *Peru* **124** E3
Panaon I. *Phil.* **61** F6
Panare *Thailand* **65** J3
Panarea *Italy* **43** D8
Panaro → *Italy* **41** D8
Panay *Phil.* **61** F5
Panay G. *Phil.* **63** B6
Panayarvi △ *Russia* **8** C24
Pančevo *Serbia* **28** F5
Panch'iao *Taiwan* **59** E13
Panciu *Romania* **29** E12
Pâncota *Romania* **28** D6
Panda *Mozam.* **89** C5
Pandan *Antique, Phil.* **61** F5
Pandan *Catanduanes, Phil.* **61** D6
Pandan, Selat *Singapore* **65** d
Pandan Tampoi = Tampoi
   Malaysia **65** d
Pandegelang *Indonesia* **63** G12
Pandhana *India* **68** J7
Pandharpur *India* **66** L9
Pando *Uruguay* **127** C4
Pando, L. = Hope, L.
   Australia **95** D2
Pandokratoras *Greece* **49** A3
Pandora *Costa Rica* **120** E3
Pandrup *Denmark* **11** G3
Panevéggio-Pale di San
   Martino △ *Italy* **41** B8
Panevėžys *Lithuania* **32** E3
Panfilovo *Russia* **34** E6
Pang-Long *Burma* **67** H21
Pang-Yang *Burma* **67** H21
Panga *Dem. Rep. of the Congo* **86** B2
Pangaíon Óros *Greece* **45** F8
Pangalanes, Canal des =
   Ampangalana,
   Lakandranon' *Madag.* **89** C8
Pangani *Tanzania* **86** D4
Pangani → *Tanzania* **86** D4
Pangar Djeréme △ *Cameroon* **83** D7
Pangfou = Bengbu *China* **57** H9
Pangil *Dem. Rep. of the Congo* **86** C2
Pangkah, Tanjung
   Indonesia **63** G15
Pangkajene *Indonesia* **63** E5
Pangkalanbrandan *Indonesia* **62** D1
Pangkalanbuun *Indonesia* **62** E4
Pangkalpinang *Indonesia* **62** E3
Pangkor, P. *Malaysia* **65** K3
Pangnirtung *Canada* **101** D18
Pangody *Russia* **52** C8
Pangong Tso = Bangong
   Co *China* **69** C8
Panguitch *U.S.A.* **109** H7
Pangutaran Group *Phil.* **61** H4
Panhandle *U.S.A.* **116** D4
Pani Mines *India* **68** H5
Pania-Mutombo
   Dem. Rep. of the Congo **86** D1
Panikota I. *India* **68** J4
Panipat *India* **68** E7
Panjal Range = Pir Panjal
   Range *India* **68** C7
Panjang, Hon *Vietnam* **65** H4
Panjgur *Pakistan* **66** F4
Panjim = Panaji *India* **66** M8
Panjin *China* **57** D12
Panjnad → *Pakistan* **68** E4
Panjnad Barrage *Pakistan* **68** E4
Panjwai *Afghan.* **68** D1
Pankshin *Nigeria* **83** D6
Panmunjŏm *N. Korea* **57** F14
Panna *India* **69** G9
Panna △ *Mexico* **119** D5
Panna Hills *India* **69** G9
Pannawonica *Australia* **92** D2

Pannga, Tanjung *Indonesia* **63** K19
Pannirtuuq = Pangnirtung
   Canada **101** D18
Pano Akil *Pakistan* **68** F3
Pano Lefkara *Cyprus* **49** E12
Pano Panayia *Cyprus* **49** E11
Panorama *Brazil* **127** A5
Panormos *Greece* **49** C9
Pansemal *India* **68** J6
Panshan = Panjin *China* **57** D12
Panshi *China* **57** C14
Pantanal *Brazil* **124** H7
Pantanos de Centla △
   Mexico **119** D6
Pantar *Indonesia* **63** F6
Pante Macassar *E. Timor* **63** F6
Pantelleria *Italy* **42** F4
Pantón *Spain* **36** C3
Pánuco *Mexico* **119** C5
Panyam *Nigeria* **83** D6
Panyu *China* **59** F9
Panzhihua *China* **58** D3
Páola *Italy* **43** C9
Paola *Malta* **49** D2
Paola *U.S.A.* **112** F6
Paonia *U.S.A.* **108** G10
Paopao *Moorea* **91** d
Paoting = Baoding *China* **56** E8
Paot'ou = Baotou *China* **56** D6
Paoua *C.A.R.* **84** C3
Pápa *Hungary* **28** C2
Papa Stour *U.K.* **13** A7
Papa Westray *U.K.* **13** B6
Papagayo → *Mexico* **119** D5
Papagayo, G. de *Costa Rica* **120** D2
Papakura *N.Z.* **91** B5
Papantla *Mexico* **119** C5
Papar *Malaysia* **62** C5
Papara *Tahiti* **91** d
Paparoa △ *N.Z.* **91** E3
Papas, Akra *Greece* **46** C3
Papeete *Tahiti* **91** d
Papenburg *Germany* **24** B3
Papenoo *Tahiti* **91** d
Papenoo → *Tahiti* **91** d
Papetoai *Moorea* **91** d
Paphlagonia *Turkey* **72** B5
Paphos *Cyprus* **49** E11
Papikio Oros *Greece* **45** E9
Paposo *Chile* **126** B1
Papoutsa *Cyprus* **49** E12
Papua □ *Indonesia* **63** E9
Papua, G. of *Papua N. G.* **90** B7
Papua New Guinea ■
   Oceania **90** B7
Papudo *Chile* **126** C1
Papuk *Croatia* **28** E2
Papun *Burma* **67** K20
Papunya *Australia* **92** D5
Pará = Belém *Brazil* **125** D9
Pará □ *Brazil* **125** D8
Paraburdoo *Australia* **92** D2
Paracale *Phil.* **61** D5
Paracatu *Brazil* **125** G9
Paracel Is. *S. China Sea* **62** A4
Parachilna *Australia* **95** E2
Parachinar *Pakistan* **68** C4
Paradas *Spain* **37** H5
Paradela *Spain* **36** C3
Paradip *India* **67** J15
Paradise *Calif., U.S.A.* **110** F5
Paradise *Nev., U.S.A.* **111** J11
Paradise → *Canada* **105** B8
Paradise Hill *Canada* **103** C7
Paradise River *Canada* **105** B8
Paradise Valley *U.S.A.* **108** F5
Paradisi *Greece* **49** C10
Parado *Indonesia* **63** F5
Paragould *U.S.A.* **117** C9
Paragua → *Venezuela* **124** B6
Paraguaçu → *Brazil* **125** F11
Paraguaçu Paulista *Brazil* **127** A5
Paraguaná, Pen. de
   Venezuela **124** A5
Paraguarí *Paraguay* **126** B4
Paraguarí □ *Paraguay* **126** B4
Paraguay ■ *S. Amer.* **126** A4
Paraguay → *Paraguay* **126** B4
Paraíba = João Pessoa
   Brazil **125** E12
Paraíba □ *Brazil* **125** E11
Paraíba do Sul → *Brazil* **127** A7
Parainen *Finland* **32** B2
Paraíso *Mexico* **119** D6
Parak *Iran* **71** E7
Parakhino Paddubye *Russia* **32** C7
Parakou *Benin* **83** D5
Paralimni *Cyprus* **49** D12
Paralio Astros *Greece* **46** D4
Paramithia *Greece* **46** B2
Páramos del Batallón y La
   Negra △ *Venezuela* **121** E5
Paramushir, Ostrov *Russia* **53** D16
Paran → *Israel* **74** E4
Paraná *Argentina* **126** C3
Paraná *Brazil* **125** F9
Paraná □ *Brazil* **127** A5
Paraná → *Argentina* **126** C4

Paranaguá *Brazil* **127** B6
Paranaíba *Brazil* **125** G8
Paranaíba → *Brazil* **125** H8
Paranapanema → *Brazil* **127** A5
Paranapiacaba, Serra do
  Brazil **127** A6
Paranas *Phil.* **61** F6
Paranavaí *Brazil* **127** A5
Parang *Maguindanao, Phil.* **63** C6
Parang *Sulu, Phil.* **61** J4
Parângul Mare, Vf. *Romania* **29** E8
Paraparaumu *N.Z.* **91** D5
Paraspóri, Ákra *Greece* **47** F9
Paray-le-Monial *France* **19** F11
Parbati → *Mad. P., India* **68** G7
Parbati → *Raj., India* **68** F7
Parbhani *India* **66** K10
Parchim *Germany* **24** B7
Parczew *Poland* **31** G9
Pardes Hanna-Karkur *Israel* **74** C3
Pardilla *Spain* **36** D7
Pardo → *Bahia, Brazil* **125** G11
Pardo → *Mato Grosso, Brazil* **127** A5
Pardoo Roadhouse *Australia* **92** D2
Pardubice *Czech Rep.* **26** A8
Pardubický □ *Czech Rep.* **26** B8
Pare *Indonesia* **63** G15
Pare Mts. *Tanzania* **86** C4
Parecis, Serra dos *Brazil* **124** F7
Paredes de Nava *Spain* **36** C6
Paren *Russia* **53** C17
Parent *Canada* **104** C5
Parent, L. *Canada* **104** C4
Parentis-en-Born *France* **20** D2
Parepare *Indonesia* **63** E5
Parfino *Russia* **32** D6
Parga *Greece* **46** B2
Pargas = Parainen *Finland* **32** B2
Pargo, Pta. do *Madeira* **48** D2
Parham *Canada* **115** B8
Paria → *U.S.A.* **109** H8
Paria, G. de *Venezuela* **125** K14
Pariaguán *Venezuela* **124** B6
Paricutín, Cerro *Mexico* **118** D4
Parigi *Indonesia* **63** E6
Parika *Guyana* **124** B7
Parikia *Greece* **47** D7
Parikkala *Finland* **32** B5
Parima, Serra *Brazil* **124** C6
Parinari *Peru* **124** D4
Pariñas, Pta. *Peru* **122** D2
Parincea *Romania* **29** D12
Parintins *Brazil* **125** D7
Pariparit Kyun *Burma* **67** M18
Paris *Canada* **114** C4
Paris *France* **19** D9
Paris *Idaho, U.S.A.* **108** E8
Paris *Ky., U.S.A.* **113** F11
Paris *Tenn., U.S.A.* **117** C10
Paris *Tex., U.S.A.* **116** E7
Paris, Ville de □ *France* **19** D9
Paris Charles de Gaulle ✈
  (CDG) *France* **19** D9
Paris Orly ✈ (ORY) *France* **19** D9
Parish *U.S.A.* **115** C8
Parishville *U.S.A.* **115** B10
Pariti *Indonesia* **92** B3
Park *U.S.A.* **110** B4
Park City *U.S.A.* **112** G5
Park Falls *U.S.A.* **112** C8
Park Head *Canada* **114** B3
Park Hills *U.S.A.* **112** G8
Park Range *U.S.A.* **108** F10
Park Rapids *U.S.A.* **112** B6
Park River *U.S.A.* **112** A5
Park Rynie *S. Africa* **89** E5
Parkā Bandar *Iran* **71** E8
Parkano *Finland* **32** A2
Parker *Ariz., U.S.A.* **111** L12
Parker *Pa., U.S.A.* **114** E5
Parker Dam *U.S.A.* **111** L12
Parkersburg *U.S.A.* **113** F13
Parkes *Australia* **95** E4
Parkfield *U.S.A.* **110** K6
Parkhill *Canada* **114** C3
Parkland *U.S.A.* **110** C4
Parkston *U.S.A.* **112** D5
Parksville *Canada* **102** D4
Parkway *U.S.A.* **110** G5
Parla *Spain* **36** E7
Pârlița *Moldova* **29** C12
Parma *Italy* **40** D7
Parma *Idaho, U.S.A.* **108** E5
Parma *Ohio, U.S.A.* **114** E3
Parma → *Italy* **40** D7
Parnaguá *Brazil* **125** F10
Parnaíba *Brazil* **125** D10
Parnaíba → *Brazil* **125** D10
Parnassós *Greece* **46** C4
Parnitha *Greece* **46** C5
Parnon Oros *Greece* **46** D4
Pärnu *Estonia* **32** C3
Paro Dzong *Bhutan* **69** F13
Paroo → *Australia* **95** E3
Páros *Greece* **47** D7
Parowan *U.S.A.* **109** H7
Parpaillon *France* **21** D10
Parral *Chile* **126** D1
Parramatta *Australia* **95** B5

Parras *Mexico* **118** B4
Parrett → *U.K.* **15** F4
Parris I. *U.S.A.* **117** E14
Parrsboro *Canada* **105** C7
Parry Channel *Canada* **101** C13
Parry I. *Canada* **114** A4
Parry Is. *Canada* **101** B10
Parry Sound *Canada* **114** A5
Parsábád *Iran* **73** C13
Parsaloi *Kenya* **86** B4
Parsberg *Germany* **25** F7
Parsęta → *Poland* **30** D2
Parsnip → *Canada* **102** B4
Parsons *U.S.A.* **112** G6
Parsons Ra. *Australia* **94** A2
Partanna *Italy* **42** E5
Partenio △ *Italy* **43** B7
Parthenay *France* **18** F6
Partinico *Italy* **42** D6
Partizansk *Russia* **54** C6
Partizánske *Slovak Rep.* **27** C11
Partridge I. *Canada* **104** A2
Partry Mts. *Ireland* **12** C2
Paru → *Brazil* **125** D8
Parvän □ *Afghan.* **66** B6
Parvatipuram *India* **67** K13
Parvatsar *India* **68** F6
Påryd *Sweden* **11** H9
Parys *S. Africa* **88** D4
Pas, Pta. des *Spain* **48** C7
Pas, The *Canada* **103** C8
Pas-de-Calais □ *France* **19** B9
Pasada *Spain* **36** B5
Pasadena *Canada* **105** C8
Pasadena *Calif., U.S.A.* **111** L8
Pasadena *Tex., U.S.A.* **116** G7
Pasaje → *Argentina* **126** B3
Pasar *Indonesia* **63** J17
Pasay *Phil.* **61** D4
Pascagoula *U.S.A.* **117** F10
Pascagoula → *U.S.A.* **117** F10
Paşcani *Romania* **29** C11
Pasco *U.S.A.* **108** C4
Pasco I. *Australia* **92** D2
Pascoag *U.S.A.* **115** E13
Pascua, I. de *Chile* **97** K17
Pasewalk *Germany* **24** B9
Pasfield L. *Canada* **103** B7
Pasha → *Russia* **32** B7
Pasinler *Turkey* **73** C10
Pasir Mas *Malaysia* **65** J4
Pasir Panjang *Singapore* **65** d
Pasir Putih *Malaysia* **65** K4
Pasirian *Indonesia* **63** H15
Pasirkuning *Indonesia* **62** E2
Påskallavik *Sweden* **11** G10
Paskūh *Iran* **71** E9
Pasłęk *Poland* **30** D6
Pasłęka → *Poland* **30** D6
Pasley, C. *Australia* **93** F3
Pašman *Croatia* **41** E12
Pasni *Pakistan* **66** G3
Paso Bravo △ *Paraguay* **126** A4
Paso Cantinela *Mexico* **111** N11
Paso de Indios *Argentina* **128** E3
Paso de los Libres *Argentina* **126** B4
Paso de los Toros *Uruguay* **126** C4
Paso Robles *U.S.A.* **110** K6
Paspébiac *Canada* **105** C6
Pasrur *Pakistan* **68** C6
Passage East *Ireland* **12** D5
Passage West *Ireland* **12** E3
Passaic *U.S.A.* **115** F10
Passau *Germany* **25** G9
Passero, C. *Italy* **43** F8
Passo Fundo *Brazil* **127** B5
Passos *Brazil* **125** H9
Passow *Germany* **24** B10
Passy *France* **21** C10
Pastavy *Belarus* **32** E4
Pastaza → *Peru* **124** D3
Pasto *Colombia* **124** C3
Pastrana *Spain* **38** E2
Pasuruan *Indonesia* **63** G15
Pasym *Poland* **30** E7
Pásztó *Hungary* **28** C4
Patagonia *Argentina* **128** F3
Patagonia *U.S.A.* **109** L8
Patambar *Iran* **71** D9
Patan = Lalitapur *Nepal* **69** F11
Patan = Somnath *India* **68** J4
Patan *India* **68** H5
Patani *Indonesia* **63** D7
Pătârlagele *Romania* **29** E11
Pataudi *India* **68** E7
Patchewollock *Australia* **95** F3
Patchogue *U.S.A.* **115** F11
Pate *Kenya* **86** C5
Patea *N.Z.* **91** C5
Pategi *Nigeria* **83** D6
Patensie *S. Africa* **88** E3
Paternion *Austria* **26** E6
Paternò *Italy* **43** E7
Pateros *U.S.A.* **108** B4
Paterson *U.S.A.* **115** F10
Paterson Ra. *Australia* **92** D3
Pathankot *India* **68** C6
Pathein = Bassein *Burma* **67** L19

Pathfinder Res. *U.S.A.* **108** E10
Pathiu *Thailand* **65** G2
Pathum Thani *Thailand* **64** E3
Pati *Indonesia* **63** G14
Patía → *Colombia* **124** C3
Patiala *Punjab, India* **68** D7
Patiala *Ut. P., India* **69** F8
Patine Kouka *Senegal* **82** C2
Patkai Bum *India* **67** F19
Patmos *Greece* **47** D8
Patna *India* **69** G11
Patnos *Turkey* **73** C10
Pato Branco *Brazil* **127** B5
Patong, Ao *Thailand* **65** a
Patonga *Uganda* **86** B3
Patos *Albania* **44** F3
Patos *Brazil* **125** E11
Patos, L. dos *Brazil* **127** C5
Patos, Río de los →
  Argentina **126** C2
Patos de Minas *Brazil* **125** G9
Patquía *Argentina* **126** C2
Patra *Greece* **46** C3
Patraikós Kólpos *Greece* **46** C3
Patras = Patra *Greece* **46** C3
Patrício *Brazil* **125** G9
Pattada *Italy* **42** B2
Pattani *Thailand* **65** J3
Pattaya *Thailand* **64** F3
Patten *U.S.A.* **113** B19
Patterson *Calif., U.S.A.* **110** H5
Patterson *La., U.S.A.* **116** G9
Patterson, Mt. *U.S.A.* **110** G7
Patti *Punjab, India* **68** D6
Patti *Ut. P., India* **69** G10
Patti *Italy* **43** D7
Pattoki *Pakistan* **68** D5
Patton *U.S.A.* **114** F6
Patuakhali *Bangla.* **67** H17
Patuanak *Canada* **103** B7
Patuca → *Honduras* **120** C3
Patuca, Punta *Honduras* **120** C3
Pătulele *Romania* **28** F7
Pátzcuaro *Mexico* **118** D4
Pau *France* **20** E3
Pau, Gave de → *France* **20** E2
Paudash *Canada* **114** B7
Pauillac *France* **20** C3
Pauk *Burma* **67** J19
Paul I. *Canada* **105** A7
Paul Smiths *U.S.A.* **115** B10
Paulatuk *Canada* **100** D7
Paulding Bay *S. Ocean* **5** C8
Paulhan *France* **20** E7
Paulistana *Brazil* **125** E10
Paulo Afonso *Brazil* **125** E11
Paulpietersburg *S. Africa* **89** D5
Pauls Valley *U.S.A.* **116** D6
Pauma Valley *U.S.A.* **111** M10
Pauri *India* **69** D8
Pāveh *Iran* **73** E12
Pavelets *Russia* **32** F10
Pavia *Italy* **40** C6
Pavilion *U.S.A.* **114** D6
Pavilly *France* **18** C7
Pāvilosta *Latvia* **30** B8
Pavlikeni *Bulgaria* **45** C9
Pavlodar *Kazakhstan* **52** D8
Pavlograd = Pavlohrad
  Ukraine **33** H8
Pavlohrad *Ukraine* **33** H8
Pavlovo *Russia* **34** C6
Pavlovsk *Russia* **34** E5
Pavlovskaya *Russia* **35** G4
Pavlovskiy-Posad *Russia* **32** E10
Pavullo nel Frignano *Italy* **40** D7
Pawai, Pulau *Singapore* **65** d
Pawayan *India* **69** E9
Pawhuska *U.S.A.* **116** C6
Pawling *U.S.A.* **115** E11
Pawnee *U.S.A.* **116** C6
Pawnee City *U.S.A.* **112** E5
Pawtucket *U.S.A.* **115** E13
Paxi *Greece* **46** B2
Paximádia *Greece* **49** E6
Paxton *U.S.A.* **112** E9
Payakumbuh *Indonesia* **62** E2
Payerne *Switz.* **25** J2
Payette *U.S.A.* **108** D5
Paymogo *Spain* **37** H3
Payne Bay = Kangirsuk
  Canada **101** F18
Payne L. *Canada* **101** F17
Paynes Find *Australia* **93** E2
Paynesville *Liberia* **82** D2
Paynesville *U.S.A.* **112** C6
Pays de la Loire □ *France* **18** E6
Paysandú *Uruguay* **126** C4
Payson *Ariz., U.S.A.* **109** J8
Payson *Utah, U.S.A.* **108** F8
Paz → *Guatemala* **120** D1
Paz, B. de la *Mexico* **118** C2
Pāzanān *Iran* **71** D6
Pazar *Turkey* **73** B9
Pazarcık *Turkey* **72** D7
Pazardzhik *Bulgaria* **45** D8

Pazarköy *Turkey* **47** B9
Pazarlar *Turkey* **47** C11
Pazaryeri *Turkey* **47** B11
Pazaryolu *Turkey* **73** B9
Pazin *Croatia* **41** C10
Pčinja → *Macedonia* **44** E5
Pe Ell *U.S.A.* **110** D3
Peabody *U.S.A.* **115** D14
Peace → *Canada* **102** B6
Peace Point *Canada* **102** B6
Peace River *Canada* **102** B5
Peach Springs *U.S.A.* **109** J7
Peachland *Canada* **102** D5
Peachtree City *U.S.A.* **117** E12
Peak, The = Kinder Scout
  U.K. **14** D6
Peak Charles △ *Australia* **93** F3
Peak District △ *U.K.* **14** D6
Peak Hill *Australia* **95** E4
Peak Ra. *Australia* **94** C4
Peake Cr. → *Australia* **95** D2
Peal de Becerro *Spain* **37** H7
Peale, Mt. *U.S.A.* **108** G9
Pearblossom *U.S.A.* **111** L9
Pearl → *U.S.A.* **117** F10
Pearl and Hermes Reef
  U.S.A. **107** K4
Pearl River = Zhu Jiang →
  China **59** F9
Pearl River *U.S.A.* **115** E10
Pearsall *U.S.A.* **116** G5
Pearson Int. Toronto ✈
  (YYZ) *Canada* **114** C5
Peary Land *Greenland* **4** A6
Pease → *U.S.A.* **116** D5
Peawanuck *Canada* **104** A2
Pebane *Mozam.* **87** F4
Pebas *Peru* **124** D4
Pebble Beach *U.S.A.* **110** J5
Peć = Kosovo *44** A4
Péccioli *Italy* **40** E7
Pechea *Romania* **29** E12
Pechenga *Russia* **8** B24
Pechenizhyn *Ukraine* **29** B9
Pechnezhskoye Vdkhr.
  Ukraine **33** G9
Pechora *Russia* **52** C6
Pechora → *Russia* **6** B16
Pechory *Russia* **32** C4
Pecica *Romania* **28** D6
Pecka *Serbia* **44** B3
Pécora, C. *Italy* **42** C1
Pecos *N. Mex., U.S.A.* **109** J11
Pecos *Tex., U.S.A.* **116** F3
Pecos → *U.S.A.* **116** G4
Pécs *Hungary* **28** D3
Pedasí *Panama* **120** E3
Pedder, L. *Australia* **95** G4
Peddie *S. Africa* **89** E4
Pedernales *Dom. Rep.* **121** C5
Pedirka Desert *Australia* **95** A1
Pedra Azul *Brazil* **125** G10
Pedra Lume → *C. Verde Is.* **78** b
Pedreguer *Spain* **39** G5
Pedreiras *Brazil* **125** D10
Pedro Afonso *Brazil* **125** E9
Pedro Cays *Jamaica* **120** C4
Pedro de Valdivia *Chile* **126** A2
Pedro Juan Caballero
  Paraguay **127** A4
Pedro Muñoz *Spain* **37** F8
Pedrógão Grande *Portugal* **36** F2
Pee Dee = Great Pee
  Dee → *U.S.A.* **117** E15
Peebinga *Australia* **95** E3
Peebles *U.K.* **13** F5
Peekskill *U.S.A.* **115** E11
Peel I. of Man *U.K.* **14** C3
Peel → *Australia* **95** E5
Peel → *Canada* **100** B6
Peel Sd. *Canada* **100** C12
Peene → *Germany* **24** A9
Peera Peera Poolanna L.
  Australia **95** D2
Peerless Lake *Canada* **102** B6
Peers *Canada* **102** C5
Pegasus Bay *N.Z.* **91** E4
Peggau *Austria* **26** D8
Pegnitz *Germany* **25** F7
Pegnitz → *Germany* **25** F6
Pego *Spain* **39** G4
Pegu *Burma* **67** L20
Pegu Yoma *Burma* **67** K20
Pehčevo *Macedonia* **44** E6
Pehlivanköy *Turkey* **45** E10
Pehuajó *Argentina* **126** D3
Pei Xian = Pizhou *China* **56** G9
Peikang *Taiwan* **59** F13
Peine *Chile* **126** A2
Peine *Germany* **24** C6
Peip'ing = Beijing *China* **56** E9
Peipus, L. = Chudskoye,
  Ozero *Russia* **32** C4
Peissenberg *Germany* **25** H7
Peitz *Germany* **24** D10
Peixe *Brazil* **125** F9
Peixe → *Brazil* **125** H8

Pek → *Serbia* **44** B5
Pekalongan *Indonesia* **62** F3
Pekan *Malaysia* **65** L4
Pekan Nenas *Malaysia* **65** d
Pekanbaru *Indonesia* **62** D2
Pekin *U.S.A.* **112** E9
Peking = Beijing *China* **56** E9
Pekutatan *Indonesia* **63** J17
Pelabuhan Klang *Malaysia* **65** L3
Pelabuhan Ratu, Teluk
  Indonesia **63** G12
Pelabuhanratu *Indonesia* **63** G12
Pélagos = Kira Panagia
  Greece **46** B5
Pelaihari *Indonesia* **62** E4
Pelat, Mt. *France* **21** D10
Peleaga, Vf. *Romania* **28** E7
Pelée, Mt. *Martinique* **120** c
Pelee, Pt. *Canada* **104** D3
Pelee I. *Canada* **114** E2
Pelekech *Kenya* **86** B4
Peleng *Indonesia* **63** E6
Pelentong *Malaysia* **65** d
Pélézi *Ivory C.* **82** D3
Pelham *U.S.A.* **117** F12
Pelican *U.S.A.* **102** B1
Pelican L. *Canada* **103** C8
Pelican Narrows *Canada* **103** B8
Pelister △ *Macedonia* **44** F5
Pelješac *Croatia* **41** F14
Pelkosenniemi *Finland* **8** C22
Pella *S. Africa* **88** D2
Pella *U.S.A.* **112** E7
Pella → *Greece* **44** F6
Pello *Finland* **8** C20
Pellworm *Germany* **24** A4
Pelly → *Canada* **102** A1
Pelly Bay *Canada* **101** D14
Peloponnese □ *Greece* **46** D4
Peloritani, Monti *Italy* **43** D8
Pelorus Sd. *N.Z.* **91** D4
Pelotas *Brazil* **127** C5
Pelotas → *Brazil* **127** B5
Pelovo *Bulgaria* **45** C8
Pelplin *Poland* **30** E5
Pelvoux, Massif du *France* **21** D10
Pemalang *Indonesia* **63** G13
Pemanggil, Pulau *Malaysia* **65** L5
Pematangsiantar *Indonesia* **62** D1
Pemba *Mozam.* **87** E5
Pemba *Zambia* **87** F2
Pemba Channel *Tanzania* **86** D4
Pemba I. *Tanzania* **86** D4
Pemberton *Australia* **93** F2
Pemberton *Canada* **102** C4
Pembina → *Canada* **102** C6
Pembroke *Canada* **104** C4
Pembroke *U.K.* **15** F3
Pembrokeshire □ *U.K.* **15** F3
Pembrokeshire Coast △ *U.K.* **15** F2
Pen-y-Ghent *U.K.* **14** C5
Peña, Sierra de la *Spain* **38** C4
Peña de Francia, Sierra de
  la *Spain* **36** E4
Peñafiel *Portugal* **36** D2
Peñafiel *Spain* **36** D6
Peñaflor *Spain* **37** H5
Penal *Trin. & Tob.* **125** K15
Peñalara *Spain* **36** E7
Penamacôr *Portugal* **36** E3
Penang = Pinang *Malaysia* **65** c
Penápolis *Brazil* **127** A6
Peñaranda de Bracamonte
  Spain **36** E5
Peñarroya *Spain* **38** E4
Peñarroya-Pueblonuevo
  Spain **37** G5
Penarth *U.K.* **15** F4
Peñas, C. de *Spain* **36** B5
Peñas, G. de *Chile* **128** F2
Peñas de San Pedro *Spain* **39** G3
Peñas del Chache *Canary Is.* **48** E6
Peñausende *Spain* **36** D5
Pench △ *India* **69** J8
Pench'i = Benxi *China* **57** D12
Pend Oreille → *U.S.A.* **108** B5
Pend Oreille, L. *U.S.A.* **108** B5
Pendalofos *Greece* **44** F5
Pendembu *Eastern, S. Leone* **82** D2
Pendembu *Northern, S. Leone* **82** D2
Pender B. *Australia* **92** C3
Pendik *Turkey* **45** F13
Pendjari △ *Benin* **83** C5
Pendjari → *Benin* **83** C5
Pendleton *U.S.A.* **108** D4
Pendra *India* **69** H9
Penedo *Brazil* **125** F11
Penelokan *Indonesia* **63** J18
Penetanguishene *Canada* **114** B5
Penfield *U.S.A.* **114** E6
Pengalengan *Indonesia* **63** G12
Penge *Kasai-Or.,
  Dem. Rep. of the Congo* **86** D1
Penge *Sud-Kivu,
  Dem. Rep. of the Congo* **86** C2
P'enghu Ch'üntou *Taiwan* **59** F12

Penglai *China* **57** F11
Pengshan *China* **58** B4
Pengshui *China* **58** C7
Penguin *Australia* **95** G4
Pengxi *China* **58** B5
Pengze *China* **59** C11
Penhalonga *Zimbabwe* **87** F3
Peniche *Portugal* **37** F1
Penicuik *U.K.* **13** F5
Penida, Nusa *Indonesia* **62** F5
Peninnes, Alpes = Pennine,
  Alpi *Alps* **25** J3
Peninsular Malaysia □
  Malaysia **65** L4
Peñíscola *Spain* **38** E5
Penitente, Serra do *Brazil* **125** E9
Pēnjwīn *Iraq* **73** E11
Penkridge *U.K.* **14** E5
Penmarch *France* **18** E2
Penmarch, Pte. de *France* **18** E2
Penn Hills *U.S.A.* **114** F5
Penn Yan *U.S.A.* **114** D7
Penna, Punta della *Italy* **41** F11
Penne *Italy* **41** F10
Penner → *India* **66** M12
Pennine, Alpi *Alps* **25** J3
Pennines *U.K.* **14** C5
Pennington *U.S.A.* **110** F5
Pennington → *Nigeria* **83** E6
Pennino, Mte. *Italy* **41** E9
Pennsburg *U.S.A.* **115** F9
Pennsylvania □ *U.S.A.* **113** E15
Penny *Canada* **102** C4
Peno *Russia* **32** D7
Penobscot → *U.S.A.* **113** C19
Penobscot B. *U.S.A.* **113** C19
Penola *Australia* **95** F3
Penong *Australia* **93** F5
Penonomé *Panama* **120** E3
Penrhyn *Cook Is.* **97** H12
Penrith *Australia* **95** E5
Penrith *U.K.* **14** C5
Penryn *U.K.* **15** G2
Pensacola *U.S.A.* **117** F11
Pensacola Mts. *Antarctica* **5** E1
Pense *Canada* **103** C7
Penshurst *Australia* **95** F3
Penticton *Canada* **102** D5
Pentland *Australia* **94** C4
Pentland Firth *U.K.* **13** C5
Pentland Hills *U.K.* **13** F5
Pentland Hills △ *U.K.* **13** F5
Penza *Russia* **34** D7
Penza □ *Russia* **34** D7
Penzance *U.K.* **15** G2
Penzberg *Germany* **25** H7
Penzhino *Russia* **53** C17
Penzhou *China* **58** B4
Penzlin *Germany* **24** B9
Peoria *Ariz., U.S.A.* **109** K7
Peoria *Ill., U.S.A.* **112** E9
Pepacton Res. *U.S.A.* **115** D10
Pepani → *S. Africa* **88** D3
Pepel *S. Leone* **82** D2
Peqin *Albania* **44** E3
Pera Hd. *Australia* **94** A3
Perabumulih *Indonesia* **62** E2
Perachora *Greece* **46** C4
Perak → *Malaysia* **65** K3
Perales del Alfambra *Spain* **38** E4
Perales del Puerto *Spain* **36** E4
Perama *Kérkyra, Greece* **49** A3
Perama *Kríti, Greece* **49** D6
Perancak *Indonesia* **63** J17
Peräpohjola *Finland* **8** C22
Perast *Montenegro* **44** D2
Percé *Canada* **105** C7
Perche *France* **18** D8
Perche → *France* **18** D7
Perchtoldsdorf *Austria* **27** C9
Percival Lakes *Australia* **92** D4
Percy *France* **18** D5
Percy Is. *Australia* **94** C5
Perdido, Mte. *Spain* **38** C5
Perdu, Mt. = Perdido, Mte.
  Spain **38** C5
Perechyn *Ukraine* **28** B7
Perehinske *Ukraine* **29** B9
Pereira *Colombia* **124** C3
Perelazovskiy *Russia* **35** F6
Perenjori *Australia* **93** E2
Peresecina *Moldova* **29** C13
Pereslavl-Zalesskiy *Russia* **32** D10
Peretu *Romania* **29** F10
Pereyaslav-Khmelnytskyy
  Ukraine **33** G6
Pereyma *Ukraine* **29** B14
Pérez, I. *Mexico* **119** C7
Perg *Austria* **26** C7
Pergamino *Argentina* **126** C3
Pérgine Valsugana *Italy* **41** B8
Pérgola *Italy* **41** E9
Perham *U.S.A.* **112** B6
Perhentian, Kepulauan
  Malaysia **65** K4
Peri → *Turkey* **73** C8
Periam *Romania* **28** D5

Péribonka → *Canada* **105** C5
Péribonka, L. *Canada* **105** B5
Perico *Argentina* **126** A2
Pericos *Mexico* **118** B3
Périers *France* **18** C5
Périgord *France* **20** D4
Périgord-Limousin △ *France* **20** C4
Périgueux *France* **20** C4
Perijá, Sierra de *Colombia* **124** B4
Perijá △ *Venezuela* **121** E5
Peristera *Greece* **46** B5
Peristerona → *Cyprus* **49** D12
Perito Moreno *Argentina* **128** F2
Perivol = Dragovishtitsa
  Bulgaria **44** D6
Perkasie *U.S.A.* **115** F9
Perković *Croatia* **41** E13
Perlas, Arch. de las *Panama* **120** E4
Perlas, Punta de *Nic.* **120** D3
Perleberg *Germany* **24** B7
Perlez *Serbia* **28** E5
Perm *Russia* **52** D6
Përmet *Albania* **44** F4
Pernambuco = Recife *Brazil*
  125 E12
Pernambuco □ *Brazil* **125** E11
Pernatty Lagoon *Australia* **95** E2
Pernik *Bulgaria* **44** D7
Peron Is. *Australia* **92** B5
Peron Pen. *Australia* **93** E1
Péronne *France* **19** C9
Perosa Argentina *Italy* **40** D4
Perow *Canada* **102** C3
Perpignan *France* **20** F6
Perris *U.S.A.* **111** M9
Perros-Guirec *France* **18** D3
Perry *Fla., U.S.A.* **117** F13
Perry *Ga., U.S.A.* **117** E13
Perry *Iowa, U.S.A.* **112** E6
Perry *N.Y., U.S.A.* **114** D7
Perry *Okla., U.S.A.* **116** C6
Perryton *U.S.A.* **116** C4
Perryville *U.S.A.* **112** G9
Persan *France* **19** C9
Persberg *Sweden* **10** E8
Perşembe *Turkey* **72** B7
Persepolis *Iran* **71** D7
Pershotravensk *Ukraine* **23** C14
Persia = Iran ■ *Asia* **71** C7
Persian Gulf *Asia* **71** E6
Perstorp *Sweden* **11** H7
Perth *Australia* **93** F2
Perth *Canada* **115** B8
Perth *U.K.* **13** E5
Perth & Kinross □ *U.K.* **13** E5
Perth Amboy *U.S.A.* **115** F10
Perth-Andover *Canada* **105** C6
Perth Basin *Ind. Oc.* **96** L2
Pertuis *France* **21** E9
Pertusato, C. *France* **21** G13
Peru *Ind., U.S.A.* **112** E10
Peru *N.Y., U.S.A.* **115** B11
Peru ■ *S. Amer.* **124** D4
Peru Basin *Pac. Oc.* **97** J18
Peru-Chile Trench *Pac. Oc.* **124** G3
Perúgia *Italy* **41** E9
Perušić *Croatia* **41** D12
Pervomaysk *Russia* **34** C6
Pervomaysk *Ukraine* **33** H6
Pervouralsk *Russia* **52** D6
Pésaro *Italy* **41** E9
Pescadores = P'enghu
  Ch'üntou *Taiwan* **59** F12
Pescara *Italy* **41** F11
Pescara → *Italy* **41** F11
Peschanokopskoye *Russia* **35** G5
Péscia *Italy* **40** E7
Pescina *Italy* **41** F10
Peshawar *Pakistan* **68** B4
Peshkopi *Albania* **44** E4
Peshtera *Bulgaria* **45** D8
Peshtigo *U.S.A.* **112** C10
Peski *Russia* **34** E6
Pêso da Régua *Portugal* **36** D3
Pesqueira *Brazil* **125** E11
Pessac *France* **20** D3
Pest □ *Hungary* **28** C4
Pestovo *Russia* **32** C8
Pestravka *Russia* **34** D9
Petah Tiqwa *Israel* **74** C3
Petalidi *Greece* **46** E3
Petaling Jaya *Malaysia* **65** L3
Petaloudes *Greece* **49** C10
Petaluma *U.S.A.* **110** G4
Pétange *Lux.* **17** E5
Petaro *Pakistan* **68** G3
Petas *Greece* **46** B3
Petatlán *Mexico* **118** D4
Petauke *Zambia* **87** E3
Petawawa *Canada* **104** C4
Petén Itzá, L. *Guatemala* **120** C2
Peter I. *Br. Virgin Is.* **121** e
Peter I. Øy *Antarctica* **5** C16
Peter Pond L. *Canada* **103** B7
Peterbell *Canada* **104** C3
Peterborough *Australia* **95** E2
Peterborough *Canada* **114** B6
Peterborough *U.K.* **15** E7
Peterborough □ *U.K.* **15** E7
Peterborough *U.S.A.* **115** D13
Peterculter *U.K.* **13** D6
Peterhead *U.K.* **13** D7
Peterlee *U.K.* **14** C6
Petermann Gletscher
  Greenland **101** A20
Petermann Ranges *Australia* **93** E5
Petermann ۞ *Australia* **93** E4
Petersburg *Alaska, U.S.A.* **100** F15
Petersburg *Pa., U.S.A.* **114** F6
Petersburg *Va., U.S.A.* **113** G15
Petersburg *W. Va., U.S.A.* **113** F14
Petersfield *U.K.* **15** F7
Petershagen *Germany* **24** C4
Petília Policastro *Italy* **43** C9
Petit-Canal *Guadeloupe* **120** b
Petit Goâve *Haiti* **121** C5
Petit Lac Manicouagan
  Canada **105** B6
Petit-Mécatina → *Canada* **105** B8
Petit-Mécatina, Î. du *Canada* **105** B8
Petit Piton *St. Lucia* **121** f
Petit Saint Bernard, Col du
  Italy **21** C10
Petit-Saguenay *Canada* **105** C5
Petite Terre, Îles de la
  Guadeloupe **120** b
Petitcodiac *Canada* **105** C6
Petitot → *Canada* **102** A4
Petitsikapau L. *Canada* **105** B6
Petlad *India* **68** H5
Peto *Mexico* **119** C7
Petone *N.Z.* **91** D5
Petorca *Chile* **126** C1
Petoskey *U.S.A.* **113** C11
Petra *Jordan* **74** F4
Petra *Spain* **48** B10
Petra, Ostrova *Russia* **53** B12
Petra Velikogo, Zaliv *Russia* **54** C6
Petre, Pt. *Canada* **114** C7
Petrel = Petrer *Spain* **39** G4
Petrella, Monte *Italy* **42** A6
Petrer *Spain* **39** G4
Petreto-Bicchisano *France* **21** G12
Petrich *Bulgaria* **44** E7
Petrified Forest △ *U.S.A.* **109** J9
Petrijanec *Croatia* **41** B13
Petrikov = Pyetrikaw
  Belarus **23** B15
Petrila *Romania* **29** E8
Petrinja *Croatia* **41** C13
Petrodvorets *Russia* **32** C5
Petrolândia *Brazil* **125** E11
Petrolia *Canada* **114** D2
Petrolina *Brazil* **125** E10
Petropavl *Kazakhstan* **52** D7
Petropavlovsk = Petropavl
  Kazakhstan **52** D7
Petropavlovsk-
  Kamchatskiy *Russia* **53** D16
Petropavlovskiy =
  Akhtubinsk *Russia* **35** F8
Petrópolis *Brazil* **127** A7
Petroşani *Romania* **29** E8
Petrova Gora *Croatia* **41** C12
Petrovac *Montenegro* **44** D2
Petrovac *Serbia* **44** B5
Petrovaradin *Serbia* **28** E4
Petrovsk *Russia* **34** D7
Petrovsk-Zabaykalskiy
  Russia **53** D11
Petrovskaya *Russia* **33** K9
Petrozavodsk *Russia* **32** B8
Petrus Steyn *S. Africa* **89** D4
Petrusburg *S. Africa* **88** D4
Petzeck *Austria* **26** E5
Peumo *Chile* **126** C1
Pevek *Russia* **53** C18
Peveragno *Italy* **40** D4
Peyrehorade *France* **20** E2
Peyruis *France* **21** D9
Pézenas *France* **20** E7
Pezinok *Slovak Rep.* **27** C10
Pfaffenhofen *Germany* **25** G7
Pfälzerwald △ *Germany* **25** F5
Pfarrkirchen *Germany* **25** G8
Pfeffenhausen *Germany* **25** G7
Pforzheim *Germany* **25** G4
Pfullendorf *Germany* **25** H5
Pfungstadt *Germany* **25** F4
Pha Taem △ *Thailand* **64** E5
Phaestos *Greece* **49** D6
Phagwara *India* **68** D6
Phala *Botswana* **88** C4
Phalera = Phulera *India* **68** F6
Phalodi *India* **68** F5
Phalsbourg *France* **19** D14
Phaluai, Ko *Thailand* **65** b
Phan *Thailand* **64** C2
Phan Rang *Vietnam* **65** G7
Phan Ri = Hoa Da *Vietnam* **65** G7
Phan Thiet *Vietnam* **65** G7
Phanae *Greece* **47** C7
Phanat Nikhom *Thailand* **64** F3
Phangan, Ko *Thailand* **65** H3
Phangnga *Thailand* **65** H2
Phangnga, Ao *Thailand* **65** a
Phanom Sarakham *Thailand* **64** F3
Phaphund *India* **69** F8
Pharenda *India* **69** F10
Pharr *U.S.A.* **116** H5
Phatthalung *Thailand* **65** J3
Phayao *Thailand* **64** C2
Phelps *U.S.A.* **114** D7
Phelps L. *Canada* **103** B8
Phenix City *U.S.A.* **117** E12
Phet Buri *Thailand* **64** F2
Phetchabun *Thailand* **64** D3
Phetchabun, Thiu Khao
  Thailand **64** D3
Phetchaburi = Phet Buri
  Thailand **64** F2
Phi Phi, Ko *Thailand* **65** J2
Phiafay *Laos* **64** E6
Phibun Mangsahan *Thailand* **64** E5
Phichai *Thailand* **64** D3
Phichit *Thailand* **64** D3
Philadelphia *Miss., U.S.A.* **117** E10
Philadelphia *N.Y., U.S.A.* **115** B9
Philadelphia *Pa., U.S.A.* **115** G9
Philip *U.S.A.* **112** C3
Philip Smith Mts. *U.S.A.* **106** B10
Philipi *Greece* **45** E8
Philippi *U.S.A.* **113** F13
Philippi L. *Australia* **94** C2
Philippeville *Belgium* **17** D4
Philippine Basin *Pac. Oc.* **96** F5
Philippine Sea *Pac. Oc.* **61** C6
Philippine Trench =
  Mindanao Trench *Pac. Oc.* **61** F7
Philippines ■ *Asia* **61** F5
Philippolis *S. Africa* **88** E4
Philippopolis = Plovdiv
  Bulgaria **45** D8
Philipsburg *Canada* **115** A11
Philipsburg *Mont., U.S.A.* **108** C7
Philipsburg *Pa., U.S.A.* **114** F6
Philipstown = Daingean
  Ireland **12** C4
Philipstown *S. Africa* **88** E3
Phillip I. *Australia* **95** F4
Phillips *U.S.A.* **112** C8
Phillipsburg *Kans., U.S.A.* **112** F4
Phillipsburg *N.J., U.S.A.* **115** F9
Philmont *U.S.A.* **115** D11
Philomath *U.S.A.* **108** D2
Phimai *Thailand* **64** E4
Phitsanulok *Thailand* **64** D3
Phnom Kulen △ *Cambodia* **64** F5
Phnom Penh *Cambodia* **65** G5
Phnum Penh = Phnom
  Penh *Cambodia* **65** G5
Phoenicia *U.S.A.* **115** D10
Phoenix *Mauritius* **85** d
Phoenix *Ariz., U.S.A.* **109** K7
Phoenix *N.Y., U.S.A.* **115** C8
Phoenix Is. *Kiribati* **96** H10
Phoenixville *U.S.A.* **115** F9
Phon *Thailand* **64** E4
Phon Tiou *Laos* **64** D5
Phong → *Thailand* **64** D4
Phong Saly *Laos* **58** G4
Phong Tho *Vietnam* **64** A4
Phonhong *Laos* **64** C4
Phonum *Thailand* **65** H2
Phra Nakhon Si Ayutthaya
  Thailand **64** E3
Phra Pradaeng *Thailand* **64** F3
Phra Thong, Ko *Thailand* **65** H2
Phrae *Thailand* **64** C3
Phrom Phiram *Thailand* **64** D3
Phrygia *Turkey* **72** C4
Phu Bia *Laos* **64** C4
Phu Chong-Na Yoi △
  Thailand **64** E5
Phu Dien *Vietnam* **64** C5
Phu Hin Rang Kla △
  Thailand **64** D3
Phu Kradung △ *Thailand* **64** D3
Phu Luang △ *Thailand* **64** D3
Phu Ly *Vietnam* **58** G5
Phu Phan △ *Thailand* **64** D4
Phu Quoc, Dao *Vietnam* **65** G4
Phu Tho *Vietnam* **58** G5
Phu Wiang △ *Thailand* **64** D4
Phuc Yen *Vietnam* **58** G5
Phuket *Thailand* **65** a
Phuket, Ko *Thailand* **65** a
Phul *India* **68** D6
Phulad *India* **68** G5
Phulchari *Bangla.* **69** G13
Phulera *India* **68** F6
Phulpur *India* **69** G10
Phun Phin *Thailand* **65** H2
Phuntsholing *Bhutan* **69** F13
Piacenza *Italy* **40** C6
Piai, Tanjung *Malaysia* **65** d
Pian Cr. → *Australia* **95** E4
Pian-Upe △ *Uganda* **86** B3
Piana *France* **21** F12
Pianella *Italy* **41** F11
Pianosa *Puglia, Italy* **41** F12
Pianosa *Toscana, Italy* **40** F7
Piapot *Canada* **103** D7
Pias *Portugal* **37** G3
Piaseczno *Poland* **31** F8
Piaski *Poland* **31** G9
Piastów *Poland* **31** F7
Piatra *Romania* **29** G10
Piatra Craiului △ *Romania* **29** E10
Piatra Neamţ *Romania* **29** D11
Piatra Olt *Romania* **29** F9
Piauí □ *Brazil* **125** E10
Piauí → *Brazil* **125** E10
Piave → *Italy* **41** C9
Piazza Ármerina *Italy* **43** E7
Pia ۞ *Australia* **93** E2
Pibor → *Sudan* **81** F3
Pibor Post *Sudan* **81** F3
Picardie □ *France* **19** C9
Picardie, Plaine de *France* **19** C9
Picardy = Picardie □ *France* **19** C10
Picayune *U.S.A.* **117** F10
Picerno *Italy* **43** B8
Pichhor *India* **69** G8
Pichilemu *Chile* **126** C1
Pichor *India* **68** G7
Pickerel L. *Canada* **104** C1
Pickering *U.K.* **14** C7
Pickering, Vale of *U.K.* **14** C7
Pickle Lake *Canada* **104** B1
Pickwick L. *U.S.A.* **117** D10
Pico *Azores* **78** a
Pico Bonito △ *Honduras* **120** C2
Pico Truncado *Argentina* **128** F3
Picos *Brazil* **125** E10
Picos de Europa △ *Spain* **36** B6
Picton *Canada* **114** B7
Picton *N.Z.* **91** D5
Pictou *Canada* **105** C7
Picture Butte *Canada* **102** D6
Pictured Rocks △ *U.S.A.* **112** B10
Picún Leufú *Argentina* **128** D3
Pidbuzh *Ukraine* **23** D12
Pidurutalagala *Sri Lanka* **66** R12
Piechowice *Poland* **31** H2
Piedmont *S. Africa* **88** E3
Piedmont = Piemonte □
  Italy **40** D5
Piedmont *Ala., U.S.A.* **117** E12
Piedmont *S.C., U.S.A.* **98** F11
Piedra → *Spain* **38** D3
Piedrabuena *Spain* **37** G6
Piedrahita *Spain* **36** E5
Piedralaves *Spain* **36** E6
Piedras Blancas △ *Spain* **36** B5
Piedras Negras *Mexico* **118** B4
Piekary Śląskie *Poland* **31** H5
Pieksämäki *Finland* **32** A4
Pielinen *Finland* **8** E23
Piemonte □ *Italy* **40** D5
Pienaarsrivier *S. Africa* **89** D4
Pieniężno *Poland* **30** D7
Pieninský △ *Europe* **27** B13
Pieńsk *Poland* **31** G2
Piercefield *U.S.A.* **115** B10
Pierceland *Canada* **103** C7
Pieria □ *Greece* **44** F6
Pierpont *U.S.A.* **114** E4
Pierre *U.S.A.* **112** C3
Pierre-Buffière *France* **20** C5
Pierre-de-Bresse *France* **19** F12
Pierrefonds *Canada* **115** A11
Pierrefontaine-les-Varans
  France **19** E13
Pierrefort *France* **20** D6
Pierrelatte *France* **21** D8
Pierreville *Trin. & Tob.* **125** K16
Piešťany *Slovak Rep.* **27** C10
Piesting → *Austria* **27** C9
Pieszyce *Poland* **31** H3
Piet Retief *S. Africa* **89** D5
Pietarsaari *Finland* **8** E20
Pietermaritzburg *S. Africa* **89** D5
Pietersburg = Polokwane
  S. Africa **89** C4
Pietragalla *Italy* **43** B8
Pietrasanta *Italy* **40** E7
Pietroşiţa *Romania* **29** E10
Pietrosul, Vf. *Maramureş,*
  Romania **29** C9
Pietrosul, Vf. *Suceava,*
  Romania **29** C10
Pieve di Cadore *Italy* **41** B9
Pieve di Teco *Italy* **40** D4
Pievepélago *Italy* **40** D7
Pigadítsa *Greece* **44** G5
Pigeon L. *Canada* **114** B6
Piges *Greece* **46** B3
Piggott *U.S.A.* **117** C9
Pigna *Italy* **40** E4
Pigüe *Argentina* **126** D3
Pihani *India* **69** F9
Pihlajavesi *Finland* **32** B5
Pijijiapan *Mexico* **119** D6
Pikalevo *Russia* **32** C8
Pikangikum *Canada* **103** C10
Pikes Peak *U.S.A.* **108** G11
Piketberg *S. Africa* **88** E2
Pikeville *U.S.A.* **113** G12
Pikou *China* **57** E12
Pikwitonei *Canada* **103** B9
Piła *Poland* **31** E3
Pila *Spain* **39** G3
Pilanesberg △ *S. Africa* **88** D4
Pilani *India* **68** E6
Pilar *Paraguay* **126** B4
Pilar de la Horadada *Spain* **39** H4
Pilat △ *France* **21** C9
Pilawa *Poland* **31** G8
Pilaya → *Bolivia* **124** H6
Pilbara *Australia* **92** D2
Pilcomaya → *Paraguay* **126** B4
Pilea *Greece* **44** F6
Pilgrim's Rest *S. Africa* **89** C5
Pilgrimstad *Sweden* **10** B9
Pili *Greece* **47** E9
Pilibhit *India* **69** E8
Pilica → *Poland* **31** G8
Pilio, Oros *Greece* **46** B5
Pilipinas = Philippines ■
  Asia **61** F5
Pilis *Hungary* **28** C4
Pilisvörösvár *Hungary* **28** C3
Pilkhawa *India* **68** E7
Pilliga *Australia* **95** E4
Pilos *Greece* **46** E3
Pilot Mound *Canada* **103** D9
Pilot Point *U.S.A.* **116** E6
Pilot Rock *U.S.A.* **108** D4
Pilštanj *Slovenia* **41** B12
Piltene *Latvia* **30** A8
Pilzno *Poland* **31** J8
Pima *U.S.A.* **109** K9
Pimba *Australia* **95** E2
Pimenta Bueno *Brazil* **124** F6
Pimentel *Peru* **124** E3
Pin Valley △ *India* **68** D7
Pina de Ebro *Spain* **38** D4
Pinamalayan *Phil.* **61** E4
Pinang *Malaysia* **65** c
Pinar, C. des *Spain* **48** B10
Pinar del Río *Cuba* **120** B3
Pınarbaşı *Çanakkale, Turkey* **47** B8
Pınarbaşı *Kayseri, Turkey* **72** C7
Pınarhisar *Turkey* **45** E11
Pinatubo, Mt. *Phil.* **61** D3
Pinawa *Canada* **103** C9
Pincehely *Hungary* **28** D3
Pinchang *China* **58** B6
Pincher Creek *Canada* **102** D6
Pinchi L. *Canada* **102** C4
Pinckneyville *U.S.A.* **112** F9
Pińczów *Poland* **31** H7
Pindar *Australia* **93** E2
Pindera Downs ۞ *Australia* **95** A3
Pindi Gheb *Pakistan* **68** C5
Pindiga *Nigeria* **83** D7
Pindos △ *Greece* **46** B3
Pindos Oros *Greece* **46** B3
Pindus Mts. = Pindos Oros
  Greece **46** B3
Pine → *B.C., Canada* **102** B4
Pine → *Sask., Canada* **103** B7
Pine Bluff *U.S.A.* **116** D8
Pine Bluffs *U.S.A.* **108** F11
Pine City *U.S.A.* **112** C7
Pine Cr. → *U.S.A.* **114** E7
Pine Creek *Australia* **92** B5
Pine Falls *Canada* **103** C9
Pine Flat L. *U.S.A.* **110** J7
Pine Grove *U.S.A.* **115** F8
Pine Hill *U.S.A.* **94** C4
Pine Pass *Canada* **102** B4
Pine Point *Canada* **102** A6
Pine Ridge *U.S.A.* **112** D2
Pine River *Canada* **103** C8
Pine River *U.S.A.* **112** B6
Pine Valley *U.S.A.* **111** N10
Pinecrest *U.S.A.* **110** G6
Pineda de Mar *Spain* **38** D7
Pinedale *Calif., U.S.A.* **110** J7
Pinedale *Wyo., U.S.A.* **108** E9
Pinega → *Russia* **52** C5
Pinehouse L. *Canada* **103** B7
Pineimuta → *Canada* **104** B1
Pinerolo *Italy* **40** D4
Pines, Akra *Greece* **45** F8
Pineto *Italy* **41** F11
Pinetop-Lakeside *U.S.A.* **109** J9
Pinetown *S. Africa* **89** D5
Pineville *U.S.A.* **116** F8
Piney *France* **19** D11
Ping → *Thailand* **64** E3
Pingaring *Australia* **93** F2
Pingba *China* **58** D6
Pingbian *China* **58** F4
Pingchuan *China* **58** D3
Pingding *China* **56** F7
Pingdingshan *China* **56** H7
Pingdong *Taiwan* **59** F13
Pingdu *China* **57** F10
Pingelly *Australia* **93** F2
Pingguo *China* **58** F6
Pinghe *China* **59** E11
Pinghu *China* **59** B13
Pingjiang *China* **59** C9
Pingle *China* **59** E8
Pingli *China* **58** A7
Pingliang *China* **56** G4
Pinglu *China* **56** E7
Pingluo *China* **56** E4
Pingnan *Fujian, China* **59** D12
Pingnan *Guangxi Zhuangzu,*
  China **59** F8
Pingquan *China* **57** D10
Pingrup *Australia* **93** F2
Pingshan *China* **58** C5
Pingtan *China* **59** E12
Pingtang *China* **58** E5
P'ingtung *Taiwan* **59** F13
Pingwu *China* **56** H3
Pingxiang *Guangxi Zhuangzu,*
  China **58** F6
Pingxiang *Jiangxi, China* **59** D9
Pingyao *China* **56** F7
Pingyi *China* **57** G9
Pingyin *China* **56** F9
Pingyuan *Guangdong, China* **59** E10
Pingyuan *Shandong, China* **56** F9
Pingyuanjie *China* **58** F4
Pinhal Novo *Portugal* **37** G2
Pinheiro *Brazil* **125** D9
Pinheiro Machado *Brazil* **127** C5
Pinhel *Portugal* **36** E3
Pini *Indonesia* **62** D1
Pinios → *Ilia, Greece* **46** D3
Pinios → *Trikala, Greece* **46** B4
Pinjarra *Australia* **93** F2
Pink Mountain *Canada* **102** B4
Pinkafeld *Austria* **27** D9
Pinnacles △ *U.S.A.* **110** J5
Pinnaroo *Australia* **95** F3
Pinneberg *Germany* **24** B5
Pinon Hills *U.S.A.* **111** L9
Pinos *Mexico* **118** C4
Pinos, Mt. *U.S.A.* **111** L7
Pinos Pt. *U.S.A.* **109** H3
Pinos Puente *Spain* **37** H7
Pinrang *Indonesia* **63** E5
Pins, Pte. aux *Canada* **114** D3
Pinsk *Belarus* **23** B14
Pintados *Chile* **124** H5
Pinyang *China* **59** D13
Pinyug *Russia* **52** C5
Pioche *U.S.A.* **109** H6
Piombino *Italy* **40** F7
Piombino, Canale di *Italy* **40** F7
Pioner, Ostrov *Russia* **53** B10
Pionerskiy *Russia* **30** D7
Pionki *Poland* **31** G8
Piopiotaki = Milford Sd. *N.Z.* **91** F1
Piorini, L. *Brazil* **124** D6
Piotrków Trybunalski
  Poland **31** G6
Piove di Sacco *Italy* **41** C9
Pīp *Iran* **71** E9
Pipar *India* **68** F5
Pipar Road *India* **68** F5
Piparia *Mad. P., India* **68** H8
Piparia *Mad. P., India* **68** J7
Piperi *Greece* **46** B6
Pipestone *U.S.A.* **112** D5
Pipestone → *Canada* **104** B2
Pipestone Cr. → *Canada* **103** D8
Piplan *Pakistan* **68** C4
Piploda *India* **68** H6
Pipmuacan, Rés. *Canada* **105** C5
Pippingarra *Australia* **92** D2
Pipriac *France* **18** E5
Piqua *U.S.A.* **113** E11
Piquiri → *Brazil* **127** A5
Pir Panjal Range *India* **68** C7
Pīr Sohrāb *Iran* **71** E9
Pira *Benin* **83** D5
Piracicaba *Brazil* **127** A6
Piracuruca *Brazil* **125** D10
Pirae *Tahiti* **91** d
Piræus = Pireas *Greece* **46** D5
Piraiévs = Pireas *Greece* **46** D5
Pirajuí *Brazil* **127** A6
Piram I. *India* **68** J5
Piran *Slovenia* **41** C10
Pirané *Argentina* **126** B4
Pirano = Piran *Slovenia* **41** C10
Pīrānshahr *Iran* **73** D11
Pirapora *Brazil* **125** G10
Pirawa *India* **68** G7
Pirdop *Bulgaria* **45** D8
Pireas *Greece* **46** D5
Pirgi *Greece* **47** C7
Pirgos, Ilia, *Greece* **46** D3
Pirgos, Kriti, *Greece* **47** F7
Pirgovo *Bulgaria* **45** C9
Piribebuy *Paraguay* **126** B4
Pirimapun *Indonesia* **63** F9
Pirin △ *Bulgaria* **44** E7
Pirin Planina *Bulgaria* **44** E7
Pirineos = Pyrénées *Europe* **20** F4
Piripiri *Brazil* **125** D10
Pirlangimpi *Australia* **92** B5
Pirmasens *Germany* **25** F3
Pirna *Germany* **24** E9
Pirot *Serbia* **44** C6
Piru *Indonesia* **63** E7
Piru *U.S.A.* **111** L8
Piryatin = Pyryatyn *Ukraine* **33** G7
Pisa *Italy* **40** E7
Pisa → *Poland* **31** E8
Pisa, Firenze ✈ (PSA) *Italy* **40** E7
Pisagne *Italy* **40** C7
Pisagua *Chile* **124** G4
Pisarovina *Croatia* **41** C12

Pisco *Peru* 124 F3
Piscu *Romania* 29 E12
Písek *Czech Rep.* 26 B7
Pishan *China* 60 C2
Pishchanka *Ukraine* 31 G10
Pishchanka *Ukraine* 29 B13
Pishin *Iran* 71 E9
Pishin *Pakistan* 68 D2
Pishin Lora → *Pakistan* 68 E1
Pisidia *Turkey* 72 D4
Pising *Indonesia* 63 F6
Pismo Beach *U.S.A.* 111 K6
Piso, L. *Liberia* 82 D2
Pissila *Burkina Faso* 83 C4
Pissis, Cerro *Argentina* 126 B2
Pissos *France* 20 D3
Pissouri *Cyprus* 49 E11
Pisticci *Italy* 43 B9
Pistóia *Italy* 40 E7
Pistol B. *Canada* 103 A10
Pisuerga → *Spain* 36 D6
Pisz *Poland* 30 E8
Pit → *U.S.A.* 108 F2
Pita *Guinea* 82 C2
Pitarpunga L. *Australia* 95 E3
Pitcairn I. *Pac. Oc.* 97 K14
Pitch L. *Trin. & Tob.* 125 K15
Piteå *Sweden* 8 D19
Piteälven → *Sweden* 8 D19
Piterka *Russia* 34 E8
Pitești *Romania* 29 F9
Pithapuram *India* 67 L13
Pithara *Australia* 93 F2
Pithio *Greece* 45 E10
Pithoragarh *India* 69 E9
Pithoro *Pakistan* 68 G3
Pitigliano *Italy* 41 F8
Pitkyaranta *Russia* 32 B6
Pitlochry *U.K.* 13 E5
Pitsilia *Cyprus* 49 E12
Pitt I. *Canada* 102 C2
Pittsburg *Calif., U.S.A.* 110 G5
Pittsburg *Kans., U.S.A.* 112 G6
Pittsburg *Tex., U.S.A.* 116 E7
Pittsburgh *U.S.A.* 114 F5
Pittsfield *Ill., U.S.A.* 112 F8
Pittsfield *Maine, U.S.A.* 113 C19
Pittsfield *Mass., U.S.A.* 115 D11
Pittsfield *N.H., U.S.A.* 115 C13
Pittston *U.S.A.* 115 E9
Pittsworth *Australia* 95 D5
Pituri → *Australia* 94 C2
Piura *Peru* 124 E2
Piva → *Montenegro* 44 C2
Piwniczna *Poland* 31 J7
Pixley *U.S.A.* 110 K7
Pizarra *Spain* 37 J6
Pizhou *China* 56 G9
Pizzo *Italy* 43 D9
Placentia *Canada* 105 C9
Placentia B. *Canada* 105 C9
Placer *Masbate, Phil.* 61 F5
Placer *Surigao N., Phil.* 61 G6
Placerville *U.S.A.* 110 G6
Placetas *Cuba* 120 B4
Plačkovica *Macedonia* 44 E6
Plainfield *N.J., U.S.A.* 115 F10
Plainfield *Ohio, U.S.A.* 114 F3
Plainfield *Vt., U.S.A.* 115 B12
Plains *Mont., U.S.A.* 108 C6
Plains *Tex., U.S.A.* 116 J3
Plainview *Nebr., U.S.A.* 112 D5
Plainview *Tex., U.S.A.* 116 D4
Plainwell *U.S.A.* 113 D11
Plaisance *France* 20 E4
Plaistow *U.S.A.* 115 D13
Plaka *Greece* 47 B7
Plaka, Akra *Greece* 49 D8
Plakenska Planina *Macedonia* 44 E5
Planá *Czech Rep.* 26 B5
Plana Cays *Bahamas* 121 B5
Planada *U.S.A.* 110 H6
Plancoët *France* 18 D4
Plandište *Serbia* 28 E6
Plano *U.S.A.* 116 E6
Plant City *U.S.A.* 117 G13
Plaquemine *U.S.A.* 116 F9
Plasencia *Spain* 36 E4
Plaški *Croatia* 41 C12
Plaster City *U.S.A.* 111 N11
Plaster Rock *Canada* 105 C6
Plastun *Russia* 54 B8
Plasy *Czech Rep.* 26 B6
Plata, Río de la → *S. Amer.* 126 C4
Plátani → *Italy* 42 E6
Platanos *Greece* 49 D5
Plateau □ *Nigeria* 83 D6
Platte *U.S.A.* 112 D4
Platte → *Mo., U.S.A.* 112 F6
Platte → *Nebr., U.S.A.* 112 E6
Platteville *U.S.A.* 112 D8
Plattling *Germany* 25 G8
Plattsburgh *U.S.A.* 115 B11
Plattsmouth *U.S.A.* 112 E6
Plau *Germany* 24 B8
Plauen *Germany* 24 E8
Plauer See *Germany* 24 B8
Plav *Montenegro* 44 D3
Plavinas *Latvia* 32 D3

Plavnica *Montenegro* 44 D3
Plavno *Croatia* 41 D13
Plavsk *Russia* 32 F9
Playa Blanca *Canary Is.* 48 F6
Playa Blanca Sur *Canary Is.* 48 F6
Playa de las Americas
Canary Is. 48 F3
Playa de Mogán *Canary Is.* 48 G4
Playa del Carmen *Mexico* 119 C7
Playa del Inglés *Canary Is.* 48 G4
Playa Esmerelda *Canary Is.* 48 F5
Playgreen L. *Canada* 103 C9
Pleasant Bay *Canada* 105 C7
Pleasant Hill *U.S.A.* 110 H4
Pleasant Mount *U.S.A.* 115 E9
Pleasanton *Calif., U.S.A.* 110 H5
Pleasanton *Tex., U.S.A.* 116 G5
Pleasantville *N.J., U.S.A.* 113 F16
Pleasantville *Pa., U.S.A.* 114 E5
Pléaux *France* 20 C6
Plei Ku *Vietnam* 64 F7
Plélan-le-Grand *France* 18 D4
Pléneuf-Val-André *France* 18 D4
Plenița *Romania* 29 F8
Plenty → *Australia* 94 C2
Plenty, B. of *N.Z.* 91 B6
Plentywood *U.S.A.* 108 B11
Plérin *France* 18 D4
Plessisville *Canada* 105 C5
Plestin-les-Grèves *France* 18 D3
Pleszew *Poland* 31 G4
Pleternica *Croatia* 28 E2
Plétipi, L. *Canada* 105 B5
Pleven *Bulgaria* 45 C8
Plevlja *Montenegro* 44 C3
Plevna *Canada* 114 B8
Plitvička Jezera △ *Croatia* 41 D12
Pljevica *Croatia* 41 D12
Ploaghe *Italy* 42 B1
Ploče *Croatia* 41 E14
Płock *Poland* 31 F6
Plöckenpass *Italy* 41 B9
Plöckenstein *Germany* 25 G9
Ploemeur *France* 18 E3
Ploërmel *France* 18 E4
Ploiești *Romania* 29 F11
Plomari *Greece* 47 C8
Plombières-les-Bains *France* 19 E13
Plomin *Croatia* 41 C11
Plön *Germany* 24 A6
Plonge, Lac la *Canada* 103 B7
Płońsk *Poland* 31 F7
Plopeni *Romania* 29 E10
Plopii-Slăvitești *Romania* 29 F9
Plopișului, Munții *Romania* 28 C7
Płoty *Poland* 30 E2
Plouaret *France* 18 D3
Plouay *France* 18 E3
Plouha *France* 18 D4
Plouhinec *France* 18 E2
Plougasnou *France* 18 D3
Plougastel-Daoulas *France* 18 D2
Plouguerneau *France* 18 D2
Plouha *France* 18 D4
Plouhinec *France* 18 E2
Ploudalmézeau *France* 18 D2
Plouescat *France* 18 D2
Plouha *France* 18 D4
Plouhinec *France* 18 E2
Plovdiv *Bulgaria* 45 D8
Plovdiv □ *Bulgaria* 45 D8
Plum *U.S.A.* 114 F5
Plum I. *U.S.A.* 115 E12
Plumas *U.S.A.* 110 F6
Plummer *U.S.A.* 108 C5
Plumridge Lakes *Australia* 93 E4
Plumtree *Zimbabwe* 87 G2
Plungė *Lithuania* 30 C8
Pluvigner *France* 18 E3
Plužine *Montenegro* 44 C2
Plymouth *Trin. & Tob.* 125 J16
Plymouth *U.K.* 15 G3
Plymouth *Calif., U.S.A.* 110 G6
Plymouth *Ind., U.S.A.* 112 E10
Plymouth *Mass., U.S.A.* 115 E14
Plymouth *N.C., U.S.A.* 117 D16
Plymouth *N.H., U.S.A.* 115 C13
Plymouth *Pa., U.S.A.* 115 E9
Plymouth *Wis., U.S.A.* 112 D10
Plympton-Wyoming =
Wyoming *Canada* 114 D2
Plynlimon = Pumlumon
Fawr *U.K.* 15 E4
Plyusa *Russia* 32 C5
Plyusa → *Russia* 32 C5
Plzeň *Czech Rep.* 26 B6
Plzeňský □ *Czech Rep.* 26 B6
Pmere Nyente ☉ *Australia* 94 C2
Pniewy *Poland* 31 F3
Pô *Burkina Faso* 83 C4
Po → *Italy* 41 D9
Po, Foci del *Italy* 41 D9
Pô △ *Burkina Faso* 83 C4
Po Hai = Bo Hai *China* 57 E10
Pobé *Benin* 83 D5
Pobé *Burkina Faso* 83 C4
Pobeda *Russia* 53 C15
Pobedy, Pik *Kyrgyzstan* 52 E8
Pobiedziska *Poland* 31 F4
Pobladura del Valle *Spain* 36 C5
Pobra de Trives *Spain* 36 C3
Pocahontas *Ark., U.S.A.* 117 C9
Pocahontas *Iowa, U.S.A.* 112 D6
Pocatello *U.S.A.* 108 E7

Počátky *Czech Rep.* 26 B8
Pochep *Russia* 33 F7
Pochinki *Russia* 34 C7
Pochinok *Russia* 32 E7
Pochutla *Mexico* 119 D5
Pocinhos *Brazil* 127 A6
Pocklington Reef *Papua N. G.* ...
Pocomoke City *U.S.A.* 113 F16
Poços de Caldas *Brazil* 127 A6
Podberezye *Russia* 32 C6
Poděbrady *Czech Rep.* 26 A6
Poddębice *Poland* 31 G5
Podensac *France* 20 D3
Podenzano *Italy* 40 D6
Podgorač *Croatia* 28 E3
Podgorica *Montenegro* 44 D3
Podgorie *Albania* 44 F4
Podilska Vysochyna
Ukraine 29 B13
Podkarpackie □ *Poland* 31 H9
Podkova *Bulgaria* 45 E9
Podlapača *Croatia* 41 D12
Podlaskie □ *Poland* 31 E10
Podoleni *Romania* 29 D11
Podolínec *Slovak Rep.* 27 B13
Podolsk *Russia* 32 E9
Podor *Senegal* 82 B1
Podporozhye *Russia* 32 B8
Podu Iloaiei *Romania* 29 C12
Podu Turcului *Romania* 29 D12
Podujevo *Kosovo* 44 D5
Podyjí △ *Czech Rep.* 26 C8
Poel *Germany* 24 B6
Pofadder *S. Africa* 88 D2
Poggiardo *Italy* 43 B11
Poggibonsi *Italy* 40 E8
Póggio Mirteto *Italy* 41 F9
Pogoanele *Romania* 29 F12
Pogorzela *Poland* 31 G4
Pogradec *Albania* 44 F4
Pogranichnyy *Russia* 54 B5
Poh *Indonesia* 63 E6
Pohang *S. Korea* 57 F15
Pohjanmaa *Finland* 8 E20
Pohnpei *Micronesia* 96 G7
Pohorelá *Slovak Rep.* 27 C13
Pohořelice *Czech Rep.* 27 C9
Pohorje *Slovenia* 41 B12
Pohri *India* 68 G6
Poiana Mare *Romania* 28 G8
Poiana Ruscăi, Munții
Romania 28 E7
Poiana Stampei *Romania* 29 C10
Poinsett, C. *Antarctica* 5 C9
Point Arena *U.S.A.* 110 G3
Point Baker *U.S.A.* 102 B2
Point Fortin *Trin. & Tob.* 125 K15
Point Hope *U.S.A.* 106 B6
Point L. *Canada* 100 D9
Point Lisas *Trin. & Tob.* 125 K15
Point Pedro *Sri Lanka* 66 Q12
Point Pelee △ *Canada* 114 E2
Point Pleasant *N.J., U.S.A.* 115 F10
Point Pleasant *W. Va.,
U.S.A.* 113 F12
Point Reyes △ *U.S.A.* 110 G2
Pointe-à-Pitre *Guadeloupe* 120 b
Pointe-au-Pic = La Malbaie
Canada 105 C5
Pointe-Claire *Canada* 115 A11
Pointe-Gatineau *Canada* 115 A9
Pointe-Noire *Congo* 84 E2
Pointe-Noire *Guadeloupe* 120 b
Poio *Spain* 36 C2
Poipet *Cambodia* 64 F4
Poirino *Italy* 40 D4
Poisonbush Ra. *Australia* 92 D3
Poissonnier Pt. *Australia* 92 C2
Poitiers *France* 18 F7
Poitou *France* 18 F6
Poitou-Charentes □ *France* 20 B4
Poix-de-Picardie *France* 19 C8
Poix-Terron *France* 19 C11
Pojoaque *U.S.A.* 109 J10
Pokataroo *Australia* 95 D4
Pokhara *Nepal* 69 E10
Pokhvistnevo *Russia* 34 D11
Poko *Dem. Rep. of the Congo* 86 B2
Poko *Sudan* 81 F3
Pokrov *Russia* 32 E10
Pokrovsk *Russia* 53 C13
Pokrovskoye *Russia* 33 J10
Pol *France* 18 F8
Pol-e Dokhtar *Iran* 73 F12
Pol-e Zahāb *Iran* 73 E11
Pola = Pula *Croatia* 41 D10
Pola *Russia* 32 D7
Pola de Allande *Spain* 36 B4
Pola de Lena *Spain* 36 B5
Pola de Siero *Spain* 36 B5
Pola de Somiedo *Spain* 36 B4
Polacca *U.S.A.* 109 J8
Polan *Iran* 71 E9
Pol'ana *Slovak Rep.* 27 C12
Poland *U.S.A.* 115 C9
Poland ■ *Europe* 31 G3
Polanica-Zdrój *Poland* 31 H3
Połaniec *Poland* 31 H8
Polanów *Poland* 30 D3
Polar Bear △ *Canada* 104 A2
Polatlı *Turkey* 72 C5

Polatsk *Belarus* 32 E5
Polcura *Chile* 126 D1
Polczyn-Zdrój *Poland* 30 E3
Poldasht *Iran* 73 C11
Poleski △ *Poland* 31 G10
Polessk *Russia* 30 D8
Polesye = Pripet Marshes
Europe 23 B15
Polgar *Hungary* 28 C6
Poli *Cameroon* 83 C7
Policastro, G. di *Italy* 43 C8
Police *Poland* 30 E1
Police, Pte. *Seychelles* 85 b
Polichnitos *Greece* 47 B8
Polička *Czech Rep.* 27 B9
Policoro *Italy* 43 B9
Poliegos *Greece* 46 E6
Poligiros *Greece* 44 F7
Polignano a Mare *Italy* 43 A9
Poligny *France* 19 F12
Polillo Is. *Phil.* 61 D5
Polillo Strait *Phil.* 61 D4
Polis *Cyprus* 49 D11
Polístena *Italy* 43 D9
Polk *U.S.A.* 114 E5
Polkowice *Poland* 31 G3
Polla *Italy* 43 B8
Pollachi *India* 66 P10
Pollença *Spain* 48 B10
Pollença, B. de *Spain* 48 B10
Póllica *Italy* 43 B8
Pollino, Mte. *Italy* 43 C9
Pollino △ *Italy* 43 C9
Polna *Russia* 32 C5
Polnovat *Russia* 52 C7
Pology *Ukraine* 33 J9
Polokwane *S. Africa* 89 C4
Polokwane → *S. Africa* 89 C5
Polonne *Ukraine* 23 C14
Polonnoye = Polonne
Ukraine 23 C14
Polski Trümbesh *Bulgaria* 45 C9
Polsko Kosovo *Bulgaria* 45 C9
Polson *U.S.A.* 108 C6
Poltár *Slovak Rep.* 27 C12
Poltava *Ukraine* 33 H8
Poltava □ *Ukraine* 33 H8
Põltsamaa *Estonia* 32 C3
Polunochnoye *Russia* 52 C7
Põlva *Estonia* 32 C4
Polyana *Ukraine* 28 B7
Polyarny *Russia* 8 B25
Polyarnyye Zori *Russia* 8 C25
Polynesia *Pac. Oc.* 97 F11
Polynésie française =
French Polynesia ☒
Pac. Oc. 97 J13
Pomarance *Italy* 40 E7
Pombal *Portugal* 36 F2
Pombia *Greece* 49 E6
Pomene *Mozam.* 89 C6
Pomeroy *S. Africa* 89 D5
Pomeroy *Ohio, U.S.A.* 113 F12
Pomeroy *Wash., U.S.A.* 108 C5
Pomézia *Italy* 42 A5
Pomichna *Ukraine* 33 H6
Pomona *Australia* 95 D5
Pomona *U.S.A.* 111 L9
Pomorie *Bulgaria* 45 D11
Pomorskie □ *Poland* 30 D5
Pomorskie, Pojezierze *Poland* 30 E3
Pomos *Cyprus* 49 D11
Pomos, C. *Cyprus* 49 D11
Pompano Beach *U.S.A.* 117 H14
Pompei *Italy* 43 B7
Pompey *France* 19 D13
Pompeys Pillar *U.S.A.* 108 D10
Pompeys Pillar △ *U.S.A.* 108 D10
Pompton Lakes *U.S.A.* 115 F10
Ponape = Pohnpei *Micronesia* 96 G7
Ponask L. *Canada* 104 B1
Ponca *U.S.A.* 112 D5
Ponca City *U.S.A.* 116 C6
Ponce *Puerto Rico* 121 d
Ponchatoula *U.S.A.* 117 F9
Poncheville, L. *Canada* 104 B4
Pond *U.S.A.* 111 K7
Pond Inlet *Canada* 101 C16
Pondicherry = Puducherry
India 66 P11
Ponds, I. of *Canada* 105 B8
Ponferrada *Spain* 36 C4
Pongo, Wadi → *Sudan* 81 F2
Poniatowa *Poland* 31 G9
Poniec *Poland* 31 G3
Ponikva *Slovenia* 41 B12
Ponnani *India* 66 P9
Ponoka *Canada* 102 C6
Ponorogo *Indonesia* 63 G14
Pons = Ponts *Spain* 38 D6
Pons *France* 20 C3
Ponsul → *Portugal* 36 F3
Pont-à-Mousson *France* 19 D13
Pont-Audemer *France* 18 C7
Pont-Aven *France* 18 E3
Pont Canavese *Italy* 40 C4
Pont-d'Ain *France* 19 F12
Pont-de-Roide *France* 19 E13
Pont-de-Salars *France* 20 D6
Pont-de-Vaux *France* 19 F11
Pont-de-Veyle *France* 19 F11

Pont-du-Château *France* 19 G10
Pont-l'Abbé *France* 18 E2
Pont-l'Évêque *France* 18 C7
Pont-St-Esprit *France* 21 D8
Pont-Ste-Maxence *France* 19 C9
Pont-St-Martin *Italy* 40 C4
Pont-sur-Yonne *France* 19 D10
Ponta Delgada *Azores* 78 a
Ponta do Sol *Madeira* 48 D2
Ponta Grossa *Brazil* 127 B5
Ponta Porã *Brazil* 127 A4
Pontacq *France* 20 E3
Pontailler-sur-Saône *France* 19 E12
Pontarlier *France* 19 F13
Pontassieve *Italy* 41 E8
Pontaumur *France* 20 C6
Pontcharra *France* 21 C10
Pontchartrain, L. *U.S.A.* 117 F9
Pontchâteau *France* 18 E4
Ponte da Barca *Portugal* 36 D2
Ponte de Sor *Portugal* 37 F2
Ponte dell'Ólio *Italy* 40 D6
Ponte di Legno *Italy* 40 B7
Ponte do Lima *Portugal* 36 D2
Ponte do Pungué *Mozam.* 87 F3
Ponte Nova *Brazil* 127 A7
Ponte-Leccia *France* 21 F13
Ponte nelle Alpi *Italy* 41 B9
Ponteareas *Spain* 36 C2
Pontebba *Italy* 41 B10
Ponteceso *Spain* 36 B2
Pontecorvo *Italy* 42 A6
Pontedeume *Spain* 36 B2
Ponteix *Canada* 103 D7
Pontevedra *Spain* 36 C2
Pontevedra □ *Spain* 36 C2
Pontevedra, R. de → *Spain* 36 C2
Pontevico *Italy* 40 C7
Pontiac *Ill., U.S.A.* 112 E9
Pontiac *Mich., U.S.A.* 113 D12
Pontian Kechil *Malaysia* 65 d
Pontianak *Indonesia* 62 E3
Pontine Is. = Ponziane,
Ísole *Italy* 42 B5
Pontine Mts. = Kuzey
Anadolu Dağları *Turkey* 72 B7
Pontínia *Italy* 42 A6
Pontivy *France* 18 D4
Pontoise *France* 19 C9
Ponton → *Canada* 102 B5
Pontorson *France* 18 D5
Pontrémoli *Italy* 40 D6
Pontrieux *France* 18 D3
Ponts *Spain* 38 D6
Pontypool *Canada* 114 B6
Pontypool *U.K.* 15 F4
Ponza *Italy* 42 B5
Ponziane, Ísole *Italy* 42 B5
Poochera *Australia* 95 E1
Poole *U.K.* 15 G6
Poole □ *U.K.* 15 G6
Poona = Pune *India* 66 K8
Pooncarie *Australia* 95 E3
Poopelloe L. *Australia* 95 E3
Poopó, L. de *Bolivia* 124 G5
Popayán *Colombia* 124 C3
Poperinge *Belgium* 17 D2
Popilta L. *Australia* 95 E3
Popina *Bulgaria* 45 B10
Popio L. *Australia* 95 E3
Poplar *U.S.A.* 108 B11
Poplar → *Canada* 103 C9
Poplar Bluff *U.S.A.* 112 G8
Poplarville *U.S.A.* 117 F10
Popocatépetl, Volcán
Mexico 119 D5
Popokabaka
Dem. Rep. of the Congo 84 F3
Pópoli *Italy* 41 F10
Popovača *Croatia* 41 C13
Popovo *Bulgaria* 45 C10
Poppberg *Germany* 25 F7
Poppi *Italy* 41 E8
Poprad *Slovak Rep.* 27 B13
Poprad → *Slovak Rep.* 27 B13
Porbandar *India* 68 J3
Porcher I. *Canada* 102 C2
Porcuna *Spain* 37 H6
Porcupine → *Canada* 103 B8
Porcupine → *U.S.A.* 100 D2
Porcupine Gorge △ *Australia* 94 C3
Pordenone *Italy* 41 C9
Pordim *Bulgaria* 45 C8
Poreč *Croatia* 41 C10
Poretskoye *Russia* 34 C8
Pori *Finland* 8 F19
Pori *Greece* 46 F5
Porlamar *Venezuela* 124 A6
Porlezza *Italy* 40 B6
Porma → *Spain* 36 C5
Pormpuraaw *Australia* 94 A3
Pormpuraaw ☉ *Australia* 94 A3
Pornic *France* 18 E4
Poronaysk *Russia* 53 E15
Poros *Greece* 46 D5
Poroshiri-Dake *Japan* 54 C11
Poroszló *Hungary* 28 C5
Poroto Mts. *Tanzania* 87 D3

Porpoise B. *Antarctica* 5 C9
Porquerolles, Î. de *France* 21 F10
Porrentruy *Switz.* 25 H3
Porreres *Spain* 48 B10
Porretta, Passo di *Italy* ...
Porsangerfjorden *Norway* 8 A21
Porsgrunn *Norway* 9 G13
Port Alberni *Canada* 102 D4
Port Alfred *S. Africa* 88 E4
Port Alice *Canada* 102 C3
Port Allegany *U.S.A.* 114 E6
Port Allen *U.S.A.* 116 F9
Port Alma *Australia* 94 C5
Port Alma *Canada* 114 D2
Port Angeles *U.S.A.* 110 B3
Port Antonio *Jamaica* 120 a
Port Aransas *U.S.A.* 116 H6
Port Arthur *Australia* 95 G4
Port Arthur *U.S.A.* 116 G8
Port au Choix *Canada* 105 B8
Port au Port B. *Canada* 105 C8
Port-au-Prince *Haiti* 121 C5
Port Augusta *Australia* 95 E2
Port Austin *U.S.A.* 114 B2
Port Bell *Uganda* 86 B3
Port Bergé Vaovao *Madag.* 89 B8
Port Blandford *Canada* 105 C9
Port-Bouët *Ivory C.* 82 D4
Port Bradshaw *Australia* 94 A2
Port Broughton *Australia* 95 E2
Port Bruce *Canada* 114 D4
Port Burwell *Canada* 114 D4
Port Canning *India* 69 H13
Port Carling *Canada* 114 A5
Port-Cartier *Canada* 105 B6
Port Chalmers *N.Z.* 91 F3
Port Charlotte *U.S.A.* 117 H13
Port Chester *U.S.A.* 115 F11
Port Clements *Canada* 102 C2
Port Clinton *U.S.A.* 113 E12
Port Colborne *Canada* 114 D5
Port Coquitlam *Canada* 110 A4
Port Credit *Canada* 114 C5
Port-Cros △ *France* 21 F10
Port Curtis *Australia* 94 C5
Port d'Alcúdia *Spain* 48 B10
Port Dalhousie *Canada* 114 C5
Port d'Andratx *Spain* 48 B9
Port Darwin *Australia* 92 B5
Port Darwin *Falk. Is.* 128 G5
Port Davey *Australia* 95 G4
Port-de-Bouc *France* 21 E8
Port-de-Paix *Haiti* 121 C5
Port de Pollença *Spain* 48 B10
Port de Sóller *Spain* 48 B9
Port Dickson *Malaysia* 65 L3
Port Douglas *Australia* 94 B4
Port Dover *Canada* 114 D4
Port Edward *Canada* 102 C2
Port Elgin *Canada* 114 B3
Port Elizabeth *S. Africa* 88 E4
Port Ellen *U.K.* 13 F2
Port-en-Bessin-Huppain
France 18 C6
Port Erin *I. of Man* 14 C3
Port Essington *Australia* 92 B5
Port Ewen *U.S.A.* 115 E11
Port Fairy *Australia* 95 F3
Port Fouâd = Bûr Fuad *Egypt* 80 H8
Port Gamble *U.S.A.* 110 C4
Port-Gentil *Gabon* 84 E1
Port Germein *Australia* 95 E2
Port Ghalib *Egypt* 70 E2
Port Gibson *U.S.A.* 116 F9
Port Glasgow *U.K.* 13 F4
Port Harcourt *Nigeria* 83 E6
Port Hardy *Canada* 102 C3
Port Harrison = Inukjuak
Canada 101 F16
Port Hawkesbury *Canada* 105 C7
Port Hedland *Australia* 92 D2
Port Henry *U.S.A.* 115 B11
Port Hood *Canada* 105 C7
Port Hope *Canada* 114 C6
Port Hope *U.S.A.* 114 C2
Port Hope Simpson *Canada* 105 B8
Port Hueneme *U.S.A.* 111 L7
Port Huron *U.S.A.* 114 D2
Port Iliç *Azerbaijan* 73 C13
Port Jefferson *U.S.A.* 115 F11
Port Jervis *U.S.A.* 115 E10
Port-Joinville *France* 18 F4
Port Katon *Russia* 33 J10
Port Kelang = Pelabuhan
Klang *Malaysia* 65 L3
Port Kenny *Australia* 95 E1
Port-la-Nouvelle *France* 20 E7
Port Laoise = Waterford
Ireland 12 D4
Port Laoise *Ireland* 12 C4
Port Lavaca *U.S.A.* 116 G6
Port Leyden *U.S.A.* 115 C9
Port Loko *S. Leone* 82 D2
Port Louis *France* 18 E3
Port-Louis *Guadeloupe* 120 b
Port Louis *Mauritius* 85 d
Port MacDonnell *Australia* 95 F3
Port McNeill *Canada* 102 C3
Port Macquarie *Australia* 95 E5
Port Maria *Jamaica* 120 a

Port Matilda *U.S.A.* **114** F6
Port McNicoll *Canada* **114** B5
Port Mellon *Canada* **102** D4
Port-Menier *Canada* **105** C7
Port Moody *Canada* **110** A4
Port Morant *Jamaica* **120** a
Port Moresby *Papua N. G.* **90** B7
Port Musgrave *Australia* **94** A3
Port-Navalo *France* **18** E4
Port Neches *U.S.A.* **116** G8
Port Nolloth *S. Africa* **88** D2
Port Nouveau-Québec =
  Kangiqsualujjuaq *Canada*
  101 F18
Port of Climax *Canada* **103** D7
Port of Coronach *Canada* **103** D7
Port of Spain *Trin. & Tob.* **121** D7
Port Orange *U.S.A.* **117** G14
Port Orchard *U.S.A.* **110** C4
Port Orford *U.S.A.* **108** E1
Port Pegasus *N.Z.* **91** G1
Port Perry *Canada* **114** B6
Port Phillip B. *Australia* **95** F3
Port Pirie *Australia* **95** E2
Port Renfrew *Canada* **110** B2
Port Roper *Australia* **94** A2
Port Rowan *Canada* **114** D4
Port Safaga = Bûr Safâga
  Egypt **70** E2
Port Said = Bûr Sa'îd *Egypt* **80** H8
Port St. Joe *U.S.A.* **117** G12
Port St. Johns =
  Umzimvubu *S. Africa* **89** E4
Port-St-Louis-du-Rhône
  France **21** E8
Port St. Lucie *U.S.A.* **117** H14
Port-Ste-Marie *France* **20** D4
Port Sanilac *U.S.A.* **114** C2
Port Severn *Canada* **114** B5
Port Shepstone *S. Africa* **89** E5
Port Simpson *Canada* **102** C2
Port Stanley = Stanley
  Falk. Is. **128** G5
Port Stanley *Canada* **114** D3
Port Sudan = Bûr Sûdân
  Sudan **80** D4
Port Sulphur *U.S.A.* **117** G10
Port-sur-Saône *France* **19** E13
Port Talbot *U.K.* **15** F4
Port Townsend *U.S.A.* **110** B4
Port-Vendres *France* **20** F7
Port Vila *Vanuatu* **90** C9
Port Vladimir *Russia* **8** B25
Port Wakefield *Australia* **95** E2
Port Washington *U.S.A.* **112** D10
Porta Orientalis *Romania* **23** F12
Portacloy *Ireland* **12** B2
Portadown *U.K.* **12** B5
Portaferry *U.K.* **12** B6
Portage *Pa., U.S.A.* **114** F6
Portage *Wis., U.S.A.* **112** D9
Portage la Prairie *Canada* **103** D9
Portageville *U.S.A.* **112** G9
Portalegre *Portugal* **37** F3
Portalegre □ *Portugal* **37** F3
Portales *U.S.A.* **109** J12
Portarlington *Ireland* **12** C4
Portbou *Spain* **38** C8
Portel *Portugal* **37** G3
Portela, Lisboa ✕ (LIS)
  Portugal **37** G1
Porter L. *N.W.T., Canada* **103** A7
Porter L. *Sask., Canada* **103** B7
Porterville *S. Africa* **88** E2
Porterville *U.S.A.* **110** J8
Portes-lès-Valence *France* **21** D8
Porthcawl *U.K.* **15** F4
Porthill *U.S.A.* **108** B5
Porthmadog *U.K.* **14** E3
Portile de Fier *Europe* **28** F7
Portimão *Portugal* **37** H2
Portishead *U.K.* **15** F5
Portiţei, Gura *Romania* **29** F14
Portknockie *U.K.* **13** D6
Portland *N.S.W., Australia* **95** E5
Portland *Vic., Australia* **95** F3
Portland *Canada* **115** B8
Portland *Conn., U.S.A.* **115** E12
Portland *Maine, U.S.A.* **113** D18
Portland *Mich., U.S.A.* **113** D11
Portland *Oreg., U.S.A.* **110** E4
Portland *Pa., U.S.A.* **115** F9
Portland, I. of *U.K.* **15** G5
Portland B. *Australia* **95** F3
Portland Bight *Jamaica* **120** a
Portland Bill *U.K.* **15** G5
Portland Canal *Canada* **102** B2
Portland Int. ✕ (PDX)
  U.S.A. **110** E4
Portland Pt. *Jamaica* **120** a
Portmadoc = Porthmadog
  U.K. **14** E3
Portmore *Jamaica* **120** a
Porto *France* **21** F12
Porto *Portugal* **36** D2
Porto □ *Portugal* **36** D2
Porto, G. de *France* **21** F12

Pôrto Alegre *Brazil* **127** C5
Porto Azzurro *Italy* **40** F7
Porto Colom *Spain* **48** B10
Porto Cristo *Spain* **48** B10
Porto de Moz *Brazil* **125** D8
Porto Empédocle *Italy* **42** E6
Porto Esperança *Brazil* **124** G7
Porto Franco *Brazil* **125** E9
Porto Inglês *C. Verde Is.* **78** b
Porto Mendes *Brazil* **127** A5
Porto Moniz *Madeira* **48** D2
Porto Murtinho *Brazil* **124** H7
Porto Nacional *Brazil* **125** F9
Porto-Novo *Benin* **83** D5
Porto Primavera, Represa
  Brazil **127** A5
Porto San Giórgio *Italy* **41** E10
Porto Sant' Elpídio *Italy* **41** E10
Porto Santo, I. de *Madeira* **78** B2
Porto Santo Stéfano *Italy* **40** F8
Porto São José *Brazil* **127** A5
Porto Seguro *Brazil* **125** G11
Porto Tolle *Italy* **41** D9
Porto Tórres *Italy* **42** B1
Porto União *Brazil* **127** B5
Pôrto Velho *Brazil* **124** E6
Porto Walter *Brazil* **124** E4
Porto-Vecchio *France* **21** G13
Portobelo *Panama* **120** E4
Portoferráio *Italy* **40** F7
Portogruaro *Italy* **41** C9
Portola *U.S.A.* **110** F6
Portomaggiore *Italy* **41** D8
Portopetro *Spain* **48** B10
Portoscuso *Italy* **42** C1
Portovénere *Italy* **40** D6
Portoviejo *Ecuador* **124** D2
Portpatrick *U.K.* **13** G3
Portree *U.K.* **13** D2
Portrush *U.K.* **12** A5
Portsmouth *Dominica* **121** C7
Portsmouth *U.K.* **15** G6
Portsmouth *N.H., U.S.A.* **115** C14
Portsmouth *Ohio, U.S.A.* **113** F12
Portsmouth *R.I., U.S.A.* **115** E13
Portsmouth *Va., U.S.A.* **113** G15
Portsmouth □ *U.K.* **15** G6
Portsoy *U.K.* **13** D6
Portstewart *U.K.* **12** A5
Porttipahdan tekojärvi
  Finland **8** B22
Portugal ■ *Europe* **36** F3
Portugalete *Spain* **38** B1
Portumna *Ireland* **12** C3
Portville *U.S.A.* **114** D6
Poruma *Australia* **94** a
Porvenir *Chile* **128** G2
Porvoo *Finland* **32** B3
Porzuna *Spain* **37** F6
Posada *Italy* **42** B2
Posada → *Italy* **42** B2
Posadas *Argentina* **127** B4
Posadas *Spain* **37** H5
Poschiavo *Switz.* **25** J6
Posets *Spain* **38** C5
Posht-e Badam *Iran* **71** C7
Posídium *Greece* **47** F9
Poso *Indonesia* **63** E6
Posof *Turkey* **73** B10
Posse *Brazil* **125** F9
Possession I. *Antarctica* **5** D11
Pössneck *Germany* **24** E7
Possum Kingdom L. *U.S.A.* **116** E5
Post *U.S.A.* **116** E4
Post Falls *U.S.A.* **108** C5
Postavy = Pastavy *Belarus* **32** E4
Poste-de-la-Baleine =
  Kuujjuarapik *Canada* **104** A4
Postmasburg *S. Africa* **88** D3
Postojna *Slovenia* **41** C11
Poston *U.S.A.* **111** M12
Postville *Canada* **105** B8
Posyet *Russia* **54** C5
Potamós *Antikythira, Greece* **46** F5
Potamós *Kythira, Greece* **46** E4
Potchefstroom *S. Africa* **88** D4
Potcoava *Romania* **29** F9
Poteau *U.S.A.* **116** D7
Poteet *U.S.A.* **116** G5
Potenza *Italy* **43** B8
Potenza → *Italy* **41** E10
Potenza Picena *Italy* **41** E10
Poteriteri, L. *N.Z.* **91** G1
Potgietersrus = Mokopane
  S. Africa **89** C4
Poti *Georgia* **35** J5
Potiskum *Nigeria* **83** C7
Potlogi *Romania* **29** F10
Potomac → *U.S.A.* **113** F14
Potosí *Bolivia* **124** G5
Potosi Mt. *U.S.A.* **111** K11
Pototan *Phil.* **61** F5
Potrerillos *Chile* **126** B2
Potsdam *Germany* **24** C9
Potsdam *U.S.A.* **115** B10
Pottenstein *Germany* **25** F7
Pottersville *U.S.A.* **115** C11
Pottstown *U.S.A.* **115** F9
Pottsville *U.S.A.* **115** F8
Pottuvil *Sri Lanka* **66** R12

P'otzu *Taiwan* **59** F13
Pouancé *France* **18** E5
Pouce Coupé *Canada* **102** B4
Poughkeepsie *U.S.A.* **115** E11
Pouilly-sur-Loire *France* **19** E10
Poulaphouca Res. *Ireland* **12** C5
Poulsbo *U.S.A.* **110** C4
Poultney *U.S.A.* **115** C11
Poulton-le-Fylde *U.K.* **14** D5
Pouso Alegre *Brazil* **127** A6
Pout *Senegal* **82** C1
Pouthisat *Cambodia* **64** F4
Pouytenga *Burkina Faso* **83** C4
Pouzauges *France* **18** F6
Pova de Santa Iria *Portugal* **37** G1
Považská Bystrica
  Slovak Rep. **27** B11
Poverty B. *N.Z.* **91** C7
Povlen *Serbia* **44** B3
Póvoa de Lanhosa *Portugal* **36** D2
Póvoa de Varzim *Portugal* **36** D2
Povorino *Russia* **34** E6
Povorotnyy, Mys *Russia* **54** C6
Povungnituk = Puvirnituq
  Canada **101** E16
Powassan *Canada* **104** C4
Poway *U.S.A.* **111** N9
Powder → *U.S.A.* **108** C11
Powder River *U.S.A.* **108** E10
Powell *U.S.A.* **108** D9
Powell, L. *U.S.A.* **109** H8
Powell River *Canada* **102** D4
Powers *U.S.A.* **112** C10
Pownal *U.S.A.* **115** D11
Powys □ *U.K.* **15** E4
Poyang Hu *China* **59** C11
Poyarkovo *Russia* **53** E13
Poysdorf *Austria* **27** C9
Poza de la Sal *Spain* **36** C7
Poza Rica *Mexico* **119** C5
Pozanti *Turkey* **72** D6
Požarevac *Serbia* **44** B5
Pozazal, Puerto *Spain* **36** C6
Požega *Croatia* **28** E2
Požega *Serbia* **44** C4
Poznań *Poland* **31** F3
Poznań ✕ (POZ) *Poland* **31** F3
Pozo *U.S.A.* **111** K6
Pozo Alcón *Spain* **37** H8
Pozo Almonte *Chile* **124** H5
Pozo Colorado *Paraguay* **126** A4
Pozoblanco *Spain* **37** G6
Pozzallo *Italy* **43** F7
Pozzomaggiore *Italy* **42** B1
Pozzuoli *Italy* **43** B7
Pra → *Ghana* **83** D4
Prabuty *Poland* **30** E6
Prača *Bos.-H.* **28** G3
Prachatice *Czech Rep.* **26** B6
Prachin Buri *Thailand* **64** F3
Prachuap Khiri Khan
  Thailand **65** G2
Pradelles *France* **20** D7
Prades *France* **20** F6
Prado *Brazil* **125** G11
Prado del Rey *Spain* **37** J5
Præstø *Denmark* **11** J6
Pragersko *Slovenia* **41** B12
Prague = Praha *Czech Rep.* **26** A7
Praha *Czech Rep.* **26** A7
Praha ✕ (PRG) *Czech Rep.* **26** A7
Prahecq *France* **20** B3
Prahova □ *Romania* **29** E10
Prahova → *Romania* **29** F10
Prahovo *Serbia* **44** B6
Praia *C. Verde Is.* **78** b
Praia a Mare *Italy* **43** C8
Praid *Romania* **29** D10
Prainha *Brazil* **125** D8
Prainha Nova *Brazil* **124** E6
Prairie *Australia* **94** C3
Prairie City *U.S.A.* **108** D4
Prairie Dog Town Fork
  Red → *U.S.A.* **116** D5
Prairie du Chien *U.S.A.* **112** D8
Prairies, L. of the *Canada* **103** C8
Pramanda *Greece* **46** B3
Prampram *Ghana* **83** D5
Pran Buri *Thailand* **64** F2
Prang *Ghana* **83** D4
Prapat *Indonesia* **62** D1
Praslin *Seychelles* **85** b
Prasonísi, Ákra *Greece* **49** D9
Prästmon *Sweden* **10** A11
Praszka *Poland* **31** G5
Prata *Brazil* **125** G9
Pratabpur *India* **69** H10
Pratapgarh *Raj., India* **68** G6
Pratapgarh *Ut. P., India* **69** G9
Pratas Is. = Dongsha Dao
  S. China Sea **59** G11
Prato *Italy* **40** E8
Prátola Peligna *Italy* **41** F10
Prats-de-Mollo-la-Preste
  France **20** F6
Pratt *U.S.A.* **112** G4
Prattville *U.S.A.* **117** E11
Pravdinsk *Kaliningrad, Russia* **30** D8
Pravdinsk *Nizhniy Novgorod,*
  Russia **34** B6

Pravets *Bulgaria* **44** D7
Pravia *Spain* **36** B4
Praya *Indonesia* **62** F5
Prayag = Allahabad *India* **69** G9
Pré-en-Pail *France* **18** D6
Preble *U.S.A.* **115** D8
Precipice △ *Australia* **95** D5
Precordillera *Argentina* **126** C2
Predáppio *Italy* **41** D8
Predazzo *Italy* **41** B8
Predeal *Romania* **29** E10
Predejane *Serbia* **44** D6
Preeceville *Canada* **103** C8
Preetz *Germany* **24** A6
Pregolya → *Russia* **30** D7
Pregrada *Croatia* **41** B12
Preiļi *Latvia* **32** D4
Preko *Croatia* **41** D12
Prelog *Croatia* **41** B13
Prémery *France* **19** E10
Premià de Mar *Spain* **38** D7
Premont *U.S.A.* **116** H5
Premuda *Croatia* **41** D11
Prentice *U.S.A.* **112** C8
Prenzlau *Germany* **24** B9
Preobrazheniye *Russia* **54** C6
Preparis North Channel
  Ind. Oc. **67** M18
Preparis South Channel
  Ind. Oc. **67** M18
Přerov *Czech Rep.* **27** B10
Prescott *Canada* **115** B9
Prescott *Ariz., U.S.A.* **109** J7
Prescott *Ark., U.S.A.* **116** E8
Prescott Valley *U.S.A.* **109** J7
Preservation Inlet *N.Z.* **91** G1
Preševo *Serbia* **44** D5
Presho *U.S.A.* **112** D3
Presicce *Italy* **43** C11
Presidencia de la Plaza
  Argentina **126** B4
Presidencia Roque Saenz
  Peña *Argentina* **126** B3
Presidente Epitácio *Brazil* **125** H8
Presidente Hayes □
  Paraguay **126** A4
Presidente Prudente *Brazil* **127** A5
Presidio *Mexico* **118** B4
Presidio *U.S.A.* **116** G2
Preslav *Bulgaria* **45** C10
Preslavska Planina *Bulgaria* **45** C10
Prešov *Slovak Rep.* **27** B14
Prešovský □ *Slovak Rep.* **27** B13
Prespa *Bulgaria* **45** E8
Prespa, L. = Prespansko
  Jezero *Macedonia* **44** F5
Prespa △ *Greece* **44** F5
Prespansko Jezero *Macedonia* **44** F5
Presque I. *U.S.A.* **114** D4
Presque Isle *U.S.A.* **113** B19
Prestatyn *U.K.* **14** D4
Prestea *Ghana* **82** D4
Presteigne *U.K.* **15** E5
Přeštice *Czech Rep.* **26** B6
Preston *Canada* **114** C4
Preston *U.K.* **14** D5
Preston *Idaho, U.S.A.* **108** E8
Preston *Minn., U.S.A.* **112** D7
Preston, C. *Australia* **92** D2
Prestonsburg *U.S.A.* **113** G12
Prestranda *Norway* **10** E3
Prestwick *U.K.* **13** F4
Pretoria *S. Africa* **89** D4
Preuilly-sur-Claise *France* **18** F7
Preveza *Greece* **46** C2
Preveza □ *Greece* **46** B2
Prey Veng *Cambodia* **65** G5
Priazovskoye *Ukraine* **33** J8
Pribilof Is. *U.S.A.* **106** D6
Priboj *Serbia* **44** C3
Příbram *Czech Rep.* **26** B7
Price *U.S.A.* **108** G8
Price I. *Canada* **102** C3
Prichard *U.S.A.* **117** F10
Priego *Spain* **38** E2
Priego de Córdoba *Spain* **37** H6
Priekule *Latvia* **30** B8
Priekule *Lithuania* **30** C8
Prien *Germany* **25** H8
Prienai *Lithuania* **30** D10
Prieska *S. Africa* **88** D3
Priest L. *U.S.A.* **108** B5
Priest River *U.S.A.* **108** B5
Priest Valley *U.S.A.* **110** J6
Prievidza *Slovak Rep.* **27** C11
Prignitz *Germany* **24** B7
Prijedor *Bos.-H.* **41** D13
Prijepolje *Serbia* **44** C3
Prikaspiyskaya
  Nizmennost = Caspian
  Depression *Eurasia* **35** G9
Prikro *Ivory C.* **82** D4
Prikubanskaya
  Nizmennost *Russia* **35** H4
Prilep *Macedonia* **44** E5
Priluki = Pryluky *Ukraine* **33** G7
Prime Seal I. *Australia* **95** G4
Primo Tapia *Mexico* **111** N10
Primorsk *Kaliningrad, Russia* **30** D6

Primorsk *St. Petersburg,*
  Russia **32** B5
Primorskiy Kray □ *Russia* **54** B7
Primorsko *Bulgaria* **45** D11
Primorsko-Akhtarsk *Russia* **33** J10
Primorskoye *Ukraine* **33** J9
Primrose L. *Canada* **103** C7
Prince Albert *Canada* **103** C7
Prince Albert *S. Africa* **88** E3
Prince Albert □ *Canada* **100** C9
Prince Albert Mts. *Antarctica* **5** D11
Prince Albert Pen. *Canada* **100** C8
Prince Albert Sd. *Canada* **100** C9
Prince Alfred, C. *Canada* **4** B1
Prince Charles I. *Canada* **101** D16
Prince Charles Mts. *Antarctica* **5** D6
Prince Edward Fracture
  Zone *Ind. Oc.* **5** A4
Prince Edward I. □ *Canada* **105** C7
Prince Edward Is. *Ind. Oc.* **3** G11
Prince George *Canada* **102** C4
Prince of Wales, C. *U.S.A.* **106** B6
Prince of Wales I. *Australia* **94** A3
Prince of Wales I. *Canada* **100** C12
Prince of Wales I. *U.S.A.* **100** F5
Prince of Wales Icefield
  Canada **101** B16
Prince of Wales Str. *Canada* **100** C8
Prince Patrick I. *Canada* **101** B8
Prince Regent Inlet *Canada* **101** C14
Prince Rupert *Canada* **102** C2
Prince William Sd. *U.S.A.* **100** E2
Princes Town *Trin. & Tob.* **125** K15
Princess Charlotte B.
  Australia **94** A3
Princess Elizabeth Trough
  S. Ocean **5** C7
Princess May Ranges
  Australia **92** C4
Princess Royal I. *Canada* **102** C3
Princeton *Canada* **102** D4
Princeton *Calif., U.S.A.* **110** F4
Princeton *Ill., U.S.A.* **112** E9
Princeton *Ind., U.S.A.* **112** F10
Princeton *Ky., U.S.A.* **112** G10
Princeton *Mo., U.S.A.* **112** E7
Princeton *N.J., U.S.A.* **115** F10
Princeton *W. Va., U.S.A.* **113** G13
Príncipe *São Tomé & Príncipe* **76** F4
Príncipe da Beira *Brazil* **124** F6
Prineville *U.S.A.* **108** D3
Prins Harald Kyst *Antarctica* **5** D4
Prinsesse Astrid Kyst
  Antarctica **5** D3
Prinsesse Ragnhild Kyst
  Antarctica **5** D3
Prinzapolca *Nic.* **120** D3
Prior, C. *Spain* **36** B2
Priozersk *Russia* **32** B6
Pripet = Prypyat → *Europe* **23** C16
Pripet Marshes *Europe* **23** B15
Pripyat = Prypyat → *Europe* **23** C16
Pripyat Marshes = Pripet
  Marshes *Europe* **23** B15
Pripyats = Prypyat →
  Europe **23** C16
Prislop, Pasul *Romania* **29** C9
Pristen *Russia* **33** G9
Priština *Kosovo* **44** D5
Pritzwalk *Germany* **24** B8
Privas *France* **21** D8
Priverno *Italy* **42** A6
Privolzhsk *Russia* **34** B5
Privolzhskaya
  Vozvyshennost *Russia* **34** E7
Privolzhskiy *Russia* **34** E8
Privolzhskiy □ *Russia* **34** B10
Privolzhye *Russia* **34** D9
Priyutnoye *Russia* **35** G6
Prizren *Kosovo* **44** D4
Prizzi *Italy* **42** E6
Prnjavor *Bos.-H.* **28** F2
Probolinggo *Indonesia* **63** G15
Prochowice *Poland* **31** G3
Proctor *U.S.A.* **115** C11
Proddatur *India* **66** M11
Prodhromos *Cyprus* **49** E11
Proença-a-Nova *Portugal* **36** F3
Profilia *Greece* **49** D9
Profondeville *Belgium* **17** D4
Progreso *Coahuila, Mexico* **118** B4
Progreso *Yucatán, Mexico* **119** C7
Progress *Antarctica* **5** C12
Progress *Russia* **53** E13
Prokhladnyy *Russia* **35** J7
Prokletije *Albania* **44** D3
Prokopyevsk *Russia* **52** D9
Prokuplje *Serbia* **44** C5
Proletarsk *Russia* **35** G5
Proletarskaya = Proletarsk
  Russia **35** G5
Prome *Burma* **67** K19
Prophet → *Canada* **102** B4
Prophet River *Canada* **102** B4
Propriá *Brazil* **125** F11
Propriano *France* **21** G12
Proserpine *Australia* **94** b
Prosna → *Poland* **31** G5
Prospect *U.S.A.* **115** C9
Prosser *U.S.A.* **108** C4

Prostějov *Czech Rep.* **27** B10
Prostki *Poland* **30** E9
Proston *Australia* **95** D5
Proszowice *Poland* **31** H7
Proti *Greece* **46** D3
Provadiya *Bulgaria* **45** C11
Provence *France* **21** E10
Provence-Alpes-Côte
  d'Azur □ *France* **21** D10
Providence *Ky., U.S.A.* **112** G10
Providence *R.I., U.S.A.* **115** E13
Providence Bay *Canada* **104** C3
Providence Mts. *U.S.A.* **111** K11
Providencia, I. de *Colombia* **120** D3
Provideniya *Russia* **53** C19
Provincetown *U.S.A.* **113** D18
Provins *France* **19** D10
Provo *U.S.A.* **108** F8
Provost *Canada* **103** C6
Prozor *Bos.-H.* **28** G2
Prrenjas *Albania* **44** E4
Prudhoe Bay *U.S.A.* **106** A10
Prudhoe I. *Australia* **94** C4
Prud'homme *Canada* **103** C7
Prudnik *Poland* **31** H4
Prüm *Germany* **25** E2
Prundu *Romania* **29** F11
Prunelli → *France* **21** G13
Pruszcz Gdański *Poland* **30** D5
Pruszków *Poland* **31** F7
Prut → *Romania* **29** E13
Pruzhany *Belarus* **23** B13
Prvić *Croatia* **41** D11
Prydz B. *Antarctica* **5** C6
Pryluky *Ukraine* **33** G7
Pryor *U.S.A.* **116** C7
Prypyat → *Europe* **23** C16
Przasnysz *Poland* **31** E7
Przedbórz *Poland* **31** G6
Przedecz *Poland* **31** F5
Przemków *Poland* **31** G2
Przemyśl *Poland* **31** J9
Przeworsk *Poland* **31** H9
Przewóz *Poland* **31** G1
Przhevalsk = Karakol
  Kyrgyzstan **52** E8
Przysucha *Poland* **31** G7
Psachná *Greece* **46** C5
Psara *Greece* **47** C7
Psathoura *Greece* **46** B5
Psel → *Ukraine* **33** H7
Psérimos *Greece* **47** E9
Psilorítis, Óros *Greece* **49** D6
Psíra *Greece* **49** D7
Pskov *Russia* **32** D5
Pskov □ *Russia* **32** D5
Pskovskoye, Ozero *Russia* **32** D5
Psunj *Croatia* **28** E2
Pteleos *Greece* **46** B4
Ptich = Ptsich → *Belarus* **23** B15
Ptichia = Vidos *Greece* **49** A3
Ptolemaída *Greece* **44** F5
Ptsich → *Belarus* **23** B15
Ptuj *Slovenia* **41** B12
Ptujska Gora *Slovenia* **41** B12
Pu Xian *China* **56** F6
Pua *Thailand* **64** C3
Puán *Argentina* **126** D3
Pu'an *China* **58** E5
Pu'apu'a *Samoa* **91** b
Pubei *China* **58** F7
Pucallpa *Peru* **124** E4
Pucheng *China* **59** D12
Pucheni *Romania* **29** E10
Puchheim *Germany* **25** G7
Puch'on = Bucheon *S. Korea* **57** F14
Púchov *Slovak Rep.* **27** B11
Pucioasa *Romania* **29** E10
Pučišća *Croatia* **41** E13
Puck *Poland* **30** D5
Pucka, Zatoka *Poland* **30** D5
Puçol *Spain* **39** F4
Pudasjärvi *Finland* **8** D22
Puding *China* **58** D5
Pudozh *Russia* **32** B9
Pudu = Suizhou *China* **59** B9
Puducherry *India* **66** P11
Pudukkottai *India* **66** P11
Puebla *Mexico* **119** D5
Puebla □ *Mexico* **119** D5
Puebla de Alcocer *Spain* **37** G5
Puebla de Don Fadrique
  Spain **39** H2
Puebla de Don Rodrigo *Spain* **37** F6
Puebla de Guzmán *Spain* **37** H3
Puebla de la Calzada *Spain* **37** G4
Puebla de Sanabria *Spain* **36** C4
Puebla de Trives = Pobra
  de Trives *Spain* **36** C3
Pueblo *U.S.A.* **108** G11
Puelches *Argentina* **126** D2
Puelén *Argentina* **126** D2
Puente Alto *Chile* **126** C1
Puente-Genil *Spain* **37** H6
Puente la Reina *Spain* **38** C3
Puente San Miguel *Spain* **36** B6
Puenteareas = Ponteareas
  Spain **36** C2
Puentedeume =
  Pontedeume *Spain* **36** B2

Puentes de Garcia
  Rodriguez = As Pontes
  de García Rodríguez *Spain* **36** B3
Pu'er *China* **58** F3
Puerca, Pta. *Puerto Rico* **121** d
Puerco → *U.S.A.* **109** J10
Puerto Aisén *Chile* **128** F2
Puerto Ángel *Mexico* **119** D5
Puerto Arista *Mexico* **119** D6
Puerto Armuelles *Panama* **120** E3
Puerto Ayacucho *Venezuela* **124** B5
Puerto Barrios *Guatemala* **120** C2
Puerto Bermejo *Argentina* **126** B4
Puerto Bermúdez *Peru* **124** F4
Puerto Bolívar *Ecuador* **124** D3
Puerto Cabello *Venezuela* **124** A5
Puerto Cabezas *Nic.* **120** D3
Puerto Cabo Gracias á Dios
  Nic. **120** D3
Puerto Carreño *Colombia* **124** B5
Puerto Castilla *Honduras* **120** C2
Puerto Chicama *Peru* **124** E3
Puerto Coig *Argentina* **128** G3
Puerto Cortés *Honduras* **120** C2
Puerto Cumarebo *Venezuela* **124** A5
Puerto de Alcudia = Port
  d'Alcúdia *Spain* **48** B10
Puerto de Cabrera *Spain* **48** B9
Puerto de Gran Tarajal
  Canary Is. **48** F5
Puerto de la Cruz *Canary Is.* **48** F3
Puerto de los Angeles △
  Mexico **118** C3
Puerto de Mazarrón *Spain* **39** H3
Puerto de Pozo Negro
  Canary Is. **48** F6
Puerto de Sóller = Port de
  Sóller *Spain* **48** B9
Puerto de Somosierra *Spain* **36** D7
Puerto del Carmen *Canary Is.* **48** F6
Puerto del Rosario *Canary Is.* **48** F6
Puerto Deseado *Argentina* **128** F3
Puerto Escondido *Mexico* **119** D5
Puerto Heath *Bolivia* **124** F5
Puerto Inírida *Colombia* **124** C5
Puerto Juárez *Mexico* **119** C7
Puerto La Cruz *Venezuela* **124** A6
Puerto Leguízamo *Colombia* **124** D4
Puerto Lempira *Honduras* **120** C3
Puerto Libertad *Mexico* **118** B2
Puerto Limón *Colombia* **124** C4
Puerto Lobos *Argentina* **128** E3
Puerto Lumbreras *Spain* **39** H3
Puerto Madryn *Argentina* **128** E3
Puerto Maldonado *Peru* **124** F5
Puerto Manatí *Cuba* **120** B4
Puerto Montt *Chile* **128** E2
Puerto Morazán *Nic.* **120** D2
Puerto Morelos *Mexico* **119** C7
Puerto Natales *Chile* **128** G2
Puerto Oscuro *Chile* **126** C1
Puerto Padre *Cuba* **120** B4
Puerto Páez *Venezuela* **124** B5
Puerto Peñasco *Mexico* **118** A2
Puerto Pinasco *Paraguay* **126** A4
Puerto Pinata *Dom. Rep.* **121** C5
Puerto Plata *Dom. Rep.* **121** C5
Puerto Pollensa = Port de
  Pollença *Spain* **48** B10
Puerto Princesa *Phil.* **61** G3
Puerto Quepos *Costa Rica* **120** E3
Puerto Real *Spain* **37** J4
Puerto Rico *Canary Is.* **48** G4
Puerto Rico ☑ *W. Indies* **121** d
Puerto Rico Trench *Atl. Oc.* **121** C6
Puerto San Julián *Argentina* **128** F3
Puerto Santa Cruz *Argentina* **128** G3
Puerto Sastre *Paraguay* **126** A4
Puerto Serrano *Spain* **37** J5
Puerto Suárez *Bolivia* **124** G7
Puerto Vallarta *Mexico* **118** C3
Puerto Varas *Chile* **128** E2
Puerto Wilches *Colombia* **124** B4
Puertollano *Spain* **37** G6
Pueu *Tahiti* **91** d
Pueyrredón, L. *Argentina* **128** F2
Púez Odle △ *Italy* **41** B8
Puffin I. *Ireland* **12** E1
Pugachev *Russia* **34** D9
Pugal *India* **68** E5
Puge *China* **58** D4
Puge *Tanzania* **86** C3
Puget Sound *U.S.A.* **108** C2
Puget-Théniers *France* **21** E10
Púglia ☑ *Italy* **43** A9
Pugōdong *N. Korea* **57** C16
Pugu *Tanzania* **86** D4
Pūgünzī *Iran* **71** E8
Pui *Romania* **28** E8
Puieşti *Romania* **29** D12
Puig Major *Spain* **48** B9
Puigcerdà *Spain* **38** C6
Puigmal *Spain* **38** C7
Puigpunyent *Spain* **48** B9
Puijiang *China* **58** B4
Puisaye, Collines de la
  France **19** E10
Puiseaux *France* **19** D9
Pujehun *S. Leone* **82** D2
Pujiang *China* **59** C12

Pujon-ho *N. Korea* **57** D14
Pukaki, L. *N.Z.* **91** F3
Pukapuka *Cook Is.* **97** J11
Pukaskwa △ *Canada* **104** C2
Pukatawagan *Canada* **103** B8
Pukchin *N. Korea* **57** D13
Pukch'ōng *N. Korea* **57** D15
Pukë *Albania* **44** D3
Pukekohe *N.Z.* **91** B5
Pukhrayan *India* **69** F8
Pukou *China* **59** A12
Pula *Croatia* **41** D10
Pula *Italy* **42** C1
Pulacayo *Bolivia* **124** H5
Pulai *Malaysia* **65** d
Pulandian *China* **57** E11
Pulaski *N.Y., U.S.A.* **115** C8
Pulaski *Tenn., U.S.A.* **117** D11
Pulaski *Va., U.S.A.* **113** G13
Pulau → *Indonesia* **63** F9
Pulawy *Poland* **31** G8
Pulga *Switz.* △ **110** F5
Pulicat L. *India* **66** N12
Pullman *U.S.A.* **108** C5
Pulog, Mt. *Phil.* **61** C4
Pultusk *Poland* **31** F8
Pülümür *Turkey* **73** C8
Pumlumon Fawr *U.K.* **15** E4
Puná, I. *Ecuador* **124** D2
Punaauia *Tahiti* **91** d
Punakaiki *N.Z.* **91** E3
Punakha Dzong *Bhutan* **67** F16
Punasar *India* **68** F5
Punata *Bolivia* **124** G5
Punch *India* **69** C6
Punch → *Pakistan* **68** C5
Punda Maria *S. Africa* **89** C5
Pune *India* **66** K8
Pungue, Ponte de *Mozam.* **87** F3
Puning *China* **59** F11
Punjab ☑ *India* **68** D7
Punjab ☑ *Pakistan* **68** E6
Puno *Peru* **124** G4
Punpun → *India* **69** G11
Punsar *India* **68** F5
Punta, La *India* **124** G5
Punta Alta *Argentina* **128** D4
Punta Arenas *Chile* **128** G2
Punta del Díaz *Chile* **126** B1
Punta del Hidalgo *Canary Is.* **48** F3
Punta Gorda *Belize* **120** D2
Punta Gorda *U.S.A.* **117** H13
Punta Prieta *Mexico* **118** B2
Punta Prima *Spain* **48** B12
Punta Umbría *Spain* **37** H4
Puntarenas *Costa Rica* **120** E3
Puntland *Somali Rep.* **75** F4
Punto Fijo *Venezuela* **124** A4
Punxsutawney *U.S.A.* **114** F6
Pupuan *Indonesia* **63** J18
Puqi *China* **59** C9
Puquio *Peru* **124** F4
Pur → *Russia* **52** C8
Puracé, Vol. *Colombia* **124** C3
Puračić *Bos.-H.* **28** F3
Puralia = Puruliya *India* **69** H12
Puranpur *India* **69** E9
Purbeck, Isle of *U.K.* **15** G5
Purcell *U.S.A.* **116** D6
Purcell Mts. *Canada* **102** D5
Purdy *Canada* **114** A7
Puri *India* **67** K14
Purmerend *Neths.* **17** B4
Purnia *India* **69** G12
Purnululu △ *Australia* **92** C4
Pursat = Pouthisat *Cambodia* **64** F4
Purukcahu *Indonesia* **62** E4
Puruliya *India* **69** H12
Purus → *Brazil* **124** D6
Puruvesi *Finland* **32** B5
Purvis *U.S.A.* **117** F10
Pŭrvomay *Bulgaria* **45** D9
Purwa *India* **69** F9
Purwakarta *Indonesia* **63** G12
Purwo, Tanjung *Indonesia* **63** K18
Purwodadi *Indonesia* **63** G14
Purwokerto *Indonesia* **63** G13
Puryōng *N. Korea* **57** C15
Pusa *India* **69** G11
Pusan = Busan *S. Korea* **57** G15
Pushkin *Russia* **32** C6
Pushkino *Moskva, Russia* **32** D9
Pushkino *Saratov, Russia* **34** E8
Püspökladány *Hungary* **28** C6
Pustoshka *Russia* **32** D5
Puszczykowo *Poland* **31** F3
Put-in-Bay *U.S.A.* **114** E2
Putahow L. *Canada* **103** B8
Putao *Burma* **67** F20
Putaruru *N.Z.* **91** C5
Putbus *Germany* **24** A9
Putian *China* **59** E12
Putignano *Italy* **43** B10
Puting, Tanjung *Indonesia* **62** E4
Putlitz *Germany* **24** B8
Putna *Romania* **29** C10
Putna → *Romania* **29** E12
Putnam *U.S.A.* **115** E13
Putnok *Hungary* **28** B5
Putorana, Gory *Russia* **53** C10

Putrajaya *Malaysia* **65** L3
Puttalam *Sri Lanka* **66** Q11
Puttgarden *Germany* **24** A7
Püttlingen *Germany* **25** F2
Putumayo → *S. Amer.* **124** D5
Putuo *China* **59** C14
Putussibau *Indonesia* **62** D4
Putyla *Ukraine* **29** B10
Puvirnituq *Canada* **101** E16
Puy-de-Dôme *France* **20** C6
Puy-de-Dôme ☑ *France* **20** C7
Puy-l'Évêque *France* **20** D5
Puyallup *U.S.A.* **110** C4
Puyang *China* **56** G8
Puylaurens *France* **20** E6
Püzeh Rīg *Iran* **71** E8
Puzhaykove *Ukraine* **29** B14
Pwani ☑ *Tanzania* **86** D4
Pweto *Dem. Rep. of the Congo* **87** D2
Pwllheli *U.K.* **14** E3
Pyana → *Russia* **34** C8
Pyaozero, Ozero *Russia* **8** C24
Pyapon *Burma* **67** L19
Pyasina → *Russia* **53** B9
Pyatigorsk *Russia* **35** H6
Pyatykhatky *Ukraine* **33** H7
Pydna *Greece* **44** F6
Pye = Prome *Burma* **67** K19
Pyeongtaek *S. Korea* **57** F14
Pyetrikaw *Belarus* **23** B15
Pyhäjoki *Finland* **8** D21
Pyinmana *Burma* **67** K20
Pyla, C. *Cyprus* **49** E12
Pymatuning Res. *U.S.A.* **114** E4
Pyŏktong *N. Korea* **57** D13
Pyŏnggang *N. Korea* **57** E14
P'yŏngsong *N. Korea* **57** E13
P'yŏngyang *N. Korea* **57** E13
Pyote *U.S.A.* **116** F3
Pyramid L. *U.S.A.* **108** F4
Pyramid Pk. *U.S.A.* **111** J10
Pyramids *Egypt* **80** J7
Pyrénées *Europe* **20** F3
Pyrénées △ *France* **20** F3
Pyrénées-Atlantiques ☑
  France **20** E3
Pyrénées-Orientales ☑
  France **20** F6
Pyryatyn *Ukraine* **33** G7
Pyrzyce *Poland* **31** E1
Pyskowice *Poland* **31** H5
Pytalovo *Russia* **32** D4
Pyu *Burma* **67** K20
Pyzdry *Poland* **31** F4

Q

Qaanaaq *Greenland* **101** B18
Qabirri → *Azerbaijan* **35** K8
Qachasnek *S. Africa* **89** E4
Qādisiyah, Buhayrat al *Iraq* **73** E10
Qa'el Jafr *Jordan* **74** E5
Qa'emābād *Iran* **71** D9
Qā'emshahr *Iran* **71** B7
Qagan Nur *China* **56** C8
Qahar Youyi Zhongqi *China* **56** D7
Qahremānshahr =
  Kermānshāh *Iran* **73** E12
Qaidam Pendi *China* **60** C4
Qaiyara *Iraq* **73** E10
Qajarīyeh *Iran* **71** D6
Qala, Ras il *Malta* **49** C1
Qala Point = Qala, Ras il
  Malta **49** C1
Qala Viala *Pakistan* **68** D2
Qala Yangi *Afghan.* **68** B2
Qal'at al Akhḍar *Si. Arabia* **70** E3
Qal'at Bīshah *Si. Arabia* **80** D5
Qal'at Dīzah *Iraq* **73** D11
Qal'at Ṣāliḥ *Iraq* **70** D5
Qal'at Sukkar *Iraq* **73** G12
Qalyūb *Egypt* **80** H7
Qamani'tuaq = Baker Lake
  Canada **100** E12
Qamdo *China* **58** B1
Qamea *Fiji* **91** a
Qamruddin Karez *Pakistan* **68** D3
Qandahār = Kandahār
  Afghan. **66** D4
Qandahār = Kandahār ☑
  Afghan. **66** D4
Qandyaghash *Kazakhstan* **52** E6
Qapān *Iran* **71** B7
Qapshaghay *Kazakhstan* **52** E8
Qaqortoq *Greenland* **4** C5
Qâra *Egypt* **80** B2
Qara Dāgh *Iraq* **73** E11
Qara Qash → *China* **69** B8
Qarabutaq *Kazakhstan* **52** E7
Qaraçala *Azerbaijan* **35** L9
Qarah *Si. Arabia* **70** D4
Qarah Āghāj *Iran* **73** D12
Qaraqosh *Iraq* **73** D10
Qaratau *Ongtüstik Qazaqstan,
  Kazakhstan* **52** E7
Qaratau *Zhambyl, Kazakhstan* **52** E8

Qarazhal *Kazakhstan* **52** E8
Qardho *Somali Rep.* **75** F4
Qardud *Sudan* **81** E2
Qareh *Iran* **73** C12
Qareh Tekān *Iran* **71** B6
Qarqan He → *China* **60** C3
Qarqaraly *Kazakhstan* **52** E8
Qarrasa *Sudan* **81** E3
Qarshi *Uzbekistan* **52** F7
Qartabā *Lebanon* **74** A4
Qaryat al Gharab *Iraq* **70** D5
Qaryat al 'Ulyā *Si. Arabia* **70** E5
Qasr 'Amra *Jordan* **70** D3
Qaşr-e Qand *Iran* **71** E9
Qaşr-e Shīrīn *Iran* **73** E11
Qasr Farâfra *Egypt* **80** B2
Qatanā *Syria* **74** B5
Qatar ■ *Asia* **71** E6
Qatlīsh *Iran* **71** B8
Qattâra *Egypt* **80** A2
Qattâra, Munkhafed el *Egypt* **80** A2
Qattâra Depression =
  Qattâra, Munkhafed el
  Egypt **80** B2
Qausuittuq = Resolute
  Canada **101** C13
Qawām al Ḥamzah = Al
  Ḥamzah *Iraq* **70** D5
Qāyen *Iran* **71** C8
Qazaqstan =
  Kazakhstan ■ *Asia* **52** E8
Qazax *Azerbaijan* **35** K7
Qazimämmäd *Azerbaijan* **35** K9
Qazvīn *Iran* **71** B6
Qazvīn ☑ *Iran* **71** B6
Qeissan *Sudan* **81** E3
Qena *Egypt* **80** B3
Qena, W. → *Egypt* **80** B3
Qeqertarsuaq *Greenland* **4** C5
Qeqertarsuaq *Greenland* **98** C14
Qeshlāq *Iran* **73** E12
Qeshm *Iran* **71** E8
Qeyḍār *Iran* **73** D13
Qeys *Iran* **71** E7
Qezel Owzen → *Iran* **71** B6
Qezi'ot *Israel* **74** E3
Qi Xian *China* **56** G8
Qian Gorlos *China* **57** B13
Qian Xian *China* **56** G5
Qiancheng *China* **58** D7
Qianjiang *Guangxi Zhuangzu,
  China* **58** F7
Qianjiang *Hubei, China* **59** B9
Qianjiang *Sichuan, China* **58** C7
Qianshan *China* **59** B11
Qianwei *China* **58** C4
Qianxi *China* **58** D6
Qianyang *Hunan, China* **59** D8
Qianyang *Shaanxi, China* **56** G4
Qianyang *Zhejiang, China* **59** B12
Qiaojia *China* **58** D4
Qichun *China* **59** B10
Qidong *Hunan, China* **59** D9
Qidong *Jiangsu, China* **59** B13
Qijiang *China* **58** C6
Qikiqtarjuaq *Canada* **101** D19
Qila Saifullāh *Pakistan* **68** D3
Qilian Shan *China* **60** C4
Qimen *China* **59** C11
Qin He → *China* **56** G7
Qin Jiang →
  Guangxi Zhuangzu, China **58** F7
Qin Jiang → *Jiangxi, China* **59** D10
Qin Ling = Qinling Shandi
  China **56** H5
Qin'an *China* **56** G3
Qing Xian *China* **56** E9
Qingcheng *China* **57** F9
Qingdao *China* **57** F11
Qingfeng *China* **56** G8
Qingpu *China* **59** B13
Qingshui *China* **56** G4
Qingshuihe *China* **56** E6
Qingtian *China* **59** C13
Qingtongxia Shuiku *China* **56** F3
Qingxi *China* **58** D7
Qingxu *China* **56** F7
Qingyang *Anhui, China* **59** B11
Qingyang *Gansu, China* **56** G4
Qingyi Jiang → *China* **58** C4
Qingyuan *Guangdong, China* **59** F9
Qingyuan *Liaoning, China* **57** C13
Qingyuan *Zhejiang, China* **59** D12
Qingyun *China* **57** F9
Qingzhen *China* **58** D6
Qinhuangdao *China* **57** E10
Qinling Shandi *China* **56** H5
Qinshui *China* **56** G7
Qinyang = Jiyuan *China* **56** G7

Qinyuan *China* **56** F7
Qinzhou *China* **58** G7
Qionghai *China* **64** C8
Qionglai *China* **58** B4
Qionglai Shan *China* **58** B4
Qiongzhou Haixia *China* **64** B8
Qiqihar *China* **53** E13
Qiraïya, W. → *Egypt* **74** E3
Qiryat Ata *Israel* **74** C4
Qiryat Gat *Israel* **74** D3
Qiryat Mal'akhi *Israel* **74** D3
Qiryat Shemona *Israel* **74** B4
Qiryat Yam *Israel* **74** C4
Qishan *China* **56** G4
Qitai *China* **60** B3
Qitaihe *China* **54** B5
Qiubei *China* **58** E5
Qiyang *China* **59** D8
Qizlağac Körfäzi *Azerbaijan* **73** C13
Qojūr *Iran* **70** B5
Qom *Iran* **71** C6
Qom ☑ *Iran* **71** C6
Qomolangma Feng =
  Everest, Mt. *Nepal* **69** E12
Qomsheh *Iran* **71** D6
Qoqek = Tacheng *China* **60** B3
Qoqon = Qŭqon *Uzbekistan* **52** E8
Qoraqalpoghistan ☑
  Uzbekistan **52** E6
Qorveh *Iran* **73** E12
Qostanay *Kazakhstan* **52** D7
Qoṭūr *Iran* **73** C11
Qu Jiang → *China* **58** B6
Qu Xian *China* **58** B6
Quabbin Res. *U.S.A.* **115** D12
Quairading *Australia* **93** F2
Quakenbrück *Germany* **24** C3
Quakertown *U.S.A.* **115** F9
Qualicum Beach *Canada* **102** D4
Quambatook *Australia* **95** F3
Quambone *Australia* **95** E4
Quamby *Australia* **94** C3
Quan Long = Ca Mau
  Vietnam **65** H5
Quanah *U.S.A.* **116** D5
Quang Ngai *Vietnam* **64** E7
Quang Tri *Vietnam* **64** D6
Quang Yen *Vietnam* **58** G6
Quannan *China* **59** E10
Quantock Hills *U.K.* **15** F4
Quanzhou *Fujian, China* **59** E12
Quanzhou
  Guangxi Zhuangzu, China **59** D8
Qu'Appelle → *Canada* **103** C8
Quaqtaq *Canada* **101** E18
Quarai *Brazil* **126** C4
Quarré-les-Tombes *France* **19** E11
Quartu Sant'Élena *Italy* **42** C2
Quartzsite *U.S.A.* **111** M12
Quatre Bornes *Mauritius* **85** d
Quatsino Sd. *Canada* **102** C3
Quba *Azerbaijan* **35** K9
Qūchān *Iran* **71** B8
Queanbeyan *Australia* **95** F4
Québec *Canada* **105** C5
Québec ☑ *Canada* **105** C6
Quebo *Guinea-Biss.* **82** C2
Quebrada del Condorito △
  Argentina **126** C3
Queen Alexandra Ra.
  Antarctica **5** E11
Queen Charlotte City
  Canada **102** C2
Queen Charlotte Is. *Canada* **102** C2
Queen Charlotte Sd. *Canada* **102** C3
Queen Charlotte Strait
  Canada **102** C3
Queen Elizabeth △ *Uganda* **86** C3
Queen Elizabeth △ *U.K.* **13** E4
Queen Elizabeth Is. *Canada* **101** B13
Queen Mary Land *Antarctica* **5** D7
Queen Maud G. *Canada* **100** D11
Queen Maud Land =
  Dronning Maud Land
  Antarctica **5** D3
Queen Maud Mts. *Antarctica* **5** E13
Queens Channel *Australia* **92** C4
Queenscliff *Australia* **95** F3
Queensland ☑ *Australia* **94** C3
Queenstown *Australia* **95** G4
Queenstown *N.Z.* **91** F2
Queenstown *Singapore* **65** d
Queenstown *S. Africa* **88** E4
Queets *U.S.A.* **110** C2
Queguay Grande →
  Uruguay **126** C4
Queimadas *Brazil* **125** F11
Quelimane *Mozam.* **87** F4
Quellón *Chile* **128** E2

Querétaro ☑ *Mexico* **118** C5
Querfurt *Germany* **24** D7
Querqueville *France* **18** C5
Quesada *Spain* **37** H7
Queshan *China* **56** H8
Quesnel → *Canada* **102** C4
Quesnel *Canada* **102** C4
Quesnel L. *Canada* **102** C4
Questa *U.S.A.* **109** H11
Questembert *France* **18** E4
Quetico △ *Canada* **104** C1
Quetta *Pakistan* **68** D2
Queyras △ *France* **21** D10
Quezaltenango *Guatemala* **120** D1
Quezon City *Phil.* **61** D4
Qufār *Si. Arabia* **70** E4
Qui Nhon *Vietnam* **64** F7
Quibala *Angola* **84** G2
Quibaxe *Angola* **84** G2
Quibdó *Colombia* **124** B3
Quiberon *France* **18** E3
Quiberon, Presqu'île de
  France **18** E3
Quickborn *Germany* **24** B5
Quiet L. *Canada* **102** A2
Quiindy *Paraguay* **126** B4
Quilá *Mexico* **118** C3
Quilán, C. *Chile* **128** E2
Quilcene *U.S.A.* **110** C4
Quilimarí *Chile* **126** C1
Quilino *Argentina* **126** C3
Quillabamba *Peru* **124** F4
Quillagua *Chile* **126** A2
Quillan *France* **20** F6
Quillota *Chile* **126** C1
Quilmes *Argentina* **126** C4
Quilon *India* **66** Q10
Quilpie *Australia* **95** D3
Quilpué *Chile* **126** C1
Quilua *Mozam.* **87** F4
Quimilí *Argentina* **126** B3
Quimper *France* **18** E2
Quimperlé *France* **18** E3
Quinault → *U.S.A.* **110** C2
Quincy *Calif., U.S.A.* **110** F6
Quincy *Fla., U.S.A.* **117** F12
Quincy *Ill., U.S.A.* **112** F8
Quincy *Mass., U.S.A.* **115** D14
Quincy *Wash., U.S.A.* **108** C4
Quines *Argentina* **126** C2
Quinga *Mozam.* **87** F5
Quingey *France* **19** E12
Quinhámel *Guinea-Biss.* **82** C1
Quintana de la Serena *Spain* **37** G5
Quintana Roo ☑ *Mexico* **119** D7
Quintanar de la Orden *Spain* **37** F7
Quintanar de la Sierra *Spain* **38** D2
Quintanar del Rey *Spain* **39** F3
Quintero *Chile* **126** C1
Quintin *France* **18** D4
Quinto *Spain* **38** D4
Quípar → *Spain* **39** G3
Quirihue *Chile* **126** D1
Quirimbas △ *Mozam.* **87** E5
Quirindi *Australia* **95** E5
Quirinópolis *Brazil* **125** G8
Quiroga *Spain* **36** C3
Quissac *France* **21** E12
Quissanga *Mozam.* **87** E5
Quissico *Mozam.* **89** C5
Quitilipi *Argentina* **126** B3
Quitman *U.S.A.* **117** F13
Quito *Ecuador* **124** D3
Quixadá *Brazil* **125** D11
Quixaxe *Mozam.* **87** F5
Qujing *China* **58** E4
Qulan *Kazakhstan* **52** E8
Qul'ān, Jazā'ir *Egypt* **70** E2
Qulsary *Kazakhstan* **52** E6
Qumbu *S. Africa* **89** E4
Quneitra *Syria* **74** B4
Qŭnghirot *Uzbekistan* **52** E6
Qu'nyido *China* **58** B1
Quoin I. *Australia* **92** B4
Quoin Pt. *S. Africa* **88** E2
Quorn *Australia* **95** E2
Qŭqon *Uzbekistan* **52** E8
Qurein *Sudan* **81** E3
Qurimbas *Mozam.* **87** E5
Qurnat as Sawdā' *Lebanon* **74** A5
Qûs *Egypt* **80** B3
Qusar *Azerbaijan* **35** K9
Quşaybā' *Si. Arabia* **70** E4
Qusaybah *Iraq* **73** E9
Quseir *Egypt* **70** D2
Qūshchī *Iran* **73** D11
Quthing *Lesotho* **89** E4
Qūṭīābād *Iran* **73** E13
Quttinirpaaq △ *Canada* **101** A17
Quwo *China* **56** G6
Quyang *China* **56** E8
Quynh Nhai *Vietnam* **64** B4
Quyon *Canada* **115** A8
Quzhou *China* **59** C12
Quzi *China* **56** F4
Qvareli *Georgia* **35** K7
Qyzylorda *Kazakhstan* **52** E7

R

Ra, Ko *Thailand* **65** H2
Raab *Austria* **26** C6
Raahe *Finland* **8** D21
Raalte *Neths.* **17** B6
Raasay *U.K.* **13** D2
Raasay, Sd. of *U.K.* **13** D2
Rab *Croatia* **41** D11
Raba *Indonesia* **63** F5
Rába → *Hungary* **28** C2
Raba → *Poland* **31** H7
Rabaçal → *Portugal* **36** D3
Rabah *Nigeria* **83** C6
Rabai *Kenya* **86** C4
Rabak *Sudan* **81** E3
Rabastens *France* **20** E5
Rabastens-de-Bigorre *France* **20** E4
Rabat = Victoria *Malta* **49** C1
Rabat *Malta* **49** D1
Rabat *Morocco* **78** B4
Rabaul *Papua N. G.* **90** B8
Rabbit Flat *Australia* **92** D5
Rabbit Lake Mine *Canada* **103** B8
Rabi *Fiji* **91** a
Rābigh *Si. Arabia* **75** C2
Rabka *Poland* **31** J6
Râbnița *Moldova* **29** C14
Rābor *Iran* **71** D8
Rabwah = Chenab Nagar
  Pakistan **68** D5
Rača *Serbia* **44** B4
Răcăciuni *Romania* **29** D11
Răcășdia *Romania* **28** F6
Racconigi *Italy* **40** D4
Race, C. *Canada* **105** C9
Rach Gia *Vietnam* **65** G5
Rachid *Mauritania* **82** B2
Raciąż *Poland* **31** F7
Racibórz *Poland* **31** H5
Racichy *Belarus* **30** E10
Racine *U.S.A.* **112** D10
Rackerby *U.S.A.* **110** F5
Radama, Nosy *Madag.* **89** A8
Radama, Saikanosy *Madag.* **89** A8
Radan *Serbia* **44** D5
Rădăuți *Romania* **29** C10
Rădăuți-Prut *Romania* **29** B11
Radbuza → *Czech Rep.* **26** B6
Radcliff *U.S.A.* **113** G11
Radeberg *Germany* **24** D9
Radebeul *Germany* **24** D9
Radeče *Slovenia* **41** B12
Radekhiv *Ukraine* **23** C13
Radekhov = Radekhiv
  Ukraine **23** C13
Radenthein *Austria* **26** E6
Radew → *Poland* **30** D2
Radford *U.S.A.* **113** G13
Radhanpur *India* **68** H4
Radhwa, Jabal *Si. Arabia* **70** E3
Radika → *Macedonia* **44** E4
Radisson *Qué., Canada* **104** A4
Radisson *Sask., Canada* **103** C7
Radium Hot Springs *Canada* **102** C5
Radlje ob Dravi *Slovenia* **41** B12
Radnevo *Bulgaria* **45** D9
Radnice *Czech Rep.* **26** B6
Radnor Forest *U.K.* **15** E4
Radolfzell *Germany* **25** H4
Radom *Poland* **31** G8
Radomir *Bulgaria* **44** D6
Radomka → *Poland* **31** G8
Radomsko *Poland* **31** G6
Radomyshl *Ukraine* **23** C15
Radomyśl Wielki *Poland* **31** H8
Radoszyce *Poland* **31** G7
Radoviš *Macedonia* **44** E6
Radovljica *Slovenia* **41** B11
Radstadt *Austria* **26** D6
Radstock, C. *Australia* **95** E1
Răducăneni *Romania* **29** D12
Raduša *Macedonia* **44** D5
Raduzhnyy *Russia* **52** C8
Radvanichy *Belarus* **23** F11
Radviliškis *Lithuania* **30** C10
Radville *Canada* **103** D8
Raḍwā, J. *Si. Arabia* **80** C4
Radymno *Poland* **31** J9
Radzanów *Poland* **31** F7
Radziejów *Poland* **31** F5
Radzyń Chełmiński *Poland* **30** E5
Radzyń Podlaski *Poland* **31** G9
Rae *Canada* **102** A5
Rae Bareli *India* **69** F9
Rae Isthmus *Canada* **101** D14
Raeren *Belgium* **17** D6
Raeside, L. *Australia* **93** E3
Raetihi *N.Z.* **91** C5
Rafaela *Argentina* **126** C3
Rafah *Gaza Strip* **74** D3
Rafai *C.A.R.* **86** B1
Raffadali *Italy* **42** E6
Raffili *Sudan* **81** F2
Rafḩā *Si. Arabia* **70** D4
Rafina *Greece* **46** C6
Rafsanjān *Iran* **71** D8
Raft Pt. *Australia* **92** C3
Râga *Sudan* **81** F2
Raga → *Sudan* **81** F2

Ragachow *Belarus* **23** B16
Ragag *Sudan* **81** E1
Ragama *Sri Lanka* **66** R11
Ragged, Mt. *Australia* **93** F3
Ragged Pt. *Barbados* **121** g
Raglan *N.Z.* **91** B5
Ragusa *Italy* **43** F7
Raha *Indonesia* **63** E6
Rahad, Nahr ed → *Sudan* **81** E3
Rahaeng = Tak *Thailand* **64** D2
Rahat, Ḥarrat *Si. Arabia* **80** C5
Rahatgarh *India* **69** H8
Rahden *Germany* **24** C4
Raheita *Eritrea* **81** E5
Rahimyar Khan *Pakistan* **68** E4
Rāhjerd *Iran* **71** C6
Rahole △ *Kenya* **86** B4
Rahon *India* **68** D7
Raiatéa, Î. *French Polynesia* **97** J12
Raichur *India* **66** L10
Raiganj *India* **69** G13
Raigarh *India* **67** J13
Raijua *Indonesia* **63** F6
Raikot *India* **68** D6
Railton *Australia* **95** G4
Rainbow Bridge △ *U.S.A.* **109** H8
Rainbow Lake *Canada* **102** B5
Rainier *U.S.A.* **110** D4
Rainier, Mt. *U.S.A.* **110** D5
Rainy L. *Canada* **103** D10
Rainy River *Canada* **103** D10
Raippaluoto *Finland* **8** E19
Raipur *India* **67** J12
Ra'is *Si. Arabia* **80** C4
Raisen *India* **68** H8
Raisio *Finland* **32** B2
Raj Nandgaon *India* **67** J12
Raj Nilgiri *India* **69** J12
Raja, Ujung *Indonesia* **62** D1
Raja Ampat, Kepulauan
  Indonesia **63** E8
Rajahmundry *India* **67** L12
Rajaji △ *India* **68** D8
Rajang → *Malaysia* **62** D4
Rajanpur *Pakistan* **68** E4
Rajapalaiyam *India* **66** Q10
Rajasthan □ *India* **68** F5
Rajasthan Canal = Indira
  Gandhi Canal *India* **68** F5
Rajauri *India* **69** C6
Rajgarh *Mad. P., India* **68** G7
Rajgarh *Raj., India* **68** F7
Rajgarh *Raj., India* **68** E6
Rajgir *India* **69** G11
Rajgród *Poland* **30** E9
Rajkot *India* **68** H4
Rajmahal Hills *India* **69** G12
Rajpipla *India* **66** J8
Rajpur *India* **68** H6
Rajpura *India* **68** D7
Rajsamand = Kankroli *India* **68** G5
Rajshahi *Bangla.* **67** G16
Rajshahi □ *Bangla.* **69** G13
Rajula *India* **68** J4
Rakaia *N.Z.* **91** E4
Rakaia → *N.Z.* **91** E4
Rakan, Ra's *Qatar* **71** E6
Rakaposhi *Pakistan* **69** A6
Rakata, Pulau *Indonesia* **62** F3
Rakbah, Sahl *Si. Arabia* **80** C5
Rakhiv *Ukraine* **29** B9
Rakhni *Pakistan* **68** D3
Rakhni → *Pakistan* **68** E3
Rakhny-Lisovi *Ukraine* **29** B13
Rakiraki *Fiji* **91** a
Rakitnoye *Russia* **54** B7
Rakitovo *Bulgaria* **45** E8
Rakiura = Stewart I. *N.Z.* **91** G1
Rakiura △ *N.Z.* **91** G1
Rakoniewice *Poland* **31** F3
Rakops *Botswana* **88** C3
Rakovica *Croatia* **41** D12
Rakovník *Czech Rep.* **26** A6
Rakovski *Bulgaria* **45** D8
Rakvere *Estonia* **32** C4
Raleigh *U.S.A.* **117** D15
Ralik Chain *Pac. Oc.* **96** G8
Ralja *Serbia* **44** B4
Ralls *U.S.A.* **116** E4
Ralston *U.S.A.* **114** E8
Ram → *Canada* **102** A4
Rām Allāh *West Bank* **74** D4
Rama *Nic.* **120** D3
Ramacca *Italy* **43** E7
Ramakona *India* **69** J8
Ramales de la Victoria *Spain* **36** B7
Rāmallāh = Rām Allāh
  West Bank **74** D4
Raman *Thailand* **65** J3
Ramanathapuram *India* **66** Q11
Ramanetaka, B. de *Madag.* **89** A8
Ramanujganj *India* **69** H10
Ramat Gan *Israel* **74** C3
Ramatlhabama *S. Africa* **88** D4
Ramban *India* **69** C6
Rambervillers *France* **19** D13
Rambi = Rabi *Fiji* **91** a
Rambipuji *Indonesia* **63** H15

Rambouillet *France* **19** D8
Rame Hd. *Australia* **95** F4
Ramechhap *Nepal* **69** F12
Ramenskoye *Russia* **32** E10
Ramganga → *India* **69** F8
Ramgarh *Jharkhand, India* **69** H11
Ramgarh *Raj., India* **68** F5
Ramgarh *Raj., India* **68** F4
Rāmhormoz *Iran* **71** D6
Ramīān *Iran* **71** B7
Ramingining *Australia* **94** A2
Ramla *Israel* **74** D3
Ramlu *Eritrea* **81** E5
Ramm = Rum *Jordan* **74** F4
Ramm, Jabal *Jordan* **74** F4
Râmna → *Romania* **29** E12
Ramnad =
  Ramanathapuram *India* **66** Q11
Ramnagar
  Jammu & Kashmir, India **69** C6
Ramnagar *Uttarakhand, India* **69** E8
Ramnäs *Sweden* **10** E10
Râmnicu Sărat *Romania* **29** E12
Râmnicu Vâlcea *Romania* **29** E9
Ramnous *Greece* **46** C6
Ramon *Russia* **33** G10
Ramona *U.S.A.* **111** M10
Ramonville-St-Agne *France* **20** E5
Ramore *Canada* **104** C3
Ramos → *Nigeria* **83** D6
Ramotswa *Botswana* **88** C4
Rampur *H.P., India* **68** D7
Rampur *Mad. P., India* **68** H5
Rampur *Ut. P., India* **69** E8
Rampur Hat *India* **69** G12
Rampura *India* **68** G6
Ramrama Tola *India* **69** J8
Ramree I. *Burma* **67** K19
Rāmsar *Iran* **71** B6
Ramsey *I. of Man* **14** C3
Ramsey *U.S.A.* **115** E10
Ramsey L. *Canada* **104** C3
Ramsgate *U.K.* **15** F9
Ramsjö *Sweden* **10** B9
Ramstein *Germany* **25** F3
Ramtek *India* **66** J11
Ramu *Kenya* **86** B5
Ramvik *Sweden* **10** B11
Rana Pratap Sagar Dam
  India **68** G6
Ranaghat *India* **69** H13
Ranahu *Pakistan* **68** G3
Ranau *Malaysia* **62** C5
Rancagua *Chile* **126** C1
Rancheria → *Canada* **102** A3
Ranchester *U.S.A.* **108** D10
Ranchi *India* **69** H11
Rancho Cordova *U.S.A.* **110** G5
Rancho Cucamonga *U.S.A.* **111** L9
Randalstown *U.K.* **12** B5
Randan *France* **19** F10
Randazzo *Italy* **43** E7
Randers *Denmark* **11** H4
Randers Fjord *Denmark* **11** H4
Randfontein *S. Africa* **89** D4
Randle *U.S.A.* **110** D5
Randolph *Mass., U.S.A.* **115** D13
Randolph *N.Y., U.S.A.* **114** D6
Randolph *Utah, U.S.A.* **108** F8
Randolph *Vt., U.S.A.* **115** C12
Randsburg *U.S.A.* **111** K9
Råneälven → *Sweden* **8** D20
Rangae *Thailand* **65** J3
Rangaunu B. *N.Z.* **91** A4
Range, The *Zimbabwe* **87** F3
Rangeley *U.S.A.* **115** B14
Rangeley L. *U.S.A.* **115** B14
Rangely *U.S.A.* **108** F9
Ranger *U.S.A.* **116** E5
Rangia *India* **67** F17
Rangiora *N.Z.* **91** E4
Rangitaiki → *N.Z.* **91** B6
Rangitata → *N.Z.* **91** E3
Rangitoto ke te tonga =
  D'Urville I. *N.Z.* **91** D4
Rangkasbitung *Indonesia* **63** G12
Rangon → *Burma* **67** L20
Rangoon *Burma* **67** L20
Rangpur *Bangla.* **67** G16
Rangsang *Indonesia* **65** M4
Rangsit *Thailand* **64** F3
Ranibennur *India* **66** M9
Raniganj *Ut. P., India* **69** F9
Raniganj *W. Bengal, India* **67** H15
Ranikhet *India* **69** E8
Raniwara *India* **68** G5
Rāniyah *Iraq* **73** D11
Ranka *India* **69** H10
Ranken → *Australia* **94** C2
Rankin *U.S.A.* **116** F4
Rankin Inlet *Canada* **100** E13
Rankins Springs *Australia* **95** E4
Rankweil *Austria* **26** D2
Rannoch, L. *U.K.* **13** E4
Rannoch Moor *U.K.* **13** E4
Ranobe, Helodranon' i
  Madag. **89** C7

Ranomafana *Toamasina,
  Madag.* **89** B8
Ranomafana *Toliara, Madag.* **89** C8
Ranomafana △ *Madag.* **89** C8
Ranomena *Madag.* **89** C8
Ranong *Thailand* **65** H2
Ranotsara Nord *Madag.* **89** C8
Ransiki *Indonesia* **63** E8
Rānsa *Iran* **71** C6
Ransiki *Indonesia* **63** E8
Rantabe *Madag.* **89** B8
Rantauprapat *Indonesia* **62** D1
Rantemario *Indonesia* **63** E5
Ranthambore △ *India* **68** F7
Rantoul *U.S.A.* **112** E9
Ranum *Denmark* **11** H3
Ranyah, W. → *Si. Arabia* **80** C5
Raohe *China* **54** A7
Raoping *China* **59** F11
Raoyang *China* **56** E8
Rap, Ko *Thailand* **65** b
Rapa *French Polynesia* **97** K13
Rapa Nui = Pascua, I. de
  Chile **97** K17
Rapallo *Italy* **40** D6
Rapar *India* **68** H4
Rāpch *Iran* **71** E8
Rapel, Lago *Chile* **126** C1
Raper, C. *Canada* **101** D18
Rapid City *U.S.A.* **112** C2
Rapid River *U.S.A.* **112** C10
Rapla *Estonia* **32** C3
Rapti → *India* **69** F10
Rapu Rapu I. *Phil.* **61** E6
Raqaba ez Zarqa → *Sudan* **81** F2
Raquette → *U.S.A.* **115** B10
Raquette Lake *U.S.A.* **115** C10
Rara △ *Nepal* **69** E10
Rarotonga *Cook Is.* **97** K12
Ras Abu Soma *Egypt* **80** B3
Ra's al 'Ayn *Syria* **73** D9
Ra's al Khaymah *U.A.E.* **71** E7
Ra's aṭ Ṭīb *Tunisia* **76** C5
Râs el Mâ *Mali* **82** B4
Râs Ghârib *Egypt* **80** B3
Râs Muhammad △ *Egypt* **80** B3
Râs Sudr *Egypt* **80** B3
Rasa, Pta. *Argentina* **126** D4
Rasca, Pta. de la *Canary Is.* **48** G3
Râşcani *Moldova* **29** C12
Raseiniai *Lithuania* **30** C10
Rashad *Sudan* **81** E3
Rashîd *Egypt* **80** H7
Rashîd, Masabb *Egypt* **80** H7
Rashmi *India* **68** G6
Rasht *Iran* **73** D13
Rasi Salai *Thailand* **64** E5
Raška *Serbia* **44** C4
Rason L. *Australia* **93** E3
Raşova *Romania* **29** F12
Rasovo *Bulgaria* **44** C7
Rasra *India* **69** G10
Rasskazovo *Russia* **34** D5
Rast *Romania* **29** G8
Rastatt *Germany* **25** G4
Rastede *Germany* **24** B4
Răstoliţa *Romania* **29** D9
Rasul *Pakistan* **68** C5
Raszków *Poland* **31** G4
Rat → *Canada* **103** D9
Rat Buri *Thailand* **64** F2
Rat Islands *U.S.A.* **106** E3
Rat L. *Canada* **103** B9
Ratak Chain *Pac. Oc.* **96** G8
Ratangarh *India* **68** E6
Raṭāwī *Iraq* **70** D5
Rath *India* **69** G8
Rathangan *Ireland* **12** C4
Rathdrum *Ireland* **12** D5
Rathenow *Germany* **24** C8
Rathkeale *Ireland* **12** D3
Rathlin I. *U.K.* **12** A5
Rathmelton *Ireland* **12** A4
Ratibor = Racibórz *Poland* **31** H5
Rätikon *Austria* **26** D2
Ratingen *Germany* **24** D2
Ratlam *India* **68** H6
Ratmanova Ostrov *Russia* **106** B6
Ratnagiri *India* **66** L8
Ratodero *Pakistan* **68** F3
Raton *U.S.A.* **109** H11
Rattaphum *Thailand* **65** J3
Ratten *Austria* **26** D8
Rattray Hd. *U.K.* **13** D7
Ratz, Mt. *Canada* **102** B2
Ratzeburg *Germany* **24** B6
Raub *Malaysia* **65** L3
Rauch *Argentina* **126** D4
Raudales *Mexico* **119** D6
Raufarhöfn *Iceland* **8** C6
Raufoss *Norway* **8** F14
Raukumara Ra. *N.Z.* **91** C6
Rauma *Finland* **32** B1
Raumo = Rauma *Finland* **32** B1
Raung, Gunung *Indonesia* **63** J17
Raurkela *India* **69** H11

Rausu-Dake *Japan* **54** B12
Răut → *Moldova* **29** C14
Rava-Ruska *Ukraine* **31** H10
Rava Russkaya =
  Rava-Ruska *Ukraine* **31** H10
Ravalli *U.S.A.* **108** C6
Ravānsar *Iran* **73** E12
Ravanusa *Italy* **42** E6
Ravar *Iran* **71** D8
Ravena *U.S.A.* **115** D11
Ravenna *Italy* **41** D9
Ravenna *Nebr., U.S.A.* **112** E4
Ravenna *Ohio, U.S.A.* **114** E3
Ravensburg *Germany* **25** H5
Ravenshoe *Australia* **94** B4
Ravensthorpe *Australia* **93** F3
Ravenswood *Australia* **94** C4
Ravenswood *U.S.A.* **113** F13
Ravi → *Pakistan* **68** D5
Ravna Gora *Croatia* **41** C11
Ravna Reka *Serbia* **44** B5
Ravne na Koroškem
  Slovenia **41** B11
Rawa Mazowiecka *Poland* **31** G7
Rawalpindi *Pakistan* **68** C5
Rawang *Malaysia* **65** L3
Rawene *N.Z.* **91** A4
Rawicz *Poland* **31** G3
Rawka → *Poland* **31** F7
Rawlinna *Australia* **93** F4
Rawlins *U.S.A.* **108** F10
Rawlinson Ra. *Australia* **93** D4
Rawson *Argentina* **128** E3
Raxaul *India* **69** F11
Ray *U.S.A.* **112** A2
Ray, C. *Canada* **105** C8
Ray Mts. *U.S.A.* **106** B9
Raya Ring, Ko *Thailand* **65** a
Rayadurg *India* **66** M10
Rayagada *India* **67** K13
Raychikhinsk *Russia* **53** E14
Rāyen *Iran* **71** D8
Rayleigh *U.K.* **15** F8
Raymond *Canada* **102** D6
Raymond *Calif., U.S.A.* **110** H7
Raymond *N.H., U.S.A.* **115** C13
Raymond *Wash., U.S.A.* **110** D3
Raymondville *U.S.A.* **116** H6
Raymore *Canada* **103** C8
Rayón *Mexico* **118** B2
Rayong *Thailand* **64** F3
Raystown L. *U.S.A.* **114** F6
Rayville *U.S.A.* **116** E9
Raz, Pte. du *France* **18** D2
Razan *Iran* **73** E13
Razāzah, Buḩayrat ar *Iraq* **73** F10
Razazah, L. = Razāzah,
  Buḩayrat ar *Iraq* **73** F10
Razdelna *Bulgaria* **45** C11
Razdel'naya = Rozdilna
  Ukraine **29** D15
Razdolnoye *Russia* **54** C5
Razdolnoye *Ukraine* **33** K7
Razeh *Iran* **71** D8
Razgrad *Bulgaria* **45** C10
Razim, Lacul *Romania* **29** F14
Razlog *Bulgaria* **44** E7
Razmak *Pakistan* **68** C3
Re, Cu Lao *Vietnam* **64** E7
Ré, Î. de *France* **20** B2
Reading *U.K.* **15** F7
Reading *U.S.A.* **115** F10
Reading □ *U.K.* **15** F7
Realicó *Argentina* **126** D3
Réalmont *France* **20** E6
Ream *Cambodia* **65** G4
Ream △ *Cambodia* **65** G4
Reay Forest *U.K.* **13** C4
Rebais *France* **19** D10
Rebecca, L. *Australia* **93** F3
Rebi *Indonesia* **63** F8
Rebiana *Libya* **79** D10
Rebiana, Sahrâ' *Libya* **79** D10
Reboly *Russia* **8** E24
Rebun-Tō *Japan* **54** B10
Recanati *Italy* **41** E10
Recaş *Romania* **28** E6
Recco *Italy* **40** D6
Recherche, Arch. of the
  Australia **93** F3
Rechna Doab *Pakistan* **68** D5
Rechytsa *Belarus* **23** B16
Recife *Brazil* **125** E12
Recife *Seychelles* **85** b
Recklinghausen *Germany* **17** C7
Reconquista *Argentina* **126** B4
Recreo *Argentina* **126** B2
Recz *Poland* **31** E2
Red → *U.S.A.* **116** F9
Red Bank *U.S.A.* **115** F10
Red Bay *Canada* **105** B8
Red Bluff *U.S.A.* **108** F2
Red Bluff Res. *U.S.A.* **109** L12
Red Cliffs *Australia* **95** E3
Red Cloud *U.S.A.* **112** E4
Red Creek *U.S.A.* **115** C8
Red Deer *Canada* **102** C6
Red Deer → *Alta., Canada* **103** C7

Red Deer → *Man., Canada* **103** C8
Red Deer L. *Canada* **103** C8
Red Hook *U.S.A.* **115** E11
Red Indian L. *Canada* **105** C8
Red L. *Canada* **103** C10
Red Lake *Canada* **103** C10
Red Lake Falls *U.S.A.* **112** B5
Red Lake Road *Canada* **103** C10
Red Lodge *U.S.A.* **108** D9
Red Mountain *U.S.A.* **111** K9
Red Oak *U.S.A.* **112** E6
Red River of the North →
  N. Amer. **112** A5
Red Rock *Canada* **104** C2
Red Rock, L. *U.S.A.* **112** E7
Red Rocks Pt. *Australia* **93** F4
Red Sea *Asia* **75** C2
Red Slate Mt. *U.S.A.* **110** H8
Red Sucker L. *Canada* **104** B1
Red Tower Pass = Turnu
  Roşu, P. *Romania* **29** E9
Red Volta → *Africa* **83** C4
Red Wing *U.S.A.* **112** C7
Reda *Poland* **30** D5
Redang *Malaysia* **65** K4
Redange *Lux.* **17** E5
Redcar *U.K.* **14** C6
Redcar & Cleveland □ *U.K.* **14** C7
Redcliff *Canada* **108** A8
Redcliffe *Australia* **95** D5
Redcliffe, Mt. *Australia* **93** E3
Reddersburg *S. Africa* **88** D4
Redding *U.S.A.* **108** F2
Redditch *U.K.* **15** E6
Redfield *U.S.A.* **112** C4
Redford *U.S.A.* **115** B11
Redhead *Trin. & Tob.* **125** K16
Redkino *Russia* **32** D9
Redlands *U.S.A.* **111** M9
Redmond *Oreg., U.S.A.* **108** D3
Redmond *Wash., U.S.A.* **110** C4
Redon *France* **18** E4
Redonda *Antigua & B.* **121** C7
Redondela *Spain* **36** C2
Redondo *Portugal* **37** G3
Redondo Beach *U.S.A.* **111** M8
Redoubt Volcano *U.S.A.* **106** C9
Redruth *U.K.* **15** G2
Redvers *Canada* **103** D8
Redwater *Canada* **102** C6
Redwood *U.S.A.* **115** B9
Redwood △ *U.S.A.* **108** F1
Redwood City *U.S.A.* **110** H4
Redwood Falls *U.S.A.* **112** C6
Ree, L. *Ireland* **12** C3
Reed City *U.S.A.* **113** D11
Reed L. *Canada* **103** C8
Reedley *U.S.A.* **110** J7
Reedsburg *U.S.A.* **112** D8
Reedsport *U.S.A.* **108** E1
Reedsville *U.S.A.* **114** F7
Reefton *N.Z.* **91** E3
Rees *Germany* **24** D2
Reese → *U.S.A.* **108** F5
Refahiye *Turkey* **73** C8
Reftele *Sweden* **11** G7
Refugio *U.S.A.* **116** G6
Rega → *Poland* **30** D2
Regalbuto *Italy* **43** E7
Regana, C. de *Spain* **48** B9
Regen *Germany* **25** G9
Regen → *Germany* **25** F8
Regensburg *Germany* **25** F8
Regenstauf *Germany* **25** F8
Reggâne = Zaouiet
  Reggâne *Algeria* **78** C6
Reggello *Italy* **41** E8
Réggio di Calábria *Italy* **43** D8
Réggio nell'Emília *Italy* **40** D7
Reghin *Romania* **29** D9
Regina *Canada* **103** C8
Regina Beach *Canada* **103** C8
Registro *Brazil* **127** A6
Reguengos de Monsaraz
  Portugal **37** G3
Rehar → *India* **69** H10
Rehli *India* **69** H8
Rehoboth *Namibia* **88** C2
Rehovot *Israel* **74** D3
Reichenbach *Germany* **24** E8
Reid *Australia* **93** F4
Reidsville *U.S.A.* **117** C15
Reigate *U.K.* **15** F7
Reillo *Spain* **38** F3
Reims *France* **19** C11
Reina Adelaida, Arch. *Chile* **128** G2
Reina Sofía, Tenerife ✈
  (TFS) *Canary Is.* **48** F3
Reinbek *Germany* **24** B6
Reindeer → *Canada* **103** B8
Reindeer I. *Canada* **103** C9
Reindeer L. *Canada* **103** B8
Reinga, C. *N.Z.* **91** A4
Reinosa *Spain* **36** B6
Reitz *S. Africa* **89** D4
Reivilo *S. Africa* **88** D3
Rejaf *Sudan* **81** F3
Rejmyre *Sweden* **11** F9
Rejowiec Fabryczny *Poland* **31** G10
Reka → *Slovenia* **41** C11

Rekovac *Serbia* **44** C5
Reliance *Canada* **103** A7
Rémalard *France* **18** D7
Remanso *Brazil* **125** E10
Remarkable, Mt. *Australia* **95** E2
Rembang *Indonesia* **63** G14
Remedios *Panama* **120** E3
Remeshk *Iran* **71** E8
Remich *Lux.* **17** E6
Remiremont *France* **19** D13
Remo *Ethiopia* **81** F5
Remontnoye *Russia* **35** G6
Remoulins *France* **21** E8
Remscheid *Germany* **17** C7
Ren Xian *China* **56** F8
Rendang *Indonesia* **63** J18
Rende *Italy* **43** C9
Rendina *Greece* **46** B3
Rendsburg *Germany* **24** A5
Renfrew *Canada* **115** A8
Renfrewshire □ *U.K.* **13** F4
Rengat *Indonesia* **62** E2
Rengo *Chile* **126** C1
Renhua *China* **59** E9
Renhuai *China* **58** D6
Reni = Taranagar *India* **68** E6
Reni *Ukraine* **29** E13
Renk *Sudan* **81** E3
Renmark *Australia* **95** E3
Rennell Sd. *Canada* **102** C2
Renner Springs *Australia* **94** B1
Rennes *France* **18** D5
Rennick Glacier *Antarctica* **5** D21
Rennie L. *Canada* **103** A7
Reno *U.S.A.* **110** F7
Reno → *Italy* **41** D9
Renovo *U.S.A.* **114** E7
Renqiu *China* **56** E9
Rens *Denmark* **11** K3
Renshou *China* **58** C5
Rensselaer *Ind., U.S.A.* **112** E10
Rensselaer *N.Y., U.S.A.* **115** D11
Renton *U.S.A.* **110** C4
Renukoot *India* **69** G10
Réo *Burkina Faso* **82** C4
Reocín = Puente San
    Miguel *Spain* **36** B6
Reotipur *India* **69** G10
Répcelak *Hungary* **28** C2
Republic *Mo., U.S.A.* **112** G7
Republic *Wash., U.S.A.* **108** B4
Republican → *U.S.A.* **112** F5
Repulse B. *Australia* **94** b
Repulse Bay *Canada* **101** D14
Requena *Peru* **124** E4
Requena *Spain* **39** F3
Réquista *France* **20** D6
Reşadiye *Muğla, Turkey* **47** E9
Reşadiye *Tokat, Turkey* **72** B7
Reşadiye Yarımadası *Turkey* **47** E9
Resavica *Serbia* **44** B5
Resen *Macedonia* **44** E5
Reserve *U.S.A.* **109** K9
Resht = Rasht *Iran* **73** D13
Resistencia *Argentina* **126** B4
Reşiţa *Romania* **28** E6
Resko *Poland* **30** E2
Reso = Raisio *Finland* **32** B2
Resolute *Canada* **101** C13
Resolution I. *Canada* **101** E19
Resolution I. *N.Z.* **91** F1
Ressano Garcia *Mozam.* **89** D5
Reston *Canada* **103** D8
Reszel *Poland* **30** D8
Retalhuleu *Guatemala* **120** D1
Retenue, L. de
    Dem. Rep. of the Congo **87** E2
Retezat, Munţii *Romania* **28** E8
Retezat △ *Romania* **28** E7
Retford *U.K.* **14** D7
Rethel *France* **19** C11
Rethem *Germany* **24** C5
Rethimno *Greece* **49** D6
Rethimno □ *Greece* **49** D6
Reti *Pakistan* **68** E3
Retiche, Alpi *Switz.* **25** J6
Retiers *France* **18** E5
Retortillo *Spain* **36** E4
Retournac *France* **21** C8
Rétság *Hungary* **28** C4
Réunion □ *Ind. Oc.* **85** c
Reus *Spain* **38** D6
Reuterstadt Stavenhagen
    Germany **24** B8
Reutlingen *Germany* **25** G5
Reutte *Austria* **26** D3
Reval = Tallinn *Estonia* **32** C3
Revel *France* **20** E6
Revelganj *India* **69** G11
Revelstoke *Canada* **102** C5
Reventazón *Peru* **124** E2
Revigny-sur-Ornain *France* **19** D11
Revillagigedo, Is. de *Pac. Oc.* **118** D2
Revin *France* **19** C11
Revúca *Slovak Rep.* **27** C13
Revuè → *Mozam.* **87** F3
Rewa *India* **69** G9
Rewari *India* **68** E7
Rexburg *U.S.A.* **108** E8

Rey *Iran* **71** C6
Rey, I. del *Panama* **120** E4
Rey, L. del *Mexico* **118** B4
Rey Malabo *Eq. Guin.* **83** E6
Reyðarfjörður *Iceland* **8** D6
Reyes, Pt. *U.S.A.* **110** H3
Reyhanlı *Turkey* **72** D7
Reykjahlíð *Iceland* **8** D5
Reykjanes *Iceland* **8** E2
Reykjavík *Iceland* **8** D3
Reynolds Ra. *Australia* **92** D5
Reynoldsville *U.S.A.* **114** E6
Reynosa *Mexico* **119** B5
Rēzekne *Latvia* **32** D4
Rezina *Moldova* **29** C13
Rezovo *Bulgaria* **45** D12
Rezvān *Iran* **71** E8
Rezvānshahr *Iran* **73** D13
Rgotina *Serbia* **44** B6
Rhayader *U.K.* **15** E4
Rheda-Wiedenbrück
    Germany **24** D4
Rhede *Germany* **24** D2
Rhein → *Europe* **17** C6
Rhein-Main-Donau-Kanal
    Germany **25** F7
Rhein-Ruhr, Düsseldorf ✈
    (DUS) *Germany* **24** D2
Rhein-Taunus △ *Germany* **25** E4
Rhein-Westerwald △
    Germany **25** E4
Rheinbach *Germany* **24** E2
Rheine *Germany* **24** C3
Rheinfelden *Germany* **25** H3
Rheinhessen-Pfalz □
    Germany **25** F3
Rheinland-Pfalz □ *Germany* **25** E2
Rhinelander *U.S.A.* **112** C9
Rhinns Pt. *U.K.* **13** F2
Rhino Camp *Uganda* **86** B3
Rhir, Cap *Morocco* **78** B4
Rho *Italy* **40** C6
Rhode Island □ *U.S.A.* **115** E13
Rhodes *Greece* **49** C10
Rhodes ✈ (RHO) *Greece* **47** E10
Rhodope Mts. = Rhodopi
    Planina *Bulgaria* **45** E8
Rhodopi Planina *Bulgaria* **45** E8
Rhön *Germany* **24** E5
Rhondda *U.K.* **15** F4
Rhondda Cynon Taff □ *U.K.* **15** F4
Rhône □ *France* **21** C8
Rhône → *France* **21** E8
Rhône-Alpes □ *France* **21** C9
Rhum *U.K.* **13** E2
Rhyl *U.K.* **14** D4
Ri-Aba *Eq. Guin.* **83** E6
Ria Formosa △ *Portugal* **37** H3
Riachão *Brazil* **125** E9
Riangnom *Sudan* **81** F3
Riano *Spain* **36** C6
Rians *France* **21** E9
Riansáres → *Spain* **37** F7
Riasi *India* **69** C6
Riau □ *Indonesia* **62** E2
Riau, Kepulauan *Indonesia* **62** D2
Riau Arch. = Riau,
    Kepulauan *Indonesia* **62** D2
Riaza *Spain* **36** D7
Riaza → *Spain* **36** D7
Riba de Saelices *Spain* **38** E2
Riba-roja de Túria *Spain* **39** F4
Ribadavia *Spain* **36** C2
Ribadeo *Spain* **36** B3
Ribadesella *Spain* **36** B5
Ribado *Nigeria* **83** D7
Ribao *Cameroon* **83** D7
Ribas = Ribes de Freser *Spain* **38** C7
Ribas do Rio Pardo *Brazil* **125** H8
Ribauè *Mozam.* **87** E4
Ribble → *U.K.* **14** D5
Ribe *Denmark* **11** J2
Ribeauvillé *France* **19** D14
Ribécourt-Dreslincourt
    France **19** C9
Ribeira = Santa Uxía de
    Ribeira *Spain* **36** C2
Ribeira Brava *Madeira* **48** D2
Ribeira Grande *C. Verde Is.* **78** b
Ribeirão Prêto *Brazil* **127** A6
Ribemont *France* **19** C10
Ribera *Italy* **42** E6
Ribérac *France* **20** C4
Riberalta *Bolivia* **124** F5
Ribes de Freser *Spain* **38** C7
Ribnica *Slovenia* **41** C11
Ribnitz-Damgarten *Germany* **24** A8
Ričany *Czech Rep.* **26** B7
Riccarton *N.Z.* **91** E4
Riccia *Italy* **43** A7
Riccione *Italy* **41** E9
Rice *U.S.A.* **111** L12
Rice L. *Canada* **114** B6

Rice Lake *U.S.A.* **112** C8
Rich, C. *Canada* **114** B4
Richard Toll *Senegal* **82** B1
Richards Bay *S. Africa* **89** D5
Richardson → *Canada* **103** B6
Richardson Lakes *U.S.A.* **113** C18
Richardson Springs *U.S.A.* **110** F5
Riche, C. *Australia* **93** F2
Richelieu → *France* **18** E7
Richey *U.S.A.* **108** C11
Richfield *U.S.A.* **108** G7
Richfield Springs *U.S.A.* **115** D10
Richford *U.S.A.* **115** B12
Richibucto *Canada* **105** C7
Richland *Ga., U.S.A.* **117** E12
Richland *Wash., U.S.A.* **108** C4
Richland Center *U.S.A.* **112** D8
Richlands *U.S.A.* **113** G13
Richmond *N.Z.* **91** D4
Richmond *U.K.* **14** C6
Richmond *Calif., U.S.A.* **110** H4
Richmond *Ind., U.S.A.* **113** F11
Richmond *Ky., U.S.A.* **113** G11
Richmond *Mich., U.S.A.* **114** D2
Richmond *Mo., U.S.A.* **112** F7
Richmond *Tex., U.S.A.* **116** G7
Richmond *Utah, U.S.A.* **108** F8
Richmond *Va., U.S.A.* **113** G15
Richmond *Vt., U.S.A.* **115** B11
Richmond Hill *Canada* **114** C5
Richmond Ra. *Australia* **95** D5
Richmondville *U.S.A.* **115** D10
Richtersveld △ *S. Africa* **88** D2
Richville *U.S.A.* **115** B9
Richwood *U.S.A.* **113** F13
Ricla *Spain* **38** D3
Riddlesburg *U.S.A.* **114** F6
Ridgecrest *U.S.A.* **111** K9
Ridgefield *Conn., U.S.A.* **115** E11
Ridgefield *Wash., U.S.A.* **110** E4
Ridgeland *Miss., U.S.A.* **117** E9
Ridgeland *S.C., U.S.A.* **117** E14
Ridgetown *Canada* **114** D3
Ridgewood *U.S.A.* **115** F10
Ridgway *U.S.A.* **114** E6
Riding Mountain △ *Canada* **103** C9
Ridley, Mt. *Australia* **93** F3
Riebeek-Oos *S. Africa* **88** E4
Ried *Austria* **26** C6
Riedlingen *Germany* **25** G5
Riedstadt *Germany* **25** F4
Rienza → *Italy* **41** B8
Riesa *Germany* **24** D9
Riesi *Italy* **43** E7
Riet → *S. Africa* **88** D3
Rietavas *Lithuania* **30** C8
Rietbron *S. Africa* **88** E3
Rietfontein *Namibia* **88** C3
Rieti *Italy* **41** F9
Rieupeyroux *France* **20** D6
Riez *France* **21** E10
Rif = Er Rif *Morocco* **78** A5
Riffe L. *U.S.A.* **110** D4
Rifle *U.S.A.* **108** G10
Rift Valley *Africa* **76** G7
Rift Valley □ *Kenya* **86** B4
Rīga *Latvia* **30** B11
Rīga ✈ (RIX) *Latvia* **30** B10
Riga, G. of *Latvia* **30** A10
Rigacikun *Nigeria* **83** C6
Rīgān *Iran* **71** D8
Rīgas Jūras Līcis = Riga, G.
    of *Latvia* **30** A10
Rigaud *Canada* **115** A10
Rigby *U.S.A.* **108** E8
Rīgestān *Afghan.* **66** D4
Riggins *U.S.A.* **108** D5
Rignac *France* **20** D6
Rigolet *Canada* **105** B8
Rigu *Ghana* **83** D4
Rihand Dam *India* **69** G10
Riihimäki *Finland* **32** B3
Riiser-Larsen-halvøya
    Antarctica **5** C4
Riiser-Larsen Ice Shelf
    S. Ocean **5** D2
Riiser-Larsen Sea *S. Ocean* **5** C4
Rijau *Nigeria* **83** C6
Rijeka *Croatia* **41** C11
Rijeka Crnojevića *Montenegro* **44** D3
Rijssen *Neths.* **17** B6
Rika → *Ukraine* **29** B8
Rike *Ethiopia* **81** E4
Rikuchū-Kaigan △ *Japan* **54** E11
Rikuzentakada *Japan* **54** E10
Rila *Bulgaria* **44** D7
Rila Planina *Bulgaria* **44** D7
Riley *U.S.A.* **108** E4
Rima → *Nigeria* **83** C6
Rimah, Wadi ar → *Si. Arabia* **70** E4
Rimau, Pulau *Malaysia* **65** c
Rimavská Sobota
    Slovak Rep. **27** C13
Rimbey *Canada* **102** C6
Rimbo *Sweden* **10** E12
Rimersburg *U.S.A.* **114** E5
Rimforsa *Sweden* **11** F9

Rimi *Nigeria* **83** C6
Rímini *Italy* **41** D9
Rimouski *Canada* **105** C6
Rimrock *U.S.A.* **110** D5
Rinca *Indonesia* **63** F5
Rincón de la Victoria *Spain* **37** J6
Rincón de Romos *Mexico* **118** C4
Rinconada *Argentina* **126** A2
Rind → *India* **69** G9
Ringarum *Sweden* **11** F10
Ringas *India* **68** F6
Ringe *Denmark* **11** J4
Ringgold Is. *Fiji* **91** a
Ringim *Nigeria* **83** C6
Ringkøbing *Denmark* **11** H2
Ringkøbing Fjord *Denmark* **11** H2
Ringsjön *Sweden* **11** J7
Ringsted *Denmark* **11** J5
Ringvassøya *Norway* **8** B18
Ringwood *U.S.A.* **115** E10
Rinia *Greece* **47** D7
Rinjani *Indonesia* **62** F5
Rinteln *Germany* **24** C5
Río, Punta del *Spain* **39** J2
Rio Branco *Brazil* **124** E5
Río Branco *Uruguay* **127** C5
Río Bravo *Mexico* **119** B5
Río Bravo → *N. Amer.* **118** B4
Río Bravo del Norte →
    Mexico **118** B4
Rio Brilhante *Brazil* **127** A5
Rio Claro *Brazil* **127** A6
Rio Claro *Trin. & Tob.* **121** D7
Río Colorado *Argentina* **128** D4
Río Cuarto *Argentina* **126** C3
Rio das Pedras *Mozam.* **89** C6
Rio de Janeiro *Brazil* **127** A7
Rio de Janeiro □ *Brazil* **127** A7
Rio do Sul *Brazil* **127** B6
Río Dulce △ *Guatemala* **120** C2
Río Gallegos *Argentina* **128** G3
Río Grande *Argentina* **128** G3
Rio Grande *Brazil* **127** C5
Río Grande *Mexico* **118** C4
Río Grande *Puerto Rico* **121** d
Rio Grande → *N. Amer.* **116** J6
Rio Grande City *U.S.A.* **116** H5
Río Grande de Santiago →
    Mexico **118** C3
Rio Grande do Norte □
    Brazil **125** E11
Rio Grande do Sul □ *Brazil* **127** C5
Río Hato *Panama* **120** E3
Río Lagartos *Mexico* **119** C7
Rio Largo *Brazil* **125** E11
Rio Maior *Portugal* **37** F2
Rio Marina *Italy* **40** F7
Río Mulatos *Bolivia* **124** G5
Río Muni □ *Eq. Guin.* **84** D2
Rio Negro *Brazil* **127** B6
Rio Pardo *Brazil* **127** C5
Río Pilcomayo △ *Argentina* **126** B4
Río Platano △ *Honduras* **120** C3
Rio Rancho *U.S.A.* **109** J10
Río Segundo *Argentina* **126** C3
Río Tercero *Argentina* **126** C3
Rio Tinto *Portugal* **36** D2
Rio Verde *Brazil* **125** G8
Río Verde *Mexico* **119** C5
Rio Vista *U.S.A.* **110** G5
Ríobamba *Ecuador* **124** D3
Ríohacha *Colombia* **124** A4
Riom *France* **20** C7
Riom-ès-Montagnes *France* **20** C6
Rion-des-Landes *France* **20** E3
Rionero in Vúlture *Italy* **43** B8
Rioni → *Georgia* **35** J5
Ríos *Spain* **36** D3
Riosucio *Colombia* **124** B3
Riou L. *Canada* **103** B7
Rioz *France* **19** E13
Ripatransone *Italy* **41** F10
Ripley *Canada* **114** B3
Ripley *Calif., U.S.A.* **111** M12
Ripley *N.Y., U.S.A.* **114** D5
Ripley *Tenn., U.S.A.* **117** D10
Ripley *W. Va., U.S.A.* **113** F13
Ripoll *Spain* **38** C7
Ripon *U.K.* **14** C6
Ripon *Calif., U.S.A.* **110** H5
Ripon *Wis., U.S.A.* **112** D9
Riposto *Italy* **43** E8
Risan *Montenegro* **44** D2
Riscle *France* **20** E3
Rishā', W. ar → *Si. Arabia* **70** E5
Rishiri-Rebun-Sarobetsu △
    Japan **54** B10
Rishiri-Tō *Japan* **54** B10
Rishon le Ziyyon *Israel* **74** D3
Risle → *France* **18** C7
Risnjak △ *Croatia* **41** C11
Rison *U.S.A.* **116** E8
Risør *Norway* **9** G13
Rita Blanca Cr. → *U.S.A.* **116** D3
Riti *Nigeria* **83** D6
Ritter, Mt. *U.S.A.* **110** H7
Rittman *U.S.A.* **114** F3
Ritzville *U.S.A.* **108** C4
Riva del Garda *Italy* **40** C7
Riva Lígure *Italy* **40** E4

Rivadavia *B. Aires, Argentina* **126** D3
Rivadavia *Mendoza,
    Argentina* **126** C2
Rivadavia *Salta, Argentina* **126** A3
Rivadavia *Chile* **126** B1
Rivarolo Canavese *Italy* **40** C4
Rivas *Nic.* **120** D2
Rive-de-Gier *France* **21** C8
River Cess *Liberia* **82** D3
River Jordan *Canada* **110** B2
Rivera *Argentina* **126** D3
Rivera *Uruguay* **127** C4
Riverbank *U.S.A.* **110** H6
Riverdale *U.S.A.* **110** J7
Riverhead *U.S.A.* **115** F12
Riverhurst *Canada* **103** C7
Rivers *Canada* **103** C8
Rivers □ *Nigeria* **83** E6
Rivers Inlet *Canada* **102** C3
Riversdale *Canada* **114** B3
Riversdale *S. Africa* **88** E3
Riverside *U.S.A.* **111** M9
Riverton *Australia* **95** E2
Riverton *Canada* **103** C9
Riverton *N.Z.* **91** G2
Riverton *U.S.A.* **108** E9
Rives *France* **21** C9
Rivesaltes *France* **20** F6
Riviera *U.S.A.* **111** K12
Riviera di Levante *Italy* **40** D6
Riviera di Ponente *Italy* **40** D5
Rivière-au-Renard *Canada* **105** C7
Rivière-du-Loup *Canada* **105** C6
Rivière-Pentecôte *Canada* **105** C6
Rivière-Pilote *Martinique* **120** c
Rivière St-Paul *Canada* **105** B8
Rivière-Salée *Martinique* **120** c
Rivne *Odesa, Ukraine* **29** D14
Rivne *Rivne, Ukraine* **23** C14
Rivne □ *Ukraine* **33** G4
Rívoli *Italy* **40** C4
Rívoli B. *Australia* **95** F3
Rixheim *France* **19** E14
Riyadh = Ar Riyāḍ *Si. Arabia* **70** E5
Riyadh al Khabrā' *Si. Arabia* **70** E4
Riza *Greece* **44** F7
Rize *Turkey* **73** B9
Rize □ *Turkey* **73** B9
Rizhao *China* **57** G10
Rizokarpaso *Cyprus* **49** D13
Rizzuto, C. *Italy* **43** D10
Rjukan *Norway* **9** G13
Rkîz *St. Mauritania* **82** B1
Ro *Greece* **47** E11
Roa *Spain* **36** D7
Road Town *Br. Virgin Is.* **121** e
Roan Plateau *U.S.A.* **108** G9
Roanne *France* **19** F11
Roanoke *Ala., U.S.A.* **117** E12
Roanoke *Va., U.S.A.* **113** G14
Roanoke → *U.S.A.* **117** D16
Roanoke I. *U.S.A.* **117** D17
Roanoke Rapids *U.S.A.* **117** C16
Roatán *Honduras* **120** C2
Robāt *Iran* **73** E12
Robāt Sang *Iran* **71** C9
Robāṭkarīm *Iran* **71** C6
Robbins I. *Australia* **95** G4
Röbel *Germany* **24** B8
Róbbio *Italy* **40** C5
Robert Bourassa, Rés.
    Canada **104** B4
Robert Lee *U.S.A.* **116** F4
Robertsdale *U.S.A.* **114** F6
Robertsganj *India* **69** G10
Robertson *S. Africa* **88** E2
Robertson I. *Antarctica* **5** C18
Robertson Ra. *Australia* **92** D3
Robertsport *Liberia* **82** D2
Robertstown *Australia* **95** E2
Roberval *Canada* **105** C5
Robeson Chan. *N. Amer.* **101** A19
Robesonia *U.S.A.* **115** F8
Robi *Ethiopia* **81** F4
Robinson *U.S.A.* **112** F10
Robinson → *Australia* **94** B2
Robinson Crusoe I. *Pac. Oc.* **122** F2
Robinson Ra. *Australia* **93** E2
Robinvale *Australia* **95** E3
Robledo *Spain* **39** G2
Roblin *Canada* **103** C8
Roboré *Bolivia* **124** G7
Robson, Mt. *Canada* **102** C5
Robstown *U.S.A.* **116** H6
Roca, C. da *Portugal* **37** G1
Roca Partida, I. *Mexico* **118** D2
Rocas, I. *Brazil* **125** D12
Rocca San Casciano *Italy* **41** D8
Roccadáspide *Italy* **43** B8
Roccastrada *Italy* **41** F8
Roccella Iónica *Italy* **43** D9
Rocciamelone, Monte =
    Roche Melon *Italy* **21** C11
Rocha *Uruguay* **127** C5
Rochdale *U.K.* **14** D5
Roche Melon *Italy* **21** C11
Rochechouart *France* **20** C4

Rochefort *Belgium* **17** D5
Rochefort *France* **20** C3
Rochefort-en-Terre *France* **18** E4
Rochelle *U.S.A.* **112** E9
Rocher River *Canada* **102** A6
Rocheservière *France* **18** F5
Rochester *U.K.* **15** F8
Rochester *Ind., U.S.A.* **112** E10
Rochester *Minn., U.S.A.* **112** C7
Rochester *N.H., U.S.A.* **115** C14
Rochester *N.Y., U.S.A.* **114** C7
Rociu *Romania* **29** F10
Rock → *Canada* **102** A3
Rock, The *Australia* **95** F4
Rock Creek *U.S.A.* **114** E4
Rock Falls *U.S.A.* **112** E9
Rock Hill *U.S.A.* **117** D14
Rock Island *U.S.A.* **112** E8
Rock Port *U.S.A.* **112** E6
Rock Rapids *U.S.A.* **112** D5
Rock Sound *Bahamas* **120** B4
Rock Springs *Mont., U.S.A.* **108** C10
Rock Springs *Wyo., U.S.A.* **108** F9
Rock Valley *U.S.A.* **112** D5
Rockall *Atl. Oc.* **6** D3
Rockdale *Tex., U.S.A.* **116** F6
Rockdale *Wash., U.S.A.* **110** C5
Rockeby = Mungkan
    Kandju △ *Australia* **94** A3
Rockefeller Plateau
    Antarctica **5** E14
Rockford *U.S.A.* **112** D9
Rockglen *Canada* **103** D7
Rockhampton *Australia* **94** C5
Rockingham *Australia* **93** F2
Rockingham *N.C., U.S.A.* **117** D15
Rockingham *Vt., U.S.A.* **115** C12
Rockingham B. *Australia* **94** B4
Rocklake *U.S.A.* **112** A4
Rockland *Canada* **115** A9
Rockland *Idaho, U.S.A.* **108** E7
Rockland *Maine, U.S.A.* **113** C19
Rockland *Mich., U.S.A.* **112** B9
Rocklin *U.S.A.* **110** G5
Rockly B. *Trin. & Tob.* **125** J16
Rockmart *U.S.A.* **117** D12
Rockport *Mass., U.S.A.* **115** D14
Rockport *Tex., U.S.A.* **116** G6
Rocksprings *U.S.A.* **116** F4
Rockville *Conn., U.S.A.* **115** E12
Rockville *Md., U.S.A.* **113** F15
Rockwall *U.S.A.* **116** E6
Rockwell City *U.S.A.* **112** D6
Rockwood *Canada* **114** C4
Rockwood *Maine, U.S.A.* **113** C19
Rockwood *Tenn., U.S.A.* **117** D12
Rocky Ford *U.S.A.* **108** G12
Rocky Gully *Australia* **93** F2
Rocky Harbour *Canada* **105** C8
Rocky Island L. *Canada* **104** C3
Rocky Lane *Canada* **102** B5
Rocky Mount *U.S.A.* **117** D16
Rocky Mountain △ *U.S.A.* **108** F11
Rocky Mountain House
    Canada **102** C4
Rocky Mts. *N. Amer.* **108** B6
Rocky Point *Namibia* **88** B2
Rocroi *France* **19** C11
Rod *Pakistan* **66** E3
Roda *Greece* **49** A3
Rødby *Denmark* **11** K5
Rødbyhavn *Denmark* **11** K5
Roddickton *Canada* **105** B8
Rødding *Denmark* **11** J3
Rødeby *Sweden* **11** H9
Rødekro *Denmark* **11** J3
Rodenkirchen *Germany* **24** B4
Rodez *France* **20** D6
Ródhos = Rhodes *Greece* **49** C10
Rodi Gargánico *Italy* **41** G12
Rodia *Greece* **49** D7
Rodna *Romania* **29** C9
Rodna □ *Australia* **92** D5
Rodnei, Munţii *Romania* **29** C9
Rodney *Canada* **114** D3
Rodney, C. *N.Z.* **91** B5
Rodniki *Russia* **34** B5
Rodolivos *Greece* **44** F7
Rodonit, Kepi i *Albania* **44** E3
Rodopi □ *Greece* **45** E9
Rodopos *Greece* **49** D5
Rodrigues *Ind. Oc.* **3** E13
Roe → *U.K.* **12** A5
Roebling *U.S.A.* **115** F10
Roebourne *Australia* **92** D2
Roebuck B. *Australia* **92** C3
Roebuck Roadhouse
    Australia **92** C3
Roermond *Neths.* **17** C6
Roes Welcome Sd. *Canada* **101** E14
Roeselare *Belgium* **17** D3
Rogachev = Ragachow
    Belarus **23** B16
Rogačica *Serbia* **44** B3
Rogagua, L. *Bolivia* **124** F5
Rogaška Slatina *Slovenia* **41** B12
Rogatec *Slovenia* **41** B12
Rogatica *Bos.-H.* **28** G4
Rogatyn *Ukraine* **23** D13
Rogers *U.S.A.* **116** C7

Rogers City *U.S.A.* **113** C12
Rogersville *Canada* **105** C6
Roggan ↣ *Canada* **104** B4
Roggan L. *Canada* **104** B4
Roggeveen Basin *Pac. Oc.* **97** L18
Roggiano Gravina *Italy* **43** C9
Rogliano *France* **21** F13
Rogliano *Italy* **43** C9
Rogoaguado, L. *Bolivia* **124** F5
Rogojampi *Indonesia* **63** J17
Rogoźno *Poland* **31** F3
Rogue ↣ *U.S.A.* **108** E1
Rohan *France* **18** D4
Rohnert Park *U.S.A.* **110** G4
Rohri *Pakistan* **68** F3
Rohri Canal *Pakistan* **68** F3
Rohtak *India* **68** E7
Roi Et *Thailand* **64** D4
Roja *Latvia* **30** A9
Rojas *Argentina* **126** C3
Rojişte *Romania* **29** F8
Rojo, C. *Mexico* **119** C5
Rokan ↣ *Indonesia* **62** D2
Rokel ↣ *S. Leone* **82** D2
Rokiškis *Lithuania* **32** E3
Rokitno *Russia* **33** G9
Rokycany *Czech Rep.* **26** B6
Rolândia *Brazil* **127** A5
Rolla *Mo., U.S.A.* **112** G8
Rolla *N. Dak., U.S.A.* **112** A4
Rolleston *Australia* **94** C4
Rollingstone *Australia* **94** B4
Rom *Sudan* **81** F3
Roma *Australia* **95** D4
Roma *Italy* **41** G9
Roma *Sweden* **11** G12
Roma Fiumicino ✈ (FCO) *Italy* **41** G9
Roma-Los Saenz *U.S.A.* **116** H5
Romain, C. *U.S.A.* **117** E15
Romaine ↣ *Canada* **105** B7
Roman *Bulgaria* **44** C7
Roman *Romania* **29** D11
Roman-Kosh, Gora *Ukraine* **33** K8
Romanche ↣ *France* **21** C9
Romang *Indonesia* **63** F7
Români *Egypt* **74** E1
Romania ■ *Europe* **29** D10
Romanija *Bos.-H.* **28** G3
Romano, Cayo *Cuba* **120** B4
Romans-sur-Isère *France* **21** C9
Romanshorn *Switz.* **25** H5
Romanzof C. *U.S.A.* **106** C6
Rombari *Sudan* **81** G3
Romblon *Phil.* **61** E5
Rome = Roma *Italy* **41** G9
Rome *Ga., U.S.A.* **117** D12
Rome *N.Y., U.S.A.* **115** C9
Rome *Pa., U.S.A.* **115** E8
Rometta *Italy* **43** D8
Romilly-sur-Seine *France* **19** D10
Romney *U.S.A.* **113** F14
Romney Marsh *U.K.* **15** F8
Romny *Ukraine* **33** G7
Rømø *Denmark* **11** J2
Romodan *Ukraine* **33** G7
Romodanovo *Russia* **34** C7
Romont *Switz.* **25** J2
Romorantin-Lanthenay *France* **19** E8
Romsdalen *Norway* **8** E12
Romsey *U.K.* **15** G6
Ron *Vietnam* **64** D6
Rona *U.K.* **13** D3
Ronan *U.S.A.* **108** C6
Roncador, Cayos *Colombia* **120** D3
Roncador, Serra do *Brazil* **125** F8
Ronciglione *Italy* **41** F9
Ronco ↣ *Italy* **41** D9
Ronda *Spain* **37** J5
Ronda, Serranía de *Spain* **37** J5
Rondane *Norway* **8** F13
Rondônia □ *Brazil* **124** F6
Rondonópolis *Brazil* **125** G8
Rondu *Pakistan* **69** B6
Rong, Koh *Cambodia* **65** G4
Rong Jiang ↣ *China* **58** E7
Rong Xian *Guangxi Zhuangzu, China* **59** F8
Rong Xian *Sichuan, China* **58** C5
Rong'an *China* **58** E7
Rongchang *China* **58** C5
Ronge, L. la *Canada* **103** B7
Rongjiang *China* **58** E7
Rongshui *China* **58** E7
Rønne *Denmark* **11** J8
Ronne Ice Shelf *Antarctica* **5** D18
Ronneby *Sweden* **11** H9
Ronnebyån ↣ *Sweden* **11** H9
Rönneshytta *Sweden* **11** F9
Ronsard, C. *Australia* **93** D1
Ronse *Belgium* **17** D3
Roodepoort *S. Africa* **89** D4
Roof Butte *U.S.A.* **109** H9
Rooiboklaagte ↣ *Namibia* **88** C3
Rooniu, Mt. *Tahiti* **91** d
Roorkee *India* **68** E7
Roosendaal *Neths.* **17** C4
Roosevelt *U.S.A.* **108** F9

Roosevelt ↣ *Brazil* **124** E6
Roosevelt, Mt. *Canada* **102** B3
Roosevelt I. *Antarctica* **5** D12
Ropczyce *Poland* **31** H8
Roper ↣ *Australia* **94** A2
Roper Bar *Australia* **94** A1
Roper River = St. Vidgeon's ☺ *Australia* **94** A1
Roque Pérez *Argentina* **126** D4
Roquefort *France* **20** D3
Roquemaure *France* **21** D8
Roquetas de Mar *Spain* **39** J2
Roquetes *Spain* **38** E5
Roquevaire *France* **21** E9
Roraima □ *Brazil* **124** C6
Roraima, Mt. *Venezuela* **124** B6
Røros *Norway* **8** E14
Rorschach *Switz.* **25** H5
Rosa *Zambia* **87** D3
Rosa, Monte *Europe* **40** C4
Rosal de la Frontera *Spain* **37** H3
Rosalia *U.S.A.* **108** C5
Rosamond *U.S.A.* **111** L8
Rosans *France* **21** D9
Rosario *Argentina* **126** C3
Rosário *Brazil* **125** D10
Rosario *Baja Calif., Mexico* **118** B1
Rosario *Sinaloa, Mexico* **118** C3
Rosario *Paraguay* **126** A4
Rosario de la Frontera *Argentina* **126** B3
Rosario de Lerma *Argentina* **126** A2
Rosario del Tala *Argentina* **126** C4
Rosário do Sul *Brazil* **127** C5
Rosarito *Mexico* **111** N9
Rosarno *Italy* **43** D8
Rosas = Roses *Spain* **38** C8
Roscoe *U.S.A.* **115** E10
Roscoff *France* **18** D3
Roscommon *Ireland* **12** C3
Roscommon □ *Ireland* **12** C3
Roscrea *Ireland* **12** D4
Rose ↣ *Australia* **94** A2
Rose, L. *Bahamas* **121** B5
Rose Belle *Mauritius* **85** d
Rose Blanche *Canada* **105** C8
Rose Hill *Mauritius* **85** d
Rose Pt. *Canada* **102** C2
Rose Valley *Canada* **103** C8
Roseau *Dominica* **121** C7
Roseau *U.S.A.* **112** A6
Rosebery *Australia* **95** G4
Rosebud *S. Dak., U.S.A.* **112** D3
Rosebud *Tex., U.S.A.* **116** F6
Roseburg *U.S.A.* **108** E2
Rosedale *U.S.A.* **117** E9
Rosehearty *U.K.* **13** D6
Roseires Res. *Sudan* **79** F12
Roseland *U.S.A.* **110** G4
Rosemary *Canada* **102** C6
Rosenberg *U.S.A.* **116** G7
Rosendaël *France* **19** A9
Rosenheim *Germany* **25** H8
Roses *Spain* **38** C8
Roses, G. de *Spain* **38** C8
Roseto degli Abruzzi *Italy* **41** F11
Rosetown *Canada* **103** C7
Rosetta = Rashîd *Egypt* **80** H7
Roseville *Calif., U.S.A.* **110** G5
Roseville *Mich., U.S.A.* **114** D2
Roseville *Pa., U.S.A.* **115** E8
Rosewood *Australia* **95** D5
Roshkhvār *Iran* **71** C8
Rosières-en-Santerre *France* **19** C9
Rosignano Maríttimo *Italy* **40** E7
Rosignol *Guyana* **124** B7
Roşiori de Vede *Romania* **29** F10
Rositsa *Bulgaria* **45** C8
Rositsa ↣ *Bulgaria* **45** C9
Roskilde *Denmark* **11** J6
Roskovec *Albania* **44** F3
Roslavl *Russia* **32** F7
Rosmaninhal *Portugal* **36** F3
Rosmead *S. Africa* **88** E4
Røsnæs *Denmark* **11** J4
Rosolini *Italy* **43** F7
Rosporden *France* **18** E3
Ross *Australia* **95** G4
Ross *N.Z.* **91** E3
Ross Béthio *Mauritania* **82** B1
Ross Dependency *Antarctica* **5** D12
Ross I. *Antarctica* **5** D11
Ross Ice Shelf *Antarctica* **5** E12
Ross L. *U.S.A.* **108** B3
Ross Mhic Thriúin = New Ross *Ireland* **12** D5
Ross-on-Wye *U.K.* **15** F5
Ross River *Australia* **94** C1
Ross River *Canada* **102** A2
Ross Sea *Antarctica* **5** D11
Roßlau *Sweden* **11** H9
Roy *Mont., U.S.A.* **108** C9
Roy *N. Mex., U.S.A.* **109** J11
Roy *Utah, U.S.A.* **108** F7
Royal Bardia △ *Nepal* **69** E9
Royal Canal *Ireland* **12** C4
Royal Chitawan △ *Nepal* **69** F11
Royal Geographical Society Is. *Canada* **100** D11
Royal Leamington Spa *U.K.* **15** E6

Rossignol L. *Canada* **105** D6
Rossiya = Russia ■ *Eurasia* **53** C11
Rossland *Canada* **102** D5
Rosslare *Ireland* **12** D5
Rosslare Harbour *Ireland* **12** D5
Rosslau *Germany* **24** D8
Rossmore *Canada* **114** B7
Rosso *Mauritania* **82** B1
Rosso, C. *France* **21** F12
Rossosh *Russia* **33** G10
Rossvatnet *Norway* **8** D16
Røst *Norway* **8** C15
Rosthern *Canada* **103** C7
Rostock *Germany* **24** A8
Rostov *Don, Russia* **33** J10
Rostov *Yaroslavl, Russia* **32** D10
Rostov □ *Russia* **35** F5
Rostrenen *France* **18** D3
Roswell *Ga., U.S.A.* **117** D12
Roswell *N. Mex., U.S.A.* **109** K11
Rota *Spain* **37** J4
Rotan *U.S.A.* **116** E4
Rotenburg *Hessen, Germany* **24** D5
Rotenburg *Niedersachsen, Germany* **24** B5
Roth *Germany* **25** F7
Rothaargebirge *Germany* **24** D4
Rothaargebirge △ *Germany* **24** E4
Rothenburg ob der Tauber *Germany* **25** F6
Rother ↣ *U.K.* **15** G8
Rothera *Antarctica* **5** C17
Rotherham *U.K.* **14** D6
Rothes *U.K.* **13** D5
Rothesay *Canada* **105** C6
Rothesay *U.K.* **13** F3
Roti *Indonesia* **63** F6
Rotja, Pta. *Spain* **39** G6
Roto *Australia* **95** E4
Rotondo, Mte. *France* **21** F13
Rotoroa, L. *N.Z.* **91** D4
Rotorua *N.Z.* **91** C6
Rotorua, L. *N.Z.* **91** C6
Rott ↣ *Germany* **25** G9
Rottenburg *Germany* **25** G4
Rottenmann *Austria* **26** D7
Rotterdam *Neths.* **17** C4
Rotterdam *U.S.A.* **115** D10
Rottne *Sweden* **11** G8
Rottnest I. *Australia* **93** F2
Rottumeroog *Neths.* **17** A6
Rottweil *Germany* **25** G4
Rotuma *Fiji* **90** C10
Roubaix *France* **19** B10
Roudnice nad Labem *Czech Rep.* **26** A7
Rouen *France* **18** C8
Rouergue *France* **20** D5
Rouillac *France* **20** C3
Rouleau *Canada* **103** C8
Roulpmaulpma ☺ *Australia* **92** D5
Round I. *Mauritius* **85** d
Round Mountain *U.S.A.* **108** G5
Round Mt. *Australia* **95** E5
Round Rock *U.S.A.* **116** F6
Roundup *U.S.A.* **108** C9
Rousay *U.K.* **13** B5
Rouses Point *U.S.A.* **115** B11
Rouseville *U.S.A.* **114** E5
Rousse = Ruse *Bulgaria* **45** C9
Roussenski Lom ↣ *Bulgaria* **45** C10
Roussillon *Isère, France* **21** C8
Roussillon *Pyrénées-Or., France* **20** F6
Rouxville *S. Africa* **88** E4
Rouyn-Noranda *Canada* **104** C4
Rovaniemi *Finland* **8** C21
Rovato *Italy* **40** C7
Rovenki *Ukraine* **33** H10
Rovereto *Italy* **40** C8
Rovigo *Italy* **41** C8
Rovinj *Croatia* **41** C10
Rovno = Rivne *Ukraine* **23** C14
Rovnoye *Russia* **34** E8
Rovuma = Ruvuma ↣ *Tanzania* **87** E5
Row'ān *Iran* **71** C6
Rowena *Australia* **95** D4
Rowley I. *Canada* **101** D16
Rowley Shoals *Australia* **92** C2
Roxa *Guinea-Biss.* **82** C1
Roxas *Capiz, Phil.* **61** F5
Roxas *Isabela, Phil.* **61** C4
Roxas *Mind. Or., Phil.* **61** E4
Roxboro *U.S.A.* **117** G7
Roxborough *Trin. & Tob.* **125** J16
Roxburgh *N.Z.* **91** F2
Roxbury *N.Y., U.S.A.* **115** D10
Roxbury *Pa., U.S.A.* **114** F7
Roxby Downs *Australia* **95** E2
Roxen *Sweden* **11** F9
Royal Natal △ *S. Africa* **89** D4
Royal Tunbridge Wells *U.K.* **15** F8
Royale, Isle *U.S.A.* **112** B9
Royan *France* **20** C2
Roye *France* **19** C9
Royston *U.K.* **15** E7
Rožaj *Montenegro* **44** D4
Rožan *Poland* **31** F8
Rozay-en-Brie *France* **19** D9
Rozdilna *Ukraine* **29** D15
Rozhishche *Ukraine* **23** C13
Rozhnyativ *Ukraine* **29** B9
Rožmitál pod Třemšínem *Czech Rep.* **26** B6
Rožňava *Slovak Rep.* **27** C13
Rozogi *Poland* **30** E8
Rozoy-sur-Serre *France* **19** C11
Roztoczański △ *Poland* **31** H10
Rozzano *Italy* **40** C6
Rrëshen *Albania* **44** E3
Rrogozhinë *Albania* **44** E3
Rtanj *Serbia* **44** C5
Rtishchevo *Russia* **34** D6
Rúa = A Rúa *Spain* **36** C3
Ruacaná *Namibia* **88** B1
Ruaha △ *Tanzania* **86** D3
Ruahine Ra. *N.Z.* **91** C6
Ruapehu *N.Z.* **91** C5
Ruapuke I. *N.Z.* **91** G2
Ruâq, W. ↣ *Egypt* **74** F2
Rub' al Khālī *Si. Arabia* **75** D4
Rubeho Mts. *Tanzania* **86** D4
Rubezhnoye = Rubizhne *Ukraine* **33** H10
Rubh a' Mhail *U.K.* **13** F2
Rubha Hunish *U.K.* **13** D2
Rubha Robhanais = Lewis, Butt of *U.K.* **13** C2
Rubí *Spain* **38** D7
Rubicon ↣ *U.S.A.* **110** G5
Rubicone ↣ *Italy* **41** D9
Rubik *Albania* **44** E3
Rubino *Ivory C.* **82** D4
Rubio *Venezuela* **124** B4
Rubizhne *Ukraine* **33** H10
Rubondo △ *Tanzania* **86** C3
Rubtsovsk *Russia* **52** D9
Ruby L. *U.S.A.* **108** F6
Ruby Mts. *U.S.A.* **108** F6
Rubyvale *Australia* **94** C4
Rucheng *China* **59** E9
Ruciane-Nida *Poland* **30** E8
Rūd Sar *Iran* **71** B6
Ruda *Sweden* **11** G10
Ruda Śląska *Poland* **31** H5
Rudall *Australia* **95** E2
Rudall ↣ *Australia* **92** D3
Rudall River △ *Australia* **92** D3
Rudbar *Iran* **71** B6
Rüdersdorf *Germany* **24** C9
Rudewa *Tanzania* **87** E3
Rudkøbing *Denmark* **11** K4
Rudky *Ukraine* **31** J10
Rudna *Poland* **31** G3
Rudnik *Bulgaria* **45** C11
Rudnik *Poland* **31** H9
Rudnik *Serbia* **44** B4
Rudnya *Russia* **32** E6
Rudnytsa *Ukraine* **29** B13
Rudnyy *Kazakhstan* **52** D7
Rudo *Bos.-H.* **28** G4
Rudolfa, Ostrov *Russia* **52** A6
Rudolstadt *Germany* **24** E7
Rudong *China* **59** A13
Rudozem *Bulgaria* **45** E8
Rudyard *U.S.A.* **113** B11
Rue *France* **19** B8
Ruenya ↣ *Africa* **87** F3
Rufa'a *Sudan* **81** E3
Ruffling Pt. *Br. Virgin Is.* **121** e
Rufiji ↣ *Tanzania* **86** D4
Rufino *Argentina* **126** C3
Rufisque *Senegal* **82** C1
Rufunsa *Zambia* **87** F2
Rugao *China* **59** A13
Rugby *U.K.* **15** E6
Rugby *U.S.A.* **112** A4
Rügen *Germany* **24** A9
Rügen ↣ *Germany* **24** A9
Rugles *France* **18** D7
Ruhengeri *Rwanda* **86** C2
Ruhla *Germany* **24** E6
Ruhland *Germany* **24** D9
Ruhnu *Estonia* **30** A10
Ruhr ↣ *Germany* **24** D2
Ruhuhu ↣ *Tanzania* **87** E3
Rui'an *China* **59** D13
Ruichang *China* **59** C10
Ruidoso *U.S.A.* **109** K11
Ruijin *China* **59** E10
Ruili *China* **58** E1
Ruivo, Pico *Madeira* **48** D3
Ruj *Bulgaria* **44** D6
Rujen *Macedonia* **44** D6
Rujm Tal'at al Jamā'ah *Jordan* **74** E4
Ruk *Pakistan* **68** F3
Rukhla *Pakistan* **68** C4
Ruki ↣ *Dem. Rep. of the Congo* **84** E3
Rukwa □ *Tanzania* **86** D3

Rukwa, L. *Tanzania* **86** D3
Rulenge *Burundi* **86** C3
Rulhieres, C. *Australia* **92** B4
Rum = Rhum *U.K.* **13** E2
Rum *Jordan* **74** F4
Rum Cay *Bahamas* **121** B5
Rum Jungle *Australia* **92** B5
Ruma *Serbia* **28** E4
Ruma △ *Kenya* **86** C3
Rumāḥ *Si. Arabia* **70** E5
Rumania = Romania ■ *Europe* **29** D10
Rumaylah *Iraq* **70** D5
Rumbêk *Sudan* **81** F2
Rumburk *Czech Rep.* **26** A7
Rumford *U.S.A.* **115** B14
Rumia *Poland* **30** D5
Rumilly *France* **21** C9
Rumoi *Japan* **54** C10
Rumonge *Burundi* **86** C2
Rumphi *Malawi* **87** E3
Rumson *U.S.A.* **115** F11
Rumuruti *Kenya* **86** B4
Runan *China* **56** H8
Runanga *N.Z.* **91** E3
Runaway, C. *N.Z.* **91** B6
Runaway Bay *Jamaica* **120** a
Runcorn *U.K.* **14** D5
Rundu *Namibia* **88** B2
Rungwa *Tanzania* **86** D3
Rungwa ↣ *Tanzania* **86** D3
Rungwa □ *Tanzania* **86** D3
Rungwe *Tanzania* **87** D3
Rungwe, Mt. *Tanzania* **84** F6
Runka *Nigeria* **83** C6
Runn *Sweden* **10** D9
Runton Ra. *Australia* **92** D3
Ruokolahti *Finland* **32** B5
Ruoqiang *China* **60** C3
Rupa *India* **67** F18
Rupar *India* **68** D7
Rupat *Indonesia* **62** D2
Rupea *Romania* **29** D10
Rupen ↣ *India* **68** H4
Rupert *U.S.A.* **108** E7
Rupert ↣ *Canada* **104** B4
Rupert B. *Canada* **104** B4
Rupert House = Waskaganish *Canada* **104** B4
Rupsa *India* **69** J12
Rur ↣ *Germany* **24** D1
Rurrenabaque *Bolivia* **124** F5
Rus ↣ *Spain* **39** F2
Rusambo *Zimbabwe* **87** F3
Rusape *Zimbabwe* **87** F3
Ruschuk = Ruse *Bulgaria* **45** C9
Ruse *Bulgaria* **45** C9
Ruse □ *Bulgaria* **45** C10
Ruşeţu *Romania* **29** F12
Rush *Ireland* **12** C5
Rushan *China* **57** F11
Rushden *U.K.* **15** E7
Rushmore, Mt. *U.S.A.* **112** D2
Rushville *Ill., U.S.A.* **112** E8
Rushville *Ind., U.S.A.* **113** F11
Rushville *Nebr., U.S.A.* **112** D2
Russas *Brazil* **125** D11
Russell *Canada* **103** C8
Russell *Kans., U.S.A.* **112** F4
Russell *N.Y., U.S.A.* **115** B9
Russell *Pa., U.S.A.* **114** E5
Russell Cave △ *U.S.A.* **117** D12
Russell L. *Man., Canada* **103** B8
Russell L. *N.W.T., Canada* **102** A5
Russellkonda *India* **67** K14
Russellville *Ala., U.S.A.* **117** D11
Russellville *Ark., U.S.A.* **116** D8
Russellville *Ky., U.S.A.* **112** G10
Rüsselsheim *Germany* **25** F4
Russi *Italy* **41** D9
Russia ■ *Eurasia* **53** C11
Russian ↣ *U.S.A.* **110** G3
Rust *Austria* **27** D9
Rustam Shahr *Pakistan* **68** F2
Rustavi *Georgia* **35** K7
Rustenburg *S. Africa* **88** D4
Ruston *U.S.A.* **116** E8
Rutana *Burundi* **86** C3
Rute *Spain* **37** H6
Rutenga *Zimbabwe* **87** G3
Ruteng *Indonesia* **63** F6
Ruth *U.S.A.* **114** C2
Rutherford *U.S.A.* **110** G4
Rutland *U.S.A.* **115** C12
Rutland □ *U.K.* **15** E7
Rutland Water *U.K.* **15** E7
Rutledge ↣ *Canada* **103** A6
Rutledge L. *Canada* **103** A6
Rutqa, W. ↣ *Syria* **73** E9
Rutshuru *Dem. Rep. of the Congo* **86** C2
Ruvo di Púglia *Italy* **43** A9
Ruvu *Tanzania* **86** D4
Ruvu ↣ *Tanzania* **86** D4
Ruvuba △ *Burundi* **86** C2
Ruvuma □ *Tanzania* **87** E4
Ruvuma ↣ *Tanzania* **87** E5
Ruwais *U.A.E.* **71** E7
Ruwenzori *Africa* **86** B2
Ruwenzori △ *Uganda* **86** B2

Ruya ↣ *Zimbabwe* **89** B5
Ruyigi *Burundi* **86** C3
Ruyuan *China* **59** E9
Ruzayevka *Russia* **34** C7
Růžhevo Konare *Bulgaria* **45** D8
Ružomberok *Slovak Rep.* **27** B12
Ruzyne, Praha ✈ (PRG) *Czech Rep.* **26** A7
Rwanda ■ *Africa* **86** C3
Ryakhovo *Bulgaria* **45** C10
Ryan, L. *U.K.* **13** G3
Ryazan *Russia* **32** E10
Ryazan □ *Russia* **34** C7
Ryazhsk *Russia* **32** F11
Rybachiy *Russia* **30** C7
Rybachiy Poluostrov *Russia* **8** B25
Rybinsk *Russia* **32** C10
Rybinskoye Vdkhr. *Russia* **32** C10
Rybnik *Poland* **31** H5
Rybnitsa = Râbniţa *Moldova* **29** C14
Rybnoye *Russia* **32** E10
Rychnov nad Kněžnou *Czech Rep.* **27** A9
Rychwał *Poland* **31** F5
Rycroft *Canada* **102** B5
Ryd *Sweden* **11** H8
Rydaholm *Sweden* **11** H8
Ryde *U.K.* **15** G6
Ryderwood *U.S.A.* **110** D3
Rydzyna *Poland* **31** G3
Rye *U.K.* **15** G8
Rye ↣ *U.K.* **14** C7
Rye Bay *U.K.* **15** G8
Rye Patch Res. *U.S.A.* **108** F4
Ryegate *U.S.A.* **108** C9
Ryley *Canada* **102** C6
Rylsk *Russia* **33** G8
Rylstone *Australia* **95** E4
Rymanów *Poland* **31** J8
Ryn *Poland* **30** E8
Ryn Peski = Naryn Qum *Kazakhstan* **35** G9
Ryōtsu *Japan* **54** E9
Rypin *Poland* **31** E6
Ryssby *Sweden* **11** H8
Ryūgasaki *Japan* **55** G10
Ryukyu Is. = Ryūkyū-rettō *Japan* **55** M3
Ryūkyū-rettō *Japan* **55** M3
Rzepin *Poland* **31** F1
Rzeszów *Poland* **31** H8
Rzhev *Russia* **32** D8

S

Sa *Thailand* **64** C3
Sa Cabaneta *Spain* **48** B9
Sa Canal *Spain* **48** C7
Sa Conillera *Spain* **48** C7
Sa Dec *Vietnam* **65** G5
Sa Dragonera *Spain* **48** B9
Sa Kaeo *Thailand* **64** F4
Sa Mesquida *Spain* **48** B11
Sa Pa *Vietnam* **64** A4
Sa Pobla *Spain* **38** F8
Sa Savina *Spain* **48** C7
Sa'ādatābād *Fārs, Iran* **71** D7
Sa'ādatābād *Hormozgān, Iran* **71** D7
Sa'ādatābād *Kermān, Iran* **71** D7
Saale ↣ *Germany* **24** D7
Saaler Bodden *Germany* **24** A8
Saalfeld *Germany* **24** E7
Saalfelden *Austria* **26** D5
Saane ↣ *Switz.* **25** H3
Saanich *Canada* **110** B3
Saar ↣ *Europe* **17** E6
Saar-Hunsrück △ *Germany* **25** F2
Saarbrücken *Germany* **25** F2
Saarburg *Germany* **25** F2
Saaremaa *Estonia* **32** C2
Saarijärvi *Finland* **8** E21
Saariselkä *Finland* **8** B23
Saarland □ *Germany* **25** F2
Saarlouis *Germany* **25** F2
Saatlı *Azerbaijan* **73** C13
Saba *W. Indies* **121** C7
Šabac *Serbia* **44** B3
Sabadell *Spain* **38** D7
Sabah □ *Malaysia* **62** C5
Sabak *Malaysia* **65** L3
Sabalān, Kūhhā-ye *Iran* **73** C12
Sabalana, Kepulauan *Indonesia* **63** F5
Sábana de la Mar *Dom. Rep.* **121** C6
Sábanalarga *Colombia* **124** A4
Sabang *Indonesia* **62** C1
Şabanözü *Turkey* **72** B5
Sābāoani *Romania* **29** C11
Sabarmati ↣ *India* **68** H5
Sabattis *U.S.A.* **115** B10
Sabáudia *Italy* **42** A6
Saberania *Indonesia* **63** E9
Sabhā *Libya* **79** C8
Sabi ↣ *India* **68** E7
Sabidana, J. *Sudan* **80** D4
Sabie *S. Africa* **89** D5
Sabinal *Mexico* **118** A3

Sabinal *U.S.A.* **116** G5
Sabiñánigo *Spain* **38** C4
Sabinar, Punta del *Spain* **39** J2
Sabinas *Mexico* **118** B4
Sabinas → *Mexico* **118** B4
Sabinas Hidalgo *Mexico* **118** B4
Sabine → *U.S.A.* **116** G8
Sabine L. *U.S.A.* **116** G8
Sabine Pass *U.S.A.* **116** G8
Sabinov *Slovak Rep.* **27** B14
Sabirabad *Azerbaijan* **35** K9
Sablayan *Phil.* **61** E4
Sable *Canada* **105** A6
Sable, C. *Canada* **105** D6
Sable, C. *U.S.A.* **120** A3
Sable I. *Canada* **105** D8
Sablé-sur-Sarthe *France* **18** E6
Sabonkafi *Niger* **83** C6
Sabor → *Portugal* **36** D3
Sabou *Burkina Faso* **82** C4
Sabres *France* **20** D3
Sabrina Coast *Antarctica* **5** C9
Sabugal *Portugal* **36** E3
Sabulubbek *Indonesia* **62** E1
Sabuncu *Turkey* **47** B10
Sabzevār *Iran* **71** B8
Sabzvārān = Jiroft *Iran* **71** D8
Sac City *U.S.A.* **112** D7
Sacedón *Spain* **38** E2
Săcele *Romania* **29** E10
Sacheon *S. Korea* **57** G15
Sachigo → *Canada* **104** A2
Sachigo, L. *Canada* **104** B1
Sachimbo *Angola* **84** F4
Sachkhere *Georgia* **35** J6
Sachsen □ *Germany* **24** E9
Sachsen-Anhalt □ *Germany* **24** D7
Sächsische Schweiz △
    Germany **24** E10
Sacile *Italy* **41** C9
Sackets Harbor *U.S.A.* **115** C8
Sackville *Canada* **105** C7
Saco *Maine, U.S.A.* **115** C14
Saco *Mont., U.S.A.* **108** B10
Sacramento → *U.S.A.* **110** G5
Sacramento → *U.S.A.* **110** G5
Sacramento Mts. *U.S.A.* **109** K11
Sacramento Valley *U.S.A.* **110** G5
Sacratif, C. *Spain* **37** J7
Săcueni *Romania* **28** C7
Sada *Spain* **36** B2
Sada-Misaki *Japan* **55** H6
Sádaba *Spain* **38** C3
Sadabad *India* **68** F8
Sadani *Tanzania* **86** D4
Sadani △ *Tanzania* **86** D4
Sadao *Thailand* **65** J3
Sadd el Aali *Egypt* **80** C3
Saddle Mt. *U.S.A.* **110** E3
Sade *Nigeria* **83** C7
Sadimi *Dem. Rep. of the Congo* **87** D1
Sadiola *Mali* **82** C2
Sa'dīyah, Hawr as *Iraq* **73** F12
Sado *Japan* **54** F9
Sado → *Portugal* **37** G2
Sadon *Russia* **35** J6
Sadovoye *Russia* **35** G7
Sadra *India* **68** H5
Sadri *India* **68** G5
Sæby *Denmark* **11** G4
Saegertown *U.S.A.* **114** E4
Saelices *Spain* **38** F2
Safaalan *Turkey* **45** E12
Safaga *Egypt* **80** B3
Şafājah *Si. Arabia* **70** E3
Šafárikovo = Tornal'a
    Slovak Rep. **27** C13
Safata B. *Samoa* **91** b
Säffle *Sweden* **10** E6
Safford *U.S.A.* **109** K9
Saffron Walden *U.K.* **15** E8
Safi *Morocco* **78** B4
Şafīābād *Iran* **71** B8
Safid Dasht *Iran* **71** C6
Safid Kūh *Afghan.* **66** B3
Safid Rūd → *Iran* **71** B6
Safipur *India* **69** F9
Şafītā *Syria* **72** E7
Safonovo *Russia* **32** E7
Safranbolu *Turkey* **72** B5
Saft Rashīn *Egypt* **80** J7
Safune *Samoa* **91** b
Şafwān *Iraq* **70** D5
Sag Harbor *U.S.A.* **115** F12
Saga *Japan* **55** H5
Saga □ *Japan* **55** H5
Sagae *Japan* **54** E10
Sagaing *Burma* **67** J19
Sagala *Mali* **82** C3
Sagamore *U.S.A.* **114** F5
Saganaga L. *Canada* **112** A8
Sagar *Karnataka, India* **66** M9
Sagar *Mad. P., India* **69** H8
Sagara, L. *Tanzania* **86** D3
Sagarejo *Georgia* **35** K7
Sagarmatha = Everest, Mt.
    Nepal **69** E12
Sagarmatha △ *Nepal* **69** F12
Sagay *Phil.* **61** F5
Saginaw *U.S.A.* **113** D12

Saginaw B. *U.S.A.* **113** D12
Sagleipie *Liberia* **82** D3
Saglouc = Salluit *Canada* **101** E16
Sagone *France* **21** F12
Sagone, G. de *France* **21** F12
Sagres *Portugal* **37** J2
Sagua la Grande *Cuba* **120** B3
Saguache *U.S.A.* **108** G10
Saguaro △ *U.S.A.* **109** K8
Saguenay → *Canada* **105** C5
Sagunt *Spain* **38** F4
Sagunto = Sagunt *Spain* **38** F4
Sagwara *India* **68** H6
Sahaba *Sudan* **80** D3
Sahagún *Spain* **36** C5
Saḥam al Jawlān *Syria* **74** C4
Sahamandrevo *Madag.* **89** C8
Sahand, Kūh-e *Iran* **73** D12
Sahara *Africa* **78** D6
Saharan Atlas = Saharien,
    Atlas *Algeria* **78** B6
Saharanpur *India* **68** E7
Saharien, Atlas *Algeria* **78** B6
Saharsa *India* **69** G12
Sahasinaka *Madag.* **89** C8
Sahaswan *India* **69** E8
Saheira, W. el → *Egypt* **74** E2
Sahel *Africa* **78** E5
Sahel, Canal du *Mali* **82** C3
Sahibganj *India* **69** G12
Şāḥilīyah *Iraq* **73** F10
Şaḥneh *Iran* **73** E12
Sahrawi = Western
    Sahara ■ *Africa* **78** D3
Sahuaripa *Mexico* **118** B3
Sahuarita *U.S.A.* **109** L8
Sahuayo de Díaz *Mexico* **118** C4
Şahy *Slovak Rep.* **27** C11
Sai → *India* **69** G10
Sai Buri *Thailand* **65** J3
Sai Twong △ *Thailand* **64** E3
Sai Yok △ *Thailand* **64** E2
Saibai I. *Australia* **94** a
Sa'id Bundās *Sudan* **79** G10
Sa'īdābād = Sīrjān *Iran* **71** D7
Sa'īdābād *Iran* **71** B7
Sa'īdīyeh *Iran* **71** B6
Saidpur *Bangla.* **67** G16
Saidpur *India* **69** G10
Saidu Sharif *Pakistan* **69** B5
Saignes *France* **20** C6
Saigō *Japan* **55** F6
Saigon = Thanh Pho Ho
    Chi Minh *Vietnam* **65** G6
Saijō *Japan* **55** H6
Saikai *Japan* **55** H4
Saikanosy Masoala *Madag.* **89** B9
Saikhoa Ghat *India* **67** F19
Saiki *Japan* **55** H5
Şā'īl *Si. Arabia* **70** E4
Sailana *India* **68** H6
Saillans *France* **21** D9
Sailolof *Indonesia* **63** E8
Saimaa *Finland* **32** B5
Saimbeyli *Turkey* **72** D7
Saimen = Saimaa *Finland* **32** B5
Sa'in Dezh *Iran* **73** D12
St. Abb's Head *U.K.* **13** F6
St-Affrique *France* **20** E6
St-Agrève *France* **21** C8
St-Aignan *France* **18** E8
St. Alban's *Canada* **105** C8
St. Albans *U.K.* **15** F7
St. Albans *Vt., U.S.A.* **115** B11
St. Albans *W. Va., U.S.A.* **113** F13
St. Alban's Head *U.K.* **15** G5
St. Albert *Canada* **102** C6
St-Amand-en-Puisaye
    France **19** E10
St-Amand-les-Eaux *France* **19** B10
St-Amand-Montrond *France* **19** F9
St-Amarin *France* **19** E14
St-Amour *France* **19** F12
St-André *Réunion* **85** c
St-André-de-Cubzac *France* **20** D3
St-André-les-Alpes *France* **21** E10
St. Andrew's *Canada* **105** C8
St. Andrews *U.K.* **13** E6
St-Anicet *Canada* **115** A10
St. Annes *Canada* **103** D9
St. Anns B. *Canada* **105** C7
St. Ann's Bay *Jamaica* **120** a
St. Anthony *Canada* **105** B8
St. Anthony *U.S.A.* **108** E8
St-Antoine *Canada* **105** C7
St-Antonin-Noble-Val *France* **20** D5
St. Arnaud *Australia* **95** F3
St-Astier *France* **20** C4
St-Aubin-du-Cormier *France* **18** D5
St-Augustin *Canada* **105** B8
St-Augustin → *Canada* **105** B8
St. Augustine *U.S.A.* **117** G14
St-Aulaye *France* **20** C4
St. Austell *U.K.* **15** G3
St-Avold *France* **19** C13
St. Barbe *Canada* **105** B8
St-Barthélemy *W. Indies* **121** C7
St-Béat *France* **20** F4
St. Bees Hd. *U.K.* **14** C4

St. Bees I. *Australia* **94** b
St-Benoît *Réunion* **85** c
St-Benoît-du-Sault *France* **20** B5
St-Bonnet-en-Champsaur
    France **21** D10
St-Brevin-les-Pins *France* **18** E4
St-Brice-en-Coglès *France* **18** D5
St. Bride's *Canada* **105** C9
St. Brides B. *U.K.* **15** F2
St-Brieuc *France* **18** D4
St-Calais *France* **18** E7
St-Cast-le-Guildo *France* **18** D4
St. Catharines *Canada* **114** C5
St. Catherines I. *U.S.A.* **117** F14
St. Catherine's Pt. *U.K.* **15** G6
St-Céré *France* **20** D5
St-Cergue *Switz.* **25** J2
St-Cernin *France* **20** C6
St-Chamond *France* **21** C8
St. Charles *Ill., U.S.A.* **112** E9
St. Charles *Md., U.S.A.* **113** F15
St. Charles *Mo., U.S.A.* **112** F8
St. Charles *Va., U.S.A.* **113** G12
St-Chély-d'Apcher *France* **20** D7
St-Chinian *France* **20** E6
St. Christopher-Nevis = St.
    Kitts & Nevis ■ *W. Indies* **121** C7
St-Ciers-sur-Gironde *France* **20** C3
St. Clair *Mich., U.S.A.* **114** D2
St. Clair *Pa., U.S.A.* **115** F8
St. Clair → *U.S.A.* **114** D2
St. Clair, L. *N. Amer.* **114** D2
St. Clairsville *U.S.A.* **114** F4
St-Claud *France* **20** C4
St. Claude *Canada* **103** D9
St-Claude *France* **19** F12
St. Clears *U.K.* **15** F3
St-Clet *Canada* **115** A10
St. Cloud *Fla., U.S.A.* **117** G14
St. Cloud *Minn., U.S.A.* **112** C6
St-Cricq, C. *Australia* **93** E1
St. Croix *U.S. Virgin Is.* **121** C7
St. Croix → *U.S.A.* **112** C7
St. Croix Falls *U.S.A.* **112** C7
St-Cyprien *France* **20** F7
St-Cyr-sur-Mer *France* **21** E9
St. David's *Canada* **105** C8
St. David's *U.K.* **15** F2
St. David's Head *U.K.* **15** F2
St-Denis *France* **19** D9
St-Denis *Réunion* **85** c
St-Denis ✈ (RUN) *Réunion* **85** c
St-Dié *France* **19** D13
St-Dizier *France* **19** D11
St. Elias, Mt. *U.S.A.* **100** B5
St. Elias Mts. *N. Amer.* **102** A1
St-Eloy-les-Mines *France* **19** F9
St-Émilion *France* **20** D3
St-Étienne *France* **21** C8
St-Étienne-de-Tinée *France* **21** D10
St-Étienne-du-Rouvray
    France **18** C8
St. Eugène *Canada* **115** A10
St. Eustatius *W. Indies* **121** C7
St-Exupery, Lyon ✈ (LYS)
    France **21** C9
St-Fargeau *France* **19** E10
St-Félicien *Canada* **104** C5
St-Florent *France* **21** F13
St-Florent, G. de *France* **21** F13
St-Florent-sur-Cher *France* **19** F9
St-Florentin *France* **19** E10
St-Flour *France* **20** C7
St. Francis *U.S.A.* **112** F3
St. Francis → *U.S.A.* **117** D9
St. Francis, C. *S. Africa* **88** E3
St. Francisville *U.S.A.* **116** F9
St-François, L. *Canada* **115** A10
St-Fulgent *France* **18** F5
St-Gabriel *Canada* **104** C5
St. Gallen = Sankt Gallen
    Switz. **25** H5
St-Galmier *France* **19** G11
St-Gaudens *France* **20** E4
St-Gaultier *France* **18** F8
St-Gengoux-le-National
    France **19** F11
St-Geniez-d'Olt *France* **20** D6
St. George *Australia* **95** D4
St. George *N.B., Canada* **105** C6
St. George *Ont., Canada* **114** C4
St. George *S.C., U.S.A.* **117** E14
St. George *Utah, U.S.A.* **109** H7
St. George, C. *Canada* **105** C8
St. George, C. *U.S.A.* **117** G12
St. George I. *U.S.A.* **106** D6
St. George Ra. *Australia* **92** C4
St. George's *Canada* **105** C8
St. George's *Grenada* **121** D7
St. George's B. *Canada* **105** C8
St. Georges Basin *N.S.W.,
    Australia* **95** F5
St. Georges Basin
    W. Austral., Australia **92** C4
St. George's Channel *Europe* **12** E6
St. George's Hd. *Australia* **95** F5
St-Georges-lès-
    Baillargeaux *France* **20** B4

St-Germain-de-Calberte
    France **20** D7
St-Germain-en-Laye *France* **19** D9
St-Germain-Lembron *France* **20** C7
St-Gervais-d'Auvergne
    France **19** F9
St-Gervais-les-Bains *France* **21** C10
St-Gildas, Pte. de *France* **18** E4
St-Gilles *France* **21** E8
St-Girons *France* **20** F5
St-Girons *Landes, France* **20** E2
St. Gotthard P. = San
    Gottardo, P. del *Switz.* **25** J4
St. Helena *Atl. Oc.* **76** H3
St. Helena *U.S.A.* **110** G4
St. Helena, Mt. *U.S.A.* **110** G4
St. Helena B. *S. Africa* **88** E2
St. Helens *Australia* **95** G4
St. Helens *U.K.* **14** D5
St. Helens *U.S.A.* **110** E4
St. Helens, Mt. *U.S.A.* **110** D4
St. Helier *U.K.* **15** H5
St-Herblain *France* **18** E5
St-Hilaire-du-Harcouët
    France **18** D5
St-Hippolyte *France* **19** E13
St-Hippolyte-du-Fort *France* **20** E7
St-Honoré-les-Bains *France* **19** F10
St-Hubert *Belgium* **17** D5
St. Hubert *U.S.A.* **115** A11
St-Hyacinthe *Canada* **104** C5
St. Ignace *U.S.A.* **113** C11
St. Ignace I. *Canada* **104** C2
St. Ignatius *U.S.A.* **108** C6
St-Imier *Switz.* **25** H2
St. Ives *Cambs., U.K.* **15** E7
St. Ives *Corn., U.K.* **15** G2
St-James *France* **18** D5
St. James *U.S.A.* **112** D7
St-Jean → *Canada* **105** B7
St-Jean, L. *Canada* **105** C5
St-Jean-d'Angély *France* **20** C3
St-Jean-de-Braye *France* **19** E8
St-Jean-de-Luz *France* **20** E2
St-Jean-de-Maurienne
    France **21** C10
St-Jean-de-Monts *France* **18** F4
St-Jean-du-Gard *France* **20** D7
St-Jean-en-Royans *France* **21** C9
St-Jean-Pied-de-Port *France* **20** E2
St-Jean-Port-Joli *Canada* **105** C5
St-Jean-sur-Richelieu
    Canada **115** A11
St-Jérôme *Canada* **104** C5
St. John *Canada* **105** C6
St. John *U.S.A.* **112** F4
St. John → *N. Amer.* **113** C20
St. John, C. *Canada* **105** C8
St. John I. *U.S. Virgin Is.* **121** e
St. John's *Antigua & B.* **121** C7
St. John's *Canada* **105** C9
St. Johns *Ariz., U.S.A.* **109** J9
St. Johns *Mich., U.S.A.* **113** D11
St. Johns → *U.S.A.* **117** F14
St. John's Pt. *Ireland* **12** B3
St. Johnsbury *U.S.A.* **115** B12
St. Johnsville *U.S.A.* **115** C10
St. Joseph *Canada* **114** C3
St-Joseph *Martinique* **120** c
St-Joseph *Réunion* **85** c
St. Joseph *La., U.S.A.* **116** F9
St. Joseph *Mo., U.S.A.* **112** F6
St. Joseph → *U.S.A.* **112** D10
St. Joseph, I. *Canada* **104** C4
St. Joseph, L. *Canada* **104** B1
St-Jovite *Canada* **104** C5
St-Juéry *France* **20** E6
St-Julien-Chapteuil *France* **21** C8
St-Julien-de-Vouvantes
    France **18** E5
St-Julien-en-Genevois
    France **19** F13
St-Junien *France* **20** C4
St-Just-en-Chaussée *France* **19** C9
St-Just-en-Chevalet *France* **20** C7
St. Kilda *U.K.* **16** C2
St. Kitts & Nevis ■ *W. Indies* **121** C7
St. Laurent *Canada* **103** C9
St-Laurent-de-la-Salanque
    France **20** F6
St-Laurent-du-Pont *France* **21** C9
St-Laurent-en-Grandvaux
    France **19** F12
St-Laurent-Médoc *France* **20** C3
St. Lawrence *Australia* **94** C4
St. Lawrence → *Canada* **105** C6
St. Lawrence *Canada* **105** C8
St. Lawrence, Gulf of *Canada* **105** C7
St. Lawrence I. *U.S.A.* **106** C5
St. Lawrence Islands △
    Canada **115** B9
St. Léonard *Canada* **105** C6
St-Léonard-de-Noblat *France* **20** C5
St-Leu *Réunion* **85** c
St. Lewis → *Canada* **105** B8
St-Lô *France* **18** C5
St-Louis *France* **19** E14
St-Louis *Guadeloupe* **120** b
St-Louis *Réunion* **85** c

St. Louis *Senegal* **82** B1
St. Louis *U.S.A.* **112** F8
St. Louis □ *Senegal* **82** B2
St. Louis → *U.S.A.* **112** B7
St-Loup-sur-Semouse
    France **19** E13
St-Luc *Canada* **115** A11
St. Lucia ■ *W. Indies* **121** f
St. Lucia, L. *S. Africa* **89** D5
St. Lucia Channel *W. Indies* **121** D7
St. Maarten ☑ *W. Indies* **121** C7
St. Magnus B. *U.K.* **13** A7
St-Maixent-l'École *France* **20** B3
St-Malo *France* **18** D4
St-Malo, G. de *France* **18** D4
St-Mandrier-sur-Mer *France* **21** E9
St-Marc *Haiti* **121** C5
St-Marcellin *France* **21** C9
St-Marcouf, Îs. *France* **18** C5
St. Maries *U.S.A.* **108** C5
St-Martin ☑ *W. Indies* **121** C7
St. Martin, C. *Martinique* **120** c
St. Martin, L. *Canada* **103** C9
St-Martin-de-Crau *France* **21** E8
St-Martin-de-Ré *France* **20** B2
St-Martin-d'Hères *France* **21** C9
St-Martin-Vésubie *France* **21** D11
St. Martins *Barbados* **121** g
St-Martory *France* **20** E4
St. Mary Pk. *Australia* **95** E2
St. Mary → *Australia* **95** G4
St-Maurice → *Canada* **104** C5
St. Mawes *U.K.* **15** G2
St-Maximin-la-Ste-Baume
    France **21** E9
St-Médard-en-Jalles *France* **20** D3
St-Méen-le-Grand *France* **18** D4
St-Mihiel *France* **19** D12
St-Nazaire *France* **18** E4
St. Neots *U.K.* **15** E7
St-Nicolas-de-Port *France* **19** D13
St-Niklaas *Belgium* **17** C4
St-Omer *France* **19** B9
St-Palais-sur-Mer *France* **20** C2
St-Pamphile *Canada* **105** C6
St-Pardoux-la-Rivière *France* **20** C4
St-Pascal *Canada* **105** C6
St. Paul *Canada* **102** C6
St-Paul *France* **21** D10
St-Paul *Réunion* **85** c
St. Paul *Minn., U.S.A.* **112** C7
St. Paul *Nebr., U.S.A.* **112** E4
St-Paul → *Canada* **105** B8
St. Paul → *Liberia* **82** D2
St. Paul, I. *Ind. Oc.* **3** F13
St-Paul-de-Fenouillet *France* **20** F6
St. Paul I. *Canada* **105** C8
St. Paul I. *U.S.A.* **106** D5
St-Paul-lès-Dax *France* **20** E2
St-Péray *France* **21** D8
St. Peter *U.S.A.* **112** C7
St-Peter-Ording *Germany* **24** A4
St. Peter Port *U.K.* **15** H5
St. Peters *N.S., Canada* **105** C7
St. Peters *P.E.I., Canada* **105** C7
St. Petersburg =
    Sankt-Peterburg *Russia* **32** C6
St. Petersburg *U.S.A.* **117** H13
St-Philbert-de-Grand-Lieu
    France **18** E5
St-Phillippe *Réunion* **85** c
St-Pie *Canada* **115** A12
St-Pierre *Martinique* **120** c
St-Pierre *Réunion* **85** c
St-Pierre *St-P. & M.* **105** C8
St-Pierre, L. *Canada* **104** C5
St-Pierre-d'Oléron *France* **20** C2
St-Pierre-en-Port *France* **18** C7
St-Pierre-et-Miquelon ☑
    N. Amer. **105** C8
St-Pierre-le-Moûtier *France* **19** F10
St-Pierre-sur-Dives *France* **18** C6
St-Pol-de-Léon *France* **18** D3
St-Pol-sur-Mer *France* **19** A9
St-Pol-sur-Ternoise *France* **19** B9
St-Pons *France* **20** E6
St-Pourçain-sur-Sioule
    France **19** F10
St-Priest *France* **21** C8
St-Quay-Portrieux *France* **18** D4
St-Quentin *Canada* **105** C6
St-Quentin *France* **19** C10
St-Rambert-d'Albon *France* **21** C8
St-Raphaël *France* **21** E10
St. Regis *U.S.A.* **108** C6
St. Regis Falls *U.S.A.* **115** B10
St-Renan *France* **18** D2
St-Saëns *France* **18** C8
St-Savin *France* **20** B4
St-Savinien *France* **20** C3

St. Sebastien, Tanjon' i
    Madag. **89** A8
St-Seine-l'Abbaye *France* **19** E11
St-Sernin-sur-Rance *France* **20** E6
St-Sever *France* **20** E3
St-Siméon *Canada* **105** C6
St. Simons I. *U.S.A.* **117** F14
St. Simons Island *U.S.A.* **117** F14
St. Stephen *Canada* **105** C6
St-Sulpice *France* **20** E5
St-Sulpice-Laurière *France* **20** B5
St-Sulpice-les-Feuilles *France* **20** B5
St-Syprien = St-Cyprien
    France **20** F7
St-Thégonnec *France* **18** D3
St. Thomas *Canada* **114** D3
St. Thomas I. *U.S. Virgin Is.* **121** e
St-Tite *Canada* **104** C5
St-Tropez *France* **21** E10
St-Troud = St. Truiden
    Belgium **17** D5
St. Truiden *Belgium* **17** D5
St-Vaast-la-Hougue *France* **18** C5
St-Valery-en-Caux *France* **18** C7
St-Valéry-sur-Somme *France* **19** B8
St-Vallier *France* **19** F11
St-Vallier-de-Thiey *France* **21** E10
St-Varent *France* **18** F6
St-Vaury *France* **20** B5
St. Vidgeon's △ *Australia* **94** A1
St. Vincent = São Vicente
    C. Verde Is. **78** b
St. Vincent *Italy* **40** C4
St. Vincent, G. *Australia* **95** F2
St. Vincent & the
    Grenadines ■ *W. Indies* **121** D7
St-Vincent-de-Tyrosse *France* **20** E2
St. Vincent Passage
    W. Indies **121** D7
St-Vith *Belgium* **17** D6
St-Vivien-de-Médoc *France* **20** C2
St. Walburg *Canada* **103** C7
St-Yrieix-la-Perche *France* **20** C5
Ste-Adresse *France* **18** C7
Ste-Agathe-des-Monts
    Canada **104** C5
Ste-Anne *Guadeloupe* **120** b
Ste-Anne *Seychelles* **85** b
Ste-Anne, L. *Canada* **105** B6
Ste-Anne-des-Monts *Canada* **105** C6
Ste-Croix *Switz.* **25** J2
Ste-Enimie *France* **20** D7
Ste-Foy-la-Grande *France* **20** D4
Ste. Genevieve *U.S.A.* **112** G8
Ste-Hermine *France* **20** B2
Ste-Livrade-sur-Lot *France* **20** D4
Ste-Marguerite → *Canada* **105** B6
Ste-Marie *Canada* **105** C5
Ste-Marie *Martinique* **120** c
Ste-Marie *Réunion* **85** c
Ste-Marie, Ile = Nosy
    Boraha *Madag.* **89** B8
Ste-Marie-aux-Mines
    France **19** D14
Ste-Maure-de-Touraine
    France **18** E7
Ste-Maxime *France* **21** E10
Ste-Menehould *France* **19** C11
Ste-Mère-Église *France* **18** C5
Ste-Rose *Guadeloupe* **120** b
Ste-Rose *Réunion* **85** c
Ste. Rose du Lac *Canada* **103** C9
Ste-Savine *France* **19** D11
Ste-Sigolène *France* **21** C8
Saintes *France* **20** C3
Saintes, Îs. des *Guadeloupe* **120** b
Stes-Maries-de-la-Mer *France* **21** E8
Saintfield *U.K.* **12** B6
Saintonge *France* **20** C3
Saipan *N. Marianas* **96** F6
Sairang *India* **67** H18
Sairecábur, Cerro *Bolivia* **126** A2
Saitama *Japan* **55** G9
Saitama □ *Japan* **55** F9
Saiteli = Kadınhanı *Turkey* **72** C5
Saiţi *Moldova* **29** D14
Saiyid *Pakistan* **68** C5
Saja-Besaya △ *Spain* **36** B6
Sajama *Bolivia* **124** G5
Sajan *Serbia* **28** E5
Sajó → *Hungary* **28** C6
Sajószentpéter *Hungary* **28** B5
Sajum *India* **69** C8
Sak → *S. Africa* **88** E3
Saka *Kenya* **86** C5
Sakaba *Nigeria* **83** C6
Sakai *Japan* **55** G7
Sakaide *Japan* **55** G6
Sakaiminato *Japan* **55** G6
Sakākah *Si. Arabia* **70** D4
Sakakawea, L. *U.S.A.* **112** B3
Sakami → *Canada* **104** B4
Sakami, L. *Canada* **104** B4
Sâkâne, 'Erg i-n *Mali* **83** A4
Sakania *Dem. Rep. of the Congo* **87** E2
Sakaraha *Madag.* **89** C7
Sakartvelo = Georgia ■ *Asia* **35** J6
Sakarya *Turkey* **72** B4
Sakarya □ *Turkey* **72** B4
Sakarya → *Turkey* **72** B4

Sakashima-Guntō *Japan* **55** M2
Sakassou *Ivory C.* **82** D3
Sakata *Japan* **54** E9
Sakchu *N. Korea* **57** D13
Sakeny → *Madag.* **89** C8
Sakété *Benin* **83** D5
Sakha □ *Russia* **53** C14
Sakhalin *Russia* **53** D15
Sakhalinskiy Zaliv *Russia* **53** D15
Şaki *Azerbaijan* **35** K8
Šakiai *Lithuania* **30** D10
Sakon Nakhon *Thailand* **64** D5
Sakrand *Pakistan* **68** F3
Sakri *India* **69** F12
Sakrivier *S. Africa* **88** E3
Sakskøbing *Denmark* **11** K5
Sakti *India* **69** H10
Sakuma *Japan* **55** G8
Sakurai *Japan* **55** G7
Saky *Ukraine* **33** K7
Sal *C. Verde Is.* **78** b
Sal → *Russia* **35** G5
Sal Rei *C. Verde Is.* **78** b
Sala *Eritrea* **81** D4
Sala Consilina *Italy* **43** B8
Sala-y-Gómez *Pac. Oc.* **97** K17
Sala y Gómez Ridge *Pac. Oc.* **97** K18
Salaberry-de-Valleyfield
    Canada **115** A10
Salacgrīva *Latvia* **30** A11
Salada, L. *Mexico* **109** K6
Saladas *Argentina* **126** B4
Saladillo *Argentina* **126** D4
Salado → *B. Aires, Argentina* **126** D4
Salado → *La Pampa,
    Argentina* **128** D3
Salado → *Santa Fe,
    Argentina* **126** C3
Salado → *Mexico* **116** H5
Salaga *Ghana* **83** D4
Sãlah *Syria* **74** C5
Şalāh ad Dīn □ *Iraq* **70** C4
Sãlaj □ *Romania* **28** C8
Salakos *Greece* **49** C9
Salala *Liberia* **82** D2
Salala *Sudan* **80** C4
Salãlah *Oman* **75** D5
Salamanca *Chile* **126** C1
Salamanca *Spain* **36** E5
Salamanca *U.S.A.* **114** D6
Salamanca □ *Spain* **36** E5
Salãmatãbãd *Iran* **70** C5
Salamina *Greece* **46** D5
Salamis *Cyprus* **49** D12
Salar de Atacama *Chile* **126** A2
Salar de Uyuni *Bolivia* **124** H5
Sãlard *Romania* **28** C7
Salas *Spain* **36** B4
Salas de los Infantes *Spain* **36** C7
Salatiga *Indonesia* **63** G14
Salaverry *Peru* **124** E3
Salawati *Indonesia* **63** E8
Salaya *India* **68** H3
Salayar *Indonesia* **63** F6
Salazar → *Spain* **38** C3
Salbris *France* **19** E9
S'Albufera *Spain* **48** B10
Salcia *Romania* **29** G9
Sãlciua *Romania* **29** D8
Salcombe *U.K.* **15** G4
Saldaña *Spain* **36** C6
Saldanha *S. Africa* **88** E2
Saldanha B. *S. Africa* **88** E2
Saldus *Latvia* **30** B9
Saldus □ *Latvia* **30** B9
Sale *Australia* **95** F4
Sale *Italy* **40** D5
Salé *Morocco* **78** B4
Sale *U.K.* **14** D5
Salekhard *Russia* **52** C7
Salelologa *Samoa* **91** b
Salem *India* **66** P11
Salem *Ill., U.S.A.* **112** F9
Salem *Ind., U.S.A.* **112** F10
Salem *Mass., U.S.A.* **115** D14
Salem *Mo., U.S.A.* **112** G8
Salem *N.H., U.S.A.* **115** D13
Salem *N.J., U.S.A.* **113** F16
Salem *N.Y., U.S.A.* **115** C11
Salem *Ohio, U.S.A.* **114** F4
Salem *Oreg., U.S.A.* **108** D2
Salem *S. Dak., U.S.A.* **112** D5
Salem *Va., U.S.A.* **113** G13
Salemi *Italy* **42** E5
Sälen *Sweden* **10** C7
Salernes *France* **21** E10
Salerno *Italy* **43** B7
Salerno, G. di *Italy* **43** B7
Salford *U.K.* **14** D5
Salgir → *Ukraine* **33** K8
Salgótarján *Hungary* **28** B4
Salgueiro *Brazil* **125** E11
Salibabu *Indonesia* **63** D7
Salibea = Salybia
    Trin. & Tob. **125** K15
Salida *U.S.A.* **107** H18
Salies-de-Béarn *France* **20** E3

Salihli *Turkey* **72** C3
Salihorsk *Belarus* **23** B14
Salima *Malawi* **85** G6
Salina *Italy* **43** D7
Salina *Kans., U.S.A.* **112** F5
Salina *Utah, U.S.A.* **108** G8
Salina Cruz *Mexico* **119** D5
Salina di Margherita di
    Savoia △ *Italy* **43** A9
Salinas *Brazil* **125** G10
Salinas *Ecuador* **124** D2
Salinas *U.S.A.* **110** J5
Salinas → *Guatemala* **119** D6
Salinas → *U.S.A.* **110** J5
Salinas, B. de *Nic.* **120** D2
Salinas, Pampa de las
    Argentina **126** C2
Salinas Ambargasta
    Argentina **126** B3
Salinas de Hidalgo *Mexico* **118** C4
Salinas Grandes *Argentina* **126** C3
Salinas Pueblo Missions △
    U.S.A. **109** J10
Salinas Valley *U.S.A.* **110** J5
Saline → *Ark., U.S.A.* **116** E8
Saline → *Kans., U.S.A.* **112** F5
Saline di Trapani =
    Paceco △ *Italy* **42** E5
Salines, C. de ses *Spain* **48** B10
Salinópolis *Brazil* **125** D9
Salins-les-Bains *France* **19** F12
Salir *Portugal* **37** H2
Salisbury *Australia* **95** E2
Salisbury *U.K.* **15** F6
Salisbury *Md., U.S.A.* **113** F16
Salisbury *N.C., U.S.A.* **117** D14
Salisbury I. *Canada* **101** E16
Salisbury Plain *U.K.* **15** F6
Sãliște *Romania* **29** E8
Salka *Nigeria* **83** C5
Salkhad *Syria* **74** C5
Salkove *Ukraine* **29** B14
Salla *Finland* **8** C23
Sallent *Spain* **38** D6
Salles *France* **20** D3
Salles-Curan *France* **20** D6
Salling *Denmark* **11** H2
Salliq = Coral Harbour
    Canada **101** E15
Sallisaw *U.S.A.* **116** D7
Sallom *Sudan* **80** D4
Salluit *Canada* **101** E16
Salmãn Pak *Iraq* **73** G11
Salmãs *Iran* **73** C11
Salmerón *Spain* **38** E2
Salmo *Canada* **102** D5
Salmon *U.S.A.* **108** D7
Salmon → *Canada* **102** C4
Salmon → *U.S.A.* **108** D5
Salmon Arm *Canada* **102** C5
Salmon Gums *Australia* **93** F3
Salmon Pt. *Canada* **114** C7
Salmon River Mts. *U.S.A.* **108** D6
Salmon River Res. *U.S.A.* **115** C9
Salo *Finland* **32** B2
Salò *Italy* **40** C7
Salobreña *Spain* **37** J7
Salome *U.S.A.* **111** M13
Salon *India* **69** F9
Salon-de-Provence *France* **21** E9
Salonica = Thessaloniki
    Greece **44** F6
Salonta *Romania* **28** D6
Salor → *Spain* **37** F3
Salou *Spain* **38** D6
Salou, C. de *Spain* **38** D6
Saloum → *Senegal* **82** C1
Salpausselkä *Finland* **32** B4
Salsacate *Argentina* **126** C2
Salses *France* **20** F6
Salsk *Russia* **35** G5
Salso → *Italy* **42** E6
Salsomaggiore Terme *Italy* **40** D6
Salt *Spain* **38** D7
Salt → *Canada* **102** B6
Salt → *U.S.A.* **109** K7
Salt Fork Red → *U.S.A.* **116** D5
Salt L. *Australia* **95** E3
Salt Lake City *U.S.A.* **108** F8
Salt Range *Pakistan* **68** C5
Salta *Argentina* **126** A2
Salta □ *Argentina* **126** A2
Saltara *Italy* **41** E9
Saltash *U.K.* **15** G3
Saltburn by the Sea *U.K.* **14** C7
Saltcoats *U.K.* **13** F4
Saltee Is. *Ireland* **12** D5
Saltfjellet *Norway* **8** C16
Saltfjorden *Norway* **8** C16
Saltholm *Denmark* **11** J6
Saltillo *Mexico* **118** B4
Salto *Argentina* **126** C3
Salto *Uruguay* **126** C4
Salto del Guaíra *Paraguay* **127** A5
Salton City *U.S.A.* **111** M11
Salton Sea *U.S.A.* **111** M11
Saltpond *Ghana* **83** D4
Saltsburg *U.S.A.* **114** F5
Saltsjöbaden *Sweden* **10** E12

Saluda → *U.S.A.* **117** D14
Salûm *Egypt* **80** A2
Salûm, Khâlig el *Egypt* **80** A2
Salur *India* **67** K13
Saluzzo *Italy* **40** D4
Salvador *Brazil* **125** F11
Salvador *Canada* **103** C7
Salvador, El ■ *Cent. Amer.* **120** D2
Salvador, L. *U.S.A.* **117** G9
Salvaterra de Magos *Portugal* **37** F2
Sálvora, I. de *Spain* **36** C2
Salween → *Burma* **67** L20
Salyan *Azerbaijan* **73** C13
Salybia *Trin. & Tob.* **125** K15
Salza → *Austria* **26** D7
Salzach → *Austria* **26** C5
Salzburg *Austria* **26** D6
Salzburg □ *Austria* **26** D6
Salzgitter *Germany* **24** C6
Salzkotten *Germany* **24** C4
Salzwedel *Germany* **24** C7
Sam *India* **68** F4
Sam Neua *Laos* **58** G5
Sam Ngao *Thailand* **64** D2
Sam Rayburn Res. *U.S.A.* **116** F7
Sam Son *Vietnam* **64** C5
Sam Teu *Laos* **64** C5
Sama de Langreo =
    Langreo *Spain* **36** B5
Samagaltay *Russia* **53** D10
Samales Group *Phil.* **61** J5
Samãlût *Egypt* **80** B3
Samana *India* **68** D7
Samana Cay *Bahamas* **121** B5
Samandağ *Turkey* **72** D6
Samandra *Turkey* **45** F13
Samanga *Tanzania* **87** D4
Samangãn □ *Afghan.* **66** B5
Samangwa
    Dem. Rep. of the Congo **86** C1
Samani *Japan* **54** C11
Samanli Dağları *Turkey* **45** F13
Samar *Phil.* **61** F6
Samara *Russia* **34** D10
Samara → *Russia* **34** D10
Samara → *Ukraine* **33** H8
Samaria = Shōmrōn
    West Bank **74** C4
Samaria △ *Greece* **49** D5
Samarinda *Indonesia* **62** E5
Samarkand = Samarqand
    Uzbekistan **52** F7
Samarqand *Uzbekistan* **52** F7
Sãmarrã' *Iraq* **73** E10
Samastipur *India* **69** G11
Samaxı *Azerbaijan* **35** K9
Samba *Dem. Rep. of the Congo* **86** C2
Samba *India* **69** C6
Sambalpur *India* **67** J14
Sambar, Tanjung *Indonesia* **62** E4
Sambas *Indonesia* **62** D3
Sambava *Madag.* **89** A9
Sambawizi *Zimbabwe* **87** F2
Sambhajinagar =
    Aurangabad *India* **66** K9
Sambhal *India* **69** E8
Sambhar *India* **68** F6
Sambhar L. *India* **68** F6
Sambiase *Italy* **43** D9
Sambir *Ukraine* **31** J10
Sambor *Cambodia* **64** F6
Samborombón, B. *Argentina* **126** D4
Sambuca di Sicília *Italy* **42** E6
Samburu □ *Kenya* **86** B4
Samcheok *S. Korea* **57** F15
Same *Tanzania* **86** C4
Samer *France* **19** B8
Samfya *Zambia* **87** E2
Sami *Greece* **46** C2
Şämkir *Azerbaijan* **35** K8
Şamlı *Turkey* **47** B9
Samnah *Si. Arabia* **70** E3
Samo Alto *Chile* **126** C1
Samoa ■ *Pac. Oc.* **91** b
Samobor *Croatia* **41** C12
Samoëns *France* **19** F13
Samokov *Bulgaria* **40** D7
Šamorín *Slovak Rep.* **27** C10
Samorogouan *Burkina Faso* **82** C4
Samos *Greece* **47** D8
Samoš *Serbia* **28** E5
Samos *Spain* **36** C3
Samos □ *Greece* **47** D8
Samothráki = Mathraki
    Greece **49** A3
Samothraki *Greece* **45** F9
Samoylovka *Russia* **34** E6
Sampa *Ghana* **82** D4
Sampacho *Argentina* **126** C3
Sampalan *Indonesia* **63** K18
Sampang *Indonesia* **63** G15
Samper de Calanda *Spain* **38** D4
Sampéyre *Italy* **40** D4
Sampit *Indonesia* **62** E4
Sampit, Teluk *Indonesia* **62** E4
Samrong *Cambodia* **64** E4
Samrong *Thailand* **64** E3
Samsø *Denmark* **11** J4
Samsø Bælt *Denmark* **11** J4
Samsun *Turkey* **72** B7

Samsun □ *Turkey* **72** B7
Samtredia *Georgia* **35** J6
Samui, Ko *Thailand* **65** b
Samur → *Russia* **35** K9
Samurskiy Khrebet *Russia* **35** K8
Samusole
    Dem. Rep. of the Congo **87** E1
Samut Prakan *Thailand* **64** F3
Samut Songkhram *Thailand* **64** F3
Samwari *Pakistan* **68** E2
San *Mali* **82** C4
San → *Cambodia* **64** F5
San → *Poland* **31** H8
San Adrián *Spain* **38** C3
San Adrián, C. de *Spain* **36** B2
San Agustin, C. *Phil.* **61** H7
San Agustín de Valle Fértil
    Argentina **126** C2
San Ambrosio *Pac. Oc.* **122** F3
San Andreas *U.S.A.* **110** G6
San Andres *Phil.* **61** E6
San Andrés, I. de *Caribbean* **120** D3
San Andrès del Rabanedo
    Spain **36** C5
San Andres Mts. *U.S.A.* **109** K10
San Andrés Tuxtla *Mexico* **119** D5
San Angelo *U.S.A.* **116** F4
San Anselmo *U.S.A.* **110** H4
San Antonio *Belize* **119** D7
San Antonio *Chile* **126** C1
San Antonio *Phil.* **61** H6
San Antonio *N. Mex., U.S.A.*
    109 K10
San Antonio *Tex., U.S.A.* **116** G5
San Antonio → *U.S.A.* **116** G6
San Antonio, C. *Argentina* **126** D4
San Antonio, C. de *Cuba* **120** B3
San Antonio, C. de *Spain* **39** G5
San Antonio, Mt. *U.S.A.* **111** L9
San Antonio de los Baños
    Cuba **120** B3
San Antonio de los Cobres
    Argentina **126** A2
San Antonio Oeste
    Argentina **128** E4
San Arcángelo *Italy* **43** B9
San Ardo *U.S.A.* **110** J6
San Agustín *Canary Is.* **48** G4
San Augustine *U.S.A.* **116** F7
San Bartolomé *Canary Is.* **48** F6
San Bartolomé de Tirajana
    Canary Is. **48** G4
San Bartolomeo in Galdo
    Italy **43** A8
San Benedetto del Tronto
    Italy **41** F10
San Benedetto Po *Italy* **40** C7
San Benedicto, I. *Mexico* **118** D2
San Benito *U.S.A.* **116** H6
San Benito → *U.S.A.* **110** J5
San Benito Mt. *U.S.A.* **110** J6
San Bernardino *U.S.A.* **111** L9
San Bernardino Mts. *U.S.A.*
    111 L10
San Bernardino Str. *Phil.* **61** E6
San Bernardo *Chile* **126** C1
San Bernardo, I. de *Colombia* **124** B3
San Blas *Mexico* **118** B3
San Blas, Arch. de *Panama* **120** E4
San Blas, C. *U.S.A.* **117** G12
San Bonifacio *Italy* **41** C8
San Borja *Bolivia* **124** F5
San Buenaventura =
    Ventura *U.S.A.* **111** L7
San Buenaventura *Mexico* **118** B4
San Carlos = Sant Carles
    Spain **48** B8
San Carlos *Argentina* **126** C2
San Carlos *Chile* **126** D1
San Carlos *Baja Calif. S.,
    Mexico* **118** C2
San Carlos *Coahuila, Mexico* **118** B4
San Carlos *Nic.* **120** D3
San Carlos *Neg. Occ., Phil.* **61** F5
San Carlos *Pangasinan, Phil.* **61** D4
San Carlos *Uruguay* **127** C5
San Carlos *U.S.A.* **109** K8
San Carlos *Venezuela* **124** B5
San Carlos de Bariloche
    Argentina **128** E2
San Carlos de Bolívar
    Argentina **126** D3
San Carlos de la Rápita =
    Sant Carles de la Ràpita
    Spain **38** E5
San Carlos del Zulia
    Venezuela **124** B4
San Carlos L. *U.S.A.* **109** K8
San Cataldo *Italy* **42** E6
San Celoni = Sant Celoni
    Spain **38** D7
San Clemente *Chile* **126** D1
San Clemente *Spain* **39** F2
San Clemente *U.S.A.* **111** M9
San Clemente I. *U.S.A.* **111** N8
San Cristóbal = Es Migjorn
    Gran *Spain* **48** B11
San Cristóbal *Argentina* **126** C3
San Cristóbal *Dom. Rep.* **121** C5
San Cristóbal *Solomon Is.* **90** C9

San Cristóbal *Venezuela* **124** B4
San Cristóbal de las Casas
    Mexico **119** D6
San Damiano d'Asti *Italy* **40** D5
San Daniele del Friuli *Italy* **41** B10
San Diego *Calif., U.S.A.* **111** N9
San Diego *Tex., U.S.A.* **116** H5
San Diego, C. *Argentina* **128** G3
San Diego de la Unión
    Mexico **118** C4
San Diego Int. ✈ (SAN)
    U.S.A. **111** N9
San Dimitri, Ras *Malta* **49** C1
San Dimitri Point = San
    Dimitri, Ras *Malta* **49** C1
San Donà di Piave *Italy* **41** C9
San Estanislao *Paraguay* **126** A4
San Esteban de Gormaz
    Spain **38** D1
San Felice Circeo *Italy* **42** A6
San Felice sul Panaro *Italy* **41** D8
San Felipe *Chile* **126** C1
San Felipe *Mexico* **118** A2
San Felipe *Venezuela* **124** A5
San Felipe → *U.S.A.* **111** M11
San Félix *Chile* **126** B1
San Félix *Pac. Oc.* **122** F2
San Fernando = Sant
    Ferran *Spain* **48** C7
San Fernando *Chile* **126** C1
San Fernando *Mexico* **119** C5
San Fernando *La Union, Phil.* **61** C4
San Fernando *Pampanga,
    Phil.* **61** D4
San Fernando *Spain* **37** J4
San Fernando *Trin. & Tob.* **121** D7
San Fernando *U.S.A.* **111** L8
San Fernando de Apure
    Venezuela **124** B5
San Fernando de Atabapo
    Venezuela **124** C5
San Francisco *Argentina* **126** C3
San Francisco *U.S.A.* **110** H4
San Francisco → *U.S.A.* **109** K9
San Francisco, C. de
    Colombia **122** C3
San Francisco, Paso de
    S. Amer. **126** B2
San Francisco de Macorís
    Dom. Rep. **121** C5
San Francisco del Monte de
    Oro *Argentina* **126** C2
San Francisco del Oro
    Mexico **118** B3
San Francisco Int. ✈ (SFO)
    U.S.A. **110** H4
San Francisco Javier = Sant
    Francesc de Formentera
    Spain **48** C7
San Fratello *Italy* **43** D7
San Gabriel *Chile* **126** C1
San Gabriel Chilac *Mexico* **119** D5
San Gabriel Mts. *U.S.A.* **111** L9
San Gavino Monreale *Italy* **42** C1
San Germán *Puerto Rico* **121** d
San Gimignano *Italy* **40** E8
San Giórgio di Nogaro *Italy* **41** C10
San Giórgio Iónico *Italy* **43** B10
San Giovanni Bianco *Italy* **40** C6
San Giovanni in Fiore *Italy* **43** C9
San Giovanni in Persiceto
    Italy **41** D8
San Giovanni Rotondo *Italy* **41** G12
San Giovanni Valdarno *Italy* **41** E8
San Giuliano Terme *Italy* **40** E7
San Gorgonio Mt. *U.S.A.* **111** L10
San Gottardo, P. del *Switz.* **25** J4
San Gregorio *Uruguay* **127** C4
San Gregorio *U.S.A.* **110** H4
San Guillermo △ *Argentina* **126** B2
San Guiseppe Jato *Italy* **42** E6
San Ignacio *Belize* **119** D7
San Ignacio *Bolivia* **124** G6
San Ignacio *Mexico* **118** B2
San Ignacio *Paraguay* **126** B4
San Ignacio, L. *Mexico* **118** B2
San Ildefonso, C. *Phil.* **61** D5
San Isidro *Argentina* **126** C4
San Isidro *Phil.* **61** H7
San Jacinto *U.S.A.* **111** M10
San Jaime = Sant Jaume
    Spain **48** B11
San Javier *Misiones,
    Argentina* **127** B4
San Javier *Santa Fe,
    Argentina* **126** C2
San Javier *Bolivia* **124** G6
San Javier *Spain* **39** H4
San Jerónimo Taviche
    Mexico **119** D5
San Joaquin *U.S.A.* **110** J6
San Joaquin → *U.S.A.* **110** G5
San Joaquin Valley *U.S.A.* **110** J6
San Jon *U.S.A.* **109** J12
San Jordi = Sant Jordi *Spain* **48** B9
San Jorge *Argentina* **126** C3
San Jorge, B. *Mexico* **118** A2
San Jorge, G. *Argentina* **128** F3

San José = San Josep *Spain* **48** C7
San José *Argentina* **126** C4
San José *Costa Rica* **120** E3
San José *Guatemala* **120** D1
San José *Mind. Occ., Phil.* **61** E4
San Jose *Nueva Ecija, Phil.* **61** D4
San Jose *U.S.A.* **110** H5
San Jose → *U.S.A.* **109** J10
San José, I. *Mexico* **118** C2
San Jose de Buenavista *Phil.* **63** B6
San José de Chiquitos
    Bolivia **124** G6
San José de Feliciano
    Argentina **126** C4
San José de Jáchal *Argentina* **126** C2
San José de Mayo *Uruguay* **126** C4
San José del Cabo *Mexico* **118** C3
San José del Guaviare
    Colombia **124** C4
San Josep *Spain* **48** C7
San Juan *Argentina* **126** C2
San Juan *Phil.* **61** F6
San Juan *Puerto Rico* **121** d
San Juan *Trin. & Tob.* **125** K15
San Juan □ *Argentina* **126** C2
San Juan → *Argentina* **126** C2
San Juan → *Nic.* **120** D3
San Juan → *U.S.A.* **109** H8
San Juan Bautista = Sant
    Joan de Labritja *Spain* **48** B8
San Juan Bautista *Paraguay* **126** B4
San Juan Bautista *U.S.A.* **110** J5
San Juan Capistrano *U.S.A.* **111** M9
San Juan Cr. → *U.S.A.* **110** J5
San Juan de Guadelupe
    Mexico **118** C4
San Juan de la Costa *Mexico* **118** C2
San Juan de los Lagos
    Mexico **118** C4
San Juan de los Morros
    Venezuela **124** B5
San Juan del Norte *Nic.* **120** D3
San Juan del Norte, B. de
    Nic. **120** D3
San Juan del Río *Mexico* **119** C5
San Juan del Sur *Nic.* **120** D2
San Juan I. *U.S.A.* **110** B3
San Juan Island △ *U.S.A.* **110** B4
San Juan Mts. *U.S.A.* **109** H10
San Just, Sierra de *Spain* **38** E4
San Justo *Argentina* **126** C3
San Kamphaeng *Thailand* **64** C2
San Lázaro, C. *Mexico* **118** C2
San Leandro *U.S.A.* **110** H4
San Leonardo de Yagüe
    Spain **38** D1
San Lorenzo = Sant Llorenç
    des Cardassar *Spain* **48** B10
San Lorenzo *Argentina* **126** C3
San Lorenzo *Ecuador* **124** C3
San Lorenzo *Paraguay* **126** B4
San Lorenzo → *Mexico* **118** C3
San Lorenzo, I. *Mexico* **118** B2
San Lorenzo, Mte. *Argentina* **128** F2
San Lorenzo de la Parrilla
    Spain **38** F2
San Lorenzo de Morunys =
    Sant Llorenç de Morunys
    Spain **38** C6
San Lucas = Cabo San
    Lucas *Mexico* **118** C3
San Lucas *Bolivia* **124** H5
San Lucas *Mexico* **118** B2
San Lucas *U.S.A.* **110** J5
San Lucas, C. *Mexico* **118** C3
San Lúcido *Italy* **43** C9
San Luis *Argentina* **126** C2
San Luis *Cuba* **120** B3
San Luis *Guatemala* **120** C2
San Luis *Ariz., U.S.A.* **109** K6
San Luis *Colo., U.S.A.* **109** H11
San Luis □ *Argentina* **126** C2
San Luis, I. *Mexico* **118** B2
San Luis, Sierra de *Argentina* **126** C2
San Luis de la Paz *Mexico* **118** C4
San Luis Obispo *U.S.A.* **111** K6
San Luis Potosí *Mexico* **118** C4
San Luis Potosí □ *Mexico* **118** C4
San Luis Res. *U.S.A.* **110** H5
San Luis Río Colorado
    Mexico **118** A2
San Manuel *U.S.A.* **109** K8
San Marco, C. *Italy* **42** C1
San Marco Argentano *Italy* **43** C9
San Marco in Lámis *Italy* **41** G12
San Marcos *Guatemala* **120** D1
San Marcos *Calif., U.S.A.* **111** M9
San Marcos *Tex., U.S.A.* **116** G6
San Marcos, I. *Mexico* **118** B2
San Marino *San Marino* **41** E9
San Marino ■ *Europe* **41** E9
San Martín *Antarctica* **5** C17
San Martín *Argentina* **126** C2
San Martín → *Bolivia* **124** F6
San Martín, L. *Argentina* **128** F2
San Martín de la Vega *Spain* **36** E7
San Martín de los Andes
    Argentina **128** E2
San Martín de
    Valdeiglesias *Spain* **36** E6

San Mateo = Sant Mateu *Baleares, Spain* **48** B7
San Mateo = Sant Mateu *Valencia, Spain* **38** E5
San Mateo *Phil.* **61** C4
San Mateo *U.S.A.* **110** H4
San Matías *Bolivia* **124** G7
San Matías, G. *Argentina* **128** E4
San Miguel = Sant Miquel *Spain* **48** B7
San Miguel *El Salv.* **120** D2
San Miguel *Panama* **120** E4
San Miguel *U.S.A.* **110** K6
San Miguel → *Bolivia* **124** F6
San Miguel de Tucumán *Argentina* **126** B2
San Miguel del Monte *Argentina* **126** D4
San Miguel I. *U.S.A.* **111** L6
San Miniato *Italy* **40** E7
San Nicolás *Canary Is.* **48** G4
San Nicolas *Phil.* **61** B4
San Nicolás de los Arroyos *Argentina* **126** C3
San Nicolas I. *U.S.A.* **111** M7
San Onofre *U.S.A.* **111** M9
San Pablo *Bolivia* **126** A2
San Pablo *Phil.* **61** D4
San Pablo *U.S.A.* **110** H4
San Páolo di Civitate *Italy* **41** G12
San Pedro *B. Aires, Argentina* **126** C4
San Pedro *Misiones, Argentina* **127** B5
San Pedro *Chile* **126** C1
San Pedro *Ivory C.* **82** E3
San Pedro *Mexico* **118** C2
San Pedro □ *Paraguay* **126** A4
San Pedro → *Chihuahua, Mexico* **118** B3
San Pedro → *Nayarit, Mexico* **118** C3
San Pedro → *U.S.A.* **109** K8
San Pedro, Pta. *Chile* **126** B1
San Pedro, Sierra de *Spain* **37** F4
San Pedro Channel *U.S.A.* **111** M8
San Pedro de Atacama *Chile* **126** A2
San Pedro de Jujuy *Argentina* **126** A3
San Pedro de las Colonias *Mexico* **118** B4
San Pedro de Macorís *Dom. Rep.* **121** C6
San Pedro del Norte *Nic.* **120** D3
San Pedro del Paraná *Paraguay* **126** B4
San Pedro del Pinatar *Spain* **39** H4
San Pedro Mártir, Sierra *Mexico* **118** A1
San Pedro Mártir △ *Mexico* **118** A1
San Pedro Ocampo = Melchor Ocampo *Mexico* **118** C4
San Pedro Pochutla *Mexico* **119** D5
San Pedro Sula *Honduras* **120** C2
San Pedro Tututepec *Mexico* **119** D5
San Pietro *Italy* **42** C1
San Pietro Vernótico *Italy* **43** B11
San Rafael *Argentina* **126** C2
San Rafael *Calif., U.S.A.* **110** H4
San Rafael *N. Mex., U.S.A.* **109** J10
San Rafael Mt. *U.S.A.* **111** L7
San Rafael Mts. *U.S.A.* **111** L7
San Ramón de la Nueva Orán *Argentina* **126** A3
San Remo *Italy* **40** E4
San Roque *Argentina* **126** B4
San Roque *Spain* **37** J5
San Rosendo *Chile* **126** D1
San Saba *U.S.A.* **116** F5
San Salvador *El Salv.* **120** D2
San Salvador de Jujuy *Argentina* **126** A3
San Salvador I. *Bahamas* **121** B5
San Salvo *Italy* **41** F11
San Sebastián = Donostia-San Sebastián *Spain* **38** B3
San Sebastián *Argentina* **128** G3
San Sebastián *Puerto Rico* **121** d
San Sebastián de la Gomera *Canary Is.* **48** F2
San Serra = Son Serra *Spain* **48** B10
San Serverino Marche *Italy* **41** E10
San Severo *Italy* **41** G12
San Simeon *U.S.A.* **110** K5
San Simon *U.S.A.* **109** K9
San Stéfano di Cadore *Italy* **41** B9
San Stino di Livenza *Italy* **41** C9
San Telmo = Sant Elm *Spain* **48** B9
San Telmo *Mexico* **118** A1
San Tiburcio *Mexico* **118** C4
San Valentin, Mte. *Chile* **128** F2
San Vicente de Alcántara *Spain* **37** F3
San Vicente de Cañete *Peru* **124** F3
San Vicente de la Barquera *Spain* **36** B6
San Vincenzo *Italy* **40** E7
San Vito *Costa Rica* **120** E3
San Vito *Italy* **42** C2
San Vito, C. *Italy* **42** D5

San Vito al Tagliamento *Italy* **41** C9
San Vito Chietino *Italy* **41** F11
San Vito dei Normanni *Italy* **43** B10
Sana' *Yemen* **75** D3
Sana → *Bos.-H.* **41** C13
Sanaba *Burkina Faso* **82** C4
Sanae IV *Antarctica* **5** D2
Sanak I. *U.S.A.* **106** E7
Sanaloa, Presa *Mexico* **118** C3
Sanana *Indonesia* **63** E7
Sanand *India* **68** H5
Sanandaj *Iran* **73** E12
Sanandita *Bolivia* **126** A3
Sanary-sur-Mer *France* **21** E9
Sanawad *India* **68** H7
Sancellas = Sencelles *Spain* **48** B9
Sancergues *France* **19** E9
Sancerre *France* **19** E9
Sancerrois, Collines du *France* **19** E9
Sancha He → *China* **58** D6
Sanchahe *China* **57** B14
Sánchez *Dom. Rep.* **121** C6
Sanchor *India* **68** G4
Sancoins *France* **19** F9
Sancti Spíritus *Cuba* **120** B4
Sancy, Puy de *France* **20** C6
Sand = Polokwane → *S. Africa* **89** C5
Sand Hills *U.S.A.* **112** D3
Sand Lakes ○ *Canada* **103** B9
Sand Springs *U.S.A.* **116** C6
Sanda *Japan* **55** G7
Sandakan *Malaysia* **62** C5
Sandan = Sambor *Cambodia* **64** F6
Sandanski *Bulgaria* **44** E7
Sandaré *Mali* **82** C2
Sandared *Sweden* **11** G6
Sandarne *Sweden* **10** C11
Sanday *U.K.* **13** B6
Sande *Norway* **10** E4
Sandefjord *Norway* **9** G14
Sanders *U.S.A.* **109** J9
Sanderson *U.S.A.* **116** F3
Sandersville *U.S.A.* **117** E13
Sandfire Roadhouse *Australia* **92** C3
Sandfly L. *Canada* **103** B7
Sandfontein *Namibia* **88** C2
Sandhammaren *Sweden* **11** J8
Sandheads, The *India* **69** J13
Sandía *Peru* **124** F5
Sandıklı *Turkey* **47** C12
Sandila *India* **69** F9
Sandnes *Norway* **9** G11
Sandnessjøen *Norway* **8** C15
Sandoa *Dem. Rep. of the Congo* **84** F4
Sandomierz *Poland* **31** H8
Sândominic *Romania* **29** D10
Sandover → *Australia* **94** C2
Sandoway = Thandwe *Burma* **67** K19
Sandoy *Færoe Is.* **8** F9
Sandpoint *U.S.A.* **108** B5
Sandray *U.K.* **13** E1
Sandringham *U.K.* **14** E8
Sandstone *Australia* **93** E2
Sandu *China* **58** E6
Sandusky *Mich., U.S.A.* **114** C2
Sandusky *Ohio, U.S.A.* **114** E2
Sandveld *Namibia* **88** C3
Sandvig *Denmark* **11** J9
Sandviken *Sweden* **10** D10
Sandwich, C. *Australia* **94** B4
Sandwich B. *Canada* **105** B8
Sandwich B. *Namibia* **88** C1
Sandy *Oreg., U.S.A.* **110** E4
Sandy *Pa., U.S.A.* **114** E6
Sandy *Utah, U.S.A.* **108** F8
Sandy Bay *Canada* **103** B8
Sandy Bight *Australia* **93** F3
Sandy C. *Queens., Australia* **94** C5
Sandy C. *Tas., Australia* **95** G3
Sandy Cay *Bahamas* **121** B4
Sandy Cr. → *Australia* **95** B4
Sandy Cr. → *U.S.A.* **108** F9
Sandy Creek *U.S.A.* **115** C8
Sandy L. *Canada* **104** B1
Sandy Lake *Canada* **104** B1
Sandy Valley *U.S.A.* **111** K11
Sånfjällets △ *Sweden* **10** B7
Sanford *Fla., U.S.A.* **117** G14
Sanford *Maine, U.S.A.* **115** C14
Sanford *N.C., U.S.A.* **117** D15
Sanford → *Australia* **93** E2
Sanford, Mt. *U.S.A.* **100** E3
Sang-i-Masha *Afghan.* **68** C2
Sanga *Mozam.* **87** E4
Sanga → *Congo* **84** E3
Sangamner *India* **66** K9
Sangán *Iran* **71** C9
Sanganeb Atoll △ *Sudan* **80** D4
Sangar *Afghan.* **68** C1
Sangar *Russia* **53** C13
Sangar Sarai *Afghan.* **68** B4
Sangaredi *Guinea* **82** C2
Sangarh → *Pakistan* **68** D4
Sangasso *Mali* **82** C3

Sangatte *France* **19** B8
Sangāw *Iraq* **73** E11
Sangay *Ecuador* **124** D3
Sangbé *Cameroon* **83** D7
Sange *Dem. Rep. of the Congo* **86** D2
Sangeang *Indonesia* **63** F5
Sângeorz-Băi *Romania* **29** C9
Sanger *U.S.A.* **110** J7
Sangerhausen *Germany* **24** D7
Sanggan He → *China* **56** E9
Sanggau *Indonesia* **62** D4
Sanghar *Pakistan* **68** G3
Sangihe, Kepulauan *Indonesia* **63** D7
Sangihe, Pulau *Indonesia* **63** D7
Sangju *S. Korea* **57** F15
Sangkapura *Indonesia* **62** F4
Sangkhla Buri *Thailand* **64** E2
Sangkulirang *Indonesia* **62** D5
Sangla *Pakistan* **68** D5
Sangli *India* **66** L9
Sangmélima *Cameroon* **83** E7
Sango *Zimbabwe* **87** F3
Sangod *India* **68** G7
Sangre de Cristo Mts. *U.S.A.* **109** H11
Sangre Grande *Trin. & Tob.* **125** K15
Sangro → *Italy* **41** F11
Sangrur *India* **68** D6
Sangudo *Canada* **102** C6
Sangue → *Brazil* **124** F7
Sangüesa *Spain* **38** C3
Sanguinaires, Îs. *France* **21** G12
Sangzhi *China* **59** C8
Sanhala *Ivory C.* **82** D3
Sanibel *U.S.A.* **117** H13
Sanikiluaq *Canada* **104** A4
Sanin-Kaigan △ *Japan* **55** G7
Sanirajak = Hall Beach *Canada* **101** D15
Sanjawi *Pakistan* **68** D3
Sanje *Uganda* **86** C3
Sanjiang *China* **58** E7
Sanjo *Japan* **54** F9
Sankh → *India* **69** H11
Sankt Andrä *Austria* **26** E7
Sankt Anton *Austria* **25** H6
Sankt Augustin *Germany* **24** E3
Sankt Blasien *Germany* **25** H4
Sankt Gallen *Switz.* **25** H5
Sankt Gallen □ *Switz.* **25** H5
Sankt Goar *Germany* **25** E3
Sankt Ingbert *Germany* **25** F3
Sankt Johann im Pongau *Austria* **26** D6
Sankt Johann in Tirol *Austria* **26** D5
Sankt Michel = Mikkeli *Finland* **32** B5
Sankt Moritz *Switz.* **25** J5
Sankt-Peterburg *Russia* **32** C6
Sankt Pölten *Austria* **26** C8
Sankt Ulrich = Ortisei *Italy* **41** B8
Sankt Valentin *Austria* **26** C7
Sankt Veit an der Glan *Austria* **26** E7
Sankt Wendel *Germany* **25** F3
Sankt Wolfgang *Austria* **26** D6
Sankuru → *Dem. Rep. of the Congo* **84** E4
Sanliurfa *Turkey* **73** D8
Sanliurfa □ *Turkey* **73** D8
Sanlúcar de Barrameda *Spain* **37** J4
Sanluri *Italy* **42** C1
Sânmartin *Romania* **29** D10
Sanmen *China* **59** C13
Sanmenxia *China* **56** G6
Sanming *China* **59** D11
Sannicandro Gargánico *Italy* **41** G12
Sânnicolau Mare *Romania* **28** D5
Sannieshof *S. Africa* **88** D4
Sannın, J. *Lebanon* **74** B4
Sanniquellie *Liberia* **82** D3
Sannûr, W. → *Egypt* **80** B3
Sanok *Poland* **31** J9
Sanquhar *U.K.* **13** F5
Sans Souci *Trin. & Tob.* **125** K16
Sansanding *Mali* **82** C3
Sansané *Niger* **83** C5
Sansepolcro *Italy* **41** E9
Sansha *China* **59** D13
Sanshui *China* **59** F9
Sanski Most *Bos.-H.* **41** D13
Sansui *China* **58** D7
Sant Antoni de Portmany *Spain* **48** C7
Sant Boi de Llobregat *Spain* **38** D7
Sant Carles *Spain* **48** B8
Sant Carles de la Ràpita *Spain* **38** E5
Sant Celoni *Spain* **38** D7
Sant Elm *Spain* **48** B9
Sant Feliu de Guíxols *Spain* **38** D8
Sant Feliu de Llobregat *Spain* **38** D7
Sant Ferran *Spain* **48** C7
Sant Francesc de Formentera *Spain* **48** C7
Sant Jaume *Spain* **48** B11

Sant Joan *Spain* **48** B10
Sant Joan d'Alacant *Spain* **39** G4
Sant Joan de Labritja *Spain* **48** B8
Sant Jordi *Ibiza, Spain* **48** C7
Sant Jordi *Mallorca, Spain* **48** B9
Sant Jordi, G. de *Spain* **38** E6
Sant Llorenç de Morunys *Spain* **38** C6
Sant Llorenç del Munt y l'Obac △ *Spain* **38** D6
Sant Llorenç des Cardassar *Spain* **48** B10
Sant Mateu *Valencia, Spain* **38** E5
Sant Miquel *Spain* **48** B7
Sant Salvador *Spain* **48** B10
Sant Vicent del Raspeig *Spain* **39** G4
Sant' Ágata Militello *Italy* **43** D7
Santa Agnés *Spain* **48** B7
Santa Ana *Bolivia* **124** F5
Santa Ana *El Salv.* **120** D2
Santa Ana *Mexico* **118** A2
Santa Ana *U.S.A.* **111** M9
Sant' Ángelo Lodigiano *Italy* **40** C6
Sant' Antíoco *Italy* **42** C1
Santa Bárbara *Chile* **126** D1
Santa Bárbara *Honduras* **120** D2
Santa Bárbara *Mexico* **118** B3
Santa Bárbara *Spain* **38** E5
Santa Barbara *U.S.A.* **111** L7
Santa Bárbara, Mt. *Spain* **39** H2
Santa Barbara Channel *U.S.A.* **111** L7
Santa Barbara I. *U.S.A.* **111** M7
Santa Catalina, Gulf of *U.S.A.* **111** N9
Santa Catalina, I. *Mexico* **118** B2
Santa Catalina I. *U.S.A.* **111** M8
Santa Catarina □ *Brazil* **127** B6
Santa Catarina, I. de *Brazil* **127** B6
Santa Caterina di Pittinuri *Italy* **42** B1
Santa Caterina Villarmosa *Italy* **43** E7
Santa Cecília *Brazil* **127** B5
Santa Clara *Cuba* **120** B4
Santa Clara *Calif., U.S.A.* **110** H5
Santa Clara *N.Y., U.S.A.* **115** B10
Santa Clara *Utah, U.S.A.* **109** H7
Santa Clara de Olimar *Uruguay* **127** C5
Santa Clara Valley *U.S.A.* **110** J5
Santa Clarita *U.S.A.* **111** L8
Santa Clotilde *Peru* **124** D4
Santa Coloma de Farners *Spain* **38** D7
Santa Coloma de Gramenet *Spain* **38** D7
Santa Comba *Spain* **36** B2
Santa Croce Camerina *Italy* **43** F7
Santa Croce di Magliano *Italy* **41** G11
Santa Cruz *Bolivia* **124** G6
Santa Cruz *Chile* **126** C1
Santa Cruz *Costa Rica* **120** D2
Santa Cruz *Madeira* **48** D3
Santa Cruz *Phil.* **61** D4
Santa Cruz *U.S.A.* **110** J4
Santa Cruz → *Argentina* **128** G3
Santa Cruz de la Palma *Canary Is.* **48** F2
Santa Cruz de la Palma ✈ (SPC) *Canary Is.* **48** F2
Santa Cruz de Mudela *Spain* **37** G7
Santa Cruz de Tenerife *Canary Is.* **48** F3
Santa Cruz del Norte *Cuba* **120** B3
Santa Cruz del Retamar *Spain* **36** E6
Santa Cruz del Sur *Cuba* **120** B4
Santa Cruz do Rio Pardo *Brazil* **127** A6
Santa Cruz do Sul *Brazil* **127** B5
Santa Cruz I. *U.S.A.* **111** M7
Santa Cruz Is. *Solomon Is.* **90** C9
Santa Cruz Mts. *Jamaica* **120** a
Santa Domingo, Cay *Bahamas* **120** B4
Sant' Egídio alla Vibrata *Italy* **41** F10
Santa Elena *Argentina* **126** C4
Santa Elena, C. *Costa Rica* **120** D2
Sant' Eufémia, G. di *Italy* **43** D9
Santa Eulària des Riu *Spain* **48** C8
Santa Fé *Argentina* **126** C3
Santa Fe *Spain* **37** H7
Santa Fe *U.S.A.* **109** J11
Santa Fé □ *Argentina* **126** C3
Santa Fé do Sul *Brazil* **125** H8
Santa Filomena *Brazil* **125** E9
Santa Fiora *Italy* **41** F8
Santa Gertrudis *Spain* **48** C7
Santa Giustina *Italy* **41** B9
Santa Inês *Brazil* **125** F11
Santa Inés *Spain* **37** G5
Santa Inés, I. *Chile* **128** G2
Santa Isabel *Argentina* **126** D2
Santa Isabel do Morro *Brazil* **125** F8

Santa Lucía *Corrientes, Argentina* **126** B4
Santa Lucía *San Juan, Argentina* **126** C2
Santa Lucía *Spain* **39** H4
Santa Lucía *Uruguay* **126** C4
Santa Lucia Range *U.S.A.* **110** K5
Santa Luzia *C. Verde Is.* **78** b
Santa Margalida *Spain* **48** B10
Santa Margarita *Argentina* **126** D3
Santa Margarita *U.S.A.* **110** K6
Santa Margarita → *U.S.A.* **111** M9
Santa Margherita *Italy* **42** C2
Santa Margherita Ligure *Italy* **40** D6
Santa Maria *Argentina* **126** B2
Santa Maria *Azores* **78** a
Santa María *Brazil* **127** B5
Santa Maria *C. Verde Is.* **78** b
Santa Maria *Phil.* **61** C4
Santa Maria *U.S.A.* **111** L6
Santa María → *Mexico* **118** A3
Santa Maria, B. de *Mexico* **118** B3
Santa Maria, C. de *Portugal* **37** J3
Santa Maria Cápua Vétere *Italy* **43** A7
Santa Maria da Feira *Portugal* **36** E2
Santa Maria da Vitória *Brazil* **125** F10
Santa María del Camí *Spain* **48** B9
Santa Maria di Léuca, C. *Italy* **43** C11
Santa María la Real de Nieva *Spain* **36** D6
Santa Marinella *Italy* **41** F8
Santa Marta *Colombia* **124** A4
Santa Marta, Sierra Nevada de *Colombia* **124** A4
Santa Marta de Tormes *Spain* **36** E5
Santa Marta Grande, C. *Brazil* **127** B6
Santa Marta Ortigueira, Ría de *Spain* **36** B3
Santa Maura = Lefkada *Greece* **46** C2
Santa Monica *U.S.A.* **111** M8
Santa Monica Mts. ○ *U.S.A.* **111** L8
Santa Olalla *Spain* **36** E6
Santa Olalla del Cala *Spain* **37** H4
Santa Paula *U.S.A.* **111** L7
Santa Pola *Spain* **39** G4
Santa Ponça *Spain* **48** B9
Santa Rosa *La Pampa, Argentina* **126** D3
Santa Rosa *San Luis, Argentina* **126** C2
Santa Rosa *Brazil* **127** B5
Santa Rosa *Calif., U.S.A.* **110** G4
Santa Rosa *N. Mex., U.S.A.* **109** J11
Santa Rosa and San Jacinto Mts. ○ *U.S.A.* **111** M10
Santa Rosa de Copán *Honduras* **120** D2
Santa Rosa de Río Primero *Argentina* **126** C3
Santa Rosa del Sara *Bolivia* **124** G6
Santa Rosa I. *Calif., U.S.A.* **111** M6
Santa Rosa I. *Fla., U.S.A.* **117** F11
Santa Rosa Range *U.S.A.* **108** F5
Santa Rosalía *Mexico* **118** B2
Santa Sylvina *Argentina* **126** B3
Santa Tecla = Nueva San Salvador *El Salv.* **120** D2
Santa Teresa *Argentina* **126** C3
Santa Teresa *Australia* **94** C1
Santa Teresa *Mexico* **119** B5
Santa Teresa △ *Uruguay* **127** C5
Santa Teresa di Riva *Italy* **43** E8
Santa Teresa Gallura *Italy* **42** A2
Santa Teresita *Argentina* **126** D4
Santa Uxía de Ribeira *Spain* **36** C2
Santa Vitória do Palmar *Brazil* **127** C5
Santa Ynez → *U.S.A.* **111** L6
Santa Ynez Mts. *U.S.A.* **111** L6
Santa Ysabel *U.S.A.* **111** M10
Santadi *Italy* **42** C1
Santaella *Spain* **37** H6
Santai *China* **58** B5
Santana *Madeira* **48** D3
Sântana *Romania* **28** D6
Santana, Coxilha de *Brazil* **127** C4
Santana do Livramento *Brazil* **127** C4
Santander *Spain* **36** B7
Santander Jiménez *Mexico* **119** C5
Santanilla, Is. *Honduras* **120** C3
Santanyí *Spain* **48** B10
Santaquin *U.S.A.* **108** G8
Santarcángelo di Romagna *Italy* **41** D9
Santarém *Brazil* **125** D8
Santarém *Portugal* **37** F2
Santarém □ *Portugal* **37** F2
Santaren Channel *W. Indies* **120** B4
Santee *U.S.A.* **111** N10
Santee → *U.S.A.* **117** E15

Santéramo in Colle *Italy* **43** B9
Santerno → *Italy* **41** D8
Santhià *Italy* **40** C5
Santi-Quaranta = Sarandë *Albania* **44** G3
Santiago = Río Grande de Santiago → *Mexico* **118** C3
Santiago = São Tiago *C. Verde Is.* **78** b
Santiago *Brazil* **127** B5
Santiago *Canary Is.* **48** F2
Santiago *Chile* **126** C1
Santiago *Panama* **120** E3
Santiago *Phil.* **61** C4
Santiago → *Peru* **124** D3
Santiago, Punta de *Eq. Guin.* **83** D6
Santiago de Compostela *Spain* **36** C2
Santiago de Cuba *Cuba* **120** C4
Santiago de los Caballeros *Dom. Rep.* **121** C5
Santiago del Estero *Argentina* **126** B3
Santiago del Estero □ *Argentina* **126** B3
Santiago del Teide *Canary Is.* **48** F3
Santiago do Cacém *Portugal* **37** G2
Santiago Ixcuintla *Mexico* **118** C3
Santiago Jamiltepec *Mexico* **119** D5
Santiago Papasquiaro *Mexico* **118** C3
Santiago Pinotepa Nacional *Mexico* **119** D5
Santiaguillo, L. de *Mexico* **118** C4
Santiguila *Mali* **82** C3
Santillana del Mar *Spain* **36** B6
Santisteban del Puerto *Spain* **37** G7
Santo Amaro *Brazil* **125** F11
Santo Anastácio *Brazil* **127** A5
Santo André *Brazil* **127** A6
Santo Ângelo *Brazil* **127** B5
Santo Antão *C. Verde Is.* **78** b
Santo Antônio do Içá *Brazil* **124** D5
Santo Antônio do Leverger *Brazil* **125** G7
Santo Domingo *Dom. Rep.* **121** C6
Santo Domingo *Baja Calif., Mexico* **118** A1
Santo Domingo *Baja Calif. S., Mexico* **118** B2
Santo Domingo *Nic.* **120** D3
Santo Domingo de la Calzada *Spain* **38** C2
Santo Domingo de los Colorados *Ecuador* **124** D3
Santo Domingo Pueblo *U.S.A.* **109** J10
Santo Stéfano di Camastro *Italy* **43** D7
Santo Tirso *Portugal* **36** D2
Santo Tomás *Mexico* **118** A1
Santo Tomás *Peru* **124** F4
Santo Tomé *Argentina* **127** B4
Santo Tomé de Guayana = Ciudad Guayana *Venezuela* **124** B6
Santomera *Spain* **39** G3
Santoña *Spain* **36** B7
Santorini *Greece* **47** E7
Santos *Brazil* **127** A6
Santos, Sierra de los *Spain* **37** G5
Santos Dumont *Brazil* **127** A7
Santuario de Aves Laguna Colorada △ *Bolivia* **126** A2
Sanur *Indonesia* **63** K18
Sanwer *India* **68** H6
Sanxenxo *Spain* **36** C2
Sanya *China* **64** C7
Sanyuan *China* **56** G5
São Bartolomeu de Messines *Portugal* **37** H2
São Bernardo do Campo *Brazil* **127** A6
São Borja *Brazil* **127** B4
São Brás de Alportel *Portugal* **37** H3
São Carlos *Brazil* **127** A6
São Cristóvão *Brazil* **125** F11
São Domingos *Brazil* **125** F9
São Domingos *Guinea-Biss.* **82** C1
São Filipe *C. Verde Is.* **78** b
São Francisco *Brazil* **125** G10
São Francisco → *Brazil* **125** F11
São Francisco do Sul *Brazil* **127** B6
São Gabriel *Brazil* **127** C5
São Gonçalo *Brazil* **127** A7
Sao Hill *Tanzania* **87** D4
São João *Guinea-Biss.* **82** C1
São João da Boa Vista *Brazil* **127** A6
São João da Madeira *Portugal* **36** E2
São João da Pesqueira *Portugal* **36** D3
São João del Rei *Brazil* **127** A7
São João do Araguaia *Brazil* **125** E9
São João do Piauí *Brazil* **125** E10
São Joaquim *Brazil* **127** B6
São Joaquim △ *Brazil* **127** B6
São Jorge *Azores* **78** a
São Jorge, Pta. de *Madeira* **48** D3
São José *Brazil* **127** B5
São José do Norte *Brazil* **127** C5

São José do Rio Preto *Brazil* **127** A6
São José dos Campos *Brazil* **127** A6
São Leopoldo *Brazil* **127** B5
São Lourenço *Brazil* **127** A6
São Lourenço ➤ *Brazil* **125** G7
São Lourenço, Pta. de
  Madeira **48** A2
São Lourenço do Sul *Brazil* **127** C5
São Luís *Brazil* **125** D10
São Luís Gonzaga *Brazil* **127** B5
São Marcos ➤ *Brazil* **125** G9
São Marcos, B. de *Brazil* **125** D10
São Martinho da Cortiça
  Portugal **36** E2
São Mateus *Brazil* **125** G11
São Mateus do Sul *Brazil* **127** B5
São Miguel *Azores* **78** a
São Miguel do Oeste *Brazil* **127** B5
São Nicolau *C. Verde Is.* **78** b
São Paulo *Brazil* **127** A6
São Paulo □ *Brazil* **127** A6
São Paulo de Olivença
  Brazil **124** D5
São Pedro do Sul *Portugal* **36** E2
São Roque *Madeira* **48** D3
São Roque, C. de *Brazil* **125** E11
São Sebastião, I. de *Brazil* **127** A6
São Sebastião do Paraíso
  Brazil **127** A6
São Teotónio *Portugal* **37** H2
São Tiago *C. Verde Is.* **78** b
São Tomé *São Tomé & Príncipe* **76** F4
São Tomé, C. de *Brazil* **127** A7
São Tomé & Príncipe ■
  Africa **77** F4
São Vicente *Brazil* **127** A6
São Vicente *C. Verde Is.* **78** b
São Vicente *Madeira* **48** D2
São Vicente, C. de *Portugal* **37** H1
Saona, I. *Dom. Rep.* **121** C6
Saône ➤ *France* **19** G11
Saône-et-Loire □ *France* **19** F11
Saonek *Indonesia* **63** E8
Sapam, Ao *Thailand* **65** a
Sapanca *Turkey* **72** B4
Saparua *Indonesia* **63** E7
Sapele *Nigeria* **83** D6
Sapelo I. *U.S.A.* **117** F14
Sapes *Greece* **45** E9
Saphane *Turkey* **47** B11
Sapi △ *Zimbabwe* **87** F2
Sapienza *Greece* **46** E3
Sapo △ *Liberia* **82** D3
Sapone *Burkina Faso* **83** C4
Saposoa *Peru* **124** E3
Sapotskina *Belarus* **30** E10
Sapouy *Burkina Faso* **83** C4
Sapozhok *Russia* **34** D5
Sapphire *Australia* **94** C4
Sappho *U.S.A.* **110** B2
Sapporo *Japan* **54** C10
Sapri *Italy* **43** B8
Sapulpa *U.S.A.* **116** D6
Saqqez *Iran* **73** D12
Sar Dasht
  Āzarbāyjān-e Gharbī, Iran **73** D11
Sar Dasht *Khuzestān, Iran* **71** C6
Sar-e Pol □ *Afghan.* **66** B4
Sar Gachīneh = Yāsūj *Iran* **71** D6
Sar Planina *Macedonia* **44** E4
Sara *Burkina Faso* **82** C4
Sara *Phil.* **61** F5
Šara △ *Serbia* **44** D5
Sara Buri = Saraburi *Thailand* **64** E3
Sarāb *Iran* **73** D12
Sarābādī *Iraq* **70** C5
Saraburi *Thailand* **64** E3
Saradiya *India* **68** J4
Saraféré *Mali* **82** B4
Saragossa = Zaragoza *Spain* **38** D4
Saraguro *Ecuador* **124** D3
Sarahs *Turkmenistan* **71** B9
Sarai Naurang *Pakistan* **68** C4
Saraikela *India* **69** H11
Saraiu *Romania* **29** F13
Sarajevo *Bos.-H.* **28** G3
Sarakhs = Sarahs
  Turkmenistan **71** B9
Saran, Gunung *Indonesia* **62** E4
Saranac Lake *U.S.A.* **115** B10
Saranac Lakes *U.S.A.* **115** B10
Saranda *Tanzania* **86** D3
Sarandë *Albania* **44** G3
Sarandí del Yí *Uruguay* **127** C4
Sarandí Grande *Uruguay* **126** C4
Sarangani B. *Phil.* **61** J6
Sarangani Is. *Phil.* **61** J6
Sarangarh *India* **67** J13
Saransk *Russia* **34** C7
Sarapul *Russia* **52** D6
Sarasota *U.S.A.* **117** H13
Sarata *Ukraine* **29** D14
Sarata ➤ *Ukraine* **29** E14
Saratoga *Calif., U.S.A.* **110** H4
Saratoga *Wyo., U.S.A.* **108** F10
Saratoga △ *U.S.A.* **115** D11
Saratoga L. *U.S.A.* **115** C11
Saratoga Springs *U.S.A.* **115** C11
Saratok *Malaysia* **62** D4

Saratov *Russia* **34** E7
Saratov □ *Russia* **34** E8
Sarāvān *Iran* **71** E9
Saravane *Laos* **64** E6
Sarawak □ *Malaysia* **62** D4
Saray *Tekirdağ, Turkey* **45** E11
Saray *Van, Turkey* **73** C11
Saraya *Senegal* **82** C2
Saraycık *Turkey* **47** B11
Sarayköy *Turkey* **47** D10
Saraylar *Turkey* **45** F11
Sarayönü *Turkey* **72** C5
Sarbāz *Iran* **71** E9
Sarbīsheh *Iran* **71** C8
Sárbogárd *Hungary* **28** D3
Sarca ➤ *Italy* **40** C7
Sarcelles *France* **19** D9
Sarda ➤ *India* **69** F9
Sardarshahr *India* **68** E6
Sardegna □ *Italy* **42** B1
Sardhana *India* **68** E7
Sardina, Pta. *Canary Is.* **48** F4
Sardinia = Sardegna □ *Italy* **42** B1
Sardis *Turkey* **47** C10
Sārdūīyeh = Dar Mazār *Iran* **71** D8
Saren *Indonesia* **63** J18
S'Arenal *Spain* **48** B9
Sarentino *Italy* **41** B8
Sarera, G. of *Indonesia* **90** B6
Saréyamou *Mali* **82** B4
Sargasso Sea *Atl. Oc.* **98** G13
Sargodha *Pakistan* **68** C5
Sarh *Chad* **79** G9
Sarhala *Ivory C.* **82** D3
Sārī *Iran* **71** B7
Sari d'Orcino *France* **21** F12
Saria *Greece* **47** F9
Saria *India* **69** J10
Sariab *Pakistan* **68** D2
Saribeyler *Turkey* **47** B9
Sarıgöl *Turkey* **72** C3
Sarıkamış *Turkey* **73** B10
Sarıkaya *Turkey* **72** C6
Sarikei *Malaysia* **62** D4
Sarila *India* **69** G8
Sarina *Australia* **94** C4
Sariñena *Spain* **38** D4
Sarıoğlan *Turkey* **72** C6
Sarita *U.S.A.* **116** H6
Sariwŏn *N. Korea* **57** E13
Sariyar Barajı *Turkey* **72** B4
Sarıyer *Turkey* **45** E13
Sarız *Turkey* **72** C7
Sarju ➤ *India* **69** F9
Sark *U.K.* **15** H5
Sarkad *Hungary* **28** D6
Sarkari Tala *India* **68** F4
Şarkışla *Turkey* **72** C7
Şarköy *Turkey* **45** F11
Sarlat-la-Canéda *France* **20** D5
Sărmăşag *Romania* **28** C7
Sărmaşu *Romania* **28** D9
Sarmi *Indonesia* **63** E9
Sarmiento *Argentina* **128** F3
Sarmizegetusa *Romania* **28** E7
Särna *Sweden* **10** C7
Sarnano *Italy* **41** E10
Sarnen *Switz.* **25** J4
Sarnia *Canada* **114** D2
Sarno *Italy* **43** B7
Sarnthein = Sarentino *Italy* **41** B8
Sarolangun *Indonesia* **62** E2
Saronikos Kolpos *Greece* **46** D5
Saronno *Italy* **40** C6
Saros Körfezi *Turkey* **45** F10
Sárospatak *Hungary* **28** B6
Sarpsborg *Norway* **9** G14
Sarqan *Kazakhstan* **52** E8
Sarracín *Spain* **36** C7
Sarralbe *France* **19** D14
Sarre = Saar ➤ *Europe* **17** E6
Sarre *Italy* **40** C4
Sarre-Union *France* **19** D14
Sarrebourg *France* **19** D14
Sarreguemines *France* **19** C14
Sarria *Spain* **36** C3
Sarrión *Spain* **38** E4
Sarro *Mali* **82** C3
Sarsing *Iraq* **73** D10
Sarstedt *Germany* **24** C5
Sartène *France* **21** G12
Sarthe □ *France* **18** D7
Sarthe ➤ *France* **18** E6
Sartilly *France* **18** D5
Saruhanlı *Turkey* **47** C9
Saruna ➤ *Pakistan* **68** F2
Sărulești *Romania* **29** F11
Sărur *Azerbaijan* **73** C11
Sárvár *Hungary* **28** C1
Sarvar *India* **68** F6
Sarvestān *Iran* **71** D7
Särvfjället *Sweden* **10** B7
Sárviz ➤ *Hungary* **28** D3
Sary-Tash *Kyrgyzstan* **52** F8
Saryagash *Kazakhstan* **52** E8
Sarzana *Italy* **40** D6
Sarzeau *France* **18** E4

Sasan Gir *India* **68** J4
Sasaram *India* **69** G11
Sasebo *Japan* **55** H4
Saser Kangri *India* **69** B7
Saskatchewan □ *Canada* **103** C7
Saskatchewan ➤ *Canada* **103** C8
Saskatoon *Canada* **103** C7
Saskylakh *Russia* **53** B12
Saslaya △ *Nic.* **120** D2
Sasolburg *S. Africa* **89** D4
Sason *Turkey* **73** C10
Sasovo *Russia* **34** C5
Sassandra *Ivory C.* **82** E3
Sassandra ➤ *Ivory C.* **82** E3
Sássari *Italy* **42** B1
Sassie *Australia* **94** a
Sassnitz *Germany* **24** A9
Sasso Marconi *Italy* **41** D8
Sassocorvaro *Italy* **41** E9
Sassoferrato *Italy* **41** E9
Sasstown *Liberia* **82** E3
Sassuolo *Italy* **40** D7
Sástago *Spain* **38** D4
Sasyk, Ozero *Ukraine* **29** E14
Sata-Misaki *Japan* **55** J5
Satadougou *Mali* **82** C2
Satakunda = Satakunta
  Finland **32** B2
Satakunta *Finland* **32** B2
Satama-Soukoura *Ivory C.* **82** D4
Satara *India* **66** L8
Satara *S. Africa* **89** C5
Satbarwa *India* **69** H11
Såtenäs *Sweden* **11** F6
Satevó *Mexico* **118** B3
Satilla ➤ *U.S.A.* **117** F14
Satmala Hills
  Andhra Pradesh, India **66** K11
Satmala Hills *Maharashtra, India* **66** J9
Satna *India* **69** G9
Šator *Bos.-H.* **41** D13
Sátoraljaújhely *Hungary* **28** B6
Satpura △ *India* **68** H8
Satpura Ra. *India* **66** J10
Satrup *Germany* **24** A5
Satsuna-Shotō *Japan* **55** K5
Sattahip *Thailand* **64** F3
Satu Mare *Romania* **28** C7
Satu Mare □ *Romania* **28** C8
Satui *Indonesia* **62** E5
Satun *Thailand* **65** J3
Satupa'itea *Samoa* **91** b
Saturnina ➤ *Brazil* **124** F7
Sauce *Argentina* **126** C4
Sauceda *Mexico* **118** B4
Saucillo *Mexico* **118** B3
Sauda *Norway* **9** G12
Sauðárkrókur *Iceland* **8** D4
Saudi Arabia ■ *Asia* **70** B3
Sauerland *Germany* **22** C4
Saugeen ➤ *Canada* **114** B3
Saugerties *U.S.A.* **115** D11
Saugues *France* **20** D7
Saugus *U.S.A.* **111** L8
Saujon *France* **20** C3
Sauk Centre *U.S.A.* **112** C6
Sauk Rapids *U.S.A.* **112** C6
Saulgau *Germany* **25** G5
Saulieu *France* **19** E11
Sault *France* **21** D9
Sault Ste. Marie *Canada* **104** C3
Sault Ste. Marie *U.S.A.* **113** B11
Saumlaki *Indonesia* **63** F8
Saumur *France* **18** E6
Saunders, C. *N.Z.* **91** F3
Saunders I. *Antarctica* **5** B1
Saunders Pt. *Australia* **93** E4
Sauri *Nigeria* **83** C6
Saurimo *Angola* **84** F4
Sausalito *U.S.A.* **110** H4
Sauveterre-de-Béarn *France* **20** E3
Sauzé-Vaussais *France* **20** B4
Savá *Honduras* **120** C2
Sava *Italy* **43** B10
Sava ➤ *Serbia* **28** F5
Savage *U.S.A.* **108** C11
Savage I. = Niue *Pac. Oc.* **97** J11
Savage River *Australia* **95** G4
Savai'i *Samoa* **91** b
Savalou *Benin* **83** D5
Savane *Mozam.* **87** F4
Savanna *U.S.A.* **112** D8
Savanna-la-Mar *Jamaica* **120** a
Savannah *Ga., U.S.A.* **117** E14
Savannah *Mo., U.S.A.* **112** F6
Savannah *Tenn., U.S.A.* **117** D10
Savannah ➤ *U.S.A.* **117** E14
Savannakhet *Laos* **64** D5
Savant L. *Canada* **104** B1
Savant Lake *Canada* **104** B1
Savarkundla = Kundla *India* **68** J4
Săvârşin *Romania* **28** D7
Savaştepe *Turkey* **47** B9
Savé *Benin* **83** D5
Save ➤ *France* **20** E5
Save ➤ *Mozam.* **89** C5
Sāveh *Iran* **71** C6
Savelugu *Ghana* **83** D4

Savenay *France* **18** E5
Săveni *Romania* **29** C11
Saverdun *France* **20** E5
Saverne *France* **19** D14
Savigliano *Italy* **40** D4
Savigny-sur-Braye *France* **18** E7
Sávio ➤ *Italy* **41** D9
Savoie □ *France* **21** C10
Savolax = Savo *Finland* **8** E22
Savona *Italy* **40** D5
Savona *U.S.A.* **114** D7
Savonlinna *Finland* **32** B5
Savoy = Savoie □ *France* **21** C10
Şavşat *Turkey* **73** B10
Sävsjö *Sweden* **11** G8
Savur *Turkey* **70** B4
Savusavu *Fiji* **91** a
Savusavu B. *Fiji* **91** a
Sawahlunto *Indonesia* **62** E2
Sawai *Indonesia* **63** E7
Sawai Madhopur *India* **68** G7
Sawaleke *Fiji* **91** a
Sawang Daen Din *Thailand* **64** D5
Sawankhalok *Thailand* **64** D2
Sawara *Japan* **55** G10
Sawatch Range *U.S.A.* **108** G10
Sawel Mt. *U.K.* **12** B4
Sawi *Thailand* **65** G2
Sawla *Ghana* **82** D4
Sawmills *Zimbabwe* **87** F2
Sawtooth △ *U.S.A.* **108** D6
Sawtooth Range *U.S.A.* **108** D6
Sawu *Indonesia* **63** F6
Sawu Sea *Indonesia* **63** F6
Saxby ➤ *Australia* **94** B3
Saxmundham *U.K.* **15** E9
Saxony = Sachsen □
  Germany **24** E9
Saxony, Lower =
  Niedersachsen □ *Germany* **24** C4
Saxton *U.S.A.* **114** F6
Say *Mali* **82** C4
Say *Niger* **83** C5
Saya *Nigeria* **83** D5
Sayabec *Canada* **105** C6
Sayaboury *Laos* **64** C3
Sayán *Peru* **124** F3
Sayan, Vostochnyy *Russia* **53** D10
Sayan, Zapadnyy *Russia* **53** D10
Sayanogorsk *Russia* **53** D10
Saydā *Lebanon* **74** C3
Sayhandulaan = Oldziyt
  Mongolia **56** B5
Sayḥūt *Yemen* **75** D5
Saykhin *Kazakhstan* **35** F8
Saylac *Somali Rep.* **75** E3
Saynshand = Buyant-Uhaa
  Mongolia **60** B6
Sayre *Okla., U.S.A.* **116** D5
Sayre *Pa., U.S.A.* **115** E8
Sayreville *U.S.A.* **115** F10
Sayula *Mexico* **118** D4
Sayward *Canada* **102** C3
Sazanit *Albania* **44** F3
Sázava ➤ *Czech Rep.* **26** B7
Sazin *Pakistan* **69** B5
Sazlıka ➤ *Bulgaria* **45** E9
Scaër *France* **18** D3
Scafell Pike *U.K.* **14** C4
Scalea *Italy* **43** C8
Scalloway *U.K.* **13** A7
Scalpay *U.K.* **13** D3
Scandia *Canada* **102** C6
Scandiano *Italy* **40** D7
Scandicci *Italy* **41** E8
Scandinavia *Europe* **8** E15
Scansano *Italy* **41** F8
Scapa Flow *U.K.* **13** C5
Scappoose *U.S.A.* **110** E4
Scarámia, Capo *Italy* **43** F7
Scarba *U.K.* **13** E3
Scarborough *Trin. & Tob.* **121** D7
Scarborough *U.K.* **14** C7
Scariff I. *Ireland* **12** E1
Scarp *U.K.* **13** C1
Scarpe-Escaut △ *France* **19** B10
Scebeli = Shabeelle ➤
  Somali Rep. **75** G3
Ščedro *Croatia* **41** E13
Schaal See *Germany* **24** B6
Schaalsee △ *Germany* **24** B6
Schaffhausen *Switz.* **25** H4
Schagen *Neths.* **17** B4
Schaghticoke *U.S.A.* **115** D11
Schärding *Austria* **26** C6
Scharhörn *Germany* **24** B4
Scheessel *Germany* **24** B5
Schefferville *Canada* **105** B6
Scheibbs *Austria* **26** C8
Schelde ➤ *Belgium* **17** C4
Schell Creek Ra. *U.S.A.* **108** G6
Schellsburg *U.S.A.* **114** F6
Schenectady *U.S.A.* **115** D11
Schenevus *U.S.A.* **115** D10
Scherfede *Germany* **24** D5
Schesslitz *Germany* **25** F7
Schiedam *Neths.* **17** C4
Schiermonnikoog *Neths.* **17** A6

Schiltigheim *France* **19** D14
Schinousa *Greece* **47** E7
Schio *Italy* **41** C8
Schiphol, Amsterdam ✈
  (AMS) *Neths.* **17** B4
Schladming *Austria* **26** D6
Schlanders = Silandro *Italy* **40** B7
Schlei ➤ *Germany* **24** A5
Schleiden *Germany* **24** E2
Schleiz *Germany* **24** E7
Schleswig *Germany* **24** A5
Schleswig-Holstein □
  Germany **24** A5
Schlüchtern *Germany* **25** E5
Schmalkalden *Germany* **24** E6
Schmölln *Germany* **24** E8
Schneeberg *Austria* **26** D8
Schneeberg *Germany* **24** E8
Schneverdingen *Germany* **24** B5
Schœlcher *Martinique* **120** c
Schoharie *U.S.A.* **115** D10
Schoharie Cr. ➤ *U.S.A.* **115** D10
Scholls *U.S.A.* **110** E4
Schönberg
  Mecklenburg-Vorpommern, Germany **24** B6
Schönberg
  Schleswig-Holstein, Germany **24** A6
Schönbuch △ *Germany* **25** G5
Schönebeck *Germany* **24** C7
Schöngau *Germany* **25** H6
Schöningen *Germany* **24** C6
Schopfheim *Germany* **25** H3
Schorndorf *Germany* **25** G5
Schortens *Germany* **24** B3
Schouten I. *Australia* **95** G4
Schouten Is. = Supiori
  Indonesia **63** E9
Schouwen *Neths.* **17** C3
Schramberg *Germany* **25** G4
Schrankogel *Austria* **26** D4
Schreiber *Canada* **104** C2
Schrems *Austria* **26** C8
Schrobenhausen *Germany* **25** G7
Schroffenstein *Namibia* **88** D2
Schroon Lake *U.S.A.* **115** C11
Schruns *Austria* **26** D2
Schuler *Canada* **103** C6
Schumacher *Canada* **104** C3
Schurz *U.S.A.* **108** G4
Schuyler *U.S.A.* **112** E5
Schuylerville *U.S.A.* **115** C11
Schuylkill ➤ *U.S.A.* **115** G9
Schuylkill Haven *U.S.A.* **115** F8
Schwabach *Germany* **25** F7
Schwaben □ *Germany* **25** G6
Schwäbisch-Fränkischer
  Wald △ *Germany* **25** G5
Schwäbisch Gmünd *Germany* **25** G5
Schwäbisch Hall *Germany* **25** F5
Schwäbische Alb *Germany* **25** G5
Schwabmünchen *Germany* **25** G6
Schwalmstadt *Germany* **24** E5
Schwandorf *Germany* **25** F8
Schwaner, Pegunungan
  Indonesia **62** E4
Schwanewede *Germany* **24** B4
Schwarmstedt *Germany* **24** C5
Schwarze Elster ➤ *Germany* **24** D8
Schwarzenberg *Germany* **24** E8
Schwarzrand *Namibia* **88** D2
Schwarzwald *Germany* **25** G4
Schwatka Mts. *U.S.A.* **106** B8
Schwaz *Austria* **26** D4
Schwechat *Austria* **27** C9
Schwechat, Wien ✈ (VIE)
  Austria **27** C9
Schwedt *Germany* **24** B10
Schweinfurt *Germany* **25** E6
Schwenningen = Villingen-
  Schwenningen *Germany* **25** G4
Schwerin *Germany* **24** B7
Schweriner See *Germany* **24** B7
Schwetzingen *Germany* **25** F4
Schwyz *Switz.* **25** H4
Schwyz □ *Switz.* **25** H4
Sciacca *Italy* **42** E6
Scicli *Italy* **43** F7
Sciliar △ *Italy* **41** B8
Scilla *Italy* **43** D8
Scilly, Isles of *U.K.* **15** H1
Ścinawa *Poland* **31** G3
Scione *Greece* **44** G7
Scioto ➤ *U.S.A.* **113** F12
Scituate *U.S.A.* **115** D14
Scobey *U.S.A.* **108** B11
Scone *Australia* **95** E5
Scone *U.K.* **13** E5
Scordia *Italy* **43** E7
Scoresbysund =
  Ittoqqortoormiit *Greenland* **4** B6
Scornicești *Romania* **29** F9
Scotia *Calif., U.S.A.* **108** F1
Scotia *N.Y., U.S.A.* **115** D11
Scotia Sea *Antarctica* **5** B18
Scotland *Canada* **114** C4
Scotland □ *U.K.* **13** E5

Scott *Antarctica* **5** D11
Scott, C. *Australia* **92** B4
Scott City *U.S.A.* **112** F3
Scott Glacier *Antarctica* **5** C8
Scott I. *Antarctica* **5** C11
Scott Is. *Canada* **102** C3
Scott L. *Canada* **103** B7
Scott Reef *Australia* **92** B3
Scottburgh *S. Africa* **89** E5
Scottdale *U.S.A.* **114** F5
Scottish Borders □ *U.K.* **13** F6
Scotts Valley *U.S.A.* **110** H4
Scottsbluff *U.S.A.* **112** E2
Scottsboro *U.S.A.* **117** D11
Scottsburg *U.S.A.* **113** F11
Scottsdale *Australia* **95** G4
Scottsdale *U.S.A.* **109** K8
Scottsville *Ky., U.S.A.* **112** G10
Scottsville *N.Y., U.S.A.* **114** C7
Scottville *U.S.A.* **112** D10
Scranton *U.S.A.* **115** E9
Scugog, L. *Canada* **114** B6
Sculeni *Moldova* **29** C12
Scunthorpe *U.K.* **14** D7
Scuol Schuls *Switz.* **25** J6
Scutari = Shkodër *Albania* **44** D3
Scutari = Üsküdar *Turkey* **45** F13
Sea Is. *U.S.A.* **117** F14
Seabrook, L. *Australia* **93** F2
Seaford *U.K.* **15** G8
Seaford *U.S.A.* **113** F16
Seaforth *Australia* **94** b
Seaforth *Canada* **114** C3
Seaforth, L. *U.K.* **13** D2
Seagraves *U.S.A.* **116** E3
Seaham *U.K.* **14** C6
Seal ➤ *Canada* **103** B10
Seal L. *Canada* **105** B7
Sealy *U.S.A.* **116** G6
Searchlight *U.S.A.* **111** K12
Searcy *U.S.A.* **116** D9
Searles L. *U.S.A.* **111** K9
Seascale *U.K.* **14** C4
Seaside *Calif., U.S.A.* **110** J5
Seaside *Oreg., U.S.A.* **110** E3
Seaspray *Australia* **95** F4
Seattle *U.S.A.* **110** C4
Seattle-Tacoma Int. ✈
  (SEA) *U.S.A.* **110** C4
Seba *Indonesia* **92** B3
Sebago L. *U.S.A.* **115** C14
Sebago Lake *U.S.A.* **115** C14
Sebastián Vizcaíno, B.
  Mexico **118** B2
Sebastopol = Sevastopol
  Ukraine **33** K7
Sebastopol *U.S.A.* **110** G4
Sebba *Burkina Faso* **83** C5
Sebderat *Eritrea* **81** D4
Sébékoro *Mali* **82** C3
Seben *Turkey* **72** B4
Sebeş *Romania* **29** E8
Sebekoro *Mali* **82** C3
Sebeşului, Munții *Romania* **29** E8
Sebewaing *U.S.A.* **113** D12
Sebezh *Russia* **32** D5
Sebha = Sabhā *Libya* **79** C8
Sébi *Mali* **82** B4
Şebinkarahisar *Turkey* **73** B8
Sebiş *Romania* **28** D7
Sebnitz *Germany* **24** E10
Sebring *Fla., U.S.A.* **117** H14
Sebring *Ohio, U.S.A.* **114** F3
Sebringville *Canada* **114** C3
Sebta = Ceuta *N. Afr.* **78** A4
Sebuku *Indonesia* **62** E5
Sebuku, Teluk *Malaysia* **62** D5
Sečanj *Serbia* **28** E5
Secchia ➤ *Italy* **40** C8
Sechelt *Canada* **102** D4
Sechura, Desierto de *Peru* **124** E2
Seclin *France* **19** B10
Secondigny *France* **18** F6
Sečovce *Slovak Rep.* **27** C14
Secretary I. *N.Z.* **91** F1
Secunderabad *India* **66** L11
Security *U.S.A.* **108** G11
Sedalia *U.S.A.* **112** F7
Sedan *France* **19** C11
Sedan *U.S.A.* **112** G6
Sedano *Spain* **36** C7
Sedbergh *U.K.* **14** C5
Seddon *N.Z.* **91** D5
Seddonville *N.Z.* **91** D4
Sedé Boqér *Israel* **74** E3
Sedeh *Fārs, Iran* **71** D7
Sedeh *Khorāsān, Iran* **71** C8
Séderon *France* **21** D9
Sederot *Israel* **74** D3
Sédhiou *Senegal* **82** C1
Sedico *Italy* **41** B9
Sedlčany *Czech Rep.* **26** B7
Sedley *Canada* **103** C8
Sedona *U.S.A.* **109** J8
Sedova, Pik *Russia* **52** B6
Sedro-Woolley *U.S.A.* **110** B4
Šeduva *Lithuania* **30** C10
Sędziszów *Poland* **31** H7
Sędziszów Małopolski *Poland* **31** H8
Seebad Ahlbeck *Germany* **24** B10
Seefeld in Tirol *Austria* **26** D4

Seehausen *Germany* **24 C7**
Seeheim *Namibia* **88 D2**
Seeheim-Jugenheim *Germany* **25 F4**
Seeis *Namibia* **88 C2**
Seekoei ➜ *S. Africa* **88 E4**
Seeley's Bay *Canada* **115 B8**
Seelow *Germany* **24 C10**
Sées *France* **18 D7**
Seesen *Germany* **24 D6**
Seevetal *Germany* **24 B6**
Seewinkel = Neusiedler
  See-Seewinkel △ *Austria* **27 D9**
Sefaatli *Turkey* **72 C6**
Seferihisar *Turkey* **47 C8**
Séfeto *Mali* **82 C3**
Sefophe *Botswana* **87 G2**
Sefwi Bekwai *Ghana* **82 D4**
Segamat *Malaysia* **65 L4**
Segarcea *Romania* **29 F8**
Ségbana *Benin* **83 C5**
Segbwema *S. Leone* **82 D2**
Segesta *Italy* **42 E5**
Seget *Indonesia* **63 E8**
Segonzac *France* **20 C3**
Segorbe *Spain* **38 F4**
Ségou *Mali* **82 C3**
Ségou □ *Mali* **82 C3**
Segovia = Coco ➜
  Cent. Amer. **120 D3**
Segovia *Spain* **36 E6**
Segovia □ *Spain* **36 E6**
Segré *France* **18 E6**
Segre ➜ *Spain* **38 D5**
Seguam I. *U.S.A.* **106 E5**
Séguéla *Ivory C.* **82 D3**
Séguélon *Ivory C.* **82 D3**
Séguénéga *Burkina Faso* **83 C4**
Seguin *U.S.A.* **116 G6**
Segundo ➜ *Argentina* **126 C3**
Segura ➜ *Spain* **39 G4**
Segura, Sierra de *Spain* **39 G2**
Seh Konj, Kūh-e *Iran* **71 D8**
Seh Qal'eh *Iran* **71 C8**
Sehitwa *Botswana* **88 C3**
Sehlabathebe △ *Lesotho* **89 D4**
Sehore *India* **68 H7**
Sehwan *Pakistan* **68 F2**
Şeica Mare *Romania* **29 D9**
Seikan Tunnel *Japan* **54 D10**
Seil *U.K.* **13 E3**
Seiland *Norway* **8 A20**
Seilhac *France* **20 C5**
Seiling *U.S.A.* **116 C5**
Seille ➜ *Moselle, France* **19 C13**
Seille ➜ *Saône-et-Loire,*
  France **19 F11**
Sein, Î. de *France* **18 D2**
Seinäjoki *Finland* **8 E20**
Seine ➜ *France* **18 C7**
Seine, B. de la *France* **18 C6**
Seine-et-Marne □ *France* **19 D10**
Seine-Maritime □ *France* **18 C7**
Seine-St-Denis □ *France* **19 D9**
Seini *Romania* **29 C8**
Seirijai *Lithuania* **30 D10**
Seistan = Sīstān *Asia* **71 D9**
Seistan, Daryācheh-ye =
  Sīstān, Daryācheh-ye *Iran* **71 D9**
Sejerø *Denmark* **11 J5**
Sejerø Bugt *Denmark* **11 J5**
Sejny *Poland* **30 D10**
Seka *Ethiopia* **81 F4**
Sekayu *Indonesia* **62 E2**
Seke *Tanzania* **86 C3**
Sekenke *Tanzania* **86 C3**
Seki *Turkey* **47 E11**
Sekondi-Takoradi *Ghana* **82 E4**
Sekota *Ethiopia* **81 E4**
Seksna *Russia* **32 C10**
Sekudai *Malaysia* **65 d**
Sekuma *Botswana* **88 C3**
Selah *U.S.A.* **108 C3**
Selama *Malaysia* **65 K3**
Selárgius *Italy* **42 C2**
Selaru *Indonesia* **63 F8**
Selatan, Selat *Malaysia* **65 c**
Selawik L. *U.S.A.* **106 B7**
Selb *Germany* **25 E8**
Selby *U.K.* **14 D6**
Selby *U.S.A.* **112 C3**
Selca *Croatia* **41 E13**
Selçuk *Turkey* **47 D9**
Selden *U.S.A.* **112 F3**
Sele ➜ *Italy* **43 B7**
Selebi-Phikwe *Botswana* **89 C4**
Selemdzha ➜ *Russia* **53 D13**
Selendi *Manisa, Turkey* **47 C10**
Selendi *Manisa, Turkey* **47 C9**
Selenga = Selenge
  Mörön ➜ *Asia* **60 A5**
Selenge Mörön ➜ *Asia* **60 A5**
Selenicë *Albania* **44 F3**
Selenter See *Germany* **24 A6**
Sélestat *France* **19 D14**
Seletan, Tanjung *Indonesia* **62 E4**
Selevac *Serbia* **44 B4**
Sélibabi *Mauritania* **82 B2**
Seliger, Ozero *Russia* **32 D7**
Seligman *U.S.A.* **109 J7**
Şelim *Turkey* **73 B10**

Selīma *Sudan* **80 C2**
Selimiye *Turkey* **47 D9**
Selinda Spillway ➜
  Botswana **88 B3**
Sélingué, L. de *Mali* **82 C3**
Selinsgrove *U.S.A.* **114 F8**
Selizharovo *Russia* **32 D7**
Selkirk *Man., Canada* **103 C9**
Selkirk *Ont., Canada* **114 D5**
Selkirk *U.K.* **13 F6**
Selkirk I. = Horse I. *Canada* **103 C9**
Selkirk Mts. *Canada* **100 G8**
Sellafield *U.K.* **14 C4**
Sellama *Sudan* **81 E2**
Sellia *Greece* **49 D6**
Sellières *France* **19 F12**
Sells *U.S.A.* **109 L8**
Sellye *Hungary* **28 E2**
Selma, Ala., *U.S.A.* **117 E11**
Selma *Calif., U.S.A.* **110 J7**
Selma *N.C., U.S.A.* **117 D15**
Selmer *U.S.A.* **117 D10**
Selongey *France* **19 E12**
Selous △ *Tanzania* **86 D4**
Selowandoma Falls *Zimbabwe* **87 G3**
Selpele *Indonesia* **63 E8**
Selsey Bill *U.K.* **15 G7**
Seltso *Russia* **32 F8**
Seltz *France* **19 D15**
Selu *Indonesia* **63 F8**
Sélune ➜ *France* **18 D5**
Selva = La Selva del Camp
  Spain **38 D6**
Selva *Argentina* **126 B3**
Selva *Spain* **48 B9**
Selva Lancandona =
  Montes Azules △ *Mexico* **119 D6**
Selvagens, Ilhas *Madeira* **78 B2**
Selvas *Brazil* **124 E5**
Selwyn L. *Canada* **103 B8**
Selwyn Mts. *Canada* **100 E5**
Selwyn Ra. *Australia* **94 C3**
Selyatyn *Ukraine* **29 C10**
Seman ➜ *Albania* **44 F3**
Semarang *Indonesia* **63 G14**
Sembabule *Uganda* **86 C3**
Sembawang *Singapore* **65 d**
Sembung *Indonesia* **63 J18**
Şemdinli *Turkey* **73 D11**
Sémé *Senegal* **82 B2**
Semeih *Sudan* **81 E3**
Semenanjung Blambangan
  Indonesia **63 K17**
Semenov *Russia* **34 B7**
Semenovka *Chernihiv, Ukraine* **33 F7**
Semenovka *Kremenchuk,*
  Ukraine **33 H7**
Semeru *Indonesia* **63 H15**
Semey *Kazakhstan* **52 D9**
Semikarakorskiy *Russia* **35 G5**
Semiluki *Russia* **33 G10**
Seminoe Res. *U.S.A.* **108 E10**
Seminole *Okla., U.S.A.* **116 D6**
Seminole *Tex., U.S.A.* **116 E3**
Seminole Draw ➜ *U.S.A.* **116 E3**
Semipalatinsk = Semey
  Kazakhstan **52 D9**
Semirara Is. *Phil.* **61 F4**
Semisopochnoi I. *U.S.A.* **106 E3**
Semitau *Indonesia* **62 D4**
Semliki ➜ *Uganda* **86 B3**
Semmering P. *Austria* **26 D8**
Semnān *Iran* **71 C7**
Semnān □ *Iran* **71 C7**
Semporna *Malaysia* **63 D5**
Semuda *Indonesia* **62 E4**
Semur-en-Auxois *France* **19 E11**
Sen ➜ *Cambodia* **64 F5**
Sená *Iran* **71 D6**
Sena *Mozam.* **87 F4**
Sena Madureira *Brazil* **124 E5**
Senador Pompeu *Brazil* **125 E11**
Senaki *Georgia* **35 J6**
Senang, Pulau *Singapore* **65 d**
Senanga *Zambia* **85 H4**
Senatobia *U.S.A.* **117 D10**
Sencelles *Spain* **48 B9**
Sendafa *Ethiopia* **81 F4**
Sendai *Kagoshima, Japan* **55 J5**
Sendai *Miyagi, Japan* **54 E10**
Sendai-Wan *Japan* **54 E10**
Senden *Bayern, Germany* **25 G6**
Senden *Nordrhein-Westfalen,*
  Germany **24 D3**
Sendhwa *India* **68 J6**
Sene ➜ *Ghana* **83 D4**
Senec *Slovak Rep.* **27 C10**
Seneca *U.S.A.* **117 D13**
Seneca Falls *U.S.A.* **115 D8**
Seneca L. *U.S.A.* **114 D8**
Senecaville L. *U.S.A.* **114 G3**
Senegal ■ *W. Afr.* **82 C2**
Sénégal ➜ *W. Afr.* **82 B1**
Senegambia *Africa* **76 E2**
Senekal *S. Africa* **89 D4**
Senftenberg *Germany* **24 D9**
Senga Hill *Zambia* **87 D3**
Sengerema *Tanzania* **86 C3**

Sengiley *Russia* **34 D9**
Sengua ➜ *Zimbabwe* **87 F2**
Senhor-do-Bonfim *Brazil* **125 F10**
Senica *Slovak Rep.* **27 C10**
Senigállia *Italy* **41 E10**
Senio ➜ *Italy* **41 D9**
Senirkent *Turkey* **47 C12**
Senise *Italy* **43 B9**
Senj *Croatia* **41 D11**
Senja *Norway* **8 B17**
Senkaku-Shotō *E. China Sea* **55 M1**
Senkuang *Indonesia* **65 d**
Senlis *France* **19 C9**
Senmonorom *Cambodia* **64 F6**
Sennâr *Sudan* **81 E3**
Sennâr □ *Sudan* **81 E3**
Senneterre *Canada* **104 C4**
Senno *Belarus* **32 E5**
Sénnori *Italy* **42 B1**
Seno *Laos* **64 D5**
Senonches *France* **18 D8**
Senorbì *Italy* **42 C2**
Senožeče *Slovenia* **41 C11**
Sentani *Indonesia* **63 E10**
Sentery = Lubao
  Dem. Rep. of the Congo **86 D2**
Sentinel *U.S.A.* **109 K7**
Šentjur *Slovenia* **41 B12**
Sentosa *Singapore* **65 d**
Senya Beraku *Ghana* **83 D4**
Seo de Urgel = La Seu
  d'Urgell *Spain* **38 C6**
Seogwipo *S. Korea* **57 H14**
Seohara *India* **69 E8**
Seonath ➜ *India* **69 J10**
Seondha *India* **69 F8**
Seongnam *S. Korea* **57 F14**
Seonsan *S. Korea* **57 F15**
Seoni *India* **69 H8**
Seoni Malwa *India* **68 H8**
Seosan *S. Korea* **57 F14**
Seoul = Soul *S. Korea* **57 F14**
Sepīdān *Iran* **71 D7**
Sep'o *N. Korea* **57 E14**
Sępólno Krajeńskie *Poland* **30 E4**
Sepone *Laos* **64 D6**
Sepopol *Poland* **30 D8**
Sept-Îles *Canada* **105 B6**
Septemvri *Bulgaria* **45 D8**
Sepúlveda *Spain* **36 D7**
Sequeros *Spain* **36 E4**
Sequim *U.S.A.* **110 B3**
Sequoia △ *U.S.A.* **110 J8**
Serafimovich *Russia* **34 F6**
Seraing *Belgium* **17 D5**
Serakhis ➜ *Cyprus* **49 D11**
Seram *Indonesia* **63 E7**
Seram Sea *Indonesia* **63 E7**
Serampore = Shrirampur
  India **69 H13**
Seranantsara *Madag.* **89 B8**
Serang *Indonesia* **63 G12**
Serangoon *Singapore* **65 d**
Serasan *Indonesia* **62 D3**
Seravezza *Italy* **40 E7**
Şerbettar *Turkey* **45 E10**
Serbia ■ *Europe* **44 C4**
Şercaia *Romania* **29 E10**
Serdar *Turkmenistan* **71 B8**
Serdo *Ethiopia* **81 E5**
Serdobsk *Russia* **34 D7**
Sered' *Slovak Rep.* **27 C10**
Seredka *Russia* **32 C5**
Serednye *Ukraine* **28 B7**
Şereflikoçhisar *Turkey* **72 C5**
Seregno *Italy* **40 C6**
Seremban *Malaysia* **65 L3**
Serengeti △ *Tanzania* **86 C3**
Serengeti Plain *Tanzania* **86 C4**
Serenje *Zambia* **87 E3**
Seret ➜ *Ukraine* **29 B10**
Sereth = Siret ➜ *Romania* **29 E12**
Sergach *Russia* **34 C7**
Sergen *Turkey* **45 E11**
Sergeya Kirova, Ostrova
  Russia **53 B10**
Sergino *Russia* **52 C7**
Sergipe □ *Brazil* **125 F11**
Sergiyev Posad *Russia* **32 D10**
Serhetabat *Turkmenistan* **71 C9**
Seria *Brunei* **62 D4**
Serian *Malaysia* **62 D4**
Seriate *Italy* **40 C6**
Seribu, Kepulauan *Indonesia* **62 F3**
Sericho *Kenya* **86 B4**
Sérifontaine *France* **19 C8**
Serifos *Greece* **46 D6**
Sérignan *France* **20 E7**
Sérigny ➜ *Canada* **105 A6**
Serik *Turkey* **72 D4**
Seringapatam Reef *Australia* **92 B3**
Serinhisar *Turkey* **47 D11**
Serinya *India* **68 H7**
Seririt *Indonesia* **63 J17**
Serishābād *Iran* **73 E12**
Serkout *Algeria* **78 D7**
Sermaize-les-Bains *France* **19 D11**
Sermata *Indonesia* **63 F7**

Sermersuaq *Greenland* **101 B19**
Sérmide *Italy* **41 D8**
Sernovodsk *Russia* **34 D10**
Sernur *Russia* **34 B9**
Serock *Poland* **31 F8**
Serón *Spain* **39 H2**
Seròs *Spain* **38 D5**
Serov *Russia* **52 D7**
Serowe *Botswana* **88 C4**
Serpa *Portugal* **37 H3**
Serpeddì, Punta *Italy* **42 C2**
Serpentara *Italy* **42 C2**
Serpentine Lakes *Australia* **93 E4**
Serpent's Mouth = Sierpe,
  Bocas de la *Venezuela* **125 L15**
Serpis ➜ *Spain* **39 G4**
Serpneve *Ukraine* **29 D14**
Serpukhov *Russia* **32 E9**
Serra da Estrela △ *Portugal* **36 E3**
Serra do Navio *Brazil* **125 C8**
Serra San Bruno *Italy* **43 D9**
Serradilla *Spain* **36 F4**
Serramanna *Italy* **42 C1**
Serramanna *Italy* **42 C1**
Serranía San Luís △
  Paraguay **126 A4**
Serranía San Rafael △
  Paraguay **127 B4**
Serras d'Aire e
  Candeeiros △ *Portugal* **37 F2**
Serravalle Scrívia *Italy* **40 D5**
Serre-Ponçon, L. de *France* **21 D10**
Serres *France* **21 D9**
Serres *Greece* **44 E7**
Serres □ *Greece* **44 E7**
Serrezuela *Argentina* **126 C2**
Serrinha *Brazil* **125 F11**
Sersale *Italy* **43 C9**
Sertã *Portugal* **36 F2**
Sertânia *Brazil* **127 A5**
Sêrtar *China* **58 A3**
Serua *Indonesia* **63 F8**
Serui *Indonesia* **63 E9**
Serule *Botswana* **88 C4**
Servia *Greece* **44 F6**
Serzedelo *Portugal* **36 D2**
Ses Salines *Spain* **48 B10**
Sese Is. *Uganda* **86 C3**
Sesepe *Indonesia* **63 E7**
Sesfontein *Namibia* **88 B1**
Sesheke *Zambia* **88 B3**
Sésia ➜ *Italy* **40 C5**
Sesimbra *Portugal* **37 G1**
S'Espalmador *Spain* **48 C7**
S'Espardell *Spain* **48 C7**
Sessa Aurunca *Italy* **42 A6**
S'Estanyol *Spain* **48 B9**
Sestao *Spain* **38 B2**
Sesto Calende *Italy* **40 C5**
Sesto San Giovanni *Italy* **40 C6**
Sestri Levante *Italy* **40 D6**
Sestriere *Italy* **40 D3**
Sestroretsk *Russia* **32 B6**
Sestrunj *Croatia* **41 D11**
Sestu *Italy* **42 C2**
Setana *Japan* **54 C9**
Sète *France* **20 E7**
Sete Lagoas *Brazil* **125 G10**
Sétif *Algeria* **78 A7**
Setit ➜ *Sudan* **81 E4**
Seto *Japan* **55 G8**
Setonaikai *Japan* **55 G6**
Setonaikai △ *Japan* **55 G6**
Settat *Morocco* **78 B4**
Séttimo Torinese *Italy* **40 C4**
Setting L. *Canada* **103 C9**
Settle *U.K.* **14 C5**
Settlement, The *Br. Virgin Is.* **121 e**
Settlers *S. Africa* **89 C4**
Setúbal *Portugal* **37 G2**
Setúbal □ *Portugal* **37 G1**
Setúbal, B. de *Portugal* **37 G2**
Seugne ➜ *France* **20 C3**
Seul, Lac *Canada* **104 B1**
Seurre *France* **19 F12**
Sevan *Armenia* **35 K7**
Sevan, Ozero = Sevana
  Lich *Armenia* **35 K7**
Sevana Lich *Armenia* **35 K7**
Sevastopol *Ukraine* **33 K7**
Seven Sisters *Canada* **102 C3**
Sever ➜ *Spain* **37 F3**
Sévérac-le-Château *France* **20 D7**
Severn ➜ *Canada* **104 A2**
Severn ➜ *U.K.* **15 F5**
Severnaya Zemlya *Russia* **53 B11**
Severo-Kurilsk *Russia* **53 D16**
Severo-Yeniseyskiy *Russia* **53 C10**
Severo-Zapadnyy □ *Russia* **52 C4**
Severobaykalsk *Russia* **53 D11**
Severočeský □ *Czech Rep.* **26 A7**
Severodonetsk =
  Syeverodonetsk *Ukraine* **33 H10**
Severodvinsk *Russia* **52 C4**
Severomoravský □
  Czech Rep. **27 B10**
Severomorsk *Russia* **8 B25**
Seversk *Russia* **52 D9**
Sevier ➜ *U.S.A.* **108 G7**
Sevier Desert *U.S.A.* **108 G7**
Sevier L. *U.S.A.* **108 G7**

Sevilla *Spain* **37 H5**
Sevilla □ *Spain* **37 H5**
Seville = Sevilla *Spain* **37 H5**
Sevlievo *Bulgaria* **45 C9**
Sevnica *Slovenia* **41 B12**
Sevsk *Russia* **33 F8**
Sewa ➜ *S. Leone* **82 D2**
Sewani *India* **68 E6**
Seward *Alaska, U.S.A.* **100 E2**
Seward *Nebr., U.S.A.* **112 E6**
Seward *Pa., U.S.A.* **114 F5**
Seward Peninsula *U.S.A.* **106 B6**
Sewell *Chile* **126 C1**
Sewer *Indonesia* **63 F8**
Sewickley *U.S.A.* **114 F4**
Sexsmith *Canada* **102 B5**
Seychelles ■ *Ind. Oc.* **85 b**
Seyðisfjörður *Iceland* **8 D7**
Seydişehir *Turkey* **72 D4**
Seydvān *Iran* **73 C11**
Seyhan ➜ *Turkey* **72 D6**
Seyhan Baraji *Turkey* **72 D6**
Seyitgazi *Turkey* **47 B12**
Seyitömer *Turkey* **47 B11**
Seym ➜ *Ukraine* **33 G7**
Seymen *Turkey* **45 E11**
Seymour *Australia* **95 F4**
Seymour *S. Africa* **89 E4**
Seymour *Conn., U.S.A.* **115 E11**
Seymour *Ind., U.S.A.* **113 F11**
Seymour *Tex., U.S.A.* **116 E5**
Seyne *France* **21 D10**
Seyssel *France* **21 C9**
Sežana *Slovenia* **41 C10**
Sézanne *France* **19 D10**
Sezze *Italy* **42 A6**
Sfântu Gheorghe *Covasna,*
  Romania **29 E10**
Sfântu Gheorghe *Tulcea,*
  Romania **29 F14**
Sfântu Gheorghe,
  Brațul ➜ *Romania* **29 F14**
Sfax *Tunisia* **79 B8**
Sha Xi ➜ *China* **59 D12**
Sha Xian *China* **59 D12**
Shaanxi □ *China* **56 G5**
Shaba = Katanga □
  Dem. Rep. of the Congo **86 D2**
Shaba △ *Kenya* **86 B4**
Shabeelle ➜ *Somali Rep.* **75 G3**
Shabestar *Iran* **73 C11**
Shabla *Bulgaria* **45 C12**
Shabogamo L. *Canada* **105 B6**
Shabunda
  Dem. Rep. of the Congo **86 C2**
Shache *China* **60 C2**
Shackleton Fracture Zone
  S. Ocean **5 B18**
Shackleton Ice Shelf
  Antarctica **5 C8**
Shackleton Inlet *Antarctica* **5 E11**
Shādegān *Iran* **71 D6**
Shadi *China* **59 D10**
Shadi *India* **69 C7**
Shadrinsk *Russia* **52 D7**
Shadyside *U.S.A.* **114 G4**
Shaffa *Nigeria* **83 C7**
Shafter *U.S.A.* **111 K7**
Shaftesbury *U.K.* **15 F5**
Shaftsbury *U.S.A.* **115 D11**
Shagamu *Nigeria* **83 D5**
Shagram *Pakistan* **69 A5**
Shah Alam *Malaysia* **65 L3**
Shah Alizai *Pakistan* **68 E2**
Shah Bunder *Pakistan* **68 G2**
Shahabad *Punjab, India* **68 D7**
Shahabad *Raj., India* **68 G7**
Shahabad *Ut. P., India* **69 F8**
Shahadpur *Pakistan* **68 G3**
Shahba' *Syria* **74 C5**
Shahdād *Iran* **71 D8**
Shahdād, Namakzār-e *Iran* **71 D8**
Shahdadkot *Pakistan* **68 F2**
Shahdol *India* **69 H9**
Shahe *China* **56 F8**
Shahganj *India* **69 F10**
Shahgarh *India* **68 F3**
Shahjahanpur *India* **69 F8**
Shahpur = Salmās *Iran* **73 C11**
Shahpur *India* **68 H7**
Shahpur *Baluchistan, Pakistan* **68 E3**
Shahpur *Punjab, Pakistan* **68 C5**
Shahpur Chakar *Pakistan* **68 F3**
Shahpura *Mad. P., India* **69 H9**
Shahpura *Raj., India* **68 G6**
Shahr-e Bābak *Iran* **71 D7**
Shahr-e Kord *Iran* **71 C6**
Shāhrakht *Iran* **71 C9**
Shahrezā = Qomsheh *Iran* **71 D6**
Shāhrūd = Emāmrūd *Iran* **71 B7**
Shahukou *China* **56 D7**
Shaikhabad *Afghan.* **68 B3**
Shajapur *India* **68 H7**
Shakargarh *Pakistan* **68 C6**
Shakawe *Botswana* **88 B3**
Shaker Heights *U.S.A.* **114 E3**
Shakhtersk *Russia* **53 E15**

Shakhty *Russia* **35 G5**
Shakhunya *Russia* **34 B8**
Shaki *Nigeria* **83 D5**
Shākir *Egypt* **80 B3**
Shala, L. *Ethiopia* **81 F4**
Shaksam Valley *Asia* **69 A7**
Shala, L. *Ethiopia* **81 F4**
Shali *Russia* **35 J7**
Shalkar Köli *Kazakhstan* **34 E10**
Shallow Lake *Canada* **114 B3**
Shalqar *Kazakhstan* **52 E6**
Shalskiy *Russia* **32 B8**
Shaluli Shan *China* **58 B2**
Shām *Iran* **71 E8**
Shām, Bādiyat ash *Asia* **70 C3**
Shamāl Bahr el Ghazal □
  Sudan **81 F2**
Shamāl Dârfûr □ *Sudan* **81 E2**
Shamāl Kordofân □ *Sudan* **81 E3**
Shamāl Sînî □ *Egypt* **74 E2**
Shamattawa *Canada* **104 A1**
Shamattawa ➜ *Canada* **104 A2**
Shambe *Sudan* **81 F3**
Shambe △ *Sudan* **81 F3**
Shambu *Ethiopia* **81 F4**
Shamīl *Iran* **71 E8**
Shamkhor = Şämkir
  Azerbaijan **35 K8**
Shāmkūh *Iran* **71 C8**
Shamli *India* **68 E7**
Shammar, Jabal *Si. Arabia* **70 E4**
Shamo = Gobi *Asia* **56 C6**
Shamo, L. *Ethiopia* **81 F4**
Shamokin *U.S.A.* **115 F8**
Shamrock *Canada* **115 A8**
Shamrock *U.S.A.* **116 D4**
Shamva *Zimbabwe* **87 F3**
Shan □ *Burma* **67 J21**
Shan Xian *China* **56 G9**
Shanan ➜ *Ethiopia* **81 F5**
Shanchengzhen *China* **57 C13**
Shāndak *Iran* **71 D9**
Shandon *U.S.A.* **110 K6**
Shandong □ *China* **57 G10**
Shandong Bandao *China* **57 F11**
Shandur Pass *Pakistan* **69 A5**
Shang Xian = Shangzhou
  China **56 H5**
Shangalowe
  Dem. Rep. of the Congo **87 E2**
Shangani *Zimbabwe* **89 B4**
Shangani ➜ *Zimbabwe* **87 F2**
Shangbancheng *China* **57 D10**
Shangcheng *China* **59 B10**
Shangchuan Dao *China* **59 G9**
Shangdu *China* **56 D7**
Shanggao *China* **59 C10**
Shanghai *China* **59 B13**
Shanghai Shi □ *China* **59 B13**
Shanghang *China* **59 E11**
Shanghe *China* **57 F9**
Shanglin *China* **58 F7**
Shangnan *China* **56 H6**
Shangqiu *China* **56 G8**
Shangrao *China* **59 C11**
Shangri-La = Zhongdian
  China **58 D2**
Shangshui *China* **60 C6**
Shangsi *China* **58 F6**
Shangyou *China* **59 E10**
Shangyu *China* **59 B13**
Shangzhi *China* **57 B14**
Shangzhou *China* **56 H5**
Shanhetun *China* **57 B14**
Shani *Nigeria* **83 C7**
Shānidar *Iraq* **73 D11**
Shanklin *U.K.* **15 G6**
Shannon *N.Z.* **91 J5**
Shannon ➜ *Ireland* **12 D2**
Shannon ✈ (SNN) *Ireland* **12 D3**
Shannon, Mouth of the
  Ireland **12 D2**
Shannon △ *Australia* **93 F2**
Shannonbridge *Ireland* **12 C3**
Shansi = Shanxi □ *China* **56 F7**
Shantar, Ostrov Bolshoy
  Russia **53 D14**
Shantipur *India* **69 H13**
Shantou *China* **59 F11**
Shantung = Shandong □
  China **57 G10**
Shanwei *China* **59 F10**
Shanxi □ *China* **56 F7**
Shanyang *China* **56 H5**
Shanyin *China* **56 E7**
Shaodong *China* **59 D8**
Shaoguan *China* **59 E9**
Shaoshan *China* **59 D8**
Shaowu *China* **59 D11**
Shaoxing *China* **59 C13**
Shaoyang *Hunan, China* **59 D8**
Shaoyang *Hunan, China* **59 D8**
Shap *U.K.* **14 C5**
Shapinsay *U.K.* **13 B6**
Shaqlāwah *Iraq* **73 D11**
Shaqq el Gi'eifer ➜ *Sudan* **81 D2**
Shaqra' *Si. Arabia* **70 E5**
Shaqrā' *Yemen* **75 E4**
Sharafa *Sudan* **81 E2**
Sharafkhāneh *Iran* **73 C11**
Sharashova *Belarus* **31 F11**

Sharbot Lake *Canada* **115** B8
Sharhorod *Ukraine* **29** B13
Shari *Japan* **54** C12
Sharjah = Ash Shāriqah
　U.A.E. **71** E7
Shark B. *Australia* **93** E1
Shark Bay △ *Australia* **93** E1
Sharm el Sheikh *Egypt* **80** B3
Sharon *Canada* **114** B5
Sharon *Mass., U.S.A.* **115** D13
Sharon *Pa., U.S.A.* **114** E4
Sharon Springs *Kans., U.S.A.* **112** F3
Sharon Springs *N.Y., U.S.A.*
　115 D10
Sharp Pt. *Australia* **94** A3
Sharpe L. *Canada* **104** B1
Sharpsville *U.S.A.* **114** E4
Sharq el Istiwa'iya □ *Sudan* **81** G3
Sharqi, Al Jabal ash *Lebanon* **74** B5
Sharya *Russia* **34** A7
Shasha *Ethiopia* **81** F4
Shashemene *Ethiopia* **81** F4
Shashi *Botswana* **89** C4
Shashi *China* **59** B9
Shashi ➤ *Africa* **87** G2
Shasta, Mt. *U.S.A.* **108** F2
Shasta L. *U.S.A.* **108** F2
Shatawi *Sudan* **81** E3
Shatsk *Russia* **34** C5
Shatsk *Ukraine* **31** G10
Shatsky Rise *Pac. Oc.* **96** D7
Shatskyi △ *Ukraine* **31** G10
Shatt al Arab *Asia* **71** D6
Shatura *Russia* **32** E10
Shaumyani = Shulaveri
　Georgia **35** K7
Shaunavon *Canada* **103** D7
Shaver L. *U.S.A.* **110** H7
Shaw ➤ *Australia* **92** D2
Shaw I. *Australia* **94** b
Shawanaga *Canada* **114** A4
Shawangunk Mts. *U.S.A.* **115** E10
Shawano *U.S.A.* **112** C9
Shawinigan *Canada* **104** C5
Shawmari, J. ash *Jordan* **74** E5
Shawnee *U.S.A.* **116** D6
Shay Gap *Australia* **92** D3
Shayang *China* **59** B9
Shaybārā *Si. Arabia* **70** E3
Shayib el Banat, Gebel *Egypt* **80** B3
Shaykh, J. ash *Lebanon* **74** B4
Shaykh Miskīn *Syria* **74** C5
Shaykh Sa'd *Iraq* **73** F12
Shāzand *Iran* **71** C6
Shchekino *Russia* **32** E9
Shchigry *Russia* **33** G9
Shchors *Ukraine* **33** G6
Shchūchīnsk *Kazakhstan* **52** D8
She Xian *Anhui, China* **59** C12
She Xian *Hebei, China* **56** F7
Shebekino *Russia* **33** G9
Shebele = Shabeelle ➤
　Somali Rep. **75** G3
Sheboygan *U.S.A.* **112** D10
Shebshi Mts. *Nigeria* **83** D7
Shediac *Canada* **105** C7
Sheelin, L. *Ireland* **12** C4
Sheenjek ➤ *U.S.A.* **106** B11
Sheep Haven *Ireland* **12** A4
Sheep Range *U.S.A.* **111** J11
Sheerness *U.K.* **15** F8
Sheet Harbour *Canada* **105** D7
Sheffield *U.K.* **14** D6
Sheffield *Ala., U.S.A.* **117** D11
Sheffield *Mass., U.S.A.* **115** D11
Sheffield *Pa., U.S.A.* **114** E5
Shehojele *Ethiopia* **81** E4
Shehong *China* **58** B5
Sheikh Zayed, Qana es *Egypt* **80** C3
Sheikh Zayed Canal =
　Sheikh Zayed, Qana es
　Egypt **80** C3
Sheikhpura *India* **69** G11
Shek Hasan *Ethiopia* **81** E4
Shekhupura *Pakistan* **68** D5
Sheki = Şaki *Azerbaijan* **35** K8
Shelburne *N.S., Canada* **105** D6
Shelburne *Ont., Canada* **114** B4
Shelburne *U.S.A.* **115** B11
Shelburne B. *Australia* **94** A3
Shelburne Falls *U.S.A.* **115** D12
Shelby *Mich., U.S.A.* **112** D10
Shelby *Miss., U.S.A.* **117** E9
Shelby *Mont., U.S.A.* **108** B8
Shelby *N.C., U.S.A.* **117** D14
Shelby *Ohio, U.S.A.* **114** F2
Shelbyville *Ill., U.S.A.* **112** F9
Shelbyville *Ind., U.S.A.* **113** F11
Shelbyville *Ky., U.S.A.* **113** F11
Shelbyville *Tenn., U.S.A.* **117** D11
Sheldon *U.S.A.* **112** D6
Sheldrake *Canada* **105** B7
Shelengo, Khawr ➤ *Sudan* **81** E2
Shelikhova, Zaliv *Russia* **53** D16
Shelikof Strait *U.S.A.* **106** D9
Shell Lakes *Australia* **93** E4
Shellbrook *Canada* **103** C7
Shellharbour *Australia* **95** E5
Shelon ➤ *Russia* **32** C6
Shelter I. *U.S.A.* **115** E12

Shelton *Conn., U.S.A.* **115** E11
Shelton *Wash., U.S.A.* **110** C3
Shemakha = Şamaxı
　Azerbaijan **35** K9
Shëmri *Albania* **44** D4
Shemsi *Sudan* **80** D2
Shen Xian *China* **56** F8
Shenandoah *Iowa, U.S.A.* **112** E6
Shenandoah *Pa., U.S.A.* **115** F8
Shenandoah *Va., U.S.A.* **113** F14
Shenandoah ➤ *U.S.A.* **113** F15
Shenandoah △ *U.S.A.* **113** F14
Shenchi *China* **56** E7
Shendam *Nigeria* **83** D6
Shendî *Sudan* **81** D3
Shenge S. *Leone* **82** D2
Shengfang *China* **56** E9
Shëngjergj *Albania* **44** E4
Shëngjin *Albania* **44** E3
Shengzhou *China* **59** C13
Shenjingzi *China* **57** B13
Shenmu *China* **56** E6
Shennongjia *China* **59** B8
Shenqiu *China* **56** H8
Shensi = Shaanxi □ *China* **56** G5
Shenyang *China* **57** D12
Shenzhen *China* **59** F10
Sheo *India* **68** F4
Sheopur Kalan *India* **68** G7
Shepetivka *Ukraine* **23** C14
Shepparton *Australia* **95** F4
Sheppey, I. of *U.K.* **15** F8
Shepton Mallet *U.K.* **15** F5
Sheqi *China* **56** H7
Sher Qila *Pakistan* **69** A6
Sherab *Sudan* **81** F1
Sherborne *U.K.* **15** G5
Sherbro I. S. *Leone* **82** D2
Sherbro ➤ *S. Leone* **82** D2
Sherbrooke *N.S., Canada* **105** C7
Sherbrooke *Qué., Canada* **115** A13
Sherburne *U.S.A.* **115** D9
Shereik *Sudan* **80** D3
Shergarh *India* **68** F5
Sherghati *India* **69** G11
Sheridan *Ark., U.S.A.* **116** D8
Sheridan *Wyo., U.S.A.* **108** D10
Sheringham *U.K.* **14** E9
Sherkin I. *Ireland* **12** E2
Sherkot *India* **69** E8
Sherlovaya Gora *Russia* **53** D12
Sherman *N.Y., U.S.A.* **114** D5
Sherman *Tex., U.S.A.* **116** E6
Sherpur *India* **69** G10
Sherridon *Canada* **103** B8
Sherwood Forest *U.K.* **14** D6
Sherwood Park *Canada* **102** C6
Sheslay ➤ *Canada* **102** B2
Shethanei L. *Canada* **103** B9
Shetland □ *U.K.* **13** A7
Shetland Is. *U.K.* **13** A7
Shetrunji ➤ *India* **68** J5
Shevchenkovo *Ukraine* **29** E14
Shevisheh *Iran* **73** E12
Shewa *Ethiopia* **81** F4
Shewa Gimira *Ethiopia* **81** F4
Shey-Phoksundo △ *Nepal* **69** E10
Sheyenne ➤ *U.S.A.* **112** B5
Shiashkotan, Ostrov *Russia* **53** E16
Shibām *Yemen* **75** D4
Shibata *Japan* **54** E9
Shibecha *Japan* **54** C12
Shibetsu *Japan* **54** B11
Shibîn el Kôm *Egypt* **80** H7
Shibîn el Qanâtir *Egypt* **80** H7
Shibing *China* **58** D7
Shibogama L. *Canada* **104** B2
Shibushi *Japan* **55** J5
Shicheng *China* **59** D11
Shickshinny *U.S.A.* **115** E8
Shickshock Mts. =
　Chic-Chocs, Mts. *Canada* **105** C6
Shidao *China* **57** F12
Shidian *China* **58** E2
Shido *Japan* **55** G7
Shiel, L. *U.K.* **13** E3
Shield, C. *Australia* **94** A2
Shīeli *Kazakhstan* **52** E7
Shifang *China* **58** B5
Shiga □ *Japan* **55** G8
Shigu *China* **58** D2
Shiguaigou *China* **56** D6
Shihchiachuangi =
　Shijiazhuang *China* **56** E8
Shihezi *China* **60** B3
Shijak *Albania* **44** E3
Shijiazhuang *China* **56** E8
Shijiu Hu *China* **59** B12
Shikarpur *India* **69** E8
Shikarpur *Pakistan* **68** F3
Shikohabad *India* **69** F8
Shikoku □ *Japan* **55** H6
Shikoku-Sanchi *Japan* **55** H6
Shikotan, Ostrov *Asia* **53** E15
Shikotsu-Ko *Japan* **54** C10
Shikotsu-Tōya △ *Japan* **54** C10
Shiliguri *India* **67** F16
Shiliu = Changjiang *China* **64** C7
Shilka *Russia* **53** D12
Shilka ➤ *Russia* **53** D13

Shillelagh *Ireland* **12** D5
Shillington *U.S.A.* **115** F9
Shillong *India* **67** G17
Shilo *West Bank* **74** C4
Shilong *China* **59** F9
Shilou *China* **56** F6
Shilovo *Russia* **34** C5
Shimabara *Japan* **55** H5
Shimada *Japan* **55** G9
Shimane □ *Japan* **55** G6
Shimanovsk *Russia* **53** D13
Shimba Hills △ *Kenya* **86** C4
Shimbiris *Somali Rep.* **75** E4
Shimen *China* **59** C8
Shimenjie *China* **59** C11
Shimian *China* **58** C4
Shimizu *Japan* **55** G9
Shimla *India* **68** D7
Shimodate *Japan* **55** F9
Shimoga *India* **66** N9
Shimoni *Kenya* **86** C4
Shimonoseki *Japan* **55** H5
Shimpuru Rapids *Namibia* **88** B2
Shimsk *Russia* **32** C6
Shin, L. *U.K.* **13** C4
Shinan *China* **58** F7
Shinano-Gawa ➤ *Japan* **55** F9
Shinās *Oman* **71** E8
Shīndand *Afghan.* **66** C3
Shinglehouse *U.S.A.* **114** E6
Shingū *Japan* **55** H7
Shingwidzi *S. Africa* **89** C5
Shinjō *Japan* **54** E10
Shinkafe *Nigeria* **83** C6
Shinkolobwe
　Dem. Rep. of the Congo **84** G5
Shinshār *Syria* **74** A5
Shinyanga *Tanzania* **86** C3
Shinyanga □ *Tanzania* **86** C3
Shio-no-Misaki *Japan* **55** H7
Shiogama *Japan* **54** E10
Shiojiri *Japan* **55** F8
Shipchenski Prokhod
　Bulgaria **45** D9
Shiping *China* **58** F4
Shippagan *Canada* **105** C7
Shippensburg *U.S.A.* **114** F7
Shippenville *U.S.A.* **114** E5
Shiprock *U.S.A.* **109** H9
Shiqian *China* **58** D7
Shiqma, N. ➤ *Israel* **74** D3
Shiquan *China* **56** H5
Shiquan He = Indus ➤
　Pakistan **68** G2
Shīr Kūh *Iran* **71** D7
Shiragami-Misaki *Japan* **54** D10
Shirakawa *Fukushima, Japan* **55** F10
Shirakawa *Gifu, Japan* **55** F8
Shirane-San *Gumma, Japan* **55** F9
Shirane-San *Yamanashi, Japan* **55** G9
Shiraoi *Japan* **54** C10
Shīrāz *Iran* **71** D7
Shirbīn *Egypt* **80** H7
Shire ➤ *Africa* **87** F4
Shiretoko-Misaki *Japan* **54** B12
Shirinab ➤ *Pakistan* **68** D2
Shiriya-Zaki *Japan* **54** D10
Shiroishi *Japan* **54** F10
Shiroro Res. *Nigeria* **83** D6
Shīrvān *Iran* **71** B8
Shirwa, L. = Chilwa, L.
　Malawi **87** F4
Shishaldin Volcano *U.S.A.* **106** E7
Shishi *China* **59** E12
Shishou *China* **59** C9
Shitai *China* **59** B11
Shithāthah *Iraq* **73** G10
Shivamogga = Shimoga
　India **66** N9
Shivpuri *India* **68** G7
Shixian *China* **57** C15
Shixing *China* **59** E10
Shiyan *China* **59** A8
Shiyata *Egypt* **80** B2
Shizhu *China* **58** C7
Shizong *China* **58** E5
Shizuishan *China* **56** E4
Shizuoka *Japan* **55** G9
Shizuoka □ *Japan* **55** G9
Shkhara *Georgia* **73** A10
Shklov = Shklow *Belarus* **23** A16
Shklow *Belarus* **23** A16
Shkodër *Albania* **44** D3
Shkumbini ➤ *Albania* **44** E3
Shmidta, Ostrov *Russia* **53** A10
Shō-Gawa ➤ *Japan* **55** F8
Shoal I. *Canada* **103** D9
Shoal Lake *Canada* **103** C8
Shōdo-Shima *Japan* **55** G7
Sholapur = Solapur *India* **66** L9
Shōmrōn *West Bank* **74** C4
Shoreham *U.S.A.* **115** C11
Shoreham by Sea *U.K.* **15** G7
Shori ➤ *Pakistan* **68** E3
Shorkot *Pakistan* **68** D4
Shorkot Road *Pakistan* **68** D5
Shoshone *Calif., U.S.A.* **111** K10
Shoshone *Idaho, U.S.A.* **108** E6
Shoshone L. *U.S.A.* **108** D8

Shoshone Mts. *U.S.A.* **108** G5
Shoshong *Botswana* **88** C4
Shoshoni *U.S.A.* **108** E9
Shostka *Ukraine* **33** G7
Shot *Iran* **73** C11
Shou Xian *China* **59** A11
Shouchang *China* **59** C12
Shouguang *China* **57** F10
Shouning *China* **59** D12
Shouyang *China* **56** F7
Show Low *U.S.A.* **109** J8
Showak *Sudan* **81** E4
Shpola *Ukraine* **33** H6
Shpykiv *Ukraine* **29** B13
Shqipëria = Albania ■
　Europe **44** E4
Shreveport *U.S.A.* **116** E8
Shrewsbury *U.K.* **15** E5
Shri Mohangarh *India* **68** F4
Shrirampur *India* **69** H13
Shropshire □ *U.K.* **15** E5
Shū *Kazakhstan* **52** E8
Shuangbai *China* **58** E3
Shuangcheng *China* **57** B14
Shuangfeng *China* **59** D9
Shuanggou *China* **57** G9
Shuangjiang *China* **58** F2
Shuangliao *China* **57** C12
Shuangyang *China* **57** C13
Shuangshanzi *China* **57** D10
Shuangyashan *China* **60** B8
Shubrā el Kheima *Egypt* **80** H7
Shubrā Khīt *Egypt* **80** H7
Shucheng *China* **59** B11
Shugozero *Russia* **32** C8
Shuguri Falls *Tanzania* **87** D4
Shuiji *China* **59** D12
Shuiye *China* **56** F8
Shujalpur *India* **68** H7
Shukpa Kunzang *India* **69** B8
Shulan *China* **57** B14
Shulaveri *Georgia* **35** K7
Shule *China* **60** C2
Shumagin Is. *U.S.A.* **106** D7
Shumen *Bulgaria* **45** C10
Shumerlya *Russia* **34** C8
Shumikha *Russia* **52** D7
Shunchang *China* **59** D11
Shunde *China* **59** F9
Shungay *Kazakhstan* **35** F8
Shungnak *U.S.A.* **106** B8
Shuo Xian = Shuozhou
　China **56** E7
Shuozhou *China* **56** E7
Shūr ➤ *Fārs, Iran* **71** D7
Shūr ➤ *Kermān, Iran* **71** D8
Shūr ➤ *Yazd, Iran* **71** D7
Shūr Āb *Iran* **71** C6
Shūr Gaz *Iran* **71** D8
Shūrāb *Iran* **71** C8
Shūrjestān *Iran* **71** D7
Shurugwi *Zimbabwe* **87** F3
Shūsf *Iran* **71** D9
Shūsh *Iran* **73** F13
Shūshtar *Iran* **71** D6
Shuswap L. *Canada* **102** C5
Shute Harbour △ *Australia* **94** b
Shuya *Russia* **34** B5
Shuyang *China* **57** G10
Shūzū *Iran* **71** D7
Shwebo *Burma* **67** H19
Shwegu *Burma* **67** G20
Shweli ➤ *Burma* **67** H20
Shymkent *Kazakhstan* **52** E7
Shyok *India* **69** B8
Shyok ➤ *Pakistan* **69** B6
Shyroke *Odesa, Ukraine* **29** E15
Shyroke *Ternopil, Ukraine* **28** B8
Si Kiang = Xi Jiang ➤ *China* **59** F9
Si Lanna △ *Thailand* **64** C2
Si Nakarin Res. *Thailand* **64** E2
Si-ngan = Xi'an *China* **56** G5
Si Prachan *Thailand* **64** E3
Si Racha *Thailand* **64** F3
Si Xian *China* **57** H9
Siachen Glacier *Asia* **69** B7
Sīah Chashmeh *Iran* **73** C11
Siahaf ➤ *Pakistan* **68** E3
Siahan Range *Pakistan* **66** F4
Siaksriindrapura *Indonesia* **62** D2
Sialkot *Pakistan* **68** C6
Siam = Thailand ■ *Asia* **64** E4
Sian = Xi'an *China* **56** G5
Sian Ka'an △ *Mexico* **119** D7
Sianów *Poland* **30** D3
Siantan *Indonesia* **62** D3
Sīāreh *Iran* **71** D9
Siargao I. *Phil.* **61** G7
Siari *Pakistan* **69** B7
Siasi *Phil.* **63** C6
Siasi I. *Phil.* **61** J4
Siatista *Greece* **44** F5
Siau *Indonesia* **63** D7
Šiauliai *Lithuania* **30** C10
Šiauliai □ *Lithuania* **30** C10
Siazan = Siyäzän *Azerbaijan* **35** K9
Sībāi, Gebel el *Egypt* **70** E2
Sibang *Indonesia* **63** K18
Sibayi, L. *S. Africa* **89** D5
Sibdu *Sudan* **81** E2

Šibenik *Croatia* **41** E12
Siberia = Sibirskiy □ *Russia* **53** D10
Siberia *Russia* **4** D13
Siberut *Indonesia* **62** E1
Sibi *Pakistan* **68** E2
Sibil = Oksibil *Indonesia* **63** E10
Sibiloi □ *Kenya* **86** B4
Sibirskiy □ *Russia* **53** D10
Sibirtsevo *Russia* **54** B5
Sibiti *Congo* **84** E2
Sibiu *Romania* **29** E9
Sibiu □ *Romania* **29** E9
Sibley *U.S.A.* **112** D6
Sibolga *Indonesia* **62** D1
Siborongborong *Indonesia* **65** L2
Sibsagar *India* **67** F19
Sibu *Malaysia* **62** D4
Sibuco *Phil.* **61** G5
Sibutu *Phil.* **63** D5
Sibutu Group *Phil.* **61** J3
Sibutu Passage *E. Indies* **61** J4
Sibuyan I. *Phil.* **61** E5
Sibuyan Sea *Phil.* **61** E5
Sic *Romania* **29** D8
Sicamous *Canada* **102** C5
Siccus ➤ *Australia* **95** E2
Sichon *Thailand* **65** H2
Sichuan □ *China* **58** B5
Sichuan Pendi *China* **58** C5
Sicilia *Italy* **43** E7
Sicily = Sicilia *Italy* **43** E7
Sicily, Str. of *Medit. S.* **42** E4
Sico ➤ *Honduras* **120** C3
Sicuani *Peru* **124** F4
Šid *Serbia* **28** E4
Sidamo *Ethiopia* **81** G4
Sidaouet *Niger* **83** B6
Sidari *Greece* **49** A3
Siddhapur *India* **68** H5
Siddipet *India* **66** K11
Sidensjö *Sweden* **10** A12
Sidéradougou *Burkina Faso* **82** C4
Siderno *Italy* **43** D9
Sideros, Akra *Greece* **49** D8
Sidhauli *India* **69** F9
Sidhi *India* **69** G9
Sīdi Abd el Rahmân *Egypt* **80** A2
Sîdi Barrâni *Egypt* **80** A2
Sidi-bel-Abbès *Algeria* **78** A5
Sīdi Haneish *Egypt* **80** A2
Sidi Ifni *Morocco* **78** C3
Sîdi Omar *Egypt* **80** A1
Sidikalang *Indonesia* **65** L2
Sidirokastro *Greece* **44** E7
Sidlaw Hills *U.K.* **13** E5
Sidley, Mt. *Antarctica* **5** D14
Sidmouth *U.K.* **15** G4
Sidmouth, C. *Australia* **94** A3
Sidney *Canada* **110** B3
Sidney *Mont., U.S.A.* **108** C11
Sidney *N.Y., U.S.A.* **115** D9
Sidney *Nebr., U.S.A.* **112** E3
Sidney *Ohio, U.S.A.* **113** E11
Sidney Lanier, L. *U.S.A.* **117** D12
Sido *Mali* **82** C3
Sidoarjo *Indonesia* **63** G15
Sidon = Saydā *Lebanon* **74** B4
Sidra, G. of = Surt, Khalīj
　Libya **79** B9
Siedlce *Poland* **31** F9
Sieg ➤ *Germany* **24** E3
Siegburg *Germany* **24** E3
Siegen *Germany* **24** E4
Siem Pang *Cambodia* **64** E6
Siem Reap = Siemreab
　Cambodia **64** F4
Siemiatycze *Poland* **31** F9
Siemreab *Cambodia* **64** F4
Siena *Italy* **41** E8
Sieniawa *Poland* **31** H9
Sieradz *Poland* **31** G5
Sieraków *Poland* **31** F3
Sierck-les-Bains *France* **19** C13
Sierning *Austria* **26** C7
Sierpc *Poland* **31** F6
Sierpe, Bocas de la *Venezuela*
　125 L15
Sierra Blanca *U.S.A.* **116** F2
Sierra Blanca Peak *U.S.A.* **109** K11
Sierra City *U.S.A.* **110** F6
Sierra Colorada *Argentina* **128** E3
Sierra de Agalta △ *Honduras* **120** C2
Sierra de Aracena y Picas
　de Aroche △ *Spain* **37** H4
Sierra de Bahoruco △
　Dom. Rep. **121** C5
Sierra de Baza △ *Spain* **39** H2
Sierra de Castril △ *Spain* **39** H2
Sierra de España △ *Spain* **39** H3
Sierra de Grazalema △ *Spain* **37** J5
Sierra de Gredos △ *Spain* **36** E5
Sierra de Hornachuelos △
　Spain **37** H5
Sierra de Huétor △ *Spain* **37** H7
Sierra de La Culata △
　Venezuela **121** E5
Sierra de Lancandón △
　Guatemala **120** C1

Sierra de las Nieves △ *Spain* **37** J6
Sierra de las Quijadas △
　Argentina **126** C2
Sierra de María-Los
　Vélez △ *Spain* **39** H2
Sierra de San Luis △
　Venezuela **121** D6
Sierra de San Pedro Mártir,
　Parque Nac. △ *Mexico* **118** A1
Sierra de Yeguas *Spain* **37** H6
Sierra del São Mamede △
　Portugal **37** F3
Sierra Gorda *Chile* **126** A2
Sierra Leone ■ *W. Afr.* **82** D2
Sierra Madre *Mexico* **119** D6
Sierra Madre Occidental
　Mexico **118** B3
Sierra Madre Oriental
　Mexico **118** C5
Sierra Mágina △ *Spain* **37** H7
Sierra Mojada *Mexico* **118** B4
Sierra Nevada *Spain* **37** H7
Sierra Nevada *U.S.A.* **110** H8
Sierra Nevada △ *Spain* **37** H7
Sierra Nevada △ *Venezuela* **121** E5
Sierra Nevada de Santa
　Marta △ *Colombia* **121** D5
Sierra Norte de Sevilla △
　Spain **37** H5
Sierra Subbéticas △ *Spain* **37** H6
Sierra Vista *U.S.A.* **109** L8
Sierras de Cardeña y
　Montoro △ *Spain* **37** G6
Sierras de Cazorla, Segura
　y las Villas △ *Spain* **39** J2
Sierraville *U.S.A.* **110** F6
Sierre *Switz.* **25** J3
Sifani *Ethiopia* **81** E5
Sifié *Ivory C.* **82** D3
Sifnos *Greece* **46** E6
Sifton *Canada* **103** C8
Sifton Pass *Canada* **102** B3
Sig *Algeria* **78** A5
Sigatoka *Fiji* **91** a
Sigean *France* **20** E6
Sighetu-Marmației *Romania* **29** C8
Sighișoara *Romania* **29** D9
Sigli *Indonesia* **62** C1
Siglufjörður *Iceland* **8** C4
Sigmaringen *Germany* **25** G5
Signa *Italy* **41** C7
Signakhi = Tsnori *Georgia* **35** K7
Signal de Botrang *Belgium* **17** D6
Signal Pk. *U.S.A.* **111** M12
Signy I. *Antarctica* **5** C18
Signy-l'Abbaye *France* **19** C11
Sígsig *Ecuador* **124** D3
Sigtuna *Sweden* **10** E11
Sigüenza *Spain* **38** D2
Siguiri *Guinea* **82** C3
Sigulda *Latvia* **32** D3
Sihora *India* **69** H9
Sihui *China* **59** F9
Siikajoki ➤ *Finland* **8** D21
Siilinjärvi *Finland* **8** E22
Siirt *Turkey* **73** D9
Siirt □ *Turkey* **73** D9
Sijarira Ra. = Chizarira
　Zimbabwe **87** F2
Sika *India* **68** H3
Sikanni Chief ➤ *Canada* **102** B4
Sikao *Thailand* **65** J2
Sikar *India* **68** F6
Sikasso *Mali* **82** C3
Sikasso □ *Mali* **82** C3
Sikeston *U.S.A.* **112** G9
Sikhote Alin, Khrebet *Russia* **54** B8
Sikhote Alin Ra. = Sikhote
　Alin, Khrebet *Russia* **54** B8
Sikia *Greece* **44** F7
Sikinos *Greece* **47** E7
Sikkim □ *India* **67** F16
Siklós *Hungary* **28** E3
Sil ➤ *Spain* **36** C3
Silacayoapan *Mexico* **119** D5
Šilalė *Lithuania* **30** C9
Silandro *Italy* **40** B7
Silawad *India* **68** J6
Silay *Phil.* **61** F5
Silba *Croatia* **41** D11
Silchar *India* **67** G18
Şile *Turkey* **45** E13
Siler City *U.S.A.* **117** D15
Silesia = Śląsk *Poland* **22** C9
Silgarhi Doti *Nepal* **69** E9
Silghat *India* **67** F18
Silhouette *Seychelles* **85** b
Sili *Burkina Faso* **82** C4
Silifke *Turkey* **72** D5
Siliguri = Shiliguri *India* **67** F16
Siling Co *China* **60** C3
Silistea Nouă *Romania* **29** F10
Silistra *Bulgaria* **45** B11
Silivri *Turkey* **45** E12
Siljan *Sweden* **10** D8
Siljansnäs *Sweden* **10** D8
Silkeborg *Denmark* **11** H3
Silkwood *Australia* **94** B4
Silla *Spain* **39** F4
Sillajhuay, Cordillera *Chile* **124** G5

Sillamäe *Estonia* **32** C4
Sillé-le-Guillaume *France* **18** D6
Silleda *Spain* **36** C2
Silloth *U.K.* **14** C4
Silo *Greece* **45** E9
Siloam Springs *U.S.A.* **116** C7
Silopi *Turkey* **73** D10
Silsbee *U.S.A.* **116** F7
Siluko *Nigeria* **83** D6
Šilutė *Lithuania* **30** C8
Silvan *Turkey* **73** C9
Silvani *India* **69** H8
Silver City *U.S.A.* **109** K9
Silver Cr. → *U.S.A.* **108** E4
Silver Creek *U.S.A.* **114** D5
Silver L. *U.S.A.* **108** E4
Silver Lake *Calif., U.S.A.* **111** K10
Silver Lake *Oreg., U.S.A.* **108** E3
Silverdalen *Sweden* **11** G9
Silvermine Mts. *Ireland* **12** D3
Silverton *Colo., U.S.A.* **109** H10
Silverton *Tex., U.S.A.* **116** D4
Silves *Portugal* **37** H2
Silvi Marina *Italy* **41** F11
Silvies → *U.S.A.* **108** E4
Silvretta *India* **26** D3
Silvrettahorn *Switz.* **40** B7
Silwa Bahari *Egypt* **80** C3
Silz *Austria* **26** D3
Simaltala *India* **69** G12
Simanggang = Sri Aman *Malaysia* **62** D4
Simao *China* **58** F3
Simard, L. *Canada* **104** C4
Şimareh → *Iran* **73** F12
Simav *Turkey* **47** B10
Simav → *Turkey* **45** F12
Simav Dağları *Turkey* **47** B10
Simba *Tanzania* **86** C4
Simbach *Germany* **25** G9
Simbirsk = Ulyanovsk *Russia* **34** C9
Simbo *Tanzania* **86** C2
Simcoe *Canada* **114** D4
Simcoe, L. *Canada* **114** B5
Simdega *India* **69** H11
Simeonovgrad *Bulgaria* **45** D9
Simeria *Romania* **28** E8
Simeto → *Italy* **43** E8
Simeulue *Indonesia* **62** D1
Simferopol *Ukraine* **33** K8
Simi *Greece* **47** E9
Simi Valley *U.S.A.* **111** L8
Simien Mts. △ *Ethiopia* **81** E4
Simikot *Nepal* **69** E9
Simineh → *Iran* **73** D11
Simitli *Bulgaria* **44** E7
Simla = Shimla *India* **68** D7
Simlångsdalen *Sweden* **11** H7
Şimleu-Silvaniei *Romania* **28** C7
Simlipal △ *India* **69** J12
Simmern *Germany* **25** F3
Simmie *Canada* **103** D7
Simmler *U.S.A.* **111** K7
Simnas *Lithuania* **30** D10
Simo älv = Simojoki → *Finland* **8** D21
Simojoki → *Finland* **8** D21
Simojovel *Mexico* **119** D6
Simonette → *Canada* **102** B5
Simonstown *S. Africa* **88** E2
Simontornya *Hungary* **28** D3
Simpang Empat *Malaysia* **65** c
Simplonpass *Switz.* **25** J4
Simplontunnel *Switz.* **25** J4
Simpson Desert *Australia* **94** D2
Simpson Desert △ *Australia* **94** C2
Simpson Pen. *Canada* **101** D14
Simrishamn *Sweden* **11** J8
Simsbury *U.S.A.* **115** E12
Simushir, Ostrov *Russia* **53** E16
Sin Cowe I. *S. China Sea* **62** C4
Sina Dhago *Somali Rep.* **75** F4
Sinabang *Indonesia* **62** D1
Sinai = Es Sînâ' *Egypt* **74** F3
Sinai, Mt. = Mûsa, Gebel *Egypt* **70** D2
Sinaia *Romania* **29** E10
Sinaloa □ *Mexico* **118** C3
Sinaloa de Leyva *Mexico* **118** B3
Sinalunga *Italy* **41** E8
Sinan *China* **58** D7
Sînandrei *Romania* **28** E6
Sinarades *Greece* **49** A3
Sincan *Turkey* **72** B5
Sincanlı *Turkey* **47** C12
Sincelejo *Colombia* **124** B3
Sinch'ang *N. Korea* **57** D15
Sinch'ŏn *N. Korea* **57** E13
Sinclair *U.S.A.* **108** F10
Sinclair Mills *Canada* **102** C4
Sinclair's B. *U.K.* **13** C5
Sinclairville *U.S.A.* **114** D5
Sincorá, Serra do *Brazil* **125** F10
Sind = Sindh □ *Pakistan* **68** G3
Sind → *Jammu & Kashmir, India* **69** B6
Sind → *Mad. P., India* **69** F8
Sind Sagar Doab *Pakistan* **68** D4
Sindal *Denmark* **11** G4
Sindangan *Phil.* **61** G5
Sindangbarang *Indonesia* **63** G12

Sinde *Zambia* **87** F2
Sindelfingen *Germany* **25** G4
Sindh = Indus → *Pakistan* **68** G2
Sindh □ *Pakistan* **68** G3
Sındırgı *Turkey* **47** B10
Sindou *Burkina Faso* **82** C3
Sindri *India* **69** H12
Sine → *Senegal* **82** C1
Sinegorskiy *Russia* **35** G5
Sinekli *Turkey* **45** E12
Sinelnikovo = Synelnykove *Ukraine* **33** H8
Sinendé *Benin* **83** C5
Sines *Portugal* **37** H2
Sines, C. de *Portugal* **37** H2
Sineu *Spain* **48** B10
Sinfra *Ivory C.* **82** D3
Sing Buri *Thailand* **64** E3
Singa *Sudan* **81** E3
Singalila △ *India* **69** F13
Singapore ■ *Asia* **65** d
Singapore, Straits of *Asia* **65** d
Singapore Changi ✈ (SIN) *Singapore* **65** M4
Singaraja *Indonesia* **62** F5
Singatoka = Sigatoka *Fiji* **91** a
Singen *Germany* **25** H4
Singida *Tanzania* **86** C3
Singida □ *Tanzania* **86** D3
Singkaling Hkamti *Burma* **67** G19
Singkang *Indonesia* **63** E6
Singkawang *Indonesia* **62** D3
Singkep *Indonesia* **62** E2
Singkil *Indonesia* **65** L1
Singleton *Australia* **95** E5
Singleton, Mt. *N. Terr., Australia* **92** D5
Singleton, Mt. *W. Austral., Australia* **93** E2
Singö *Sweden* **10** D12
Singoli *India* **68** G6
Singora = Songkhla *Thailand* **65** J3
Sinhung *N. Korea* **57** D14
Siniscóla *Italy* **42** B2
Sinj *Croatia* **41** E13
Sinjai *Indonesia* **63** F6
Sinjār *Iraq* **73** D9
Sinjar, Jabal *Iraq* **73** D9
Sinkat *Sudan* **80** D4
Sinkiang = Xinjiang Uygur Zizhiqu □ *China* **60** B3
Sinko *Guinea* **82** D3
Sinmak *N. Korea* **57** E14
Sinmi-do *N. Korea* **57** E13
Sínnai *Italy* **42** C2
Sinnamary *Fr. Guiana* **125** B8
Sinni → *Italy* **43** B9
Sinnuris *Egypt* **80** J7
Sinoie, Lacul *Romania* **29** F13
Sinop *Turkey* **72** A6
Sinop □ *Turkey* **72** B6
Sinor *India* **68** J5
Sinp'o *N. Korea* **57** E15
Sinsheim *Germany* **25** F4
Sinsk *Russia* **53** C13
Sintang *Indonesia* **62** D4
Sinton *U.S.A.* **116** G6
Sintra *Portugal* **37** G1
Sintra-Cascais △ *Portugal* **37** G1
Sinŭiju *N. Korea* **57** D13
Sinyukha → *Ukraine* **33** H6
Sinzig *Germany* **24** E3
Sio → *Hungary* **28** D3
Siocon *Phil.* **61** H5
Siófok *Hungary* **28** D3
Sion *Switz.* **25** J3
Sion Mills *U.K.* **12** B4
Sionainn = Shannon → *Ireland* **12** D5
Sioux Center *U.S.A.* **112** D5
Sioux City *U.S.A.* **112** D5
Sioux Falls *U.S.A.* **112** D5
Sioux Lookout *Canada* **104** B1
Sioux Narrows *Canada* **103** D10
Sipadan *Malaysia* **63** D5
Sipalay *Phil.* **61** G5
Šipan *Croatia* **44** D1
Siparia *Trin. & Tob.* **125** K15
Sipil Dağı △ *Turkey* **47** C9
Siping *China* **57** C13
Sipiwesk L. *Canada* **103** B9
Siple *Antarctica* **5** D7
Sipra → *India* **68** H6
Sipura *Indonesia* **62** E1
Siquia → *Nic.* **120** D3
Siquijor *Phil.* **61** G6
Siquirres *Costa Rica* **120** D3
Şır Abu Nu'ayr *U.A.E.* **71** E7
Şır Banī Yās *U.A.E.* **71** E7
Sir Edward Pellew Group *Australia* **94** B2
Sir Graham Moore Is. *Australia* **92** B4
Sir James MacBrien, Mt. *Canada* **100** E6
Sira → *Norway* **9** G12
Siracusa *Italy* **43** E8
Sirajganj *Bangla.* **69** G13

Sirakoro *Mali* **82** C3
Şiran *Turkey* **73** B8
Sirasso *Ivory C.* **82** D3
Sirathu *India* **69** G9
Sīrdān *Iran* **73** D13
Sire *Ethiopia* **81** F4
Siren *U.S.A.* **112** C7
Sirente-Velino △ *Italy* **41** F10
Sirer *Spain* **48** C7
Siret *Romania* **29** C11
Siret → *Romania* **29** E12
Sirghāyā *Syria* **74** B5
Şiria *Romania* **28** D6
Sirinat △ *Thailand* **65** a
Sirino, Mte. *Italy* **43** B8
Şırjān *Iran* **71** D7
Sirmaur *India* **69** G9
Sirmilik △ *Canada* **101** C15
Sirna *Greece* **47** E8
Şırnak *Turkey* **73** D10
Sirohi *India* **68** G5
Sironj *India* **68** G7
Síros = Ermoupoli *Greece* **46** D6
Sirr, Nafud as *Si. Arabia* **70** E5
Sirretta Pk. *U.S.A.* **111** K8
Sīrrī *Iran* **71** E7
Sirsa *India* **68** E6
Sirsa → *India* **69** F8
Siruela *Spain* **37** G5
Sirvän → *Iran* **73** E12
Sisak *Croatia* **41** C13
Sisaket *Thailand* **64** E5
Sisante *Spain* **39** F2
Sisargas, Is. *Spain* **36** B2
Sishen *S. Africa* **88** D3
Sishui *Henan, China* **56** G7
Sishui *Shandong, China* **57** G9
Sisian *Armenia* **73** C12
Sisipuk L. *Canada* **103** B8
Sisophon *Cambodia* **64** F4
Sisseton *U.S.A.* **112** C5
Sissonne *France* **19** C10
Sīstān *Asia* **71** D9
Sīstān, Daryācheh-ye *Iran* **71** D9
Sīstān va Balūchestān □ *Iran* **71** E9
Sisteron *France* **21** D9
Sisters *U.S.A.* **108** D3
Sisters, The *Seychelles* **85** b
Siswa Bazar *India* **69** F10
Sitakili *Mali* **82** C3
Sitamarhi *India* **69** F11
Sitampiky *Madag.* **89** B8
Sitapur *India* **69** F9
Siteki *Swaziland* **89** D5
Sitges *Spain* **38** D6
Sithonia *Greece* **44** F7
Sitia *Greece* **49** D8
Sitito-Ozima Ridge *Pac. Oc.* **96** E6
Sitka *U.S.A.* **102** B1
Sitoti *Botswana* **88** B3
Sitra *Egypt* **80** B2
Sittang Myit → *Burma* **67** L20
Sittard *Neths.* **17** C5
Sittensen *Germany* **24** B5
Sittingbourne *U.K.* **15** F8
Sittona *Eritrea* **81** E4
Sittoung = Sittang Myit → *Burma* **67** L20
Sittwe *Burma* **67** J18
Situbondo *Indonesia* **63** G16
Si'umu *Samoa* **91** b
Siuna *Nic.* **120** D3
Siuri *India* **69** H12
Siutghiol, Lacul *Romania* **29** F13
Sīvand *Iran* **71** D7
Sivas *Turkey* **72** C7
Sivas □ *Turkey* **72** C7
Sivash *Turkey* **47** C11
Siverek *Turkey* **73** D8
Sivrihisar *Turkey* **72** C4
Sîwa *Egypt* **80** B2
Sîwa, El Wâhât es *Egypt* **80** B2
Sîwa Oasis = Sîwa, El Wâhât es *Egypt* **80** B2
Siwalik Range *Nepal* **69** F10
Siwan *India* **69** F11
Siwana *India* **68** G5
Six Cross Roads *Barbados* **121** g
Sixmilebridge *Ireland* **12** D3
Sixth Cataract *Sudan* **81** D3
Siyah Kuh, Kavīr-e *Iran* **71** C7
Siyâl, Jazâ'ir *Egypt* **80** C4
Siyäzän *Azerbaijan* **35** K9
Siziwang Qi *China* **56** D6
Sjælland *Denmark* **11** J5
Sjælland □ *Denmark* **11** J5
Sjællands Odde *Denmark* **11** J5
Sjenica *Serbia* **44** C3
Sjöbo *Sweden* **11** J7
Sjötofta *Sweden* **11** G7
Sjötorp *Sweden* **11** F7
Sjumen = Shumen *Bulgaria* **45** C10
Sjuntorp *Sweden* **11** F6
Skadarsko Jezero *Europe* **44** D3
Skadarsko Jezero △ *Montenegro* **44** D3
Skadovsk *Ukraine* **33** J7
Skælskør *Denmark* **11** J5
Skærbæk *Denmark* **11** J2

Skaftafell *Iceland* **8** D5
Skaftafell △ *Iceland* **8** D5
Skagafjörður *Iceland* **8** D4
Skagastølstindane *Norway* **8** F12
Skagaströnd *Iceland* **8** D3
Skagen *Denmark* **11** G4
Skagern *Sweden* **10** E8
Skagerrak *Denmark* **11** G2
Skagit → *U.S.A.* **110** B4
Skagway *U.S.A.* **100** F4
Skala-Podilska *Ukraine* **29** B11
Skalat *Ukraine* **23** D13
Skalbmierz *Poland* **31** H7
Skälderviken *Sweden* **11** H6
Skalica *Slovak Rep.* **27** C10
Skalni Dol = Kamenyak *Bulgaria* **45** C10
Skanderborg *Denmark* **11** H3
Skåne *Sweden* **11** J7
Skåne län □ *Sweden* **11** H7
Skaneateles *U.S.A.* **115** D8
Skaneateles L. *U.S.A.* **115** D8
Skänninge *Sweden* **11** F9
Skänör med Falsterbo *Sweden* **11** J6
Skantzoura *Greece* **46** B6
Skara *Sweden* **11** F7
Skärblacka *Sweden* **11** F9
Skardu *Pakistan* **69** B6
Skåre *Sweden* **10** E7
Skärhamn *Sweden* **11** G5
Skarszewy *Poland* **30** D5
Skaryszew *Poland* **31** G8
Skarżysko-Kamienna *Poland* **31** G7
Skattkärr *Sweden* **10** E7
Skattungbyn *Sweden* **10** C8
Skawina *Poland* **31** J6
Skebobruk *Sweden* **10** E12
Skeena → *Canada* **102** C2
Skeena Mts. *Canada* **102** B3
Skegness *U.K.* **14** D8
Skeldon = Corriverton *Guyana* **124** B7
Skeleton Coast *Namibia* **85** J2
Skeleton Coast △ *Namibia* **88** C1
Skellefteå *Sweden* **8** D19
Skellefteälven → *Sweden* **8** D19
Skelleftehamn *Sweden* **8** D19
Skender Vakuf *Bos.-H.* **28** F2
Skerries, The *U.K.* **14** D3
Skhidnytsya *Ukraine* **31** J10
Skhiza *Greece* **46** E3
Ski *Norway* **9** G14
Skiathos *Greece* **46** B5
Skibbereen *Ireland* **12** E2
Skiddaw *U.K.* **14** C4
Skidegate *Canada* **102** C2
Skidra *Greece* **44** F6
Skien *Norway* **9** G13
Skierniewice *Poland* **31** G7
Skihist, Mt. *Canada* **102** C4
Skikda *Algeria* **78** A7
Skillingaryd *Sweden* **11** G8
Skillinge *Sweden* **11** J8
Skilloura *Cyprus* **49** D12
Skinari, Akra *Greece* **46** D2
Skinnskatteberg *Sweden* **10** E9
Skipton *U.K.* **14** D5
Skiring, C. *Senegal* **82** C1
Skirmish Pt. *Australia* **94** A1
Skíros = Skiros *Greece* **46** C6
Skiropoula *Greece* **46** C6
Skiros *Greece* **46** C6
Skivarp *Sweden* **11** J7
Skive *Denmark* **11** H3
Skjálfandafljót → *Iceland* **8** D5
Skjálfandi *Iceland* **8** C5
Skjern *Denmark* **11** J2
Škofja Loka *Slovenia* **41** B11
Skoghall *Sweden* **10** E7
Skogstorp *Sweden* **10** E10
Skoki *Poland* **31** F4
Skole *Ukraine* **23** D12
Skopelos *Greece* **46** B5
Skopi *Greece* **49** D8
Skopin *Russia* **32** F10
Skopje *Macedonia* **44** D5
Skopje ✈ (SKP) *Macedonia* **44** E5
Skórcz *Poland* **30** E5
Skovorodino *Russia* **53** D13
Skowhegan *U.S.A.* **113** C19
Skradin *Croatia* **41** E12
Skrea *Sweden* **11** H6
Skrunda *Latvia* **30** B9
Skrwa → *Poland* **31** F6
Skuleskogen △ *Sweden* **10** A12
Skull *Ireland* **12** E2
Skultorp *Sweden* **11** F7
Skultuna *Sweden* **10** E10
Skunk → *U.S.A.* **112** E9
Skuodas *Lithuania* **30** B8
Skurup *Sweden* **11** J7
Skutskär *Sweden* **10** D11
Skvyra *Ukraine* **23** D15
Skwierzyna *Poland* **31** F2
Skye *U.K.* **13** D2
Skykomish *U.S.A.* **108** C3
Skyros = Skiros *Greece* **46** C6

Skyttorp *Sweden* **10** D11
Slade Point *Australia* **94** b
Slade Pt. *Australia* **94** b
Slættaratindur *Færoe Is.* **8** E9
Slagelse *Denmark* **11** J5
Slamet *Indonesia* **63** G13
Slane *Ireland* **12** C5
Slaney → *Ireland* **12** D5
Slangberge *S. Africa* **88** E3
Slănic *Romania* **29** E11
Slano *Croatia* **44** D1
Slantsy *Russia* **32** C5
Slaný *Czech Rep.* **26** A7
Śląsk *Poland* **22** C3
Śląskie □ *Poland* **31** H6
Slätbaken *Sweden* **11** F10
Slate Is. *Canada* **104** C2
Slatina *Croatia* **28** E2
Slatina *Romania* **29** F9
Slatina Timiş *Romania* **28** E7
Slatington *U.S.A.* **115** F9
Slaton *U.S.A.* **116** E4
Slave → *Canada* **102** A6
Slave Coast *W. Afr.* **83** D5
Slave Lake *Canada* **102** B6
Slave Pt. *Canada* **102** A5
Slavgorod *Russia* **52** D8
Slavinja *Serbia* **44** C6
Slavkov u Brna *Czech Rep.* **27** B9
Slavkovský Les △ *Czech Rep.* **26** A5
Slavonia = Europe **28** E2
Slavonski Brod *Croatia* **28** E3
Slavsk *Russia* **30** C8
Slavska *Ukraine* **29** B8
Slavskoye *Russia* **30** D7
Slavuta *Ukraine* **23** C14
Slavyanka *Russia* **54** C5
Slavyanovo *Bulgaria* **45** C8
Slavyansk = Slovyansk *Ukraine* **33** H9
Slavyansk-na-Kubani *Russia* **33** K10
Sława *Poland* **31** G3
Slawharad *Belarus* **23** B16
Sławno *Poland* **30** D3
Sławoborze *Poland* **30** E2
Sleaford *U.K.* **14** D7
Sleaford B. *Australia* **95** E2
Sleat, Sd. of *U.K.* **13** D3
Sleeper Is. *Canada* **101** F15
Sleeping Bear Dunes △ *U.S.A.* **112** C10
Sleepy Eye *U.S.A.* **112** C6
Slemon L. *Canada* **102** A5
Ślesin *Poland* **31** F5
Slide Mt. *U.S.A.* **115** E10
Slidell *U.S.A.* **117** F10
Sliema *Malta* **49** D2
Sligo *Ireland* **12** B3
Sligo *U.S.A.* **114** E5
Sligo □ *Ireland* **12** B3
Sligo B. *Ireland* **12** B3
Slippery Rock *U.S.A.* **114** E4
Slite *Sweden* **11** G12
Slīteres △ *Latvia* **30** A9
Sliven *Bulgaria* **45** D10
Slivnitsa *Bulgaria* **44** D7
Sljeme *Croatia* **41** C12
Sloan *U.S.A.* **111** K11
Sloansville *U.S.A.* **115** D10
Slobidka *Ukraine* **29** C14
Slobozia *Moldova* **29** D14
Slobozia *Argeş, Romania* **29** F10
Slobozia *Ialomiţa, Romania* **29** F12
Slocan *Canada* **102** D5
Słomniki *Poland* **31** H7
Slonim *Belarus* **23** B13
Slough *U.K.* **15** F7
Slough □ *U.K.* **15** F7
Sloughhouse *U.S.A.* **110** G5
Slovak Rep. ■ *Europe* **27** C13
Slovakia = Slovak Rep. ■ *Europe* **27** C13
Slovakian Ore Mts. = Slovenské Rudohorie *Slovak Rep.* **27** C12
Slovenia ■ *Europe* **41** C11
Slovenija = Slovenia ■ *Europe* **41** C11
Slovenj Gradec *Slovenia* **41** B12
Slovenska = Slovak Rep. ■ *Europe* **27** C13
Slovenska Bistrica *Slovenia* **41** B12
Slovenské Konjice *Slovenia* **41** B12
Slovenské Rudohorie *Slovak Rep.* **27** C12
Slovenský Raj △ *Slovak Rep.* **27** C13
Slovyansk *Ukraine* **33** H9
Słowiński △ *Poland* **30** D4
Słubice *Poland* **31** F1
Sluch → *Ukraine* **23** C14

Sluis *Neths.* **17** C3
Slŭnchev Bryag *Bulgaria* **45** D11
Slunj *Croatia* **41** C12
Słupca *Poland* **31** F4
Słupia → *Poland* **30** D4
Słupsk *Poland* **30** D4
Slurry *S. Africa* **88** D4
Slutsk *Belarus* **23** B14
Slyne Hd. *Ireland* **12** C1
Slyudyanka *Russia* **53** D11
Småland *Sweden* **11** G9
Smålandsfarvandet *Denmark* **11** J5
Smålandsstenar *Sweden* **11** G7
Smalltree L. *Canada* **103** A8
Smallwood Res. *Canada* **105** B7
Smarhon *Belarus* **23** A14
Smarje *Slovenia* **41** B12
Smartt Syndicate Dam *S. Africa* **88** E3
Smartville *U.S.A.* **110** F5
Smeaton *Canada* **103** C8
Smedby *Sweden* **11** H10
Smederevo *Serbia* **44** B4
Smederevska Palanka *Serbia* **44** B4
Smedjebacken *Sweden* **10** D9
Smela = Smila *Ukraine* **33** H6
Smerwick Harbour *Ireland* **12** D1
Smethport *U.S.A.* **114** E6
Smidovich *Russia* **53** E14
Śmigiel *Poland* **31** F3
Smila *Ukraine* **33** H6
Smilyan *Bulgaria* **45** E8
Smith *Canada* **102** B6
Smith Center *U.S.A.* **112** F4
Smith I. *Canada* **101** E16
Smith Islands △ *Australia* **94** b
Smith River *Canada* **102** F2
Smithburne → *Australia* **94** B3
Smithers *Canada* **102** C3
Smithfield *S. Africa* **89** E4
Smithfield *N.C., U.S.A.* **117** D15
Smithfield *Utah, U.S.A.* **108** F8
Smiths Falls *Canada* **115** B9
Smithton *Australia* **95** G4
Smithville *Canada* **114** C5
Smithville *U.S.A.* **116** F6
Smoke Creek Desert *U.S.A.* **108** F4
Smoky → *Canada* **102** B5
Smoky Bay *Australia* **95** E1
Smoky Hill → *U.S.A.* **112** F5
Smoky Hills *U.S.A.* **112** F4
Smoky Lake *Canada* **102** C6
Smøla *Norway* **8** E13
Smolensk *Russia* **32** E7
Smolensk □ *Russia* **32** E7
Smolikas, Oros *Greece* **44** F4
Smolník *Slovak Rep.* **27** C13
Smolyan *Bulgaria* **45** E8
Smooth Rock Falls *Canada* **104** C3
Smoothstone L. *Canada* **103** C7
Smorgon = Smarhon *Belarus* **23** A14
Smotrych *Ukraine* **29** B11
Smotrych → *Ukraine* **29** B11
Smulţi *Romania* **29** E12
Smyadovo *Bulgaria* **45** C11
Smygehamn *Sweden* **11** J7
Smyrna = İzmir *Turkey* **47** C9
Smyrna *U.S.A.* **113** F16
Snæfell *Iceland* **8** D6
Snaefell *I. of Man* **14** C3
Snæfellsjökull *Iceland* **8** D2
Snake → *U.S.A.* **108** C4
Snake I. *Australia* **95** F4
Snake Range *U.S.A.* **108** G6
Snake River Plain *U.S.A.* **108** E7
Snasahögarna *Sweden* **10** A6
Snåsavatnet *Norway* **8** D15
Snedsted *Denmark* **11** H2
Sneek *Neths.* **17** A5
Sneem *Ireland* **12** E2
Sneeuberge *S. Africa* **88** E3
Snejbjerg *Denmark* **11** H2
Snelling *U.S.A.* **110** H6
Snezhnoye *Ukraine* **33** J10
Snežka *Europe* **31** A8
Sneznik *Slovenia* **41** C11
Śniadowo *Poland* **31** E8
Sniardwy, Jezioro *Poland* **30** C9
Śnieżka *Europe* **26** A8
Snigirevka = Snihurivka *Ukraine* **33** J7
Snihurivka *Ukraine* **33** J7
Snina *Slovak Rep.* **27** C15
Snizort, L. *U.K.* **13** D2
Snøhetta *Norway* **8** E13
Snohomish *U.S.A.* **110** C4
Snoul *Cambodia* **65** F6
Snover *U.S.A.* **114** C2
Snow Hill *U.S.A.* **113** F16
Snow Lake *Canada* **103** C8
Snow Mt. *Calif., U.S.A.* **110** F4
Snow Mt. *Maine, U.S.A.* **115** A14
Snow Shoe *U.S.A.* **114** E7
Snowbird L. *Canada* **103** A8
Snowdon *U.K.* **14** D3
Snowdonia △ *U.K.* **14** D4
Snowdrift = Łutsel K'e *Canada* **103** A6

Snowdrift ⇜ *Canada* **103** A6
Snowflake *U.S.A.* **109** J8
Snowshoe Pk. *U.S.A.* **108** B6
Snowtown *Australia* **95** E2
Snowville *U.S.A.* **108** F7
Snowy ⇜ *Australia* **95** F4
Snowy Mt. *U.S.A.* **115** C10
Snowy Mts. *Australia* **95** F4
Snug Corner *Bahamas* **121** B5
Snug Harbour *Canada* **114** A4
Snyatyn *Ukraine* **29** B14
Snyder *Okla., U.S.A.* **116** D5
Snyder *Tex., U.S.A.* **116** E4
Soahanina *Madag.* **89** B7
Soalala *Madag.* **89** B8
Soaloka *Madag.* **89** B8
Soamanonga *Madag.* **89** C7
Soan ⇜ *Pakistan* **68** C4
Soanierana-Ivongo *Madag.* **89** B8
Soanindrariny *Madag.* **89** B8
Şoarş *Romania* **29** E9
Soavina *Madag.* **89** C8
Soavinandriana *Madag.* **89** B8
Sob ⇜ *Ukraine* **29** B14
Soba *Nigeria* **83** C6
Sobat, Nahr ⇜ *Sudan* **81** F3
Soběslav *Czech Rep.* **26** B7
Sobhapur *India* **68** H8
Sobinka *Russia* **32** C11
Sobótka *Poland* **31** H3
Sobra *Croatia* **41** F14
Sobradinho, Represa de
　Brazil **125** E10
Sobral *Brazil* **125** D10
Sobrance *Slovak Rep.* **27** C15
Sobreira Formosa *Portugal* **36** F3
Soc Giang *Vietnam* **58** F6
Soc Trang *Vietnam* **65** H5
Soča ⇜ *Europe* **26** C6
Socastee *U.S.A.* **117** E15
Sochaczew *Poland* **31** F7
Soch'e = Shache *China* **60** C2
Sochi *Russia* **35** J4
Sochos *Greece* **44** F7
Société, Îs. de la
　French Polynesia **97** J12
Society Is. = Société, Îs. de
　la *French Polynesia* **97** J12
Socompa, Portezuelo de
　Chile **126** A2
Socorro *N. Mex., U.S.A.* **109** J10
Socorro *Tex., U.S.A.* **116** F1
Socorro, I. *Mexico* **118** D2
Socotra *Yemen* **75** E5
Socovos *Spain* **39** G3
Socuéllamos *Spain* **39** F2
Soda L. *U.S.A.* **109** J5
Soda Plains *India* **69** B8
Soda Springs *U.S.A.* **108** E8
Sodankylä *Finland* **8** C22
Soddy-Daisy *U.S.A.* **117** D12
Söderala *Sweden* **10** C10
Söderåsen △ *Sweden* **11** H7
Söderbärke *Sweden* **10** D9
Söderfors *Sweden* **10** D11
Söderhamn *Sweden* **10** C11
Söderköping *Sweden* **11** F10
Södermanland *Sweden* **9** G17
Södermanlands län □
　Sweden **10** E10
Södertälje *Sweden* **10** E11
Sodiri *Sudan* **81** E2
Sodo *Ethiopia* **81** F4
Södra Dellen *Sweden* **10** C10
Södra Finnskoga *Sweden* **10** D6
Södra Sandby *Sweden* **11** J7
Södra Ulvön *Sweden* **10** B12
Södra Vi *Sweden* **11** G9
Sodražica *Slovenia* **41** C11
Sodus *U.S.A.* **114** C7
Sodwana Bay △ *S. Africa* **89** D5
Soe *Indonesia* **92** A3
Soekmekaar = Morebeng
　S. Africa **89** C4
Soest *Germany* **24** D4
Soest *Neths.* **17** B5
Sofades *Greece* **46** B4
Sofala □ *Mozam.* **89** B5
Sofara *Mali* **82** C4
Sofia = Sofiya *Bulgaria* **44** D7
Sofia ⇜ *Madag.* **89** B8
Sofievka *Ukraine* **33** H7
Sofiko *Greece* **46** D5
Sofiya *Bulgaria* **44** D7
Sofiya □ *Bulgaria* **44** D7
Sofiya ✈ (SOF) *Bulgaria* **44** D7
Sofrana *Greece* **47** E8
Sōfu-Gan *Japan* **55** K10
Sogakofe *Ghana* **83** D5
Sogamoso *Colombia* **124** B4
Sogār *Iran* **71** E8
Sögel *Germany* **24** C3
Sogndalsfjøra *Norway* **8** F12
Søgne *Norway* **9** G12
Sognefjorden ⇜ *Norway* **8** F11
Söğüt *Bilecik, Turkey* **47** A12
Söğüt *Burdur, Turkey* **47** D11
Söğüt Dağı *Turkey* **47** D11
Söğütköy *Turkey* **47** E10
Soh *Iran* **71** C6

Sohâg *Egypt* **80** B3
Sohagpur *India* **68** H8
Soignies *Belgium* **17** D4
Soin *Burkina Faso* **82** C4
Soira *Eritrea* **81** E4
Soissons *France* **19** C10
Sōja *Japan* **55** G6
Sojat *India* **68** G5
Sok ⇜ *Russia* **34** D10
Sokal *Ukraine* **23** C13
Sokcho *S. Korea* **57** E15
Söke *Turkey* **47** D9
Sokelo *Dem. Rep. of the Congo* **87** D1
Sokhumi *Georgia* **35** J5
Soko Banja *Serbia* **44** C5
Sokodé *Togo* **83** D5
Sokol *Russia* **32** C11
Sokolac *Bos.-H.* **28** G3
Sokólka *Poland* **30** E10
Sokolo *Ségou, Mali* **82** C3
Sokolo *Sikasso, Mali* **82** C3
Sokolov *Czech Rep.* **26** A5
Sokolów Małopolski *Poland* **31** H9
Sokołów Podlaski *Poland* **31** F9
Sokoly *Poland* **31** F9
Sokoto *Nigeria* **83** C6
Sokoto □ *Nigeria* **83** C6
Sokoto ⇜ *Nigeria* **83** C5
Sokyrnytsya *Ukraine* **29** B8
Sokyryany *Ukraine* **29** B12
Sol Iletsk *Russia* **52** D6
Sola ⇜ *Poland* **31** H6
Solai *Kenya* **86** B4
Solan *India* **68** D7
Solana Beach *U.S.A.* **111** N9
Solano *Phil.* **61** C4
Solapur *India* **66** L9
Solca *Romania* **29** C10
Solda Gölü *Turkey* **47** D11
Soldānești *Moldova* **29** C13
Soldeu *Andorra* **38** C6
Soldotna *U.S.A.* **100** E1
Soléa *Cyprus* **49** D12
Solec Kujawski *Poland* **31** E5
Soledad *Colombia* **124** A4
Soledad *U.S.A.* **110** J5
Soledad *Venezuela* **124** B6
Solent, The *U.K.* **15** G6
Solenzara *France* **21** G13
Solesmes *France* **19** B10
Solfonntaggen *Norway* **9** F12
Solhan *Turkey* **73** C9
Soligorsk = Salihorsk
　Belarus **23** B14
Solihull *U.K.* **15** E6
Solikamsk *Russia* **52** D6
Solila *Madag.* **89** C8
Solimões = Amazonas ⇜
　S. Amer. **125** D8
Solin *Croatia* **41** E13
Solingen *Germany* **24** D3
Söll *Austria* **25** H8
Sollebrunn *Sweden* **11** F6
Sollefteå *Sweden* **10** A11
Sollentuna *Sweden* **10** E11
Sóller *Spain* **48** B9
Sollerön *Sweden* **10** D8
Solling *Germany* **24** D5
Solling-Vogler △ *Germany* **24** D5
Solnechnogorsk *Russia* **32** D9
Solo ⇜ *Indonesia* **63** G15
Solofra *Italy* **43** B7
Sologne *France* **19** E8
Solok *Indonesia* **62** E2
Sololá *Guatemala* **120** D1
Sololo *Kenya* **86** B4
Solomon, N. Fork ⇜ *U.S.A.* **112** F4
Solomon, S. Fork ⇜ *U.S.A.* **112** F4
Solomon Is. ■ *Pac. Oc.* **90** B8
Solomon Rise *Pac. Oc.* **96** G7
Solon *China* **60** B7
Solon Springs *U.S.A.* **112** B8
Solor *Indonesia* **63** F6
Solotcha *Russia* **32** E10
Solothurn *Switz.* **25** H3
Solothurn □ *Switz.* **25** H3
Solotvyn *Ukraine* **29** B9
Solsona *Spain* **38** C6
Solt *Hungary* **28** D4
Šolta *Croatia* **41** E13
Solṭānābād *Khorāsān, Iran* **71** C8
Solṭānābād *Khorāsān, Iran* **71** C8
Soltau *Germany* **24** C5
Soltsy *Russia* **32** C6
Solunska Glava *Macedonia* **44** E5
Solvang *U.S.A.* **111** L6
Solvay *U.S.A.* **115** D8
Sölvesborg *Sweden* **11** H8
Solwezi *Zambia* **87** E2
Sōma *Japan* **54** F10
Soma *Turkey* **47** B9
Somabhula *Zimbabwe* **89** B4
Somali Pen. *Africa* **76** F8
Somali Rep. ■ *Africa* **75** F4
Somalia = Somali Rep. ■
　Africa **75** F4
Somaliland □ *Somali Rep.* **75** F4
Sombernon *France* **19** E11

Sombor *Serbia* **28** E4
Sombra *Canada* **114** D2
Sombrerete *Mexico* **118** C4
Sombrero *Anguilla* **121** C7
Şomcuta Mare *Romania* **29** C8
Somdari *India* **68** G5
Someido △ *Spain* **36** B4
Somers *U.S.A.* **108** B6
Somerset *Ky., U.S.A.* **113** G11
Somerset *Mass., U.S.A.* **115** E13
Somerset *Pa., U.S.A.* **114** F5
Somerset □ *U.K.* **15** F5
Somerset East *S. Africa* **88** E4
Somerset I. *Canada* **100** C13
Somerset West *S. Africa* **88** E2
Somersworth *U.S.A.* **115** C14
Somerton *U.S.A.* **109** K6
Somerville *U.S.A.* **115** F10
Someş ⇜ *Romania* **28** C7
Someşul Mare ⇜ *Romania* **29** C8
Somme □ *France* **19** C9
Somme ⇜ *France* **19** B8
Somme, B. de la *France* **18** B8
Sommen *Jönköping, Sweden* **11** F8
Sommen *Östergötland, Sweden* **11** F9
Sommepy-Tahure *France* **19** C11
Sömmerda *Germany* **24** D7
Sommesous *France* **19** D11
Sommières *France* **21** E8
Somnath *India* **68** J4
Somogy □ *Hungary* **28** D2
Somogyszob *Hungary* **28** D2
Somosomo *Fiji* **91** a
Somosomo Str. *Fiji* **91** a
Somoto *Nic.* **120** D2
Sompolno *Poland* **31** F5
Somport, Tunnel de *Spain* **38** C4
Son ⇜ *India* **69** G11
Son Ha *Vietnam* **64** E7
Son Hoa *Vietnam* **64** F7
Son La *Vietnam* **58** G4
Son Morrell *Spain* **48** B10
Son Rapinya *Spain* **48** B9
Son Sardina *Spain* **48** B9
Son Serra *Spain* **48** B10
Son Servera *Spain* **38** F8
Son Tay *Vietnam* **58** G5
Soná *Panama* **120** E3
Sonamarg *India* **69** B6
Sonamukhi *India* **69** H12
Sonar ⇜ *India* **69** G8
Sŏnch'ŏn *N. Korea* **57** E13
Sondags ⇜ *S. Africa* **88** E4
Sóndalo *Italy* **40** B7
Sondar *India* **69** C6
Sønder Felding *Denmark* **11** J2
Sønder Omme *Denmark* **11** J2
Sønderborg *Denmark* **11** K3
Sondershausen *Germany* **24** D6
Sóndrio *Italy* **40** B6
Sone *Mozam.* **87** F3
Sonepur *India* **67** J13
Song *Nigeria* **83** D7
Song *Thailand* **64** C3
Song Cau *Vietnam* **64** F7
Song Hong = Hong ⇜ *Vietnam* **58** F5
Song Xian *China* **56** G7
Songan *Indonesia* **63** J18
Songea *Tanzania* **87** E4
Songeons *France* **19** C8
Songhua Hu *China* **57** C14
Songhua Jiang ⇜ *China* **60** B8
Songimvelo △ *S. Africa* **89** D5
Songjiang *China* **59** B13
Songjin = Kimch'aek
　N. Korea **57** D15
Songkan *China* **58** C6
Songkhla *Thailand* **65** J3
Songming *China* **58** E4
Songnim *N. Korea* **57** E13
Songo *Mozam.* **87** F3
Songo *Sudan* **79** G10
Songpan *China* **58** A4
Songtao *China* **58** C7
Songwe *Dem. Rep. of the Congo* **86** C2
Songwe ⇜ *Africa* **87** D3
Songxi *China* **59** D12
Songzi *China* **59** B8
Sonhat *India* **69** H10
Sonid Youqi *China* **56** C7
Sonipat *India* **68** E7
Sonkach *India* **68** H7
Sonkovo *Russia* **32** D9
Sonmiani *Pakistan* **68** G2
Sonmiani B. *Pakistan* **68** G2
Sonnino *Italy* **42** A6
Sono ⇜ *Brazil* **125** E9
Sonoma *U.S.A.* **110** G4
Sonora *Calif., U.S.A.* **110** H6
Sonora *Tex., U.S.A.* **116** F4
Sonora □ *Mexico* **118** B2
Sonora ⇜ *Mexico* **118** B2
Sonoran Desert *U.S.A.* **111** L12
Sonoyta *Mexico* **118** A2
Sonqor *Iran* **73** E12
Sonseca *Spain* **37** F7
Sonsonate *El Salv.* **120** D2
Sonstorp *Sweden* **11** F9
Sonthofen *Germany* **25** H6
Soochow = Suzhou *China* **59** B13

Sooke *Canada* **110** B3
Soomaaliya = Somali
　Rep. ■ *Africa* **75** F4
Sop Hao *Laos* **58** G5
Sop Prap *Thailand* **64** D2
Sopelana *Spain* **38** B2
Sopi *Indonesia* **63** D7
Sopo, Nahr ⇜ *Sudan* **81** F2
Sopot *Bulgaria* **45** D8
Sopot *Poland* **31** D5
Sopot *Serbia* **44** B4
Sopotnica *Macedonia* **44** E5
Sopron *Hungary* **28** C1
Sopur *India* **69** B6
Sør-Rondane *Antarctica* **5** D4
Sora *Italy* **41** G10
Sorah *Pakistan* **68** F3
Söråker *Sweden* **10** B11
Sorano *Italy* **40** C6
Soraon *India* **69** G9
Sorbas *Spain* **39** H2
Sörbygden *Sweden* **10** B10
Sord = Swords *Ireland* **12** C5
Sore *France* **20** D3
Sorel-Tracy *Canada* **104** C5
Soresina *Italy* **40** C6
Sörforsa *Sweden* **10** C10
Sórgono *Italy* **42** B2
Sorgues *France* **21** D8
Sorgun *Turkey* **72** C6
Soria *Spain* **38** D2
Soria □ *Spain* **38** D2
Soriano *Uruguay* **126** C4
Soriano nel Cimino *Italy* **41** F9
Sorkh, Kuh-e *Iran* **71** C8
Sorø *Denmark* **11** J5
Soro *Guinea* **82** C3
Soroca *Moldova* **29** B13
Sorocaba *Brazil* **127** A6
Soroki = Soroca *Moldova* **29** B13
Sorong *Indonesia* **63** E8
Soroni *Greece* **49** C10
Soroti *Uganda* **86** B3
Sørøya *Norway* **8** A20
Sørøysundet *Norway* **8** A20
Sorraia ⇜ *Portugal* **37** G2
Sorrell *Australia* **95** G4
Sorrento *Italy* **43** B7
Sorsele *Sweden* **8** D17
Sörsjön *Sweden* **10** C7
Sorso *Italy* **42** B1
Sorsogon *Phil.* **61** E6
Sortavala *Russia* **32** B6
Sortino *Italy* **43** E8
Sortland *Norway* **8** B16
Sortot *Sudan* **80** D3
Sorvizhi *Russia* **34** B9
Sos del Rey Católico *Spain* **38** C3
Soscumica, L. *Canada* **104** B4
Sösdala *Sweden* **11** H7
Sosna ⇜ *Russia* **33** F10
Sosnovka *Kirov, Russia* **34** B10
Sosnovka *Tambov, Russia* **34** D5
Sosnovyy Bor *Russia* **32** C5
Sosnowiec *Poland* **31** H6
Sospel *France* **21** E11
Sossus Vlei *Namibia* **88** C2
Šoštanj *Slovenia* **41** B12
Sōsura *N. Korea* **57** C16
Sot ⇜ *India* **69** F8
Sotavento *C. Verde Is.* **78** b
Sotik *Kenya* **86** C4
Sotkamo *Finland* **8** D23
Soto del Barco *Spain* **36** B4
Soto la Marina *Mexico* **119** C5
Soto la Marina ⇜ *Mexico* **119** C5
Soto y Amío *Spain* **36** C5
Sotouboua *Togo* **83** D5
Sotrondio *Spain* **36** B5
Sotuta *Mexico* **119** C7
Souanké *Congo* **84** D2
Soubré *Ivory C.* **82** D3
Souda *Greece* **49** D6
Soudas, Ormos *Greece* **49** D6
Souderton *U.S.A.* **115** F9
Soufli *Greece* **45** E10
Soufrière *Guadeloupe* **120** b
Soufrière *St. Lucia* **121** f
Soufrière Bay *Dominica* **121** f
Souillac *France* **20** D5
Souilly *France* **19** C12
Soukhouma *Laos* **64** E5
Sŏul = Seoul *S. Korea* **57** F14
Soulac-sur-Mer *France* **20** C2
Soulougou *Burkina Faso* **83** C5
Soultz-sous-Forêts *France* **19** D14
Sound, The = Øresund
　Europe **11** J6
Sound, The *U.K.* **15** G3
Sounio, Akra *Greece* **46** D6
Sources, Mt. aux *Lesotho* **89** D4
Soure *Brazil* **125** D9
Soure *Portugal* **36** E2
Souris *Man., Canada* **103** D8
Souris *P.E.I., Canada* **105** C7
Souris ⇜ *N. Amer.* **112** A4
Sourou *Africa* **82** C4
Sourpi *Greece* **46** B4
Sousa *Brazil* **125** E11
Sousel *Portugal* **37** G3

Sousse *Tunisia* **79** A8
Soustons *France* **20** E2
Sout ⇜ *S. Africa* **88** E2
South Africa ■ *Africa* **88** E3
South America **122** E5
South Aulatsivik I. *Canada* **105** A7
South Australia □ *Australia* **95** E2
South Australian Basin
　Ind. Oc. **96** L4
South Ayrshire □ *U.K.* **13** F4
South Baldy Pk. *U.S.A.* **109** J10
South Bass I. *U.S.A.* **114** E2
South Bend *Ind., U.S.A.* **112** E10
South Bend *Wash., U.S.A.* **110** D3
South Boston *U.S.A.* **113** G14
South Branch *Canada* **105** C8
South Brook *Canada* **105** C8
South Bruny I. *Australia* **95** G4
South Carolina □ *U.S.A.* **117** E14
South Charleston *U.S.A.* **113** F13
South China Sea *Asia* **62** C4
South Cumberland Is. △
　Australia **94** b
South Dakota □ *U.S.A.* **112** C4
South Dayton *U.S.A.* **114** D5
South Deerfield *U.S.A.* **115** D12
South Downs *U.K.* **15** G7
South East C. *Australia* **95** G4
South East Is. *Australia* **93** F3
South Esk ⇜ *U.K.* **13** E6
South Fiji Basin *Pac. Oc.* **96** K9
South Foreland *U.K.* **15** F9
South Fork American ⇜
　U.S.A. **110** G5
South Fork Feather ⇜
　U.S.A. **110** F5
South Fork Grand ⇜
　U.S.A. **112** C2
South Fork Milk ⇜ *U.S.A.* **108** B10
South Fork Republican ⇜
　U.S.A. **112** E3
South Georgia *Antarctica* **128** G9
South Gloucestershire □
　U.K. **15** F5
South Hadley *U.S.A.* **115** D12
South Haven *U.S.A.* **112** D10
South Henik L. *Canada* **103** A9
South Horr *Kenya* **86** B4
South I. *Kenya* **86** B4
South I. *N.Z.* **91** F3
South Indian Lake *Canada* **103** B9
South Invercargill *N.Z.* **91** G2
South Island △ *Kenya* **86** B4
South Kitui △ *Kenya* **86** C4
South Knife ⇜ *Canada* **103** B10
South Koel ⇜ *India* **69** H11
South Korea ■ *Asia* **57** G15
South Lake Tahoe *U.S.A.* **110** G6
South Lanarkshire □ *U.K.* **13** F5
South Loup ⇜ *U.S.A.* **112** E4
South Luangwa △ *Zambia* **87** E3
South Magnetic Pole
　Antarctica **5** C9
South Milwaukee *U.S.A.* **112** D10
South Molton *U.K.* **15** F4
South Moose L. *Canada* **103** C8
South Nahanni ⇜ *Canada* **102** A4
South Nation ⇜ *Canada* **115** A9
South Natuna Is. = Natuna
　Selatan, Kepulauan
　Indonesia **62** D3
South Negril Pt. *Jamaica* **120** a
South Orkney Is. *Antarctica* **5** C18
South Ossetia □ *Georgia* **35** J7
South Ostselic *U.S.A.* **115** D9
South Pagai, I. = Pagai
　Selatan, Pulau *Indonesia* **62** E2
South Paris *U.S.A.* **115** B14
South Pittsburg *U.S.A.* **117** D12
South Platte ⇜ *U.S.A.* **112** E3
South Pole *Antarctica* **5** E
South Porcupine *Canada* **104** C3
South Portland *U.S.A.* **113** D18
South Pt. *Barbados* **121** g
South Pt. *U.S.A.* **114** B1
South River *Canada* **104** C4
South River *U.S.A.* **115** F10
South Ronaldsay *U.K.* **13** C6
South Rukuru ⇜ *Malawi* **87** E3
South Sandwich Is. *Antarctica* **5** B1
South Sandwich Trench
　Atl. Oc. **5** B1
South Saskatchewan ⇜
　Canada **103** C7
South Seal ⇜ *Canada* **103** B9
South Shetland Is. *Antarctica* **5** C18
South Shields *U.K.* **14** C6
South Sioux City *U.S.A.* **112** D5
South Sister *U.S.A.* **108** D3
South Talpatti = New
　Moore I. *India* **69** J13
South Taranaki Bight *N.Z.* **91** E4
South Tasman Rise *S. Ocean* **5** A10
South Thompson ⇜ *Canada* **102** C4
South Twin I. *Canada* **104** B4
South Tyne ⇜ *U.K.* **14** C5
South Uist □ *U.K.* **13** D1
South Valley *U.S.A.* **109** J10
South Wellesley Is. *Australia* **94** B2
South West C. *Australia* **95** G4

South West C. *N.Z.* **91** G1
South Williamsport *U.S.A.* **114** E8
South Yorkshire □ *U.K.* **14** D6
Southampton *Canada* **114** B3
Southampton *U.K.* **15** G6
Southampton *U.S.A.* **115** F12
Southampton □ *U.K.* **15** G6
Southampton I. *Canada* **101** E15
Southaven *U.S.A.* **117** D9
Southbank *Canada* **102** C3
Southbridge *N.Z.* **91** E4
Southbridge *U.S.A.* **115** D12
Southend *Canada* **103** B8
Southend-on-Sea *U.K.* **15** F8
Southend-on-Sea □ *U.K.* **15** F8
Southern = Janub □ *Sudan* **81** F2
Southern = Yedebub
　Biheroch Bihereseboch
　na Hizboch □ *Ethiopia* **81** F4
Southern = Yuzhnyy □
　Russia **35** H5
Southern □ *Malawi* **87** F4
Southern □ *S. Leone* **82** D2
Southern □ *Zambia* **87** F2
Southern Alps *N.Z.* **91** E3
Southern Cross *Australia* **93** F2
Southern Indian L. *Canada* **103** B9
Southern Lau Group *Fiji* **91** a
Southern Ocean *Antarctica* **5** C6
Southern Pines *U.S.A.* **117** D15
Southern Uplands *U.K.* **13** F5
Southington *U.S.A.* **115** E12
Southland □ *N.Z.* **91** F1
Southold *U.S.A.* **115** E12
Southport *Australia* **95** D5
Southport *U.K.* **14** D4
Southport *U.S.A.* **114** D8
Southwest △ *Australia* **95** G4
Southwest Pacific Basin
　Pac. Oc. **5** A12
Southwold *U.K.* **15** E9
Southwood △ *Australia* **95** D5
Soutpansberg *S. Africa* **89** C4
Souvigny *France* **19** F9
Sovata *Romania* **29** D10
Soverato *Italy* **43** D9
Sovetsk *Kaliningrad, Russia* **30** C8
Sovetsk *Kirov, Russia* **34** B9
Sovetskaya Gavan *Russia* **53** E15
Sovicille *Italy* **41** E8
Soweto *S. Africa* **89** D4
Sowma'eh Sarā *Iran* **73** D13
Soyaux *France* **20** C4
Soyo *Angola* **84** F2
Sozh ⇜ *Belarus* **23** B16
Sozopol *Bulgaria* **45** D11
Spa *Belgium* **17** D5
Spain ■ *Europe* **7** H5
Spalding *Australia* **95** E2
Spalding *U.K.* **14** E7
Spanaway *U.S.A.* **110** C4
Spangler *U.S.A.* **114** F6
Spanish *Canada* **104** C3
Spanish Fork *U.S.A.* **108** F8
Spanish Town *Br. Virgin Is.* **121** e
Spanish Town *Jamaica* **120** a
Sparks *U.S.A.* **110** F7
Sparreholm *Sweden* **10** E10
Sparta = Sparti *Greece* **46** D4
Sparta *Mich., U.S.A.* **113** D11
Sparta *N.J., U.S.A.* **115** E10
Sparta *Wis., U.S.A.* **112** D8
Spartanburg *U.S.A.* **117** D14
Sparti *Greece* **46** D4
Spartivento, C. *Calabria, Italy* **43** F3
Spartivento, C. *Sard., Italy* **42** D1
Sparwood *Canada* **102** D6
Spas-Demensk *Russia* **32** E7
Spas-Klepiki *Russia* **32** E11
Spassk Dalniy *Russia* **54** B6
Spassk-Ryazanskiy *Russia* **32** E11
Spatha, Akra *Greece* **49** D5
Spatsizi ⇜ *Canada* **102** B3
Spatsizi Plateau
　Wilderness △ *Canada* **102** B3
Spean ⇜ *U.K.* **13** E4
Spearfish *U.S.A.* **112** C2
Spearman *U.S.A.* **116** C4
Speculator *U.S.A.* **115** C10
Speia *Moldova* **29** D14
Speightstown *Barbados* **121** g
Speke Gulf *Tanzania* **86** C3
Spello *Italy* **41** F9
Spence Bay = Taloyoak
　Canada **100** D13
Spencer *Idaho, U.S.A.* **108** D7
Spencer *Iowa, U.S.A.* **112** D6
Spencer *N.Y., U.S.A.* **115** D8
Spencer *Nebr., U.S.A.* **112** D4
Spencer, C. *Australia* **95** F2
Spencer B. *Namibia* **88** D1
Spencer G. *Australia* **95** E2
Spencerville *Canada* **115** B9
Spences Bridge *Canada* **102** C4
Spennymoor *U.K.* **14** C6
Spenser Mts. *N.Z.* **91** E4
Spentrup *Denmark* **11** H4

Sperchios → Greece 46 C4
Sperrin Mts. U.K. 12 B5
Spessart Germany 25 F5
Spetses Greece 46 D3
Spey → U.K. 13 D5
Speyer Germany 25 F4
Spezand Pakistan 68 E2
Spezzano Albanese Italy 43 C9
Spiddle Ireland 12 C2
Spiekeroog Germany 24 B3
Spiez Switz. 25 J3
Spili Greece 49 D6
Spilimbergo Italy 41 B9
Spinazzola Italy 43 B9
Spineni Romania 29 F9
Spinifex ☼ Australia 93 E4
Spirit Lake U.S.A. 110 D4
Spirit River Canada 102 B5
Spiritwood Canada 103 C7
Spišská Nová Ves
  Slovak Rep. 27 C13
Spišské Podhradie
  Slovak Rep. 27 B13
Spital Austria 26 D7
Spithead U.K. 15 G6
Spittal an der Drau Austria 26 E6
Spitzbergen = Svalbard Arctic 4 B8
Spjelkavik Norway 8 E12
Split Croatia 41 E13
Split ✈ (SPU) Croatia 41 E13
Split L. Canada 103 B9
Split Lake Canada 103 B9
Splitski Kanal Croatia 41 E13
Splügenpass Switz. 25 J5
Spofford U.S.A. 116 G4
Spokane U.S.A. 108 C5
Spoleto Italy 41 F9
Spooner U.S.A. 112 C8
Sporyy Navolok, Mys Russia 52 B7
Sprague U.S.A. 108 C5
Spratly I. S. China Sea 62 C4
Spratly Is. S. China Sea 62 C4
Spray U.S.A. 108 D4
Spreča → Bos.-H. 28 F3
Spree → Germany 24 C9
Spreewald Germany 24 D9
Spremberg Germany 24 D10
Sprengisandur Iceland 8 D4
Spring City U.S.A. 115 F9
Spring Creek U.S.A. 108 F6
Spring Garden U.S.A. 110 F6
Spring Hall Barbados 121 g
Spring Hill U.S.A. 117 G13
Spring Mts. U.S.A. 111 J11
Spring Valley Calif., U.S.A. 111 N10
Spring Valley Nev., U.S.A. 111 J11
Springbok S. Africa 88 D2
Springboro U.S.A. 114 E4
Springdale Canada 105 C8
Springdale U.S.A. 116 C7
Springe Germany 24 C5
Springer U.S.A. 109 H11
Springerville U.S.A. 109 J9
Springfield Canada 114 D4
Springfield N.Z. 91 E3
Springfield Colo., U.S.A. 109 H12
Springfield Ill., U.S.A. 112 F9
Springfield Mass., U.S.A. 115 D12
Springfield Mo., U.S.A. 112 G7
Springfield Ohio, U.S.A. 113 F12
Springfield Oreg., U.S.A. 108 D2
Springfield Tenn., U.S.A. 117 C11
Springfield Vt., U.S.A. 115 C12
Springfontein S. Africa 88 E4
Springhill Canada 105 C7
Springhill U.S.A. 116 E8
Springhouse Canada 102 C4
Springs S. Africa 89 D4
Springsure Australia 94 C4
Springvale U.S.A. 115 C14
Springville Calif., U.S.A. 110 J8
Springville N.Y., U.S.A. 114 D6
Springville Utah, U.S.A. 108 F8
Springwater U.S.A. 114 D7
Spruce-Creek U.S.A. 114 F6
Spruce Knob-Seneca
  Rocks △ U.S.A. 113 F14
Spruce Mt. U.S.A. 115 B12
Sprucedale Canada 114 A5
Spur U.S.A. 116 E4
Spurn Hd. U.K. 14 D8
Spuž Montenegro 44 D3
Spuzzum Canada 102 D4
Squam L. U.S.A. 115 C13
Squamish Canada 102 D4
Square Islands Canada 105 B8
Squillace, G. di Italy 43 D9
Squinzano Italy 43 B11
Squires, Mt. Australia 93 E4
Srbac Bos.-H. 28 E7
Srbica Kosovo 44 D4
Srbija = Serbia ■ Europe 44 C4
Srbobran Serbia 28 E4
Sre Ambel Cambodia 65 G4
Sre Khtum Cambodia 65 F6
Sre Umbell = Sre Ambel
  Cambodia 65 G4

Srebrenica Bos.-H. 28 F4
Sredinny Ra. = Sredinnyy
  Khrebet Russia 53 D17
Sredinnyy Khrebet Russia 53 D17
Središče Slovenia 41 B13
Sredna Gora Bulgaria 45 D8
Srednekolymsk Russia 53 C16
Sredni Rodopi Bulgaria 45 E8
Srednogorie Bulgaria 45 D8
Śrem Poland 31 F4
Sremska Mitrovica Serbia 28 F4
Sremski Karlovci Serbia 28 E4
Srepok → Cambodia 64 F6
Sretensk Russia 53 D12
Sri Aman Malaysia 62 D4
Sri Lanka ■ Asia 66 R12
Srikakulam India 67 K13
Srinagar India 69 B6
Środa Śląska Poland 31 G3
Środa Wielkopolski Poland 31 F4
Srono Indonesia 63 J17
Srpska Crnja Serbia 28 E5
Srpski Itebej Serbia 28 E5
Ssese Is. = Sese Is. Uganda 86 C3
Staaten → Australia 94 B3
Staaten River △ Australia 94 B3
Staberhuk Germany 24 A7
Stade Germany 24 B5
Stadskanaal Neths. 17 A6
Stadtallendorf Germany 24 E5
Stadthagen Germany 24 C5
Stadtlohn Germany 24 D2
Stadtroda Germany 24 E7
Staffa U.K. 13 E2
Staffanstorp Sweden 11 J7
Stafford U.K. 14 E5
Stafford U.S.A. 112 G4
Stafford Springs U.S.A. 115 E12
Staffordshire □ U.K. 14 E5
Stagnone Italy 42 E5
Stagnone di Marsala △ Italy 42 E5
Staines U.K. 15 F7
Stainz Germany 26 E8
Stakhanov Ukraine 33 H10
Stalać Serbia 44 C5
Stalida Greece 49 D7
Stallarholmen Sweden 10 E11
Ställdalen Sweden 10 E8
Stalowa Wola Poland 31 H9
Stalybridge U.K. 14 D5
Stamford Australia 94 C3
Stamford U.K. 15 E7
Stamford Conn., U.S.A. 115 E11
Stamford N.Y., U.S.A. 115 D10
Stamford Tex., U.S.A. 116 E5
Stampriet Namibia 88 C2
Stamps U.S.A. 116 E8
Stančevo = Kalipetrovo
  Bulgaria 45 B11
Standerton S. Africa 89 D4
Standish U.S.A. 113 D12
Stanford S. Africa 88 E2
Stanford U.S.A. 108 C8
Stånga Sweden 11 G12
Stanger S. Africa 89 D5
Stängselsän =
  Salpausselkä Finland 32 B4
Stanišić Serbia 28 E4
Stanislaus → U.S.A. 110 H5
Stanisławów Poland 31 F8
Stanley Australia 95 G4
Stanley Falk. Is. 128 G5
Stanley U.K. 14 C6
Stanley Idaho, U.S.A. 108 D6
Stanley N. Dak., U.S.A. 112 A2
Stanley N.Y., U.S.A. 114 D7
Stanley Mission Canada 103 B8
Stannards U.S.A. 114 D7
Stanovoy Khrebet Russia 53 D14
Stanovoy Ra. = Stanovoy
  Khrebet Russia 53 D14
Stansmore Ra. Australia 92 D4
Stansted, London ✈ (STN)
  U.K. 15 F8
Stanthorpe Australia 95 D5
Stanton U.S.A. 116 E4
Stanwood U.S.A. 110 B4
Staples Canada 114 D2
Staples U.S.A. 112 B6
Stapleton U.S.A. 112 E3
Stąporków Poland 31 G7
Star City Canada 103 C8
Star Lake U.S.A. 115 B9
Stará L'ubovňa Slovak Rep. 27 B13
Stara Moravica Serbia 28 E4
Stara Pazova Serbia 28 F5
Stara Planina Bulgaria 44 C7
Stara Sil Ukraine 31 J9
Stará Turá Slovak Rep. 27 C10
Stara Ushytsya Ukraine 29 B12
Stara Zagora Bulgaria 45 D9
Starachowice Poland 31 G8
Staraya Russa Russia 32 D6
Starbuck I. Kiribati 97 H12
Starchiojd Romania 29 E11
Starcke △ Australia 94 A4
Stargard Szczeciński Poland 30 E2
Stari Bar Montenegro 44 D3
Stari Trg Slovenia 41 C12
Staritsa Russia 32 D8

Starke U.S.A. 117 G13
Starkville U.S.A. 117 E10
Starnberg Germany 25 H7
Starnberger See Germany 25 H7
Starobilsk Ukraine 33 H10
Starodub Russia 33 F7
Starogard Gdański Poland 30 E5
Starokonstantinov =
  Starokonstyantyniv
  Ukraine 23 D14
Starokonstyantyniv Ukraine 23 D14
Starokozache Ukraine 29 D14
Starominskaya Russia 33 J10
Staroshcherbinovskaya
  Russia 33 J10
Start Pt. U.K. 15 G4
Stary Sącz Poland 31 J7
Staryy Biryuzyak Russia 35 H8
Staryy Chartoriysk Ukraine 23 C13
Staryy Krym Ukraine 33 K8
Staryy Oskol Russia 33 G9
Staryy Sambir Ukraine 31 J9
Stassfurt Germany 24 D7
Staszów Poland 31 H8
State College U.S.A. 114 F7
Stateline U.S.A. 110 G7
Staten, I. = Estados, I. de
  Los Argentina 128 G4
Staten I. U.S.A. 115 F10
Statesboro U.S.A. 117 E14
Statesville U.S.A. 117 D14
Statia = St. Eustatius
  W. Indies 121 C7
Stauffer U.S.A. 111 L7
Staunton Ill., U.S.A. 112 F9
Staunton Va., U.S.A. 113 F14
Stavanger Norway 9 G11
Staveley N.Z. 91 E3
Stavelot Belgium 17 D5
Stavern Norway 9 G14
Stavoren Neths. 17 B5
Stavropol Russia 35 H6
Stavropol □ Russia 35 G6
Stavros Cyprus 49 D11
Stavros Kriti, Greece 49 D6
Stavros Thessaloniki, Greece 44 F7
Stavros, Akra Greece 49 D6
Stavroupoli Greece 45 E8
Stawell Australia 95 F3
Stawell → Australia 94 C3
Stawiski Poland 30 E9
Stawiszyn Poland 31 G5
Stayner Canada 114 B4
Stayton U.S.A. 108 D2
Steamboat Springs U.S.A. 108 F10
Steblevë Albania 44 E4
Steele U.S.A. 112 B4
Steelton U.S.A. 114 F8
Steen River Canada 102 B5
Steens Mt. U.S.A. 108 E4
Steenwijk Neths. 17 B6
Steep Pt. Australia 93 E1
Steep Rock Canada 103 C9
Ştefan Vodă Moldova 29 D14
Ştefăneşti Romania 29 C12
Stefanie = Ethiopia 81 G4
Stefanie L. = Chew Bahir
  Ethiopia 81 G4
Stefansson Bay Antarctica 5 C5
Stefansson I. Canada 101 C10
Stege Denmark 11 K6
Steiermark □ Austria 26 D8
Steigerwald Germany 25 F6
Steigerwald △ Germany 25 F6
Steilacoom U.S.A. 110 C4
Steilrandberge Namibia 88 B1
Steinbach Canada 103 D9
Steinfurt Germany 24 C3
Steinhausen Namibia 88 C2
Steinheim Germany 24 D5
Steinhuder Meer Germany 24 C5
Steinhuder Meer △ Germany 24 C5
Steinkjer Norway 8 D14
Steinkopf S. Africa 88 D2
Steinwald △ Germany 25 F8
Stellarton Canada 105 C7
Stellenbosch S. Africa 88 E2
Stelvio, Paso dello Italy 40 B7
Stenay France 19 C12
Stendal Germany 24 C7
Stende Latvia 30 A9
Stenhamra Sweden 10 E11
Stenshuvud △ Sweden 11 J8
Stenstorp Sweden 11 F7
Stenungsund Sweden 11 F5
Steornabhaigh =
  Stornoway U.K. 13 C2
Stepanakert = Xankändi
  Azerbaijan 73 C12
Stepanavan Armenia 35 K7
Stephens Creek Australia 95 E3
Stephens I. Canada 102 C2
Stephens L. Canada 103 B9
Stephenville Canada 105 C8
Stephenville U.S.A. 116 E5
Stepnica Poland 30 E1
Steppe Asia 50 C7
Sterea Ellas □ Greece 46 C4
Sterkstroom S. Africa 88 E4

Sterling Colo., U.S.A. 108 F12
Sterling Ill., U.S.A. 112 E9
Sterling Kans., U.S.A. 112 F4
Sterling City U.S.A. 116 F4
Sterling Heights U.S.A. 113 D12
Sterling Run U.S.A. 114 E6
Sterlitamak Russia 52 D6
Sternberg Germany 24 B7
Šternberk Czech Rep. 27 B10
Sterzing = Vipiteno Italy 41 B8
Stettin = Szczecin Poland 30 E1
Stettiner Haff Germany 24 B10
Stettler Canada 102 C6
Steubenville U.S.A. 114 F4
Stevenage U.K. 15 F7
Stevens Point U.S.A. 112 C9
Stevenson U.S.A. 110 E5
Stevenson → Australia 95 D2
Stevenson L. Canada 103 C9
Stevensville U.S.A. 108 C6
Stevns Klint Denmark 11 J6
Stewart Canada 102 B3
Stewart U.S.A. 110 F7
Stewart → Canada 100 E4
Stewart, C. Australia 94 A1
Stewart, I. Chile 128 G2
Stewart I. N.Z. 91 G1
Stewarts Point U.S.A. 110 G3
Stewartville U.S.A. 112 D7
Stewiacke Canada 105 C7
Steynsburg S. Africa 88 E4
Steyr Austria 26 C7
Steyr → Austria 26 C7
Steytlerville S. Africa 88 E3
Stia Italy 41 E8
Stigler U.S.A. 116 D7
Stigliano Italy 43 B9
Stigtomta Sweden 11 F10
Stikine → Canada 102 B2
Stilfontein S. Africa 88 D4
Stilida Greece 46 C4
Stillwater N.Z. 91 E3
Stillwater N.Y., U.S.A. 115 D11
Stillwater Okla., U.S.A. 116 D6
Stillwater Range U.S.A. 108 G4
Stillwater Res. U.S.A. 115 C9
Stilo, Pta. Italy 43 D9
Stilwell U.S.A. 116 D7
Ştînga Nistrului □ Moldova 29 C14
Štip Macedonia 44 E6
Stira Greece 46 C6
Stirling Canada 114 B7
Stirling U.K. 13 E5
Stirling □ U.K. 13 E4
Stirling Ra. Australia 93 F2
Stirling Range △ Australia 93 F2
Stittsville Canada 115 A9
Stjernøya Norway 8 A20
Stjørdalshalsen Norway 8 E14
Stockach Germany 25 H5
Stockaryd Sweden 11 G8
Stockerau Austria 27 C9
Stockholm Sweden 10 E12
Stockholm Arlanda ✈
  (ARN) Sweden 10 E11
Stockholms län □ Sweden 10 E12
Stockport U.K. 14 D5
Stocksbridge U.K. 14 D6
Stockton Calif., U.S.A. 110 H5
Stockton Kans., U.S.A. 112 F4
Stockton Mo., U.S.A. 112 G7
Stockton-on-Tees U.K. 14 C6
Stockton-on-Tees □ U.K. 14 C6
Stockton Plateau U.S.A. 116 F3
Stoczek Łukowski Poland 31 G8
Stöde Sweden 10 B10
Stoeng Treng = Stoeng
  Treng Cambodia 64 F5
Stoer, Pt. of U.K. 13 C3
Stogovo Macedonia 44 E4
Stoholm Denmark 11 H3
Stoke-on-Trent U.K. 14 D5
Stoke-on-Trent □ U.K. 14 D5
Stokes △ Australia 93 F3
Stokes Bay Canada 114 B3
Stokes Pt. Australia 95 G3
Stokes Ra. Australia 92 C5
Stokksnes Iceland 8 D6
Stokmarknes Norway 8 B16
Stolac Bos.-H. 44 C1
Stolberg Germany 24 E2
Stolbovoy, Ostrov Russia 53 B14
Stolbtsy = Stowbtsy Belarus 23 B14
Stolin Belarus 23 C14
Stolnici Romania 29 F9
Stomio Greece 49 D5
Ston Croatia 41 F14
Stone U.K. 14 E5
Stoneboro U.S.A. 114 E4
Stonehaven U.K. 13 E6
Stonehenge Australia 94 C3
Stonehenge U.K. 15 F6
Stonewall Canada 103 C9
Stony I. U.S.A. 115 C8
Stony L. Man., Canada 103 B9
Stony L. Ont., Canada 114 B6
Stony Point U.S.A. 115 E11
Stony Pt. U.S.A. 115 C8
Stony Rapids Canada 103 B7

Stony Tunguska =
  Tunguska,
  Podkamennaya →
  Russia 53 C10
Stonyford U.S.A. 110 F4
Stopnica Poland 31 H7
Storå Sweden 10 E9
Storå → Denmark 11 H2
Stora Gla Sweden 10 E6
Stora Le Sweden 10 E5
Stora Lulevatten Sweden 8 C18
Storavan Sweden 8 D18
Stord Norway 9 G11
Store Bælt Denmark 11 J4
Store Heddinge Denmark 11 J6
Store Mosse △ Sweden 11 G7
Storebro Sweden 11 G9
Storfors Sweden 10 E8
Storkerson Pen. Canada 100 C10
Storlien Sweden 10 A6
Storm B. Australia 95 G4
Storm Lake U.S.A. 112 D6
Stormberge S. Africa 88 E4
Stormsrivier S. Africa 88 E3
Stornoway U.K. 13 C2
Storo Italy 40 C7
Storozhinets =
  Storozhynets Ukraine 29 B10
Storozhynets Ukraine 29 B10
Storrs U.S.A. 115 E12
Storsjön Gävleborg, Sweden 10 D10
Storsjön Jämtland, Sweden 10 B7
Storsjön Jämtland, Sweden 10 A8
Storuman Sweden 8 D17
Storuman, L. Sweden 8 D17
Storvik Sweden 10 D10
Storvreta Sweden 10 E11
Storvätteshågna Sweden 10 B6
Stouffville Canada 114 C5
Stoughton Canada 103 D8
Stour → Dorset, U.K. 15 G6
Stour → Kent, U.K. 15 F9
Stour → Suffolk, U.K. 15 F9
Stourbridge U.K. 15 E5
Stout L. Canada 103 C10
Stove Pipe Wells Village
  U.S.A. 111 J9
Støvring Denmark 11 H3
Stow U.S.A. 114 E3
Stowbtsy Belarus 23 B14
Stowmarket U.K. 15 E9
Strabane U.K. 12 B4
Stracin Macedonia 44 D6
Stradella Italy 40 C6
Strahan Australia 95 G4
Strajitsa Bulgaria 45 C9
Strakonice Czech Rep. 26 B6
Straldzha Bulgaria 45 D10
Stralsund Germany 24 A9
Strand S. Africa 88 E2
Stranda Møre og Romsdal,
  Norway 8 E12
Stranda Nord-Trøndelag,
  Norway 8 E14
Strandby Denmark 11 G4
Strangford L. U.K. 12 B6
Strängnäs Sweden 10 E11
Stranorlar Ireland 12 B4
Stranraer U.K. 13 G3
Strasbourg Canada 103 C8
Strasbourg France 19 D14
Strasburg Germany 24 B9
Strășeni Moldova 29 C13
Strässa Sweden 10 E9
Stratford Canada 114 C4
Stratford N.Z. 91 C5
Stratford Calif., U.S.A. 110 J7
Stratford Conn., U.S.A. 115 E11
Stratford Tex., U.S.A. 116 C3
Stratford-upon-Avon U.K. 15 E6
Strath Spey U.K. 13 D5
Strathalbyn Australia 95 F2
Strathaven U.K. 13 F4
Strathcona △ Canada 102 D3
Strathmore Canada 102 C6
Strathmore U.K. 13 E5
Strathmore U.S.A. 110 J7
Strathnaver Canada 102 C4
Strathpeffer U.K. 13 D4
Strathroy Canada 114 D3
Strathy Pt. U.K. 13 C4
Strattanville U.S.A. 114 E5
Stratton U.S.A. 115 A14
Stratton Mt. U.S.A. 115 C12
Straubing Germany 25 G8
Straumnes Iceland 8 C2
Strausberg Germany 24 C9
Strawberry → U.S.A. 108 F8
Strážnice Czech Rep. 27 C10
Streaky B. Australia 95 E1
Streaky Bay Australia 95 E1
Streator U.S.A. 112 E9
Středočeský □ Czech Rep. 26 B7
Streetsboro U.S.A. 114 E3
Streetsville Canada 114 C5
Strehaia Romania 29 F8
Strelcha Bulgaria 45 D8
Streng → Cambodia 64 F4
Stresa Italy 40 C5
Streymoy Færoe Is. 8 E9

Strezhevoy Russia 52 C8
Stříbro Czech Rep. 26 A6
Strilky Ukraine 31 J9
Strimonas → Greece 44 F7
Strofades Greece 46 D3
Strokestown Ireland 12 C3
Stroma U.K. 13 C5
Stromberg-Heuchelberg △
  Germany 25 F4
Strómboli Italy 43 D8
Stromeferry U.K. 13 D3
Stromness U.K. 13 C5
Strömsbruk Sweden 10 C11
Stromsburg U.S.A. 112 E5
Strömsnäsbruk Sweden 11 H7
Strömstad Sweden 11 F5
Strömsund Sweden 8 E16
Strongili Greece 47 E11
Stróngoli Italy 43 C10
Strongsville U.S.A. 114 E3
Stronie Śląskie Poland 31 H3
Stronsay U.K. 13 B6
Stropkov Slovak Rep. 27 B14
Stroud U.K. 15 F5
Stroud Road Australia 95 E5
Stroudsburg U.S.A. 115 F9
Stroumbi Cyprus 49 E11
Štrpce Kosovo 44 D5
Struer Denmark 11 H2
Struga Macedonia 44 E4
Strugi Krasnyye Russia 32 C5
Strumica Macedonia 44 E6
Strumica → Europe 44 E7
Strumok Ukraine 29 E14
Struthers U.S.A. 114 E4
Stryama Bulgaria 45 D8
Stryker U.S.A. 108 B6
Strykow Poland 31 G6
Stryy Ukraine 23 D12
Strzegom Poland 31 H3
Strzelce Krajeńskie Poland 31 F2
Strzelce Opolskie Poland 31 H5
Strzelecki Cr. → Australia 95 D2
Strzelecki Desert Australia 95 D3
Strzelin Poland 31 H4
Strzelno Poland 31 F5
Strzybnica Poland 31 H5
Strzyżów Poland 31 J8
Stuart Fla., U.S.A. 117 H14
Stuart Nebr., U.S.A. 112 D4
Stuart → Canada 102 C4
Stuart Bluff Ra. Australia 92 D5
Stuart I. U.S.A. 106 C7
Stuart L. Canada 102 C4
Stuart Ra. Australia 95 D1
Stubbekøbing Denmark 11 K6
Stuben Austria 26 D3
Studen Kladenets, Yazovir
  Bulgaria 45 E9
Studenka Czech Rep. 27 B11
Stugun Sweden 10 A9
Stuhr Germany 24 B4
Stull L. Canada 104 B1
Stung Treng = Stoeng
  Treng Cambodia 64 F5
Stupart → Canada 104 A1
Stupava Slovak Rep. 27 C10
Stupino Russia 32 E10
Sturge I. Antarctica 5 C11
Sturgeon B. Canada 103 C9
Sturgeon Bay U.S.A. 112 C10
Sturgeon Falls Canada 104 C4
Sturgeon L. Alta., Canada 102 B5
Sturgeon L. Ont., Canada 104 C1
Sturgeon L. Ont., Canada 114 B6
Sturgis Canada 103 C8
Sturgis Mich., U.S.A. 113 E11
Sturgis S. Dak., U.S.A. 112 C2
Sturkö Sweden 11 H9
Sturt △ Australia 95 D3
Sturt Cr. → Australia 92 C4
Sturt Stony Desert Australia 95 D3
Stutterheim S. Africa 88 E4
Stuttgart Germany 25 G5
Stuttgart U.S.A. 116 D9
Stuttgart Echterdingen ✈
  (STR) Germany 25 G5
Stuyvesant U.S.A. 115 D11
Stykkishólmur Iceland 8 D2
Styria = Steiermark □
  Austria 26 D8
Styrsö Sweden 11 G5
Su Xian = Suzhou China 56 H9
Suakin Sudan 80 D4
Suakin Archipelago Sudan 80 D4
Suan N. Korea 57 E14
Suar India 69 E8
Şubā Si. Arabia 70 E2
Subang Indonesia 63 G12
Subansiri → India 67 F18
Subarnarekha → India 69 H12
Subay', Urūq Si. Arabia 80 C5
Subayhah Si. Arabia 70 D3
Subcetate Romania 28 E8
Subi Indonesia 62 D3
Subiaco Italy 41 G10
Subotica Serbia 28 D4
Suca Ethiopia 81 F4

Suceava *Romania* **29** C11
Suceava □ *Romania* **29** C10
Suceava → *Romania* **29** C11
Sucha-Beskidzka *Poland* **31** J6
Suchan = Partizansk *Russia* **54** C6
Suchań *Poland* **31** E2
Suchedniów *Poland* **31** G7
Suchil *Mexico* **118** C4
Suchou = Suzhou *China* **59** B13
Süchow = Xuzhou *China* **57** G9
Suchowola *Poland* **30** E10
Suck → *Ireland* **12** C3
Sucre *Bolivia* **124** G5
Sućuraj *Croatia* **41** E14
Sucuriú → *Brazil* **125** H8
Sud □ *Cameroon* **83** E7
Sud, Pte. du *Canada* **105** C7
Sud-Kivu □
  Dem. Rep. of the Congo **86** C2
Sud-Ouest □ *Cameroon* **83** D6
Sud-Ouest, Pte. *Canada* **105** C7
Sud Ouest, Pte. *Mauritius* **85** d
Suda → *Russia* **32** C9
Sudak *Ukraine* **33** K8
Sudan *India* **116** D3
Sudan ■ *Africa* **81** E3
Sudbury *Canada* **104** C3
Sudbury *U.K.* **15** E8
Sûdd *Sudan* **81** F3
Sudeifel = Deutsch-
  Luxemburgischer △
  Germany **25** F2
Süderbrarup *Germany* **24** A5
Süderlügum *Germany* **24** A4
Süderoogsand *Germany* **24** A4
Sudeten Mts. = Sudety
  Europe **27** A9
Sudety *Europe* **27** A9
Südheide △ *Germany* **24** C6
Suðuroy *Færoe Is.* **8** F9
Sudi *Tanzania* **87** E4
Sudirman, Pegunungan
  Indonesia **63** E5
Sudiţi *Romania* **29** F12
Sudogda *Russia* **34** C5
Sudong, Pulau *Singapore* **65** d
Sudova Vyshnya *Ukraine* **31** J10
Sudzha *Russia* **33** G8
Sue → *Sudan* **81** F2
Sueca *Spain* **39** F4
Süedinenie *Bulgaria* **45** D8
Suemez I. *U.S.A.* **102** B2
Suez = El Suweis *Egypt* **80** J8
Suez, G. of = Suweis,
  Khalîg el *Egypt* **80** J8
Suez Canal = Suweis, Qanâ
  es *Egypt* **80** H8
Suffield *Canada* **102** C6
Suffolk *U.S.A.* **113** G15
Suffolk □ *U.K.* **15** E9
Şufian *Iran* **73** C11
Şugag *Romania* **29** E8
Sugar Grove *U.S.A.* **114** E5
Sugarcreek *U.S.A.* **114** E5
Sugarive → *India* **69** F12
Suğla Gölü *Turkey* **72** D5
Sugluk = Salluit *Canada* **101** E16
Suhaia, Lacul *Romania* **29** G10
Şuhār *Oman* **71** E8
Sühbaatar □ *Mongolia* **56** B8
Suhl *Germany* **24** E6
Şuhut *Turkey* **47** C12
Sui *Pakistan* **68** E3
Sui Xian *China* **56** G8
Šuica *Bos.-H.* **28** G2
Suichang *China* **59** C12
Suichuan *China* **59** D10
Suide *China* **56** F6
Suifenhe *China* **57** B16
Suihua *China* **60** B7
Suijiang *China* **58** C4
Suining *Hunan, China* **59** D8
Suining *Jiangsu, China* **57** H9
Suining *Sichuan, China* **58** B5
Suiping *China* **56** H7
Suippes *France* **19** C11
Suir → *Ireland* **12** D4
Suisse = Switzerland ■
  Europe **25** J4
Suisun City *U.S.A.* **110** G4
Suixi *China* **59** G8
Suiyang *Guizhou, China* **58** D6
Suiyang *Heilongjiang, China* **57** B16
Suizhong *China* **57** D11
Suizhou *China* **59** B9
Sujangarh *India* **68** F6
Sukabumi *Indonesia* **63** G12
Sukadana *Indonesia* **62** E4
Sukagawa *Japan* **55** F10
Sukaraja *Indonesia* **62** E4
Sukawati *Indonesia* **63** K18
Sukch'ŏn *N. Korea* **57** E13
Sukhindol *Bulgaria* **45** C9
Sukhinichi *Russia* **32** E8
Sukhona → *Russia* **52** D4
Sukhothai *Thailand* **64** D2
Sukhumi = Sokhumi *Georgia* **35** J5
Sukkur *Pakistan* **68** F3
Sukkur Barrage *Pakistan* **68** F3

Sukovo *Serbia* **44** C6
Sukri → *India* **68** G4
Sukumo *Japan* **55** H6
Sukunka → *Canada* **102** B4
Sula → *Ukraine* **33** H7
Sula, Kepulauan *Indonesia* **63** E7
Sulaco → *Honduras* **120** C2
Sulaiman Range *Pakistan* **68** D3
Sulak → *Russia* **35** J8
Sulakyurt *Turkey* **72** B5
Sūlār *Iran* **71** D6
Sulawesi *Indonesia* **63** E6
Sulawesi Barat □ *Indonesia* **63** E5
Sulawesi Sea = Celebes Sea
  Indonesia **63** D6
Sulawesi Selatan □ *Indonesia* **63** E6
Sulawesi Tengah □ *Indonesia* **63** E6
Sulawesi Tenggara □
  Indonesia **63** E6
Sulawesi Utara □ *Indonesia* **63** D6
Sulechów *Poland* **31** F2
Sulęcin *Poland* **31** F2
Suleja *Nigeria* **83** D6
Sulejów *Poland* **31** G6
Sulejówek *Poland* **31** F8
Süleymanlı *Turkey* **47** C9
Sulima *S. Leone* **82** D2
Sulina *Romania* **29** E14
Sulina, Braţul → *Romania* **29** E14
Sulingen *Germany* **24** C4
Suliţa *Romania* **29** C11
Sulitjelma *Norway* **8** C17
Sułkowice *Poland* **31** J6
Sullana *Peru* **124** D2
Süller *Turkey* **47** C11
Sullivan *Ill., U.S.A.* **112** F9
Sullivan *Ind., U.S.A.* **112** F10
Sullivan *Mo., U.S.A.* **112** F8
Sullivan Bay *Canada* **102** C3
Sullivan I. = Lanbi Kyun
  Burma **65** G2
Sullom Voe *U.K.* **13** A7
Sully-sur-Loire *France* **19** E9
Sulmierzyce *Poland* **31** G4
Sulmona *Italy* **41** F10
Süloğlu *Turkey* **45** E10
Sulphur *La., U.S.A.* **116** F8
Sulphur *Okla., U.S.A.* **116** D6
Sulphur Pt. *Canada* **102** A6
Sulphur Springs *U.S.A.* **116** E7
Sultan *Canada* **104** C3
Sultan *U.S.A.* **110** C5
Sultan Dağları *Turkey* **72** C4
Sultan Hamud *Kenya* **86** C4
Sultanābād = Arāk *Iran* **71** C6
Sultanhisar *Turkey* **47** D10
Sultaniça *Turkey* **45** F10
Sultaniye *Turkey* **45** F12
Sultanpur *Mad. P., India* **68** H8
Sultanpur *Punjab, India* **68** D6
Sultanpur *Ut. P., India* **69** F10
Sulu Arch. *Phil.* **61** J4
Sulu Sea *E. Indies* **61** H4
Sülüklü *Turkey* **72** C5
Sululta *Ethiopia* **81** F4
Suluova *Turkey* **72** B6
Sulūq *Libya* **79** B10
Sulzbach *Germany* **25** F3
Sulzbach-Rosenberg
  Germany **25** F7
Sulzberger Ice Shelf
  Antarctica **5** E13
Sumalata *Indonesia* **63** D6
Sumampa *Argentina* **126** B3
Sumatera *Indonesia* **62** D2
Sumatera Barat □ *Indonesia* **62** E2
Sumatera Utara □ *Indonesia* **62** D1
Sumatra = Sumatera
  Indonesia **62** D2
Sumava △ *Czech Rep.* **26** C6
Sumba *Indonesia* **63** F5
Sumba, Selat *Indonesia* **63** F5
Sumbawa *Indonesia* **62** F5
Sumbawa Besar *Indonesia* **62** F5
Sumbawanga □ *Tanzania* **84** F6
Sumbe *Angola* **84** G2
Sumbu △ *Zambia* **87** D3
Sumburgh Hd. *U.K.* **13** B7
Sumdeo *India* **69** D8
Sumdo *China* **69** B8
Sumedang *Indonesia* **63** G12
Sumenep *Indonesia* **63** G15
Sümeg *Hungary* **28** D2
Sumeih *Sudan* **81** F2
Šumen = Shumen *Bulgaria* **45** C10
Sumenep *Indonesia* **63** G15
Sumgait = Sumqayıt
  Azerbaijan **35** K9
Summer L. *U.S.A.* **108** E3
Summerland *Canada* **102** D5
Summerside *Canada* **105** C7
Summersville *U.S.A.* **113** F13
Summerville *Ga., U.S.A.* **117** D12
Summerville *S.C., U.S.A.* **117** E14
Summit Lake *Canada* **102** C4
Summit Peak *U.S.A.* **109** H10
Sumner *Iowa, U.S.A.* **112** D7
Sumner *Wash., U.S.A.* **110** C4
Sumoto *Japan* **55** G7
Šumperk *Czech Rep.* **27** B9

Sumqayıt *Azerbaijan* **35** K9
Sumter *U.S.A.* **117** E14
Sumy *Ukraine* **33** G8
Sumy □ *Ukraine* **33** G7
Sun City *S. Africa* **88** D4
Sun City *Ariz., U.S.A.* **109** K7
Sun City *Calif., U.S.A.* **111** M9
Sun City Center *U.S.A.* **117** H13
Sun Lakes *U.S.A.* **109** K8
Sun Valley *U.S.A.* **108** E6
Sunagawa *Japan* **54** C10
Sunan *N. Korea* **57** E13
Sunart, L. *U.K.* **13** E3
Sunburst *U.S.A.* **108** B8
Sunbury *Australia* **95** F3
Sunbury *U.S.A.* **115** F8
Sunchales *Argentina* **126** C3
Suncheon *S. Korea* **57** G14
Suncho Corral *Argentina* **126** B3
Sunch'on *N. Korea* **57** E13
Suncook *U.S.A.* **115** C13
Sunda, Selat *Indonesia* **62** F3
Sunda Is. *Indonesia* **96** H2
Sunda Str. = Sunda, Selat
  Indonesia **62** F3
Sunda Trench = Java
  Trench *Ind. Oc.* **62** F3
Sundance *Canada* **103** B10
Sundance *U.S.A.* **108** D11
Sundar Nagar *India* **68** D7
Sundarbans *India* **67** J16
Sundarbans △ *India* **69** J13
Sundargarh *India* **67** H14
Sundays = Sondags →
  S. Africa **88** E4
Sunderland *Canada* **114** B5
Sunderland *U.K.* **14** C6
Sundown △ *Australia* **95** D5
Sundre *Canada* **102** C6
Sunds *Denmark* **11** H3
Sundsvall *Sweden* **10** B11
Sundsvallsbukten *Sweden* **10** B11
Sung Hei *Vietnam* **65** G6
Sungai Acheh *Malaysia* **65** c
Sungai Kolok *Thailand* **65** J3
Sungai Lembing *Malaysia* **65** L4
Sungai Petani *Malaysia* **65** K3
Sungaigerong *Indonesia* **62** E2
Sungailiat *Indonesia* **62** E3
Sungaipenuh *Indonesia* **62** E2
Sungari = Songhua
  Jiang → *China* **60** B8
Sunghua Chiang =
  Songhua Jiang → *China* **60** B8
Sungikai *Sudan* **81** E2
Sungurlu *Turkey* **72** B6
Sunja *Croatia* **41** C13
Sunland Park *U.S.A.* **109** L10
Sunnansjö *Sweden* **10** D8
Sunndalsøra *Norway* **8** E13
Sunne *Sweden* **10** E7
Sunnemo *Sweden* **10** E7
Sunnyside *U.S.A.* **108** C4
Sunnyvale *U.S.A.* **110** H4
Sunrise Manor *U.S.A.* **111** J11
Suntar *Russia* **53** C12
Sunyani *Ghana* **82** D4
Suomenselkä *Finland* **8** E21
Suomi = Finland ■ *Europe* **8** E22
Suomussalmi *Finland* **8** D23
Suoyarvi *Russia* **32** A7
Supai *U.S.A.* **109** H7
Supaul *India* **69** F12
Superior *Ariz., U.S.A.* **109** K8
Superior *Mont., U.S.A.* **108** C6
Superior *Nebr., U.S.A.* **112** E4
Superior *Wis., U.S.A.* **112** B7
Superior, L. *N. Amer.* **104** C2
Supetar *Croatia* **41** E13
Suphan Buri *Thailand* **64** E3
Suphan Dağı *Turkey* **73** C10
Supiori *Indonesia* **63** E9
Supraśl *Poland* **31** E10
Supraśl → *Poland* **31** E9
Supung Shuiku *China* **57** D13
Süq ash Shuyūkh *Iraq* **70** D5
Süq Suwayq *Si. Arabia* **70** E3
Suqian *China* **57** H10
Suqutra = Socotra *Yemen* **75** E5
Sūr *Lebanon* **74** B4
Şūr *Oman* **71** C6
Sur, Pt. *U.S.A.* **110** J5
Sura → *Russia* **34** C8
Surab *Pakistan* **68** E2
Surabaja = Surabaya
  Indonesia **62** F4
Surabaya *Indonesia* **62** F4
Surahammar *Sweden* **10** E10
Suraia *Romania* **29** E12
Surakarta *Indonesia* **62** F4
Šurany *Slovak Rep.* **27** C11
Surat *Australia* **95** D4
Surat *India* **66** J8
Surat Thani *Thailand* **65** H2
Suratgarh *India* **68** E5
Suraxanı *Azerbaijan* **35** K10
Şūraymilā *Si. Arabia* **70** E5
Suraż *Poland* **31** F9
Surazh *Belarus* **32** E6

Surazh *Russia* **33** F7
Surduc *Romania* **29** C8
Surduc Pasul *Romania* **29** E8
Surdulica *Serbia* **44** D6
Surendranagar *India* **68** H4
Surf *U.S.A.* **111** L6
Surfers Paradise *Australia* **95** D5
Surgères *France* **20** B3
Surgut *Russia* **52** C8
Sùria *Spain* **38** D6
Suriapet *India* **66** L11
Surigao *Phil.* **61** G6
Surigao Strait *Phil.* **61** F6
Surin *Thailand* **64** E4
Surin Nua, Ko *Thailand* **65** H1
Surinam = Suriname ■
  S. Amer. **125** C7
Suriname ■ *S. Amer.* **125** C7
Suriname → *Suriname* **125** B7
Sūrmaq *Iran* **71** D7
Sürmene *Turkey* **73** B9
Surovikino *Russia* **35** F6
Surrey *Canada* **110** A4
Surrey □ *U.K.* **15** F7
Sursand *India* **69** F11
Sursar → *India* **69** F12
Sursee *Switz.* **25** H4
Sursk *Russia* **34** D8
Surskoye *Russia* **34** C8
Surt *Libya* **79** B9
Surt, Khalīj *Libya* **79** B9
Surtanahu *Pakistan* **68** F4
Surte *Sweden* **11** G6
Surtsey *Iceland* **8** E3
Sürüç *Turkey* **73** D8
Suruga-Wan *Japan* **55** G9
Susa *Italy* **40** C4
Susa → *Denmark* **11** J5
Sušac *Croatia* **41** F13
Sušak *Croatia* **41** D11
Susaki *Japan* **55** H6
Susanville *U.S.A.* **108** F3
Susch *Switz.* **25** J6
Suşehri *Turkey* **73** B8
Susleni *Moldova* **29** C13
Susner *India* **68** H7
Susong *China* **59** B11
Susquehanna *U.S.A.* **115** E9
Susquehanna → *U.S.A.* **115** G8
Susques *Argentina* **126** A2
Sussex *Canada* **105** C6
Sussex *U.S.A.* **115** E10
Sussex, E. □ *U.K.* **15** G8
Sussex, W. □ *U.K.* **15** G7
Sustut → *Canada* **102** B3
Susuman *Russia* **53** C15
Susunu *Indonesia* **63** E8
Susurluk *Turkey* **47** B10
Susuz *Turkey* **73** B10
Susz *Poland* **30** E6
Sütçüler *Turkey* **72** D4
Şuţeşti *Romania* **29** E12
Sutherland *S. Africa* **88** E3
Sutherland *U.K.* **13** C4
Sutherland *U.S.A.* **112** E3
Sutherland Falls *N.Z.* **91** F1
Sutherlin *U.S.A.* **108** E2
Suthri *India* **68** H3
Sutjeska △ *Bos.-H.* **28** G3
Sutlej → *Pakistan* **68** E4
Sutter *U.S.A.* **110** F5
Sutter Buttes *U.S.A.* **110** F5
Sutter Creek *U.S.A.* **110** G6
Sutton *Canada* **115** A12
Sutton *Nebr., U.S.A.* **112** E5
Sutton *W. Va., U.S.A.* **113** F13
Sutton → *Canada* **104** A3
Sutton Coldfield *U.K.* **15** E6
Sutton L. *Canada* **104** B3
Suttor → *Australia* **94** C4
Suttsu *Japan* **54** C10
Sutwik I. *U.S.A.* **106** D8
Suva *Fiji* **91** a
Suva Gora *Macedonia* **44** E5
Suva Planina *Serbia* **44** C6
Suva Reka *Kosovo* **44** D4
Suvorov *Russia* **32** E9
Suvorov Is. = Suwarrow Is.
  Cook Is. **97** J11
Suvorove *Ukraine* **29** E13
Suvorovo *Bulgaria* **45** C11
Suwałki *Poland* **30** D9
Suwana *Indonesia* **63** K18
Suwannaphum *Thailand* **64** E4
Suwannee → *U.S.A.* **117** G13
Suwanose-Jima *Japan* **55** K4
Suwarrow Is. *Cook Is.* **97** J11
Suwayqīyah, Hawr as *Iraq* **73** G12
Suweis, Khalîg el *Egypt* **80** J8
Suweis, Qanâ es *Egypt* **80** H8
Suwon *S. Korea* **57** F14
Suzdal *Russia* **32** D11
Suzhou *Anhui, China* **56** H9
Suzhou *Jiangsu, China* **59** B13
Suzu *Japan* **55** F8
Suzu-Misaki *Japan* **55** F8

Suzuka *Japan* **55** G8
Suzzara *Italy* **40** D7
Svalbard *Arctic* **4** B8
Svalbard Radio =
  Longyearbyen *Svalbard* **4** B8
Svalöv *Sweden* **11** J7
Svalyava *Ukraine* **28** B7
Svaneke *Denmark* **11** J9
Svansko *Sweden* **10** E6
Svappavaara *Sweden* **8** C19
Svärdsjö *Sweden* **10** D9
Svartå *Sweden* **10** E8
Svartisen *Norway* **8** C15
Svartvik *Sweden* **10** B11
Svatove *Ukraine* **33** H10
Svatovo = Svatove *Ukraine* **33** H10
Svay Chek *Cambodia* **64** F4
Svay Rieng *Cambodia* **65** G5
Svealand *Sweden* **10** D9
Svedala *Sweden* **11** J7
Sveg *Sweden* **10** B8
Svendborg *Denmark* **11** J4
Svenljunga *Sweden* **11** G7
Svenstavik *Sweden* **10** B8
Svenstrup *Denmark* **11** H3
Sverdlovsk *Ukraine* **33** H10
Sverdrup Chan. *Canada* **101** B12
Sverdrup Is. *Canada* **98** B10
Sverige = Sweden ■ *Europe* **9** H16
Svetac *Croatia* **40** E12
Sveti Nikola, Prokhad *Europe* **44** C6
Sveti Nikole *Macedonia* **44** E5
Sveti Rok *Croatia* **41** D12
Svetlaya *Russia* **54** A9
Svetlogorsk =
  Svyatlahorsk *Belarus* **23** B15
Svetlogorsk *Russia* **30** D7
Svetlograd *Russia* **35** H6
Svetlovodsk = Svitlovodsk
  Ukraine **33** H7
Svetlyy *Russia* **30** D7
Svetozarevo = Jagodina
  Serbia **44** C5
Svidník *Slovak Rep.* **27** B14
Svilaja Planina *Croatia* **41** E13
Svilajnac *Serbia* **44** B5
Svilengrad *Bulgaria* **45** E10
Svir → *Russia* **32** B7
Sviritsa *Russia* **32** B7
Svishtov *Bulgaria* **45** C9
Svislach *Belarus* **31** E11
Svitava → *Czech Rep.* **27** B9
Svitavy *Czech Rep.* **27** B9
Svitlovodsk *Ukraine* **33** H7
Svizzera = Switzerland ■
  Europe **25** J4
Svobodnyy *Russia* **53** D13
Svoge *Bulgaria* **44** D7
Svolvær *Norway* **8** B16
Svratka → *Czech Rep.* **27** B9
Svrljig *Serbia* **44** C6
Svyetlahorsk *Belarus* **23** B15
Swabian Alps =
  Schwäbische Alb *Germany* **25** G5
Swaffham *U.K.* **15** E8
Swains I. *Amer. Samoa* **97** J11
Swainsboro *U.S.A.* **117** E13
Swakop → *Namibia* **88** C2
Swakopmund *Namibia* **88** C2
Swale → *U.K.* **14** C6
Swan → *Australia* **93** F2
Swan → *Canada* **103** C8
Swan Hill *Australia* **95** F3
Swan Hills *Canada* **102** C5
Swan Is. = Santanilla, Is.
  Honduras **120** C3
Swan L. *Man., Canada* **103** C8
Swan L. *Ont., Canada* **104** B1
Swan Ra. *Canada* **102** B5
Swan River *Canada* **103** C8
Swanage *U.K.* **15** G6
Swansea *Australia* **95** G4
Swansea *Canada* **114** C5
Swansea *U.K.* **15** F4
Swansea □ *U.K.* **15** F3
Swartberge *S. Africa* **88** E3
Swartmodder *S. Africa* **88** D3
Swartnossob → *Namibia* **88** C2
Swartruggens *S. Africa* **88** D4
Swarzędz *Poland* **31** F3
Swastika *Canada* **104** C3
Swat → *Pakistan* **69** B5
Swatow = Shantou *China* **59** F11
Swaziland ■ *Africa* **89** D5
Sweden ■ *Europe* **9** H16
Swedru *Ghana* **83** D4
Sweet Grass *U.S.A.* **108** B8
Sweet Home *U.S.A.* **108** D2
Sweetwater *Nev., U.S.A.* **110** G7
Sweetwater *Tenn., U.S.A.* **117** D12
Sweetwater *Tex., U.S.A.* **116** E4
Sweetwater → *U.S.A.* **108** E10
Swellendam *S. Africa* **88** E3
Swider → *Poland* **31** F8
Świdnica *Poland* **31** H3
Świdnik *Poland* **31** G9
Świdwin *Poland* **30** E2
Świebodzice *Poland* **31** H3
Świebodzin *Poland* **31** F2
Świecie *Poland* **30** E5
Świerzawa *Poland* **31** G2

Świętokrzyski △ *Poland* **31** H7
Świętokrzyskie □ *Poland* **31** H7
Świętokrzyskie, Góry *Poland* **31** H7
Swift Current *Canada* **103** C7
Swift Current → *Canada* **103** C7
Swilly, L. *Ireland* **12** A4
Swindon *U.K.* **15** F6
Swindon □ *U.K.* **15** F6
Swinemünde =
  Świnoujście *Poland* **30** E1
Swinford *Ireland* **12** C3
Świnoujście *Poland* **30** E1
Świnoujście *Europe* **25** J4
Switzerland ■ *Europe* **25** J4
Swords *Ireland* **12** C5
Swoyerville *U.S.A.* **115** E9
Syasstroy *Russia* **32** B7
Sychevka *Russia* **32** E8
Syców *Poland* **31** G4
Syddanmark □ *Denmark* **11** J2
Sydenham → *Canada* **114** D2
Sydney *Australia* **95** E5
Sydney *Canada* **105** C7
Sydney L. *Canada* **103** C10
Sydney Mines *Canada* **105** C7
Sydprøven = Alluitsup Paa
  Greenland **4** C5
Sydra, G. of = Surt, Khalīj
  Libya **79** B9
Syeverodonetsk *Ukraine* **33** H10
Syke *Germany* **24** C4
Sykesville *U.S.A.* **114** E6
Syktyvkar *Russia* **52** C6
Sylacauga *U.S.A.* **117** E11
Sylarna *Sweden* **8** E15
Sylhet *Bangla.* **67** G17
Sylhet □ *Bangla.* **67** G17
Sylt *Germany* **24** A4
Sylvan Beach *U.S.A.* **115** C9
Sylvan Lake *Canada* **102** C6
Sylvania *Ga., U.S.A.* **117** E14
Sylvania *Ohio, U.S.A.* **113** E12
Sylvester *U.S.A.* **117** F13
Sym *Russia* **52** C9
Synelnykove *Ukraine* **33** H8
Synevyr △ *Ukraine* **29** B8
Synevyrska Polyana *Ukraine* **29** B8
Synnak *Ukraine* **29** B7
Synnot Ra. *Australia* **92** C4
Syowa *Antarctica* **5** C5
Syracuse *Kans., U.S.A.* **112** G3
Syracuse *N.Y., U.S.A.* **115** C8
Syracuse *Nebr., U.S.A.* **112** E5
Syrdarya → *Kazakhstan* **52** E7
Syria ■ *Asia* **73** E8
Syrian Desert = Shām,
  Bādiyat ash *Asia* **70** C3
Syros = Ermoupoli *Greece* **46** D6
Syssleback *Sweden* **10** D6
Syzran *Russia* **34** D9
Szabolcs-Szatmár-Bereg □
  Hungary **28** B6
Szadek *Poland* **31** G5
Szamocin *Poland* **31** E4
Szamos → *Hungary* **28** B7
Szamotuły *Poland* **31** F3
Szárasz → *Hungary* **28** D5
Szarvas *Hungary* **28** D5
Százhalombatta *Hungary* **28** C3
Szczawnica *Poland* **31** J7
Szczebrzeszyn *Poland* **31** H9
Szczecin *Poland* **30** E1
Szczecinek *Poland* **30** E3
Szczeciński, Zalew =
  Stettiner Haff *Germany* **24** B10
Szczekociny *Poland* **31** H6
Szczucin *Poland* **31** H8
Szczuczyn *Poland* **30** E9
Szczyrk *Poland* **31** J6
Szczytna *Poland* **31** H3
Szczytno *Poland* **30** E7
Szechuan = Sichuan □
  China **58** B5
Szechwan = Sichuan □
  China **58** B5
Szécsény *Hungary* **28** B4
Szeged *Hungary* **28** D5
Szeghalom *Hungary* **28** C6
Székesfehérvár *Hungary* **28** C3
Szekszárd *Hungary* **28** D3
Szendrő *Hungary* **28** B5
Szentendre *Hungary* **28** C4
Szentes *Hungary* **28** D5
Szentgotthárd *Hungary* **28** D1
Szentlörinc *Hungary* **28** D3
Szerencs *Hungary* **28** B5
Szigetszentmiklós *Hungary* **28** C4
Sziksző *Hungary* **28** B5
Szigetvár *Hungary* **28** D2
Szklarska Poreba *Poland* **31** H2
Szkwa → *Poland* **31** E8
Szlichtyngowa *Poland* **31** G3
Szob *Hungary* **28** C3
Szolnok *Hungary* **28** C5
Szombathely *Hungary* **28** C1
Szprotawa *Poland* **31** G2
Sztum *Poland* **30** E6
Sztutowo *Poland* **30** D6
Szubin *Poland* **31** E4
Szydłowiec *Poland* **31** G7
Szypliszki *Poland* **30** D10

T

Ta Khli *Thailand* **64** E3
Ta Khli Khok *Thailand* **64** E3
Ta Lai *Vietnam* **65** G6
Tab *Hungary* **28** D3
Tabacal *Argentina* **126** A3
Tabaco *Phil.* **61** E5
Tabagné *Ivory C.* **82** D4
Țābah *Si. Arabia* **70** E4
Tabanan *Indonesia* **63** K18
Tabankort *Niger* **83** B5
Țabas *Khorāsān, Iran* **71** C9
Țabas *Yazd, Iran* **71** C8
Tabasará, Serranía de
  Panama **120** E3
Tabasco □ *Mexico* **119** D6
Tabāsīn *Iran* **71** D8
Tabatinga, Serra da *Brazil* **125** F10
Tabayin *Burma* **67** H19
Tabāzīn *Iran* **71** D8
Tabelbala *Algeria* **78** C5
Taber *Canada* **104** D6
Taberg *Sweden* **11** G8
Tabla *Niger* **83** C5
Tablas *Phil.* **61** E5
Tablas de Daimiel △ *Spain* **37** F7
Tablas Strait *Phil.* **61** E4
Table, Pte. de la *Réunion* **85** c
Table B. *Canada* **105** B8
Table B. *S. Africa* **88** E2
Table Mountain △ *S. Africa* **88** E2
Table Mt. *S. Africa* **88** E2
Table Rock L. *U.S.A.* **112** G7
Tabletop, Mt. *Australia* **94** C4
Tábor *Czech Rep.* **26** B7
Tabora *Tanzania* **86** D3
Tabora □ *Tanzania* **86** D3
Tabou *Ivory C.* **82** E3
Tabrīz *Iran* **73** C12
Tabuaeran *Kiribati* **97** G12
Tabuenca *Spain* **38** D3
Tabūk *Si. Arabia* **70** D3
Tabūk □ *Si. Arabia* **70** E3
Taburno-Camposauro △
  Italy **43** A7
Täby *Sweden* **10** E12
Tacámbaro de Codallos
  Mexico **118** D4
Tacheng *China* **60** B3
Tach'i *Taiwan* **59** E13
Tachia *Taiwan* **59** E13
Tach'ing Shan = Daqing
  Shan *China* **56** D6
Tachov *Czech Rep.* **26** B5
Tácina → *Italy* **43** D9
Tacloban *Phil.* **61** F6
Tacna *Peru* **124** G4
Tacoma *U.S.A.* **110** C4
Tacuarembó *Uruguay* **127** C4
Tademaït, Plateau du *Algeria* **78** C6
Tadio, L. *Ivory C.* **82** D3
Tadjoura *Djibouti* **81** E5
Tadjoura, Golfe de *Djibouti* **81** E5
Tadmor *N.Z.* **91** D4
Tadoule L. *Canada* **103** B9
Tadoussac *Canada* **105** C6
Tadrés △ *Niger* **83** B6
Tadzhikistan =
  Tajikistan ■ *Asia* **52** F8
Taegu = Daegu *S. Korea* **57** G15
Taegwan *N. Korea* **57** D13
Taejŏn = Daejeon *S. Korea* **57** F14
Taen, Ko *Thailand* **65** b
Tafalla *Spain* **38** C3
Tafar *Sudan* **81** F2
Tafelbaai = Table B. *S. Africa* **88** E2
Tafermaar *Indonesia* **63** F8
Tafi Viejo *Argentina* **126** B2
Tafīhān *Iran* **71** D7
Tafiré *Ivory C.* **82** D3
Tafo *Ghana* **83** D4
Tafresh *Iran* **71** C6
Taft *Iran* **71** D7
Taft *Phil.* **61** F6
Taft *U.S.A.* **111** K7
Taftan *Pakistan* **66** E2
Taftān, Kūh-e *Iran* **71** D9
Taga *Samoa* **91** b
Taga Dzong *Bhutan* **67** F16
Taganrog *Russia* **33** J10
Taganrogskiy Zaliv *Russia* **33** J10
Tagânt □ *Mauritania* **82** B3
Tagatay *Phil.* **61** D4
Tagbilaran *Phil.* **61** G5
Tággia *Italy* **40** E4
Tagish *Canada* **102** A2
Tagish L. *Canada* **102** A2
Tagliacozzo *Italy* **41** F10
Tagliamento → *Italy* **41** C10
Táglio di Po *Italy* **41** D9
Tago *Phil.* **61** G7
Tagomago *Spain* **48** B8
Tagouraret *Mauritania* **82** B3
Taguatinga *Brazil* **125** F10
Tagudin *Phil.* **61** C4
Tagum *Phil.* **61** H6
Tagus = Tejo → *Europe* **37** F2
Tahakopa *N.Z.* **91** G2
Tahan, Gunung *Malaysia* **65** K4
Tahat *Algeria* **78** D7
Tāherī *Iran* **71** E7
Tahiti *French Polynesia* **91** d

Tahiti, I. *Tahiti* **91** d
Tahlequah *U.S.A.* **116** D7
Tahoe, L. *U.S.A.* **110** G6
Tahoe City *U.S.A.* **110** F6
Tahoka *U.S.A.* **116** E4
Taholah *U.S.A.* **110** C2
Tahoua *Niger* **83** C6
Tahrūd *Iran* **71** D8
Tahsis *Canada* **102** D3
Tahta *Egypt* **80** B3
Tahtaköprü *Turkey* **45** G13
Tahtalı Dağları *Turkey* **72** C7
Tahulandang *Indonesia* **63** D7
Tahuna *Indonesia* **63** D7
Taï *Ivory C.* **82** D3
Taï △ *Ivory C.* **82** D3
Tai Hu *China* **59** B12
Tai Rom Yen △ *Thailand* **65** H2
Tai Shan *China* **57** F9
Tai'an *China* **57** F9
Taiarapu, Presqu'île de *Tahiti* **91** d
Taibei = T'aipei *Taiwan* **59** E13
Taibique *Canary Is.* **48** G2
Taibus Qi *China* **56** D8
Taicang *China* **59** B13
T'aichung *Taiwan* **59** E13
Taieri → *N.Z.* **91** G3
Taigu *China* **56** F7
Taihang Shan *China* **56** G7
Taihape *N.Z.* **91** C5
Taihe *Anhui, China* **56** H8
Taihe *Jiangxi, China* **59** D10
Taihu *China* **59** B11
Taijiang *China* **58** D7
Taikang *China* **56** G8
Tailem Bend *Australia* **95** F2
Tailfingen *Germany* **25** G5
T'ailuko *Taiwan* **59** E13
Taimyr Peninsula =
  Taymyr, Poluostrov
  Russia **53** B11
Tain *U.K.* **13** D4
T'ainan *Taiwan* **59** F13
Taining *China* **59** D11
T'aipei *Taiwan* **59** E13
Taiping *China* **59** B12
Taiping *Malaysia* **65** K3
Taipingzhen *China* **56** H6
Tairbeart = Tarbert *U.K.* **13** D2
Taishan *China* **59** F9
Taishun *China* **59** D12
Taita Hills *Kenya* **86** C4
Taitao, Pen. de *Chile* **128** F2
T'aitung *Taiwan* **59** F13
Taivalkoski *Finland* **8** D23
Taiwan ■ *Asia* **59** F13
Taiwan Strait *China* **59** E12
Taixing *China* **59** A13
Taiyara *Sudan* **81** E3
Taiyiba *Israel* **74** C4
Taiyuan *China* **56** F7
Taizhong = T'aichung
  Taiwan **59** E13
Taizhou *China* **59** A12
Taizhou Liedao *China* **59** C13
Ta'izz *Yemen* **75** E3
Tājābād *Iran* **71** D7
Tajikistan ■ *Asia* **52** F8
Tajima *Japan* **55** F9
Tajo = Tejo → *Europe* **37** F2
Tajrīsh *Iran* **71** C6
Tak *Thailand* **64** D2
Takāb *Iran* **73** C12
Takachiho *Japan* **55** H5
Takachu *Botswana* **88** C3
Takada *Japan* **55** F9
Takahagi *Japan* **55** F10
Takaka *N.Z.* **91** D4
Takamaka *Seychelles* **85** b
Takamatsu *Japan* **55** G7
Takaoka *Japan* **55** F8
Takapuna *N.Z.* **91** B5
Takasaki *Japan* **55** F9
Takatsuki *Japan* **55** G7
Takaungu *Kenya* **86** C4
Takayama *Japan* **55** F8
Take-Shima *Japan* **55** J5
Takefu *Japan* **55** G8
Takengon *Indonesia* **62** D1
Takeo *Japan* **55** H5
Tåkern *Sweden* **11** F8
Takeshima = Tokdo *Asia* **55** F5
Tākestān *Iran* **71** C6
Taketa *Japan* **55** H5
Takev *Cambodia* **65** G5
Takh *India* **69** C7
Takhmau *Cambodia* **65** G5
Takht-Sulaiman *Pakistan* **68** D3
Takiéta *Niger* **83** C6
Takikawa *Japan* **54** C10
Takla L. *Canada* **102** B3
Takla Landing *Canada* **102** B3
Takla Makan *China* **60** C3
Taklamakan Shamo =
  Takla Makan *China* **60** C3
Taksimo *Russia* **53** D12
Taku → *Canada* **102** B2
Takua Pa *Thailand* **65** H2
Takua Thung *Thailand* **65** a
Takum *Nigeria* **83** D6

Tal Halāl *Iran* **71** D7
Tala *Uruguay* **127** C4
Talachyn *Belarus* **32** E5
Talacogan *Phil.* **61** G6
Talagang *Pakistan* **68** C5
Talagante *Chile* **126** C1
Talak *Niger* **83** B6
Talamanca, Cordillera de
  Cent. Amer. **120** E3
Talampaya △ *Argentina* **126** B2
Talant *France* **19** E11
Talara *Peru* **124** D2
Talas *Kyrgyzstan* **52** E8
Talas *Turkey* **72** C6
Talâta *Egypt* **74** E1
Talata Mafara *Nigeria* **83** C6
Talaud, Kepulauan *Indonesia* **63** D7
Talaud Is. = Talaud,
  Kepulauan *Indonesia* **63** D7
Talavera de la Reina *Spain* **36** F6
Talavera la Real *Spain* **37** G4
Talayan *Phil.* **61** H6
Talayuela *Spain* **36** F5
Talbandh *India* **69** H12
Talbert, Sillon de *France* **18** D3
Talbot, C. *Australia* **92** B4
Talbragar → *Australia* **95** E4
Talca *Chile* **126** D1
Talcahuano *Chile* **126** D1
Talcher *India* **67** J14
Talcho *Niger* **83** C5
Taldy Kurgan =
  Taldyqorghan *Kazakhstan* **52** E8
Taldyqorghan *Kazakhstan* **52** E8
Tälesh *Iran* **73** D13
Tälesh, Kühhä-ye *Iran* **73** D13
Talguharai *Sudan* **80** D4
Tali Post *Sudan* **81** F3
Taliabu *Indonesia* **63** E6
Talibon *Phil.* **63** B6
Talihina *U.S.A.* **116** D7
Talisayan *Phil.* **61** G6
Taliwang *Indonesia* **62** F5
Talkha *Egypt* **80** H7
Tall 'Afar *Iraq* **73** D10
Tall Kalakh *Syria* **74** A5
Tall Kayf *Iraq* **73** D10
Talla *Egypt* **80** B3
Talladega *U.S.A.* **117** E11
Tallahassee *U.S.A.* **117** F12
Tallangatta *Australia* **95** F4
Tallard *France* **21** D10
Tällberg *Sweden* **10** D9
Tallering Pk. *Australia* **93** E2
Talli *Pakistan* **68** E3
Tallinn *Estonia* **32** C3
Tallmadge *U.S.A.* **114** E3
Tallulah *U.S.A.* **116** E9
Tălmaciu *Romania* **29** E9
Talmont-St-Hilaire *France* **20** B2
Talnakh *Russia* **53** C9
Talne *Ukraine* **33** H6
Talnoye = Talne *Ukraine* **33** H6
Talodi *Sudan* **81** E3
Talovaya *Russia* **34** E5
Taloyoak *Canada* **100** D13
Talpa de Allende *Mexico* **118** C4
Talparo *Trin. & Tob.* **125** K15
Talsi *Latvia* **30** A9
Talsi = Talsi *Latvia* **30** A9
Taltal *Chile* **126** B1
Taltson → *Canada* **102** A6
Talwood *Australia* **95** D4
Talyawalka Cr. → *Australia* **95** E3
Tam Ky *Vietnam* **64** E7
Tam Quan *Vietnam* **64** E7
Tama *U.S.A.* **112** E8
Tama → *Ethiopia* **81** F4
Tama Abu, Banjaran
  Malaysia **62** D5
Tamale *Ghana* **83** D4
Taman *Russia* **33** K9
Taman Negara △ *Malaysia* **65** K4
Tamani *Mali* **82** C3
Tamano *Japan* **55** G6
Tamanrasset *Algeria* **78** D7
Tamaqua *U.S.A.* **115** F9
Tamar → *U.K.* **15** G3
Tamarin *Mauritius* **85** d
Tamarinda *Spain* **48** B10
Tamarite de Litera *Spain* **38** D5
Tamashima *Japan* **55** G6
Tamási *Hungary* **28** D2
Tamaské *Niger* **83** C6
Tamatave = Toamasina
  Madag. **89** B8
Tamaulipas □ *Mexico* **119** C5
Tamaulipas, Sierra de
  Mexico **119** C5
Tamazula *Mexico* **118** C3
Tamazunchale *Mexico* **119** C5
Tamba-Dabatou *Guinea* **82** C2
Tambach *Kenya* **86** B4
Tambacounda *Senegal* **82** C2
Tambacounda □ *Senegal* **82** C2
Tambelan, Kepulauan
  Indonesia **62** D3
Tambellup *Australia* **93** F2
Tambo *Australia* **94** C4
Tambo de Mora *Peru* **124** F3

Tambohorano *Madag.* **89** B7
Tambora *Indonesia* **62** F5
Tamboura *C.A.R.* **81** F2
Tambov *Russia* **34** D5
Tambov □ *Russia* **34** D5
Tambre → *Spain* **36** C2
Tambuku *Indonesia* **63** G15
Tamburà *Sudan* **81** F2
Tâmchekket *Mauritania* **82** B2
Tâmega → *Portugal* **36** D2
Tamenglong *India* **67** G18
Tamgak, Massif du *Niger* **83** B7
Tamgué, Massif du *Guinea* **82** C2
Tamiahua, L. de *Mexico* **119** C5
Tamil Nadu □ *India* **66** P10
Tamis → *Serbia* **28** F5
Tamiya *Egypt* **80** J7
Tamluk *India* **69** H12
Tammerfors = Tampere
  Finland **32** B2
Tammisaari *Finland* **32** B2
Tämnaren *Sweden* **10** D11
Tampa *U.S.A.* **117** H13
Tampa, Tanjung *Indonesia* **63** K19
Tampa B. *U.S.A.* **117** H13
Tampere *Finland* **32** B2
Tampico *Mexico* **119** C5
Tampin *Malaysia* **65** L4
Tampoi *Malaysia* **65** d
Tampoi *Indonesia* **65** d
Tamsweg *Austria* **26** D6
Tamu *Burma* **67** G19
Tamuja → *Spain* **37** F4
Tamworth *Australia* **95** E5
Tamworth *Canada* **114** B8
Tamworth *U.K.* **15** E6
Tan An *Vietnam* **65** G6
Tan Chau *Vietnam* **65** G5
Tan-Tan *Morocco* **78** C3
Tana → *Kenya* **86** C5
Tana → *Norway* **8** A23
Tana, L. *Ethiopia* **81** E4
Tana River Primate △ *Kenya* **86** C5
Tanabe *Japan* **55** H7
Tanafjorden *Norway* **8** A23
Tanaga I. *U.S.A.* **106** E4
Tanahbala *Indonesia* **62** E1
Tanahgrogot *Indonesia* **62** E5
Tanahjampea *Indonesia* **63** F6
Tanahmasa *Indonesia* **62** E1
Tanahmerah *Indonesia* **63** F10
Tanakpur *India* **69** E9
Tanakura *Japan* **55** F10
Tanami Desert *Australia* **92** C5
Tanana *U.S.A.* **106** B9
Tanana → *U.S.A.* **100** D1
Tananarive =
  Antananarivo *Madag.* **89** B8
Tánaro → *Italy* **40** D5
Tancheng *China* **57** G10
Tanch'ŏn *N. Korea* **57** D15
Tanda *Ut. P., India* **69** F10
Tanda *Ut. P., India* **69** E8
Tanda *Ivory C.* **82** D4
Tandag *Phil.* **61** G7
Tandaia *Tanzania* **87** D3
Tăndărei *Romania* **29** F12
Tandaué *Angola* **88** B2
Tandil *Argentina* **126** D4
Tandil, Sa. del *Argentina* **126** D4
Tandlianwala *Pakistan* **68** D5
Tando Adam *Pakistan* **68** G3
Tando Allahyar *Pakistan* **68** G3
Tando Bago *Pakistan* **68** G3
Tando Mohommed Khan
  Pakistan **68** G3
Tandou L. *Australia* **95** E3
Tandoureh △ *Iran* **71** B8
Tandragee *U.K.* **12** B5
Tandsjöborg *Sweden* **10** C8
Tane-ga-Shima *Japan* **55** J5
Taneatua *N.Z.* **91** C6
Tanen Tong Dan = Dawna
  Ra. *Burma* **64** D2
Tanew → *Poland* **31** H9
Tanezrouft *Algeria* **78** D6
Tang, Koh *Cambodia* **65** G4
Tang, Ra's-e *Iran* **71** E8
Tang Krasang *Cambodia* **64** F5
Tanga *Tanzania* **86** D4
Tanga □ *Tanzania* **86** D4
Tanganyika, L. *Africa* **86** D3
Tangaza *Nigeria* **83** C5
Tanger *Morocco* **78** A4
Tangerang *Indonesia* **63** G12
Tangerhütte *Germany* **24** C7
Tangermünde *Germany* **24** C7
Tanggu *China* **57** E9
Tanggula Shan *China* **60** C4
Tanghe *China* **56** H7
Tanghla Range =
  Tanggula Shan *China* **60** C4
Tangier = Tanger *Morocco* **78** A4
Tangorin *Australia* **94** C3
Tangorombohitr'i Makay
  Madag. **89** C8
Tangshan *China* **57** E10
Tangtou *China* **57** G10
Tanguen-Dassouri
  Burkina Faso **83** C4
Tanguiéta *Benin* **83** C5
Tangxi *China* **59** C12

Tangyan He → *China* **58** C7
Tanimbar, Kepulauan
  Indonesia **63** F8
Tanimbar Is. = Tanimbar,
  Kepulauan *Indonesia* **63** F8
Taninthari = Tenasserim
  Burma **65** F2
Tanjay *Phil.* **61** G5
Tanjong Malim *Malaysia* **65** L3
Tanjong Pelepas *Malaysia* **65** d
Tanjore = Thanjavur *India* **66** P11
Tanjung *Bali, Indonesia* **63** J19
Tanjung *Kalimantan, Indonesia* **62** E5
Tanjung Tokong *Malaysia* **65** c
Tanjungbalai *Indonesia* **62** D1
Tanjungbatu *Indonesia* **62** D5
Tanjungkarang
  Telukbetung = Bandar
  Lampung *Indonesia* **62** F3
Tanjungpandan *Indonesia* **62** E3
Tanjungpinang *Indonesia* **62** D2
Tanjungredeb *Indonesia* **62** D5
Tanjungselor *Indonesia* **62** D5
Tank *Pakistan* **68** C4
Tankhala *India* **68** J5
Tankwa-Karoo △ *S. Africa* **88** E2
Tännäs *Sweden* **10** B6
Tannersville *U.S.A.* **115** E9
Tannis Bugt *Denmark* **11** G4
Tannu Ola *Asia* **53** D10
Tannum Sands *Australia* **94** C5
Tano → *Ghana* **82** D4
Tanon Str. *Phil.* **61** F5
Tanout *Niger* **83** C6
Tanshui *Taiwan* **59** E13
Tansilla *Burkina Faso* **82** C4
Tanta *Egypt* **80** H7
Tantoyuca *Mexico* **119** C5
Tantung = Dandong *China* **57** D13
Tanumshede *Sweden* **11** F5
Tanunda *Australia* **95** E2
Tanus *France* **20** D6
Tanzania ■ *Africa* **86** D3
Tanzilla → *Canada* **102** B2
Tao, Ko *Thailand* **65** G2
Tao'an = Taonan *China* **57** B12
Tao'er He → *China* **57** B13
Taohua Dao *China* **59** C14
Taolanaro *Madag.* **89** D8
Taole *China* **56** E4
Taonan *China* **57** B12
Taormina *Italy* **43** E8
Taos *U.S.A.* **109** H11
Taoudenni *Mali* **78** D5
Taoyuan *China* **59** C8
T'aoyüan *Taiwan* **59** E13
Tapa *Estonia* **32** C3
Tapa Shan = Daba Shan
  China **58** B7
Tapachula *Mexico* **119** E6
Tapah *Malaysia* **65** K3
Tapajós → *Brazil* **125** D8
Tapaktuan *Indonesia* **62** D1
Tapanahoni → *Suriname* **125** C8
Tapanui *N.Z.* **91** F2
Tapauá *Brazil* **124** E6
Tapauá → *Brazil* **124** E6
Tapes *Brazil* **127** C5
Tapeta *Liberia* **82** D3
Tapi → *India* **66** J8
Tapia de Casariego *Spain* **36** B4
Tapirapecó, Serra *Venezuela* **124** C6
Tapo-Capara △ *Venezuela* **121** E5
Tapolca *Hungary* **28** D2
Tapti → *India* **66** J8
Tapuae-o-Uenuku *N.Z.* **91** E4
Tapul Group *Phil.* **61** J4
Tapurucuará *Brazil* **124** D5
Taquara *Brazil* **127** B5
Taquari → *Brazil* **124** G7
Tara *Australia* **95** D5
Tara *Canada* **114** B3
Tara *Russia* **52** D8
Tara *Zambia* **87** F2
Tara → *Montenegro* **44** C2
Tara △ *Serbia* **44** C3
Taraba □ *Nigeria* **83** D7
Taraba → *Nigeria* **83** D7
Țarābulus *Lebanon* **74** A4
Țarābulus *Libya* **79** B8
Țarābulus N. Afr. **79** B8
Taracahi *India* **69** H8
Taraclia *Taraclia, Moldova* **29** E13
Taraclia *Tighina, Moldova* **29** D14
Taradehi *India* **69** H8
Tarajalejo *Canary Is.* **48** F5
Tarakan *Indonesia* **62** D5
Tarakit, Mt. *Kenya* **86** B4
Tarama-Jima *Japan* **55** M2
Taran, Mys *Russia* **30** D7
Taranagar *India* **68** E6
Taranaki □ *N.Z.* **91** C5
Taranaki, Mt. *N.Z.* **91** C5
Tarancón *Spain* **38** E1
Tarangire △ *Tanzania* **86** C4
Taransay *U.K.* **13** D1
Táranto *Italy* **43** B10
Táranto, G. di *Italy* **43** B10
Tarapacá *Colombia* **124** D5
Tarapacá □ *Chile* **126** A2
Tarapoto *Peru* **124** E3

Tarare *France* **21** C8
Tararua Ra. *N.Z.* **91** D5
Tarascon *France* **21** E8
Tarascon-sur-Ariège *France* **20** F5
Tarashcha *Ukraine* **23** D16
Tarauacá *Brazil* **124** E4
Tarauacá → *Brazil* **124** E5
Taravao *Tahiti* **91** d
Taravao, Isthme de *Tahiti* **91** d
Taravo → *France* **21** G12
Tarawa *Kiribati* **96** G9
Tarawera *N.Z.* **91** C6
Tarawera, L. *N.Z.* **91** C6
Taraz *Kazakhstan* **52** E8
Tarazona *Spain* **38** D3
Tarazona de la Mancha
  Spain **39** F3
Tarbagatay, Khrebet
  Kazakhstan **52** E9
Tarbat Ness *U.K.* **13** D5
Tarbela Dam *Pakistan* **68** B5
Tarbert *Ireland* **12** D2
Tarbert *Argyll & Bute, U.K.* **13** F3
Tarbert *W. Isles, U.K.* **13** D2
Tarbes *France* **20** E4
Tarboro *U.S.A.* **117** D16
Tărcău, Munții *Romania* **29** D11
Tarcento *Italy* **41** B10
Tarcoola *Australia* **95** E1
Tarcoon *Australia* **95** E4
Tardets-Sorholus *France* **20** E3
Tardoire → *France* **20** C4
Taree *Australia* **95** E5
Tarfa, W. el → *Egypt* **80** B3
Tarfaya *Morocco* **78** C3
Târgoviște *Romania* **29** F10
Târgu Bujor *Romania* **29** E12
Târgu Cărbunești *Romania* **29** F8
Târgu Frumos *Romania* **29** C12
Târgu Jiu *Romania* **29** E8
Târgu Lăpuș *Romania* **29** C8
Târgu Mureș *Romania* **29** D9
Târgu Neamț *Romania* **29** C11
Târgu Ocna *Romania* **29** D11
Târgu Secuiesc *Romania* **29** E11
Târgușor *Romania* **29** F13
Tărhăus, Vf. *Romania* **29** D11
Țarif *U.A.E.* **71** E7
Tarifa *Spain* **37** J5
Tarija *Bolivia* **126** A3
Tarija □ *Bolivia* **126** A3
Tariku → *Indonesia* **63** E9
Tarim Basin = Tarim Pendi
  China **52** F9
Tarim He → *China* **60** C3
Tarim Pendi *China* **52** F9
Taritatu → *Indonesia* **63** E9
Tarka → *S. Africa* **88** E4
Tarka La *Bhutan* **69** F13
Tarkastad *S. Africa* **88** E4
Tarkhankut, Mys *Ukraine* **33** K7
Tarko Sale *Russia* **52** C8
Tarkwa *Ghana* **82** D4
Tarlac *Phil.* **61** D4
Tarm *Denmark* **11** J2
Tarma *Peru* **124** F3
Tarmiya *Iraq* **73** G11
Tarn □ *France* **20** E6
Tarn → *France* **20** D5
Tarn-et-Garonne □ *France* **20** D5
Tarna → *Hungary* **28** C4
Târnava Mare → *Romania* **29** D8
Târnava Mică → *Romania* **29** D8
Târnăveni *Romania* **29** D9
Tarnica *Poland* **31** J9
Tarnobrzeg *Poland* **31** H8
Tarnogród *Poland* **31** H9
Tarnos *France* **20** E2
Târnova *Moldova* **29** B12
Târnova *Romania* **28** E6
Tarnów *Poland* **31** H8
Tarnowskie Góry *Poland* **31** H5
Tärnsjö *Sweden* **10** D10
Táro → *Italy* **40** C7
Țārom *Iran* **71** D7
Taroom *Australia* **95** D4
Taroudannt *Morocco* **78** B4
Tarp *Germany* **24** A5
Tarpon Springs *U.S.A.* **117** G13
Tarquínia *Italy* **41** F8
Tarrafal *C. Verde Is.* **78** b
Tarragona *Spain* **38** D6
Tarragona □ *Spain* **38** D6
Tarraleah *Australia* **95** G4
Tarrasa = Terrassa *Spain* **38** D7
Tàrrega *Spain* **38** D6
Tarrytown *U.S.A.* **115** E11
Tårs *Denmark* **11** G4
Tarshiha = Me'ona *Israel* **74** B4
Tarsus *Turkey* **72** D6
Tartagal *Argentina* **126** A3
Tärtär *Azerbaijan* **35** K8
Tärtär → *Azerbaijan* **35** K8
Tartas *France* **20** E3
Tartu *Estonia* **32** C4
Țarṭūs *Syria* **72** E6
Țarṭūs □ *Syria* **72** E7
Tarumizu *Japan* **55** J5
Tarussa *Russia* **32** E9

Tarutao = Ko Tarutao △ *Thailand* 65 J2
Tarutao, Ko *Thailand* 65 J2
Tarutung *Indonesia* 62 D1
Tarutyne *Ukraine* 29 D14
Tarvísio *Italy* 41 B10
Taseko ➤ *Canada* 102 C4
Tash-Kömür *Kyrgyzstan* 52 E8
Tash-Kumyr = Tash-Kömür *Kyrgyzstan* 52 E8
Tashauz = Dashoguz *Turkmenistan* 52 E6
Tashi Chho Dzong = Thimphu *Bhutan* 67 F16
Ţashk, Daryācheh-ye *Iran* 71 D7
Tashkent = Toshkent *Uzbekistan* 52 E7
Tashtagol *Russia* 52 D9
Tasiilaq *Greenland* 4 C6
Tasik Kenyir *Malaysia* 65 K4
Tasikmalaya *Indonesia* 63 G13
Tåsinge *Denmark* 11 J4
Tåsjön *Sweden* 8 D16
Task *Niger* 83 C7
Taskan *Russia* 53 C16
Taşkent *Turkey* 72 D5
Taşköprü *Turkey* 72 B6
Taşlâc *Moldova* 29 C14
Taşliçay *Turkey* 73 C10
Tasman B. *N.Z.* 91 D4
Tasman Basin *Pac. Oc.* 96 M7
Tasman Mts. *N.Z.* 91 D4
Tasman Pen. *Australia* 95 G4
Tasman Sea *Pac. Oc.* 90 E9
Tasmania □ *Australia* 95 G4
Tasmanian Wilderness World Heritage Area △ *Australia* 95 G4
Tăşnad *Romania* 28 C7
Taşova *Turkey* 72 B7
Tassili n'Ajjer *Algeria* 78 C7
Tassili-Oua-n-Ahaggar *Algeria* 78 D7
Tassili Tin-Rerhoh *Algeria* 83 A5
Tasuj *Iran* 73 C11
Tat Ton △ *Thailand* 64 E4
Tata *Hungary* 28 C3
Tata *Morocco* 78 C4
Tatabánya *Hungary* 28 C3
Tatahouine *Tunisia* 79 B8
Tataouine *Tunisia* 79 B8
Tatar Republic = Tatarstan □ *Russia* 34 C10
Tatarbunary *Ukraine* 29 E14
Tatarsk *Russia* 52 D8
Tatarskiy Proliv *Russia* 53 E15
Tatarstan □ *Russia* 34 C10
Tatatua, Pte. *Tahiti* 91 d
Tateyama *Japan* 55 G9
Tathlina L. *Canada* 102 A5
Tathra *Australia* 95 F4
Tatinnai L. *Canada* 103 A9
Tatla Lake *Canada* 102 C4
Tatlısu *Turkey* 45 F11
Tatnam, C. *Canada* 103 B10
Tatra = Tatry *Slovak Rep.* 27 B13
Tatranský △ *Slovak Rep.* 27 B13
Tatry *Slovak Rep.* 27 B13
Tatshenshini ➤ *Canada* 102 B1
Tatsuno *Japan* 55 G7
Tatta *Pakistan* 68 G2
Tatuī *Brazil* 127 A6
Tatum *U.S.A.* 109 K12
Tat'ung = Datong *China* 56 D7
Tatvan *Turkey* 73 C10
Ta'ū *Amer. Samoa* 91 b
Taubaté *Brazil* 127 A6
Tauberbischofsheim *Germany* 25 F5
Taucha *Germany* 24 D8
Tauern *Austria* 22 E7
Tauern-tunnel *Austria* 26 D6
Taufikia *Sudan* 81 F3
Taulé *France* 18 D3
Taumarunui *N.Z.* 91 C5
Taumaturgo *Brazil* 124 E4
Taung *S. Africa* 88 D3
Taungdwingyi *Burma* 67 J19
Taunggyi *Burma* 67 J20
Taungup *Burma* 67 K19
Taunsa *Pakistan* 68 D4
Taunsa Barrage *Pakistan* 68 D4
Taunton *U.K.* 15 F4
Taunton *U.S.A.* 115 E13
Taunus *Germany* 25 E4
Taupo *N.Z.* 91 C6
Taupo, L. *N.Z.* 91 C5
Tauragė *Lithuania* 30 C9
Tauragė *Lithuania* 30 C9
Tauranga *N.Z.* 91 B6
Tauranga Harb. *N.Z.* 91 B6
Taureau, Rés. *Canada* 104 C5
Taurianova *Italy* 43 D9
Taurus Mts. = Toros Dağları *Turkey* 72 D5
Tauste *Spain* 38 D3
Tautira *Tahiti* 91 d
Tauyskaya Guba *Russia* 53 D16
Tauz = Tovuz *Azerbaijan* 35 K7
Tavas *Turkey* 47 D11

Tavastehus = Hämeenlinna *Finland* 32 B3
Tavda *Russia* 52 D7
Tavda ➤ *Russia* 52 D7
Taverner B. *Canada* 101 D17
Tavernes de la Valldigna *Spain* 39 F4
Taveta *Kenya* 86 C4
Taveuni *Fiji* 91 a
Taviano *Italy* 43 C11
Tavira *Portugal* 37 H3
Tavistock *Canada* 114 C4
Tavistock *U.K.* 15 G3
Tavolara *Italy* 42 B2
Távora ➤ *Portugal* 36 D3
Tavoy *Burma* 64 E2
Tavrichanka *Russia* 54 C5
Tavropos ➤ *Greece* 46 B3
Tavşanlı *Turkey* 47 B11
Tavua *Fiji* 91 a
Tavuki *Fiji* 91 a
Taw ➤ *U.K.* 15 F3
Tawa ➤ *India* 68 H8
Tawas City *U.S.A.* 113 C12
Tawau *Malaysia* 62 D5
Tawi-Tawi *Phil.* 63 C6
Tawu *Taiwan* 59 F13
Tāwūq *Iraq* 73 E11
Taxco *Mexico* 119 D5
Taxila *Pakistan* 68 C5
Tay ➤ *U.K.* 13 E5
Tay, Firth of *U.K.* 13 E5
Tay, L. *Australia* 93 F3
Tay, L. *U.K.* 13 E4
Tay ➤ *U.K.* 13 E5
Tay Ninh *Vietnam* 65 G6
Tayabamba *Peru* 124 E3
Tayabas Bay *Phil.* 61 E4
Taygetos Oros *Greece* 46 D4
Taylakova *Russia* 52 D8
Taylor *Canada* 102 B4
Taylor *Nebr., U.S.A.* 112 E4
Taylor *Pa., U.S.A.* 115 E9
Taylor *Tex., U.S.A.* 116 F6
Taylor, Mt. *U.S.A.* 109 J10
Taylorville *U.S.A.* 112 F9
Taymā *Si. Arabia* 70 E3
Taymyr, Oz. *Russia* 53 B11
Taymyr, Poluostrov *Russia* 53 B11
Tayport *U.K.* 13 E6
Tayrona △ *Colombia* 121 D5
Tayshet *Russia* 53 D10
Taytay *Phil.* 61 F3
Tăyyebād *Iran* 71 C9
Tāyyebād □ *Iran* 71 C9
Taz ➤ *Russia* 52 C8
Taza *Morocco* 78 B5
Tāza Khurmātū *Iraq* 73 E11
Tazawa-Ko *Japan* 54 E10
Tazerbo *Libya* 79 C10
Tazin ➤ *Canada* 103 B7
Tazin L. *Canada* 103 B7
Tazovskiy *Russia* 52 C8
Tbilisi *Georgia* 35 K7
Tchad = Chad ■ *Africa* 79 F8
Tchad, L. *Chad* 79 F8
Tchaourou *Benin* 83 D5
Tch'eng-tou = Chengdu *China* 58 B5
Tchentlo L. *Canada* 102 B4
Tchetti *Benin* 83 D5
Tchibanga *Gabon* 84 E2
Tchien *Liberia* 82 D3
Tchin Tabaraden *Niger* 83 B6
Tch'ong-k'ing = Chongqing *China* 58 C6
Tczew *Poland* 30 D5
Te Anau, L. *N.Z.* 91 F1
Te Aroha *N.Z.* 91 B5
Te Awamutu *N.Z.* 91 C5
Te Ika a Maui = North I. *N.Z.* 91 C5
Te Kuiti *N.Z.* 91 C5
Te-n-Dghâmcha, Sebkhet *Mauritania* 82 B1
Te Puke *N.Z.* 91 B6
Te Waewae B. *N.Z.* 91 G1
Te Wai Pounamu = South I. *N.Z.* 91 F3
Teaca *Romania* 29 D9
Teague *U.S.A.* 116 F6
Teahupoo *Tahiti* 91 d
Teano *Italy* 43 A7
Teapa *Mexico* 119 D6
Teba *Spain* 37 J6
Tebakang *Malaysia* 62 D4
Tébarat *Niger* 83 C5
Teberda *Russia* 35 J5
Teberu *Malaysia* 65 d
Tébessa *Algeria* 78 A7
Tebicuary ➤ *Paraguay* 126 B4
Tebingtinggi *Riau, Indonesia* 62 E2
Tebingtinggi *Sumatera Utara, Indonesia* 62 D1
Tebulos *Georgia* 35 J7
Tecate *Mexico* 111 N10
Tecer Dağları *Turkey* 72 C7
Tech ➤ *France* 20 F7

Techiman *Ghana* 82 D4
Techirghiol *Romania* 29 F13
Tecka *Argentina* 128 E2
Tecomán *Mexico* 118 D4
Tecopa *U.S.A.* 111 K10
Tecoripa *Mexico* 118 B3
Tecuala *Mexico* 118 C3
Tecuci *Romania* 29 E12
Tecumseh *Canada* 114 D2
Tecumseh *Mich., U.S.A.* 113 D12
Tecumseh *Okla., U.S.A.* 116 D6
Tedzhen = Tejen *Turkmenistan* 52 F7
Tees ➤ *U.K.* 14 C6
Tees B. *U.K.* 14 C6
Teeswater *Canada* 114 C3
Tefé *Brazil* 124 D6
Tefenni *Turkey* 47 D11
Tegal *Indonesia* 62 F3
Tegallalang *Indonesia* 63 J18
Tegalsari *Indonesia* 63 J17
Tegel, Berlin ✈ (TXL) *Germany* 24 C9
Tegernsee *Germany* 25 H7
Teggiano *Italy* 43 B8
Tegid, L. = Bala, L. *U.K.* 14 E4
Tegina *Nigeria* 83 C6
Tegucigalpa *Honduras* 120 D2
Teguidda i-n-Tessoum *Niger* 83 B6
Tehachapi *U.S.A.* 111 K8
Tehachapi Mts. *U.S.A.* 111 L8
Tehamiyam *Sudan* 80 D4
Teheran = Tehrān *Iran* 71 C6
Tehilla *Sudan* 80 D4
Téhini *Ivory C.* 82 D4
Tehoru *Indonesia* 63 E7
Tehrān *Iran* 71 C6
Tehrān □ *Iran* 71 C6
Tehri *India* 69 D8
Tehuacán *Mexico* 119 D5
Tehuantepec *Mexico* 119 D5
Tehuantepec, G. de *Mexico* 119 D5
Tehuantepec, Istmo de *Mexico* 119 D6
Teide, Pico de *Canary Is.* 48 F3
Teifi ➤ *U.K.* 15 E3
Teigebyen *Norway* 10 D5
Teign ➤ *U.K.* 15 G4
Teignmouth *U.K.* 15 G4
Teiuş *Romania* 29 D8
Teixeira Pinto *Guinea-Biss.* 82 C1
Tejakula *Indonesia* 63 J18
Tejam *India* 69 E9
Tejen *Turkmenistan* 52 F7
Tejen ➤ *Turkmenistan* 71 B9
Tejo ➤ *Europe* 37 F2
Tejon Pass *U.S.A.* 111 L8
Tekamah *U.S.A.* 112 E5
Tekapo, L. *N.Z.* 91 E3
Tekax *Mexico* 119 C7
Teke ➤ *S. Arabia* 45 E13
Tekeli *Kazakhstan* 52 E8
Tekeze ➤ *Ethiopia* 81 E4
Tekija *Serbia* 44 B6
Tekirdağ *Turkey* 45 F11
Tekirdağ □ *Turkey* 45 E11
Tekirova *Turkey* 47 E12
Tekkali *India* 67 K14
Tekke *Turkey* 72 B7
Tekman *Turkey* 73 C9
Tekoa *U.S.A.* 108 C5
Tekong Besar, Pulau *Singapore* 65 d
Tel Aviv ✈ (TLV) *Israel* 74 C3
Tel Aviv-Yafo *Israel* 74 C3
Tel Lakhish *Israel* 74 D3
Tel Megiddo *Israel* 74 C4
Tela *Honduras* 120 C2
Telanaipura = Jambi *Indonesia* 62 E2
Telašćica △ *Croatia* 41 E12
Telavi *Georgia* 35 J7
Telč *Czech Rep.* 26 B8
Telciu *Romania* 29 C9
Telde *Canary Is.* 48 G4
Telegraph Creek *Canada* 102 B2
Telekhany = Tsyelyakhany *Belarus* 23 B13
Telemark *Norway* 9 G12
Télemsès *Niger* 83 B5
Telén *Argentina* 126 D2
Teleneşti *Moldova* 29 C13
Teleng *Iran* 71 E9
Teleño *Spain* 36 C4
Teleorman □ *Romania* 29 G10
Teleorman ➤ *Romania* 29 G10
Teles Pires ➤ *Brazil* 124 E7
Telescope Pk. *U.S.A.* 111 J9
Teletaye *Mali* 83 B5
Telford *U.K.* 15 E5
Telford and Wrekin □ *U.K.* 14 E5
Telfs *Austria* 26 D4
Télimélé *Guinea* 82 C2
Teljo, J. *Sudan* 81 E2
Telkwa *Canada* 102 C3
Tell City *U.S.A.* 113 G10
Teller *U.S.A.* 106 B6
Tellicherry *India* 66 P9
Telluride *U.S.A.* 109 H10
Teloloapán *Mexico* 119 D5
Telpos Iz *Russia* 6 C17

Telsen *Argentina* 128 E3
Telšiai *Lithuania* 30 C9
Telšiai □ *Lithuania* 30 C9
Teltow *Germany* 24 C9
Teluk Anson = Teluk Intan *Malaysia* 65 K3
Teluk Bahang *Malaysia* 65 c
Teluk Betung = Bandar Lampung *Indonesia* 62 F3
Teluk Intan *Malaysia* 65 K3
Teluk Kumbar *Malaysia* 65 c
Telukbutun *Indonesia* 62 D3
Telukdalem *Indonesia* 62 D1
Tema *Ghana* 83 D5
Temagami, L. *Canada* 104 C3
Temax *Mexico* 119 C7
Temba *S. Africa* 89 D4
Tembagapura *Indonesia* 63 E9
Tembe ➤ *Dem. Rep. of the Congo* 86 C2
Tembe ➤ *S. Africa* 89 D5
Tembleque *Spain* 36 F7
Temblor Range *U.S.A.* 111 K7
Teme ➤ *U.K.* 15 E5
Temecula *U.S.A.* 111 M9
Temengor, Tasik *Malaysia* 65 K3
Temerloh *Malaysia* 65 L4
Temir *Kazakhstan* 52 E6
Temirtau *Russia* 52 D9
Témiscamie ➤ *Canada* 105 B5
Témiscaming *Canada* 104 C4
Témiscamingue, L. *Canada* 104 C4
Temnikov *Russia* 34 C6
Temo ➤ *Italy* 42 B1
Tempe *U.S.A.* 109 K8
Tempe *U.S.A.* 109 K8
Témpio Pausánia *Italy* 42 B2
Templemore *Ireland* 12 D4
Templeton *U.S.A.* 110 K6
Templeton ➤ *Australia* 94 C2
Templin *Germany* 24 B9
Tempoal de Sánchez *Mexico* 119 C5
Temryuk *Russia* 33 K9
Temska ➤ *Serbia* 44 C5
Temuco *Chile* 128 D2
Temuka *N.Z.* 91 F3
Tenabo *Mexico* 119 C6
Tenaha *U.S.A.* 116 F7
Tenakee Springs *U.S.A.* 102 B1
Tenali *India* 67 L12
Tenancingo de Degollado *Mexico* 119 D5
Tenango del Valle *Mexico* 119 D5
Tenaro, Akra *Greece* 46 E4
Tenasserim *Burma* 65 F2
Tenasserim □ *Burma* 64 F2
Tenby *U.K.* 15 F3
Tenda, Colle di *France* 21 D11
Tendaho *Ethiopia* 81 E5
Tende *France* 21 D11
Tendelti *Sudan* 81 E3
Tendrovskaya Kosa *Ukraine* 33 J6
Tendukhera *India* 69 H8
Teneguía, Volcanes de *Canary Is.* 48 F2
Teneida *Egypt* 80 B3
Tenenkou *Mali* 82 C4
Ténéré *Niger* 83 B7
Ténéré, Erg du *Niger* 79 E8
Tenerife *Canary Is.* 48 F3
Tenerife, Pico *Canary Is.* 48 G1
Tenerife Norte ✈ (TFN) *Canary Is.* 48 F3
Tenerife Sur ✈ (TFS) *Canary Is.* 48 F3
Teng Xian *Guangxi Zhuangzu, China* 59 F8
Teng Xian *Shandong, China* 57 G9
Tengah, Kepulauan *Indonesia* 62 F5
Tengchong *China* 58 E2
Tengchowfu = Penglai *China* 57 F11
Tenggarong *Indonesia* 62 E5
Tenggol, Pulau *Malaysia* 65 K4
Tengiz Köli *Kazakhstan* 52 D7
Tenhult *Sweden* 11 G8
Teniente Enciso △ *Paraguay* 126 A3
Teniente Rodolfo Marsh *Antarctica* 5 C18
Tenino *U.S.A.* 110 D4
Tenkasi *India* 66 Q10
Tenke *Katanga, Dem. Rep. of the Congo* 87 E2
Tenke *Katanga, Dem. Rep. of the Congo* 87 E2
Tenkodogo *Burkina Faso* 83 C4
Tenna ➤ *Italy* 41 E10
Tennant Creek *Australia* 94 B1
Tennessee □ *U.S.A.* 117 D11
Tennessee ➤ *U.S.A.* 117 C10
Teno, Pta. de *Canary Is.* 48 F3
Tenom *Malaysia* 62 C5
Tenosique *Mexico* 119 D6
Tenryū-Gawa ➤ *Japan* 55 G8
Tenterden *U.K.* 15 F8
Tenterfield *Australia* 95 D5
Teo = A Ramallosa *Spain* 36 C2

Teófilo Otoni *Brazil* 125 G10
Tepa *Indonesia* 63 F7
Tepalcatepec ➤ *Mexico* 118 D4
Tepecik *Bursa, Turkey* 45 F12
Tepecik *Kütahya, Turkey* 47 B11
Tepehuanes *Mexico* 118 C4
Tepelenë *Albania* 44 F4
Tepetongo *Mexico* 118 C4
Tepic *Mexico* 118 C4
Teplá *Czech Rep.* 26 B5
Teplice *Czech Rep.* 26 A6
Teplyk *Ukraine* 29 B14
Tepoca, C. *Mexico* 118 A2
Tequila *Mexico* 118 C4
Ter ➤ *Spain* 38 C8
Ter Apel *Neths.* 17 B7
Téra *Niger* 83 C5
Tera ➤ *Spain* 36 D5
Teraina *Kiribati* 97 G12
Terakeka *Sudan* 81 F3
Téramo *Italy* 41 F10
Terang *Australia* 95 F3
Terang, Teluk *Indonesia* 63 K19
Terazit, Massif de *Niger* 83 A6
Tercan *Turkey* 73 C9
Terceira *Azores* 78 a
Tercero ➤ *Argentina* 126 C3
Terebovlya *Ukraine* 23 D13
Teregova *Romania* 28 E8
Tereida *Sudan* 81 E3
Terek ➤ *Russia* 35 J8
Terepaima △ *Venezuela* 121 E6
Teresa *Brazil* 125 E10
Teresina *Brazil* 125 E10
Terespol *Poland* 31 F10
Teresva *Ukraine* 29 B8
Terewah, L. *Australia* 95 D4
Terges ➤ *Portugal* 37 H3
Tergnier *France* 19 C10
Teridgerie ➤ *Australia* 95 E4
Terlizzi *Italy* 43 A9
Termas de Río Hondo *Argentina* 126 B3
Terme *Turkey* 72 B7
Termez = Termiz *Uzbekistan* 52 F7
Términi Imerese *Italy* 42 E6
Términos, L. de *Mexico* 119 D6
Termiz *Uzbekistan* 52 F7
Térmoli *Italy* 41 F12
Ternate *Indonesia* 63 D7
Terneuzen *Neths.* 17 C3
Terney *Russia* 54 B8
Terni *Italy* 41 F9
Ternitz *Austria* 26 D9
Ternivka *Ukraine* 29 B14
Ternopil *Ukraine* 23 D13
Ternopil □ *Ukraine* 33 H3
Ternopol = Ternopil *Ukraine* 23 D13
Terowie *Australia* 95 E2
Terpeni *Greece* 44 F7
Terra Bella *U.S.A.* 111 K7
Terra Nova △ *Canada* 105 C9
Terrace *Canada* 102 C3
Terrace Bay *Canada* 104 C2
Terracina *Italy* 42 A6
Terralba *Italy* 42 C1
Terrassini *Italy* 42 D6
Terrassa *Spain* 38 D7
Terrasson-la-Villedieu *France* 20 C5
Terre Haute *U.S.A.* 112 F10
Terrebonne B. *U.S.A.* 117 G9
Terrecht *Mali* 83 B5
Terrell *U.S.A.* 116 E6
Terrenceville *Canada* 105 C9
Terry *U.S.A.* 108 C11
Terryville *U.S.A.* 115 E11
Terschelling *Neths.* 17 A5
Tersko-Kumskiy Kanal *Russia* 35 H7
Tertenía *Italy* 42 C2
Terter = Tärtär ➤ *Azerbaijan* 35 K8
Teruel *Spain* 38 E3
Teruel □ *Spain* 38 E4
Tervel *Bulgaria* 45 C11
Tervola *Finland* 8 C21
Teryaweynya L. *Australia* 95 E3
Tešanj *Bos.-H.* 28 F3
Teseney *Eritrea* 81 D4
Teshio *Japan* 54 B10
Teshio-Gawa ➤ *Japan* 54 B10
Tešica *Serbia* 44 C5
Tesiyn Gol ➤ *Mongolia* 60 A4
Teslić *Bos.-H.* 28 F2
Teslin *Canada* 102 A2
Teslin ➤ *Canada* 102 A2
Teslin L. *Canada* 102 A2
Tessalit *Mali* 83 A5
Tessaoua *Niger* 83 C6
Tessin *Germany* 24 A8
Tessit *Mali* 83 B5
Test ➤ *U.K.* 15 G6
Testa del Gargano *Italy* 41 G13
Testigos, Is. Los *Venezuela* 121 D7
Testuch L. *Canada* 102 C3
Tetas, Pta. *Chile* 126 A1
Tete *Mozam.* 87 F3
Tete □ *Mozam.* 87 F3

Teterev ➤ *Ukraine* 23 C16
Teterow *Germany* 24 B8
Teteven *Bulgaria* 45 D8
Tethul ➤ *Canada* 102 A6
Tetiyev *Ukraine* 23 D15
Teton ➤ *U.S.A.* 108 C8
Tétouan *Morocco* 78 A4
Tetovo *Macedonia* 44 D4
Tetufera, Mt. *Tahiti* 91 d
Tetyushi *Russia* 34 C9
Teuco ➤ *Argentina* 126 B3
Teulada *Italy* 42 D1
Teulon *Canada* 103 C9
Teun *Indonesia* 63 F7
Teuri-Tō *Japan* 54 B10
Teutoburger Wald *Germany* 24 C4
Tevere ➤ *Italy* 41 G9
Tevere △ *Italy* 41 F9
Teverya *Israel* 74 C4
Teviot ➤ *U.K.* 13 F6
Tewantin *Australia* 95 D5
Tewkesbury *U.K.* 15 F5
Texada I. *Canada* 102 D4
Texarkana *Ark., U.S.A.* 116 E7
Texarkana *Tex., U.S.A.* 116 E7
Texas *Australia* 95 D5
Texas □ *U.S.A.* 116 F5
Texas City *U.S.A.* 116 G7
Texel *Neths.* 17 A4
Texline *U.S.A.* 116 C3
Texoma, L. *U.S.A.* 116 E6
Teyateyaneng *Lesotho* 85 K5
Teykovo *Russia* 32 D11
Teza ➤ *Russia* 34 B5
Tezin *Afghan.* 68 B3
Tezpur *India* 67 F18
Tezzeron L. *Canada* 102 C4
Tha-anne ➤ *Canada* 103 A10
Tha Deua *Laos* 64 D4
Tha Deua *Laos* 64 D4
Tha Li *Thailand* 64 D3
Tha Pla *Thailand* 64 D3
Tha Rua *Thailand* 64 E3
Tha Sala *Thailand* 65 H2
Tha Song Yang *Thailand* 64 D1
Thaba Putsoa *Lesotho* 89 D4
Thabana Ntlenyana *Lesotho* 89 D4
Thabazimbi *S. Africa* 89 C4
Thādiq *Si. Arabia* 70 E5
Thai Binh *Vietnam* 58 G6
Thai Muang *Thailand* 65 H2
Thai Nguyen *Vietnam* 58 G5
Thailand ■ *Asia* 64 E4
Thailand, G. of *Asia* 65 G3
Thakhek *Laos* 64 D5
Thal *Pakistan* 68 C4
Thal Desert *Pakistan* 68 D4
Thala La = Hkakabo Razi *Burma* 67 E20
Thalabarivat *Cambodia* 64 F5
Thalassery = Tellicherry *India* 66 P9
Thallon *Australia* 95 D4
Thalu, Ko *Thailand* 65 b
Thalwil *Switz.* 25 H4
Thames *N.Z.* 91 B5
Thames ➤ *Canada* 114 D2
Thames ➤ *U.K.* 15 F8
Thames ➤ *U.S.A.* 115 E12
Thames Estuary *U.K.* 15 F8
Thamesford *Canada* 114 C4
Thamesville *Canada* 114 D3
Than *India* 68 H4
Than Uyen *Vietnam* 64 B4
Thana Gazi *India* 68 F7
Thandla *India* 68 H6
Thandwe *Burma* 67 K19
Thane *India* 66 K8
Thanesar *India* 68 D7
Thanet, I. of *U.K.* 15 F9
Thangool *Australia* 94 C5
Thanh Hoa *Vietnam* 64 C5
Thanh Hung *Vietnam* 65 H5
Thanh Pho Ho Chi Minh *Vietnam* 65 G6
Thanh Thuy *Vietnam* 64 A5
Thanjavur *India* 66 P11
Thanlwin = Salween ➤ *Burma* 67 L20
Thann *France* 19 E14
Thano Bula Khan *Pakistan* 68 G2
Thaolintoa L. *Canada* 103 A9
Thaon-les-Vosges *France* 19 D13
Thap Lan △ *Thailand* 64 E4
Thap Sakae *Thailand* 65 G2
Thap Than *Thailand* 64 E2
Thar Desert *India* 68 F5
Tharad *India* 68 G4
Thargomindah *Australia* 95 D3
Tharrawaddy *Burma* 67 L19
Tharthar, Buḩayrat ath *Iraq* 73 E10
Tharthar, L. = Tharthār, Buḩayrat ath *Iraq* 73 E10
Tharthār, W. ath ➤ *Iraq* 73 E10
Thasopoula *Greece* 45 F8
Thasos *Greece* 45 F8
That Khe *Vietnam* 58 F6

Thatcher *Ariz., U.S.A.* **109** K9
Thatcher *Colo., U.S.A.* **109** H11
Thaton *Burma* **67** L20
Thau, Bassin de *France* **20** E7
Thaungdut *Burma* **67** G19
Thayer *U.S.A.* **112** G8
Thayetmyo *Burma* **67** K19
Thazi *Burma* **67** J20
Thbeng Meanchey *Cambodia* **64** F5
The Broads *U.K.* **14** E9
The Everglades *U.S.A.* **117** J14
The Gulf = Persian Gulf *Asia* **71** E6
The Hague =
   's-Gravenhage *Neths.* **17** B4
The Pas *Canada* **103** C8
The Wash *U.K.* **14** E8
The Weald *U.K.* **15** F8
Thebes = Thiva *Greece* **46** C5
Thebes *Egypt* **80** B3
Thedford *U.S.A.* **112** E3
Theebine *Australia* **95** D5
Thekulthili L. *Canada* **103** A7
Thelon → *Canada* **103** A8
Thénezay *France* **18** F6
Thenon *France* **20** C5
Theodore *Australia* **94** C5
Theodore *Canada* **103** C8
Theodore *U.S.A.* **117** F10
Theodore Roosevelt △
   U.S.A. **112** B2
Theodore Roosevelt L.
   U.S.A. **109** K8
Thepha *Thailand* **65** J3
Thérain → *France* **19** C9
Theresa *U.S.A.* **115** D9
Thermopolis *U.S.A.* **108** E9
Thermopylae *Greece* **45** F8
Thesprotia □ *Greece* **46** B2
Thessalon *Canada* **104** C3
Thessalonica, Gulf of =
   Thessaloniki Kolpos *Greece* **44** F6
Thessaloniki *Greece* **44** F6
Thessaloniki □ *Greece* **44** F7
Thessaloniki ✈ (SKG) *Greece* **44** F7
Thessaloniki Kolpos *Greece* **44** F6
Thessaly □ *Greece* **46** B4
Thetford *U.K.* **15** E8
Thetford Mines *Canada* **105** C5
Theun → *Laos* **64** C5
Theunissen *S. Africa* **88** D4
Thevenard *Australia* **95** E1
Thiamis → *Greece* **46** B2
Thiberville *France* **18** C4
Thibodaux *U.S.A.* **117** G9
Thicket Portage *Canada* **103** B9
Thief River Falls *U.S.A.* **112** A5
Thiel Mts. *Antarctica* **5** E16
Thiene *Italy* **41** C8
Thiérache *France* **19** C10
Thiers *France* **20** C7
Thiès *Senegal* **82** C1
Thiès □ *Senegal* **82** C1
Thiesi *Italy* **42** B1
Thika *Kenya* **86** C4
Thille-Boubacar *Senegal* **82** B1
Thimphu *Bhutan* **67** F16
Thina → *S. Africa* **89** E4
Þingvallavatn *Iceland* **8** D3
Thionville *France* **19** C13
Thira = Santorini *Greece* **47** E7
Thirasia *Greece* **47** E7
Third Cataract *Sudan* **80** D3
Thirsk *U.K.* **14** C6
Thiruvananthapuram =
   Trivandrum *India* **66** Q10
Thisted *Denmark* **11** H2
Thistle I. *Australia* **95** F2
Thithia = Cicia *Fiji* **91** a
Thiva *Greece* **46** C5
Thiviers *France* **20** C4
Thizy *France* **19** F11
Þjórsá → *Iceland* **8** E3
Thlewiaza → *Canada* **103** A10
Thmar Puok *Cambodia* **64** F4
Tho Vinh *Vietnam* **64** C5
Thoa → *Canada* **103** A7
Thoen *Thailand* **64** C2
Thoeng *Thailand* **64** C3
Thohoyandou *S. Africa* **85** J6
Tholdi *Pakistan* **69** B7
Thomas *U.S.A.* **116** D5
Thomas, L. *Australia* **95** D2
Thomas Hubbard, C. *Canada*
   101 A13
Thomaston *U.S.A.* **117** E12
Thomasville *Ala., U.S.A.* **117** F11
Thomasville *Ga., U.S.A.* **117** F13
Thomasville *N.C., U.S.A.* **117** D14
Thompson *Canada* **103** B9
Thompson *U.S.A.* **115** E9
Thompson → *Canada* **102** C4
Thompson → *U.S.A.* **112** F7
Thompson Falls *U.S.A.* **108** C6
Thompson Pk. *U.S.A.* **108** F2
Thompson Springs *U.S.A.* **108** G9
Thompsontown *U.S.A.* **114** F7
Thomson *U.S.A.* **117** E13
Thomson → *Australia* **94** C3
Thônes *France* **21** C10
Thong Yang *Thailand* **65** b

Thonon-les-Bains *France* **19** F13
Thoothukudi = Tuticorin
   India **66** Q11
Þórisvatn *Iceland* **8** D4
Thornaby on Tees *U.K.* **14** C6
Thornbury *Canada* **114** B4
Thorne *U.K.* **14** D7
Thornton *Canada* **114** B5
Thornton *U.S.A.* **108** G11
Thorold *Canada* **114** C5
Þórshöfn *Iceland* **8** C6
Thouarcé *France* **18** E6
Thouars *France* **18** F6
Thouet → *France* **18** E6
Thouin, C. *Australia* **92** D2
Thousand Islands *U.S.A.* **115** B9
Thousand Oaks *U.S.A.* **111** L8
Thrace *Turkey* **45** F10
Thrace, Sea of *Greece* **45** F8
Three Forks *U.S.A.* **108** D8
Three Gorges Dam *China* **59** B8
Three Hills *Canada* **102** C6
Three Hummock I. *Australia* **95** G3
Three Pagodas Pass *Asia* **64** E2
Three Points, C. *Ghana* **82** E4
Three Rivers *Calif., U.S.A.* **110** J8
Three Rivers *Tex., U.S.A.* **116** G5
Three Springs *Australia* **93** E2
Thrissur = Trichur *India* **66** P10
Throssell, L. *Australia* **93** E3
Throssell Ra. *Australia* **92** D3
Thrushton △ *Australia* **95** D4
Thua → *Kenya* **86** C4
Thuan Hoa *Vietnam* **65** H5
Thubun Lakes *Canada* **103** A6
Thueyts *France* **21** D8
Thuin *Belgium* **17** D4
Thuir *France* **20** F6
Thule = Qaanaaq *Greenland*
   101 B18
Thule Air Base =
   Uummannaq *Greenland* **101** B18
Thun *Switz.* **25** J3
Thunder B. *U.S.A.* **114** B1
Thunder Bay *Canada* **104** C2
Thunersee *Switz.* **25** J3
Thung Salaeng Luang △
   Thailand **64** D3
Thung Song *Thailand* **65** H2
Thunkar *Bhutan* **67** F17
Thuong Tra *Vietnam* **64** D6
Thur → *Switz.* **25** H5
Thurgau □ *Switz.* **25** H5
Thüringen □ *Germany* **24** D6
Thüringer Wald *Germany* **24** E6
Thuringowa △ *Australia* **94** B4
Thurles *Ireland* **12** D4
Thurn P. *Austria* **26** D5
Thurrock □ *U.K.* **15** F8
Thursday I. *Australia* **94** A3
Thurso *Canada* **104** C4
Thurso *U.K.* **13** C5
Thurso → *U.K.* **13** C5
Thurston I. *Antarctica* **5** D16
Thury-Harcourt *France* **18** D6
Thutade L. *Canada* **102** B3
Thy *Denmark* **11** H2
Thyborøn *Denmark* **11** H2
Thyolo *Malawi* **87** F4
Ti-n-Amzi → *Niger* **83** B5
Ti-n-Barraouene, O. →
   Africa **83** B5
Ti-n-Zaouatene *Algeria* **83** B5
Ti-Tree *Australia* **94** C1
Tiadiaye *Senegal* **82** C1
Tian Shan *Asia* **60** B3
Tianchang *China* **59** A12
Tiandeng *China* **58** F6
Tiandong *China* **58** F6
Tian'e *China* **58** E6
Tianhe *China* **58** E7
Tianjin *China* **57** E9
Tiankoura *Burkina Faso* **82** C4
Tianlin *China* **58** E6
Tianmen *China* **59** B9
Tianquan *China* **58** B4
Tianshifu *China* **57** D13
Tianshui *China* **56** G3
Tiantai *China* **59** C13
Tianyang *China* **58** F6
Tianyar *Indonesia* **63** J18
Tianzhen *China* **56** D8
Tianzhu *China* **58** D7
Tianzhuangtai *China* **57** D12
Tiarei *Tahiti* **91** d
Tiaret *Algeria* **78** A6
Tiassalé *Ivory C.* **82** D4
Tibagi *Brazil* **127** A5
Tibagi → *Brazil* **127** A5
Tibastī, Sarīr *Libya* **79** D9
Tibati *Cameroon* **83** D7
Tibe *Ethiopia* **81** F4
Tiber = Tevere → *Italy* **41** G9
Tiber Res. = *U.S.A.* **108** B8
Tiberias = Teverya *Israel* **74** C4
Tiberias, L. = Yam
   Kinneret *Israel* **74** C4
Tibesti *Chad* **79** D9

Tibet = Xizang Zizhiqu □
   China **60** C3
Tibet, Plateau of *Asia* **50** E10
Tibiao *Phil.* **61** F5
Tibiri *Niger* **83** C6
Tiblès, Vf. *Romania* **29** C9
Tiblèsului, Munţii *Romania* **29** C9
Tibnī *Syria* **73** E8
Tibooburra *Australia* **95** D3
Tibro *Sweden* **11** F8
Tiburón, I. *Mexico* **118** B2
Ticao I. *Phil.* **61** E5
Tîchît *Mauritania* **82** B3
Ticho *Ethiopia* **81** F4
Ticino □ *Switz.* **25** J4
Ticino → *Italy* **25** J4
Ticleni *Romania* **29** F8
Ticonderoga *U.S.A.* **115** C11
Ticul *Mexico* **119** C7
Tidaholm *Sweden* **11** F7
Tidan *Sweden* **11** F8
Tiddim *Burma* **67** H18
Tidioute *U.S.A.* **114** E5
Tidjikja *Mauritania* **82** B2
Tidore *Indonesia* **63** D7
Tiébissou *Ivory C.* **82** D3
Tiefa *China* **57** C12
Tiel *Neths.* **17** C5
Tiel *Senegal* **82** C1
Tieling *China* **57** C12
Tielt *Belgium* **17** C3
Tien Shan = Tian Shan *Asia* **60** B3
Tien-tsin = Tianjin *China* **57** E9
Tien Yen *Vietnam* **64** B6
T'ienching = Tianjin *China* **57** E9
Tienen *Belgium* **17** D4
Tiénigbé *Ivory C.* **82** D3
Tientsin = Tianjin *China* **57** E9
Tieri *Australia* **94** C4
Tierp *Sweden* **10** D11
Tierra Amarilla *Chile* **126** B1
Tierra Amarilla *U.S.A.* **109** H10
Tierra Colorada *Mexico* **119** D5
Tierra de Barros *Spain* **37** G4
Tierra de Campos *Spain* **36** C6
Tierra del Fuego, I. Grande
   de *Argentina* **128** G3
Tiétar → *Spain* **36** F4
Tieté → *Brazil* **127** A5
Tiffin *U.S.A.* **113** E12
Tifton *U.S.A.* **117** F13
Tifu *Indonesia* **63** E7
Tiga Res. *Nigeria* **83** C6
Tighina *Moldova* **29** D14
Tigil *Russia* **53** D16
Tignish *Canada* **105** C7
Tigray □ *Ethiopia* **81** E4
Tigre → *Peru* **124** D4
Tigre → *Venezuela* **124** B6
Tigris = Dijlah, Nahr →
   Asia **70** D5
Tigveni *Romania* **29** E9
Tigyaing *Burma* **67** H20
Tîh, Gebel el *Egypt* **80** B3
Tihāmah *Asia* **75** D3
Tijara *India* **68** F7
Tijuana *Mexico* **111** N9
Tikal *Guatemala* **120** C2
Tikal △ *Guatemala* **120** C2
Tikamgarh *India* **69** G8
Tikaré *Burkina Faso* **83** C4
Tikchik Lakes *U.S.A.* **106** D8
Tikhoretsk *Russia* **35** H5
Tikhvin *Russia* **32** C7
Tikirarjuaq = Whale Cove
   Canada **103** A10
Tikmehdāsh *Iran* **73** D12
Tiko *Cameroon* **83** E6
Tikrīt *Iraq* **73** E10
Tiksi *Russia* **53** B13
Tilamuta *Indonesia* **63** D6
Tilburg *Neths.* **17** C5
Tilbury *Canada* **114** D2
Tilbury *U.K.* **15** F8
Tilcara *Argentina* **126** A2
Tilden *U.S.A.* **112** D5
Tilemsi, Vallée du *Mali* **83** B5
Tilhar *India* **69** F8
Tilichiki *Russia* **53** C17
Tilissos *Greece* **49** D7
Till → *U.K.* **14** B5
Tillabéri *Niger* **83** C5
Tillamook *U.S.A.* **108** D2
Tillberga *Sweden* **10** E10
Tillia *Niger* **83** B5
Tillsonburg *Canada* **114** D4
Tillyeria *Cyprus* **49** D11
Tilogne *Senegal* **82** B2
Tilos *Greece* **47** E9
Tilpa *Australia* **95** E3
Tilt → *U.K.* **13** E5
Tilton *U.S.A.* **115** C13
Tiltonsville *U.S.A.* **114** F4
Tim *Denmark* **11** H2
Tima *Egypt* **80** B3
Timanfaya △ *Canary Is.* **48** F6
Timaru *N.Z.* **91** F3
Timashevo *Russia* **34** D10
Timashevsk *Russia* **35** H4
Tirodi *India* **66** J11
Timau *Kenya* **86** B4

Timbaki *Greece* **49** D6
Timbedgha *Mauritania* **82** B3
Timber Creek *Australia* **92** C5
Timber Lake *U.S.A.* **112** C3
Timber Mt. *U.S.A.* **110** H10
Timbo *Guinea* **82** C2
Timbo *Liberia* **82** D3
Timbué, Ponta *Mozam.* **87** F4
Timbuktu = Tombouctou
   Mali **82** B4
Timeïaouine *Algeria* **83** A5
Timétrin *Mali* **83** B4
Timfi Oros *Greece* **46** B2
Timfristos, Oros *Greece* **46** C3
Timi *Cyprus* **49** E11
Tîmia *Niger* **83** B6
Timimoun *Algeria* **78** C6
Timiris, Râs *Mauritania* **82** B1
Timiş □ *Romania* **28** E6
Timiş = Tamiš → *Serbia* **28** F5
Timişoara *Romania* **28** E6
Timmersdala *Sweden* **11** F7
Timmins *Canada* **104** C3
Timok → *Serbia* **28** F6
Timoleague *Ireland* **12** E3
Timor *Asia* **63** F7
Timor Leste = East
   Timor ■ *Asia* **63** F7
Timor Sea *Ind. Oc.* **92** B4
Timrå *Sweden* **10** B11
Tin Can Bay *Australia* **95** D5
Tin Ethisane *Mali* **83** B4
Tin Gornai *Mali* **83** B4
Tin Mt. *U.S.A.* **110** J9
Tina = Thina → *S. Africa* **89** E4
Tîna, Khalîg el *Egypt* **74** D1
Tinaca Pt. *Phil.* **61** J6
Tinajo *Canary Is.* **48** E6
Tinca *Romania* **28** D6
Tindal *Australia* **92** B5
Tindouf *Algeria* **78** C4
Tinée → *France* **21** E11
Tineo *Spain* **36** B4
Tinfunque △ *Paraguay* **126** A3
Ting Jiang → *China* **59** E11
Tinggi, Pulau *Malaysia* **65** L5
Tingi Mts. *S. Leone* **82** D2
Tinglev *Denmark* **11** K3
Tingo María *Peru* **124** E3
Tingrela *Ivory C.* **82** C3
Tingsryd *Sweden* **11** H9
Tingstäde *Sweden* **11** G12
Tinh Bien *Vietnam* **65** G5
Tinian *N. Marianas* **96** F6
Tinkisso → *Guinea* **82** C3
Tinnevelly = Tirunelveli
   India **66** Q10
Tinogasta *Argentina* **126** B2
Tinos *Greece* **47** D7
Tiñoso, C. *Spain* **39** H3
Tinpahar *India* **69** G12
Tîntâne *Mauritania* **82** B2
Tintina *Argentina* **126** B3
Tintinara *Australia* **95** F3
Tintioulé *Guinea* **82** C3
Tinto → *Spain* **37** H4
Tiobraid Árran = Tipperary
   Ireland **12** D3
Tioga *N. Dak., U.S.A.* **112** A2
Tioga *Pa., U.S.A.* **114** E7
Tioman, Pulau *Malaysia* **65** L5
Tione di Trento *Italy* **40** B7
Tionesta *U.S.A.* **114** E5
Tior *Sudan* **81** F3
Tipperary *Ireland* **12** D3
Tipperary □ *Ireland* **12** D4
Tipton *Calif., U.S.A.* **110** J7
Tipton *Iowa, U.S.A.* **112** E8
Tipton Mt. *U.S.A.* **111** K12
Tiptonville *U.S.A.* **117** C10
Tīrān *Iran* **71** C6
Tīrān *Si. Arabia* **80** B3
Tiranë *Albania* **44** E3
Tiranë ✈ (TIA) *Albania* **44** E3
Tirano *Italy* **40** B7
Tiraspol *Moldova* **29** D14
Tirari Desert *Australia* **95** D2
Tirdout *Mali* **83** B4
Tire *Turkey* **47** C9
Tirebolu *Turkey* **73** B8
Tiree *U.K.* **13** E2
Tiree, Passage of *U.K.* **13** E2
Tîrgovişte = Târgovişte
   Romania **29** F10
Tîrgu Jiu = Târgu Jiu
   Romania **29** E8
Tîrgu Mureş = Târgu
   Mureş *Romania* **29** D9
Tirich Mir *Pakistan* **66** A7
Tiriolo *Italy* **43** D9
Tiriro *Guinea* **82** C3
Tiritiri o te Moana =
   Southern Alps *N.Z.* **91** E3
Tirnavos *Greece* **46** B4
Tirodi *India* **66** J11
Tirol □ *Austria* **26** D3

Tirschenreuth *Germany* **25** F8
Tirso → *Italy* **42** C1
Tirstrup *Denmark* **11** H4
Tiruchchirappalli *India* **66** P11
Tirunelveli *India* **66** Q10
Tiruppur *India* **66** P10
Tiruvannamalai *India* **66** N11
Tisa *India* **68** C7
Tisa → *Serbia* **28** E5
Tisdale *Canada* **103** C8
Tishomingo *U.S.A.* **116** D6
Tisjön *Sweden* **10** D7
Tisnaren *Sweden* **11** F9
Tišnov *Czech Rep.* **27** B9
Tisovec *Slovak Rep.* **27** C12
Tisza = Tisa → *Serbia* **28** E5
Tiszaföldvár *Hungary* **28** D5
Tiszafüred *Hungary* **28** C5
Tiszalök *Hungary* **28** B6
Tiszavasvári *Hungary* **28** C6
Tit-Ary *Russia* **53** B13
Titaguas *Spain* **38** F3
Titao *Burkina Faso* **83** C4
Titel *Serbia* **28** E5
Tithwal *Pakistan* **69** B5
Titicaca, L. *S. Amer.* **124** G5
Titiwa *Nigeria* **83** C7
Tito *Italy* **43** B8
Titova Korenica *Croatia* **41** D12
Titu *Romania* **29** F10
Titule *Dem. Rep. of the Congo* **86** B2
Titusville *Fla., U.S.A.* **117** G14
Titusville *Pa., U.S.A.* **114** E5
Tivaouane *Senegal* **82** C1
Tivat *Montenegro* **44** D2
Tivedens △ *Sweden* **11** F8
Tiverton *Canada* **114** B3
Tiverton *U.K.* **15** G4
Tivoli *Italy* **41** G9
Tiwi ☉ *Australia* **92** B5
Tiyo *Eritrea* **81** E5
Tizi-Ouzou *Algeria* **78** A6
Tizimín *Mexico* **119** C7
Tiznit *Morocco* **78** C4
Tjæreborg *Denmark* **11** J2
Tjällmo *Sweden* **11** F9
Tjeggelvas *Sweden* **8** C17
Tjeggelvas = Tjeggelvas
   Sweden **8** C17
Tjirebon = Cirebon *Indonesia* **62** F3
Tjirrkarli ☉ *Australia* **93** E4
Tjluring *Indonesia* **63** J17
Tjörn *Sweden* **11** F5
Tjukayirla Roadhouse
   Australia **93** E4
Tjurabalan ☉ *Australia* **92** C4
Tkibuli = Tqibuli *Georgia* **35** J6
Tkvarcheli = Tqvarcheli
   Georgia **35** J5
Tlacotalpan *Mexico* **119** D5
Tlahualilo de Zaragoza
   Mexico **118** B4
Tlaquepaque *Mexico* **118** C4
Tlaxcala *Mexico* **119** D5
Tlaxcala □ *Mexico* **119** D5
Tlaxiaco *Mexico* **119** D5
Tlemcen *Algeria* **78** B5
Tlumach *Ukraine* **29** B10
Tluszcz *Poland* **31** F8
Tlyarata *Russia* **35** J8
To Bong *Vietnam* **64** F7
Toa Payoh *Singapore* **65** d
Toad → *Canada* **102** B4
Toad River *Canada* **102** B3
Toamasina *Madag.* **89** B8
Toamasina □ *Madag.* **89** B8
Toay *Argentina* **126** D3
Toba *China* **58** B1
Toba *Japan* **55** G8
Toba, Danau *Indonesia* **62** D1
Toba Kakar *Pakistan* **68** D3
Toba Tek Singh *Pakistan* **68** D5
Tobago *Trin. & Tob.* **121** D7
Tobarra *Spain* **39** G3
Tobelo *Indonesia* **63** D7
Tobermory *Canada* **114** A3
Tobermory *U.K.* **13** E2
Tobi *Pac. Oc.* **63** D8
Tobi-Shima *Japan* **54** D9
Tobin, L. *Australia* **92** D4
Tobin L. *Canada* **103** C8
Toblach = Dobbiaco *Italy* **41** B9
Toboali *Indonesia* **62** E3
Tobol → *Russia* **52** D7
Toboli *Indonesia* **63** E6
Tobolsk *Russia* **52** D7
Tobor *Senegal* **82** C1
Tobruk = Tubruq *Libya* **79** B10
Tobyhanna *U.S.A.* **115** E9
Tobyl = Tobol → *Russia* **52** D7
Tocantinópolis *Brazil* **125** E9
Tocantins □ *Brazil* **125** F9
Tocantins → *Brazil* **125** D9
Toccoa *U.S.A.* **117** D13
Toce → *Italy* **40** C5
Tochi → *Pakistan* **68** C4
Tochigi *Japan* **55** F9
Tochigi □ *Japan* **55** F9

Tocina *Spain* **37** H5
Töcksfors *Sweden* **10** E5
Toco *Trin. & Tob.* **125** K16
Toconao *Chile* **126** A2
Tocopilla *Chile* **126** A1
Tocumwal *Australia* **95** F4
Tocuyo → *Venezuela* **124** A5
Todd → *Australia* **94** C2
Todeli *Indonesia* **63** E6
Todenyang *Kenya* **86** B4
Todgarh *India* **68** G5
Todi *Italy* **41** F9
Todos os Santos, B. de *Brazil*
   125 F11
Todos Santos *Mexico* **118** C2
Todtnau *Germany* **25** H3
Toe Hd. *U.K.* **13** D1
Toecé *Burkina Faso* **83** C4
Tofield *Canada* **102** C6
Tofino *Canada* **102** D3
Töfsingdalens △ *Sweden* **10** B6
Tofua *Tonga* **91** c
Tōgane *Japan* **55** G10
Togba *Mauritania* **82** B2
Togian, Kepulauan *Indonesia* **63** E6
Togliatti *Russia* **34** D9
Togo ■ *W. Afr.* **83** D5
Togtoh *China* **56** D6
Tohiea, Mt. *Moorea* **91** d
Tohma → *Turkey* **72** C8
Tōhoku □ *Japan* **54** E10
Töhöm *Mongolia* **56** B5
Toinya *Sudan* **81** F2
Toiyabe Range *U.S.A.* **108** G5
Tojikiston = Tajikistan ■
   Asia **52** F8
Tojo *Indonesia* **63** E6
Tōjō *Japan* **55** G6
Tok *U.S.A.* **100** E3
Tokachi-Dake *Japan* **54** C11
Tokachi-Gawa → *Japan* **54** C11
Tokaj *Hungary* **28** B6
Tokala *Indonesia* **63** E6
Tōkamachi *Japan* **55** F9
Tokanui *N.Z.* **91** G2
Tokar *Sudan* **80** D4
Tokara-Rettō *Japan* **55** K4
Tokarahi *N.Z.* **91** F3
Tokashiki-Shima *Japan* **55** L3
Tokat *Turkey* **72** B7
Tokat □ *Turkey* **72** B7
Tŏkch'ŏn *N. Korea* **57** E14
Tokdo *Asia* **55** F5
Tokeland *U.S.A.* **110** D3
Tokelau Is. *Pac. Oc.* **96** H10
Tokmak *Kyrgyzstan* **52** E8
Tokmak *Ukraine* **33** J8
Toko Ra. *Australia* **94** C2
Tokoro-Gawa → *Japan* **54** B12
Toku *Tonga* **91** c
Tokuno-Shima *Japan* **55** L4
Tokushima *Japan* **55** G7
Tokushima □ *Japan* **55** H7
Tokuyama *Japan* **55** G5
Tōkyō *Japan* **55** G9
Tolaga Bay *N.Z.* **91** C7
Tolbukhin = Dobrich
   Bulgaria **45** C11
Toledo *Brazil* **127** A5
Toledo *Spain* **36** F6
Toledo *Ohio, U.S.A.* **113** E12
Toledo *Oreg., U.S.A.* **108** D2
Toledo *Wash., U.S.A.* **108** C2
Toledo, Montes de *Spain* **37** F6
Toledo Bend Res. *U.S.A.* **116** F8
Tolentino *Italy* **41** E10
Tolfa *Italy* **41** F8
Tolga *Australia* **94** B4
Toliara *Madag.* **89** C7
Toliara □ *Madag.* **89** C8
Tolima *Colombia* **124** C3
Tolitoli *Indonesia* **63** D6
Tolkmicko *Poland* **30** D6
Tollarp *Sweden* **11** J7
Tollensesee *Germany* **24** B9
Tollhouse *U.S.A.* **110** H7
Tolmachevo *Russia* **32** C5
Tolmezzo *Italy* **41** B10
Tolmin *Slovenia* **41** B10
Tolna *Hungary* **28** D3
Tolna □ *Hungary* **28** D3
Tolo, Teluk *Indonesia* **63** E6
Tolochin = Talachyn *Belarus* **32** E5
Tolosa *Spain* **38** B2
Tolox *Spain* **37** J6
Toluca *Mexico* **119** D5
Tolyatti = Togliatti *Russia* **34** D9
Tom Burke *S. Africa* **89** C4
Tom Price *Australia* **92** D2
Toma *Burkina Faso* **82** C4
Tomah *U.S.A.* **112** D8
Tomahawk *U.S.A.* **112** C9
Tomaini *Moldova* **29** D13
Tomales *U.S.A.* **110** G4
Tomales B. *U.S.A.* **110** G3
Tomanivi *Fiji* **91** a
Tomar *Portugal* **37** F2
Tomaros, Oros *Greece* **46** B2
Tomarza *Turkey* **72** C6

Tomashevka *Belarus* **31** G10
Tomashpil *Ukraine* **29** B13
Tomaszów Lubelski *Poland* **31** H10
Tomaszów Mazowiecki
   Poland **31** G7
Tomatlán *Mexico* **118** D3
Tombadonkéa *Guinea* **82** C2
Tombador, Serra do *Brazil* **124** F7
Tombe *Sudan* **81** F3
Tombigbee → *U.S.A.* **117** F11
Tombouctou *Mali* **82** B4
Tombouctou □ *Mali* **82** B4
Tombstone *U.S.A.* **109** L8
Tombua *Angola* **88** B1
Tomé *Chile* **126** D1
Tomelilla *Sweden* **11** J7
Tomelloso *Spain* **37** F7
Tomini *Indonesia* **63** D6
Tomini, Teluk *Indonesia* **63** E6
Tominian *Mali* **82** C4
Tomiño *Spain* **36** C2
Tomintoul *U.K.* **13** D5
Tomislavgrad *Bos.-H.* **28** G2
Tomkinson Ranges *Australia* **93** E4
Tommot *Russia* **53** D13
Tomnop Ta Suos *Cambodia* **65** G5
Tomo → *Colombia* **124** B5
Toms Place *U.S.A.* **110** H8
Toms River *U.S.A.* **115** G10
Tomsk *Russia* **52** D9
Tomtabacken *Sweden* **11** G8
Tona *Spain* **38** D7
Tonalá *Chiapas, Mexico* **119** D6
Tonalá *Jalisco, Mexico* **118** C4
Tonale, Passo del *Italy* **40** B7
Tonantins *Brazil* **124** D5
Tonasket *U.S.A.* **108** B4
Tonawanda *U.S.A.* **114** D6
Tonb *Iran* **71** E7
Tonbridge *U.K.* **15** F8
Tondano *Indonesia* **63** D6
Tondela *Portugal* **36** E2
Tønder *Denmark* **11** K2
Tondi Kiwindi *Niger* **83** C5
Tondibi *Mali* **83** B4
Tondoro *Namibia* **88** B2
Tone → *Australia* **93** F2
Tone-Gawa → *Japan* **55** F9
Tonekābon *Iran* **71** B6
Tong Xian *China* **56** E9
Tong-Yeong *S. Korea* **57** G15
Tonga *Cameroon* **83** E7
Tôngâ *Sudan* **81** F3
Tonga ■ *Pac. Oc.* **91** c
Tonga Trench *Pac. Oc.* **96** J10
Tongaat *S. Africa* **89** D5
Tong'an *China* **59** E12
Tongareva = Penrhyn
   Cook Is. **97** H12
Tongariro △ *N.Z.* **91** C5
Tongatapu *Tonga* **91** c
Tongatapu Group *Tonga* **91** c
Tongbai *China* **59** A9
Tongcheng *Anhui, China* **59** B11
Tongcheng *Hubei, China* **59** C9
Tongchuan *China* **56** G5
Tongdao *China* **58** D7
Tongeren *Belgium* **17** D5
Tonggu *China* **59** C10
Tongguan *China* **56** G6
Tonghai *China* **58** E4
Tonghua *China* **57** D13
Tongjiang *China* **58** B6
Tongjosŏn Man *N. Korea* **57** E15
Tongking, G. of = Tonkin,
   G. of *Asia* **64** C7
Tongliang *China* **58** C6
Tongliao *China* **57** C12
Tongling *China* **59** B11
Tonglu *China* **59** C12
Tongnan = Anyue *China* **58** B5
Tongobory *Madag.* **89** C7
Tongoy *Chile* **126** C1
Tongren *China* **58** D7
Tongres = Tongeren *Belgium* **17** D5
Tongsa Dzong *Bhutan* **67** F17
Tongshi *China* **64** C7
Tongue *U.K.* **13** C4
Tongue → *U.S.A.* **108** C11
Tongwei *China* **56** G3
Tongxiang *China* **59** B13
Tongxin *China* **56** F3
Tongyang *N. Korea* **57** E14
Tongyu *China* **57** B12
Tongzi *China* **58** C6
Tonj *Sudan* **81** F2
Tonj → *Sudan* **81** F2
Tonk *India* **68** F6
Tonkawa *U.S.A.* **116** C6
Tonkin = Bac Phan *Vietnam* **58** G5
Tonkin, G. of *Asia* **64** C7
Tonle Sap *Cambodia* **64** F5
Tonnay-Charente *France* **20** C3
Tonneins *France* **20** D4
Tonnerre *France* **19** E10
Tönning *Germany* **24** A4
Tono *Japan* **54** E10
Tonopah *U.S.A.* **109** G5
Tonosí *Panama* **120** E3
Tons → *Haryana, India* **68** D7

Tons → *Ut. P., India* **69** F10
Tønsberg *Norway* **9** G14
Tonto → *U.S.A.* **109** K8
Tonumea *Tonga* **91** c
Tonya *Turkey* **73** B8
Toobanna *Australia* **94** B4
Toodyay *Australia* **93** F2
Tooele *U.S.A.* **108** F7
Toompine *Australia* **95** D3
Toora *Australia* **95** F4
Toora-Khem *Russia* **53** D10
Toowoomba *Australia* **95** D5
Top Springs *Australia* **92** C5
Topalu *Romania* **29** F13
Topaz *U.S.A.* **110** G7
Topeka *U.S.A.* **112** F6
Topľa → *Slovak Rep.* **27** C14
Topley *Canada* **102** C3
Toplica → *Serbia* **44** C5
Topliţa *Romania* **29** D10
Topocalma, Pta. *Chile* **126** C1
Topock *U.S.A.* **111** L12
Topol'čany *Slovak Rep.* **27** C11
Topola *Serbia* **44** B4
Topolčani *Macedonia* **44** E5
Topolnitsa → *Bulgaria* **45** D8
Topolobampo *Mexico* **118** B3
Topoloveni *Romania* **29** F10
Topolovgrad *Bulgaria* **45** D10
Topolváţu Mare *Romania* **28** E6
Topozero, Ozero *Russia* **8** C5
Toppenish *U.S.A.* **108** C3
Topraisar *Romania* **29** F13
Topusko *Croatia* **41** C12
Torà *Spain* **38** D6
Tora Kit *Sudan* **81** E3
Toraka Vestale *Madag.* **89** B7
Torata *Peru* **124** G4
Torbalı *Turkey* **47** C9
Torbat-e Heydārīyeh *Iran* **71** C8
Torbat-e Jām *Iran* **71** C9
Torbay *Canada* **105** C9
Torbay □ *U.K.* **15** G4
Torbjörntorp *Sweden* **11** F7
Tordesillas *Spain* **36** D6
Töreboda *Sweden* **11** F8
Torekov *Sweden* **11** H6
Torelló *Spain* **38** C7
Toreno *Spain* **36** C4
Torfaen □ *U.K.* **15** F4
Torgau *Germany* **24** D8
Torgelow *Germany* **24** B10
Torhamn *Sweden* **11** H9
Torhout *Belgium* **17** C3
Torhovytsya *Ukraine* **29** B10
Tori *Ethiopia* **81** F3
Tori-Shima *Japan* **55** J10
Torigni-sur-Vire *France* **18** C6
Torija *Spain* **38** E1
Torilla Pen. *Australia* **94** C5
Torino *Italy* **40** C4
Torit *Sudan* **81** G3
Torkamān *Iran* **73** D12
Torkovichi *Russia* **32** C6
Tormac *Romania* **28** E6
Tormes → *Spain* **36** D4
Tornado Mt. *Canada* **102** D6
Tornal'a *Slovak Rep.* **27** C13
Torneå = Tornio *Finland* **8** D21
Torneälven → *Europe* **8** D21
Torneträsk *Sweden* **8** B18
Torngat Mts. *Canada* **101** F19
Tornio *Finland* **8** D21
Tornionjoki =
   Torneälven → *Europe* **8** D21
Tornquist *Argentina* **126** D3
Toro *Baleares, Spain* **48** B11
Toro *Zamora, Spain* **36** D5
Torö *Sweden* **11** F11
Toro, Cerro del *Chile* **126** B2
Toro → *Uganda* **86** C3
Toro Pk. *U.S.A.* **111** M10
Torodi *Niger* **83** C5
Törökszentmiklós *Hungary* **28** C5
Toronto *Canada* **114** C5
Toronto *U.S.A.* **114** F4
Toronto Lester B. Pearson
   Int. ✈ (YYZ) *Canada* **114** C5
Toropets *Russia* **32** D6
Tororo *Uganda* **86** B3
Toros Dağları *Turkey* **72** D5
Torpa *India* **69** H11
Torquay *U.K.* **15** G4
Torquemada *Spain* **36** C6
Torrance *U.S.A.* **111** M8
Torrão *Portugal* **37** G2
Torre Annunziata *Italy* **43** B7
Torre del Campo *Spain* **37** H7
Torre del Greco *Italy* **43** B7
Torre del Mar *Spain* **37** J6
Torre-Pacheco *Spain* **39** H4
Torre Péllice *Italy* **40** D4
Torreblanca *Spain* **38** E5
Torrecampo *Spain* **37** G6
Torrecilla en Cameros *Spain* **38** C2
Torredembarra *Spain* **38** D6
Torredonjimeno *Spain* **37** H7
Torrejón de Ardoz *Spain* **36** E7
Torrejoncillo *Spain* **36** F4
Tons → *Ut. P., India* **69** F10

Torrelaguna *Spain* **36** E7
Torrelavega *Spain* **36** B6
Torremaggiore *Italy* **41** G12
Torremolinos *Spain* **37** J6
Torrens, L. *Australia* **95** E2
Torrens Cr. → *Australia* **94** C4
Torrens Creek *Australia* **94** C4
Torrent *Spain* **39** F4
Torrenueva *Spain* **37** G7
Torreón *Mexico* **118** B4
Torreperogil *Spain* **37** G7
Torres *Brazil* **127** B5
Torres *Mexico* **118** B2
Torres Novas *Portugal* **37** F2
Torres Strait *Australia* **94** a
Torres Vedras *Portugal* **37** F1
Torrevieja *Spain* **39** H4
Torrey *U.S.A.* **108** G8
Torridge → *U.K.* **15** G3
Torridon, L. *U.K.* **13** D3
Torrijos *Spain* **36** F6
Tørring *Denmark* **11** J3
Torrington *Conn., U.S.A.* **115** E11
Torrington *Wyo., U.S.A.* **108** E11
Torroella de Montgrí *Spain* **38** C8
Torrox *Spain* **37** J7
Torsås *Sweden* **11** H9
Torsby *Sweden* **10** D6
Torshälla *Sweden* **10** E10
Tórshavn *Færoe Is.* **8** E9
Torslanda *Sweden* **11** G5
Torsö *Sweden* **11** F7
Tortola *Br. Virgin Is.* **121** e
Tórtoles de Esgueva *Spain* **36** D6
Tortolì *Italy* **42** C2
Tortona *Italy* **40** C5
Tortorici *Italy* **43** D7
Tortosa *Spain* **38** E5
Tortosa, C. *Spain* **38** E5
Tortosendo *Portugal* **36** E3
Tortue, Î. de la *Haiti* **121** B5
Tortuguero △ *Costa Rica* **120** D3
Tortum *Turkey* **73** B9
Ţorūd *Iran* **71** C7
Torul *Turkey* **73** B8
Toruń *Poland* **31** E5
Torun *Ukraine* **29** B8
Tory Hill *Canada* **114** B6
Tory I. *Ireland* **12** A3
Torysa → *Slovak Rep.* **27** C14
Torzhok *Russia* **32** D9
Torzym *Poland* **31** F2
Tosa *Japan* **55** H6
Tosa-Shimizu *Japan* **55** H6
Tosa-Wan *Japan* **55** H6
Toscana □ *Italy* **40** E8
Toscano, Arcipelago *Italy* **40** F7
Toshka, Buheirat en *Egypt* **80** C3
Toshka Lakes = Toshka,
   Buheirat en *Egypt* **80** C3
Toshkent *Uzbekistan* **52** E7
Tosno *Russia* **32** C6
Tossa de Mar *Spain* **38** D7
Tösse *Sweden* **11** F6
Tostado *Argentina* **126** B3
Tostedt *Germany* **24** B5
Tostón, Pta. de *Canary Is.* **48** F5
Tosu *Japan* **55** H5
Tosya *Turkey* **72** B6
Totana *Spain* **39** H3
Totebo *Sweden* **11** G10
Toteng *Botswana* **88** C3
Tôtes *France* **18** C8
Tótkomlós *Hungary* **28** D5
Totma *Russia* **32** D5
Totnes *U.K.* **15** G4
Totness *Suriname* **125** B7
Toto *Nigeria* **83** D6
Totonicapán *Guatemala* **120** D1
Totoya, I. *Fiji* **91** a
Totten Glacier *Antarctica* **5** C8
Tottenham *Australia* **95** E4
Tottenham *Canada* **114** B5
Tottori *Japan* **55** G7
Tottori □ *Japan* **55** G7
Touáret *Niger* **83** A6
Touba *Ivory C.* **82** D3
Touba *Senegal* **82** C1
Toubkal, Djebel *Morocco* **78** B4
Toucy *France* **19** E10
Tougan *Burkina Faso* **82** C4
Touggourt *Algeria* **78** B7
Tougouri *Burkina Faso* **83** C4
Tougué *Guinea* **82** C2
Toukoto *Mali* **82** C3
Toul *France* **19** D12
Toulepleu *Ivory C.* **82** D3
Toulon *France* **21** E9
Toulouse *France* **20** E5
Toulouse Blagnac ✈ (TLS)
   France **20** E5
Toummo *Niger* **79** D8
Toumodi *Ivory C.* **82** D3
Tounan *Taiwan* **59** F13
Toungo *Nigeria* **83** D7
Toungoo *Burma* **67** K20
Touques → *France* **18** C7

Touraine *France* **18** E7
Tourcoing *France* **19** B10
Touriñán, C. *Spain* **36** B1
Tournai *Belgium* **17** D3
Tournan-en-Brie *France* **19** D9
Tournay *France* **20** E4
Tournon-St-Martin *France* **18** F7
Tournon-sur-Rhône *France* **21** C8
Tournus *France* **19** F11
Tours *France* **18** E7
Toussoro, Mt. *C.A.R.* **84** C4
Touws → *S. Africa* **88** E3
Touwsrivier *S. Africa* **88** E3
Tovarkovskiy *Russia* **32** F10
Tovste *Ukraine* **29** B10
Tovuz *Azerbaijan* **35** K7
Towada *Japan* **54** D10
Towada-Hachimantai △
   Japan **54** D10
Towada-Ko *Japan* **54** D10
Towanda *U.S.A.* **115** E8
Tower *U.S.A.* **112** B7
Towerhill Cr. → *Australia* **94** C3
Towner *U.S.A.* **112** A3
Townsend *U.S.A.* **108** C8
Townshend I. *Australia* **94** C5
Townsville *Australia* **94** B4
Towot *Sudan* **81** F3
Towraghondī *Afghan.* **66** B3
Towson *U.S.A.* **113** F15
Towuti, Danau *Indonesia* **63** E6
Toya-Ko *Japan* **54** C10
Toyama *Japan* **55** F8
Toyama □ *Japan* **55** F8
Toyama-Wan *Japan* **55** F8
Toyapakeh *Indonesia* **63** K18
Toyohashi *Japan* **55** G8
Toyokawa *Japan* **55** G8
Toyonaka *Japan* **55** G7
Toyooka *Japan* **55** G7
Toyota *Japan* **55** G8
Tozeur *Tunisia* **78** B7
Tqibuli *Georgia* **35** J6
Tqvarcheli *Georgia* **35** J5
Trá Lí = Tralee *Ireland* **12** D2
Trá Mhór = Tramore *Ireland* **12** D4
Tra On *Vietnam* **65** H5
Trabancos → *Spain* **36** D5
Traben-Trarbach *Germany* **25** F3
Trabzon *Turkey* **73** B8
Tracadie *Canada* **105** C7
Tracy *Canada* **104** C5
Tracy *Calif., U.S.A.* **110** H5
Tracy *Minn., U.S.A.* **112** C6
Tradate *Italy* **40** C5
Trade Town *Liberia* **82** D3
Trafalgar, C. *Spain* **37** J4
Tragonhisi *Greece* **47** D7
Traian *Brăila, Romania* **29** E12
Traian *Tulcea, Romania* **29** E13
Trail *Canada* **102** D5
Trainor L. *Canada* **102** A4
Trakai △ *Lithuania* **9** J21
Trákhonas *Cyprus* **49** D12
Tralee *Ireland* **12** D2
Tralee B. *Ireland* **12** D2
Tramore *Ireland* **12** D4
Tramore B. *Ireland* **12** D4
Tranås *Sweden* **11** F8
Tran Ninh, Cao Nguyen *Laos* **64** C4
Tranbjerg *Denmark* **11** H4
Trancas *Argentina* **126** B2
Trancoso *Portugal* **36** E3
Tranebjerg *Denmark* **11** J4
Tranemo *Sweden* **11** G7
Trang *Thailand* **65** J2
Trangahy *Madag.* **89** B7
Trangan *Indonesia* **63** F8
Trangie *Australia* **95** E4
Trångsviken *Sweden* **10** A7
Trani *Italy* **43** A9
Tranoroa *Madag.* **89** C8
Tranqueras *Uruguay* **127** C4
Transantarctic Mts.
   Antarctica **5** E12
Transcarpathia =
   Zakarpattya □ *Ukraine* **29** B8
Transilvania *Romania* **29** D9
Transilvanian Alps =
   Carpaţii Meridionali
   Romania **29** E9
Transnistria = Stînga
   Nistrului □ *Moldova* **29** C14
Transtrand *Sweden* **10** C7
Transtrandsfjällen *Sweden* **10** C6
Transvase Tajo-Segura,
   Canal de *Spain* **38** E2
Transylvania =
   Transilvania *Romania* **29** D9
Trápani *Italy* **42** D5
Trapper Pk. *U.S.A.* **108** D6
Traralgon *Australia* **95** F4
Trarza □ *Mauritania* **82** B2
Trasacco *Italy* **41** G10
Trăscău, Munţii *Romania* **29** D8
Trasimeno, L. *Italy* **41** E9
Träslövsläge *Sweden* **11** G6
Trasvase Tajo-Segura,
   Canal de *Spain* **38** E2
Trat *Thailand* **65** F4

Tratani → *Pakistan* **68** E3
Traun *Austria* **26** C7
Traunreut *Germany* **25** H8
Traunsee *Austria* **26** D6
Traunstein *Germany* **25** H8
Travellers L. *Australia* **95** E3
Travemünde *Germany* **24** B6
Travers, Mt. *N.Z.* **91** E4
Traverse City *U.S.A.* **113** C11
Travis, L. *U.S.A.* **116** F6
Travnik *Bos.-H.* **28** F2
Trawbreaga B. *Ireland* **12** A4
Trbovlje *Slovenia* **41** B12
Trbušani → *Russia* **32** F10
Trebbia → *Italy* **40** C6
Trebel → *Germany* **24** B9
Trébeurden *France* **18** D3
Trebević △ *Bos.-H.* **28** G3
Třebíč *Czech Rep.* **26** B8
Trebinje *Bos.-H.* **44** D2
Trebisacce *Italy* **43** C9
Trebišov *Slovak Rep.* **27** C14
Trebižat → *Bos.-H.* **41** E14
Trebnje *Slovenia* **41** C12
Třeboň *Czech Rep.* **26** B7
Trebonne *Australia* **94** B4
Třebon △ *Czech Rep.* **26** B7
Trebujena *Spain* **37** J4
Trecate *Italy* **40** C5
Tregaron *U.K.* **15** E4
Tregnago *Italy* **41** C8
Tregrosse Is. *Australia* **94** B5
Tréguier *France* **18** D3
Trégunc *France* **18** E3
Treherne *Canada* **103** D9
Tréia *Italy* **41** E10
Treignac *France* **20** C5
Treinta y Tres *Uruguay* **127** C5
Treis-karden *Germany* **25** E3
Treklyano *Bulgaria* **44** D6
Trelawney *Zimbabwe* **89** B5
Trélazé *France* **18** E6
Trelew *Argentina* **128** E3
Trélissac *France* **20** C4
Trelleborg *Sweden* **11** J7
Tremadog Bay *U.K.* **14** E3
Tremonton *U.S.A.* **108** F7
Tremp *Spain* **38** C5
Trenche → *Canada* **104** C5
Trenčiansky □ *Slovak Rep.* **27** C11
Trenčín *Slovak Rep.* **27** C11
Trenggalek *Indonesia* **63** H14
Trenque Lauquen *Argentina* **126** D3
Trent → *Canada* **114** B7
Trent → *U.K.* **14** D7
Trentino-Alto Adige □ *Italy* **41** B8
Trento *Italy* **40** B8
Trenton *Canada* **114** B7
Trenton *Mo., U.S.A.* **112** E7
Trenton *N.J., U.S.A.* **115** F10
Trenton *Nebr., U.S.A.* **112** E3
Trepassey *Canada* **105** C9
Trepuzzi *Italy* **43** B11
Tres Arroyos *Argentina* **126** D3
Três Corações *Brazil* **127** A6
Três Lagoas *Brazil* **125** H8
Tres Lomas *Argentina* **126** D3
Tres Montes, C. *Chile* **128** F1
Tres Pinos *U.S.A.* **110** J5
Três Pontas *Brazil* **127** A6
Tres Puentes *Chile* **126** B1
Tres Puntas, C. *Argentina* **128** F3
Três Rios *Brazil* **127** A7
Tres Valles *Mexico* **119** D5
Tresco *U.K.* **15** H1
Treska → *Macedonia* **44** E5
Treskavica *Bos.-H.* **28** G3
Trespaderne *Spain* **36** C7
Tresticklan △ *Sweden* **11** F5
Trets *France* **21** E9
Treuchtlingen *Germany* **25** G6
Treuenbrietzen *Germany* **24** C8
Trevi *Italy* **41** F9
Trévieso, Peña *Spain* **36** C4
Treviso *Italy* **41** C9
Trévoux *France* **21** C8
Trgovište *Serbia* **44** D6
Triabunna *Australia* **95** G4
Trianda *Greece* **49** C10
Triangle *Zimbabwe* **89** C5
Triaucourt-en-Argonne
   France **19** D12
Tribal Areas □ *Pakistan* **68** C4
Tribsees *Germany* **24** A8
Tribulation, C. *Australia* **94** B4
Tribune *U.S.A.* **112** F3
Tricárico *Italy* **43** B9
Tricase *Italy* **43** C11
Trichinopoly =
   Tiruchchirappalli *India* **66** P11
Trichonida, L. *Greece* **46** C3
Trichur *India* **66** P10
Trichy = Tiruchchirappalli
   India **66** P11
Trida *Australia* **95** E4
Trier *Germany* **25** F2
Trieste *Italy* **41** C10
Trieste, G. di *Italy* **41** C10

Trieux → *France* **18** D3
Triggiano *Italy* **43** A9
Triglav *Slovenia* **41** B10
Triglavski △ *Slovenia* **41** B10
Trigno → *Italy* **41** F11
Trigueros *Spain* **37** H4
Trikala *Greece* **46** B3
Trikala □ *Greece* **46** B3
Trikeri *Greece* **46** B5
Trikomo *Cyprus* **49** D12
Trikora, Puncak *Indonesia* **63** E9
Trilj *Croatia* **41** E13
Trillo *Spain* **38** E2
Trim *Ireland* **12** C5
Trimmu Dam *Pakistan* **68** D5
Trincomalee *Sri Lanka* **66** Q12
Trindade *Brazil* **125** E9
Trindade, I. *Atl. Oc.* **2** F8
Třinec *Czech Rep.* **27** B11
Trinidad *Bolivia* **124** F6
Trinidad *Cuba* **120** B4
Trinidad *Trin. & Tob.* **121** D7
Trinidad *Uruguay* **126** C4
Trinidad *U.S.A.* **109** H11
Trinidad → *Mexico* **119** D5
Trinidad & Tobago ■
   W. Indies **121** D7
Trinitápoli *Italy* **43** A9
Trinity *Canada* **105** C9
Trinity *U.S.A.* **116** F7
Trinity → *Calif., U.S.A.* **108** F2
Trinity → *Tex., U.S.A.* **116** G7
Trinity B. *Canada* **105** C9
Trinity Hills *Trin. & Tob.* **125** K15
Trinity Is. *U.S.A.* **106** D9
Trinity Range *U.S.A.* **108** F4
Trinkitat *Sudan* **80** D4
Trino *Italy* **40** C5
Trinway *U.S.A.* **114** F2
Triolet *Mauritius* **85** d
Trionto, C. *Italy* **43** C9
Triora *Italy* **40** D4
Tripoli = Tarābulus *Lebanon* **74** A4
Tripoli = Tarābulus *Libya* **79** B8
Tripoli *Greece* **46** D4
Tripolitania = Tarābulus
   N. Afr. **79** B8
Tripura □ *India* **67** H18
Triplos *Cyprus* **49** E11
Trischen *Germany* **24** A4
Tristan da Cunha *Atl. Oc.* **77** K2
Trisul *India* **69** D8
Trivandrum *India* **66** Q10
Trivento *Italy* **41** G11
Trizin *Greece* **46** D5
Trnava *Slovak Rep.* **27** C10
Trnavský □ *Slovak Rep.* **27** C10
Troarn *France* **18** C6
Trochu *Canada* **102** C6
Trodely I. *Canada* **104** B4
Troglav *Croatia* **41** E13
Trogir *Croatia* **41** E13
Tróia *Italy* **43** A8
Troilus, L. *Canada* **104** B5
Troina *Italy* **43** E7
Trois-Pistoles *Canada* **105** C6
Trois-Rivières *Canada* **104** C5
Trois-Rivières *Guadeloupe* **120** b
Troisdorf *Germany* **24** E3
Troitsk *Russia* **52** D7
Troitsko Pechorsk *Russia* **52** C6
Troitskoye *Russia* **35** G7
Trölladyngja *Iceland* **8** D5
Trollhättan *Sweden* **11** F6
Trollheimen *Norway* **8** E13
Trombetas → *Brazil* **125** D7
Tromsø *Norway* **8** B18
Tron *Thailand* **64** D3
Trona *U.S.A.* **111** K9
Tronador, Mte. *Argentina* **128** E2
Trøndelag *Norway* **8** D14
Trondheim *Norway* **8** E14
Trondheimsfjorden *Norway* **8** E14
Trönninge *Sweden* **11** H6
Tronto → *Italy* **41** F10
Troodos *Cyprus* **49** E11
Troon *U.K.* **13** F4
Tropea *Italy* **43** D8
Tropic *U.S.A.* **109** H7
Tropojë *Albania* **44** D4
Trosa *Sweden* **11** F11
Trostan *U.K.* **12** A5
Trostberg *Germany* **25** G8
Trostyanets *Sumy, Ukraine* **33** G8
Trostyanets *Vinnytsya,
   Ukraine* **29** B14
Trou Gras Pt. *St. Lucia* **121** f
Trout → *Canada* **102** A5
Trout L. *N.W.T., Canada* **102** A4
Trout L. *Ont., Canada* **103** C10
Trout Lake *Canada* **102** B6
Trout Lake *U.S.A.* **110** E5
Trout River *Canada* **105** C8
Trout Run *U.S.A.* **114** E7
Trouville-sur-Mer *France* **18** C7
Trowbridge *U.K.* **15** F5
Troy *Turkey* **47** B8
Troy *Ala., U.S.A.* **117** F12
Troy *Kans., U.S.A.* **112** F6
Troy *Mo., U.S.A.* **112** F8

Troy Mont., U.S.A. 108 B6
Troy N.Y., U.S.A. 115 D11
Troy Ohio, U.S.A. 113 E11
Troy Pa., U.S.A. 115 E8
Troyan Bulgaria 45 D8
Troyes France 19 D11
Trpanj Croatia 41 E8
Trstenik Serbia 44 C5
Truchas Pk. U.S.A. 109 J11
Trucial States = United
   Arab Emirates ■ Asia 71 F7
Truckee U.S.A. 110 F6
Trudfront Russia 35 H8
Trudovoye Russia 54 C6
Trujillo Honduras 120 C2
Trujillo Peru 124 E3
Trujillo Spain 37 F5
Trujillo U.S.A. 109 J11
Trujillo Venezuela 124 B4
Truk Micronesia 96 G7
Trumann U.S.A. 117 D9
Trumansburg U.S.A. 115 D8
Trumbull, Mt. U.S.A. 109 H7
Trůn Bulgaria 44 D6
Trun France 18 D7
Trundle Australia 95 E4
Trung-Phan = Annam
   Vietnam 64 E7
Truro Canada 105 C7
Truro U.K. 15 G2
Truskavets Ukraine 23 D12
Trustrup Denmark 11 H4
Trutch Canada 102 B4
Truth or Consequences
   U.S.A. 109 K10
Trutnov Czech Rep. 26 A8
Truyère → France 20 D6
Tryavna Bulgaria 45 D9
Tryonville U.S.A. 114 E5
Trzcianka Poland 31 E3
Trzciel Poland 31 F2
Trzcińsko Zdrój Poland 31 F1
Trzebiatów Poland 30 D2
Trzebiez Poland 30 E1
Trzebnica Poland 31 G4
Trzemeszno Poland 31 F4
Tržič Slovenia 41 B11
Tsagan Aman Russia 35 G8
Tsamandas Greece 46 B2
Tsandi Namibia 88 B1
Tsaratanana Madag. 89 B8
Tsaratanana, Mt. de =
   Maromokotro Madag. 89 A8
Tsaratanana △ Madag. 89 A8
Tsarevo Bulgaria 45 D9
Tsaritsani Greece 46 B4
Tsau Botswana 88 C3
Tsavo Kenya 86 C4
Tsavo East △ Kenya 86 C4
Tsavo West △ Kenya 86 C4
Tsebrykove Ukraine 33 J6
Tsentralnyy □ Russia 34 D4
Tses Namibia 88 D2
Tsetserleg Mongolia 60 B5
Tsévié Togo 83 D5
Tshabong Botswana 88 D3
Tshane Botswana 88 C3
Tshela Dem. Rep. of the Congo 84 E2
Tshesebe Botswana 89 C4
Tshibeke
   Dem. Rep. of the Congo 86 C2
Tshibinda
   Dem. Rep. of the Congo 86 C2
Tshikapa
   Dem. Rep. of the Congo 84 F4
Tshilenge
   Dem. Rep. of the Congo 86 D1
Tshinsenda
   Dem. Rep. of the Congo 87 E2
Tshofa Dem. Rep. of the Congo 86 D2
Tshwane = Pretoria S. Africa 89 D4
Tshwane Botswana 88 C3
Tsigara Botswana 88 C4
Tsihombe Madag. 89 D8
Tsiigehtchic Canada 100 D5
Ts'il-os △ Canada 102 C4
Tsimlyansk Russia 35 G6
Tsimlyansk Res. =
   Tsimlyanskoye Vdkhr.
   Russia 35 F6
Tsimlyanskoye Vdkhr.
   Russia 35 F6
Tsinan = Jinan China 56 F9
Tsineng S. Africa 88 D3
Tsinghai = Qinghai □ China 60 C4
Tsingtao = Qingdao China 57 F11
Tsingy de Bemaraha △
   Madag. 89 B8
Tsingy de Namoraka △
   Madag. 89 B8
Tsinjoarivo Madag. 89 B8
Tsinjomitondraka Madag. 89 B8
Tsirigo = Kythira Greece 46 E5
Tsiroanomandidy Madag. 89 B8
Tsiteli-Tsqaro Georgia 35 K8
Tsitondroina Madag. 89 C8
Tsitsikamma △ S. Africa 88 E3
Tsivilsk Russia 34 C8

Tsivory Madag. 89 C8
Tskhinvali Georgia 35 J7
Tsna → Russia 34 C6
Tsnori Georgia 35 K7
Tso Moriri, L. India 69 C8
Tsobis Namibia 88 B2
Tsodilo Hill Botswana 88 B3
Tsogttsetsiy = Baruunsuu
   Mongolia 56 C3
Tsolo S. Africa 89 E4
Tsomo S. Africa 89 E4
Tsu Japan 55 G8
Tsu L. Canada 102 A6
Tsuchiura Japan 55 F10
Tsuen Wan China 59 F10
Tsugaru-Kaikyō Japan 54 D10
Tsumeb Namibia 88 B2
Tsumis Namibia 88 C2
Tsuruga Japan 55 G8
Tsurugi-San Japan 55 H7
Tsuruoka Japan 54 E9
Tsushima Gifu, Japan 55 G8
Tsushima Nagasaki, Japan 55 G4
Tsuyama Japan 55 G7
Tsvetkovo Ukraine 33 H6
Tsyelyakhany Belarus 23 B13
Tua → Portugal 36 D3
Tuaim = Tuam Ireland 12 C3
Tual Indonesia 63 F8
Tualatin U.S.A. 110 E4
Tuam Ireland 12 C3
Tuamotu, Îs.
   French Polynesia 97 J13
Tuamotu Arch. =
   Tuamotu, Îs.
   French Polynesia 97 J13
Tuamotu Ridge Pac. Oc. 97 K14
Tuan Giao Vietnam 64 B4
Tuanfeng China 59 B10
Tuanxi China 58 D6
Tuao Phil. 61 C4
Tuapse Russia 35 H4
Tuas Singapore 65 d
Tuatapere N.Z. 91 G1
Tuba City U.S.A. 109 H8
Tuban Indonesia 63 G15
Tubani Botswana 88 C3
Tubarão Brazil 127 B6
Tūbās West Bank 74 C4
Tubas → Namibia 88 C2
Tübingen Germany 25 G5
Tubou Fiji 91 a
Tubruq Libya 79 B10
Tubuaï, Îs. French Polynesia 97 K13
Tuc Trung Vietnam 65 G6
Tucacas Venezuela 124 A5
T'uch'ang Taiwan 59 E13
Tuchitua Canada 102 A3
Tuchodi → Canada 102 B4
Tuchola Poland 30 E4
Tuchów Poland 31 J8
Tuckanarra Australia 93 E2
Tucson U.S.A. 109 K8
Tucumán □ Argentina 126 B2
Tucumcari U.S.A. 109 J12
Tucupita Venezuela 124 B6
Tucuruí Brazil 125 D9
Tucuruí, Represa de Brazil 125 D9
Tuczno Poland 31 E3
Tudela Spain 38 C3
Tudmur Syria 73 E8
Tudor, L. Canada 105 A6
Tudora Romania 29 C11
Tuela → Portugal 36 D3
Tufanbeyli Turkey 72 C7
Tugela → S. Africa 89 D5
Tuguegarao Phil. 61 C4
Tugur Russia 53 D14
Tui Spain 36 C2
Tuineje Canary Is. 48 F5
Tukangbesi, Kepulauan
   Indonesia 63 F6
Tukarak I. Canada 104 A4
Tukayyid Iraq 70 D5
Tũkh Egypt 80 H7
Tukhlya Ukraine 29 B8
Tukobo Ghana 82 D4
Tuktoyaktuk Canada 100 D5
Tuktut Nogait △ Canada 100 D7
Tukums Latvia 30 B10
Tukums □ Latvia 30 B10
Tukuyu Tanzania 87 D3
Tula Hidalgo, Mexico 119 C5
Tula Tamaulipas, Mexico 119 C5
Tula Nigeria 83 D7
Tula Russia 32 E9
Tula □ Russia 32 F9
Tulach Mhór = Tullamore
   Ireland 12 C4
Tulancingo Mexico 119 C5
Tulare Serbia 44 D5
Tulare U.S.A. 110 J7
Tulare Lake Bed U.S.A. 110 K7
Tularosa U.S.A. 109 K10
Tulbagh S. Africa 88 E2
Tulcán Ecuador 124 C3
Tulcea Romania 29 D13
Tulcea □ Romania 29 E13
Tulchyn Ukraine 29 B13
Tũledi Araldary Kazakhstan 35 H10

Tũleh Iran 71 C7
Tulemalu L. Canada 103 A9
Tulgheş Romania 29 D10
Tuli Zimbabwe 87 G2
Tulia U.S.A. 116 D4
Tuliszków Poland 31 F5
Tulita Canada 100 E6
Ţülkarm West Bank 74 C4
Tulla Ireland 12 D3
Tullahoma U.S.A. 117 D11
Tullamore Australia 95 E4
Tullamore Ireland 12 C4
Tulle France 20 C5
Tulln Austria 26 C9
Tullow Ireland 12 D5
Tullus Sudan 81 E1
Tully Australia 94 B4
Tully U.S.A. 115 D8
Tulnici Romania 29 E11
Tulovo Bulgaria 45 D9
Tulsa U.S.A. 116 C7
Tulsequah Canada 102 B2
Tulu Milki Ethiopia 81 F4
Tulu Welel Ethiopia 81 F3
Tuluá Colombia 124 C3
Tulucești Romania 29 E13
Tulun Russia 53 D11
Tulungagung Indonesia 63 H14
Tuma Russia 32 E11
Tuma → Nic. 120 D3
Tumaco Colombia 124 C3
Tumacacori △ U.S.A. 109 L8
Tumakuru = Tumkur India 66 N10
Tumatumari Guyana 124 B7
Tumba Sweden 10 E11
Tumba, L.
   Dem. Rep. of the Congo 84 E3
Tumbarumba Australia 95 F4
Tumbaya Argentina 126 A2
Tumbes Peru 124 D2
Tumbler Ridge Canada 102 B4
Tumbwe
   Dem. Rep. of the Congo 87 E2
Tumby Bay Australia 95 E2
Tumd Youqi China 56 D6
Tumen China 54 C4
Tumen Jiang → China 57 C16
Tumeremo Venezuela 124 B6
Tumkur India 66 N10
Tump Pakistan 66 F3
Tumpat Malaysia 65 J4
Tumu Ghana 82 C4
Tumucumaque, Serra
   Brazil 125 C8
Tumut Australia 95 F4
Tumwater U.S.A. 110 C4
Tuna India 68 H4
Tunadal Sweden 10 B11
Tunapuna Trin. & Tob. 125 K15
Tunas de Zaza Cuba 120 B4
Tunbridge Wells = Royal
   Tunbridge Wells U.K. 15 F8
Tunçbilek Turkey 47 B11
Tunceli Turkey 73 C8
Tunceli □ Turkey 73 C8
Tuncurry Australia 95 E5
Tundla India 68 F8
Tundubai Sudan 80 D2
Tunduru Tanzania 87 E4
Tundzha → Bulgaria 45 E10
Tungabhadra → India 66 M11
Tungaru Sudan 81 E3
Tungla Nic. 120 D3
Tungsha Tao = Dongsha
   Dao S. China Sea 59 G11
Tungshih Taiwan 59 E13
Tungsten Canada 102 A3
Tunguska, Nizhnyaya →
   Russia 53 C9
Tunguska,
   Podkamennaya →
   Russia 53 C10
Tunica U.S.A. 117 D9
Tunis Tunisia 78 A7
Tunis ✈ (TUN) Tunisia 42 F3
Tunisia ■ Africa 79 A7
Tunja Colombia 124 B4
Tunkhannock U.S.A. 115 E9
Tunliu China 56 F7
Tunnel Creek △ Australia 92 C4
Tunnsjøen Norway 8 D15
Tunø Denmark 11 J4
Tunnewun Mexico 119 C5
Tunuyán Argentina 126 C2
Tunuyán → Argentina 126 C2
Tunxi = Huangshan China 59 B12
Tuo Jiang → China 58 C5
Tuolumne U.S.A. 110 H6
Tuolumne → U.S.A. 110 H5
Tūp Āghāj Iran 73 D12
Tupã Brazil 127 A5
Tupelo U.S.A. 117 D10
Tupik Russia 53 D12
Tupinambarana, I. Brazil 124 D7
Tupiza Bolivia 126 A2
Tupižnica Serbia 44 C6
Tupman U.S.A. 111 K7
Tupper Canada 102 B4
Tupper L. U.S.A. 115 B10

Tupper Lake U.S.A. 115 B10
Tüpqaraghan Muyis
   Kazakhstan 35 H10
Tupungato, Cerro S. Amer. 126 C2
Tuquan China 57 B11
Tuquerres Colombia 124 C3
Tura Russia 53 C11
Turabah Ḥāʾil, Si. Arabia 70 D4
Turabah Makkah, Si. Arabia 80 C5
Tūrān Iran 71 C8
Turan Russia 53 D10
Turayf Si. Arabia 70 D3
Turbacz Poland 31 J7
Turbe Bos.-H. 28 F2
Turčianske Teplice
   Slovak Rep. 27 C11
Turcoaia Romania 29 E13
Turda Romania 29 D8
Turek Poland 31 F5
Turén Venezuela 124 B5
Turfan = Turpan China 60 B3
Turgeon → Canada 104 C4
Türgovishte Bulgaria 45 C10
Turgut Turkey 47 D10
Turgutlu Turkey 47 C9
Turgwe → Zimbabwe 89 C5
Turhal Turkey 72 B7
Turia → Spain 39 F4
Turiaçu Brazil 125 D9
Turiaçu → Brazil 125 D9
Turiec → Slovak Rep. 27 C11
Turin = Torino Italy 40 C4
Turistan □ Türkistan
   Kazakhstan 52 E7
Túrkeve Hungary 28 C5
Turkey ■ Eurasia 72 C7
Turkey Creek = Warmun
   Australia 92 C4
Turki Russia 34 D6
Türkistan Kazakhstan 52 E7
Türkmenabat Turkmenistan 71 B9
Türkmenbashi Turkmenistan 71 A7
Turkmenistan ■ Asia 52 F6
Türkmenli Turkey 47 B8
Türkoğlu Turkey 72 D7
Turks & Caicos Is. ☑
   W. Indies 121 B5
Turks Island Passage
   W. Indies 121 B5
Turku Finland 32 B2
Turkwel → Kenya 86 B4
Turlock U.S.A. 110 H6
Turnagain → Australia 94 a
Turnagain → Canada 102 B3
Turnagain, C. N.Z. 91 D6
Turneffe Is. Belize 119 D7
Turner U.S.A. 108 B9
Turner Pt. Australia 94 A1
Turner Valley Canada 102 C6
Turners Falls U.S.A. 115 D12
Turner's Pen. S. Leone 82 D2
Turnhout Belgium 17 C4
Türnitz Austria 26 D8
Turnor L. Canada 103 B7
Turnov Czech Rep. 26 A8
Tūrnovo = Veliko Tŭrnovo
   Bulgaria 45 C9
Turnu Măgurele Romania 29 G9
Turnu Roşu, P. Romania 29 E9
Turobin Poland 31 H9
Turpan China 60 B3
Turrës, Kala e Albania 44 E3
Turriff U.K. 13 D6
Tursāq Iraq 73 F11
Tursi Italy 43 B9
Turtle Head I. Australia 94 A3
Turtle Is. S. Leone 82 D2
Turtle L. Canada 103 C7
Turtle Lake U.S.A. 112 B3
Turtleford Canada 103 C7
Turuépano △ Venezuela 121 D7
Turukhansk Russia 53 C9
Turzovka Slovak Rep. 27 B11
Tuscaloosa U.S.A. 117 E11
Tuscánia Italy 41 F8
Tuscany = Toscana □ Italy 40 E8
Tuscarawas → U.S.A. 114 F3
Tuscarora Mt. U.S.A. 114 F7
Tuscola Ill., U.S.A. 114 F1
Tuscola Tex., U.S.A. 116 E5
Tuscumbia U.S.A. 117 D11
Tuskegee U.S.A. 117 E12
Tuszyn Poland 31 G6
Tutak Turkey 73 C10
Tutatyev Russia 32 D7
Tuticorin India 66 Q11
Tutin Serbia 44 D4
Tutóia Brazil 125 D10
Tutong Brunei 62 D4
Tutova → Romania 29 D12
Tutrakan Bulgaria 45 B10
Tuttle Creek L. U.S.A. 112 F5
Tuttlingen Germany 25 H4
Tutuala E. Timor 63 F7
Tutuila Amer. Samoa 91 b
Tutume Botswana 85 J5
Tutun Egypt 80 J7

Tuva □ Russia 53 D10
Tuvalu ■ Pac. Oc. 90 B10
Tuvuca Fiji 91 a
Tuxer Alpen Austria 26 D4
Tuxpan Mexico 119 C5
Tuxtla Gutiérrez Mexico 119 D6
Tuy = Tui Spain 36 C2
Tuy An Vietnam 64 F7
Tuy Duc Vietnam 65 F6
Tuy Hoa Vietnam 64 F7
Tuy Phong Vietnam 65 G7
Tuya L. Canada 102 B2
Tuyen Hoa Vietnam 64 D6
Tuyen Quang Vietnam 58 G5
Tūysarkān Iran 73 E13
Tuz Gölü Turkey 72 C5
Ţūz Khurmātū Iraq 73 E11
Tuzi Montenegro 44 D3
Tuzigoot △ U.S.A. 109 J7
Tuzla Bos.-H. 28 F3
Tuzla Turkey 73 B10
Tuzlov → Russia 33 J10
Tuzly 29 E15
Tvååker Sweden 11 G6
Tvardița Moldova 29 D13
Tver Russia 32 D8
Tver □ Russia 32 D8
Tvrdošin Slovak Rep. 27 B12
Tvrdošovce Slovak Rep. 27 C11
Tvŭrditsa Bulgaria 45 D9
Twain U.S.A. 110 E5
Twain Harte U.S.A. 110 G6
Twardogóra Poland 31 G4
Tweed Canada 114 B7
Tweed → U.K. 13 F6
Tweed Heads Australia 95 D5
Tweedsmuir △ Canada 102 C3
Twentynine Palms U.S.A. 111 L10
Twillingate Canada 105 C9
Twin Bridges U.S.A. 108 D7
Twin Falls Canada 105 B7
Twin Falls U.S.A. 108 E6
Twin Valley U.S.A. 112 B5
Twinsburg U.S.A. 114 E3
Twistringen Germany 24 C4
Twitchell Res. U.S.A. 111 L6
Two Harbors U.S.A. 112 B8
Two Hills Canada 102 C6
Two Rivers U.S.A. 112 C10
Two Rocks Australia 93 F2
Twofold B. Australia 95 F4
Tyachiv Ukraine 23 D12
Tychy Poland 31 H5
Tyczyn Poland 31 J9
Tykocin Poland 31 E9
Tyler Minn., U.S.A. 112 C5
Tyler Tex., U.S.A. 116 E7
Tyligul → Ukraine 33 J6
Tymankivka Ukraine 29 B13
Týn nad Vltavou Czech Rep. 26 B7
Tynda Russia 53 D13
Tyndall U.S.A. 112 D5
Tyne → U.K. 14 C6
Tyne & Wear □ U.K. 14 B6
Týnec nad Sázavou
   Czech Rep. 26 B7
Tynemouth U.K. 14 B6
Tyre = Ṣūr Lebanon 74 B4
Tyresta △ Sweden 10 E12
Tyrifjorden Norway 9 F14
Tyringe Sweden 11 H7
Tyrnyauz Russia 35 J6
Tyrol = Tirol □ Austria 26 D3
Tyrone U.S.A. 114 F6
Tyrone □ U.K. 12 B4
Tyrrell → Australia 95 F3
Tyrrell, L. Australia 95 F3
Tyrrell L. Canada 103 A7
Tyrrhenian Sea Medit. S. 6 G8
Tysfjorden Norway 8 B17
Tysmenytsya Ukraine 29 B9
Tystberga Sweden 11 F11
Tytuvėnai Lithuania 30 C10
Tyub Karagan, Mys =
   Tüpqaraghan Muyis
   Kazakhstan 35 H10
Tyuleni, Ostrova = Tüledi
   Araldary Kazakhstan 35 H10
Tyuleniy, Mys Azerbaijan 35 K10
Tyumen Russia 52 D7
Tywi → U.K. 15 F3
Tywyn U.K. 15 E3
Tzaneen S. Africa 89 C5
Tzermiado Greece 49 D7
Tzoumérka, Óros =
   Athamanon Oros Greece 46 B3
Tzukong = Zigong China 58 C5

U

U.S.A. = United States of
   America ■ N. Amer. 107 H20
U.S. Virgin Is. ☑ W. Indies 121 e
Uanle Uen = Wanleweyne
   Somali Rep. 75 G3
Uatumã → Brazil 124 D7
Uaupés Brazil 124 D5
Uaupés → Brazil 124 C5
Uaxactún Guatemala 120 C2

Ub Serbia 44 B4
Ubá Brazil 127 A7
Uba Nigeria 83 C7
Ubaitaba Brazil 125 F11
Ubangi = Oubangi →
   Dem. Rep. of the Congo 84 E3
Ubauro Pakistan 68 E3
Ubaye → France 21 D10
Ube Japan 55 H5
Úbeda Spain 37 G7
Uberaba Brazil 125 G9
Uberlândia Brazil 125 G9
Überlingen Germany 25 H5
Ubin, Pulau Singapore 65 d
Ubly U.S.A. 114 C2
Ubolratna Res. Thailand 64 D4
Ubombo S. Africa 89 D5
Ubon Ratchathani Thailand 64 E5
Ubondo Dem. Rep. of the Congo 86 C2
Ubort → Belarus 23 B15
Ubrique Spain 37 J5
Ubud Indonesia 63 J18
Ubundu Dem. Rep. of the Congo 86 C2
Ucar Azerbaijan 73 B12
Ucayali → Peru 124 D4
Uchab Namibia 88 B2
Uchiura-Wan Japan 54 C10
Uchquduq Uzbekistan 52 E7
Uchte Germany 24 C4
Uchur → Russia 53 D14
Uda → Russia 53 D14
Udachnyy Russia 53 C12
Udagamandalam India 66 P10
Udainagar India 68 H7
Udaipur India 68 G5
Udaipur Garhi Nepal 69 F12
Udala India 69 J12
Udbina Croatia 41 D12
Uddeholm Sweden 10 D8
Uddevalla Sweden 11 F5
Uddjaure Sweden 8 D17
Uden Neths. 17 C5
Udgir India 66 K10
Udhampur India 69 C6
Udi Nigeria 83 D6
Údine Italy 41 B10
Udintsev Fracture Zone
   S. Ocean 5 B13
Udmurtia □ Russia 52 D6
Udon Thani Thailand 64 D4
Udong Cambodia 65 G5
Udskaya Guba Russia 53 D14
Udu Pt. Fiji 91 a
Udupi India 66 N9
Udvoy Balkan Bulgaria 45 D10
Udzungwa △ Tanzania 86 D4
Udzungwa Range Tanzania 87 D4
Ueckermünde Germany 24 B10
Ueda Japan 55 F9
Uedineniya, Os. Russia 4 B12
Uele → Dem. Rep. of the Congo 84 D4
Uelen Russia 53 C19
Uelzen Germany 24 C6
Uetersen Germany 24 B5
Uetze Germany 24 C6
Ufa Russia 52 D6
Uffenheim Germany 25 F6
Ugab → Namibia 88 C1
Ugalla → Tanzania 86 D3
Ugalla River △ Tanzania 86 D3
Uganda ■ Africa 86 B3
Ugento Italy 43 C11
Ugep Nigeria 83 D6
Ughelli Nigeria 83 D6
Ugie S. Africa 89 E4
Ugíjar Spain 39 J7
Ugine France 21 C10
Uglegorsk Russia 53 E15
Uglich Russia 32 D10
Ugljan Croatia 41 D12
Ugljane Croatia 41 E13
Ugolnye Kopi Russia 53 C18
Ugra → Russia 32 E9
Uğurchin Bulgaria 45 C8
Uh → Slovak Rep. 27 C15
Uherské Hradiště Czech Rep. 27 B9
Uherský Brod Czech Rep. 27 B10
Úhlava → Czech Rep. 26 B6
Uhlenhorst Namibia 88 C2
Uhniv Ukraine 31 H10
Uhrichsville U.S.A. 114 F3
Uibhist a Deas = South Uist
   U.K. 13 D1
Uibhist a Tuath = North
   Uist U.K. 13 D1
Uig U.K. 13 D2
Uíge Angola 84 F2
Uiha Tonga 91 c
Uijeongbu S. Korea 57 F14
Ŭiju N. Korea 57 D13
Uinta Mts. U.S.A. 108 F8
Uis Namibia 88 C1
Uiseong S. Korea 57 F15
Uitenhage S. Africa 88 E4
Uithuizen Neths. 17 A6
Ujazd Poland 31 H5

Újfehértó *Hungary* **28** C6
Ujh → *India* **68** C6
Ujhani *India* **69** F8
Uji-guntō *Japan* **55** J4
Ujjain *India* **68** H6
Ujście *Poland* **31** E3
Újszász *Hungary* **28** C5
Ujung Pandang *Indonesia* **63** F5
Uka *Russia* **53** D17
Ukara I. *Tanzania* **86** C3
Uke-Shima *Japan* **55** K4
Ukerewe I. *Tanzania* **86** C3
Ukholovo *Russia* **34** D5
Ukhrul *India* **67** G19
Ukhta *Russia* **52** C6
Ukiah *U.S.A.* **110** F3
Ukmergė *Lithuania* **32** E3
Ukraine ■ *Europe* **33** H7
Ukwi *Botswana* **88** C3
Ula *Turkey* **72** D3
Ulaan-Uul *Mongolia* **56** B6
Ulaanbaatar *Mongolia* **53** E11
Ulaangom *Mongolia* **60** A4
Ulaanjirem *Mongolia* **56** B3
Ulak I. *U.S.A.* **106** E4
Ulamba *Dem. Rep. of the Congo* **87** D1
Ulan Bator = Ulaanbaatar
  Mongolia **53** E11
Ulan Erge *Russia* **35** G7
Ulan Khol *Russia* **35** H8
Ulan Ude *Russia* **53** D11
Ulanhad = Chifeng *China* **57** C10
Ulanów *Poland* **31** H9
Ulaş *Sivas, Turkey* **72** C7
Ulaş *Tekirdağ, Turkey* **45** E11
Ulaya *Morogoro, Tanzania* **86** D4
Ulaya *Tabora, Tanzania* **86** C3
Ulcinj *Montenegro* **44** E3
Ulco *S. Africa* **88** D3
Ule älv = Oulujoki →
  Finland **8** D21
Ule träsk = Oulujärvi *Finland* **8** D22
Uleåborg = Oulu *Finland* **8** D21
Ulefoss *Norway* **9** G13
Ulëz *Albania* **44** E3
Ulfborg *Denmark* **11** H2
Ulhasnagar *India* **66** K8
Uliastay *Mongolia* **60** B4
Uljin *S. Korea* **57** F15
Uljma *Serbia* **28** E6
Ulla → *Spain* **36** C2
Ulladulla *Australia* **95** F5
Ullapool *U.K.* **13** D3
Ullared *Sweden* **11** G6
Ulleungdo *S. Korea* **55** F5
Ullswater *Canada* **114** A5
Ullswater *U.K.* **14** C5
Ulm *Germany* **25** G5
Ulmarra *Australia* **95** D5
Ulmeni *Buzău, Romania* **29** E11
Ulmeni *Maramureș, Romania* **29** C8
Ulonguè *Mozam.* **87** E3
Ulricehamn *Sweden* **11** G7
Ulrika *Sweden* **11** F9
Ulsan *S. Korea* **57** G15
Ulsta *U.K.* **13** A7
Ulster □ *U.K.* **12** B5
Ulstrem *Bulgaria* **45** D10
Ulubat Gölü *Turkey* **45** F12
Ulubey *Turkey* **47** C11
Uluborlu *Turkey* **47** C12
Uluçinar *Turkey* **72** D6
Uludağ *Turkey* **45** F13
Uludağ △ *Turkey* **45** F13
Uludere *Turkey* **73** D10
Uluguru Mts. *Tanzania* **86** D4
Ulukışla *Turkey* **72** D6
Ulungur He → *China* **60** B3
Uluru *Australia* **93** E5
Uluru-Kata Tjuta △ *Australia* **93** E5
Ulutau *Kazakhstan* **52** E7
Uluwatu *Indonesia* **63** K18
Ulva *U.K.* **13** E2
Ulverston *U.K.* **14** C4
Ulverstone *Australia* **95** G4
Ulya *Russia* **53** D15
Ulyanovo *Russia* **30** D9
Ulyanovsk *Russia* **34** C9
Ulyanovsk □ *Russia* **34** C9
Ulyasutay = Uliastay
  Mongolia **60** B4
Ulysses *Kans., U.S.A.* **112** G3
Ulysses *Pa., U.S.A.* **114** E7
Ulysses, Mt. *Canada* **102** B4
Umag *Croatia* **41** C10
Umala *Bolivia* **124** G5
'Umān = Oman ■ *Asia* **75** C6
Uman *Ukraine* **23** D16
Umaria *India* **69** H9
Umarkot *Pakistan* **68** G3
Umarpada *India* **68** J5
Umatilla *U.S.A.* **108** D4
Umbagog L. *U.S.A.* **115** B13
Umbakumba *Australia* **94** A2
Umbértide *Italy* **41** E9
Umbrella Mts. *N.Z.* **91** F2
Umbria □ *Italy* **41** F9
Umeå *Sweden* **8** E19
Umeälven → *Sweden* **8** E19

Umera *Indonesia* **63** E7
Umfuli → *Zimbabwe* **87** F2
Umfurudzi ○ *Zimbabwe* **87** F3
Umgusa *Zimbabwe* **87** F2
Umgwenya → *Mozam.* **89** D5
Umiujaq *Canada* **104** A4
Umka *Serbia* **44** B4
Umkomaas *S. Africa* **89** E5
Umlazi *S. Africa* **85** L6
Umm ad Daraj, J. *Jordan* **74** C4
Umm al Khashab *Si. Arabia* **80** D5
Umm al Qaywayn *U.A.E.* **71** E7
Umm al Qittayn *Jordan* **74** C5
Umm Arda *Sudan* **81** D3
Umm Bāb *Qatar* **71** E6
Umm Badr *Sudan* **81** E2
Umm Bel *Sudan* **81** E2
Umm Birkah *Si. Arabia* **80** B4
Umm Boim *Sudan* **81** E2
Umm Dam *Sudan* **81** E3
Umm Debi *Sudan* **81** E2
Umm Dubban *Sudan* **81** D3
Umm Durman =
  Omdurman *Sudan* **81** D3
Umm el Fahm *Israel* **74** C4
Umm Gafala *Sudan* **81** E2
Umm Gimala *Sudan* **81** E2
Umm Inderaba *Sudan* **80** D3
Umm Keddada *Sudan* **81** E2
Umm Koweika *Sudan* **81** E3
Umm Lajj *Si. Arabia* **70** E3
Umm Merwa *Sudan* **80** D3
Umm Qantur *Sudan* **81** E3
Umm Qasr *Iraq* **70** D5
Umm Qurein *Sudan* **81** F2
Umm Ruwaba *Sudan* **81** E3
Umm Saiyala *Sudan* **81** E3
Umm Shutur *Sudan* **81** F3
Umm Sidr *Sudan* **81** E2
Umm Urūmah *Si. Arabia* **80** B4
Umm Zehetir *Egypt* **80** J8
Umnak I. *U.S.A.* **106** E6
Umniati → *Zimbabwe* **87** F2
Umpang *U.S.A.* **106** C9
Umpqua → *U.S.A.* **108** E1
Umreth *India* **68** H5
Umtata = Mthatha *S. Africa* **89** E4
Umuahia *Nigeria* **83** D6
Umuarama *Brazil* **127** A5
Umurbey *Turkey* **45** F10
Umvukwe Ra. *Zimbabwe* **87** F3
Umzimkulu *S. Africa* **89** E4
Umzingwane → *Zimbabwe* **87** G2
Umzinto = eMuziwezinto
  S. Africa **89** E5
Una *India* **68** D7
Una → *Bos.-H.* **41** D13
Unac → *Bos.-H.* **41** D13
Unadilla *U.S.A.* **115** D9
Unalakleet *U.S.A.* **106** C7
Unalaska *U.S.A.* **106** E6
Unalaska I. *U.S.A.* **106** E6
'Unayzah *Si. Arabia* **70** E4
'Unayzah, J. *Iraq* **73** F8
Uncastillo *Spain* **38** C3
Uncía *Bolivia* **124** E5
Uncompahgre Peak *U.S.A.* **108** G10
Uncompahgre Plateau
  U.S.A. **108** G9
Undara Volcanic △ *Australia* **94** B3
Unden *Sweden* **11** F8
Underbool *Australia* **95** F3
Undersaker *Sweden* **10** A7
Underwood *Canada* **114** B3
Unecha *Russia* **33** F7
Ungarie *Australia* **95** E4
Ungarra *Australia* **95** E2
Ungava, Pén. d' *Canada* **101** F17
Ungava B. *Canada* **101** F18
Ungeny = Ungheni *Moldova* **29** C12
Unggi *N. Korea* **57** C16
Ungheni *Moldova* **29** C12
Unguala → *Ethiopia* **81** F5
Ungwana B. *Kenya* **86** C5
Ungwatiri *Sudan* **81** D4
Uni *Russia* **34** B10
União da Vitória *Brazil* **127** B5
Uničov *Czech Rep.* **27** B10
Uniejów *Poland* **31** G5
Unije *Croatia* **41** D11
Unimak I. *U.S.A.* **106** E7
Unimak Pass. *U.S.A.* **106** E7
Union *Miss., U.S.A.* **117** E10
Union *Mo., U.S.A.* **112** F8
Union *S.C., U.S.A.* **117** D14
Union City *Calif., U.S.A.* **110** H4
Union City *N.J., U.S.A.* **115** F10
Union City *Pa., U.S.A.* **114** E5
Union City *Tenn., U.S.A.* **117** C10
Union Dale *U.S.A.* **115** E9
Union Gap *U.S.A.* **108** C3
Union Springs *Ala., U.S.A.* **117** E12
Union Springs *N.Y., U.S.A.* **115** D8
Uniondale *S. Africa* **88** E3
Uniontown *U.S.A.* **113** F5
Unionville *U.S.A.* **112** E7
Unirea *Romania* **29** F12
United Arab Emirates ■ *Asia* **71** F7
United Kingdom ■ *Europe* **16** E6
United States of America ■
  N. Amer. **107** H20

Unity *Canada* **103** C7
Universales, Mtes. *Spain* **38** E3
University Park *U.S.A.* **109** K10
University Place *U.S.A.* **110** C4
Unjha *India* **68** H5
Unna *Germany* **24** D3
Unnao *India* **69** F9
Uno, Ilha *Guinea-Biss.* **82** C1
Unsengedsi → *Zimbabwe* **87** F3
Unst *U.K.* **13** A8
Unstrut → *Germany* **24** D7
Unterfranken □ *Germany* **25** F5
Unterschleissheim *Germany* **25** G7
Unuk → *Canada* **102** B2
Ünye *Turkey* **72** B7
Unzen-Amakusa △ *Japan* **55** H5
Unzha *Russia* **34** B6
Unzha → *Russia* **34** B6
Uozu *Japan* **55** F8
Upata *Venezuela* **124** B6
Upemba, L.
  Dem. Rep. of the Congo **87** D2
Upemba △
  Dem. Rep. of the Congo **87** D2
Upernavik *Greenland* **4** B5
Upington *S. Africa* **88** D3
Upleta *India* **68** J4
Upper □ *Ghana* **83** C4
Upper Alkali L. *U.S.A.* **108** F3
Upper Arrow L. *Canada* **102** C5
Upper Daly ○ *Australia* **92** B5
Upper Darby *U.S.A.* **115** F11
Upper Foster L. *Canada* **103** B7
Upper Hutt *N.Z.* **91** D5
Upper Klamath L. *U.S.A.* **108** E3
Upper Lake *U.S.A.* **110** F4
Upper Liard *Canada* **102** A3
Upper Manzanilla
  Trin. & Tob. **125** K15
Upper Missouri Breaks △
  U.S.A. **108** C9
Upper Musquodoboit
  Canada **105** C7
Upper Red L. *U.S.A.* **112** A6
Upper Sandusky *U.S.A.* **113** E12
Upper Volta = Burkina
  Faso ■ *Africa* **82** C4
Upphärad *Sweden* **11** F6
Uppland *Sweden* **10** D12
Upplands-Väsby *Sweden* **10** E11
Uppsala *Sweden* **10** E11
Uppsala län □ *Sweden* **10** D11
Upshi *India* **69** C7
Upton *U.S.A.* **108** D11
Uqsuqtuuq = Gjoa Haven
  Canada **100** D12
Ur *Iraq* **70** D5
Urad Qianqi *China* **56** D5
Urakawa *Japan* **54** C11
Ural = Uralskiy □ *Russia* **52** C7
Ural → *Zhayyq →
  Kazakhstan* **6** F16
Ural *Australia* **95** E4
Ural Mts. = Uralskie Gory
  Eurasia **6** C17
Uralla *Australia* **95** E5
Uralsk = Oral *Kazakhstan* **34** E10
Uralskie Gory *Eurasia* **6** C17
Uralskiy □ *Russia* **52** C7
Urambo *Tanzania* **86** D3
Urandangi *Australia* **94** C2
Uranium City *Canada* **103** B7
Urapuntja = Utopia *Australia* **94** C1
Uraricoera → *Brazil* **124** C6
Urasoe *Japan* **55** L3
Urawa = Saitama *Japan* **55** G9
Uray *Russia* **52** C7
'Uray'irah *Si. Arabia* **71** E6
Urbana *Ill., U.S.A.* **112** E9
Urbana *Ohio, U.S.A.* **113** E12
Urbandale *U.S.A.* **112** E7
Urbánia *Italy* **41** E9
Urbel → *Spain* **36** C7
Urbino *Italy* **41** E9
Urbión, Picos de *Spain* **38** C2
Urcos *Peru* **124** F4
Urdinarrain *Argentina* **126** C4
Urdos *France* **20** F3
Ure → *U.K.* **14** C6
Uren *Russia* **34** B7
Urengoy *Russia* **52** C8
Ures *Mexico* **118** B2
Urewera △ *N.Z.* **91** C6
Urfa = Şanlıurfa *Turkey* **73** D8
Urganch *Uzbekistan* **52** E7
Urgench = Urganch
  Uzbekistan **52** E7
Ürgüp *Turkey* **72** C6
Uri *India* **69** B6
Uri □ *Switz.* **25** J4
Uribia *Colombia* **124** A4
Uricani *Romania* **28** E8
Uriondo *Bolivia* **126** A3
Urique *Mexico* **118** B3
Urique → *Mexico* **118** B3
Urk *Neths.* **17** B5
Urkiola △ *Spain* **38** B3
Urla *Turkey* **47** C8
Urlați *Romania* **29** F11
Urmia = Orūmīyeh *Iran* **73** D11

Uromi *Nigeria* **83** D6
Uroševac *Kosovo* **44** D5
Uroyan, Montanas de
  Puerto Rico **121** d
Urrampinyi Iltjiltarri ○
  Australia **92** D5
Urshult *Sweden* **11** H8
Uruaçu *Brazil* **125** F9
Uruapan *Mexico* **118** D4
Urubamba → *Peru* **124** F4
Urucará *Brazil* **124** D7
Uruçuí *Brazil* **125** E10
Uruguai → *Brazil* **127** B5
Uruguaiana *Brazil* **126** B4
Uruguay ■ *S. Amer.* **126** C4
Uruguay → *S. Amer.* **126** C4
Urumchi = Ürümqi *China* **52** E9
Ürümqi *China* **52** E9
Uruna ○ *Australia* **92** D5
Urup → *Russia* **35** H5
Urup, Ostrov *Russia* **53** E16
Uryupinsk *Russia* **34** E5
Urzhum *Russia* **34** B9
Urziceni *Romania* **29** F11
Usa → *Russia* **52** C6
Uşak *Turkey* **47** C11
Uşak □ *Turkey* **47** C11
Usakos *Namibia* **88** C2
Ušće *Serbia* **44** C4
Usedom *Germany* **24** B10
Usedom ○ *Germany* **24** B10
Useless Loop *Australia* **93** E1
Ushakova, Ostrov *Russia* **53** A8
Ushakovo *Russia* **30** D7
Ushant = Ouessant, Î. d'
  France **18** D1
Ushashi *Tanzania* **86** C3
Ushat *Sudan* **81** F2
'Ushayrah *Ar Riyāḍ, Si. Arabia* **70** E5
'Ushayrah *Makkah, Si. Arabia* **80** C5
Ushibuka *Japan* **55** H5
Ushuaia *Argentina* **128** G3
Ushumun *Russia* **53** D13
Ushytsya → *Ukraine* **29** B12
Usinsk *Russia* **52** C6
Usk *Canada* **102** C3
Usk → *U.K.* **15** F5
Uska *India* **69** F10
Üsküdar *Turkey* **45** F13
Uslar *Germany* **24** D5
Usman *Russia* **33** F10
Usoke *Tanzania* **86** D3
Usolye-Sibirskoye *Russia* **53** D11
Usoro *Nigeria* **83** D6
Uspallata, P. de *Argentina* **126** C2
Ussel *France* **20** C6
Usson-du-Poitou *France* **20** B4
Ussuriysk *Russia* **54** C5
Ussurka *Russia* **54** B6
Ust-Buzulukskaya *Russia* **34** E6
Ust-Chaun *Russia* **53** C18
Ust-Chorna *Ukraine* **29** B8
Ust-Donetskiy *Russia* **35** G5
Ust-Ilimsk *Russia* **53** D11
Ust-Ishim *Russia* **52** D8
Ust-Kamchatsk *Russia* **53** D17
Ust-Kamenogorsk =
  Öskemen *Kazakhstan* **52** E9
Ust-Khayryuzovo *Russia* **53** D16
Ust-Kut *Russia* **53** D11
Ust-Kuyga *Russia* **53** B14
Ust-Labinsk *Russia* **35** H4
Ust-Luga *Russia* **32** C5
Ust-Maya *Russia* **53** C14
Ust-Mil *Russia* **53** D14
Ust-Nera *Russia* **53** C15
Ust-Nyukzha *Russia* **53** D13
Ust-Olenek *Russia* **53** B12
Ust-Omchug *Russia* **53** C15
Ust-Port *Russia* **52** C9
Ust-Tsilma *Russia* **52** C6
Ust-Urt = Ustyurt Plateau
  Asia **52** E6
Ustaritz *France* **20** E2
Ustecký □ *Czech Rep.* **26** A7
Uster *Switz.* **25** H4
Ústí nad Labem *Czech Rep.* **26** A7
Ústí nad Orlicí *Czech Rep.* **27** B9
Ústica *Italy* **42** E6
Ustinov = Izhevsk *Russia* **52** D6
Ustka *Poland* **30** D3
Ustroń *Poland* **31** J5
Ustrzyki Dolne *Poland* **31** J9
Ustyluh *Ukraine* **31** H11
Ustyurt Plateau *Asia* **52** E6
Ustyuzhna *Russia* **32** C9
Usu *China* **60** B3
Usuki *Japan* **55** H5
Usulután *El Salv.* **120** D2
Usumacinta → *Mexico* **119** D6
Usumbura = Bujumbura
  Burundi **86** C2
Usure *Tanzania* **86** C3
Usutuo → *Mozam.* **89** D5
Uta *Indonesia* **63** E9
Utah □ *U.S.A.* **108** G8
Utah L. *U.S.A.* **108** F8

Utansjö *Sweden* **10** B11
Utara, Selat *Malaysia* **65** c
Utarni *India* **68** F4
Utatlan *Guatemala* **120** C1
Ute Creek → *U.S.A.* **109** J12
Utebo *Spain* **38** D4
Utena *Lithuania* **32** E3
Utete *Tanzania* **86** D4
Uthai Thani *Thailand* **64** E3
Uthal *Pakistan* **68** G2
Utiariti *Brazil* **124** F7
Utica *N.Y., U.S.A.* **115** C9
Utica *Ohio, U.S.A.* **114** F2
Utiel *Spain* **39** F3
Utikuma L. *Canada* **102** B5
Utila *Honduras* **120** C2
Utō *Sweden* **10** F12
Utopia *Australia* **94** C1
Utraula *India* **69** F10
Utrecht *Neths.* **17** B5
Utrecht *S. Africa* **89** D5
Utrecht □ *Neths.* **17** B5
Utrera *Spain* **37** H5
Utsjoki → *Finland* **8** B22
Utsunomiya *Japan* **55** F9
Uttar Pradesh □ *India* **69** F9
Uttaradit *Thailand* **64** D3
Uttarakhand □ *India* **69** D8
Utterson *Canada* **114** A5
Uttoxeter *U.K.* **14** E6
Utuado *Puerto Rico* **121** d
Uummannaq *Avannaarsua,
  Greenland* **101** B18
Uummannaq *Kitaa, Greenland* **4** B5
Uummannarsuaq = Nunap
  Isua *Greenland* **98** D15
Uva → *Russia* **52** C6
Uvac → *Serbia* **44** C3
Uvalde *U.S.A.* **116** G5
Uvarovo *Russia* **34** E6
Uvat *Russia* **52** D7
Uvinza *Tanzania* **86** D3
Uvira *Dem. Rep. of the Congo* **86** C2
Uvs Nuur *Mongolia* **60** A4
'Uwairidh, Ḥarrat al
  Si. Arabia **70** E4
Uwajima *Japan* **55** H6
Uwanda ○ *Tanzania* **86** D3
Uweinat, Jebel *Sudan* **80** C1
Uxbridge *Canada* **114** B5
Uxin Qi *China* **56** E5
Uxmal *Mexico* **119** C7
Üydzin *Mongolia* **56** B4
Uyo *Nigeria* **83** D6
Uyûn Mûsa *Egypt* **74** F1
Uyuni *Bolivia* **124** H5
Uzbekistan ■ *Asia* **52** E7
Uzboy → *Turkmenistan* **71** B7
Uzen, Bolshoi = Uzen,
  Mal → *Kazakhstan* **35** F9
Uzen, Mal → *Kazakhstan* **35** F9
Uzerche *France* **20** C5
Uzès *France* **21** D8
Uzh → *Ukraine* **23** C16
Uzhgorod = Uzhhorod
  Ukraine **28** B7
Uzhhorod *Ukraine* **28** B7
Uzhok *Ukraine* **28** B7
Užice *Serbia* **44** C3
Uzlovaya *Russia* **32** F10
Üzümlü *Turkey* **47** E11
Uzunköprü *Turkey* **45** E10
Uzunkuyu *Turkey* **47** C8

V

Vaal → *S. Africa* **88** D3
Vaal Dam *S. Africa* **89** D4
Vaalbos △ *S. Africa* **88** D3
Vaalwater *S. Africa* **89** C4
Vaasa *Finland* **8** E19
Vabre *France* **20** E6
Vác *Hungary* **28** C9
Vacaria *Brazil* **127** B5
Vacata *Fiji* **91** a
Vacaville *U.S.A.* **110** G5
Vaccarès, Étang de *France* **21** E8
Vach = Vakh → *Russia* **52** C8
Vache, Î. à *Haiti* **121** C5
Väckelsång *Sweden* **11** H8
Vacoas *Mauritius* **85** d
Vadakara = Badagara *India* **66** P9
Väddö *Sweden* **10** D12
Väderstad *Sweden* **11** F8
Vadnagar *India* **68** H5
Vado Lígure *Italy* **40** D5
Vadodara *India* **68** H5
Vadsø *Norway* **8** A23
Vadstena *Sweden* **11** F8
Vaduz *Liech.* **25** H5
Værøy *Norway* **8** C15
Vágar *Færoe Is.* **8** E9
Vaggeryd *Sweden* **11** G8
Vaghia, Akra *Greece* **49** C10
Vagia *Greece* **46** C5
Vaghia, Akra *Greece* **49** C10
Vagney *France* **19** D13
Vagnhärad *Sweden* **11** F11

Vagos *Portugal* **36** E2
Vågsfjorden *Norway* **8** B17
Váh → *Slovak Rep.* **27** D11
Vahsel B. *Antarctica* **5** D1
Váhtjer = Gällivare *Sweden* **8** C19
Vaï *Greece* **49** D8
Vaiges *France* **18** D6
Vaihingen *Germany* **25** G4
Vaihiria, L. *Tahiti* **91** d
Vail *U.S.A.* **107** H18
Vailly-sur-Aisne *France* **19** C10
Vairao *Tahiti* **91** d
Vaisali → *India* **69** F8
Vaison-la-Romaine *France* **21** D9
Vaitogi *Amer. Samoa* **91** b
Vakarel *Bulgaria* **44** D7
Vakfıkebir *Turkey* **73** B8
Vakh → *Russia* **52** C8
Vakhtan *Russia* **34** B8
Vál *Hungary* **28** C3
Val-de-Marne □ *France* **19** D9
Val-d'Isère *France* **21** C10
Val-d'Oise □ *France* **19** C9
Val-d'Or *Canada* **104** C4
Val Grande △ *Italy* **40** B5
Val Marie *Canada* **103** D7
Val Thorens *France* **21** C10
Valaam *Russia* **32** B6
Valadares *Portugal* **36** D2
Valahia *Romania* **29** F9
Valais □ *Switz.* **25** J3
Valais, Alpes du *Switz.* **25** J3
Valandovo *Macedonia* **44** E6
Valašské Meziříčí *Czech Rep.* **27** B10
Valatie *U.S.A.* **115** D11
Valaxa *Greece* **46** C6
Vålberg *Sweden* **10** D10
Valbo *Sweden* **10** D10
Valbondione *Italy* **40** B7
Vălcani *Romania* **28** D5
Vâlcea □ *Romania* **29** F9
Valcheta *Argentina* **128** E3
Valdagno *Italy* **41** C8
Valdahon *France* **19** E13
Valdai Hills = Valdayskaya
  Vozvyshennost *Russia* **32** D7
Valday *Russia* **32** D7
Valdayskaya
  Vozvyshennost *Russia* **32** D7
Valdeazogues → *Spain* **37** G6
Valdecañas, Embalse de
  Spain **36** F5
Valdemarsvik *Sweden* **11** F10
Valdemoro *Spain* **36** E7
Valdepeñas *Spain* **37** G7
Valderaduey → *Spain* **36** D5
Valdérice *Italy* **42** D5
Valderrobres *Spain* **38** E5
Valdés, Pen. *Argentina* **128** E4
Valdez *U.S.A.* **100** C2
Valdivia *Chile* **128** D2
Valdivia Abyssal Plain
  S. Ocean **5** C6
Valdobbiádene *Italy* **41** C8
Valdosta *U.S.A.* **117** F13
Valdoviño *Spain* **36** B2
Valdres *Norway* **8** F13
Vale *Georgia* **35** K6
Vale *U.S.A.* **108** E5
Vale of Glamorgan □ *U.K.* **15** F4
Valea lui Mihai *Romania* **28** C7
Valea Mărului *Romania* **29** E12
Valemount *Canada* **102** C5
Valença *Brazil* **125** F11
Valença *Portugal* **36** C2
Valença do Piauí *Brazil* **125** E10
Valençay *France* **19** E8
Valence *France* **21** D8
Valence d'Agen *France* **20** D4
Valencia *Phil.* **61** H6
Valencia *Spain* **39** F4
Valencia *Trin. & Tob.* **125** K15
Valencia *U.S.A.* **109** J10
Valencia *Venezuela* **124** A5
Valencia □ *Spain* **39** F4
Valencia ✈ (VLC) *Spain* **39** F4
Valencia, G. de *Spain* **39** F5
Valencia de Alcántara *Spain* **37** F3
Valencia de Don Juan *Spain* **36** C5
Valencia I. *Ireland* **12** E1
Valenciennes *France* **19** B10
Văleni *Romania* **29** F9
Vălenii de Munte *Romania* **29** E11
Valensole *France* **21** E9
Valentano *Italy* **41** F8
Valentigney *France* **19** E13
Valentim, Sa. do *Brazil* **125** E10
Valentin *Russia* **54** C7
Valentine *Nebr., U.S.A.* **112** D3
Valentine *Tex., U.S.A.* **116** F2
Valenza *Italy* **40** C5
Valera *Venezuela* **124** B4
Valga *Estonia* **32** D4
Valguarnera Caropepe *Italy* **43** E7
Valier *U.S.A.* **108** B7
Valinco, G. de *France* **21** G12
Valjevo *Serbia* **44** B3
Valka *Latvia* **32** D3
Valkeakoski *Finland* **32** B2
Valkenswaard *Neths.* **17** C5

Vall de Uxó = La Vall d'Uixó *Spain* **38** F4
Valla *Sweden* **10** E10
Valladolid *Mexico* **119** C7
Valladolid *Spain* **36** D6
Valladolid □ *Spain* **36** D6
Vallata *Italy* **43** A8
Valldemossa *Spain* **48** B9
Valle d'Aosta □ *Italy* **40** C4
Valle de Aran *Spain* **38** C5
Valle de la Pascua *Venezuela* **124** B5
Valle de las Palmas *Mexico* **111** N10
Valle de Santiago *Mexico* **118** C4
Valle de Zaragoza *Mexico* **118** B3
Valle del Ticino △ *Italy* **40** C6
Valle Fértil, Sierra del *Argentina* **126** C2
Valle Gran Rey *Canary Is.* **48** F2
Valle Hermoso *Mexico* **119** B5
Valle Nacional *Mexico* **119** D5
Valledupar *Colombia* **124** A4
Vallehermoso *Canary Is.* **48** F2
Vallejo *U.S.A.* **110** G4
Vallenar *Chile* **126** B1
Vallentuna *Sweden* **10** E12
Valleraugue *France* **20** D7
Vallet *France* **18** E5
Valletta *Malta* **49** D2
Valley Center *U.S.A.* **111** M9
Valley City *U.S.A.* **112** B5
Valley Falls *Oreg., U.S.A.* **108** E3
Valley Falls *R.I., U.S.A.* **115** E13
Valley of Flowers △ *India* **69** D8
Valley of the Kings *Egypt* **80** B3
Valley Springs *U.S.A.* **110** G6
Valley View *U.S.A.* **115** F8
Valley Wells *U.S.A.* **111** K11
Valleyview *Canada* **102** C5
Valli di Comácchio *Italy* **41** D9
Vallimanca, Arroyo *Argentina* **126** D4
Vallo della Lucánia *Italy* **43** B8
Vallon-Pont-d'Arc *France* **21** D8
Vallorbe *Switz.* **25** J2
Valls *Spain* **38** D6
Valmaseda = Balmaseda *Spain* **38** B1
Valmiera *Latvia* **32** D3
Valnera *Spain* **36** B7
Valognes *France* **18** C5
Valona = Vlorë *Albania* **44** F3
Valongo *Portugal* **36** D2
Valozhyn *Belarus* **23** A14
Valpaços *Portugal* **36** D3
Valparaíso *Chile* **126** C1
Valparaíso *Mexico* **118** C4
Valparaiso *U.S.A.* **112** E10
Valparaíso □ *Chile* **126** C1
Valpovo *Croatia* **28** E3
Valréas *France* **21** D9
Vals *Switz.* **25** J5
Vals → *S. Africa* **88** D4
Vals, Tanjung *Indonesia* **63** F9
Vals-les-Bains *France* **21** D8
Valsad *India* **66** J8
Valtellina *Italy* **40** B6
Valuyki *Russia* **33** G10
Valverde *Canary Is.* **48** G2
Valverde del Camino *Spain* **37** H4
Valverde del Fresno *Spain* **36** E4
Vama *Romania* **29** C10
Vamdrup *Denmark* **11** J3
Vámhus *Sweden* **10** C8
Vamizi, I. *Mozam.* **87** E5
Vammala *Finland* **32** B2
Vamos *Greece* **49** D6
Van *Turkey* **73** C10
Van □ *Turkey* **73** C10
Van, L. = Van Gölü *Turkey* **73** C10
Van Alstyne *U.S.A.* **116** E6
Van Blommestein Meer *Suriname* **125** C7
Van Buren *Canada* **105** C6
Van Buren *Ark., U.S.A.* **116** D7
Van Buren *Maine, U.S.A.* **113** B20
Van Buren *Mo., U.S.A.* **112** G9
Van Canh *Vietnam* **64** F7
Van Diemen, C. *N. Terr., Australia* **92** B4
Van Diemen, C. *Queens., Australia* **94** B2
Van Diemen G. *Australia* **92** B5
Van Gölü *Turkey* **73** C10
Van Horn *U.S.A.* **116** F2
Van Ninh *Vietnam* **64** F7
Van Rees, Pegunungan *Indonesia* **63** E9
Van Wert *U.S.A.* **113** E11
Van Yen *Vietnam* **58** G5
Van Zylsrus *S. Africa* **88** D3
Vanadzor *Armenia* **35** K7
Vanavara *Russia* **53** C11
Vancouver *Canada* **110** A3
Vancouver *U.S.A.* **110** E4
Vancouver, C. *Australia* **93** G2
Vancouver I. *Canada* **110** D3
Vancouver Int. ✈ (YVR) *Canada* **110** A3
Vanda = Vantaa *Finland* **32** B3
Vandalia *Ill., U.S.A.* **112** F9

Vandalia *Mo., U.S.A.* **112** F8
Vandenberg Village *U.S.A.* **111** L6
Vandergrift *U.S.A.* **114** F5
Vanderhoof *Canada* **102** C4
Vanderkloof Dam *S. Africa* **88** E3
Vanderlin I. *Australia* **94** B2
Vanderlin I. *Canada* **101** D15
Vänern *Sweden* **11** F7
Vänersborg *Sweden* **11** F6
Vang Vieng *Laos* **64** C4
Vanga *Kenya* **86** C4
Vangaindrano *Madag.* **89** C8
Vanguard *Canada* **103** D7
Vânju Mare *Romania* **28** F7
Vankleek Hill *Canada* **115** A10
Vännäs *Sweden* **8** E18
Vannes *France* **18** E4
Vannøya *Norway* **8** A18
Vanoise, Massif de la *France* **21** C10
Vanrhynsdorp *S. Africa* **88** E2
Vansbro *Sweden* **10** D8
Vansittart B. *Australia* **92** B4
Vansittart I. *Canada* **101** D15
Vantaa *Finland* **32** B3
Vanua Balavu *Fiji* **91** a
Vanua Levu *Fiji* **91** a
Vanua Vatu *Fiji* **91** a
Vanuatu ■ *Pac. Oc.* **90** C9
Vanwyksvlei *S. Africa* **88** E3
Vapnyarka *Ukraine* **29** B13
Var □ *France* **21** E10
Var → *France* **21** E11
Vara *Sweden* **11** F6
Varades *France* **18** E5
Varáita → *Italy* **40** D4
Varalé *Ivory C.* **82** D4
Varallo *Italy* **40** C5
Varāmīn *Iran* **71** C6
Varāmīn □ *Iran* **71** B6
Varanasi *India* **69** G10
Varangerfjorden *Norway* **8** A23
Varangerhalvøya *Norway* **8** A23
Varano, Lago di *Italy* **41** G12
Varaždin *Croatia* **41** B13
Varazze *Italy* **40** D5
Varberg *Sweden* **11** G6
Vardak □ *Afghan.* **66** B6
Vardar = Axios → *Greece* **44** F6
Varde *Denmark* **11** J2
Varde Å → *Denmark* **11** J2
Vardenis *Armenia* **35** K7
Vardø *Norway* **8** A24
Varel *Germany* **24** B4
Varella, Mui *Vietnam* **64** F7
Varèna *Lithuania* **32** E3
Vareš *Bos.-H.* **28** F3
Varese *Italy* **40** C5
Vârfurile *Romania* **28** D7
Vårgårda *Sweden* **11** F6
Varginha *Brazil* **127** A6
Vargön *Sweden* **11** F6
Varillas *Chile* **126** A1
Varkaus *Finland* **32** A4
Värmdölandet *Sweden* **10** E12
Värmeln *Sweden* **10** E6
Värmlands län □ *Sweden* **10** E6
Värmlandsbro *Sweden* **10** E7
Varna *Bulgaria* **45** C11
Varna □ *Bulgaria* **45** C11
Värnamo *Sweden* **11** G8
Varnsdorf *Czech Rep.* **26** A7
Várpalota *Hungary* **28** C3
Vars *Canada* **115** A9
Vars *France* **21** D10
Varto *Turkey* **73** C9
Varvarin *Serbia* **44** C5
Varysburg *U.S.A.* **114** D6
Varzaneh *Iran* **71** C7
Varzağan *Iran* **73** C12
Varzi *Italy* **40** D6
Varzo *Italy* **40** B5
Varzy *France* **19** E10
Vas □ *Hungary* **28** C1
Vasa = Vaasa *Finland* **8** E19
Vasa Barris → *Brazil* **125** F11
Vásárosnamény *Hungary* **28** B7
Vascão → *Portugal* **37** H3
Vaşcău *Romania* **28** D7
Vascongadas = País Vasco □ *Spain* **38** C2
Vashkivtsi *Ukraine* **29** B10
Vasht = Khāsh *Iran* **71** D9
Vasilevichi *Belarus* **23** B15
Vasiliki *Greece* **46** C2
Vasilkov = Vasylkiv *Ukraine* **23** C16
Vaslui *Romania* **29** D12
Vaslui □ *Romania* **29** D12
Väsman *Sweden* **10** D9
Vassar *Canada* **103** D9
Vassar *U.S.A.* **113** D12
Västerås *Sweden* **10** E10
Västerbotten *Sweden* **8** D19
Västerdalälven → *Sweden* **10** D8
Västergötland *Sweden* **11** F7
Västerhaninge *Sweden* **10** E12
Västervik *Sweden* **11** G10
Västmanland *Sweden* **9** G17

Västmanlands län □ *Sweden* **10** E10
Vasto *Italy* **41** F11
Västra Götalands Län □ *Sweden* **11** F6
Vasvár *Hungary* **28** C1
Vasylivka *Ukraine* **29** E13
Vasylkiv *Ukraine* **23** C16
Vatan *France* **19** E8
Vatersay *U.K.* **13** E1
Vathia *Greece* **46** E4
Vati *Greece* **49** C9
Vatican City ■ *Europe* **41** G9
Vaticano, C. *Italy* **43** D8
Vatili *Cyprus* **49** D12
Vatin *Serbia* **28** E6
Vatiu = Atiu *Cook Is.* **97** J12
Vatnajökull *Iceland* **8** D5
Vatolakkos *Greece* **44** F5
Vatoloha *Madag.* **89** B8
Vatomandry *Madag.* **89** B8
Vatra-Dornei *Romania* **29** C10
Vatrak → *India* **68** H5
Vättern *Sweden* **11** F8
Vatu Vara *Fiji* **91** a
Vatulele *Fiji* **91** a
Vaucluse □ *France* **21** E9
Vaucouleurs *France* **19** D12
Vaud □ *Switz.* **25** J2
Vaudreuil-Dorion *Canada* **115** A10
Vaughn *Mont., U.S.A.* **108** C8
Vaughn *N. Mex., U.S.A.* **109** J11
Vaujours L. *Canada* **104** A5
Vaupés → *Brazil* **124** C5
Vaupés □ *Colombia* **124** C4
Vauvert *France* **21** E8
Vauxhall *Canada* **102** C6
Vav *India* **68** G4
Vavatenina *Madag.* **89** B8
Vava'u *Tonga* **91** c
Vava'u Group *Tonga* **91** c
Vavoua *Ivory C.* **82** D3
Vawkavysk *Belarus* **23** B13
Vaxholm *Sweden* **10** E12
Växjö *Sweden* **11** H8
Våxtorp *Sweden* **11** H7
Vaygach, Ostrov *Russia* **52** C7
Veaikevárri = Svappavaara *Sweden* **8** C19
Vechelde *Germany* **24** C6
Vechta *Germany* **24** C4
Vechte → *Neths.* **17** B6
Vecsés *Hungary* **28** C4
Veddige *Sweden* **11** G6
Vedea → *Romania* **29** G10
Vedi *Armenia* **73** C11
Vedia *Argentina* **126** C3
Vedrette di Ries-Aurina △ *Italy* **41** B9
Vedum *Sweden* **11** F7
Veendam *Neths.* **17** A6
Veenendaal *Neths.* **17** B5
Vefsna → *Norway* **8** D15
Vega *Norway* **8** D14
Vega *U.S.A.* **116** D3
Vega Baja *Puerto Rico* **121** d
Vegadeo *Spain* **36** B3
Vegoritida, L. *Greece* **44** F5
Vegreville *Canada* **102** C6
Veinge *Sweden* **11** H7
Veisiejai *Lithuania* **30** D10
Vejbystrand *Sweden* **11** H6
Vejen *Denmark* **11** J3
Vejer de la Frontera *Spain* **37** J5
Vejle *Denmark* **11** J3
Vejle Fjord *Denmark* **11** J3
Vela Luka *Croatia* **41** F13
Velas, C. *Costa Rica* **120** D2
Velasco, Sierra de *Argentina* **126** B2
Velay, Mts. du *France* **20** D7
Velbert *Germany* **24** D3
Velddrif *S. Africa* **88** E2
Velebit *Croatia* **41** D12
Velebit Planina *Croatia* **41** D12
Velebitski Kanal *Croatia* **41** D11
Veleka → *Bulgaria* **45** D11
Velencei-tó *Hungary* **28** C3
Velenje *Slovenia* **41** B12
Veles *Macedonia* **44** E5
Velestino *Greece* **46** B4
Vélez-Málaga *Spain* **37** J6
Vélez Rubio *Spain* **39** H2
Velhas → *Brazil* **125** G10
Velika *Croatia* **28** E2
Velika Gorica *Croatia* **41** C13
Velika Kapela *Croatia* **41** C12
Velika Kladuša *Bos.-H.* **41** C12
Velika Kruša *Kosovo* **44** D5
Velika Morava → *Serbia* **44** B5
Velika Plana *Serbia* **44** B5
Velikaya → *Russia* **32** D5
Velikaya Kema *Russia* **54** B8
Velikaya Lepetikha *Ukraine* **33** J7
Veliké Kapušany *Slovak Rep.* **27** C15
Velike Lašče *Slovenia* **41** C11
Veliki Jastrebac *Serbia* **44** C5
Veliki Kanal *Serbia* **28** E4
Veliki Popović *Serbia* **44** B5
Velikiye Luki *Russia* **32** D6
Veliko Gradište *Serbia* **44** B5
Veliko Tŭrnovo *Bulgaria* **45** C9

Velikonda Range *India* **66** M11
Vélingara *Kolda, Senegal* **82** C2
Vélingara *Louga, Senegal* **82** B2
Velingrad *Bulgaria* **44** D7
Velino, Mte. *Italy* **41** F10
Velizh *Russia* **32** E6
Velké Karlovice *Czech Rep.* **27** B11
Velké Meziříčí *Czech Rep.* **26** B9
Vel'ký Javorník *Slovak Rep.* **27** B11
Vel'ký Krtíš *Slovak Rep.* **27** C12
Vel'ký Meder *Slovak Rep.* **27** D10
Vel'ký Tribeč *Slovak Rep.* **27** C11
Velletri *Italy* **42** A5
Vellinge *Sweden* **11** J6
Vellmar *Germany* **24** D5
Vellore *India* **66** N11
Velopoula *Greece* **46** E5
Velsk *Russia* **32** B11
Velten *Germany* **24** C9
Veluwezoom △ *Neths.* **17** B6
Velva *U.S.A.* **112** A3
Velvendos *Greece* **44** F6
Velyka Mykhaylivka *Ukraine* **29** C14
Velyki Luchky *Ukraine* **28** B7
Velykyy Bereznyy *Ukraine* **28** B7
Velykyy Bychkiv *Ukraine* **29** C9
Vemb *Denmark* **11** H2
Vemdalen *Sweden* **10** B7
Ven *Sweden* **11** J6
Venaco *France* **21** F13
Venado *Mexico* **118** C4
Venado Tuerto *Argentina* **126** C3
Venafro *Italy* **43** A7
Venarey-les-Laumes *France* **19** E11
Venaría *Italy* **40** C4
Venčane *Serbia* **44** B4
Vence *France* **21** E11
Venda Novas *Portugal* **37** G2
Vendas Novas *Portugal* **37** G2
Vendée □ *France* **18** F5
Vendée → *France* **18** F5
Vendéen, Bocage *France* **20** B2
Vendeuvre-sur-Barse *France* **19** D11
Vendôme *France* **18** E8
Vendrell = El Vendrell *Spain* **38** D6
Vendsyssel *Denmark* **11** G4
Vendychany *Ukraine* **29** B12
Venelles *France* **21** E9
Véneta, L. *Italy* **41** C9
Véneto □ *Italy* **41** C9
Venev *Russia* **32** E10
Venézia *Italy* **41** C10
Venézia, G. di *Italy* **41** C10
Venezuela ■ *S. Amer.* **124** B5
Venezuela, G. de *Venezuela* **124** A4
Vengurla *India* **66** M8
Venice = Venézia *Italy* **41** C10
Venice *U.S.A.* **117** H14
Vénissieux *France* **21** C8
Venjansjön *Sweden* **10** D8
Venkatapuram *India* **67** K12
Venlo *Neths.* **17** C6
Vennachar Junction *Canada* **114** A7
Vennesla *Norway* **9** G12
Venosa *Italy* **43** B8
Venray *Neths.* **17** C6
Venta *Lithuania* **30** B9
Venta → *Latvia* **30** A8
Venta de Baños *Spain* **36** D6
Venta de Cardeña = Cardeña *Spain* **37** G6
Ventana, Punta de la *Mexico* **118** A1
Ventana, Sa. de la *Argentina* **126** D3
Ventersburg *S. Africa* **88** D4
Venterstad *S. Africa* **88** E4
Ventimíglia *Italy* **40** E4
Ventnor *U.K.* **15** G6
Ventotene I. *Italy* **42** B6
Ventoux, Mt. *France* **21** D9
Ventspils *Latvia* **30** A8
Ventspils □ *Latvia* **30** A8
Ventuarí → *Venezuela* **124** C5
Ventucopa *U.S.A.* **111** L7
Ventura *U.S.A.* **111** L7
Vénus, Pte. *Tahiti* **91** d
Venus B. *Australia* **95** F4
Venustiano Carranza *Mexico* **118** A1
Vera *Argentina* **126** B3
Vera *Spain* **39** H3
Veracruz *Mexico* **119** D5
Veracruz □ *Mexico* **119** D5
Veral → *India* **68** J4
Verbánia *Italy* **40** C5
Verbicaro *Italy* **43** C8
Verbier *Switz.* **25** J3
Vercelli *Italy* **40** C5
Verchovchevo *Ukraine* **33** H8
Vercors △ *France* **21** D9
Verdalsøra *Norway* **8** E14
Verde → *Argentina* **128** E3
Verde → *Goiás, Brazil* **125** G8
Verde → *Mato Grosso do Sul, Brazil* **125** H8
Verde → *Chihuahua, Mexico* **118** B3
Verde → *Oaxaca, Mexico* **119** D5
Verde → *Veracruz, Mexico* **118** C4
Verde → *Paraguay* **126** A4

Verde → *U.S.A.* **106** J17
Verde, Cay *Bahamas* **120** B4
Verde Island Pass *Phil.* **61** E4
Verden *Germany* **24** C5
Verdi *U.S.A.* **110** F7
Verdikoussa *Greece* **46** B3
Verdon → *France* **21** E9
Verdon △ *France* **21** E10
Verdun *France* **19** C12
Verdun-sur-le-Doubs *France* **19** F12
Vereeniging *S. Africa* **89** D4
Verga, C. *Guinea* **82** C2
Vergara *Uruguay* **127** C5
Vergato *Italy* **40** D8
Vergemont Cr. → *Australia* **94** C3
Vergennes *U.S.A.* **115** B11
Vergt *France* **20** C4
Veria *Greece* **44** F6
Verín *Spain* **36** D3
Verkhnedvinsk = Vyerkhnyadzvinsk *Belarus* **32** E4
Verkhnetulomskoye Vdkhr. *Russia* **8** B24
Verkhneuralsk *Russia* **52** D6
Verkhniy Baskunchak *Russia* **35** F8
Verkhovye *Russia* **33** F9
Verkhovyna *Ukraine* **29** B9
Verkhoyansk *Russia* **53** C14
Verkhoyansk Ra. = Verkhoyanskiy Khrebet *Russia* **53** C13
Verkhoyanskiy Khrebet *Russia* **53** C13
Vermenton *France* **19** E10
Vermilion *Canada* **103** C6
Vermilion *U.S.A.* **114** E2
Vermilion → *Canada* **103** C6
Vermilion B. *U.S.A.* **116** G9
Vermilion Bay *Canada* **103** D10
Vermilion L. *U.S.A.* **112** B7
Vermillion *U.S.A.* **112** D5
Vermillion → *Canada* **104** C5
Vermont □ *U.S.A.* **115** C12
Vermosh *Albania* **44** D3
Vernadsky *Antarctica* **5** C17
Vernal *U.S.A.* **108** F9
Vernalis *U.S.A.* **110** H5
Vernazza *Italy* **40** D6
Verner *Canada* **104** C3
Verneuil-sur-Avre *France* **18** D7
Verneukpan *S. Africa* **88** E3
Vernier *Switz.* **25** J2
Vernio *Italy* **40** D8
Vernon *Canada* **102** C5
Vernon *France* **18** C8
Vernon *U.S.A.* **116** D5
Vernonia *U.S.A.* **110** E3
Vero Beach *U.S.A.* **117** H14
Véroia = Veria *Greece* **44** F6
Véroli *Italy* **41** G10
Verona *Canada* **115** B8
Verona *Italy* **40** C7
Verrès *Italy* **40** C4
Versailles *France* **19** D9
Versmold *Germany* **24** C4
Vert, C. *Senegal* **82** C1
Vertou *France* **18** E5
Vertus *France* **19** D11
Verulam *S. Africa* **89** D5
Verviers *Belgium* **17** D5
Vervins *France* **19** C10
Veržej *Slovenia* **41** B13
Verzy *France* **19** C11
Vescovato *France* **21** F13
Veselí nad Lužnicí *Czech Rep.* **26** B7
Veselie *Bulgaria* **45** D11
Veselovskoye Vdkhr. *Russia* **35** G5
Veshenskaya *Russia* **34** F5
Vesle → *France* **19** C10
Vesoul *France* **19** E13
Vessigebro *Sweden* **11** H6
Vesterålen *Norway* **8** B16
Vestfjorden *Norway* **8** C16
Vestmannaeyjar *Iceland* **8** E3
Vestspitsbergen *Svalbard* **4** B8
Vestvågøya *Norway* **8** B15
Vesuvio *Italy* **43** B7
Vesuvius, Mt. = Vesuvio *Italy* **43** B7
Vesyegonsk *Russia* **32** C9
Veszprém *Hungary* **28** C2
Veszprém □ *Hungary* **28** C2
Vésztő *Hungary* **28** D6
Vetlanda *Sweden* **11** G9
Vetluga *Russia* **34** B7
Vetlugu → *Russia* **34** B8
Vetluzhskiy *Kostroma, Russia* **34** A7
Vetluzhskiy *Nizhniy Novgorod, Russia* **34** B7
Vetovo *Bulgaria* **45** C10
Vetralla *Italy* **41** F9
Vetren *Bulgaria* **45** D8
Vettore, Mte. *Italy* **41** F10
Veurne *Belgium* **17** C2
Veveno → *Sudan* **81** F3
Vevey *Switz.* **25** J2
Vevi *Greece* **44** F5
Vevil → *Russia* **34** B7
Veynes *France* **21** D9
Veys *Iran* **71** D6

Vézelay *France* **19** E10
Vézelise *France* **19** D13
Vézère → *France* **20** D4
Vezhen *Bulgaria* **45** D8
Vezirköprü *Turkey* **72** B6
Vezzani *France* **21** F13
Vi Thanh *Vietnam* **65** H5
Viacha *Bolivia* **124** G5
Viadana *Italy* **40** D7
Viamão *Brazil* **127** C5
Viana *Brazil* **125** D10
Viana *Spain* **38** C2
Viana do Alentejo *Portugal* **37** G3
Viana do Bolo *Spain* **36** D3
Viana do Castelo *Portugal* **36** D2
Viana do Castelo □ *Portugal* **36** D2
Vianden *Lux.* **17** E6
Viangchan = Vientiane *Laos* **64** D4
Vianópolis *Brazil* **125** G9
Vianos *Greece* **49** D7
Viar → *Spain* **37** H5
Viaréggio *Italy* **40** E7
Viaur → *France* **20** D5
Vibble *Sweden* **11** G12
Vibo Valéntia *Italy* **43** D9
Viborg *Denmark* **11** H3
Vibraye *France* **18** D7
Vic *Spain* **38** D7
Vic, Étang de *France* **20** E7
Vic-en-Bigorre *France* **20** E4
Vic-Fezensac *France* **20** E4
Vic-le-Comte *France* **19** G10
Vic-sur-Cère *France* **20** D6
Vícar *Spain* **39** J2
Vicenza *Italy* **41** C8
Vich = Vic *Spain* **38** D7
Vichada → *Colombia* **124** C5
Vichuga *Russia* **34** B5
Vichy *France* **19** F10
Vicksburg *Ariz., U.S.A.* **111** M13
Vicksburg *Miss., U.S.A.* **117** E9
Vico *France* **21** F12
Vico, L. di *Italy* **41** F9
Vico del Gargano *Italy* **41** G12
Vicovu de Sus *Romania* **29** C10
Victor *India* **68** J4
Victor Harbor *Australia* **95** F2
Victoria *Argentina* **126** C3
Victoria *Canada* **110** B3
Victoria *Chile* **128** D2
Victoria *Guinea* **82** C2
Victoria *Malta* **49** C1
Victoria *Phil.* **61** D4
Victoria *Romania* **28** E9
Victoria *Seychelles* **85** b
Victoria *Kans., U.S.A.* **112** F4
Victoria *Tex., U.S.A.* **116** G6
Victoria □ *Australia* **95** F3
Victoria → *Australia* **92** C4
Victoria, Grand L. *Canada* **104** C4
Victoria, L. *Africa* **86** C3
Victoria, L. *Australia* **95** E3
Victoria, Mt. *Burma* **67** J18
Victoria Beach *Canada* **103** C9
Victoria de Durango = Durango *Mexico* **118** C4
Victoria de las Tunas = Las Tunas *Cuba* **120** B4
Victoria Falls *Zimbabwe* **87** F2
Victoria Harbour *Canada* **114** B5
Victoria I. *Canada* **100** C9
Victoria L. *Canada* **105** C8
Victoria Ld. *Antarctica* **5** D11
Victoria Nile → *Uganda* **86** B3
Victoria Pk. *Belize* **119** D7
Victoria River *Australia* **92** C5
Victoria Str. *Canada* **100** D11
Victoria West *S. Africa* **88** E3
Victorias *Phil.* **61** F5
Victoriaville *Canada* **105** C5
Victorica *Argentina* **126** D2
Victorville *U.S.A.* **111** L9
Vicuña *Chile* **126** C1
Vicuña Mackenna *Argentina* **126** C3
Vidal *Calif., U.S.A.* **111** L12
Vidal *Calif., U.S.A.* **111** L12
Vidalia *U.S.A.* **117** E13
Vidamlya *Belarus* **31** F10
Vidauban *France* **21** E10
Videbæk *Denmark* **11** H2
Videle *Romania* **29** E11
Vidigueira *Portugal* **37** G3
Vidin *Bulgaria* **44** C6
Vidio, C. *Spain* **36** B4
Vidisha *India* **68** H7
Vidos *Greece* **49** A3
Vidra *Romania* **29** E11
Viduša *Bos.-H.* **44** D2
Vidzy *Belarus* **32** E4
Viechtach *Germany* **25** F8
Viedma *Argentina* **128** E4
Viedma, L. *Argentina* **128** F2
Vieira do Minho *Portugal* **36** D2
Vielha *Spain* **38** C5
Vielha = Vielha *Spain* **38** C5
Vielsalm *Belgium* **17** D5
Vienenburg *Germany* **24** D6
Vieng Pou Kha *Laos* **58** G3
Vienna = Wien *Austria* **27** C9

Vienna *Canada* **114** D4
Vienna *Ill., U.S.A.* **112** G9
Vienna *Mo., U.S.A.* **112** F8
Vienne *France* **21** C8
Vienne □ *France* **20** B4
Vienne ➝ *France* **18** E7
Vientiane *Laos* **64** D4
Vientos, Paso de los
  Caribbean **121** C5
Vieques *Puerto Rico* **121** d
Vierge Pt. *St. Lucia* **121** f
Viernheim *Germany* **25** F4
Viersen *Germany* **24** D2
Vierwaldstättersee *Switz.* **25** J4
Vierzon *France* **19** E9
Vieste *Italy* **41** G13
Viet Tri *Vietnam* **64** B5
Vietnam ■ *Asia* **64** C6
Vieux-Boucau-les-Bains
  France **20** E2
Vieux Fort *St. Lucia* **121** f
Vif *France* **21** C9
Vigan *Phil.* **61** C4
Vigévano *Italy* **40** C5
Vigia *Brazil* **125** D9
Viglas, Akra *Greece* **49** D9
Vignemalle *France* **20** F3
Vigneulles-lès-
  Hattonchâtel *France* **19** D12
Vignola *Italy* **40** D8
Vigo *Spain* **36** C2
Vigo, Ría de *Spain* **36** C2
Vigsø Bugt *Denmark* **11** G2
Vihiers *France* **18** E6
Vihowa *Pakistan* **68** D4
Vihowa ➝ *Pakistan* **68** D4
Vijayawada *India* **67** L12
Vijosë ➝ *Albania* **44** F3
Vík *Iceland* **8** E4
Vika *Sweden* **10** D8
Vikarbyn *Sweden* **10** D9
Vikeke = Viqueque *E. Timor* **63** F7
Viken *Skåne, Sweden* **11** H6
Viken *Västra Götaland, Sweden* **11** F8
Viking *Canada* **102** C6
Vikmanshyttan *Sweden* **10** D9
Vikna *Norway* **8** D14
Vikos-Aoos △ *Greece* **46** B2
Vila da Maganja *Mozam.* **87** F4
Vila da Ribeira Brava
  C. Verde Is. **78** b
Vila de Rei *Portugal* **36** F2
Vila do Bispo *Portugal* **37** H2
Vila do Conde *Portugal* **36** D2
Vila Franca de Xira *Portugal* **37** G2
Vila Gamito *Mozam.* **87** E3
Vila Gomes da Costa *Mozam.* **89** C5
Vila Machado *Mozam.* **87** F3
Vila Mouzinho *Mozam.* **87** E3
Vila Nova de Famalicão
  Portugal **36** D2
Vila Nova de Fos Côa
  Portugal **36** D3
Vila Nova de Gaia *Portugal* **36** D2
Vila Nova de Ourém *Portugal* **36** F2
Vila Pouca de Aguiar
  Portugal **36** D3
Vila Real *Portugal* **36** D3
Vila-Real *Spain* **38** F4
Vila Real □ *Portugal* **36** D3
Vila Real de Santo António
  Portugal **37** H3
Vila-seca *Spain* **38** D6
Vila Vasco da Gama *Mozam.* **87** E3
Vila Velha *Brazil* **127** A7
Vila Viçosa *Portugal* **37** G3
Vilafranca del Maestrat *Spain* **38** E4
Vilafranca del Penedès *Spain* **38** D6
Vilagarcía de Arousa *Spain* **36** C2
Vilaine ➝ *France* **18** E4
Vilanandro, Tanjona *Madag.* **89** B7
Vilanculos *Mozam.* **89** C6
Vilanova i la Geltrú *Spain* **38** D6
Vilar Formosa *Portugal* **36** E4
Vilaseca-Salou = Vila-seca
  Spain **38** D6
Vilbjerg *Denmark* **11** H2
Vilcheka, Ostrov *Russia* **52** B6
Vilcheka, Zemlya *Russia* **4** A11
Vilches *Spain* **37** G7
Vileyka *Belarus* **23** A14
Vilhelmina *Sweden* **8** D17
Vilhena *Brazil* **124** F6
Viliya = Neris ➝ *Lithuania* **32** E3
Viljandi *Estonia* **32** C3
Vilkaviškis *Lithuania* **30** D10
Vilkija *Lithuania* **30** C10
Vilkitskogo, Proliv *Russia* **53** B11
Vilkovo = Vylkove *Ukraine* **29** E14
Villa Abecia *Bolivia* **126** A2
Villa Ana *Argentina* **126** B4
Villa Ángela *Argentina* **126** B3
Villa Bella *Bolivia* **124** F5
Villa Cañás *Argentina* **126** C3
Villa Constitución *Argentina* **126** C3
Villa de Arriaga *Mexico* **118** C4
Villa de María *Argentina* **126** B3
Villa de Méndez *Mexico* **119** B5
Villa del Rio *Spain* **37** H6
Villa Dolores *Argentina* **126** C2

Villa Frontera *Mexico* **118** B4
Villa Gesell *Argentina* **126** D4
Villa Guillermina *Argentina* **126** B4
Villa Hayes *Paraguay* **126** B4
Villa Hidalgo *Mexico* **119** C5
Villa Iris *Argentina* **126** D3
Villa María *Argentina* **126** C3
Villa Mazán *Argentina* **126** B2
Villa Minozzo *Italy* **40** D7
Villa Montes *Bolivia* **126** A3
Villa Ocampo *Argentina* **126** B4
Villa Ocampo *Mexico* **118** B3
Villa Ojo de Agua *Argentina* **126** B3
Villa San Giovanni *Italy* **43** D8
Villa San Martín *Argentina* **126** B3
Villa Santina *Italy* **41** B9
Villa Unión *Mexico* **118** C3
Villablino *Spain* **36** C4
Villacarlos *Spain* **48** B11
Villacarriedo *Spain* **36** B7
Villacarrillo *Spain* **37** G7
Villacastín *Spain* **36** E6
Villach *Austria* **26** E6
Villacidro *Italy* **42** C1
Villada *Spain* **36** C6
Villadiego *Spain* **36** C6
Villadóssola *Italy* **40** B5
Villafeliche *Spain* **38** D3
Villafranca *Spain* **38** C3
Villafranca de Bonany *Spain* **48** B10
Villafranca de los Barros
  Spain **37** G4
Villafranca de los
  Caballeros *Spain* **37** F7
Villafranca del Cid =
  Vilafranca del Maestrat
  Spain **38** E4
Villafranca del Panadés =
  Vilafranca del Penedès
  Spain **38** D6
Villafranca di Verona *Italy* **40** C7
Villafranca Tirrena *Italy* **43** D8
Villagrán *Mexico* **119** C5
Villaguay *Argentina* **126** C4
Villaharta *Spain* **37** G6
Villahermosa *Mexico* **119** D6
Villahermosa *Spain* **39** G2
Villaines-la-Juhel *France* **18** D6
Villajoyosa *Spain* **39** G4
Villalba *Spain* **36** B3
Villalba de Guardo *Spain* **36** C6
Villalón de Campos *Spain* **36** C5
Villalpando *Spain* **36** D5
Villaluenga de la Sagra *Spain* **36** E7
Villamanán *Spain* **36** C5
Villamartín *Spain* **37** J5
Villamayor de Santiago *Spain* **38** F2
Villamblard *France* **20** C4
Villanova Monteleone *Italy* **42** B1
Villanueva *U.S.A.* **109** J11
Villanueva de Castellón *Spain* **39** F4
Villanueva de Córdoba *Spain* **37** G6
Villanueva de la Fuente
  Spain **39** G2
Villanueva de la Serena
  Spain **37** G5
Villanueva de la Sierra *Spain* **36** E4
Villanueva de los Castillejos
  Spain **37** H3
Villanueva de los Infantes
  Spain **37** G7
Villanueva del Arzobispo
  Spain **39** G2
Villanueva del Fresno *Spain* **37** G3
Villanueva y Geltrú =
  Vilanova i la Geltrú *Spain* **38** D6
Villaputzu *Italy* **42** C2
Villaquilambre *Spain* **36** C5
Villar del Arzobispo *Spain* **38** F4
Villar del Rey *Spain* **37** F4
Villard-de-Lans *France* **21** C9
Villarramiel *Spain* **36** C6
Villarreal = Vila-Real *Spain* **38** F4
Villarrica *Chile* **128** D2
Villarrica *Paraguay* **126** B4
Villarrobledo *Spain* **39** F2
Villarroya de la Sierra *Spain* **38** D3
Villarrubia de los Ojos *Spain* **37** F7
Villars-les-Dombes *France* **19** F12
Villasayas *Spain* **38** D2
Villaseco de los Gamitos
  Spain **36** D4
Villasimíus *Italy* **42** C2
Villastar *Spain* **38** E4
Villatobas *Spain* **36** F7
Villavicencio *Argentina* **126** C2
Villavicencio *Colombia* **124** C4
Villaviciosa *Spain* **36** B5
Villazón *Bolivia* **126** A2
Ville-Marie *Canada* **104** C4
Ville Platte *U.S.A.* **116** F8
Villedieu-les-Poêles *France* **18** D5
Villefort *France* **20** D7
Villefranche-de-Lauragais
  France **20** E5
Villefranche-de-Rouergue
  France **20** D6
Villefranche-du-Périgord
  France **20** D5

Villefranche-sur-Saône
  France **21** C8
Villel *Spain* **38** E3
Villemur-sur-Tarn *France* **20** E5
Villena *Spain* **39** G4
Villenauxe-la-Grande
  France **19** D10
Villenave-d'Ornon *France* **20** D3
Villeneuve-d'Ascq *France* **19** B10
Villeneuve-l'Archevêque
  France **19** D10
Villeneuve-lès-Avignon
  France **21** E8
Villeneuve-sur-Allier *France* **19** F10
Villeneuve-sur-Lot *France* **20** D4
Villeneuve-sur-Yonne
  France **19** D10
Villeréal *France* **20** D4
Villers-Bocage *France* **18** C6
Villers-Cotterêts *France* **19** C10
Villers-sur-Mer *France* **18** C6
Villersexel *France* **19** E13
Villerupt *France* **19** C12
Villeurbanne *France* **21** C8
Villiers *S. Africa* **89** D4
Villingen-Schwenningen
  Germany **25** G4
Villmanstrand =
  Lappeenranta *Finland* **32** B5
Vilna *Canada* **102** C6
Vilnius *Lithuania* **32** E3
Vils *Austria* **26** D3
Vils ➝ *Bayern, Germany* **25** G9
Vils ➝ *Bayern, Germany* **25** F7
Vilsbiburg *Germany* **25** G8
Vilshofen *Germany* **25** G9
Vilusi *Montenegro* **44** D2
Vilvoorde *Belgium* **17** D4
Vilyuchinsk *Russia* **53** D16
Vilyuy ➝ *Russia* **53** C13
Vilyuysk *Russia* **53** C13
Vimianzo *Spain* **36** B1
Vimioso *Portugal* **36** D4
Vimmerby *Sweden* **11** G9
Vimoutiers *France* **18** D7
Vimperk *Czech Rep.* **26** B6
Viña del Mar *Chile* **126** C1
Vinaròs *Spain* **38** E5
Vincennes *U.S.A.* **112** F10
Vincennes Bay *S. Ocean* **5** C8
Vincent *U.S.A.* **111** L8
Vinchina *Argentina* **126** B2
Vindelälven ➝ *Sweden* **8** E18
Vindeln *Sweden* **8** D18
Vinderup *Denmark* **11** H2
Vindhya Ra. *India* **68** H7
Vineland *U.S.A.* **113** F16
Vinga *Romania* **28** D6
Vingåker *Sweden* **10** E9
Vinh *Vietnam* **64** C5
Vinh Linh *Vietnam* **64** D6
Vinh Long *Vietnam* **65** G5
Vinh Yen *Vietnam* **58** G5
Vinhais *Portugal* **36** D3
Vinica *Croatia* **41** B13
Vinica *Macedonia* **44** E6
Vinica *Slovenia* **41** C12
Vinita *U.S.A.* **116** C7
Vinkovci *Croatia* **28** E3
Vinnitsa = Vinnytsya
  Ukraine **23** D15
Vinnytsya *Ukraine* **23** D15
Vinnytsya □ *Ukraine* **33** H5
Vinslöv *Sweden* **11** H7
Vinson Massif *Antarctica* **5** D16
Vintjärn *Sweden* **10** D10
Vinton *Calif., U.S.A.* **110** F6
Vinton *Iowa, U.S.A.* **112** D7
Vinton *La., U.S.A.* **116** F8
Vinţu de Jos *Romania* **29** D8
Viöl *Germany* **24** A5
Violet Valley ✺ *Australia* **92** C4
Viotia □ *Greece* **46** C5
Vipava *Slovenia* **41** C10
Vipiteno *Italy* **40** B7
Viqueque *E. Timor* **63** F7
Vir *Croatia* **41** D12
Virac *Phil.* **61** E6
Virachey *Cambodia* **64** F6
Virachey △ *Cambodia* **64** E6
Virago Sd. *Canada* **102** C2
Viramgam *India* **68** H5
Viranşehir *Turkey* **73** D8
Virawah *Pakistan* **68** G4
Virbalis *Lithuania* **30** D9
Virden *Canada* **103** D8
Vire *France* **18** D6
Vire ➝ *France* **18** C5
Vírgenes, C. *Argentina* **128** G3
Virgin ➝ *U.S.A.* **109** H6
Virgin Gorda *Br. Virgin Is.* **121** e
Virgin Is. (British) ☑
  W. Indies **121** e
Virgin Is. (U.S.) ☑ *W. Indies* **121** e
Virgin Islands △
  U.S. Virgin Is. **121** C7
Virginia *S. Africa* **88** D4
Virginia *U.S.A.* **112** B7
Virginia □ *U.S.A.* **113** G14

Virginia Beach *U.S.A.* **113** F16
Virginia City *Mont., U.S.A.* **108** D8
Virginia City *Nev., U.S.A.* **110** F7
Virginia Falls *Canada* **102** A3
Virginiatown *Canada* **104** C4
Virje *Croatia* **41** B13
Viroqua *U.S.A.* **112** D8
Virovitica *Croatia* **28** E2
Virpazar *Montenegro* **44** D3
Virpur *India* **68** J4
Virserum *Sweden* **11** G9
Virton *Belgium* **17** E5
Virudunagar *India* **66** Q10
Virunga △
  Dem. Rep. of the Congo **86** B2
Vis *Croatia* **41** E13
Visalia *U.S.A.* **110** J7
Visayan Sea *Phil.* **61** F5
Visby *Sweden* **11** G12
Viscount Melville Sd.
  Canada **101** C10
Visé *Belgium* **17** D5
Vise, Ostrov *Russia* **52** B8
Višegrad *Bos.-H.* **28** G4
Viseu *Brazil* **125** D9
Viseu *Portugal* **36** E3
Viseu □ *Portugal* **36** E3
Vişeu de Sus *Romania* **29** C9
Vishakhapatnam *India* **67** L13
Vişina *Romania* **29** F9
Vişineşti *Moldova* **29** D13
Vişineşti *Prahova, Romania* **29** E10
Visingsö *Sweden* **11** F8
Viskafors *Sweden* **11** G6
Viskan ➝ *Sweden* **11** G6
Viški Kanal *Croatia* **41** E13
Vislanda *Sweden* **11** H8
Visnagar *India* **68** H5
Višnja Gora *Slovenia* **41** C11
Viso, Mte. *Italy* **40** D4
Viso del Marqués *Spain* **37** G7
Visoko *Bos.-H.* **28** G3
Visokoi I. *Antarctica* **5** B1
Visp *Switz.* **25** J3
Vissefjärda *Sweden* **11** H9
Visselhövede *Germany* **24** C5
Vissenbjerg *Denmark* **11** J4
Vista *U.S.A.* **111** M9
Vistonida, L. *Greece* **45** E9
Vistonikos, Ormos =
  Vistonida, L. *Greece* **45** E9
Vistula = Wisła ➝ *Poland* **30** D5
Vit ➝ *Bulgaria* **45** C8
Vitanje *Slovenia* **41** B12
Vitebsk = Vitsyebsk *Belarus* **32** E6
Viterbo *Italy* **41** F9
Vitez *Bos.-H.* **28** F2
Viti Levu *Fiji* **91** a
Vitigudino *Spain* **36** D4
Vitim *Russia* **53** D12
Vitim ➝ *Russia* **53** D12
Vitina *Bos.-H.* **41** E14
Vitina *Greece* **46** D4
Vítkov *Czech Rep.* **27** B10
Vitória *Brazil* **125** H10
Vitória da Conquista *Brazil* **125** F10
Vitória de Santo Antão
  Brazil **125** E11
Vitoria-Gasteiz *Spain* **38** C2
Vitosha △ *Bulgaria* **44** D7
Vitré *France* **18** D5
Vitry-le-François *France* **19** D11
Vitry-sur-Seine *France* **19** D9
Vitsand *Sweden* **10** D7
Vitsi, Oros *Greece* **44** F5
Vitsyebsk *Belarus* **32** E6
Vitsyebsk □ *Belarus* **32** E5
Vittangi *Sweden* **11** H7
Vitteaux *France* **19** E11
Vittel *France* **19** D12
Vittória *Italy* **43** F7
Vittório Véneto *Italy* **41** C9
Vittsjö *Sweden* **11** H7
Volkach *Germany* **25** F6
Völkermarkt *Austria* **26** E7
Volkhov *Russia* **32** C7
Volkhov ➝ *Russia* **32** B7
Völklingen *Germany* **25** F2
Volkovysk = Vawkavysk
  Belarus **23** B13
Volksrust *S. Africa* **89** D4
Volnansk *Ukraine* **33** H8
Volochanka *Russia* **53** B10
Volodarsk *Russia* **34** B6
Volodymyr-Volynskyy
  Ukraine **23** C13
Vologda *Russia* **32** C10
Vologda □ *Russia* **32** B10
Volokolamsk *Russia* **32** D8
Volokonovka *Russia* **33** G9
Volos *Greece* **46** B4
Volosovo *Russia* **32** C5
Volovets *Ukraine* **29** B8
Volovo *Russia* **32** F10
Volozhin = Valozhyn
  Belarus **23** A14
Volsk *Russia* **34** D8
Volta ➝ *Ghana* **83** D5
Volta, L. *Ghana* **83** D5
Volta Blanche = White
  Volta ➝ *Ghana* **83** D4
Volta Redonda *Brazil* **127** A7
Voltaire, C. *Australia* **92** B4

Vladimirovo *Bulgaria* **44** C7
Vladislavovka *Ukraine* **33** K8
Vladivostok *Russia* **54** C5
Vlăhiţa *Romania* **29** D11
Vlasenica *Bos.-H.* **28** F3
Vlašić *Bos.-H.* **28** F2
Vlašim *Czech Rep.* **26** B7
Vlasinsko Jezero *Serbia* **44** D6
Vlasotince *Serbia* **44** D6
Vlieland *Neths.* **17** A4
Vlissingen *Neths.* **17** C3
Vlorë *Albania* **44** F3
Vlorës, Gjiri i *Albania* **44** F3
Vltava ➝ *Czech Rep.* **26** A7
Vo Dat *Vietnam* **65** G6
Vobarno *Italy* **40** C7
Voćin *Croatia* **28** E2
Vodňany *Czech Rep.* **26** B7
Vodnjan *Croatia* **41** D10
Voe *U.K.* **13** A7
Vogan *Togo* **83** D5
Vogel Pk. *Nigeria* **83** D7
Vogelkop = Doberai,
  Jazirah *Indonesia* **63** E8
Vogelsberg *Germany* **24** E5
Voghera *Italy* **40** D6
Vohibinany *Madag.* **89** B8
Vohilava *Madag.* **89** C8
Vohimarina = Iharana
  Madag. **89** A9
Vohimena, Tanjon' i *Madag.* **89** D8
Vohipeno *Madag.* **89** C8
Voi *Kenya* **86** C4
Void-Vacon *France* **19** D12
Voineşti *Iaşi, Romania* **29** C12
Voineşti *Prahova, Romania* **29** E10
Voinjama *Liberia* **82** D3
Voiron *France* **21** C9
Voisey B. *Canada* **105** A7
Voitsberg *Austria* **26** D8
Vojens *Denmark* **11** J3
Vojmsjön *Sweden* **8** D17
Vojnić *Croatia* **41** C12
Vojnik *Italy* **41** B12
Vojvodina □ *Serbia* **28** E5
Vóikha *Russia* **32** E10
Vokhtoga *Russia* **32** C11
Volary *Czech Rep.* **26** C6
Volborg *U.S.A.* **108** D11
Volcán de Colima △ *Mexico* **118** D4
Volcano Is. = Kazan-Rettō
  Pac. Oc. **96** E6
Volcans △ *Rwanda* **86** C2
Volcans d'Auvergne △
  France **20** C6
Volchansk = Vovchansk
  Ukraine **33** G9
Volchya ➝ *Ukraine* **33** H8
Volda *Norway* **8** E12
Volga = Privolzhskiy □
  Russia **34** B10
Volga *Russia* **32** C10
Volga ➝ *Russia* **35** G9
Volga Hts. = Privolzhskaya
  Vozvyshennost *Russia* **34** E7
Volgo-Baltiyskiy Kanal
  Russia **32** B9
Volgo-Donskoy Kanal *Russia* **35** F7
Volgodonsk *Russia* **35** G6
Volgograd *Russia* **35** F7
Volgograd □ *Russia* **34** F7
Volgogradskoye Vdkhr.
  Russia **34** E8
Volgorechensk *Russia* **34** B5

Volterra *Italy* **40** E7
Voltri *Italy* **40** D5
Volturno ➝ *Italy* **42** A6
Volvi, L. *Greece* **44** F7
Volyn □ *Ukraine* **33** G3
Volyně *Czech Rep.* **26** B6
Volzhsk *Russia* **34** C9
Volzhskiy *Russia* **35** F7
Vomo *Fiji* **91** a
Vondrozo *Madag.* **89** C8
Vonitsa *Greece* **46** C2
Vopnafjörður *Iceland* **8** D6
Vorarlberg □ *Austria* **26** D2
Voras Oros *Greece* **44** F5
Vorbasse *Denmark* **11** J3
Vorchdorf *Austria* **26** D6
Vorderrhein ➝ *Switz.* **25** J5
Vordingborg *Denmark* **11** J5
Vorë *Albania* **44** E3
Voreio Aigaio □ *Greece* **47** C7
Voreppe *France* **21** C9
Vori *Greece* **46** F6
Vorios Evoikos Kolpos *Greece* **46** C5
Vorkuta *Russia* **52** C7
Vormsi *Estonia* **32** C2
Vorona ➝ *Russia* **34** E6
Voronezh *Russia* **33** G10
Voronezh *Ukraine* **33** G7
Voronezh □ *Russia* **34** E4
Voronezh ➝ *Russia* **33** G10
Vorontsovo-
  Aleksandrovskoye =
  Zelenokumsk *Russia* **35** H6
Vorpommersche
  Boddenlandschaft △
  Germany **24** A8
Vorskla ➝ *Ukraine* **33** H8
Võrts Järv *Estonia* **32** C4
Võru *Estonia* **32** D4
Vosges *France* **19** D14
Vosges □ *France* **19** D13
Vosges du Nord △ *France* **19** D14
Voskopojë *Albania* **44** F4
Voskresensk *Russia* **32** E10
Voskresenskoye *Russia* **34** B7
Voss *Norway* **8** F12
Vostok *Antarctica* **5** D8
Vostok I. *Kiribati* **97** J12
Votice *Czech Rep.* **26** B7
Votsuri-Shima *Japan* **55** M1
Vouga ➝ *Portugal* **36** E2
Vouillé *France* **18** F7
Vouxa, Akra *Greece* **49** D5
Vouzela *Portugal* **36** E2
Vouziers *France* **19** C11
Vovchansk *Ukraine* **33** G9
Vowchyn *Belarus* **31** F10
Voyageurs △ *U.S.A.* **112** A7
Voynitsa *Russia* **8** D24
Voyvozh *Russia* **52** C6
Vozhe, Ozero *Russia* **32** B10
Vozhega *Russia* **32** B10
Voznesensk *Ukraine* **33** J6
Voznesenye *Russia* **32** B8
Vrå *Denmark* **11** G3
Vráble *Slovak Rep.* **27** C11
Vraćevšnica *Serbia* **44** B4
Vrachneika *Greece* **46** C3
Vrancea □ *Romania* **29** E11
Vrancei, Munţii *Romania* **29** E11
Vrangel *Russia* **54** C6
Vrangelya, Ostrov *Russia* **53** B18
Vranica *Bos.-H.* **28** G2
Vranje *Serbia* **44** D5
Vranjska Banja *Serbia* **44** D6
Vranov nad Topl'ou
  Slovak Rep. **27** C14
Vransko *Slovenia* **41** B11
Vransko Jezero *Croatia* **41** E12
Vrapčište *Macedonia* **44** E4
Vratsa *Bulgaria* **44** C7
Vrbas *Serbia* **28** E4
Vrbas ➝ *Bos.-H.* **28** E2
Vrbnik *Croatia* **41** C11
Vrbovec *Croatia* **41** C13
Vrbovsko *Croatia* **41** C12
Vrchlabí *Czech Rep.* **26** A8
Vrede *S. Africa* **89** D4
Vredefort *S. Africa* **88** D4
Vreden *Germany* **24** C2
Vredenburg *S. Africa* **88** E2
Vredendal *S. Africa* **88** E2
Vretstorp *Sweden* **10** E8
Vrgorac *Croatia* **41** E14
Vrhnika *Slovenia* **41** C11
Vriddhachalam *India* **66** P11
Vrīdi *Ivory C.* **82** D4
Vrigstad *Sweden* **11** G8
Vrindavan *India* **68** F7
Vrisses *Greece* **49** D6
Vrnograč *Bos.-H.* **41** C12
Vrondados *Greece* **47** C8
Vrpolje *Croatia* **28** E3
Vršac *Serbia* **28** E6
Vršacki Kanal *Serbia* **28** E5
Vrútky *Slovak Rep.* **27** B11
Vryburg *S. Africa* **88** D3
Vryheid *S. Africa* **89** D5
Vsetín *Czech Rep.* **27** B11
Vu Liet *Vietnam* **64** C5
Vŭcha ➝ *Bulgaria* **45** D8

Vučitrn *Kosovo* **44** D4
Vukovar *Croatia* **28** E3
Vuktyl *Russia* **52** C6
Vulcan *Canada* **102** C6
Vulcan *Romania* **29** E8
Vulcaneşti *Moldova* **29** E13
Vulcano *Italy* **43** D7
Vúlchedruma *Bulgaria* **44** C7
Vulkaneshty = Vulcaneşti
　Moldova **29** E13
Vunduzi → *Mozam.* **87** F3
Vunidawa *Fiji* **91** a
Vunisea *Fiji* **91** a
Vürbitsa *Bulgaria* **45** D10
Vurshets *Bulgaria* **44** C7
Vutcani *Romania* **29** D12
Vuya *Sudan* **81** F2
Vuzlove *Ukraine* **28** B7
Vwaza △ *Malawi* **87** E3
Vyartsilya *Russia* **32** A6
Vyatka = Kirov *Russia* **52** D5
Vyatka → *Russia* **34** C10
Vyatskiye Polyany *Russia* **34** B10
Vyazemskiy *Russia* **53** E14
Vyazma *Russia* **32** E8
Vyazniki *Russia* **34** B6
Vyborg *Russia* **32** B5
Vychegda → *Russia* **52** C5
Východné Beskydy *Europe* **27** B15
Vyerkhnyadzvinsk *Belarus* **32** E4
Vyhoda *Ukraine* **29** B8
Vyksa *Russia* **34** C6
Vylkove *Ukraine* **29** E14
Vylok *Ukraine* **28** B7
Vynohradiv *Ukraine* **28** B8
Vyrnwy, L. *U.K.* **14** E4
Vyshkiv *Ukraine* **29** B8
Vyshkove *Ukraine* **29** B8
Vyshniy Volochek *Russia* **32** D8
Vyshzha = imeni 26
　Bakinskikh Komissarov
　Turkmenistan **71** B7
Vyškov *Czech Rep.* **27** B9
Vysokaye *Belarus* **31** F10
Vysoké Mýto *Czech Rep.* **27** B9
Vysokovsk *Russia* **32** D9
Vyšší Brod *Czech Rep.* **26** C7
Vytegra *Russia* **32** B9
Vyzhnytsya *Ukraine* **29** B10
Vyzhnytsya → *Ukraine* **29** B10

W

W du Benin △ *Benin* **83** C5
W du Burkina Faso △
　Burkina Faso **83** C4
W du Niger △ *Niger* **83** C5
W.A.C. Bennett Dam
　Canada **102** B4
Wa *Ghana* **82** C4
Waal → *Neths.* **17** C5
Waalwijk *Neths.* **17** C5
Waanyi-Garawa ☼ *Australia* **94** B2
Waat *Sudan* **81** F3
Wabakimi △ *Canada* **104** B2
Wabana *Canada* **105** C9
Wabasca → *Canada* **102** B5
Wabasca-Desmarais *Canada* **102** B6
Wabash *U.S.A.* **113** E11
Wabash → *U.S.A.* **112** G9
Wabi → *Ethiopia* **81** F5
Wabigoon L. *Canada* **103** D10
Wabowden *Canada* **103** C7
Wąbrzeźno *Poland* **31** E5
Wabu Hu *China* **59** A11
Wabuk Pt. *Canada* **104** A2
Wabush *Canada* **105** B6
Wąchock *Poland* **31** G8
Wächtersbach *Germany* **25** E5
Waco *U.S.A.* **116** F6
Waconichi, L. *Canada* **104** B5
Wad Ban Naqa *Sudan* **81** D3
Wad Banda *Sudan* **81** E2
Wad el Haddad *Sudan* **81** E3
Wad en Nau *Sudan* **81** E3
Wad Hamid *Sudan* **81** D3
Wad Medanî *Sudan* **81** E3
Wad Thana *Pakistan* **68** F2
Wadai *Africa* **76** E5
Wadayama *Japan* **55** G7
Waddeneilanden *Neths.* **17** A5
Waddenzee *Neths.* **17** A5
Waddi, Chappal *Nigeria* **83** D7
Waddington *U.S.A.* **115** B9
Waddington, Mt. *Canada* **102** C3
Waddy Pt. *Australia* **95** C5
Wadebridge *U.K.* **15** G3
Wadena *Canada* **103** C8
Wadena *U.S.A.* **112** B6
Wädenswil *Switz.* **25** H4
Wadern *Germany* **25** F2
Wadeye *Australia* **92** B4
Wadhams *Canada* **102** C3
Wadhwan *India* **68** H4
Wādī as Sīr *Jordan* **74** D4
Wâdi Gemâl, J. *Egypt* **80** C4
Wadi Halfa *Sudan* **80** C3
Wadi Rum △ *Jordan* **74** F4
Wadian *China* **59** A9

Wadlew *Poland* **31** G6
Wadowice *Poland* **31** J6
Wadsworth *Nev., U.S.A.* **108** G4
Wadsworth *Ohio, U.S.A.* **114** E3
Waegwan *S. Korea* **57** G15
Wafangdian *China* **57** E11
Wafrah *Kuwait* **70** D5
Wagait ☼ *Australia* **92** B5
Wageningen *Neths.* **17** C5
Wager B. *Canada* **101** D14
Wagga Wagga *Australia* **95** F4
Waghete *Indonesia* **63** E9
Wagin *Australia* **93** F2
Wagner *U.S.A.* **112** D4
Wagon Mound *U.S.A.* **109** H11
Wagoner *U.S.A.* **116** D7
Wągrowiec *Poland* **31** F4
Wah *Pakistan* **68** C5
Wahai *Indonesia* **63** E7
Wâḩid *Egypt* **74** E1
Wahnian *Afghan.* **68** C1
Wahni *Ethiopia* **81** E4
Wahoo *U.S.A.* **112** E5
Wahpeton *U.S.A.* **112** B5
Waialua *U.S.A.* **107** L8
Waiau → *N.Z.* **91** E4
Waibeem *Indonesia* **63** E8
Waiblingen *Germany* **25** G5
Waidhofen an der Thaya
　Austria **26** C8
Waidhofen an der Ybbs
　Austria **26** D7
Waigeo *Indonesia* **63** E8
Waihi *N.Z.* **91** B5
Waihou → *N.Z.* **91** B5
Waika *Dem. Rep. of the Congo* **86** C2
Waikabubak *Indonesia* **63** F5
Waikaremoana, L. *N.Z.* **91** C6
Waikari *N.Z.* **91** E4
Waikato → *N.Z.* **91** B5
Waikelo *Indonesia* **92** A2
Waikerie *Australia* **95** E3
Waikokopu *N.Z.* **91** C6
Waikouaiti *N.Z.* **91** F3
Waimakariri → *N.Z.* **91** E4
Waimate *N.Z.* **91** F3
Wainganga → *India* **66** K11
Waingapu *Indonesia* **63** F6
Waini → *Guyana* **124** B7
Wainwright *Canada* **103** C6
Wainwright *U.S.A.* **106** A7
Waiouru *N.Z.* **91** C5
Waipara *N.Z.* **91** E4
Waipawa *N.Z.* **91** C6
Waipiro *N.Z.* **91** C7
Waipoua Forest *N.Z.* **91** A4
Waipu *N.Z.* **91** A5
Waipukurau *N.Z.* **91** D6
Wairakei *N.Z.* **91** C6
Wairarapa, L. *N.Z.* **91** D5
Wairoa *N.Z.* **91** C6
Waitaki → *N.Z.* **91** F3
Waitangi *N.Z.* **91** A5
Waitara *N.Z.* **91** C5
Waitomo Caves *N.Z.* **91** C5
Waitsburg *U.S.A.* **108** C4
Waiuku *N.Z.* **91** B5
Wajima *Japan* **55** F8
Wajir *Kenya* **86** B5
Waka *Ethiopia* **81** F4
Wakasa *Japan* **55** G7
Wakasa-Wan *Japan* **55** G7
Wakatipu, L. *N.Z.* **91** F2
Wakaw *Canada* **103** C7
Wakaya *Fiji* **91** a
Wakayama *Japan* **55** G7
Wakayama □ *Japan* **55** H7
Wake Forest *U.S.A.* **117** D15
Wake I. *Pac. Oc.* **96** F8
WaKeeney *U.S.A.* **112** F4
Wakefield *Jamaica* **120** a
Wakefield *N.Z.* **91** D4
Wakefield *U.K.* **14** D6
Wakefield *Mass., U.S.A.* **115** D13
Wakefield *Mich., U.S.A.* **112** B9
Wakkanai *Japan* **54** B10
Wakkerstroom *S. Africa* **89** D5
Wakool *Australia* **95** F3
Wakool → *Australia* **95** F3
Wakre *Indonesia* **63** E8
Wakuach, L. *Canada* **105** A6
Walagunya ☼ *Australia* **92** D3
Walamba *Zambia* **87** E2
Wałbrzych *Poland* **31** H3
Walbury Hill *U.K.* **15** F6
Walcha *Australia* **95** E5
Walcott *U.S.A.* **108** F10
Wałcz *Poland* **31** E3
Waldbröl *Germany* **24** E3
Waldburg Ra. *Australia* **93** D2
Waldeck *Germany* **24** D5
Walden *Colo., U.S.A.* **108** F10
Walden *N.Y., U.S.A.* **115** E10
Waldkirch *Germany* **25** G3
Waldkirchen *Germany* **25** G9
Waldkraiburg *Germany* **25** G8
Waldport *U.S.A.* **108** D1
Waldron *U.S.A.* **116** D7
Waldviertel *Austria* **26** C8

Walebing *Australia* **93** F2
Walembele *Ghana* **82** C4
Walensee *Switz.* **25** H5
Wales □ *U.K.* **15** E3
Wales I. *Canada* **101** D14
Walewale *Ghana* **83** C4
Walgett *Australia* **95** E4
Walgreen Coast *Antarctica* **5** D15
Walker *U.S.A.* **112** B6
Walker, L. *Canada* **105** B6
Walker L. *Canada* **103** C9
Walker L. *U.S.A.* **108** G4
Walkerston *Australia* **94** b
Walkerton *Canada* **114** B3
Wall *U.S.A.* **112** C2
Walla Walla *U.S.A.* **108** C4
Wallace *Idaho, U.S.A.* **108** C6
Wallace *N.C., U.S.A.* **117** D16
Wallaceburg *Canada* **114** D2
Wallachia = Valahia
　Romania **29** F9
Wallal *Australia* **95** D4
Wallam Cr. → *Australia* **95** D4
Wallambin, L. *Australia* **93** F2
Wallangarra *Australia* **95** D5
Wallaroo *Australia* **95** E2
Walldürn *Germany* **25** F5
Wallenhorst *Germany* **24** C4
Wallenpaupack, L. *U.S.A.* **115** E9
Wallingford *U.S.A.* **115** E12
Wallingford *Vt., U.S.A.* **115** C12
Wallis & Futuna, Is. *Pac. Oc.* **90** C11
Wallowa *U.S.A.* **108** D5
Wallowa Mts. *U.S.A.* **108** D5
Walls *U.K.* **13** A7
Walls of Jerusalem △
　Australia **95** G4
Wallula *U.S.A.* **108** C4
Wallumbilla *Australia* **95** D4
Walmsley L. *Canada* **103** A7
Walney, I. of *U.K.* **14** C4
Walnut Canyon △ *U.S.A.* **109** J8
Walnut Creek *U.S.A.* **110** H4
Walnut Ridge *U.S.A.* **117** C9
Walpole *Australia* **93** F2
Walpole *U.S.A.* **115** D13
Walpole-Nornalup △
　Australia **93** G2
Wals *Austria* **26** D5
Walsall *U.K.* **15** E6
Walsenburg *U.S.A.* **109** H11
Walsh *U.S.A.* **109** H12
Walsh → *Australia* **94** B3
Walsingham *Canada* **114** D4
Walsrode *Germany* **24** C5
Walter F. George Res.
　U.S.A. **117** F12
Walterboro *U.S.A.* **117** E14
Walters *U.S.A.* **116** D5
Waltershausen *Germany* **24** E6
Waltham *U.S.A.* **115** D13
Waltman *U.S.A.* **108** E10
Walton *U.S.A.* **115** D9
Walton-on-the-Naze *U.K.* **15** F9
Walvis Bay *Namibia* **88** C1
Walvisbaai = Walvis Bay
　Namibia **88** C1
Wamba *Dem. Rep. of the Congo* **86** B2
Wamba *Kenya* **86** B4
Wamba *Nigeria* **83** D6
Wambardi ☼ *Australia* **92** C5
Wamego *U.S.A.* **112** F5
Wamena *Indonesia* **63** E9
Wampana Karlantijpa ☼
　Australia **92** C5
Wampaya ☼ *Australia* **94** B2
Wampsville *U.S.A.* **115** C9
Wamsutter *U.S.A.* **108** F10
Wamulan *Indonesia* **63** E7
Wan Xian *China* **56** E8
Wana *Pakistan* **68** C3
Wanaaring *Australia* **95** D3
Wanaka *N.Z.* **91** F2
Wanaka, L. *N.Z.* **91** F2
Wan'an *China* **59** D10
Wanapitei L. *Canada* **104** C3
Wandel Sea = McKinley
　Sea *Arctic* **4** A7
Wandérama *Ivory C.* **82** D4
Wanderer *Zimbabwe* **87** F3
Wandhari *Pakistan* **68** F2
Wanding *China* **58** E2
Wandoan *Australia* **95** D4
Wanfu *China* **57** D12
Wang → *Thailand* **64** D2
Wang Kai *Sudan* **81** F2
Wang Noi *Thailand* **64** E3
Wang Saphung *Thailand* **64** D3
Wang Thong *Thailand* **64** D3
Wanga *Dem. Rep. of the Congo* **86** B2
Wangal *Indonesia* **63** F8
Wanganella *Australia* **95** F3
Wanganui *N.Z.* **91** C5
Wangaratta *Australia* **95** F4
Wangary *Australia* **95** E2
Wangcang *China* **58** A6
Wangcheng *China* **59** C9
Wangdu *China* **56** E8
Wangen *Germany* **25** H5
Wangerooge *Germany* **24** B3

Wangiwangi *Indonesia* **63** F6
Wangjiang *China* **59** B11
Wangmo *China* **58** E6
Wangolodougou *Ivory C.* **82** D3
Wangqing *China* **57** C15
Wanimiyn ☼ *Australia* **92** C5
Wanjina Wunggurr
　Wilinggin ☼ *Australia* **92** C4
Wankaner *India* **68** H4
Wanless *Canada* **103** B8
Wanleweyne *Somali Rep.* **75** G3
Wanneroo *Australia* **93** F2
Wannian *China* **59** C11
Wanning *China* **64** C8
Wannoo Billabong
　Roadhouse *Australia* **93** E2
Wanon Niwat *Thailand* **64** D4
Wanquan *China* **56** D8
Wanrong *China* **56** G6
Wanshan *China* **58** D7
Wanshengchang *China* **58** C6
Wantage *U.K.* **15** F6
Wanxian *China* **58** B7
Wanyuan *China* **58** A7
Wanzai *China* **59** C10
Wapakoneta *U.S.A.* **113** E11
Wapato *U.S.A.* **108** C3
Wapawekka L. *Canada* **103** C8
Wapikopa L. *Canada* **104** B2
Wapiti → *Canada* **102** B5
Wappingers Falls *U.S.A.* **115** E11
Wapsipinicon → *U.S.A.* **112** E8
Wapusk △ *Canada* **103** B10
Warab *Sudan* **81** F2
Warab □ *Sudan* **81** F2
Warakurna *Australia* **93** D4
Warangal *India* **66** L11
Waraseoni *India* **69** J9
Waratah *Australia* **95** G4
Waratah B. *Australia* **95** F4
Warburg *Germany* **24** D5
Warburton *Vic., Australia* **95** F4
Warburton *W. Austral.,
　Australia* **93** E4
Warburton → *Australia* **95** D2
Warburton Groove *Australia* **95** A2
Warburton Ra. *Australia* **93** E4
Warburton ☼ *Australia* **93** E4
Ward *N.Z.* **91** D5
Ward → *Australia* **95** D4
Ward Mt. *U.S.A.* **110** H8
Warden *S. Africa* **89** D4
Wardha *India* **66** J11
Wardha → *India* **66** K11
Wardsville *Canada* **114** D3
Ware *U.K.* **15** F8
Ware *U.S.A.* **115** D12
Waregem *Belgium* **17** D3
Wareham *U.S.A.* **115** E14
Waremme *Belgium* **17** D5
Waren *Germany* **24** B8
Warendorf *Germany* **24** D4
Warialda *Australia* **95** D5
Wariap *Indonesia* **63** E8
Warin Chamrap *Thailand* **64** E5
Warka *Poland* **31** G8
Warkopi *Indonesia* **63** E8
Warm Springs *U.S.A.* **109** G5
Warman *Canada* **103** C7
Warmbad = Bela Bela
　S. Africa **89** C4
Warmbad *Namibia* **88** D2
Warmińsko-Mazurskie □
　Poland **30** D8
Warminster *U.K.* **15** F5
Warminster *U.S.A.* **115** F9
Warmun *Australia* **92** C4
Warnemünde *Germany* **24** A8
Warner Mts. *U.S.A.* **108** F3
Warner Robins *U.S.A.* **117** E13
Warnow → *Germany* **24** A8
Waroona *Australia* **93** F2
Warrabri ☼ *Australia* **94** C1
Warracknabeal *Australia* **95** F3
Warragul *Australia* **95** F4
Warrego → *Australia* **95** E4
Warrego Ra. *Australia* **94** C4
Warren *Australia* **95** E4
Warren *Ark., U.S.A.* **116** E8
Warren *Mich., U.S.A.* **113** D12
Warren *Minn., U.S.A.* **112** A5
Warren *Ohio, U.S.A.* **114** E4
Warren *Pa., U.S.A.* **114** E5
Warrenpoint *U.K.* **12** B5
Warrensburg *Mo., U.S.A.* **112** F7
Warrensburg *N.Y., U.S.A.* **115** C11
Warrenton *S. Africa* **88** D3
Warrenton *U.S.A.* **110** D3
Warri *Nigeria* **83** D6
Warrington *U.K.* **14** D5
Warrington *U.S.A.* **117** F11
Warrington □ *U.K.* **14** D5
Warrnambool *Australia* **95** F3
Warroad *U.S.A.* **112** A7
Warruwi *Australia* **94** A1
Warsa *Indonesia* **63** E9
Warsak Dam *Pakistan* **68** C4
Warsaw = Warszawa *Poland* **31** F8
Warsaw *Ind., U.S.A.* **113** E11
Warsaw *N.Y., U.S.A.* **114** D6

Warsaw *Ohio, U.S.A.* **114** F3
Warstein *Germany* **24** D4
Warszawa *Poland* **31** F8
Warszawa ✈ (WAW) *Poland* **31** F7
Warta *Poland* **31** F1
Warta → *Poland* **31** F1
Warthe = Warta → *Poland* **31** F1
Waru *Indonesia* **63** E8
Warwick *Australia* **95** D5
Warwick *U.K.* **15** E6
Warwick *N.Y., U.S.A.* **115** E10
Warwick *R.I., U.S.A.* **115** E13
Warwickshire □ *U.K.* **15** E6
Wasaga Beach *Canada* **114** B4
Wasagaming *Canada* **103** C9
Wasatch Ra. *U.S.A.* **108** F8
Wasbank *S. Africa* **89** D5
Wasca *Calif., U.S.A.* **111** K7
Wasco *Oreg., U.S.A.* **108** D3
Waseca *U.S.A.* **112** C7
Wasekamio L. *Canada* **103** B7
Wash, The *U.K.* **14** E8
Washago *Canada* **114** B5
Washburn *N. Dak., U.S.A.* **112** B3
Washburn *Wis., U.S.A.* **112** B8
Washim *India* **66** J10
Washington *U.K.* **14** C6
Washington *D.C., U.S.A.* **113** F15
Washington *Ga., U.S.A.* **117** E13
Washington *Ind., U.S.A.* **112** F10
Washington *Iowa, U.S.A.* **112** E8
Washington *Mo., U.S.A.* **112** F8
Washington *N.C., U.S.A.* **117** D16
Washington *N.J., U.S.A.* **115** F10
Washington *Pa., U.S.A.* **114** F4
Washington *Utah, U.S.A.* **109** H7
Washington □ *U.S.A.* **108** C3
Washington, Mt. *U.S.A.* **115** B13
Washington Court House
　U.S.A. **113** F12
Washington I. *U.S.A.* **112** C10
Washougal *U.S.A.* **110** E4
Washpool △ *Australia* **95** D5
Wasian *Indonesia* **63** E8
Wasilków *Poland* **31** E10
Wasilla *U.S.A.* **100** C2
Wasini Marine △ *Kenya* **86** C5
Wasior *Indonesia* **63** E8
Wāsiţ □ *Iraq* **73** F11
Waskaganish *Canada* **104** B4
Waskaiowaka L. *Canada* **103** B9
Waskesiu Lake *Canada* **103** C7
Wasserburg *Germany* **25** G8
Wasserkuppe *Germany* **24** E5
Wassy *France* **19** D11
Waswanipi *Canada* **104** C4
Waswanipi, L. *Canada* **104** C4
Watampone *Indonesia* **63** E6
Watamu *Kenya* **86** C5
Watarrka △ *Australia* **92** D5
Water Park Pt. *Australia* **94** C5
Water Valley *U.S.A.* **117** D10
Waterberg Plateau △
　Namibia **88** C2
Waterberge *S. Africa* **89** C4
Waterbury *Conn., U.S.A.* **115** E11
Waterbury *Vt., U.S.A.* **115** B12
Waterbury L. *Canada* **103** B8
Waterdown *Canada* **114** C5
Waterford *Ireland* **12** D4
Waterford *Calif., U.S.A.* **110** H6
Waterford *Pa., U.S.A.* **114** E5
Waterford □ *Ireland* **12** D4
Waterford Harbour *Ireland* **12** D5
Waterhen L. *Canada* **103** C9
Waterloo *Belgium* **17** D4
Waterloo *Ont., Canada* **114** C4
Waterloo *Qué., Canada* **115** A12
Waterloo *S. Leone* **82** D2
Waterloo *Ill., U.S.A.* **112** F8
Waterloo *Iowa, U.S.A.* **112** D7
Waterloo *N.Y., U.S.A.* **114** D8
Watersmeet *U.S.A.* **112** B9
Waterton Lakes △ *Canada* **102** D6
Watertown *Conn., U.S.A.* **115** E11
Watertown *N.Y., U.S.A.* **115** C9
Watertown *S. Dak., U.S.A.* **112** C5
Watertown *Wis., U.S.A.* **112** D9
Waterval-Boven *S. Africa* **89** D5
Waterville *Canada* **115** A13
Waterville *Maine, U.S.A.* **113** C19
Waterville *N.Y., U.S.A.* **115** D9
Waterville *Pa., U.S.A.* **114** E7
Waterville *Wash., U.S.A.* **108** C3
Watervliet *U.S.A.* **115** D11
Wates *Indonesia* **63** G14
Watford *Canada* **114** D3
Watford *U.K.* **15** F7
Watford City *U.S.A.* **112** B2
Wathaman → *Canada* **103** B8
Wathaman L. *Canada* **103** B8
Watheroo *Australia* **93** F2
Watheroo △ *Australia* **93** F2
Wating *China* **56** G4
Watkins Glen *U.S.A.* **114** D8
Watling I. = San Salvador
　I. *Bahamas* **121** B5

Watonga *U.S.A.* **116** D5
Watrous *Canada* **103** C7
Watrous *U.S.A.* **109** J11
Watsa *Dem. Rep. of the Congo* **86** B2
Watseka *U.S.A.* **112** E10
Watson *Canada* **103** C8
Watson Lake *Canada* **102** A3
Watsontown *U.S.A.* **114** E8
Watsonville *U.S.A.* **110** J5
Wattiwarriganna Cr. →
　Australia **95** D2
Wattwil *Switz.* **25** H5
Watuata = Batuata *Indonesia* **63** F6
Watubela, Kepulauan
　Indonesia **63** E8
Watubela Is. = Watubela,
　Kepulauan *Indonesia* **63** E8
Wau = Wâw *Sudan* **81** F2
Waubamik *Canada* **114** A4
Waubay *U.S.A.* **112** C5
Wauchope *N.S.W., Australia* **95** E5
Wauchope *N. Terr., Australia* **94** C1
Wauchula *U.S.A.* **117** H14
Waukarlycarly, L. *Australia* **92** D3
Waukegan *U.S.A.* **112** D10
Waukesha *U.S.A.* **112** D9
Waukon *U.S.A.* **112** D8
Waupaca *U.S.A.* **112** C9
Waupun *U.S.A.* **112** D9
Waurika *U.S.A.* **116** D6
Wausau *U.S.A.* **112** C9
Wautoma *U.S.A.* **112** C9
Wauwatosa *U.S.A.* **112** D9
Wave Hill = Kalkarindji
　Australia **92** C5
Wave Rock *Australia* **93** F2
Waveney → *U.K.* **15** E9
Waverley *N.Z.* **91** C5
Waverly *Iowa, U.S.A.* **112** D7
Waverly *N.Y., U.S.A.* **115** E8
Wavre *Belgium* **17** D4
Wâw *Sudan* **81** F2
Wâw al Kabîr *Libya* **79** C9
Wawa *Canada* **104** C3
Wawa *Nigeria* **83** D5
Wawa *Sudan* **80** C3
Wawanesa *Canada* **103** D9
Wawona *U.S.A.* **110** H7
Waxahachie *U.S.A.* **116** E6
Way, L. *Australia* **93** E3
Waya *Fiji* **91** a
Waycross *U.S.A.* **117** F13
Wayi *Sudan* **81** F3
Wayland *U.S.A.* **114** D7
Wayne *Nebr., U.S.A.* **112** D5
Wayne *W. Va., U.S.A.* **113** F12
Waynesboro *Ga., U.S.A.* **117** E13
Waynesboro *Miss., U.S.A.* **117** F10
Waynesboro *Pa., U.S.A.* **113** F15
Waynesboro *Va., U.S.A.* **113** F14
Waynesburg *U.S.A.* **113** F13
Waynesville *U.S.A.* **117** D13
Waynoka *U.S.A.* **116** C5
Wazirabad *Pakistan* **68** C6
Waziristan *Pakistan* **68** C4
Wda → *Poland* **30** E5
We *Indonesia* **62** C1
Weald, The *U.K.* **15** F8
Wear → *U.K.* **14** C6
Weatherford *Okla., U.S.A.* **116** D5
Weatherford *Tex., U.S.A.* **116** E6
Weaverville *U.S.A.* **108** F2
Webb City *U.S.A.* **112** G6
Webequie *Canada* **104** B2
Webo = Nyaake *Liberia* **82** D3
Webster *Mass., U.S.A.* **115** D13
Webster *N.Y., U.S.A.* **114** C7
Webster *S. Dak., U.S.A.* **112** C5
Webster City *U.S.A.* **112** D7
Webster Springs *U.S.A.* **113** F13
Webuye *Kenya* **86** B3
Weda *Indonesia* **63** D7
Weda, Teluk *Indonesia* **63** D7
Weddell Abyssal Plain
　S. Ocean **5** C2
Weddell I. *Falk. Is.* **128** G4
Weddell Sea *Antarctica* **5** D1
Wedderburn *Australia* **95** F3
Wedel *Germany* **24** B5
Wedemark *Germany* **24** C5
Wedgeport *Canada* **105** D6
Wedza *Zimbabwe* **87** F3
Wee Waa *Australia* **95** E4
Weed *U.S.A.* **108** F2
Weed Heights *U.S.A.* **110** G7
Weedsport *U.S.A.* **115** C8
Weedville *U.S.A.* **114** E6
Weenen *S. Africa* **89** D5
Weener *Germany* **24** B3
Weert *Neths.* **17** C5
Węgierska-Górka *Poland* **31** J6
Węgliniec *Poland* **31** G2
Węgorzewo *Poland* **30** D8
Węgorzyno *Poland* **30** E2
Węgrów *Poland* **31** F9
Wehda □ *Sudan* **81** F3
Wei He → *Hebei, China* **56** F8
Wei He → *Shaanxi, China* **56** G6
Weichang *China* **57** D9
Weichuan *China* **56** G7

Weida *Germany* **24** E8
Weiden *Germany* **25** F8
Weifang *China* **57** F10
Weihai *China* **57** F12
Weil *Germany* **25** H3
Weilburg *Germany* **24** E4
Weilheim *Germany* **25** H7
Weimar *Germany* **24** E7
Weinan *China* **56** G5
Weingarten *Germany* **25** F4
Weinheim *Germany* **25** F4
Weining *China* **58** D5
Weipa *Australia* **94** A3
Weir → *Australia* **95** D4
Weir → *Canada* **103** B10
Weir River *Canada* **103** B10
Weirton *U.S.A.* **114** F4
Weiser *U.S.A.* **108** D5
Weishan *Shandong, China* **57** G9
Weishan *Yunnan, China* **58** E3
Weissenburg *Germany* **25** F6
Weissenfels *Germany* **24** D7
Weisswasser *Germany* **24** D10
Wéitra *Austria* **26** C7
Weixi *China* **58** D2
Weixin *China* **58** D5
Weiyuan *China* **56** G3
Weiz *Austria* **26** D8
Weizhou Dao *China* **58** G7
Wejherowo *Poland* **30** D5
Wekusko L. *Canada* **103** C9
Welch *U.S.A.* **113** G13
Weldya *Ethiopia* **81** E4
Welega *Ethiopia* **81** F3
Welford △ *Australia* **94** D3
Welkite *Ethiopia* **81** F4
Welkom *S. Africa* **88** D4
Welland *Canada* **114** D5
Welland → *U.K.* **15** E7
Wellesley Is. *Australia* **94** B2
Wellesley Islands ◎ *Australia* **94** B2
Wellingborough *U.K.* **15** E7
Wellington *Australia* **95** E4
Wellington *Canada* **114** C7
Wellington *N.Z.* **91** D5
Wellington *S. Africa* **88** E2
Wellington *Somst., U.K.* **15** G4
Wellington *Telford & Wrekin, U.K.* **15** E5
Wellington *Colo., U.S.A.* **108** F11
Wellington *Kans., U.S.A.* **112** G5
Wellington *Nev., U.S.A.* **110** G7
Wellington *Ohio, U.S.A.* **114** E2
Wellington *Tex., U.S.A.* **116** D4
Wellington, I. *Chile* **128** F2
Wellington, L. *Australia* **95** F4
Wellington Chan. *Canada* **101** C13
Wells *U.K.* **15** F5
Wells *Maine, U.S.A.* **115** C14
Wells *N.Y., U.S.A.* **115** C10
Wells *Nev., U.S.A.* **108** F6
Wells, L. *Australia* **93** E3
Wells, Mt. *Australia* **92** C4
Wells Gray △ *Canada* **102** C4
Wells-next-the-Sea *U.K.* **14** E8
Wells River *U.S.A.* **115** B12
Wellsboro *U.S.A.* **114** E7
Wellsburg *U.S.A.* **114** F4
Wellsville *N.Y., U.S.A.* **114** D7
Wellsville *Ohio, U.S.A.* **114** F4
Wellsville *Utah, U.S.A.* **108** F8
Wellton *U.S.A.* **109** K6
Welmel, Wabi → *Ethiopia* **81** F5
Welo *Ethiopia* **81** E4
Wels *Austria* **26** C7
Welshpool *U.K.* **15** E4
Welwyn Garden City *U.K.* **15** F7
Wem *U.K.* **14** E5
Wembere → *Tanzania* **86** C3
Wemindji *Canada* **104** B3
Wemyss *Canada* **115** B8
Wen Xian *China* **56** G7
Wenatchee *U.S.A.* **108** C3
Wenchang *China* **64** C8
Wencheng *China* **59** D13
Wenchi *Ghana* **82** D4
Wenchow = Wenzhou *China* **59** D13
Wenchuan *China* **58** B4
Wenden *U.S.A.* **111** M13
Wendeng *China* **57** F12
Wendesi *Indonesia* **63** E8
Wendo *Ethiopia* **81** F4
Wendover *U.S.A.* **108** F6
Weng'an *China* **58** D6
Wengcheng *China* **59** E9
Wengen *Switz.* **19** F14
Wengyuan *China* **59** E10
Wenjiang *China* **58** B4
Wenling *China* **59** C13
Wenlock → *Australia* **94** A3
Wenshan *China* **58** F5
Wenshang *China* **56** G9
Wenshui *China* **56** F7
Wensleydale *U.K.* **14** C6
Wensu *China* **60** B3
Wensum → *U.K.* **14** E8
Wentworth *Australia* **95** E3
Wentzel L. *Canada* **102** B6
Wenut *Indonesia* **63** E8

Wenxi *China* **56** G6
Wenxian *China* **56** H3
Wenzhou *China* **59** D13
Weott *U.S.A.* **108** F2
Wepener *S. Africa* **88** D4
Werda *Botswana* **88** D3
Werdau *Germany* **24** E8
Werder *Germany* **24** C8
Werdohl *Germany* **24** D3
Wereilu *Ethiopia* **81** E4
Weri *Indonesia* **63** E8
Werneck *Germany* **25** F6
Wernigerode *Germany* **24** D6
Werra → *Germany* **24** D5
Werrimull *Australia* **95** E3
Werris Creek *Australia* **95** E5
Wertach → *Germany* **25** G6
Wertheim *Germany* **25** F5
Wertingen *Germany* **25** G6
Wesel *Germany* **24** D2
Weser → *Germany* **24** B4
Weser-Ems □ *Germany* **24** C3
Weserbergland *Germany* **24** C5
Weserbergland Schaumburg Hameln △ *Germany* **24** C5
Wesiri *Indonesia* **63** F7
Weslaco *U.S.A.* **116** H6
Weslemkoon L. *Canada* **114** A7
Wesleyville *Canada* **105** C9
Wesleyville *U.S.A.* **114** D4
Wessel, C. *Australia* **94** A2
Wessel Is. *Australia* **94** A2
Wesselburen *Germany* **24** A4
Wessington Springs *U.S.A.* **112** C4
West □ *U.S.A.* **116** F6
West → *U.S.A.* **115** D12
West Allis *U.S.A.* **112** D9
West Antarctica *Antarctica* **5** D15
West Baines → *Australia* **92** C4
West Bank ■ *Asia* **74** C4
West Bend *U.S.A.* **112** D9
West Bengal □ *India* **69** H13
West Berkshire □ *U.K.* **15** F6
West Beskids = Západné Beskydy *Europe* **27** B12
West Branch *U.S.A.* **113** C11
West Branch Susquehanna → *U.S.A.* **115** F8
West Bromwich *U.K.* **15** E6
West Burra □ *U.K.* **13** A7
West Canada Cr. → *U.S.A.* **115** C10
West Caroline Basin *Pac. Oc.* **96** G5
West Chazy *U.S.A.* **115** B11
West Chester *U.S.A.* **115** G9
West Coast △ *Namibia* **88** C1
West Coast △ *S. Africa* **88** E2
West Columbia *U.S.A.* **116** G7
West Covina *U.S.A.* **111** L9
West Des Moines *U.S.A.* **112** E7
West Dunbartonshire □ *U.K.* **13** F4
West End *Bahamas* **120** A4
West Falkland *Falk. Is.* **128** G4
West Fargo *U.S.A.* **112** B6
West Fiji Basin *Pac. Oc.* **96** J9
West Fjord = Vestfjorden *Norway* **8** C16
West Fork Trinity → *U.S.A.* **116** E6
West Frankfort *U.S.A.* **112** G9
West Grand L. *U.S.A.* **113** C20
West Hartford *U.S.A.* **115** E12
West Haven *U.S.A.* **115** E12
West Hazleton *U.S.A.* **115** F9
West Helena *U.S.A.* **117** D9
West Hurley *U.S.A.* **115** E10
West Ice Shelf *Antarctica* **5** C7
West Indies *Cent. Amer.* **121** D7
West Jordan *U.S.A.* **108** F8
West Linn *U.S.A.* **110** E4
West Lorne *Canada* **114** D3
West Lothian □ *U.K.* **13** F5
West Lunga → *Zambia* **87** E1
West MacDonnell △ *Australia* **92** D5
West Mariana Basin *Pac. Oc.* **96** F5
West Memphis *U.S.A.* **117** D9
West Midlands □ *U.K.* **15** E6
West Mifflin *U.S.A.* **114** F5
West Milford *U.S.A.* **115** E10
West Milton *U.S.A.* **114** E8
West Monroe *U.S.A.* **116** E8
West Newton *U.S.A.* **114** F5
West Nicholson *Zimbabwe* **87** G2
West Odessa *U.S.A.* **116** F3
West Palm Beach *U.S.A.* **117** H14
West Plains *U.S.A.* **112** G8
West Point *Miss., U.S.A.* **117** E10
West Point *N.Y., U.S.A.* **115** E11
West Point *Nebr., U.S.A.* **112** E5
West Point *Va., U.S.A.* **113** G15
West Point L. *U.S.A.* **117** E12
West Pt. = Ouest, Pte. de l' *Canada* **105** C7
West Pt. *Australia* **95** F2
West Road → *Canada* **102** C4
West Rutland *U.S.A.* **115** C11
West Schelde = Westerschelde → *Neths.* **17** C3
West Seneca *U.S.A.* **114** D6

West Siberian Plain *Russia* **50** B9
West Sussex □ *U.K.* **15** G7
West-Terschelling *Neths.* **17** A5
West Valley City *U.S.A.* **108** F8
West Virginia □ *U.S.A.* **113** F13
West-Vlaanderen □ *Belgium* **17** D2
West Walker → *U.S.A.* **110** G7
West Wyalong *Australia* **95** E4
West Yellowstone *U.S.A.* **108** D8
West Yorkshire □ *U.K.* **14** D6
Westall, Pt. *Australia* **95** E1
Westbrook *U.S.A.* **113** D18
Westbury *Australia* **95** G4
Westby *U.S.A.* **108** B11
Westend *U.S.A.* **111** K9
Westerland *Germany* **24** A4
Westerly *U.S.A.* **115** E13
Western □ *Ghana* **82** D4
Western □ *Kenya* **86** B3
Western □ *S. Leone* **82** D2
Western □ *Zambia* **87** F1
Western Australia □ *Australia* **93** E2
Western Cape □ *S. Africa* **88** E3
Western Dvina = Daugava → *Latvia* **32** D3
Western Ghats *India* **66** N9
Western Isles □ *U.K.* **13** D1
Western Sahara ■ *Africa* **78** D3
Western Samoa = Samoa ■ *Pac. Oc.* **91** b
Western Sierra Madre = Madre Occidental, Sierra *Mexico* **118** B3
Westernport *U.S.A.* **113** F14
Westerschelde → *Neths.* **17** C3
Westerstede *Germany* **24** B3
Westerwald *Germany* **24** E3
Westfield *Mass., U.S.A.* **115** D12
Westfield *N.Y., U.S.A.* **114** D5
Westfield *Pa., U.S.A.* **114** E7
Westhill *U.K.* **13** D6
Westhope *U.S.A.* **112** A3
Westland △ *N.Z.* **91** E2
Westland Bight *N.Z.* **91** E3
Westlock *Canada* **102** C6
Westmar *Australia* **95** D4
Westmeath □ *Ireland* **12** C4
Westminster *Calif., U.S.A.* **111** M8
Westminster *Colo., U.S.A.* **108** G11
Westminster *Md., U.S.A.* **113** F15
Westmont *U.S.A.* **114** F6
Westmoreland *Barbados* **121** g
Westmorland *U.S.A.* **111** M11
Weston *Oreg., U.S.A.* **108** D4
Weston *W. Va., U.S.A.* **113** F13
Weston I. *Canada* **104** B4
Weston-super-Mare *U.K.* **15** F5
Westover *U.S.A.* **114** F6
Westport *Canada* **115** B8
Westport *Ireland* **12** C2
Westport *N.Z.* **91** D3
Westport *N.Y., U.S.A.* **115** B11
Westport *Oreg., U.S.A.* **110** D3
Westport *Wash., U.S.A.* **110** D2
Westray *Canada* **103** C8
Westray *U.K.* **13** B5
Westree *Canada* **104** C3
Westville *U.S.A.* **110** F6
Westwood *U.S.A.* **108** F3
Wetar *Indonesia* **63** F7
Wetaskiwin *Canada* **102** C6
Wete *Tanzania* **84** F7
Wetherby *U.K.* **14** D6
Wethersfield *U.S.A.* **115** E12
Wetteren *Belgium* **17** D3
Wetzlar *Germany* **24** E4
Wewoka *U.S.A.* **116** D6
Wexford *Ireland* **12** D5
Wexford □ *Ireland* **12** D5
Wexford Harbour *Ireland* **12** D5
Weyburn *Canada* **103** D8
Weyer Markt *Austria* **26** D7
Weyhe *Germany* **24** C4
Weyib → *Ethiopia* **81** F5
Weymouth *Canada* **105** D6
Weymouth *U.K.* **15** G5
Weymouth *U.S.A.* **115** D14
Weymouth, C. *Australia* **94** A3
Wha Ti *Canada* **100** E8
Whakaari *N.Z.* **91** B6
Whakatane *N.Z.* **91** B6
Whale = Baleine → *Canada* **105** A6
Whale Cove *Canada* **103** A10
Whales, B. of *Antarctica* **5** D12
Whalsay *U.K.* **13** A8
Whangamata *N.Z.* **91** B5
Whangamomona *N.Z.* **91** C5
Whanganui △ *N.Z.* **91** C5
Whangarei *N.Z.* **91** A5
Whangarei Harb. *N.Z.* **91** A5
Wharekauri = Chatham Is. *Pac. Oc.* **96** M10
Wharfe → *U.K.* **14** D6
Wharfedale *U.K.* **14** C5
Wharton *N.J., U.S.A.* **115** F10
Wharton *Pa., U.S.A.* **114** E6
Wharton *Tex., U.S.A.* **116** G6
Wharton Basin *Ind. Oc.* **96** K1
Wheatland *Calif., U.S.A.* **110** F5

Wheatland *Wyo., U.S.A.* **108** E11
Wheatley *Canada* **114** D2
Wheaton *Md., U.S.A.* **113** F15
Wheaton *Minn., U.S.A.* **112** C5
Wheelbarrow Pk. *U.S.A.* **110** H10
Wheeler *Oreg., U.S.A.* **108** D2
Wheeler *Tex., U.S.A.* **116** D4
Wheeler → *Canada* **105** A6
Wheeler L. *U.S.A.* **117** D11
Wheeler Pk. *N. Mex., U.S.A.* **109** H11
Wheeler Pk. *Nev., U.S.A.* **108** G6
Wheeler Ridge *U.S.A.* **111** L8
Wheelersburg *U.S.A.* **113** F12
Wheeling *U.S.A.* **114** F4
Whernside *U.K.* **14** C5
Whiddy I. *Ireland* **12** E2
Whim Creek *Australia* **92** D2
Whiskey Jack L. *Canada* **103** B8
Whiskeytown-Shasta-Trinity △ *U.S.A.* **108** F2
Whistleduck Cr. → *Australia* **94** C2
Whistler *Canada* **102** C4
Whitby *Canada* **114** C6
Whitby *U.K.* **14** C7
White → *Ark., U.S.A.* **116** E9
White → *Ind., U.S.A.* **112** F10
White → *S. Dak., U.S.A.* **112** D4
White → *Tex., U.S.A.* **116** E4
White → *Utah, U.S.A.* **108** F9
White → *Vt., U.S.A.* **115** C12
White → *Wash., U.S.A.* **110** C4
White, L. *Australia* **92** D4
White B. *Canada* **105** C8
White Bird *U.S.A.* **108** D5
White Butte *U.S.A.* **112** B2
White City *U.S.A.* **108** E2
White Cliffs *Australia* **95** E3
White Desert = Sahrā al Beida *Egypt* **80** B2
White Hall *U.S.A.* **112** F8
White Haven *U.S.A.* **115** E9
White Horse, Vale of *U.K.* **15** F6
White I. = Whakaari *N.Z.* **91** B6
White L. *Canada* **115** A8
White L. *U.S.A.* **116** G8
White Lake *Canada* **115** A8
White Mountain Peak *U.S.A.* **109** H4
White Mts. *Calif., U.S.A.* **110** H8
White Mts. *N.H., U.S.A.* **115** B13
White Mts. △ *Australia* **94** C4
White Nile = Nîl el Abyad → *Sudan* **81** D3
White Nile Dam = Khazzân Jabal al Awliyâ *Sudan* **81** D3
White Otter L. *Canada* **104** C1
White Pass *U.S.A.* **110** D5
White Plains *U.S.A.* **115** E11
White River *Canada* **104** C2
White River *U.S.A.* **112** D3
White Rock *Canada* **110** A4
White Rock *U.S.A.* **109** J10
White Russia = Belarus ■ *Europe* **23** B14
White Sands △ *U.S.A.* **109** K10
White Sea = Beloye More *Russia* **8** C25
White Sulphur Springs *Mont., U.S.A.* **108** C8
White Sulphur Springs *W. Va., U.S.A.* **113** G13
White Swan *U.S.A.* **110** D6
White Volta → *Ghana* **83** D4
Whitecliffs *N.Z.* **91** E3
Whitecourt *Canada* **102** C5
Whiteface Mt. *U.S.A.* **115** B11
Whitefield *U.S.A.* **115** B13
Whitefish *U.S.A.* **108** B6
Whitefish B. *U.S.A.* **104** C3
Whitefish L. *Canada* **103** A7
Whitefish Pt. *U.S.A.* **113** B11
Whitegull, L. = Goélands, L. aux *Canada* **105** A7
Whitehall *Mich., U.S.A.* **112** D10
Whitehall *Mont., U.S.A.* **108** D7
Whitehall *N.Y., U.S.A.* **115** C11
Whitehall *Wis., U.S.A.* **112** C8
Whitehaven *U.K.* **14** C4
Whitehorse *Canada* **102** A1
Whitemark *Australia* **95** G4
Whiteplains *Liberia* **82** D2
Whiteriver *U.S.A.* **109** K9
Whitesand → *Canada* **102** A5
Whitesands *S. Africa* **88** E3
Whitesboro *N.Y., U.S.A.* **115** C9
Whitesboro *Tex., U.S.A.* **116** E6
Whiteshell △ *Canada* **103** D9
Whiteville *U.S.A.* **117** D15
Whitewater *U.S.A.* **112** D9
Whitewater Baldy *U.S.A.* **109** K9
Whitewater L. *Canada* **104** B2
Whitewood *Australia* **94** C3
Whitewood *Canada* **103** C8
Whithorn *U.K.* **13** G4
Whitianga *N.Z.* **91** B5
Whitman *U.S.A.* **115** D14
Whitney *Canada* **114** A6
Whitney, Mt. *U.S.A.* **110** J8
Whitney Point *U.S.A.* **115** D9

Whitstable *U.K.* **15** F9
Whitsunday I. *Australia* **94** b
Whitsunday Islands △ *Australia* **94** b
Whittier *Alaska, U.S.A.* **106** C10
Whittier *Calif., U.S.A.* **111** M8
Whittlesea *Australia* **95** F4
Wholdaia L. *Canada* **103** A8
Whyalla *Australia* **95** E2
Whyjalla *Australia* **95** E2
Wiang Kosai △ *Thailand* **64** D2
Wiang Sa *Thailand* **64** C3
Wiarton *Canada* **114** B3
Wiawso *Ghana* **82** D4
Wiay *U.K.* **13** D1
Wiązów *Poland* **31** H4
Wibaux *U.S.A.* **108** C11
Wichian Buri *Thailand* **64** E3
Wichita *U.S.A.* **112** G5
Wichita Falls *U.S.A.* **116** E5
Wick *U.K.* **13** C5
Wickenburg *U.S.A.* **109** K7
Wickepin *Australia* **93** F2
Wickham *Australia* **92** D2
Wickham, C. *Australia* **95** F3
Wickliffe *U.S.A.* **114** E3
Wicklow *Ireland* **12** D5
Wicklow □ *Ireland* **12** D5
Wicklow Hd. *Ireland* **12** D6
Wicklow Mts. *Ireland* **12** C5
Wicklow Mts. △ *Ireland* **12** C5
Widawa *Poland* **31** G5
Widawka → *Poland* **31** G5
Widgeegoara Cr. → *Australia* **95** D4
Widgiemooltha *Australia* **93** F3
Widnes *U.K.* **14** D5
Więcbork *Poland* **31** E4
Wiehengebirge = Nördlicher Teutoburger Wald-Wiehengebirge △ *Germany* **24** C4
Wiehl *Germany* **24** E3
Wiek *Germany* **24** A9
Wielbark *Poland* **30** E7
Wieleń *Poland* **31** F3
Wielichowo *Poland* **31** F3
Wieliczka *Poland* **31** J7
Wielkopolski △ *Poland* **31** F3
Wielkopolskie □ *Poland* **31** F4
Wieluń *Poland* **31** G5
Wien *Austria* **27** C9
Wien-Schwechat ✈ (VIE) *Austria* **27** C9
Wiener Neustadt *Austria* **27** D9
Wieprz → *Poland* **31** G8
Wieprza → *Poland* **30** D3
Wieruszów *Poland* **31** G5
Wiesbaden *Germany* **25** E4
Wiesental *Germany* **25** F4
Wiesloch *Germany* **25** F4
Wiesmoor *Germany* **24** B3
Wieżyca *Poland* **30** D5
Wiggins *Colo., U.S.A.* **108** F11
Wiggins *Miss., U.S.A.* **117** F10
Wight, I. of *U.K.* **15** G6
Wigierski △ *Poland* **30** D10
Wigry, Jezioro *Poland* **30** D10
Wigston *U.K.* **15** E6
Wigton *U.K.* **14** C4
Wigtown *U.K.* **13** G4
Wigtown B. *U.K.* **13** G4
Wik and Wikway People ◎ *Australia* **94** A3
Wil *Switz.* **25** H5
Wilamowice *Poland* **31** J6
Wilber *U.S.A.* **112** E5
Wilberforce *Canada* **114** A6
Wilberforce, C. *Australia* **94** A2
Wilburton *U.S.A.* **116** D7
Wilcannia *Australia* **95** E3
Wilcox *U.S.A.* **114** E6
Wildbad *Germany* **25** G4
Wildeshausen *Germany* **24** C4
Wildeshauser Geest △ *Germany* **24** C4
Wildon *Austria* **26** E8
Wildrose *U.S.A.* **111** J9
Wildspitze *Austria* **26** E3
Wilga → *Poland* **31** G8
Wilge → *S. Africa* **89** D4
Wilhelm II Coast *Antarctica* **5** C7
Wilhelmsburg *Austria* **26** C8
Wilhelmshaven *Germany* **24** B4
Wilhelmstal *Namibia* **88** C2
Wilkes-Barre *U.S.A.* **115** E9
Wilkes Land *Antarctica* **5** D9
Wilkie *Canada* **103** C7
Wilkinsburg *U.S.A.* **114** F5
Wilkinson Lakes *Australia* **93** E5
Willandra Creek → *Australia* **95** E4
Willapa B. *U.S.A.* **108** C1
Willapa Hills *U.S.A.* **110** D3
Willard *U.S.A.* **114** E2
Willare Bridge Roadhouse *Australia* **92** C3
Willcox *U.S.A.* **109** K9
Willemstad *Neth. Ant.* **121** D6
William → *Canada* **103** B7

William 'Bill' Dannelly Res. *U.S.A.* **117** E11
William Creek *Australia* **95** D2
Williams *Australia* **93** F2
Williams *Ariz., U.S.A.* **109** J7
Williams *Calif., U.S.A.* **110** F4
Williams Harbour *Canada* **105** B8
Williams Lake *Canada* **102** C4
Williamsburg *Ky., U.S.A.* **113** G11
Williamsburg *Pa., U.S.A.* **114** F6
Williamsburg *Va., U.S.A.* **113** G15
Williamson *N.Y., U.S.A.* **114** C7
Williamson *W. Va., U.S.A.* **113** G12
Williamsport *U.S.A.* **114** E7
Williamston *U.S.A.* **117** D16
Williamstown *Australia* **95** F3
Williamstown *Ky., U.S.A.* **113** F11
Williamstown *Mass., U.S.A.* **115** D11
Williamstown *N.Y., U.S.A.* **115** C9
Willimantic *U.S.A.* **115** E12
Willingboro *U.S.A.* **113** E16
Williston *S. Africa* **88** E3
Williston *Fla., U.S.A.* **117** G13
Williston *N. Dak., U.S.A.* **112** A2
Williston L. *Canada* **102** B4
Willits *U.S.A.* **108** G2
Willmar *U.S.A.* **112** C6
Willmore Wilderness △ *Canada* **102** C5
Willoughby *U.S.A.* **114** E3
Willow Bunch *Canada* **103** D7
Willow L. *Canada* **102** A5
Willow Wall, The *China* **57** C12
Willowick *U.S.A.* **114** E3
Willowlake → *Canada* **102** A4
Willowmore *S. Africa* **88** E3
Willows *U.S.A.* **110** F4
Willowvale = Gatyana *S. Africa* **89** E4
Wills, L. *Australia* **92** D4
Wills Cr. → *Australia* **94** C3
Willsboro *U.S.A.* **115** B11
Willunga *Australia* **95** F2
Wilmette *U.S.A.* **112** D10
Wilmington *Australia* **95** E2
Wilmington *Del., U.S.A.* **113** F16
Wilmington *N.C., U.S.A.* **117** D16
Wilmington *Ohio, U.S.A.* **113** F12
Wilmington *Vt., U.S.A.* **115** D12
Wilmslow *U.K.* **14** D5
Wilpena Cr. → *Australia* **95** E2
Wilsall *U.S.A.* **108** D8
Wilson *N.C., U.S.A.* **117** D16
Wilson *N.Y., U.S.A.* **114** C6
Wilson *Pa., U.S.A.* **115** F9
Wilson → *Australia* **92** C4
Wilson Bluff *Australia* **93** F4
Wilson Inlet *Australia* **93** G2
Wilsons Promontory *Australia* **95** F4
Wilster *Germany* **24** B5
Wilton *U.S.A.* **112** B3
Wilton → *Australia* **94** A1
Wiltshire □ *U.K.* **15** F6
Wiltz *Lux.* **17** E5
Wiluna *Australia* **93** E3
Wimborne Minster *U.K.* **15** G6
Wimereux *France* **19** B8
Wimmera → *Australia* **95** F3
Winam G. *Kenya* **86** C3
Winburg *S. Africa* **88** D4
Winchendon *U.S.A.* **115** D12
Winchester *U.K.* **15** F6
Winchester *Conn., U.S.A.* **115** E11
Winchester *Idaho, U.S.A.* **108** C5
Winchester *Ind., U.S.A.* **113** E11
Winchester *Ky., U.S.A.* **113** G11
Winchester *N.H., U.S.A.* **115** D12
Winchester *Nev., U.S.A.* **111** J11
Winchester *Tenn., U.S.A.* **117** D11
Winchester *Va., U.S.A.* **113** F14
Wind → *U.S.A.* **108** E9
Wind Cave △ *U.S.A.* **112** D2
Wind River Range *U.S.A.* **108** E9
Windamere, L. *Australia* **95** B4
Windau = Ventspils *Latvia* **30** A8
Windber *U.S.A.* **114** F6
Winder *U.S.A.* **117** D13
Windermere *U.K.* **14** C5
Windhoek *Namibia* **88** C2
Windidda ◎ *Australia* **93** E3
Windischgarsten *Austria* **26** D7
Windjana Gorge △ *Australia* **92** C3
Windom *U.S.A.* **112** D6
Windorah *Australia* **94** D3
Window Rock *U.S.A.* **109** J9
Windrush → *U.K.* **15** F6
Windsor *Australia* **95** E5
Windsor *N.S., Canada* **105** D7
Windsor *Ont., Canada* **114** D2
Windsor *U.K.* **15** F7
Windsor *Calif., U.S.A.* **108** G2
Windsor *Colo., U.S.A.* **108** F11
Windsor *Conn., U.S.A.* **115** E12
Windsor *Mo., U.S.A.* **112** F7
Windsor *N.Y., U.S.A.* **115** D9
Windsor *Vt., U.S.A.* **115** C12
Windsor & Maidenhead □ *U.K.* **15** F7

Windsorton *S. Africa* **88** D3
Windward Is. *W. Indies* **121** D7
Windward Passage = Vientos, Paso de los *Caribbean* **121** C5
Winefred L. *Canada* **103** B6
Winejok *Sudan* **81** F2
Winfield *U.S.A.* **112** G5
Wingate Mts. *Australia* **92** B5
Wingellina = Irrunytju *Australia* **93** E4
Wingham *Australia* **95** E5
Wingham *Canada* **114** C3
Winisk → *Canada* **104** A2
Winisk L. *Canada* **104** B2
Wink *U.S.A.* **116** F3
Winkler *Canada* **103** D9
Winklern *Austria* **26** E5
Winlock *U.S.A.* **110** D4
Winneba *Ghana* **83** D4
Winnebago, L. *U.S.A.* **112** D9
Winnecke Cr. → *Australia* **92** C5
Winnemucca *U.S.A.* **108** F5
Winnemucca L. *U.S.A.* **108** F4
Winner *U.S.A.* **112** D4
Winnett *U.S.A.* **108** C9
Winnfield *U.S.A.* **116** F8
Winnibigoshish, L. *U.S.A.* **112** B6
Winnipeg *Canada* **103** D9
Winnipeg → *Canada* **103** C9
Winnipeg, L. *Canada* **103** C9
Winnipeg Beach *Canada* **103** C9
Winnipegosis *Canada* **103** C9
Winnipegosis L. *Canada* **103** C9
Winnipesaukee, L. *U.S.A.* **115** C13
Winnisquam L. *U.S.A.* **115** C13
Winnsboro *La., U.S.A.* **116** F9
Winnsboro *S.C., U.S.A.* **117** D14
Winnsboro *Tex., U.S.A.* **116** E7
Winokapau, L. *Canada* **105** B7
Winona *Minn., U.S.A.* **112** C8
Winona *Miss., U.S.A.* **117** E10
Winooski *U.S.A.* **115** B11
Winooski → *U.S.A.* **115** B11
Winschoten *Neths.* **17** A7
Winsen *Germany* **24** B6
Winsford *U.K.* **14** D5
Winslow = Bainbridge Island *U.S.A.* **110** C4
Winslow *U.S.A.* **109** J8
Winsted *U.S.A.* **115** E11
Winston-Salem *U.S.A.* **117** C14
Winter Garden *U.S.A.* **117** G14
Winter Haven *U.S.A.* **117** G14
Winter Park *U.S.A.* **117** G14
Winterberg *Germany* **24** D4
Winterhaven *U.S.A.* **111** N12
Winters *U.S.A.* **110** G5
Winterset *U.S.A.* **112** E6
Wintersville *U.S.A.* **114** F4
Winterswijk *Neths.* **17** C6
Winterthur *Switz.* **25** H4
Winthrop *U.S.A.* **108** B3
Winton *Australia* **94** C3
Winton *N.Z.* **91** G2
Wipper → *Germany* **24** D7
Wirlyajarrayi ◉ *Australia* **92** D5
Wirrulla *Australia* **95** E1
Wisbech *U.K.* **15** E8
Wisconsin □ *U.S.A.* **112** C9
Wisconsin → *U.S.A.* **112** D8
Wisconsin Rapids *U.S.A.* **112** C9
Wisdom *U.S.A.* **108** D7
Wiseman *U.S.A.* **106** B9
Wishaw *U.K.* **13** F5
Wishek *U.S.A.* **112** B4
Wisła *Poland* **31** J5
Wisła → *Poland* **30** D5
Wisłok → *Poland* **31** H9
Wisłoka → *Poland* **31** H8
Wismar *Germany* **24** B7
Wisner *U.S.A.* **112** E5
Wissant *France* **19** B8
Wissembourg *France* **19** C14
Wisznice *Poland* **31** G10
Witbank = eMalahleni *S. Africa* **89** D4
Witdraai *S. Africa* **88** D3
Witham *U.K.* **15** F8
Witham → *U.K.* **14** E7
Withernsea *U.K.* **14** D8
Witjira △ *Australia* **95** D2
Witkowo *Poland* **31** F4
Witless Bay *Canada* **105** C9
Witney *U.K.* **15** F6
Witnica *Poland* **31** F1
Witossob → *Namibia* **88** D3
Witrivier *S. Africa* **89** D5
Wittdün *Germany* **24** A4
Witten *Germany* **24** D3
Wittenberge *Germany* **24** B7
Wittenburg *Germany* **24** B7
Wittenheim *France* **19** E14
Wittenoom *Australia* **92** D2
Wittingen *Germany* **24** C6
Witlich *Germany* **25** F2
Wittmund *Germany* **24** B3
Wittow *Germany* **24** A9
Wittstock *Germany* **24** B8

Witvlei *Namibia* **88** C2
Witzenhausen *Germany* **24** D5
Wiwon *N. Korea* **57** D14
Wkra → *Poland* **31** F7
Władysławowo *Poland* **30** D5
Wleń *Poland* **31** G2
Wlingi *Indonesia* **63** H15
Włocławek *Poland* **31** F6
Włodawa *Poland* **31** G10
Włoszczowa *Poland* **31** H6
Woburn *U.S.A.* **115** D13
Wodian *China* **56** H7
Wodonga *Australia* **95** F4
Wodzisław Śląski *Poland* **31** H5
Wœrth *France* **19** D14
Woinbogoin *China* **58** A2
Woippy *France* **19** C13
Wojcieszow *Poland* **31** H2
Wokam *Indonesia* **63** F8
Woking *U.K.* **15** F7
Wokingham *U.K.* **15** F7
Wokingham □ *U.K.* **15** F7
Wolbrom *Poland* **31** H6
Wolczyn *Poland* **31** G5
Woldegk *Germany* **24** B9
Wolf → *Canada* **102** A2
Wolf Creek *U.S.A.* **108** C7
Wolf L. *Canada* **102** A2
Wolf Point *U.S.A.* **108** B11
Wolfe Creek Crater △ *Australia* **92** C4
Wolfe I. *Canada* **115** B8
Wolfeboro *U.S.A.* **115** C13
Wolfen *Germany* **24** D8
Wolfenbüttel *Germany* **24** C6
Wolfratshausen *Germany* **25** H7
Wolfsberg *Austria* **26** E7
Wolfsburg *Germany* **24** C6
Wolgast *Germany* **24** A9
Wolhusen *Switz.* **25** H4
Wolin *Poland* **30** E1
Woliński △ *Poland* **30** E1
Wollaston, Is. *Chile* **128** H3
Wollaston L. *Canada* **103** B8
Wollaston Lake *Canada* **103** B8
Wollaston Pen. *Canada* **100** D9
Wollongong *Australia* **95** E5
Wolmaransstad *S. Africa* **88** D4
Wolmirstedt *Germany* **24** C7
Wołomin *Poland* **31** F8
Wolseley *S. Africa* **88** E2
Wolsey *U.S.A.* **112** C4
Wolstenholme, C. *Canada* **98** C12
Wolsztyn *Poland* **31** F3
Wolvega *Neths.* **17** B6
Wolverhampton *U.K.* **15** E5
Wondai *Australia* **95** D5
Wongalarroo L. *Australia* **95** E3
Wongan Hills *Australia* **93** F2
Wonju *S. Korea* **57** F14
Wonosari *Indonesia* **63** G14
Wonosobo *Indonesia* **63** G13
Wonowon *Canada* **102** B4
Wŏnsan *N. Korea* **57** E14
Wonthaggi *Australia* **95** F4
Wood Buffalo △ *Canada* **102** B6
Wood Is. *Australia* **92** C3
Wood L. *Canada* **103** B8
Woodah, I. *Australia* **94** A2
Woodbourne *U.S.A.* **115** E10
Woodbridge *Canada* **114** C5
Woodbridge *U.K.* **15** E9
Woodburn *Australia* **95** A5
Woodburn *U.S.A.* **108** D2
Woodenbong *Australia* **95** D5
Woodend *Australia* **95** F3
Woodford *Australia* **95** D5
Woodfords *U.S.A.* **110** G7
Woodlake *U.S.A.* **110** J7
Woodland *Calif., U.S.A.* **110** G5
Woodland *Maine, U.S.A.* **113** C20
Woodland *Pa., U.S.A.* **114** F6
Woodland *Wash., U.S.A.* **110** E4
Woodland Caribou △ *Canada* **103** C10
Woodlands *Singapore* **65** d
Woodlands, The *U.S.A.* **116** F7
Woodonga *Australia* **95** F4
Woodridge *Canada* **103** D9
Woodroffe, Mt. *Australia* **93** E5
Woods, L. *Australia* **94** B1
Woods, L. of the *Canada* **103** D10
Woods, L. of the *U.S.A.* **107** F21
Woods Bay *Canada* **114** A5
Woodstock *Australia* **94** B4
Woodstock *N.B., Canada* **105** C6
Woodstock *Ont., Canada* **114** C4
Woodstock *U.K.* **15** F6
Woodstock *Ill., U.S.A.* **112** D9
Woodstock *N.Y., U.S.A.* **115** D10
Woodstock *Vt., U.S.A.* **115** C12
Woodsville *U.S.A.* **115** B13
Woodview *Canada* **114** B6
Woodville *N.Z.* **91** D5
Woodville *Miss., U.S.A.* **116** F9
Woodville *Tex., U.S.A.* **116** F7
Woodward *U.S.A.* **116** C5
Woody *U.S.A.* **111** K8
Woody → *Canada* **103** C8

Woolacombe *U.K.* **15** F3
Woolamai, C. *Australia* **95** F4
Woolgoolga *Australia* **95** E5
Woomera *Australia* **95** E2
Woonsocket *R.I., U.S.A.* **115** E13
Woonsocket *S. Dak., U.S.A.* **112** C4
Wooramel → *Australia* **93** E1
Wooramel Roadhouse *Australia* **93** E1
Wooroonooran △ *Australia* **94** B4
Wooster *U.S.A.* **114** F3
Worcester *S. Africa* **88** E2
Worcester *U.K.* **15** E5
Worcester *Mass., U.S.A.* **115** D13
Worcester *N.Y., U.S.A.* **115** D10
Worcestershire □ *U.K.* **15** E5
Wörgl *Austria* **26** D5
Workington *U.K.* **14** C4
Worksop *U.K.* **14** D6
Workum *Neths.* **17** B5
Worland *U.S.A.* **108** D10
Wormhout *France* **19** B9
Worms *Germany* **25** F9
Worsley *Canada* **102** B5
Wortham *U.S.A.* **116** F6
Wörther See *Austria* **26** E7
Worthing *Barbados* **121** g
Worthing *U.K.* **15** G7
Worthington *Minn., U.S.A.* **112** D6
Worthington *Pa., U.S.A.* **114** F5
Wosi *Indonesia* **63** E7
Wote *Kenya* **86** C4
Wotjalum ◉ *Australia* **92** C3
Wotjobaluk = *Australia* **95** C3
Wou-han = Wuhan *China* **59** B10
Wousi = Wuxi *China* **59** B13
Wowoni *Indonesia* **63** E6
Wrangel I. = Vrangelya, Ostrov *Russia* **53** B18
Wrangell *U.S.A.* **102** B2
Wrangell Mts. *U.S.A.* **100** E3
Wrath, C. *U.K.* **13** C3
Wray *U.S.A.* **108** E3
Wrekin, The *U.K.* **15** E5
Wrens *U.S.A.* **117** E13
Wrexham *U.K.* **14** D5
Wrexham □ *U.K.* **14** D5
Wriezen *Germany* **24** C10
Wright = Paranas *Phil.* **61** F6
Wright *Fla., U.S.A.* **117** F11
Wright *Wyo., U.S.A.* **108** E11
Wright Pt. *Canada* **114** C3
Wrightson, Mt. *U.S.A.* **109** L8
Wrightwood *U.S.A.* **111** L9
Wrigley *Canada* **100** E7
Wrocław *Poland* **31** G4
Wronki *Poland* **31** F3
Września *Poland* **31** F4
Wschowa *Poland* **31** G3
Wu Jiang → *China* **58** C6
Wu'an *China* **56** F8
Wubalawun ◉ *Australia* **92** C5
Wubin *Australia* **93** F2
Wubu *China* **56** F6
Wuchang *China* **57** B14
Wucheng *China* **56** F9
Wuchuan *Guangdong, China* **59** G8
Wuchuan *Guizhou, China* **58** C7
Wuchuan *Nei Monggol Zizhiqu, China* **56** D6
Wudi *China* **57** F9
Wuding *China* **58** E4
Wuding He → *China* **56** F6
Wudinna *Australia* **95** E2
Wudu *China* **56** H3
Wufeng *China* **59** B8
Wugang *China* **59** D8
Wugong Shan *China* **59** D9
Wugullar = Beswick *Australia* **92** B5
Wuhan *China* **59** B10
Wuhe *China* **57** H9
Wuhsi = Wuxi *China* **59** B13
Wuhu *China* **59** B12
Wujiang *China* **59** B13
Wukari *Nigeria* **83** D6
Wulajie *China* **57** B14
Wulanbulang *China* **56** D6
Wular L. *India* **69** B6
Wulehe *Ghana* **83** D5
Wulian *China* **57** G10
Wuliang Shan *China* **58** E3
Wuliaru *Indonesia* **63** F8
Wuling Shan *China* **58** C7
Wulong *China* **58** C6
Wulumuchi = Ürümqi *China* **52** B3
Wum *Cameroon* **83** D7
Wuming *China* **58** F7
Wun Rog *Sudan* **81** F2
Wundanyi *Kenya* **86** C4
Wuning *China* **59** C10
Wunnummin L. *Canada* **104** B2
Wunsiedel *Germany* **25** E8
Wunstorf *Germany* **24** C5
Wuntho *Burma* **67** H19
Wupatki △ *U.S.A.* **109** J8
Wuping *China* **59** E11
Wuppertal *Germany* **24** D3

Wuppertal *S. Africa* **88** E2
Wuqing *China* **57** E9
Wurralibi ◉ *Australia* **94** B2
Wurtsboro *U.S.A.* **115** E10
Würzburg *Germany* **25** F5
Wurzen *Germany* **24** D8
Wushan *China* **56** G3
Wushishi *Nigeria* **83** D6
Wutach → *Germany* **25** H4
Wutai *China* **56** E7
Wuting = Huimin *China* **57** F9
Wutong *China* **59** E8
Wutonghaolai *China* **57** C11
Wutongqiao *China* **58** C4
Wuwei *Anhui, China* **59** B11
Wuwei *Gansu, China* **60** C5
Wuxi *Jiangsu, China* **59** B13
Wuxi *Sichuan, China* **58** B7
Wuxiang *China* **56** F7
Wuxuan *China* **58** F7
Wuxue *China* **59** C10
Wuyang *China* **56** H7
Wuyi *Hebei, China* **56** F8
Wuyi *Zhejiang, China* **59** C12
Wuyi Shan *China* **59** D11
Wuyishan *China* **59** D12
Wuyo *China* **83** C7
Wuyuan *Nei Monggol Zizhiqu, China* **56** D5
Wuyuan *Jiangxi, China* **59** C11
Wuzhai *China* **56** E6
Wuzhi Shan *China* **64** C7
Wuzhong *China* **56** E4
Wuzhou *China* **59** F8
Wyaaba Cr. → *Australia* **94** B3
Wyalkatchem *Australia* **93** F2
Wyalusing *U.S.A.* **115** E8
Wyandotte *U.S.A.* **113** D12
Wyandra *Australia* **95** D4
Wyangala, L. *Australia* **95** E4
Wyara, L. *Australia* **95** D3
Wycheproof *Australia* **95** F3
Wycliffe Well *Australia* **94** C1
Wye → *U.K.* **15** F5
Wyemandoo *Australia* **93** E2
Wyk *Germany* **24** A4
Wymondham *U.K.* **15** E9
Wymore *U.S.A.* **112** E5
Wyndham *Australia* **92** C4
Wyndham *N.Z.* **91** G2
Wynne *U.S.A.* **117** D9
Wynyard *Australia* **95** G4
Wynyard *Canada* **103** C8
Wyola L. *Australia* **95** E5
Wyoming *Canada* **114** D2
Wyoming □ *U.S.A.* **108** E10
Wyomissing *U.S.A.* **115** F9
Wyong *Australia* **95** E5
Wyrzysk *Poland* **31** F4
Wyśmierzyce *Poland* **31** G7
Wysoka *Poland* **31** E4
Wysokie *Poland* **31** H9
Wysokie Mazowieckie *Poland* **31** F9
Wyszków *Poland* **31** F8
Wyszogród *Poland* **31** F7
Wytheville *U.S.A.* **113** G13
Wyżyna Małopolska *Poland* **31** H7

X

Xaafuun *Somali Rep.* **75** E5
Xaafuun, Ras *Somali Rep.* **75** E5
Xaçmaz *Azerbaijan* **35** K9
Xai-Xai *Mozam.* **89** D5
Xainza *China* **60** C3
Xalapa *Mexico* **119** D5
Xallas → *Spain* **36** C1
Xangongo *Angola* **88** B2
Xankändi *Azerbaijan* **73** C12
Xanlar *Azerbaijan* **35** K8
Xanten *Germany* **24** D2
Xanthi *Greece* **45** E8
Xanthi □ *Greece* **45** E8
Xanthos *Turkey* **47** E11
Xanxerê *Brazil* **127** B5
Xapuri *Brazil* **124** F5
Xar Moron He → *China* **57** C11
Xarrë *Albania* **44** G4
Xátiva *Spain* **39** G4
Xau, L. *Botswana* **88** C3
Xavantina *Brazil* **127** A5
Xenia *U.S.A.* **113** F12
Xeropotamos → *Cyprus* **49** E11
Xertigny *France* **19** D13
Xhora *S. Africa* **89** E4
Xhumo *Botswana* **88** C3
Xi Jiang → *China* **59** F9
Xi Xian *Henan, China* **59** A10
Xi Xian *Shanxi, China* **56** F6
Xia Xian *China* **56** G6
Xiachengzi *China* **57** B16
Xiachuan Dao *China* **59** G9
Xiaguan *China* **60** D5
Xiajiang *China* **59** D10
Xiajin *China* **56** F9
Xiamen *China* **59** E12
Xi'an *China* **56** G5
Xian Xian *China* **56** E9
Xianfeng *China* **58** C7

Xiang Jiang → *China* **59** C9
Xiangcheng *Henan, China* **56** H8
Xiangcheng *Henan, China* **56** H7
Xiangcheng *Sichuan, China* **58** C2
Xiangdu *China* **58** F6
Xiangfan *China* **59** A9
Xianggang = Hong Kong □ *China* **59** F10
Xianghuang Qi *China* **56** C7
Xiangning *China* **56** G6
Xiangquan *China* **56** F7
Xiangquan He = Sutlej → *Pakistan* **68** E4
Xiangshan *China* **59** C13
Xiangshui *China* **57** G10
Xiangtan *China* **59** D9
Xiangxiang *China* **59** D9
Xiangyin *China* **59** C9
Xiangyun *China* **58** E3
Xiangzhou *China* **58** F7
Xianju *China* **59** C13
Xianning *China* **59** C10
Xiantao *China* **59** B9
Xianyang *China* **56** G5
Xianyou *China* **59** E12
Xiao Hinggan Ling *China* **60** B7
Xiao Xian *China* **56** G9
Xiaofeng *China* **59** B12
Xiaogan *China* **59** B9
Xiaojin *China* **58** B4
Xiaolan *China* **59** F9
Xiaoshan *China* **59** B13
Xiaoyi *China* **56** F6
Xiapu *China* **59** D12
Xiawa *China* **57** C11
Xiayi *China* **56** G9
Xichang *China* **58** D4
Xichong *China* **58** B5
Xichou *China* **58** E5
Xichuan *China* **56** H6
Xide *China* **58** C4
Xiemahe *China* **59** B8
Xieng Khouang *Laos* **64** C4
Xifei He → *China* **56** H9
Xifeng *Gansu, China* **56** G4
Xifeng *Guizhou, China* **58** D6
Xifeng *Liaoning, China* **57** C13
Xifengzhen = Xifeng *China* **56** G4
Xigazê *China* **60** D3
Xihe *China* **56** G3
Xihua *China* **56** H8
Xilagani *Greece* **45** F9
Xiliao He → *China* **57** C12
Xilin *China* **58** E5
Xilinhot *China* **56** C9
Xilokastro *Greece* **46** C4
Ximana *Mozam.* **87** F3
Xime *Guinea-Biss.* **82** C2
Ximeng *China* **58** F2
Xin Jiang → *China* **59** C11
Xin Xian = Xinzhou *China* **56** E7
Xinavane *Mozam.* **89** D5
Xinbin *China* **57** D13
Xincai *China* **59** A10
Xinchang *China* **59** C13
Xincheng *Guangxi Zhuangzu, China* **58** E7
Xincheng *Jiangxi, China* **59** D10
Xincun *China* **57** E9
Xindu *China* **58** B5
Xinfeng *Guangdong, China* **59** E10
Xinfeng *Jiangxi, China* **59** D11
Xinfeng *Jiangxi, China* **59** D10
Xinfengjiang Shuiku *China* **59** F10
Xing Xian *China* **56** E6
Xing'an *Guangxi Zhuangzu, China* **59** E8
Xingan *Jiangxi, China* **59** D10
Xingcheng *China* **57** D11
Xingguo *China* **59** D10
Xinghe *China* **56** D7
Xinghua *China* **57** H10
Xinghua Wan *China* **59** E12
Xinglong *China* **57** D9
Xingning *China* **59** E10
Xingping *China* **56** G5
Xingren *China* **58** E5
Xingshan *China* **59** B8
Xingtai *China* **56** F8
Xingu → *Brazil* **125** D8
Xingwen *China* **58** C5
Xingyang *China* **56** G7
Xinhe *China* **56** F8
Xinhua *China* **59** D8
Xinhuang *China* **58** D7
Xinhui *China* **59** F9
Xining *China* **60** C5
Xinjian *China* **59** C10
Xinjiang *China* **56** G6
Xinjiang Uygur Zizhiqu □ *China* **60** B3
Xinjie *China* **58** D3
Xinjin = Pulandian *China* **57** E11
Xinjin *China* **58** B4
Xinkai He → *China* **57** C12
Xinle *China* **56** E8
Xinlitun *China* **57** D12
Xinlong *China* **58** B3
Xinmin *China* **57** D12

Xinning *China* **59** D8
Xinping *China* **58** E3
Xinshao *China* **59** D8
Xintai *China* **57** G9
Xintian *China* **59** E9
Xinxian *China* **59** B10
Xinxiang *China* **56** G7
Xinxing *China* **59** F9
Xinyang *China* **59** A10
Xinye *China* **59** A9
Xinyi *China* **57** F8
Xinyu *China* **59** D10
Xinzhan *China* **57** C14
Xinzheng *China* **56** G7
Xinzhou *Hainan, China* **64** C7
Xinzhou *Hubei, China* **59** B10
Xinzhou *Shanxi, China* **56** E7
Xinzo de Limia *Spain* **36** C3
Xiongyuecheng *China* **57** D12
Xiping *Henan, China* **56** H8
Xiping *Henan, China* **56** H6
Xiping *Zhejiang, China* **59** D12
Xique-Xique *Brazil* **125** F10
Xisha Qundao = Paracel Is. *S. China Sea* **62** A4
Xishui *Guizhou, China* **58** C6
Xishui *Hubei, China* **59** B10
Xitole *Guinea-Biss.* **82** C2
Xiu Shui → *China* **59** C10
Xiuning *China* **59** C12
Xiuren *China* **59** E8
Xiushan *China* **58** C7
Xiushui *China* **59** C10
Xiuwen *China* **58** D6
Xiuyan *China* **57** D12
Xixabangma Feng *China* **69** E11
Xixia *China* **56** H6
Xixiang *China* **56** H4
Xixón = Gijón *Spain* **36** B5
Xiyang *China* **56** F7
Xizang Zhizhiqu □ *China* **60** C3
Xlendi *Malta* **49** C1
Xochob *Mexico* **119** D7
Xu Jiang → *China* **59** D11
Xuan Loc *Vietnam* **65** G6
Xuan'en *China* **58** C7
Xuanhan *China* **58** B6
Xuanhua *China* **56** D8
Xuanwei *China* **58** C5
Xuanzhou *China* **59** B12
Xuchang *China* **56** G7
Xudat *Azerbaijan* **35** K9
Xuefeng Shan *China* **59** D8
Xuejiaping *China* **59** B8
Xun Jiang → *China* **59** F8
Xun Xian *China* **56** G8
Xundian *China* **58** E4
Xunwu *China* **59** E10
Xunyang *China* **56** H5
Xunyi *China* **56** G5
Xupu *China* **59** D8
Xúquer → *Spain* **39** F4
Xushui *China* **56** E8
Xuwen *China* **59** G8
Xuyen Moc *Vietnam* **65** G6
Xuyong *China* **58** C5
Xuzhou *China* **57** G9
Xylophagou *Cyprus* **49** E12

Y

Ya Xian = Sanya *China* **64** C7
Yaamba *Australia* **94** C5
Ya'an *China* **58** C4
Yaapeet *Australia* **95** F3
Yabassi *Cameroon* **83** E6
Yabayo *Ivory C.* **82** D3
Yabelo *Ethiopia* **81** G4
Yabelo △ *Ethiopia* **81** F4
Yablanitsa *Bulgaria* **45** C8
Yablonovyy Khrebet *Russia* **53** D12
Yablonovyy Ra. = Yablonovyy Khrebet *Russia* **53** D12
Yabluniv *Ukraine* **29** B9
Yablunytsya *Ukraine* **29** B9
Yabrai Shan *China* **56** E2
Yabrūd *Syria* **74** B5
Yabucoa *Puerto Rico* **121** d
Yacambú △ *Venezuela* **121** E6
Yacheng *China* **64** C7
Yacuiba *Bolivia* **126** A3
Yacuma → *Bolivia* **124** F5
Yadgir *India* **66** L10
Yadkin → *U.S.A.* **117** D14
Yadrin *Russia* **34** C8
Yadua *Fiji* **91** a
Yaeyama-Rettō *Japan* **55** M1
Yagaba *Ghana* **83** C4
Yagasa Cluster *Fiji* **91** a
Yağcılar *Turkey* **47** B10
Yagodnoye *Russia* **53** C15
Yahila *Dem. Rep. of the Congo* **86** B1
Yahk *Canada* **102** D5
Yahotyn *Ukraine* **33** G6
Yahuma *Dem. Rep. of the Congo* **84** D4
Yahyalı *Turkey* **72** C6
Yaita *Japan* **55** F9
Yaiza *Canary Is.* **48** F6

Yajiang *China* **58** B3
Yajua *Nigeria* **83** C7
Yakima *U.S.A.* **108** C3
Yakima → *U.S.A.* **108** C4
Yakishiri-Jima *Japan* **54** B10
Yako *Burkina Faso* **82** C4
Yakobi I. *U.S.A.* **102** B1
Yakoruda *Bulgaria* **44** D7
Yakovlevka *Russia* **54** B6
Yaku-Shima *Japan* **55** J5
Yakumo *Japan* **54** C10
Yakutat *U.S.A.* **100** F4
Yakutat B. *U.S.A.* **106** D11
Yakutia = Sakha □ *Russia* **53** C14
Yakutsk *Russia* **53** C13
Yala *Thailand* **65** J3
Yalata *Australia* **93** F5
Yalata ☺ *Australia* **93** F5
Yalboroo *Australia* **94** b
Yale *U.S.A.* **114** C2
Yalgorup △ *Australia* **93** F2
Yalinga *C.A.R.* **84** C4
Yalkabul, Pta. *Mexico* **119** C7
Yalleroi *Australia* **94** C4
Yalobusha → *U.S.A.* **117** E9
Yalong Jiang → *China* **58** D3
Yalova *Turkey* **45** F13
Yalpirakinu ☺ *Australia* **92** D5
Yalpuh, Ozero *Ukraine* **29** E13
Yalta *Ukraine* **33** K8
Yalu Jiang → *China* **57** E13
Yalvaç *Turkey* **72** C4
Yam *Australia* **94** a
Yam Ha Melah = Dead Sea
  Asia **74** D4
Yam Kinneret *Israel* **74** C4
Yamada *Japan* **55** H5
Yamagata *Japan* **54** E10
Yamagata □ *Japan* **54** E10
Yamaguchi *Japan* **55** G5
Yamaguchi □ *Japan* **55** G5
Yamal, Poluostrov *Russia* **52** B8
Yamal Pen. = Yamal,
  Poluostrov *Russia* **52** B8
Yamanashi □ *Japan* **55** G9
Yamato Ridge *Sea of Japan* **54** E7
Yamba *Australia* **95** D5
Yambarran Ra. *Australia* **92** C5
Yambéring *Guinea* **82** C2
Yâmbiô *Sudan* **81** G2
Yambol *Bulgaria* **45** D10
Yamburg *Russia* **52** C8
Yamdena *Indonesia* **63** F8
Yame *Japan* **55** H5
Yamethin *Burma* **67** J20
Yamma Yamma, L. *Australia* **95** D3
Yamoussoukro *Ivory C.* **82** D3
Yampa → *U.S.A.* **108** F9
Yampi Sd. *Australia* **92** C3
Yampil *Moldova* **23** D15
Yampol = Yampil *Moldova* **23** D15
Yamrat *Russia* **30** D6
Yamrukchal = Botev
  Bulgaria **45** D8
Yamuna → *India* **69** G9
Yamunanagar *India* **68** D7
Yamzho Yumco *China* **60** D4
Yan *Nigeria* **83** C7
Yana → *Russia* **53** B14
Yanagawa *Japan* **55** H5
Yanai *Japan* **55** H6
Yan'an *China* **56** F5
Yanbian *China* **58** D3
Yanbu 'al Baḥr *Si. Arabia* **70** F3
Yanchang *China* **56** F6
Yancheng *Henan, China* **56** H8
Yancheng *Jiangsu, China* **57** H11
Yanchep *Australia* **93** F2
Yanchi *China* **56** F4
Yanchuan *China* **56** F6
Yanco Cr. → *Australia* **95** F4
Yandeyarra ☺ *Australia* **92** D2
Yandicoogina *Australia* **92** D2
Yandoon *Burma* **67** L19
Yanfeng *China* **58** E3
Yanfolila *Mali* **82** C3
Yang Xian *China* **56** H4
Yang-yang *S. Korea* **57** E15
Yang-Yang *Senegal* **82** B1
Yangambi
  Dem. Rep. of the Congo **86** B1
Yangbi *China* **58** E2
Yangcheng *China* **56** G7
Yangch'ü = Taiyuan *China* **56** F7
Yangchun *China* **59** F8
Yanggao *China* **56** D7
Yanggu *China* **56** F8
Yangjiang *China* **59** G8
Yangliuqing *China* **57** E9
Yangon = Rangoon *Burma* **67** L20
Yangping *China* **59** B12
Yangpingguan *China* **56** H4
Yangquan *China* **56** F7
Yangshan *China* **59** E9
Yangshuo *China* **59** E8
Yangtse = Chang Jiang →
  China **59** B13
Yangtze Kiang = Chang
  Jiang → *China* **59** B13
Yangudi Rassa △ *Ethiopia* **81** E5
Yangxin *China* **59** C10

Yangyuan *China* **56** D8
Yangzhong *China* **59** A12
Yangzhou *China* **59** A12
Yanhe *China* **58** C7
Yanji *China* **57** C15
Yanjin *China* **58** C5
Yanjing *China* **58** C2
Yankari △ *Nigeria* **83** D7
Yankton *U.S.A.* **112** D5
Yankunytjatjara-
  Antakirinja ☺ *Australia* **95** A1
Yanonge
  Dem. Rep. of the Congo **86** B1
Yanqi *China* **60** B3
Yanqing *China* **56** D9
Yanshan *Hebei, China* **57** E9
Yanshan *Jiangxi, China* **59** C11
Yanshan *Yunnan, China* **58** F5
Yanshou *China* **57** B15
Yantai *China* **57** F11
Yantarnyy *Russia* **30** D6
Yanting *China* **58** B5
Yantra → *Bulgaria* **45** C9
Yanuca *Fiji* **91** a
Yanwa *China* **58** D2
Yanyuan *China* **58** D3
Yanzhou *China* **56** G9
Yao Noi, Ko *Thailand* **65** a
Yao Xian *China* **56** G5
Yao Yai, Ko *Thailand* **65** a
Yao'an *China* **58** E3
Yaodu *China* **58** A5
Yaowan *China* **57** G10
Yaoundé *Cameroon* **83** E7
Yap *Pac. Oc.* **96** G5
Yapei *Ghana* **83** D4
Yapen *Indonesia* **63** E9
Yapen, Selat *Indonesia* **63** E9
Yapero *Indonesia* **63** E9
Yappar → *Australia* **94** B3
Yapuparra ☺ *Australia* **93** E4
Yaqaga *Fiji* **91** a
Yaqui → *Mexico* **118** B2
Yar-Sale *Russia* **52** C8
Yaraka *Australia* **94** C3
Yaransk *Russia* **34** B8
Yarbasan *Turkey* **47** C10
Yardımcı Burnu *Turkey* **47** E12
Yare → *U.K.* **15** E9
Yaremcha *Ukraine* **29** B9
Yarensk *Russia* **52** C5
Yarfa *Si. Arabia* **80** C4
Yarí → *Colombia* **124** D4
Yarkand = Shache *China* **60** C2
Yarker *Canada* **115** B8
Yarkhun → *Pakistan* **69** A5
Yarlung Ziangbo Jiang =
  Brahmaputra → *Asia* **69** H13
Yarmouth *Canada* **105** D6
Yarmūk → *Syria* **74** C4
Yaroslavl *Russia* **32** D10
Yaroslavl □ *Russia* **32** C10
Yarqa, W. → *Egypt* **74** F2
Yarra Yarra Lakes *Australia* **93** E2
Yarram *Australia* **95** F4
Yarraman *Australia* **95** D5
Yarras *Australia* **95** E5
Yarrie *Australia* **92** D3
Yartsevo *Sib., Russia* **53** C10
Yartsevo *Smolensk, Russia* **32** E7
Yarumal *Colombia* **124** B3
Yasawa *Fiji* **91** a
Yasawa Group *Fiji* **91** a
Yaselda *Belarus* **23** B14
Yasen *Ukraine* **29** B9
Yashi *Nigeria* **83** C6
Yashikera *Nigeria* **83** D5
Yashkul *Russia* **35** G7
Yasin *Pakistan* **69** A5
Yasinovataya *Ukraine* **33** H9
Yasinski, L. *Canada* **104** B4
Yasinya *Ukraine* **29** B9
Yasothon *Thailand* **64** E5
Yass *Australia* **95** E4
Yāsūj *Iran* **71** D6
Yatağan *Turkey* **47** D10
Yatakala *Niger* **83** C5
Yates Center *U.S.A.* **112** G6
Yathkyed L. *Canada* **103** A9
Yatsushiro *Japan* **55** H5
Yatta Plateau *Kenya* **86** C4
Yauco *Puerto Rico* **121** d
Yavarí → *Peru* **124** D4
Yávaros *Mexico* **118** B3
Yavatmal *India* **66** J11
Yavne *Israel* **74** D3
Yavoriv *Ukraine* **31** J10
Yavorov = Yavoriv *Ukraine* **31** J10
Yavuzeli *Turkey* **73** D8
Yawatahama *Japan* **55** H6
Yawri B. *S. Leone* **82** D2
Yaxi *China* **58** D6
Yaxian = Sanya *China* **64** C7
Yayladağı *Turkey* **72** E7
Yazd *Iran* **71** D7
Yazd □ *Iran* **71** D7
Yazd-e Khvāst *Iran* **71** D7
Yazıköy *Turkey* **47** E9
Yazman *Pakistan* **68** E4
Yazoo → *U.S.A.* **117** E9

Yazoo City *U.S.A.* **117** E9
Ybbs *Austria* **26** C8
Ybycuí △ *Paraguay* **126** B4
Ybytyruzú △ *Paraguay* **127** B4
Ye *Burma* **64** E1
Ye Xian *China* **56** H7
Yebyu *Burma* **64** E2
Yecheon *S. Korea* **57** F15
Yecla *Spain* **39** G3
Yécora *Mexico* **118** B3
Yedebub Biheroch
  Biheresebochna
  Hizboch □ *Ethiopia* **81** F4
Yedigöller △ *Turkey* **72** B4
Yedseram → *Nigeria* **83** C7
Yefremov *Russia* **32** F10
Yeghegnadzor *Armenia* **73** C11
Yegorlyk → *Russia* **35** G5
Yegorlykskaya *Russia* **35** G5
Yegoryevsk *Russia* **32** E10
Yegros *Paraguay* **126** B4
Yehbuah *Indonesia* **63** J17
Yehuda, Midbar *Israel* **74** D4
Yei *Sudan* **81** G3
Yei, Nahr → *Sudan* **81** F3
Yeji *Ghana* **83** D4
Yejmiadzin *Armenia* **35** K7
Yekaterinburg *Russia* **52** D7
Yelabuga *Russia* **34** C11
Yelan *Russia* **34** E6
Yelarbon *Australia* **95** D5
Yelatma *Russia* **34** C5
Yelets *Russia* **33** F10
Yélimané *Mali* **82** B2
Yelizavetgrad =
  Kirovohrad *Ukraine* **33** H7
Yelizovo *Russia* **53** D16
Yell *U.K.* **13** A7
Yell Sd. *U.K.* **13** A7
Yellow = Huang He →
  China **57** F10
Yellow Sea *China* **57** G12
Yellowhead Pass *Canada* **102** C5
Yellowknife *Canada* **102** A6
Yellowknife → *Canada* **102** A6
Yellowstone → *U.S.A.* **108** C12
Yellowstone △ *U.S.A.* **108** D8
Yellowstone L. *U.S.A.* **108** D8
Yelnya *Russia* **32** E7
Yelsk *Belarus* **23** C15
Yelwa *Nigeria* **83** C5
Yemen ■ *Asia* **75** E3
Yen Bai *Vietnam* **58** G5
Yenagoa *Nigeria* **83** E6
Yenakiyeve *Ukraine* **33** H10
Yenakiyevo = Yenakiyeve
  Ukraine **33** H10
Yenangyaung *Burma* **67** J19
Yenbo = Yanbu 'al Baḥr
  Si. Arabia **70** F3
Yenda *Australia* **95** E4
Yende Millimou *Guinea* **82** D2
Yendéré *Burkina Faso* **82** C4
Yendi *Ghana* **83** D4
Yéni *Niger* **83** C5
Yeni Erenköy = Yialousa
  Cyprus **49** D13
Yenice *Ankara, Turkey* **72** C5
Yenice *Aydın, Turkey* **47** D10
Yenice *Çanakkale, Turkey* **47** B9
Yenice *Edirne, Turkey* **45** F10
Yenice → *Turkey* **72** D6
Yenifoça *Turkey* **47** C8
Yenihisar *Turkey* **47** D9
Yeniköy *Bursa, Turkey* **45** F13
Yeniköy *Çanakkale, Turkey* **47** B8
Yeniköy *Kütahya, Turkey* **47** C11
Yenipazar *Turkey* **47** D10
Yenişehir *Turkey* **45** F13
Yenisey → *Russia* **52** B9
Yeniseysk *Russia* **53** D10
Yeniseyskiy Zaliv *Russia* **52** B9
Yenne *France* **21** C9
Yenotayevka *Russia* **35** G8
Yenyuka *Russia* **53** D13
Yeo → *U.K.* **15** G5
Yeo, L. *Australia* **93** E3
Yeo I. *Canada* **114** A3
Yeoju *S. Korea* **57** F14
Yeola *India* **66** J9
Yeong-wol *S. Korea* **57** F15
Yeongcheon *S. Korea* **57** G15
Yeongdeok *S. Korea* **57** F15
Yeongdeungpo *S. Korea* **57** F14
Yeongdong *S. Korea* **57** F14
Yeongju *S. Korea* **57** F15
Yeosu *S. Korea* **57** G14
Yeotmal = Yavatmal *India* **66** J11
Yeovil *U.K.* **15** G5
Yepes *Spain* **36** F7
Yeppoon *Australia* **94** C5
Yerbent *Turkmenistan* **52** F6
Yerbogachen *Russia* **53** C11
Yerevan *Armenia* **35** K7
Yerköy *Turkey* **72** C6
Yerington *U.S.A.* **108** G4
Yerkesik *Turkey* **47** D10
Yerköy *Turkey* **72** C6
Yermak *Kazakhstan* **52** D8
Yermo *U.S.A.* **111** L10
Yerólakkos *Cyprus* **49** D12

Yeropol *Russia* **53** C17
Yeroskipos *Cyprus* **49** E11
Yershov *Russia* **34** E9
Yerushalayim = Jerusalem
  Israel/West Bank **74** D4
Yerville *France* **18** C7
Yes Tor *U.K.* **15** G4
Yesan *S. Korea* **57** F14
Yeşilhisar *Turkey* **72** C6
Yeşilırmak → *Turkey* **72** B7
Yeşilkent *Turkey* **72** D7
Yeşilköy *Turkey* **45** F12
Yeşilova *Turkey* **47** D11
Yeşilyurt *Manisa, Turkey* **47** C10
Yeşilyurt *Muğla, Turkey* **47** D10
Yesnogorsk *Russia* **32** E9
Yeso *U.S.A.* **109** J11
Yessentuki *Russia* **35** H6
Yessey *Russia* **53** C11
Yeste *Spain* **39** G2
Yetman *Australia* **95** D5
Yeu, Î. d' *France* **18** F4
Yevlakh = Yevlax *Azerbaijan* **35** K8
Yevlax *Azerbaijan* **35** K8
Yevpatoriya *Ukraine* **33** K7
Yeya → *Russia* **33** J10
Yeysk *Russia* **33** J10
Yezd = Yazd *Iran* **71** D7
Yezerishche *Belarus* **32** E5
Ygatimi *Paraguay* **127** A4
Yhati *Paraguay* **126** B4
Yhú *Paraguay* **127** B4
Yí → *Uruguay* **126** C4
Yi 'Allaq, G. *Egypt* **74** E2
Yi He → *China* **57** G10
Yi Xian *Anhui, China* **59** C11
Yi Xian *Hebei, China* **56** E8
Yi Xian *Liaoning, China* **57** D11
Yialiás → *Cyprus* **49** D12
Yialousa *Cyprus* **49** D13
Yibin *China* **58** C5
Yichang *China* **59** B8
Yicheng *Henan, China* **59** B9
Yicheng *Shanxi, China* **56** G6
Yichuan *China* **56** F6
Yichun *Heilongjiang, China* **60** B7
Yichun *Jiangxi, China* **59** D10
Yidu *China* **57** F10
Yidun *China* **58** B2
Yifag *Ethiopia* **81** E4
Yifeng *China* **59** C10
Yihuang *China* **59** D11
Yijun *China* **56** G5
Yilan *China* **57** B15
Yıldız Dağları *Turkey* **45** E11
Yıldızeli *Turkey* **72** C7
Yiliang *Yunnan, China* **58** D5
Yiliang *Yunnan, China* **58** E4
Yilong *China* **58** B6
Yimen *China* **58** E4
Yimianpo *China* **57** B15
Yinchuan *China* **56** E4
Yindarlgooda, L. *Australia* **93** F3
Yindjibarndi ☺ *Australia* **92** D2
Ying He → *China* **56** H9
Ying Xian *China* **56** E7
Yingcheng *China* **59** B9
Yingde *China* **59** E9
Yingjiang *China* **58** E1
Yingjing *China* **58** C4
Yingkou *China* **57** D12
Yingshan *Henan, China* **59** B9
Yingshan *Hubei, China* **59** B10
Yingshan *Sichuan, China* **58** B6
Yingshang *China* **59** A11
Yingtan *China* **59** C11
Yingualyarra ☺ *Australia* **92** C4
Yining *China* **52** E9
Yiningarra ☺ *Australia* **92** D2
Yinjiang *China* **58** C7
Yinmabin *Burma* **67** H19
Yioúra = Giaros *Greece* **46** D6
Yipinglang *China* **58** E3
Yirba Muda *Ethiopia* **81** F4
Yirga Alem *Ethiopia* **81** F4
Yirol *Sudan* **81** F3
Yirrkala *Australia* **94** A2
Yishan *China* **58** E7
Yishui *China* **57** G10
Yishun *Singapore* **65** d
Yitong *China* **57** C13
Yiwu *China* **59** C13
Yixing *China* **59** B12
Yiyang *Henan, China* **56** G7
Yiyang *Hunan, China* **59** C9
Yiyang *Jiangxi, China* **59** C11
Yizhang *China* **59** E9
Yizheng *China* **59** A12
Yli-Kitka *Finland* **8** C23
Yliki, L. *Greece* **46** C5
Ylitornio *Finland* **8** C20
Ylivieska *Finland* **8** D21
Yngaren *Sweden* **11** F10
Yoakum *U.S.A.* **116** G6
Yob △ *Eritrea* **81** D4
Yobe □ *Nigeria* **83** C7
Yoboki *Djibouti* **81** E5
Yog Pt. *Phil.* **63** B6
Yoğuntaş *Turkey* **45** E11
Yogyakarta *Indonesia* **62** F4
Yogyakarta □ *Indonesia* **63** G14
Yoho △ *Canada* **102** C5

Yojoa, L. de *Honduras* **120** D2
Yok Don △ *Vietnam* **64** F6
Yokadouma *Cameroon* **84** D2
Yokkaichi *Japan* **55** G8
Yoko *Cameroon* **83** D7
Yokohama *Japan* **55** G9
Yokosuka *Japan* **55** G9
Yokote *Japan* **54** E10
Yola *Nigeria* **83** D7
Yolaina, Cordillera de *Nic.* **120** D3
Yólöten *Turkmenistan* **71** B9
Yom → *Thailand* **64** E3
Yonago *Japan* **55** G6
Yonaguni-Jima *Japan* **55** M1
Yŏnan *N. Korea* **57** F13
Yonezawa *Japan* **54** F10
Yong Peng *Malaysia* **65** M4
Yong Sata *Thailand* **65** J2
Yongamp'o *N. Korea* **57** E13
Yong'an *China* **59** E11
Yongcheng *China* **56** H9
Yongchuan *China* **58** C5
Yongchun *China* **59** E12
Yongde *China* **58** E2
Yongdeng *China* **56** F2
Yongding *China* **59** E11
Yongfeng *China* **59** D10
Yongfu *China* **58** E7
Yonghe *China* **56** F6
Yŏnghŭng *N. Korea* **57** E14
Yongji *China* **56** G6
Yongjia *China* **59** C13
Yongkang *Yunnan, China* **58** E2
Yongkang *Zhejiang, China* **59** C13
Yongnian *China* **56** F8
Yongning *Guangxi Zhuangzu,
  China* **58** F7
Yongning *Ningxia Huizu,
  China* **56** E4
Yongping *China* **58** E2
Yongqing *China* **58** D3
Yongren *China* **58** D3
Yongshan *China* **58** C4
Yongsheng *China* **58** D3
Yongshun *China* **58** C7
Yongtai *China* **59** E12
Yongxin = Jinggangshan
  China **59** D10
Yongxing *China* **59** D9
Yongxiu *China* **59** C10
Yongzhou *China* **59** D8
Yonibana *S. Leone* **82** D2
Yonkers *U.S.A.* **115** F11
Yonne □ *France* **19** F9
Yonne → *France* **19** D9
York *Australia* **93** F2
York *U.K.* **14** D6
York *Ala., U.S.A.* **117** E10
York *Nebr.., U.S.A.* **112** E6
York *Pa., U.S.A.* **113** F15
York, C. *Australia* **94** A3
York, City of □ *U.K.* **14** D6
York, Kap *Greenland* **101** B18
York, Vale of *U.K.* **14** C6
York Sd. *Australia* **92** C4
Yorke Pen. *Australia* **95** E2
Yorkshire Dales △ *U.K.* **14** C5
Yorkshire Wolds *U.K.* **14** C7
Yorkton *Canada* **103** C8
Yorkville *U.S.A.* **110** G3
Yoro *Honduras* **120** C2
Yoron-Jima *Japan* **55** L4
Yorosso *Mali* **82** C4
Yos Sudarso, Pulau =
  Dolak, Pulau *Indonesia* **63** F9
Yosemite △ *U.S.A.* **110** H7
Yosemite Village *U.S.A.* **110** H7
Yoshino-Kumano △ *Japan* **55** H8
Yoshkar Ola *Russia* **34** B8
Yotvata *Israel* **74** C4
You Jiang → *China* **58** F6
You Xian *China* **59** D9
Youbou *Canada* **110** B2
Youghal *Ireland* **12** E4
Youghal B. *Ireland* **12** E4
Youkounkoun *Guinea* **82** C2
Young *Australia* **95** E4
Young *Canada* **103** C7
Young *Uruguay* **126** C4
Young I. *Antarctica* **5** C11
Younghusband, L. *Australia* **95** E2
Younghusband Pen.
  Australia **95** F2
Youngstown *Canada* **103** C6
Youngstown *N.Y., U.S.A.* **114** C5
Youngstown *Ohio, U.S.A.* **114** E4
Youngsville *U.S.A.* **114** E5
Youngwood *U.S.A.* **114** F5
Youxi *China* **59** D12
Youyang *China* **58** C7
Youyu *China* **56** D7

Ythan → *U.K.* **13** D7
Ytterhogdal *Sweden* **10** B8
Ytyk-Kyuyel *Russia* **53** C14
Yu Jiang → *China* **58** F7
Yü Shan *Taiwan* **59** F13
Yu Xian = Yuzhou *China* **56** G7
Yu Xian *Hebei, China* **56** E8
Yu Xian *Shanxi, China* **56** E7
Yuan Jiang → *Hunan, China* **59** C8
Yuan Jiang → *Yunnan, China* **58** F4
Yuan'an *China* **59** B8
Yuanjiang *Hunan, China* **59** C9
Yuanjiang *Yunnan, China* **58** F4
Yüanli *Taiwan* **59** E13
Yüanlin *Taiwan* **59** F13
Yuanling *China* **59** C8
Yuanmou *China* **58** E3
Yuanqu *China* **56** G6
Yuanyang *Henan, China* **56** G7
Yuanyang *Yunnan, China* **58** F4
Yuba → *U.S.A.* **110** F5
Yuba City *U.S.A.* **110** F5
Yūbari *Japan* **54** C10
Yubdo *Ethiopia* **81** F4
Yūbetsu *Japan* **54** B11
Yubo *Sudan* **81** F2
Yucatán □ *Mexico* **119** C7
Yucatán, Canal de *Caribbean* **120** B2
Yucatán, Península de
  Mexico **98** H11
Yucatan Basin *Cent. Amer.* **119** D7
Yucatan Channel =
  Yucatán, Canal de
  Caribbean **120** B2
Yucca *U.S.A.* **111** L12
Yucca Valley *U.S.A.* **111** L10
Yucheng *China* **56** F9
Yuci = Jinzhong *China* **56** F7
Yudu *China* **59** E10
Yuechi *China* **58** B6
Yuendumu *Australia* **92** D5
Yuendumu ☺ *Australia* **92** D5
Yueqing *China* **59** C13
Yueqing Wan *China* **59** D13
Yuexi *Anhui, China* **59** B11
Yuexi *Sichuan, China* **58** C4
Yueyang *China* **59** C9
Yugan *China* **59** C11
Yugorenok *Russia* **53** D14
Yuhuan *China* **59** C13
Yuhuan Dao *China* **59** C13
Yujiang *China* **59** C11
Yukhnov *Russia* **32** E8
Yukon *U.S.A.* **116** D6
Yukon → *U.S.A.* **106** C7
Yukon Flats *U.S.A.* **106** B10
Yukon Territory □ *Canada* **100** E5
Yüksekova *Turkey* **73** D11
Yukta *Russia* **53** C11
Yukuhashi *Japan* **55** H5
Yulara *Australia* **93** E5
Yule → *Australia* **92** D2
Yuleba *Australia* **95** D4
Yuli *Nigeria* **83** D7
Yüli *Taiwan* **59** F13
Yulin *Guangxi Zhuangzu, China* **59** F8
Yulin *Hainan, China* **64** C7
Yulin *Shaanxi, China* **56** E5
Yuma *Ariz., U.S.A.* **111** N12
Yuma *Colo., U.S.A.* **108** F12
Yuma, B. de *Dom. Rep.* **121** C6
Yumbe *Uganda* **86** B3
Yumbi *Dem. Rep. of the Congo* **86** C2
Yumen *China* **60** C4
Yumurtalık *Turkey* **72** D6
Yun Gui Gaoyuan *China* **58** E3
Yun Ling *China* **58** D2
Yun Xian *Hubei, China* **59** A8
Yun Xian *Yunnan, China* **58** E3
Yuna *Australia* **93** E2
Yunak *Turkey* **72** C4
Yunan *China* **59** F8
Yuncheng *Henan, China* **56** G8
Yuncheng *Shanxi, China* **56** G6
Yunfu *China* **59** F9
Yungas *Bolivia* **124** G5
Yungay *Chile* **126** D1
Yunhe *China* **59** C12
Yunkai Dashan *China* **59** F8
Yunkanjini ☺ *Australia* **92** D5
Yunlong *China* **58** E2
Yunmeng *China* **59** B9
Yunnan □ *China* **58** E4
Yunquera de Henares *Spain* **38** E1
Yunt Dağı *Turkey* **47** C9
Yunta *Australia* **95** E2
Yunxi *China* **59** H6
Yunxiao *China* **59** F11
Yupanqui Basin *Pac. Oc.* **97** J17
Yuping *China* **58** D7
Yuraygir △ *Australia* **95** D5
Yurga *Russia* **52** D9
Yurimaguas *Peru* **124** E3
Yurkivka *Ukraine* **29** B13
Yurubí △ *Venezuela* **121** D6
Yuryev-Polskiy *Russia* **32** D10
Yuryevets *Russia* **34** B6
Yuscarán *Honduras* **120** D2
Yūsef, Baḥr → *Egypt* **80** B3
Yushan *China* **59** C12

Yushanzhen *China* **58** C7
Yushe *China* **56** F7
Yushu *Jilin, China* **57** B14
Yushu *Qinghai, China* **60** C4
Yusufeli *Turkey* **73** B9
Yutai *China* **56** G9
Yutian *China* **57** E9
Yuxarı Qarabağ =
  Nagorno-Karabakh □
  Azerbaijan **73** C12
Yuxi *China* **58** E4
Yuyao *China* **59** B13
Yuza *Russia* **34** B6
Yuzhno-Kurilsk *Russia* **53** E15
Yuzhno-Sakhalinsk *Russia* **53** E15
Yuzhno-Sukhokumsk
  Russia **35** H7
Yuzhnyy ◯ *Russia* **35** H5
Yvelines □ *France* **19** D8
Yverdon-les-Bains *Switz.* **25** J2
Yvetot *France* **18** C7
Yzeure *France* **19** F10

Z

Zaanstad *Neths.* **17** B4
Zāb al Kabīr ➤ *Iraq* **73** D10
Zāb aş Şaghīr ➤ *Iraq* **73** E10
Žabalj *Serbia* **28** E5
Žabari *Serbia* **44** B5
Zabarjad *Egypt* **80** C4
Zabaykalsk *Russia* **53** E12
Zabki *Poland* **31** F8
Ząbkowice Śląskie *Poland* **31** H3
Žabljak *Montenegro* **44** C3
Zabłudów *Poland* **31** F9
Zabno *Poland* **31** H7
Zabol *Iran* **71** D9
Zābol □ *Afghan.* **66** D5
Zābolī *Iran* **71** E9
Zabolotiv *Ukraine* **29** B10
Zabolottya *Ukraine* **31** G11
Zabré *Burkina Faso* **83** C4
Zábřeh *Czech Rep.* **27** B9
Zabrze *Poland* **31** H5
Zabuzhzhya *Ukraine* **31** G10
Zabzuga *Ghana* **83** D5
Zacapa *Guatemala* **120** D2
Zacapu *Mexico* **118** D4
Zacatecas *Mexico* **118** C4
Zacatecas □ *Mexico* **118** C4
Zacatecoluca *El Salv.* **120** D2
Zacháro *Greece* **46** D3
Zachary *U.S.A.* **116** F9
Zachodnio-Pomorskie □
  Poland **30** E2
Zacoalco de Torres *Mexico* **118** C4
Zacualtipán *Mexico* **119** C5
Zadar *Croatia* **41** D12
Zadawa *Nigeria* **83** C7
Zadetkyi Kyun *Burma* **65** G2
Zadonsk *Russia* **33** F10
Zafarqand *Iran* **71** C7
Zafra *Spain* **37** G4
Žagań *Poland* **31** G2
Zagaoua *Chad* **79** E10
Žagarė *Lithuania* **30** B10
Zagazig *Egypt* **80** H7
Zāgheh *Iran* **71** C6
Zagnanado *Benin* **83** D5
Zagora *Greece* **46** B5
Zagorje *Slovenia* **41** B11
Zagórów *Poland* **31** F4
Zagórz *Poland* **31** J9
Zagreb *Croatia* **41** C12
Zagreb ✈ (ZAG) *Croatia* **41** C13
Zāgros, Kūhhā-ye *Iran* **71** C6
Zagros Mts. = Zāgros,
  Kūhhā-ye *Iran* **71** C6
Žagubica *Serbia* **44** B5
Zaguinaso *Ivory C.* **82** C3
Zagyva ➤ *Hungary* **28** C5
Zahamena △ *Madag.* **89** B8
Zāhedān *Fārs, Iran* **71** D7
Zāhedān
  Sīstān va Balūchestān, Iran **71** D9
Zahlah *Lebanon* **74** B4
Zahna *Germany* **24** D8
Záhony *Hungary* **28** B7
Zainsk *Russia* **34** C11
Zaïre = Congo ➤ *Africa* **84** F2
Zaječar *Serbia* **44** C6
Zaka *Zimbabwe* **89** C5
Zakamensk *Russia* **53** D11
Zakarpattya □ *Ukraine* **29** B8
Zakataly = Zaqatala
  Azerbaijan **35** K8
Zakhodnaya Dzvina =
  Daugava ➤ *Latvia* **32** D3
Zākhū *Iraq* **73** D10
Zakinthos = Zakynthos
  Greece **46** D2
Zakopane *Poland* **31** J6
Zakroczym *Poland* **31** F7
Zákros *Greece* **49** D8
Zakynthos *Greece* **46** D2
Zakynthos □ *Greece* **46** D2
Zala *Ethiopia* **81** F4
Zala □ *Hungary* **28** D1

Zala ➤ *Hungary* **28** D2
Zalaegerszeg *Hungary* **28** D1
Zalakomár *Hungary* **28** D2
Zalalövő *Hungary* **28** D1
Zalamea de la Serena *Spain* **37** G5
Zalamea la Real *Spain* **37** H4
Zalari *Russia* **53** D11
Zalău *Romania* **28** C8
Žalec *Slovenia* **41** B12
Zaleshchiki = Zalishchyky
  Ukraine **29** B10
Zalesye *Russia* **30** D8
Zalew Wiślany *Poland* **30** D6
Zalewo *Poland* **30** E6
Zalingei *Sudan* **79** F10
Zalishchyky *Ukraine* **29** B10
Zama L. *Canada* **102** B5
Zambeke
  Dem. Rep. of the Congo **86** B2
Zambeze ➤ *Africa* **87** F4
Zambezi = Zambeze ➤ *Africa* **87** F4
Zambezi *Zambia* **85** G4
Zambezi △ *Zimbabwe* **87** F2
Zambézia □ *Mozam.* **87** F4
Zambia ■ *Africa* **87** F2
Zamboanga *Phil.* **61** H5
Zambrów *Poland* **31** F9
Zametchino *Russia* **34** D6
Zamfara □ *Nigeria* **83** C6
Zamfara ➤ *Nigeria* **83** C5
Zamora *Mexico* **118** D4
Zamora *Spain* **36** D5
Zamora □ *Spain* **36** D5
Zamość *Poland* **31** H10
Zamtang *China* **58** A3
Zan *Ghana* **83** D4
Záncara ➤ *Spain* **39** F1
Zandvoort *Neths.* **17** B4
Zanesville *U.S.A.* **114** G2
Zangābād *Iran* **70** B5
Zangliveri *Greece* **44** F7
Zangoza = Sangüesa *Spain* **38** C3
Zangue ➤ *Mozam.* **87** F4
Zanjān *Iran* **73** D13
Zanjān □ *Iran* **71** B6
Zanjān ➤ *Iran* **71** B6
Zannone *Italy* **42** B6
Zante = Zakynthos *Greece* **46** D2
Zanthus *Australia* **93** F3
Zanzibar *Tanzania* **86** D4
Zaouiet El-Kala = Bordj
  Omar Driss *Algeria* **78** C7
Zaouiet Reggâne *Algeria* **78** C6
Zaoyang *China* **59** A9
Zaozhuang *China* **57** G9
Zap Suyu = Zāb al Kabīr ➤
  Iraq **73** D10
Zapadna Morava ➤ *Serbia* **44** C5
Zapadnaya Dvina =
  Daugava ➤ *Latvia* **32** D3
Zapadnaya Dvina *Russia* **32** D7
Západné Beskydy *Europe* **27** B12
Zapadni Rodopi *Bulgaria* **44** E7
Západočeský □ *Czech Rep.* **26** B6
Zapala *Argentina* **128** D2
Zapaleri, Cerro *Bolivia* **126** A2
Zapata *U.S.A.* **116** H5
Zapatón ➤ *Spain* **37** F4
Zapolyarnyy *Russia* **8** B24
Zapopán *Mexico* **118** D4
Zaporizhzhya *Ukraine* **33** J8
Zaporizhzhya □ *Ukraine* **33** J8
Zaporozhye =
  Zaporizhzhya *Ukraine* **33** J8
Zaqatala *Azerbaijan* **35** K8
Zara *Turkey* **72** C7
Zaragoza *Coahuila, Mexico* **118** B4
Zaragoza *Nuevo León, Mexico* **119** C5
Zaragoza *Spain* **38** D4
Zaragoza □ *Spain* **38** D4
Zarand *Kermān, Iran* **71** D8
Zarand *Markazī, Iran* **71** C6
Zaranj *Afghan.* **66** D2
Zarasai *Lithuania* **32** E4
Zárate *Argentina* **126** C4
Zarautz *Spain* **38** B2
Zaraysk *Russia* **32** E10
Zard, Kūh-e *Iran* **71** C6
Zāreh *Iran* **71** C6
Zari *Nigeria* **83** C7
Zaria *Nigeria* **83** C6
Zarīneh ➤ *Iran* **73** D12
Żarki *Poland* **31** H6
Zarko *Greece* **46** B4
Zarneh *Iran* **70** C5
Zărnești *Romania* **29** E10
Żarów *Poland* **31** H3
Zarqā', Nahr az ➤ *Jordan* **74** C4
Zarrīn *Iran* **71** C7
Zarrīnābād *Iran* **71** D13
Zaruma *Ecuador* **124** D3
Żary *Poland* **31** G2
Zarza de Granadilla *Spain* **36** E4
Zarzis *Tunisia* **79** B8
Zas *Spain* **36** B2
Zaskar ➤ *India* **69** B7
Zaskar Mts. *India* **69** C7
Zastavna *Ukraine* **29** B10
Zastron *S. Africa* **88** E4

Žatec *Czech Rep.* **26** A6
Zaterechnyy *Russia* **35** H7
Zator *Poland* **31** J6
Zatyshshya *Ukraine* **29** C14
Zavala *Bos.-H.* **44** D1
Zavārēh *Iran* **71** C7
Zave *Zimbabwe* **89** B5
Zavetnoye *Russia* **35** G6
Zavidovići *Bos.-H.* **28** F3
Zavitinsk *Russia* **53** D13
Zavodovski, I. *Antarctica* **5** B1
Zavolzhsk *Russia* **34** B6
Zavolzhye *Russia* **34** B6
Zawadzkie *Poland* **31** H5
Zawichost *Poland* **31** H8
Zawidów *Poland* **31** G2
Zawiercie *Poland* **31** H6
Zāwiyat al Baydā = Al
  Baydā *Libya* **79** B10
Zâwyet Shammas *Egypt* **80** A2
Zâwyet Um el Rakham *Egypt* **80** A2
Zâwyet Ungeîla *Egypt* **80** A2
Zāyā *Iraq* **70** C5
Zāyandeh ➤ *Iran* **71** C7
Zaysan *Kazakhstan* **52** E9
Zaysan Köli *Kazakhstan* **52** E9
Zayü *China* **58** C1
Zazafotsy *Madag.* **89** C8
Zázrivá *Slovak Rep.* **27** B12
Zbarazh *Ukraine* **23** D13
Zbąszyń *Poland* **31** F2
Zbąszynek *Poland* **31** F2
Zblewo *Poland* **30** E5
Zbruch ➤ **29** B11
Žďár nad Sázavou *Czech Rep.* **26** B8
Zdolbuniv *Ukraine* **23** C14
Ždrelo *Serbia* **44** B5
Zduńska Wola *Poland* **31** G5
Zduny *Poland* **31** G4
Zeballos *Canada* **102** D3
Zebdiela *S. Africa* **89** C4
Zebila *Ghana* **83** C5
Zeebrugge *Belgium* **17** C3
Zeehan *Australia* **95** G4
Zeeland □ *Neths.* **17** C3
Zeerust *S. Africa* **88** D4
Zefat *Israel* **74** C4
Zege *Ethiopia* **81** E4
Zeggerene, Iracher *Mali* **83** B5
Zégoua *Mali* **82** C3
Zehak *Iran* **71** D9
Zehdenick *Germany* **24** C9
Zeil, Mt. *Australia* **92** D5
Zeila = Saylac *Somali Rep.* **75** E3
Zeist *Neths.* **17** B5
Zeitz *Germany* **24** D8
Żelechów *Poland* **31** G8
Zelena *Ukraine* **29** B9
Zelengora *Bos.-H.* **44** C2
Zelenodolsk *Russia* **34** C9
Zelenogorsk *Russia* **32** B5
Zelenograd *Russia* **32** D9
Zelenogradsk *Russia* **30** D7
Zelenokumsk *Russia* **35** H6
Železná Ruda *Czech Rep.* **26** B6
Zelienople *U.S.A.* **114** F4
Železiovce *Slovak Rep.* **27** C11
Zelina *Croatia* **41** C13
Zell *Baden-W., Germany* **25** H3
Zell *Rhld-Pfz., Germany* **25** E3
Zell am See *Austria* **26** D5
Zella-Mehlis *Germany* **24** E6
Zelów *Poland* **31** G6
Zeltweg *Austria* **26** D7
Żemaitijos △ *Lithuania* **30** B8
Zémio *C.A.R.* **86** A2
Zempléni-hegység *Hungary* **28** B6
Zemplínska šírava
  Slovak Rep. **27** C15
Zempoala *Mexico* **119** D5
Zemun *Serbia* **44** B4
Zengbé *Cameroon* **83** D7
Zengcheng *China* **59** F9
Zenica *Bos.-H.* **28** F2
Žepče *Bos.-H.* **28** F3
Zeraf, Bahr ez ➤ *Sudan* **81** F3
Zerbst *Germany* **24** D8
Żerków *Poland* **31** F4
Zermatt *Switz.* **25** J3
Zernez *Switz.* **25** J6
Zernograd *Russia* **35** G5
Zerqan *Albania* **44** E4
Zestaponi *Georgia* **35** J6
Zetel *Germany* **24** B3
Zeulenroda *Germany* **24** E7
Zevenaar *Neths.* **17** C6
Zévio *Italy* **40** C8
Zeya *Russia* **53** D13
Zeya ➤ *Russia* **53** D13
Zeytinbaği *Turkey* **45** F12
Zeytindağ *Turkey* **47** C9
Zghartā *Lebanon* **74** A4
Zgierz *Poland* **31** G6
Zgorzelec *Poland* **31** G2
Zguriţa *Moldova* **29** B13
Zhabinka *Belarus* **31** F11
Zhabokrych *Ukraine* **29** B13
Zhalpaqtal *Kazakhstan* **34** F7
Zhambyl = Taraz *Kazakhstan* **52** E8

Zhangaly *Kazakhstan* **35** G10
Zhangaqala *Kazakhstan* **35** F9
Zhangaqazaly *Kazakhstan* **52** E7
Zhangbei *China* **56** D8
Zhangguangcai Ling *China* **57** B15
Zhangjiagang *China* **59** B13
Zhangjiakou *China* **56** D8
Zhangping *China* **59** E11
Zhangpu *China* **59** E11
Zhangshu *China* **59** C10
Zhangye *China* **60** C5
Zhangzhou *China* **59** E11
Zhanhua *China* **57** F10
Zhänibek *Kazakhstan* **34** F8
Zhanjiang *China* **59** G8
Zhannetty, Ostrov *Russia* **53** B16
Zhanyi *China* **58** E4
Zhanyu *China* **57** B12
Zhao Xian *China* **56** F8
Zhao'an *China* **59** F11
Zhaocheng *China* **56** F6
Zhaojue *China* **58** C4
Zhaoping *China* **59** E8
Zhaoqing *China* **59** F9
Zhaotong *China* **58** D4
Zhaoyuan *Heilongjiang, China* **57** B13
Zhaoyuan *Shandong, China* **57** F11
Zharkent *Kazakhstan* **52** E9
Zharkovskiy *Russia* **32** E7
Zhashkiv *Ukraine* **23** D16
Zhashui *China* **56** H5
Zhayylma *Kazakhstan* **52** D7
Zhayyq ➤ *Kazakhstan* **6** F16
Zhdanov = Mariupol *Ukraine* **33** J9
Zhecheng *China* **56** G8
Zhegao *China* **59** B11
Zhejiang □ *China* **59** C13
Zheleznodorozhnyy *Russia* **30** D8
Zheleznogorsk *Russia* **33** F8
Zheleznogorsk-Ilimskiy
  Russia **53** D11
Zheltyye Vody = Zhovti
  Vody *Ukraine* **33** H7
Zhen'an *China* **56** H5
Zhenba *China* **58** A6
Zhenfeng *China* **58** E5
Zheng'an *China* **58** C6
Zhengding *China* **56** E8
Zhenghe *China* **59** D12
Zhengyang *China* **59** A10
Zhengyangguan *China* **59** A11
Zhengzhou *China* **56** G7
Zhenhai *China* **59** C13
Zhenjiang *China* **59** A12
Zhenkang *China* **58** F2
Zhenlai *China* **57** B12
Zhenning *China* **58** D5
Zhenping *Henan, China* **56** H7
Zhenping *Shaanxi, China* **58** B7
Zhenxiong *China* **58** D5
Zhenyuan *Gansu, China* **56** G4
Zhenyuan *Guizhou, China* **58** D7
Zherdevka *Russia* **34** E5
Zherebkove *Ukraine* **29** C14
Zherong *China* **59** D12
Zhetiqara *Kazakhstan* **52** D7
Zhezqazghan *Kazakhstan* **52** E7
Zhicheng *China* **59** B8
Zhidan *China* **56** F5
Zhigansk *Russia* **53** C13
Zhigulevsk *Russia* **34** D9
Zhijiang *Hubei, China* **59** B8
Zhijiang *Hunan, China* **58** D7
Zhijin *China* **58** D5
Zhilinda *Russia* **53** C12
Zhilino *Russia* **30** D8
Zhirnovsk *Russia* **34** E7
Zhitomir = Zhytomyr
  Ukraine **23** C15
Zhizdra *Russia* **32** F8
Zhlobin *Belarus* **23** B16
Zhmerynka *Ukraine* **23** D15
Zhob *Pakistan* **68** D3
Zhob ➤ *Pakistan* **68** C3
Zhodzina *Belarus* **23** A15
Zhokhova, Ostrov *Russia* **53** B16
Zhongdian *China* **58** D2
Zhongdong *China* **58** F6
Zhongdu *China* **58** E7
Zhongning *China* **56** F3
Zhongshan *Antarctica* **5** C6
Zhongshan *Guangdong, China* **59** F9
Zhongshan
  Guangxi Zhuangzu, China **59** E8
Zhongtiao Shan *China* **56** G6
Zhongwei *China* **56** F3
Zhongxiang *China* **59** B9
Zhongyang *China* **56** F6
Zhorany *Ukraine* **31** G10
Zhosaly *Kazakhstan* **52** E7
Zhouning *China* **59** D12
Zhoucun *China* **57** F9
Zhoushan *China* **59** B14
Zhoushan Dao *China* **59** C14
Zhouzhi *China* **56** G5
Zhovti Vody *Ukraine* **33** H7
Zhovtneve *Ukraine* **31** H11
Zhovtneve *Mykolayiv, Ukraine* **33** J7
Zhu Jiang ➤ *China* **59** F9

Zhuanghe *China* **57** E12
Zhucheng *China* **57** G10
Zhugqu *China* **56** H3
Zhuhai *China* **59** F9
Zhuji *China* **59** C13
Zhujiang ➤ *China* **59** D8
Zhumadian *China* **56** H8
Zhuo Xian = Zhuozhou
  China **56** E8
Zhuolu *China* **56** D8
Zhuozhou *China* **56** E8
Zhuozi *China* **56** D7
Zhushan *China* **59** A8
Zhuxi *China* **58** A7
Zhuzhou *China* **59** D9
Zhvanets *Ukraine* **29** B11
Zhytomyr *Ukraine* **23** C15
Zhytomyr □ *Ukraine* **33** G5
Zi Shui ➤ *China* **59** D9
Zia L. *China* **58** E4
Zibo *China* **57** F10
Zichang *China* **56** F5
Zidarovo *Bulgaria* **45** D11
Zidi = Wandhari *Pakistan* **68** F2
Ziębice *Poland* **31** H4
Zielona Góra *Poland* **31** G2
Zierikzee *Neths.* **17** C3
Ziesar *Germany* **24** C8
Zifta *Egypt* **80** H7
Zigong *China* **58** C5
Ziguéy *Chad* **79** F9
Ziguinchor *Senegal* **82** C1
Ziguinchor □ *Senegal* **82** C1
Zihuatanejo *Mexico* **118** D4
Zijin *China* **59** F10
Zile *Turkey* **72** B6
Žilina *Slovak Rep.* **27** B11
Žilinský □ *Slovak Rep.* **27** B12
Zillah *Libya* **79** C9
Zillertaler Alpen *Austria* **26** D4
Zima *Russia* **53** D11
Zimapán *Mexico* **119** C5
Zimba *Zambia* **87** F2
Zimbabwe *Zimbabwe* **87** G3
Zimbabwe ■ *Africa* **87** F3
Zimmi *S. Leone* **82** D2
Zimnicea *Romania* **29** G10
Zimovniki *Russia* **35** G6
Zinave △ *Mozam.* **89** C5
Zinder *China* **83** C6
Zinder □ *Niger* **83** C7
Zinga *Tanzania* **87** D4
Zingaro △ *Italy* **42** D5
Zingst *Germany* **24** A8
Ziniaré *Burkina Faso* **83** C4
Zinnowitz *Germany* **24** A9
Zion △ *U.S.A.* **109** H7
Zirbitzkogel *Austria* **26** D7
Zirc *Hungary* **28** C2
Žiri *Slovenia* **41** B11
Žirje *Croatia* **41** E12
Zirl *Austria* **26** D4
Zirndorf *Germany* **25** F6
Ziros *Greece* **49** D8
Zirreh, Gowd-e *Afghan.* **66** E3
Zisterdorf *Austria* **27** C9
Zitácuaro *Mexico* **118** D4
Žitava ➤ *Slovak Rep.* **27** C11
Žitište *Serbia* **28** E5
Zitong *China* **58** B5
Zitsa *Greece* **46** B2
Zittau *Germany* **24** E10
Zitundo *Mozam.* **89** D5
Zixi *China* **59** D11
Zixing *China* **59** D9
Ziyang *Shaanxi, China* **56** H5
Ziyang *Sichuan, China* **58** B5
Ziyuan *China* **59** D8
Ziyun *China* **58** E6
Zizhong *China* **58** C5
Zizur Mayor *Spain* **38** C3
Zlarin *Croatia* **41** E12
Zlatar *Croatia* **41** B13
Zlatar *Serbia* **44** C3
Zlataritsa *Bulgaria* **45** C9
Zlatibor *Serbia* **44** C3
Zlatitsa *Bulgaria* **45** D8
Zlatna *Romania* **29** D8
Zlatna Panega *Bulgaria* **45** C8
Zlatni Pyasŭtsi *Bulgaria* **45** C12
Zlatograd *Bulgaria* **45** E9
Zlatoust *Russia* **52** D6
Zletovo *Macedonia* **44** E6
Zlín *Czech Rep.* **27** B10
Zlínský □ *Czech Rep.* **27** B10
Złocieniec *Poland* **30** E3
Złoczew *Poland* **31** G5
Zlot *Serbia* **44** B5
Złotoryja *Poland* **31** G2
Złotów *Poland* **30** E4
Zmeinogorsk *Kazakhstan* **52** D9
Zmiyev *Ukraine* **33** H9

Znamenka = Znamyanka
  Ukraine **33** H7
Znamensk *Russia* **30** D8
Znamyanka *Ukraine* **33** H7
Żnin *Poland* **31** F4
Znojmo *Czech Rep.* **26** C9
Zobeyrī *Iran* **70** C5
Zobia *Dem. Rep. of the Congo* **86** B2
Zoetermeer *Neths.* **17** B4
Zogang *China* **58** C1
Zogno *Italy* **40** C6
Zogqên *China* **58** A2
Zohreh ➤ *Iran* **71** D6
Zolochiv *Ukraine* **23** D13
Zolotonosha *Ukraine* **33** H7
Zolotyy Potik *Ukraine* **29** B10
Zomba *Malawi* **87** F4
Zongo *Dem. Rep. of the Congo* **84** D3
Zonguldak *Turkey* **72** B4
Zonguldak □ *Turkey* **72** B4
Zongyang *China* **59** B11
Zonqor Pt. *Malta* **49** D2
Zonza *France* **21** G13
Zorgo *Burkina Faso* **83** C4
Zorita *Spain* **37** F5
Zorleni *Romania* **29** D12
Zornitsa *Bulgaria* **45** D10
Zorritos *Peru* **124** D2
Żory *Poland* **31** H5
Zorzor *Liberia* **82** D3
Zossen *Germany* **24** C9
Zou Xiang *China* **56** G9
Zouan-Hounien *Ivory C.* **82** D3
Zouar *Chad* **79** D9
Zouérate = Zoûîrât
  Mauritania **78** D3
Zoûîrât *Mauritania* **78** D3
Zourika *Niger* **83** B6
Zourma *Burkina Faso* **83** C4
Zoutkamp *Neths.* **17** A6
Zrenjanin *Serbia* **28** E5
Zuarungu *Ghana* **83** C4
Zuba *Nigeria* **83** D6
Zubayr *Yemen* **81** D5
Zubin Potok *Kosovo* **44** D4
Zubtsov *Russia* **32** D8
Zuénoula *Ivory C.* **82** D3
Zuera *Spain* **38** D4
Zufār *Oman* **75** D5
Zug *Switz.* **25** H4
Zugdidi *Georgia* **35** J5
Zugersee *Switz.* **25** H4
Zugspitze *Germany* **25** H6
Zuid-Holland □ *Neths.* **17** C4
Zuidbeveland *Neths.* **17** C3
Zuidhorn *Neths.* **17** A6
Zújar *Spain* **37** H8
Zújar ➤ *Spain* **37** G5
Żukowo *Poland* **30** D5
Zula *Eritrea* **81** D4
Zülpich *Germany* **24** E2
Zumaia *Spain* **38** B2
Zumárraga *Spain* **38** B2
Zumbo *Mozam.* **87** F3
Zummo *Nigeria* **83** D7
Zumpango *Mexico* **119** D5
Zungeru *Nigeria* **83** D6
Zunhua *China* **57** D9
Zuni Pueblo *U.S.A.* **109** J9
Zunyi *China* **58** D6
Zuo Jiang ➤ *China* **58** F6
Zuozhou *China* **58** F6
Županja *Croatia* **28** E3
Žur *Kosovo* **44** D4
Zurbāṭīyah *Iraq* **73** F12
Zürich *Switz.* **25** H4
Zürich □ *Switz.* **25** H4
Zürichsee *Switz.* **25** H4
Żuromin *Poland* **31** F6
Żut *Croatia* **41** E12
Zutphen *Neths.* **17** B6
Zuurberg △ *S. Africa* **88** E4
Zuwārah *Libya* **79** B8
Žūzan *Iran* **71** C8
Žužemberk *Slovenia* **41** C11
Zvečan *Kosovo* **44** D4
Zvenigorodka =
  Zvenyhorodka *Ukraine* **33** H6
Zvenyhorodka *Ukraine* **33** H6
Zvezdets *Bulgaria* **45** D11
Zvishavane *Zimbabwe* **87** G3
Zvolen *Slovak Rep.* **27** C12
Zvonce *Serbia* **44** D6
Zvornik *Bos.-H.* **28** F4
Zwedru = Tchien *Liberia* **82** D3
Zweibrücken *Germany* **25** F3
Zwenkau *Germany* **24** D8
Zwettl *Austria* **26** C8
Zwickau *Germany* **24** E8
Zwierzyniec *Poland* **31** H9
Zwiesel *Germany* **25** F5
Zwolen *Poland* **31** G8
Zwolle *Neths.* **17** B6
Zwolle *U.S.A.* **116** F8
Żychlin *Poland* **31** F6
Żyrardów *Poland* **31** F7
Żyrzyn *Poland* **31** G8
Żyryan *Kazakhstan* **52** D9
Zyryanka *Russia* **53** C16
Zyryanovsk = Žyryan
  Kazakhstan **52** D9
Żywiec *Poland* **31** J6

KEY TO EUROPEAN MAP PAGES

 Large scale maps
(>1:2 500 000)

 Medium scale maps
(1: 2 800 000 — 1:9 900 000)

 Small scale maps
(<1:10 000 000)

Arctic Circle

8

ICELAND

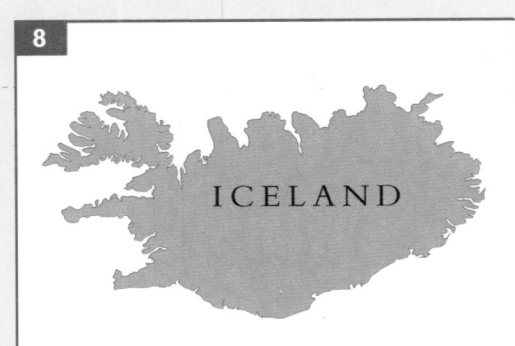

WORLD COUNTRY INDEX

Afghanistan	66	**G**ermany	24—25	**O**man	75
Albania	44	Ghana	82—83		
Algeria	78	Greece	44—47	**P**akistan	66, 68
Angola	84—85	Greenland	4	Panama	120
Argentina	126, 128	Guadeloupe	120	Papua New Guinea	96
Armenia	73	Guatemala	120	Paraguay	126—127
Australia	92—95	Guinea	82	Peru	124
Austria	26—27	Guinea-Bissau	82	Philippines	61
Azerbaijan	73	Guyana	124	Poland	30—31
				Portugal	36—37
Bahamas	120—121	**H**aiti	121	Puerto Rico	121
Bahrain	71	Honduras	120		
Bangladesh	67	Hungary	28	**Q**atar	71
Barbados	121				
Belarus	32—33	**I**celand	8	**R**omania	28—29
Belgium	17	India	66—69	Russia	32—35, 52—53
Belize	120	Indonesia	62—63	Rwanda	86
Benin	83	Iran	70—71, 73		
Bhutan	67	Iraq	70—71, 73	**S**t. Lucia	121
Bolivia	124	Irish Republic	12	Samoa	91
Bosnia-Herzegovina	41, 44	Israel	74	Saudi Arabia	70—71, 75
Botswana	88	Italy	40—43	Scotland	13
Brazil	124—125, 127	Ivory Coast	82	Senegal	82
Brunei	62			Serbia	28, 44
Bulgaria	44—45	**J**amaica	120	Sierra Leone	82
Burkina Faso	82—83	Japan	54—55	Singapore	65
Burma (Myanmar)	67	Jordan	74	Slovak Republic	27
Burundi	86			Slovenia	41
		Kazakhstan	52	Solomon Is.	96
Cambodia	64—65	Kenya	86	Somali Republic	75
Canary Is.	48	Korea, North	57	South Africa	88—89
Cameroon	83, 84	Korea, South	57	Spain	36—39
Canada	100—105	Kosovo	44	Sri Lanka	66
Central African Republic	84	Kuwait	70—71	Sudan	80—81
Chad	79	Kyrgyzstan	52	Suriname	124—125
Chile	126, 128			Swaziland	89
China	56—60	**L**aos	64	Sweden	8—9
Colombia	124	Latvia	32	Switzerland	25
Congo	84	Lebanon	74	Syria	70, 72—73
Congo, Dem. Rep.		Lesotho	89		
of the	84—85, 86—87	Liberia	82	**T**aiwan	59
Costa Rica	120	Libya	79	Tajikistan	52
Croatia	41	Lithuania	32	Tanzania	86—87
Cuba	120—121	Luxembourg	17	Thailand	64—65
Cyprus	49			Togo	83
Czech Republic	26—27	**M**acedonia	44	Tonga	91
		Madagascar	89	Trinidad and Tobago	125
Denmark	11	Malawi	87	Tunisia	78—79
Djibouti	81	Malaysia	62—63, 65	Turkey	72—73
Dominican Republic	121	Mali	78, 82—83	Turkmenistan	52
		Malta	49		
East Timor	63	Martinique	120	**U**ganda	86
Ecuador	124	Mauritania	78, 82	Ukraine	33
Egypt	80	Mexico	118—119	United Arab Emirates	75
El Salvador	120	Moldova	29	United Kingdom	12—16
England	14—15	Mongolia	60	USA	106—117
Equatorial Guinea	84	Montenegro	44	Uruguay	126—127
Eritrea	80—81	Morocco	78	Uzbekistan	52
Estonia	32	Mozambique	87, 89		
Ethiopia	75, 81			**V**anuatu	96
		Namibia	88	Venezuela	124
Fiji	91	Nepal	69	Vietnam	64—65
Finland	8—9	Netherlands	17		
France	18—21	New Zealand	91	**W**ales	14—15
French Guiana	125	Nicaragua	120		
		Niger	78—79, 83	**Y**emen	75
Gabon	84	Nigeria	83		
Gambia	82	Northern Ireland	12	**Z**ambia	85, 87
Georgia	35	Norway	8—9	Zimbabwe	87

8

16 **13**

13

13

14

12 **22**

17

IRELAND

UNITED KINGDOM

N

18

B

20 FRAN

36 **38**

ANDORRA

PORTUGAL SPAIN **48**

MOROCCO ALG